Exposure
A GUIDE TO SOURCES OF INFECTIONS

Exposure
A GUIDE TO SOURCES OF INFECTIONS

Dieter A. Stürchler, M.D., M.P.H.
Department of Social and Preventive Medicine
Basel University
and Sturchler Epidemiologics,
Büren, Switzerland

With contributions by
Matius P. Stürchler, M.D.
Marjam S. Rüdiger-Stürchler, M.D.
and Nikolas J. Stürchler, Ph.D., LL.M.

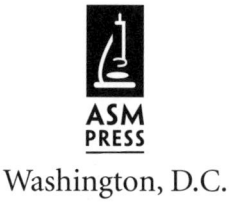

Washington, D.C.

Address editorial correspondence to ASM Press, 1752 N St. NW, Washington, DC 20036-2904, USA

Send orders to ASM Press, P.O. Box 605, Herndon, VA 20172, USA
Phone: (800) 546-2416 or (703) 661-1593
Fax: (703) 661-1501
E-mail: books@asmusa.org
Online: estore.asm.org

Copyright © 2006   ASM Press
American Society for Microbiology
1752 N Street NW
Washington, DC 20036-2904

Library of Congress Cataloging-in-Publication Data
Stürchler, Dieter.
  Exposure : a guide to sources of infections / Dieter A. Stürchler ; with contributions by Matius P. Stürchler, Marjam S. Rüdiger-Stürchler, and Nikolas J. Stürchler.
    p. ; cm.
  Includes bibliographical references and index.
  ISBN-13: 978-1-55581-376-5 (alk. paper)
  ISBN-10: 1-55581-376-3 (alk. paper)
1. Infection—Handbooks, manuals, etc.   2. Infection—Etiology—Handbooks, manuals, etc.
   [DNLM: 1. Infection—diagnosis.   2. Infection—epidemiology.
3. Environmental Exposure. WC 195 S935e 2006]   I. Title.

RB153.S78 2006
616.9—dc22

2006006130

10 9 8 7 6 5 4 3 2 1

All Rights Reserved
Printed in the United States of America

The image font used throughout the book and on the cover is SignPix, designed by James M. Harris, and is a trademark of Harris Design.
Cover and interior design by Susan Brown Schmidler.

Contents

Preface xi
Acknowledgments xiii

Introduction 1

SECTION I ## Animals 5

1 Animal Bites 7
1.1 Rabies 7
1.2 Other systemic infections from bites 9
1.3 Bite wound infections 10

2 Domestic Mammals 13
2.1 Dogs 13
2.2 Cats 18
2.3 Domestic bovids 21
2.4 Suids 27
2.5 Equids 31
2.6 Camelids 34

3 Wild Vertebrates 37
3.1 Wild herbivores 37
3.2 Carnivores 40
3.3 Rodents 42
3.4 Lagomorphs 49
3.5 Primates 51
3.6 Bats 53
3.7 Birds 55
3.8 Reptiles and amphibians 60
3.9 Fish 61

4 Invertebrates 65
- 4.1 Hard ticks and vector mites 66
- 4.2 Diurnal fleas and flies 71
- 4.3 Mainly diurnal mosquitoes 73
- 4.4 Mainly nocturnal mosquitoes 76
- 4.5 Nocturnal bugs and soft ticks 82
- 4.6 Ectoparasites (lice, fly larvae, and scabies mites) 83

SECTION II Environment 87

5 Natural Environments 89
- 5.1 Marine habitats 89
- 5.2 Freshwater habitats and floods 92
- 5.3 Soil and plants 98
- 5.4 Terrestrial Biomes 100
- 5.5 Dust and winds 116
- 5.6 Seasons 118

6 Human-Made Environments 125
- 6.1 Dams and irrigation 125
- 6.2 Buildings, sanitation, and wastewater 128
- 6.3 Cities 132
- 6.4 Utensils and belongings 138

SECTION III Foods 143

7 Animal-Derived Foods 149
- 7.1 Milk and Dairy Products 149
- 7.2 Eggs and Egg Products 156
- 7.3 Poultry 157
- 7.4 Meat and Meat Products 159
- 7.5 Seafood, fish, and molluscs 166

8 Plant-Derived Foods 175
- 8.1 Cereals, pasta, bakery, and sweets 175
- 8.2 Vegetables, salads, fruits, and spices 177

9 Finished Foods 187
- 9.1 Snacks and sandwiches 187
- 9.2 Menus and ethnic foods 188

10 Drinking Water and Other Beverages 193
- 10.1 Bottled waters and ice 194

10.2 Municipal high-income tap water 197
10.3 Private and low-income water supplies 200

SECTION IV Humans 205

11 Human Domiciles 207
11.1 Regular domiciles 207
11.2 Substandard domiciles 214
11.3 Homeless persons 223
11.4 Refugees and relief camps 225
11.5 Orphans and adoptees 230
11.6 Adults in long-term care 233
11.7 Detention facilities 237
11.8 Hotel accommodation 241

12 Human Work 247
12.1 Construction and mining 248
12.2 Manufacture and maintenance 251
12.3 Military, police, and guards 253
12.4 Field, forest, herd, and abattoir 264
12.5 Catering 276
12.6 Health and laboratory work 281
12.7 Cleaning and waste work 296
12.8 Transportation work 299
12.9 Clerk, class, and sales work 300

13 Human Leisure and Lifestyle 303
13.1 Fairs and mass gatherings 303
13.2 Catered events and restaurants 307
13.3 Swimming pools and spas 310
13.4 Outdoor sports and hobbies 314
13.5 Indoor sports and hobbies 320
13.6 Female prostitution 323
13.7 Sex among men 326
13.8 Injection drug use 330

14 Human Community 335
14.1 Colonization, carriage, and contact 335
14.2 Age 347
14.3 Day care 353
14.4 Schools and training 358
14.5 Minorities 365
14.6 Latency, reactivation, and immune impairment 370
14.7 Community-acquired syndromes 376

SECTION V Travel and Transport 393

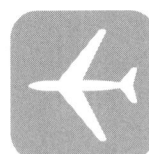

15 Human Travel 395
15.1 Local travel 395
15.2 Ships and seaports 398
15.3 Aircraft and airports 401
15.4 International short-term travel 404
15.5 Expatriates 416
15.6 Immigrants and migrants 420

16 Transported Animals and Goods 427
16.1 Migrating and transported vertebrates 427
16.2 Transported invertebrates 430
16.3 Transported goods 432

SECTION VI Nosocomial Infections 437

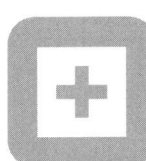

17 Noninvasive Procedures 441
17.1 Hands 441
17.2 Materials and machines 443
17.3 Endoscopy 446
17.4 Bladder catheters and UTI 447
17.5 Intubation and nosocomial pneumonia 448
17.6 Drugs, bioproducts, and nosocomial diarrhea 449
17.7 Hospital air, water, and surfaces 458
17.8 Viral hemorrhagic fevers in hospitals 464

18 Invasive Procedures 467
18.1 Instantly invasive procedures 467
18.2 Intravascular devices and bloodstream infections 471
18.3 Surgical site and wound infections 474
18.4 Transfusions 477
18.5 Transplants 482
18.6 Implants 489
18.7 Dialysis 492
18.8 Intensive care 494

SECTION VII Agents 495
19 Taxonomic Overview 497
20 Genera A to Z 499

APPENDIX 1 **Exposure Checklist** 591

APPENDIX 2 **Acronyms** 595

Glossary 599
References 605
Index 869

Preface

All interest in disease and death is only another expression of interest in life.
T. Mann (1875-1955), *The Magic Mountain*

What do a tick in the scalp of a child, a man with a boil after an adventure trip to Kenya, and a febrile elderly person reporting the death of her pet bird have in common? The answer is exposure: the critical first step in infection. Like light impacts on a film, exposure impacts on hosts.

Exposure embraces all agents (prions to parasites), ages (embryo to elderly), and habitats (city to coast). Exposure is the key to directed search for causative agents, characterization of infection severity and stage, interpretation of laboratory test results, and preventive and public health action. Determining the exposure history should be a part of any patient evaluation. You might take the table of contents or the checklist in the appendix as a starting point. By generating a reduced list of agents to consider for priority laboratory work up, treatment, and prevention, the exposure history can curb health care costs. I grouped the diverse methods of exposure into chapters and sections in a way that I felt would be useful for clinicians, public health officers, and microbiologists.

Infections are still with us. Worldwide in 2002, infectious diseases accounted for nearly 25% of disability-adjusted life years (DALYs) (350 of 1,490 million) and nearly 20% (11 of 57 million) of deaths. Impact is considerably greater in low-income than high-income countries (causing 2% of DALYS and 4% of deaths in high-income countries versus 10 and 50% in low-income countries). Despite these gradients, infections remain significant in high-income countries. In the United States in 2001, about 3% of outpatients (23.8 million of 880.5 million) were diagnosed infectious diseases, and about 9% of all prescriptions were antimicrobials (114 million of 1,314 million). Exposure helps a physician decide whether a patient's illness is likely to be infectious. Further evidence comes from symptoms and signs. Infectious diseases cause localized (organ-related, calor, rubor, dolor, or tumor), regional (migrating lesions or adenopathy), or systemic (fever, rash, somnolence, or shock) signs.

The scope of the book is epidemiologic rather than clinical. For reasons of space, I had to omit many details and simplify a number of complex issues. I regret any oversimplifications, inconsistencies, or errors. Please contact me through ASM Press for your comments or suggestions (books@asmusa.org).

Nonetheless I hope that practitioners, infectious disease specialists, travel clinic managers, clinical and environmental microbiologists, and public health promoters will benefit from working with the book, without the feeling "I understand it, so it must be wrong."

DIETER STÜRCHLER
Büren, Switzerland
2 December 2005

As the epidemiologic situation, recommended treatments, and preventive measures can change rapidly, readers are urged to consult national guidelines and formularies before administering any vaccines or medications.

Acknowledgments

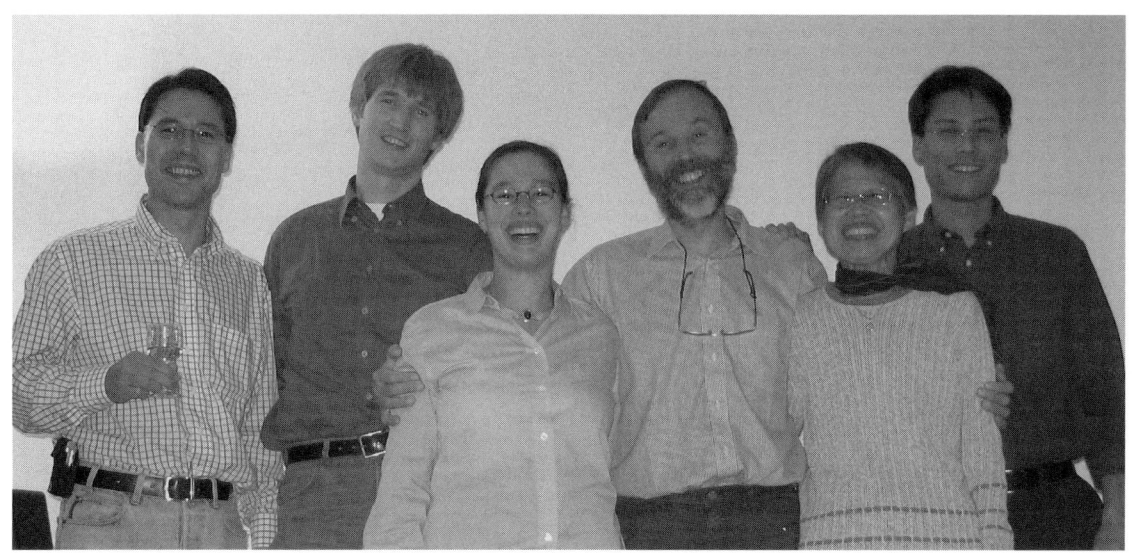

From left to right, Matius Stürchler, Jochen and Marjam Rüdiger-Stürchler, Dieter and Tjoek Stürchler, and Nikolas Stürchler.

I am deeply grateful to my wife Tjoek and to our three children who supported me in the 5 years I was laboring on this book. All gave valuable input to make the book practical.

Matius P. Stürchler (M.D., M.B.A.) graduated from the University of Basel Medical School in Switzerland in 1998, with a thesis on occupational *Toxoplasma* and *Hantavirus* infections. He worked at the WHO Collaboration Centre for Travellers' Health of the University of Zürich and at the medical department of the Liestal University Hospital. From 2003 to 2005 he completed an M.B.A. at the Robert Emmett McDonough School of Business, Georgetown University, Washington, D.C.

Marjam S. Rüdiger-Stürchler (M.D.) graduated from the University of Basel Medical School in 1999, with a thesis on usage of antibiotics and antimicrobial resistance in outpatients. She worked at the Basel University Hospital, including the intensive care unit and the emergency and medical departments.

Nikolas J. Stürchler (Ph.D., LL.M., M.A.) obtained degrees from Basel University (law licentiate), King's College of the University of Cambridge, United Kingdom (LL.M.), and the University of Stanford, Calif. (Master's degree in international policy studies). With support from the National Science Foundation, he completed a Ph.D. thesis on the threat of force in international law in 2005.

Introduction

Better to be approximately right than exactly wrong.
Attributed to J. W. Tukey (1915–2000)

CONVENTIONS AND METHODS
ACRONYMS
Acronyms are introduced in chapters and listed in the appendix.

TERMS
Terms are explained in the glossary and in chapters. I aimed to distinguish colonization and infection from disease and to avoid ambiguous terms, e.g., "ascariasis," which could mean infection or disease. Country names are for geographic reference only and do not imply political or legal status. For brevity, prefixes such as "Republic" are omitted. For practical purposes, high-income (industrial) countries here include those in North America and Europe and Australia, Japan, and New Zealand, while low-income (developing) countries are all remaining countries of Africa, Latin America, Asia, and the Pacific. A "tree of life" is presented in Table 20.1.

NUMBERS
Numbers are generally rounded to a full digit. I aimed to provide magnitude and range rather than precision. For the same reason, confidence limits are preferred over significances. Attack rates are per 100 exposed persons, and infection and disease rates are per 1,000 person-years or 10^5 population. In general, "infrequent" refers to a prevalence <1–5% or a rate <$100/10^5$ and year. International units are used, including meter and centigrade. Season is a diagnostically useful, perhaps underrated variable that I have emphasized whenever possible.

EVIDENCE
This book is based on evidence and my own clinical and epidemiological experience. For years, I have watched journals (e.g., *American Journal of Tropical*

Medicine and Hygiene, Clinical Infectious Diseases, Emerging Infectious Diseases, Epidemiology and Infection, Journal of the American Medical Association, Journal of Clinical Microbiology, Lancet, Trends in Parasitology) and visited governmental websites, mainly of the Centers for Disease Control and Prevention of the United States (CDC, for *Morbidity and Mortality Weekly Report* at http://www.cdc.gov/), *Communicable Disease Intelligence of Australia* (http://www.health.gov.au/internet/wcms/publishing.nsf/Content/cda-pubs-cdipubs.htm), *Communicable Disease Report of the United Kingdom* (http://www.hpa.org.uk/), Eurosurveillance (http://www.eurosurveillance.org), and World Health Organization (WHO, for *Weekly Epidemiological Record* at http://www.who.int/). Via PubMed (http://www.ncbi.nlm.nih.gov/), I searched for habitats, agents, names of authors, and diseases. To evaluate evidence, I considered the source (peer-reviewed journal, expert committee), purpose, sampling method and sample (size and case mix), findings, and conclusions. Of course, I had a preference for random, large (>100/group), or "representative" (national) samples and for control (placebo) or low-risk groups in comparative or prospective clinical or epidemiological studies.

REFERENCES

I reviewed >13,000 publications. Only a fraction could be cited (using EndNote version 7.0), however. I selected only the most recent publications in a series, although I aimed to represent a mix of review and original work from all continents.

EXPOSURE HISTORY

Goal: *To efficiently recognize and manage infectious agents and diseases.*

INTERVIEW

An exposure interview should be part of the medical history. At least the following topics should be covered: susceptibility (past infectious diseases, vaccines, and immune impairments), time and place of exposure (home, work, leisure, and travel), possible sources (humans, animals, foods, and environment), and preventive measures.

TIME AND DOSE

Exposure can be instantaneous (e.g., a date marked by a meal, injection, or a flight), seasonal (e.g., tick emergence in spring or swimming in summer), continuous (e.g., hours spent in a closed room or days on assisted ventilation), or intermittent (e.g., frequent drinks of raw milk or drug injections). The infective dose can be estimated from microbiological (e.g., from leftover foods) or entomological (e.g., from vectors) data, experimental studies (animal or human volunteer), or epidemiologic data (e.g., number of cups of tap water consumed per day). Intensity is a measure of exposure that aggregates dose over time. Intensity helps to interpret laboratory findings (e.g., a single water contact is incompatible with a heavy *Schistosoma mansoni* egg output) and to assess causality.

RECALL

Memory of many exposing events is lost within days. A few measures may assist recall. Ask your patient for vaccination, travel, and other records. Recounting life around the clock ("from breakfast to bed") in the last 24 h before the visit may bring back memories of routine activities, meals, drinks, and exposures from work or leisure. Habitat photos could also enhance recall. Alternatively, you may obtain a structured exposure interview (appendix 1).

Some events are remembered for life, typically deliveries, abortions, owned pet animals, continents visited, past and current sex partners, some diagnoses and treatments (e.g., tuberculosis, AIDS, and sexually transmitted infections [STI]), injection drug use, general anesthesia for major surgery, stays in an intensive care unit, organ transplants, and implants.

MODES OF SPREAD AND AGENT CLUSTERS

Humans acquire agents from animals, from the environment, from foods or objects, from other humans (including by droplets, by close and sexual contact, and transplacentally), and nosocomially, including by injection drug use and invasive health procedures. Agents may use several modes. Direction of spread can be opposite, from humans to animals (e.g., *Mycobacterium tuberculosis* from caretaker to captive primate), to the environment (e.g., *Giardia* from hiker to mountain creek), or to foods (e.g., *Salmonella enterica* serovar Typhi from carrier to food). Agents can be taken up from ingestion, inhalation, inoculation, or contact. These portals can be difficult to identify clinically. Fecally polluted foods and hands could result in uptake by ingestion. Skin contact could result from touching water, soil, or other skin and from human or animal droplets settling on hands or conjunctiva.

About 300 agents commonly infect humans. For convenience, this list is broken down into five arbitrary "eco-transmission" clusters and further into seven agent classes (prions, viruses, bacteria, fungi, protozoa, helminths, ectoparasites). For acronyms of viruses, see appendix 2, and for agent taxonomy, see Table 21.1.

DROPLET-AIR CLUSTER (~40 agents or 13%)

Viruses. Vaccine-preventable viruses include *Influenzavirus*; mumps, measles, and rubella viruses; poliovirus; and varicella-zoster virus. Others include adenovirus, Epstein-Barr virus, *Enterovirus*, parainfluenza virus, parvovirus B19, *Rhinovirus*, and respiratory syncytial virus.

Bacteria. Vaccine-preventable bacteria include *Bordetella pertussis, Corynebacterium diphtheriae, Haemophilus influenzae* b (Hib), *Mycobacterium tuberculosis, Neisseria meningitidis, Streptococcus pneumoniae*, and the "four pneumos" (*Chlamydia pneumoniae, Klebsiella pneumoniae, Legionella pneumophila,* and *Mycoplasma pneumoniae*).

Fungi. Fungi from air include, e.g., *Aspergillus, Blastomyces, Cryptococcus, Histoplasma, Paracoccidioides,* and *Pneumocystis*.

FECES-FOOD CLUSTER (~70 agents or 24%)

Agents in this cluster are found in foods, beverages, and drinking water and on objects.

Prions. Prions from foods are those associated with variant Creutzfeldt-Jakob disease.

Viruses. Viruses include astrovirus, hepatitis viruses A and E, *Norovirus,* and *Rotavirus*.

Bacteria. Bacteria include all Enterobacteriaceae (e.g., *Escherichia, Salmonella,* and *Shigella*), *Bacteroides, Clostridium* (*C. botulinum, C. difficile,* and *C. perfringens*), *Helicobacter, Listeria,* and *Vibrio* (*V. cholerae* and *V. parahaemolyticus*).

Fungi. Fungi from foods include Microsporidia, e.g., *Encephalitozoon* and *Enterocytozoon*.

Protozoa. Protozoa include *Cryptosporidium, Cyclospora, Entamoeba, Giardia, Sarcocystis,* and *Toxoplasma*.

Helminths. Helminths from foods include *Anisakis, Ascaris, Fasciola, Paragonimus, Taenia, Trichinella,* and *Trichuris*.

ZOONOTIC CLUSTER (~100 agents or 34%)

Viruses. Viruses from mammals include *Lyssavirus* and *Hantavirus*. Many zoonotic viruses are vectorborne, including, for example, dengue virus.

Bacteria. Bacteria include *Bacillus anthracis, Borrelia, Brucella, Coxiella, Francisella, Rickettsia,* and *Yersinia pestis*.

Fungi. Fungi include zoophilic dermatophytes, e.g., *Microsporum canis*.

Protozoa. Protozoa include *Babesia, Leishmania, Plasmodium,* and *Trypanosoma*.

Helminths. Helminths from animals include *Echinococcus granulosus, E. multilocularis,* and filariae (e.g., *Onchocerca, Wuchereria*).

ENVIRONMENTAL CLUSTER (~45 agents or 15%)

Bacteria. Bacteria from water and soil include *Acinetobacter, Burkholderia cepacia, Clostridium tetani,* mycobacteria, *Leptospira,* and *Pseudomonas aeruginosa*.

Fungi. Fungi from soil and plants include *Acremonium, Fonsecaea, Fusarium, Penicillium marneffei, Sporothrix,* and *Trichosporon*.

Protozoa. Protozoa include *Rhinosporidium seeberi* and free-living amebas (e.g., *Acanthamoeba* and *Naegleria*).

Helminths. Helminths from water and soil include hookworms (*Ancylostoma* and *Necator*), *Schistosoma, Strongyloides,* and *Toxocara*.

Ectoparasites. Ectoparasites from soil include *Tunga penetrans*.

SKIN-BLOOD CLUSTER (~40 agents or ~14%)

Prions. Prions from blood include those causing sporadic Creutzfeldt-Jakob disease.

Viruses. Viruses from skin, sexual transmission (STI), or blood include cytomegalovirus, hepatitis viruses B and C, herpes simplex virus, human immunodeficiency virus, human papillomavirus, human T-lymphotropic virus, molluscum contagiosum, and vaccinia virus.

Bacteria. Bacteria from skin, or STI, include *Chlamydia trachomatis* (ocular and genital), *Mycobacterium leprae, Neisseria gonorrhoeae, Staphylococcus aureus, Streptococcus pyogenes,* and *Treponema pallidum pallidum*.

Fungi. Fungi include anthropophilic dermatophytes, e.g., *Candida, Epidermophyton, Malassezia,* and *Trichophyton*.

Protozoa. Protozoa include *Trichomonas vaginalis*.

Helminths. Helminths from contact include *Enterobius vermicularis* and *Hymenolepis nana*.

Ectoparasites. Ectoparasites from contact include *Pediculus humanus* (var. *capitis,* var. *corporis*) and *Sarcoptes scabiei*.

DIAGNOSTIC WORKUP

Probable impossibilities are to be preferred to improbable possibilities.
  Aristotle of Stagira (384–322 BC)

A targeted microbiologic workup should be attempted from the exposure history and clinical examination. If

> **Box I.1** Suggested vertebrate animal exposure history
>
> **Right now,** name all pet animals that you own, including dogs, cats, birds, reptiles, and fish.
>
> **In the past week:**
> - Have you touched a farm, pet, sick, or dead animal, including bird, reptile, fish, or rodent?
> - Have you been near a sick or parturient animal, including a sneezing cat or a dog with diarrhea?
>
> **In the past 3–12 months:**
> - Have you sustained bites or scratches by animals, including pets, livestock, bats, mosquitoes, or ticks?
> - Have you seen rats, foxes, bugs, or other animals in or on your premises, or seen birds, horses, or rats die?
> - Have you cleaned animals, handled manure, removed bugs from an animal, or worked with bones or wool?
>
> **In your lifetime:**
> - Has any of your jobs involved contact with animals, including at zoos, research facilities, or abattoirs?
> - Name all the kinds of animals that you have ever kept at home.

more than a dozen agents are tentatively included in the differential diagnosis, priority should be given to infections with high lethality (e.g., >5%), high potential for spread (e.g., 2° attack rates >5% or R_0 >2), or rapid response to locally available, presumptive antimicrobials (e.g., antimalarials). In the chapter on agents (see chapter 21), impact variables are summarized by agent genus. Taxonomy (Table 20.1) helps to explain serologic cross-reactivities.

Clinical materials for laboratory workup should be commensurate with the natural history of the disease concerned (prepatent and incubation periods, time to appearance of immunoglobulins M and G). At an early disease stage, immunoglobulin M may not yet be detectable. A "null" serum sample can then be stored for antibody determination with a second sample obtained 2–3 weeks later ("paired" sera). Tests with high (>95%) sensitivity, specificity, and predictive values are ideal, because they substantially increase the pretest to posttest disease certainty. In general, the preferred test is culture. If clinical material cannot be obtained, consider surrogates such as leftover foods, tap or recreational water, removed ectoparasites, samples from pet or domestic animals, soil from flower arrangements or gardens, or home or office dust. Archived specimens may still be available (e.g., null sera at work places or aliquots at diagnostic laboratories).

A colonized, infected, or ill person points to agents that circulate in the source community. Clinicians and microbiologists should therefore always keep in mind the "three I's" of information: inform yourself (epidemic situation, test methods), inform the patient (what to expect and do), and inform health authorities (reporting).

SECTION I
Animals

1 **Animal Bites**
2 **Domestic Mammals**
3 **Wild Vertebrates**
4 **Invertebrates**

Of >2 million animal species catalogued, most (>98%) are invertebrates (e.g., molluscs, worms, and arthropods); only ~40,000 (<2%) are vertebrates, including ~4,500 species of mammals in ~16 orders (mainly ~2,000 rodent species and ~950 bat species). In high-income countries, 50–60% of households keep pet animals.

Zoonoses (695, 5694, 7371). Animals can be reservoirs, sources, or vectors of infections in humans (zoonoses). Arguments in favor of zoonotic spread include an animal exposure history that fits with the incubation period and clinical presentation, isolation of identical agents from patients and animals, and evidence of animal-to-human spread from ecologic, epidemiologic, and experimental studies. Uptake is by inoculation (via bite, scratch, licking of abraded skin, or splash into eye or mouth), ingestion (via foods, hands, or objects), inhalation of animal dust or aerosols (from fur shaking, skin scaling, urination, birth, or slaughter), or contact (e.g., petting, cleaning, milking, or moving carcasses).

Exposure History. The exposure history should address bites and work and leisure contacts with animals (Box I.1).

Antimicrobials (334, 1405, 1660, 4896, 5127, 6905, 7987). Fifty to 85% of antimicrobial sales are for animals, mainly feeds. Antimicrobials licensed for feeds in the United States include amoxicillin (cattle and swine), erythromycin and fluoroquinolones (cattle and poultry), and oxytetracycline (fish). Some countries permit use of streptomycin in agriculture; for instance, in Belgium it is used for spraying flowering apple and pear trees against fire blight. A complex web (food chain) links antimicrobials in animal feeds with humans via livestock waste, dust, contact, carcasses, meat, wildlife, and pets. Antibiotics in poultry feed have been shown to alter the gut flora of attending farmers. There is a demonstrated chain for *Salmonella enterica* serovar Newport from beef to hamburgers and humans. Antimicrobials of related structure (class) or activity that are used in humans and in animal feeds are likely to select for resistant enteric agents that animals share with humans (cross-resistance). Examples are avoparcin- and vancomycin-resistant *Enterococcus*, quinolone-resistant *S. enterica* serovars Choleraesuis and Typhimurium, and macrolide-resistant *Staphylococcus aureus*. Proposed targets for veterinary surveillance include animals (cattle, pig, poultry, and fish), antimicrobial classes (aminoglycosides, β-lactams, macrolides, quinolones, and tetracyclines), and agents (*Campylobacter*, *Enterococcus*, *Escherichia*, and *Salmonella*).

1

Animal Bites

1.1 Rabies
1.2 Other systemic infections from bites
1.3 Bite wound infections

Animal trauma (1212, 2374, 2429, 7857). Virtually any wild or domestic vertebrate animal can inflict bite, scratch, or other wounds to humans. By setting, culprits are mainly dogs (in 66–95% of cases) and cats (5–15%), infrequently (2–15%) other animals, including cattle, rodents, wild carnivores, bats, snakes, fish, and birds. Main considerations from animal-related injuries are rabies, wound infection, and systemic bacterial infections.

Risks (1212, 1324, 2374, 2429, 3042, 4838). By location and surveillance, reported rates of vertebrate-related injuries are 40–700/10^5 and year. In the United States in 2001, ~368,000 persons were treated for dog-related injuries, for a rate of 129 (95% confidence interval [95% CI] 116–143)/10^5. Rates peaked in children of age 5–9 years with 278 (95% CI 235–322)/10^5 and decreased with increasing age (Fig. 1.1). The main injured body parts were arm and hand (in 45%), leg and foot (in 26%), and head and neck (in 23%). Dogs in the United States cause 10–20 deaths each year, mainly in children.

In rural tropical areas, rates of snake bites can reach 500/10^5 per year.

1.1 RABIES
RABID MAMMALS (4103, 5988, 6158)
Most mammals are susceptible to rabies virus, including domestic mammals, bats, and terrestrial wildlife.

Of rabid animals in North America, >90% are wildlife, mainly raccoons, skunks, bats, and foxes, and 6–9% are domestic mammals, mainly cats, dogs, and cattle (Fig. 1.2). Raccoon (*Procyon lotor*) rabies is enzootic in the eastern United States, skunk (*Mephitis mephitis*) rabies is enzootic in the central prairie states and California, red fox (*Vulpes vulpes*) and Arctic fox (*Alopex lagopus*) rabies is enzootic in Alaska, gray fox (*Urocyon cinereoargenteus*) rabies is enzootic in the southwestern United States, coyote (*Canis latrans*) rabies is enzootic along the Texas-Mexico border, and mongoose (*Herpestes javanicus*) rabies is enzootic in Puerto Rico.

In Europe, 41,530 domestic animals were diagnosed with rabies infections in 1990–2002 (nearly 3,200/year), including dogs, cats, cattle, sheep, and goats (Fig. 1.3). In Lithuania in 2003, 19% (2,268/11,797) of animals that had injured people were rabid, 6% (449) of dogs, 9% (9) of rats, 15% (290) of cats, 50%

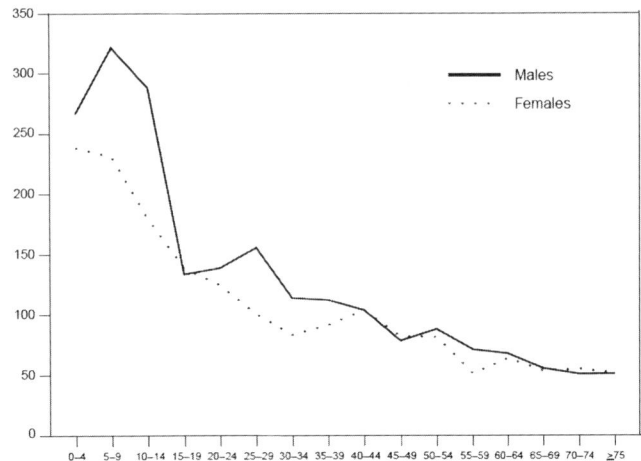

Figure 1.1 Dog-related injuries treated in United States hospital emergency departments, 2001. Rates are number per 10^5 populations (y axis) and are shown by age group (x axis, in years) and sex (females, dotted lines; males, solid lines). From reference 1212.

(88) of other domestic animals, 72% (849) of other wild animals, and 81% (643) of cattle. In Russia in 1980–1998, reindeer accounted for 3% of rabies in animals.

HUMAN RISKS

Any terrestrial mammal that is not validly vaccinated or any bat species can be a source of human rabies (1319, 2374, 6470, 8106). Main source animals vary locally and over time. Suspected or confirmed rabid animals that have caused visits for risk evaluation or postexposure prophylaxis (PEP) include dogs (see Fig. 2.1), cats, cattle, goats, horses, foxes, skunks, and other mammals. In New York state in 1993–1998, 29% (2,556/8,858) of animals confirmed rabid caused 6,139 PEP (1–465 [mean 2–3] /event): 23% (266/1,161) of skunks, 25% (1,666/6,649) of raccoons, 45% (184/405) of bats, 56% (127/228) of foxes,

Figure 1.2 Reported cases of animal rabies in the United States, 1972–2002. Results are given as number of cases (y axis) by year (x axis) and type of animal (wildlife and domestic animals). From reference 2956.

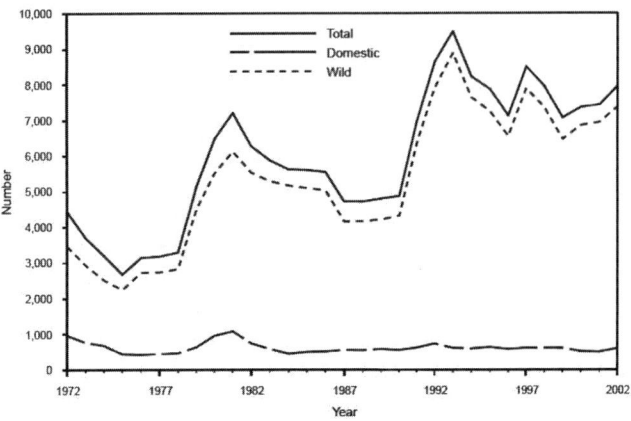

and 80–100% of domestic animals, including dogs, cats, cows, goats, and horses. From a random sample of health centers in Uganda, the risk of death from rabies in the absence of PEP was estimated to be 1 (95% CI 0.7–2)/10^5 population and year.

TRAVELERS

Rabies has been reported in international travelers (272, 1169, 2152, 3181, 3719, 4100, 4322, 5709, 6319, 6985). In the United States in 1980–1997, 33% (12/36) of rabies cases in humans could be attributed to virus variants from outside the United States. In Europe in 1977–1996, of 214 reported cases, 192 (90%) were contracted domestically (in 17 countries), and 24 (11%) were imported. Sources abroad are mainly donated or ownerless puppies or stray dogs, but also monkeys and other wild or peridomestic mammals. On a beach in Agadir, Morocco, two Austrian tourists were bitten while playing with a puppy; the woman remained healthy, but her boyfriend developed signs of rabies and died 3 weeks later.

With PEP as proxy, the risk of exposure is estimated to be 0.5–3.5/1,000 travelers and month. In Nepal in 1996–1998, with bites as proxy, risk estimates per 1,000 per year ranged from 1.9 for tourists to 5.7 for expatriates. Short-term travelers likely exposed to vertebrates, e.g., children, bikers, hunters, trekkers, and expatriates, should be offered preexposure vaccine.

RABID DOGS

Most reported human deaths from rabies are due to dogs: ≥95% in China and India and >90% worldwide (2206, 2601, 5708, 7232, 8106, 8376). Similarly, most visits for

Figure 1.3 Rabies in domestic animals in Europe, 1990–2002. Results are given as number of cases (y axis) by year (x axis) and type of animal (dogs, cats, cattle, sheep, and goats). Reproduced from reference 5988 with permission.

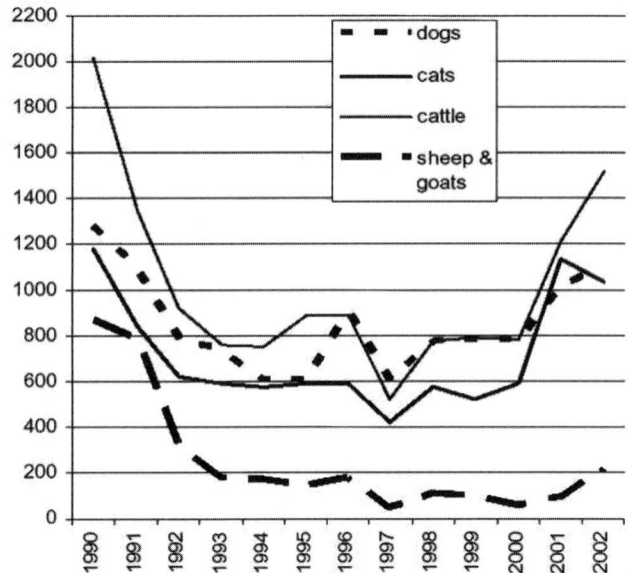

risk evaluation or PEP are due to suspected or confirmed rabid dogs: >50% in the Philippines, >85% in Thailand, and >90% worldwide. By location, owned dogs or stray dogs are the main culprits. In Thailand, children are exposed to dogs mainly in or around their homes. Rabid dogs have been reported to expose up to 11 persons. In Hermosillo, Mexico, in July 1987–December 1988, during an urban epizootic with >280 rabid dogs, ~2.5% of residents were bitten. Catching or eliminating rabid dogs should be left to experts. Vaccination has significantly reduced the importance of dogs as rabies vectors in high-income countries. Nonvaccinated dogs, including puppies, illegally imported into high-income countries from enzootic areas are an emerging source of rabies.

RABID CATS

Cats (1319, 1870, 5708, 8106) can be sources of rabies in humans. Worldwide, ~1% of reported human rabies deaths are due to cats. Of visits for risk evaluation or PEP, 10% (2,622 in 1994) were due to suspected or confirmed rabid cats in children in Thailand, 14% (844/6,139 PEP in 1993–1998) in New York state, 14% (43/315) of visits and 19% (15/79) of PEP at a United States navy facility in the Philippines, and 3–4% worldwide.

RABID MONKEYS

In tropical countries, exposure to monkeys (2333, 5709) may cause 5–40% of visits for rabies risk evaluation and 10–25% of PEP. In Kathmandu, Nepal, in 1996–1998, monkeys inhabiting temples were responsible for 43% (24/56) of bites or scratches in tourists who consulted for risk evaluation. In Brazil in 1991–1998, rabid marmosets ("saguí," *Callithrix jacchus*, small, insect-eating primates kept as pets) caused eight human deaths from rabies.

RABID BATS

Outdoor or indoor bat (2723, 3122, 5009, 5720, 6428, 7963) encounters include touching for curiosity, contact for removal from a structure, picking up a grounded bat, and "landings" on sleeping or awakening persons. However, a majority of exposures are without reported physical contact. The risk of nocturnal bat exposure is reduced by bat-proofed houses and mosquito nets. Worldwide, bats account for ~0.5% (4/1,001 in 1997) of human rabies deaths and ~0.5% of PEP.

In the Americas, classical rabies virus circulates in bats. In the United States in 1970–2000, exposure or molecular fingerprinting linked >50% of human rabies deaths to bats (30% in 1970–1989, 75% (24/32) in 1990–2000). In Latin America, rural residents can be exposed to vampire bats. In a Venezuelan gold mine village in 4 months, bites by *Desmodus rotundus* were diagnosed from bite marks or blood-stained bedding in >8% (145/~1,650) of residents. The high biting rate was explained by bats using mines as caves, and by a bat migratory corridor (1071). In a gold prospector settlement of the Brazilian Amazon, 23% (30/129) inhabitants reported vampire bat attacks in the previous year, for an average of three bites per person (6693). In Costa Rica, in an area where *D. rotundus* feeds on cattle at a rate of 3.5/100 each year, two humans contracted bat-derived rabies from a cat after 31 years without human rabies (378). A municipality in Bahia state, Brazil, with ~16,000 inhabitants recorded 308 vampire bat attacks and three rabies deaths in 1992, and another municipality of similar size recorded five attacks and two deaths (2830). In two settlements in the Amazon of northern Peru in 1990, *D. rotundus* was implicated in 29 rabies deaths; 96% (22/29) of cases and 22% (66/301) of unaffected inhabitants gave a history of bat bites (mostly on the head), and identical virus variants were isolated from bats and the brain of one deceased inhabitant (4505).

In Australia, Australian bat lyssavirus circulates in bats; 2 human deaths due to Australian bat lyssavirus have been reported. Adults exposed to bats and Australian bat lyssavirus are mainly volunteer and professional bat handlers.

In Europe, European bat lyssaviruses 1 and 2 circulate in bats; at least 4 human deaths due to European bat lyssavirus have been documented: in Ukraine in 1977 (a girl bitten in the finger), in Finland in 1985 (a bat handler), in Russia in 1985 (a girl bitten on the lip by *Eptesicus serotinus*), and in Scotland in 2002 (a bat handler bitten by *Myosotis daubentonii*).

RABID OTHER MAMMALS

In central Romania in October 2004, a bear killed a man who was picking mushrooms deep in the forest and wounded 11 others; the bear was confirmed to be rabid, and the 11 wounded and 86 other people received PEP (6076). In Iran in 1954, a rabid wolf attacked 29 persons.

1.2 OTHER SYSTEMIC INFECTIONS FROM BITES

BACTERIA

Itching at an injured site or neurological manifestations point to rabies virus or *Clostridium tetani* as causative agents. Fever or an immune impaired (e.g., splenectomized or human immunodeficiency virus-infected) victim point to invasive disease (e.g., bacteremia or septic arthritis) (Box 1.1).

Clostridium tetani **(3042, 7312, 7635).** *C. tetani* can be isolated from soil, dog feces, horse manure, and cow and sheep dung. Although poorly documented, soil-polluted beaks of birds and claws of reptiles and mammals are likely sources of *C. tetani*. Dirty or puncture wounds are particularly hazardous. While none of 50 dog or 57 cat

> **Box 1.1** Systemic agents from vertebrate animal bite or scratch
>
> **Any vertebrate:** *Clostridium tetani, Francisella, Leptospira, Pasteurella; Sporothrix*
> **Any mammal:** also rabies virus
> **Cats:** also *Bartonella*
> **Dogs:** also *Capnocytophaga*
> **Rodents:** also *Spirillum, Streptobacillus moniliformis*
> **Monkeys:** also simian herpesviruses and retroviruses

bite wounds grew *C. tetani*, *C. sordellii* was isolated from 2% of cat bite wounds. Tetanus should be considered after any vertebrate injury, including snake bites and bird pickings. Inappropriate first aid (e.g., "black stones" for snake bites) increases the risk of tetanus in nonvaccinated persons.

Francisella tularensis (260, 346, 2172, 2347, 4333). An array of vertebrates can be infected. Cats can serve as a reservoir and source of human infections. In southern Canada in 1995, 4% (9/242) of farm cats were seroreactive. Cats preying on rodents can carry *F. tularensis* on teeth or claws. Acquisition from cats via bite, scratch, or casual contact is well documented, and in a case-control study, cat ownership was a significant risk. A veterinary surgeon contracted ulceroglandular tularemia from cutting his finger while operating on a cat. Occasional other sources of human tularemia are bites by squirrels, prairie dogs, raccoons, and other wild mammals.

Pasteurella (2232, 3457, 4493, 7312, 7889). The mouths of dogs (in 50–65%), cats (in 50–90%), and laboratory rodents (e.g., mice and guinea pigs) can be colonized with *P. multocida*. By geography, dogs are implicated in ~50% of bite wounds that yield *P. multocida*, cats in 20–80%. Of 767 *Pasteurella* infections acquired from animals in France in 1985–1992, most (98.5%) had dogs or cats as sources; nearly 50% of infections were in age groups 0–20 years. In contrast, of 302 laboratory-confirmed cases in the United Kingdom (200 due to *P. multocida* and 102 due to other *Pasteurella* spp.), 67% were in people >45 years of age; only 22% (59) of cases reported animal contacts. *P. multocida* can cause invasive disease, mainly at the extremes of age. Of 23 infants with *P. multocida* meningitis, about half (12) had a history of exposure to dogs. Other vertebrate sources of *P. haemolytica*, *P. multocida*, and *P. pneumotropica* that are infrequently reported include cattle, sheep, goats, wild pigs, rodents, captive felines, and snakes.

Streptobacillus moniliformis (1243). Bites by laboratory or pet rats are a cause of rat bite (Haverhill) fever. However, bites are not a requirement for transmission (for the nonbite mode, see section 3.3).

Sporothrix schenckii (5668, 6613). Animal injury is a source. In a sporothrichosis outbreak in Rio de Janeiro in 1998–2000, 79% (52/66) of patients reported cat contacts, and 47% (31) reported scratches or bites. Cases have also been reported following injury from rodents, birds, reptiles, and fish. A male adult developed sporotrichosis 6 weeks after a squirrel bite (probably *Sciurus carolinensis*).

1.3 BITE WOUND INFECTIONS

Risks and management (1939, 2429, 2935, 7312, 7857). About 5–50% of bite wounds become infected (up to 85% are colonized). Infections seem more frequent in cat bites (30–50%) than dog bites (5–20%). Of 734 patients with dog bite wounds, 2.5% had infected wounds initially, and another 2% developed infection on follow-up. Wounds should be promptly cleaned with water and soap and evaluated for rabies, tetanus, need for débridement, and wound infection. Lymphangitis and regional adenopathy point to dissemination or invasive disease. Wound culture is recommended for bites by research, zoo, and wild animals, and a specialist's advice may be needed. Antibiotic prophylaxis is not routinely indicated. For human bites, see section 13.5.

Agents (2819, 7312, 7989). Bite and scratch wound infections reflect buccal, skin, or claw flora. Infections are typically polymicrobial and grow three to five (range, 0–16) bacterial species per culture. The spectrum varies with test method and animal species.

Main agents from dog and cat bite wounds are *Streptococcus* (in ~50%), including *S. agalactiae*, *S. equinus*, *S. mitis*, and *S. pyogenes*, and *Staphylococcus* (in 35–50%), including *S. aureus*, *S. epidermidis*, and *S. saprophyticus*.

Other aerobes (by frequency) from infected animal wounds include *Corynebacterium* (12–28%), *Neisseria* (16–19%), *Moraxella* (10–35%, cat), *Bacillus* (10%), *Enterococcus* (~10%), *Acinetobacter* (7%, cat), *Actinomyces* (5%), *Pseudomonas* (5%), *Alcaligenes* (4%, cat), *Citrobacter* (4%, dog), *Enterobacter* (4%, cat), *Capnocytophaga* (2–7%), *Aeromonas* (2%, cat), *Eikenella* (2%), *Erysipelothrix* (4%, cat), *Gemella* (5%), *Klebsiella* (2–4%), *Lactobacillus* (2–4%), *Rhodococcus* (2%, cat), and *Streptomyces* (2%, cat).

Anaerobes recovered from animal wounds include *Fusobacterium* (33%), *Bacteroides* (30%), *Porphyromonas* (30%), *Propionibacterium* (20%), *Prevotella* (19–28%, dog), *Peptostreptococcus* (5–16%, dog), and *Veillonella* (2%).

"WET" AGENTS AND FISH TRAUMA

Agents following fish trauma include *Aeromonas*, environmental mycobacteria, *Erysipelothrix rhusiopathiae*, *Streptococcus iniae*, and *Vibrio* (333, 666, 1110, 4323, 8017).

Mycobacterium marinum. *M. marinum* has been isolated from marine and freshwater fish. *M. marinum* infections (fish tank granuloma) typically follow exposure to aquarium water or fish, rarely shellfish. Exposure may involve skin trauma, for example, abrasions. In France in 1996–1998, 63 cases of *M. marinum* infection were identified, including 53 (84%) in hobbyists exposed to fish tanks. Of 72 lesions, 67% (48) were located on the hands, 22% (16) on the arms, and 11% (8) on the other sites. In Spain in 1991–1998, of 39 confirmed cases, 90% (35) were fish related and most lesions were located on the hand.

Streptococcus iniae. *S. iniae* invasive disease was diagnosed in Toronto in 1995–1996, in four patients (clustered cases) who had handled farmed, fresh fish. Surveillance for 1 year detected eight cases of cellulitis of the hand and one case of *S. iniae* endocarditis; all eight had handled live or freshly killed fish, including tilapia (*Oreochromis*), which is used in Asian cuisine.

Vibrio vulnificus. *V. vulnificus* has caused skin infections from fish injury. In Israel in 1996–1997, *V. vulnificus* was reported in 62 people who had recently purchased and handled live fish from inland ponds (57 had cellulitis, 4 had necrotizing fasciitis, and 1 had osteomyelitis); before the outbreak, fishpond managers had changed selling practices from selling fish packed in ice to selling live fish.

2

Domestic Mammals

2.1 Dogs
2.2 Cats
2.3 Domestic bovids
2.4 Suids
2.5 Equids
2.6 Camelids

For bites, see chapter 1; for work with animals, see chapter 12; for wild vertebrates, see chapter 3, and for animal-derived foods, see chapter 7.

Domesticated mammals include dogs, cats, cattle, sheep, goats, pigs, horses, donkeys, and camels. Agents are acquired from domestic animals by contact, ingestion, inhalation, or inoculation. Some agents are host specific and do not readily cross species, in particular, some zoonotic viruses. Other agents have a broader host range, for instance, *Lyssavirus*, *Brucella*, *Francisella*, *Salmonella*, microsporidia, and *Toxoplasma*. In rare instances of species jumps from mammals to receptive humans, severe (virgin territory) epidemics can result. Examples include human immunodeficiency virus, *Henipavirus*, and severe acute respiratory syndrome-associated coronavirus.

2.1 DOGS

The domestic dog (*Canis familiaris*) and dingo (*C. dingo*) are members of Canidae (order Carnivora).

Canine zoonoses (3457, 4462, 4630) (Box 2.1). Dogs have been "close" to humans since their domestication about 12,000 years ago. The current world dog population is estimated to be ~500 million. In the United States, about every third household owns ≥1 dog, and the dog population is ~40–50 million (~15/100 population). In the United Kingdom in 2001, there were 6.1 million dogs (~10/100 population). Healthy, incubating, or ill owned or stray dogs can spread infections to humans.

CANINE DROPLET-AIR CLUSTER
Dog-to-human spread via respiratory secretions is unusual.

Viruses
Humans do not seem susceptible to canine respiratory viruses such as canine parainfluenza virus, canine parvovirus, and canine distemper virus.

Bacteria (2104, 5540)
Dogs can harbor *Bordetella bronchiseptica* in the pharynx, and dogs are a source of this agent for individuals infected with human immunodeficiency virus. Dogs seem susceptible to *Mycobacterium bovis*.

> **Box 2.1** Agents from dogs, by cluster
>
> For bites, see chapter 1.
>
> | | |
> |---|---|
> | Droplet-air | *Bordetella bronchiseptica* |
> | Feces-food | *Campylobacter*; microsporidia; *Giardia* |
> | Zoonotic | Rabies virus, *Borrelia burgdorferi* sl, *Brucella canis*, *C. burnetii*, rickettsiae, *Y. pestis*; *Babesia* (*B. canis* and *B. microti*-like), *Leishmania* (cutaneous and visceral), *T. cruzi*; *E. granulosus*, *E. multilocularis* |
> | Environmental | *Leptospira*, hookworms (cutaneous larva migrans), *T. canis* |
> | Skin-blood | *S. aureus* (including methicillin-resistant *S. aureus*), dermatophytes (*Malassezia* and *Microsporum*), mites (*Sarcoptes scabiei* subsp. *canis*), attached ectoparasites |

Fungi (1109)
Soil-borne fungi such as *Cryptococcus neoformans* and *Blastomyces dermatitidis* can infect dogs. Illness in dogs can point to an environmental focus, but dogs are not considered sources for humans.

CANINE FECES-FOOD CLUSTER
Viruses
Dogs can harbor rotaviruses, but spread from dog to human is not well documented. In children in Mexico City, 1 of 39 sequenced *Rotavirus* isolates exhibited a VP7 gene sequence that was homologous with a canine strain, suggesting possible and hitherto unrecognized dog-to-human spread (4188).

Bacteria
Dogs seem infrequent sources for humans (1727, 2841, 3031, 6592, 6753, 7536).

Campylobacter. Dogs can harbor *C. coli*, *C. jejuni*, and *C. upsaliensis*, and all three species can cause diarrhea in dogs. By age, the fecal prevalence in healthy dogs is ~5–30%. Risks are contacts with puppies and dogs that have diarrhea. Some 2–6% of sporadic human infections are attributed to contacts with pet animals or diarrheic animals.

Escherichia coli. Enterohemorrhagic *E. coli* (EHEC) are isolated from dogs, as well as enteropathogenic *E. coli* (EPEC), including plasmid-negative (atypical) serotypes such as O111:H25, O119:H2, and O128:H2. The epidemiologic and clinical significance of these findings is unclear.

Helicobacter. Dogs are a suspected source of nonpylori *Helicobacter*, e.g., *H. canis*.

Plesiomonas shigelloides. *P. shigelloides* is recovered from up to 4% of dog feces, and dogs are a potential source.

Salmonella. Dogs can carry *Salmonella*. The fecal prevalence in domestic, healthy dogs is 1–30%. Although humans can acquire *Salmonella* from dogs, dog-to-human spread seems unusual.

Yersinia. Dogs can carry *Y. enterocolitica*, including serogroups infective to humans, e.g., O:3, O:8, and O:9, and *Y. pseudotuberculosis*. Fecal prevalence can reach 5–30%. Dog-to-human spread seems unusual. In the United States in the 1970s, a sick bitch and her puppies were the source of an outbreak that propagated person-to-person and ultimately infected 18 (86%) of 21 members from two families.

Protozoa
Dogs are sources mainly of *Cryptosporidium* and *Giardia* (2519, 4441, 4443, 7452, 7542).

Cryptosporidium canis. *C. canis* (formerly *C. parvum* genotype 3) is prevalent in ~10–20% of stray and domestic dogs, and there is evidence for infection with this agent in humans. In a cryptosporidiosis outbreak among veterinary students, dogs were the implicated source. Immune-impaired persons should be aware of this risk.

***Cyclospora* spp.** *Cyclospora* spp. are detected in the feces of dogs. Infectivity for humans is not reported.

Entamoeba. Although dogs can host *E. histolytica/dispar*, dogs do not constitute a significant source of *Entamoeba* for humans.

Giardia. Dogs can harbor human-infective *G. lamblia* genotypes and dog-specific *G. canis*. By sampling and test, the fecal, microscopic prevalence of *Giardia* spp. in dogs is ~1–70% (typically ~5%). According to molecular and household studies, dogs are increasingly accepted as a source of human infections.

Isospora. Dogs can harbor and shed *I. canis* and *I. belli*. By dog age and provenance, 2–9% of dogs shed *Isospora* in feces. Dogs seem an unlikely source of infections in humans.

Toxoplasma gondii. Dogs do not shed oocysts. In Panama, dogs are a source of *T. gondii* in children, presumably from exposure to the fur of dogs that have rolled in cat feces.

Fungi
The microsporidia *Encephalitozoon cuniculi*, *E. intestinalis*, and *Enterocytozoon bieneusi* are reported in dogs. In

Slovakia, 73 (38%) of 193 dogs were reactive to *E. cuniculi* in immunofluorescence assay (IFA). Dog owners are at risk of infection (1924, 3076).

Helminths
Free-roaming (hunting and fish-eating) dogs can be naturally infected by an array of helminths, including *Angiostrongylus*, *Ascaris lumbricoides* (species confirmed by molecular fingerprinting; prevalence in endemic areas up to 30%), *Diphyllobothrium*, *Clonorchis sinensis* (prevalence in Vietnam and People's Republic of China, 5–100%), *Echinostoma*, *Fasciolopsis*, *Gnathostoma*, *Heterophyes*, *Metagonimus*, *Opistorchis*, *Paragonimus* (prevalence in Vietnam, 3–63%), *Trichinella* (*T. britovi*, prevalence in Italy, 0–1%; *T. nativa* and *T. spiralis*, prevalence in People's Republic of China, 21% or 4,151 of 19,662), and *Trichuris vulpis* (human infections documented in urban slums) (1672, 1818, 2074, 4570, 6017, 7165, 7542). Dog meat is popular in parts of East Asia and a potential source for gnathostomiasis or trichinellosis.

CANINE ZOONOTIC CLUSTER
Dogs can lead humans to foci, attract arthropods, and bring ticks or other ectoparasites into houses, kennels, and barns, exposing owners, friends, and other animals. Ectoparasites should be removed from dogs with instruments and not be crushed by bare hands (1300, 2856, 7663).

Viruses
Crimean-Congo hemorrhagic fever virus (CCHFV) (6746, 6844). Dogs can contract CCHFV from animal contacts or ticks. In South Africa, the reported seroprevalence in domestic dogs is 6% (118/1,978). *Rhipicephalus sanguineus* is suspected to carry CCHFV to humans. Removing ticks from dogs could be hazardous.

Powassan virus. Ticks can carry Powassan virus to dogs. Canine infections have been reported.

Rabies virus (4103, 5988, 7404, 8106, 8149). For bites, see chapter 1. Worldwide, about one-third of animals with confirmed rabies are dogs. In Santa Cruz city, Bolivia, in 1972–1997, 50% (4,694/9,308) of dog brain samples tested positive for rabies virus, and in 1997 the rate of dog rabies was ~$44/10^5$ (120/276,034). In Africa, Latin America, Asia, and eastern Europe, nonvaccinated dogs are major rabies reservoirs. Incubating dogs shed virus in saliva some days before becoming symptomatic. Almost all rabid dogs die within an observation period of 10 days. Vaccination has significantly reduced dog rabies in North America and western Europe. In the United States, 6,949 dog rabies cases were reported in 1947, but only 114 were reported in 2000 (1.6% of all rabid animals), 89 (1.2%) in 2001, 99 (1.2%) in 2002, and 117 (1.6%) in 2003 (Fig. 1.2). In Europe in 1990–2002, 11,065 dogs (8.5% of all rabid animals) were diagnosed as rabid (851 per year), principally in eastern Europe and Turkey (Fig. 1.3). In Greenland, where the Arctic fox maintains rabies, epizootic rabies can affect sledge dogs.

Tick-borne encephalitis virus (TBEV) (1664, 7305). Ticks can carry TBEV to dogs. Dogs and other medium-sized mammals are hosts for *Ixodes* nymphs. Reported seroprevalences in dogs are 5–15%.

West Nile virus (WNV). Mosquitoes carry WNV to dogs. Canine infections are reported.

Bacteria
Anaplasma phagocytophilum **(6040).** Ticks carry *A. phagocytophilum* to dogs. Infections are reported in dogs. In Switzerland, 3% (22/642) of healthy dogs are seroreactive.

Bacillus anthracis. Dogs are susceptible to cutaneous and gastrointestinal *B. anthracis*, and dog epizootics have occurred. Human risks seem to be limited to contacts with ill animals.

Bartonella **(852, 1316, 3003).** *B. clarridgeiae*, *B. henselae*, and *B. vinsonii berkhoffii* have been isolated in dogs. Hematophagous arthropods (including *Ixodes* ticks) are suspected vectors to dogs. The reported prevalence of anti-*Bartonella* immunoglobulin G in healthy dogs is 4–10%.

Borrelia burgdorferi **sensu lato (sl) (2983, 5457).** Ticks carry *B. burgdorferi* to dogs. Dogs are competent reservoir hosts. By the time spent outdoors and testing, 10–55% of dogs can be seroreactive. Dog owners are at increased risk of infection (because of increased outdoor exposure or by ticks that dogs bring home). In The Netherlands, seroprevalence is 15% in 440 owners of hunting dogs versus 9% in 1,052 blood donors.

Brucella **(2637, 4552, 6223).** *B. melitensis*, *B. abortus*, *B. suis*, and *B. canis* have been reported from dogs, but only *B. canis* is enzootic in some dog populations, e.g., stray and kennel dogs. In India, the anti-*Brucella* prevalence in dogs is ~2%. Dogs have a role in the dispersal of *Brucella* between farms. Dogs are a source of *B. canis* in humans. Because of diagnostic difficulties, infections in humans are likely underrated. Contact with dogs is a risk, in particular, among dog owners and handlers.

Coxiella burnetii **(966, 3319, 7258).** By geography, seroprevalence in dogs is 0–45% (0% in 12,556 sheep dogs in New Zealand, 10–45% in dogs in Europe, 28% in Thailand). Dogs can carry ticks infective to humans and become a source of sporadic infections in humans. Dogs can become involved in a peridomestic cycle. Three family members contracted Q fever 8–12 days after exposure to an infected parturient dog.

***Ehrlichia* (2067, 4404).** *E. canis*, *E. chaffeensis*, and *E. ewingii* have been reported in dogs. Whether these represent true species has not been confirmed. Ticks are vectors to dogs. By geography, 0.2–63% of dogs are seroreactive to *E. canis* antigen. In Vietnam in 1968, an *E. canis* epizootic caused hundreds of canine cases.

***Francisella tularensis* (4333, 4787, 5562, 7418).** Of farm dogs in enzootic areas, 14–16% can be seroreactive to *F. tularensis*. Reactive roaming dogs can point to enzootic foci. Dogs can infect humans via aerosols or attached ticks. On Martha's Vineyard, Mass., in 1978, seven persons contracted tularemia, likely from two free-roaming dogs that shook off moisture inside the house on a rainy day. In Washington, D.C., in 1978, three men developed pneumonic tularemia 3–4 days after familiarizing hunting dogs with the scent of a rabbit previously caught by another dog that had died. *F. tularensis*-infected ticks have been recovered from dogs close to human cases, and owners who removed and crushed ticks from dogs have contracted tularemia.

***Rickettsia* (4333, 4472, 6455, 6795, 7485).** *R. australis*, *R. conorii*, *R. rickettsii*, and *R. typhi* have been reported in dogs. Dogs are sentinels of enzootic rickettsiae.

Dogs can bring ticks and rickettsiae close to humans: in North America, mainly *Dermacentor variabilis*; in the Mediterranean, mainly *Rhipicephalus sanguineus*; and in Russia, mainly *D. reticulatus*. *D. variabilis* (American dog tick) carries *R. rickettsii* to dogs. In Ohio, 0.6% (1/155) of *D. variabilis* collected from dogs was infected. In enzootic areas, 3–8% of dogs are seroreactive (the reported seroprevalence of 60–75% is likely confounded by cross-reactivity or selective sampling). *R. sanguineus* (brown dog tick) is a vector of *R. conorii* to dogs and humans. Up to 80–90% of human Mediterranean spotted fever cases have a history of exposure to dogs. Traveled dogs have brought *R. sanguineus* and *R. conorii* back from the Mediterranean to central Europe, causing infections in owners and friends. In the Mediterranean, by sample (stray or owned) 25–90% of dogs are seroreactive to *R. conorii*. *D. reticulatus* is a vector of *R. sibirica*.

***Yersinia pestis* (1643, 4333, 6974).** Fleas are vectors of *Y. pestis* to dogs. Dogs seem relatively resistant to plague. In enzootic areas, <1% (pet) to 4–10% (farm) of dogs are seroreactive to *Y. pestis* antigen. Dogs and their fleas can be a source of human plague. Dog ownership in enzootic areas is considered a risk for plague in humans.

Protozoa

***Babesia* (1633, 3558, 3658).** *B. canis*, *B. gibsoni*, and emerging species have been isolated in dogs. *Babesia* is difficult to separate morphologically from *Theileria*, which has also been reported from dogs. Vector ticks of *B. canis* to dogs include *R. sanguineus* (worldwide), *D. reticulatus* (Europe), and *Haemaphysalis* (southern Africa and Japan). Dogs and their ticks seem to be an underrated hazard for human infections with *B. canis* and *B. microti*-like babesiae.

***Leishmania* (1021, 1077, 1895, 2216, 3211, 6210).** Sandflies are vectors of *Leishmania* to dogs. Domestic dogs are suspected to maintain and contribute to the peridomestic spread of zoonotic cutaneous leishmaniasis. Dermotropic *Leishmania* recovered from dogs include *L. major* and *L. tropica* in the Old World and *L. braziliensis* and *L. peruviana* in Latin America. By focus and test, the prevalence of zoonotic cutaneous leishmaniasis in dogs in South America is 5–25%. Dogs are the principal reservoir of zoonotic visceral leishmaniasis in the Old and New Worlds. Viscerotropic *L. infantum* (*L. chagasi*) has been isolated in dogs. Seroprevalence in healthy or mildly symptomatic dogs is ~5–45%. In northern Portugal, 20% of 294 dogs are seroreactive, and 3% have evidence of visceral leishmaniasis disease. Infected pet, stray, and herd dogs can introduce *L. infantum* in new areas, including North America. In 1999–2000, epizootic *L. infantum* affected hunting dogs in 21 states of the United States and in Ontario, Canada. The presence of dogs in or near houses is a risk. Synanthropic sandflies feeding on dogs are likely to transfer *L. infantum* from dog to human.

***Trypanosoma* (502, 1114, 1936, 8090, 8099).** *T. brucei* sl, *T. cruzi*, *T. evansi*, *T. rangeli*, and *T. vivax* have been diagnosed in dogs. Tsetse flies are vectors of *T. brucei* sl to dogs. Dogs are highly susceptible to *T. brucei brucei* (to which humans are refractory). Dogs are a putative host for (human-infective) *T. brucei rhodesiense*. *T. brucei gambiense* does not seem to be reported in dogs. Triatomine bugs are vectors of *T. cruzi* to dogs. Dogs are a major peridomestic reservoir, constitute a ready source of *T. cruzi* for bugs, and are indicators of active transmission (from Argentina to Texas). By sample and enzooticity, 0–50% of dogs are parasitemic, and 0–65% are seroreactive. Dog ownership is likely to increase human risks.

Helminths

***Dipylidium caninum* (5130, 7542).** Dogs are final hosts of *D. caninum*. They acquire the tapeworm by biting infective fleas or lice. *D. caninum* is enzootic in neglected dogs parasitized by fleas (*Ctenocephalides felis* and *C. canis*) or lice (*Trichodectes canis*). Humans acquire *D. caninum* by the same mode as dogs, by biting on dog ectoparasites.

Dirofilaria **(1357, 2307, 5269, 5556, 6068, 7431).** Dogs are final hosts for *D. immitis*, *D. reconditum*, and *D. repens*. Dogs that attract infective mosquitoes are a suspected hazard for humans. *D. immitis* (canine heartworm) is enzootic in dogs in warm climates. By geography and test, 0–90% (typically 1–15%) of dogs are microfilaremic. Traveled dogs can carry *D. immitis* away from enzootic areas. Peridomestic mosquitoes can carry *D. immitis* from infected dogs to humans. *D. repens* is enzootic in dogs in the Old World, including in the Mediterranean. By geography and test, 0–20% of dogs are microfilaremic.

Echinococcus **(968, 1887, 2119, 2869, 3901, 4225, 6140, 7454, 7950, 8320).** Dogs are synanthropic final hosts of *E. granulosus*, including the sheep (genotype G1), cattle (G5), pig (G7), horse (G4), camel (G6), and Nordic-cervid (G8) strains. In Australia, dingos replace dogs as the final, "sylvatic" host of a strain that circulates in wallabies. Slaughter and abattoir offal are important sources for dogs, including sled, herding, rural, and city dogs. By sample (stray or pet) and test (autopsy, purgation, or fecal antigen capture), prevalence in dogs is 0–70% (typically 5–35%). In Libya, prevalence is 10% in urban pet dogs, 30% in urban stray dogs, and up to 60% in rural dogs. In Uruguay, worm loads in 44 purged dogs were 1–4,331 (median, 8–10) per dog. Keeping dogs is a risk: humans infected with *E. granulosus* report dog ownership significantly more often than uninfected controls, and risks tend to increase with increasing numbers of dogs in the household and with increasing contact time. In Spain, compared with nonowners, infection odds were 1.2 (95% confidence interval [95% CI] 0.4–3.5) for ownership of 1–10 years, 3.5 (1.2–9.8) for ownership of 11–30 years, and 5 (2–14) for ownership of >30 years. The relationship is not always straightforward, however. Because the incubation period is years, past dog ownership reflects exposure better than current ownership. By setting and *E. granulosus* strain, infections in humans result from short contacts (with strays) or year-long contacts (with pets). Dog feces on the premises, kissing dogs, letting dogs lick utensils or children, and feeding raw offal to dogs are peridomestic "infection short circuits."

Dogs are also susceptible to *E. multilocularis*, and they can become natural, synanthropic, final hosts. The prepatent period in dogs is ~4 weeks. In Europe, 0.3–7% of dogs are infected. Dog ownership is a risk. Other domestic animals and access of wildlife (e.g., foxes) to the premises can confound risk evaluation.

CANINE ENVIRONMENTAL CLUSTER
Roaming dogs can acquire agents via ingestion or contact from water, soil, plants, rodents, and larger mammals.

Bacteria
Leptospira **(1450, 4279, 4369, 7678).** *Leptospira* serovars demonstrated in dogs include Canicola, Icterohaemorrhagiae, Grippotyphosa, and Pomona. Infections in dogs are frequently inapparent. Dogs recovered from disease can shed *Leptospira* in urine for life. Vaccines do not prevent shedding in urine. Reported seroprevalence in roaming dogs is ~20–80%.

Dogs are important for the spread of *Leptospira* to humans by contact or by polluting water or soil. In enzootic, rural areas, ownership of (seroreactive) dogs is a risk. In the United States in 1950–2000, four leptospirosis outbreaks were linked to pet dogs: 1950 in North Dakota (nine human cases), 1971 in Texas (seven human cases), 1972 in Oregon (nine human cases), and 1972 in Missouri (five human cases). In the Missouri outbreak, a previously vaccinated pet dog was implicated. In Italy in 1994–1996, 1% (1/126) of leptospirosis cases identified dogs as the source.

Fungi
Sporothrix schenckii infections have been reported from dogs.

Helminths
Hookworms (1638, 2578, 7794). Dogs can harbor and shed eggs of *Ancylostoma braziliense*, *A. caninum*, and *A. ceylanicum*. In Townsville, Australia, the prevalence of *A. caninum* in dogs by necropsy is 50%. *A. ceylanicum* occasionally completes its life cycle in humans, causing eosinophilic enteritis and anemia. All three species can cause cutaneous larva migrans in humans. Contact of bare skin with polluted soil is a hazard, including construction work, gardening, playing, and barefoot walking at beaches, in parks, and on public or private lawns.

Strongyloides stercoralis. Dogs can acquire *S. stercoralis* larvae percutaneously and via the transmammary route. Whether dogs are a significant source for humans is not known.

Schistosoma **(4830, 6417).** Dogs in enzootic areas can harbor *S. japonicum* and *S. mekongi*, which are infective to humans, and *Heterobilharza americana*, which can cause cercarial dermatitis in humans.

Toxocara canis **(3540, 4392, 4581, 5662, 6450, 6515, 7542).** Dogs are final hosts of *T. canis*. Transmammary transmission from bitches to puppies is the main mode of spread among dogs. The dog prepatent period is 3–4 weeks. By age, deworming, and geography, the overall infection prevalence in dogs is ~15% (~5–30% in North America and western Europe, 10–40% in Africa, 10–80% in Australasia). Mainly puppies shed eggs with feces; up to

85% of puppies can shed eggs with feces. Eggs are not immediately infective when passed. Despite this, ownership of dogs, in particular of puppies, is a risk, presumably from embryonated eggs in the fur, dust, or puppy litter.

CANINE SKIN-BLOOD CLUSTER
Bacteria (4712, 8338)
Methicillin-resistant *Staphylococcus aureus* has been reported from the nares of dogs. Pet dogs can be a household reservoir, and the potential exists for spread in veterinary clinics (animal-to-human and human-to-animal). Dogs can also carry *Streptococcus agalactiae* (group B *Streptococcus*) and *S. canis* (mainly group C or group G *Streptococcus*).

Fungi (1020, 1320, 3457, 5208)
Malassezia pachydermatis is part of the skin flora of dogs. By test (culture and PCR), the skin prevalence in healthy dogs is ~10–85%. In dogs with atopic dermatitis, colonization is intense and extends into ear canals. Pet dogs can be a source of *M. pachydermatis* in owners. By test and dog infection status, ~5–90% of dog owners are colonized. *M. pachydermatis* is a cause of fungemia in immune-impaired hosts. Dogs are a reservoir of *Microsporum canis*, and this agent is a main cause of tinea in dogs. The skin of dogs can also grow *M. gypseum* acquired from soil. Dogs are sources of *M. canis* and *M. gypseum* in humans. Where dogs and humans live close together, *M. canis* is a frequent cause of tinea capitis. The skin of dogs can grow *Trichophyton mentagrophytes* var. *mentagrophytes*. Reported yield is 5–15%. Pet dogs are a source of *T. mentagrophytes* var. *mentagrophytes* in humans.

Ectoparasites (5445, 7445, 7933)
A range of fleas can dwell on dogs, including "dog" flea (*Ctenocephalides canis*), "cat" flea (*Ctenocephalides felis*), "rabbit" flea (*Spilopsyllus cuniculi*), and "human" flea (*Pulex irritans*). How dog fleas affect human health is not well known. Dogs can harbor *Sarcoptes*, *Cheyletiella*, and *Otodectes* mites. Molecular studies suggest that *Sarcoptes scabiei* of dogs and humans constitute distinct populations and that a species barrier exists. Humans can acquire the mites above from dogs, mainly *S. scabiei* subsp. *canis*, however, and in patients with unexplained prurigo or allergy, examination of home dogs for ectoparasites is advised. Roaming or traveling dogs can bring ticks and their agents to homes (see "Canine Zoonotic Cluster" above). Depending on sample (kennel and farm dogs), some 20% of dogs can be tick infested. Tick genera found on dogs include *Boophilus*, *Ixodes*, and *Rhipicephalus*.

2.2 CATS
Domestic cats (*Felis catus*) and wild cats (*F. silvestris*) belong to Felidae (order Carnivora).

Feline zoonoses (3457, 4462, 5694) (Box 2.2). Healthy, incubating, or ill, pet or stray, kittens or older cats can be sources of infections in humans. Cats have been associated with humans since their domestication 5,000 years ago. In the United States, 25–33% of households own ≥1 cat, and the cat population is .55 million (,19/100 population). In the United Kingdom in 2001, there were 7.5 million cats (,13/100 population).

FELINE DROPLET-AIR CLUSTER
Cat-to-human spread is unusual (2104, 2277, 6996).

Viruses
Feline respiratory viruses such as feline calicivirus, feline herpesvirus, and feline rhinotracheitis virus are enzootic among cats, especially kittens and sheltered cats. There is no indication that these viruses cross species. However, the severe acute respiratory syndrome pandemic has taught us to keep an eye on felid viruses.

Bacteria
B. bronchiseptica is part of the respiratory flora of cats. Cats are an occasional source of pertussis-like illness in children and of pneumonia in individuals infected with human immunodeficiency virus. *Chlamydophila felis* and *C. psittaci* are enzootic in household cats and breeding catteries. *C. felis* is a cause of feline conjunctivitis and rhinitis. Human infections with *C. felis* and *C. psittaci* acquired from cats have been reported. Cats are susceptible to *M. bovis*; spread to humans is not reported. For *Y. pestis*, see "Feline Zoonotic Cluster" below.

Fungi
Although soil-borne fungi such as *C. neoformans* and *Histoplasma capsulatum* can infect cats as they can humans, cats are not a known source for humans.

FELINE FECES-FOOD CLUSTER
Cat-to-human spread seems unusual.

Box 2.2 Agents from cats, by cluster

For bites, see chapter 1.

Droplet-air	*B. bronchiseptica*
Feces-food	*Campylobacter* (drug-resistant); microsporidia; *Cryptosporidium*, *Giardia*, *Toxoplasma*
Zoonotic	Hantavirus, rabies virus; *B. henselae*, *C. burnetii*, *Y. pestis*; *T. cruzi*, *E. multilocularis*
Environmental	*Leptospira*; *Sporothrix schenckii*; *T. cati*
Skin-blood	Cowpox virus; dermatophytes (*Microsporum canis*); ectoparasites

Prions
In the United Kingdom in 1990–1998, commercial pet feed was associated with >80 cases of feline spongiform encephalopathy. Hazardous bovine materials are now banned from pet feeds (5767).

Viruses
Although feline enteric coronavirus and feline parvovirus circulate among cats that shed these viruses with feces, there is little indication that they could cross species.

Bacteria
Cats can harbor *Anaerobiospirillum succiniciproducens*, *Campylobacter* spp., *E. coli* (EHEC), *Helicobacter* spp., *P. shigelloides*, *Salmonella* spp., and *Yersinia* spp. (553, 1727, 2553, 3633, 5373, 6592).

Campylobacter. Cats can harbor *C. coli*, *C. jejuni*, and *C. upsaliensis*. By age and provenance, the prevalence in cats is ~5–30%, with a high prevalence in kittens and young cats. Antimicrobial resistance is an issue. Cats are a potential source for humans. Risks include contacts with kittens or diarrheic cats and living in a household with a cat.

Helicobacter. Cats can harbor *H. bizzozeronii* (*H. heilmannii*), *H. felis*, and *H. pylori*. Whereas the prevalence of *H. felis* and *H. bizzozeronii* in cats is 50–100%, *H. pylori* in cats seems sporadic, and its epidemiological significance is uncertain.

Salmonella **(7737).** The prevalence of *Salmonella* in healthy house cats is low, typically 0.5–3%, with a high prevalence in kittens and ill and ownerless cats. Antimicrobial resistance is an issue.

Yersinia. Cats can carry *Y. enterocolitica* (including human-infective serogroups) and *Y. pseudotuberculosis*. In cats in Japan, the fecal prevalence of *Y. pseudotuberculosis* is 4% (13/318).

Fungi
The microsporidia *E. cuniculi* and *E. bieneusi* are reported in cats. Cat owners seem to be at risk of infection (1924, 6700).

Protozoa
Cats can be sources of *Cryptosporidium* spp., *G. lamblia*, *T. gondii*, *E. histolytica/dispar*, *Isospora felis* (but not *I. belli*), and *Sarcocystis* (cats can be final or intermediate hosts).

Cryptosporidium **(4900, 5618).** Cats can harbor *Cryptosporidium* spp., including *C. felis*. In western Australia, the prevalence in domestic cats by PCR is 10%. Infected cats are an occasional source of *C. felis* in humans.

Giardia **(4900, 7452, 7738).** Cats can harbor cat-specific *G. cati* and *G. lamblia* genotypes pathogenic to humans. *Giardia* is enzootic and mostly inapparent in cats. In western Australia, the prevalence in domestic cats is 80% by PCR.

Toxoplasma gondii **(2051, 2519, 2672, 3756, 4063, 4790, 7238).** Cats are intermediate and definitive hosts of *T. gondii*. The prepatent period in cats is 5–19 days. Few cats (0–1%, typically kittens) shed oocysts, and shedding is limited to about 1–2 weeks. In contrast, oocysts are hardy and survive in soil for years. Cat age, feed (cooked or raw), and coinfection with feline immunodeficiency virus influence seroreactivity in cats. The reported seroprevalence in domestic cats is 5–70%. Risks for humans include cat ownership, cleaning cat litter boxes, cat contacts, and earthen courtyards frequented by stray cats. The association seems stronger for cat feces and litter trays than for contact with the fur of cats, which is perhaps noninfective. On a farm in Illinois, in 1979, 6 of 13 household members contracted acute toxoplasmosis, and three others seroconverted; sick cats were the likely source of the outbreak (6840).

Helminths
Free-roaming (rodent-hunting and fish-eating) cats can be naturally infected with *Capillaria hepatica*, *Clonorchis sinensis* (prevalence in People's Republic of China, up to 50–100%), *Diphyllobothrium* spp., *D. caninum* (mainly flea-infested neglected cats), *Echinostoma* spp., *Heterophyes* spp., *Metagonimus* spp., *Opistorchis felineus* (prevalence in Brandenburg, Germany, 16%), *O. viverrini* (prevalence in Laos, 20%), *Paragonimus* spp., and *T. nativa* (3767, 4570, 5130, 6633, 6717, 7299).

FELINE ZOONOTIC CLUSTER
Roaming cats can acquire zoonotic agents from prey (e.g., mice) or from picked-up vectors.

Viruses
Hantavirus **(4333, 5491, 8294).** Cats seem an underrated source. Hantaan virus, Puumala virus, and Sin Nombre virus are reported in cats. In southern Canada in 1995, 3% (7/242) of farm cats were seroreactive to Sin Nombre virus. In Shanghai, compared with 136 matched controls, cat ownership was a risk in 111 cases of hemorrhagic fever with renal syndrome due to Hantaan virus. In Austria, 5% of 200 cats were reactive to *Hantavirus* in IFA (with high titers to Puumala virus).

Rabies (4103, 5988, 7404, 8106). (For bites, see chapter 1.) Worldwide, cats account for 4–5% of confirmed rabid animals. Virtually all rabid cats die within an observation period of 10 days. In the United States, 249 cat rabies cases were reported in 2000 (3.4% of all rabid animals), 270 (3.6%) in 2001, 299 (3.8%) in 2002, and 321 (4.5%) in 2003 (Fig. 1.2). In those 4 years, cat rabies cases (1,139) outnumbered dog rabies cases (419) >2.5-fold. In such situations, cats should be vaccinated like dogs. In Europe in 1990–2002, 9,277 cats were diagnosed with rabies (714/year, 7.2% of all rabid animals) (Fig. 1.3).

Bacteria
B. anthracis. *B. anthracis* has been reported in cats.

***Bartonella* (694, 1414, 2283, 3013, 3348, 4060, 4790, 6382, 6594).** *B. clarridgeiae*, *B. elizabethae*, *B. henselae*, and *B. koehlerae* have been reported in cats. In Paris, France, 5% (23/436) of domestic cats have *B. clarridgeiae* bacteremia. In Sweden, 25% of 292 domestic cats are reactive to *B. elizabethae*. Cats support inapparent, persistent *B. henselae* bacteremia and are a major reservoir. By sample and setting, ~5–50% of cats have *B. henselae* bacteremia, and 1–80% are reactive to the *B. henselae* antigen. Risks for infections in cats include young age, short ownership, free roaming, flea infestation, housing with other cats, and cats in or from pounds or catteries. Fleas are important for cat-to-cat spread. Cat owners are at risk of cat scratch disease and bacillary angiomatosis. Saliva from kittens with inapparent bacteremia can be infective and is a likely source for humans. In the United States, the cats of patients with cat scratch disease were more frequently bacteremic (17/19 or 89%) than the cats of unaffected owners (7/25 or 28%). In Spain, anti-*B. henselae* immunoglobulin G were nearly five times more frequent in cat owners than blood donors. In Germany, high immunoglobulin G titers (>1:128 in indirect IFA) were more frequent in 63 current (13%) than in 207 past or never owners (2%).

***Brucella* (2637, 6225).** *Brucella* seems rare in cats. In France in 1980–2000, only 1 of 1,298 animal isolates was recovered from a cat (*B. melitensis* biovar 3). In Siberia, six human cases were linked to a domestic cat infected by *B. suis* serovar 5.

***Coxiella burnetii* (4045, 4757).** Cats can be infected with *C. burnetii* and become a source for human infections. By type (pet or stray), 2–40% of cats can be seroreactive. Several cat-related outbreaks have been reported. In Nova Scotia, Canada, in 1995, 25 of 32 Q fever cases were linked to a parturient cat that had a stillborn kitten.

***Rickettsia* (762, 4840).** *R. conorii*, *R. felis*, and *R. typhi* have been reported in cats. Cats have been used as sentinels for the presence of rickettsiae. Cats can contract latent or manifest infections. By type (pet or stray) and location, 0–90% of cats are seroreactive. Although cats are not established reservoir hosts, they are a suspected source for spotted fever rickettsiae in humans. Species identification requires culture or nucleic acid amplification tests. In Corpus Christi, Tex., in 1997–1998, 13% of 39 murine typhus fever cases had a history of exposure to cats.

***Yersinia pestis* (1643, 5633, 5844).** Roaming, flea-infested cats in enzootic areas are at risk of infection with *Y. pestis*. Unlike dogs, cats can become ill and shed *Y. pestis* in respiratory secretions (similar to humans with pneumonic plague). Cat-to-human spread results in lethal, easily overlooked primary pneumonic plague. Spread can also occur via fleas from cats. Cat ownership is a risk. In the United States, in 1977–2001, 6% (23/377) of reported plague cases were cat associated. Six were veterinary staff and 17 were owners or other persons who handled a sick cat; 5 (22%) of the 23 died.

Protozoa
Leishmania infantum (in France, Italy), *L. mexicana* (in Texas), and *L. braziliensis* (in Brazil) have been diagnosed in cats (6704). Cats are a domestic reservoir for *T. cruzi* (8099). The prevalence of parasitemia in house cats can be 3–30%. The role of cats in peridomestic transmission remains to be determined for both protozooses.

Helminths
Cats, dogs, and wild carnivores can carry *Brugia pahangi* and subperiodic *B. malayi*. Cats can be final hosts for *E. multilocularis*. In Europe, the prevalence in cats is 0.2–3%. Cat ownership is a risk (2119, 2869).

FELINE ENVIRONMENTAL CLUSTER
Bacteria
Leptospira can infect cats (4279, 5348). The reported seroprevalence in cats is 13–67%. Cats are usually considered insignificant sources. In rural Mexico, cat ownership is a reported risk.

Fungi
Sporothrix schenckii can infect cats (1810, 5668). In Rio de Janeiro, of 184 cats with sporotrichosis, all yielded *S. schenckii* from cutaneous lesions, 66% from the nose, 42% from the mouth, and 40% from nails. In addition, the oral cavity of 4% (3/84) of apparently healthy cats yielded *S. schenckii*. Cats are a source of human infections, either via injury (see chapter 1) or contact.

Helminths (2415, 3945, 4581, 6417)
Cats can harbor *A. ceylanicum* and perhaps other *Ancylostoma* spp. How cat feces contribute to cutaneous larva migrans is not known (for dogs, see section 2.1). Cats can harbor *S. japonicum*.

Cats are a final host for *Toxocara cati*. By type (pet or stray), age, and test, 1–90% of cats test positive for eggs in feces, typically 20% of domestic or pet cats, and 50% of farm or feral cats. Patent infections are more prevalent in kittens than in older cats. Eggs are not immediately infective when passed. Human infections are suspected but mostly unconfirmed, and compared with dogs, cats are considered a minor source. Indeed, cat breeders are not at increased risk of infection, and in Iceland, when dogs were prohibited for control of cystic echinococcosis, no infections were detected. In contrast, an epidemiologic study in Germany found an infection risk for kitten or cat ownership.

FELINE SKIN-BLOOD CLUSTER
Viruses (1996, 4790, 5491)
Humans seem nonreceptive to feline immunodeficiency virus and feline leukemia virus. Infection prevalence in cats is 3–12% (feline leukemia virus) to ~10% (feline immunodeficiency virus). Cowpox virus can occur in Old World cats that hunt for rodents. In Austria, 4% of 200 free-roaming cats had antibodies to *Orthopoxvirus*, including cowpox virus. Cats can be a source of cowpox virus in humans.

Bacteria (7358, 8338)
Corynebacterium ulcerans, *S. agalactiae* (group B *Streptococcus*) and *S. canis* (group C or group G *Streptococcus*) have been isolated from cats. Whether colonized cats are a hazard for humans is uncertain.

Fungi (834, 2041, 3457)
M. canis, *M. gypseum*, *T. mentagrophytes*, and *T. terrestre* have been isolated from cats. Cats are a principal reservoir for *M. canis*. Yield by culture from cats is 20–35%. Stray and pet animals, including cats in urban areas, are main sources of tinea capitis in humans. Five neonates acquired tinea corporis due to *M. canis* from a nurse whose infection came from her cat. Cats are also sources of *T. mentagrophytes* var. *mentagrophytes* in humans.

Ectoparasites
S. scabiei mites are diagnosed in cats. A potential exists for human infections.

2.3 DOMESTIC BOVIDS
Domesticated cattle (*Bos taurus*), zebu (*B. indicus*), yak (*B. grunniens*), sheep (*Ovis aries*), goat (*Capra hircus*), and water buffalo (*Bubalus bubalus*) are members of the Bovidae (order Artiodactyla). Worldwide, there are ~1.4 billion cattle (16% in India and 13% in Brazil), 1 billion sheep (13% in People's Republic of China and 11% in Australia), 0.7 billion goats (23% in People's Republic of China and 18% in India), and 170 million buffaloes (>50% in India) (Food and Agriculture Organization of the United Nations [FAO] at http://apps.fao.org/).

Bovine zoonoses (4896, 5694, 8039) (http://www.oie.int) (Box 2.3). International organizations, ministries, veterinarians, and food industries aim to contain agents of bovids such as bluetongue virus (an *Orbivirus*: Reoviridae), foot-and-mouth-disease virus (FMDV, an *Aphthovirus*: Picornaviridae), and rinderpest virus (a *Morbillivirus*: Paramyxoviridae). Obstacles to control include persisting agents (e.g., *Brucella* spp., *M. bovis*, and *M. avium* subsp. *paratuberculosis*), emerging agents (e.g., prions, *E. coli* O157, and multidrug-resistant [MDR] *Campylobacter* and *Salmonella*), trade of infected herds, antimicrobials in feeds, agents in feeds, and agents transferred from wildlife.

BOVINE DROPLET-AIR CLUSTER
Viruses
Humans seem nonreceptive to some respiratory viruses that are enzootic in bovids, e.g., FMDV, vesicular stomatitis virus (VSV, *Vesiculovirus*: Rhabdoviridae), and infectious bovine rhinotracheitis virus (α-Herpesviridae).

Bacteria
Mycoplasma can colonize bovids, including *M. bovis*. Spread to humans is not known. For mycobacteria, see "Bovine Zoonotic Cluster" below.

Box 2.3 Agents from bovids, by cluster

For bites, see chapter 1; for milk, see section 7.1; and for animal work, see section 12.4.

Feces-food	Variant Creutzfeldt-Jakob disease; *C. jejuni* (MDR), *E. coli* O157; *Salmonella* (MDR), *L. monocytogenes*; microsporidia; *C. parvum*, Giardia, *Sarcocystis hominis*, *T. gondii*; *Taenia saginata*
Zoonotic	Rabies virus, viral hemorrhagic fever (e.g., CCHFV); *A. phagocytophila*, *B. anthracis*, *B. abortus*, *C. burnetii*, *M. bovis*; Babesia, *T. brucei* sl; *E. granulosus*
Environmental	Leptospira, *M. avium* subsp. *paratuberculosis*
Skin-blood	Pseudocowpox virus; *C. abortus*, *C. ulcerans*, mastitis (*S. aureus*, *Streptococcus bovis*); dermatophytes; myiases, bovids attract mosquitoes and flies

Fungi (446)

Soil-borne fungi such as *C. neoformans* can naturally infect bovids. However, domestic bovids are not considered a source for humans. *Pneumocystis carinii* is diagnosed in cattle and sheep, but unlike *P. jiroveci*, this agent does not seem to infect humans.

BOVINE FECES-FOOD CLUSTER

Manure can yield bovine viruses (e.g., bovine viral disease virus [BVDV] and corona-, entero-, and parvoviruses), bacteria (e.g., *Campylobacter*, *E. coli* O157, *Listeria*, *M. bovis*, and *Salmonella*), and protozoa (e.g., *C. parvum*).

Prions

Bovine spongiform encephalopathy (BSE) and variant Creutzfeldt-Jakob disease (1224, 1526, 5767, 6995). High-risk tissues from cows with BSE that have entered the food chain are the most likely source of variant Creutzfeldt-Jakob disease in humans.

Incompletely inactivated sheep offal fed to cows (industrial cannibalism) likely sparked the BSE epizootic in the United Kingdom that in 1986–2003 caused ~200,000 BSE cases in that country. Modeling suggests that 2 million cattle were infected and that 0.4–1.6 million entered the human food chain. By a similar mode (infective meat and bones), zoo animals contracted BSE in the United Kingdom in 1986–1992, including mouflon (*Ovis musimon*) and antelopes (*Oryx leucoryx*, *O. gazella*, *Tragelaphus angasi*, *T. strepsiceros*, and *Taurotragus oryx*). The epizootic highlighted veterinary health and industry deficiencies. Although banned in 1988, renderers continued to export hazardous feeds from the United Kingdom until 1996. BSE was reported in Ireland (1989), Portugal and Switzerland (1990), France (1991), Benelux countries (1997), Denmark, Germany, and Spain (2000), and much of remaining western and central Europe (2001), but also in Israel and Japan, and North America. In Washington state in 2003, a dairy cow was diagnosed with BSE; although "downer," its carcass was released for consumption, and the remaining beef from that slaughterhouse had to be recalled. The cow had been imported from Alberta, Canada, in 2001, from a herd cleared for human consumption. Feeds from rendered cattle have been prohibited in the United States since 1997, and foods for human consumption from downer cattle have been prohibited since 2004.

Scrapie (2909, 3384). Scrapie is enzootic in sheep in many countries. It is infectious to sheep and goats but apparently not to humans. Sheep and goats experimentally fed brain from cattle with BSE can contract a disease that is clinically and histopathologically indistinguishable from scrapie. In France in 2002, naturally occurring BSE was confirmed in a goat (which did not enter the human food chain).

Viruses

Humans seem nonreceptive to enteric viruses that bovids shed with feces, e.g., BVDV (*Flaviviridae: Pestivirus*), bovine parvovirus, and bovine (non-A) rotavirus.

Bacteria

***Campylobacter* (384, 2207, 3457, 6992).** Calves, cattle, lambs, sheep, and goats can shed *Campylobacter*, mainly *C. jejuni* but also *C. coli*. By age and crowding, reported fecal prevalence is 0–70%. In Australia, 14 (74%) of 19 herds were infected with *C. jejuni*, and by 475 random fecal samples, median prevalence was 0% in mutton sheep, 8% in prime lamb, 2% in pasture beef cattle, 6% in dairy cattle, and 58% in feedlot beef cattle. In the United Kingdom in 1999–2000, the prevalence at slaughter was 25% in cattle and 17% in sheep. Contact with cattle, in particular calves, is an established hazard for humans. A threat is the spread of quinolone- and macrolide-resistant strains from cattle to humans.

***Escherichia coli* (1089, 1660, 2129, 3457, 5998, 6992, 7160, 7685).** *E. coli* is part of the bovid enteric flora. *E. coli* O157 (EHEC) is recovered from cattle, sheep, and goats. In sheep at slaughter, the prevalence can be 2%, and sheep have been implicated in an EHEC outbreak at a scout camp.

The main concern, however, is cattle that are a major reservoir and source of diarrheagenic *E. coli*, including EHEC and EPEC. By age and setting 0–60% (often, 3–35%) of cattle test positive for *E. coli* O157 in high-income countries, with a peak in heifers and calves. A majority of bovine isolates may not be human pathogenic. Feed (from hay to grain) and other industry changes may have an impact on gut flora and favor overgrowth of diarrheagenic *E. coli* in cattle.

In Ireland, 2% (32/1,351) of beef trimmings and 3% of carcasses (4/132) grew *E. coli* O157. At slaughter, beef can become polluted by EHEC, making raw beef unsafe. Risks for the acquisition of EHEC include visits to farms, contacts with farm animals, density of cattle, and the application of manure to land. In Swaziland in 1992, a cattle epizootic preceded an EHEC epidemic with >40,000 cases of diarrhea; the same *E. coli* O157 clone was isolated from cattle, water sources, and patients, and eating beef was a risk.

***Listeria* (4915, 6354).** Bovine listeriosis is mainly fodder borne. Feeding of silage seems a hazard, in particular bale silage that favors growth of *L. monocytogenes*. At slaughter, the bowel of 10–50% of cattle is colonized, and 25% of tonsil samples grow *L. monocytogenes*. The main risk for humans is food rather than contact.

***Salmonella* (156, 1660, 2231, 3457).** In high-income countries, 0.2–5% of cattle and 20–70% of herds are infected. In the United States, ~55% of larger (≥400 cows) herds are infected. In the United Kingdom in 2002, the prevalence at slaughter was 0.2% in cattle ($n = 891$) and 0.1% in sheep ($n = 973$). Serovars indicative of bovine source are *S. enterica* serovar Dublin and to a lesser extent serovar Typhimurium. *S. enterica* serovar Dulin can be maintained on Alpine pastures where cows from various herds congregate. Routes into human foods are multiple, but main vehicles are unpasteurized cow's milk, and veal from home butchering. Of concern are MDR serotypes that spread to humans via beef, e.g., quinolone-resistant *S. enterica* serovar Dublin and MDR serovar Typhimurium DT 104.

Other bacteria (793, 1080, 2849). *Clostridium perfringens* is prevalent in the intestinal tract of cattle and sheep. Cattle can acquire *C. botulinum* and develop botulism; in France, a likely source for types C and D are cattle feeds from nearby poultry farms. Sheep contact is a risk for *Helicobacter pylori* infection in children from Chile. Cattle, sheep, and goats can harbor *Y. enterocolitica* and *Y. pseudotuberculosis*. Cattle can harbor *Vibrio fetus*.

Fungi
Microsporidia (1924, 6700). Cows can harbor *E. intestinalis* and *E. bieneusi*, and sheep and goats can harbor *E. intestinalis* and *E. cuniculi*.

Protozoa
***Blastocystis hominis* (16).** *Blastocystis hominis* is prevalent in cattle, and several genotypes are identified. Cattle-to-human spread is possible but unconfirmed.

***Cryptosporidium* (2813, 5608).** Cattle can shed *C. andersoni* (for months or years, noninfective to humans) and *C. parvum* (for 1–2 weeks, infective to humans). *C. parvum* (genotype 2) is enzootic in cattle, sheep, and goats, with higher prevalence in calves and lambs than adult animals. Tap water that is polluted by livestock feces is a suspected major source of cryptosporidiosis in humans. Cattle-to-human and sheep-to-human spread has also been reported, including among nomadic shepherds.

***Giardia* (5608, 7452, 7738).** Livestock can carry *G. bovis* (noninfective to humans) and closely related *G. lamblia* (including "assemblage A" infective to humans). Cattle can shed *G. lamblia* for >30 weeks. *Giardia* is prevalent in beef and dairy cattle worldwide (in up to 100% of calves). Cattle-to-human spread seems insignificant, but cattle herds are a conceivable hazard for municipal water supplies.

***Sarcocystis* (2554, 4235).** Bovids are intermediate hosts for *Sarcocystis* spp., cattle, zebu, water buffalo, and yak for *S. hominis*. The prevalence of muscular sarcocystosis is 10–100%; in sheep and goats locally, it is up to 80–95%.

***Toxoplasma gondii* (2380, 3756, 8286).** Cattle, sheep, and goats are intermediate hosts harboring tissue cysts. Seroprevalence is 3–25% in cattle, 10–40% in sheep, and ~20% in goats. Handling tissues and undercooked meat is hazardous. In cattle, related *Neospora caninum* should be differentiated from *T. gondii*.

Helminths
Bovids can maintain synanthropic cycles of *Fasciola*, *Taenia*, and *Trichinella*.

***Fasciola* (1723).** Cattle, sheep, goats, and buffalo are final hosts for *F. hepatica*. By geography, test, and interventions, prevalence is 0–100% (typically 15%) in cattle, 1–30% (15%) in sheep, and ~20% in goats. Cattle, sheep, goats, and buffalo are also hosts for *F. gigantica*. Prevalence is 5–65% (typically 20–25%) in cattle, 2–70% (30%) in buffalo, 1–80% (10%) in sheep, and 1–55% in goats.

***Taenia* (1997, 3593, 8192).** Cattle and yak are intermediate hosts for *T. saginata* (bovine cysticercosis); in East Asia, cattle and goats are intermediate hosts for *T. asiatica*. Infected feedlot workers have caused epizootics in cattle in the United States. Classical meat inspection detects only a fraction of bovine cysticercosis. In Belgium in 1997–1995, 3% (36/1,164) of cattle were antigenemic at slaughter, but meat inspection detected cysticercosis in only 0.3% (3) of carcasses. The prevalence of cysticercosis in cattle slaughtered in Hanoi, Vietnam, in 1989–1993 was 0.03% (39/144,390). Undercooked "measly" beef is the principle source of intestinal *T. saginata* infection in humans.

***Trichinella spiralis* (7952).** *T. spiralis* is reported in cattle and goats. In Henan province, People's Republic of China, in the 1980s, the microscopic prevalence in cattle at slaughter was 0.1–0.7%.

BOVINE ZOONOTIC CLUSTER
Cattle can attract mosquitoes, flies, and ticks and bring ectoparasites to farms. In Thailand in 2000–2001, 43% of 450 zebus and 33% of 189 cattle carried *R. sanguineus* or *Boophilus microplus* ticks (5445). Ticks and other ectoparasites removed from goats, sheep, and cattle, herd dust, birth products, and carcasses are potential sources of human infections.

Viruses
Humans seem refractory to Bluetongue virus that is carried to cattle by midges, and FMDV that is aerosol borne.

Humans are insensitive to louping ill virus (*Flaviviridae*) that is carried to sheep by *Ixodes* ticks, and VSV (*Coronaviridae*) that is contact or insect borne; sporadic louping ill virus or VSV infections are reported in exposed workers. Zoonotic spread is not known for *Bornavirus* (BDV, *Bornaviridae*) that infects cattle, sheep, and goats.

CCHFV (3168, 5303, 7277, 8075). Ticks carry CCHFV to livestock and maintain it in tick-livestock-tick cycles in the Old World, including in cattle, sheep, goats, camels, and wild ungulates. While most infections are not apparent, epizootics have been reported. Seroprevalence in cattle, sheep, and goats from enzootic areas is 1–58%. Ticks, blood, and tissue from viremic animals are a hazard for workers, including handling for vaccination, delivery, castration, ear tagging, and slaughter.

TBEV (6218, 6268). *Ixodes* ticks carry TBEV to cows, sheep, and goats. Seroprevalence in enzootic areas in Europe is 0–40% in cattle, 15–45% in sheep, and 20–65% in goats. Ticks from livestock and milk from viremic animals are a hazard. Infected animals can shed TBEV in milk for 5–25 days.

Japanese encephalitis virus (JEV) (5814). Mosquitoes carry JEV to livestock, and mosquitoes attracted to homes by livestock are a potential hazard. Livestock participates in maintenance of JEV. Seroprevalence in enzootic areas is 25–60% in cattle, 23–68% in goats, and 36% in sheep.

Rift Valley fever virus (RVFV) (5304, 6278, 6868, 8263). RVFV affects cattle, sheep, and goats in Africa and the Arabian peninsula, causing disease, abortions, and epizootics at intervals. Abortion storms and animal deaths can herald epizootics and epidemics. During epizootics, abortion rates can reach 40–80%. In the East African epizootic of 1997–1998, owners lost ~70% of sheep and goats and 20–30% of cattle and camels. In the Mauritanian epizootic of 1998, 35% of sheep, 16% of goats, and 2% of cattle had evidence of acute infection. By enzooticity, seroprevalence ranges from 0–10% to 30–60%. Movement of livestock during epizootics must be restricted. Hazards for humans include mosquitoes that are attracted to livestock, microtrauma, raw milk from viremic animals, and sheltering of livestock on the premises during floods.

Rabies virus (1319, 4103, 5988). (For bites, see chapter 1.) Worldwide, 12–14% of rabid animals are ruminants. In the United States, 83 cattle rabies cases were reported in 2000 (1.1% of all animal rabies cases), 82 (1.1%) in 2001, 116 (1.5%) in 2002, and 98 (1.4%) in 2003 (Fig. 1.2). In Europe in 1990–2002, 13,168 rabies cases were reported in cattle (1,013/year, 10% of all rabid animals) and 3,348 in sheep and goats (258/year, 2.6%) (Fig. 1.3). In New York state in 1993–1998, exposure to goats caused 8% (476/6,139) of all PEP; in 1996, a single rabid goat at a county fair caused PEP in 465 attendees.

Bacteria

***Anaplasma* (2629, 6039, 7215).** *Ixodes* ticks carry *A. phagocytophila* to livestock. The agent is enzootic in Europe, in cattle, sheep, and goats. In Switzerland, 17% (12/70) of cattle tested positive in nucleic acid amplification tests, and >40% seroconverted after returning from pasturing. In countries with warm climates *Boophilus* ticks carry *A. marginale* to cattle (in North America the vector is *Dermacentor*). *A. marginale* can infectd sheep, bighorn sheep (*Ovis canadensis*), goats, water buffalo, and wildlife. It can cause severe disease in cattle.

***B. anthracis* (2022, 4358, 6865, 7682, 8264).** Herds can acquire anthrax via grazing or dust. In France in 1980–2000, 114 anthrax foci were identified, most (>95%) with cattle, only 2% (2) with sheep. Vaccination prevents anthrax in livestock. Affected herds should be quarantined. Carcasses and contaminated bedding should be incinerated. Products such as bone meal should be autoclaved. Humans can acquire anthrax via inhalation, microtrauma, contact, or ingestion. Exposed workers should receive antibiotic prophylaxis. *B. anthracis* has caused epizootics and outbreaks. In Gambia in 1970–1974, epizootics in sheep and goats preceded four epidemics with 448 human cases. In Mali in 1978, a cattle epizootic preceded an outbreak with 84 human cases (all males), for an estimated attack rate of 5.6% in the affected ethnic group. In Zimbabwe in 1979–1980, a cattle epizootic preceded an epidemic with 9,711 human cases (mostly cutaneous) and 151 (1.6%) deaths. In Australia in 1997, *B. anthracis* caused 80 cattle cases (in 38 herds), and one human (cutaneous) case. In North Dakota, in 2000, a livestock epizootic caused 157 animal deaths on 31 farms; 1.6% (1/62) of exposed persons (including animal health workers) developed cutaneous anthrax.

***Brucella* (126, 2790, 4882, 6181, 6223, 6658, 6808).** *Brucella* has a great impact on animal health, including by rejected milk and meat, infertility, and epizootic abortions.

Some countries have controlled or eliminated bovine brucellosis, but nearly 60 countries reported infected cattle in 2003, mainly Africa, Latin America, and Asia, but also southern Europe, the United Kingdom, and the United States. Cattle, sheep, goat, and water buffalo are sources of human brucellosis. Risks are intensified in areas where livestock is kept on the premises. In cattle, *B. abortus* is the main species while *B. melitensis* and *B. suis* are sporadic (spill over from coherding of cattle with sheep or swine). By rearing and herd size, seroprevalences in cattle are 0.3–45% (typically 10%) in Africa, 3–5% in Latin America, 1–3% in southern Europe, and 0–30% (4–7%) in Asia. Benelux countries, Germany, Austria, and Scandinavia are officially free of bovine brucellosis.

In sheep and goats, *B. melitensis* is the main agent, but *B. ovis* occurs frequently in sheep as well. By test, seroprevalences are 4–6% in Africa, 0–15% in southern Europe, and 0–30% in Asia and Latin America. Much of western and northern Europe is officially free of ovine and caprine brucellosis. In low-income countries, contact with infected goats is a risk.

Brucellosis in domestic buffalo and yak resemble bovine brucellosis, with reported seroprevalence of 1.5–15%.

C. burnetii **(2085, 3243, 4080, 4707, 4932, 6658, 6778, 7434).** *C. burnetii* is enzootic and epizootic in cattle, sheep, and goats worldwide. Infections are also documented in yak, buffalo, and wild bovids. Prevalence in animals should be interpreted with caution because data are fragmentary. Worldwide, 2–50% of herds can be infected. Seroprevalence is 0–40% in cattle (3% in the United States, 0–30% in Europe, 1–40% in Africa, 25% in India 25%), 0–75% in sheep (17% in the United States, 0–75% in Europe, 4–11% in Africa), and 0–90% (generally highest) in goats (40% in the United States, up to 90% in Europe, and 10–15% in Africa). Animal dust, aerosols from parturient animals, contact with birth products, ticks attached to animals, milk, and urine can all be sources for infections in humans. In central France in 1991–1992, the seroprevalence (acute phase II antibody titer ≥1:320) was <5% (>1,000 sera) in the gerneral population, 25% (3/12) in veterinarians, and 37% (62/168) in goat farmers and their families.

Outbreaks   Cattle have caused occasional outbreaks in humans. In Germany in 1947–1999, 6 (15%) of 40 Q fever outbreaks were due to cattle. Sheep have caused many outbreaks. In Germany in 1947–1999, sheep were implicated in 24 (60%) of 40 outbreaks. In the Alps in central Europe, pasturing sheep have caused outbreaks in Italy (58 human cases) and Switzerland (415 cases). In Slovakia in 1993, aborting goats caused an outbreak with 113 cases (103 males).

Mycobacterium. Both *M. bovis* (*M. tuberculosis* complex) and *M. avium* subsp. *paratuberculosis* (MAP) can circulate in domestic bovids. **M. bovis (256, 1589, 3116, 6686, 6996).** Cattle are the main host, but zebu, buffalo, and wildlife are also susceptible. Bovine tuberculosis is sporadic or enzootic in much of the Americas, Africa, and Eurasia. Its prevalence can exceed 1%, e.g., in parts of Argentina, Brazil, Spain, and the United Kingdom. Bovine tuberculosis seems to reemerge in the United Kingdom, with ~9,000 cases in 2000. Strategies for control include vaccination or tuberculin testing and culling of reactors. Infected wildlife and imported livestock are obstacles to control. Bovids are a continued source of zoonotic tuberculosis in humans. Modes of spread include droplets, aerosols, and unpasteurized milk. In occupationally exposed persons, pulmonary rather than alimentary tuberculosis dominates. **MAP (296, 1905, 3918, 5232, 8080).** MAP can cause disease (cachexia, inflammatory bowel disease, or Johne's disease) in cattle, sheep, and goats. Infected animals shed MAP with feces, milk, and sperma. Cattle can shed MAP for 1–2½ years before Johne's disease becomes manifest. Bovid-to-bovid spread is mainly oral, including from grass, water, and colostrum. In North America, up to 3% of cattle, and ≥20% of dairy herds can be infected. In Austria in 2002–2004, lymph nodes of 24% (80/338) of cattle or 25% (77/303) of herds yielded MAP by PCR. Although increasingly likely, MAP as a zoonosis is unconfirmed.

Other bovine bacterioses (1315, 2060, 2708). In the United States, *Bartonella* was isolated from the blood of 49% (63/128) of cattle, 15% (15/100) of elk (*Cervus elaphus*), and 90% (38/42) of mule deer (*Odocoileus hemionus*). Whether bovine bartonellae are pathogenic to humans and how humans could become infected are not known. Ungulates can become infected with *Borrelia burgdorferi* sl, but ungulates are not considered reservoirs. *Amblyomma* ticks carry *E. chaffeensis* to livestock; in the United States, seroprevalence in cattle and goats can reach >70%. Livestock can be seroreactive to *F. tularensis*; die-offs can herald epizootics and outbreaks in humans. In enzootic areas, up to 40-70% of cattle, sheep, and goats can be seroreactive to *Rickettsia* spp., e.g., *R. conorii* in the Mediterranean. In Tibet, sheep and goats are sporadic sources of *Y. pestis* and plague in humans, apparently via contact rather than fleas.

Protozoa
***Babesia* spp. (1633, 4861, 8415).** *Babesia* sp. are enzootic in bovids in Africa, Latin America, and Eurasia, including *B. bigemina*, *B. bovis*, *B. divergens*, *B. major*, and *B. ovis* in cattle. In Egypt in 2001, *B. ovis* was detected in 3% (13/475) of sheep, 7% (14/200) of goats, and 10% (13/135) of cattle. Little is known about babesiae in cattle in the United States; in Europe, the main species in cattle is *B. divergens*. *Babesia* spp. are difficult to differentiate microscopically from *Theileria* spp. that naturally infect cattle, sheep, and goats and coinfect the same hosts. Ticks carry *Babesia* to bovids. In Europe, *Ixodes ricinus* is the principal vector. Epizootics have occurred in cattle. Ticks attached to livestock are a putative hazard for humans.

***Trypanosoma* (3517, 4842, 7899, 7900).** In Africa, *T. congolense*, *T. vivax*, and *T. brucei* sl are all diagnosed in cattle and other herbivores. Mixed infections compound diagnostic difficulties. N'dama (West Africa) and Orma Boran (East Africa) breeds, and wild ungulates are relatively resistant to *T. brucei* sl (trypotolerant) and its disease (nagana). The crude prevalence of *Trypanosma* in cattle in tropical Africa is ~5–45%. Of this burden, a variable fraction is attributed to *T. brucei rhodesiense* (infective in humans). Cattle, sheep, goats, and wild ungulates are reservoirs of *T. brucei rhodesiense*. In East Africa, cattle-to-human carriage via tsetse flies is considered significant, and tsetse-borne sheep-to-human transmission is postulated. In postwar Uganda, restocking of zebus was associated with an epidemic in humans that has been ongoing since 1998. In contrast to *T. brucei rhodesiense*, *T. brucei gambiense* is unusual in cattle and sheep, and these animals are not considered maintenance hosts.

Helminths
***Echinococcus* (2119, 2187).** Sheep, cattle, and goats are intermediate hosts for *E. granulosus*, maintaining the common "sheep" (genotype G1) strain in Africa, America, and Eurasia. Cattle can also harbor "cattle" (G5) and "camel" (G6) strains. By test, farming practice, and public health measures, prevalences in enzootic areas are 3–55% in cattle, 1–87% in sheep, and 1–20% in goats.

***Onchocerca* (37).** *O. gutturosa*, *O. lienalis*, and *O. ochengi* can infect cattle in countries with warm climates. Human-infective *O. volvulus* does not naturally infect cattle.

BOVINE ENVIRONMENTAL CLUSTER
Bacteria
***Burkholderia pseudomallei* (1421, 1683).** Goats and sheep are highly susceptible, and the agent can appear in milk. Nonetheless, the risk of zoonotic spread seems small.

***Clostridium tetani* (2117).** Cattle and sheep can shed the agent with feces. Reported shedding prevalences are 4% for cows in sheds, 8% for cows on pasture, and 25% for sheep on pasture.

***Leptospira* (4279, 4369, 4989, 5348).** Bovids, mainly cattle, are a major reservoir. Serovars Grippotyphosa, Hardjo, and Pomona are associated with dairy cattle, Hardjo and Pomona with sheep and goats. By herd size and vaccination, the seroprevalence reported in cattle is 5–50%. Cattle ownership increases the risk of human infection. In New Caledonia in 1989–1993, 36% (69/192) leptospirosis patients mentioned cattle as the source of their infections.

Helminths
***S. japonicum* (6417).** *S. japonicum* has a major reservoir in cattle and buffaloes.

***Toxocara vitulorum* (4392).** *T. vitulorum* infects water buffalo. In Egypt, the prevalence in buffalo is 1–80%. A potential for human infections exists, e.g., when water from buffalo wallows is used for washing vegetables and when parathenic hosts, such as rabbits or ducks, are kept together with buffaloes.

BOVINE SKIN-BLOOD CLUSTER
Blood and tissues from viremic bovids are potentially infective, and bovids can shed agents with milk (see section 7.1), urine, and genital secretions.

Viruses
Humans seem refractory to bovine leucosis virus that is enzootic in cattle. Occasional human infections are reported with FMDV, which is enzootic in cattle, sheep, and goats in low-income countries, causing intermittent epizootics, with pseudocowpox virus (milker's nodules), which is enzootic in cattle (rodents and cats rather than cattle are source for cowpox virus) (6714, 8053), and VSV that is enzootic in cattle in Latin America, causing epizootics.

Bacteria
***Chlamydophila* (4959, 5975).** *C. abortus* and *C. pecorum* are enzootic in cattle, sheep, and goats. *C. abortus* is a significant cause of stillbirth in sheep and goats. Aborting animals remain carriers that shed the agent from the reproductive tract during estrus. The seroprevalence in ruminants is 3–24%, with a high seroprevalence in aborted animals and a low seroprevalence in healthy animals. Sheep, goats, and cattle occasionally spread *C. abortus* to humans. Aborting ruminants and their products are a risk for pregnant women. *C. pecorum* is a cause of keratoconjunctivitis in sheep and goats.

***Corynebacterium* (296, 1274, 3174, 5800, 8335).** *C. pseudotuberculosis* is a cause of granulomatous, ulcerative, or caseous lesions of skin, lymph nodes, udder, and visceral organs of cows, sheep, and goats. In epizootics, attack rates can exceed 5%, and the prevalence in culled animals can exceed 20%. Contact with cattle is an occupational risk, and the spread by milk is suspected. *C. ulcerans* is a cause of mastitis in cows and goats and is recovered from cow milk. Raw milk is a source for zoonotic, diphtheria-like human infections. Contact with infected animals is a suspected risk. While disease is usually milder than that caused by *C. diphtheriae*, strains of *C. ulcerans* can produce diphtheria toxin.

***Staphylococcus* (2694, 6324, 8365).** Up to 25–30% of heifers and dairy cows can be colonized. *S. aureus* and coagulase-negative staphylococci are frequently recovered from cows with (manifest or inapparent) mastitis, milk, and milk equipment. An infection scenario is from the dairy cow over the farmer's hands to equipment and milk. Methicillin-resistant *S. aureus* have also been detected in cattle.

***Streptococcus* (3167, 4778, 6421).** Cattle, sheep, and goats can carry or shed into milk a bewildering array of *Streptococcus* spp., including *S. agalactiae* (group B *Streptococcus*), *S. bovis*, *S. canis*, *S. equi* subsp. *zooepidemicus*, *S. dysgalactiae* subsp. *dysgalactiae*, and *S. dysgalactiae* subsp. *equisimilis*.

Other bacteria. *Erysipelothrix rhusiopathiae* infects sheep and cattle. Animal-to-human spread seems rare. *Ureaplasma diversum* causes endometritis in cattle, but humans seem refractory.

Dermatophytes
Zoophilic and geophilic dermatophytes have been recovered from bovids and their environment, including *Aspergillus* (*A. flavus*, *A. fumigatus*, *A. niger*, and *A. terreus*), *Microsporum* (*M. gypseum*), and *Trichophyton* (*T. mentagrophytes* var. *mentagrophytes*, *T. rubrum*, *T. verrucosum*, and *T. violaceum*). Contact with livestock or its environment is a source of *T. verrucosum* and *T. mentagrophytes* in farmers and their families (1020, 2132, 3457).

Ectoparasites
Myiasis (2563, 4245, 7345). Livestock attracts flies. Herdsmen are at increased risk of myiasis. Transportation is suspected to have spread myiasis (see section 16.1). In the 1970s, *Chrysomya* invaded the Americas, perhaps with domestic animals from Africa or in the cargo holds of aircraft; *Chrysomya* larvae have been intercepted in dried meat and fish at the Houston airport in Texas. Perhaps by a similar mechanisms, *Cochliomyia* appeared in Libya. Imported cattle are the accepted source of *Hypoderma* in Africa and Latin America.

2.4 SUIDS
Domesticated pig, wild boar (both *Sus scrofa*), bush pig (*Potamochoerus porcus*), warthog (*Phacochoerus aethiopicus*), and babirusa (*Babyrousa babyroussa*) are members of the Suidae (order Artiodactyla). Worldwide in 2001, there were 0.9 billion pigs (49% in People's Republic of China, 7% in United States, and 3% in Brazil).

Porcine zoonoses (756, 3058, 5428) (http://www.oie.int) (Box 2.4). International organizations, ministries, veterinary services, and food industry aim to contain porcine agents such as classical swine fever virus (*Pestivirus*: *Flaviviridae*), FMDV, swine vesicular disease virus (*Enterovirus*: *Picornaviridae*), and VSV (*Vesicolovirus*: *Rhabdoviridae*). Some countries in the Americas, Europe, and the Pacific Rim are committed to or have achieved control of porcine brucellosis, tuberculosis, and trichinellosis. A challenge are MDR salmonellae in human foods. A research topic is porcine xenografts.

PORCINE DROPLET-AIR CLUSTER
Viruses
Humans are not usually susceptible to VSV and FMDV that are enzootic in pigs; infections with these viruses are rare in humans.

***Influenzavirus* (5420, 5595, 8278).** *Influenzavirus* in pigs is a public health concern. Pigs are natural hosts for porcine, avian, and human subtypes of influenza A virus. Of 2,375 pigs tested at slaughter in the United States in 1997–1998, ~8% were seroreactive to avian and human subtypes. Epizootics have occurred. Although infectivity of porcine subtypes for humans is limited, swine-to-human spread (swine flu) is documented. In 1988, an index pregnant woman, one or two health care workers, and 19 (76%) of 25 swine exhibitors contracted swine flu virus at a county fair where many of the exhibited swine were ill. Work with pigs is a risk. Coinfected pigs can "mix" (reassort) H1-15 and N1-9 genes, releasing new (shifted) strains with potential for pandemics.

Box 2.4 Agents from pigs, by cluster

For bites, see chapter 1; for pork, see section 7.4; for work, see section 12.4.

Droplet-air	*Influenzavirus*; *B. bronchiseptica*
Feces-food	HEV; *E. coli*, *Helicobacter* spp., *L. monocytogenes*, *Salmonella*, *Y. enterocolitica*; microsporidia; *B. coli*, *B. hominis*, *C. parvum*; *Ascaris suum*, *Gnathostoma*, *Taenia solium*, *Trichinella*
Zoonotic	JEV, Nipahvirus, rabies virus, VSV; *Brucella suis*, *M. bovis*; *T. brucei rhodesiense*; *E. granulosis*
Environmental	*Leptospira*, *C. tetani*, *M. avium*; *S. japonicum*
Skin-blood	*E. rhusiopathiae*, *Streptococcus suis*; dermatophytes

Bacteria

Humans seem naturally resistant to *Actinobacillus pleuropneumoniae* and *Mycoplasma hyopneumoniae* that are enzootic in swine worldwide. *B. bronchiseptica* commonly colonizes the upper respiratory tract of swine. *P. multocida* infects the upper respiratory tract of swine, causing progressive atrophic rhinitis.

Fungi

Fungi reported in pigs include *Aspergillus, Coccidioides immitis, Cryptococcus neoformans* var. *neoformans*, and *Histoplasma capsulatum*. Pigs are unlikely sources for humans. *P. carinii* is diagnosed in pigs, but does not cross species; the human-infective species is *P. jiroveci*.

PORCINE FECES-FOOD CLUSTER

Agents to be expected from swine manure include hepatitis E virus (HEV), *Campylobacter, Clostridium botulinum, E. coli* O157, *Listeria, Salmonella, Yersinia, B. coli, Blastocystis hominis, Cryptosporidium*, and *Ascaris suum*.

Viruses

Hepatitis E virus (HEV) (94, 426, 4985, 8145). Strains of HEV circulate in pigs. In Bali, Indonesia, 72% (71/99) of pigs are seropositive. The evidence is growing that HEV is zoonotic and that pigs can transmit HEV to humans via contact, manure, or polluted tap water. In the United Kingdom, a woman, who used to eat raw sausage and bacon and had not traveled in the past 10 years, contracted hepatitis E with a strain identical to two United Kingdom pig strains.

Bacteria

Humans seem naturally resistant to *Brachyspira hyodysenteriae*, which causes swine dysentery.

***Campylobacter* (3457, 5382).** Piglets and swine can harbor *Campylobacter*, mainly *C. coli*, less often *C. jejuni*, and occasionally *C. lari*. Including extraintestinal sites, prevalence can reach 100%; in the United Kingdom in 1999–2000, the fecal prevalence in 860 pigs at slaughter was 95% (84% *C. coli*, 3% *C. jejuni*, and 8% other species). Contact infections are possible, but pork seems to be an insignificant vehicle.

***E. coli* (753, 3457).** EHEC and ETEC are recovered from pig excreta. In pigs at slaughter in Europe, the prevalence of *E. coli* O157 is 0.3–0.7%. Contact infections are possible, but pork seems an insignificant vehicle.

***Helicobacter* (3633).** Pigs are a suspected source of zoonotic *Helicobacter* spp. in humans.

***Listeria monocytogenes* (6354).** *L. monocytogenes* is enzootic in swine. At slaughter, 10–50% of pigs yield the agent from the intestine, and 45% yield it from the tonsils. In French cuisine, pork belly (rillettes) is a vehicle for humans.

***Salmonella* (428, 753, 3077, 3457, 5127).** Pigs are a major reservoir. Typical serotypes are Agona, Choleraesuis, Derby, Enteritidis, Infantis, and Typhimurium (including DT104 that is MDR). Pigs carry *Salmonella* inapparently. By sampling site (feces and extraintestinal), reported prevalence is 2–37%. In the United Kingdom in 2002, the fecal prevalence in 2,509 pigs at slaughter was 5% from carcass swab and 23% from caecum (*S. enterica* serovar Typhimurium, 11%; serovar Derby, 6%; serovar Enteritidis, 0.1%; and others, 5.9%). *Salmonella* is also widespread in the pig environment, including pen surfaces, flies, and the boots and hands of workers. Fecal shedding during transportation cross-infects skin and mouth, and cross-infection is enhanced during slaughter. *Salmonella* has multiple routes into the food supply. *Salmonella* is recovered in ~1% of fresh pork, and ground pork is a reported outbreak vehicle (see section 7.4).

***Yersinia* (489, 720, 753, 4242, 5382, 7802).** *Y. enterocolitica* is enzootic in pigs, including serogroups infective to humans (e.g., O:3, O:5,27, and O:9). For these, pigs are a major reservoir, mainly their tonsils, while porcine bowels can grow apathogenic or virulent biovars. In Belgium, serogroups in humans correlated with porcine serogroups. By sampling (feces and extraintestinal), the reported prevalence is 5–15%; >50% of piggeries can be infected. Shift from small-scale family pig farming to large-scale industrial production seems to have increased enzootic occurrence. Pigs also contribute to maintenance of *Y. pseudotuberculosis*.

Fungi

Pigs can harbor *Encephalitozoon cuniculi, E. intestinalis*, and *Enterocytozoon bieneusi* (1924, 6700).

Protozoa

***Balantidium coli* (1909, 3336).** Domestic and wild pigs are the principal reservoir. Pigs shed cysts with feces. The prevalence in pigs is 20–100%, including in high-income countries. Humans can acquire *B. coli* directly, via uptake of cysts.

***Blastocystis hominis* (16, 7428).** Pigs harbor the agent. In Japan, the prevalence in pigs is 95%. The spread from pigs to humans is likely.

***Cryptosporidium* (3607, 5398, 6491).** Pigs can harbor *C. parvum* and *C. suis* and pass infective oocysts. Fecal prevalences are 0–20%; in piglets they are up to 70%; >50% of herds can be infected. Humans can acquire *Cryptosporidium* from contact with pigs or from polluted tap water. Pig-to-human spread is a particular hazard in areas where pigs are kept in domiciles, e.g., periurban slums.

Isospora suis. *I. suis* is recovered from pigs but not *I. belli*.

Sarcocystis. Pigs are intermediate hosts for *S. suihominis* and other *Sarcocystis* spp. The prevalence in pigs is 0–30%. Muscle and raw meat are a potential hazard.

***Toxoplasma gondii* (2049, 2573, 5155).** Suids are intermediate hosts. By geography, feed, sample, and test, seroprevalences in pigs are 0.5–95%. In North America and western Europe, ≥3% of pigs are reactive. Of seroreactive pigs, 0–90% harbor infective cysts. In the United States, 93% (51/55) of pigs raised on farms for human consumption are tissue infective by bioassay. In contrast, in Canada, 9% (240/2,800) of market-age pigs are reactive in the commercial latex agglutination test, 25% (9/36) are positive by nucleic acid amplification tests, but all bioassays are negative. New World feral pigs (e.g., peccary and *Tayassu tajacu*), which are important game animals, can also be infected. Overall, pork is considered an unusual source of human infections, unless consumed raw or rare.

Helminths

A. Of main concern are helminths that are spread via raw pork or the handling of infective porcine tissues. These include *Echinococcus*, *Gnathostoma*, *Taenia*, and *Trichinella*.

***Echinococcus* (2119, 5779, 7454, 8320).** Handling of infective tissues is a risk. The *E. granulosus* genotype G7 strain is enzootic in domestic pigs in Europe and Argentina. Near Poznan, Poland, ~14% of pigs are infected, and G7 dominates human infections. Warthogs can be intermediate hosts for other strains. Domestic and wild pigs can be intermediate hosts for *E. multilocularis*. In Hokkaido, Japan, rearing pigs is a significant risk, presumably because afterbirths and other swine offal attract foxes to the premises.

***Gnathostoma* (1708, 3582).** Raw pork is a risk. Pigs are final hosts for *G. hispidum* and *G. doloresi* and paratenic hosts for *G. spinigerum*. In Southeast Asia and parts of Japan, *G. doloresi* is widespread in domestic pigs and wild boars. In Miyazaki prefecture, Japan, 31 of 32 wild boars harbor adult worms.

***Paragonimus* (7631).** Raw boar meat is a risk, because immature stages can persist in boar muscle.

***Spirometra* (561).** Raw pork is a risk. In Florida in 1999, the prevalence of larval infection in feral pigs was 2–22%.

***Taenia solium* (2211, 2440, 2621, 3593, 5872, 6086, 8418).** Raw pork is a risk. Domestic and wild pigs are intermediate hosts for *T. solium* (and *T. asiatica*). Larvae locate in muscle, tongue, skin, eye, and brain (porcine cysticercosis). *T. solium* is enzootic in parts of Africa, Asia, and Latin America, in particular, free-roaming pigs that have access to human feces. By test method, the prevalence of porcine cysticercosis is 0–55% in Africa (often 10%; "active," 0.4–3%), 1–75% in Latin America (often 15–30%), and 0.02–40% in Asia east of Pakistan (often <1%).

***Trichinella* (638, 2824, 4224, 5611, 5996, 6107, 7049).** Raw pork is a risk. Pigs can host *T. britovi*, *T. nativa*, *T. papuae*, *T. pseudospiralis*, and *T. spiralis*. **T. spiralis.** Pigs are the principal domestic reservoir for *T. spiralis*. The domestic cycle is based on raw offal feed, scavenging on garbage and cadavers, crowding and biting, clandestine slaughtering, import of infected pigs, and contact of domestic pigs with rats, foxes, and mustelids. *T. spiralis* is enzootic in pigs in parts of Argentina, Chile, Mexico, East Europe, Finland, Spain, Israel, Lebanon, and People's Republic of China. Carcasses are screened by digestion assay or microscopy ("trichinoscopy", since the 1860s). By geography and test, infection prevalences are 0.003–24%; in enzootic areas, typically 0.15–1.5%. In North America and West Europe, pigs are virtually kept free of *Trichinella*. **T. britovi.** *T. britovi* infects pigs and wild boars. In Romania in 1990–1999, 0.3% (1/319) of boars tested positive. **T. nativa.** *T. nativa* is diagnosed in pigs (in People's Republic of China), and boars (in Estonia). **T. nelsoni.** *T. nelsoni* is diagnosed in Africa, in warthog and bush pig (*Potamochoerus porcus*). **T. pseudospiralis.** *T. pseudospiralis* is diagnosed in domestic and wild pigs. This agent has caused pork-borne outbreaks in humans in Thailand and France.

B. Some helminths can be acquired from pig manure, soiled tools, or polluted pigsties. This mode of spread applies to *Ascaris* and *Oesophagostomum*.

***Ascaris suum* (1098, 4521, 5823).** *A. suum* is prevalent in many pig populations. In Denmark in 1999, prevalences were 4% in sows, 28% in weaning sucklings, and 33% in fattening pigs. Eggs are recovered from feces, liquid manure, skin of sows, pigsty walls, drinking troughs, and tools. Despite the abundance of eggs in the environment, pig-to-human spread is unusual, and *A. suum* circulates in pigs largely separate from humans.

C. For a last group of helminths, pigs are intermediate hosts and stages of worms need to go through further hosts before being infective to humans. Examples are *Clonorchis*, *Diphyllobothrium*, *Fasciolopsis*, *Opisthorchis*, and *Paragonimus* (1368, 4570). For *Fasciolopsis buski*, pigs are principal hosts. Aquatic green fodder and canal water bring *F. buski* to pig farms. In Vietnam, the prevalence in 891 pigs from 12 provinces at necropsy was 3% (1818, 2885).

PORCINE ZOONOTIC CLUSTER
Viruses
Pigs can aquire viruses from contacts in crowded pigsties or from vectors. Pigs can attract mosquitos to domiciles.

Nipahvirus (1440, 2804). In Malaysia in 1998–1999, an epizootic of Nipahvirus in pigs and an outbreak among pig farmers led to the discovery of this virus. Fruit bats may be a source of infection for pigs while resting on trees or when eaten by pigs. Initially, in the belief that JEV was the culprit, and with the aim to contain the epizootic, ~1.1 million pigs were culled (up to 35,000/day).

JEV (358, 5814, 5895). *Culex* mosquitoes carry JEV to pigs and from pigs to humans. Pigs are a major reservoir and amplification host in rural Asia. Viremia in pigs lasts 2–4 days and is high enough to infect mosquitoes. By season and location, seroprevalences in pigs in enzootic areas are ~15–80%. Continuous slaughtering maintains a large, young, and susceptible swine population. In Sri Lanka, monsoonal infection waves in pigs were correlated with high seroprevalence in cattle, goats, and humans. Proximity to pigs is a hazard. In Japan, vaccinations and relocation of pig farms away from residential areas led to decreased JEV circulation.

Rabies virus (4103, 5988). (For bites, see chapter 1). Pigs are sporadically affected and account for <1% of rabid animal cases in North America and western Europe.

Bacteria
***B. anthracis* (6232, 7682, 8181).** Pigs are susceptible to *B. anthracis*. Infections can be sporadic or epizootic. Porcine disease can be protracted. In Burkina Faso, an epizootic in pigs in 1977 was followed by an outbreak with ≥80 human cases.

***Brucella* (2637, 2790, 4882, 5949, 6181, 6223, 6808).** Porcine brucellosis is less well understood and controlled than bovine brucellosis. *Brucella* seems enzootic in feral and domestic pig populations. *B. suis* seems to be the main species. Reported seroprevalences are 0–10% in domestic pigs and up to 10–45% in feral pigs. Porcine brucellosis is rare in domestic pigs in western Europe but is reemerging locally, likely as a result of spillover from wild boar. Pigs are a confirmed source of human brucellosis. In People's Republic of China in the 1990s, *B. suis* accounted for 0.5% of human brucellosis cases.

***C. burnetii* (4852).** *C. burnetii* has been reported in swine. Whether pigs contribute to human infection is uncertain.

***M. bovis* (256).** *M. bovis* has been detected in wild swine in Australia, New Zealand, Italy, and Spain. Spread to humans has not been reported.

***Pasteurella multocida* (7457).** *P. multocida* has been isolated from the tonsils and nares of healthy and ill swine. *P. multocida* in swine can cause progressive atrophic rhinitis.

***Rickettsia* (3276).** In an enzootic area of Spain (Salamanca province), all of 15 pigs were seroreactive to *R. conorii*.

Protozoa
***Trypanosoma* (1127, 1599, 7900, 8090).** *T. brucei* sl, *T. congolense*, *T. cruzi*, and other trypanosomes are diagnosed in pigs.

In East Africa, domestic pigs and wild suids (e.g., warthog, *Phacochoerus aethiopicus*) are likely reservoirs for *T. brucei rhodesiense*, and spread from pig to tsetse to humans seems important. In Uganda, the prevalence of *T. brucei* sl in pigs is 14% (164/1,181); by the blood incubation infectivity test, 30% (16/53) of isolates were determined to be *T. brucei rhodesiense*.

In West Africa, pigs are considered marginal for the maintenance of *T. brucei gambiense*.

Pigs are naturally infected with *T. cruzi*. In the Amazon, triatomine bugs (*Panstrongylus geniculatus*) from armadillo burrows have invaded pigsties adjacent to houses with a risk of spread to pigs and humans.

PORCINE ENVIRONMENTAL CLUSTER
Roaming pigs can acquire agents from the environment or pollute the environment.

Bacteria
Environmental bacteria diagnosed in pigs include *Burkholderia pseudomallei* (1421), *Clostridium tetani*, *Leptospira*, and environmental mycobacteria.

***Leptospira* (1044, 1450, 4279, 4369, 4989, 7678).** Pigs are a reservoir. Serovars suggestive of porcine source are Bratislava, Pomona, and Tarassovi. By geography, reported seroprevalences in pigs are 25–60%. Captive pigs kept in zoos can also be infected. Contact with pigs is a risk, including for owners and workers. By setting, 3% (Italy, $n = 126$) to 35% (New Caledonia, $n = 192$) of leptospirosis patients mention pigs as source of their infection.

***Mycobacterium* (256, 4044, 4770).** Pigs can be infected with *M. avium* and *M. intracellulare*; boars can also be infected with *M. bovis* (see above) and *M. caprae*. Pigs are likely sources of *M. avium* in humans or share (unknown) sources with humans. In The Netherlands in

1996, caseous lymph nodes were detected in 0.5% (856/158,763) of slaughtered pigs, and 54% (219/402) of cultured nodes grew *M. intracellulare*.

Helminths
S. japonicum has a major reservoir in pigs (6417). For *T. canis*, pigs can be parathenic hosts (7173). Whether larvae-containing, undercooked pork is a source for human infections is uncertain.

PORCINE SKIN-BLOOD CLUSTER
Viruses
Porcine endogenous retrovirus (*Gammaretrovirus*: *Retroviridae*) (2180, 3254) and encephalomyocarditis virus (870) can be prevalent in swine and are of interest in xenotransplantation. Of 10 recipients of porcine fetal islet xenotransplants, none had evidence of porcine endogenous retrovirus infection.

Bacteria
Chlamydophila abortus, *C. pecorum*, and *Chlamydia suis* can infect swine (3370). Spread to humans has not been reported.

***Erysipelothrix rhusiopathiae* (183, 897, 8319).** This agent is recovered from the tonsils of 30–50% of healthy pigs. It can cause swine erysipelas and has caused epizootics among nonvaccinated swine. Antibiotics in feeds may jeopardize sensitivity of this agent to penicillin. *E. rhusiopathiae* is hardy in the environment. Infections in humans are mainly occupational.

***S. aureus*.** *S. aureus* has been isolated in the tonsils of healthy pigs (7307).

***Streptococcus* (6546, 7188, 7343, 7825).** Healthy and ill swine can harbor *S. dysgalactiae* subsp. *dysgalactiae*, *S. dysgalactiae* subsp. *equisimilis*, *S. equi* subsp. *zooepidemicus*, and *S. suis*. *S. suis* colonizes the nose, tonsils, bowel, and genital tract of swine. In Spain, 81 (35%) of 234 tonsils from apparently healthy pigs at slaughter grew *S. suis*. *S. equi* subsp. *zooepidemicus* can infect pigs and humans. Pig-to-human spread of streptococci is via contact, cuts, or pork meat.

Dermatophytes
Isolates from pigs include *Candida albicans*, *Microsporum*, and *Trichophyton*.

2.5 EQUIDS
Domestic horse (*Equus caballus*), donkey (*E. asinus*), mule (*E. asinus* jackass × *E. caballus* mare), wild ass (*E. africanus*), and zebra (*E. zebra*) are members of Equidae (order Perissodactyla). Worldwide in 2001, there were 58 million horses (16% in People's Republic of China and 11% in Mexico), 43 million asses (21% in People's Republic of China and 12% in Ethiopia), and 13.5 million mules (FAO at http://apps.fao.org/).

Equine zoonoses (555) (Box 2.5). Agents can spread from horses to humans via contact, inhalation, ingestion, or inoculation.

EQUINE DROPLET-AIR CLUSTER
Information is scant. Horses can shed agents with respiratory secretions.

Viruses
Humans seem refractory to equine herpesvirus (EHV1, EHV4), which causes equine rhinopneumonitis. Horses are susceptible to influenza A virus (H3N8, H7N7), which has caused epizootics in the Americas. Probable horse-to-human spread is reported in a veterinary student in Chile (1725, 5760). Hendravirus has emerged in horses in Australia, causing work-related, sporadic human cases (5755).

Bacteria
An equine biovar of *Chlamydophila pneumoniae* has been isolated from horses (2277).

Fungi
Air-borne spores can infect horses similarly to humans. *C. neoformans* var. *neoformans* is isolated from ill horses.

Box 2.5 Agents from horses, by cluster

For bites, see chapter 1, and for work, see section 12.4.

Droplet-air	*Influenzavirus*
Feces-food	*Salmonella*; microsporidia; *Trichinella*
Zoonotic	Arboviruses (CCHFV, VEEV, WNV), rabies virus; *Burkholderia mallei*, *Rhodococcus equi*; *Trypanosoma* spp.; *E. granulosus*
Environmental	*Leptospira*, *C. tetani*; *S. japonicum*
Skin-blood	*S. aureus* (including methicillin-resistant *S. aureus*), *Streptococcus*; dermatophytes

EQUINE FECES-FOOD CLUSTER

Agents to be expected in horse excreta (1889) or manure include *Rotavirus*, *Clostridium difficile*, *C. tetani*, *E. coli*, *Salmonella*, *Rhodococcus equi*, *Y. enterocolitica*, microsporidia (*E. cuniculi* and *E. intestinalis*), *B. hominis*, *C. parvum*, *Giardia*, and eggs of *S. japonicum*. Undercooked horse meat is a potential health hazard.

Bacteria
***E. coli* (1294, 3307).** *E. coli* is isolated from the excreta of horses and ponies, including *E. coli* O157 (EHEC). However, EHEC in horses is an unusual source of human infections.

***Neorickettsia risticii* (441, 3245).** The agent of Potomac horse fever is enzootic in horses in North America. In New York state, 7% of randomly selected nonvaccinated horses were seroreactive. *N. risticii* has been identified in freshwater snails (*Juga* and *Pleuroceridae*) and aquatic insects (caddisflies, mayflies, damselflies, dragonflies, and stoneflies). Horses might acquire *N. risticii* by swallowing infected insects or snails. Raw horse meat might constitute a hazard for human infections.

***Salmonella* (2229, 7543, 7728).** Reported prevalences are 0.8% in healthy horses and >10% in horses with enteric disease. Serotypes recovered include Anatum, Enteritidis, Newport, and Typhimurium. *Salmonella* tends to persist in the veterinary hospital environment. Shedding risks are increased in foals and after recent use of antibiotics. Humans in contact with horses can become infected.

Protozoa
Horses and donkeys are intermediate hosts for *Sarcocystis* spp. (2554). Handling muscle and eating rare horse meat are potential hazards. Horses can also be intermediate hosts for *T. gondii*, presumably in settings that horses share with parturient cats. In North America, 7% (124/1,788) of horses slaughtered for food were seroreactive (2052).

Helminths
***Trichinella* (733, 5995).** Horses can be infected with *T. britovi*, *T. murelli*, and *T. spiralis*. The prevalence of *Trichinella* infection in horses is usually low: by digestion assay, 0/315,000 in Canada, to 3/600,000 in Italy, and to 2/59,600 in France. In Mexico in 1995, however, 5% (4/80) of horses at the abattoir were infected. Larvae of all three horse-infective species but mainly *T. spiralis* have been diagnosed in human outbreaks due to horse meat (see section 7.4).

EQUINE ZOONOTIC CLUSTER
Domestic equids can attract mosquitoes and flies and can carry ticks. "Bridge" mosquitoes and flies can carry agents from peridomestic horses to humans. Handling viremic horses is a potential health hazard.

Viruses
A. Humans are refractory to African horse sickness virus (*Orbivirus*: *Reoviridae*) that circulates in tropical Africa, in horses and donkeys, and in *Culicoides* and occasionally other arthropods (*Culex*, *Anopheles*, *Aedes*, *Hyalomma*, and *Rhipicephalus*). Although enzootic in equids, spread of *Bornavirus* to humans has not been documented.

Rabies virus (4103, 8106). (For bites, see chapter 1). Equids can contract rabies. In the United States and worldwide, horses account for ≤1% of animals confirmed rabid. Horses have caused PEP in humans.

VSV (6195). VSV can affect horses in the Americas. Spread is via droplets or bite by *Lutzomyia* sandflies. In a United States epizootic in 1982–1983, the attack rate in horses was 45%. Infected horses can be an occupational hazard for humans.

B. For some mosquito-borne viruses, equids, like humans, are marginal rather than maintenance hosts. Horses that attract mosquitoes are a potential hazard. Epizootics may herald cases in humans. Encephalitis viruses that equids share with humans include eastern equine encephalitis virus, JEV, Venezuelan equine encephalitis virus, St. Louis encephalitis virus, western equine encephalitis virus, and WNV.

Eastern equine encephalitis virus (839, 2503). Eastern equine encephalitis virus circulates in the Americas. Equine lethality is 40–90%, and epizootics recur at intervals.

Venezuelan equine encephalitis virus (6288, 7985). Venezuelan equine encephalitis virus circulates in Latin America. Equine lethality is 30–80%. During epizootics, equids develop high viremia and serve as amplification hosts. In Colombia in 1995, an epizootic killed 4,000 horses and caused 75,000 human cases.

Western equine encephalitis virus (1035, 3602). Western equine encephalitis virus circulates in the Americas. Equine lethality is 20–50%. In 1987, an epizootic caused 132 equine cases in 11 states of the United States and in Manitoba, Canada. In the Pantanal area of Brazil in 1992, when unexplained horse deaths occurred, 1% of 432 equids had neutralizing antibodies to western equine encephalitis virus.

West Nile virus (WNV) (345, 684, 1198, 2087, 5267). WNV circulates in the Old and New Worlds. Equine lethality is 30–45%. Infections in horses signal viral activity. Recent epizootics occurred in Morocco in 1996 (94 equine cases, 42 [45%] deaths), Italy in 1998 (14 [2.8%] cases in 498 horses and 6 [43%] deaths), and Camargue, southern France, in IX/2000 (131 equine cases). In Camargue, epizootics in horses are separated by long silent periods; the area has large marshes and hosts >300 species of resident and migratory birds, mostly water birds. After WNV appeared in the United States in 1999, epizootic waves caused 733 equine cases in 2001 (in 19 states) and 8,130 cases in 2002 (in 36 states).

C. For tick-borne viruses, too, equids seem largely dead-end hosts. Removing attached ticks or handling viremic horses are potential hazards. Tick-borne viruses that equids are suspected or confirmed to share with humans include New World Powassanvirus and Old World CCHFV and TBEV. In Iraq in 1980, 59% (148/252) of horses were seroreactive to CCHFV (7329).

Bacteria
***A. phagocytophilum* (973).** Ticks carry the agent to horses in the United States and Europe. Attached ticks are a potential hazard.

***B. anthracis* (7682, 8264).** Horses are susceptible. In France in 1980–2000, 4 of 114 anthrax foci concerned horses. Horses are a source of anthrax in humans.

***Burkholderia mallei* (7083).** *B. mallei* is enzootic in equids in warm climates. This agent causes glanders in horses, mules, and donkeys. Contact with infected horses is a hazard. Infections in humans have been reported.

***Brucella* (6181, 6808).** Horses can become infected with *B. abortus* and *B. suis*. In Egypt, seroprevalence was ~6% in horses, ~20% in donkeys, and ~70% in mules. Although secretions and aerosols are a potential hazard, *Brucella* rarely spreads from horses to humans.

C. burnetii. Equids can become infected but seem an insignificant source.

***Rhodococcus equi* (4927, 7809).** *R. equi* is enzootic on some horse-breeding farms. Seroprevalence in horses is 0–80% (often 0.5–10%). Epizootics can occur. *R. equi* has been isolated from respiratory secretions, feces, and soil. Spread to humans has been documented. Suspected modes include inhalation, microtrauma, contact, or ingestion.

Protozoa
***Babesia* (1633, 8292).** *B. caballi*, *B. canis*, and *Theileria equi* (*B. equi*) have been isolated in horses. These species may be difficult to separate morphologically. Ticks attached to horses are a potential hazard.

***Trypanosoma* (24, 2335).** *T. brucei* sensu lato, *T. congolense*, and *T. vivax* (all carried by tsetse flies in Africa) and *T. evansi* (carried by tabanid flies in countries with warm climates), have been reported in equids; all four can cause equine trypanosomiasis (surra). In Gambia in 1997–1998, 4 (6%) of 67 donkeys and 5 (46%) of 11 horses were infected, mostly by *T. vivax* or *T. congolense*. In an area of Jordan, 27 (33%) of 83 horses were parasitemic, and 8 (10%) had evidence of surra. In Latin America, horses are putative hosts of *T. cruzi*.

Helminths
Horses can become infected with *Angiostrongylus cantonensis* (6017). Equids of Eurasia can be intermediate hosts for the genotype G4 strain of *E. granulosus* (2119). Equids can be final host for *Fasciola hepatica* and *F. gigantica* (1723).

EQUINE ENVIRONMENTAL CLUSTER
Bacteria
***Clostridium tetani* (2117, 8169).** Horses can shed the agent and pollute soil, including pasture and play fields. The reported shedding prevalence is 1–6%.

***Leptospira* (4989).** Horses and donkeys can be naturally infected. Serovars recovered from horses include Canicola, Icterohaemorrhagiae, and Pomona. In New Caledonia in 1989–1993, 46 (24%) of 192 leptospirosis patients indicated horses as the source. Aerosols and environmental contamination are potential hazards.

Helminths
Horses, mules, and donkeys can become naturally infected with *S. japonicum*. In mountainous Yunnan province, People's Republic of China, reported prevalences are 10–30%. Trade in infected horses contributes to spread of the infection.

EQUINE SKIN-BLOOD CLUSTER
Bacteria
***S. aureus* (8000).** In Ontario, Canada, in 2000–2002, epidemic methicillin-resistant *S. aureus* was recovered from the nares of horses in hospital and clinic workers, thoroughbreds on farms, and farm workers. There is a risk of spread between horses and humans.

***Streptococcus* (2191).** Groups D and S streptococci have been recovered from healthy and ill horses, including *S. equi* subsp. *equi* (causes "strangles" in young horses, a mainly respiratory disease), *S. equi* subsp. *zooepidemicus*, and *S. dysgalactiae* subsp. *equisimilis*. Horse-to-human spread has been reported.

Dermatophytes (1020)
Trichophyton mentagrophytes var. *mentagrophytes* is a common agent of ringworm in horses. *M. equinum*,

M. gypseum, and *T. equinum* have also been isolated from horses. Via contact, these dermatophytes can spread from horse to humans.

2.6 CAMELIDS

Domestic camel (*Camelus bactrianus*, two humps), dromedary (*C. dromedarius*, one hump), llama (*Lama glama*), and alpaca (*L. pacos*) are members of Camelidae (order Artiodactyla), as are wild guanaco (*L. guanicoe*) and vicuña (*Vicugna vicugna*).

Camelid zoonoses. Putative hazards include animal dust (anthrax and Q fever), excrements (brucellosis and leptospirosis), milk (brucellosis), and ectoparasites (CCHFV). In herdsmen, camels can be sources of viral hemorrhagic fevers, brucellosis, and plague. Camel milk should not be consumed raw. Camel rides are popular among tourists visiting the north edge of the Sahara. Worldwide in 2001, there were 19 million camels, 15 million in Africa (Somalia, Sudan, and Ethiopia) and 4 million in Asia (FAO at http://apps.fao.org/).

CAMELID DROPLET-AIR CLUSTER

Information is scant. An epizootic of influenza (A/H1N1) has been reported in camels from Mongolia, and aspergillosis has been reported in camels in Australia.

CAMELID FECES-FOOD CLUSTER
Bacteria
E. coli has been isolated from diarrheic camels. *Salmonella* (5133) is enzootic in camels, including MDR serovars of Braenderup, Hadar, Heidelberg, and Typhimurium.

Protozoa
***Sarcocystis* (2554, 4235).** Camels are intermediate hosts for *S. cameli* and other species. The prevalence of muscular sarcocystosis in camels can reach 100%. Handling flesh and eating undercooked meat are potential hazards.

***Toxoplasma gondii* (2166).** Camels are intermediate hosts. Reported seroprevalence in pastoral camels is 15–75%. Raw milk and undercooked liver or meat are potential hazards.

Helminths
Camels can harbor intestinal nematodes, including species of *Strongyloides* and *Trichostrongylus*. Camels can be final hosts for *Fasciola hepatica* and *F. gigantica*.

CAMELID ZOONOTIC CLUSTER
Viruses
***Bornavirus*.** Bornavirus has been documented in alpacas and llamas.

CCHFV (2159, 4740). Camels are a suspected maintenance host. Reported seroprevalence in camels is 23–54%. In Saudi Arabia, 97% (107/110) of camels carry known vector ticks (mostly *Hyalomma dromedarii*), including on the udder and scrotum; average load is 53 ticks/camel.

RVFV (5304). RVFV is enzootic and epizootic in camels. In Niger in 1984–1988, 48% (67/141) of camels had neutralizing antibodies to RVFV. In the 1998 Mauritania epizootic, the clinical attack rate in camels was 3% (1/39).

Bacteria
***A. phagocytophilum*.** Llamas are a putative reservoir.

***B. anthracis*.** Camels are susceptible.

***B. melitensis* (8, 6181, 6658, 6808).** *B. melitensis* is isolated from camels. Brucellosis is enzootic in *Camelus bactrianus* in central Asia and *C. dromedarius* in Arabia. By setting (nomadic, dairy farms, and domestic corrals), seroprevalence in camels is 0–15% (often 5%). Camels are a source of human brucellosis via unpasteurized dairy products and excretions.

***C. burnetii* (4852, 6658).** *C. burnetii* is diagnosed in camels. In Chad, 80% of 142 camels were seroreactive, and camel breeders are at increased risk of infection.

***Mycobacterium microti*.** *M. microti* (of the *M. tuberculosis* complex) is diagnosed in llamas. Infections in humans are reported (although not from contact with llamas).

***Y. pestis* (5633, 8093).** Camels and llamas can contract plague. In central Asia, slaughtering of sick camels and camel meat are sources of plague in humans.

Protozoa
***Babesia ovis* and *Theileria ovis*.** *B. ovis* and *T. ovis* have been isolated from blood of camels. In Egypt, the reported prevalence is 10–13% (4861).

***Trypanosoma evansi* (24, 1860).** *T. evansi* that is carried by tabanid flies is enzootic in camels, causing surra. By age, geography, and test, 5–30% of animals and 30–90% of herds are infected (parasitemic), and up to 8% of animals have signs of surra. Humans are believed to be naturally resistant, but a human case has been documented.

Helminths
***Echinococcus* (1933, 2119, 2187, 4182).** *C. bactrianus*, *C. dromedarius*, and *Lama pacos* are intermediate hosts for sheep (genotype G1) and camel (G6) strains of *E.*

granulosus. G1 and G6 strains are infective for cattle and humans. G1 infections in humans have been confirmed in East Africa. Raw offall from camelids available to canids sustains a synanthropic cycle. Reported prevalence in camels is 1–80%.

Mansonella. Microfilariae of *Mansonella* sp. have been isolated from blood of camels. Camels are hosts of tegumentary *Onchocerca fasciata* and *O. gutturosa*.

CAMELID ENVIRONMENTAL CLUSTER
Camels are susceptible to *Burkholderia pseudomallei*, but it is an unlikely source for humans. Camels are naturally infected with *Leptospira*.

CAMELID SKIN-BLOOD CLUSTER
Viruses
Camelpox virus (*Orthopoxvirus*) is diagnosed in camels.

Bacteria
S. aureus has been isolated from infected camel udders. *S. agalactiae* is the most frequent cause of manifest and inapparent mastitis in camels. Reported herd prevalence is ~25%. By source, *S. agalactiae* is recovered from 50–90% of raw camel milk (2318).

Dermatophytes
M. gypseum is prevalent in camels.

3

Wild Vertebrates

3.1 Wild herbivores
3.2 Carnivores
3.3 Rodents
3.4 Lagomorphs
3.5 Primates
3.6 Bats
3.7 Birds
3.8 Reptiles and amphibians
3.9 Fish

For animal bites, see chapter 1; for animal transports, see section 16.2; and for invertebrate vectors, see chapter 4.

The phylum Vertebrata includes mammals, birds, reptiles, amphibians, and fish.

Zoonoses from wild (free roaming) and captive (zoos and research facilities) vertebrates (1736, 1812, 6383) include microbial and parasitic diseases. Global trade, hunting safaris, sileage feeding, and habitat reduction increase chances of encounters with wild vertebrates, infections that cross from wildlife to livestock (e.g., *Mycobacterium bovis*), and jumps of agents across species to humans, e.g., human immunodeficiency virus (from primates in Africa), monkeypox virus (from Gambian giant rats imported into the United States), and severe acute respiratory syndrome coronavirus (SARS-CoV) (from carnivores in China).

Feeds stored on farms attract wildlife, with a risk of fecal pollution. On Scottish farms in the winter of 1998–1999, rodent droppings were identified on stored feeds at a rate of 80/m^2 per month, and bird guano was identified at a rate of 25/m^2 per month. In Amboseli National Park, Kenya, enteric bacteria resistant to antimicrobials were significantly more frequent in baboons (*Papio cynocephalus*) that lived close to a tourist lodge with daily access to human refuse than in the wild.

Wildlife-to-human agent spread is via contact (e.g., *Bacillus anthracis* and *Francisella*), inhalation (e.g., *Hantavirus*, *B. anthracis*, *Coxiella*), ingestion (foods or hands, e.g., *Hantavirus*, *B. anthracis*, *Escherichia coli*, *Salmonella*, *Trichinella*, and *Diphyllobothrium*), or inoculation (e.g., rabies). Agents with a broad host range include *Lyssavirus*, *Babesia*, *Diphyllobothrium*, and *Trichinella*.

3.1 WILD HERBIVORES

The order Artiodactyla includes wild Bovidae and Cervidae, notably black-tailed deer (*Odocoileus hemionus columbianus*), caribou (wild) and reindeer (domesticated, both *Rangifer tarandus*), fallow deer (*Dama dama*), mule deer (*O. hemionus*), moose ("elk," *Alces alces*), red deer ("elk," *Cervus elaphus*), Rocky Mountain elk (*Cervus elaphus nelsoni*), roe deer (*Capreolus capreolus*), wapiti (*Cervus canadensis*), and white-tailed deer (*O. virginianus*). These and grazing wild herd mammals from other mammalian orders (herbivores) are reviewed next.

Zoonoses from herbivores can result from contact (trapping and skinning), ingestion (undercooked game, soiled hands), inoculation (bite, microtrauma, attached ectoparasites, and attracted mosquitoes), or inhalation (droplets, mainly mycobacteria).

HERBIVOROUS DROPLET-AIR CLUSTER
Knowledge is scant. For mycobacteria, see "Herbivorous Zoonotic Cluster" and "Herbivorous Environmental Cluster" below.

HERBIVOROUS FECES-FOOD CLUSTER
Poorly cooked game and unwashed hands are potential health hazards.

Prions
Chronic wasting disease (CWD) (4123, 5054). CWD affects captive and free-ranging cervids in North America, including mule deer, white-tailed deer, and red deer. By species, sampling, and disease stage, 0.001–15% of animals may test positive. In northern Colorado in 1996–2004, 15% (25/171, 95% confidence interval [95% CI] 10–21%) of vehicle-killed mule deer (*O. hemionus*) and 7.5% (173/2,317, 6–9%) of deer sampled in their vicinity tested positive for CWD in immunohistochemistry of lymphatic tissues, and 60% and 44% of subsamples, respectively, had brain lesions of spongiform encephalopathy. Infected deer seemed more vulnerable to vehicle collision than uninfected deer. Unlike bovine spongiform encephalopathy (BSE), deer-to-deer spread of CWD is likely. Although prions have not been demonstrated in feces or soil, a worrisome possibility is spread via feces from naturally infected deer or decomposing carcasses. Commercial transports are thought to contribute to its spread.

Bacteria
***E. coli* (3878).** An enterohemorrhagic *E. coli* (EHEC) outbreak carried in mule deer (*O. hemionus*) jerky prompted an environmental investigation during which *E. coli* O157 was recovered from 9% (3/32) of deer pellets from a forest close to the outbreak site. Deer were suspected of having acquired EHEC from a pasture shared with infected cattle.

Protozoa
***Cryptosporidium parvum* (5618).** *C. parvum* has been diagnosed in deer ("bovine" and "cervine" genotypes). Wildlife-to-human spread seems plausible in areas where drinking water is drawn unfiltered from remote watersheds.

***Toxoplasma gondii* (3445).** Many ungulates can be intermediate hosts of *T. gondii*, including deer, caribou, and African game animals.

HERBIVOROUS ZOONOTIC CLUSTER
By habitat and invertebrate vector, wild herbivores maintain zoonotic viruses, bacteria, and protozoa. Blood and tissues from viremic animals and attached ectoparasites are potential hazards. Findings from animals submitted by hunters are likely confounded by hunting prescriptions (bucks and hunting season).

Viruses
Crimean-Congo hemorrhagic fever virus (CCHFV) (6844). CCHFV is tick borne. In Africa, ungulates contribute to the reservoir. In southern Africa, antibodies to CCHFV are detected in 47% (59/127) of eland (*Taurotragus oryx*), 20% (56/287) of buffalo (*Syncerus caffer*), 22% (17/78) of kudu (*Tragelaphus strepsiceros*), and 17% (16/93) of zebra (*Equus burchelli*).

***Ebolavirus* (EBOV) (4352).** In the African rain forest, hunters handling dead duikers (*Cephalophus*, a small forest herbivore) are suspected of triggering infection chains and outbreaks.

***Hantavirus* (89).** In central Sweden in 1995–1997, antibodies to Puumala virus (PUUV) were detected in 5 of 427 wild-living moose (*A. alces*).

Inkoo virus (INKV) (*Orthobunyavirus*). INKV in Eurasia circulates in *Aedes* mosquitoes and reindeer.

Jamestown Canyon virus (JCV) (*Orthobunyavirus*). JCV is mosquito borne (7932). In Alaska, moose (*A. alces*), caribou (*Rangifer tarandus granti*), and white-tailed deer are putative reservoirs and amplifying hosts. The presence of these herbivores is significantly associated with seroreactivity in Alaskan residents.

Rift Valley Fever virus (RVFV) (207). RVFV is mosquito borne. There is evidence for infection in African wildlife, including buffalo (*S. caffer*), waterbuck (*Kobus ellipsiprymnus*), and black (*Diceros bicornis*) and white rhinoceros (*Ceratotherium simum*).

Tick-borne encephalitis virus (TBEV) (6945). Roe deer (*C. capreolus*) is an important host for all stages of *Ixodes ricinus*, and the density of this tick is strongly related to roe deer abundance. In Denmark, 7% of 237 roe deer were heavily infested, that is, with >100 engorged ticks per deer. However, although neutralizing antibodies have been found in roe deer, whether roe deer are a reservoir is uncertain.

Bacteria
***Anaplasma* (133, 2949, 5555, 6945, 7182).** *A. phagocytophilum* is tick borne. In North America, small mammals

rather than deer are thought to constitute the reservoir. In Europe, roe deer are a significant reservoir. By season, sampling, and test, reported seroprevalence is 25–95%, and 10–85% of roe deer test positive by nucleic acid amplification test (NAT). Of *I. ricinus* from deer, >80% can be infected. *A. marginale* is enzootic in cervids worldwide, including in black-tailed, white-tailed, and mule deer and Rocky Mountain elk. *A. marginale* has also been recovered from pronghorn (*Antilocapra americana*).

***Bacillus anthracis* (2022, 6865, 6993).** *B. anthracis* circulates in herbivores and soil. Deer, bison (*Bison bison*), antelopes, and elephants are among the susceptible herbivores. Epizootics can occur at intervals. In Wood Buffalo National Park in northern Canada in 2001, an epizootic killed 92 bison and 1 moose. After epizootics, the soil around carcasses can remain spore laden for a long time. In Kruger National Park in South Africa, *B. anthracis* was recovered from animals, carcasses, dung, bone, soil, and water.

***Bartonella* (6945).** In Denmark, 237 roe deer tested negative for *B. quintana* and *B. henselae* by indirect immunofluorescence assay (IFA).

***Borrelia burgdorferi* sensu lato (sl) (1680, 6273, 6945, 7128).** *B. burgdorferi* sl is tick borne. In North America, deer (*O. virginianus* and *O. hemionus*) are blood sources for *Ixodes* adults but unlikely reservoir hosts. However, the proliferation of deer has contributed to the emergence of Lyme disease in periurban areas. In Delaware, during the hunting season of 1998, 84% (212/252) of white-tailed deer brought in by hunters carried a total of 1,480 ticks (seven per deer), of which 98% were *Ixodes scapularis*. Of 150 ticks, 14 (9%) tested positive for *B. burgdorferi* sl by NAT. In Europe, roe deer, although important for *I. ricinus* maintenance and frequently (in 10–50%) seroreactive, are unlikely to be maintenance hosts for *B. burgdorferi*. However, up to 20–30% of ticks removed from deer are reported to amplify *B. burgdorferi* sl (*B. afzelii*, *B. burgdorferi* sensu stricto [ss], and *B. garinii*).

***Brucella* (1766, 2637, 4978, 6077, 6181, 6808).** *B. abortus*, *B. melitensis*, and *B. suis* can infect wild herbivores. *B. abortus* is recovered from water buck (*K. ellipsiprymnus*) and buffalo (*S. caffer*) in Africa, bison in North America, and roe deer (biovar 3) and chamois (*Rupicapra rupicapra*, biovar 1) in Europe. In Yellowstone National Park, *B. abortus* has spilled from bison to elk (*A. alces*). *B. suis* has been recovered from caribou and domesticated reindeer (biovar 4). *B. melitensis* has been recovered from chamois (biovar 3).

***Coxiella burnetii* (4932, 6293).** *C. burnetii* is enzootic in wild herbivores. Hosts include deer and moose. In Baden-Württemberg, Germany, in 1997, an epizootic on a farm for fallow deer caused 34 animal cases, 2 human cases (the owner and a relative), and 12 inapparent infections among 13 contact persons of infected animals, for a manifestation index of 14% (2/14).

***Ehrlichia chaffeensis* (1872, 7182, 8297).** *E. chaffeensis* is tick borne. In North America, white-tailed deer (*O. virginianus*) are thought to be the major vertebrate reservoir. In 1981–2001, 47% (984/2,101) of deer from 18 U.S. states were reactive, and nearly half of reactive animals tested positive for *E. chaffeensis* by PCR or culture.

Mycobacterium. *M. avium* subsp. *paratuberculosis* and *M. bovis* are enzootic in wild herbivores that are a potential source for infections in livestock. ***M. avium* subsp. *paratuberculosis* (1905).** In Austria in 2002–2004, lymph nodes from 26 (36%) of 73 hunted or dead wild red deer, 76 (37%) of 206 roe deer, 12 (20%) of 59 chamois, as well as muflon, fallow deer, and ibex yielded *M. avium* subsp. *paratuberculosis* by PCR. ***M. bovis* (256, 2315, 6686, 6996).** Wild and farmed cervids are susceptible, including white-tailed deer, red deer, and fallow deer (*D. dama*). High deer densities and bait feeding for hunting are implicated in the introduction of tuberculosis in free-ranging deer in North America that now is self-sustained. In Alberta, Canada, in 1990, an epizootic affected domesticated red deer; one active *M. bovis* infection was diagnosed in a veterinary surgeon, and 6 of 106 workers converted to tuberculin (two rendering plant workers, two necropsy technicians, one herd inspector, and one meat inspector).

Protozoa

***Babesia* (2062).** *Babesia* is emerging in cervids. In the United States, *B. odocoilei*, which is transmitted by *I. scapularis*, has been isolated from white-tailed deer (*O. virginianus*), elk (*Cervus elaphus elaphus*), and caribou (*Rangifer tarandus caribou*). In Europe, *B. divergens*, likely transmitted by *I. ricinus*, has been isolated from roe deer (*C. capreolus*), red deer (*C. elaphus*), and reindeer (*Rangifer tarandus tarandus*). *B. capreoli* has been isolated from red deer and sika deer (*Cervus nippon*), and a *B. odocoilei*-like *Babesia* has been isolated from roe deer.

***Leishmania* (3622).** In Africa and Southwest Asia, hyraxes (*Procavia* and *Heterohyrax*) are natural hosts of *L. aethiopica*. In an emerging focus in Israel, *Leishmania* DNA was amplified from 3 (10%) of 29 *Procavia capensis*.

***Trypanosoma* (5448, 8090, 8099).** In Africa, the situation is complicated by the occurrence of *T. brucei* sl

(*T. brucei brucei* and *T. brucei rhodesiense*), *T. congolense*, and *T. vivax* in herbivores, notably duikers (*Cephalophus*). *T. brucei rhodesiense* naturally infects wild bovids such as bushbuck (*Tragelaphus scriptus*), hartebeest (*Alcelaphus buselaphus*), reedbuck (*Redunca redunca*), and waterbuck (*Kobus defassa*). In Latin America, *T. cruzi* naturally infects >100 species of mammals from 25 families and 7 orders.

Helminths
Cervids can be intermediate hosts for the Nordic biotype or cervid (G8) genotype of *Echinococcus granulosus* that circulates in North America and Eurasia (198, 2119, 6140). Susceptible species include caribou and domesticated reindeer (infection prevalence, 2–25%), moose (10–80%), red deer (≤5%), mule deer, white-tailed deer, and ibex (*Capra sibirica*). Reindeer and caribou are intermediate hosts for *Taenia saginata* in Siberia.

HERBIVOROUS ENVIRONMENTAL CLUSTER
Bacteria
Deer can be infected with *Leptospira*. In Czechia in 1987–1989, 4% of 398 captive red deer and 7% of 136 captive roe deer were reactive to serotype Grippotyphosa (7548). In Spain, red deer and fallow deer have yielded *Mycobacterium avium* subsp. *avium* (256).

Helminths
Species of *Schistosoma* reported in ungulates include *S. bovis* and *S. mattheei* in Africa and *S. japonicum*, *S. nasale*, and *S. spindale* in Asia. Infections by nonjaponicum, zoonotic schistosomes in humans should be questioned critically (3953). However, animal schistosomes are recognized causes of cercarial dermatitis in humans.

3.2 CARNIVORES
The mammalian order Carnivora has ~230 species, including foxes and wolves of Canidae, wild cats of Felidae, bears of Ursidae, raccoons of Procyonidae, badgers, skunks, and weasels of Mustelidae, hyenas of Hyaenidae, and mongooses of Viverridae. Some wild carnivores have adapted well to humans, around parks, dump sites, and urban areas, e.g., the raccoon (*Procyon lotor*) in North America and the red fox (*Vulpes vulpes*) in western Europe.

Zoonoses from carnivores. Who is exposed to wild carnivores? Occupationally exposed groups include zoo and circus workers, hunters and wildlife rangers, pelt ranchers, quarantine station officers, police officers dealing with wildlife road accidents, and veterinary staff. Exposure can result from contact (handling, trapping, and skinning), inoculation (bite or microtrauma), ingestion (excreta on berries and mushrooms), or inhalation (droplets from captive carnivores).

CARNIVOROUS DROPLET-AIR CLUSTER
Ferrets (*Mustela* sp.) are susceptible to *Influenzavirus* and used in the laboratory for vaccine research (5081). In the United States, raccoon hunters and their dogs have contracted *Blastomyces dermatitidis*, likely from the environment rather than raccoons (279).

CARNIVOROUS FECES-FOOD CLUSTER
Prions
Transmissible mink encephalopathy is sporadically diagnosed in farmed mink (*Mustela vison*) (4763). Captive carnivores in the United Kingdom, likely through risky feeds from infected cattle, have contracted bovine spongiform encephalopathy (BSE), including cheetah (*Acinonyx jubatus*), cougar (*Felis concolor*), ocelot (*Felis pardalis*), and tiger (*Panthera tigris*) (5767).

Bacteria
Wild, zoo, and laboratory carnivores can be expected to shed enteric agents similar to dogs (see section 2.1). *Campylobacter jejuni* and *C. coli* were identified in laboratory ferrets (7377).

Fungi
Foxes are reported to harbor microsporidia (*Encephalitozoon cuniculi*).

Protozoa
Sarcocystis. Coyote, wolf, and other carnivores are final hosts.

Toxoplasma gondii **(255, 2501, 6980).** Besides cats, wild felids can be final hosts, including the lynx (*Lynx canadiensis*) in the Arctic, the cougar (*F. concolor*) in North America, and probably the jaguar (*Panthera onca*) and ocelot (*F. pardalis*) in South America. Numerous carnivores are intermediate hosts, including canids, ursids, and mustelids, with reported prevalence of 22–66%. Felids can pollute water supplies with oocysts. In Wisconsin in 1999, an epizootic caused litter loss in 26% of farmed female mink (*M. vison*), and >10,000 kits died.

Helminths
Wild carnivores can be naturally infected with *Diphyllobothrium*, *Clonorchis*, *Gnathostoma*, *Taenia solium* cysticeri, and *Trichinella* larvae. Carnivores can fecally pollute foods (e.g., fallen fruits and berries). Meat from undercooked game carnivores can be a hazard.

Diphyllobothrium. *Diphyllobothrium* ranges broadly in fish-eating mammals, including wolf, brown bear, and black bear in the Northern Hemisphere, and marine mammals such as seals in the Southern Hemisphere.

Trichinella* (2457, 5279, 5995, 6657, 7888).** The genus ranges broadly in carnivores. ***T. britovi. *T. britovi* is enzootic in Eurasia, in canids, mustelids, and ursids. In Italy, virtually all infections in red foxes are due to *T. britovi*, for an overall prevalence of 4% (155/3,565), with a range of 0% in the lowlands to 60% in mountainous areas. ***T. nativa.*** *T. nativa* is enzootic in the Arctic, in ursids, mustelids, canids, and felids, including the Arctic fox (*Alopex lagopus*), black bear (*Ursus americanus*), and polar bear (*U. maritimus*). ***T. nelsoni.*** *T. nelsoni* is enzootic in Africa, in hyaenids and felids, with spotted hyena (*Crocuta crocuta*) as a major reservoir host. ***T. spiralis.*** *T. spiralis* is enzootic in canids and ursids in Eurasia. In Brandenburg, Germany, in 1993–1995, the prevalence in wild red foxes was 3–18% (mean, 8%, 255/3,295) by serology and 0.07% (5/7,103) by demonstration of larvae (confirmed as *T. spiralis* by molecular fingerprinting).

CARNIVOROUS ZOONOTIC CLUSTER
Viruses
Seroreactivity in carnivores may merely reflect past exposure to arthropod-borne viruses. Seroreactivity is reported to Sindbis virus in brown bear (*Ursus arctos*) and wolf (*Canis lupus*) in Finland (946) and to TBEV in red foxes (*V. vulpes*) in southern Germany (8279).

Reservoir carnivores should carry viremia of an intensity and duration sufficient to infect a significant fraction of invertebrate vectors.

Powassan virus. Skunks, weasles, raccoons, and red and gray foxes are presumed reservoir hosts of Powassan virus.

Rabies virus (1319, 2276, 2345, 4103, 5988, 8106, 8283). (For bites, see chapter 1.) Most wild mammals are susceptible to rabies and are potential sources for humans. Worldwide, wild mammals account for 43–48% of animals rabies cases, mainly foxes (13–16%), raccoons (13–16%), skunks (8–10%), bats (4–5%), and mongoose (0.3–0.6%), and remaining wildlife accounts for ~3%.

In the United States in 2001–2003 (1996–2000, mean), raccoons (*P. lotor*) accounted for 36–37% (45%) of animal rabies cases, skunks (mainly *Mephitis mephitis*) accounted for 29–31% (27%), and foxes accounted for 6% (6%). Human encounters with raccoons were frequent in rural and urban areas, for postexposure prohylaxis (PEP) rates of 32–123/10^5 per year. In New York state in 1993–1998, rabid raccoons caused 48% (2,944/6,139) of PEP (1–25/event), and rabid skunks caused 8% (470; 1–8/event). In the Caribbean, the introduced mongoose (*Herpestes auropunctatus*) has become a potential vector to humans.

In Europe, red (*V. vulpes*) and Arctic (*A. lagopus*) foxes are reservoirs for sylvatic rabies. Fox rabies has been controlled by bait vaccines in western Europe. In eastern Europe, the percentage of raccoon dogs (*Nyctereutes procyonoides*) with wildlife rabies is increasing, in Russia from 0.4% (1980–1998) to 1.9% (2003, 53/2,863), while wolves have a share of <1%. In Ethiopia, 1% (487/62,751) of PEP was caused by wild mammals, mostly jackals (78%, 381/487) and hyenas (13%, 63).

SARS-CoV (2975). SARS-CoV is assumed to have jumped species in People's Republic of China in 2003. Candidate source hosts are the palm civet (*Paguma larvata*), raccoon dog (*N. procyonoides*), ferret badger (*Melogale moschata*), ferret (*Mustela furo*), or domestic cat. This conclusion is based on virus isolations, culinary habits in People's Republic of China, early SARS cases among restaurant workers who handled such animals, and high seroreactivities among traders of such animals.

Bacteria
Agent recovery may reflect incidental exposure. *E. chaffeensis*, *E. ewingii*, and *Yersinia pestis* have been recovered in carnivores in North America. Seroreactivity is reported for *A. phagocytophilum* in red foxes in Switzerland and for *C. burnetii* in coyotes, foxes, skunks, and raccoons in the United States. While incidental or amplifying hosts, carnivores are believed to be able to carry ectoparasites (ticks and fleas) into new territory.

***Francisella tularensis* (3672).** Natural infections with *F. tularensis* have been reported in a number of wild and captive carnivorous species, mainly predators of rabbits and hares such as the coyote (*Canis latrans*) and foxes (*Vulpes fulva* and *Urocyon cinereoargenteus*). Feeding infective rabbit meat to minks (*M. vison*) has caused epizootics among ranched minks. Occupational infections have resulted from bites, skinning, and fleas.

***M. bovis* (949, 2642, 6996).** Susceptible carnivores include the red fox (*V. vulpes*), the coyote (*Canis latrans*), and the raccoon (*P. lotor*) in North America and the badger (*Meles meles*) in Europe. Carnivores can acquire *M. bovis* through uptake of infective prey or carcasses. Badgers that visit farms can become a source of tuberculosis in livestock, thereby expanding the zoonotic reservoir; infected badgers have been observed to search barns, haystacks, and silage, to fecally pollute feeds, and to come into close contact with cattle.

Protozoa
***Leishmania* (424, 1895).** Wild canids are a sylvatic reservoir for zoonotic visceral leishmaniasis (VL), including the jackal (*Canis aureus*) and raccoon dog (*N. procyonoides*) in

Asia, the red fox (*V. vulpes*) in southern Europe, and foxes (*Lycalopex vetulus* and *Cerdocyon thous*) in South America. In an emerging focus of zoonotic VL in Israel, 8% (4/53) of jackals and 5% (1/20) of red foxes were seroreactive. Risk for humans is limited, as this cycle involves "sylvatic" sandflies. However, wild canids are suspected to disseminate zoonotic VL.

***Trypanosoma* (3291, 5448, 8099).** *T. brucei* sl is identified in various carnivores in Africa, including civets (*Nandinia binotata* and *Viverra civetta*), genet (*Genetta servalina*), and mongoose (*Crossarchus obscurus*). In Latin America, *T. cruzi*-infected carnivores include "foxes" (*Dusicyon griseus*), coatis (*Nasua nasua*), and ferrets (*Galictis cuja*). In rural Tennessee, in 1998, two of three raccoons trapped in the vicinity of locally acquired human cases tested positive for *T. cruzi*.

Helminths
***Dirofilaria* (1079, 6068).** Cats, red and gray foxes, and other carnivores are natural hosts for *D. immitis* (canine heartworm) in Old and New Worlds. Raccoons are reservoirs for *D. tenuis* in the New World. Cats and foxes are natural hosts for *D. repens* in the Old World.

***Dipylidium caninum* (1887).** Red foxes are natural hosts. In Switzerland, the prevalence in 548 urban foxes is 0.5–2.5%.

***Echinococcus* (474, 1125, 2119, 3374, 6140).** Dingo, jackal (*Canis mesomelas, C. aureus*), coyote (*C. latrans*), red fox (*V. vulpes*), and hyena are major sylvatic final hosts for the sheep (G1) genotype of *E. granulosus* that is enzootic on all continents. The wolf (*C. lupus*) is host for the Nordic biotype or cervid (G8) genotype in the Arctic and Sub-Arctic. Foxes (*V. vulpes* and *A. lagopus*) and wolf (*C. lupus*) are major sylvatic final hosts for *E. multilocularis*. By test, 0.5–70% of foxes from enzootic areas are infected. In Europe, enzootic areas are expanding from the core Alpine areas into Benelux and eastern European countries and into cities that support infected fox populations such as Stuttgart, Germany, and Zürich, Switzerland. Neotropical wild felids are final hosts for *E. oligarthrus*. The neotropical bush dog (*Speothos venaticus*) is a final host for *E. vogeli*.

CARNIVOROUS ENVIRONMENTAL CLUSTER
Bacteria
Carnivores (foxes, raccoons, and skunks) can harbor *Leptospira* (2358, 7548, 8091). In the United States in 1979, the seroprevalence in striped skunks (*M. mephitis*) removed from public places was 47% (21/45). In Czechia in 1987–1989, 5% of red foxes in zoos were reactive to serotype Grippotyphosa.

Helminths
In North America, *Baylisascaris procyonis* is enzootic in raccoons (6434). Peridomestic raccoons are a hazard, because they defecate in "latrines" such as rooftops, attics, woodpiles, decks, and lawns near trees. Of 215 raccoon latrines in three Californian cities (Carmel, Pacific Grove, and San Jose), 44–53% tested positive for *B. procyonis*. Humans contract invasive baylisascariasis via polluted hands. *Toxocara canis* and related *Toxascaris leonina* are enzootic in foxes (3812, 4581). In western and eastern Europe, 15–70% of red foxes are infected with *T. canis*. In the Arctic, the Arctic fox (*A. lagopus*) carries *T. leonina*. Whether foxes are sources for humans is not known, but red foxes that adapt to urban living are a hazard.

CARNIVOROUS SKIN-BLOOD CLUSTER
Corynebacterium ulcerans has been isolated from free-ranging otter (*Lutra*) (2468).

3.3 RODENTS
The mammalian order Rodentia includes suborders hystricomorphs, with agoutis (Dasyproctidae), chinchillas (Chinchillidae), guinea pigs (Caviidae), nutrias (Myocastoridae), pacas (Agoutidae), and porcupines (Hystricidae), and sciuromorphs, with beavers (Castoridae), Muridae, and squirrels, chipmunks, prairie dogs, and marmots (Sciuridae). Of particular interest are Muridae, with subfamilies Murinae (*Apodemus, Bandicota, Mus,* and *Rattus*), Arvicolinae (voles: *Arvicola, Clethrionomys,* and *Microtus*; muskrat), Sigmodontinae (New World *Calomys, Neotoma, Oryzomys,* and *Sigmodon*), Gerbillinae (gerbils and jirds), and Cricetinae (hamsters).

Exposure. Exposure to rodents can be on premises (wild rodents) or fur farms (chinchillas and nutrias), in zoos, laboratories, and houses (pets and food rodents). Rats are cosmopolitan. The brown or canal rat (*Rattus norvegicus*; body, 19–25 cm; tail, 16–20 cm) lives indoors and outdoors, including in (port) cities and sewers. It can burrow, gnaw, and swim. Black, roof, or ship rat (*R. rattus*; body, 17–20 cm; tail, 20–25 cm) lives around houses, including in tree holes, barns, and huts. Its burrows can be 20–70 cm deep, with several openings. Mice have a more patchy range. The house mouse (*Mus musculus*, body and tail each 9 cm long) lives indoors and outdoors, in rural and urban areas. It can gnaw, burrow, and climb. Popular pet rodents include gerbils, guinea pigs, hamsters, and albino varieties of rats and mice. In the United Kingdom in 2001, there were 0.9 million pet hamsters and 0.7 million guinea pigs (overall, ~2–3/100 population).

Rodent zoonoses (394, 3457) (Box 3.1 and Table 3.1). Spread to humans is through contact (petting, breeding,

Table 3.1 Hantaviruses reported in humans, by geography and rodent host

World[a]	Rodent	Virus	Disease[b]
Old	Rats (*Rattus norvegicus*, *R. rattus*)	Seoul (SEOV)	HFRS
	Bank vole (*Clethrionomys glareolus*)	Puumala (PUUV)	Epidemic nephropathy
	Common vole (*Microtus arvalis*)	Tula (TULV)	Fever, rash
	Striped field mouse (*Apodemus agrarius*, *R. norvegicus*)	Hantaan (HTNV)	HFRS
	Yellow-neck field mouse (*Apodemus flavicollis*)	Dobrava (DOBV)	HFRS
New	Deer mouse (*Peromyscus maniculatus*)	Sin Nombre (SNV)	HPS
	Pygmy rice rats (*Oligoryzomys*)	Andes (ANDV)	HPS
	Vesper and grass mice (*Calomys*, *Akodon*)	Laguna Negra (LNV)	HPS

[a]Old World is Africa, Australasia, and Europe. New World is the Americas.
[b]HFRS, hemorrhagic fever with renal syndrome; HPS, *Hantavirus* (cardio)pulmonary syndrome.

and trapping), inhalation (secretions and aerosols from urine), ingestion (rodent-polluted foods and rodents for food), or inoculation (research with viremic animals and ectoparasites on rodents). Rodents readily infest substandard or abandoned housings. A patient with diabetic neuropathy is reported to have sustained rat bites while asleep (1563). Rodent die-offs can signal epizootics and pending epidemics. In central Asia, abundance of the great gerbil (*Rhombomys opimus*) paralleled the plague in that animal (1773). The exposure history should address pets and contacts with dead rodents (Box I.1).

RODENT DROPLET-AIR CLUSTER
Viruses
Humans seem refractory to some viruses that circulate in laboratory mice and rats, including murine adenovirus, murine parvovirus, and Sendai virus (*Paramyxoviridae*: *Respirovirus*).

Box 3.1 Agents from rodents, by cluster

For bites, see chapter 1; for work, see section 12.4; and for domicile, see section 11.2. Typical hosts are given in parentheses.

Feces-food	HEV, *Rotavirus* (rat, mouse); *Campylobacter*, *Salmonella*, *Yersinia*; *Cryptosporidium muris* (mouse), *Toxoplasma* (agouti), *Trichinella*
Zoonotic	CCHFV, *Filovirus*, *Hantavirus*, LCMV (mouse, hamster), TBEV, rabies virus; *Anaplasma*, *Bartonella* (mouse, vole), *Borrelia*, *Brucella*, *Francisella* (hamster, prairie dog, beaver), *Orientia* (rat), *Rickettsia* (squirrel), *Streptobacillus moniliformis*, *Y. pestis*; *Babesia* (vole), *Leishmania* (gerbil, jird), *Trypanosoma*; *E. multilocularis* (vole)
Environmental	*Leptospira*
Skin-blood	Cowpox virus (rat), monkeypox virus; *C. ulcerans*; dermatophytes; ectoparasites (fleas, mites, ticks)

Bacteria
Wild or laboratory rodents are reported to be naturally colonized or infected with *Chlamydophila caviae* (guinea pigs), *Klebsiella pneumoniae*, *Mycoplasma pulmonis* (black rats), and *Streptococcus pneumoniae*. However, rodent-to-human spread is not reported.

Fungi
Two healthy adults have contracted *B. dermatitidis* pneumonia while relocating prairie dogs in a range management project outside known endemic areas (1160). *Pneumocystis carinii* has been isolated in *Apodemus*, *Clethrionomys*, *Microtus*, *Mus*, *Rattus*, and other rodents. Reported microscopic prevalence is 6–22%. However, rodent-to-human spread does not seem to occur (the human-infective species is *P. jirovecii*).

RODENT FECES-FOOD CLUSTER
Viruses
Hepatitis E virus (HEV) (2334, 3777). Strains of HEV circulate in rodents. In the United States, seroreactive rodents include *M. musculus* (14%), *R. rattus* (38–90%), and *R. norwegicus* (44–94%). Zoonotic spread has been suggested.

Rotavirus. Mice and rats are frequently infected with highly rodent-infective types, mice with group A viruses that are common in humans, and rats with group B viruses that are infrequent in humans.

Bacteria
Enteric bacteria that are presumed or confirmed enzootic in rodents (720, 3213, 4455, 7377) include *Campylobacter* (*C. jejuni*, *C. coli*), *Helicobacter* spp., *Salmonella* (e.g., serotypes Enteritidis and Typhimurium), and *Yersinia*. In general, rodent-to-human spread seems infrequent. *Y. enterocolitica* is widely enzootic in rodents. *Y. pseudotuberculosis* is enzootic in wild rodents (mice and rats), farmed rodents (nutrias *Myocastor* and chinchillas *Chinchilla*) and laboratory rodents (guinea pigs *Cavia*

and hamster *Mesocricetus*). In the Brazilian Amazon, 0.6% (5/819) of *Oryzomys capito* and 0.6% (2/319) of *Proechimys guyanensis* grow *Salmonella*.

Fungi
Rodents can harbor microsporidia, including *E. cuniculi* (laboratory mice and rats) and *Enterocytozoon bieneusi* (muskrat and beaver) (1924).

Protozoa
***Cryptosporidium muris* (5692).** *C. muris* infects mice and other rodents. It can be transmitted to dogs, cats, lambs, and humans.

***Giardia* (2072, 3570, 7019, 7452).** Rodents harbor rodent-specific *G. muris* and *G. microti* and human genotypes of *G. lamblia*. Reported *G. lamblia* hosts include *R. rattus*, muskrat (*Ondatra zibethica*), beaver (*Castor canadensis*), nutria (*Myocastor coypus*), and water rat (*Nectomys squamipes*). By species and test (mucosal scraping or feces), microscopic prevalence is ~10–100%. Beavers (in North America) and water rats (in Brazil) are suspected of polluting pristine waters and domestic or municipal water supplies.

***T. gondii* (1084, 2519, 5612).** Rodents are intermediate hosts, including mice, rats, and squirrels. Rodents are sources of *T. gondii* for hunting cats. Rodents for food are sources of toxoplasmosis in humans; in West Africa this includes rats and in South America this includes paca (*Agouti paca*) and agouti (*Dasyprocta agouti*).

Helminths
Mice are natural hosts for *Capillaria hepatica* and *T. spiralis*. Rats are natural hosts for *Angiostrongylus*, *C. hepatica*, *Clonorchis sinensis*, *Fasciola hepatica*, *Gnathostoma*, *Metagonimus*, *Paragonimus*, and *T. spiralis*.

***Angiostrongylus* (3765, 3934, 4442, 5926, 6070).** Wild rats are hosts for *A. cantonensis*, including *Rattus*, *Bandicota*, and in Louisiana likely the wood rat (*Neotoma floridanus*). By location, the reported prevalence is 1% (*Bandicota indica*, Thailand), 0–20% (*R. rattus*), and 5–75% (*R. norvegicus*). Hosts for *A. costaricensis* include the cotton rat (*Sigmodon hispidus*), rice rat (*Oryzomys*), common rat (*R. norvegicus* and *R. rattus*), and pocket mice (*Liomys*).

***Trichinella* (638, 4224, 5994).** *Rattus* and *M. musculus* are natural hosts for *T. spiralis*. In Henan province, People's Republic of China, 0.5% of rats captured in farm households and 4% of rats from around abattoirs were infected. *R. norvegicus* is also a natural host for *T. britovi*.

RODENT ZOONOTIC CLUSTER
Habitats such as crowded burrows, tick-infested grasslands, trees with canopy-dwelling mosquitoes, and peridomestic food stores influence the agent spectrum in rodents and potential human risks. Seasonal abundance can parallel the number of human cases. Rodents that range beyond sites where humans have acquired infections delineate vulnerable areas. Rodents attract arthropods to burrows, bring ticks to cabins or summer vacation homes, and defecate and urinate on foods. Hazards include handling, ectoparasites (fleas, ticks, and mites), excrements (droppings and urine), cleaning out of cabins or basements, and using rodents for food (498, 2103, 4022, 5061, 7406).

Viruses
Rodents harbor zoonotic viruses from at least 10 genera, including viruses that cause hemorrhagic fever or encephalitis.

Alphavirus. For Sindbis virus (SINV) (946), Castoridae are suspected hosts, e.g., the beaver (*Castor fiber*). For Venezuelan equine encephalitis virus (6545, 7985), hosts are Muridae, e.g., rice rat (*Oryzomys*), deer mouse (*Peromyscus*), cotton rat (*Sigmodon*), and cane mouse (*Zygodontomys*), and hystricognaths, e.g., the spiny rat (*Proechimys*).

Arenavirus. For Guanarito virus (7416), hosts are Muridae, e.g., the cotton rat (*Sigmodon alstoni*) and cane mouse (*Zygodontomys brevicauda*). For Junín virus (5061), hosts are Muridae, e.g., *Calomys musculinus* and *Calomys laucha*. For Machupo virus (7828), hosts are Muridae, e.g., *Calomys callosus*. For Lassa virus (6256), hosts are Muridae, e.g., multimammate rat (*Mastomys natalensis*).

For lymphocytic choriomeningitis virus (LCMV) (41, 642, 1249, 1386, 2107, 6433), the house mouse (*M. musculus*) is the primary reservoir. Pet hamsters (*Mesocricetus*), guinea pigs, and rats are not known to be reservoirs but can become infected on contact with house mice, e.g., in homes and pet shops. By focus, the prevalence of infection in house mice is 3–40%. In Baltimore, in 1984–1989, 4–13% of 480 mice were seroreactive; in the inner city, high mouse densities (274/1,000 trap nights) were correlated with high murine seroprevalence (11–13%). Epizootics have occurred in mice at research facilities. Mice in houses and laboratories, and pet hamsters have been sources of LCMV in workers and pet owners in North America and western Europe. In the United States in 1973–1974, pet hamsters from one supplier were the source for an epidemic with >180 human LCM cases in 12 states. In Germany in the early 1970s, 47 pet hamster-associated human cases were reported. In France, a

30-year-old woman had kept a Syrian hamster (*M. auratus*) in the kitchen for many months before she fell ill with LCM.

Coltivirus. For Colorado tick fever virus, suspected hosts are Muridae, e.g., wood rat (*Neotoma*), deer mouse (*Peromyscus maniculatus*), and voles, and Sciuridae, e.g., ground squirrel (*Spermophilus*) and chipmunk (*Eutamias*).

Filovirus. For EBOV (5221), suspected hosts are African rain forest Muridae, e.g., *Mus setulosus* and *Praomys*.

Flavivirus. For Chikungunya virus (1917), hosts are Sciuridae, e.g., palm squirrel (*Xerus erythropus*). For Omsk hemorrhagic fever virus, hosts are Muridae, e.g., muskrat (*Ondatra zibethica*). For POWV, hosts are Muridae, e.g., rats and white-footed mice, and Sciuridae, e.g., red and gray squirrels, chipmunks, and woodchuck (*Marmota monax*). For TBEV (4022, 4172, 7305), hosts are young, viremic (nonimmune) Muridae that harbor *Ixodes* ticks (mainly small, larval stages). TBEV has been isolated from *Apodemus flavicollis* (in Austria), *A. speciosis*, and *Clethrionomys rufocanus* (in Japan). Reported seroprevalences are ~15–50% in *A. flavicollis*, ~20% in *A. speciosis*, ~15–30% in *C. glareolus*, ~20% in *C. rufocanus*, and 25% in *Rattus norvegicus*. For West Nile virus (WNV) (1198), suspected hosts are Sciuridae, e.g., squirrels. For yellow fever virus (YFV) (1841), hosts are hystricognaths, e.g., New World porcupine (*Coendou*) and agouti (*Dasyprocta leporine*).

Hantavirus (1347, 3311, 4494, 5063). *Hantavirus* has diversified in Muridae (Table 3.1), in Old World Murinae and Arvicolinae (Dobrava-Belgrade [DOBV], Hantaan [HTNV], Puumala [PUUV], and Saaremaa [SAAV] viruses), in New World Sigmodontinae (Sin Nombre [SNV], Andes [ANDV], and Laguna Negra [LNV] viruses), and in rats (Seoul virus [SEOV]) in both Old and New Worlds. In the United States, seroreactive Sciuridae (chipmunks, *Tamias minimus*) were also reported. **Old and New Worlds.** Rats (*R. rattus* and *R. norvegicus*) (1390, 3810, 4295) are main hosts of SEOV. Alternative hosts are bandicots (*Bandicota indica* and *B. bengalensis*). Besides SEOV, HTNV seems to occur in *R. norvegicus*, and in parts of People's Republic of China, SEOV and HTNV may cocirculate in rats. In the 1980s, global SEOV seroprevalence was 10% (36/370 *R. rattus*) to 27% (243/910 *R. norvegicus*). In Taiwan, seroprevalence was higher in *R. norvegicus* from international seaports (20%) than from rural areas (~5%). **Old World Murinae and Arvicolinae (88, 636, 4574, 5609, 6405, 6712, 6877, 6944, 7765).** The striped field mouse (*Apodemus agrarius*) is main host for HTNV in Eurasia; in the Balticum, it may also host SAAV. The yellow-necked mouse (*A. flavicollis*) is main host for DOBV in northern, eastern, and southeastern Europe. The bank vole (*Clethrionomys glareolus*) is the main host for PUUV in northern, western, eastern, and southeastern Europe, mainly in beech (*Fagus*) forest with bushes, and in periurban gardens. *Microtus arvalis* is host for TULV. Further hantaviruses have been identified in *M. musculus* and *Lemmus sibiricus*. DOBV, HTNV, SAAV, PUUV, and TULV are reported to infect humans. In autumn, when voles (*C. clareolus*) abandon territories, there is a risk of house infestation. Harsh winters and scarce snow cover reinforce this risk. In northern Sweden, the anti-PUUV prevalence was ~16% in voles from around epidemic nephropathy cases, but only ~6% in voles from randomly selected controls residing 10 km away from cases. In Anhui province of People's Republic of China, the rate of hemorrhagic fever with renal syndrome (due to HTNV) was correlated with precipitations, fall crop production, and density of mice (*A. agrarius*); this was explained by the habit of farmers for harvest to sleep in huts on the farmland and outdoor exposure to mice. **New World Sigmodontinae (498, 4132, 4378, 5922, 7268, 7519, 8312).** Confirmed or suspected hosts include in the United States *Peromyscus maniculatus* for Sin Nombre Virus (SNV), in Central and South America *Oligoryzomys* for Andes (ANDV) and Juquitiba (JUQV) viruses, in the Atlantic rain forest of Brazil *Bolomys lasiurus* for Araraquara virus (ARAV), in croplands, pastures, and thorn scrubs ("Chaco") of Paraguay and Argentina *Calomys callosus* for Laguna Negra (LNV), and in Argentina *Akodon simulator* for Oran virus (ORNV). Reported seroprevalence is 7–25% in *P. maniculatus*, 10–13% in *Oligoryzomys* (*O. longicaudatus* in Chile, *O. fulvescens* in Panama), and 5–12% in *C. callosus*. Besides SNV, ANDV, ARAV, LNV, JUQV, and ORNV are reported to cause febrile illness or hantavirus (cardio)pulmonary syndrome in humans.

Lyssavirus. Any rodent species can be infective for rabies virus (for bites, see chapter 1). In the United States, rabies is diagnosed annually in ~50 rodents, mainly beaver (*C. canadensis*) and woodchuck (*M. monax*) (1199, 4103).

Nairovirus. For CCHFV, Muridae are hosts, e.g., gerbils (*Gerbillus*) and jirds (*Meriones*).

Orthobunyavirus. For snowshoe hare virus (SSHV) (7932), hosts are Muridae, e.g., *A. agrarius*, *A. sylvaticus*, *Clethrionomys rutilus*, and *Microtus arvalis*, and Sciuridae, e.g., *Spermophilus parryii* and *Tamiasciurus hudsonicus*. For La Crosse virus (1035), Sciuridae are hosts, e.g., *Tamias striatus* and *Sciurus carolinensis*.

Phlebovirus. For RVFV (2854, 6012), Muridae are hosts, e.g., rock rat (*Aethomys namaquensis*), multimammate rat

(*Mastomys huberti*), grass rat (*Arvicanthis niloticus*), and possibly *R. rattus*. For sandfly fever virus, Muridae are suspected hosts, e.g., gerbils (*Psammomys obesus* and *Rhombomys opimus*).

Bacteria

Rodents harbor zoonotic bacteria from at least 10 genera.

***A. phagocytophilum* (816, 1124, 1872, 4469).** Ticks carry the agent to rodents that are suspected reservoirs. In the eastern United States, the white-footed mouse (*Peromyscus leucopus*) is considered the major vertebrate reservoir. Other candidates in the United States are the deer mouse (*P. maniculatus*) and wood rat (*Neotoma fuscipes*). Of rodent hosts, 10–40% are seroreactive, and a subset is positive in NAT. In western Europe, candidate reservoirs include bank vole (*Clethrionomys glareolus*) and wood mouse (*Apodemus sylvaticus*); 2–11% of rodents and 4–12% of attached *Ixodes* ticks are positive for *A. phagocytophilum* by PCR. In the United Kingdom, rodent bacteremia is short-lived and *I. trianguliceps* ticks rather than rodents are suspected of maintaining *A. phagocytophilum* over the winter.

***Bartonella* (852, 3397, 4070).** Arthropods are suspected of carrying *Bartonella* to rodents (and humans). For *B. elisabethae* and *B. grahamii*, rodents are significant reservoirs, including *M. musculus*, *R. norvegicus*, and *R. rattus* worldwide, cotton rat (*Sigmodon hispidus*), white-footed mouse (*P. maniculatus*), cotton mouse (*P. gossypinus*), and rice rat (*Oryzomys palustris*) in the New World, and yellow-neck mouse (*A. flavicollis*), wood mouse (*A. sylvaticus*), bank vole (*C. glareolus*), and field vole (*Microtus agrestis*) in the Old World. Bacteremia is prevalent, typically in 10–20% of rodents.

***Borrelia* (978, 2708, 7128, 7553).** Ticks carry agents of Lyme disease and relapsing borrelioses to rodents. New World rodent hosts for *B. burgdorferi* ss are mainly white-footed mouse (*P. leucopus*), but also dusky-footed woodrat (*N. fuscipes*), eastern chipmunk (*T. striatus*), and gray squirrel (*S. carolinensis*). Reported infection prevalence in *P. leucopus* is 40–90%, and infection (seroconversion) rates (in trapped, ear-tagged, and retrapped mice) are 0.2/mouse per week. In Eurasia, confirmed or suspected reservoirs of *B. burgdorferi* sl include mainly *A. flavicollis*, *A. sylvaticus*, and *C. glareolus*, but also *M. musculus*, *R. norvegicus*, *R. rattus*, red squirrel (*Sciurus vulgaris*), and dormice (*Glis glis*).

Rodent hosts for relapsing borreliae include *M. musculus* and *R. rattus*, as well as *Peromyscus*, *Eutamias*, and *Tamiasciurus* in the New World, and rats (*Arvicanthis*, *Mastomys*, and *Cricetomys*) and gerbils (*Tatera gambiana*) in the Old World. Agents include *B. hermsii*, *B. turicatae*, and *B. venezuelensis* in the New World and *B. crocidurae*, *B. hispanica*, and *B. persica* in the Old World.

***Brucella* (4978, 5535).** Aerosols are a potential hazard. Human-infective *B. suis* (biovar 5) and apparently human noninfective *B. neotomae* have been isolated from rodents.

C. burnetii. *C. burnetii* is maintained in rodents in a sylvatic cycle that involves inhalation, ingestion, and ticks. Infected rodents include rats, mice, and marmosets (*Marmota himalayana*).

***F. tularensis* (346, 1256, 4367, 5849, 6202).** *F. tularensis* reservoirs are aquatic rodents such as the muskrat (*O. zibethicus*) and beaver (*C. canadensis*), and terrestrial rodents such as *M. musculus*, ground vole (*Arvicola terrestris*), and common vole (*Microtus arvalis*). Infected *R. norvegicus*, *R. rattus*, squirrels, hamsters (*Cricetus cricetus*), and prairie dogs (*Cynomys ludovicianus*) can carry the agent to humans. Rodents can shed *F. tularensis* from excreta. In pet shops, pet animals could acquire the agent from wild rodents that enter shops and urinate or defecate on cages. Contact, microtrauma, or polluted surface water are potential sources for tularemia in humans. In Texas, in 2002, a tularemia epizootic among wild-caught prairie dogs kept at a commercial distributor killed ~250 of ~3,600 animals. Seroconversion in a prairie dog handler confirmed that the infection could spread to humans. Of 20 exposed prairie dog handlers, 6 (32%) reported recent bites, 7 (37%) ate or drank without handwashing after contact, and 13 (67%) handled animals or cages with bare hands. Owners should know the risks from scratches or inhalation of dust when cleaning litter. Wild or dead rodents should not be handled without gloves.

***Orientia tsutsugamushi* (1521, 4467, 6172, 7031).** Chigger mites (*Leptotrombidium deliense*) carry the agent to rodents (and humans). Peridomestic rodents are a hazard. Suspected or confirmed reservoirs include *Apodemus agrarius*, *B. indica*, *M. musculus*, *Tupaia glis*, and rats (*Rattus exulans*, *R. losea*, *R. norvegicus*, *R. rattus*, and *R. tiomanicus*). Prevalence in rodents from enzootic areas is ~5–75% by serology, 1–23% by bioassay (with a high prevalence in *R. rattus*), and up to 46% by NAT. In People's Republic of China, ~75–90% of trapped, living *A. agrarius* and *Cricetulus triton* were chigger infested.

Rickettsia. *Rickettsia* spp. identified in rodents include *R. akari* (1534), *R. conorii*, *R. prowazekii* (6235), and *R. typhi* (2728, 3539, 7042, 7590). For mite-borne *R. akari*, *M. musculus* is the main reservoir. LCMV in mice is suspected to cause mites to seek alternative hosts, with a risk of *R. akari* spread to humans. For tick-borne *R. conorii*, *R. norvegicus* and *R. rattus* are putative hosts. For louse-borne *R. prowazekii*, the classic reservoir is humans. An alternative reservoir in the eastern United States is the flying squirrel (*Glaucomys volans*) and its ectoparasites (squirrel-specific *Neohaematopinus sciuropteri* louse and the promiscuous *Orchopeas howardii* squirrel flea). In 1977–1980, at least seven human cases of "epidemic" typhus were linked to squirrels. For tick-borne *R. rickettsii*, *P. leucopus* is a putative host. For tick-borne *R. sibirica*, *A. agrarius*, *Clethrionomys rufocanus*, and *O. zibethicus* are putative hosts. For flea-borne *R. typhi*, the classic reservoir is *Rattus*, and an alternative reservoir is *Mus*. In enzootic areas, ~5–25% of *M. musculus* and 5–90% of *R. norvegicus* and *R. rattus* are seroreactive. In Greece in 1993, 4% (8/226) of fleas (*Xenopsylla cheopis*) collected from *R. norvegicus* amplified *R. typhi* DNA. Also in Greece in 1993–1997, over 50% (45/83) of the cases of murine typhus had a history of rat contact. In contrast in suburban Los Angeles in 1984–1988, none of 35 *R. norvegicus* and only 6% (2/36) of *R. rattus* trapped in the neighborhood with human cases were seroreactive.

Streptobacillus moniliformis (1243, 5570, 6875).
From 10 to 100% of laboratory rats and 50–100% of wild rats are reported to carry *S. moniliformis*. Bites (see chapter 1) are not a requirement for spread; about 30% of patients with rat bite fever do not recall a bite. Risks include ownership of pet rodents, work in pet shops, and petting, handling, or breeding rodents.

Y. pestis (735, 1773, 2570, 5633, 5860, 8109).
Rodents, fleas, and soil maintain *Y. pestis* in natural foci that exist in America, Africa, and Asia. While *Y. pestis* can infect numerous rodent species, only a few species are true maintenance hosts. Cosmopolitan rats (acutely ill *R. rattus* and more chronically ill *R. norvegicus*) are sources rather than reservoirs of plague. Infected rodents and their fleas carry *Y. pestis* to humans. Epizootics and die-offs among rodents (rats and prairie dogs) can herald epidemics.

In Africa, likely reservoirs are multimammate rat (*Mastomys natalensis*), swamp rat (*Pelomys fallax*), and vlei rat (*Otomys*). Other infected rodents include *Arvicanthis*, *Lophuromys*, *Grammomys*, and *Tatera*. Of trapped rodents, ~5–20% are seroreactive.

In the Americas, likely reservoirs are the deer mouse (*P. maniculatus*) and California vole (*Microtus californicus*). Other infected rodents include *Akodon*, *Callomys*, *Cavia* (guinea pigs, a food source), *Cynomys* (prairie dog), *Dipodomys*, *Neotoma*, *Oryzomys*, *Sigmodon*, chipmunks (*Tamias*), and squirrels (*Citellus*, *Sciurus*, and *Spermophilus*). In the United States, squirrels (with the flea *Oropsylla montanus*) were sources for 44% of plague cases reported in 1970–1994, and prairie dogs were for 6%.

In Asia, likely reservoirs are gerbils (*Meriones meridianus* and *Rhombomys optimus*), marmots (*Marmota sibirica*), and little suslik (*Spermophilus pygmaeus*). In Iran, plague maintenance involves *Meriones* that succumb to or resist plague, fleas that survive host die-offs by starving, and *Y. pestis* that persists in the soil around burrows. In central Asia, marmots are an important source of plague in hunters.

Protozoa
Ectoparasites and arthropods attracted to rodent burrows are hazards for infections in humans with *Babesia*, *Leishmania*, and *Trypanosoma*.

Babesia (992, 2063, 5572, 7152).
Babesia is tick borne. Rodents are reservoirs. In the United States, hosts of *B. microti* include white-footed mouse (*P. leucopus*, up to 40–60% parasitemic) and meadow vole (*Microtus pennsylvanicus*, up to ~20% parasitemic) in the northeastern and upper midwestern states, and prairie vole (*M. ochrogaster*, up to 87% PCR positive) in Colorado. In Europe, hosts of *B. microti* and related species include yellow-neck mouse (*A. flavicollis*, 12% PCR positive), bank vole (*Clethrionomys glareolus*, 16% PCR positive), and field vole (*Microtus agrestis*, 25% parasitemic). In Japan, a *B. microti*-like agent was detected by PCR in 23% of 47 *A. speciosus* and 4% of 50 *C. rufocanus*.

Leishmania (835, 1065, 2377, 3627, 7199).
Leishmania is sandfly borne. *R. rattus* and *Arvicanthis niloticus* are suspected reservoirs for the zoonotic form of VL.

Rodents are reservoirs for the zoonotic form of cutaneous leishmaniasis (CL). In arid areas of the Old World (North Africa, Southwest Asia, agent *L. major*), this includes fat sand rat (*Psammomys obesus*), jird (e.g., *Meriones crassus* and *M. libycus*), and gerbils (*Rhombomys opimus* and *Gerbillus dasyurus*). In West and East Africa, Nile grass rat (*Arvicanthis niloticus*) and Senegal gerbil (*Tatera gambiana*) are hosts of zoonotic CL, in central Asia and northern India, the great gerbil (*R. opimus*). By season, habitat, and test (e.g., amastigotes in ear smear), the prevalence of infection in rodents is 1–60%. Findings of human-infective *L. major* in rodents can be confounded by human noninfective species (e.g., *L. turanica*) that appear to support maintenance of *L. major* in gerbils. In the New World, confirmed or suspected reservoir rodents for *L. mexicana* sl include in Arizona and Texas wood rat (*Neotoma albugula* and *N. micropus*), in Mexico *Peromyscus yucatanicus*, *Sigmodon hispidus*, *Oryzomys melanotis*, and *Ototylomys phyllotis*, and in Brazilean 2° forest and plantations, *Proechimys guyannensis*. For *L. braziliensis* in Brazil, suspected reservoirs include the black rat (*R. rattus*), water rat (*Nectomys squamipes*), and grass mouse (*Bolomys lasiurus*). Amastigotes were seen in blood films from 6% of these latter animals, and 1% was culture positive.

***Trypanosoma* (1599, 5448, 7834, 8099).** In Africa, *T. brucei brucei*, *T. brucei rhodesiense*, *T. congolense*, and *T. vivax* are identified in rodents, notably the giant rat (*Cricetomys gambianus*) and brush-tailed porcupine (*Atherurus africanus*).

In Latin America, the New World porcupine (*Coendu*) is a main reservoir for *T. cruzi*. Other infected rodents include *R. rattus*, *R. norvegicus*, *M. musculus*, and species of *Agouti*, *Akodon*, *Baiomys*, *Dasyprocta*, *Echimys*, *Nectomys*, *Oryzomys*, *Peromyscus*, *Proechimys*, *Sciurus*, and *Spermophilus*.

Helminths
***E. multilocularis* (2119, 2869, 3374, 6113, 7947).** Infected dense rodent populations that are continuously available to predators (foxes, dogs, and cats) maintain sylvatic cycles and bridge sylvatic with domestic cycles. Rodent hosts include Arvicolinae (*Arvicola*, *Clethrionomys*, *Lemmus*, *Microtus*, *O. zibethica*), Murinae (*A. agrarius*, *M. musculus*, and *R. norvegicus*), Gerbillinae (*Meriones* and *Rhombomys*), and Sciuridae (*Sciurus vulgaris* and *Citellus undulates*). Reported prevalence ranges from 0.01% (1/6,890 *M. musculus*) to ≥25% (*Microtus* species in People's Republic of China and Alaska). Rodents can establish urban foci, for instance, in Zurich, Switzerland (prevalence, 9–20% in *Arvicola terrestris*), and Freiburg, Switzerland (prevalence, 9–39% in *A. terrestris* and 10–21% in *M. arvalis*).

Neotropical rodents are intermediate hosts for *E. oligarthrus* (e.g., agoutis, *Dasyprocta*) and *E. vogeli* (e.g., pacas, *Cuniculus paca*) (474).

RODENT ENVIRONMENTAL CLUSTER
Bacteria
Except *Leptospira*, the role of rodents for environmental bacteria such as *Burkholderia pseudomallei* and *Pseudomonas aeruginosa* is largely unknown.

***Leptospira* (74, 1450, 3718, 5341, 6899, 7552, 7613, 7838).** Numerous rodent species can be infected. The main reservoirs are Muridae: cosmopolitan *Mus* and *Rattus*; in the New World also *Akodon*, *Nectomys*, *Oryzomys*, and *Zygodontomys*; in the Old World also *Apodemus*, *Arvicanthis*, *Bandicota*, *Clethrionomys*, *Cricetomys*, *Mastomys*, and *Ondatra*. Serovars that point to rodent sources include Autumnalis, Ballum, Grippotyphosa, Icterohaemorrhagia, and Sejroe.

Prevalence of infection in mice, rats, and other rodents is roughly 5–20% by tissue culture, 10–50% by serology, and 5–90% by NAT. In informal settlements around Iquitos in the Peruvian Andes, 5% (7/151) of trapped *R. rattus* and 16% (20/124) of *R. norvegicus* tested positive by PCR. In the alleys of Baltimore, where patients had contracted leptospirosis, 90% (19/21) of trapped *R. norvegicus* were PCR positive. In Zurich, Switzerland, 10% (5/50) of trapped *C. glareolus* were PCR positive, as were 12% (7/60) of *A. sylvaticus* and 13% (8/60) of *A. terrestris*.

Urine of rats and other rodents is a significant source of environmental and crop pollution, including during floods. Rodents are a well-recorded source of infections in humans. In Italy, 4% (5/126) of leptospirosis cases had a history of exposure to mice or rats. In a case-control study in Nicaragua, having rodents in the household was a risk. In Guyana, men who hunted, prepared, and ate *A. paca* were at increased risk. Cases of Weil's disease have followed consumption of rat meat.

Fungi
Relationships between rodents and soil-dwelling fungi are largely unexplored. Bamboo rats (*Cannomys* and *Rhizomys*) are natural hosts for *Penicillium marneffei* (1341).

Helminths
***Schistosoma* (1700).** Mice and rats are natural hosts for *S. japonicum*. In Brazil, water rats (*Nectomys squamipes*) have been found naturally infected with *S. mansoni*.

***Toxocara canis* (2053).** Squirrels and chipmunks are suspected to spread eggs. Synanthropic rodents such as *M. musculus* and *A. agrarius* are likely to act as paratenic hosts.

RODENT SKIN-BLOOD CLUSTER
Viruses
Viruses reported in laboratory rodents include cytomegalovirus and ectromelia virus.

Cowpox virus (CPXV) (5817, 8245). Rodents are reservoirs of the cowpox virus, including the bank vole (*C. glareolus*) and gerbil (*Citellus fulvus*). In Finland, 4.5% (41/902) of wild rodents (mainly *C. glareolus*) had antibodies to Orthopoxvirus in IFA. Spread of CPXV from rodents to humans has been reported. A 14-year-old girl who cared for a wild, ill *R. norvegicus* contracted a CPXV eyelid infection.

Monkeypox virus (MPXV) (1221). Rodents in Africa, including squirrels (*Funisciurus* and *Heliosciurus*) and Gambian rats (*Cricetomys emini*), are likely reservoirs of MPXV. In 2003, imported Gambian rats introduced MPXV into the United States, causing an epizootic that spread to pet prairie dogs and further to humans.

Bacteria
Bacteria reported in rodents include *Corynebacterium ulcerans* and *Staphylococcus aureus*.

***C. ulcerans* (5607).** During an epizootic of gangrenous dermatitis, this agent was isolated from 63 of 350 wild ground squirrels (*Spermophilus richardsonii*). Handling ground squirrels can expose humans to *C. ulcerans*, which can cause diphtheria-like disease.

Dermatophytes
Microsporum canis, *M. gypseum*, and *Trichophyton mentagrophytes mentagrophytes* are recovered from rodents, including laboratory rats and mice and pet hamsters and guinea pigs.

Helminths
Rats and mice can be infected with both *Hymenolepis diminuta* and *H. nana*.

***H. nana* (4626).** Although infective when shed, molecular evidence suggests that *H. nana* circulates in rodents separately from humans.

Ectoparasites
Besides notorious rat flea (*Xenopsylla cheopis*, vector of *R. typhi* and *Y. pestis*) and house mouse mite (*Allodermanyssus sanguineus*, vector of *R. akari*), rodents harbor an array of fleas, ticks, and mites.

3.4 LAGOMORPHS
The mammalian order Lagomorpha includes hares and rabbits (Leporidae) and pikas (Ochotonidae). Of note among leporids are the snowshoe hare (*Lepus amercanus*), black-tailed jackrabbit (*L. californicus*), and eastern cottontail (*Sylvilagus floridanus*) in North America, and the brown hare (*L. europaeus*) and European rabbit (*Oryctolagus cuniculus*) in Europe. In contrast, mice, guinea pigs, and hamsters are rodents (see section 3.3).

Lagomorph zoonoses (394, 2618, 3457) (Box 3.2). Spread is by contact (petting, hunting, skinning, and roadside cadavers), inhalation (pets, laboratories, and rabbitries), ingestion (litter-soiled hands and lagomorphs for food), or inoculation (skinning and laboratory). In the United States in 2000, 0.25 million rabbits were used in laboratories, 2 million were raised for food, and 9 million were kept domestically (~3/100 population). In the United Kingdom in 2001, households kept about 1.1 million pet rabbits (~2/100).

LAGOMORPH DROPLET-AIR CLUSTER
Bordetella bronchiseptica and *Pasteurella multocida* (2158) commonly colonize the upper respiratory tract of laboratory and wild lagomorphs. Infections in humans can result from handling living or dead animals.

Box 3.2 Agents from rabbits and hares, by cluster

For bites, see chapter 1.

Feces-food	*Rotavirus*, *E. coli*, *Salmonella*, *Yersinia*, and *Toxoplasma*
Zoonotic	*C. burnetii*, *F. tularensis*, *Y. pestis*
Environmental	*Toxocara*
Skin-blood	Dermatophytes and ectoparasites

LAGOMORPH FECES-FOOD CLUSTER
Viruses
Coronavirus and *Rotavirus* (1929) are prevalent in rabbitries and laboratory rabbits. In particular, human-infective serotypes of group A rotavirus have been reported in laboratory rabbits.

Bacteria (660, 720, 998, 2618, 3057, 8280)
Domestic and commercial rabbits can be naturally infected with *Escherichia coli*, including EHEC (*E. coli* O157:H7) and enteropathogenic *E. coli* (including "atypical" serotypes, e.g., O128:H2), posing risks for humans. *Listeria monocytogenes* is recovered from rabbits and hares. The prevalence in perished hares (*Lepus europaeus*) in Switzerland is 0.6%. *Salmonella* seems poorly documented in lagomorphs. In Italy in 1999–2001, of 92 isolates from rabbits, most were MDR. Also in Italy, roast rabbit caused an outbreak of *S. enterica* serovar Hadar with 29 human cases, but epidemiological evidence pointed to contamination at the restaurant, not the producing farm. Hares contribute to maintain *Y. enterocolitica*, including serogroups pathogenic to humans. The prevalence in perished hares in Germany is 0.5%. Rabbits and hares are considered the principal reservoir for *Y. pseudotuberculosis*. In Switzerland, the prevalence in perished hares is 3%.

Fungi (3076, 3137)
Pet and research rabbits can harbor microsporidia (*E. cuniculi* and *E. bieneusi*). *E. cuniculi* is enzootic in rabbitries, with reported seroprevalence of up to 20–40%.

Protozoa (2120, 2538, 3057, 6980)
C. parvum is reported in laboratory rabbits. *Eimeria* spp. cause intestinal coccidiosis in rabbits (infections in humans have not been reported).

Toxoplasma. Rabbits and hares are intermediate hosts and potential sources. Reported seroprevalence is 18% (*S. floridanus*) to ~2–45% (*L. europaeus*).

LAGOMORPH ZOONOTIC CLUSTER
Viruses (1347, 7932)
Lagomorphs are suspected or confirmed reservoirs or amplifying hosts for at least five zoonotic virus genera.

Alphavirus. SINV has been isolated in the mountain hare (*Lepus timidus*) in northern Scandinavia.

Coltivirus. Eyach virus has been isolated in *O. cuniculus*.

Flavivirus. POWV has been isolated in *L. americanus* and TBEV in *L. europaeus*.

Nairovirus. CCHFV has been isolated in Old World hares (*L. europaeus* and *L. capensis*).

Orthobunyavirus. Snowshoe hare virus has been isolated from snowshoe hares (*L. americanus*), California encephalitis virus has been identified in jackrabbits (*L. californicus*) and desert cottontails (*Sylvilagus auduboni*), and Tahyna virus has been isolated from *O. cuniculus*.

Bacteria
Knowledge is rather patchy.

Bartonella alsatica. *B. alsatica* has been isolated from wild *O. cuniculus* in northeastern France (3246).

B. suis. *B. suis* has been isolated from *L. europaeus* in Switzerland (3057).

C. burnetii (4760, 6188). *C. burnetii* is enzootic in lagomorphs, including *L. americanus* in North America, pika (*Ochotona thibetana*) in Asia, and *L. europaeus* in Europe. In Nova Scotia, Canada, a rabbit snarer and three other persons who had contact with wild rabbits contracted atypical pneumonia. Of 2,180 *L. europaeus* hunted in Bohemia, Czechia, 2.8% are seroreactive to *C. burnetii*. Of *L. europaeus* imported into Italy from eastern Europe for hunting, 17% are seroreactive.

F. tularensis (1272, 3030, 3205, 4270, 5200, 5562). *F. tularensis* is enzootic or epizootic in wild lagomorphs but rare in domestic and laboratory rabbits. Natural infections have been documented in North America, in the mountain cottontail (*Sylvilagus nuttalli*), snowshoe hare (*L. americanus*), and white-tailed jackrabbit (*L. townsendii*); in Japan, in the Japanese hare (*L. brachyurus*); and in Europe, in the brown (*L. europaeus*) and mountain (*L. timidus*) hare. Birds migrating from Finland were suspected of having introduced *F. tularensis* on an island off Sweden in the fall of 1983, which resulted in an epizootic among *L. timidus*. Hares are considered terminal rather than reservoir hosts that fall victim to epizootics. Tularemia in hares is seasonal, with peaks in fall, winter, or spring that follow vector tick activity. Infected hares are suspected to pollute unprotected water supplies. Lagomorphs are important sources of tularemia in humans. In North America, rabbits are the main source (rabbit fever), in particular, *S. nuttalli*, and >15% of cases have reported skinning. In Eurasia, hares are the main source. In Castilla y León, Spain, in 1997, an outbreak caused 513 tularemia cases among hunters who had handled hares. In Czechia in 1959–1999, contact with hares accounted for ~$\frac{1}{3}$ of 577 tularemia cases.

***R. conorii* and *R. rickettsii*.** *R. conorii* and *R. rickettsii* naturally infected lagomorphs (1449, 2550). In Costa Rica, 55% (26/47) of wild *Sylvilagus braziliensis* were seroreactive, and *R. rickettsii* was isolated from attached *Haemaphysalis leporispalustris* ticks. In Tuscany, Italy, 79% of *O. cuniculus* were seroreactive, and *R. conorii* was identified by biotest from attached *Rhipicephalus pusillus* ticks.

Y. pestis (2570, 5844, 7867). *Y. pestis* naturally infects over 10 species of lagomorphs. Rabbits, and in central Asia pikas, are suspected reservoirs. Lagomorphs are an established source of plague in humans. Rabbits were sources for 7% of human plague cases reported in the United States in 1970–1994. The main risks are hunting and skinning wild rabbits, tasks that are typical for winter and men.

Protozoa (3979)
In the eastern United States, the microscopic prevalence of *Babesia microti* in *S. floridanus* is 4%.

Helminths (1620, 7947)
Pikas (*Ochotona daurica* and *O. curzoniae*) and the Tibetan hare (*Lepus oiostolus*) can be intermediate hosts for *E. multilocularis*.

LAGOMORPH ENVIRONMENTAL CLUSTER
Bacteria
Lagomorphs can be naturally infected with *Burkholderia pseudomallei* and *Leptospira*.

Helminths
Baylisascaris procyonis. In a small wildlife park in Japan, an epizootic among *O. cuniculus* kept in the vicinity of caged raccoons (*P. lotor*) was traced to a raccoon that had been donated to the park 8 weeks previously (6624). Antihelminthic treatment of raccoons, and flaming of cages and park dirt floor were insufficient to eradicate *B. procyonis* in raccoons.

Rabbits are suspected transport hosts for *T. canis* or *T. cati*, and undercooked rabbit meat is a suspected source for humans (7222).

LAGOMORPH SKIN-BLOOD CLUSTER
Viruses
Humans seem refractory to rabbit oral papilloma virus (*Papillomavirus*) and Myxomavirus (*Leporipoxvirus*) (4988) that are enzootic in wild and domestic rabbits.

Bacteria
S. aureus can colonize the skin and respiratory and digestive tracts of rabbits.

Dermatophytes
M. canis, *M. gypseum*, and *T. mentagrophytes* are frequently isolated from rabbits (1020, 2132). Lagomorphs are a known source of tinea in humans.

3.5 PRIMATES

The order Primates comprises >200 species in >10 families, notably New World Cebidae (*Alouatta*, *Aotus*, *Ateles*, *Cebus*, and *Saimiri*), and Old World Cercopithecidae (*Cercopithecus*, *Colobus*, *Macaca*, *Mandrillus*, *Papio*, and *Presbytis*), Hylobatidae (gibbons) and Pongidae (chimpanzee, *Pan troglodytes*; gorilla, *Gorilla gorilla*; orangutan, *Pongo pygmaeus*). Monkey is the term for long-tailed primates, and ape is the term for Hylobatidae and Pongidae.

Simian zoonoses (822, 1144, 6701) (Box 3.3). Primates host >180 species of infectious disease agents. Monkey-to-human spread can be by contact (e.g., petting and logging), inoculation (for bites, see chapter 1), inhalation (holding stations, zoos, and laboratories), or ingestion (hunt and rural markets). Some 40,000 live primates are estimated to be traded annually. Of 22,913 primates shipped to the United States in 1990–1993, 90% (20,580) were cynomolgus (*Macaca fascicularis*), 7% (1,621) were rhesus (*Macaca mulatta*), and 3% (712) were African greens (*Cercopithecus aethiops*). Adherence to national or professional guidelines can reduce transmission risks.

SIMIAN DROPLET-AIR CLUSTER
Monkeys in holding stations and pet shops can acquire respiratory tract infections from caretakers ("reverse" spread), with a risk of recirculation to humans.

Viruses
Simian parvovirus (SPV) (922) behaves in cynomolgus (*M. fascicularis*) as parvovirus B19 (PVB19) does in humans. Handlers of an SPV-seropositive macaque are more often seroreactive (51% or 33/65) than nonhandling workers (38% or 9/24) or blood donors (34% or 34/100).

Bacteria
Mycobacterium tuberculosis (1144). *Macaca* is particularly susceptible. In the United States, infection has been diagnosed in 0.4% (81/20,580) of captive cynomolgus (*M. fascicularis*) and 0.6% (9/1,621) of rhesus (*M. mulatta*), with high variability in between shipments.

SIMIAN FECES-FOOD CLUSTER
Mainly captive primates have been studied. Coprophagia in primates increases the risk for enteric infections.

Box 3.3 Agents from primates, by cluster

For bites, see chapter 1; for work, see section 12.4; and for bioproducts, see section 17.6.

Droplet-air	*M. tuberculosis* complex
Feces-food	HEV, *Rotavirus*; *Campylobacter*, *Salmonella*, *Shigella*, *Yersinia*; microsporidia; *C. parvum*, *Entamoeba histolytica*, *G. lamblia*; *Strongyloides fuelleborni*
Zoonotic	CeHV1, *Filovirus* (Ebola, Marburg), *Flavivirus* (DENV, YFV), rabies virus, simian foamy virus, SIV, simian virus 40; *Plasmodium brasilianum*, *P. knowlesi*
Environmental	*S. fuelleborni*
Skin-blood	Monkeypox virus; *Enterobius vermicularis*

Workers can infect primates, and handling captive or pet primates is a risk, with a potential for "ping-pong" (back and forth) infections that can be difficult to control.

Viruses (224, 257, 3699)
Captive primates are susceptible to hepatitis A virus (HAV), hepatitis B virus (HEV), and *Rotavirus*. Natural HEV infections have been reported in wild rhesus (*M. mulatta*), bonnet (*M. radiata*), and langur (*Presbytes entellus*) in India. At a primate field station in Atlanta, Ga., of 109 primates (capuchins, chimpanzees, mangabey, pigtail, and rhesus), 76% had antibodies to *Norovirus*, and 89% had antibodies to *Rotavirus*.

Bacteria (425, 3790, 3889)
Primates in zoos and research facilities (e.g., *Ateles*, *Callithrix*, *Cercopithecus*, *Erythrocebus*, *Galago*, *Macaca*, and *Saimiri*) are susceptible to *Campylobacter* (*C. jejuni* and *C. coli*), *E. coli* (e.g., atypical enteropathogenic *E. coli*), *Salmonella* (virtually any serotype except Typhi and Paratyphi), *Shigella*, and *Yersinia* (*Y. enterocolitica* and *Y. pseudotuberculosis*). *Shigella* spreads easily but is particularly difficult to control.

Fungi
E. bieneusi has been reported in *Macaca*.

Protozoa (14, 4004, 4443, 5334, 7025, 7810)
Captive primates (including pongids) can shed *Balantidium coli*, *Blastocystis hominis*, *C. parvum*, *Entamoeba histolytica* ss (in Old and New World primates, often inapparent; in pongids, often invasive), *G. lamblia*, *Isospora* (e.g., *I. cebi* and *I. paponis*, but apparently not *I. belli*), and *Sarcocystis* (*S. hominis* and *S. suihominis*).

Helminths (4004, 7025)
Information is patchy. *Trichuris trichiura* is consistently reported from captive and semicaptive primates (e.g., *Macaca* and *Papio*).

SIMIAN ZOONOTIC CLUSTER

Wild or captive primates can expose humans to zoonotic agents, including by logging (via canopy-dwelling mosquitoes) or in zoos and holding stations (via ectoparasites).

Viruses

Bites or mucosal splash should prompt evaluation for rabies virus (see chapter 1). Wild primates are suspected or confirmed sylvatic reservoir hosts for at least four genera of viruses.

Alphavirus **(1917, 7313, 8242).** For Chikungunya virus (CHIKV), primates are major reservoirs. CHIKV has been isolated from African greens (or vervets, *Cercopithecus aethiops*), baboons (*Papio papio*), patas (*Erythrocebus patas*), and bush babies (*Galago senegalensis*). For Mayaro virus, candidate reservoir species are howlers (*Alouatta seniculus*), tamarins (*Saguinus midas*), and squirrels (*Saimiri sciureus*). Primates are reservoirs for Sindbis virus.

Filovirus **(2461, 3629, 4353, 5074, 8110).** Primates are a suspected reservoir for EBOV. At Reston, Va., in 1989, EBOV-Reston caused epizootics in cynomolgus (*M. fascicularis*) from the Philippines. Infected monkeys were again detected in Italy in 1992 and the United States in 1996. At the provider facility in the Philippines, 3 (0.2%) of 1,732 monkeys were seroreactive. In Tai National Park, Côte d'Ivoire, in 1994, an epizootic of EBOV-Ivory Coast affected wild chimpanzees. In central Africa in 2001–2002, EBOV was detected in the carcass of a gorilla butchered by a hunter who initiated an outbreak. Nonlethal EBOV infections are now documented in wild-born chimpanzees and *Mandrillus* in central Africa. In African rain forest, hunters of primates seem part of an infection chain that leads to village and hospital outbreaks. **Marburgvirus (MARV).** MARV was introduced into Marburg, Germany, in 1967 by vervets (*C. aethiops*) from Uganda. Greens are not considered reservoir hosts, however.

Flavivirus **(859, 1833, 1841, 7079, 8242).** For dengue virus (DENV), candidate reservoir hosts include pongids and *Macaca*. For Japanese encephalitis virus (JEV), orangutan is a likely reservoir. Epizootics of Kyasanur Forest disease virus (KFDV) have occurred in langurs (*Presbytis entellus*) and bonnets (*Macaca radiata*). **YFV.** In African rain forest, suspected reservoirs of YFV include species of *Cercopithecus*, *Colobus*, *Erythrocebus*, and *Papio*. In the East African dry savanna, *Galago* is a suspected reservoir. In South America, suspected reservoirs include species of *Alouatta*, *Ateles*, *Cebus*, *Pithecia*, and *Saguinus*. Epizootics and die-offs have been observed among *Aotus*, *Callithrix*, and *Saimiri*. For Zikavirus, primates are likely reservoir hosts.

Orthobunyavirus. Primates are likely reservoirs for oropouche virus.

Bacteria

Zoonotic bacteria are poorly documented in wild primates.

Protozoa

Plasmodium **(1787, 1850, 2310, 3745, 5590, 6918, 7861).** Primates host >25 species of plasmodia, most are vivax-like (tertian), e.g., *P. cynomolgi*, *P. simiovale*, and *P. simium*, few are malariae-like (quartan); e.g., *P. brasilianum* (seems conspecific with *P. malariae*), and one is unique ("quotidian," *P. knowlesi*). Reservoir primates are reported in South America and Southeast Asia but apparently not in Africa.

Of wild monkeys examined in Brazil and French Guiana, 6–57% (typically 10–15%) were parasitemic, including *Alouatta*, *Ateles*, *Pithecia*, and *Saguinus*. Whether primate malaria is pre-Columbian or a result of human-to-monkey "reverse" spread is controversial.

In Southeast Asia, *P. knowlesi* is enzootic in *M. fascicularis*, *M. nemestrina*, and *Presbytis melalophos*.

Human infections are documented, in research laboratories with *P. cynomolgi* and *P. knowlesi*, in South America with *P. brasilianum* (in native Amerindians) and *P. simium* (in a forest guard and in Southeast Asia with *P. cynomolgi*, *P. knowlesi*, and *P. simiovale*. In Sarawak (Malaysian Borneo), 120 human cases of *P. knowlesi* malaria that were initially misdiagnosed as quartan malaria have been confirmed by microscopy and PCR.

Trypanosoma **(1599, 5448, 8099).** In Africa, *T. brucei brucei*, *T. brucei rhodesiense*, *T. congolense*, and *T. vivax* have been identified in primates, notably *Cercopithecus nictitans* and *C. mona*. In Latin America, peridomestic primates that attract triatomine bugs are potential hazards for infections with *T. cruzi*. Natural infections have been reported in *Alouatta*, *Ateles*, *Cebus*, *Saguinus*, and *Saimiri sciureus*.

Helminths

Leaf monkeys (*Presbytis*) are a reservoir host for subperiodic *Brugia malayi* in Southeast Asia. Monkeys are naturally infected with human noninfective *B. pahangi*.

SIMIAN ENVIRONMENTAL CLUSTER

Shared habitats (common grounds) are potential sources for infections in humans.

Ancylostoma. *Ancylostoma* has been isolated in captive primates.

Schistosoma mansoni. Natural infections are reported in primates in Africa.

Strongyloides **(317, 7025).** *S. fuelleborni* and *S. stercoralis* can infect wild and captive primates. In Africa, natural *S. fuelleborni* infections are reported in chimpanzees, gorillas, and baboons. Spread to humans is possible via contact, feces, or soil. In Uganda, *S. fuelleborni* is the only intestinal helminth common in mountain gorillas (*G. gorilla beringei*; 10/41) and humans (game guards and families, and pygmies; 2/35) living in the same habitat.

SIMIAN SKIN-BLOOD CLUSTER
Knowledge of skin flora of wild primates is marginal.

Viruses
Blood, simian cell lines, and xenotransplants can expose humans to zoonotic viruses.

MPXV (276). MPXV was diagnosed in Copenhagen, Denmark, in 1958, in *M. cynomolgus* from Singapore. As we now know, its reservoir is rodents rather than primates. However, ill primates are a potential source for humans.

Papillomavirus. *Papillomavirus* DNA has been amplified from the skin of pongids and other primates.

Retroviruses (5805). Primates can be sources of several retroviruses. **Baboon endogenous virus (BaEV) (150).** BaEV (a *Gammaretrovirus*) has been identified in Old World monkeys, including African greens (*C. aethiops*), baboon (e.g., *Papio cynocephalus*), gelada (*Theropithecus gelada*), and mangabey (e.g., *Cercocebus torquatus* and *C. aterrimus*). Contaminated cell lines are a theoretical hazard. **Simian T-lymphotropic virus (STLV).** STLV (a *Deltaretrovirus*) by species crossing is the likely ancestor of HTLV1 and HTLV2 in humans. **Simian immunodeficiency virus (SIV) (5806, 6608).** SIV (a *Lentivirus*), by species crossing, is likely the ancestor of HIV1 and HIV2 in humans. Surprisingly, HIV1 and HIV2 are phylogenetically further apart than HIV1 and SIV from chimpanzee (SIV_{cpz}), or HIV2 and SIV from *Macaca* (SIV_{mac}). At Cameroon markets in 1999–2001, of 573 primates sold for meat and 215 pet primates, 21% (165/788) were reactive to HIV antigen, including members of *Cercocebus*, *Cercopithecus*, *Colobus*, *Lophocebus*, *Mandrillus*, and *Papio*. Of 550 persons who worked with primates in the United States, 2 (0.4%) were seroreactive to SIV. Needlesticks and mucosal exposures were reported by 6–36% of workers. Accidental SIV infection has been reported in laboratory workers who handled monkey blood or tissues. **Simian retrovirus D (4350).** Simian retrovirus D is enzootic in Old World monkeys, including captive and wild *Macaca*. Inapparent infections have been reported in laboratory workers. **Simian foamy virus (SiFV) (150, 3253, 3743, 4958, 8243).** SiFV (a *Spumavirus*) is isolated in pongids, *Ateles* (spider), *Cebus* (capuchin), *C. aethiops* (African greens), *C. neglectus* (guenon), *Galago crassicaudatus*, *M. mulatta* (rhesus), *Mandrillus sphinx*, *Papio* (baboon), and *S. sciureus* (squirrel). Infections from captive and free-ranging monkeys have been reported in occupationally exposed persons, likely from droplets or contact. Infected macaques (*M. fascicularis*) at Sangeh temple in central Bali are a potential source not only for workers but also for monks, nuns, worshippers, and tourists.

Simian herpes viruses (SHV) (1510, 2209, 2516, 3681, 5408). Infected primates carry SHV for life, shedding SHV silently, from secretions or from herpetiform lesions. In Quebec, ~50% (264/519) of captured primates were seroreactive to SHV, despite being caged singly and having submitted to quarantine for 2–8 weeks.

Of concern is cercopithecine herpesvirus 1 (CeHV1) that is enzootic in *Macaca* in Asia and in laboratories, including rhesus (*M. mulatta*) and cynomolgus (*M. fascicularis*). In humans, CeHV1 can cause encephalomyelitis that is fatal in ~70%. In contrast, CeHV1 does not appear to cause latent infections in humans; none of 321 primate handlers, including many with repeated *Macaca* injuries, were seroreactive. Recommended PEP is to immediately wash the exposed site thoroughly with water and soap (or detergent). Sangeh forest in Bali, Indonesia, hosts a population of *M. fascicularis* that frequently scratch or bite visitors, with a risk of CeHV1 transmission to visitors or temple workers.

Simian virus 40 (SV40) (1002, 2213). *Macaca* in Asia are natural hosts, especially *M. mulatta*, but in captivity, related species are easily infected, including *M. fascicularis* or African greens (*C. aethiops*). Zoo workers are at risk of zoonotic SV40 infections.

Fungi
T. mentagrophytes is occasionally reported in primates.

Helminths
Enterobius vermiculars (5329) is reported in captive chimpanzees. Coprophagia, geophagia, and abundance of infective eggs in the environment are risks for caretakers at zoos and research facilities.

3.6 BATS
The mammalian order Chiroptera (bats) includes ~1,000 species in >15 families, notably vesper bats (Vespertilionidae, ~300 species) that occur worldwide and are mostly insectivorous, and hematophagous vampire bats (Phyllostomidae) that occur in the New World. Bats are active at night, resting in enclosed spaces during the day.

Chiropteran zoonoses. By geography and exposure, major agents acquired from bats are rabies virus and histoplasmosis.

CHIROPTERAN DROPLET-AIR CLUSTER

By excreta and secretions, visits to bat resting sites are a potential hazard.

Histoplasma capsulatum **(313, 1060, 2226, 7374).** Soil enriched with bat guano is a major substrate for this fungus. Unlike birds, *H. capsulatum* infects bats, mainly New World insectivorous (e.g., *Myotis californicus*: Vespertilionidae) and fructivorous (e.g., *Artibeus hirsutus*: Phyllostomidae) species.

In a sandstone cave in Nigeria, one *Nycteris hispida* (Nycteridae) grew *H. capsulatum* var. *duboisii* from intestinal contents.

By shedding *H. capsulatum* with guano, migratory bats can establish new foci in enclosed places. Bat-inhabited caves (see section 5.4), abandoned mines, remote buildings, and hollow trees are well-known sources of *H. capsulatum*. Aerosols stirred up by walking, working, or machines in enclosed places have caused outbreaks, including inside buildings. In Illinois, in 1980, big brown bats (*Eptesicus fuscus*) in the attic of a 100-year-old school building caused an outbreak of 20 histoplasmosis cases. In Cuba, six of eight German scientists contracted clinical histoplasmosis from investigating bats in caves, although all had worn respiration masks; the six who became ill had occasionally removed their masks while in the cave.

CHIROPTERAN FECES-FOOD CLUSTER

Although poorly documented, mammalian enteric agents such as *Salmonella* are expected from bat feces.

CHIROPTERAN ZOONOTIC CLUSTER
Viruses

Bat landings and unusual bat activity during the daytime should prompt rabies evaluation.

Lyssavirus **(902, 5988, 7963, 7966).** (For bites, see chapter 1). Virus species reported in bats are Duvenhage virus in *Nycteris thebaica* in Zimbabwe, Lagos bat virus in insectivorous bats in Africa, rabies virus in insectivorous and hematophagous bats in New World, Australian bat lyssavirus (ABLV) in (frugivorous) bats in Australia, and European bat lyssaviruses (EBLV1, EBLV2) in insectivorous bats in Europe, e.g., *Eptesicus serotinus* and *Myotis daubentonii*. Bats seem to maintain *Lyssavirus* largely independently from terrestrial mammals, but EBLV has been isolated in five sheep in Denmark (in 1998 and 2002) and a stone marten (*Martes foina*) in Germany (in 2001). **Rabies virus (2830, 4103, 5009, 5720, 6374).** Bats account for 3% of confirmed animal rabies cases worldwide. In the United States in 1996–2000, the mean number of bats confirmed rabid was 984/year, and the mean proportion among animal rabies cases was 13%. The respective numbers of cases (and proportions) were 1,281 (17%) in 2001, 1,373 (17%) in 2002, and 1,212 (17%) in 2003. Sampling influences the proportion of bats found rabid: the percentage is <1% in randomly sampled bats, 3–25% in submitted bats, and 30% in bats that have exposed people. In Colorado, of 210 biting bats, 58% were big browns (*E. fuscus*), 21% were *Myotis*, 13% (28) were silver-haired (*Lasionycteris noctivagans*), and 8% were other species. In Texas, submitted bats that most often test positive for rabies virus were hoaries (*L. cinereus*, 26%), free-tails (*Tadarida brasiliensis*, 16%), and northern yellows (*L. intermedius*, 9%). In Latin America, vampire bats can be vectors, mainly *Desmodus rotundus* that has a preference for mammals, rarely *Diaemus youngi* and *Diphylla ecaudata* that have a preference for birds. **ABLV (7965).** ABLV circulates in flying foxes (*Pteropus* spp). In Queensland in 2000–2001, 7% (8/119) of submitted bats tested positive for ABLV, including 12% (6/50) of *P. alecto*, 1 of 8 *P. poliocephalus*, and 1 of 5 *Pteropus* sp. **EBLV1 and EBLV2 (902, 5988).** EBLV1 and EBLV2 have emerged in regions that have eliminated terrestrial rabies through vaccination of foxes and dogs. In 1990–2002, Europe reported a total of 314 rabid bats (7–42 [mean 24]/year). EBLV is isolated in bats from northern, western, and eastern Europe, including the United Kingdom. Most cases (95%) are in serotine bats (*E. serotinus*, Vespertilionidae). In Scotland in 2003, the seroprevalence of EBLV2 in mainly *M. daubentonis* was estimated at 0.05–3.8%.

Bats can be sources of zoonotic viruses from at least six virus genera, by arthropods that are associated with bats, or by secretions.

Alphavirus **(1917, 3146).** In Senegal, West Africa, CHIKV was isolated from a vespertilionid bat (*Scotophilus* sp.). Around Cairns in Queensland, Australia, Ross River virus (RRV) was isolated from a pteropodid flying fox (*Pteropus conspicillatus*), which is a candidate reservoir host.

Filovirus. MARV (612, 5138) has occurred in bat-inhabited environments. In East Africa, >10 species of cave-dwelling bats are considered potential sources of MARV. Bats were a suspected source for gold miners who likely introduced the disease into Congo in 1998–2000.

Flavivirus. DENV (5939) genome was amplified from bats in Hainan, southern People's Republic of China, and neutralizing antibodies were detected in bats from Costa Rica (23% or 12/53) and Ecuador (30% or 3/10).

***Henipavirus* (3099, 3707)**. In Australia, Hendra virus was isolated from flying foxes (*Pteropus* spp.) that seem to be reservoir hosts. In Malaysia, neutralizing antibodies to Nipah virus were detected in wild-caught bats of several species: the fruit bats *Cynopterus brachyotis* (4%, 2/56) and *Eonycteris spelaea* (5%, 2/38), the flying foxes *Pteropus hypomelanus* (31%, 11/35) and *P. vampyrus* (17%, 5/29), and the insectivorous bat *Scotophilus kuhlii* (3%, 1/33).

Phlebovirus. In Guinea, West Africa, RVFV (734) was isolated from *Micropteropus pusillus* (Pteropodidae) and *Hipposideros abae* (Hipposideridae).

Rubulavirus. Menangle virus (4618) was isolated in Australia in pigs with reproductive failure from an intensive piggery and in 34% (42/125) of flying foxes from a roost near the piggery; infection was also diagnosed in two workers.

Protozoa
Natural infections with *T. cruzi* or *T. cruzi*-like agents have been reported in bats, including species of *Artibeus*, *Carollia*, *Choeroniscus*, *Desmodus*, *Glossophaga*, *Leptonycteris*, *Lonchophylla*, *Micronycteris*, *Molossus*, *Noctilio*, *Phyllostomus*, *Saccopterix*, and *Sturnira*.

CHIROPTERAN ENVIRONMENTAL CLUSTER
Environmental contamination by bats is a potential hazard.

***Leptospira* (981)**. Around Iquitos, Peru, in 1997–1998, 40% (14/35) of bats tested positive for *Leptospira* DNA by NAT, including species of *Artibeus*, *Carollia*, *Platyrhinus*, and *Sturnira*.

***T. pteropodis* (5175)**. On Palm Island, off Townsville in Queensland, Australia, a fruit bat (*Pteropus alecto*) was suspected to have contaminated mango fruits with eggs of *T. pteropodis* and to have caused an outbreak of hepatitis-like illness among Aborigines.

3.7 BIRDS
Class Aves (birds) has ~9,000 species in ~30 orders, notably Anseriformes (e.g., goose, *Anser anser*; duck, *Anas domesticus*), Charadriiformes (shorebirds), Galliformes (e.g., chicken, *Gallus gallus*; turkey, *Meleagris pallopavo*), Passeriformes (song birds, e.g., sparrow, *Passer domesticus*; canary, *Serinus canaries*), and Psittaciformes (e.g., budgerigar, *Melopsittacus undulatus*). Poultry is the term for domesticated birds that are raised for food, mainly chicken, turkey, goose, and duck, but also ostrich (*Struthio camelus*: Struthiformes).

Avian zoonoses (2403, 3457, 5694, 5825) (Box 3.4). (www.oie.int) Spread of agents from birds to humans occurs by contact (handling, clothes, and carcasses), inhalation (droplets, feather dust, and aerosolized feces), ingestion (hands, cage cleaning, and poultry meat), or inoculation (ectoparasites, associated mosquitoes, and slaughter).

Worldwide in 2000, there were >14 billion chickens (25% in People's Republic of China and 12% in United States), nearly 0.9 billion ducks (69% in People's Republic of China and 6% in Vietnam), and >0.2 billion geese (87% in People's Republic of China and 4% in Egypt). Pet bird trade focuses on canaries and psittaciformes. Some 4 million live birds are estimated to be traded annually. In the United Kingdom in 2001, there were ~2.1 million pet birds (~1/3 budgerigars, 3–4/100 population).

International institutions, governments, and industry aim to limit infections in commercial birds, including early detection of epizootics, elimination of infected herds, vaccination programs, and international surveillance and reporting. However, influenza A/H5N1 that is brewing in birds and humans reminds us of remaining threats. In the United Kingdom, peanuts fed to garden birds total 15,000 tons/year; feeding appears to contribute to the emergence of *Salmonella enterica* serovar Typhimurium DT40 in birds in Europe and of *Mycoplasma gallisepticum* in birds in North America. Migratory birds can carry agents and ectoparasites over continents.

AVIAN DROPLET-AIR CLUSTER
Birds shed agents from sneezed droplets, aerosolized feather dust (shaking, plucking), or liquid feces.

Viruses
Humans seem refractory to avian infectious bronchitis virus (AIBV) and gallid herpesvirus 1 that causes avian infectious laryngotracheitis.

Box 3.4 Agents from birds, by cluster

For trauma, see chapter 1; for work, see section 12.4; and for migrating birds, see section 16.1.

Droplet-air	Avian influenza viruses, NDV; mycobacteria; *Cryptococcus*, *Histoplasma*
Feces-food	*Campylobacter* (*C. jejuni*, *C. coli*, *C. lari*, and macrolide resistance), *Clostridium* (*C. perfringens* and *C. botulinum*), *Enterococcus* (including VRE), *Salmonella*, *Yersinia*; microsporidia; *Cryptosporidium melagridis*, *Toxoplasma*
Zoonotic	*Alphavirus* (EEEV, SINV, WEEV), *Flavivirus* (JEV, MVEV, SLEV, WNV), *Nairovirus* (CCHFV); *Borrelia burgdorferi* sl, *Chlamydophila psittaci*, *C. burnetii*, *E. rhusiopathiae*
Skin-blood	*Candida*; attached ticks and mites

***Influenzavirus* (2472, 4056, 4977, 5813, 7622, 7648, 8113, 8278).** The guts of wild aquatic birds are a natural reservoir for all subtypes of influenza A virus (H1-15 and N1-9). Over 80 bird species from 12 orders can yield A virus subtypes. In Germany in 1977–1989, influenza A virus was isolated from ~10% of birds (38% of 193 sentinel Peking ducks, 9% of 236 wild ducks, and 1% of 89 other wild birds). Frequent subtypes were A/H6N1 (24%) and A/H4N6 (11%). In poultry, some subtypes (e.g., A/H9N2) are enzootic, while others (A/H5N1, A/H7N7) are epizootic and highly virulent, causing die-offs. In Hong Kong in 1997, migratory birds were suspected to have introduced A/H5N1 to poultry farms. Attack rates were 20% in chickens, 3% in geese, and 2% in ducks; >1 million chickens were slaughtered to control the epizootic. Another A/H5N1 epizootic hit nine Asian countries in 2003–2005, resulting in death or slaughter of >100 million chickens. Time and geography suggested spread by transported chickens rather than migratory birds. In Asia, chickens are typically brought to market alive and in close contact with other birds and food animals, creating opportunities for species jumps. Another opportunity for virus mixing exists in Malaysia, where duck feces are scavenged by pigs.

Infected birds also shed virus fecally. Risks for humans are mainly from handling poultry, but poultry heated throughout to 70°C is safe for consumption.

Outbreaks Avian subtypes that have been documented in humans include:

- A/H5N1 in Hong Kong in 1997 (18 cases with 6 [33%] deaths), Hong Kong in 2003 (2 cases with 1 (50%) death), and in Eurasia (beginning in Cambodia, Thailand, and Vietnam) in 2004–2006 (>100 cases);
- A/H7N2 in New York in XI/2003 (one case of mild respiratory illness);
- A/H7N3 in Canada in 2004 (two cases of conjunctivitis);
- A/H7N7 in United Kingdom in 1995 (one case of conjunctivitis) and in The Netherlands in 2003 (85 cases of conjunctivitis, and one respiratory illness that was fatal);
- A/H9N2 in Hong Kong in 1999 (11 mild cases) and in 2003 (one case);
- A/H10N7 in Egypt in 2004 (two cases).

Secondary human-to-human spread, although unlikely, is a continuous threat, with a risk of pandemic spread. In Hong Kong in 1997, none of 399 controls were seroreactive to H5N1, while reactivity was 0.8% (3/365) in contacts of cases, 1.4% (1/71) in laboratory workers, and 2.5% (1/40) in persons exposed to poultry. Travelers should avoid visits to poultry farms and living animal markets and consumption of foods that include undercooked poultry. Workers should wear protective gear (gown, footwear, gloves, face mask, and goggles), wash hands, and receive vaccine. Neuraminidase inhibitors are available for PEP.

Newcastle disease virus (NDV) (3747, 5284). NDV can infect wild and domestic birds worldwide, including chickens and parrots. Birds shed NDV with respiratory secretions and feces. Epizootics and panzootics have occurred. In Denmark in 1996, an epizootic affected pheasants (*Phasianus colchicus*) that were free living on an island, for a lethality of 56%. NDV has occasionally spread to humans. Potential sources include feces, clothes, and soiled hands. In hen's eggs, NDV survives at ambient temperature for several months and at 4°C for 12 months.

Bacteria

Humans seem refractory to *M. gallisepticum*.

***Mycobacterium* (4770, 5970, 6097).** *M. avium* subsp. *avium* and *M. genavense* have been isolated from birds. In Germany, 130–230 cases of avian tuberculosis are reported annually, mainly in private flocks (with <20 birds) and zoos. *M. avium* subsp. *avium* is shed via feces; it has rarely been spread to humans. *M. genavense* has been isolated from psittaciform pets (*Amazona* and *Melopsittacus*) and passeriform pets (*S. canarius*), and from birds in zoos.

Fungi

Immune compromised persons are at increased risk and should avoid feather dust from pigeons and pet birds.

Aspergillus. *Aspergillus* has been recovered from birds, in particular, *A. fumigatus* from water fowl.

***Cryptococcus neoformans* (696, 1026, 4141, 6128).** Birds are the reservoir and shed the yeast with feces. *C. neoformans* is isolated from droppings and dust in the surroundings of birds (e.g., roosts). Epizootics have occurred in aviaries. Sources for humans are feather dust and aerosols rather than close contact. Infections have been reported in bird fanciers and in a person who helped to dismantle an aviary that had been unused for 10 years. Implicated source birds include chickens, pigeons, starlings (*Sturnus vulgaris*), zoo birds (e.g., caracara, *Polyborus plancus*; cockatoo, *Probosciger aterrimus*), and pet birds (e.g., budgerigar, *M. undulatus*).

***H. capsulatum* (1060, 5214).** Birds do not get ill but carry the agent, including on feathers and feet. Bird droppings are optimal for growth of the agent. *H. capsulatum* has been recovered from roosts and coops and from birds such as starlings and petrels (Procellariidae: Ciconiiformes).

Outbreaks have been associated with chickens, pigeons, black birds (Icteridae: Passeriformes), and sea gulls (Laridae: Lariformes). Soil samples from roost sites can remain contaminated for >10 years.

AVIAN FECES-FOOD CLUSTER

Bird intestines and feces grow a rich enteric flora. After evisceration, ~1–10% of poultry carcasses can be visibly fecally polluted.

Viruses

Humans seem refractory to duck hepatitis virus (DHV, *Enterovirus*) that circulates in birds. *Rotavirus* is recovered from chicken.

Bacteria

Campylobacter **(1011, 1880, 2527, 3297, 4489, 6182, 7795, 7910).** *Campylobacter* colonizes the intestinal tract of pet, zoo, and wild birds (e.g., seagulls) and poultry. Of 1,794 migrating birds trapped in southern Sweden, 5.6% grew *C. lari*, 5% grew *C. jejuni*, 0.9% grew *C. coli*, and 10.7% grew *Campylobacter* spp. The main concerns, however, are infections in poultry and transfer of macrolide resistance. By setting and sampling, 0–100% of flocks are infected. In the United States, *C. jejuni*, *C. coli*, *C. fetus*, *C. lari*, and *C. upsaliensis* were isolated from 30–40% of turkey processed at two plants. In Europe, ~20–80% of flocks are infected. In the United Kingdom in 1989–1994, *C. jejuni* was isolated from 27% (3,304/12,233) of random samples from 1.4 million broiler chickens. In The Netherlands, *Campylobacter* has been recovered from ~80% (153/187) of broiler flocks, with a peak of 100% in summer and a low of 50% in spring. All stages of production can become contaminated, including dressing in water baths. In a French "farm-to-fork" study, *Campylobacter* was detected by NAT in 66% (201/303) of the samples, including poultry houses (79%), chicken droppings (44%), carcasses at the slaughterhouse (6%), and supermarkets (18%).

Risks for humans include ownership of three or more caged birds, work in the poultry industry, consumption of undercooked chicken, and cross-contaminated foods. Poultry as a vehicle for human infections was underscored during a dioxin incident in Belgium in 1999 that prompted withdrawal of chicken and eggs from market; in the 4 weeks after withdrawal, the *Campylobacter* case rate in humans fell by 40% (from 153 to 94/week).

Clostridium **(1080, 7736).** In Europe, ducks and other waterfowl are regular victims of *C. botulinum* type C, which was isolated from carcasses at ponds and swamps. Poultry is a reservoir for *C. botulinum* type D, and hens, pheasants, and turkeys can contract type C or D botulism. Contaminated feeds are a likely source. *C. perfringens* seems to emerge in countries that have banned antibiotic growth promoters. *C. perfringens* can cause silent infections and necrotic enteritis in poultry.

Enterococcus **(772, 3282, 5950, 7712).** Commensals in poultry include *E. faecalis*, *E. faecium*, other *Enterococcus* spp., and vancomycin-resistant *Enterococcus* (VRE). In The Netherlands in 1997, VRE was isolated from 60% (21/35) of turkey flocks fed avoparcin, 8% (1/12) of flocks not on avoparcin, 39% (18/47) of turkey farmers, 20% of turkey slaughterers, and 14% of residents in the area, suggesting spread of VRE from turkeys to farmers. In Norway, after the European Union banned avoparcin in 1997, broiler flocks and houses continued to yield VRE, suggesting enzootic persistence. In Portugal in 2003, 9% (7/76) of poultry fecal samples tested positive for VRE gene A, underscoring enzooticity. In contrast, VRE is absent from the animal food chain in the United States to date. Instead, in 1996–2003, 85% (62/73) of *E. faecium* isolates from chicken farms and 52% (74/142) from turkey farms were resistant to quinupristin-dalfopristin, a compound analogous to virginiamycin that has been used in feeds for more than two decades.

***Enterobacter sakazakii*.** *E. sakazakii* has been recovered from chicken carcasses (3704).

E. coli **(119, 1334, 3704, 5349).** *E. coli* has been isolated from poultry and wild birds. Antibiotics in feeds can select for resistant *E. coli* in poultry and exposed workers. In Saudi Arabia, ampicillin-resistant *E. coli* was prevalent in 89% (102/115) of chicken at slaughter, 54% (63/117) of workers, and 71% (70/99) of hospitalized patients. In contrast, EHEC is rare in chicken or wild birds. In the United Kingdom, none of 1,000 chicken feces collected immediately after slaughter grew EHEC.

Salmonella **(3269, 3312, 3473, 5384, 6166, 6183, 8001, 8173).** *Samonella* is commonly isolated from poultry, pet birds, and wild birds. Risks include contact with birds or their droppings, pet chicks and ducklings, raw hen's eggs, undercooked poultry meat, contaminated commercial and home bird feeds, untreated (rain) water for drinking, and birds scavenging human waste.

Poultry flocks, feces, feeds, and water frequently grow *Salmonella*. Poultry flocks are an important reservoir of *Salmonella*. Typically 25–80% of flocks are infected. In Belgium in 1998–2000, 18 broiler flocks were monitored from hatchery to slaugtherhouse; 3,150 samples were taken. The proportion of infected flocks was 5% (1/18) at hatchery, 11% (2/18) after chick transport, 56% (10/18) after rearing in broiler houses, 75% (12/16) after transport to the abattoir, and 94% (17/18) after slaughter. Denmark in a decade has controlled *Salmonella* in broiler production.

In the 1970s, parrots (*Psittacus erithacus*) imported from Africa into the United Kingdom were found to harbor *S. enterica* serovar Typhimurium. Children who handle pet birds are at increased risk of salmonellosis, including chicks and ducklings. Playing and geophagia at places polluted by bird droppings are further hazards.

As a rule of thumb, the more remote the bird populations are the less frequently they will carry *Salmonella*. In Spain, 7% (21/264) of captive raptors and 4% (13/297) of free-ranging raptors grew *Salmonella* serovars Typhimurium, Enteritidis, and others. Infected wild raptors included Accipitriformes (*Accipiter*, *Buteo*, and *Gyps*), Falconiformes (*Falco*), and Strigiformes (*Asio*, *Athene*, and *Tyto*). In Czechia, 5% (40/756) synanthropic wild birds from 57 species grew *Salmonella*; 80% (32/40) of isolates were *Salmonella* serovar Typhimurium, and most (95% or 38/40) isolates were from gulls (*Larus ridibundus*). In contrast, on remote Öland island off the Swedish coast, only 1 of 2,377 migratory birds tested positive, a thrush (*Turdus viscivorus*) that grew *Salmonella* servovar Schleissheim. In Norway, 65% (94/145) of passeriformes found dead at feeding places grew *Salmonella* serovar Typhimurium, compared with 2% (40/1,990) of apparently healthy passeriformes caught at feeding places set up for bird ringing. There is evidence that synanthropic wild birds spread *Salmonella* in the environment. In Norway, fingerprinting suggested a link of *Salmonella* in gulls with fish-meal factories.

***Yersinia* (720).** Wild birds contribute to the animal reservoir of *Y. pseudotuberculosis*, together with rodents and lagomorphs. This agent can also infect farmed birds (chicken, ducks, pheasants, and doves) and pet birds (canaries). In contrast, *Y. enterocolitica* seems very rare in birds.

Fungi
Ostrich and parrots can harbor microsporidia such as *Encephalitozoon hellem*.

Protozoa
***Blastocystis* (14).** By microscopy, *B. hominis* has been identified in ducks and pheasants in zoos.

***Cryptosporidium* (5618).** *C. meleagridis* has been identified in turkeys and other birds, and occasionally in children and immune impaired persons.

***Sarcocystis* (4160).** *Sarcocystis* spp. have been isolated in tissues from birds, including chickens, ducks, egrets, and Passeriformes.

***T. gondii* (2519).** Birds are intermediate hosts, including chickens, game birds such as partridge (*Perdix perdix*) and pheasant (*P. colchicus*), and wild Passeriformes. Undercooked poultry meat is a hazard.

Helminths
***Capillaria philippensis*.** Fish-eating birds are a putative reservoir.

***Gnathostoma* (1920, 6380).** Many species of birds can be transporters or intermediate hosts of *G. spinigerum* and related species, including fish-eating birds such as herons, egrets, and pelicans.

***T. spiralis* (5994).** *T. spiralis* is isolated in Accipitriformes (e.g., eagle, *Aquila*), Strigiformes (e.g., owl, *Athene*), Ciconiiformes (e.g., black vulture, *Coragyps atratus*), and Passeriformes (e.g., rook, *Corvus frugilegus*).

AVIAN ZOONOTIC CLUSTER
Viruses
Zoonotic viruses (675, 7027). Mosquitoes can be pests to birds in marshlands; ground-feeding and migratory birds can be infested by ticks. In the delta of the Volga River, *Hyalomma marginatum* was isolated from 93% (431/461) of rooks (*C. frugilegus*, 69 ticks/bird), 81% (73/90) of crows (*C. corone*, 41 ticks/bird), 77% (85/111) of starlings (*S. vulgaris*, 5 ticks/bird), and 66% (21/32) of magpies (*Pica pica*, 28 ticks/bird). In Sweden, 2% (73/3,054) of migrating birds carried *I. ricinus*, for a density of about two ticks per infected bird. Birds are significant reservoirs for arboviruses, mainly from genera *Alphavirus* (Eastern equine encephalitis virus [EEEV], SINV, Western equine encephalitis virus [WEEV]), *Flavivirus* (JEV, Murray Valley encephalitis virus [MVEV], Saint Louis encephalitis virus [SLEV], WNV), and *Nairovirus* (CCHFV). **CCHFV (1042, 6842).** Ticks carry CCHFV in the Old World. Birds can be naturally infected and are suspected of contributing to virus reservoir. In South Africa in November 1984 after a worker contracted CCCHF when slaughtering ostriches (*S. camelus*), farmed ostriches were screened and 24% (22/92) were seroreactive. **EEEV (1035, 1626, 4040).** Mosquitoes carry EEEV in North America. Birds maintain EEEV enzootically, mainly Passeriformes. Of resident birds surveyed in marshlands, ~1% are seroreactive. In Florida in 1965–1974, 1.3% (70/5,295) of birds were seroreactive, including the blue jay (*Cyanocitta cristata*), mockingbird (*Mimus polyglottos*), and cardinal (*Richmondena cardinalis*). The Native American robin (*Turdus migratorius*) and introduced European starling (*S. vulgaris*) are experimentally competent reservoir hosts. EEEV can cause epizootics and die-offs in nonreservoir birds, e.g., pen-raised pheasants (*P. colchicus*) and partridges (*Alectoris graeca*). **JEV (3635, 5773).** Mosquitoes

carry JEV in Asia. Domestic and migrating birds are reservoir and amplifying hosts. Chickens are used for sentinel surveillance. In People's Republic of China, 1% of hens have been reported seroreactive. In India, reported seroprevalence in birds ranges from 0.002 to 35%. Ciconiiformes, mainly cattle egret (*Bubulcus ibis*) and pond heron (*Ardeola grayii*) are likely reservoir hosts. Migratory viremic birds were the source implicated in an outbreak on Saipan Island in 1990. **MVEV (7065).** Mosquitoes carry MVEV in Australia. Wading birds are reservoirs, including herons (*Ardea novaehollandiae* and *Nycticorax caledonicus*) and domestic birds. **SLEV (2971, 6206, 6805).** Mosquitoes carry SLEV in the New World. Birds, including sparrows, finches, jays, robins, pigeons, and doves, are reservoirs and amplifying hosts. Chickens are used for sentinel surveillance. In 1987–1996, among 52,589 peridomestic birds tested, 1% of finches (*Carpodacus mexicanus*), 1% of sparrows, and ~4% of doves (*Columbia livia*) were seroreactive. In Arkansas, after an outbreak of 25 human cases, 43% of 54 American robins (*Turdus migratorius*) and 42% of 129 house sparrows were seroreactive. At wetland sites in California in 1996–1998, 0.1% (27/20,192) of wild birds from 149 species were seroreactive. In southern Florida, ingredients for annual epizootics were droughts that drove mosquitoes and birds to densely vegetated "hammock" habitats, amplification of SLEV in birds, and abundant rains in the summer and early fall. **SINV (946).** Mosquitoes carry SINV in the Old World, mainly to marsh-nesting and shore birds. In Finland, seroreactive birds included Anseriformes (teal, *Anas crecca*; goldeneye, *Bucephala clangula*) and Galliformes (grouse, *Tetrao tetrix*; capercaillie, *T. urogallus*). **TBEV (3775).** Ticks carry TBEV in the Old World. By breeding and feeding pattern, seroprevalences reported for wild Passeriformes in central Europe were 1–7%. Because attempts to isolate the virus have failed, seroreactions are likely confounded by cross-reactivity (e.g., WNV). **WEEV (2971, 3206, 6206).** Mosquitoes carry WEEV in the New World. Some nesting birds are likely reservoirs, including house sparrows (*P. domesticus*), in North America also house finches (*C. mexicanus*). Others develop sufficient viremia to infect feeding mosquitoes. By age and enzooticity, 0–15% of birds can be seroreactive. In 1987–1996, seroprevalence was negligible in 52,589 birds, except rock doves (*C. livia*) of which 0.4% (219/5,481) were reactive. In 1996–1998, 0.7% (143/20,192) of wild birds in California wetland sites were seroreactive, including the house finch, house sparrow, quails, and doves. Reactive birds typically roosted or nested in upland vegetation where *Culex tarsalis* females hunted most frequently. Unlike in sentinel chickens, seroprevalence in wild birds did not herald pending epizootics, because spring findings reflected infections acquired during the previous season. **WNV (684, 2112, 3635, 3774, 4041, 4089, 4693, 4922, 8386).** Mosquitoes carry WNV in the Old and New Worlds. Natural and experimental infections suggest reservoir competence for synanthropic Passeriformes, e.g., sparrow, crow, and blue jay (*C. cristata*), Columbiformes, e.g., doves, and Galliformes, e.g., quails. In the Old World, house sparrows seem to maintain an urban cycle. By enzooticity, domestic fowl are silently infected or overtly ill. In Romania in 1996, 37% (19/52) of chickens, 38% (5/13) of ducks, and four of six turkeys had neutralizing antibodies. In Israel in 1997–1999, an epizootic affected hundreds of farmed geese. In India, 21% (178/859) of wild birds were reactive to WNV. Migratory birds are strongly suspected to periodically introduce WNV from core areas in tropical Africa to fringe areas in Southwest Asia and southern Europe.

In 1999, WNV reached North America, causing crows and other birds to "drop dead from the sky." In New York in 1999, wild-caught and frequently (>10%) seroreactive birds included the house sparrow, Canada goose (*Branta canadensis*), and rock dove (*C. livia*). In 2000, surveillance identified 1,203 WNV-positive dead birds representing 63 species in 30 bird families. High avian lethality suggested enhanced virulence, or "virgin territory" infection. By 2001, antibodies were detected in 23 species from 12 orders, including the sparrow, crow, starling (*S. vulgaris*), rock dove, wild turkey (*Meleagris gallopavo*), and domestic goose, but crows, blue jays, and other species continued to suffer from high lethality. Related to WNV is Kunjin virus that circulates in Australia, with wading birds as a putative reservoir.

Bacteria

***B. burgdorferi* sl (2709, 3037, 5593, 6259).** Ticks carry the agent in the Old and New Worlds. Birds are presumptive reservoir hosts, in North America robin (*T. migratorius*) and thrush (*Turdus iliacus*), in Europe blackbird (*Turdus merula*), pheasant (*P. colchicus*), and razorbill (*Alca torda*). Seabirds can carry *B. garinii* and *I. uriae* ticks to and from islands, in the Northern Hemisphere, e.g., Iceland, Faroe, and the Aleutian Islands, and in the Southern Hemisphere, e.g., Crozet Island off Antarctica. Birds in Europe also host *B. valaisiana*.

***Chlamydophila psittaci* (1166, 3792, 4892, 5594).** Birds shed *C. psittaci* in secretions, excreta, and feather dust. Shipping, crowding, and other forms of stress increase shedding and susceptibility.

C. psittaci colonizes or infects >450 species of birds, mainly Psittaciformes (45% or 153/307 species, serovars A and F), e.g., amazons, budgerigars, cockatoos, lovebirds, parrots; Lariformes (28% or 26/92 species), e.g., gulls; Anseriformes (21% or 33/157 species, serovars C and D), e.g., duck, goose; less consistently Columbiformes (6% or 17/307 species, serovar B), e.g., pigeon and dove; Galliformes (5% or 14/259 species, serovars C and D), e.g., hen, turkey, quail; and Passeriformes (2% or 90/~4,000 species), e.g., finch, sparrow.

By test and species, *C. psittaci* is isolated in 0–57% (typically 3–10%) of submitted birds or bird feces. Pet psittaciformes and poultry are the most frequent sources of ornithosis in humans. In the United States in 1988–1998, of 813 human cases with a known source, ~70% resulted from exposure to infected pet birds. However, urban pigeons seem to be an underrecognized source. Pigeon fanciers, pet bird owners, poultry farm workers, and abattoir workers are at risk. Settings for outbreaks include aviaries and pet shops. In contrast in Sweden, none of 65 ringers of wild birds was seroreactive.

***C. burnetii* (6188, 6435, 7140).** Wild and domestic birds seem to participate in a "sylvatic" cycle that includes inhalation, ingestion, and tick bites. Infections are reported in chickens, ducks, geese, turkeys, pigeons, and other birds. In Provence, France, in 1996, a farm family of 5 contracted Q fever from exposure to pigeon feces and ticks. In Bratislava, Slovakia, ~10% of urban pigeons were seroreactive; their infections were likely from a farm ~30 km outside the city where cattle were *C. burnetii*-infected and rats infested the corn silage.

***Erysipelothrix rhusiopathiae* (1397, 3393, 5285).** *E. rhusiopathiae* is recovered from poultry and captive wild birds, and epizootics are reported in flocks. The red mite (*Dermanyssus gallinae*) is a suspected vector of *E. rhusiopathiae* in poultry. Two attendants who handled dead birds during an outbreak developed lesions typical of erysipeloid.

***P. multocida* (6575).** *P. multocida* can colonize the upper respiratory tract of birds and cause avian bloodstream infections and "fowl cholera." By test (culture and serology) and season, <0.1–8% of birds may test positive. However, in general, *P. multocida* in birds seems to circulate separately from humans.

Protozoa
***Babesia*.** Ticks carry *Babesia* spp. to birds. Over 10 species of *Babesia* from birds have been reported. Avian *Babesia* has not been documented in humans.

***Plasmodium*.** Mosquitoes carry *Plasmodium* spp. to birds. Numerous species of *Plasmodium* have been reported in >50 species of birds, in particular, from orders Passeriformes (e.g., *P. cathemerium* and *P. relictum* in house sparrows) and Galliformes (e.g., *P. gallinaceum* in chickens and *P. lophurae* in pheasants). Avian *Plasmodium* has not been documented in humans.

AVIAN SKIN-BLOOD CLUSTER
Viruses
Avian leukosis virus (ALV) (7586). Chicken cells have tested positive for an endogenous subgroup (E) of ALV. However, ALV from avian cells seems noninfectious, and recipients of contaminated cell lines have tested negative for proviral sequences in peripheral blood cells.

***Avipoxvirus*.** Poultry, pet, and wild birds can be infected with canarypox virus (CNPV), fowlpox virus (FWPV), and quailpox virus (QUPV). However, humans seem refractory to *Avipoxvirus*.

Marek's disease virus (MDV) (4247). MDV circulates in chickens worldwide. MDV seems able to jump species. However, equal proportions of persons tested positive for MDV by NAT whether exposed to chicken (19%, 26/137) or not (23%, 15/65).

Fungi (4700)
Columbiformes, Psittaciformes, and other birds can harbor opportunistic yeasts. In Turin, Italy, pigeon (*C. livia*) droppings obtained from densely populated areas grew *Candida*, including *C. albicans*, *C. krusei*, *C. parapsilosis*, and *C. tropicalis*. In central Italy, 49% (160/325) of fresh droppings from parrots (mainly *Amazona* and *Ara*), parakeets (mainly *Pionites* and *Psittacula*), budgerigars, and other pet birds grew yeasts, including *C. albicans*, *C. krusei*, and *C. parapsilosis*. Note that *C. neoformans* was not isolated.

Ectoparasites (6743, 6966, 7020, 7974)
Passeriformes and other birds can harbor larvae, nymphs, and adults of *Amblyomma*, *Haemaphysalis*, *Ixodes*, and other hard ticks, as well as *Argas* and *Ornithodorus* soft ticks. Domestic birds (Galliformes), pet and zoo birds (Psittaciformes), wild birds, and bird surroundings can host mites. *Dermanyssus gallinae* feeds on poultry only at night while *Ornithonyssus* species remain on birds. Humans can be bitten when handling birds. An allergenic, bird-related mite is *Acarus immobilis*.

3.8 REPTILES AND AMPHIBIANS
The vertebrate class Reptilia has 6,000 species (crocodiles, iguanas, lizards, skinks, snakes, tortoises, and turtles), and the class Amphibia has 2,800 species (frogs, salamanders, and toads).

Reptilian and amphibian zoonoses (996, 1219). Reptiles can shed agents infective to humans and disperse attached ectoparasites. Spread to humans is mainly via contact (handling and excreta) or inoculation (microtrauma). At least 0.6 million live reptiles are traded annually worldwide. Some 1.7 million United States households keep reptiles. Pet reptiles in the United Kingdom are estimated at 5 million (8/100 population).

Bacteria
Bacteria isolated from amphibians and reptiles include *Aeromonas*, *Campylobacter*, and *Salmonella*.

Salmonella (1219, 3625, 4995, 5112, 7082, 8037).
Snakes, land and pond turtles, lizards, iguanas, and ornamental frogs and toads are significant sources of *Salmonella* in humans, including from the intestine, body surface, or eggs.

Reported *Salmonella* prevalence is 10–85% in turtles, 15–90% in snakes, and 15–75% in lizards. Of 28 lots of eggs from red-eared turtle (*Pseudemys scripta-elegans*) imported into Canada from Louisiana in 1988, 6 (21%) grew *Salmonella*. Use of gentamicin on turtle farms to produce *Salmonella*-free eggs for export is a potential source of resistant *Salmonella* in humans.

By age and geography, 3–14% of human salmonellosis in high-income countries follows exposure to reptiles or amphibians. Mainly children and household members are affected. Agents include ubiquitous *Salmonella* serovars Enteritidis and Typhimurium, as well as unusual, reptile-related serovars such as Chameleon, Javiana, Poona, and Stanley. Risks for humans include touching or owning reptiles or amphibians and not washing hands after handling or feeding animals or cleaning out terraria or aquaria. An unusual infection chain went from an *Salmonella* serovar Enteritidis-infected pet boa, to a subclinically bacteremic owner who donated blood and a recipient of platelets who developed sepsis. In Canada in 1996, turtle tank water caused an outbreak of *Salmonella* serovar Paratyphi B.

3.9 FISH
The class Pisces has >26,000 species, including Cyclostomata (scaleless, e.g., lamprey), Chondrichthyes (cartilaginous, e.g., sharks), and Osteichthyes (bony) with >30 orders, including Clupeiformes (e.g., herring), Cypriniformes (e.g., carp), Perciformes (e.g., perch), and Salmoniformes (e.g., trout).

Zoonoses from fish (2670, 3227, 3457). Spread to humans is mainly via contact (handling and polluted water), inoculation (microtrauma), or ingestion. In 2000, world commercial (marine and freshwater) fishery production was 95 billion kg by capture (92 billion kg in 1995, up 3%), and 35 billion kg by aquaculture (25 billion kg in 1995, up 45%) (www.fao.org). For fish as food, see section 7.5; for occupational fish contact, see section 12.4. Trade in living fish (eggs, larvae, and adults), and fish products can disperse agents (see chapter 16). Some 350 million live tropical fish are estimated to be traded worldwide each year. About 12 million aquarium owners are estimated in the United States (4/100 population) and 1 million in Canada (3/100). The pet fish population in the United Kingdom is estimated at 25 million.

Fish Viruses
Viruses (5273) identified in farmed or ornamental fish include infectious pancreatic necrosis virus (IPNV, *Aquabirnavirus*: Birnaviridae) and iridovirus (an iridescent insect virus). These have not been isolated in humans.

Fish Bacteria
Bacteria of interest in aquaculture include *Flavobacterium psychrophilum* and *Piscirickettsia salmonis*. Human-infective bacteria isolated from fish include *Aeromonas hydrophila*, *E. coli*, *Listeria monocytogenes*, *Mycobacterium marinum*, *Plesiomonas shigelloides*, *Salmonella*, *Streptococcus iniae*, and *Vibrio*. Hazards are trauma (see chapter 1), consumption of undercooked fish (see section 7.5), and soiled hands. Ice containing chlorine dioxide (ClO_2) seems able to control surface contaminants of fresh fish (6864).

Plesiomonas shigelloides (252).
In Japan, *P. shigelloides* has been isolated from 10% (25/246) of freshwater fish.

Salmonella (2670, 2982).
Main sources are handled fish and polluted aquarium waters. In Canada in 2000, aquarium water and fish caused seven *Salmonella* serovar Paratyphi B infections; aquarium water (and fish food secondarily contaminated) grew the agent. In Scandinavia in 2001, *Salmonella* serovar Livingstone in processed fish caused 60 cases and 3 (5%) deaths.

Vibrio (1470).
V. cholerae has been isolated from fish; *V. parahaemolyticus* has been isolated from fresh, cured, and dried fish. In Japan in 1950, sardines were the vehicle for an outbreak with 272 cases and 20 (7%) deaths.

Fish Parasites
Fish are (intermediate) hosts for many parasites, including protozoa (*Cryptosporidium* and *Eimeria*), nematodes, trematodes, and cestodes. The focus is on parasites infective to humans (for seafood, see section 7.5).

Nematodes
Anisakis and ***Pseudoterranova*** (336, 1606, 1806, 4178, 4877). Over 100 species of marine fish from 10 orders are secondary intermediate hosts for *A. simplex* and *P. decipiens*, including Clupeiformes (herring), Gadiformes (cod), and Perciformes (mackerel). Larvae of *A. simplex* prefer visceral locations but are able to invade muscle, even in dead fish. Gutting at sea may prevent flesh

invasion. At processing plants, fillets and napes of groundfish are screened for parasites on light tables ("candling"), but this method is inefficient unless fillets are cut into flat slices (which is economically unattractive). Freezing ($-20°C$ for ≥ 7 days) kills anisakid larvae.

Fish implicated epidemiologically or parasitologically in infections in humans include:

- North America. Atlantic cod (*Gadus morhua*), coho salmon (*Oncorhynchus kisutch*), and chum salmon (*O. keta*).
- Newfoundland, Canada. In 1984–1985, the larval prevalence in cod was 9–51%, and the larval density was 0.2–9/kg of fillet. Of wild-caught coho or chum, up to 100% can harbor larvae.
- Latin America. Barracuda (*Sphyraena barracuda*) and grouper (*Epinephelus morio*). In Yucatan, Mexico, the larval prevalence is 33–83%, and larval density is 7–10/fish.
- Asia. Bonito, Pacific cod (*Gadus morhua macrocephala*), halibut (*Hippoglossus stenolepis*), mackerels (*Scomber scombrus* and *S. japonicus*), Japanese anchovy (*Engraulis japonica*). Larval prevalence in fish from markets in Jakarta and Tokyo is 13% to close to 100%.
- Europe. Atlantic salmon (*Salmo salar*), anchovy (*Engraulis encrasicolus*), Atlantic cod (*Gadus morhua*), herring (*Clupea harengus*), sardines (*Sardina pilchardus*), mackerel (*S. scombrus*), and hake (*Merlucius merlucius*). Larval prevalence is 15% to close to 100%.

Gnathostoma (105, 1287, 1920, 3579, 6380, 6540). Freshwater fish from numerous species, as well as water snakes and frog-eating snakes can harbor larvae.

- Southeast Asia. In Thailand, swamp eel (*Monopterus albus*, Anguilliformes) seems to be the main host for *G. spinigerum*. Larvae can be recovered from all parts of the body. By provenance (wild-caught or farmed), the prevalence of infective larvae (L3) in eels from Southeast Asia is ~9–69%. In Thailand, in the rainy season of 1999, 12% (97/785) of livers of swamp eels from large Bangkok markets yielded *G. spinigerum* L3, for densities of 1–17 (mean, 3)/liver.
- East Asia. In Japan, reported hosts include brook trout (*Oncorhynchus masou masou*) for *G. doloresi*, largemouth bass (*Micropterus salmoides*) for *G. nipponicum*, and kokanee (*Salmo nerka*), carp (*Cyprinus carpio*), and loach (*Misgurnus anguillicaudatus*) for *G. hispidum* or *G. nipponicum*.
- Latin America. In South America, larvae are identified in freshwater fish of several species that can be eaten raw. In Mexico, a main host for *Gnathostoma* (*G. spinigerum* and *G. doloresi*) is perch ("alahuate" *Eleotris pictus*, a sleeper of Perciformes), for a larval prevalence of 32%, and a larval density of ~0–3 (mean, 1)/fish.

Trematodes

Clonorchis **(1818, 3779, 4570).** *Clonorchis* is reported in >130 species of fish from >40 genera. Examples are cypriniformes such as common carp (*Cyprinus*), crucian carp (*Carassius*), and bighead carp (*Hypophthalmichthys*), and the perciform *Tilapia mossambica*. Infection prevalence can reach 40%, and numbers of metacercariae can range from 50 to 1,600/fish.

Heterophyes **(1289, 1818).** Hosts include brackish water fish of Perciformes such as grey mullet (*Mugil cephalus*) and sea bass (*Lateolabrax japonicus*).

Opistorchis **(1818, 3779, 8347).** Cypriniformes (carps and barbs) are the main intermediate hosts. For *O. viverrini*, examples are carp (*Cyclocheilichthys*) and barb (*Puntius*). For *O. felineus*, examples are crucian carp (*Carassius*) and grass carp (*Tinca*). Metacercariae are found in various parts of the fish body, mainly the muscles. Reported infection prevalence in enzootic areas is 13–97%.

Cestodes

Diphyllobothrium **(218, 1923, 2549, 2832, 6141, 6570, 7408).** At least 30 species of freshwater and marine fish are reported to host plerocercoid *Diphyllobothrium* larvae. *D. pacificum* infects marine fish, *D. latum* infects fish that spent at least part of life in freshwater. However, the distinction of freshwater and marine cycles is not absolute. Salmon caught at sea can carry *Diphyllobothrium* from freshwater lakes and rivers. Burbots, that live in freshwater can aquire marine parasites by feeding on marine fish in brackish waters.

Larval prevalences in trouts from Lake Morena, southern Argentina were 28% (*D. latum*) to 58% (*D. dendriticum*), and larval densities were one to seven per fish. In marine fish from the Peruvian coast, larval prevalences were 5–14%.

Location of larvae in fish influences infection risks. However, larvae of all tapeworms can excyst, move, and contaminate fish flesh after capture. Larvae are inactivated by heat (56°C throughout for 5 min), freezing ($-18°C$ for 24 h, or $-10°C$ for 72 h), salting (10–20% brine for 1 h), smoking, and canning. Refrigerated (5°C) or chilled (0.5°C) fish remain infective for ≥ 6 days.

Fish hosts implicated parasitologically or epidemiologically are briefly reviewed by location.

- North America. Hosts include the following: *D. alascense*, burbots (*Lota lota*, Gadiformes); *D. ursi*, chinook salmon (*Oncorhynchus tshawytscha*), sockeye salmon (*O. nerka*), rainbow trout (*O. mykiss*), and dolly varden

(*Salvelinus malma*, all Salmoniformes); *D. dendriticum*, *O. mykiss*, *O. nerka*, Arctic char (*S. alpinus*), lake trout (*S. namaycush*), and *S. malma*; and *D. latum* (likely brought to North America by immigrants), pike (*Esox lucius*, Esociformes), yellow perch (*Perca flavescens*), sauger (*Sander canadensis*, both Perciformes), and walleye (*Theragra chalcogramma*, Gadiformes).

- South America. Hosts include the following: *D. dendriticum*, *O. mykiss* and brook trout (*S. fontinalis*); *D. latum*, *O. mykiss*, *S. fontinalis*, and perca (*Percichthys*, Perciformes); and *D. pacificum*, marine fish that can be part of cebiche, such as: "lorna" (*Sciaena deliciosa*), "bagre marino" (*Galeichthys jordani*), "pampanito" (*Trachinotus paitensis*), "lenguado" (*Paralichthys adspersus*), and "cojinoba" (*Seriolella violacea*).
- Asia. A host for *D. latum* and *D. nihonkaiense* is cherry salmon (*O. masou*). *D. latum*-infected salmon may have been caught in the Ochotskian sea, off the coast of far eastern Russia.
- West Europe. Only *D. latum* seems present. Hosts include *E. lucius*, perch (*Perca fluviatilis*, Perciformes), and *S. alpinus*.

4

Invertebrates

4.1 Hard ticks and vector mites
4.2 Diurnal fleas and flies
4.3 Mainly diurnal mosquitoes
4.4 Mainly nocturnal mosquitoes
4.5 Nocturnal bugs and soft ticks
4.6 Ectoparasites (lice, fly larvae, and scabies mites)

It is well to be up before daybreak, for such habits contribute to health, wealth, and wisdom.

Aristotle of Stagira (384–322 BC)

For invertebrates at domiciles, see sections 11.1 and 11.2; for exposure at work, see sections 12.1 and 12.4; for seasonality, see section 5.6.

Invertebrates comprise >2 million species, mainly molluscs, helminths, and arthropods (with insects, spiders, and crustaceans). Some arthropods are efficient vectors of diseases (3425, 5679, 6449) (Table 4.1). In cyclic vectors, agents invade or develop internally (intrinsic incubation) before being infective through saliva, feces, or coaxial fluid. In mechanical vectors, agents are transported on the outside and immediately infective if viable. Arguments for an arthropod being a vector to humans include regular feeding on reservoir hosts and humans (bridging), consistent yield of infective stages, and experimental transmission competence; additionally, infections in humans are correlated with its abundance and territory. Infected vector biomass contributes to the infection reservoir. Maintenance may include transstadial and transovarial agent passage.

One way to group vectors is by morphology of adults (Table 4.1). Mosquitoes and flies (Arthropoda; Insecta; order Diptera) have one pair of wings. Mosquitoes (suborder Nematocera) are slender and bear long, multisegmented antennae. They include families Culicidae, Psychodidae, and Simuliidae. Flies (suborder Brachycera) are stocky and bear short antennae with few segments. Flies carry *Trypanosoma brucei* and *Loa loa* cyclically, and enterobacteria, fungal spores, protozoal cysts, and helminth eggs mechanically. Other important insect orders include fleas (Siphonaptera, which carry *Rickettsia typhi* and *Yersinia pestis*), lice (Anoplura, which carry *R. prowazekii*, *Borrelia recurrentis*, and *Bartonella quintana*), bugs (Hemiptera, which carry *Trypanosoma cruzi*), bedbugs (also Hemiptera, a nuisance), and cockroaches (Dictyoptera, putative mechanical vectors). Ticks and mites (Arthropoda: Acari) are spiderlike. Unlike insects, adults have four leg pairs.

Another way to group vectors is by activity (Table 4.2). Hard ticks, vector mites, fleas, vector flies (*Glossina* and *Chrysops*), and some mosquitoes (*Aedes*, *Culicoides*, and *Simulium*) mainly seek hosts during the day, while other mosquitoes (*Anopheles*, *Culex*, *Lutzomyia*, and *Phlebotomus*), bugs, and bedbugs

Table 4.1 Arthropod disease vectors: distinguishing features of adults

Vector	Order (family)	Leg pairs	Wing pairs	Size (mm)	Body and behavior
Mosquito	Diptera (Culicidae)	3	1	2–12	Slender, fly, antennae multisegmented
Fly	Diptera (e.g., Simuliidae, Tabanidae)	3	1	1–30	Squat, fly, antennae 3–segmented
Bug	Hemiptera (Reduviidae)	3	2	≤40	Oval, snout-like head, prominent eyes
Bedbug	Hemiptera (Cimicidae)	3	0	4–7	Oval, walk, yellow-brown
Lice	Anoplura	3	0	2–5	Dorsoventrally flat, crawl, legs clawed
Flea	Siphonaptera	3	0	1–9	Laterally flat, jump, powerful legs
Tick	Parasitiformes	4	0	≤25	Oval, walk, pincer mouth (chelicerae)
Mite	Acariformes	4	0	0.2–2	Tiny, run, pincer mouth (chelicerae)

seek hosts at night. For most diurnal and nocturnal vectors, contact time is minutes to hours; contact lasts days or indefinitely with lice and ectoparasites. Fleas are recognized as "bugs that jump" at humans during the day, from animals, their pens, or rags. Diurnal, straight, solitary, "bomberlike" attacks suggest flies (*Glossina* and *Chrysops*), and diurnal swarms suggest midges (*Culicoides*). Nocturnal "buzz" is typical for *Anopheles* and *Culex*, while *Phlebotomus*, triatomines, and bedbugs attack silently, being noticed only the following day from marks. Because vectors are often not available for morphological identification, classification by host seeking is preferred here.

Clinical evaluation (2437, 7209). The exposure history should address diurnal and nocturnal bites and removals of ticks or ectoparasites, including from domestic animals (Box 4.1). Pictures of vectors are likely to enhance recall of recent exposures (see Fig. 4.1 to 4.4).

Examine the head, armpits, wrists, pubic region, legs, and feet for ticks, lice, mites, and skin lesions. Examine clothes for body lice. Scratches and papules at exposed parts of the body suggest mosquito bites, grouped lesions at the neck suggest lice bites, grouped or linear weals at sites in contact with mattresses or chairs (household urticaria) suggest bedbugs, nocturnal itch at the wrists and genitals suggest scabies mites, small ulcers (eschars) suggest tick bites, boils suggest *Glossina* bites or myiasis, and a painful subungual swelling suggests *Tunga*. Attached and recovered vectors can be useful for laboratory investigation.

Control and prevention (1358, 3207, 3855, 4446, 5871). Control measures include community participation for key habitat elimination (resting and peridomestic breeding sites), water management (intermittent irrigation), and chemical (insecticides against larvae and adults), physical (fly traps), and biological (larvivorous predators and sterile males) measures, and good housing (durable construction materials, screened openings, and keeping out mammals and garbage). Regularly used and impregnated bednets reduce all-cause mortality in preschool children. Cleaned surfaces, rubbish removal, and sanitation reduce filth flies, diarrhea in infants, and trachoma. Long clothes and repellents prevent bites outdoors. After excursions, clothes and body should be screened for ticks.

4.1 HARD TICKS AND VECTOR MITES

Hard ticks and vector mites are mainly active during the day. Developmental stages are eggs, larvae (three leg pairs), nymphs, and adults (four leg pairs). In "three-host" ticks, larvae, nymphs, and adults each seek a different host species. Climate and land use modulate abundance.

HARD (IXODID) TICKS

Hard ticks (Acari; order Parasitiformes; family Ixodidae; >680 species) (675, 2787, 3425, 4991, 5371, 5739) feature a hard body shield and protruding biting parts (false heads). Ixodid ticks congregate in foci. The main means of dispersal is by attachment to hosts (for mammals and birds, see section 16.8). Number and proximity of foci, species abundance and aggressiveness, the infective proportion, and avoidance behavior influence risks for humans. In central Spain, of 185 ticks removed from 179 persons visiting health care centers, 56% were identified

Table 4.2 Host seeking and feeding behavior of main arthropod disease vectors

Contact time	Diurnal and free roaming	Nocturnal and free roaming	Residual and ectoparasitic
Minutes	*Aedes, Culicoides, Simulium, Chrysops, Glossina, Tabanus*	*Anopheles, Culex, Mansonia, Lutzomyia, Phlebotomus*	
Hours	Hard ticks, vector mites, fleas	Soft ticks, bugs, bed bug	
Days			Fly larvae (myiasis), lice, *Tunga*, scabies mites

> **Box 4.1** Suggested vector exposure history and evaluation
>
> **In the past month:**
> - Have you participated in any nighttime outdoor activity such as strolling in shorts or dining on the porch?
> - Have you had any accommodation in a remote cabin or a non-mosquito-proofed shelter, under a mosquito net, or in the open?
>
> **In the past week:**
> - Have you had any bites by a fly, a bug, a tick, or another "insect," singly or in swarms, during the day or at night?
> - Did you notice any beetlelike "bugs" running over the bed or furniture or hear any mosquito-like buzzing?
> - Have you removed any ticks, "bugs," or other "insects" from furniture, body, clothes, or animals?
>
> **Right now:**
> - Are you aware of any itchy skin lesions?
>
> **Check** status of current vaccinations (JEV, TBEV, and YFV), malaria chemoprophylaxis, mosquito exposure prophylaxis. Note the season your patient is in (monsoon or summer).

as *Dermacentor marginatus*, 12% as *Ixodes ricinus*, 12% as *Rhipicephalus bursa*, and 20% as six other species. Ticks are generally infective through saliva and infrequently through feces (e.g., *Coxiella*). Antibodies to tick saliva are a surrogate measure of exposure. Humans are largely incidental hosts.

Amblyomma (>100 species) (996, 1872, 2251, 3256, 3683, 5184, 5363, 5808, 6455). *Amblyomma* can carry viruses (Crimean-Congo hemorrhagic fever virus [CCHFV]) and *Borrelia*, *Coxiella*, *Ehrlichia*, *Francisella*, and *Rickettsia*. **A. americanum.** *A. americanum* (lone star tick) ranges in southeastern and southcentral United States and Mexico, in 2° forest with dense understory. It feeds on humans, mammals, and land birds. It is the main vector for *Ehrlichia chaffeensis*, and it harbors *Borrelia burgdorferi* sensu lato (sl), *Coxiella burnetii*, *Francisella tularensis*, and *Rickettsia* species. **A. cajennense.** *A. cajennense* (Cayenne tick) ranges from Texas to northern Argentina. It avoids cool mountain areas. It feeds on humans, mammals, and land birds. It carries *R. rickettsii*. **A. hebraeum.** *A. hebraeum* (bont tick) ranges in sub-Saharan Africa, in tall-grass prairie, bush savanna, and farms. It feeds on humans and large mammals (e.g., rhinos). It carries *R. africae*. **A. variegatum.** *A. variegatum* (tropical bont tick) ranges in Africa, the Caribbean, and Southwest Asia, in tall-grass prairie, bush savanna, and farmland. By stage, hosts include reptiles (lizards, snakes, and tortoises) and mammals (rhinos, cattle, horses, sheep, goats, and dogs). It escaped from cattle imported into the Caribbean during the eighteenth and nineteenth centuries; it has been eliminated from some Caribbean islands. It is reported to have escaped locally from reptiles imported into Florida. *A. variegatum* carries CCHFV and *R. africae* (and *Cowdria ruminantium* = *E. chaffeensis* to cattle). In Cameroon, 75% (62/83) of *A. variegatum* adults removed from cattle tested positive for *R. africae* by PCR.

Dermacentor (>30 species) (1347, 1439, 2696, 3256, 3981, 4991, 5184, 6455, 6794). *Dermacentor* can carry viruses (CTFV, OHFV, Powassan virus [POWV], and TBEV), *Borrelia*, *Coxiella*, *Francisella*, *Rickettsia*, and *Babesia*. **D. andersoni.** *D. andersoni* (wood tick) ranges in western North America, in sagebrush near streams. It feeds on rodents and larger mammals. It is the main vector for Colorado tick fever virus (CTFV) and *R. rickettsii*, and it carries other rickettsiae. **D. marginatus.** *D. marginatus* ranges in the Mediterranean and Asia, in steppe, pasture, shrubs, and temperate forest. It feeds on dogs, sheep, swine, cattle, camels, and humans. It carries Omsk hemorrhagic fever virus (OHFV), *R. conorii*, *R. slovaca*, and *R. sibirica*, likely also *Anaplasma phagocytophilum*. **D. nuttalli.** *D. nuttalli* ranges in Eurasia. It carries *R. sibirica* (in Mongolia also *B. caballi* and *B. equi*). **D. reticulatus.** *D. reticulatus* ranges in Eurasia. It feeds on mammals and birds. It carries OHFV, *F. tularensis*, and *R. sibirica*, and it is a suspected vector of tick-borne encephalitis virus (TBEV) and *Borrelia* (it carries *B. canis* to dogs). **D. variabilis.** *D. variabilis* (American dog tick) ranges from eastern North America to Mexico, in brushland and clearings around houses. It feeds on rodents, dogs, and large mammals. It is a main vector of *R. rickettsii*, and it carries other rickettsiae, and *B. burgdorferi* sl.

Haemaphysalis (>165 species) (1367, 3018, 6455). *Haemaphysalis* carries viruses (KFDV and TBEV), *Coxiella*, *Francisella*, and *Rickettsia* (*Babesia* to dogs). **H. concinna.** *H. concinna* ranges in Eurasia in temperate forest. It carries

F. tularensis and *R. sibirica*. **H. leachi.** *H. leachi* (yellow dog tick) ranges in Africa. It feeds on rodents, dogs, and humans. **H. longicornis.** *H. longicornis* ranges in Asia. It carries *R. japonica*. **H. spinigera.** *H. spinigera* ranges in Asia, in forests. It feeds on small mammals, monkeys, tiger, cattle, and birds. It carries Kyasanur forest disease virus (KFDV).

Hyalomma **(30 species) (2362, 6455).** Ticks of this genus carry viruses (CCHFV and West Nile virus [WNV]), *Coxiella*, Rickettsiales, and *Babesia*. This hardy genus survives heat, cold, and dry. **H. anatolicum.** *H. anatolicum* ranges in the Mediterranean, Africa, and West Asia, in dry areas. It feeds on rodents, hares, cats, and dogs. It carries CCHFV and is a putative vector of *Babesia* to goats. **H. marginatum.** *H. marginatum* ranges in the Old World (Africa, the Mediterranean, and central Asia), in semiarid areas and steppes. It feeds on birds, hares, and hedgehogs, domestic animals (cattle, horses, and dogs), and humans. It is a major vector of CCHFV. It also carries *R. aeschlimanni*.

Ixodes **(>240 species) (68, 777, 1067, 1872, 2144, 3395, 4817, 7080).** *Ixodes* carries viruses (OHFV, POWV, and TBEV), *Anaplasma*, *Bartonella*, *B. burgdorferi* sl, *Coxiella*, *Francisella*, *Rickettsia*, and *Babesia*. The genus feeds on >100 species of mammals and birds. Activity is seasonal; adults are most abundant in spring, with densities of up to 0.2/m of standard flagging. **I. cookie.** *I. cookie* (woodchuck tick) ranges in North America. Macroscopically it is indistinguishable from *I. scapularis*. It feeds on groundhogs (*Marmota monax*) and other mammals, mainly around burrows. It carries POWV. **I. dendatus.** *I. dendatus* ranges in the eastern United States. It carries *B. burgdorferi* sensu stricto (ss), *C. burnetii*, and *F. tularensis*. **I. holocyclus.** *I. holocyclus* ranges in Australia and Papua New Guinea, in rain forest. It is suspected vector of *R. australis*. **I. ovatus.** *I. ovatus* ranges in central Asia and Japan. In Japan, its range overlaps with *I. persulcatus*. It carries *R. japonica* and *Borrelia sinica* to humans and *Babesia* to dogs. **I. pacificus.** *I. pacificus* (western black-leg tick) ranges from coastal British Columbia to Baja California. It maintains *B. burgdorferi* ss enzootically and carries it to humans. It also carries *A. phagocytophilum* to humans, and likely *B. henselae* cat to cat. In northern California in 1997–2001, densities of nymphs was 3–17/100 m², that of *B. burgdorferi*-infected nymphs was 0.06–2.4/100 m². **I. persulcatus.** *I. persulcatus* ranges in forest in eastern Europe to northern Asia and Japan. It is abundant in northeastern People's Republic of China. In the Balticum and around Moscow its range overlaps with *I. ricinus*. It is the main vector of TBEV and *B. burgdorferi* sl to humans, and it carries *A. phagocytophilum* and *R. helvetica*. In Japan, it transmits *B. afzelii* and *B. garinii*. **I. ricinus.** *I. ricinus* (castor bean tick) ranges in Europe and North Africa, in grassy woodlands. It feeds on birds, small mammals, deer, domestic mammals, and humans. It is the main vector for TBEV and *B. burgdorferi* sl, and it carries Eyach virus, *A. phagocytophilum*, *B. henselae*, *F. tularensis*, *R. helvetica*, *B. divergens*, and likely other *Babesia* spp. **I. scapularis.** *I. scapularis* (black-legged tick) ranges in the eastern United States and Mexico, in coastal woodlands. It feeds on lizards, small mammals, deer, domestic mammals, and humans. It maintains *B. burgdorferi* ss enzootically and carries it to humans. It also carries *A. phagocytophilum* and *B. microti* to humans, perhaps also *Bartonella* spp.

Rhipicephalus **(80 species, incorporates ex-*Boophilus*) (1873, 4601, 6031, 6493).** *Rhipicephalus* carries *Babesia*, *Coxiella*, *Ehrlichia*, and *Rickettsia*. **R. appendiculatus.** *R. appendiculatus* (brown ear tick) ranges in Africa, in the savanna. It feeds on antelopes and cattle. It occasionally carries *R. africae* (and likely carries *B. ovata* to sheep and *Theileria parva* to cattle). **R. sanguineus.** *R. sanguineus* (brown dog tick) is the only cosmopolitan tick. It feeds on dogs, typically in kennels, but also on sheep, goat, and cattle. It is the main vector of *R. conorii* to humans, and it carries *B. canis* and *B. gibsoni* to dogs. In a focus in Arizona in 2002–2004, it carried *R. rickettsii* to humans, causing 16 infections (11 confirmed and 5 probable). Given the tick's cosmopolitan range, the regional limitation of agents is somewhat surprising, e.g., the absence from North America of *R. conorii*.

AGENTS FROM IXODID TICKS

Ixodids can carry viruses, bacteria, and protozoa to humans (284, 1634, 2113, 3683, 3841, 4062, 4098, 6455) (Box 4.2).

An individual tick can carry more than one agent, and a particular agent can use more than one tick species as a vector. Mixed infections are normal in ticks from natural foci. The probability for two agents to co-occur is the product of single probabilities. If, for instance, 30% of *I. ricinus* would carry *B. burgdorferi* sl and 1% would carry TBEV, the theoretical risk of cocarriage is 0.3% (0.3 × 0.01). Of 28 Slovenian children with febrile illnesses following tick bites, 34 had tick-borne infections, and 6 (21%) had coinfections.

Flat (questing) ticks need hours or days to become activated and engorged. As a rule of thumb, the longer the attachment, the higher is the risk of transmission. This attachment rule seems applicable to *A. phagocytophilum*, *B. burgdorferi* sl, *R. rickettsii*, and *Babesia microti*. However, *B. burgdorferi* sl can be transmitted in <24 h, *R. rickettsii* in 6–24 h, and POWV in <1 h.

Viruses

By area, ixodid ticks can be sources of viruses from at least three genera that cause flulike illness, viral hemorrhagic fever (VHF), or encephalitis.

> **Box 4.2** Agents or infections from ticks. Except when noted, vectors are hard (ixodid) ticks
>
> Viruses *Coltivirus* (CTFV), *Nairovirus* (CCHFV), *Flavivirus* (KFDV, OHFV, POWV, and TBEV)
> Bacteria *B. burgdorferi* sl, relapsing borrelia (by soft ticks), *Coxiella*, *Francisella*, Rickettsiales (*A. phagocytophilum, E. chaffeensis, R. africae, R. australis, R. conorii, R. helveticae, R. japonica, R. rickettsii,* and *R. sibirica*)
> Protozoa *Babesia* (several species in North America, mainly *B. microti*; in western Europe, mainly *B. divergens*)

Coltivirus. CTFV circulates in western North America. The principal vector is *D. andersoni*. Eyach virus circulates in Europe. The principal vector is *I. ricinus*.

Nairovirus (1042, 2419, 3414, 8385). CCHFV circulates in the Old World. Principal vectors are *H. marginatum* in Eurasia and *H. truncatum* and *A. variegatum* in Africa. Species of *Amblyomma, Dermacentor, Haemaphysalis, Ixodes,* and *Rhipicephalus* can also carry CCHFV. Some species of *Amblyomma, Hyalomma,* and *Rhipicephalus* pass CCHFV transovarially.

Flavivirus (777, 1178, 1348, 4357, 7262, 8147, 8386). Alkhurma virus (ALKV) circulates in Southwest Asia. KFDV circulates in India, likely in *Haemaphysalis*. OHFV circulates in central Asia, in *Dermacentor* and *Ixodes*. ALKV, KFDV, and OHFV are causes of VHF. POWV circulates in North America and eastern Russia, in *I. cookie, I. scapularis,* and *D. andersoni*. TBEV circulates in Eurasia, in *I. ricinus* and *I. persulcatus*. POWV and TBEV are causes of encephalitis. TBEV spreads transstadially in 10–50% of *I. ricinus*, and transovarially in 1–10%. By area, tick stage, and test, 0–27% (typically 0.5–5%) of *I. ricinus* and 0–40% (typically 10–20%) of *I. persulcatus* are infective. Fewer than 50% of pediatric patients notice a tick bite. Although carried by mosquitoes, WNV has been detected in *Argas* and *Hyalomma*.

Bacteria

Tick-borne agents and causes of febrile illness include *B. burgdorferi* sl, *C. burnetii, F. tularensis,* and members of the Rickettsiales (e.g., *Anaplasma, Ehrlichia* and *Rickettsia*).

A. phagocytophilum (68, 1067, 3395, 4991, 7080, 7203). In North America, the agent circulates in *I. scapularis* and *I. pacificus*. By area, tick stage, and sampling (vegetation, healthy hosts, and infected hosts), the reported infection prevalence is <1% (*I. pacificus*) to 0–50% (*I. scapularis*, typically 1–10%). In Eurasia, the agent circulates in *I. persulcatus, I. ricinus,* and *I. trianguliceps*, probably also in *D. marginatus*. Infection prevalence is 0.5–30% (*I. ricinus*, typically 1–3%) to 1–5% (*I. persulcatus*). There is no transovarial passage. Ticks need to be attached for >36 h to efficiently transmit *A. phagocytophilum*. Of patients with human granulocytic anaplasmosis, 45–85% recall a recent tick bite.

Bartonella (68, 1316, 6605). Ticks are suspected vectors. *B. henselae, B. quintana,* and *B. vinsonii berkhoffii* DNA has been amplified from *I. pacificus*, and *B. henselae* DNA from *I. ricinus*, for prevalence of 2–35% by nucleic acid amplication test (NAT). Tick bites could explain *Bartonella* infections in humans with a blank exposure history for cats, fleas, or lice.

***B. burgdorferi* sl** (68, 777, 1439, 2144, 3395, 4716, 4817, 5314). Ixodids are vectors in the Old and New Worlds (for relapsing borreliae by soft ticks, see section 4.5).

In North America, *B. burgdorferi* ss circulates in *I. pacificus* and *I. scapularis*. By area, tick stage, and test, the reported infection prevalence is 1–10% (*I. pacificus*) to 30–35% (*I. scapularis*). In Eurasia, *B. burgdorferi* sl circulates in *I. ricinus* and *I. persulcatus*.

In Europe, the *B. burgdorferi* complex cocirculates, including *B. afzelii* (frequent), *B. burgdorferi* ss (infrequent), *B. garinii, B. lusitaniae,* and *B. valaisiana*. By area, tick stage, and test, the reported infection prevalence is 0.5–50% (*I. ricinus*, typically 15–35%) to 25–50% (*I. persulcatus*).

In Asia, the situation may be even more complex. *B. afzelii* and *B. garinii* circulate in far eastern Russia, northern and western People's Republic of China, Korea, and Japan. *B. sinica* circulates in central China and Nepal. *B. valaisiana*-related species circulate in southern People's Republic of China, South Korea, Okinawa, and Thailand. *B. japonica* circulates in Japan.

Ticks in periurban areas, e.g., parks, can be highly infective, too. Nymphs are less often infected than adults, in part, because immature stages feed on reservoir-incompetent hosts such as lizards. At variance with this observation are the higher transmission rates reported for nymphs than for adult ticks.

By area and disease stage, 25–80% of patients with Lyme disease recall tick bites; nymphs that are small may be more difficult to notice than adults that are larger. Once attached, ticks need hours to become engorged. Of 212 adults with erythema migrans, most (68%) reported attachment for >12–24 h, but 18% reported 7–12 h, and

14% reported ≤6 h. By area, tick stage, feeding time, and test, the risk of erythema migrans from a tick bite is 1–2%, the untreated infection (seroconversion) risk is 1–15%, and the risk from a confirmed infective tick is 30–45%, a steep gradient implying that many infections are subclinical.

***C. burnetii* (4852, 6189).** More than 40 tick species are naturally infected, including cosmopolitan *Rhipicephalus sanguineus, A. americanum, D. andersoni, Haemaphysalis leporis-palustris,* and *I. dentatus* in North America; *Amblyomma triguttatum, H. humerosa* (both on marsupials), and *Hyalomma asiaticum* in Australasia; and *D. marginatus, D. reticulatus, H. concinna,* and *I. ricinus* in Europe. In Slovakia in 1987–1989, *C. burnetii* was isolated in 0.7% (10/1,469) of adult ticks, including *I. ricinus* (0.6%, 6/1,090) and *H. concinna* (0.8%, 1/126). Ticks remain infected for life and transfer the agent transovarially. The proportion of Q fever that is acquired from ticks is not known but probably small.

***E. chaffeensis* (989, 7182, 7209).** This agent circulates in *A. americanum.* The reported infection prevalence in *A. americanum* is 5–17%. Of patients with monocytic ehrlichiosis, 70–90% recall a recent tick bite.

***F. tularensis* (827, 1272, 3018, 3205, 3472, 8147).** *F. tularensis* circulates in ixodids of the Northern Hemisphere. Vector ticks include *A. americanum, Dermacentor* (*D. andersoni, D. marginatus, D. reticulatus,* and *D. variabilis*), *H. concinna,* and *Ixodes* (*I. dentatus* and *I. ricinus*). In the United States, bites from ticks are a comon mode of transmission (in perhaps one-third of cases), and ticks collected from dogs have yielded *F. tularensis.* In Europe, ticks account for only ~1% of cases, but in eastern Europe, this fraction may be increasing. By area, tick stage, and test, reported infection prevalence in ticks in Europe is 0.1–0.4% (*I. ricinus*) to 1–3% (*D. reticulates* and *H. concinna*).

***Rickettsia* (6455).** The list of tick-borne rickettsiae is long and expanding. Rickettsiae of the spotted fever group are transmitted transstadially and transovarially at rates of ~40–100%. Agents listed below have caused febrile illness in humans. Some rickettsiae (e.g., *R. aeschlimanni, R. helvetica, R. mongolotimonae,* and *R. slovaca*) are considered opportunists. **R. africae (3683, 4601, 5739).** *R. africae* circulates in Africa and the Caribbean, in *A. hebraeum* and *A. variegatum.* Virtually none of the immature, but 15–70% of the adult, *Amblyomma* ticks test positive for *R. africae.* Close to foci, >80% of residents can be seroreactive. Of patients, 50–60% recall a tick bite. **R. australis (6793).** *R. australis* circulates in Australia, likely in *I. holocyclus* and *I. australis.* Of patients, 75% recall a tick bite. **R. conorii (1439, 3663, 5739, 6493).** *R. conorii* circulates in the Old World, principally in *R. sanguineus,* but also in *R. pumilio,* and perhaps *R. bursa, Boophilus annulatus, D. marginatus,* and *Hyalomma.* By area, tick stage, sampling, and test, 2–20% of *R. sanguineus* are infected. Around Astrakhan on the Caspian Sea, 3% (2/65) of *R. pumilio* adults from dogs amplified DNA of the Astrakhan fever agent that is related to *R. conorii.* Affinity of *R. sanguineus* for humans is low and it needs to be attached for many (>20) hours before transmitting *R. conorii.* Of patients, 10–35% recall a recent tick bite or removal of ticks from animals. **R. helvetica (504, 5437, 6455).** *R. helvetica* circulates in Europe, in *I. ricinus, I. persulcatus,* and *D. marginatus.* Reported prevalence in free-ranging *I. ricinus* is 6–37%. **R. japonica (4649, 7630).** *R. japonica* circulates in Japan, in *Dermacentor taiwanensis, Haemaphysalis* (*H. flava* and *H. longicornis*), and *Ixodes* (*I. ovatus,* likely also *I. persulcatus*). **R. rickettsii (3683, 5184, 6794, 7209).** *R. rickettsii* circulates in the New World, mainly in *D. andersoni* (mountainous North America), *D. variabilis* (eastern United States and the Pacific coast), *R. sanguineus* (Mexico), and *A. cajennense* (South America). Nonpathogenic *R. montana* was amplified from 4% (13/308) of *D. variabilis* isolated from humans, but the prevalence of *R. rickettsii* in vector ticks is typically low, <0.1% (*A. cajennense* and *D. andersoni*) to 0.5% (*D. variabilis*). However, low prevalence is counterbalanced by high anthropophily. Of patients, 60–80% recall a recent tick bite or tick removal. The time *D. andersoni* needs to transmit *R. rickettsii* is 6–24 h. **R. sibirica (1367, 6455, 6493).** *R. sibirica* circulates in the Eurasian steppes, in *Dermacentor* (e.g., *D. marginatus, D. nutallii, D. reticulatus, D. silvarum,* and *D. sinicus*), and *Haemaphysalis* (e.g., *H. concinna* and *H. yeni*). In the Altai Mountains in 1994, 12% (12/101) of *D. nutallii* adults amplified *R. sibirica* DNA by NAT. **R. slovaca (504, 6118, 6870).** *R. slovaca* circulates in Eurasia, in *D. marginatus.* Of free-ranging *D. marginatus,* 2% (forest-steppe zone of southwestern Russia) to 30% (Switzerland) test positive for *R. slovaca* by NAT.

Protozoa
***Babesia* (68, 2455, 3395, 3410, 4949, 6953).** *Babesia* is transmitted by ixodid ticks. The picture is complex, because species identification requires molecular methods, species that are noninfective to humans seem enzootic in domestic mammals, the same species can use several tick vectors, an individual tick can host more than one species, and new species seem to emerge in humans. *Ixodes* is considered the principal vector to humans. After full engorgement, *Ixodes* ticks may have injected several 1,000 sporozoites. Nearly two-thirds of patients do not recall a recent tick bite. In North America, *B. microti* is the

main species reported in humans, and 0–8% (typically 3–5%) of *I. scapularis* test positive for *B. microti* by NAT. In Europe, *B. divergens* and *B. bovis* are the main species reported in humans, but *B. microti* is emerging. Of *I. ricinus*, 3–16% amplify *Babesia* DNA by NAT.

VECTOR MITES

Mites (Acari; order Acariformes; family Prostigmata; >1,000 species) are microscopic or just-visible (0.15–2 mm) arthropods. Mites occupy various habitats. In houses live house dust mites (*Dermatophagoides* spp). In grasslands live straw itch mites (*Pyemotes ventricosus* and *P. tritici*) and grass itch mite (*Trombicula autumnalis*), while the oak leaf gall mite *P. herfsi* lives on oak leaves in Europe and North America; these itch mites prey on insect larvae, occasionally on humans, causing pruritic skin eruptions. Mites of birds that occasionally bite humans include *Dermanyssus gallinae* (on chickens) and *Ornithonyssus bursa* (on tropical fowl). Mites of mammals include *Ornithonyssus bacoti* (on tropical rats), *Sarcoptes bovis*, and *S. equi* (on domestic mammals; these cause mange). Animal *Sarcoptes*, but mainly *S. scabiei* of humans causes scabies. Only *Leptotrombidium* and *Liponyssoides* mites are vectors.

Leptotrombidium (1521, 5866, 6172, 6892). The classical vector for *Orientia tsutsugamushi* is *L. akamushi* (red mite, Trombiculidae). Suspected alternative vectors include *L. chiangraiensis*, *L. deliense*, *L. pallidum*, and *L. scutellare*. Mites maintain *O. tsutsugamushi* transstadially and transovarially. In South Korea, 0.5% (6/1,142) of *L. scutellare* tested positive for *O. tsutsugamushi* by immunofluorescence assay (IFA) in 1991–1992, and 41/104 pools tested positive by NAT in 1997–1999. Similarly in southwestern Japan, 7/234 pools of free-ranging *L. scutellare* and 4/43 pools of *L. pallidum* amplified *O. tsutsugamushi* DNA. Only larvae (chiggers) feed on humans. Exposure is outdoors. Chiggers wait in ambush on vegetation, typically 2° growth, in foci such as clearings, plantations, and overgrowth between houses and fields. Attachment is for hours to 2–3 days. In Thailand, only 1% (1/71) of pediatric patients with scrub typhus had a history of mite bite.

Liponyssoides (1534, 4124). *L. sanguineus*, the house mouse mite, is the vector of *R. akari* to mice and humans. Patients are usually unaware of mite bites and an inoculation eschar.

AGENTS FROM MITES

Mites are confirmed vectors of *O. tsutsugamushi* and *R. akari*. Mites are suspected vectors of prions (scrapie) (8226), viruses (e.g., TBEV) (4022), and *Bartonella vinsonii*.

4.2 DIURNAL FLEAS AND FLIES
VECTOR FLEAS

Fleas (360, 5633, 6114, 6449, 6849) (Siphonaptera, 2,000–3,000 species) are laterally flattened insects (Table 4.1). Adults hide in rodent borrows, swine pens, dog carpets, and dust in vacant houses, temporarily also in feathers, hair, and clothes. Starving, hiding adults survive for months. Both males and females suck blood. Eggs are deposited in filth near hosts. In a rural community of the Andes, 8% (16/194) of inhabitants were found flea infested.

A few flea species *frequently* attack humans. These include *Xenopsylla cheopis* ("rat" flea, Leptophyllidae), *Ctenocephalides canis*, *C. felis*, and *Pulex irritans* ("human" flea, all Pulicidae). The epithets "rat," "dog," "cat," and "human" are misleading, as host specificity is low and host range is broad, e.g., *C. felis* feeds on domestic mammals, and hosts of *P. irritans* include dogs, swine, goats, and rodents. Preventive and control measures include personal hygiene, regular washing of clothes and bedding, livestock shelters away from domiciles, rat proofing, flea collars for pets, and residual insecticides on home surfaces.

AGENTS FROM FLEAS

Fleas are known vectors of bacterial zoonoses. Furthermore, humans can contract *Dipylidium caninum* when swallowing or crushing infective fleas from cats or dogs.

Bartonella (852, 2283, 3885). *C. felis* carries *B. henselae* to cats and humans. *C. felis* is also a suspected vector of *B. clarridgeiae*.

Rickettsia. *C. felis* carries *R. felis* to humans (762, 3885, 4746, 5584). Of *C. felis* isolated from opossums (Texas), cats, and dogs (Spain and New Zealand), 2–33% tested positive for *Rickettsia* by NAT. *C. felis*, *X. cheopis*, *Neopsyllus fasciatus* from rats, and *Leptopsylla segnis* from mice can carry *R. typhi* to humans (360, 762, 7590). *R. typhi* is spread via bite or feces. Dry feces apparently remain infectious for days to years. In *X. cheopis*, transovarial passage of *R. typhi* seems possible. By location and test, 4–18% of *X. cheopis* collected from rats tested positive for *R. typhi*. Of patients with murine typhus, <15% to nearly 40% had recent flea bites, attacks, or removals.

Yersinia (3338, 5633, 6463). Some 30–80 flea species are putative vectors of *Y. pestis*, including from squirrels, prairie dogs, and other rodents, and including *X. cheopis* (cosmopolitan and efficient), *C. felis*, *C. canis*, and *P. irritans* (all inefficient). Vector fleas attempt to regurgitate the bacterial bolus that blocks their feeding. Fleas that cannot regurgitate will starve and die. Following an epizootic, 48% (21/44) of fleas from prairie dogs amplified *Y. pestis* by NAT, but concentrations were below the infective threshold.

VECTOR FLIES

***Chrysops* and *Tabanus* (1396, 5463, 7955).** *Chrysops* and *Tabanus* (both Diptera; order Brachycera; family Tabanidae, ~3,000 species) are flies with large, iridescent eyes, *downward*-pointing mouthparts, and nonfeathery antenna segments. Tabanids are cosmopolitan. They are strong fliers that hunt by sight during the day. *Chrysops* (mangrove fly) is highly anthropophilic: 90% of its meals are from humans; only 10% are from mammals (including hippopotamus!). It readily enters sunlit houses. *Tabanus* (horsefly) mainly feeds on mammals.

***Glossina* (tsetse fly).** *Glossina* (Diptera; Brachycera; Muscidae, >30 species) are pale-brown flies with forward-pointing mouthparts that measure 6–15 mm. Tsetses are curiously limited to sub-Saharan Africa. Both males and females take blood from humans, ruminants, and even reptiles. Tsetses hunt during the day from ambush, requiring free vision over 150–200 m. Tsetses are strong fliers, able to cover up to 17 km in 3 days. Tsetses can be dispersed by winds, floating vegetation, and animals. Females have a life span of 6 months.

***Musca* ("house fly") and *Stomoxys* ("stable fly").** *Musca* and *Stomoxys* (both Diptera; Brachycera; Muscidae) are day-active, peridomestic flies with feathery antenna segments. *Musca* (*M. domestica* and *M. sorbens*) seeks dirt, dung, feces, and faces for food. Both male and female adults of *Stomoxys calcitrans* take blood from domestic animals and humans, mainly around farms.

AGENTS FROM FLIES

Muscids are effective mechanical vectors of enteric bacteria, protozoa, and helminths. Tabanids are suspected or confirmed mechanical vectors of some systemic bacteria. *Glossina* is a significant, cyclic vector of *Trypanosoma*. *Chrysops* is a significant cyclic vector of *L. loa*. Fly control measures include sanitation, waste disposal, field traps, residual insecticides, and personal cleanliness. Fly control can reduce rates of diarrheal disease, trachoma, and trypanosomiasis.

Viruses
Musca is a putative, mechanical vector of enteric viruses such as *Rotavirus*. There is experimental evidence for *Stomoxys* to carry capripox virus and African swine fever virus to animals mechanically.

Bacteria
Enteric bacteria (1506, 3307, 6621). *Musca* is an effective mechanical carrier, including of *Campylobacter*, *Escherichia coli* (e.g., EHEC), *Salmonella*, *Shigella*, *Vibrio cholerae*, and *V. parahaemolyticus*. *Helicobacter pylori* DNA has been amplified from *M. domestica* on all continents, but whether flies are an effective mechanical vector is uncertain.

***Bacillus anthracis*.** *Stomoxys* is a suspected mechanical vector.

***B. burgdorferi* sl (4639, 7204).** *Chrysops* is strongly suspected to carry the agent to humans mechanically. In central Europe (e.g., Austria and Slovenia), 6–16% of patients with early Lyme borreliosis recall a recent insect bite.

***Chlamydia trachomatis* (2200, 6659).** Filth flies are major mechanical vectors of ocular serovars (A–C). In Gambia, 2 (0.5%) of 395 flies caught from eyes of children with active trachoma amplified *C. trachomatis* by PCR. Flies visited eyes typically 12 times per hour, and children with ocular or nasal discharge had twice as many fly-eye contacts as children without discharge. In a trial on 6,087 residents in Gambia in 1999–2001, compared with no intervention, insecticides reduced the number of *M. sorbens* caught from eyes by 88% (95% confidence interval [95% CI] 64–100%), and the age-standardized prevalence of active trachoma by 56% (19–93%). Pit latrines reduced fly numbers by 30% (7–52%) and active trachoma by 30% (the difference was not significant).

***F. tularensis* (1257, 3998).** In North America, *Chrysops discalis* is a likely vector of *F. tularensis* from rabbits to humans. In a tularemia outbreak in Utah that followed an epizootic in rabbits, 72% (28/39) of cases were attributed to bites by deerflies, 18% (7) to mosquitoes, 5% (2) to handling of dead rabbits, and 5% (2) to cat bites. In Wyoming in 2001–2003, 7 of 11 tularemia cases were attributed to bites by deerflies, horseflies, or other flies. In Europe, *Stomoxys* and *Tabanus* are suspected mechanical vectors.

Fungi
Musca is a putative, mechanical vector of *Aspergillus* and *Fusarium*.

Protozoa
Enteric protozoa (2883). *Musca* can shuttle cysts of *Entamoeba histolytica/dispar* and oocysts of *Cryptosporidium parvum* mechanically, from feces to foods.

***Trypanosoma* (1127, 1601, 2847, 3517, 5375, 8090).** Tsetse flies carry *T. brucei brucei*, *T. congolense*, and *T. vivax* to animals, and *T. brucei gambiense* and *T. brucei rhodesiense* to humans. Of 2,153 *Glossina palpalis* collected in Côte d'Ivoire, 10% carried *T. congolense*, 8% *T. vivax*, and 0.7% *T. brucei* sl. In the town of Bonon, Côte d'Ivoire, of 152 trapped *G. palpalis palpalis*, 39 (26%) carried *Trypanosoma* spp., 11 (7%) tested positive for *T. brucei* sl, and 3 (2%) for *T. brucei gambiense* by NAT.

An obstacle to ecological understanding is our inability to reliably distinguish zoonotic *T. brucei brucei* from anthroponotic *T. brucei gambiense* and *T. brucei rhodesiense*. Major carriers of human African trypanosomiasis (HAT) are *Glossina morsitans* sl, *G. pallidipes*, *G. palpalis* sl, *G. fuscipes* sl, and *G. tachinoides*. Traditionally, cases of HAT due to *T. brucei gambiense* have been associated with tsetses of a "palpalis group" that lives around settlements, plantations, forest galleries, and water sites, and HAT by *T. brucei rhodesiense* with a "morsitans group" that lives in the savanna and thornbush areas, near wild ungulates. This concept seems outdated in Uganda, where both morsitans and palpalis groups are reported to transmit *T. brucei rhodesiense* and *T. brucei gambiense*.

There is experimental and epidemiological evidence for tabanids and *Stomoxys* as a mechanical vector of *T. brucei* sl and *T. evansi* to animals.

Helminths

Enteric helminths. *Musca* can shuttle eggs of *Ascaris lumbricoides*, *Taenia solium*, and *T. trichiura* and larvae of hookworms mechanically from feces to foods.

L. loa (1396, 7531, 7955). In tropical Africa, *Chrysops* is cyclic vector to humans, mainly *C. dimidiata* and *C. silacea*. Of *Chrysops* females, 1.5–10% carry *L. loa* larvae of any stage (L1–3), and 0.5–4.5% are infective (carrying L3). By habitat and species, the calculated transmission potential is 116–433,000 L3 per person per year.

4.3 MAINLY DIURNAL MOSQUITOES (5628)

Predominantly diurnal mosquito genera are *Aedes*, *Simulium* (black flies), and *Culicoides* (midges).

AEDES FAUNA

Aedes (3208, 4220, 5147, 5919, 6199, 7419, 8369). *Aedes* (Diptera; order Nematocera; family Culicidae, >950 species) is a day-active, exophilic mosquito. *Aedes* is a paraphyletic assemblage. The taxonomy has been revised, and familiar *A. aegypti* and *A. albopictus* have been renamed *Stegomyia aegypti* and *S. albopicta*. To avoid confusion, the traditional names have been retained here.

Breeding sites are tiny water collections, including tree and rock holes, bromelias, papaya stumps, coconut and conch shells, burrows of land crabs, as well as cans, bottles, flower receptacles, cisterns, roof gutters, and used tires. By location, 10–60% of peridomestic water containers can yield larvae and pupae. Females deposit eggs below the water line or onto mud or damp soil. "Floodwater species" are adapted to rising and falling water levels. Their drought-resistant eggs (and the viruses that are passed transovarially) survive dry seasons, hatching only when rains and floods return. This mechanism can explain the recurring epizootics of Rift valley fever.

The flight range of adults is short (≤50 m). Aircraft, railway, boats, and trucks can disperse adults, mainly along traffic routes (see section 16.2). Species that are resistant to insecticides have increased >7–fold from 1950 to 1990, and pyrethroid-resistant *A. aegypti* is now widespread in Southeast Asia and Latin America.

A. (Stegomyia) aegypti (1283, 1788, 3208, 3855, 4219, 7419, 7766, 7815). *A. aegypti* was described by Linné in 1762. It ranges in countries with warm climates. Nearly eliminated in the Americas by 1970, this vector has regained most of its territory between latitudes 35°N and 35°S, including urban areas. Adult females are restless, take 0.6–0.8 meals/day, preferably on humans, mainly around daybreak, before noon, and at sunset, probe many (≤20) times, and interrupt feeding at the slightest disturbance (Fig. 4.1). *A. aegypti* breeds in water containers, natural water collections in city gardens, cemeteries, and ornamental bromelias such as *Alcantarea extensa*. Sites with taller trees less exposed to bright sunlight are preferred for breeding. City lights appear to extend its activity into the night. *A. aegypti* is the main vector of DENV, YFV, and CHIKV to humans, and a vector for Semliki forest virus (SFV), VEEV, WNV, and *Dirofilaria immitis*.

Figure 4.1 Feeding adult *Aedes aegypti* female. From WHO-TDR. Reproduced with permission. © WHO/TDR 2003.

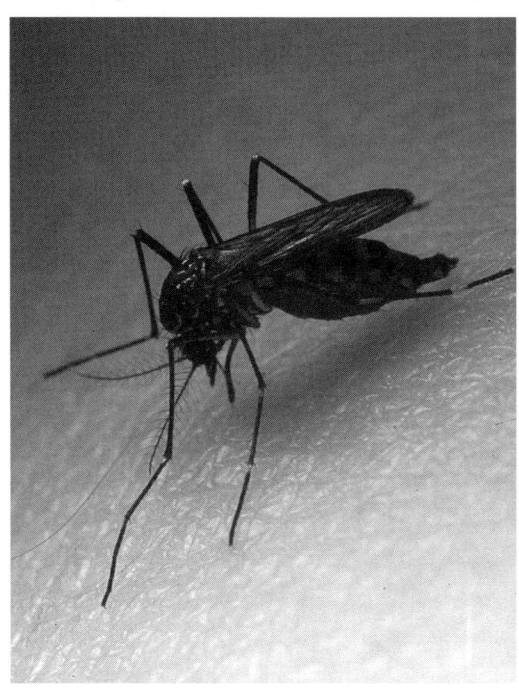

A. africanus. *A. africanus* (*S. africana*) ranges in western and central Africa. It feeds on primates and humans. It is a vector of CHIKV, SFV, YFV, and Zika virus.

***A. albopictus* ("tiger mosquito," *S. albopicta*) (2976, 2998, 5163, 7419).** *A. albopictus* has expanded its range from Asia to Africa, America, and Europe (see Table 16.2). Adult females aggressively bite during the day, carrying viruses (DENV and WNV, possibly CHIKV, LACV, and JEV, experimentally also EEEV, Mayaro virus, Rift Valley fever virus [RVFV], Ross River virus [RRV], SLEV, VEEV, WEEV, and YFV), and *Dirofilaria*. Field observations suggest that *A. albopictus* is a less efficient vector of urban, epidemic DENV than *A. aegypti*.

***A.* (*Ochlerotatus*) *albifasciatus* (2777, 7024).** *A.* (*Ochlerotatus*) *albifasciatus* is a floodwater species that ranges in wet grasslands and prairies of Latin America, as far south as Tierra del Fuego, Argentina. It feeds on birds, livestock, and humans. It is a competent vector of WEEV.

***A.* (*Stegomyia*) *polynesiensis* (991, 4220, 5422).** *A.* (*Stegomyia*) *polynesiensis* populates Pacific islands. Females bite outdoors during the day, avoiding open, sunlit areas. Its flight range is short, rarely >100 m. Breeding sites include temporarily flooded burrows of land crabs. *A. polynesiensis* is a vector of DENV, *D. immitis*, and *Wuchereria bancrofti*, experimentally also of RRV and *Brugia malayi*.

A. vexans. *A. vexans* ranges in North America, including Alaska, southwestern United States, and Hawaii. Its abdomen is striped golden-brown. *A. vexans* is a strong flyer with a reported flight range of up to 20 km. It is a floodwater species that breeds in rain pools and irrigated areas. It is a vector of EEEV, LACV, SLEV, WEEV, and WNV.

AGENTS FROM *AEDES*

Aedes carries an array of viruses, few bacteria and helminths, and apparently no fungi or protozoa.

Viruses

Aedes carries viruses from at least four genera that cause fever, encephalitis, or bleeding (VHF) in humans (Box 4.3).

***Alphavirus* (CHIKV, EEV, RRV, SFV, SINV, VEEV, WEEV). CHIKV (3656, 4219, 7762).** CHIKV circulates in the Old World, in forest *Aedes* (e.g., *A. africanus* and *A. furcifer* in Africa, *A. aegypti* in Asia), primates, and birds. *A. aegypti* is the main, urban vector to humans. **EEEV (1679, 5641).** Though species of *Culiseta* (in North America) and *Culex* (in South America) maintain EEEV enzootically, *Aedes*, *Anopheles*, and *Culex* carry EEEV to

Box 4.3	Agents from day-active mosquitoes
Aedes	*Alphavirus* (CHIKV, EEEV, RRV, SFV, SINV, VEEV, and WEEV), *Orthobunyavirus* (CALV, INKV, LACV, TAHV), *Flavivirus* (DENV, WNV, and YFV), and *Phlebovirus* (RVFV); *F. tularensis*, *D. immitis*, *W. bancrofti*
Culicoides	*Orthobunyavirus* (OROV); *M. ozzardi*, *M. perstans*, and *M. streptocerca*
Simulium	*M. ozzardi* and *O. volvulus*

horses and humans. In Alabama, 2% of 1,357 *A. vexans* were infective for EEEV by NAT. This vector breeds in coastal saltwater marshes. EEEV has also been isolated from *A. albopictus* and *A.* (*Ochlerotatus*) *taeniorhynchus*. **RRV (6477).** In coastal areas of Australia, *A. camptorhynchus* (in the south) and *A. vigilax* (in the north) are the main vectors. In the Pacific, RRV has also been isolated from *A. polynesiensis*. **SFV (4821).** SFV has been isolated from *A. africanus* and *A. aegypti* in Africa. **Sindbis virus (SINV) (4575).** In the Old World, *Aedes* is a likely vector. In Scandinavia, SINV has been isolated from *A. cinereus*. **VEEV (456, 7985).** Many mosquitoes are involved in enzootic transmission. An important epizootic vector is *A.* (*Ochlerotatus*) *taeniorhynchus* that is abundant in coastal South America. A potential vector to humans is *A. aegypti*. **WEEV (2777, 6205).** Likely vectors are *A. dorsalis* in coastal Californian salt marshes, *A. campestris* in New Mexico, and *A.* (*Ochlerotatus*) *albifasciatus* in South America. Low infection rates were reported in southern California in 1994–1996, where WEEV was not found in any of 245 pools from 10,804 *A. dorsalis*.

***Flavivirus* (DENV, WNV, WSLV, YFV). DENV (1444, 2977, 3208, 7419).** DENV circulates in countries with warm climates, in lower primates, and *Aedes* species that pass DENV transovarially. The main vector to humans is *A. aegypti*. An emerging alternative is *A. albopictus*. By test, 0.2–7% of females are infected (*A. albopictus*, up to 3%; *A. aegypti*, up to 7%). Multiple, interrupted feedings seem to facilitate spread in crowded settings. During a DENV2 epidemic in El Salvador in 2000, infested breeding sites correlated with human infections. **WNV (1198, 8386).** WNV has been recovered from *A. aegypti*, *A. albopictus*, and *Ochlerotatus*. *Aedes* is suspected to carry WNV to humans. **WSLV (Wesselbron virus).** WSLV has been isolated from *A. vexans* in West Africa (1916). **YFV (6325, 6335, 7777).** Canopy-dwelling mosquitoes maintain YFV in forest, forest fringe, and tree savanna habitats: in Latin America, mainly species of *Aedes*, *Haemagogus*, and *Sabethes*, and in Africa, mainly *Aedes*, e.g., *A. africanus*, *A. furcifer*, *A. luteocephalus*, and *A. vittatus*. In Brazil in

1993–1994, the proportion of infected females was 0.2–1.3% (*H. janthinomys*) to 1.7% (*S. chloropterus*). In Burkina Faso for 4 years, the proportion of infected females was 0.04–4% (*A. luteocephalus*) to 5–6% (*A. furcifer*). *A. aegypti* is the main carrier to and among humans; in Latin America it is mainly in periurban areas, and in Africa it is in towns *and* rural areas.

***Orthobunyavirus* (CALV, INKV, LACV, TAHV) (2169, 2230, 2705, 4575). Bunyamwera group.** Cache Valley virus (CVV) has been isolated from *Aedes*. **California group.** California encephalitis virus (CALV), La Crosse encephalitis virus (LACV), Inkoo virus (INKV), and Tahyna virus (TAHV) can be carried by *Aedes*. LACV circulates in the United States, mainly in *A. (Ochlerotatus) triseriatus* that breeds in tree holes in hardwood forest and passes LACV transovarially. LACV is also identified in *A. albopictus* (minimum infection prevalence, 0.03–0.07%). INKV and TAHV circulate in Eurasia. Likely vectors to humans are *A. vexans*, and *A. (Ochlerotatus) communis*.

Phlebovirus. *Aedes* maintains RVFV enzootically (5047, 8208). Zoophilic species do not necessarily carry RVFV to humans. A potential epizootic and endemic vector is the floodwater species *A. vexans arabiensis* that inhabits arid, rocky areas in Saudi Arabia.

Bacteria
***F. tularensis* (2172, 3474).** Evidence in Scandinavia shows that Aedes and other mosquitoes can carry the agent to humans. In Sweden, 202 epidemic tularemia cases significantly more often reported mosquito bites than age-, sex-, and residence-matched controls. In contrast, in Czechia in 1994–1995, F. tularensis was not isolated from any of 718 Aedes spp.

Helminths
***Dirofilaria immitis* (6068, 6566).** *Aedes* carries the agent to dogs. *A. aegypti* can carry the agent to humans. In Samoa, larvae of *D. immitis* were identified in *A. polynesiensis*; the proportion that carried infective larvae (L3) was ~0.3%.

***W. bancrofti* (991, 6872).** *Aedes* is estimated to transmit 1% of the global lymphatic filariasis disease burden. Main vectors are *A. polynesiensis* in the South Pacific (e.g., Cook Islands, French Polynesia, Fiji, Samoa), *A. poicilius* in the Philippines, *Ochlerotatus (A.) niveus* in Thailand and the Nicobar Islands, and *O. vigilax* in New Caledonia and Fiji. *O. niveus* bites throughout the day, but mainly early in the morning and toward dusk. On the Nicobars over 12 months, 2.7% (96/3,625) of adult females carried larvae by dissection, and 0.5% carried L3. *O. vigilax* bites outdoors, day and night, with a peak in the evening. It breeds in saltwater marshes. Its flight range is far (>10 km).

SIMULIUM BLACKFLIES
***Simulium* (Diptera; order Nematocera; family Simuliidae; 1,300 species) (1578, 2463, 2939, 5628, 6449).** These tiny (1–4 mm) mosquitoes are characterized by a hump and large eyes. Adult females are active during the day and feed outdoors, on birds, mammals, and humans. Breeding sites include fast-flowing, perennial rivers, spillways of dams, and waterfalls, also blackwater rivers in South America that are low in organic matter and acidic. The main species that feed on humans include *S. damnosum* sl (preferrably bites at legs) in West and Central Africa and *S. ochraceum* (preferrably bites at upper body parts) in Central America. Bites can be irritating for days to weeks.

Agents from *Simulium* (Box 4.3). *Simulium* carries helminths to humans, but apparently not viruses. ***Mansonella ozzardi* (6835).** *M. ozzardi* circulates in South America. Vectors include *S. exiguum* and *S. oyapockense* sl. In northern Argentina, 1% (1/97) of *S. exiguum* isolated on humans were infected. ***Onchocerca volvulus* (472, 2939, 4120, 5628, 6247, 7819, 7850, 8087, 8206).** *O. volvulus* circulates in West, Central, and East Africa, and in foci in Latin America and on the Arabian peninsula. *S. damnosum* sl is a main vector in Africa, but species composition varies by habitat, modulating transmission intensity, and disease expression (e.g., eye lesions). In savanna areas, *S. damnosum* ss and *S. sirbanum* prevail, for mean larval loads of two per infected female. In forest areas, *S. sanctipauli* ss and *S. yahense* prevail, for mean larval loads of four to five per infected female. In parts of Central and East Africa, *S. neavei* sl is a major vector. Of *S. damnosum* sl females in Uganda, 2–15% carried larvae (L1–3), and 0.1–3% carried infective (L3) larvae. In a rain forest area of Nigeria, of 5,452 *S. damnosum* sl dissected, 2.9% (159) were infected (L1–3) with *O. volvulus*, 1% (53) were infective (L3), and the transmission potential (TP) at two sites was 419–427 L3/person per year. Infection prevalence and intensity nonlinearly increase with increasing TP. A TP ≥100 L3/person per year predicts prevalence of ≥60%, and densities in adolescents and adults of ≥20 microfilariae/mg skin. In West Africa, control efforts have reduced TP from >5,000 (precontrol) to <100 (in 2000s) L3/person per year. In Central and South America, habitats for *O. volvulus* include forested lowlands, riversides, and coffee and tea plantations. By habitat, vectors include *S. exiguum* sl, *S. guianense* sl, *S. ochraceum* sl, *S. quadrivittatum* sl, and *S. oyapockense* sl. In Colombia, 2% (3/133) of *S. exiguum* females carried larvae (L1–3) of *O. volvulus*, and 1.5% (2) were infective (L3). In Ecuador, by location, season, and vector species, 0.2–3.7% of females were infective, and the transmission potential was 385–733 L3/person per year.

CULICOIDES MIDGES

***Culicoides* (Diptera; order Nematocera; family Ceratopogonidae; >1,400 species) (4975, 6449).** Midges are tiny (1–3 mm) biting mosquitoes that range from tundra to the tropics, and from sea level to altitudes of 4,000 m. Midges bite in swarms, day and night. Midges breed in marshes and mangrove swamps, at sandy beaches, and in banana plantations. They frequently enter tents of campers.

Agents from *Culicoides* (Box 4.3). Midges carry viruses to humans (OROV) and animals (African horse sickness virus [AHSV, *Reoviridae*] to horses in Africa and bluetongue virus [BTV, *Reoviridae*] to ruminants between latitudes 40°N and 35°S). Midges also carry helminths (*Mansonella*) to humans. **OROV (391, 843, 4975).** OROV circulates in forests in Central (Panama) and South (Brazil and Peru) America. A suspected epidemic and peridomestic vector is *C. paraensis*. Larvae inhabit rotting plants such as cacao husks and banana stumps. Dense populations can exist in cacao or banana plantations and urban gardens that grow banana plants. **Mansonella (466, 5464, 6835).** Midges carry *M. ozzardi*, *M. perstans*, and *M. streptocerca* to humans. Vectors for *M. ozzardi* include *C. barbosai* and *C. furens* in the Caribbean and *C. insinuatus* and *C. lahillei* in South America. In Haiti, *C. barbosai* preferably bites at head and arms, and *C. furens* bites at lower legs. In northern Argentina, the proportion of infected *C. lahillei* collected from humans is 0.8% (2/263). A vector for *M. perstans* in central African forest is *C. grahamii*, which bites during the day. The reported proportion of infective females is 0.8%.

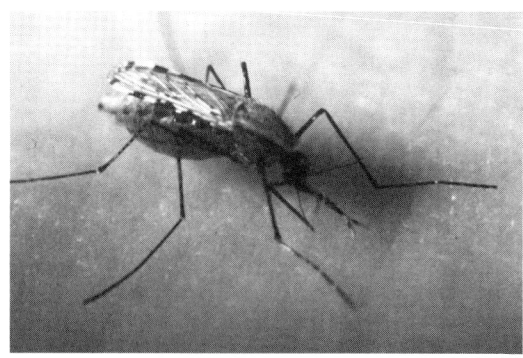

Figure 4.2 Feeding adult *Anopheles gambiae* female. © WHO/TDR 2003. Reproduced with permission.

4.4 MAINLY NOCTURNAL MOSQUITOES

Predominantly nocturnal genera are *Anopheles*, *Culex*, *Lutzomyia*, and *Phlebotomus*.

ANOPHELES FAUNA

***Anopheles* (Diptera; order Nematocera; family Culicidae; 400–500 species) (617, 3887, 4750, 6665, 7532, 7886).** Females feed at night, from sunset to sunrise, outdoors and indoors. They are characterized by palps that are longer than feathery antennas and a resting position that is at an angle to the surface (Fig. 4.2). Flight range is short (a few 100 m), but adults can be carried by wind, vehicles, and baggage (see chapter 16). Of >400 species that populate temperate and tropical climates, only few are effective malaria vectors (Table 4.3).

Unlike *Culex*, *Anopheles* needs clean water for breeding, but habitat requirements vary by species. Breeding

Table 4.3 Some *Anopheles* vectors of *Plasmodium*: habitats by continent

Continent and species	Range, habitats, breeding sites, season
Africa	
A. funestus	Widespread. Shaded freshwater bodies, e.g., swamps, ditches, wet fields
A. gambiae sl	
A. arabiensis	Savannah, arid areas. Sunlit pools, irrigated fields. Abundant in dry season
A. gambiae ss	Widespread. Sunlit pools, irrigated fields. Abundant in wet season
A. melas/A. merus	Western and eastern coasts. Lagoons, mangrove swamps, brackish waters
Americas	
A. albimanus	Texas to Ecuador. Fresh or brackish water, e.g., ditches, pools, lagoons
A. darlingi	Warm, humid forests, Mexico to Argentina. Waters with floating vegetation
Asia	
A. culicifacies sl	Arabia to Southeast and East Asia. River pools, rice fields, gem mines
A. dirus/A. balabacensis	Eastern India to Southeast Asia. Forests, camps, shady pools. Monsoonal
A. minimus	Central to Southeast Asia. Flowing waters, e.g., ditches, streams. Perennial
A. stephensi	Cities, Egypt to East Asia. Wells, cisterns, and other man-made waters
A. sundaicus	India to Southeast Asia, on coasts and in mangrove forests
Pacific	
A. punctulatus sl	Southeast Asia, Queensland, Southwest Pacific. Fresh and brackish waters

sites include seasonal or perennial water collections such as pools, canals, wet fields, cisterns, cans, and bromelias. Females lay single, floating eggs on water. Irrigation and deforestation have a profound impact on breeding habitats. Residual insecticides miss species that bite outdoors. Resistance to DDT, organophosphates (e.g., malathion), and pyrethroids (e.g., deltamethrin) is of concern, because the number of resistant species and the extent of resistance within species are increasing.

AGENTS FROM *ANOPHELES*

Although *Anopheles* can carry viruses, protozoa, and helminths to humans, the focus is on malaria (Box 4.4).

Viruses

Anopheles is a confirmed carrier to humans of fewer viruses than *Aedes*.

Alphavirus (EEEV, ONNV, WEEV) (4579, 5141, 7762). In the United States, *A. quadrimaculatus* can carry EEEV to humans. In Africa, *A. gambiae* and *A. funestus* are supplementary vectors of O'nyong-nyong virus (ONNV) to humans. In Argentina, WEEV has been isolated from *A. albitarsis*.

Flavivirus (JEV, WNV) (684, 5606). In Indonesia, JEV has been isolated from *A. vagus* (one isolate in 42 pools from 2,700) and *A. annularis* (one isolate in 28 pools from 250). In Florida, in 2001, WNV was isolated from *A. atropos* and *A. crucians*.

Orthobunyavirus. Cache Valley virus (CVV) has been isolated from *Anopheles*.

Protozoa

The only protozoon known to be carried to humans by *Anopheles* is *Plasmodium* (1339, 2023, 3264, 3965, 4750, 5870, 6326). By human blood index, highly anthropophilic species are *A. funestus* (index >0.95), *A. gambiae* ss (~0.95), *A. arabiensis* (0.9), *A. punctulatus* sl (0.85), *A. melas* (0.7), *A. farauti* (0.65), and *A. sundaicus* (0.6). Feeding and breeding sites are variable (Table 4.3).

By season, area, species, and test, 0–17% of females are infective (sporozoite index) for *Plasmodium*, and typically 0.5–10% are infective for *P. falciparum*. By season and area, entomological inoculation rates (EIR) are 0.1–700 infective bites per person per year; in holo- and hyperendemic areas, often 1 per person per *night*. Long-term malaria control incorporates mosquito control by removing peridomestic breeding sites, residual indoor insecticides, mosquito-proofed domiciles, and bednets. For decades, Hong Kong, Singapore, and Thailand have run exemplary control programs. Obstacles include insecticide resistance and modified mosquito behavior (endophilic species that become exophilic).

Africa (2023, 4169, 4375, 6858, 7532). Principal vectors are *A. funestus* and *A. gambiae* sl. *A. funestus* sl ranges in savanna; irrigation schemes and raising groundwater levels are expanding its range. *A. gambiae* sl is a complex that includes *A. arabiensis* and *A. gambiae* ss. Subspecies differ for anthropophily and resistance to dryness. *A. gambiae* ss needs more mean precipitations (surplus of ~600 mm/year) and higher annual mean temperatures (surplus of ~2°C) than *A. arabiensis*. In villages in Eritrea in 1999–2002, the EIR by antigen test for *P. falciparum* from *A. arabiensis* was 2–70 infective bites per person per year, and the time to receive another infective bite was 2–203 days.

Americas (1040, 1208, 4264, 4602, 5678, 6416, 7255, 8423). Principal vectors in malarious areas are *A. albimanus*, *A. darlingi*, and *A. pseudopuctipennis*. *A. darlingi* is anthropophilic and endophagic, ranging in warm and humid lowland forests. It bites throughout the night, with locally variable activity peaks. It breeds in sunlit or partially shaded stagnant-water bodies that can be covered by floating vegetation, e.g., water hyacinth.

Malaria has been eliminated from Chile (in the 1940s) and North America (in the 1950s to 1960s). However, controlled areas remain vulnerable. In the southern United States, competent vectors are widely available, including *A. albimanus*, *A. quadrimaculatus*, and *A. punctipennis*. In

Box 4.4 Agents from night-active mosquitoes	
Anopheles	*Alphavirus* (EEEV and ONNV) and *Flavivirus* (JEV? and WNV?); *P. falciparum*, *P. malariae*, *P. ovale*, and *P. vivax*; *D. immitis*, *B. malayi*, and *W. bancrofti*
Culex	*Alphavirus* (EEEV, RRV, SINV, and WEEV); *Flavivirus* (JEV, MVEV, SLEV, and WNV); and *Phlebovirus* (RVFV); *D. immitis* and *W. bancrofti*
Lutzomyia	*B. bacilliformis*; *Leishmania* (visceral and cutaneous)
Phlebotomus	*Phlebovirus* (SFNV, SFSV, and TOSV); *Leishmania* (visceral and cutaneous, including anthroponotic)
Mansonia	*Alphavirus* (WEEV) and *Flavivirus* (JEV and WNV); *B. malayi*

1957–2000, 60 small outbreaks borne by local mosquitoes were reported, most (~80%) due to *P. vivax*. Local outbreaks have been reported as far north as Michigan and New York.

Asia (1340, 2043, 2095, 3887, 5002, 6502, 6923, 7576, 7886). Principal vectors are *A. culicifacies*, *A. dirus*, *A minimus*, and *A. stephensi*. In Southeast Asia, by location and season, the EIR is 0–60 per person per year. *A. culicifacies* is widespread in rural and industrial Southwest and Southcentral Asia. In Pakistan it occurs at an elevation up to 1,750 m. It is mainly active at 2200–2300 h. In India, reported indoor landing rates are 5–200 (mean 50)/person per hour. In Sri Lanka, *A. culicifacies* resistance to DDT (in the 1970s), malathion (in the 1980s), and pyrethroids (since 1995, e.g., permethrin and deltamethrin) is documented.

A. dirus ranges in eastern India and Southeast Asia. It is predominantly endophagic, biting as early as 1900 h and throughout the night until 0600 h. In Laos in 2002–2004, 1% of 1,413 *A. dirus* tested positive for *P. falciparum* in enzyme-linked immunosorbent assay (ELISA) (0.2–1% in the wet season and 1–2.7% in the transition and dry season). *A. minimus* sl ranges in central and Southeast Asia. It feeds on humans outdoors and indoors, throughout the night, with peaks after sunset and before sunrise. It is more abundant during the wet than the dry season. *A. sundaicus* sl ranges from India to Southeast Asia. It breeds on coasts, in lagoons, brackish waters, and mangrove forests. Larvae tolerate salinity ranging from <0.05% (freshwater) to 3.5% (seawater), by evaporation even up to 11%. In the Mekong Delta, biting rates reach 190 bites per person per night. High densities have been attributed to a shift from rice to shrimp farming.

Malaria has been eliminated in Japan. With civil unrest and population movements, malaria has reemerged in central Asia. In the late 1990s, local malaria cases were reported in Kazakhstan, Tajikistan, Turkmenistan, and Uzbekistan, most (~85%) due to *P. vivax*. In southwestern Anatolia, Turkey, vivax malaria persists in irrigation areas on the Mediterranean coast.

Pacific (559, 991, 7066). A principal vector is *A. punctulatus* sl that ranges in Southeast Asia and the Southwest Pacific. The species complex includes *A. farauti*, *A. koliensis*, and *A. punctulatus* ss. *A. punctulatus* sl bites in- and outdoors, at night, with peaks at 1800–2400 h (*A. farauti*) to 0200–0600 h (*A. punctulatus* ss). Breeding sites include brackish water, swamps, puddles, and streams. Their flight range is 2–3 km.

Malaria was eliminated from mainland Australia in 1962. However, the country remains vulnerable, given the presence of *A. punctulatus* in northern Queensland.

Europe (408, 1668, 4121, 6396, 6502). Malaria was eliminated from western Europe in the 1950s to 1960s. However, controlled areas remain vulnerable. Historically, *A. maculipennis* sl (a complex of competent *A. sacharovi* and *A. labranchiae*, poorly competent *A. atroparvus*, and incompetent *A. maculipennis* ss) has ranged from the Mediterranean to Scandinavia and Russia and from the southern United Kingdom to the Caucasus. Competent vectors remain available in southern Europe during the summer. In the late 1990s, countries that reported locally acquired cases included Armenia, Grece, and Russia. In August 1997, *P. vivax* was transmitted locally in Tuscany, Italy, most likely by *A. labranchiae*. In Germany in the summer of 1997, *P. falciparum* was transmitted locally, likely by *A. plumbeus*. In central Spain in 2001, a woman without any known risk contracted "cryptic" *P. ovale* locally.

Helminths

Anopheles can carry *Dirofilaria immitis* from dogs to humans (6068). *Anopheles* transmits ~39% of the lymphatic filariasis (due to *Wuchereria* and *Brugia*) disease burden worldwide (249, 719, 2406, 3865, 8366).

A. funestus and *A. gambiae* are main vectors of *W. bancrofti* in Africa. In Ghana, 0.3–3% of females carried larvae (L1–3, load 1–2 larvae/infected female), and the transmission potential was 0.5–14 L3/person per year.

A. barbirostris is the principal vector of periodic *Brugia malayi* in central and Southeast Asia, and the only vector of *B. timori* in Indonesia. It is active in coastal lowlands and in rice-farming areas up to elevations of 800 m.

A. punctulatus sl (*A. farauti*, *A. koliensis*, and *A. punctulatus* ss) is the major vector of *W. bancrofti* in Papua New Guinea, the Solomon islands, and Vanuatu. In Papua New Guinea, 2.7% of females carried larvae, and 0.5% were infective (L3). By mass treatments for 4 years, the transmission potential was reduced by ~90%, from 45–2,518 to 23–234 L3/person per year.

CULEX FAUNA

Culex (Diptera; order Nematocera; family Culicidae; ~550 species) (1017, 1314, 4418, 6449, 6987). *Culex* is a cosmopolitan mosquito. Adults rest with the body parallel to the surface. Females are mainly night active, feeding on birds, mammals, and humans, in- and outdoors. Virtually any water collection can serve as breeding site, including cans, water tanks, rain barrels, drains, containers, latrine pits, septic tanks, and open sewers. Females deposit egg rafts on water. Insecticide resistance is of concern, because the number of resistant species and the extent of resistance within a species are increasing. Pyrethroid-resistant Culex has been reported in Africa.

C. pipiens sl. *C. pipiens* sl (includes *C. pipiens* ss, *C. quinquefasciatus*, and hybrids) ranges worldwide, with a northern limit in Canada, Scandinavia, and Siberia. This "house mosquito" feeds on birds, mammals, and humans.

A colony has been reported in London subways since the nineteenth century that subsists on rodents and maintenance workers. In cool climates the complex hibernates, or survives through eggs. In warmer climates, activity is perennial. Flight range is about 200–1,000 m. *C. pipiens* is widespread in expanding urban areas where sanitation is poor. Improved sanitation can reduce its density. It is a vector of JEV, SLEV, and WNV.

C. quinquefasciatus. The "southern house mosquito" is highly anthropophilic. It ranges in North America and tropical countries, including Pacific islands. Females bite after dusk and in the first part of the night. They are vectors of SLEV, WNV, and bird plasmodia.

C. tarsalis. *C. tarsalis* ranges in America, from southern Canada to northern Mexico (including Baja California). Its dark proboscis bears a white band. It is a strong flyer, with a reported range of up to 20 km. It is vector of SLEV, WEEV, and WNV.

AGENTS FROM *CULEX*
Culex carries viruses and helminths to humans, but apparently neither protozoa nor bacteria or fungi (Box 4.4).

Viruses
Culex is an efficient vector of *Alphavirus*, *Flavivirus*, and *Phlebovirus* that cause fever or encephalitis in humans.

Alphavirus **(BFV, EEEV, RRV, SINV, and WEEV). Barmah forest virus (BFV).** BFV has been isolated from *C. annulirostris* (3656). **EEEV (5141, 7911).** Species such as *C. panocossa* and *C. taeniopus* maintain EEEV enzootically. In an interepizootic period in Venezuela, by location and based on 33,541 individuals, 0.06–0.13% of *C. panocossa* females were infected. *C. salinarius* can carry EEEV to horses and humans. **RRV (3146, 6477).** RRV has been isolated from >30 mosquito species from six genera, including *Culex* and *Aedes*. In inland Australia, the freshwater breeder *C. annulirostris* is the main vector. **SINV (946, 4154).** SINV has been isolated from *C. pipiens* in Scandinavia. *Culex* is a likely vector to humans. **VEEV (7985).** Although *Culex* maintains VEEV enzootically in jungle and swamp habitats, it is unlikely to carry VEEV to humans. **WEEV (6206).** *C. tarsalis* is the main vector in North America. At California wetlands in 1996–1998, WEEV was isolated in 74 (0.03%) of 4,988 pools from 222,455 host-seeking *C. tarsalis* females.

Flavivirus **(JEV, MVEV, SLEV, WNV). JEV (3165, 7027).** *C. tritaeniorhynchus* is the principal vector to humans. Alternative vectors include *C. pipiens*, and *C. vishnui*. The proportion of infected *Culex* is typically low (0.001–0.1%), but during outbreaks it can reach 10%. Incursions of JEV into Australia suggest that winds can carry *Culex* for up to 650 km. **Murray Valley encephalitis virus (MVEV) (907).** In Australia, the freshwater mosquito *C. annulirostris* is the main vector, but *Aedes* can become involved in transmission as well. In areas with rainfall >800 mm/year, billabongs (pools), water birds, and *C. annulirostris* can maintain MVEV enzootically. In more arid areas, MVEV probably needs to be reintroduced by viremic water birds, or it persists in *Aedes* eggs that resist desiccation. **SLEV (4418, 6206, 6804).** In the United States, main vectors are *C. pipiens* sl and *C. tarsalis* in the North, *C. nigripalpus* in Florida, and *C. quinquefasciatus* in Texas. Infection rates are low ($\leq$0.01%) in wild-caught *C. quinquefasciatus* females from around Houston, Tex., and *C. tarsalis* from California wetland sites. Droughts can force *C. tarsalis* and nestling birds to the same refuge sites, thereby amplifying SLEV. **WNV (1198, 1201, 1345, 2904, 3206, 3471, 4418, 6395, 8386).** WNV has been isolated in *Aedes*, *Anopheles*, *Culex*, and *Mansonia* mosquitoes. *Culex* is the principal genus for bird-to-bird, bird-to-mammal, and bird-to-human transmission, however. By area and host, important species are: in Africa, *C. pipiens* sl and *C. univitattus*; in North America, *C. pipiens* sl, *C. quinquefasciatus*, and *C. tarsalis*; in Asia, *C. vishnui* sl; and in Europe, *C. pipiens* sl, *C. modestus*, and *C. impudicus*. Reported infection prevalence (minimum infection rates) in field-caught *Culex* is 0.07–5.7%, typically 0.5–1%. In marshland in central Italy, after a WNV outbreak among race horses, *C. impudicus* densities peaked in the spring and fall, and spring peaks coincided with migratory bird arrival from Africa. *C. univittatus* probably carried WNV from bird to horse, and *C. pipiens* could carry the virus further to humans. For WNV-related Kunjinvirus, freshwater *C. annulirostris* is the main vector.

Phlebovirus. *C. pipiens* is suspected to carry RVFV to humans (8208). In West Africa, following an outbreak in 1998, RVFV was isolated from *C. poicilipes* (1916).

Protozoa
Culex is a vector of avian plasmodia to birds.

Helminths
Culex is a vector of *D. immitis* to animals and humans (6068).

W. bancrofti **(991, 3797, 6090, 8366).** *Culex* transmits ~57% of the lymphatic filariasis disease burden worldwide, in Southeast Asia 85%. In Africa, Latin America, and Asia, *C. pipiens* sl (*C. quinquefasciatus*) is principal vector of *W. bancrofti*. In contrast, it is less significant in the Pacific. In Egypt by PCR, the minimum prevalence of *W. bancrofti* in *C. pipiens* sl is 2.8%. In India by area, 0–18% of females harbor larvae (L1–3), and 0–4.5% are infective (L3). In larger Calcutta in the 1980s, the transmission potential was 137–177 L3/person per year. In Pondicherry, India, the transmission potential was 1,120–2,690 L3/person per year, by six rounds of mass chemotherapy it was reduced to 0–482 L3/person per year.

MANSONIA MOSQUITOES

Mansonia (Diptera; order Nematocera; family Culicidae) are tropical marshland mosquites. Females bite at night, mostly outdoors. Females depost single eggs on water. Larvae live submerged, obtaining air via a tube that is connected to emerged water plants.

Viruses (4579, 5085, 5815, 8386) isolated from *Mansonia* include JEV (in Sri Lanka, in 0.03% of females), ONNV virus (from *M. uniformis* in Africa), WEEV (in Argentina), and WNV.

Mansonia is a vector of *B. malayi* to humans (4116, 8366). It carries ~3% of the global lymphatic filariasis disease burden. In India and Southeast Asia, *M. annulata*, *M. annulifera*, and *M. uniformis* are main vectors of the periodic strain of *B. malayi* to humans, and *M. annulata*, *M. bonneae*, and *M. dives* are vectors of the zoonotic, subperiodic strain.

COQUILLETTIDIA MOSQUITOES

Coquillettidia (Diptera; order Nematocera; family Culicidae) (781, 1679) are large, yellow mosquitoes related to *Mansonia* that have been reported in the Americas, Europe, and Australia. Females deposit egg rafts on water.

Viruses isolated from *Coquillettidia* include EEEV, RRV, and BFV. In the United States, ornithophilic and swamp-breeding *C. perturbans* is a long-distance flyer (up to 10 km) and able to carry EEEV away from enzootic foci to horses and humans. In Alabama, the field EEEV infection rate in *C. perturbans* is close to 10%.

CULISETA MOSQUITOES

Culiseta (Diptera; order Nematocera; family Culicidae) (684, 4154) are large, grayish mosquitoes that range in the temperate Old World and New World areas. Females deposit single eggs on water.

Viruses (1679, 5641) that have been isolated from *Culiseta* include WNV, as well as EEEV and WEEV in North America and SINV in Scandinavia. In North America, ornithophilic *C. melanura* maintains EEEV enzootically. Preferred habitats are hardwood swamp and saltwater. Large *C. melanura* populations can amplify EEEV among wild birds. Spillovers to bridge mosquitoes can cause epizootics and epidemics. By location, season, and endemicity, reported minimum EEEV infection rates in *C. melanura* are 0.4–20%.

HAEMAGOGUS MOSQUITOES

Haemagogus (Diptera; order Nematocera; family Culicidae) are mosquitoes with colorful, "metallic" thoracic scales that range in Central and South America. Females lay eggs below the water line, in tree holes, or in damp soils. *Haemagogus* is an enzootic vector of sylvatic YFV.

SANDFLIES

Phlebotomus and *Lutzomyia* (Diptera; order Nematocera; family Psychodidae, ~600 species) (2351, 7010, 7273, 8105, 8303) are tiny (1–3 mm) and hairy mosquitoes that thrive in countries with warm climates, *Phlebotomus* in the Old World and *Lutzomyia* in the New World (Fig. 4.3). Flight is silent and weak, for a horizontal range of 50–300 m, and a vertical range of few meters. In Kabul, Afghanistan, the prevalence of active *Leishmania* skin lesions in children decreased by increasing building level, from 15% (23/157) at ground level, to 9% (13/148) on the first floor, and 4% (12/208) on the second through fourth floors.

Females feed between dusk and dawn, on cattle, horses, pigs, dogs, and humans, both out- and indoors. They seek sheltered, damp sites for breeding, e.g., rodent burrows, basements, earthen house floors, or cattle or chicken dung in animal sheds. Large populations can build up where livestock is kept in or near the premises. Some species occupy niches such as caves (*P. longipes* in East Africa), termite hills (*P. celiae* in Kenya), and tree buttresses (*L. ovallesi* in Panama). Impregnated curtains help to decimate adults.

***Lutzomyia* (406, 1093, 1819, 3275, 6560).** Species range from the southwestern United States to northern Argentina and Paraguay. **L. flaviscutellata.** *L. flaviscutellata* ranges in South American 2° forest, from eastern Venezuela and Peru to much of Brazil. It is a vector of the *Leishmania mexicana* complex. **L. longipalpis.** *L. longipalpis* ranges from central Mexico, over Colombia, south to northern Argentina and Paraguay, in 2° forest, farmland, around houses, and in urban areas. It is mainly active before midnight. Populations peak after rains. It is principal vector of *Leishmania infantum* (*L. chagasi*). **L. peruensis.** *L. peruensis* ranges in the Andes. It is a likely

Figure 4.3 Tiny *Phlebotomus duboscii*. Hairs are clearly visible. © WHO/TDR 2003. Reproduced with permission.

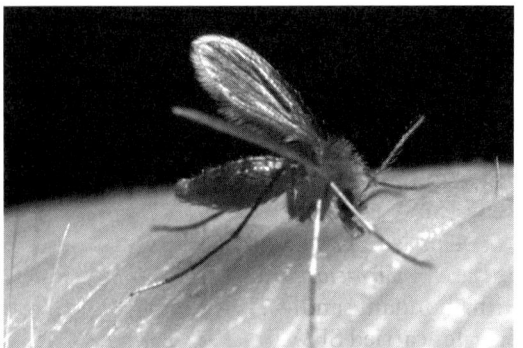

vector of *Bartonella bacilliformis*, and main vector of *L. peruviana*. It is competent even at altitudes of 2750 m. **L. umbratilis.** *L. umbratilis* ranges in the Amazon from French Guiana, Suriname, and Venezuela into Peru and Brazil. **L. verrucarum sl.** *L. verrucarum* sl ranges in the Andes. It is a likely vector of *B. bacilliformis*, and a domestic vector of *Leishmania*.

Phlebotomus **(1326, 1932, 2162, 5350, 7273, 8105).** Species range from the southern slopes of the Alps to Central and East Africa, and from Portugal to People's Republic of China (*P. mascittii* has been captured in southern Germany, at latitude 48°, north of the Alps). Species diversity is high. **P. argentipes.** *P. argentipes* ranges in India and Southeast Asia. Peak activity is at about midnight. It is the main vector of *L. donovani* in India where it is abundant. Resistance to permethrin is reported. **P. neglectus.** *P. neglectus* ranges in Greece where it is abundant in quarries, sheep and goat corrals, animal shelters, and inside houses. **P. papatasi.** *P. papatasi* ranges in the Mediterranean, Africa, and West Asia. Females feed on poultry, mice, rats, sheep, goat, cattle, horses, and humans. It carries sandfly fever virus and is the main vector of *Leishmania major*. Resistance to permethrin has been reported. **P. perniciosus.** *P. perniciosus* ranges in the western Mediterranean, from Portugal and Spain to Morocco and Tunisia. It prefers to feed on humans and dogs. It is a vector of sandfly fever virus and the main vector of *L. infantum*. **P. sergenti.** *P. sergenti* ranges in the Mediterranean and Asia, from Spain and Morocco to Greece and Egypt, and further to Southwest and central Asia and Pakistan. It is the main vector of *L. tropica* and a putative vector of *L. infantum*. At a focus in Turkey, it accounted for 65% of the sandfly fauna. Abundance was highest in animal sheds and lower in yards, basements, and rooms. By ELISA from gut content, sources of blood included poultry (in about two-thirds), mice and rats (in about one-fourth), sheep, goat and cattle, and humans (in 2%).

AGENTS FROM SANDFLIES
Old World *Phlebotomus* can carry viruses and protozoa to humans, New World *Lutzomyia* bacteria and protozoa.

Viruses
Phlebotomus is a vector of Chandipura virus (*Rhabdoviridae*: *Vesiculovirus*) and sandfly fever virus (*Bunyaviridae*: *Phlebovirus*).

Phlebovirus **(1326, 1910, 7413).** The principal vector of Sicilian (SFSV) and Naples (SFNV) serotypes of sandfly fever virus is *P. papatasi*. Vectors of Toscana (TOSV) serotype are *P. perniciosus* and *P. perfiliewi*. In an area of Iran with abundant sandfly fauna, 1 (0.5%) of 221 *P. papatasi* females carried SFSV.

Bacteria
Staphylococcus, *Stenotrophomonas*, and other gram-negative bacteria have been isolated from trapped sandflies. The epidemiological significance of this finding is uncertain.

B. bacilliformis **(2182, 7010).** In foci in Latin America, species of *Lutzomyia* (*L. verrucarum* and *L. peruensis*) carry the agent to humans. During an outbreak, 2 (2%) of 104 *L. peruensis* tested positive for *Bartonella* DNA by NAT (including one individual that tested positive for *B. bacilliformis*).

Protozoa
Some 30–50 species of *Lutzomyia* and *Phlebotomus* carry *Leishmania* of various affinities for skin and mucosa (cutaneous leishmaniasis, CL), and hemopoietic cells (visceral leishmaniasis, VL).

Zoonotic CL. In the New World (1895, 2352, 3843), the main agents are the *L. braziliensis* and *L. mexicana* complexes, but also *L. guyanensis* and *L peruvianum* ("uta"). The main vectors to humans are *L. flaviscutellata*, *L. ovallesi*, *L. umbratilis*, and *L. verrucanum*. By location and test, 2–4% of *Lutzomyia* females carry promastigotes of *L. braziliensis* sl or *L. mexicana* sl.

In the Old World (1203, 2546, 3641, 8304), the principal agent is *L. major*, and the principal vector to humans is *P. papatasi*. By geography, season, and test, 0–11% of *P. papatasi* females are infected. *Phlebotomus* peak infectivity can precede by 2–3 months the zoonotic CL peak disease rate. In Iraq in 2003, in an area where skin lesions in soldiers yielded *L. major*, 1.4% of 23,877 *Phlebotomus* females by NAT yielded *L. infantum* rather than *L. major*.

Anthroponotic CL. Anthroponotic CL is restricted to the Old World (1895, 3622, 5571), mainly West Asia and North and East Africa. The agent is *L. tropica*. The typical urban vector is *P. sergenti*. Other vectors include *P. perfiliewi*, *P. guggisbergi* (Kenya), and *P. orientalis* (Sudan). In an emerging focus in Israel, 1% (2/162) of *P. sergenti* females tested positive for *L. tropica*. In Sudan, 2–5% of *P. orientalis* females were infected.

Zoonotic VL. In the New World (5156, 7010, 8105), *L. chagasi* (conspecific with *L. infantum*) is the agent, and *L. longipalpis* is the main vector to humans. An alternative vector is *L. evansi*. By location and test, 0.2–7% of *L. longipalpis* females are infected.

In the Old World (1895, 2826) (the Mediterranean and Asia), the agent is *L. infantum*, and the main vectors are *P. ariasi* and *P. perniciosus*. Suspected alternative vectors include *P. papatasi*, *P. perfiliewi*, and *P. sergenti*. In southern Europe, *P. ariasi* and *P. perniciosus* maintain a suburban cycle that involves dogs and small gardens. In the enzootic areas of France, Italy, Portugal, and Spain, ~0.5–5% of *P. ariasi* or *P. perniciosus* females are infective.

Anthroponotic VL. Anthroponotic VL is restricted to the Old World (1895, 4140), mainly Southcentral Asia and East Africa. The agent is *L. donovani*. In India, the main vector is *P. argentipes*. In an endemic area of Bihar, the microscopic prevalence of *L. donovani* promastigotes in *P. argentipes* is 0.1%.

4.5 NOCTURNAL BUGS AND SOFT TICKS

Mainly nocturnal vectors include triatomine bugs, *Cimex* bedbugs, and *Ornithodoros* soft ticks.

TRIATOMINE BUGS

Triatomines (Insecta; order Hemiptera; family Reduviidae, subfamily Triatominae) (1599, 3268, 5460, 8099). Triatomines are large (10–40 mm) insects with a long head (snout) that bears antennae, eyes, and a proboscis (Table 4.1 and Fig. 4.4).

Triatomines are limited to the New World. Adults feed on birds, wild and domestic mammals, and humans. By flight or migration, they invade new habitats. Sylvatic triatomines may enter houses and adapt to peridomestic habitats. During the day, peridomestic triatomines hide in crevices. At night, hiding places are left for mainly indoor feeding (kissing bugs). Feeding takes 10–30 min. Triatomines frequently defecate while feeding. In heavily infested houses, *Rhodnius prolixus* can draw 3 (extreme 17) ml of blood per person per day. **T. cruzi.** The agent spectrum seems limited to *T. cruzi* (2938, 3035, 5140, 8099), which triatomines maintain in sylvatic and peridomestic cycles and carry to humans. *T. cruzi* is shed with bug feces. Humans inoculate the agent by scratching or rubbing the site. A history of bite or bug encounter in or around the premises is diagnostically useful. In Venezuela in 1988–1996, 48% (28/59) of patients with acute Chagas disease presented with an inoculation site reaction (e.g., edema), and 58% (34) reported bugs in the house. In the Amazon region of Ecuador, 51% (68/133) of seroreactive individuals compared with 37% (1,652/4,439) of seronegative controls reported bug bites. By habitat, species, and test, 5–85% (typically 20–60%) of triatomines carry *T. cruzi*.

Only three bug genera (*Panstrongylus*, *Rhodnius*, and *Triatoma*) are important vectors to domestic mammals and humans (1936, 3015, 3035, 5140, 7834, 8099). *P. megistus* ranges in Brazil, while *R. prolixus* (Fig. 4.4) occupies sylvatic and peridomestic habitats, ranging from Mexico to Venezuela.

Triatoma also occupies sylvatic and peridomestic habitats. *T. barberi* is the main vector of *T. cruzi* in Mexico. It

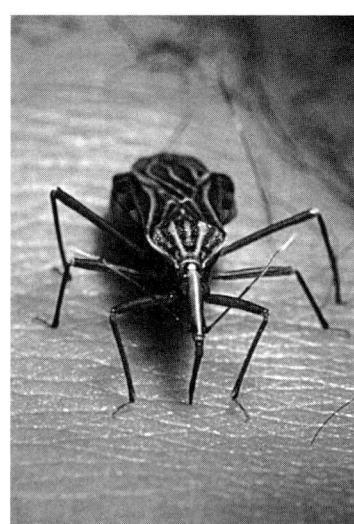

Figure 4.4 *Rhodnius prolixus* bug. © WHO/TDR 2003. Reproduced with permission.

infests house walls and poultry yards. In central Mexico, 69% (87/127) of domiciliary *T. barberi* yielded *T. cruzi*. *T. dimidiata* ranges from Mexico to Peru. *T. infestans* ranges in much of South America. It is domestic, and the principal vector in Argentina, Bolivia, Brazil, Paraguay, and Peru. By decreasing preference, it feeds on humans, dogs, chickens, cats, and goats. In northern Argentina, human blood sources peaked in winter (80%) when people slept indoors and not on verandas. In a house survey in Chaco province, Argentina, in 1999–2002, 30% (59/196) of *T. infestans* tested positive for *T. cruzi*.

CIMEX BEDBUGS

Cimex **(Hemiptera: Cimicidae) (2437, 2680, 3526, 5291, 5769).** *Cimex* is a globular, wingless, peridomestic insect of 4–7 mm. The life span of adults is 6–12 months. During the day, bedbugs hide in cracks, furniture, and mattresses. At night, they come out for feeding. Bites can cause clustered or linear, pruritic papules or wheals. *C. lectularis* is cosmopolitan and *C. hemipterus* is tropical. Substandard and unsanitary domiciles are a hazard, including refugee camps and homeless shelters. *Cimex* is readily dispersed by infested personal belongings, furniture, or luggage, less frequently by clothing. In Toronto, Canada, in 2003–2004, infestation reports included apartment units, hotels, and dormitories. Control includes building repair and maintenance, dismantling and cleaning of furniture and beds followed by residual insecticides, and installation of laundry machines. Resistance to permethrin has been reported. Development of bedbugs is arrested in cool rooms (<13°C).

Agents (708, 3526). Although not an established vector, *Cimex* in theory could carry hepatitis B and C viruses, human immunodeficiency virus, and *Bartonella* mechanically.

SOFT TICKS
Soft ticks (Acari; order Parasitiformes; family Argasidae, >180 species) are leathery, and the biting parts are hidden when viewed from above (Table 4.1). The main genera are *Argas* (>50 species) and *Ornithodoros* (>35 species).

Argas
Argas feeds on birds, inhabiting their nests. Although WNV and *Borrelia anserine* (an agent of avian borreliosis) have been recovered from *Argas*, these ticks are not known vectors to humans.

Ornithodoros (1768, 2103, 7315)
Ornithodoros inhabits fields, rodent burrows, corrals, cabins, and huts (see section 11.2). Rodents can carry ticks to premises. *Ornithodorus* feeds at night, rapidly (15–90 min) and repeatedly (2–10 times). Bites are painless and hardly noticed. It survives starvation for months. Preventive measures include the rodent proofing of houses and treating houses with acaricides. *Ornithodoros* carries *Borrelia* to humans that causes tick-borne relapsing fever (TBRF). Tick saliva alone or saliva and coaxal fluid can be infective.

New World. New World vectors include *O. hermsi*, *O. rudis*, and *O. turicata* (1023, 2255, 6726, 7111). **O. hermsi.** *O. hermsi* ranges in western North America (British Columbia to California), in coniferous forest at elevations >500 m. Hosts include chipmunks and squirrels. It dwells in crevices of cabins and at night enters beds, cots, and sleeping bags. It is vector of *Borrelia hermsii*. **O. rudis.** *O. rudis* ranges in northwestern and central South America. Although it feeds on rodents, it is highly anthropophilic. It is vector of *B. venezuelensis*. **O. turicata.** *O. turicata* ranges in southwestern North America and northern Mexico. Hosts are reptiles, birds, rodents, sheep, pigs, cattle, horses, and humans. *O. turicata* can inhabit caves. It is a vector of *Borrelia turicatae*. Of TBRF cases due to *B. turicatae*, 27–80% are complicated by meningism or facial palsy.

Old World. Old World vectors include *O. erraticus*, *O. moubata*, and *O. tholozani* (1023, 3962, 4289, 5739, 7315). **O. erraticus.** *O. erraticus* ranges in the western Mediterranean (Portugal, Spain, and North Africa), West Africa, and western Asia. In the western Mediterranean, *O. erraticus* subsp. *erraticus* carries *B. hispanica* to humans. Of TBRF cases due to *B. hispanica*, 14% are complicated by iritis or optic neuritis. In West Africa, *O. erraticus* subsp. *sonrai* carries *B. crocidurae* to humans. This subspecies feeds on small field mammals, in rodent burrows, and around houses. Its territory seems to expand, likely because of drought conditions. **O. moubata.** *O. moubata* ranges in East and southern Africa. It is peridomestic, preferring houses with earth floors, grass huts, or mud-brick houses. Humans are its principal host, and it is the principal vector of *B. duttoni*. In endemic villages in Tanzania, ≥60% of *Ornithodoros* can be infective. Of TBRF cases due to *B. duttonii*, 9–80% are complicated by meningism or facial palsy, and 11% are complicated by iritis or optic neuritis. **O. tholozani.** *O. tholozani* ranges from Egypt and Greece over the Caucasus and Southwest Asia to Southcentral Asia, Kashmir, and western People's Republic of China. It feeds mainly on rodents. It carries *B. persica* to humans.

SAUCER BUGS
Naucoris cimicoides (Insecta; order Hemiptera; family Naucoridae) is an aquatic insect that carries *Mycobacterium ulcerans* in the salivary gland. Experimentally, it can transmit *M. ulcerans* (7722).

4.6 ECTOPARASITES (LICE, FLY LARVAE, AND SCABIES MITES)
Temporary ectoparasites are fly larvae and sandfleas that leave hosts after weeks. Residual ectoparasites are lice (*Pediculus* and *Phthirus*) and scabies mites that maintain themselves by continued autoinfection (Table 4.2).

FLY LARVAE (MYIASIS)
Myiasis (513, 1129, 1866, 2126, 2341, 2613, 3667, 4898, 6709). Myiasis are soft tissue infections by invasive fly larvae (Diptera: Brachycera). About 50 fly species from many genera can cause myiasis in humans, including *Calliphora*, *Chrysomyia*, *Cochliomyia*, *Cordylobia*, and *Lucilia* (all Calliphoridae), *Fannia* (Muscidae), and *Dermatobia*, *Gasterophilus*, *Hypoderma*, and *Oestrus* (all Oestridae).

Acquisition is by flies that deposit eggs on skin (or to the body of "mosquito intermediaries"), or contact with egg-infested objects such as underwear, towels, or porch chair cloths. Risks include proximity to livestock, stays in enzootic areas, and poor personal hygiene. The main clinical manifestation is a solitary, painful lesion of the skin (dermomyiasis), eye (ophthalmomyiasis), nose, ear, or throat. In dermomyiasis, lesions are furuncle-like, and larvae are visible within the lesion. Larvae remain on hosts for 1–12 weeks. Rarely, in debilitated patients, fly larvae invade necrotic wounds (facultative myiasis). Incidental swallowing of larvae can result in harmless, intestinal larval passage. Case reports apart, impact is poorly documented. In Israeli travelers to the Amazon in 1999, the myiasis attack rate was ~0.5% (7/1,351). Of 269 travelers (¾ of tourists) presenting in Paris, France, for skin problems from tropical countries, 9% were diagnosed with myiasis. In Nigeria, cutaneous myiasis due to *Cordylobia anthropophaga* was diagnosed in 5% (48/976) of rural residents. **C. anthropophaga (tumbu fly) (5613).** *C. anthropophaga* occurs in Africa and Southwest Asia. It deposits eggs on smelly clothes or soiled laundry. This fly is the main agent of cutaneous myiasis in travelers to Africa. **Chrysomya bezziana. (Old World screwworm).** *C. bezziana* is a pest in latrines, markets, and domestic animals in the Old World tropics (sub-Saharan Africa, Southwest Asia, the Indian subcontinent, and Southeast Asia). Occasional myiasis cases are reported in local populations. **Cochliomyia hominivorax. (New World screwworm) (6777).** *C. hominivorax* is a pest in latrines, markets, and domestic animals in the New World. Sterile male technique has eliminated *C. hominivorax* in the United States and most of Central America. However, cases have been reported in travelers to South America, including adventure travelers. **Dermatobia hominis (bot fly) (1284, 6730).** *D. hominis* is a pest to domestic mammals and humans in the New World. Females deposit eggs on "slave" mosquitoes or flies that carry them ("torpedo" eggs) to hosts. *D. hominis* is the most frequent cause of myiasis in travelers to Latin America, and it causes myiasis in residents. **Hypoderma lineatum.** *H. lineatum* infests livestock in the Old World, mainly in late spring and early summer. Myiasis cases are reported in travelers and residents. In France, >200 myiasis cases have been reported in humans in 35 years. **Oestrus ovis (4806, 6888).** *O. ovis* infests sheep and goats in countries with warm climates. Myiasis cases have been reported in travelers to Africa, and in occupationally exposed residents in the Mediterranean, Southwest Asia, and the southern United States. In North Africa and Southwest Asia, most (≥95%) cases occur in men. Cases occurring in women in the United States and France, which were acquired far away from livestock, suggest that *Oestrus* can be dispersed by winds.

SANDFLEAS (TUNGIASIS)
Tunga penetrans **(Insecta: order Siphonaptera) (1129, 1280, 2143, 2970, 3303, 5238).** The sandflea (jigger or chigoe) occurs in tropical Africa and America. It parasitizes rodents, domestic mammals, and humans. Gravid females release eggs onto soil and dung. In the environment, eggs develop to larvae, pupae, and adults. Acquisition is by contact with soil or infected animals. Risks include poor living conditions and walking barefoot. Sandfleas borrow underneath the skin. Clinical manifestations are painful, up to pea-sized nodules that contain gravid females, typically at the feet, between toes or under nails, and in children also at other parts of the body. The number of lesions can range from 1–10, occasionally >100. Superinfection is a complication from scratching or improper attempts at removal. Females live for 4–6 weeks. Sandfleas are not known disease vectors. In foci, the prevalence can reach 15–30% (Trinidad) to 35–50% (Brazil and Nigeria). Cases have been reported in travelers. Of 269 travelers from tropical countries presenting in Paris, France, for skin problems, 6% were diagnosed with tungiasis.

LICE (PEDICULOSIS)
Pediculus and *Phthirus* **(order Anoplura) (258, 986, 3303, 5343, 6120).** Lice are cosmopolitan, wingless, dorsoventrally flattened insects (Table 4.1). Humans are natural hosts. Spread is by contact. Infestation of humans is perpetuated by autoreinfection. Females and males suck blood. Although head lice (*P. humanus capitis*) and body lice (*P. humanus corporis*) are morphologically identical, habitats predict species: *P. humanus capitis* inhabits scalp hair, and *P. humanus corporis* inhabits clothes (underwear, shirts; mainly over crotch, waist, and armpits; clings to hair for feeding only) and blankets, and *P. pubis* inhabits pubic hair (rarely strong body hair). Clinical examination should include inspection of hair *and* clothes for lice and their eggs. Treatment options include washing clothes, topical insecticides, and oral ivermectin. Eggs are inherently resistant to pyrethroids.

P. humanus capitis **(head louse) (963, 990, 2504, 3304, 8186).** *P. humanus capitis* is not known to transmit disease. Unhatched eggs and adults are infective, hatched (empty) eggs are not (can be confused with dandruff). Development from egg to adult takes 7–8 days. Head lice crawl (about 23 cm/min). Life span is ~30 days. **Spread.** Spread is mainly via contact (head-to-head), e.g., in kindergarten, primary schools, and households, infrequently via objects, e.g., pillows and combs. Lice do not survive on objects for >24 h. **Risks** include sparse use or availability of water. Many infestations are inapparent. Manifestations include pruriginous papules (typically nuchal) and scratched skin. A complication is bacterial superinfection. Confirmation is by combing dry hair (dry combing) or after conditioning with gel (wet combing). In high-income countries, endemic prevalences are 0.5–3%, focally >50%. In Atlanta, in 1998, 5% (91/1,729) of elementary school children had signs of infestation: 2% (28) had lice, and 4% (63) had nits only. Of 50 children with nits only, 18% (9) carried lice 2 weeks later. In Poland in 1996–2000, the prevalence in schoolchildren was 1% (934/95,153); with a high (1.6% or 682/42,759) in rural and a low (0.5% or 252/52,394) in urban children. In low-income countries, the prevalence was higher. In Fortaleza, Brazil, in 2001, 43% (95% CI 41–46%) of 1,185 inhabitants from a randomly selected favela block were infested.

***P. humanus corporis* (body louse) (3303, 6120, 6494).** *P. humanus corporis* is a known disease vector (see below). It survives focally, in East African, Andean, and homeless populations. **Spread** is via contact or shared, unwashed clothes. **Risks** include poor personal hygiene, crowding (displacement camps, homeless shelters, and prisons), and cold climate. **Clinical** manifestations are itching, scratch marks, and papulous skin eruptions at sites under clothes (axillae or waist). **Impact.** In Russia, the prevalence is 0.2–0.3%; in Moscow homeless it is 19% (57/300). In 54 infested Moscow homeless, louse density was 3–25/person. In a rural Andean community, 19% (36/194) harbored lice. **Agents (2477, 4165).** Agents from body lice include *B. quintana*, *B. recurrentis*, and *Rickettsia prowazekii*. *Acinetobacter* and *Serratia* have been isolated from body lice. Body lice have not been reported to transmit viruses such as HBV.

- ***B. quintana* (2470, 4851, 6114, 6494).** Body lice shed this agent with feces. Inoculation is via scratching or crushing lice. Manifestations include trench fever and endocarditis. *B. quintana* bacteremia can persist for >1½ years. An emerged risk group are homeless people. In the Peruvian Andes, 12% (24/194) of self-selected villagers had antibodies to *B. quintana*, and *B. quintana* DNA was amplified from lice. In Marseille, France, 43% (18/42) of homeless with *B. quintana* bacteremia were louse infested, compared with 21% (18/84) of nonbacteremic control homeless. By location, 1–26% of body lice recovered from infested humans amplify *B. quintana* by NAT.
- ***B. recurrentis* (6114).** This agent of louse-borne relapsing fever (LBRF) persists focally in humans and body lice. In the Peruvian Andes, 1% (2/194) of self-selected villagers had antibodies to *B. recurrentis*.
- ***R. prowazekii* (360, 2477, 2957, 6114).** This agent of louse-borne typhus (LBT) persists focally in humans and body lice. Infected lice die within 2 weeks; before death, lice change color to red and excrete millions of *R. prowazekii* in "powdery" feces. In Peru, 20% (39/194) of self-selected villagers had antibodies to *R. prowazekii*. Louse infestation correlated with seroreactivity and fever in the last 6 months. In 1997–2001, 7% (19/262) of body lice from Rwanda, and 9% (31/346) from Burundi tested positive for *R. prowazekii* by NAT, in contrast to none of head and body lice from Europe, North Africa, Latin America, and Australasia.

***P. pubis* (pubic louse) (3160, 7767).** *P. pubis* is not known to transmit disease. **Spread.** Spread is via intimate contact or sex. **Risks.** Risks include multiple sex partners, being unmarried, sex among men, and age <25 years. The main **clinical** manifestation is genital itch. **Impact** is not known. Phthirosis is not notifiable in many countries. At an STI clinic in northeastern Spain, in 1988–2001, 1.3–4.6% (overall, 2.2% or 197) of attendees had pubic lice, for a male:female ratio of 1.8:1. Nearly 8% of patients became reinfected, mainly men who had sex with men. At a sexually transmitted infection (STI) clinic in South Australia in 1988–1991, pubic lice were isolated in 1% (65/6,125) of females and nearly 2% (205/12,170) of males.

SCABIES MITES

***Sarcoptes scabiei* (Acari; order Acariformes; family Astigmata) (197, 2014, 3160, 3229, 3304, 4226, 4259, 4349, 4651, 8042).** Scabies mites are not known to transmit disease. Humans are the only hosts. **Spread.** Spread is via skin contact (e.g., massage) or sex. Infection is perpetuated through autoreinfection. *S. scabiei* takes 30–60 days to complete its life cycle. Risks include large households, crowding, poor living conditions, lack of water, being a child, being unemployed, and belonging to a minority community. The more mites a person carries, the greater the risk of spread. Crusted (Norwegian) scabies is highly infectious. Mites count 5–10/immune-competent host, but >10^3–10^6/immune impaired host. **Clinical.** The incubation period is 4–6 weeks in 1° infestation, to 5–47 (typically 12) days in outbreaks, or 1 day in reinfestation. Long incubation periods make contact tracing impractical. Manifestations include nocturnal itch and papulous skin eruptions, typically interdigitally, at wrists, axillae, breast areoles, and genitals. Itch in other household members is suggestive. Complications include dissemination (in immunocompromised hosts) and streptococcal pyoderma (in tropical countries). Treatment and control options include permethrin cream, lindane lotion, and oral ivermectin. Lindane resistance has been reported, but failures are mainly due to reinfestation including from inadequately treated households. **Impact.** By age and sampling, the reported prevalence is 0.5–15% (focally 20–30%) in low-income countries, and 0.1–0.5% in STI clinic attendees in high-income countries (2–4% in HIV-infected individuals). The endemic disease rate per 10^5 per year is 500 globally (50–500 in high-income countries to 1,000 in rural areas of low-income countries). Epidemics (or pandemics) are recognized at intervals of ~15–30 years. Outbreak settings include the community, prisons, hospitals, and nursing homes.

SECTION II
Environment

- 5 Natural Environments
- 6 Human-Made Environments

Wilderness is a resource which can shrink but cannot grow.
A. Leopold in "A Sand County Almanac," 1949

Natural environments (ecosystems and biomes) (266, 7473, 7929) include aquatic habitats (marine and freshwater), terrestrial habitats (soils and vegetation cover), and air (dust). The seasons and patterns of rainfall profoundly influence the natural occurrence of infectious agents and vectors. Human-made environments include cities, industrial plants, highways, deforested farm- and croplands, jetties, dams, and irrigation canals.

Exposure. Agents can be acquired from the environment by contact with water or soil, inoculation through minor trauma, inhalation of dust and environmental aerosols, or ingestion of surface water or soil (via dirty hands or geophagia). The exposure history should address these modes (Box II.1). Arguments for environmental acquisition of an agent include: the exposing site is a known or suspected disease focus or transmission site; the implicated habitat generates more than one disease case in a defined period (e.g., 3–12 months); date and intensity of environmental exposure are compatible with the incubation period and disease manifestations; and identical agents are recovered from patient and the environment.

Box II.1 Suggested environmental exposure history

Your **domicile** right now:
- Does it have tap water and a flush toilet in the house, municipal garbage service?

In the past week, has there been any **contact** with:
- Freshwater, e.g., at ponds, lakes, rivers, lagoons, or beaches, including swimming and diving?
- Soil, e.g., at playgrounds or beaches, in gardens, on farms, from barefoot walking; any injury, e.g., from a thorn?
- Dust, e.g., in open spaces or closed rooms?
- Patients, e.g., babies (changing diapers) or the elderly (incontinent, in nursing home)?

Your **activities** in the past 3–12 months:
- Have you had any work with natural materials, e.g., water, rock, soil, plants, waste, or animals?
- Have you had any leisure activities outdoors, e.g., gardening, mowing the lawn, hiking, camping, hunting, or fishing?
- For body care, did you share objects (e.g., nail clipper), visit cosmetic salons, or use tampons?

Your **lifetime** experience:
- Have you ever visited a cave, island, oasis, or another continent?
- Have you ever stayed in a domicile without a toilet?
- Have you ever eaten earth inadvertently?

5

Natural Environments

5.1 Marine habitats
5.2 Freshwater habitats and floods
5.3 Soil and plants
5.4 Terrestrial biomes
5.5 Dust and winds
5.6 Seasons

5.1 MARINE HABITATS

Oceans (4501, 7473) cover ~70% (360/510 million km^2) of the surface of the earth. Gradients of water depth (shallow shelf or deep benthic ocean), light, temperature, salinity, and marine life (phytoplankton, zooplankton, and macrobionta), as well as currents and mixing patterns (upwellings) are used to define >50 oceanic biomes.

Coral reefs, lagoons, estuaries, and beaches (7061, 7647) are part of the transition from sea to land. Coral reefs, formed by ~790 coral species, cover ~284,000 km^2, essentially between latitudes 30°N and 30°S where water temperatures remain above 16-18°C. Of the world population, about 40% live within 100 km from the sea.

Agents (2338, 3858, 6554, 8340) (Box 5.1). Raw sewage and farm waste that flows into coastal waters pollutes beaches, lagoons, and life at sea. Coasts can be sources of toxic algal blooms (e.g., by *Pfiesteria*), polluted seafoods and beach sands, and infections in humans. Marine recreational water quality is monitored microbiologically, including instantaneous or monthly geometric mean counts of indicator agents (e.g., *Enterococcus*). The U.S. Environmental Protection Agency (http://www.epa.gov/beaches/) and the European Union (http://www.europa.eu.int/water/water-bathing/index_en.html) issue reports on beach-water quality. The expected diarrhea rate from exposure to polluted coastal waters is 2–4/100 exposed persons. If the origin of life on earth is marine, oceans are likely to hold hitherto undescribed species of microorganisms.

FECES-FOOD CLUSTER
Viruses

Swallowed polluted beach water is a potential source of *Enterovirus*, hepatitis A virus (HAV), *Norovirus*, and *Rotavirus* (1893, 5897, 6554, 6850).

***Enterovirus* (EV).** In the Alabama section of the Gulf of Mexico, oysters relocated to coastal waters that had received municipal sewage accumulated EV identified by nucleic acid amplification test (NAT). In Italy, 33% (47/144) of water samples taken from the Adriatic coast over 12 months yielded EV.

Box 5.1 Agents or infections from marine habitats, by cluster	
Feces-food	*Enterovirus*, HAV, *Norovirus*, *Rotavirus*; *Campylobacter*, *Escherichia*, *Salmonella* (including serovar Typhi), *Vibrio* (including *V. cholerae* and *V. parahaemolyticus*); *Cryptosporidium*, *Giardia*
Zoonotic	Mosquito-breeding sites, arboviruses (EEEV, VEEV), *Plasmodium*
Environmental	*A. braziliense* (cutaneous larva migrans), *A. duodenale*, *N. americanus* (intestinal hookworms), *Strongylodes*, zoonotic *Schistosoma* (cercarial dermatitis)

HAV. Around Panama City, Fla., following an oyster-borne HA outbreak in 1988, inspection of bays identified failing septic tanks, boat sewage disposal, and sewage treatment sludge close to unapproved oyster beds, and marine patrols uncovered nocturnal, illegal oyster harvesting.

Norovirus. Oysters from the Alabama coastal waters also amplified *Norovirus* by NAT.

Bacteria

Sewage fosters growth of algae, bivalves, crustaceans, and fish. Filter feeders and predator fish can accumulate and recycle enteric agents to humans via food (see section 7.5). Swallowed beach water and raw seafood are potential sources of *Campylobacter*, *Escherichia coli*, *Salmonella* (including *Salmonella enterica* serovar Typhi), *Shigella*, *Vibrio* spp., and *Yersinia enterocolitica* (6554). *Vibrio* can also be acquired from marine microtrauma (5586).

***Clostridium botulinum* (3536).** *C. botulinum* is prevalent in aquatic sediments, mainly type E, whose natural habitat is the sea.

***Campylobacter* (746).** Recreational activities contribute to peaks of infection in the summer. At bathing beaches in the United Kingdom, *Campylobacter* has been isolated from 45% (82/182) of sand samples. *C. jejuni* and *C. coli* are more prevalent at beaches not meeting standards, and *C. lari* is more prevalent at beaches that meet standards.

***E. coli* (948, 3159).** In Montreal, Canada, in 2001, four boys contracted *E. coli* O157:H7 from swimming at a public beach that yielded the agent. At a Devon, United Kingdom, award-winning coastal resort in summer 1999, four cases of *E. coli* O157 diarrhea had as their sole risk use of the same beach section on the same day; sand samples yielded *E. coli* O157 of different phage types.

***Plesiomonas shigelloides* (4942).** Near Amsterdam, The Netherlands, in 1990, an outbreak of *P. shigelloides* occurred at a recreational beach.

***Salmonella* (746, 6291).** At bathing beaches in the United Kingdom, *S. enterica* serovars Enteritidis and Typhimurium, as well as other serotypes, were isolated from 6% (10/182) of sand samples, including from dry sands and from beaches that met quality standards. In Italy, polluted coastal waters seem to maintain serovar Typhi endemically. While the typhoid fever rate per 10^5 per year was ~1 nationwide, it was ~7 in Puglia (southern Italy), with particularly high rates in coastal cities such as Bari and Brindisi.

***Vibrio* (1006, 2070, 5586).** Coastal waters are natural reservoirs, including for *V. vulnificus* and *V. cholerae*. *Vibrio* seems to contribute to the degradation and recycling of marine biomass. Its growth is influenced by water temperature (ideally 10–30°C), salinity (ideally 0.5–3%), and organic material. In southern Italy, 42% (70/167) of samples from Tyrrhenian and Ionian coastal waters grow *Vibrio*, including *V. cholerae* non-O1, *V. parahaemolyticus*, and *V. alginolyticus*. ***V. alginolyticus* (2825, 3431).** *V. alginolyticus* is recovered from coastal waters, aquaculture pond water, and aquacultured clams and shrimps. This agent can cause wound infections and rarely otitis media (mainly in persons with perforated ear drum). ***V. cholerae* (779, 3698, 6194).** Fecally polluted as well as pristine river deltas, lagoons, brackish pools, and coastal waters support *V. cholerae* O1 and O139, either free living or in biofilms that form on phytoplankton or zooplankton (copepods). Warmer waters are conducive, e.g., the Gulf of Mexico, rivers in Queensland, Australia, and the Danube River delta in Romania. While *V. cholerae* O1 is a well-known cause of diarrhea, *V. cholerae* non-O1 can also cause wound and bloodstream infections. ***V. parahaemolyticus* (721, 1740, 3431, 4916).** *V. parahaemolyticus* thrives in warm and moderately saline coastal waters, including estuaries and lagoons, and it has been recovered from seafood, including oysters. An outbreak in Alaska in 2004 with demonstration of the agent in patients, oysters, and water and sediment of oyster farms in Prince William Sound east of Anchorage extended the northern latitudinal occurrence limit to ~61°N. In West Africa, *V. parahaemolyticus* yields were greater in fish, crustaceans, and bivalves from lagoons (47% or 26/55 specimens) and markets (44% or 99/224) than from the ocean (0.5% or 1/206). *V. parahaemolyticus* can cause enteric, ear, eye, wound, and bloodstream infections. In Texas in 1998, warm seawater and a virulent (O3:K6) clone contributed to a large gastroenteritis outbreak borne by oysters harvested from a monitored bed at Galveston Bay. *V. vulnificus* (3464, 6469). *V. vulnificus* thrives in warm (>20°C), pristine estuarine waters of moderate (0.5–2.5%) salinity, and it has been recovered from oysters, clams, prawns, and shrimps. Suppurative keratitis, wound infection, primary or secondary sepsis, and metastatic fasciitis of high lethality can result from swallowing, undercooked seafood, injury, or contact, mainly in men of >50 years of age and in patients with comorbidities (cirrhosis and hemochromatosis).

Protozoa
Swallowed seawater and raw seafoods from polluted coastal waters are potential sources of *Cryptosporidium*, *Entamoeba*, and *Giardia* (2338, 6554).

Giardia. *Giardia* has been detected in coastal waters and marine mammals, e.g., seals (*Phoca groenlandica* and *P. hispida*) and sea lion (*Zalophus californianus*).

Cryptosporidium. *Cryptosporidium* oocysts have been identified in estuaries and ocean waters: in North America, from oysters (*Crassostrea virginica*), mussels (*Ischadium recurvum*), and marine mammals such as seals (*P. hispida*) and sea lions (*Z. californianus*); in Australia, from dugong (*Dugong dugong*); and in Europe, from oysters (*Ostrea edulis*), mussels (*Mytilus edulis* and *M. galloprovincialis*), clams (*Venerupis pullastra* and *Venus verrucosa*), and cockles (*Cerastoderma edule*).

ZOONOTIC CLUSTER
Brackish waters and mangroves are breeding sites for coastal mosquitoes, with a risk of mosquito-borne infections.

Viruses (2515, 7911, 7934)
Freshwater and saltwater swamps are suitable habitats for eastern equine encephalitis virus (EEEV) in North America. Habitats for enzootic Venezuelan equine encephalitis virus (VEEV) include jungle, swamps, and mangroves. In contrast, epizootic VEEV emerges in areas with a marked dry season, e.g., dry forest or tropical thornbrush.

Protozoa (457, 1088, 2973, 3026, 4747)
Contrary to common belief, coasts *can* be malarious. Although coastal winds can blow mosquitoes inland, brackish lagoons, mangrove swamps, and tropical river deltas are breeding sites for salt-tolerant *Anopheles*, e.g., *A. melas*, *A. pharoensis*, and *A. aquasalis*. Malarious coasts include coasts of the Atlantic and Indian oceans in Africa, the coast of Hispaniola (Haiti and Dominican Republic) in the Caribbean, and the coast of the Pacific Ocean in parts of South America.

Helminths
In East Africa, coastal environments are favorable for the transmission of *Wuchereria bancrofti*.

ENVIRONMENTAL CLUSTER
Bacteria
Contact of intact or broken skin with coastal water and microtrauma in or near water can expose an individual to *Aeromonas*, environmental mycobacteria, *Erysipelothrix*, and *Vibrio* (see "Food-Feces Cluster" above), by lacerations from a beach rock or dock, cuts from oyster shucking or evisceration of fish, or bites by crabs (5586).

Aeromonas (2070). *Aeromonas* is ubiquitous in brackish and seawater. In southern Italy, 62% (104/167) of samples from Tyrrhenian and Ionian coastal waters grow *Aeromonas*, mostly *A. hydrophila* and *A. caviae*. *Aeromonas* can cause wound, eye, urinary tract, and bloodstream infections and diarrheal disease.

Mycobacterium marinum (5586). *M. marinum* can be acquired from contact with marine waters, including marine fish tanks. Like *V. vulnificus*, this agent can cause solitary skin lesions. Typically, the lesions are indolent.

Erysipelothrix rhusiopathiae (5586). *E. rhusiopathiae* is widespread in seawater and marine life. Erysipeloid has been isolated in seafood packers and shrimp pickers.

Helminths
Beach areas can be fecally polluted by humans, by domestic mammals such as cattle, stray dogs, and cats, and by wildlife. Contact with bare skin is a hazard.

Ancylostoma (132, 687, 2244, 4598, 7547). Polluted sand is a source of *A. braziliense* and *A. caninum* that cause cutaneous larva migrans in humans. In Guadeloupe, in the Caribbean, in 1982, *Ancylostoma* larvae were isolated in samples from three of six beaches; densities were 16–66 larvae/kg sand. Tourists have contracted cutaneous larva migrans at tropical and temperate climate beaches. In Italy, cutaneous larva migrans has been increasingly diagnosed at polluted beaches. Coastal sands are also a source of *A. duodenale* and *Necator americanus*, which cause intestinal infections. Sandy soils seem conducive for hookworm larvae but clayey, water-clogged soils seem unfavorable.

Schistosoma (2886). Although schistosomes infective to humans are limited to freshwater, avian or mammalian cercariae can survive in coastal waters, causing dermatitis (sea-bath itch or clam-digger disease) in exposed persons.

Strongyloides. Fecally polluted sands are a source of *S. stercoralis.*

***Toxocara* (2244).** In Guadeloupe, Caribbean, in 1982, eggs of *T. canis* were identified in two of six beach sand samples, for densities of 8–40 eggs/kg of sand.

5.2 FRESHWATER HABITATS AND FLOODS

Freshwater (307, 3429, 7890, 8340). Freshwater includes rain water and water from rivers, lakes, ponds, marshes, bogs, and hot springs. Indicators of water quality are fecal agents (e.g., *E. coli* and *Enterococcus*). The concentration of enteric agents in freshwater varies seasonally, with a low in winter. In the United States, limits for recreational freshwaters (monthly geometric mean numbers of CFU/100 ml) are ≤ 126 for *E. coli* or ≤ 33 for *Enterococcus*. By site and season, up to 50–90% of freshwaters are polluted fecally, at least temporarily.

Risks (1697, 5735, 7890, 8340) (Table 5.1 and Box 5.2). Unlike pool water, natural waters are untreated, and recreational users are at risk of enteric and other infections. Risks are increased near large settlements, in summer, and for children (by swallowing) and athletes (by frequency). Recreational water-related disease outbreaks peak in the summer (Fig. 13.3). In the United States in 1990–2002, most cases in outbreaks from recreational use of natural waters were due to *Shigella* and *Cryptosporidium* (Table 5.1). Drug-resistant agents recovered from freshwaters include ampicillin-resistant *Acinetobacter, Alcaligenes, Citrobacter, Enterobacter, Pseudomonas,* and *Serratia.*

Floods (4925, 5465). Floods are masses of water that overflow lands, seasonally or from natural disasters. Floods are the most frequent natural disasters. El Niño and Southern-Oscillation events (ENSO) are likely to have an impact on timing and intensity of torrential rains and floods.

Risks (1247, 1253, 7336, 7891, 8128). Floods can damage utilities (tap water, sewerage, and electricity), crops, and buildings, force people and animals to move, leave behind corpses and cadavers, and create vector-breeding sites. The 26 December 2004 tsunami struck eight countries around the Indian Ocean, causing >0.2 million deaths and making >1.5 million homeless. Hurricane Katrina of 29 August 2005 displaced ~ 1 million persons.

Floods most frequently result in increased rates of enteric illness (diarrhea, dysentery, cholera, typhoid fever, and hepatitis A and E [HA and HE]), wound infections, respiratory tract infections, leptospirosis, and arthropod-borne diseases (Box 5.3). In the United States after the Midwest flood in 2001, rates of gastrointestinal complaints per person per year increased from 1.4–2.3 preflood to 2.8 (95% confidence interval [95% CI] 2.5–3.1), and diarrhea rates increased from 0.5–0.8 preflood to 0.9 (0.7–1.0). In 3 weeks after hurricane Katrina, the main reported conditions were diarrhea ($\sim 1,000$ cases) and skin infections (>50 cases due to *V. vulnificus, V. parahaemolyticus,* and methicillin-resistant *Staphylococcus aureus* [MRSA]).

Preventive measures. Preventive measures include the boiling of water for drinking, the provison of safe food rations, shelter, and temporary installations for personal hygiene, mass vaccination, and protective clothing for removal of mud, rubble, and corpses (see section 12.7).

DROPLET-AIR CLUSTER

Floods may force people into crowded shelters, exposing them to respiratory droplets. Environmental aerosols

Table 5.1 Outbreaks from natural freshwaters (lakes and ponds) by known infectious disease agents: United States, 1990–2002[a]

Illness	Agent	No. of outbreaks	No. of cases	Mean no. of cases/outbreak
Pharyngitis	Adenovirus	1	595	
Diarrhea	*Escherichia coli*[b]	16	416	26
	Shigella[c]	13	1,256	97
	Norovirus	6	336	56
	Giardia lamblia	6	85	14
	Cryptosporidium	6	654	109
Fever	*Leptospira*	3	402	134
Meningoencephalitis	*Naegleria fowleri*	29	29	1
Dermatitis	*Schistosoma* (avian)	11	234	21
	Pseudomonas aeruginosa	1	50	

[a]Data from references 4310 and 8340 and previous issues.
[b]Including O157:H7.
[c]*S. sonnei* in 12/13 outbreaks

> **Box 5.2** Agents and infections from freshwater, by cluster
>
> For swimming pools, see section 13.3; for work water contact, see section 12.3; for domestic water, see section 10.2.
>
> | | |
> |---|---|
> | Droplet-air | *Legionella* and *Blastomyces* |
> | Feces-food | *Enterovirus*, HAV, HEV, *Norovirus*; *E. coli*, *Shigella*, *Vibrio*; *Cryptosporidium*, *Giardia*; trematodes and *Diphyllobothrium* need freshwater for life cycles |
> | Zoonotic | Breeding and transmission sites (malaria, human African trypanosomiasis; *Onchocerca*) |
> | Environmental | *Aeromonas* (dermatitis), *Leptospira*, *B. pseudomallei*, mycobacteria (granulomas and skin ulcers), *Pseudomonas* (dermatitis and otitis); *Rhinosporidium*; *Naegleria*; *Schistosoma* (infective to humans and zoonotic) |

(generated by wind or waves) are a putative source of *Legionella* and *Blastomyces*. *Pneumocystis carinii*, but not *P. jirovecii* infective to humans, has been isolated from freshwater. Human-infective "wet agents" include *Proteus*, *Klebsiella*, and *Pseudomonas*. In Thailand in 2005, these were mainly responsible for posttsunami wound infections (1253).

Legionella **(427, 778, 5642, 6349, 7149).** *Legionella* thrives in freshwater, including *L. bozemanii*, *L. longbeachae*, *L. micdadei*, and *L. pneumophila* in lakes, rivers, ground water, hot springs, spas, thermally polluted water, even sewage-polluted coastal water. In Puerto Rican rain forest, water from tree epiphytes at 9 m above the ground yielded *Legionella*. Of natural waters, 50–100% yield *Legionella*, usually at low concentrations. Warm (35–55°C) and organically rich waters, free-living amebas, and plastic tubings (biofilms) promote growth. *Legionella* concentrations of 10^3–10^5 CFU/liter are reported for hot spring spas, and 10^7 cells/liter for tropical waters. Free-living amebas that support intracellular *Legionella* include species of *Acanthamoeba*, *Hartmanella*, *Naegleria*, and *Vahlkampfia*.

Blastomyces dermatitidis **(2099, 3987).** Outbreaks suggest that *B. dermatitidis* thrives in moist soil near water, and that activities near or in water such as strolling along riverbanks, camping on lakeshores, logging near lakes, hunting in marshland, fishing, and canoeing are risks. In Wisconsin in 1984, 48 (47%) of 95 camp attendees contracted blastomycosis; soil from a nearby beaver lodge grew *B. dermatitidis*. In Ontario, Canada, in 1997–1999, 61 infections were diagnosed at Lake of the Woods district hospital; 35 (67%) of 52 persons interviewed reported exposure to shorelines.

FECES-FOOD CLUSTER

The main theme is fecal pollution by sewage from nearby settlements and by animal waste from nearby herds or farms. Agent-specific evidence for floods is fragmentary, in part because microbiological confirmation is impractical in flooded, remote areas. Boiling raw freshwater is advised for drinking, preparing foods, and washing dishes.

Viruses

Viruses (1215, 4873, 6724, 7732, 7741) (Table 5.1), including human enteric adenoviruses, *Enterovirus*, HAV, and *Norovirus*, have been detected in natural freshwaters. Recreational use is a source of *Enterovirus*, HAV, hepatitis E virus (HEV), and *Norovirus*. Floods have been associated with outbreaks of HEV, *Norovirus*, poliomyelitis, and *Rotavirus*.

Enterovirus **(1697, 3185, 3197).** In Kassel, Germany, in July–October 2001, a renaturalized swimming pond was the source for 215 cases of aseptic meningitis due to echoviruses 30 and 13. In Wisconsin in 1977, preschool children swimming at lake beaches were at increased risk of *Enterovirus* infection. At a camp in Vermont, in 1972, 21 boys were diagnosed with coxsackievirus group B5 infections; the outbreak was explained by human-to-human spread and the swallowing of lake water.

HAV (952, 7372). Freshwater-related outbreaks have become rare in high-income countries. In South Carolina, in 1969, after camping near a lake, 13 camp participants contracted HAV from swimming or consuming lake water. In contrast, HAV is detected in river water from low-income countries.

HEV (1588, 4873). Freshwater-related HEV is a hazard in low-income countries. In Southeast Asia, outbreaks

> **Box 5.3** Agents from floods, by cluster
>
> | | |
> |---|---|
> | Feces-food | HAV, HEV; *V. cholerae*, *S. enterica* serovar Typhi |
> | Zoonotic | Mosquito breeding, viral encephalitis, *Plasmodium* |
> | Environmental | *Leptospira*, *Pseudomonas* (wound infection) |

concentrate along rivers. Using river water for drinking, cooking, bathing, laundering, and personal hygiene is considered hazardous. In Kalimantan, Indonesia, in 1991, HE attack rates during outbreak decreased downriver, as the water became deeper and the current swifter. In Sudan in 1988, severe floods caused an outbreak of acute HE with at least 32 cases (confirmed by anti-HEV immunoglobulin M [IgMI]).

Norovirus (448, 1247, 3429, 8340). *Norovirus* is a significant cause of freshwater-related diarrhea (Table 5.1). At a recreational park in Michigan in 1979, ≥121 swimmers contracted diarrheal disease; *Norovirus* was implicated serologically, and by a secondary attack rate of 19% (62/326) in contacts of index cases. In southwestern Finland in 2000–2001, 9% (13/139) of surface-water samples from 7 lakes and 15 rivers tested positive for *Norovirus* (3 for genogroup I and 10 for genogroup II). *Norovirus* was implicated in diarrheal disease observed after hurricane Katrina.

Poliomyelitis virus (791, 4721, 5627, 7741). Preelimination, wild-type virus was recovered from sewage in Finland (after a type 3 outbreak in 1984–1985), Israel (from 0.7% or 17 of 2,294 routine samples in 1989–1997), and Sweden (after a paralytic type 2 case in 1977), as well as from one river-water sample and sewage in The Netherlands (in a type 3 outbreak in 1992–1993, from 9% or 14/153 sewage samples). In South Africa in 1987–1988, flood-associated surface-water pollution was the suggested trigger for a type 1 outbreak with 412 cases and 34 (8%) deaths. Pockets of wild virus continue to circulate in parts of Africa (notably Nigeria) and Asia.

Rotavirus (1215). In Jamaica in 2003, in a diarrhea outbreak among preschool children that was unusual for season (summer) and lethality (high), heavy spring rains and flooded latrines in crowded urban areas were the implicated cause.

Bacteria
Polluted recreational waters are a source of *Campylobacter*, *E. coli* (including enterohemorrhagic *E. coli* [EHEC]), *Shigella*, and *V. cholerae* (Table 5.1).

Campylobacter (3429). In southwestern Finland in 2000–2001, 24 (17%) of 139 surface-water samples from 7 lakes and 15 rivers grew *Campylobacter*, including *C. jejuni* (11 or 46% of isolates), *C. lari* (6 or 25%), and *C. coli* (1 or 4%).

E. coli (3877, 5775, 8340). Near Portland, Oreg., swimming in a lakeside park was associated with an outbreak of bloody diarrhea due to *E. coli* O157:H7 (and *Shigella sonnei*). In Finland, swimming in a lake was the suspected source for an *E. coli* O157:H8 outbreak.

Helicobacter pylori (2849). Infections have been linked to swimming in rivers, streams, and pools. Associations with freshwater may be confounded by long latency and diagnostic difficulties.

Shigella (1181, 2433, 3603, 3877). Venues for reported outbreaks include lakes, a reservoir, a recreational spray fountain, and an unchlorinated wading pool. In Georgia, in 2003, 17 (25%) of 69 visitors to a park contracted *S. sonnei* disease from swimming in a lake during Memorial Day weekend. The risk of illness was greatest for swimmers who reported to get lake water in the mouth.

Vibrio. *V. cholerae* (46, 659, 803, 7887). Domestic and recreational uses of river and lake waters in endemic areas are risks for the acquisition of cholera. Toxigenic *V. cholerae* O1 has been isolated in nonendemic areas, e.g., in an area between Townsville and Brisbane in Queensland, Australia, from both residents and river water. Likely sources of infections in residents were vegetables that were washed with or dishes that were cooled in river water.

Floods can trigger explosive cholera epidemics (1380, 6878, 7259). In Orissa, India, in 1999, torrential rains in the wake of a cyclone caused seawater to advance up to 30 km inland, >97,000 diarrhea cases, and 81 deaths; of 107 patients hospitalized with diarrhea, 83 (77%) grew *V. cholerae* O1, 7 (7%) grew *V. cholerae* O139, 16 (15%) grew *E. coli*, and 1 (1%) grew *Shigella flexneri*. In Bangladesh in 1985, a cyclone flooded large parts of Sandwip Island in the Ganges Delta, causing 12,194 diarrhea cases and 51 deaths. Houses in the area were built from mud, straw, and bamboo, and latrines were open pits. **Other vibrios (1247).** In the United States in 2005, 24 cases of likely hematogenous *Vibrio* wound infections were diagnosed in evacuees from hurricane Katrina (>80% by *V. vulnificus* and a few by *V. parahaemolyticus*), including six deaths.

Yersinia enterocolitica (4807). Surface river and lake waters seem suitable habitats for *Y. enterocolitica*, including serogroups infective to humans.

Fungi
Microsporidia (1924). Spores survive well in surface water. *Encephalitozoon intestinalis* has been isolated from ground and surface water, sewage effluent, and irrigation water, and *Enterocytozoon bieneusi* has been isolated from surface water, river water, and pool water.

Protozoa
Polluted recreational waters are sources of *Cryptosporidium* and *Giardia* (Table 5.1).

***Balantidium coli* (7935).** In the wake of a severe typhoon that hit Truk Island in 1971, 110 persons contracted *B. coli* diarrheal disease, for an attack rate of 1.2%. The vehicle implicated epidemiologically was drinking water polluted by pig feces.

***Cryptosporidium* (3429, 4092, 5620).** In Japan in 1998–1999, ~50% (74/156) of samples from 18 different rivers yielded oocysts identified as *C. parvum* or *C. hominis*. In Finland in 2000–2001, 10% (14/139) of surface-water samples tested positive for *Cryptosporidium*. In New Jersey, in the summer of 1994, *Cryptosporidium* caused an outbreak of diarrhea among visitors of a shallow lake in a state park. Likely sources of lake pollution were rainwater runoff and infected bathers. In 4 weeks, ~2,070 persons were affected, for attack rates of ~20% among one-time visitors, 40% among overnighting visitors, and 60% among multiple-time visitors. Small children wearing diapers were reported to be in the water, and parents were rinsing soiled diapers in the swimming area.

***Giardia lamblia* (3429, 7213, 7738, 8048).** Cysts of genotypes infective to humans have been recovered from water sediments. In Finland in 2000–2001, 14% (19/139) of surface-water samples tested positive for *Giardia*. In New Hampshire, in 1984–1985, significant risks in 273 cases compared with 375 controls included swimming in a lake or pond (odds of 5; 95% CI, 2–86). Similarly in the United Kingdom in 1998–1999, having recreational freshwater contact was a significant risk in 192 giardiasis cases compared with 492 age-, sex-, and location-matched community controls. In Montana, in May 1980, ashfall from the Mount St. Helens volcanic eruption darkened snow; as a result, sunny summer weather caused snow melt and water runoff that contaminated the unfiltered and inadequately chlorinated surface-water supply of a city, and two giardiasis outbreaks ensued, with a total of about 780 cases.

Helminths

Nematodes. *Dracunculus medinensis* (1028, 3419) is acquired from drinking infective copepods in unfiltered water collected at stagnant bodies of shallow water in tropical Africa and Central Asia. People with Guinea worm leg lesions, when stepping into unprotected surface water, release larvae that seek copepodes, completing the cycle.

Trematodes (2885, 4298, 5044, 7793). Freshwater is critical for trematodes' life cycles. By defecation, drainage, or rains, eggs are flushed into freshwater. Miracidia from hatched eggs of *Clonorchis, Fasciola, Fasciolopsis, Opisthorchis, Paragonimus,* and *Schistosoma* seek aquatic or amphibious snails as first intermediate hosts. Suitable snail habitats include ditches, edges of ponds, banks of slow-flowing rivers, lakeshores, and wet fields. Cercariae of *Schistosoma* that snails release into freshwater are immediately infective for humans (see "Environmental Cluster" below). Other trematodes use second intermediate hosts for the production of infective metacercariae. *Clonorchis* and *Opisthorchis* use freshwater fish (see section 3.9), *Paragonimus* uses freshwater crabs, and *Fasciola* and *Fasciolopsis* use water plants. In Cuba, 9–11 months after heavy rains had flooded lettuce fields close to a cattle pasture, 82 fascioliasis cases were diagnosed in the area, presumably because waters had flushed eggs from cattle dung onto lettuce fields.

Cestodes. *Diphyllobothrium* is limited by a need for surface water. Eggs in water develop into coracidia that seek copepodes as first intermediate hosts. Freshwater and marine fish serve as second intermediate hosts.

ZOONOTIC CLUSTER

Wetlands and freshwater bodies are common breeding sites for mosquitoes. Floods can have ramified impacts, including the flushing out of rodent burrows and the creation of new breeding sites.

Viruses

Arboviruses (5342). Arboviruses that have been associated with rains and floods include Murray Valley encephalitis virus (MVEV), Rift Valley fever virus (RVFV), St. Louis encephalitis virus (SLEV), and western equine encephalitis virus (WEEV). Of 10 natural disasters that were monitored in the United States in 1975–1997, arboviral infections were detected in humans in 1 and in sentinel mosquitoes or flocks in seven. **MVEV (906).** In Northwest Australia, outbreaks typically follow heavy rains and extensive floods. **RVFV (1157, 4456).** In East Africa in 1950–1998, all known epizootics followed periods of heavy rainfall. In particular, in 1997–1998, torrential rains and flooding caused an epidemic of RVF with 170 deaths. In Mauritania, West Africa, dam construction and flooding of the lower Senegal River was associated with an outbreak of RVF. **SLEV and WEEV.** In North Dakota in 1975, the Red River flood was associated with 55 WEE cases and 12 SLE cases in humans.

Protozoa

Plasmodium. River shores are malaria transmission sites (1040, 2223, 3762, 4833). In the Amazon, sedentary, riverine populations stably maintain transmission throughout the year. Malarious river valleys include the Congo, Nile, Niger, Senegal, and Zambezi in Africa; the Amazon with its tributaries and the Paraguay in South America; and the Ganges, Irawadi, and Mekong in Asia. There is astonishingly little evidence for increased malaria transmission and case rates after heavy rains (4801). Two to 3 months after hurricane Flora hit Haiti in 1963, the area experienced some 75,000 malaria cases in 4 months, mainly due to *Plasmodium falciparum*.

***Trypanosoma brucei* (3316, 7113).** Riparian and gallery forests are good hiding places for *Glossina*. River fords and washing and bathing places in West and Central Africa are transmission sites for *T. brucei gambiense*. Tsetse-infested river valleys include the Congo-Zaire, Logone (drains into Lake Chad), Niger, upper Nile, Senegal, Volta, and Zambezi. In Uganda, East Africa, the arm of the Nile that drains Lake Victoria into Lake Kyoga is sluggish, passing in over 100 km an elevation gradient of not more than 110 m. This area of forested marshes is prone to trypanosomiasis outbreaks; in Busoga on the northern shore of Lake Victoria, six epidemics of *T. brucei rhodesiense* occurred in 1900–1992.

Helminths
***Onchocerca volvulus* (1578, 4607, 7850, 8087, 8102).** Permanent rivers with good flow are ideal breeding sites for *Simulium* blackflies (see section 4.3), and riverine domiciles are a significant source of infections in humans. A high (>5%) blindness prevalence has forced people away from agriculturally favorable lands along rivers, to safer but less fertile lands away from rivers. The West African onchocerciasis control program required almost weekly application of larvicides to up to 50,000 km of rivers in 11 countries for a period matching or exceeding the life span of adult worms, which can approach 30 years (1974–2002).

ENVIRONMENTAL CLUSTER
Bacteria
Surface waters can be sources of "wet agents," including *Acinetobacter* (7740), *Aeromonas*, *Burkholderia*, environmental mycobacteria, *Leptospira*, *Plesiomonas*, and *Pseudomonas*. Contact can result in dermatitis, and contact with broken skin, microtrauma, or swallowing can result in systemic illness.

***Aeromonas* (5745, 6766, 7694).** *Aeromonas* is ubiquitous in freshwater, including lakes, rivers, springs, rainwater, and aquatic plants. In tropical climates, *Aeromonas* is present in water throughout the year. Most *Aeromonas* skin infections result from exposure to freshwater. Abrasions from swimming, boating, or other activities can be a portal of entry.

***Burkholderia pseudomallei* (1371).** Swallowing surface water is a source. In North Australia, the timing and location of melioidosis cases usually correlates with rainfall, and flooding after tropical cyclones can result in an increase of cases.

***Leptospira* (4369, 5894, 7325).** For occupational water contacts, see section 12.4; for leisure water contacts, see section 13.4. Lakes, streams, and other freshwater bodies can harbor *Leptospira*. Irrigation and perennial farming support high rodent densities and increase risks. Serovars recovered in U.S. waters include Ballum, Grippotyphosa, Icterohaemorrhagiae, and Pomona. Confirmed exposing activities include washing and walking in water.

Floods (314, 3718, 4279, 6595, 7552, 8095) are an additional risk for people in tropical lowlands. Leptospirosis is underrecognized after floods, however, probably because of diagnostic difficulties. Some 2 weeks after a cyclone brought heavy rains and floods to Orissa, India, in 1999, cases of febrile illness rose, and in a sample of 142 village residents, 14% (20) had a history of fever and anti-*Leptospira* IgM suggestive of recent infection. In Puerto Rico in 1996, when hurricane Hortense brought heavy rains and floods, 17 *Leptospira* infections were laboratory confirmed, and the *Leptospira* seroprevalence in dengue virus (DENV)-seronegative patients rose from 6% (4/72) prehurricane to 24% (17/70). In Nicaragua in 1995, after heavy rains and floods, an outbreak of unexplained febrile illness initially diagnosed as dengue occurred; eventually, leptospirosis was confirmed or suspected in 2,259 patients. Floodwaters contaminated with animal urine were the most likely vehicle. Risks include having ever walked in creeks or owning seroreactive dogs.

Mycobacteria (97, 2297, 3543, 3693, 4835, 8107). *M. avium*, *M. intracellulare*, and other environmental mycobacteria can inhabit acidic (pH 3.5–4.5) swamp sediments, peatlands, and *Sphagnum* mosses. Examples are the Okefenokee and Great Dismal swamps and Cranberry Glades in the eastern United States and the peatlands in Finland. Salt, brackish, aquarium, or pool waters are habitats for *M. marinum*. Tropical water courses and flooded areas are habitats for *M. ulcerans*. Regular swimming in rivers seems to increase the risks of *M. ulcerans*, infections and Buruli ulcers; this risk could be confounded by being exposed to biting insects while resting on riverbanks after swimming. Floods are suspected to create new habitats for *M. ulcerans*, resulting in increased disease rates. Water seems a reservoir and source of *M. leprae* as well. In highly endemic villages in Indonesia, *M. leprae* DNA was amplified from 21 of 44 daily used water sources, and the prevalence of leprosy was higher among villagers who used contaminated water for bathing or washing than among users of DNA-negative water.

***Plesiomonas shigelloides* (2841, 4119).** *P. shigelloides* is widespread in surface waters, including lakes and rivers, and sewage. Likely risks include contact with aquarium and irrigation waters and swimming in untreated waters.

***Pseudomonas aeruginosa* (7699).** *P. aeruginosa* is a cause of dermatitis in swimmers (Table 5.1). In The Netherlands in the summer of 1994, bathing in recreational freshwater lakes was the likely source for 98 cases of *P. aeruginosa* otitis externa. Risks of otitis increased with increasing days of swimming. Although lake water quality met national and European standards, samples yielded *P. aeruginosa* at concentrations of <1–17 (median 2) CFU/100 ml.

Fungi
***Rhinosporidium seeberi* (2513, 5224, 7882).** The putative habitat is stagnant freshwater, and bathing or swimming is a risk. In Tamil Nadu, India, in 1984–1988, most of >200 ocular cases had a history of bathing in ponds. In Serbia in 1995, all 17 cases reported bathing in a stagnant lake, but only 3 of 32 age- and sex-matched controls.

Protozoa
The free-living amebas (3708, 4777, 4911, 4957, 5306) *Acanthamoeba*, *Balamuthia*, *Hartmannella*, and *Naegleria* inhabit human-made (see section 6.1) and natural water bodies, including ponds, hot springs, lakes, and coastal waters. Although *Naegleria fowleri* naturally inhabits soil, rains flush it into surface waters. Waters warmed up by summer heat or thermal pollution enhance amebic growth. In Oklahoma water samples, the concentration was three amebas per 10 liters. Free-living amebas are hosts for bacteria such as *Legionella*, *Mycobacterium*, and *Pseudomonas*, and they are suspected of contributing to the survival and spread of these bacteria.

Swimming in freshwater is the principal mode of acquisition of primary amebic meningoencephalitis (PAM, Table 5.1) due to *N. fowleri*. Risks increase with frequent submersions, and in shallow, stagnant waters that may concentrate free-living amebas. In the United States in 1990–2000, 41% (7/17) of reported PAM cases were acquired from lakes, 24% (4) from rivers, 18% (3) from ponds, and one each from a hot spring, a canal, and a puddle.

In Iowa in 1993–1994, a link was established between an outbreak of *Acanthamoeba* keratitis among wearers of contact lenses and a flood that contaminated tap water used to rinse lenses.

Helminths
Cercarial dermatitis (swimmer's itch) (1131, 4368, 8340). Cercariae of schistosomes are acquired from skin contact with snail-inhabited freshwaters, for work, leisure, or domestic purposes. Cercariae infective to both vertebrates and humans can cause cercarial dermatitis that resolves spontaneously. However, although humans are dead-end hosts for vertebrate-infective (avian, mammalian) schistosomes enzootic in countries with warm and temperate climates, human-infective schistosomes endemic in countries with warm climates will develop to fertile adults in humans. Birds, ungulates, and rodents are sources of vertebrate-infective cercariae and swimmer's itch. In temperate climates, birds are the principal source. In the United States in 1990–2002, 11 outbreaks of cercarial dermatitis were reported, with a total of 234 cases (21 per outbreak, Table 5.1). At a lake in Oregon in July 2002, 19 persons contracted avian schistosomes and swimmer's dermatitis.

Schistosomes infective to humans (429, 1794, 2163, 2227, 3318, 3776, 4398, 4654, 7062). *Schistosoma haematobium* adults locate in genitourinary venules, *S. mansoni* and *S. intercalatum* locate in mesenteric venules, and *S. japonicum* and *S. mekongi* locate in hepatomesenteric venules. Risks of schistosomiasis increase with increasing the skin surface that is submerged, and with increasing duration and frequency of contact.

Transmission sites include snail-inhabited lakeshores, ponds, and other stagnant or sluggish freshwater bodies, typically within or near settlements. Sites are typically focal, and vary with season, vector snail and *Schistosoma* fauna, human use (work, leisure, children, and adults), and control measures. The presence and density of cercariae in freshwaters can be determined by microscopy or bioassay.

The cercarial density in infective waters is generally low (<1–3 cercariae per liter). Cercariae tend to cluster at favorable sites. Free cercariae survive in water for <24 h. Free chlorine (1 mg/liter for 30 min at 28°C) can inactivate cercariae.

Rivers. Rivers with past or current transmission sites include the Congo, Nile, Niger, Senegal, and Zambezi in Africa, the Capibaribe, São Francisco, Paraiba, and Paraná in Brazil, and the Changjiang, Euphrates, Jordan, Mekong, and Tigris in Asia. Along the Mekong River, transmission concentrates during the dry season, when river depth is low and host snails are available. In the Nile delta in Egypt, *S. mansoni* has replaced *S. haematobium*.

Lakes and dams. Lakes and dams with past or current transmission sites include the Albert, Chad, Kainji, Kariba, Kyoga, Malawi, Nasser, Tana, Tanganyika, Victoria, and Volta in Africa and Dongting in China. In an irrigated area of Sudan, 32 (65%) of 49 sites studied yielded *Biomphalaria pfeifferi* snails, and *S. mansoni*-infected snails were found at 12 (24%) sites. On Dongting Lake in central People's Republic of China in 1997, 415 (29%) of 1,440 spots surveyed yielded *Oncomelania hupensis hupensis* snails.

Floods. In central People's Republic of China, floods can periodically drown intermediate host snails. In Pernambuco, Brazil, in 2000, after rains flooded the Ipojuca River and flushed *Biomphalaria glabrata* snails into family yards, 662 *S. mansoni* infections were diagnosed in residents, including 412 (62%) cases of acute schistosomiasis.

5.3 SOIL AND PLANTS

Soil (879) is the uppermost cover of Earth's surface (skin) that consists of layers (horizons) of weathering bedrock, mineral and organic particles of various sizes and textures, water, air, roots, manure, and mulch. Soil types range from calcareous rendzina to acidic peat and from fertile brown earth and loess to permafrost and salty playas. Soil is a reservoir for microorganisms and macroorganisms, such as slugs, nematodes, and arthropods. Land makes up 29% (148/510 million km^2) of the surface of the Earth.

Plants (3759, 5930) are multicellular, photosynthetic eukaryotes. Plant cell walls contain cellulose. There are 310,000–420,000 species, including nonvascular (nontracheophytic) liverworts, hornworts, and mosses, and vascular (tracheophytic) club mosses, horsetails, ferns, gymnosperms, and angiosperms (flowering plants, ~250,000 species).

Terrestrial agents (5357, 6499) (Box 5.4) are acquired from contact (walking barefoot, working soil with bare hands, and lying on the beach), inoculation (thorn and splinter), ingestion (via soiled hands, foods, utensils, or geophagia), or inhalation of aerosolized particles (see section 5.5). Among large series of school children in South Africa and Zambia, 47–74% reported geophagia, in Zambia at a volume of 25 g of earth/day. Manure is a source of enteric agents on pasture and freshwater. Bone fertilizer from sheep or cattle is a source of *Bacillus anthracis* and a presumed source of prions in the environment.

DROPLET-AIR CLUSTER
Bacteria

Klebsiella is present in soil (5948). For *Legionella* (1170, 4033, 7125), soil is a likely natural habitat, and handling soil is a risk. In California, Oregon, and Washington states in 2000, *L. longbeachae* infections were linked to contaminated potting soil. In Australia, *L. longbeachae*, *L. bozemanii*, other legionellae, and free-living amebas have been isolated in potting mixes made of composted wood, sawdust, and shredded bark; legionellae have survived in dry potting mix for up to 20 months. *L. longbeachae* has also been isolated from potting soil in Japan.

Fungi (3703, 7758)

A variety of fungi thrives in soil, manure, and rotting wood. A subset is readily aerosolized and predominantly acquired via inhalation of spores (see section 5.5). Fungi can enter homes and hospitals with soil at shoes and in planting pots. Spores can be carried by winds.

Terrestrial, aerosolized fungi include cosmopolitan *Aspergillus* spp. and *Cryptococcus neoformans*, warm-climate *B. dermatitidis* and *Histoplasma capsulatum*, and New World *Coccidioides immitis* and *Paracoccidioides brasiliensis*. *C. immitis* tolerates arid soils of the lower Sonoran Desert, but its terrestrial territory extends to woods in northern California and tropical Central and South America.

FECES-FOOD CLUSTER
Bacteria

Clostridium **(3364, 6362).** *C. botulinum* and *C. perfringens* are ubiquitous in soil. *C. botulinum* can be recovered from ~25% of soil samples. Soil that adheres to vegetables and salads can carry these agents to food production lines.

E. coli **(1624, 3584, 5554, 7554).** Livestock, manure, contaminated compost, and irrigation waters charge pastures and fields with *E. coli* (including *E. coli* O157:H7), resulting in meadow or crop contamination, or leaching into groundwater. At a site in the United Kingdom, where sheep grazed and EHEC caused an outbreak in a scout camp, *E. coli* O157 survived in loamy sand for 15 weeks. At an open-air music festival in the United Kingdom in 1997, cattle dung on soil was the implicated source for an EHEC outbreak. On farms in the United Kingdom where cases in humans had been detected, EHEC was isolated from cowpats.

Yersinia pseudotuberculosis **(5509).** *Y. pseudotuberculosis* has been isolated from soil and irrigation water.

Box 5.4 Agents from soil or plants, by cluster

For dust, see section 5.5.

Feces-food	*C. botulinum, C. perfringens, E. coli; Cyclospora, Cryptosporidium, Toxoplasma; Ascaris, Trichuris*
Environmental	*Aeromonas, B. pseudomallei, C. tetani,* mycobacteria, *Nocardia* (actinomycetoma); *Blastomyces, Sporothrix,* agents of eumycetoma; free-living amebas; *Ancylostoma, Necator, Strongyloides, Toxocara; Tunga*

Protozoa

Cysts of *Entamoeba* and *Giardia* and oocysts of *Cryptosporidium*, *Isospora*, and *Toxoplasma* reside in various types of soils, including dairy farms and public squares. Recovery seems increased from topsoil and reduced during cold winters.

***Cryptosporidium* (470).** In New York State, oocysts were detected in 17% of 782 soil samples from 37 dairy farms.

***Cyclospora cayetanensis* (594, 4076).** Although *C. cayetanensis* has not been isolated from soil, contact with soil is an infection risk confirmed in a case-control study among raspberry farm workers in Guatemala and among consumers of fresh raspberries and strawberries in an outbreak in Florida.

***Giardia* (470).** In New York State, *Giardia* cysts were detected in 4% of 782 soil samples from 37 dairy farms.

***Toxoplasma gondii* (1554, 2519, 6590, 7101).** *T. gondii* oocysts in the soil can be identified by bioassay. They are resilient, surviving in the soil for years. By place, season, soil sample, and test, 1–40% of soil samples yield *T. gondii* oocysts. Ingestion of soil is a risk. In Alabama, in 1976, in an outbreak with seven acute cases and nine infections among 30 members of a large household, a high manifestation index in children, a history of geophagia, and concomitant *Toxocara*, *Giardia*, and *Ascaris* infections pointed to soil from the household yard as the most likely source.

Helminths

Soil is a reservoir for the thick-shelled eggs of *Ascaris*, *Capillaria*, *Echinococcus*, *Taenia*, and *Trichuris*. Climate and soil type modify the abundance of viable eggs in the soil. Mammals (soil on fur and hooves), birds, insects, rains, and perhaps winds can disperse eggs.

***Ascaris* (1098, 2299, 8252).** Human feces, pig waste, and untreated sewage are sources of eggs of *A. lumbricoides* and *A. suis*) in soil. Ingestion of eggs via vegetables, unwashed hands, or geophagia is a risk. In play areas around homes for children in Jamaica, eggs in the soil were clustered, with mean densities of 6–100 eggs/100 g. In Hamadan, Iran, eggs were found in 79% of 259 soil samples collected from 19 public parks over 12 months. In Denmark, eggs were found in 14–35% of soil samples from pig pastures, and infective eggs were abundant in summer.

***Trichuris* (6590, 8252).** Humans, dogs, and foxes can contaminate soils with *T. trichiura* and *T. vulpis*. Ingestion of soil is a risk. In Jamaica, in play areas around homes for children, *Trichuris* eggs in the soil were clustered, with mean densities of 3–270 eggs/100 g. In city public squares of Patagonia, Argentina, *Trichuris* eggs were identified in 1 (0.4%) of 226 topsoil samples.

ZOONOTIC CLUSTER
Bacteria

In soil polluted with animal excreta or birth secretions, *Coxiella burnetii* can survive for up to 150 days (6435).

Helminths

Soil polluted with *Echinococcus multilocularis* eggs is a potential source for infection in humans, in particular, farm and garden soils. In city squares in Patagonia, Argentina, *Taenia-Echinococcus* eggs have been isolated in topsoil through all seasons, with an overall prevalence of 2% (5/226 samples) (6590).

ENVIRONMENTAL CLUSTER
Bacteria

The great majority of bacteria in soil are apathogenic. However, soils of various types are reservoirs for bacteria infective to humans and animals, which humans can acquire from microtrauma. Soil-dwelling bacteria include *Acinetobacter* (7740), *Aeromonas* (7694), *B. anthracis*, *B. pseudomallei*, *Clostridium tetani*, and environmental mycobacteria.

***B. pseudomallei* (1730, 5300, 7432).** Ingestion of muddy soil is a hazard. Moist surface soils, rice paddies, newly planted fields, and sediments in canals, drains, and lakes, as well as garden soils and playgrounds, all yield *B. pseudomallei*. In endemic areas, 4% to >50% of soil samples test positive. However, earlier findings may have been confounded by avirulent *B. thailandensis* that was described only in 1998.

***C. tetani* (7635, 8169).** *C. tetani* is ubiquitous in soil. Some 10–65% of soil samples test positive. *C. tetani* has also been isolated from horse manure. Microtrauma inoculates the *C. tetani* into the skin.

Mycobacteria (1290, 3961, 5281, 8313). *Mycobacteria* with a confirmed or likely reservoir in moist soil include *M. avium*, *M. intracellulare*, *M. fortuitum*, *M. scrofulaceum*, and *M. leprae*. In San Francisco, 55% of potted-plant soils from homes of 290 persons infected by human immunodeficiency virus (HIV) yielded MAC, compared with 0.3% (1/397) of food samples and 0.8% (4/528) of water samples. From stepping on nails, four children were reported to contract *M. fortuitum* soft-tissue infection. In Louisiana, gardening on grounds visited by free-living armadillos was the only risk from the exposure history of a 27-year-old kidney transplant recipient who developed multibacillary leprosy.

Nocardia (3782, 4550, 6629). *Nocardia* inhabits soil, beach sands, decaying plants, and house dust. In low-income countries, *Nocardia* is mainly acquired percutaneously, from thorns, splinters, or bites by mammals, insects, or ticks, resulting in subcutaneous abscesses or actinomycetoma. This mode is rare in high-income countries in which *Nocardia* is mainly acquired through inhalation of aerosols. Dry, windy weather facilitates aerosolization.

Rhodococcus equi (7300). *R. equi* inhabits soil and cattle and horse manure.

Protozoa
Free-living amebas (436, 4777, 6716, 7844). Gardens, fields, and pristine soils harbor *Acanthamoeba*, *Balamuthia*, *Hartmannella*, *Naegleria*, and *Vahlkampfia*. Free-living amebas have been detected in soil from the Antarctic and the Andean Altiplano (at 3,800 m) and in sewage, dust, and air-conditioning filters. Free-living amebas are potential vectors of *Legionella* and likely other intracellular agents. Putative modes of acquisition are inhalation of dust and ingestion of runoff water.

Fungi
Numerous fungi thrive in soil, on plant roots (mycorrhiza), decaying or living wood, plants, manure, and keratin. Soil-dwelling fungi can produce potent antibiotics.

A virulent subset (geofungi) is mainly acquired from trauma, causing localized superficial or deep infections, including septic arthritis, chromomycosis, and eumycetoma (5861, 6551, 7143, 7928). Geofungi include species of *Acremonium*, *Absidia*, *Cladophialophora*, *Cladosporium*, *Fonsecaea*, *Fusarium*, *Madurella*, *Penicillium*, *Rhinosporidium*, *Rhizopus*, *Rhodotorula*, *Scedosporium*, and *Sporothrix*.

Sporothrix schenckii (1522, 3070, 5338, 5721, 6613). Reservoirs include water, soil, mosses, grasses, hay, wood, thorn plants, leaves, and potting soil. *Sphagnum* (peat moss) seems a preferred substrate, and it is a well-documented vehicle. At a tree nursery in Florida in 1994, 14% (9/65) of workers developed sporotrichosis from working with *Sphagnum*. In a U.S. multistate outbreak in 1988, 84 persons exposed to *Sphagnum* from packing tree seedlings contracted clinical sporotrichosis. Most infections are acquired via microtrauma from work or leisure outdoor activities. Unusual modes of acquisition are inhalation of conidia from the environment or laboratory and contact with or trauma by cats, squirrels, or fish (e.g., *Tilapia mozambica*). Sporotrichosis is an occupational hazard for plant and wood workers, miners, and farmers. Children have contracted clinical sporotrichosis from playing in hay bales or piles of old prairie hay. In Peru in 1995–1997, 60% of 238 cases were children ≤14 years of age, for a peak disease rate of 1/1,000 per year in this age group.

Helminths
Hookworms (*Ancylostoma* and *Necator*) (1638, 4598, 6500, 7634, 8152). Hookworm larvae are acquired percutaneously, both of *A. duodenale* and *N. americanus*, which cause intestinal infection, and of *A. braziliense* and *A. caninum*, which cause cutaneous larva migrans. Unlike thick-shelled *Ascaris* and *Toxocara* eggs, hookworm eggs and larvae are sensitive to desiccation and cold. Warm, sandy (porous), moist soils are optimal for larval development and high prevalence. In contrast, clay soils seem unfavorable. In rural Nigeria, *N. americanus* larvae were monitored by marking fecal deposits with metal stickers. During the dry season, infective larvae (L3) retreated to deeper soil, and density was low (<250/0.5 kg), while in the wet season, L3 aggregated in topsoil (0–5 cm) at high density (up to 1,500/0.5 kg).

Strongyloides (6925). Soil can harbor infective (L3) *Strongyloides* larvae and free-living adults. Although their presence in soil is poorly documented, skin contacts with soil are a risk, including by bare feet and hands. While most human infections are reported as *S. stercoralis*, animal feces in soil are potential sources of zoonotic *Strongyloides*.

Toxocara (1442, 2778, 6590, 7638). Ingestion of soil is a risk for *Toxocara*. Eggs of *T. canis* or *T. cati* are readily recovered from soils, including backyards, sandboxes, playgrounds, parks, and flower beds, typically (>12 reports) in 5–40% of samples. Eggs are hardy and remain viable in the soil for up to 2 years, including through cold winters. Dogs are not the only culprits. Video records in Japan have implicated nocturnal cats as a major source of eggs in public parks.

SKIN-BLOOD CLUSTER
Candida albicans has been isolated from soil and pigeon droppings.

5.4 TERRESTRIAL BIOMES
Biomes (266, 7929). People exploring the remotest corners on the Earth, from Alaska to Patagonia, and from Galapagos to Guam, are being exposed to virtually all ecosystems. Broadly grouped biomes are the topic of this chapter: tropical forests, other woodlands, grasslands, islands, arid lands, desert oases, barren lands (highlands and Arctic tundra), and caves.

Biome-related agents (Box 5.5). Many zoonoses have "sylvatic" cycles that involve wild animals in various biomes. Agents can spread to humans via contact (e.g., skin-

> **Box 5.5** Agents and infections from biomes, by agent clusters
>
> For bites, see chapter 1; for vectors, see chapter 4; for freshwater, see section 5.2; for livestock, see section 2.3; and for work, see section 12.4.
>
> **Tropical forests and forest savannas**
> Droplet-air *Cryptococcus, Paracoccidioides*
> Zoonotic *Alphavirus* (e.g., CHIKV, RRV, and VEEV), *Arenavirus* (e.g., Lassa, JUNV), *Filovirus* (EBOV and MARV), *Flavivirus* (e.g., DENV, WNV, and YFV), *Orthobunyavirus* (OROV), *Orthopoxvirus* (MPXV); *Orientia*, *Leishmania, P. falciparum, T. cruzi, T. brucei* sl; *Loa, Wuchereria, Onchocerca*
> Environmental *Leptospira; F. pedrosoi; S. fuelleborni*
> Skin-blood *Treponema pertenue*
>
> **Sclerophyll, temperate, and boreal forests**
> Droplet-air *Histoplasma*
> Zoonotic *Alphavirus* (EEEV, SINV, and WEEV), *Flavivirus* (e.g., SLEV, TBEV, and WNV), *Hantavirus* (e.g., DOBV, HTNV, SNV, PUUV, and SEOV), *Orthobunyavirus* (e.g., INKV, LACV, and TAHV), *Phlebovirus* (sandfly fever virus); *B. burgdorferi*, relapsing borreliae, *R. conorii, R. rickettsii; E. multilocularis*
>
> **Grasslands**
> Zoonotic *Arenavirus* (South American VHF), *Flavivirus* (JEV and WNV), *Hantavirus* (e.g., ANDV and SNV), *Nairovirus* (CCHFV), *Orthobunyavirus* (TAHV), *Phlebovirus* (RVFV); *B. anthracis, C. burnetii, F. tularensis, R. sibirica, Y. pestis; Leishmania, T. cruzi, T. brucei rhodesiense; E. granulosus, O. volvulus*
>
> **Arid lands**
> Droplet-air Conjunctivitis, ocular *C. trachomatis, N. meningitidis* meningitis; respiratory mycoses
> Zoonotic *Y. pestis; L. donovani, T. cruzi*
> Skin-blood Pyodermia, nonvenereal *T. pallidum*; ectoparasites (pediculosis and scabies)

ning), inoculation (e.g., bites by invertebrates), inhalation (e.g., environmental aerosols), or ingestion (e.g., unwashed fruits).

TROPICAL FORESTS AND SAVANNAS

Tropical forests (266, 7503) aggregate rain forests, cloud forests, monsoonal forests, gallery forests along rivers, mangrove forests, and tropical tree savannas. The latter are parklike transition zones, from closed-canopy forests to prairies, dotted by solitary trees. Mangrove forests (60–180,000 km^2) are essentially tropical, lining coasts in western, eastern and southern Africa, the Americas (from Baja California to northern Peru, and from the Gulf of Mexico to Brazil), Southwest, Southcentral, and Southeast Asia, Australia (to nearly latitude 39°S), southern Japan (to latitude 31°N), and many Pacific islands.

Agents from tropical forests (Box 5.5). Bites by forest and canopy arthropods are a major hazard. At risk are residents in forest areas and workers such as loggers and miners. Invertebrate sylvatic vectors can enter villages or urban areas, causing outbreaks or, worse, initiating peridomestic cycles. For bites by mammals, see chapter 1.

Viruses

The tropics are a transmission epicenter for many enteric and respiratory viral infections (e.g., measles), many of which are preventable by vaccines. Of note are viruses that by their vectors or sylvatic cycles are associated with tropical forest habitats.

Africa. Viruses from ≥7 genera circulate in tropical forests of Africa: (i) *Alphavirus* (Chikungunya virus [CHIKV] and O'nyong-nyong virus [ONNV]), (ii) *Arenavirus* (Lassa virus), (iii) *Filovirus* (Ebola virus [EBOV], and Marburg virus [MARV]), (iv) *Flavivirus* (DENV, West Nile virus [WNV], and yellow fever virus [YFV]), (v) *Lyssavirus* (rabies virus in mammals, locally Duvenhage virus in bats), (vi) *Orthopoxvirus* monkeypox virus (MPXV), and (vii) *Phlebovirus* (RVFV). **CHIKV (69, 1917).** Habitats suitable for CHIKV transmission include rain, swamp, gallery forests, and tree savannas. **MPXV (4281).** MPXV is enzootic in forested areas of West and Central Africa. **RVFV (1760).** Vector mosquitoes seem to prefer transition zones between forests and savannas that receive intermittent heavy rains or become flooded intermittently.

America. Viruses from ≥5 genera circulate in tropical forests of Latin America: (i) *Alphavirus* (Mayaro virus [MAYV], and VEEV), (ii) *Arenavirus* (Guanarito virus [GUAV], Junin virus [JUNV], and Machupo virus [MACV]), (iii) *Flavivirus* (DENV, YFV, perhaps SLEV), and (iv) *Lyssavirus* (rabies virus in mammals and bats),

(v) *Orthobunyavirus* (Oropouche [OROV]). **DENV and YFV.** DENV and YFV circulate in canopy-dwelling mammals such as monkeys and their mosquitoes (1841). **MAYV (1842, 7313, 7517).** MAYV circulates in Amazon rain forest. In French Guiana in 1994–1995, residents of Cayenne City had a significantly lower seroprevalence (0.7% or 6/873) than residents along rivers and forest fringes (11% or 118/1,089). Ecosystem disturbances are likely to increase human risks. In northcentral Venezuela, MAYV has been reported in cacao (*Theobroma*) plantations that are interspersed with preserved indigenous tall trees, such as *Bauhinia* and *Erythrina* (both Fabaceae), *Ceiba* (Bombacaceae), and *Ficus* (Moraceae). **OROV.** OROV circulates in rain forest areas, in midges (*Coquillettidia*) and sloths (*Bradypus*), possibly monkeys (7397). **VEEV (456, 2365).** VEEV circulates in South American lowland tropical and subtropical forests and swamps. In Venezuela, trees indicative for VEEV circulation include *Attalea* (Arecaceae), *Copaifera* (Fabaceae), *Ficus*, *Jacaranda* (Bignoniaceae), *Licania* (Chrysobalanaceae), and *Protium* (Burseraceae).

Asia. Viruses from ≥2 genera circulate in tropical forests of Asia: CHIKV from *Alphavirus* and DENV and Kyasanur Forest disease virus (KFDV) from *Flavivirus*.

Australia. Viruses from ≥3 genera circulate in tropical forests of Australia: the Barmah Forest disease virus (BFDV) and Ross River virus (RRV) from *Alphavirus*, MVEV from *Flavivirus*, and Australian bat lyssavirus (ABLV) from *Lyssavirus*.

Bacteria

The tropics are a transmission epicenter for enteric and some systemic bacterial infections. In particular, associated with tropical forest habitats are *Leptospira*, *M. ulcerans* (for Buruli ulcer, see section 5.2), *Orientia tsutsugamushi* (scrub typhus), and *Treponema pallidum pertenue* (yaws).

***Leptospira* (314).** *Leptospira* can be shed by tropical rodents and bats. In Nicaragua, wood gathering is a risk for residents to contract leptospirosis.

***O. tsutsugamushi* (1681, 2308, 3606).** *O. tsutsugamushi* is the agent of scrub typhus. Vector (larval) mites prefer tropical vegetation, including scrub and clearings left by logging and "slash-and-burn" agriculture, secondary growth forest, and riverine forests. Outliers exist in semidesert and subtropical climate areas. In Hiroshima prefecture, Japan, in 1990–1999, 55 (87%) of 63 scrub typhus cases were contracted in the Oota River valley.

***T. pallidum pertenue* (237, 1817, 3043, 6739).** *T. pallidum pertenue*, the agent of yaws, has been reduced to pockets in South America, Africa, and the Southwest Pacific. Of historical note, in an outbreak in the South African Witwatersrand mines of 1942, yaws was transmitted deep underground (−1,630 m) under tropical climate conditions, by skin contacts among workers, but not on the surface, where weather conditions were less favorable.

Fungi

The tropics are a transmission epicenter for deep-seated fungi, in particular, tropical Latin America. A speculative explanation for this peculiar pattern is the affinity of fungi for particular woods or soil types.

***Cryptococcus* (2184, 4266, 5015, 7282).** Wood is a natural habitat. In Australia, *C. neoformans gattii* seems associated with debris of river red gum (*Eucalyptus camaldulensis*, Myrtaceae) and forest red gum (*E. tereticornis*). Koalas, which feed on red gum, might play the role birds assume in other parts of the world for *C. neoformans neoformans*. Infection rates seem higher in Native Australians than in the general population, perhaps because Aborigines used to shelter under red gum ("don't sit under a red gum tree"). In South America, native trees from various genera can host *C. neoformans* (var. *gattii* or *neoformans*), including *Ficus* (Moraceae), *Guettarda* (Rubiaceae), *Moquilea* (Chrysobalanaceae), and *Terminalia* (Combretaceae). In Brazil, *C. neoformans* has been isolated from 19% (6/32) of hollow trees.

***Fonsecaea pedrosoi* (2245, 4497, 6894).** *F. pedrosoi* has a reservoir in the evergreen forest. In Madagascar, thorny *Solanum macrocarpum* is a traditionally incriminated source of chromomycosis in wood cutters. In Maranhao, Brazil, two palm cutters contracted *F. pedrosoi* gluteal chromoblastomycosis from sitting on fruit shells of babaçu palm (*Attalea phalerata*), which grows in gallery and disturbed forests. The link of chromomycosis and rain forest might be confounded by frequent barefoot walking of people in the rural tropics.

***P. brasiliensis* (707, 1036).** In endemic areas of Argentina, Brazil, Colombia, and Venezuela, the fungus is associated with middle-altitude (500–1,800 m) humid forests that have precipitations of 1,000–2,000 mm per year. Most case reports are from Brazil.

Protozoa

The tropics are a transmission epicenter for enteric protozoa (*Entamoeba* and *Giardia*) and tissue protozoa (*Leishmania*, *Plasmodium*, and *Trypanosoma*). Explanations for enteric protozoa include hygienic conditions, and for tissue protozoa, climatic restrictions of arthropod vectors.

***Leishmania*. Cutaneous leishmaniasis (CL) (5154, 6163).** Causative agents of cutaneous leishmaniasis include *Leishmania braziliensis* sensu lato (sl), *L. mexi-*

cana sl, and *L. panamensis*. In a coffee-growing area of Colombia, an outbreak of zoonotic CL caused 27 cases among 1,127 inhabitants, for an attack rate of 2%. In the Brazilean Amazon, *Lutzomyia flaviscutellata* and *Proechimys guyannensis* maintain *L. mexicana* sl in deforested areas, plantations, and secondary forest. Humans acquire zoonotic CL when residing in forests or engaging in nocturnal forest work such as hunting. **Visceral leishmaniasis (VL) (2188, 8411).** The zoonotic agent of visceral leishmaniasis is *L. infantum* (*L. chagasi*). Habitats in South America include primary and secondary forests. In Sudan, the main habitat is savanna woodland that features termite hills and *Acacia seyal* (Fabaceae) and *Balanites aegyptiaca* (Zygophyllaceae) trees. At a focus in Dinder National Park, 10% of *Phlebotomus orientalis* sandflies tested positive for *Leishmania*. At risk are wood cutters, shepherds, game wardens, and military personnel. In the Sudan, VL could be anthroponotic, as human reservoirs are available, or zoonotic, as cases occur in remote areas.

***Plasmodium* (2093, 2224, 5524, 5678, 6821).** Tropical forests are core habitats for *P. falciparum* and other plasmodia infective to humans that are endemic in West and Central Africa, the Amazon, Southcentral and Southeast Asia, and the Southwest Pacific (for vectors see section 4.5). Malaria in tropical forests is transmitted year-round.

- Africa. Tropical game preserves and national parks within or adjacent to malarious areas include Amboseli (Kenya), Caprivi (Namibia), Etosha (Namibia), Krüger (South Africa), Luangwa (Zambia), Ngorongoro and Serengeti (both Tanzania), Omo (Ethiopia), and Victoria Falls (Zimbabwe). In Krüger National Park, the risk of falciparum malaria for visitors on chloroquine plus proguanil chemoprophylaxis was ~0.8/1,000 per month.
- South America. Tree bromeliads are breeding sites for *Anopheles* (*Kerteszia*). In the nine countries that share the Amazon rainforest (Bolivia, Brazil, Colombia, Ecuador, French Guiana, Guyana, Peru, Surinam, and Venezuela), 70 million people are exposed to the infection, and in 2002 these nine countries reported 0.8 million cases (90% of the Latin American total). Of reported cases, 30% were due to *P. falciparum*.
- Asia. In Orissa, India, where most infections are due to *P. falciparum*, the parasitemia prevalence was five times higher (19.1%) in forest residents than in the plains (2.8%), and disease rates exhibited a similar gradient (348 versus 61/1,000 per year).
- Plantations (1568, 2800, 5517, 6809, 6928). *Anopheles* thrives in commercial fruit orchards and in tea, coffee, sugar, cotton, and rubber plantations. On a sugar estate in Malawi (located at 60 m above sea level), the *P. falciparum* parasitemia point prevalence was 15%. In plantations in western Kenya at 1,700 m above sea level, the proportion of malaria among all hospital admissions increased from 5–11% in 1965–1989 to 20–33% in 1990–1997, and lethality increased from 1% to 6%. This increase was likely due to the introduction of chloroquine-resistant *P. falciparum*. On a tea estate in Assam, India, in 1991–1993, the infection rate was 0.5–30/100 per year; 69% of infections were due to *P. falciparum*. In Thailand in 1996–1997, malaria cases from plantations accounted for 10–35% of all cases from districts listing plantations. *Anopheles dirus* and *A. minimus* seemed well adapted to this habitat.

Trypanosoma. Human African trypanosomiasis (HAT) and Chagas disease are adapted to tropical forests and forest savannas. ***T. brucei* sl. *T. brucei gambiense* (1127, 2919, 3802, 5375, 8090).** In West and Central Africa, habitats suitable for *Glossina* and *T. brucei gambiense* include forests near settlements and fields, forest galleries along rivers where people defecate and wash, coffee, cocoa, and oil palm plantations, including the paths frequented by humans, secondary forests, and mangrove forests. In Guinea, mangrove cleared for a golf course became a human-made hunting ground for *Glossina*. ***T. brucei rhodesiense* (3661, 4523, 5298, 7063).** Reported sites where tourists acquired *T. brucei rhodesiense* and HAT include in Botswana the Okavango Park, in Rwanda the Kagera Park, and in Tanzania the Serengeti, Ngorongoro, and Tarangire parks. ***T. cruzi* (225, 3014, 5462, 6391, 7395, 8099).** Habitats that host sylvatic bugs (for *Triatoma* and *Rhodnius*, see section 4.7) and small host mammals include tree epiphytes in rain forests, mosaics of gallery forests with shrub savanna (Brazilean "cerrado"), subtropical Gran Chaco woodland (with "quebracho" trees, *Schinopsis*: Anacardiaceae), hollow trees in Bolivian Chaco (typically *Ruprechtia*: Polygonaceae), and palm tree crowns in tropical dry forests (e.g., American oil palm, *Attalea butyracea*: Arecaceae). Large-scale deforestation for cattle ranching, e.g., in Panama and Brazil, has favored *A. butyracea* forests and *Rhodnius pallescens*, a main vector of *T. cruzi*. *A. butyracea* can harbor high numbers of *R. pallescens* (in a survey in Colombia, on average, ~20/palm). When cut for thatch, bugs from fronds can become a source for infections in humans. In Panama, corozo palms (*Scheelea zonensis*) were found to provide excellent shelter for *R. pallescens* and *T. dimidiata*. ***T. rangeli* (225, 3014).** *T. rangeli* ranges in Latin America, in forest and peridomestic habitats that overlap with *T. cruzi*. Although innocuous for humans, *T. rangeli* can confound parasitological and serological surveys in animals and humans.

Helminths

The tropics are a transmission epicenter for enteric nematodes (*Ascaris*, hookworms, and *Trichuris*) and filariae (*Loa*, *Onchocerca*, and *Wuchereria*). Explanations for the former include hygienic conditions, and for the latter, climatic restrictions of arthropod vectors.

***Loa loa* (7460, 7953).** *Chrysops* vector flies inhabit closed-canopy forest and forest fringes in equatorial Africa. In Cameroon in 2001, 42 villages and 4,532 inhabitants were examined for microfilariae of *L. loa*. Microfilariae prevalence and density were 0 in eight villages ($n = 1,167$) in grass savanna at 1500–2200 m, 3% and 167/ml in eight villages ($n = 878$) in savanna-forest patches at 900–1,100 m, 33% and 3,125/ml in ten villages ($n = 1,029$) in savanna-forest mosaics with swamps and sluggish streams at 750–800 m, 7% and 325/ml in seven villages ($n = 818$) in deciduous rain forest at 100–500 m, and 10% and 433/ml in nine villages ($n = 640$) in humid rain forest also at 100–500 m.

***O. volvulus* (1707, 5628).** *O. volvulus* is endemic in uncontrolled areas of tropical Africa, Latin America, and Southwest Asia. Control activities have changed endemicity. In Latin America, former habitats included forests and coffee and tea plantations. In Africa, the remaining habitats include rain forest, tree savanna, and secondary forests along river basins.

***S. fuelleborni* (316, 5701).** *S. fuelleborni* is enzootic in *Pongidae* and endemic in forest peoples of tropical Africa and Papua New Guinea. In Papua New Guinea, endemic areas are lowland swamps that grow nipa palms (*Nypa fruticans*) and sago palms (*Metroxylon sagu*, both Arecaceae) and receive abundant rainfall ($>$1,500–3,000 mm/year).

***Trichinella nativa*.** *T. nativa* is enzootic in tropical Africa.

***W. bancrofti* and *Brugia malayi* (4116, 5234).** Vector mosquitoes inhabit tropical and subtropical forests of Africa, Latin America, Asia, and the Pacific, including jungle, swamps, mangroves, ricefields, and banana, rubber, and coconut plantations, provided that stagnant freshwater is available for breeding. In the Philippines, the occurrence of bancroftian filariasis is linked to cultivation of Manila hemp ("abaca," *Musa textiles*, Zingiberaceae), water-filled leaf axils of which are breeding sites for *Aedes poicilius*. Though banana (*Musa sapientum*), taro (*Clocasia esculenta*, Araceae), and *Pandanus* also offer breeding sites, abaca supports the largest *A. poicilius* populations.

MEDITERRANEAN, TEMPERATE, AND BOREAL FORESTS

Forests are major biomes, covering 15–20% (20–30/148 million km^2) of the land surface of the earth (266, 1718, 6742). Mediterranean vegetation is characterized by plants with evergreen, hard leaves, in particular, in shrublands occurring in the Cape Province of South Africa (fynbos), lowland California (chapparal), central Chile (matorral), southwestern Australia (kwongan), and the Mediterranean (maquis). Temperate vegetation is characterized by deciduous, broad leaf forests that were the original cover of much of eastern North America, the southern Andes, western Europe, and East Asia. Boreal forests (taiga) are characterized by coniferous trees, mainly species of *Abies*, *Larix*, *Picea*, and *Pinus*. Taiga covers vast pre-Arctic areas, in North America from Alaska to the Great Lakes and Newfoundland, in Eurasia from Scandinavia to Siberia and Hokkaido.

Agents from nontropical forests (Box 5.5). Mediterranean, temperate, and boreal forests support an amazing variety of sylvatic cycles and vector-borne agents. Whereas Mediterranean and temperate forest areas are densely populated, the vast taiga in the Northern Hemisphere is scarcely populated.

Viruses
The focus here is on viruses with sylvatic cycles in various forest biomes.

North America (2230, 4920, 4921, 5062, 7932). Viruses from at least six genera circulate in North American forests: (i) *Alphavirus* (EEEV, WEEV), (ii) *Coltivirus* (Colorado tick fever virus [CTFV]), (iii) *Flavivirus* (Powassan virus [POWV], SLEV, and WNV), (iv) *Hantavirus* (Sin Nombre virus [SNV]), (v) *Lyssavirus*, and (vi) *Orthobunyavirus* (Inkoo virus [INKV], Jamestown Canyon virus [JCV], LaCrosse encephalitis virus [LACV], and snowshoe hare virus [SSHV]). **Pinyon-juniper.** Pinyon-juniper (*Pinus edulis-Juniperus osteosperma*) forests of the arid southwestern United States (four-corner area of Arizona, Colorado, New Mexico, and Utah) are a core enzootic area of SNV, although infected reservoir mice (*Peromyscus maniculatus* and *P. leucopus*) have been captured in at least six other states. **Ponderosa pine.** Open stands of ponderosa (*Pinus ponderosa*) and shrubs on rocky surfaces are the preferred habitat for CTFV that circulates in *Dermacentor andersoni* ticks, small rodents, and porcupines (*Erethizon dorsatum*). **Eastern hardwood.** Eastern hardwood forests and woodlots of the upper midwestern United States maintain LACV and its vector mosquitoes. A risk for LACV infection is a domicile within 100 m from a hollow tree. **Boreal forest.** In boreal forest, the risk for residents to contract INKV, JCV, or SSHV is 23 times greater than for people who live in areas of tundra or permafrost. Likely vectors are Arctic *Aedes* species. Snow-melting pools maintain high densities of *Aedes* that are counterbalanced only by cold summer winds.

Eurasia (4113, 4149, 4575, 7262). Viruses from at least six genera circulate in Eurasian forests: (i) *Alphavirus*

(Sinbis virus [SINV]), (ii) *Flavivirus* (WNV, tick-borne encephalitis virus [TBEV]), (iii) *Hantavirus* (Dobrawa-Belgrade virus [DOBV], Hantaan virus [HTNV], Puumala virus [PUUV], and Seoul viru [SEOV]), (iv) *Lyssavirus*, (v) *Phlebovirus* (sandfly fever Naples virus [SFNV], sandfly fever Sicilian virus [SFSV], sandfly fever Toscana virus [TOSV]), and (vi) *Orthobunyavirus* (INKV, and Tahyna virus [TAHV]).

Mediterranean. Mediterranean vegetation is suitable for the circulation of WNV, as well as the serotypes of sandfly fever virus (Naples [SFNV], Sicilian [SFSV], and Toscana [TOSV]) that are carried by species of *Phlebotomus*.

Beech forest. Beech forests (*Fagus sylvatica*) with a well-developed brush layer are habitat for PUUV. Years with rich beech fruiting are likely to result in expanding host rodent (*Clethrionomys clareolus*) populations and intensified transmission. Beech forests seem to be natural habitat for mosquito-borne TAHV. Beech forests support foci and enzootic patches of TBEV. Ideal habitats for *Ixodes ricinus* ticks are warm, moderately humid, lowland broadleaf forests with clearings and well-developed understory that offers shelter for small mammals. Vector ticks avoid farmland, open fields, and dry slopes that are devoid of trees, as well as coniferous mountain forests. For reasons not well known, foci can be stable, expand, merge, contract, or become dormant or reactivated. In northern Bohemia in the 1950s–1960s, brown coal mining and environmental degradation went along with an extinction of TBEV foci. With vegetation recovering in the 1990s–2000s, foci of TBEV seem to have become reestablished.

Northern forests. Coniferous northern forests are habitats for INKV and SINV. For INKV, the main northern vector is *Aedes communis*. Taiga and northern broadleaf forests are also habitat for *Ixodes persulcatus* and the Eurasian variant of TBEV.

Bacteria

The focus here is on bacteria with sylvatic cycles in temperate forest biomes.

Lyme borreliosis (3773, 4232, 4292, 6333, 7097). *Borrelia burgdorferi* sl, by its vector ticks, is associated with forests in the Northern Hemisphere. In the eastern United States, changes of land use have led to increased peridomestic risks of Lyme disease. In the 1900s, when people moved to cities, cleared land was abandoned and populated by secondary forest, mice, deer, and ticks. Since the 1980s, when people returned to periurban housing, proximity to deer and ticks facilitated transmission.

Foci have emerged in periurban parks and recreational areas in North America and western Europe. In the Boston, Mass., area, an outbreak of Lyme disease in 1980–1987 affected 35% of residents who lived within 5 km of a nature preserve. In the Helsinki, Finland, area, 32% (234/726) of *I. ricinus* ticks from four heavily used recreational areas tested positive for *B. burgdorferi* sl, and tick density was 16/100 m. In a recreational area in southern England covered with beech, oak, maple, pine, spruce, and larch trees, and with dense undergrowth harboring squirrels (*Sciurus carolinensis*), hedgehogs (*Erinaceus europaeus*), and deer (*Capreolus capreolus*), the average *I. ricinus* density from vegetation was 0.5–4.4 (mean, 1.4)/m2. In 2 years, 1,082 visitors reported to a local clinic for removal of 1,366 *I. ricinus* (82% nymphs, 15% larvae, and 3% adults). Children were more frequently attacked than adults. In children, 48% of bites were at the head and axilla; in adults, 48% of bites were at the lower leg. Tick attacks were highly seasonal. *Borrelia* was prevalent in 6–10% of nymphs by PCR, and in 5–17% by immunofluorescence assay. Genospecies typing identified *B. garinii* and *B. valaisiana*.

Tick-borne relapsing fever (TBRF) (2103). In the United States, TBRF is associated by its *Ornithodoros* vector tick with forested, mountainous habitats, typically at elevations of 650–2,300 m.

Rickettsia **(2750, 6794).** Recent data on the ecology of *R. rickettsii* in North America and *R. conorii* in the Mediterranean are surprisingly scarce. In the United States, *R. rickettsii* circulates mainly in *D. andersoni* and small mammals predominantly in woodland areas in the East. Suspected habitats for an enzootic cycle of *R. conorii* carried by *Rhipicephalus sanguineus* sl ticks are maquis and garrigue formations.

Fungi

Some fungi are associated with decaying woods (see section 5.3).

Protozoa

The focus here is on protozoa with sylvatic cycles in Mediterranean vegetation.

Leishmania **(2591, 3932, 6004).** Mediterranean vegetation characterized by olive (Olea europaea), pine (*Pinus halepensis*), oaks (*Quercus coccifera*, *Q. ilex*, and *Q. pubescens*), strawberry tree (*Arbutus unedo*), and rock roses (*Cistus albidus* and *C. salviifolius*) is favorable for *Phlebotomus ariasi* and *P. perniciosus* that carry *Leishmania infantum* from dogs and small mammals (rats and foxes) to humans in whom it causes VL, and infrequently cutaneous lesions. Typical foci are reported in France (Provence, Côte d'Azur, and Corse), Italy (Sicily and Toscana), and Spain (Priorat in Catalonia).

Plasmodium. Before elimination in the 1950s, the Mediterranean was home for *P. vivax* and *P. falciparum*. Countries with Mediterranean climates remain vulnerable to introduction and local transmission by suitable *Anopheles*.

Helminths
T. nativa and *E. multilocularis* are enzootic in temporal and boreal forest biomes of the Northern Hemisphere.

GRASSLANDS
Grasslands (266, 3738, 7929) are natural cover for ~37% (55/148 million km^2) of the world's terrestrial surface. Grassland biotopes include tropical savannas (bush savanna, grass savanna, e.g., Sahel), and temperate to cold prairies (e.g., Pampas, North American tall- and short-grass prairies, and central Asian steppes). However, ~60% (33 million km^2) of natural grassland has become farmland, including for livestock grazing, crops, and fallow fields.

Agents from grasslands (Box 5.5). Infectious disease hazards in grasslands include livestock (cattle, sheep, goats, and camels), rodents and their ectoparasites, and winds that carry particles from soil or animals.

Viruses
Viruses that are maintained in farmed grasslands include: (i) *Arenavirus* (GUAV, JUNV, MACV), (ii) *Flavivirus* (Japanese encephalitis virus [JEV], and WNV), (iii) *Hantavirus* (e.g., Andes virus [ANDV], HTNV, and SNV), (iv) *Nairovirus* (Crimean-Congo hemorrhagic fever virus [CCHFV]), (v) *Orthobunyavirus* (TAHV), and (vi) *Phlebovirus* (RVFV). Farm and crop workers are at risk of rodent contacts, in particular, during harvest when outbreaks of viral hemorrhagic fever (VHF) may occur, in South America: Argentinian, Bolivian, and Venezuelan VHF. Rainfall may bring abundant mosquitoes and outbreaks of encephalitis (JEV and WNV).

***Hantavirus* (636, 2363).** *Hantavirus* is enzootic in grasslands, including SNV in the southwestern United States; ANDV in northern Argentina and adjacent Chile, Bolivia, and Uruguay; Laguna Negra virus (LNV) in the Gran Chaco; and HTNV in People's Republic of China. In Anhui Province, People's Republic of China, cases of hemorrhagic fever with renal syndrome (HFRS, due to HTNV) correlated with rainfall and crop production.

JEV (5137, 5814). Wet rice fields are breeding sites for vector mosquitoes and foster epidemics. In Sri Lanka, the seroprevalence in children 8–15 years of age is 2% (3/129) in a high-altitude wet zone, 3% (10/339) in a mid-altitude zone, 17% (85/506) in a low-altitude, irrigated rice-growing zone, and 28% (48/172) in a low-altitude semi-urban area. Pesticides and habitat destruction seem to contribute to decreased disease rates.

TAHV and WNV are associated with mosquitoes that breed in cold, central Asian steppes.

Bacteria
Small mammals and grazing livestock maintain grassland cycles of *B. anthracis*, *Brucella*, *Coxiella*, *Francisella*, *Rickettsia sibirica*, and *Yersinia pestis*.

***B. anthracis* (2022, 6678).** Corpses of infected herbivores (cattle, sheep, and bison) are involved in a biological grassland cycle: decomposing corpses release spores that contaminate soil for months.

***C. burnetii* (6435).** *C. burnetii* naturally circulates in herbivores in grasslands, including sheep. After parturition, *C. burnetii* survives in air for 2 weeks and in soil for 6 months.

***Francisella tularensis* (346, 2347).** *F. tularensis* circulates in grasslands, in ticks, birds, rodents, rabbits, and herbivores such as sheep. In Texas in 2002, a tularemia epizootic affected wild-caught prairie dogs (*Cynomys ludovicianus*) kept at a pet trade facility, and an exposed person contracted tularemia.

***R. sibirica* (405, 4388, 6455, 6493).** Siberian tick typhus is widely distributed in Central Asia, including Armenia, Russia (Siberia, from Krasnojarsk in the west to the Altai and the Far East), Kazakhstan, Mongolia, and the northern People's Republic of China. It is seasonally (March–October) transmitted by ixodid ticks, in particular, *Dermacentor* (e.g., *D. marginatus*) and *Haemaphysalis* (e.g., *H. concinna*). Habitats are steppes, forest-steppes, meadows, and swampy tussocks. Hosts are rodents and larger wild and domestic mammals.

***V. cholerae* (80).** An association has been suggested for *V. cholerae* with sugar cane (*Saccharum officinarum*) plantations in tropical areas. Cholera endemicity and sugar cane stands are reported to overlap on the Gulf coast of the United States, in northern India, and in Queensland, Australia.

***Y. pestis* (98, 2570, 8109).** Plague foci exist in grasslands in African savanna, North American prairies and semi-deserts, inter-Andean highlands, and Central Asian steppes, with rodents as likely reservoir hosts (see section 3.3). In the North American prairies, a cycle involves prairie dogs, their mounds of bare earth, and vertebrates associated with them. In Asia, foci exist in deserts (gerbil type), steppes (suslik and pika types), meadows (marmot type), and alpine tundra (vole type). In Kazakhstan in 1990–2002, 19 cases of bubonic or bubonic-septic plague were recorded, 14 (74%) in men and 5 (26%) in women. Exposures included flea bites in 11 (58%) and slaughter of ill camels in 5 (26%).

Protozoa

Grass- and farmlands offer microhabitats for *Babesia*, *Leishmania*, and *Trypanosoma*.

***Babesia microti* (992).** In Colorado in the foothills of the Rocky Mountains, *B. microti* was amplified from prairie voles (*Microtus ochrogaster*) by NAT, a rodent that inhabits tall-grass prairies in underground burrows.

Leishmania. *Leishmania* occupies a variety of ecosystems, including farmlands and arid areas. **Cutaneous leishmaniasis (CL).** Old World zoonotic CL (1746, 2174, 4269). Small mammals and *Phlebotomus* maintain cycles in arid areas of North Africa and Southwest and Central Asia. In Central Asia, *P. papatasi* is abundant along river valleys and foothills (1–100/trap) and in oases ($\geq$100/trap). **New World zoonotic CL (1759, 4549, 4903, 8303).** In Texas, zoonotic CL (due to *L. mexicana* sl) circulates in wood rats (*Neotoma micropus*) and *Lutzomyia*, in stands of mesquite (*Prosopis glandulosa*) and cacti (*Opuntia*). In Andean and inter-Andean valleys at 900–3,000 m, zoonotic CL (uta, due to *L. peruviana*) is prevalent, carried by *L. peruensis*, *L. verrucarum*, and other sandflies. These vectors enter houses and temporary shelters near croplands. Enzootic areas extend into northern Argentina and southern Paraguay. No data are available on grasslands in the Pampas further south. **Visceral leishmaniasis (VL, kala azar), Old World (7459).** *P. perniciosus*, a major vector of zoonotic VL in Spain, France, and Italy, is well adapted to *Quercus* shrub, maquis, hill country, farmland, and isolated houses and stables. In southern and eastern Sudan, *P. orientalis* is abundant in tree savanna during the dry season when it carries VL to humans. Indicative trees are *Acacia seyal* (Fabaceae) and *Balanites aegyptiaca* (desert date, Zygophyllaceae). **Visceral leishmaniasis, New World (2366, 6560).** *L. longipalpis*, a major vector of zoonotic VL, is abundant in secondary forest, cultivated areas, pigsties, and cattle corrals. Its range extends into northern Argentina.

***Trypanosoma. T. brucei* (1127, 3517, 8090).** In East Africa, suitable habitats for *Glossina* and *T. brucei rhodesiense* include tree and shrub savannas grazed by game herds and mopane (*Colophospermum mopane*: Fabaceae) forests. Risks for humans include hunting, herding, visits to cattle markets, and safari tourism. ***T. cruzi* (2363).** The Paraguayan Gran Chaco seems suitable for transmission.

Helminths

Irrigation and green meadows point to conditions that favor helminth larvae in soil and ongoing transmission, while parched grass and recent fire suggest interruption of transmission from soil. Reported tissue helminths in grasslands include *Echinococcus* and *Onchocerca*.

***Echinococcus granulosus* (2119, 4223, 6043, 7510, 7950).** *E. granulosus* is well documented in pastoral communities in savanna, prairie, and steppe areas of Africa, the Americas (southwestern United States to Argentina), and Eurasia. By close association with infected dogs and livestock, members of up to 6–9% of East African pastoralist communities can be infected. In temperate climates, enzootic areas of *E. granulosus* may overlap with *E. multilocularis*, including in Alaska, Central Asia, and glacial relict areas of western Europe (Austria and Switzerland).

***O. volvulus* (3861, 5266, 8206).** *O. volvulus* is endemic in savanna areas of sub-Saharan Africa. Before elimination programs were instituted, onchocercal blindness tended to be more prevalent in the savanna (up to 15%) than the rain forest (<2%), forcing people away from rivers and fertile lands. However, features of savanna and forest onchocerciasis can overlap, and in parts of West Africa, *Simulium* spp. typical for savanna (e.g., *S. damnosum* sl) have been reported in originally forested but now deforested, urbanized areas.

ISLANDS

Islands are land that is secluded by water. Islands are attractive tourist destinations. Large islands include Greenland (2.1 million km^2) and Great Britain (0.2 million km^2) in the Atlantic, Cuba (0.1 million km^2) and Hispaniola (75,000 km^2) in the Caribbean, Borneo (0.7 million km^2) and Madagascar (0.6 million km^2) in the Indian Ocean, New Guinea (0.8 million km^2) and Honshu (0.2 million km^2) in the Pacific Ocean, and Sicily (25,500 km^2) and Sardinia (23,800 km^2) in the Mediterranean.

Infections on islands (1662, 5042, 5954). Island ecosystems typically include a high number of endemic flora and fauna ("splendid isolation") that are vulnerable to intruders. The same mechanism is true for infectious diseases. Agents or vectors newly introduced to naturally free islands (virgin territory) can cause devastating epidemics. Examples include dengue, *Enterovirus* infections, influenza, and cholera. Once faded, introduced agents do not seem to readily establish themselves on islands.

Endemic infections can be overdispersed by household, village, or island (in an archipelago). While latent infections can survive in small populations, acute infections may depend on a continued supply of susceptible individuals from large populations for maintenance. Stable and defined populations make islands attractive models for control programs.

Droplet-Air Cluster

Intrinsic sources include individuals not reached by vaccination programs and untreated patients with chronic respiratory illness. Extrinsic sources are carriers and incubating individuals arriving by aircraft or ferryboat.

Viruses (598, 960, 5832, 5867, 7380). Viruses introduced to islands include respiratory *Enterovirus*, *Influenzavirus*, measles virus, and mumps virus. By disease, reported attack rates can reach 40–58%. **Influenzavirus.** In V–VI/1983, A/H3N3 virus was introduced from New Zealand to the Pacific Island of Niue, causing an attack rate of 41%. **Measles virus.** Measles virus was introduced to the Faroe Islands in 1846, resulting in 6,000 cases and 255 deaths in a population of 8,000–30,000. From that outbreak, P. L. Panum (1820–1885) was able to determine the incubation period. **Mumps virus.** On St. Lawrence Island, Alaska, mumps was not known until 1956, when a boy introduced it from Fairbanks, causing an epidemic with 363 cases among the Inuit.

Bacteria. *Haemophilus influenzae* b **(6474).** *H. influenzae* b circulates at a high rate on some Pacific islands. *Mycobacterium tuberculosis* **(1043).** In 1993, an African refugee introduced the Beijing strain to Gran Canaria in the Atlantic; subsequently, 74 residents acquired this strain.

Feces-Food Cluster

Intrinsic sources include raw sewage that is discharged into lagoons and scarce domestic water supplies. Extrinsic sources include carriers or incubating individuals arriving by ferryboat or aircraft, and imported foods.

Viruses. *Norovirus* **(915, 2469).** *Norovirus* can spread rapidly on islands. At a resort hotel in Bermuda in 1998, *Norovirus* gastroenteritis affected >440 persons, including 122 staff. *Rotavirus.* Introduced to Truk Atoll in the northwestern Pacific by a Japanese fishing vessel in 1964, *Rotavirus* caused an epidemic with 3,439 cases from all 14 inhabited islands of the atoll, for attack rates of 6–25%.

Bacteria. Outbreaks reported on islands include *Campylobacter*, *Escherichia*, and *Vibrio*. *Campylobacter* **(4999).** Rainwater tanks polluted by wildlife were the source implicated in an outbreak on an island resort off North Queensland, Australia. *E. coli* **(741).** On Prince Edward Island, Canada, sandwiches or salads from a hospital vending machine were likely vehicles for an outbreak of *E. coli* O157:H7 with 109 infectons and 2 (2%) deaths. *V. cholerae* **(505, 1030, 7236).** On Ebeye Island in the northwestern Pacific in 2000–2001, polluted drinking water transported from Kwajalein caused a cholera outbreak with 103 cases, for an attack rate of 1% (103/9,345). On Pohnpei in the northwestern Pacific, mass oral vaccination helped to control a cholera outbreak in 2000–2001 with nearly 3,400 clinical cases. For the first time in October 2002, cholera hit three of the Nicobar Islands in the Indian Ocean, for an attack rate of 13% in 16 of the 45 inhabited villages; traveling persons contributed to the spread of the disease among villages, and the suspected source of *V. cholerae* O1 El Tor was the effluent from ships.

Protozoa. *T. gondii* **(2050, 7918).** Risks vary significantly between islands, by climate, locally available animal hosts, and community dietary habits. On some Pacific islands, rats and cats apparently are sufficient to maintain an enzootic cycle. In contrast, on an island off Georgia, United States, endemicity did not seem to require domestic cats.

Helminths. *Angiostrongylus cantonensis* **(306, 3993, 6070).** *A. cantonensis* is enzootic on many islands in the Pacific and Southeast Asia. The worm was likely disseminated between islands by infected rats shipped with goods and, in World War II, war materials. Cases of eosinophilic meningitis have been reported in Indonesia (Java, Kalimantan, and Sumatra), the Philippines, as well as Guam, Hawaii, Hong Kong, Japan (Honshu, Kyushu, and Okinawa), Micronesia (Ponape and Saipan), New Caledonia, Rarotonga, Samoa (American and Western), the Solomons, Tahiti, Taiwan, and Vanuatu. A more recent development is the expansion of both *A. cantonensis* and *A. costaricensis* in the Caribbean.

Zoonotic Cluster

Intrinsic sources include infected domestic and wild mammals. Competent vectors may or may not be available on islands. Extrinsic sources include arthropods carried to islands by winds, migratory birds, boats, imported livestock, and aircraft (see chapter 16).

Viruses. DENV **(1585, 2130, 4588, 6631, 7564).** Outbreaks of DENV are well documented on many islands, including in the Caribbean and the Indian and Pacific Oceans. On Tortola, British Virgin Islands, in 1995, DENV hit participants in a community-assistance program, for an attack rate of 69%. Locally contracted dengue was reported in Hawaii in 1944 and again in 2001; the latter seemed to originate from Tahiti. While *Aedes albopictus* was identified on Oahu, Maui, and Kaui, *A. agypti* was not found. **Rabies virus (8106, 8213).** Rabies virus is enzootic on many islands. Islands that are kept or are naturally rabies free include the Bermudas, Cape

Verde, Iceland, Ireland, and Sao Tome in the Atlantic; Antigua, Barbados, and Montserrat in the Caribbean; Mauritius, Reunion, and the Seychelles in the Indian Ocean; Hawaii, Japan, New Caledonia, New Zealand, and many small islands in the Pacific; and Cyprus, Malta, and the Greek and Italian islands in the Mediterranean. The United Kingdom is free from terrestrial but not from bat rabies. With three dogs from Sulawesi, canine rabies came to Flores, both Indonesia, in 1997. Despite massive killing of dogs in 1998, rabies persisted in dogs, and in 1998–2002, >3,300 people required postexposure prophylaxis (PEP). **RRV (7, 3980, 5042, 6406).** During the widespread 1979–1980 epidemic in the South Pacific, attack rates in Fiji reached 23%. The epidemic failed to establish RRV enzootically. From travelers returning from Fiji to Canada with confirmed disease, it must be assumed that RRV reappeared in Fiji in 2003–2004. **TBEV (4112).** In Denmark, TBEV is curiously limited to Bornholm Island, 100 km east from the mainland. After 40 years of silence, foci became reactivated, with two cases in 1998, three in 1999, and three in 2000. Some 2% of *Ixodes* ticks on the island carry TBEV.

Bacteria. *Anaplasma phagocytophilum* **(6610).** *A. phagocytophilum* is present on Madeira Island, which is located 800 km off Africa and 1,000 km off Europe. Of *I. ricinus* nymphs collected from vegetation, 4% amplified the *A. phagocytophilum* by NAT. **Borrelia (2426).** A park ranger returning from the U.S. Virgin Islands to mainland United States in 1991 was diagnosed TBRF, signaling ongoing transmission on these Caribbean islands. *O. tsutsugamushi* **(2086, 2282, 4394).** Islands with reported foci include the Maldives, Torres Strait Islands (off northern Australia), Pescadores (off Taiwan), and Palau (in the Northwest Pacific). In Palau, of 15 patients diagnosed in October 2001, 14 lived on Sonsoral Island, which has only 40 inhabitants. *Rickettsia typhi* **(1211, 3271).** *R. typhi* is enzootic on the Hawaii archipelago, including on Kauai, Maui, and Oahu, likely maintained by a rodent-flea cycle. *R. typhi* has also been reported on the Canary Islands.

Protozoa. *Babesia* **(2795, 6459).** On Nantucket Island off Massachusetts, foci of both *B. divergens* and *B. microti* seem to exist. Foci of babesiosis likely exist on some of the outer islands off the United States Atlantic Coast, for instance, Long Island. *Leishmania* **(1111, 2497, 3211).** Cases of CL or VL have been reported in residents of many Mediterranean islands, including Cephalonia, Crete, Cyprus, Corfu, Elba, Mallorca, Malta, Samos, Sardinia, Sicily, and Zakinthos. *Plasmodium* **(5253, 6955).** Malaria in returned visitors signals ongoing island transmission, e.g., in Australian travelers with malaria from Bali and East Timor. Islands that are naturally or are kept free from malaria include:

- Atlantic Ocean: Canary Islands, Bermudas
- Caribbean (1208, 1281, 1282, 5678, 5953): all, except Hispaniola. Vigilance is required, however, to keep islands malaria free. In Trinidad, surveillance in 1968–1997 identified 168 imported cases, mainly at port cities: 47% (80) from Africa, 27% (45) from South America, and 23% (39) from Asia. Autochthonous cases occurred in Grenada in 1978 (*P. malariae*), Trinidad in 1991 (*P. vivax*), and 1994–1995 (*P. malariae*, after ~30 years), and mainland Florida in 1996 (*P. vivax*) and 2003 (*P. vivax*). Also, falciparum malaria was diagnosed in tourists returning to France from apparently "malaria-free" Guadeloupe. Suggested modes of introduction included gametocytemic migrant workers or wind-blown infective *Anopheles*.
- Indian Ocean (2673, 2763): Maldives, Mauritius, Reunion, and Seychelles.
- Pacific Ocean (8305): outside the Southwest all, including French Polynesia, Hawaii, Hong Kong Island, Micronesia, Okinawa and all other Japanese islands, and Taiwan.
- Mediterranean: all, including Corsica, Cyprus, Sardinia, and Sicily.

Known malarious islands include:

- Atlantic Ocean (3062): São Tomé and Príncipe (all four anthroponotic species occur).
- Caribbean (5678): Hispaniola (Haiti and Dominican Republic). All malaria on Hispaniola is due to *P. falciparum*, and parasitemia prevalence is 0.2–1%.
- Indian Ocean (1691, 3761, 7719): Comoros (all four species), Madagascar and Sri Lanka.
- Pacific Ocean (830, 3144, 4111, 6955, 7066): The island archipelagos of Indonesia, Philippines, Solomons, and Vanuatu and islands of Borneo (Kalimantan, Sabah, and Sarawak), East Timor, Hainan (People's Republic of China), and Torres (Australia; mainland Australia has been declared malaria-free since 1981). In Indonesia, most islands are partly or generally malarious, including Bali, Flores, Java, Kalimantan, Lombok (all four species), Papua (formerly Irian Jaya), Sulawesi, Sumatra, and the Lesser Sunda Islands. Similarly, much of the Philippines is malarious (72 of 75 provinces), including Luzon, Mindanao, Mindoro, and Palawan, for an overall parasitemia prevalence of ~12%. *T. brucei gambiense* **(324).** A focus of human African trypanosomiasis is reported on Bioko Island, Equatorial Guinea.

Helminths. *Echinococcus* **(2119, 6142).** *E. granulosis* has been controlled on some islands. Islands free (or "provisonally free," that is, with sporadic cases only) include southern Cyprus, Iceland, Greenland, New Zealand, and Tasmania. E. multilocularis has been controlled on St. Lawrence Island in the Bering Sea. **Wuchereria and Brugia (991, 2406, 4220, 6096, 6150).** The islands of Trinidad and Tobago have interrupted transmission of lymphatic filariasis. Lymphatic filariasis is endemic on Nicobar Islands, Indonesia (W. bancrofti, B. malayi, and B. timori), the Philippines (W. bancrofti, B. malayi), and many Pacific islands (periodic and subperiodic W. bancrofti). Control attempts have a long history in the Pacific. Endemic islands include Fiji, French Polynesia, New Caledonia, Papua New Guinea, and Vanuatu. On neighboring islands or even the same island, transmission can be strikingly disjunct. Java harbors W. bancrofti only. On Kalimantan, Sulawesi, and Sumatra, B. malayi and W. bancrofti coexist, with B. malayi dominating.

Environmental Cluster

Intrinsic sources are water and soil. Extrinsic sources are dust winds and infected small mammals.

Bacteria. *Leptospira*. Rodents are likely to have brought the agent to many islands, including Hawaii and the Azores. **Mycobacterium (7789).** In 1992–1995, M. ulcerans emerged on Phillip Island, southeast of Melbourne, Australia, likely in association with an irrigated golf course.

Helminths. *Schistosoma* (4344, 5955). Establishment on islands needs human carriers and suitable snail intermediate hosts. These conditions have been met for S. mansoni in the Caribbean, on islands such as Guadeloupe, Martinique, and St. Lucia. Meanwhile, transmission has been or is being interrupted. Zoonotic reservoirs complicate control of S. japonicum, which is enzootic and endemic in the Philippines, with an overall prevalence of 4–5%. Although most of Luzon is free of transmission, prevalence is above average on Mindanao and Samar. ***Strongyloides stercoralis* (7496).** In a chemotherapy control project on Kume Island, Okinawa, in 1994–1997, the prevalence was reduced from 6.5% (95/1,468) to 2.7% (33/1,217).

Skin-Blood Cluster

Intrinsic sources include unsafe procedures such as tattooing, with consequences that are manifest after years only. Extrinsic sources include sex tourists and imported unsafe health care products.

Viruses. Epstein-Barr virus (EBV) (4157). On Faroe Island, clusters of cases of multiple sclerosis in native-born residents suggested a link with EBV and introduction of EBV by British troops in World War II. **Hepatitis C virus (HCV) (2861).** On Zakinthos Island, Greece, the seroprevalence is 1.3%, compared with 0.2–0.4% in the general population. The likely explanation is substandard inoculation techniques on this island. **Human papillomavirus (HPV) (3978).** The rate of cervical cancer in women 20–39 years of age is more than five times higher in Greenland than Denmark. While the seroprevalence of HPV was higher (8–13%) in 661 women from Denmark than in 586 women (7–9%) from Greenland; the opposite was true for Herpes simplex virus 2 (HSV2), with prevalence of 68% in Greenland and 31% in Denmark. The authors explained their findings based on the different sexual behaviors of Danish and Greenland women.

Bacteria. *Mycobacterium* (402). Leprosy was or is endemic on some islands. Father Damian (1840–1889) is known for having taken care of leprosy patients segregated on Molokai, Hawaii. On five small islands off South Sulawesi, Indonesia, 96 leprosy patients (85 new and 11 known) were identified among 4,140 of 4,774 screened inhabitants, for a case detection rate and prevalence of 2%. Susceptibility genes may possibly be perpetuated among remote, small island populations.

Arthropods. Scabies (4259). Scabies is endemic on many small tropical islands. Island scabies can be controlled by mass treatment, surveillance, and, if feasible, preemptive oral treatment of returning residents and visitors.

ARID LANDS

> . . .a land parched, weary and waterless.
>
> Psalm 63:1

Arid lands (266, 7183, 7929) include deserts, semideserts, and eroded lands (Table 5.2). In deserts, precipitations (fog, rain, and snow) is unpredictable (0–2/year), scarce (decade-long average, <250 mm/year), and lost quickly (evaporation and percolation). In semideserts, precipitations reach 250–400 mm/year. Desert vegetation is spare, ephemeral, and tolerant of drought (xerophytic and succulent) and salt (halophytic). Arid lands cover 20–45 million km^2 (14–30% of 148 million km^2 terrestrial surface).

Infections in arid lands (898, 3613, 4209, 4925) (Box 5.5). Population density in arid lands is generally low ($\leq$1/km^2). Typical inhabitants are nomad communities (see section 14.5). Exceptions are desert cities, e.g., Las Vegas in the Mojave Desert, Phoenix and Tucson in the Sonora Desert, Damascus in the Syrian Desert, and Alice Springs near the Simpson Desert. Hazards include dust (see section 5.5), infections from livestock (see section 2.3), and lack of water for personal hygiene. In the Mojave Desert, hospitalizations for respiratory illnesses (mainly

Table 5.2 Characteristics of major deserts of the world

Desert, by type	Area (km²) (10^6)	Precipitations (mm/yr)	No. of plant species; examples; comments
Hot			
Arabian-Negev-Syrian	2	Rain (100)	800; *Phoenix*, *Pistacia atlantica*, *P. vera*
Atacama-Sechura	0.3	Fog (0–25)	*Tillandsia*
Chihuahua-Mohave-Sonora	1	Rain (40–400)	2,000; cacti (*Carnegia*), *Agave*, *Yucca*
Great Sandy-Gibson-Simpson	2	Rain (100–200)	1,200; *Triodia*, nullarbor plain, 60% sand
Kalahari-Karoo-Namib	0.5	Rain, fog (100–250)	5,000; *Aloe*, *Welwitschia*
Sahara	8–9	Rain (0-25-50)	1,400; *Ziziphus lotus*, salt flats, hot ghibli
Thar	0.3	Rain (100–400)	Irrigation projects
Cold			
Gobi-Taklimakan	2	Snow (50–200)	*Nitraria*, barchan dunes, 50% sand
Great Basin	0.5	Snow (100–300)	*Artemisia*, chinook wind
Karakum-Kysylkum	0.5	Snow, rain (135)	*Haloxylon*, Amudarya, Syrdarya rivers

pneumonia and influenza) were more frequent in soldiers who had undergone desert military training ($n = 21{,}543$) than in matched controls who had never had such training ($n = 86{,}172$), for a rate ratio of 1.3 (95% CI 1.1–1.6). Lack of water fosters eye and skin infections, ectoparasites, and louse-borne infections. Paradoxically, it may increase leptospirosis transmission in some settings, perhaps by concentrating viable agents in scarce water bodies. Deserts, in general, are unfavorable for soil-borne helminths (*Ascaris*, hookworms, and *Trichuris*). Exceptions are irrigated (see section 6.1) areas, e.g., the Thar Desert in India and Pakistan.

Bacteria

***Chlamydia trachomatis* (2199, 6659).** Trachoma is endemic in arid areas, including North Africa, the Sahel, the Ethiopian highland, Southern Africa, Latin America, and Australasia. Lack of water helps to explain current occurrence. (In the nineteenth century, trachoma was observed in London.)

***Neisseria meningitidis* (1793).** In the African meningitis belt, meningococcal meningitis is strikingly seasonal, with epidemics toward the end of the dry season (December–May), when dry and hot harmattan winds calm. Rates $>5/10^5$ for three consecutive weeks seem to reliably predict outbreaks.

***T. pallidum endemicum* (4689).** Bejel is endemic among nomads in Africa and West Asia. Spread is by skin contact and shared objects.

***Y. pestis* (98, 735, 8093).** Plague foci exist in arid lands, including the cold deserts of Central Asia. In Madagascar in 1995–1998, three-fourths of 1,702 plague cases consistently occurred during the dry season (August–October).

Fungi

Perhaps surprisingly, fungi can thrive in arid soils (2245, 6245). Environmental dust (see section 5.5) is a vehicle for coccidioidomycosis. In arid areas of Madagascar *Cladophialophora carrionii* is a cause of chromomycosis in barefooted wood cutters, by injury from cactuslike plants such as *Euphorbia* and endemic *Didierea madagascariensis* (octopus tree, Didiereaceae). A similar situation exists in Venezuela in xerophytic thornbush habitats.

Protozoa

***Leishmania* (2974).** VL can be transmitted in arid areas. In People's Republic of China, VL has largely been controlled, but competent vectors persist, e.g., *Phlebotomus chinensis* in the mountaineous northwest and Taklimakan desert, *P. major wui* in the Gobi sand desert, and *P. alexandri* in stony deserts. In the precontrol period of the 1970s–1980s, prevalence of *L. donovani* promastigotes in female sandflies was ~1%.

***T. cruzi* (5043, 8099).** Arid habitats in inter-Andean valleys include burrows and rock crevices.

DESERT OASES

Oases are "green patches in a sea of sand," or places that receive sufficient moisture for permanent vegetation. Historically, oases have been crossroads in harsh environments. This role has become outdated by modern traffic. Examples of oases include in Al Liwa in Abu Dhabi, Biskra in Algeria, El Fayoum and Feiran in Egypt, Aït Bekka in Morocco, Al Hasa in Saudi Arabia, and Tozeur in Tunisia. Much of what is true for islands is applicable to oases.

Infections in oases. Health hazards include crowded housing, polluted domestic water, dust, and irrigation farming that favors vector breeding. Priority conditions are diarrhea, respiratory infections, trachoma, schistosomiasis, malaria, leishmaniasis, and ectoparasitoses.

Viruses
HIV (2888). Bilma Oasis, Chad, is a crossroads for camel caravans and trucks; in 1995, the seroprevalence of HIV1 among prostitutes was 28% (34/122).

PROTOZOA
Leishmania **(1907, 3119, 7199, 7665).** CL is enzootic in semiarid agricultural areas and oases of central and eastern Saudi Arabia, where *L. major* circulates in *Phlebotomus papatasi* and desert rodents (*Psammomys obesus* and *Meriones libycus*). In Al Hasa Oasis in 1986, 2.8% of the inhabitats had active skin lesions. In and around oases in the steppes of Turkmenistan and Uzbekistan in Central Asia, *L. major* was identified in ~23% of *Rhombomys opimus*, with a low in the spring and a high in the fall. VL is also transmitted in oases. Examples of desert foci are Tabuk in northwestern Saudi Arabia, and Iferouane in the Aïr Mountains of northwestern Niger.

Plasmodium **(165, 575, 1906, 3888, 6750, 7624).** *P. falciparum*, *P. vivax*, and *P. malariae* can be transmitted in oases. A likely oasis vector is *Anopheles sergentii*. Oases along truck routes are at risk for introduced malaria. Malarious oases have been reported in Algeria (Heiha, Yakou, Iherir, and In-Salah), Egypt (El Gara, 120 km northeast of Siwa), Niger (Bilma), and Saudi Arabia (now inactive, Al Hasa and Qatif; probably active, Jazan in the southwest). In India, irrigation schemes of the Thar Desert have changed malaria ecology. Preirrigation, the main vector was *A. stephensi*, which was limited to breeding sites in households and community underground reservoirs. With irrigation, *A. culicifacies* has become more prominent, expanding into the desert interior. With the intrusion of *A. culicifacies*, *P. falciparum* is emerging in the Thar.

Helminths
Fasciola **(3107).** In Tozeur Oasis, southwest Tunisia, cattle, sheep and goats, and lymneid snails in irrigation canals maintain *F. hepatica* in an oasis cycle. In 1997–1998, 26% (272/1,041) of snails from five of eight sites tested positive for larvae of *F. hepatica*.

Schistosoma **(725, 2163, 8421).** Irrigation farming supports oasis foci. In North Africa, oasis foci are reported in Egypt (*S. mansoni* and *S. haematobium* in El Fayoum), Morocco (*S. haematobium* in Akka) where aquatic plants (*Potamogeton*) support host snails (*Bulinus truncatus*), and Tunisia (*S. haematobium*). Tunisian foci were eliminated in the 1980s.

ALPINE AND BOREAL TUNDRA
Tundra (266, 6742). Squeezed between tree line and snow line, alpine and boreal tundra is a "biome *in extremis*." Sunlight and permafrost may limit plant growth to 6–8 weeks. Living cover is characterized by microbial mats, lichens, mosses, grasses, and dwarf shrubs, including of genera *Arctostaphylos*, *Empetrum*, *Ledum*, *Rhododendron*, *Vaccinium* (all Ericales), *Dryas* (Rosaceae), *Salix* (Salicaceae). Tundra occupies ~17% (25/148 million km^2) of terrestrial surface, mainly in the Northern Hemisphere.

Infections in tundra (7216). Life in tundra endures freezing and thawing (ecocryosystem), short growing seasons, and scarce precipitations, mainly as meltwater (cold desert). Alpine tundra marks altitudinal limits of agent transmission; polar tundras mark latitudinal limits.

Alpine Tundra
Alpine tundra is a surrogate for elevational transmission limits. By distance from the equator and mode of spread, infectious agents reach altitudes of 2,500–4,300 m (Table 5.3). Food-borne (e.g., *Toxoplasma* and *Fasciola*) and contact-borne (e.g., *Enterobius*) agents seem to go higher up than vector-borne agents. On Mount Denali, Alaska, precarious hygiene on routes and in camps and frequent diarrhea among climbers suggest possible interpersonal spread even at elevatons of >5,000 m (4917). High-altitude cities include Wenquan in Qinghai Province, People's Republic of China (at 5,100 m), Lhasa in Tibet (at 3,680 m), La Paz in Bolivia (at 3,630 m), and Leadville in Colorado (at 3,095 m).

During summer months, cows, sheep, and goats from various farms are traditionally herded together on Alpine pastures (transhumance), creating opportunities for cross-infection. *S. enterica* serovar Dublin can be maintained by this mode in cattle herds (156). Livestock and wildlife can graze on the same Alpine pastures and exchange agents, e.g., *Pestivirus* and *Mycoplasma conjunctivae*. *M. conjunctivae* from sheep and goats can cause epizootics of blindness in chamois and ibex (7588). Some parasites are adapted to overwinter in Alpine tundra, e.g., *Giardia lamblia* (in small rodents), *F. hepatica* (in snails), and *Ostertagia ostertagia* (in soil).

Bacteria. *C. trachomatis* (ocular) (139). In Ethiopia, the prevalence of active trachoma decreased with altitude, from ~70% at 2,000 m to ~10% at 3,000 m. While species of *Musca* became sparce above 2,500 m, cases occurred above 3,000 m. ***Mycobacterium* (5580).** In Peru, the prevalence of tuberculin skin reactivity was 6–8% in two high-altitude villages (at 3,340–3,500 m) compared with 25–33% in three villages at sea level, for significant odds ratios of 4.5–6 after adjustment for age, Bacillus Calmette Guerin (BCG) vaccination, and exposure.

Table 5.3 Elevational limits of human-infective agents, by agent cluster and class

Cluster	Agent	km[b]	Location	Remarks	Reference
Zoonotic	DENV	1.7	Mexico	Outbreak	3274
	B. quintana	4.3	Peru	Louse-infested people	6114
	R. prowazekii	4.3	Peru	Louse-infested people	6114
	Y. pestis	3.3	Andes	Outbreak	2564
	L. aethiopica	2.6	Mt. Elgon, Kenya	By *Phlebotomus*	4268
	L. tropica	1.8	Afghanistan	Outbreak	6233
	P. falciparum	2.2	East Africa	*Anopheles*	6665
	P. vivax	2.3	Andes	*A. pseudopunctopennis*	6485
	P. vivax	2.5	Yunnan, China		1363
	E. multilocularis	4.2	Sichuan, China	Transmission	7947
	E. granulosus	3	Altai, Mongolia	Transmission	7976
	E. granulosus	4.2	Sichuan, China	Prevalence, 4.7%	7947
	E. granulosus	3.6-4.3	Andes	Prevalence, 9%	5204
	O. volvulus	1.2	Yemen	Transmission	1009
	O. volvulus	2.2	Guatemala	Onchocercoma carriers	8318
	T. cruzi	2.5	Andes	Triatomine bugs	5462
Environmental	*S. schenckii*	2.3	Andes, Peru	Sporotrichosis in children	1550
	Hookworm	3.9	Andes	Prevalence, 0.6%	2240
	S. mansoni	1.9	East Africa	Transmission	3128
	S. stercoralis	3.9	Andes	Prevalence, 0.9%	2240
Feces-food	*Cryptosporidium*	4.2	Andes	Prevalence, 32%	2239
	F. hepatica	4.1	Andes	Snails, infected children	4793
	G. lamblia	2.5	Colorado	Outbreak	3590
	T. gondii	4.3	Andes	Seroprevalence, 7%	1064
	A. lumbricoides	3.9	Andes	Prevalence, 8%	2240
	T. trichiura	3.9	Andes	Prevalence, 18%	2240
Droplet-air, skin-blood	*M. tuberculosis*	3.5	Andes	Skin reactivity, 6–8%	5580
	C. trachomatis	3	East Africa	Prevalence, ~10%	139
	E. histolytica sl	3.9	Andes	Prevalence, 38%	2240
	Enterobius	3.9	Andes	Prevalence, 1.5%	2240

[a]Kilometers above sea level.

Reduced viability of *Mycobacterium* at high altitude seemed to better explain study findings, rather than decreased human susceptibility counterbalanced by increased crowding. **Rickettsia prowazekii (5126).** *R. prowazekii* and epidemic typhus have retreated to 3,800–4,300 m in North and East Africa, Central Asia, and the Andes.

Protozoa. *Cryptosporidium* **(2239).** In Aymara communities in the Bolivian Altiplano at 3,800–4,200 m (between La Paz and Lake Titicaca), the prevalence by single stool specimens from randomly selected asymptomatic students 5–19 years of age was 32% (119/377). Poor sanitation, polluted water, crowding, and proximity to domestic animals likely explained the high prevalence. **G. lamblia.** In the Cascades of North America, enzootic *G. lamblia* from rodents has been reported at altitudes of 1,800 m (5667). **Leishmania (4268, 5218, 6603).** In East African highlands, *L. aethiopica* has been demonstrated at 1,600–2,600 m, in *Phlebotomus* and rock hyraxes. In Africa and Southwest Asia, hyraxes (*Procavia habessinica* and *Heterohyrax brucei*) occur up to 3,000 m, in rocks, boulder fields, and rocks growing trees such as species of *Ficus* (Moraceae). **Plasmodium.** While, as a general rule, transmission becomes unstable above 1,600 m, elevational transmission limits vary by vector and distance of the highlands from the equator.

- East Africa. In East African highlands (899, 2452, 2643), *Anopheles* and *P. falciparum* can reach 1,800–2,000 m, occasionally even higher elevations. In Kenya in 1941, a falciparum malaria outbreak was reported at 2,280–2,380 m. In 1958, a falciparum malaria epidemic occurred in Ethiopia at 1,600–2,150 m, with >3 million cases and >0.15 million deaths. The Madagascar highlands (700–2,000 m) (1691, 3634, 4252) had been traditionally malaria free. Rice farming brought a change. In 1985–1990, the highlands experienced a falciparum malaria epidemic, with 40,000 deaths. Meanwhile, control has been restored. In

Zimbabwe (7378), *A. gambiae* sl populates the lowveld (<600 m) year-round while, during the hot season, it invades the highveld (>1,100 m).

- American Andes (6485). In Bolivia in 1998, a vivax malaria outbreak occurred in a community living at 2,300 m. Of 199 residents, 63 were symptomatic, and 52 had blood smears positive for *P. vivax*; none recalled travel to malarious areas, but all recalled mosquito bites. The most likely vector is *A. pseudopunctopennis*, which in Bolivia thrives at up to 2,500–3,000 m. In the Bolivian Altiplano in the 1940s, malaria was recorded at 2,440–2,770 m, carried by mosquitoes that bred in thermal springs.
- Asia. Presumed transmission limits are 2,250–2,400 m for *P. falciparum* in central Afghanistan during the short summer months (13), 1,300–1,750 m for *P. falciparum* in Pakistan (798), 2,500 m for *P. vivax* in Yunnan, People's Republic of China (1363), and 1,400–1,700 m for *P. falciparum* and *P. vivax* in Papua New Guinea (5239). There, work and overnighting in coffee and tea plantations at lower (1,200–1,400 m) elevations, shift from traditional to modern housing with gutters and drainage ditches, standing pools of water at the end of the rainy season, lack of vector control in remote areas, and an increase of mean temperature by 0.6–0.9°C in the past 40 years all contribute to epidemic malaria at high altitude. **T. cruzi (5462).** In the Andes, *T. cruzi* can survive in *Triatoma infestans* that hide in rock piles at up to 2,400–2,600 m.

Helminths. *Echinococcus* **(1125, 7947).** In central Europe, core enzootic areas of *E. multilocularis* are the Alpine areas of Austria, France, Germany, and Switzerland. In the Italian Alps, *E. multilocularis* has recently been isolated in red foxes at altitudes up to 2,000 m. On the Tibetan plateau in Sichuan Province, both *E. granulosus* and *E. multilocularis* are enzootic and endemic, in winter camps up to 4,200 m, on summer pastures perhaps even at 4,300–4,800 m.

Boreal Tundra

Because the Northern Hemisphere has more land mass and more people than the Southern Hemisphere, agents reach higher latitudes in the North (beyond the Arctic Circle at 66½°) than in the South (longitude 40°S, which dissects Patagonia, Tasmania, and New Zealand) (7216) (Table 5.4). The latitudinal amplitude is particularly broad for contact-spread *Enterobius vermicularis* (from 70°N to 50°S), but particularly narrow for vector-borne YFV (essentially intertropical, from 23.5°N to 23.5°S).

Infections at high latitudes (4914, 5638, 6007, 7352). Tundra is a natural habitat for rabies virus, *F. tularensis*, *T. nativa*, *Diphyllobothrium*, and *Echinococcus*. In the growing season, mosquitoes that transmit arboviruses abound. Crowding, inadequate sanitation, and undercoverage with vaccines predispose to enteric, respiratory, and contact infections, including by HAV, HBV, and cytomegalovirus; by genital *Chlamydia*, *Haemophilus influenzae* b, *Neisseria gonorrhoeae*, and *Streptococcus pneumoniae*; and *Sarcoptes scabiei*. At latitude 78°N, Longyearbyen on Svalbard (Spitzbergen) is likely the most northerly city in the world. From Longyearbyen cemeteries, the virus that caused the 1918 Spanish flu was unraveled by molecular archeology.

Viruses. *Flavivirus* **(5084).** I could not locate information on the northern limit of viruses in this genus, in particular, POWV in the Nearctic, and TBEV and Omsk hemorrhagic fever virus (OHFV) in the Palearctic. **Hepatitis viruses (4923).** HAV, HBV, and HCV circulate at high rates in Arctic communities, including in Alaska, the Northwest Territories, and Greenland. *Orthobunyavirus.* The genus is transmitted throughout the Arctic. In the Nearctic, the main risk is SSHV. In the Palearctic, INKV, TAHV, and SSHV circulate. In Siberia, temperature gradients along the Ob River can exceed 80°C, from +38°C in the summer to −50°C in the winter. **Rabies virus (6010).** Arctic hosts include the Arctic fox (*Alopex lagopus*) and wolf. On Svalbard (78–80°N), rabies virus was detected in Arctic foxes for the first time in 1980.

Bacteria. *Campylobacter.* An outbreak in northern Norway in 1988 occurred at latitude 70°N (4968). *F. tularensis. F. tularensis* is enzootic in northern wildlife. In North America, this includes rodents, rabbits, hares (*Lepus americanus*), and ticks (*Haemaphysalis leporispalustris*). *H. pylori* **(4914).** *H. pylori* is endemic in traditional Inuit communities. In the Canadian Arctic, water from lakes and a delivery truck for local supplies tested positive by PCR, suggesting a reservoir in water or pollution from human sewage. **S. enterica serovar Enteritidis and *Y. pseudotuberculosis*.** *S. enterica* serovar Enteritidis and *Y. pseudotuberculosis* were isolated from a fox on Svalbard (78–80°N) (7036).

Microsporidia. *E. cuniculi* has been reported in Arctic lemmings (*Dicrostonyx stevensoni*).

Protozoa. *T. gondii* has been isolated in Arctic foxes on the Svalbard Archipelago (78–80°N) (7036).

Helminths. *Diphyllobothrium* **(6141).** *Diphyllobothrium* species are enzootic in the Arctic. *Echinococcus* **(2119, 3265, 6140).** *E. multilocularis* and *E. granulosus* are enzootic in the Holarctic. *E. multilocularis* circulates in the Arctic fox (*A. lagopus*) and Tundra vole (*Microtus oeconomus*). Eggs survive to −50°C and need −70°C for 96 h for inactivation. *E. granulosus* (Nordic strain or genotype 8) circulates in wolf and wild reindeer, wolf and elk

5 ▪ Natural Environments

Table 5.4 Latitudinal limits of human-infective agents, by agent clusters and class

Agent clusters[a]	Agents reaching latitude, by class[b]
	≥70° north
Zoonotic, environmental	Rabies virus, *Francisella tularensis*; *Echinococcus granulosus*, *Echinococcus multilocularis*
Feces-food, human	*Campylobacter*, *Yersinia pseudotuberculosis*, *Toxoplasma*, *Trichinella nativa*, *Diphyllobothrium*, *Enterobius*
	66½° north (Arctic circle)
Zoonotic, environmental	Hantavirus, tick-borne encephalitis virus; *Bacillus anthracis*, *Borrelia burgdorferi*, *Coxiella burnetii*; *Sporothrix schenckii*; (*Plasmodium vivax*); *Toxocara canis*
Feces-food, human	HAV, HBV; *Salmonella enterica* serovar Typhi, *Vibrio parahaemolyticus*; *Cryptosporidium*, *Giardia lamblia*, *Entamoeba histolytica*, *Toxoplasma gondii*; *Anisakis*, *Ascaris lumbricoides*, *Taenia saginata*, *Taenia solium*
	50° north (Winnipeg, Frankfurt, Kiev)
Zoonotic, environmental	CCHFV, sandfly fever virus, St. Louis encephalitis virus; *Leptospira*, *Orientia*, *Rickettsia typhi*, *Yersinia pestis*; *Rhinosporidium*; *Leishmania*, (*Plasmodium falciparum*), hookworm, *Strongyloides*
Feces-food, human	*Vibrio cholerae*; *Histoplasma*; *Trichuris*, *Paragonimus*, *Hymenolepis*
	40° north (Philadelphia, Madrid, Beijing)
Zoonotic, environmental	CHIKV, JEV, RVFV, VEEV; *Schistosoma haematobium*, *S. japonicum*, *S. mansoni*, *Wuchereria*
Feces-food, human	*Mycobacterium leprae*, *Coccidioides immitis*
	23½° north (Tropic of Cancer)
Zoonotic, environmental	DENV, YFV; *Burkholderia pseudomallei*; *Trypanosoma brucei gambiense*, *T. cruzi*, *Loa*, *Onchocerca*
Feces-food, human	*Treponema pallidum pertenue*, *Paracoccidioides*
	23½° south (Tropic of Capricorn)
Zoonotic, environmental	CHIKV, VEEV; *Rhinosporidium*, *Sporothrix*, (*Plasmodium falciparum*, *Plasmodium vivax*), *Leishmania* (cutaneous); *Schistosoma haematobium*, *S. mansoni*, *Wuchereria*
Feces-food, human	*Vibrio cholerae*, *V. parahaemolyticus*; *Blastomyces dermatitidis*
	30° south (Porto Alegre, Durban, Perth)
Zoonotic, environmental	CCHFV, HFRS, RVFV, SLEV; *Coxiella burnetii*, *Leptospira*, *Rickettsia typhi*, *Yersinia pestis*; *Leishmania* (visceral), *Trypanosoma cruzi*; hookworm, *Strongyloides*
Feces-food, human	*S. enterica* serovar Typhi; *Coccidioides immitis*, *Histoplasma capsulatum*, *Paracoccidioides brasiliensis*; *Anisakis*
	40° south (Valdivia, Flinders island, Wellington)
Zoonotic, environmental	*Echinococcus granulosus*, *Bacillus anthracis*, *Toxocara canis*
Feces-food, human	*Mycobacterium leprae*, *Cryptosporidium*, *Entamoeba histolytica*, *Giardia lamblia*, *Toxoplasma gondii*; *Ascaris lumbricoides*, *Diphyllobothrium*, *Enterobius*, *Hymenolepis*, *Trichinella*, *Trichuris*, *Taenia saginata*, *Taenia solium*
	50° south (Patagonia)

[a]Human for droplet-air and skin-blood clusters.
[b]Agents in parentheses indicate maximum range (19th to early 20th centuries). Cities in parentheses indicate location of latitude.

(moose, *Alces alces*), sled dog and wild reindeer, and dog and domesticated reindeer. When Alaskan natives turned from nomadic to sedentary lifestyle, dogs could fecally pollute villages, and humans contracted cystic echinococcosis. Since snow mobiles have replaced sled dogs, cases of cystic enchinococcosis have become rare in Alaska. On Svalbard (78–80°N), *E. multilocularis* made its unwanted appearance in 1999. **Toxocara (3812).** *T. canis* is well adapted to cold. Even better adapted is related *Toxascaris leonina*. In Greenland, its prevalence in 254 Arctic foxes (*A. lagopus*) from several locations was 39–68%. *Baylisascaris* has been isolated from grizzly bear. **Trichinella (4625, 5134, 5994, 6011).** *T. nativa* is enzootic throughout the Arctic, including Greenland and Svalbard. Raw or cured meat from terrestrial and marine mammals is a source of acute trichinellosis and outbreaks in native communities, including by walrus (*Odobenus rosmarus*) and polar bear (*Ursus maritimus*). On Svalbard (78–80°N) in 1983–1989, diaphragms of 9% (59/697) of Arctic foxes tested positive for *Trichinella* larvae.

CAVES

Caves are hollow spaces in rock, typically in limestone (Karst), with particular conditions of light, temperature, and humidity. In human-made mines, tunnels, subways, and catacombs, similar conditions may exist (for mining, see section 12.1). Unusually long caves include Mammoth and Jewel in the United States, Optimisticeskaja in the

Ukraine, and Hölloch in Switzerland. Unusually deep caves include Krubera in Abkhazia, Lamprechtsofen in Austria, and Gouffre Mirolda in France.

Speleological agents (2103, 3721, 4086). Diverse micro- and macroorganisms thrive in caves, including "bacteria, butterflies, and bats." In Texas, *Ornithodoros turicata* ticks that inhabit caves are implicated in TBRF. In Kenya, *Phlebotomus guggisbergi*, a vector of *Leishmania tropica*, has adapted to caves. However, the main concerns are bat-associated agents.

Rabies virus (2723, 8217). Bats in caves could expose spelunkers to rabies virus. A theoretical hazard is inhalation of concentrated bat dust. In Texas in 1956, two men apparently died of inhalational rabies after exploring Frio Cave near Uvalde, Tex., in which Mexican free-tailed bats (*Tadarida braziliensis*) resided. Subsequently, rabies virus was detected in air from the cave by bioassay. Of 392 spelunkers attending a national convention, 99% confirmed having seen bats on caving trips (29% sometimes, 43% often, and 5% always).

Histoplasma **(313, 4590, 5347, 6507, 7686).** There is a well-known association of *H. capsulatum* with cave-dwelling bats and their guano. Up to 1985, 42 histoplasmosis outbreaks were summarized among spelunkers and cave visitors. Cave-associated histoplasmosis has been reported from North, Central, and South America, Africa, and the Pacific. At a speleological society meeting in Texas in 1994, 18 attendees contracted confirmed acute histoplasmosis from cave exploration and six had an illness suspected to be acute histoplasmosis. Risks include limited caving experience, spending long periods in caves, and crawling into a particular cave space. In Costa Rica in 1998–1999, San Jose residents and American tourists contracted acute histoplasmosis from visiting a cave, for attack rates of 59% (44/75) and 64% (9/14), respectively. *H. capsulatum* was isolated in bat guano from inside the cave. Risks included crawling in the cave and the visit of a wet room. Washing hands after leaving the cave had a preventive effect.

5.5 DUST AND WINDS

Winds (4434) are air parcels that move along atmospheric pressure gradients. Many winds have names, including breeze, cyclone ("cycles" along low-pressure isobars), hurricane (Atlantic tropical cyclones), typhoon (Pacific tropical cyclones), föhn (downhill warming wind), and monsoon (wind of seasonally changing direction). Dust (1329, 6026) is fine, dry particles (e.g., sand, eroded soil, and ashes) in air that are raised and carried by winds or fires. Winds regularly carry large amounts of dust over the Atlantic from Africa to the Caribbean. Wind blows dust into houses, office buildings, and hospitals. Mist is moist particles suspended from winds over water, heavy rains, or landslides. Human-made (1096, 5520, 5898) dust clouds and aerosols can be generated by farm machines, bulldozers, helicopters, all-terrain vehicles, spray and sprinkler irrigation, vacuum cleaners, vaporizers, and showerheads (for aerosols in buildings, see section 6.2).

Infections from dust (1096, 4735, 7684, 8065). Respiratory agents from dust include viruses and bacteria, but mainly fungi (Box 5.6). The exposure history (Box II.1) should include season and weather around the exposure time. Dust storms and dry, windy weather are favorable for aerosolization. Weaponized agents should be considered in cases unexpected for season, age, or occupational group. In Victoria, British Columbia, in 1999, *Bacillus thuringiensis* aerosols were air sprayed to control gypsy moth (*Lymantria dispar*); subsequently, *B. thuringiensis* was recovered from air, water, and nasal swabs of residents (77% or 131/171). Particles of diameter >10 μm are retained in the nose, while small (1–5 μm) particles reach the lung alveoli (surface, ~ 140 m^2).

VIRUSES FROM DUST

Natural dust (including nonintentional, human-generated) (945, 1650, 2779, 4272, 8003). Dust is a potential source of *Arenavirus* (e.g., Lassa, JUNV), *Hantavirus* (e.g., PUUV, HTNV, and SNV), and perhaps *Phlebovirus* (RVFV) in humans, and of *Aphthovirus* (foot-and-mouth disease virus, FMDV) in animals.

Dust from military field exercise or forest work is suspected to increase PUUV infection risks in exposed individuals. Historically, dust has been a vehicle of smallpox. During the epizootic in the United Kingdom in 2001, air was the most likely mode of spread for 1% (18/1,849) of reported FMDV animal cases. From epidemiological evidence FMDV is likely to be carried by winds over ~ 1–10 km, perhaps even over oceans.

Weaponized viruses (2505, 5469) with potential for intentional release as aerosols include *Alphavirus* (EEEV,

---

Box 5.6 Wind- and dust-borne agents

For hospital air, see section 5.1; for human-made aerosols, see section 6.2.

Viruses	*Arenavirus* (Lassa and JUNV), *Hantavirus* (PUUV and SNV)
Bacteria	*Brucella, B. pseudomallei, Coxiella, Francisella, Nocardia*
Fungi	*Blastomyces, Coccidioides, Cryptococcus, Histoplasma, Pneumocystis*

VEEV, and WEEV), *Arenavirus* (GUAV, Lassa, JUNV, and MACV), *Filovirus* (EBOV and MARV), *Hantavirus*, and *Orthopoxvirus* (variola virus).

BACTERIA FROM DUST

Bacteria (810, 4023, 8422). Spores readily get airborne, and viable bacteria are recovered from open air and air in cities, houses, and hospitals (see section 17.7). Reported concentratons range broadly, from 0–4,000 bacteria/m^3 in open rural or urban air to 7,000–106,000 CFU/m^3 in animal houses. Animal house air has yielded *E. coli*, *Pseudomonas aeruginosa*, and other agents. Dust is a vehicle mainly of *Coxiella*, *Francisella*, and *Nocardia* in humans. There is a theoretical risk for humans to inhale enteric bacteria that animals shed with excrements.

***Brucella* (7921).** Although aerosols are vehicles of brucellosis in laboratories and abattoirs and *Brucella* survives in soil and animal excreta for many weeks, contact rather than dust is the most likely mode of spread in open-air settings and brucellosis in farm workers.

***B. pseudomallei* (3448).** In the Vietnam War, cases of *B. pseudomallei* in humans were associated with the inhalation of dust or water particles around helicopter-landing areas.

***C. botulinum* (1080).** *C. botulinum* spores can get airborne by winds over dry soil or manure and have been recovered from vacuum cleaner dust. Inhalational botulism seems exceedingly rare, however.

***C. burnetii* (910, 1096, 2085, 3191, 7484).** Dust is a major, well-established vehicle for sporadic and epidemic cases of *C. burnetii*, in particular, in western Europe. In the Swiss Alps in 1983, sheep returning from pastures caused an epidemic of 415 Q fever cases, for attack rates of 21% among residents along the sheep treck and 3% among villagers away from the treck. Winds can blow the agent away from the source. In southern France over 5 years, Q fever rates were three to five times lower in Aix-en-Provence (11/10^5) and Marseille (7/10^5) than Martigues (35/10^5), likely because "mistral" winds passed over sheep pasture before blowing into Martigues. In the French Alps in 1996, in an outbreak with 29 acute cases near a slaughterhouse, sheep waste aerosolized by a nearby helicopter-landing area was the suspected source. In an urban epidemic in Birmingham, United Kingdom, in 1989, with 147 cases, domiciles of cases corresponded to the direction of stormy winds that had passed over sheep farms.

***F. tularensis* (1272, 1714).** In northern Sweden in 1966, airborne *F. tularensis* caused an outbreak with 676 tularemia cases; dust from hay polluted by vole feces was the implicated vehicle. In Czechia in 1959–1999, about one-fourth of 577 reported cases were inhalational.

***Nocardia asteroides* (6028).** Dust containing *N. asteroides* from soil is a likely vehicle for pulmonary nocardiosis.

Weaponized bacteria (285, 788, 2505, 5008, 5469). Weaponized bacteria with potential for intentional release as aerosols include *B. anthracis* (the infective dose [ID] is 8,000–50,000 spores), *C. botulinum* (LD$_{50}$, the dose that is lethal for 50% of exposed persons, is 0.003 µg/kg body weight), *C. burnetii*, *F. tularensis* (ID 10–50 bacteria), and *Y. pestis* (ID, 100–500 bacteria). In Russia in 1979, spores that were carried downwind from a production facility to Sverdlovsk caused an anthrax epizootic and epidemic with ~3,000 cases in humans, including 1,000 deaths. In the United States in 2001, spores that were intentionally delivered through U. S. postal services caused five anthrax deaths. In Japan in 1990–1995, several attempts were made to release *C. botulinum* toxin, including in downtown Toyko.

FUNGI FROM DUST

Fungi (1329, 5023, 6179). Fungal spores readily get airborne, being recovered from air in cities and buildings. Recovery is typically perennial in tropical climates and seasonal in temperate climates. On floors of Boston office buildings, the mean concentration *Aspergillus*, *Fusarium*, and other fungi was ~41,000 CFU/m^2.

Spores and viable fungi can contaminate surfaces or cause colonization, allergic reaction, infection, or invasive disease. Dust is a confirmed or suspected vehicle of *Blastomyces*, *Coccidioides*, *Cryptococcus*, *Histoplasma*, and *Pneumocystis* in humans. In the San Francisco area in 1992–1993, the invasive fungal disease rate was 18/10^5 per year. The most frequent agents were *Candida*, *Cryptococcus*, *Aspergillus*, and *Histoplasma*.

Fungi apparently are considered unsuitable for weaponizing and intentional release.

***Aspergillus* (1882, 5023).** Spores are frequently reported from out- and indoor air samples. In outdoor air, *Aspergillus* can account for 15% of all identified spores. Concentrations outdoors are typically 2–30 conidia/m^3, while inside a barn after hay or straw had been stirred, concentration is increased >1 million-fold (68 million conidia/m^3). Despite epizootics in birds and ample opportunities for human exposure, community-acquired disease outbreaks have not been reported.

***B. dermatitidis* (488, 3970).** In North America, dust from construction sites has been linked with cases of *B. dermatitidis* infection in Chicago (five in 1974–1975) and Wisconsin (four confirmed and 18 suspected in 1988).

C. immitis **(2445, 6691).** Dust is an established risk. In coastal California in 1994, a dust cloud from a landslide caused by an earthquake was source for 203 coccidioidomycosis cases. In San Joaquin Valley, Calif., in 1977, high-speed winds caused 115 acute cases and ~7,000 infections. For military work, see section 12.3.

Cryptococcus **(1026, 3358, 6464).** Spores can be recovered from dust and debris, including in buildings. In the United States, floor debris (3 million cells/g) and air samples (45 cells/100 liters) of a vacant tower that had once been inhabited by pigeons grew *C. neoformans*; 60% of cells were smaller than 5 μm. Despite conceivably ample exposure, community-acquired outbreaks have rarely been reported, and sources of many infections remain obscure.

H. capsulatum **(1296, 1698, 6670, 8065).** Dust stirred up by construction work or tilling of soil is a confirmed risk in North America. In 1962 in Mason City, Ia., bulldozing stirred up dust, causing ~8,400 infections with *H. capsulatum*. Of children living within one block from the epicenter of earth movements, 77% were skin reactive, compared with 20% of children living 1–2 miles away.

Pneumocystis **(5056, 7903).** Spores appear to constitute part of the "air flora." In rural Oxfordshire, United Kingdom, *P. carinii* and *P. jirovecii* DNA were amplified from air. In Middlesex, United Kingdom, cases of *Pneumocystis pneumonia* varied seasonally, suggesting an environmental source. Inhalation is supported by experiments with *P. carinii* and nosocomial outbreaks, but community-acquired outbreaks have not been reported in the past one to two decades.

PROTOZOA FROM DUST
Free-living amebas (26, 436, 6748). Free-living amebas have been recovered from dust and nasal mucosa of healthy people. In West Africa, colonization seemed related to "harmattan" winds, with nasal prevalence of 2–3% in the rainy season, but 4–8% in the dry season, when PAM occurred. There is controversy whether cysts of free-living amebas can resist desiccation.

T. gondii **(7417).** In Georgia, in 1977, an outbreak in a riding stable caused 37 infections in patrons; because a source could not be identified, inhalation of oocysts from stable dust was assumed.

HELMINTHS FROM DUST
E. granulosus **(198).** In arid Africa, hot winds (e.g., gibli, sirocco, and harmattan) are suspected of disseminating eggs, with the possibility of acquisition by inhalation and the formation of pulmonary cysts.

T. canis **(3389).** Dust is an unconfirmed source, although "flying worm eggs" could explain cases in adults without exposure to dogs. However, in Dublin County, Ireland, eggs were not detected in household dust, including from households with seroreactive members or back gardens positive for *T. canis* eggs.

ARTHROPODS AND WINDS
Mosquitoes (3856) typically fly at speeds of ~1 m/s. Winds can reduce flight speed or carry mosquitoes and flies over long distances (for aircraft, boats, and motor vehicles, see section 16.2). Mosquitoes (mainly *Culex*, but also *Anopheles* and *Aedes*) collected in New South Wales, Australia, in 1979–1984, by aerial kite traps demonstrated mean ($\pm$SD) dispersal distances of 24 ($\pm$15) km by day, and 152 ($\pm$116) km by night.

Infections from windblown mosquitoes (3856, 5231, 6765, 8087). **JEV.** JEV was introduced to the Torres Islands, Australia, in 1995, and to mainland Australia in 1998, likely from Papua New Guinea by mosquitoes blown by winds over 200 km. **WEEV.** In the 1980s, WEEV in Minnesota, North Dakota (United States), and Manitoba (Canada) was explained by winds that had blown infective *Culex tarsalis* mosquitoes from Texas and Oklahoma, assuming that these mosquitoes could cover 1,250–1,350 km in 24 h, at heights of $\leq$1.5 km and temperatures $\geq$13°C. **P. falciparum.** In 1989, a Frenchman contracted *P. falciparum* on malaria-free Guadeloupe, likely from *Anopheles* mosquitoes blown to the island by a cyclone that had hit the island 1 week previously. **O. volvulus.** In West Africa, infective *Simulium* blackflies blown from endemic to controlled areas are continuously threatening to reintroduce *O. volvulus* in the latter. Distances from source breeding sites were estimated to 400 km.

5.6 SEASONS

> *Whoever wishes to investigate medicine properly, should proceed thus: in the first place to consider the seasons of the year, and what effects each of them produces.*
>
> Hippocrates, ~400 BC, in On Airs, Waters, and Places

Seasons (4434) are characterized by day length and temperature at high and mid latitudes and by rainfall at low latitudes. Human activities vary with seasons, confounding climate effects on infectious disease transmission (Table 5.5).

Infections and seasons (2956, 5105, 6318, 6350, 8342). Season is diagnostically useful for infections that exhibit

Table 5.5 Four seasons: meteorologic and biologic characteristics and human activities

Variable	Winter	Spring	Summer	Fall
Months				
North	December to February	March to May	June to August	September to November
South	June to August	September to November	December to February	March to May
Daylight (h)				
Equator	12	12	12	12
Lat. 40°	9-11	11½-14½	15-13½	13-10
Lat. 70°	0–7	10–22	24–18	15-2
Weather	Ice forming	Snow melting	Dust and storms	Fires and frosts
Fauna	Protozoa encyst, vertebrates hibernate	Arthropods emerge, birds migrate to poles, kidding, lambing	Bacterial growth, arthropods bite	Arthropods pupate, birds migrate to equator
Human activities	Indoor life, crowding, heated dry rooms, peak antibiotic use	Schools open	School breaks, swimming, travel	School resumes, harvest
Foods	Home-canned	Asparagus, strawberry	Ice cream	Cider, grapes, venison

broad, recurring seasonal amplitudes, that is, high ratios of high-to-low seasonal rates (Table 5.6). Representative data may or may not be available from national surveillance systems. Long delays between onset of exposure (e_0) and disease (d_0) may obscure seasonal influences, e.g., late manifestations of tick-borne diseases. Delays vary with host susceptibility, infective dose, and incubation period.

Season is of limited diagnostic value for infections with perennial transmission. Perennially transmitted infections that are endemic in mid-latitudes and exhibit narrow seasonal amplitudes include sexually transmitted infections, blood-borne infections (e.g., due to HBV and HCV), nosocomial infections, some community-acquired enteric infections (e.g., due to *E. coli*, *Shigella*), as well as respiratory infections, both vaccine-preventable (e.g., measles, mumps, and rubella viruses, VZV; *Bordetella pertussis*, *H. influenzae* b) and vaccine nonpreventable agents (e.g., EBV, PVB19, and *Rhinovirus* and *Legionella* and *M. tuberculosis*).

Infections out of season are suspicious of importation by regional or international travel, incipient outbreaks, or intentional release.

COLD-WEATHER PEAKS
Infections in cold weather (1385). Crowding, heated rooms, and dry, stagnant air favor respiratory tract infections such as acute (rhino)sinusitis. These conditions might also explain the winter peaks observed with viral diarrheal disease. Winter survival strategies for vector-borne and environmental agents include latent stages in mammals, hardy spores, cysts, or eggs, and transovarial passage.

Table 5.6 Agents and infections prevailing in cold or warm seasons, by agent cluster

Agent cluster	Cold weather (winter) peaks	Warm weather (spring-summer-fall) peaks
Droplet-air, skin-blood	*Influenzavirus*, RSV, hMPV; *N. meningitidis*, *S. pneumoniae*, *S. pyogenes*; *Sarcoptes scabiei*	*Enterovirus*, parainfluenzavirus, *Rhinovirus*; *Mycoplasma pneumoniae*; *Coccidioides immitis*
Feces-food	Diarrhea by *Norovirus*, *Rotavirus*	Diarrhea due to *Campylobacter*, *Salmonella*, *Vibrio parahaemolyticus*; *Cryptosporidium*, *Cyclospora*, *Giardia*
	Botulism by home-preserved foods	Food poisoning by *S. aureus*
Zoonotic, environmental	Hantavirus (HTNV, PUUV) Relapsing borreliae in heated cabins, *Francisella* in fur trappers	Arthropod-borne *Alphavirus*, *Flavivirus*, *Orthobunyavirus*; *Borrelia burgdorferi* sl (early Lyme), *Orientia*, *Rickettsia*; *Babesia*, *Leishmania*
		Mammal-borne *Brucella*, *Coxiella*, *Francisella*, *Yersinia pestis*, *Leptospira*; *Naegleria* (primary amebic meningoencephalitis)

Droplet-Air Cluster

Viruses. Human metapneumovirus (hMPV) (479, 7715, 8185). hMPV infections and outbreaks peak in cooler months. **Influenzavirus (3152, 6350, 7672, 8342, 8350).** Recurring winter waves are widely known in countries with temperate climates (Fig. 5.1). Threshold algorithms are conceived to identify epidemic periods and excess deaths. In the United States in 1976–2005, influenza activity peaked in February in 45% (13/29) of seasons, in January in 21% (6/29), in December in 14% (4/29), and in other months (September, March–May) in 19%. Cases out of season were likely imported, posing a risk for seeding outbreaks. In tropical climates, transmission can be year-round. In Australia, a summer (January) outbreak occurred in a prison. **Respiratory syncytial virus (RSV) (6350, 7156).** Infections have a marked winter peak, including bronchiolitis in infants, and exacerbation of chronic obstructive pulmonary disease in the elderly. In western Europe and North America, the RSV season starts in November, typically in coastal areas and ahead of the influenza winter wave. **Rhinovirus (5150).** Rhinovirus dominates viral respiratory tract infections in spring, summer, and autumn, *except* in winter, when it is surpassed by *Influenzavirus*, RSV, and parainfluensa virus (PIV).

Bacteria. *N. meningitidis* (396, 6350, 7078). Sporadic meningitis cases can occur anytime. However, a majority of invasive disease cases in temperate climate countries occur in winter. In New Zealand in 1991–1998, two-thirds of 2,563 serogroup B cases occurred in winter (June–August in the Southern Hemisphere) and spring (September–November). ***S. pneumoniae* (2012, 3793, 3938)** invasive disease and streptococcal otitis media peaks in winter.

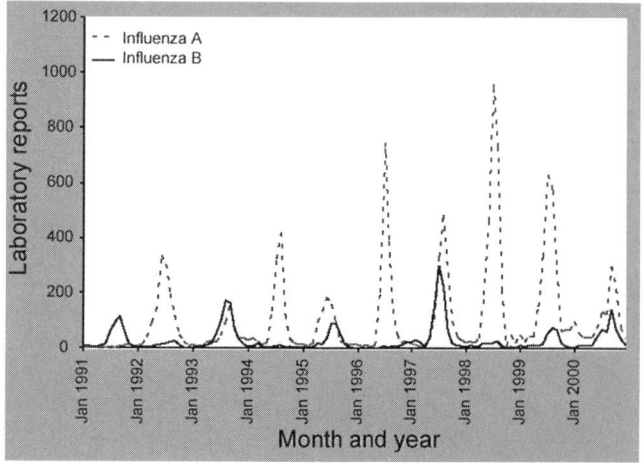

Figure 5.1 Laboratory reports of *Influenzavirus* A and B infections in Australia, 1991–2000 (10 years). The number of reports (y axis) is given by month of specimen collection (x axis) and type (A virus, dotted line [$n = 13{,}191$]; B virus, solid line [$n = 3{,}614$]). From reference 6350. Copyright by Commonwealth of Australia. Reproduced with permission.

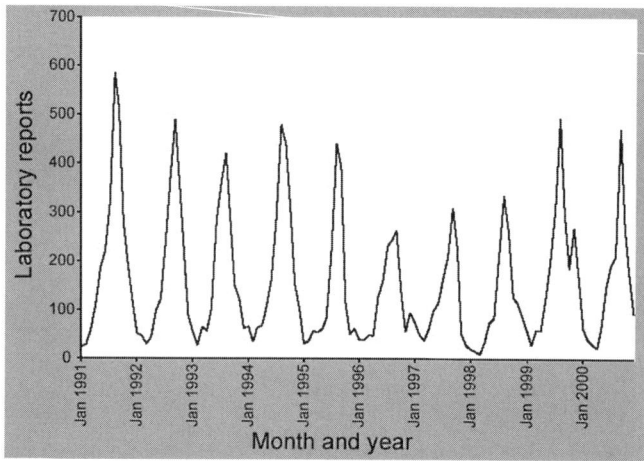

Figure 5.2 Laboratory reports of *Rotavirus* infection in Australia, 1991–2000 (10 years; $n = 18{,}968$). The number of reports (y axis) is given by month of specimen collection (x axis). From reference 6350. Copyright by Commonwealth of Australia. Reproduced with permission.

Feces-Food Cluster

Viruses. *Norovirus* (3226, 3559, 3565). Infections and outbreaks peak in winter (winter vomiting disease). In Sweden, outbreaks have a second peak in spring. ***Rotavirus* (3559, 4055, 6350, 7513).** Although transmission can be year-round in tropical areas, there are poorly understood, but predictable, strong winter peaks in areas with temperate climates in North America, Australia (Fig. 5.2), Japan, and West Europe. In North America, waves start in Mexico and the southwestern United States in October–November, move across the continent in winter, and end in the northeastern United States and maritime Canada by April–May. In Europe, waves typically begin in Spain in October, move through France and the United Kingdom in winter, and end in The Netherlands and Finland in March. In Japan, outbreaks of rotavirus diarrhea also peak in winter.

Bacteria. *C. botulinum* (7774). In the Republic of Georgia, most cases of food botulism were due to homemade vegetables, and >75% of the 329 reported incidences occurred in winter or spring.

Zoonotic Cluster

Indoor rodents and ticks can cause cold-weather clusters.

Rodents (4397, 5609, 6405). In East Asia, HTNV has a major peak in fall, when the proportion of infected *Apodemus* mice is high. In rural Scandinavia, bank vole populations peak in fall. As soil freezes, voles seek shelter in houses, thereby increasing human exposure to PUUV. Infections in humans and epidemic nephropathy peak in late fall and early winter.

Ticks (2103). Cases of TBRF can cluster in winter, by ticks that are attracted to fire in a cold cabin.

Skin-Blood Cluster
Streptococcus pyogenes (group A *Streptococcus*) isolates from throat and nose, and group A *Streptococcus* pharyngitis have been reported to peak in winter (239).

In temperate climates, scabies can be seasonal, with a peak rate in winter (8042).

WARM-WEATHER PEAKS
Infections in warm weather (405, 1368, 4023, 4306, 4310, 4315, 7261).
In spring, birds migrate from low latitudes toward middle latitudes, and arthropods become active (Table 5.5). Ticks in temperate climates emerge in March–May, when snow has melted and temperatures remain >5–7°C. Humans resume outdoor activities, including swimming in pools (Fig. 13.1). Vector snails release cercariae during May–October. Bacterial growth rate in food and tap water is accelerated. The density of fungal and bacterial spores in air reaches a high in spring and summer. Tick activity extends into October–November, until temperatures fall <5–7°C.

The transmission of arthropod-borne agents is strikingly seasonal. Some enteric and respiratory agents in temperate climates have marked warm-weather peaks (Table 5.6).

Droplet-Air Cluster
Viruses (2484, 5149). Viral respiratory tract infections in temperate climates trending toward warm-weather (spring to fall) peaks include *Enterovirus*, parainfluenzavirus, and *Rhinovirus*. **Enterovirus (EV) (1378, 6095, 6350).** EV infections, in general, peak in summer and fall, including aseptic meningitis. In summer and fall, 25–50% of febrile illness in hospitalized infants is attributed to EV. Pollution of coastal waters with EV also peaks in the summer. Spring isolates can predict >50% of serotypes likely to circulate in the summer and fall. However, coxsackie A and B viruses, and echovirus tend to occur in outbreaks rather than seasonal waves. **PIV (4249, 6350, 8185).** Transmission is year-round, but there are strong, predictable peaks, including of PIV-associated croup. PIV3 has annual peaks in late fall; PIV1 and PIV2 have biennial peaks in late fall. **Rhinovirus.** Although transmitted year-round, *Rhinovirus* seems to have a curious summer transmission peak.

Bacteria. Although not well documented, *M. pneumoniae* infections tend to peak in late summer and fall, unlike pneumonia that peaks in winter.

Fungi. Transmission of *C. immitis* (4042) is seasonal, in general, with peaks in fall that correlate with drought, dust, and winds (Fig. 5.3).

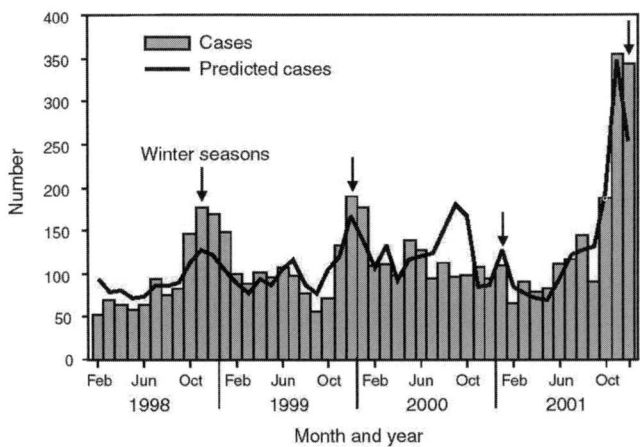

Figure 5.3 Reported coccidioidomycosis cases in Arizona, 1998–2001 ($n = 1,551$ in 1998; $n = 2,203$ in 2001). The number of reports (y axis) is given by month (x axis). Actual reports are shown as bars, and predicted numbers are shown as a line. From reference 4042.

Feces-Food Cluster
Bacteria (167, 1006, 1150, 2413, 5522, 5998, 6681, 7591). Predictable, annual warm-weather peaks are documented in countries with temperate climates for diarrhea due to *Campylobacter*, *P. shigelloides*, *Salmonella*, *Staphylococcus aureus* food poisoning, and *Vibrio* (*V. parahaemolyticus* and *V. vulnificus*). Possible explanations include human activities (e.g., barbecueing, drinking from wells, and swimming), and enhanced microbial growth and survival in foods (e.g., ice cream, cheese, oysters, and beef), reservoir animals (e.g., cattle and broiler flocks), and the environment (e.g., sewage).

Protozoa (597, 2558, 3285, 3352, 3423, 6446). Predictable, annual warm-weather peaks are documented in countries with temperate climates for diarrhea due to *Cryptosporidium*, *Cyclospora*, and *Giardia*. In the United States, *Cryptosporidium* case reports increase 5–6-fold during April–October, most markedly in children (Fig. 5.4). The same explanations can be offered as for bacterial diarrhea agents.

Figure 5.4 Reported cryptosporidiosis cases in the United States, 1999–2002 ($n = 7,270$). The number of reports (y axis) is given by month of illness (x axis) for selected age groups (lines). From reference 3352.

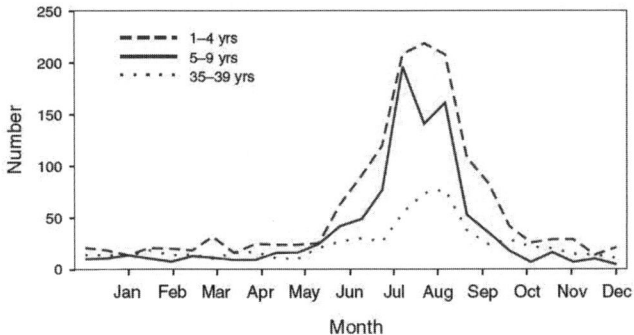

Zoonotic Cluster

Arthropod- and rodent-borne infections can exhibit striking seasonal peaks.

Viruses (1435, 2956, 3403, 6350, 6932). Examples of warm-weather peaks in countries with temperate climates include encephalitis viruses of California serogroup (e.g., LACV, *Orthobunyavirus*) (Fig. 5.5; note interrupted transmission in winter) and WNV (July to October) in the United States, RRV (*Alphavirus*) in Australia, and TBEV (*Flavivirus*) in Eurasia. Even in tropical climates, rains can dictate seasonal patterns. An example is DENV (*Flaviviridae*) in Brazil (Fig. 5.6).

Bacteria. Livestock and rodents are important sources of *Brucella*, *Coxiella*, *Francisella*, and *Y. pestis* in warm months (Table 5.6). **B. melitensis (6808).** In People's Republic of China in 1950–1999, 62% (3,862/6,212) of infections occurred in February–June, during the lambing season. **C. burnetii (2085, 3243).** In Europe, Q fever peaks in spring (lambing and kidding) and again in fall (livestock returning from alpine pastures). **F. tularensis (2172, 3205).** Vector-borne tularemia is limited to summer and fall. In contrast, occupational tularemia can occur year-round, with a peak in fall and winter that coincides with hunting. **Y. pestis (1004, 5844).** Plague seasonality is explained by epizootics that spill over to humans, for instance, when rodents awake from hibernation and leave burrows. Most human cases occur in May–October in North America, January–April in East Africa and Southeast Asia, and July–August on the Tibetan plateau.

In warm months, ticks are important sources of *Borrelia* and Rickettsiales (*Anaplasma*, *Ehrlichia*, *Orientia*, and *Rickettsia*). **B. burgdorferi sl (2103, 2291, 6315).** Acute infections and early Lyme disease (erythema migrans) follow tick activity. In Germany, >90% of acute Lyme disease cases are reported in March–October. On

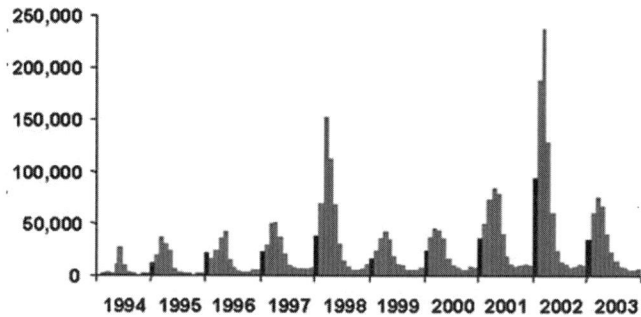

Figure 5.6 Reported dengue fever cases in Brazil, 1994–2003 (*n* = 2.8 million). The number of reports (*y* axis) is given by month of reporting (*x* axis). January: dark bars. From reference 6932.

the contrary, late-stage Lyme disease tends to occur year-round. Similarly, TBRF in temperate climates peaks in summer. ***A. phagocytophilum*** **(human granulocytic ehrlichiosis) and *Ehrlichia chaffeensis* (human monocytic ehrlichiosis) (1872).** *A. phagocytophilum* and *E. chaffeensis* are strongly seasonal, with most cases of human granulocytic and monocytic ehrlichioses having onset in May–August. ***O. tsutsugamushi*** **(3884).** Scrub typhus peaks in spring, summer, or fall, in parallel with vector mite activity. In South Korea in the 1980s, ~90% of reported (8,200) cases occurred in October–November. ***Rickettsia*** **(86, 600, 7545).** Warm-weather peaks are documented for *R. conorii* (80–90% of Mediterranean spotted fever occur in summer or fall), *R. rickettsii* (~90% of Rocky Mountain spotted fever cases in the United States occur in April–September), and *R. typhi* (about two-thirds of murine typhus cases in North America and western Europe occur in April–September).

Protozoa (805, 2546, 6459). Transmission of *Babesia* (by ticks) and *Leishmania* (by sandflies) in temperate climates is strongly seasonal, typically in April–November. ***Leishmania*.** In Marrakech, Morocco, *P. papatasi* was active throughout the year, with peaks in June and November that related to human risks of *L. major* cutaneous infections. In the Sinai, Egypt, in 1990, *P. papatasi* activity peaked in July, when human landing rates reached 95/person per hour, and promastigote infection rates reached 2.4%. In Turkmenistan and Uzbekistan, gerbils (*Rhombomys opimus*) carry *L. major* through the cold season when sandflies are inactive.

Environmental Cluster

Leptospira **(3387, 4369).** Cases peak in summer and fall. In Denmark in 1970–1996, of 118 confirmed cases, 72% occurred in July–September.

Free-living amebas (4911). Cases of PAM peak in summer. Explanations include leisure activities in freshwater (see section 5.2) and enhanced growth of free-living amebas in warm water.

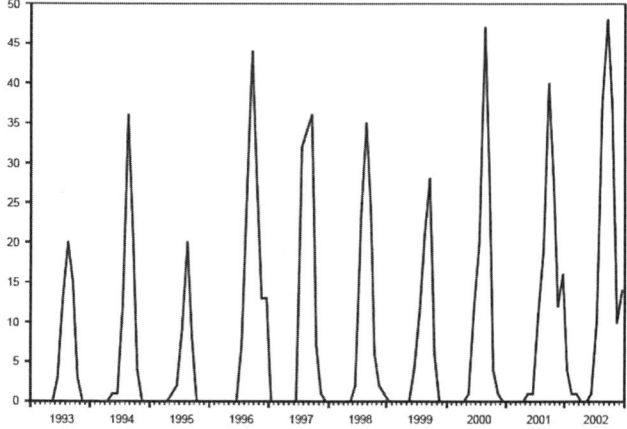

Figure 5.5 California serogroup encephalitis laboratory reports in the United States, 1993–2002. The number of reports (*y* axis, *n* > 640) is given by month of onset (*x* axis). From reference 2956.

RAINY SEASONS

Humid soils, abundant freshwater, and little variations of water and air temperatures make the tropics ideal for survival and year-round transmission of microorganisms, worm larvae and eggs, and vector arthropods and snails. However, droughts that follow rainy periods (monsoons) can generate seasonal patterns (for floods, see section 5.2).

Droplet-Air Cluster

For reasons not well understood, tropical climates seem less favorable for the transmission of varicella-zoster virus (VZV) than temperate climates. In Thailand, anti-VZV prevalence was higher in the cooler parts of the country than in the tropical parts (4495).

Feces-Food Cluster

The transmision of food-borne agents in the tropics and subtropics can vary seasonally, including HEV, *S. enterica* serovar Typhi, *V. cholerae*, *Cryptosporidium*, *Cyclospora*, *A. cantonensis*, *Dracunculus medinensis*, and *Fasciolopsis buski* (482, 595, 1028, 1588, 5397, 6528). Possible explanations include rains that flush out feces and sewers and droughts that concentrate agents in residual waters. In Bangladesh, transmission of *F. buski* is interrupted in the dry season (November–June), when fields dry out and water plants are no longer available for consumption. *D. medinensis* is well adapted to seasons; during rains, females release larvae, during droughts, copepods concentrate in shallow ponds; ultimately, when ponds have dried up, humans are the only reservoir that carries the worm over the dry season.

Periodicity can be quite remarkable, as *V. cholerae* isolates in Calcutta demonstrate (Fig. 5.7).

Zoonotic Cluster

Viruses. Monsoonal swings are reported for *Alphavirus* (e.g., CHIKV and RRV) and *Flavivirus* (e.g., DENV, JEV, and MVEV) (914, 5895, 7291, 7422). **RRV (4619, 7291).** In Australia, RRV typically accompanies wet seasons. After droughts, RRV is reactivated by drought-resistant mosquito eggs or reintroduced by viremic migratory birds. Rains after droughts carry a risk of outbreaks. **DENV (6932).** In Brazil in 1994–2003, although transmission was year-round and DENV 1–3 serotypes cocirculated nationwide, steep seasonal effects were observed, with a peak in the rainy season (December–May) (Fig. 5.6).

Protozoa. *Leishmania* **(220).** In the subtropical forest on the Yucatan Peninsula, Mexico, transmission of zoonotic CL was seasonal, with a peak in winter (November–March) that coincided with abundance of infective sandfly vectors (rodentophilic *Lutzomyia olmeca*, anthropophilic *L. cruciata*) and overnight human forest activities. **Plasmodium (367, 930, 1039, 3930, 4059, 4445, 6858, 7328).** In general, malaria transmission peaks during rainy seasons. However, paradoxically, transmission can be intense in the dry season, for instance, when receding rivers leave pools for breeding. In Africa, transmission periods can last 7–12 months (in the rain forest of equatorial Africa and on the East African coast), 4–6 months (in the south Sahel and in savanna areas of East and southern Africa), 1–3 months (in

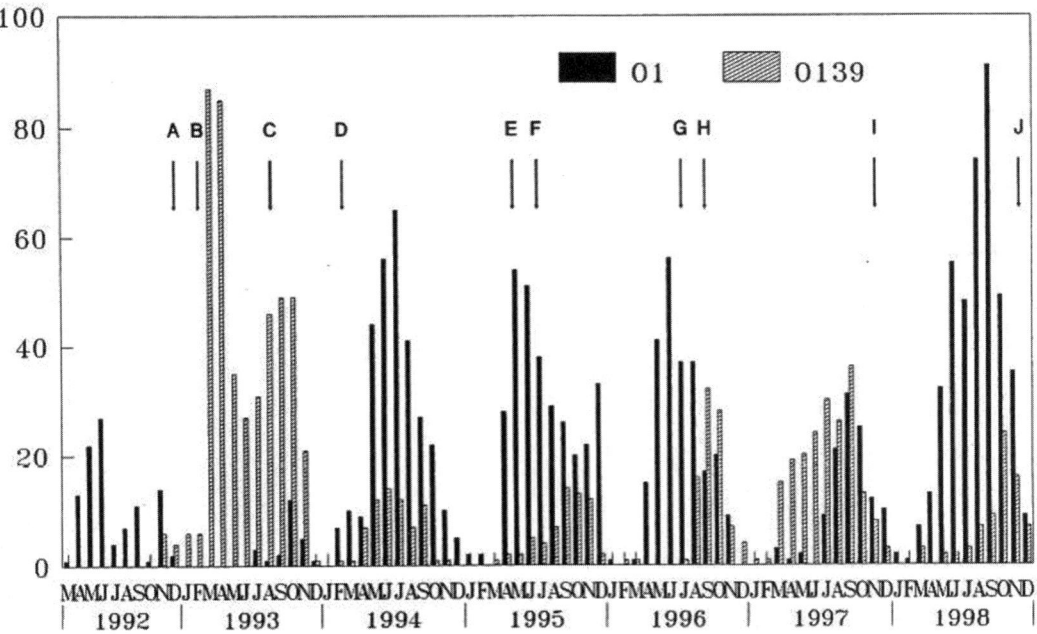

Figure 5.7 Isolates of *Vibrio cholerae* in Calcutta, India, March 1992–December 1998 (n = 2,404). The number of isolates (y axis) is given by month (x axis) and serogroup (black, group O1, n = 1491; hatched, group O139, n = 913). Letters A–J mark changes of dominant serogroup. From reference 482.

the north Sahel), or 0 months (in the Sahara, except oases; see section 5.4).

In East Sudan, where transmission lasts 2–3 months/year, residents with subpatent parasitemia carry *P. falciparum* through the dry season. In areas with intermittent transmission, including highlands and arid lands, where parasitemia prevalence fluctuates from troughs of 5–50% (typically 20%) in the dry season to 40–80% (typically 60%) in the rainy season, outbreaks are a constant threat.

Effects of ENSO events are unpredictable. In the Usambara Mountains, Tanzania, although the 1997–1998 ENSO event more than doubled the usual amount of rains, fewer malaria cases were observed. In Uganda, rains with the 1997 ENSO event more than doubled the malaria rate. In Kenya in January–May 1998, floods after long droughts caused a major falciparum malaria epidemic among nonimmune people in the northeast of the country. **T. cruzi (2754, 7786).** In areas with subtropical or cooler climates, the abundance and infectivity of *Triatoma infestans* may vary seasonally. In northwestern Argentina, houses were found to smoothen temperature at vector microhabitats (thatched roofs, storerooms, and living rooms) by as much as 8°C compared with exterior habitats (goat and pig corrals and chicken coops).

Environmental Cluster

Rains significantly affect environmental conditions for bacteria, helminths, and snails (gardeners will know).

Bacteria. ***Burkholderia* (1685).** Rainfall in the 2 weeks before admission is a risk, perhaps because rains and monsoonal winds shift transmission from inoculation to inhalation. In northern Australia, 85% (215/252) of melioidosis cases are seen during the rainy season (November–April). ***Leptospira* (5894, 7678).** Warm weather, abundant rains, and perennial water courses increase transmission risks. Serovar diversity peaks during rains. In Yucatán, Mexico, about 75% of leptospirosis cases occur in the rainy season.

Helminths. **Hookworms (7632, 7634).** Larvae of *A. duodenale* and *N. americanus* seasonally fluctuate in soil, with peaks during the rainy season and troughs in the dry season. ***Schistosoma* (3910).** Transmission in subtropical countries can vary seasonally, in parallel with the abundance of vector snails and snail infectivity. ***Toxocara* (3702).** On Canary Islands, seroprevalence is low on dry, east sides of islands, and high on humid, west sides.

6

6.1 Dams and irrigation
6.2 Buildings, sanitation, and wastewater
6.3 Cities
6.4 Utensils and belongings

Human-Made Environments

ENVIRONMENT

Human impact (2696), http://www.wri.org/wr2000. At least 3% (4.7 million/148 million km^2) of the world's land surface is built up. Human impact on the environment includes roads, agglomerations, and dams; pollution of soil, water, and air with household, traffic, farm, and industrial emissions; and degradation of land, forest, streams, and oceans by farming, logging, and fisheries.

Infections from human-made environments (7501). Modes of spread are inhalation (e.g., aerosols from sprinkler irrigation and cooling towers, dust from bed linen), ingestion (e.g., unclean hands), inoculation (e.g., shared personal objects), and contact (e.g., waste, clothes). Proof for objects (fomites) as vehicles of infections in humans is difficult. In general, high-income populations seem to overrate the importance of daily objects (e.g., toilet seats) as vehicles, but to underrate kitchen and food hygiene and municipal services of tap water, sewerage, and garbage disposal. Routine use of disinfectants (or even antibiotics) in households is discouraged.

6.1 DAMS AND IRRIGATION

Dams and irrigation (5977). Large dams are defined by wall height >15 m, or water capacity >3 million m^3. Worldwide, there were 5,000 large dams in 1950, but 45,000 in 2000. The number of small dams is estimated at 0.8 million. Many large dams are intended for irrigation. Worldwide, irrigated areas covered 1.4 million km^2 in 1961, but 2.7 million in 2001. Countries with large areas under irrigation include People's Republic of China, India (each 0.5 million km^2), and the United States (0.2 million km^2). Soil salinization can be a consequence of irrigation. Large areas of salinized lands exist in India (70,000 km^2, 17% of irrigated area), People's Republic of China (6,700 km^2, 15%), Pakistan (4,200 km^2, 26%), and the United States (4,200 km^2, 23%). How salinized soils affect soil-dwelling agents is not known.

Infections from dams and irrigation projects (872, 1389, 3995, 3996, 5299, 6283, 7057). Dams and irrigation schemes have health benefits and risks. Here, the focus is on infectious disease risks. Evidence is limited as most reports are descriptive or cross-sectional, and few studies are prospective, comparing preconstruction with operative conditions. Health risks during construction include infections by crowding and STI. Risks from established schemes are water that is fecally polluted by livestock, water fowl, and informal settlements; immigrated fish that serve as intermediate hosts; and new breeding sites for vector snails, mosquitoes, and flies (Box 6.1).

DAM-RELATED FECES-FOOD CLUSTER
Like tap water (see sections 10.2 and 10.3), fecally polluted dam and irrigation waters can be vehicles of enteric agents (for wastewater, see section 6.2 below). At low wind velocity, infective aerosols from irrigation sprinklers can be carried up to 160 m (on occasion, 300 m) away from spray sprinklers (92). On the other hand, adequate amounts of safe domestic water reduce risks of diarrheal disease (7718).

Viruses (7372)
Enteric viruses have been infrequently reported from dam or irrigation waters, but these waters are likely to contain *Enterovirus* and hepatitis A virus (HAV). In South Africa, HAV and human astrovirus have been amplified in water samples from a dam and a river, HAV in 37% (19/51) of dam and 35% (18/51) of river water samples, and human astrovirus in 6% (3/51) of dam and 22% (11/51) of river water samples.

Bacteria (2056)
Bacteria recovered from irrigation water include *Escherichia coli* and *Salmonella*.

Helminths (1028, 2127, 3107)
In Tozeur Oasis, Tunisia, lymnaeid snails harboring *Fasciola hepatica* or *F. gigantica* have been shown to invade irrigation canals and irrigated fields. In rural Africa, most *Dracunculus medinensis* transmission sites are made by humans. In Nigeria in 1983, a dam was implicated in an outbreak of dracunculiasis in a nearby community.

DAM-RELATED ZOONOTIC CLUSTER
It is widely recognized that dams and irrigation canals offer breeding sites for vector mosquitoes. In particular, in Africa, *Anopheles gambiae* sensu lato (sl) and *A. funestus* are more abundant in irrigated than nonirrigated areas (249).

Viruses (440, 3192, 3754)
Irrigation areas are a reported venue for transmission of arboviruses. In North Queensland, Australia, although dam-breeding mosquitoes (e.g., *Culex annulirostris*, *Anopheles annulipes* sl, and *Mansonia uniformis*) were more abundant near Ross River dam than in zones away from the dam, surveillance of sentinel chicken flocks for Ross River virus and Sindbis virus did not demonstrate increased risks near the dam. In Mauritania in 1987, a dam on the Senegal River was venue for an outbreak of Rift Valley fever virus with 200 human deaths.

Protozoa
The focus of dam-related vector-borne protozoa is malaria.

Leishmania. **Visceral leishmaniasis (VL) (547).** In central Tunisia, an irrigation scheme with ~10,000 wells and intensive agriculture was suspected of maintaining *Phlebotomus perniciosus* and year-round, low-level transmission of *L. infantum*. **Cutaneous leishmaniasis (CL) (2174, 2546).** In the Old World, irrigation has been reported to affect rodent burrows and vector composition. Cooler conditions in irrigated areas seem to favor *Phlebotomus papatasi* and transmission of *L. major*. In the Sinai Desert, Egypt, construction of the El Ruafa Dam appeared to result in high *P. papatasi* densities.

Plasmodium **(1088, 1389, 3995, 4750, 6789, 6922).** Hazards from irrigation schemes include poorly maintained canals that become clogged and waterlogged, abandoned reservoirs and dead-end canals that become breeding sites, shifts in *Anopheles* species composition, and nonimmune immigrants who settle near water. In Zimbabwe, malaria risks were higher with sprinkler irrigation than surface irrigation, likely because equipment was poorly maintained. In the Punjab, Pakistan, irrigation went along with a shift from *Anopheles culicifacies* to the more salt-tolerant *A. stephensi*. Net effects of irrigation on malaria risks vary by location, maintenance, principal vector, and population mix.

Box 6.1 Hazards from dams and water irrigation projects, by agent clusters

Feces-food	Enteric viruses and bacteria; *A. lumbricoides*; food-borne trematodes
Zoonotic	Breeding sites for mosquitoes; arboviruses; *Leishmania, Plasmodium*; *Wuchereria*
Environmental	*Leptospira*, mycobacteria; *S. haematobium, S. mansoni* (endemic areas)

Stable or decreased transmission have been reported from projects in West Africa: Côte d'Ivoire (3264), Mali (1970, 6939), and Senegal (2337); East Africa: Kenya (5287) and Tanzania (3547); and Central Asia: Pakistan (3995) and Sri Lanka (3996). In semiarid Mali, rice cultivation altered transmission from seasonal to perennial, but reduced clinical malaria rates (per 1,000 children per day), from 0.6 (dry season) and 3.2 (rainy season) in the unirrigated area to 0.7 (throughout the year) in the irrigated area (6939). Explanations included more cattle and more zoophilic *Anopheles* in the irrigated area and increased use of bednets (1970). In Kenya, *A. arabiensis* was 30–300 times more abundant in villages with rice irrigation that in nonirrigation villages, but the prevalence of parasitemia was lower in the former (0–9%) than in the latter (17–54%). This so-called paddy paradox has been attributed to cattle raised in irrigation areas (5287).

Increased transmission or outbreaks have been reported in West Africa: urban Ghana (79); East Africa: Burundi (1568), Ethiopia (2713), Madagascar (4252, 4750), and Sudan (4); and Central Asia: Afghanistan (6440) and India (6922, 7624–7626). In southern Madagascar, entomological inoculation rates (EIR, infective bites per person per year) are 0.4 in a nonirrigated arid area, but 41 in an irrigated, humid area and 60 in an irrigated, arid area (4750). In Ethiopia, clinical malaria rates are higher in children residing near small dams than in children away from dams (2713). In Afghanistan, irrigated rice fields are major breeding sites for *A. stephensi* (6440). On the Narmada River in westcentral India, malaria was rare before the Bargi dam was completed in 1988; in 1996–1997, epidemics occurred, and the prevalence of *Plasmodium falciparum* parasitemia in the district doubled. In parallel, numbers of *A. culicifacies* decreased, while *A. fluviatilis* increased (6922). In Thar Desert, Northwest India, malaria epidemics recur. Stagnant canal water and waterlogged fields are breeding sites for *A. stephensi* and *A. culicifacies*. Reasons for outbreaks are variously attributed to heavy rains from El Niño events, or irrigation canals (total length, 9,000 km) (799, 7625, 7626).

Helminths (249, 6283)

In Cameroon, spillways from small dams are good breeding sites for *Simulium damnosum* sl, and transmission sites for *Onchocerca volvulus*. In Ghana, dams and irrigation schemes have an impact on *Wuchereria bancrofti* transmission. In irrigated areas, *A. gambiae* sensu stricto (ss) females are carrying larvae significantly more often than those away from irrigated areas (2–3% versus 0.3%), and the transmission potential has increased >25-fold (13–14 versus 0.5).

DAM-RELATED ENVIRONMENTAL CLUSTER
Bacteria

***Leptospira* (222, 5840).** A serosurvey among French canal and locks workers suggested a reservoir for *Leptospira* in human-made water bodies, similar to natural waters (see section 5.2). Bathing in canals is a risk.

***Mycobacterium* (4391, 8107).** Stagnant artificial waters such as fish tanks and dams are a reservoir for environmental mycobacteria, mainly *M. marinum*, likely also *M. ulcerans*. *M. ulcerans* can attach to aquatic plants, and its spread by aquatic insects or snails has been proposed.

Helminths

The focus of dam-related environmental helminths is *Schistosoma*.

Schistosoma. Poorly planned or managed dams and irrigation schemes are hazards for newly exposed communities, mainly in Africa (584, 7057). Mechanized irrigation farming in Brazil seems appreciably less hazardous than labor-intensive irrigation farming in Africa (4782). In Zimbabwe, the schistosomiasis rate is higher in canal than sprinkler irrigation areas, perhaps because poor drainage from surface irrigation creates snail-breeding sites (1389). Effects of the three-gorge dam in People's Republic of China on *S. japonicum* will need monitoring. **West Africa.** In Côte d'Ivoire, Kossou Dam (height, 58 m) and Taabo Dam (height, 34 m) were monitored for schistosomiasis from construction to operation. *S. haematobium* prevalence increased from 14 to 53% (Kossou Lake) and from 0 to 73% (Taabo Lake). In contrast, *S. mansoni* prevalence remained low at Taabo Lake (3–2%; data for Kossou Lake are not available) (5299). In northern Ghana, after the Tono irrigation scheme became operational in 1977, *S. mansoni* and *S. haematobium* became highly prevalent in school children. While *Bulinus globosus* snails and *S. mansoni* transmission sites were limited to the main canal, *Biomphalaria pfeifferi* snails and *S. haematobium* were rampant in the whole scheme (181). In Mali, data from 225 villages and 34,000 persons were analyzed for small-dam effects and irrigation: compared with savanna areas without irrigation, irrigation farming increased the risk of *Schistosoma* infection 6-fold (885). Completion of the Diama Dam on the Senegal River in 1986 was followed by the emergence of *S. mansoni* and later *S. haematobium*; in 1988–1989, an outbreak caused 1,935 *S. mansoni* infections (7057, 7317). **Central and East Africa.** In small dams in Cameroon, *S. haematobium* transmission is highest in secondary and tertiary drainage channels choked by vegetation and populated by *B. globosus* and *Bulinus truncatus* vector snails (6283). In Ethiopia, the prevalence of *S. mansoni* is 48% (165/341) near small dams and 30% (100/337) far away from dams (2714).

6.2 BUILDINGS, SANITATION, AND WASTEWATER

A 1918 survey of urban housing in the United States found that nearly one-fifth of all apartments and two-fifths of all houses had outside privies

(p. 185) (7501)

Sanitation (235, 1980, 2375, 7650, 7984). Flush toilets became popular only after World War I. Broadly defined, "improved" sanitary installations include municipal sewerage, septic tanks, pour-flush toilets, or ventilated-improved or simple pit latrines. More narrowly defined, "adequate" sanitation requires well-maintained toilets within walking distance that safely dispose of waste. By definition of sanitation, worldwide about 60% of people have access to sanitation (35–75% in Africa and Asia and 50–75% in Latin America).

Main sources of infections from building environments are cooling systems and open sewers (Box 6.2). Multistorage buildings should have plans for dealing with the intentional release of weaponized agents.

AIR IN BUILDINGS

Air quality (216, 2865, 5014, 5940, 6725). Wooden materials in water-damaged buildings can grow molds and release bacteria and fungi (e.g., *Aspergillus*, *Penicillium*, and *Stachybotrys*) that have been implicated in respiratory tract disease and "sick building syndrome." In Poland, 32% of indoor air samples in >100 flats from 15 towns grew *Nocardia*, 40% grew *Aeromonas*, and 62% grew *Aspergillus*. Fungal concentrations were 0–2,000/m^3 in nonmoldy flats, and 50–17,000/m^3 in moldy flats. Confounders to consider in cross-sectional studies include crowding, smokers in households, and past respiratory illnesses.

***Bacillus anthracis* (1183, 6969, 8021).** Weaponized *B. anthracis* is a potential hazard in multistory buildings (elevator shafts and air-management systems). In the United States in 2001, government buildings became contaminated with *B. anthracis* by spores intentionally sent by mail. In 3 weeks in October, seven inhalational anthrax cases and eight cutaneous cases resulted from this release. Of the seven inhalational cases, five were postal workers, and one was a mail sorter from a news company. Of >7,000 building occupants, nasal swabs from 20 of 38 in the mail room grew *B. anthracis*. Two other letters containing *B. anthracis* spores were mailed. In one office, four inhalational anthrax cases occurred, and sampling by surface wipe, vacuum cleaning, and air pump filtering provided evidence of ample contamination with spores. Operation of mail machinery and pressured air cleaning were suspected to have spread spores further. Usual office activities can re-aerosolize spores and increase counts in the air up to 65-fold.

SANITARY INSTALLATIONS IN BUILDINGS

Although sinks, toilet seats, and other surfaces readily grow microorganisms, sanitary installations in buildings are rarely sources of infections (1955, 3780, 6741). An exception are showers and baths (wet cells) that can be sources of tinea pedis, *Legionella* (mainly in immune-impaired individuals), and exit-site and bloodstream infections (in persons who carry devices). For diaper-changing areas and kitchen utensils, see "Utensils and Belongings" below.

Viruses

There is limited evidence for enteric viruses and human papillomavirus (HPV) as sanitary hazards.

HAV (3120). In Queensland, Australia, in 1992, early in a protracted school outbreak with 23 (5%) cases among 500 students, poorly maintained toilets without soap or towels and four of eight nonworking handbasins contributed to person-to-person spread.

***Norovirus* (716, 4163, 5520).** Aerosols from polluted tap water are a risk, including from domestic showers and from showers at a beach. In an outbreak at a rehabilitation center in Finland, identical *Norovirus* was amplified from patients, a bathroom door handle, and two toilet

---

Box 6.2 Agents from buildings, installations, and waste, by agent cluster

Hazards are in parentheses.

Droplet-air	*L. pneumophila* (aerosols from showers and air conditioners, cooling towers), *P. aeruginosa* (baths), medical device exit-site infections (baths and showers); fungi
Feces-food	(Raw waste): HAV, HEV; *Salmonella*; *Cryptosporidium*, *Cyclospora*, *Giardia*; *Ascaris*, *Taenia*
Zoonotic	(Intentional release of weaponized agents): e.g., *B. anthracis*
Environmental	Environmental mycobacteria (tap water); *Acanthamoeba* (tap water); hookworm (raw waste)
Skin-blood	(Public wet floors): HPV (plantar warts); dermatophytes

seats, but environmental contamination was the result of the outbreak rather than its source.

Rotavirus **(1010).** In two day-care centers in the United States, 19% (18/96) of objects sampled for 6 months yielded *Rotavirus* by nucleic acid amplification test (NAT), including a drinking fountain, toilet handles, and a telephone receiver. These were suggested as sources of *Rotavirus* in that center.

HPV (6036, 6697). In high-income countries, there is no evidence for the acquisition of genital HPV at indoor pools, saunas, decks, or dressing rooms. In contrast, HPV-associated plantar warts can be contracted from floors at wet places such as public showers.

Bacteria

There is good evidence for *Legionella* as a sanitary hazard, and limited evidence for mycobacteria, mycoplasms, *Pseudomonas*, and *Salmonella*.

Legionella pneumophila **(1876, 1967, 2625, 5887, 7149).** For hotels, see section 11.8. Up to 60% of building and public water supplies grow *Legionella*, including drinking and decorative fountains, faucets, taps, showers, cooling towers, air conditioners, boilers, water valves, swimming pools, whirlpools, and thermal spas. Recovered species include *L. anisa*, *L. londiniensis*, *L. micdadei*, and serogroups of *L. pneumophila*. In general, clinical isolates do not parallel environmental isolates; *L. pneumophila* serogroup 1 is overrepresented in the former, *L. anisa* in the latter. Infective aerosols can be generated by fountains, air conditioners, mist machines, evaporative coolers, and cooling towers. Infective aerosols can be released into buildings and street environments. **Cooling towers (427, 635, 921, 2395, 5073, 5105).** By season, 15–50% of water samples from cooling towers grow *L. pneumophila*. Growth is slowed at <16.5°C, but exponential at 20–30°C. In Singapore in 2000, 113 (60%) of 190 cooling towers in 107 buildings grew *Legionella*, 8 (4%) with counts of $\geq 10^5$ CFU/liter. Good engineering and maintenance practices can minimize outbreak risks. Hazards include poor design and repair and cleaning work. By weather conditions, infective aerosols can disperse over 0.3–10 km. In Glasgow, United Kingdom, in 1978–1986, cooling towers and home places of 107 patients with Legionnaires' disease clustered in the city center and along the river Clyde; persons who lived within 0.5 km from a tower had a 3-times-greater risk than persons who lived >1 km away from a tower. The infective dose and the duration of exposure needed to cause illness are unknown.

Outbreaks Cooling towers are well-documented sources of legionellosis outbreaks in high-income countries:

- North America (63, 916). In Wisconsin in 1986, an outbreak of Legionnaires' disease was linked to a cooling tower from which *L. pneumophila* serogroup 1 was isolated; of 29 confirmed cases, 21 lived or worked close (≤ 1.6 km) to the tower, and 7 had visited a perimeter (1.6–3.2 km) in 3–7 days before the onset of illness. Attack rates were highest in the core area (≤ 0.8 km from the tower). In Delaware in 1994, hospital cooling towers caused a community outbreak with 29 cases; for persons who lived, worked, or visited in the hospital perimeter, the risk of illness decreased by 20% for each 160 m away from the hospital.
- Australia (4396). In 1991–2000, cooling towers were likely sources for three outbreaks, all at shopping centers.
- Western Europe (2360, 3645, 5073). In northwestern France in November 2003–January 2004, the cooling tower and sludge of a petrochemical plant was source of an outbreak with 86 confirmed cases of *L. pneumophila* serogroup 1, including 18 (21%) deaths, for an attack rate of 0.04% in affected communities and of 0.17% at the epicenter. Spill into the environment and secondary aerosols explained the epidemic waves, including one after high-pressure cleaning and disinfection of the tower. Water from the source tower, another plant, and a car-wash station, and surface air from a nearby lagoon into which sludge was discharged, all yielded the outbreak strain. Epidemiological data and modeling delineated a perimeter of ~10 km in which infections occurred. In southwestern Spain in 1999–2000, three *Legionella* genotypes released from ≥ 2 cooling towers caused a protracted epidemic with >200 patients, most of whom required hospitalization. In Barcelona, Spain, in 2000, an outbreak in the inner city linked to a cooling tower caused 54 cases of disease; attack rates were 0.6% close to the cooling tower and 0.2% in remaining census tracts.

Large buildings (682, 1552). In the United States in 2001–2002, six legionellosis outbreaks were related to drinking water that resulted in 80 cases (with 41 hospitalizations and 4 deaths). All outbreaks occurred in large buildings with water-distribution systems that supported agent multiplication. At an office building in San Francisco in 1980, 14 persons contracted legionellosis, for attack rates of 1.6% (age <50 years) to 5.5% (age ≥ 50 years). **Homes (427, 769, 3301, 5797, 7186).** In high-income countries, *Legionella* has been isolated from 5–65% of domestic supplies, including faucets, shower heads, and water tanks. Around Pittsburgh, Pa., by area 0–22% (6% or 14/218) of home supplies grew *L. pneumophila*. In Italy in 2002, 23% (33/146) of private-home, hot-water samples from six cities yielded *Legionella*, mainly (76% or 25/33) *L. pneumophila* (6 serogroup 1; 19 serogroups 2–14). Hazards include central hot-water supply, old (>10 years) supply, long (>10 m) way from heating to outlet, low (35–50°C) temperature, and infrequent flow. Home legionellosis (1370, 3301, 5797, 6636, 7149) can be acquired via aspiration or inhalation. Aerosol generators include shower heads, tap-water faucets, air conditioners, humidifiers, and sprinklers. Sporadic, home-acquired infections, Pontiac fever and Legionnaires' disease have been recognized since the 1980s. In Germany, in 52 households with a central hot-water supply and mean *Legionella* counts of 6,049 CFU/liter, seroreactivity was significantly higher than in 92 control households with decentralized hot-water supply and mean counts of 244 CFU/liter. Overall, however, disease risks from home hot-water supplies are considered low for immune competent persons.

Mycobacteria (216, 2197, 4709). Home hot water and water-damaged building materials can grow and aerosolize environmental mycobacteria. Hot tubs and shower heads were suspected sources of environmental mycobacteria in immune-competent individuals with pulmonary disease whose home installations grow *M. avium* complex or *M. fortuitum*.

Mycoplasms (5978). In Israel, *Ureaplasma urealyticum* was detected by PCR or culture from 8% (4/50) of toilet bowls in public restrooms, and *Mycoplasma hominis* was detected in 6% (3). This finding does not imply object-to-human transfer, however.

***Pseudomonas* (769, 7854, 8406).** Home hot-water samples grow *P. aeruginosa*, for instance, in Italy 38% (56/146) of samples from six cities. The agent can survive in biofilms on tube surfaces. Showers, baths, and humidifiers are occasional sources of *P. aeruginosa* infections, e.g., folliculitis. A woman in labor took a 30-min home tub bath for relaxation; her newborn baby developed *P. aeruginosa* meningitis and bacteremia. Blood, cerebrospinal fluid, bath shower head, and a skin cream used on the infant all yielded identical *P. aeruginosa* strains.

***Salmonella* (437, 6720).** *Salmonella* can persist in biofilms underneath the rim of toilet bowls and inside toilet walls below the water line. However, *Salmonella* is not isolated from well-maintained toilet seats, flush handles, or door handles, and from dry surfaces or objects in households with a recent case. In contrast, *Salmonella* is frequently isolated from members of households with children newly diagnosed with *Salmonella*, including pets and pests.

Fungi
Fungi (5861, 6067) can be ubiquitous in the environment, e.g., *Rhodotorula* on shower curtains, bathtub grouts, and toothbrushes, or *Microsporum audouinii* on backs of seats in theaters. However, there is little evidence for infections in humans from contaminated objects. In Durban, South Africa, the prevalence of microscopy- and culture-confirmed tinea pedis and onychomycosis was 85% among 78 randomly selected adult Muslim males regularly attending mosques, but only 41% among 72 non-Muslim male control office workers. Dermatophytes from carpets and floors of mosques suggested spread in mosques, in ablution areas, and on prayer carpets.

Protozoa
Free-living amebas (6748). *Acanthamoeba*, *Balamuthia*, *Hartmannella*, and *Naegleria* inhabit natural and human-made freshwaters, such as canal water, power plant effluent, aquaria, poorly maintained pools, cooling towers, condensed water from air conditioners, and even tap water. Rinsing contact lenses under water has caused keratitis in wearers. Home water supplies of 50 contact lens wearers were examined, and *Acanthamoeba* was cultured from six bathroom cold-water taps and one kitchen cold-water tap.

Trichomonas vaginalis (4109) is unlikely to be transmitted at wet sites, such as bath benches, decks that are wet from swimming suits, or contaminated douche nozzles.

Helminths
***Enterobius vermicularis* (1443).** *E. vermicularis* is frequently recovered from the close environment of infected individuals, e.g., bed linen. In Taipei, Taiwan, orphanages, 8% (32/398) of stair rails and nearly 80% (89/115) of toilets tested positive for eggs of *E. vermicularis*. Infections could be acquired from unwashed hands.

SEWAGE, WASTE
Exposure (1027, 1456, 6531). Nonenveloped viruses, bacterial and fungal spores, cysts of protozoa, and worm eggs survive in animal and human biowaste. *Enterovirus*, spores of *Clostridium* (*C. botulinum* and *C. tetani*), and eggs of *Ascaris* are resilient, *Campylobacter*, environmental mycobacteria, *E. coli*, *Listeria monocytogenes*, *Salmonella*, and *Yersinia enterocolitica* are well documented, and prions are an emerging hazard from biowaste. Wastewater treatment and composting can reduce or eliminate infection hazards. For safe inactivation, thick-shelled eggs require composting at ≥42°C for 1 year.

Infections from waste (127, 180, 713, 1456, 2056, 2218, 2328, 3041, 5898) (Box 6.2). For waste work, see section 12.7. Exposure to raw waste is a hazard for farm workers, close-by residents, and consumers, including from open drainage and wastewater irrigation:

- Farm workers are at risk of diarrheal disease and infections by helminths with soil passage (*Ascaris*, *Trichuris*, and hookworm). In Mexico, 1,768 households using wastewater for irrigation were compared with 928 households practicing rainwater agriculture. Infectious diarrhea was 1.4-fold more frequent in wastewater users (9.5% of 3,075) than in rainwater users (6.9% of 3,181).

- Residents. Children of wastewater-irrigation farmers are at increased risk of enteric helminths. In Riyadh, Saudi Arabia, in 1999, the type of sewage disposal impacted the prevalence of intestinal parasites in residents, which was 28% (377/1,347) in sectors with municipal sewerage, 33% (1,508/4,563) in sectors with septic tanks, and 47% (48/102) in sectors with open sewers. In Israel, residents in 11 kibbutzim ($n = 3,000$) were studied. Compared with clean water, wastewater sprinkling resulted in a ~2-fold excess risk of enteric infections; risks were limited to summer and children 0–4 years of age.
- For consumers, produce from raw-waste farming intended to be eaten unwashed or raw is a hazard, e.g., fruits, berries, and root vegetables. In Morocco, crops such as potatoes grown from raw sewage yielded *Giardia* cysts, and *Ascaris* unlike crops grown from treated sewage that did not.

Viruses
Risks (6724, 6986). Viruses detected (by NAT) in wastewater are typically nonenveloped (see Table 19.1) and include enteric adenovirus, *Enterovirus*, HAV, hepatitis E virus (HEV) (in raw and treated wastewater), *Norovirus*, and *Rotavirus*. A source of HEV in wastewater besides humans is swine manure.

Bacteria
Bacteria (92, 2056, 5898) recovered from wastewater or soils irrigated with filtrated wastewater include genera *Acinetobacter*, *Alcaligenes*, *Aeromonas*, *Citrobacter*, *Escherichia*, *Klebsiella*, *Plesiomonas*, *Proteus*, *Providencia*, *Salmonella*, and *Serratia*. In Italy in 2001, 27% (14/52) of irrigation water samples grew *Aeromonas*, mainly *A. caviae*, *A. sobria*, and *A. hydrophila*. Presence of *Aeromonas* in water did not correlate with indicators of fecal pollution (e.g., total coliforms or *Enterococcus*).

In Marrakesh, Morocco, *Salmonella* was prevalent in 21% of children from areas that used untreated wastewater in agriculture, compared with 1% in control children (4976).

Protozoa
Enteric protozoa recovered from biowaste water include *Cryptosporidium* (*C. hominis* and *C. parvum*) (8404) and *Giardia*. In the outskirts of Marrakesh, Morocco, use of untreated wastewater in agriculture is associated with excess infections of *Giardia lamblia* and *Entamoeba histolytica* in children (4976). Outbreaks in the United States suggest that *Cyclospora cayetanensis* can be spread by raw-waste irrigation farming in countries with warm climates.

G. lamblia (180, 1456, 4976, 7738) has been isolated in sewage and effluents from water-treatment plants, including genotypes pathogenic to humans. In Mexico, wastewater contained 50–300 *Giardia* cysts per liter. Retention in reservoirs for 3–7 months reduced levels to ≤5 cysts/liter. In residents, however, *G. lamblia* prevalence was comparable, whether villages used raw wastewater for irrigation (8%, 184/2,257), wastewater from reservoirs (11%, 234/2,147), or rainwater only (8%, 183/2,344). In Morocco, on potatoes from fields irrigated with raw sewage, *Giardia* cysts were isolated at concentrations of 5 cysts/kg.

Helminths
Worm eggs identified in wastewater include nematodes (e.g., *Ascaris*), trematodes (e.g., *Fasciola*), and cestodes (e.g., *Taenia*). Animal manure for fertilizer and raw wastewater are likely risks for workers and residents (children) in waste-irrigation areas (795, 1723, 5474).

Ascaris lumbricoides (180, 713, 2218, 3041, 5535).
In Mexico, 1,768 households using wastewater for irrigation were compared with 928 households practicing rainwater agriculture. *A. lumbricoides* was 16-fold more prevalent in wastewater users (6.5%, 5161) than rainwater users (0.4%, 2379). In Morocco, *A. lumbricoides* was 5 times more prevalent in 740 randomly selected children (20.5%) from five communities that used raw wastewater for irrigation than in 603 children (3.8%) from four control communities that did not practice wastewater irrigation.

Carriers worldwide are estimated to discharge 10^{14} eggs/day into the environment. Eggs are sticky, adhering to vegetables, hands, utensils, door handles, and money. In Morocco, eggs were identified on crops irrigated with raw sewage at concentrations of 0.2 eggs/kg (potatoes) to 0.3 eggs/kg (turnips).

Hookworm (2218).
In Faisalabad, Pakistan, a city with ~2 million inhabitants, wastewater is disposed at a rate of ~0.55 million m³/day; 32% (~0.18 million m³) of this wastewater is used untreated for crop irrigation. In 2002–2003, wastewater farmers, area residents (textile workers), and control farmers (using regular irrigation water) were examined for hookworms and other enteric helminths. Hookworm prevalence was 0% in regular farmers ($n = 167$), 3.5% in textile workers ($n = 254$), and 13.6% in wastewater farmers ($n = 176$). In children from the three groups, respectively, prevalence was 0.6% ($n = 309$), 4.9% ($n = 488$), and 6.1% ($n = 310$). Both trends were significant. A significant risk was lack of toilets.

Trichuris trichiura (2218, 7165).
Risks for *T. trichiura* include crop irrigation with raw wastewater, domicile in

wastewater irrigation areas, use of feces as fertilizer, and domicile near urban refuse dumps.

***Taenia* (6261).** *Taenia* eggs survive in raw waste. In Australia, 8% of 300 cattle reared on sewage-irrigated pastures harbored viable *T. saginata* cysticerci.

6.3 CITIES

[In 2007] for the first time in human history, the majority of the world's population will live in urban areas.

(6737)

Cities (4292, 6737, 7350, 8105) (http://www.unhabitat.org.). A consensus definition for cities does not exist. Here, urban means human-made habitats with a high density of people, businesses, and traffic, and cities are urban areas delineated by municipal (utility) boundaries. Economy and crises force people into cities. Of the world population <2% lived in cities in 1800, 10% in 1900, and 33% in 1970; the current proportion is 50% or 3 billion. There were five megacities (>10 million inhabitants) in 1975, but 19 in 2001, including Tokyo (26 million), New York (17 million), and Los Angeles (13 million) in high-income countries, and Mexico City (18 million), Mumbai (18 million), São Paulo (17–18 million), and Shanghai (17 million) in low-income countries.

Infections (1533, 7984) (http://econ.worldbank.org/wdr/wdr2004/text-30023/). Low-income cities face immense health problems, including slums (see section 11.2), lack of sewerage and food hygiene, street prostitution, and injection drug use (Box 6.3). In 2001, >920 million people lived in slums, almost all (95%) in low-income countries. In low-income cities, ≥25% of piped water is lost through leaks, and full-pressure, 24-h, 7-day supplies are a "pipe dream." Low-income cities differ from high-income cities by incorporating rural sectors, with farming plots and grazing animals.

Exposure history. Exposure history should address neighborhood (inner city, slum, or suburban), municipal services (tap water, sewerage, and garbage), and health services (vaccinations, mosquito and pest control) (Box II.1).

URBAN DROPLET-AIR CLUSTER

Commuting workers and arriving international travelers can carry respiratory agents to and from cities. Crowding and failure to vaccinate predispose inner city populations to outbreaks by vaccine-preventable agents. Winds can blow agents (e.g., *Coxiella* and spores of *Histoplasma*) into cities. Air pollution (particles, O_3 and NO_2) may aggravate respiratory tract disease burden in urban populations, mainly children.

Viruses

Nonvaccinated urban minorities are vulnerable to or reservoirs of vaccine-preventable viruses such as measles and mumps. Reasons for undercoverage include health care disparities, failed vaccine cool chain, failure to reach, and noncompliance.

Cities have been venues for viral respiratory outbreaks. Examples are *Enterovirus* conjunctivitis in Delhi (5354), influenza in London (6185), measles in Tokyo (5321) and Los Angeles (4805), mumps virus parotitis in Madrid (1814), and severe acute respiratory syndrome (SARS) in Beijing (8276), Hong Kong (4236), and Singapore (2803).

Bacteria

Nonvaccinated urban minorities are vulnerable to or reservoirs of vaccine-preventable bacteria such as *Bordetella* and *Corynebacterium*. Nondetected or noncomplying tuberculosis cases are an urban hazard.

***Bordetella pertussis* (7196).** An outbreak of *B. pertussis* in Cape Town in 1988–1989 caused 292 pediatric cases; vaccination coverage with required doses was ~80–95% by age 13 months.

Box 6.3 Agents from urbanization, by cluster

For slums, see section 11.2; for street life, see section 11.3; for STI, see sections 13.6 and 13.7; for IDU, see section 13.8.

Droplet-air	Vaccine-preventable agents; *Enterovirus*, SARS-associated coronavirus; *Coxiella* (dust), *Legionella* (cooling towers), *M. tuberculosis* (inner city and crowding), *Histoplasma capsulatum* (dust)
Feces-food	*Giardia*, *Cryptosporidium*; by city sector also *Salmonella*, *Shigella*, *Vibrio cholerae*; *Ascaris*, *Trichuris*
Zoonotic	Hantavirus, rabies, and many arboviruses (e.g., CHIKV, DENV, CCHFV, JEV, SLEV, TBEV, WNV, YFV); *Anaplasma phagocytophilum*, *Bartonella*, *B. burgdorferi* sl, *Rickettsia*; *Leishmania*, *Plasmodium*, *T. brucei gambiense*, *T. cruzi*; *E. granulosus*, *E. multilocularis*, *W. bancrofti*
Environmental	*Leptospira*; *Toxocara*, *Schistosoma*
Skin-blood	STI

Corynebacterium diphtheriae **(2579, 8352).** Venues for diphtheria outbreaks have included cities in Russia in the 1990s, slums in northern India in the 1990s (4481), and a city in Hubei Province, People's Republic of China, in 1988–1989, where commuters were suspected to have exported diphtheria to the less crowded countryside.

Coxiella burnetii. Dust from herds, farms, and helicopters has been implicated in urban outbreaks of Q fever, for instance, in Los Angeles in the late 1940s (~50,000 cases) (1533); Birmingham, United Kingdom, in 1989 (147 cases) (3191); Briançon, France, in 1996 (29 cases) (278); and the German cities of Berlin, Dortmund, Düsseldorf, and Freiburg (3243).

L. pneumophila **(2507, 3751).** For buildings, see "Buildings, Sanitation, and Wastewater" above. Venues for urban outbreaks include Philadelphia in 1976 (182 cases), and more recently cities in Spain in 2000 (70 cases) and again in 2001 (>400 cases) and the United Kingdom in 2002 (137 cases).

M. tuberculosis **(3020, 7386, 7807).** *M. tuberculosis* can be hyperendemic among residents in inner cities in high-income countries and in slums in low-income countries. In some cities in Africa, the disease rate can exceed 300–450/10^5 per year.

Fungi
Winds can blow spores into cities. Immune-impaired individuals are vulnerable to invasive disease.

Cryptococcus **(7442).** High urban disease rates are explained by the presence of human immunodeficiency virus (HIV)-infected groups in cities rather than by environmental hazards.

Histoplasma. Cities have been venues for outbreaks mainly in the United States. In Mason, Ia., in 1962, ~8,400 infections resulted from bulldozing in a park. The overall infection rate was 25%. Of children living within one block from the park, 77% were skin test positive, compared with 20% who lived 1–2 miles away (1698). In 1964, a second epidemic hit the city when trees with starling roosts were removed from the park. Despite precautions, 270 cases were diagnosed, for an attack rate of 0.9% (7523). In Indianapolis in 1978–1979, an epidemic caused 435 cases and ~100,000 infections. Attack rates were highest (0.1%) in the city center. Construction of a tennis complex was the likely source (8066). A second epidemic of similar magnitude hit the city in 1980, this time because of work on a swimming pool (8065). A further source of dust and urban histoplasmosis is earth for growing plants (3703).

URBAN FECES-FOOD CLUSTER
Tap water in low-income cities, in general, is not safe for drinking. City sectors not serviced by municipal water supply, sewerage, or drainage are a particular hazard. Domiciles on steep hillsides are difficult to service, including water trucks and sewage purification. In Salvador, Brazil, in 1989–1990, diarrhea rates per preschool child and year were 5.6 in sectors that lacked sewerage or drainage, but 1.7 in sectors that were served (5177).

Viruses
Since the sanitation era, waterborne HAV outbreaks have become rare in high-income cities. In some low-income cities, in particular, in Central Asia, HEV is endemic or epidemic. Reports of waterborne HEV outbreaks include cities in India (e.g., Delhi and Kanpur) (6153, 8269) and Pakistan (e.g., Islamabad) (6063). Of note for visitors is the HEV endemicity in Kathmandu, Nepal (1477).

Bacteria
Urban facilities (e.g., prisons and schools), and sections (e.g., neighborhoods and slum areas) can be venues for diarrheal disease outbreaks (136, 4660), including *Salmonella*, *Shigella*, and *Vibrio*.

Vibrio cholerae. The waterborne cholera epidemics in London of 1849–1854 (7004) and Hamburg of 1892 (nearly 17,000 cases and ~8,600 [50%] deaths) (2428) are well known. To date, cholera remains endemic or epidemic in several low-income cities in sub-Saharan Africa, Central Asia (Fig. 5.7), and Latin America. In Kampala, Uganda, in December 1997–March 1998, an outbreak caused 6,228 reported cases (18% in children <5 years of age), for an attack rate of 0.6%. Cases concentrated in slums with living conditions resembling refugee camps (4321). In Lusaka, Zambia, in November 2003–March 2004, an outbreak caused 4,630 cases and 153 (3%) deaths (6931). During civil war in Liberia in 2003, when ~300,000 displaced persons fled into Monrovia, lack of clean water and sanitation set off an epidemic with ≥17,000 clinical cases (874).

Protozoa
G. lamblia. *G. lamblia* can be endemic in city populations, e.g., Mexico City (1457), Salvador (Brazil) (6000), and Zimbabwe (4803). Polluted municipal water supplies have caused urban outbreaks. Examples are Rome, N.Y., in 1974–1975 (350 cases) (6824); Berlin, N.H., in 1977 (213 cases) (4509); Bristol, United Kingdom, in 1985 (108 cases) (3689); Pittsfield, Mass., in 1985–1986 (~3,800 cases) (3896); and Penticton, British Columbia, in 1986 (362 cases) (5174).

C. parvum. *C. parvum* can be endemic in city populations, e.g., Albuquerque (2540) and Fortaleza (Brazil) (5399). Polluted water supplies have caused urban outbreaks. A notable example is Milwaukee, Wis., in 1993, with ~403,000 cases (4600).

Helminths
Urban transmission of food-borne helminths is by unwashed or inadequately cooked foods.

***A. lumbricoides* (304, 5176, 5535).** *A. lumbricoides* is endemic in slums, where residents are forced to defecate around houses. In Salvador, Brazil, in 1989, prevalence by city sector was 38% in 631 school-age children served by sewers, 47% in 631 children served by rainwater drains, but 66% in 631 children not served by sanitation.

***T. trichiura* (5176, 7165).** Risks for *T. trichiura* include residing in a slum, living close to a dump site, and lack of indoor sanitation. The prevalence can exceed 60–90% in children in slums.

URBAN ZOONOTIC CLUSTER
Risks (361, 2068, 7042). Rodents and arthropods thrive in cities. Rats infest port cities, dump sites, store rooms, and sewers. Mosquitoes breed in open drains, cisterns, and containers. Habitats for ticks include periurban parks and suburban residential areas adjacent to brush or forest. Ticks commonly bite humans in the backyards of houses, for instance, while the individuals are playing or gardening. Cold weather in cities at high altitudes or high latitudes may reduce the burden of arthropod-borne diseases. At least six capital cities are situated above 2,000 m: La Paz (Bolivia, 3,600 m), Quito (Ecuador, 2,800 m), Bogota (Colombia, 2,650 m), Addis Ababa (Ethiopia, 2,400 m), Mexico City (2,300 m), and Thimphu (Bhutan, 2,400 m).

Viruses
Urban cycles exist in enzootic-endemic areas, including Chikungunya virus (CHIKV), dengue virus (DENV), Crimean-Congo hemorrhagic fever virus (CCHFV), *Hantavirus*, Japanese encephalitis virus (JEV), rabies virus, St. Louis encephalitis virus (SLEV), tick-borne encephalitis virus (TBEV), West Nile virus (WNV), and yellow fever virus (YFV).

CHIKV (5973). The urban vector for CHIKV is *Aedes aegypti*. CHIKV has been reported in the following cities: Barsi (Maharashtra, India) in the 1970s, Vellore (Madras, India) in the 1960s, and Yogyakarta (Java, Indonesia) in the 2000s.

DENV (146, 2712, 2806, 7815). Urban vectors for DENV are *A. aegypti* and *A. albopictus*. Both breed around houses, including in cans, tires, and vases. *A. aegypti* has been reported to breed in a cemetery in Buenos Aires (at latitude 35°S). Singapore has had an *Aedes*-control program since 1970. In 2000, 0.6% (3,265/583,916) of premises tested positive for *A. aegypti*-breeding sites, and 0.8% (4,853) for *A. albopictus*.

Urban transmission can be intense in uncontrolled areas, and infection risks can be high (1338, 3204, 4014, 6933). Recently in Thailand, disease rates in rural areas ($102/10^5$) surpassed the rates in urban areas ($95/10^5$). Reported seroprevalence in city residents is 30–65% compared with 25–40% in rural areas. Infections can cluster in the outskirts, low-lying areas, or sectors with open ditches or sewers. In contrast, mosquito screens or air conditioning are protective.

Urban outbreaks are frequent, and dengue hemorrhagic fever (DHF) or shock syndrome (DSS) are frequent complications (1585, 1745, 2977, 4869, 6933, 7195). Dengue virus hit Durban (South Africa), Dakar (Senegal), and Athens (Greece) in 1927–1928, and Cairo (Egypt) and Miami (Florida) in 1934–1936. DHF appeared in Manila (Philippines) and Bangkok (Thailand) in 1956–1958.

In the 1980s–2000s, DENV, DHF, or DSS affected many cities, e.g., Belém, Rio de Janeiro, and Cali in Latin America, and Bangkok, Calcutta, Delhi, Karachi, Manila, and Singapore in Asia. In Townsville (Australia) in 1992, an outbreak caused 652 cases (421 confirmed and 231 clinical); of these, 54% resided in a 2.5-km radius from the index case, and 74% within 5 km. In Charters Towers (Australia) in 1993, an outbreak caused 190 cases. According to a serosurvey, ~25% of 10,000 citizens had been infected. In Delhi (India), in 1996, an outbreak caused 8,900 cases of DHF-DSS, for an overall lethality of 4%. In Palembang (Sumatra and Indonesia) in 1998, 2,439 DEN cases (two-thirds DHF) were diagnosed, for an attack rate of 3.6% and a lethality of 4%.

CCHFV (5305). Ticks are vectors for CCHFV, but under favorable conditions, person-to-person spread seems possible. In Nouakchott, Mauritania, when drought and lack of pastures forced tick-infested animals into the city, an outbreak resulted with 28 cases confirmed by anti-CCHFV immunoglobulin M(IgM) and reverse transcriptase-PCR. Sheep, goats, and ticks (*Rhipicephalus evertsi*) also tested positive for CCHFV. Population density was high, and there was a risk for interhuman spread.

***Hantavirus* (274, 1390, 1480, 4295).** Seoul virus is enzootic in urban rats (*Rattus norvegicus* and *R. rattus*), and seroreactive rats have been reported from many cities, e.g., in Africa, in Alexandria (Egypt) and Mombasa (Kenya); in the Americas in Baltimore, Md., Buenos Aires (Argentina), Philadelphia, Pa., Recife (Brazil), and Sao Paulo (Brazil); in Asia, in Bangkong (Thailand), Hong Kong (People's Republic of China), Manila (Philippines), Singapore, Taichung (Taiwan), and Tokyo (Japan).

Reported seroprevalence in urban rats is 5–30% (5–10% in *R. rattus*, 20–30% in *R. norvegicus*, 15–25% in *Bandicota indica*). Evidence for spread to humans is limited, however.

Urban hemorrhagic fever with renal syndrome (1480, 6505) is easily confused with urban leptospirosis. Both mainly affect occupationally exposed males with a history of "rats and rains," and they are manifest with febrile jaundice, oliguria, and acute renal failure. This striking overlap and diagnostic difficulties could account for underrecognition. Recently, a U.S. soldier contracted hemorrhagic fever with renal syndrome in Seoul, Korea.

JEV (2751, 4048, 6109, 7201, 7683, 7780). Mosquitoes are JEV vectors. Although JE is essentially rural, city residents can be at risk. Reports of JE outbreaks with spill into Asian cities include Bangkok (in the 1980s), Beijing (in the 1980s), Rourkela (India, in IX–XI/1989, with 41 cases and 15 [37%] deaths), and Tokyo (up to the 1960s).

Rabies virus (3175, 6919, 7516, 8149). Puppies and adult stray dogs are the main causes of rabies evaluation visits and postexposure prophylaxis (PEP) in urban residents, in particular, children. Urbanization, unwanted dogs, and food waste support stray-dog populations that bridge rabies in wild carnivores and domestic dogs, maintaining urban rabies cycles. Reports of cities with canine rabies include Freetown (Sierra Leone) in Africa, Hermosillo (Mexico), Ribeirão Preto (Brazil), and Santa Cruz (Bolivia) in the Americas, and Bangalore (India), Bangkok (Thailand), Delhi (India), and Manila (Philippines) in Asia.

In the city of Olinda, in northeastern Brazil, in 2004, *Desmodus rotundus* was observed to feed on an owned dog, which points to bats as potential vectors of urban rabies.

SLEV (4418). SLEV is enzootic in the greater Houston, Tex., area, in *Culex quinquefasciatus* and wild birds, notably shrikes (*Lanius ludovicianus*, 13% of 379 seroreactive in 1989–2001), blue jays (*Cyanocitta cristata*, 11% of 5,800), and a dozen other bird species. In 1990–2001, 86 cases in humans, (7/year) were reported in the area.

TBEV (4046). Although vector ticks have invaded periurban parks in Europe, city-acquired TBEV is exceedingly rare in western Europe. An urban focus is reported in Tomsk, central Siberia.

WNV (4418, 5344). *Culex pipiens* (common house mosquito) is a likely urban vector. WNV was recognized for the first time in the United States in August–September 1999, when an outbreak in New York City caused 59 cases. Since then, it has swept the continent, and WNV has become enzootic in greater Houston, in *C. quinquefasciatus* and birds such as the house sparrow (*Passer domesticus*) and blue jay (*C. cristata*).

YFV (113, 5345, 6335, 8112). The urban vector for YFV is *A. aegypti*; hosts are susceptible urban residents. The risk for outbreaks increases with increasing numbers of premises that test positive for *A. aegypti* larvae; a reported threshold is a Breteau index of 1–5%. In 1798, yellow fever apparently hit New York City. Since the 1970s, *A. agypti* has reinvaded cities in Bolivia, the Guyanas, and Venezuela, as well as in West Africa, e.g., in Côte d'Ivoire and Nigeria. In western Nigeria in April–May 1987 an outbreak of urban yellow fever caused 805 reported cases and 416 (52%) deaths (the true clinical attack rate was close to 3%). Cities in endemic areas close to forests are vulnerable, and residents would benefit from YFV vaccination.

Bacteria

Vectors include ectoparasites from dogs and cats. Urban reservoirs include small mammals in gardens, parks, and forests.

***Anaplasma phagocytophilum* (1533, 7107).** Rodents and *Ixodes* ticks can maintain urban cycles. Examples are New York City and cities in Poland.

***Bartonella* (1533).** Urban hosts for *B. quintana* are louse-infested homeless, for *B. henselae*, domestic cats, and for *B. elizabethae*, rats.

***Borrelia burgdorferi* sensu lato (sl) (3773, 4046, 4844, 6178, 7107).** Rodents and ticks can maintain urban cycles. Examples are Baltimore, Boston, Bridgeport (Conn.), and Lyme in North America, and Helsinki (Finland), London (United Kingdom), Magdeburg (Germany), and Tomsk (central Siberia, Russia) in Europe. There is evidence from London that park workers are at risk of infection.

***Rickettsia* (48, 1533, 1735, 4471, 5671, 6246, 6756).** *R. akari*. *R. akari* circulates in house mice and their mites. House mice are strongly synanthropic and do not readily leave houses. Urban foci of rickettsial pox have been reported in Boston, Cleveland, New York, and Philadelphia. *R. conorii*. Domestic dogs and their ticks are likely urban sources of *R. conorii*. Although mainly rural, urban infections occur. Reported seroprevalence in Mediterranean urban populations are 5–7%, compared with 11–14% in rural residents. *R. felis*. Domestic cats and their fleas are a potential source of urban infections with *R. felis*. *R. prowazekii*. Flying squirrels and their lice are a potential urban source of "sporadic epidemic" typhus. *R. typhi*. Domestic cats and their fleas are a potential urban source of murine typhus. Seroprevalence of 17–42% has been reported in urban populations in low-income cities such as Mexico City and Malang (Indonesia). In contrast, in central Spain, reactivity was greater in rural (10%) than urban (1.7%) residents.

Protozoa

Urban cycles exist for *Leishmania*, *Plasmodium*, and *Trypanosoma*. Carriers may cause infections to cluster in households.

***Babesia* (7107).** Periurban cycles are likely to exist in North America and Europe, mainly among *Ixodes* ticks and rodents, with *B. microti* as the main agent.

***Leishmania* (8105).** Urban vector sandflies readily breed in excreta from dogs, chicken, pigs, or cattle. Both mammals and humans can be the reservoir for cutaneous (CL) or visceral leishmaniasis (VL). **Anthroponotic CL (121, 2000, 3310, 6233, 7273, 8105).** Anthroponotic CL is endemic in crowded cities in Southwest and Southcentral Asia. The main vector is *Phlebotomus sergenti*. Reported urban foci include Afghanistan (Herat, Kabul, and Kandahar), Iran (Bam, Shiraz, and Teheran), Iraq (Mosul), Syria (Aleppo, since 1745), and Turkey (Sanliurfa, border to Syria). In Kabul, in a population of <2 million, >14,000 CL cases were recorded in 1994–1995, and ~270,000 infections in 1996. At the height of this epidemic in the mid-1990s, 4.7% of the city population had active CL. In Jericho, CL due to *L. tropica* has been reported in displaced Palestinians, but local transmission is unconfirmed. **Zoonotic CL.** Proximity of informal housing to forests and brushland that support foci are hazards for city dwellers.

- New World (1825, 2839, 5582, 6209, 8105). Deforestation and demographic shifts have promoted domestication of *Lutzomyia* and establishment of urban cycles. In Brazil, infected cities include Manaus, Rio de Janeiro, and Belo Horizone. In Rio de Janeiro, the main vector is *Lutzomyia intermedia*, and ~2% are infective for *Leishmania braziliensis*. In Manaus, zoonotic CL involves *Lutzomyia umbratilis*, small mammals (e.g., opossums, sloths, and anteaters), and *Leishmania guyanensis*. In São Miguel, Brazil, an outbreak in 1987 established zoonotic CL in the city, shifting risks from rural workers to periurban residents. In Venezuela, urban zoonotic CL occurs in Barcelona on the Caribbean coast, in disturbed, dry tropical forest.
- Old World (121, 2986, 3627, 8105). Causative *L. major* circulates in *P. papatasi* and rodents. In 1995, cases of zoonotic CL emerged in suburban Taza, northern Morocco. Around Jericho and in the Negev Desert, zoonotic foci are a hazard for nearby urbanites. In eastern Saudi Arabia, cities at risk (bordering on foci) are Hofuf and Al Hasa. **Anthroponotic VL (8105).** Anthroponotic VL is endemic in India. Urban foci are reported in Madras City (Madras), Mumbai (Bombay, West Bengal), and Patna (Bihar). **Zoonotic VL.** Again, New and Old World cities can be affected.
- New World (1677, 2839, 7010, 7415, 8105). Zoonotic VL has become urbanized in some cities in Brazil, Colombia, and Venezuela. Affected cities include in Brazil the state capitals Belo Horizonte (Minas Gerais), Fortaleza (Ceará), Natal (Rio Grande do Norte), Rio de Janeiro, Salvador (Bahia), São Luís (Maranhão), and Teresina (Piauí). Typically, informal (rural-like) suburbs are most heavily affected. The main vector is *Lutzomyia longipalpis*. It is abundant in non-mosquito proofed houses. In Natal, northeastern Brazil, an epidemic in 1991 caused >100 VL cases (>two-thirds in children <15 years of age), for a rate of $19/10^5$. The epicenter was 15 km away from the city, in sand dunes cleared from vegetation for housing.
- Old World (424, 1326, 1896, 3627, 8105). In the 1980s, cases in a resort town near Alexandria, Egypt, suggested a risk for zoonotic VL to become urbanized. In Israel in 1994–1995, zoonotic VL emerged in settlements between Jerusalem and Tel-Aviv, close to urban centers, and canine leishmaniasis has now been observed in urban areas. In northwestern Saudi Arabia, the city of Tabuk is expanding into areas that are natural habitats for zoonotic VL. In the area surrounding Athens, Greece, abandoned quarries are a habitat for a VL cycle in sandflies and stray dogs. In the southwestern Mediterranean, injection drug users (IDU) in cities such as Genova, Lisboa, Madrid, Marseille, Milano, Nice, and Sevilla, and sandflies coexist, increasing the risk of VL and HIV coinfections. Of >1,900 coinfections reported from this area up to early 2001, ~80% were acquired in urban areas.

***Plasmodium*.** "Cans, cisterns, and gutters" are breeding sites for urban *Anopheles*, although pollution of water and air and intense crowding seem unfavorable for malaria mosquitoes, and transmission seems, in general, less intense in urban than in rural areas. **Malaria free.** City centers in North Africa, Central America, and Southwest Asia are kept free or are naturally malaria free. **Malarious.** There is urban or periurban malaria in sub-Saharan Africa, parts of South America, Asia, and the Southwest Pacific, and in some port cities.

- Sub-Saharan Africa (79, 244, 1031, 3863, 3879, 5616, 5729, 6326, 7095, 7350). About 200 million city dwellers are exposed to malaria in Africa. *P. falciparum* EIRs (per person per year) are 0.1–46 (typically 7–14) in cities, but ~10 times higher (0.1–884, typically 146–168) in rural areas. Similarly, parasitemia prevalence is somewhat lower in urban (24–34%, typically 30%) than in rural areas (36–43%, typically 40%). In Kinshasa in 2000, parasitemia (>97% *P. falciparum*) prevalence was 14% in the city center and up to 65% in the periphery. In a city north of Mogadishu (Somalia), an outbreak increased rates of falciparum malaria (per 100/year) from 0.5–1 in

1982–1986 to 8–14 in 1987–1988. Malarious cities include Accra, Bamako, Bobo Dioulasso, Cotonou, Dakar, Kumasi, Niamey, and Ouagadougou in West Africa; Bangui, Brazzaville, Khartoum, and Yaounde in Central Africa; Antananarivo, Dar es Salaam, Kampala, Kinshasa, Lusaka, Maputo, Mombasa, and Nairobi in East Africa.

- South America (254, 1094, 5646, 7289). Malarious cities are located in the South American lowlands, mainly the Amazon River basin. Examples of malarious cities are Buenaventura (Colombia, on the Pacific), Iquitos (Peru, in the Amazon), Manaus (Brazil, in the Amazon), and Quidbo (in northwestern Colombia). After elimination in 1976, *Anopheles darlingi* reinvaded Manaus in 1988; in 1993, a malaria outbreak affected >23,000 persons.
- Southwest and Southeast Asia (55, 3799, 4645, 4702, 8301). Malarious cities in India include Ahmedabad (Gujarat, with seasonal *P. falciparum* and *P. vivax* transmission, and a disease rate of $1,220/10^5$ per year), Mumbai, Calcutta, Delhi (seasonal transmission in April–May and July–December), and Goa. In Indonesia, *P. falciparum* and *P. vivax* have reemerged near Jakarta, in the coastal Thousand Island district visited by tourists.
- Malarious port cities (4264, 5816). Malaria can occur outside malarious areas (for "airport malaria," see section 15.3). "Port malaria" is malaria in residents of port cities that is acquired from infective *Anopheles* females having been imported by cargo or sea-going vessels. Gametocytemic migrants who arrive during the warm season are a further source of malaria in cities in which competent local *Anopheles* fauna is available. An example is New York City.

Trypanosoma. Urban foci are suspected for human African trypanosomiasis (HAT) due to *T. brucei gambiense*, and for Chagas disease due to *T. cruzi*. ***T. brucei gambiense* (1601, 2111, 2474, 5026, 6323).** Trees along watercourses or vegetable gardens in cities are suitable for *Glossina* and potential sites for urban HAT in equatorial Africa. Examples are the the "rural" town of Bonon west of Yamoussoukro in Côte d'Ivoire, the Brazzaville Zoo area, a mangrove forest near Conakry, and gardening plots in periurban Kinshasa. In Daloa, Côte d'Ivoire, *Glossina* was trapped in the city, with average densities of one fly/trap/day in the city center, and 10–12 flies/trap/day in the outskirts. In Kinshasa in 1970–1995, 1,025 HAT cases were reported (39/year); there were 254 cases in 1996, 226 in 1997, 433 in 1998, and 912 in 1999. Of 42,746 inhabitants screened, 3,165 (7%) were reactive in card agglutination test, and 875 (2%) infections were confirmed parasitologically. ***T. cruzi* (3035, 5625, 8099).** Bugs such as *Triatoma dimidiata* readily invade and colonize urban areas. The risk exists for Chagas disease to become urbanized in several Latin American countries, including cities in Mexico and Paramaribo in Suriname.

Helminths
Local transmission is supported by infections in urban residents who have not left the area, as well by seasonally persistent findings in locally trapped mammalian hosts or arthropod vectors.

Echinococcus. Both *E. granulosus* and *E. multilocularis* appear to have established urban cycles. ***E. granulosus* (5203).** An urban cycle that involves stray dogs and abattoir offal has been described in Chincha, a coastal city south of Lima, Peru. Infection prevalence is 12% (3/25) in abattoir workers, and 6% (3/48) in stray dogs around the abattoir; workers have reported observing hydatid cysts in slaughtered animals. ***E. multilocularis* (1887).** Foxes and rodents can maintain an urban "sylvatic" cycle, for instance, in parks ("urban wilderness"). Urban fox populations exist in cities in Canada (Toronto), Japan (Sapporo), and Europe (e.g., Geneva, Oslo, Stuttgart, and Zürich). In West Europe, foxes have appeared in cities in areas freed from fox rabies and where fox populations have expanded. The reported prevalence of *E. multilocularis* in urban foxes is high (17–44%).

***W. bancrofti* (1704, 2679, 4551, 6673, 6819, 7999).** *C. quinquefasciatus* mosquito vectors breed well in polluted city waters. Lymphatic filariasis was endemic in Charleston, S.C., up to the 1930s. Municipal sanitation started in the 1900s is believed to have eliminated transmission in that city. In Calcutta in the 1980s, the transmission potential (infective *W. bancrofti* larvae per person per year) was 177, compared with 137 in the countryside. Cities with suspected or confirmed, inactive or active foci include Secondi-Takoradi (Ghana) in Africa; Maceio (northeastern Brazil), Port-au-Prince (Haiti), Puerto Limon (Costa Rica), Recife (northeastern Brazil), and Georgetown (Guyana) in Latin America; Calcutta (India), Dhaka (Bangladesh), and Varanasi (India) in Southcentral Asia; and townships in several Indian states and coastal Sri Lanka. By neighborhood, reported microfilaremia prevalence in city residents is 0.5–15%.

URBAN ENVIRONMENTAL CLUSTER
Bacteria
Urban leptospirosis (4012, 6616, 7838) is an emerging infection. In Baltimore, Md., inner city residents have been reported to have contracted leptospirosis from exposure to rat urine. In Salvador, Brazil, urban outbreaks caused 326 clinical cases (193 laboratory confirmed) in 1996, and 157 clincal cases (66 confirmed) in 2000.

Helminths
Hookworm (5176). In informal housing areas of low-income cities, conditions are favorable for the

transmission of hookworm. In children in slums, the infection prevalence can reach 10–25%.

Schistosoma **(2227, 2400, 4809, 5578, 8289).** In some cities located in endemic areas, urban foci exist. *S. haematobium* transmission is suspected or confirmed in cities in Africa, including Bamako (Mali), Dar es Salam (Tanzania), Harare (Zimbabwe), Ibadan (Nigeria), Kinshasa (Congo), Lusaka (Zambia), and Niamey (Niger). *S. mansoni* transmission is suspected or confirmed in cities in Brazil, including Belo Horizonte, Fortaleza, Rio de Janeiro, and São Paulo. Settlement of carriers in urban wet habitats that support vector snails can open up new foci.

Strongyloides **(3083).** In informal housing areas of low-income cities, conditions are favorable for the transmission of *S. stercoralis*. By age and number of stools tested, the infection prevalence in children in slums exceeds 5–15%.

Toxocara **(1497, 1887, 7637).** Pollution of city squares and public parks by eggs of *Toxocara canis* or *T. cati* from dogs and cats is well documented. Locally, every other park soil sample can yield embryonated (infective) eggs. More recent is the pollution hazard by urban foxes. In the cities of Geneva, Stuttgart, and Zürich, the prevalence of *T. canis* among urban foxes (*Vulpes vulpes*, n = 1,040) is ~15–70%.

URBAN SKIN-BLOOD CLUSTER
Streets, parks, and run-down flats in inner cities are domiciles for the urban poor and homeless (see section 11.3) and venues for IDU (see section 13.8) and sex workers (see sections 13.6 and 13.7).

Chlamydia trachomatis **L1–L3 (7710).** Lymphogranuloma venereum reemerged in Rotterdam, The Netherlands, in 2003, among homosexual men with proctitis, most coinfected with HIV. Meanwhile, cases or clusters have been observed in other cities in western Europe, including Antwerp (Belgium), Barcelona (Spain), Geneva (Switzerland), Hamburg (Germany), Paris (France), and Stockholm (Sweden).

Haemophilus ducreyi **(2442, 3697).** Urban chancroid outbreaks have been reported, including in Winnipeg (Canada, 135 cases in 1975–1977, 14 cases in 1987), San Francisco (1989–1991, 54 cases), and Jackson, Miss. (in 1994–1995).

Neisseria gonorrhoeae **(515, 6240).** In U.S. cities such as Baltimore, New York, Miami, San Francisco, and Seattle, rates of reported gonorrhea peak in the inner cities and decrease toward the peripheries. At highest risk of gonorrhea are female black teenagers residing in inner cities.

Treponema pallidum pallidum **(1965, 3228, 5762, 6211, 8187).** Outbreaks of syphilis have been reported in heterosexual city populations in Vancouver (Canada) and Bristol (United Kingdom), in homosexual men in Los Angeles, Miami, New York, San Francisco, Seattle (all United States), Brighton, and Manchester (both United Kingdom), and in IDU in Baltimore and Philadelphia. In Vancouver in 1996–1999, rates of infectious syphilis rose from <0.5 to >$3/10^5$ per year, with cases concentrating in a 10-block downtown (eastside) area where sex trade work was common. Only 54% (232/429) of named sex partners had evidence of treatment. In residents of inner cities in North America of the 1990s, reported syphilis (primary, secondary, and latent) rates could reach $99–126/10^5$ per year.

6.4 UTENSILS AND BELONGINGS
Utensils are objects for cooking, bedding, clothing, body care, and daily necessities, such as purchased in grocery stores or shopping malls.

Infections from utensils (824, 3088, 7093). The focus is on infections in humans rather than microbial contamination. The evidence is rather anecdotal. Although handled objects such as telephone receivers, remote control sets, money, door-push plates, or medical charts can yield microorganisms such as hepatitis B virus (HBV), respiratory syncytial virus (RSV), and parainfluenza virus (PIV); *Acinetobacter baumannii*, *Salmonella*, and *Staphylococcus* (*S. aureus*, coagulase-negative *Staphylococcus*), recovery of microorganisms does not imply spread (function as "fomites"). Contact with daily objects rarely results in infection. Exceptions include kitchen utensils, diaper-changing areas, and shared personal objects (Box 6.4).

COOKING UTENSILS
Cooking utensils include cups, grinders, pans, pots, and many other instruments and machines used in bakeries, butcher shops, and kitchens.

Infection hazards (1485, 3780, 6196). The main sources of agents in kitchens are soil from root vegetables and fruits, raw foods (eggs, meats, seafoods, and "all that drips"), human hands and respiratory droplets, and household pests (flies, cockroaches, and rodents).

The principal hazards are mishandling (working with foods with unwashed hands), cross-contamination (safe foods that touch unclean surfaces), undercooking (heat in the food core is inadequate and meat remains red), and misstoring (cooked foods that stand at room temperature). Further hazards include aerosols, dust, or pests in kitchens and food storage rooms, defective packaging, and home-preserved foods.

Raw vegetables and fruits should be considered contaminated and washed, pealed, or heated for eating. Raw foods

> **Box 6.4** Agents or infections from daily objects
>
> | | |
> |---|---|
> | Kitchen | Enteric agents, e.g., HAV; *E. coli*, *Salmonella*. For food-borne agents, see section III; for food handlers, see section 12.5. |
> | Bedding | HAV, *E. coli*, *Salmonella*, *Pseudomonas*; dermatophytes; *E. vermicularis* |
> | Body care | Eye care: *Pseudomonas* or *A. keratitis*; tampons: menstrual TSS; shared objects: HBV, HCV; conjunctivitis, pyodermia; dermatophytes |
> | Baby care | Diapers: *Norovirus*; *E. coli* (EPEC); *Candida*; *Cryptosporidium*; toys: PIV, RSV, *Pseudomonas* |
> | Clothes | If shared unwashed: body lice, with *B. recurrentis*, or *R. typhi* |
> | Others | Leather and wool souvenirs: *B. anthracis* |

should be prepared separate from cooked or ready-to-eat items. In households with an index case or incubating cook, good personal and kitchen hygiene are generally adequate means to prevent spread, and particular measures such as individual cutlery is not necessary. In special circumstances, e.g., tuberculosis in the household, dishwashers that achieve 70–80°C for ≥1 min have been recommended.

Viruses

Unclean cups and cutlery were occasionally suspected to transmit HAV, Epstein-Barr virus (EBV), *Enterovirus*, and *Norovirus*. In the United Kingdom in 1998–1999, a barman who incubated icteric hepatitis A was the source for infections in eight patrons, likely via contaminated drinking glasses (7251). In an outbreak of EBV in an obstetric and gynecology clinic, poorly washed coffee cups were the suspected vehicle (2752).

Bacteria

Dirty utensils (1420, 3807, 4573, 5836, 7435) such as uncleaned grinders and aprons were suspected or confirmed to transmit *Enterobacter sakazakii*, *E. coli*, *Helicobacter pylori*, *L. monocytogenes*, *M. tuberculosis*, *Salmonella*, and *T. pallidum endemicum* (nonvenereal bejel).

***E. coli* (418, 5191).** In Connecticut, in 1994, an outbreak of *E. coli* O157:H7 was traced to unclean meat grinders and utensils in supermarkets. In the United Kingdom in 1991, an outbreak of *E. coli* O157:H7 from yogurt was traced to cross-contamination of a milk pump by raw milk.

***Salmonella*.** In Ontario, Canada, in 1994, an outbreak of *Salmonella enterica* serovar Berta from soft cheese was traced to cross-contamination from cheese buckets with raw poultry (2181). In Wisconsin, in 1994, the meat grinder in a butcher shop was source for serovar Typhimurium in raw ground meat and an outbreak with 158 cases (6370). In the United States in 1994, an outbreak of serovar Enteritidis from ice cream was traced to cross-contamination in a tanker trailer that transported raw eggs, then ice cream premix (3259). In Wales, United Kingdom, an outbreak of serovar Typhimurium was traced to cross-contamination of ham containers by raw pork (4473).

Protozoa

Not washing utensils after working with raw meat is suspected to spread *Toxoplasma gondii* (3816).

Helminths

Worm infective stages (eggs, metacercariae) that stick to hands, utensils, or surfaces were suspected to transmit *A. lumbricoides* (304), *Clonorchis sinensis* (1368), *F. hepatica* (5044), and *Paragonimus* (1674).

BEDDING

Vomit, feces, and urine can soil bed linen, mattresses, and frames. Mattresses can hide bedbugs (see section 4.5) and grow bacteria and molds (5932). Washing clothes in washing machines is safe when followed by drying, as this is effective against resilient agents such as HAV and *M. fortuitum*. Hospital laundry should not be shaken or sorted in rooms, but collected in bags. Vegetative bacteria in laundry are killed by hot water (76° for 25 minutes).

Viruses

Laundry (771) is an occasional, suspected or confirmed vehicle of HAV, *Norovirus*, and historically also of variola virus. In Malta, hospital laundry workers have been at increased risk of HAV infection. Smallpox is said to have been spread by linen or blankets, including by American settlers in the eighteenth century, for biowarfare against Native Americans.

Bacteria

Bedding (2552, 5360) may transmit *E. coli*, *Salmonella*, *S. aureus*, and *Pseudomonas aeruginosa*, mainly in hospital habitats.

***Enterococcus* (including vancomycin resistant) (760, 1986).** *Enterococcus* is readily recovered from soil linen, gowns, bedrails, blood-pressure cuffs, and other objects from the surroundings of colonized patients. However, hands rather than objects are the main vehicles of transmission.

***E. coli* (5349).** Linen, towels, and other objects are vehicles for enteropathogenic *E. coli* (EPEC) in nurseries, day care centers, and pediatric wards.

***Salmonella* (5599, 7109).** In nursing home outbreaks in Oregon, vehicle-to-patient transmission of fluoroquinolone-resistant *S. enterica* serovar Schwarzengrund was suspected, and the agent was isolated from a foam mattress. In a nursing home in the United States, handling of soiled linen was the implicated source in an outbreak of serovar Hadar among laundry staff.

Fungi
Bedding may transmit dermatophytes (289, 2526, 6800). *Trichophyton tonsurans* was isolated from pillow covers, and, less commonly, mattresses, blankets, and curtains. Linen was the suspected vehicle of *T. tonsurans* in 2 of 10 health care workers on a pediatric ward. In a nosocomial outbreak, *Microsporum canis* infected 13 staff and 11 patients, likely by person-to-person spread and the handling of contaminated laundry.

Helminths
Linen and underwear are widely accepted vehicles of eggs of *E. vermicularis*. In Taipei orphanages, eggs were found on nearly 80% (51/65) of linen and 7% (11/150) of bedposts (1443).

Ectoparasites and Vectors
Bedding may transmit arthropods. Impregnated bed nets and bedding materials (sheets and blankets) can prevent arthropod nuisance.

Bed bugs. See section 4.5. Beds and sleeping bags are hiding places for bed bugs (*Cimex*) during the daytime.

Lice (3303). Pillow cases occasionally appear to transmit head lice (*Pediculus humanus capitis*). Body lice (*P. humanus corporis*) are acquired from sharing unwashed clothes or blankets.

Mites (1790, 4855, 6615). Dust mites (*Dermatophagoides farinae* and *D. pteronyssinus*) are readily recovered from mattresses. Scabies mites (*Sarcoptes scabiei*) survive on inanimate surfaces for a maximum of 2–3 days. Spread by shared bedding has been demonstrated experimentally but is epidemiologically insignificant.

Ticks (2103). Fully engorged *Ornithodoros hermsi* ticks may not be able to leave beds or sleeping bags; instead, ticks may be found the following morning.

BODY CARE
Body care includes skin, nails, hair, eyes, buccal cavity, genitals, and anus. Toilet paper came into use in the 1910s, tampons in the 1930s, detergent-based toothpaste in the 1940s, and soft contact lenses in the 1970s. Personal care is good for body and soul. It prevents infections and is rarely a source for infections. Plain soap is adequate for daily use in households; disinfective soap is unnecessary. For cosmetic invasive procedures, see section 18.1.

Infections (7501, 7557) (Box 6.4). Dirty hands can contaminate reused cosmetic products. Shared toothbrushes, nail clippers, and other sharp objects are a risk among household members and sportive teams. Rings on the hands of health workers are a microhabitat for nosocomial agents, including *Acinetobacter*, *Candida*, *Enterobacter*, *Escherichia*, *Klebsiella*, *Proteus*, *Pseudomonas*, and *Serratia*. Washing hands interrupts spread.

Viruses
Although poorly documented, blood-tainted, shared sharp objects (e.g., razors, tooth brushes, and nail clippers) are widely accepted vehicles of hepatitis B and C viruses (HBV and HCV). Viruses demonstrated in menstrual blood include cytomegalovirus (CMV), herpes simplex virus (HSV), and HPV. Tampons are not known to have transmitted infections (568, 5230, 7505).

HBV (4785, 5499). Among 1,385 residents of rural Ghana (75% with markers of HBV), shared bath towels, dental cleaning materials, chewing gum, and partially eaten candies were significant risks. Compared with 1,750 hepatitis B surface antigen-negative control donors, risks in 876 hepatitis B surface antigen-positive Thai blood donors included shared nail clippers and tooth brushes.

HCV (7606). In psychiatric patients in Japan, razor sharing has been a significant infection risk (6635). In Sicily, Italy, barbers who shaved themselves with reusable, unsterilized blades had a HCV seroprevalence of 38% (14/37), compared with 0.9–1.4% in the general population.

Bacteria
Body care. Shared towels and cosmetic products (eye makeup and lubricant) can be vehicles for conjunctivitis or pyodermias, including due to *Chlamydia trachomatis* (ocular serovar A–C) (2199, 3012), *Moraxella catarrhalis* (mascara conjunctivitis) (6729), *S. aureus* ("athlete's folliculitis," including methicillin-resistant *S. aureus*) (2615), and *Streptococcus pneumoniae* (conjunctivitis) (1656).

Eye care. Home-prepared contact lense rinsing fluid is a likely vehicle for *P. aeruginosa* keratitis among contact lens wearers (8205). Use of nonprescribed, cosmetic (colored) contact lenses may lead to ocular infections, including by *P. aeruginosa* (7147). In an outbreak of *S. pneumoniae* conjunctivitis among college students, the students were advised to avoid the sharing of towels, drinking glasses, and other utensils (7611). Nondisposed mascara applicators could become vehicles of infection.

Oral care. *Corynebacterium*, *Pseudomonas*, *Staphylococcus*, and *Streptococcus* have been isolated from toothbrushes

(7293), but the significance of this finding is uncertain. However, flora from toothbrushes used by children in day care included, besides *S. epidermidis*, oral streptococci, and molds, *Haemophilus influenzae* (4694). In a Norway hospital, a moist foam swab used for mouth care in patients unable to drink or brush their teeth was a suspected source of increased colonizations and infections with *P. aeruginosa* in patients (3601).

Feminine care. During menstruation, women may be at increased risk of *S. aureus* colonization and ascending infections.

The only significant, although rare, infection risk associated with tampons is menstrual toxic shock syndrome (TSS), initially recognized in healthy young women using superabsorbent tampons (2600, 3071, 3588, 4433). For TSS to occur, *S. aureus* needs to produce TSS toxin 1 (TSST1). In the United States in 1979–1996, menstrual TSS accounted for 74% (3,921/5,296) of reported TSS cases. However, standards for absorbency and labeling have lowered this proportion. In France in 1994–1997, none of 39 reported cases of TSS was related to the use of tampons. Tampons are an emerging, convenient laboratory material for the diagnosis of HPV, *C. trachomatis*, *N. gonorrhoeae*, and *T. vaginalis* by NAT (4011, 7223).

Fungi
Hair care (178, 2526, 7310). Used combs, brushes, hats, and towels can be vehicles of anthropophilic fungi that cause tinea capitis (*T. tonsurans* and *Microsporum audouinii*), in particular, in institutions that host tinea capitis index cases. In one instance, barber instruments were a suspected vehicle of *M. canis*.

Oral care (30, 7293). *C. albicans* was found to colonize the buccal cavity of 78% (180/230) of denture wearers, compared with 37% (70/190) of control nonwearers. *Candida* has been isolated from toothbrushes. How toothbrushes contribute to oral colonization is unclear.

Protozoa
Eye care (3442, 4139, 6653). Wearers of contact lenses are at risk of *Acanthamoeba* keratitis, initially observed in the 1980s, when contact lenses became popular. Most (85–90%) cases of *Acanthamoeba* keratitis report wearing of contact lenses. Today, mainly soft lenses are used. Risks include rinsing lenses with tap water or nonsterile, home-prepared solutions, and wearing lenses while swimming. Commercially prepared disinfectants overcome risks associated with home-prepared disinfectant solutions.

Ectoparasites
Spread of head lice (*P. humanus capitis*) (990, 2504, 3303, 5343, 6329, 8186) via shared combs, hairbrushes, hats, helmets, earphones, or other objects is controversial; although it may occur, instances seem rare. Combing and static electricity can eject adult lice >1 m away from the scalp, and nymphs and adult lice survive on bedding, upholstery, and rugs for ≤3 days.

BABY CARE AND TOYS
Vehicles (3386, 5976, 7746). Pacifiers are suspected vehicles of infections. Shared toys in day care centers can grow enteric agents. Diaper-changing areas can be sources of fecal agents on surfaces and the hands of parents, and of staff in day care centers. Squeezed diapers may be a noninvasive source of urine for laboratory tests, including from babies and disabled elderly patients.

Viruses
PIV (828). PIV can be cultured for up to 4 h from absorptive surfaces, and for up to 10 h from nonabsorptive surfaces. As PIV circulates among infants, spread via contaminated objects is a likely risk.

RSV (3087). RSV survives on surfaces, including on cloth gowns, paper tissues (for 30–45 min), rubber gloves (1–2 h), and countertops (for up to 6 h). RSV transmission has been demonstrated in hospital staff who cuddled infected infants or touched contaminated toys and their eyes or nose, but not in staff who just sat near an infected infant.

Rhinovirus **(6628).** Although less important than droplets and hands, the spread of *Rhinovirus* via objects is suspected.

Bacteria
E. coli **(5349).** On pediatric wards, EPEC readily contaminates toys, tabletops, and scales. Past EPEC outbreaks suggest the environment as a possible source.

P. aeruginosa **(1008).** In Melbourne, Australia, multidrug-resistant *P. aeruginosa* in water-retaining bath toys caused an outbreak on a pediatric oncology unit.

Serratia marcescens **(2427).** Contaminated milk bottles were the vehicles implicated in an outbreak in the pediatric department of a university hospital.

Fungi
Candida colonizes the wet or fecally polluted skin of babies. Skin rash and dermatitis can result. Disposable diapers reduce the risk of diaper- and diarrhea-associated *Candida* dermatitis (110, 1995).

Protozoa
Changing diapers is a risk for the acquisition of *C. parvum* (3505).

CLOTHES

Clothes and shoes can protect the public from mosquitoes, ticks, *Tunga*, mycetoma, and hookworms and professionals from zoonotic and nosocomial infections.

Hazards (662, 712, 4490, 5473, 7602). Hazards include the sharing of unwashed clothes, washing clothes at freshwater sites that are foci of tropical disease transmission, and carrying dirt into homes and hospitals. Because professional clothes are readily contaminated, including by *S. aureus*, they should be changed frequently.

Viruses
Contaminated clothes or shoes are suspected vehicles, including for foot-and-mouth disease virus (on farms, by workers and visitors) (6764), *Norovirus* (by food handlers) (4478), and RSV (by health workers) (4285).

Bacteria
Bacillus anthracis **(411, 881, 8248).** Sweaters and other textiles from sheep, goat, or camel wool have occasionally transmitted *B. anthracis*, causing cutaneous anthrax. In North Carolina, in 1978, when two workers at a textile mill contracted anthrax, home dust from one of four vacuum cleaner samples yielded *B. anthracis*, suggesting that workers had brought spores home on their clothes.

Chlamydia. Cloths used for nose blowing and face cleaning are sources of *C. trachomatis* eye infection and trachoma (7367). In a woman with preterm stillbirth due to *Chlamydophila abortus*, her husband's farm clothes were a proposed source (4959).

C. burnetii. In Nitra district, Slovakia, in 1993, 103 males and 10 females contracted Q fever, 16% (18) from assisting in abortions and births of goats, and 84% (95) from visits to the same local pub, where contaminated clothes of workers were likely to have generated infective aerosols (7768).

Fungi
M. audouinii and *T. tonsurans* have been isolated from clothes. The observed increase of *T. rubrum* in tinea pedis and onychomycoses has been ascribed to the popularity of athletic (tennis) shoes (177).

Ectoparasites
Body lice (*P. humanus corporis*) (662, 2957, 4435, 8086). Dirty clothes can be infested, with a risk of louse-borne relapsing fever and louse-borne (epidemic) typhus. Dry (powdery) louse feces sticking to clothes are highly infectious; when rubbed into eye or skin, a minimum amount can transmit *R. prowazekii*. Infested clothes should be boiled for 30 min, burned, or treated with insecticides (e.g., 0.5–1% permethrin, or DDT). For treatment, persons should remain fully clothed, to simultaneously treat clothing and skin. Insecticide-treated persons should receive a preemptive, single dose of tetracycline.

Scabies mites (*S. scabiei*) (712, 4226). Clothes are an unlikely vehicle, but children who exchange clothes with friends have occasionally contracted scabies by this mode.

CARPETS AND OTHER OBJECTS
Hazards (6, 233, 5168, 5379). Vomit, feces, and secretions can contaminate carpets and rugs. Sweat and other body secretions can contaminate upholstery and sportive equipment. Saliva can contaminate the mouthpieces of wind music instruments. Sportive equipment should be periodically cleaned, and hazardous equipment such as mattresses should be cleaned or disinfected regularly and whenever blood spots are seen. The advice for music instruments is to "bring your own trumpet."

Viruses
Adenovirus. In Nepal, during an epidemic of hemorrhagic conjunctivitis, adenovirus was detected on paper money (3017).

HSV (5984). A 14-year-old boy was reported to have contracted labial herpes from exchanging a mouthpiece for scuba diving.

Norovirus **(1362).** In an outbreak in a United Kingdom hotel in 1996, after environmental contamination by feces and vomiting, carpets were found by NAT to have the highest *Norovirus* load.

SARS-associated coronavirus (6072). In a Hong Kong hotel, where the SARS epidemic started in 2003, the carpet in front of the room of the index patient still amplified SARS-associated coronavirus RNA 3 months after the patient had left.

Bacteria
B. anthracis **(411, 8133).** Yarn, rags, and leather objects such as saddle pads are potential sources of *B. anthracis*. In 1974, 25% (96/368) of Haitian goatskin souvenirs imported into the United States grew *B. anthracis*, including drums, rugs, dolls, and purses (for *B. anthracis* in the mail, see "Buildings, Sanitation, and Wastewater" above).

Fungi
M. canis **(7448).** *M. canis* was isolated from the scalp of a 5-year-old boy who did not have contact with cats or dogs; his tinea capitis developed a few weeks after the family had bought a used car from a dog owner, and *M. canis* was grown from the interior of the car.

SECTION III
Foods

7 Animal-Derived Foods
8 Plant-Derived Foods
9 Finished Foods
10 Drinking Water and Other Beverages

Food is "all you can eat"—legally, this includes drinking water and chewing gum (cooking is the art of serving *and* preparing tasty *and* safe food). Items are consumed singly (e.g., fruit), or combined (meals and menus).

Infections (1227, 3091, 3364, 6559). Food-borne illness follows minutes to weeks after exposure (Table III.1). Manifestations are gastrointestinal (vomiting, diarrhea, and acute abdomen) or invasive (neurological and fever). Exposure history (Box III.1), key signs (Box III.2), the number of cases (sporadic or outbreak), and consumed items help to implicate the likely agents (for food work, see section 12.5; for carriers, see section 14.1).

Impact (54, 2962, 4939, 6356, 6683, 8150). The impact of food-borne illness is substantial. In the United States, of the approximately 76 million people who contract food-borne illness each year 5,000 die (mainly of *Salmonella*, *Listeria*, and *Toxoplasma*). In Australia there are 5 million (95% confidence interval [95% CI] 4–7 million) cases of food-borne illness and 80 deaths per year, and in the United Kingdom there are 1.7 million cases and nearly 700 deaths. Reported rates of food-borne illness in high-income countries are $20–120/10^5$ per year.

Arguments for foods as vehicles include: (i) hazardous foods in the history (Box III.1); (ii) ≥2 persons ill from the same food or meal (clusters from shared meals are highly suggestive); (iii) manifestations, incubation period, and infective dose (if determined) fit with a known food-borne agent; (iv) identical agents or toxins are identified in patients (feces, vomit, and blood), foods (leftover and unopened) and environment (handlers and utensils); and (v) excreting (intensity and timing) fits with natural disease history.

Causality (2603, 2757, 2849, 3585, 3840). Causality is well established for classical food-borne agents (Table III.1). Prospective freezing (food archiving) has established a relationship between *Salmonella* dose and attack rates in outbreaks. Causality is controversial for some enteric microorganisms (*Aeromonas*, *Blastocystis*, *Candida*, *Enterococcus*, *Helicobacter*, and *Plesiomonas*) and for light-burden

Table III.1 Foodborne agents, by incubation period

Incubation period	Agent[a]	Growth in food	Source[b]	Vehicle(s) and comments
Hours				
1–4	*Staphylococcus aureus* (vomitoxin)	+	H, A	Handled: pastry, ham, meats, salads
1–6, 6–24	*Bacillus cereus* (vomi-, enterotoxin)	+	E	Poorly cooled: rice, pasta, pastry, meat
2–48	*Vibrio parahaemolyticus*	+	E	Raw seafood
4–24	*Clostridium perfringens*	+	E, A	Poorly cooled meat, poultry, gravy
Days				
½–2	*Norovirus*	No	H	Handled: sandwich; tap water, person-to-person spread
1 (¼–8)	*Clostridium botulinum* (neurotoxin)	+	E	Poorly preserved or reopened fish, honey
½–1½ (to 3)	*Salmonella* (non-Typhi)	+	A, H	Any fecally polluted food, tap water
½–3	Adenovirus (enteric)	No	H	Handled
1–3	Rotavirus	No	H	Handled, salad, fruit; person-to-person spread
1–3	ETEC	+	H	Tap water, handled, salad bar
1–3 (to 5)	*Vibrio cholerae* O1 (enterotoxin)	+	E, H	Tap water, seafood; washed, handled
1–3 (½–7)	*Shigella*	+	H	Tap water, handled; person-to-person spread
1–7	*Vibrio vulnificus*	+	E	Raw seafood
1–7	*Yersinia enterocolitica*	at 4°C	A	Cold food, pork, tofu, milk
1–8	EHEC	+	A	Beef, sprouts, milk, tap water; person-to-person spread
2–5 (1–10)	*Campylobacter jejuni*	Rare	A, H	Poultry, milk, tap water
2 (to 56)	*Trichinella*	No	A	Pork, horse meat, fermented game
2 (1–90)	*Listeria*	at 4°C	E, A	Dairy, deli, seafoods, ready-to-eat
2 (to many)	*Bacillus anthracis*	+	A	Home-butchered meat
2 (to many)	*Entamoeba histolytica*	No	H	Tap water, handled, fruit, ice cream
7 (1–14)	*Cryptosporidium*	No	A, H	Tap water, milk, handled; animal-to-person spread
7 (2–14)	*Cyclospora*	No	H, E	Berries, lettuce (difficult to wash)
Weeks				
1–2 (½–4)	*Giardia*	No	A, H	Tap water, handled
1–3	*Brucella*	+	A	Milk, soft cheese
1–3	*Toxoplasma*	No	A	Meat (pork, lamb), vegetables
1–5	*Salmonella enterica* serovar Typhi	+	H	Tap water, handled, street food
2–7	Hepatitis A virus (HAV)	No	H	Seafood, tap water, pastry, person-to-person spread
2–9	Hepatitis E virus (HEV)	No	H, A	Tap water
Many	*Taenia solium* cysticercosis	No	H	Food fecally polluted from carrier

[a]ETEC, enterotoxigenic *Escherichia coli*; EHEC, enterohemorrhagic *E. coli*.
[b]Source: H, humans; A, animals; E, environmental.

enteric helminths (*Ascaris*, *Diphyllobothrium*, and *Trichuris*). Although frequently (in ~25% of samples) recovered from fish, meats, and fresh vegetables, *Aeromonas* is rarely implicated in food-borne outbreaks. The focus on food-borne *Enterococcus* is on antimicrobial resistance that can be prevalent in Europe in isolates from raw meat and milk. In particular, vancomycin-resistant *E. faecium* and *E. faecalis* (VRE) are identified from raw and processed poultry, beef, and pork. Raw vegetables produced with wastewater irrigation are a suspected vehicle of *Helicobacter pylori*.

Preventive measures. Preventive measures include good production practice (herding, cultivation, and harvest), good processing practice (slaughter, critical processing points, and pasteurization), good sales practice (hygienic installations and handling), and good kitchen practice, including clean hands (against hepatitis A virus [HAV], *Norovirus*, and *Shigella*), good heat (against *Campylobacter*, *Escherichia*, *Salmonella*, and *Toxoplasma*), separation of raw and heated items (against cross-contamination), and safe keeping temperature (against *Bacillus cereus* and *Clostridium perfringens*).

ACUTE VOMITING (GASTRITIS AND FOOD POISONING)
VIRUSES (54, 4518, 6356)

Vomiting is a prominent feature of viral gastroenteritis, in particular, *Norovirus* (winter vomiting disease). However, only some 10–40% of all *Norovirus* infections are food-borne (person-to-person spread is more significant). In

> **Box III.1** Suggested food exposure history
>
> **Your diet.** In the past 2–3 days, did you consume any of the following:
>
> - Raw milk, "runny" eggs, tartar or "saignant" beef, red hamburger, or raw seafood (crustaceans and bivalves)?
> - Barbecued chicken, privately butchered meat, game meat, "souvenir sausages," cold meat, or any fish?
> - Seed sprouts or other raw vegetables, tropical or dried fruits, home-canned vegetables, or creams from reopened cans?
> - Water from a tap or drinking fountain, mineral water, fresh juice or cider, or ice cubes?
>
> **Food basket.** In the past 2–3 days, did you purchase any food from:
>
> - Bakery (e.g., rolls or pastry), grocery (e.g., snack or sandwich), butcher (e.g., ground or cold meat), street vendor (e.g., ice cream or cold drink), outlet (e.g., ethnic food), or farm (e.g., milk, eggs, or meat)?
>
> **Meals.** In the past 2–3 days, did you eat any meals away from home?
>
> - Meals from street vendors, cafeterias, snack bars, canteens, restaurants, salad bars, cold buffets, or parties?
> - Meals shared with friends or colleagues?
>
> **Food watch.** In the past few days, did you notice:
>
> - Malodorous or brown tap water or any interruption with your home water supply?
> - Moldy, spoiled, or outdated foods, including cheese and home-preserved vegetables?
>
> **Food work.** Your work right now, does it involve:
>
> - Food in any way, including animals, plants, food processing, preparing, or serving?
> - Drinking water, including maintenance?

high-income countries, rates per 10^5 per year are <1 for astrovirus, 6–17 for *Norovirus*, and <1 to >60 for *Rotavirus*. In the United Kingdom, astrovirus, *Norovirus*, and *Rotavirus* account for at least 1%, 3.5%, and 0.5% of food-borne disease cases, respectively. Vehicles for *Norovirus* are diverse, including handled foods, snacks, fruit, salads, vegetables, soups, poultry, meat, oysters, desserts, and tap water.

BACTERIA (2961, 4986, 6356, 7880)

(Table III.1) Vomiting within hours of exposure is the hallmark of toxins preformed in foods by *B. cereus* or *Staphylococcus aureus*.

B. cereus (1927). Sources of toxins that induce (early) vomiting or (later) diarrhea are spores that withstand heat and by heating and cooling are induced to germinate. In a family outbreak from pasta salad in Belgium, 1 of 5 affected children died of *B. cereus* intoxication. In Accra, Ghana, 6% (28/511) of foods sold by street vendors grow *B. cereus*. The median reported rate in high-income countries is $\sim 0.5/10^5$ per year.

> **Box III.2** Food-borne syndromes or agents, by lead symptom
>
> **Vomiting:** *Norovirus* ("winter vomiting"), food poisoning (*S. aureus* toxin or *B. cereus* toxin)
> **Dehydrating diarrhea:** *Vibrio cholerae*; in infants, *Rotavirus* or ETEC
> **Bloody diarrhea:** *Campylobacter*, EHEC, EIEC, *Shigella*, *Yersinia*, or *Entamoeba*
> **Neurosyndrome:** Botulism, *Listeria* or *Angiostrongylus* meningitis, or *Toxoplasma* brain abscess
> **Acute abdomen:** *Rotavirus* intussusception, *Yersinia* pseudoappendicitis, obstructive *Ascaris*, *Anisakis* larvae
> **Fever:**
>   - Acute: invasive enterobacteria: *Campylobacter*, *Salmonella*, or *Shigella*
>   - Acute plus pharyngitis: food-borne streptococcal infection
>   - Persistent: HAV, *Brucella*, *S. enterica* serovar Typhi, or amebic liver abscess
>
> **Outbreak:** *Norovirus*, *Salmonella*, *C. perfringens*, or *S. aureus*

S. aureus. Sources of preformed enterotoxin are toxigenic strains of *S. aureus* in food handlers with pyodermia or infected wounds. In Accra, Ghana, 32% (163/511) food items sold on streets by vendors grow *S. aureus*. For food poisoning to occur, a typical level of *S. aureus* in food is 30 million CFU/g. The median reported rate in high-income countries is $0.2/10^5$ per year. Main vehicles are chicken and meat products (e.g., ham).

ACUTE DIARRHEA (ENTERITIS)

Acute diarrhea (54, 2961, 2962, 3364, 3457, 6356, 6559, 7880) should be considered infectious unless good evidence suggests otherwise. In Australia, about one-third (95% CI, 28–38%) of acute gastroenteritis is food borne. Most salmonellosis is food borne.

Watery stools are a hallmark of acute enteritis that typically occurs one-half to three days after exposure to foods (Table III.1). Watery stools (and cramps) are nonspecific and do not reveal food-borne viruses, bacteria, fungi (microspiridia), protozoa, and possibly helminths. However, frequent agents in *sporadic* cases are *Campylobacter* and *Salmonella*.

Dehydrating food-borne diarrhea (standing skin fold and cold periphery) points to *Vibrio cholerae*, *Rotavirus* (infants), or *Escherichia coli* (enterotoxigenic *E. coli* [ETEC] in infants).

Dysenteric diarrhea (visible or microscopic blood) points to enteroinvasive agents, mainly *Campylobacter*, *E. coli* (enterohemorrhagic *E. coli* [EHEC], enteroinvasive *E. coli* [EIEC]), *Salmonella*, *Shigella*, or *Entamoeba histolytica* (Box III.2), infrequently to *Yersinia enterocolitica* or heavy loads of *Capillaria* or *Trichuris*.

BACTERIA

Bacteria that form toxins on mucosa rather than foods include *C. perfringens*, *E. coli*, and *V. cholerae*.

***Campylobacter* (2962).** Most (75–80%) infections are food borne. About 20% of food-borne disease cases and 10% of deaths are attributed to *Campylobacter*. Reported food-borne disease rates per 10^5 per year in high-income countries range from ~10–40 (North America), to 20–120 (western Europe), and >115 (Australia and New Zealand), for a median of 60.

***C. perfringens* (3415).** Virtually all (100%) infections are food borne. In western Europe, ~10% of food-borne disease cases and 25% of deaths are attributed to *C. perfringens*. The median food-borne disease rate reported in high-income countries is ~$0.5/10^5$ per year. Hazardous meals are lukewarm inside, prepared well in advance, kept at room temperature for >2 h, and served cold. Precooked and handled foods should be reheated (70°C throughout for ≥2 min) and held hot (63°C) if not served immediately.

***E. coli* (3838, 6105).** The majority (50–80%) of EHEC infections are food borne. In West Europe, ~5% of food-borne disease cases and deaths are attributed to EHEC. Reported food-borne disease rates per 10^5 per year in high-income countries range from ~1 (United States) to 2–10 (United Kingdom) and 5 (Canada). Typical vehicles for *E. coli* O157 are bovine-derived foods (e.g., ground or roast beef, or raw milk), or bovine-polluted foods (e.g., lettuce or alfalfa sprouts, or apple cider).

***Salmonella* (2962, 3258).** Most (80–95%) salmonellosis is food borne. In western Europe, ~5% of food-borne disease cases but 30% of deaths are due to *Salmonella* non-Typhi serovars. Reported food-borne disease rates per 10^5 per year in high-income countries range from 4 (Japan), to 15–18 (North America), 39 (Australia), and 476 (Czechia), for a median of 40. In the United Kingdom in 2002, reported rates for the two most frequent isolates were 6–19 /10^5 (*Salmonella enterica* serovar Enteritidis) and 4/10^5 (*S. enterica* serovar Typhimurium). Virtually any food can be a vehicle. For *S. enterica* serovar Enteritidis, typical (albeit nonexclusive) vehicles are raw eggs and egg products; typical for *S. enterica* serovar Heidelberg are eggs, cheese, chicken, and pork.

***Shigella* (2962).** A smaller fraction (10–15%) of all shigellosis is food borne; a majority is spread person-to-person. Reported food-borne disease rates per 10^5 per year in high-income countries range from <3 (Australia), to 4–10 (North America), and 20 (Slovakia), for a median of 3.

***Vibrio* (3587, 4049, 6814).** Most (~90%) cases of sporadic, endemic, and epidemic cholera, and a majority (55–90%) of *V. parahaemolyticus* infections are food borne. Hazards include seafoods from coastal waters and estuaries that receive raw city waste, handled foods from street vendors, and food shared with a person suffering from diarrhea.

***Yersinia* (793, 2962, 7242).** Most (90%) *Y. enterocolitica* infections are food borne. The reported food-borne disease rate in high-income countries is ~1/10^5 per year. In the United Kingdom, *Yersinia* causes 7.5% of food-borne disease cases. Vehicles include dairy products, meats, seafoods, and vegetables. Although 3–18% of ready-to-eat or environmental samples can grow *Yersinia*, in >50% of outbreaks, a vehicle is not identified.

PROTOZOA

Food-borne diarrheagenic protozoa include *Balantidium*, *Cryptosporidium*, *Cyclospora*, *E. histolytica*, *Giardia*, and

Isospora. In high-income countries, reported food-borne disease rates per 10^5 per year are <1 for *Cyclospora*, 0.5–45 (typically 10) for *Giardia*, and 1–30 (typically 5) for *Cryptosporidium*.

ACUTE AND SUBACUTE FOOD-BORNE NEUROSYNDROMES

Major neurotropic food-borne agents are *Clostridium botulinum*, *Listeria monocytogenes*, and *Toxoplasma gondii*.

C. botulinum (285, 1080, 2961, 3054, 3364, 6356, 7880, 8254). Blurred vision, diplopia, dysphagia, and other acute neurosymptoms and signs are suggestive of food-borne botulism. The median reported rate of botulism in high-income countries is $0.2/10^5$ per year.

Germination of spores and production of botulinum toxin are promoted by pH >4.6, temperature >3°C, watery content, and occlusion (vacuum, can, and low O_2). For safe destruction of spores, home canning of nonacidic foods (e.g., vegetables) requires pressure cooking and heat (116°C) for 20–100 min. Traditional vehicles of botulism (e.g., beans and peppers) are increasingly replaced by commercial (vacuum-packaged or deep-frozen) or catered foods.

L. monocytogenes (2962, 3673, 4915, 5034, 5483, 5484, 6356, 7880). Besides acute diarrhea, this agent can cause meningoencephalitis. Virtually all listeriosis is food borne. The median reported food-borne incidence in high-income countries is about $0.3/10^5$ per year. The agent is isolated from a variety of foods, including raw, stored, and ready-to-eat foods. Accepted levels are controversial. If the limit is set at ≤100 CFU/g for the time of consumption, this means zero tolerance for the time of purchase, for foods that support growth during storage (Table III.1). In Denmark, the proportion of ready-to-eat retail samples that grew >100 CFU/g was ~1%. *Listeria* is widespread in the environment, and food-processing plants frequently yield *Listeria*, including *L. monocytogenes*. *Listeria* can persist in environmental niches for years.

T. gondii. *T. gondii* from undercooked meat, unwashed vegetables, raw milk, or tap water is a cause of brain abscess or encephalitis in immune-impaired hosts. In Czechia, where food-borne toxoplasmosis is reportable, the reported rate was $8/10^5$ per year (6356).

Infrequent causes. In countries with temperate climates, *Baylisascaris procyonis* from dirty hands and tick-borne encephalitis virus from raw goat milk are causes of acute neurosyndromes. Space-occupying lesions (cyst and granuloma) can be caused by cysticercosis (from eggs of *Taenia solium* on foods fecally polluted by human carriers), *Echinococcus granulosus* (from eggs on berries, fallen-down fruits, or mushrooms fecally polluted by dogs), or *Toxocara* (from eggs on raw vegetables fecally polluted by dogs or cats, or from larvae in undercooked viscera). In countries with warm climates, *Angiostrongylus cantonensis* from snails as food, snail slime on unwashed salads, or cross-contaminated foods can cause eosinophilic meningitis.

ACUTE ABDOMINAL INFECTIONS

Abdominal cramps are a frequent, but agent nondiscriminative symptom of diarrheal disease. In contrast, few agents cause an acute (surgical) abdomen that may or may not be accompanied by perforation (peritonitis)

Intussusception is a rare complication of *Rotavirus* infections in infants (6910). Pseudoappendicitis (mesenteric adenitis) can complicate food-borne yersiniosis (typically *Yersinia pseudotuberculosis* and infrequently *Y. enterocolitica*) (720). Food-borne invasive helminth larvae can also cause acute abdomen, including *Anisakis* from raw fish, *A. costaricensis* from slugs or unwashed, slime-polluted salads, and *Fasciola* from privately collected, unwashed field salads. Migrating juveniles of *Ascaris lumbricoides* can enter bile or pancreatic ducts, causing acute syndromes, while heavy loads of adults can cause obstructive small bowel ileus.

FOOD-BORNE FEBRILE ILLNESS

Food-borne febrile diarrhea is suggestive of enteroinvasive agents, mainly *Campylobacter*, *E. coli* (hemolytic-uremic syndrome), *Salmonella*, *Shigella*, and *Yersinia*.

Food-borne febrile diarrhea with facial edema is suggestive of acute trichinellosis. *Trichinella* (2961, 6356, 7880) is acquired from undercooked pork, boar, and game meats. The reported disease rate in high-income countries is typically $<0.1/10^5$ per year (0.2 in Italy and up to 7 in Slovakia).

Case clusters and outbreaks of food-borne fever with pharyngitis are suggestive of food-borne *Streptococcus pyogenes* group A (GAS) pharyngitis (3849, 4832). Source are colonized or infected individuals who handle foods, typically cold items. In Japan in 1996, food-borne GAS caused pharyngitis in 192 (75%) of 255 employees attending a sports meeting.

Agents and typical vehicles of nondiarrheic food-borne fevers (2961, 6356, 7880) include HAV, HEV, *S. enterica* serovar Typhi, and *E. histolytica* (amebic liver abscess) from tap water (see chapter 10) or handled foods (see section 12.5), *Brucella*, mycobacteria, and *Streptococcus bovis* from raw milk products (see section 7.1), *Vibrio vulnificus* from seafood (see section 7.5), and

Lassa fever virus or *Leptospira* from rodent-polluted foods. The incubation period is typically weeks, and a link with food is difficult to find. These fevers typically persist for days or weeks. In high-income countries, reported food-borne disease rates per 10^5 per year are 0.3 for typhoid fever, 0.3–0.4 for brucellosis, and 1–20 for acute HAV infection.

FOOD-BORNE OUTBREAKS

Food-borne disease outbreaks are reviewed in brief (1721, 1878, 2330, 2961, 3051, 3457, 5602, 5763, 6105, 6355, 6986, 8150).

Impact. Impact is significant. In the United States in 1991–2000, 8,271 food-borne disease outbreaks were reported; 1,414 were reported in 2000, for a rate of 0.5 outbreak/10^5. In Lazio, Italy, in 1996–2000, active surveillance detected 410 food-borne outbreaks, for rates of one to two outbreaks per 10^5 per year. Average cases/outbreak ratios are 50 in North America and Australia, and 15 in western Europe, with broad ranges by cause, from 1–3 with *C. botulinum* and 8 with *E. coli*, to 35 with *S. enterica* serovar Enteritidis, and 100–200 with *Norovirus*.

Causes. By diagnostic workup and location, a causative agent is identified in 30–90% (typically two thirds) of outbreaks. In pre-2000 statistics, because of diagnostic difficulties, viruses were likely underrepresented. In high-income countries, *Norovirus* is the principal causative virus, and food-borne HAV or *Rotavirus* outbreaks are rare. In the United States, the proportion of outbreaks confirmed due to *Norovirus* has increased from 1% in 1991 to 12% in 2000.

The main bacterial causes of outbreaks are *Salmonella* (in 10–45% of outbreaks versus 30–60% of cases), *C. perfringens* (13–16% versus 10–20%), and *S. aureus* (4–12% versus 1–14%). Other bacteria have been identified in <5% of outbreaks. *S. enterica* serovar Typhi outbreaks through polluted foods have been reported sporadically (7681, 7687), including in France in 2003 (7 cases) and 1998 (27 cases).

The main food-borne parasites confirmed in outbreaks are *Cryptosporidium*, *Cyclospora*, and *Giardia*. A single, likely food-borne *E. histolytica* outbreak has been reported in an Israeli kibbutz (3161). Other parasites infrequently implicated in food-borne outbreaks are *Toxoplasma* and *Trichinella*.

Venues. Venues in high-income countries are catering facilities (in 20–60%, e.g., restaurants, cafeterias, and pubs), hospitals and long-term care facilities (in 5–60%), domiciles (in 5–30%), and schools (in 3–9%, including boarding schools and camps).

Vehicles. Commonly implicated are eggs and egg products, meats and meat products, seafood, poultry, pastry, fruits and vegetables, and milk and dairy products. In about 10%, the implicated vehicles are compound (menus) or multiple. *Salmonella* uses a broad range of vehicles, including eggs, dairy products, desserts, sauces, poultry, meats, seafood, and vegetables.

Sources. Sources to consider for backtracing (Table III.1) include soil (e.g., *Bacillus*, *Clostridium*, and *Vibrio*), animals (e.g., *Brucella*, *Listeria*, and *Salmonella*), and humans (e.g., HAV, *Norovirus*, *S. enterica* serovar Typhi, *S. aureus*, and *Shigella*). Foods can become polluted at any point in the farm-to-table food chain, including at production ("field-and-feed"), during processing ("slaughter-and-slice"), and at serving ("cook-and-kitchen").

Emerging hazards. Emerging hazards include industrial production, long-distance transportation, international distribution with complex backtracing, consumer preferences for raw foods, and antimicrobial resistance. In low-income countries, benefits of small-scale production and short circuits to consumers are offset by lack of hygiene and enforced regulations.

7

Animal-Derived Foods

7.1 Milk and dairy products
7.2 Eggs and egg products
7.3 Poultry
7.4 Meat and meat products
7.5 Seafood, fish, and molluscs

Surveillance data from the United Kingdom permit the calculation of attack rates per 10^5 servings (54). Rates by increasing order are 0.4 for milk, 2 for meat (bacon or ham, 0.8; pork, 2; beef, 4; mutton, 4), 4 for seafood (fish, 0.8; shellfish, 65), 5 for eggs, and 10 for poultry.

7.1 MILK AND DAIRY PRODUCTS

Milk from cows, sheep, goats, and other mammals is part of the human diet. Dairy products include butter, cheese, cream (light, heavy, or sour), ice cream, milk powder, and yogurt.

Exposure. In the United States, consumption of beverage milks per person per year was 105 liters in 1980, 85 liters in 2000, and 83 liters in 2001. In 2001, the top-ranking milk beverages were plain whole milk, reduced fat (2%) milk, and light and skim milk (http://www.census.gov/prod/2004pubs/03statab/health.pdf). In a U.S. survey of eight states in 2000, 0.6–1.2% of 13,113 respondents reported consumption of unpasteurized milk in the week that preceded the interview.

Infections (1721, 1738, 1953, 2738, 6356) (Box 7.1). In high-income countries, milk and dairy products account for ~2% of food-borne disease outbreaks. In U.S. schools, this proportion is 5% when excluding ice cream. The median duration of milk-borne disease outbreaks is 2 weeks. In the United Kingdom, 27 milk-borne outbreaks were recorded in 1992–2000 (three per year), with a total of 662 cases (25 per outbreak). In half of the outbreaks (14/27), unpasteurized milk was involved.

Exposure history (Box III.1). Inquire about the consumption of raw, powdered, and pasteurized milk and dairy products and about where brands were purchased (grocery store or farm).

RAW MILK

Infections. Raw milk is a health hazard. In the United States in 20 years (1973–1992), raw milk caused 46 outbreaks (two per year) with 1,733 cases (38 per outbreak) (3212). In the United Kingdom in 30 years (1951–1980), raw cow

> **Box 7.1** Agents from milk or cheese, by cluster
>
> For dairy herds, see section 2.3; for work, see sections 12.4 and 12.5.
>
> | | |
> |---|---|
> | Feces-food | *Campylobacter* (milk), EHEC (cheese), *Listeria* (cheese), *Salmonella* (milk, cheese), *Yersinia* (milk) |
> | Zoonotic | TBEV (milk); *Brucella* (cheese), *Mycobacterium bovis* (milk), *M. avium parainfluenzae* (milk) |
> | Environmental | *E. sakazakii* (formula milk) |
> | Skin-blood | *S. aureus* enterotoxin |

milk caused 174 outbreaks (six per year) and 3,658 cases (21 per outbreak) (2581).

Viremic or bacteremic milk cows can excrete agents into milk. Unclean udders, farm workers, or equipment can contaminate fresh milk extrinsically.

Prions

Experimental and epidemiological evidence suggests that milk is not a vehicle of bovine spongiform encephalopathy (BSE) prions to humans.

Viruses

Knowledge of viruses from raw milk is limited (576, 1435, 1976, 2031, 4171, 4845, 6268).

Hepatitis A virus (HAV). A milk-borne outbreak of HAV was reported in the 1940s.

Hepatitis E virus (HEV). In Moldavia, drinking raw milk is a risk for HEV infections in swine farmers.

Foot-and-mouth disease virus. During epizootics, milk can spread foot-and-mouth disease virus animal-to-animal, but milk-borne infections in humans seem unlikely.

Tick-borne encephalitis virus (TBEV). Viremic cows, goats, and sheep can shed TBEV from milk, and dairy products from raw cow, goat, and sheep milk can be vehicles. Cases of food-borne TBEV have been reported from enzootic areas in Europe, including Austria, Germany, Hungary, Litvania, Poland, Russia, and Slovakia. Milk-borne TBEV outbreaks were reported in Lithuania in 2003 (22 cases from unpasteurized goat milk), in Poland in 1995 (48 cases from goat milk), and in Slovakia (up to 660 suspected cases).

Bacteria

Bacillus cereus, Brucella, Campylobacter, Corynebacterium ulcerans, Coxiella, Escherichia coli, Listeria, Mycobacterium, Salmonella, Staphylococcus aureus (enterotoxin), *Yersinia enterocolitica*, and other bacteria have been reported to be carried by raw milk (886, 1171, 1953, 2581, 3052, 3212, 6822, 7016). The main agents in high-income countries are *Campylobacter*, mycobacteria, *Salmonella, S. aureus*, and *Yersinia* (Box 7.1).

Brucella **(169, 886, 1115, 2581, 4971, 4978, 5424).** In 1904–1905, T. Zammit (1864–1935) established goat milk as a vehicle of *Brucella* in Malta. *Brucella* has been isolated in milk from cows, goats, sheep, buffalos, camels, and yaks. *Brucella* in milk survives at pH of 4.0–5.9 and temperatures of 0–71°C (25–37°C for 24 h and 71°C for 5–15 s). Pasteurization inactivates *Brucella*. In milk allowed to sour for several days, the number of *Brucella* is reduced. In the United Kingdom in 30 years, 1% (2/233) of milk-borne outbreaks were due to *Brucella*. Reported vehicles include raw milk, fresh cheese, and other unpasteurized dairy products.

Campylobacter **(157, 168, 1192, 1953, 2738, 3212, 5791).** Milk is a significant vehicle of *Campylobacter*. By geography and workup, *Campylobacter* has been implicated in 25–40% of milk-borne outbreaks. In the United States in 20 years (1973–1992), *Campylobacter* caused 26 milk-related outbreaks (one per year) and 1,100 cases (42 per outbreak). In the United Kingdom in 1992–1996, *Campylobacter* caused five outbreaks (one per year) and 262 cases (52 per outbreak). Reported attack rates in milk-borne outbreaks are 7–79% (typically 47%). Raw milk is particularly hazardous. In ~20–40% of milk-borne outbreaks in the United States and the United Kingdom, the implicated milk was raw or poorly pasteurized.

Many milk-borne outbreaks have been reported, including the following. In the United States in 2001, during a "cow-leasing program" intended to circumvent prohibition of raw milk, 75 consumers of raw milk contracted campylobacteriosis (1192). In the United Kingdom, 72 attendees of a large festival contracted *Campylobacter* likely from unpasteurized milk sold at the event (5190). In a day nursery in the United Kingdom, a *C. jejuni* outbreak was traced to milk bottles pecked by magpies; milk from a pecked bottle yielded *C. jejuni* (~6 cells/500 ml) (6281).

Coxiella **(2411, 2581, 2690, 3176, 3939).** Raw milk is a vehicle of *Coxiella*. In the United States in I/2002–XII/2003, 94% (298/316) of nationwide bulk-tank milk samples tested positive for *C. burnetii* by nucleic acid amplification test (NAT). In the United Kingdom in 1951–1980, *C. burnetii* was implicated in 0.4% (1/233) of milk-borne outbreaks (with 29 cases). Of Swiss blood donors, 9.2% of 131 regular consumers of raw milk were seroreactive, compared with 2.9% of 1,717 controls who were nonconsumers. Risks identified in Q fever outbreaks included raw consumption of goat milk and of raw and pasteurized goat cheese.

***Escherichia* (639, 1722, 2738, 3306, 5998, 6105).** Raw milk and dairy products are occasional vehicles of *E. coli* O157 (enterohemorrhagic *E. coli* [EHEC]) and enterotoxigenic *E. coli* (ETEC). *E. coli* O157 has been isolated from equipment on dairy farms with infected cows, but rarely (in <0.7%) from unpasteurized milk samples. Milk-borne outbreaks have been reported in North America and West Europe. In the United States in 1982–2002, *E. coli* O157 caused four outbreaks in consumers of raw milk. In the United Kingdom in 1992–2000, *E. coli* O157:H7 was implicated in 33% (9/27) of milk-borne outbreaks. In Czechia in 1995, raw goat milk was implicated in a cluster of four cases of hemolytic-uremic syndrome (HUS) and in regular goat milk drinkers with inapparent EHEC infection.

***Listeria monocytogenes* (886, 2876, 4592, 4915, 6354).** Raw milk and milk products can be vehicles of *L. monocytogenes*, including chocolate milk, soft cheese, and butter. About 0.5–2% of raw milk samples and 1–10% of dairy products grow *L. monocytogenes*, usually at a low level, but in 0.5–1.5% of samples at >100 CFU/g. The gradient between raw milk and dairy products suggests secondary contamination from the environment. Substantial numbers of *L. monocytogenes* survive cheese ripening, including blue, brick, Camembert, cheddar, cottage, feta, and Trappist cheeses. Immune-impaired patients are advised to consume pasteurized dairy products only and to discard soft cheese crust.

***Mycobacterium*.** Milk is a historical and current vehicle of *Mycobacterium*. **M. tuberculosis complex (256, 619, 886, 2581, 3866, 5540).** Infected cows shed *M. bovis* in milk. Although tuberculosis in dairy herds can be controlled, illegal imports of infected herds and *M. bovis* from wildlife are a continuous threat. Mandatory pasteurization could eliminate milk-borne tuberculosis. In the prepasteurization era, ~10% of tuberculosis (including abdominal) and ~1% of pulmonary tuberculosis were milk-borne. In the United Kingdom in 1951–1980, one of 233 milk-borne outbreaks (with three cases) was attributed to *Mycobacterium* spp. (not typed). Recently in California, one third of isolates from children with tuberculosis were typed *M. bovis*. **Environmental mycobacteria (2297, 2902, 2926, 3866, 4572).** Environmental mycobacteria recovered from raw milk include *M. avium* complex (MAC), *M. fortuitum*, *M. gordonae*, and *M. kansasii*. In Tanzania, in a community that traditionally consumes raw milk, mycobacteria were isolated in 31 (4%) of 805 milk samples, including *M. bovis*, *M. fortuitum*, and *M. gordonae*. *M. avium paratuberculosis* is an agent of inflammatory bowel disease in cattle and is suspected to cause similar disease in humans. *M. avium paratuberculosis* is not reliably killed by pasteurization (see "Pasteurized Milk" below).

***Salmonella* (156, 1210, 2738, 3212, 5605, 6970).** Raw milk is a significant vehicle, including in outbreaks. In the United States in 20 years (1973–1992), *Salmonella* caused 12 milk-borne outbreaks with 331 cases (28 per outbreak). In the United Kingdom in 1992–2000, *Salmonella enterica* serovars caused 10 milk-borne outbreaks, 6 from serovar Typhimurium, 2 from serovar Enteritidis, and 1 each from serovars Anatum and Java. In the United States in 2002–2003, serovar Typhimurium in raw milk caused a multistate outbreak with 62 confirmed cases, comprising 40 customers who purchased raw milk from a working dairy farm, 16 dairy workers, and 6 household contacts. Among dairy workers, the attack rate was 8% (16/211); in addition, four barn workers who milked cows, bottled milk, and made ice cream were subclinically infected. Five of 32 food samples tested positive for serovar Typhimurium: three raw skim milk, one butter, and one cream. After the outbreak, the dairy discontinued selling raw milk. Serovar Dublin is suggestive of bovine sources. In Europe in the 1970s, serovar Dublin in unpasteurized milk caused an outbreak with ≥700 cases. In 2000, 181 serovar Dublin infections were reported in Europe, for a rate of 0.05 (range, 0–0.3)/10^5.

***Staphylococcus* (303, 2274, 2581, 3212).** Milk is a vehicle for *S. aureus* enterotoxin A. In leftover samples from outbreaks (low-fat milk in Japan and chocolate milk in the United States), enterotoxin concentration was 0.1–0.7 ng/ml. In Japan, intake has been estimated at 20–100 ng/person. Enterotoxin A is heat stable, retaining immunological and biological activity when pasteurized (at 130°C for 2–4 s). In the United States in 20 years (1973–1992), 1 (2%) of 46 raw milk outbreaks was due to staphylococcal enterotoxin. In the United Kingdom in 30 years (1951–1980), *S. aureus* caused 46 (20% of 233) milk-borne outbreaks (1–2 per year), and 2,406 (26% of 9,411) cases (52 per outbreak). In Kansai district, Japan, in 2000, low-fat milk, yogurt drink, and powdered skim milk manufactured in Hokkaido caused 13,420 cases of staphylococcal food poisoning, for attack rates of 0.2–10%; 62,000 (16%) of 380,000 milk cartons were recalled.

***Stenotrophomonas maltophilia* (1886).** *S. maltophilia* has been recovered from milk, but the epidemiological significance of this finding is unclear.

***Streptococcus* (2128, 4379).** Milk is a rare vehicle of *Streptococcus* spp. In 1941, tinned milk contaminated by an infected worker was implicated in outbreaks of group A *Streptococcus* (GAS) tonsillopharyngitis. Group C *Streptococcus* (GCS) in raw milk has caused an outbreak with 11 cases of invasive GCS disease, including seven deaths.

Yersinia. *Y. enterocolitica* **(44, 680, 3102, 3364, 7242).** *Y. enterocolitica* has been isolated from milk. In Morocco, 11 (37%) of 30 raw milk samples, 15 (24%) of 63 traditionally fermented milk samples, 1 (5%) of 20 pasteurized milk samples, 1 (5%) of 20 cream samples, and 7 (7%) of 94 cheese samples yielded *Y. enterocolitica*. Raw, pasteurized, and chocolate milk have been implicated in outbreaks. In New York State in 1976, an increased number of appendectomies prompted an investigation that identified 38 confirmed *Y. enterocolitica* cases and chocolate milk served at a school cafeteria as the vehicle, for attack rates of 11% among students and 3% among employees. The milk was probably contaminated during hand mixing in an open vat. *Y. pseudotuberculosis* **(6009).** *Y. pseudotuberculosis* can also be milk borne. In British Columbia, Canada, in 1998, an outbreak caused 74 confirmed cases; a single brand of homogenized milk was the vehicle.

Protozoa

Cryptosporidium **(1, 1953).** Milk is a likely vehicle for *Cryptosporidium*. In an outbreak in the United Kingdom with 67 cases, milk was the implicated vehicle. Of 120 cryptosporidiosis cases in the United Kingdom, 10% admitted to drinking raw milk in the month before disease onset.

Toxoplasma gondii **(1381, 1554, 6511, 6950).** Raw milk is a vehicle. *T. gondii* has been isolated in goat milk by bioassay. In Europe, 96 (46%) of 210 seroreactive pregnant women reported drinking raw milk, compared with 75 (10%) of 746 seronegative controls. In California in 1978, 10 (one manifest and nine inapparent) of 24 members of a large family contracted *T. gondii* from goat milk.

PASTEURIZED MILK

Contamination after pasteurization is the main hazard. Such incidences have been reported for *E. coli*, *Listeria*, *Salmonella*, and *Yersinia*.

E. coli **(7652).** In the United Kingdom in 1994, pasteurized milk in cartons or bottles from a local dairy caused an EHEC outbreak with >100 cases, including nine cases of HUS. EHEC was isolated from a pipe that carried milk from the pasteurizer to the bottling machine.

L. monocytogenes **(1720, 2436).** In Illinois in 1994, serotype 1/2b in pasteurized chocolate milk served at a picnic caused 45 listeriosis cases, for an attack rate of 75% among 60 consumers. No defects in pasteurization were detected, but in the circuit that led to a holding tank, a pool of sequestered, unrefrigerated milk was detected. In Massachusetts in 1983, a brand of pasteurized milk was epidemiologically implicated in an outbreak of serotype 4b that affected 42 immune-suppressed adults and 7 fetuses or infants.

Salmonella **(5605, 6488).** In the United States in 1960–2000, pasteurized milk was implicated in 12 outbreaks, including one in Pennsylvania and New Jersey in 2000 in which *S. enterica* serovar Typhimurium caused 93 cases; possible sources were machines leaking raw milk into pasteurized milk. In Illinois in 1985, serovar Typhimurium in a cross-contaminated brand of pasteurized low-fat milk caused 169,000–198,000 clinical cases, including 16,000 culture confirmed.

Y. enterocolitica **(44, 7288).** In Vermont and New Hampshire in 1995, 10 patients became ill after consuming bottled, pasteurized milk; *Y. enterocolitica* O:8 was isolated from all patients, one retail milk sample, and a pig from the local dairy farm. Pasteurization was not deficient, but returned milk bottles were rinsed by workers with untreated well water before being filled with pasteurized milk. In a United States multistate outbreak in 1982, pasteurized milk caused 312–1,289 clinical cases, including 172 confirmed cases, for an overall attack rate of 8%. Outbreak milk was not available, but the same *Y. enterocolitica* serotype was recovered from cases and a farm that fed outdated milk from the implicated dairy plant to pigs.

Few agents may resist usual pasteurization. These include spores of *Bacillus* and *M. avium paratuberculosis*.

B. cereus **(7384).** *B. cereus* enters milk from soil at teats. Of 334 pasteurized, low-fat milk samples from household refrigerators in The Netherlands, 40% (133) grew *B. cereus*; in general, the counts were low.

M. avium paratuberculosis **(MAP) (2902, 2926, 5045).** MAP withstands standard pasteurization (at 73°C for 15–25 s). In one study, 7% (4/60) of raw cow milk samples, and 7% (10/144) of pasteurized samples grew MAP. In the United Kingdom in 1991–1993, MAP DNA was amplified in milk from ill cows, subclinically infected cows, pasteurized milk from retail outlets, cream, and whey; overall, 7% (22/312) of samples tested positive, and 50% (9/18) of DNA-positive milk samples and 16% (6/36) of DNA-negative samples grew MAP, after incubation for 13–40 months! Subclinically infected cows can secrete the agent into milk, and there is a risk that pasteurized retail products remain infective.

DRIED AND FORMULA MILK

Infections. Dried products can be polluted at the processing plant or when handled for consumption. Whenever safe handling is in doubt, breastfeeding is preferred over formula feeding. Spores may occasionally resist pasteurization and drying.

***B. cereus* (514).** *B. cereus* is a contaminant of dried-milk products and infant food. In one study, 54% of 261 samples from 17 countries grew *B. cereus*, at levels of 0.3–600 counts/g.

***Campylobacter* (5104).** In Singapore in 1994–2000, among campylobacteriosis cases reported in patients <5 years of age, failure by caregivers to wash their hands before preparing milk formula was a significant risk.

***Enterobacter* (1185, 3807, 7698).** Powdered infant formula contaminated during factory production or bottle preparation has been a reported source in infants. In The Netherlands, *E. sakazakii* was isolated from 14 (21%) of 68 environmental samples from four milk-powder factories.

***Salmonella* (6437, 7470, 7662).** Dried products have caused several outbreaks. Salmonellosis in infants can be serious. In the United States, an outbreak of *S. enterica* serovar Newbrunswick was traced to contaminated powdered milk. In 1996–1997, serovar Anatum in a brand of formula-dried milk caused an international outbreak, with cases in infants in the United Kingdom (15) and France (2). In Spain in 1994, serovar Virchow in a brand of powdered infant formula milk caused 48 cases in infants <7 months of age from 14 of 17 regions. In the United Kingdom in 1985, serovar Ealing in a dried-milk product from one manufacturer caused a geographically widespread outbreak in infants; the source was defective machinery at the production plant.

***S. aureus*.** Reconstitution of dried products can introduce *S. aureus* from infected hands. For an extended outbreak by milk and powdered skim milk in Japan see "Raw Milk" above.

CHEESE

Cheese brands are diverse, totaling 750 varieties in France and 400 in Italy. Cow milk is material for Dutch (Edam and Gouda), English (blue and cheddar), French (bleu, Brie, Camembert, and Muenster), Italian (Bel Paese, Gorgonzola, mascarpone, parmigiana, and ricotta), and Swiss (Appenzell, Emmental, Gruyère, Sbrinz, and Tilsit) brands. Roquefort and Peccorino are made from sheep milk, mozzarella is made from buffalo milk, and feta is from cow, sheep, or goat milk. Cheeses traditionally made from raw milk include Brie, cheddar, mozzarella, and Vacherin.

Exposure. In the United States, consumption of cheese per person per year was 8 kg in 1980, 13.5 kg in 2000, and 13.6 kg in 2001. In 2001, the top-ranking brands included American cheddar, Italian mozzarella, and Swiss cheese (http://www.census.gov/prod/2004pubs/03statab/health.pdf). In the United States in 2000, 4–15% of 13,113 respondents from eight states reported consumption of soft cheese from unpasteurized milk in the week before the interview.

Infections. The main hazards are cheese made from raw milk and contamination after pasteurization (169). Cheese is not a reported vehicle for viruses, protozoa, or helminths infective to humans.

BACTERIA

Most bacteria are killed during curing, but curing alone may not be sufficient to eliminate *Salmonella*, *Listeria*, and *E. coli* O157:H7 from cheese (169). Bacterial counts can be low (e.g., <10 *Salmonella*/100 g of cheese), or agents such as *Brucella* may not be isolated from implicated items. The epidemiological significance of some bacteria in cheese such as *Enterococcus* (2757) is uncertain. For mascarpone cream cheese, see "Ice Cream" below. *Brucella*, *Listeria*, and *Salmonella* (Box 7.1) are the major agents from cheese.

***B. cereus* (3400, 5928).** *B. cereus* can be present in raw milk, and new strains from the processing plant can contaminate whey. Cheese was implicated epidemiologically and microbiologically in an outbreak of emetic *B. cereus* food poisoning.

***Brucella* (1115, 4978, 4983, 6124, 7425, 8135).** Unpasteurized cheese from enzootic areas is a significant vehicle of human brucellosis. Counts in cheese decrease during maturation, but it may take months for ripening cheese to become safe. *B. melitensis* survives in feta for 4–16 days, in other cheeses for up to 100 days. *B. abortus* survives in Roquefort for 20–60 days, in cheddar for 6 months, and in other cheeses for 6–60 days.

Outbreaks have been reported in North America and Europe. In Houston, Tex., in 1983, *B. melitensis* disease was diagnosed in 31 residents of a predominantly Hispanic neighborhood; the vehicle was unpasteurized goat milk cheese from Mexico. In Malta in 1995, soft cheese was the vehicle for 135 brucellosis cases, including two diagnosed in United Kingdom with recovery of *B. melitensis*. In Andalusia, Spain, in 2002, *B. melitensis* in raw goat cheese caused an outbreak with 11 cases (two confirmed and nine suspected); the same serovar was isolated from patients, goat milk, and goats. In Castilla-La Mancha, Spain, homemade, unpasteurized cottage cheese caused an outbreak with 81 cases; livestock in the affected county yielded *B. melitensis*.

***E. coli* (1171, 3413, 5998, 6105).** Fresh cheese, cheese curd, and unpasteurized hard (Gouda) cheese are reported vehicles of *E. coli* O157 (EHEC). In Auvergne, France, in 1997–1998, *E. coli* O157 was isolated from 1% (5/603) of cheese samples purchased from retail stores, and Shiga toxin gene was amplified in 10% (60/603) of samples. However, the majority of EHEC isolates were considered nonpathogenic. In Edmonton, Alberta, in 2002–2003, a cluster of hemorrhagic colitis cases revealed an outbreak with 13 cases. *E. coli* O157:H7 was isolated from patients and 2 of 26 cheese samples, up to 104 days after production, despite the fact that microbiological and ripening requirements had been met.

***L. monocytogenes* (970, 3778, 4452, 4606, 4679, 5683).** Cheese is a significant vehicle of *L. monocytogenes*. The agent is recovered from surfaces and utensils in cheese factories, and from soft and hard cheeses. In Switzerland in 1990–1999, 5% (3,722/76,271) of samples grew *L. monocytogenes*, including factory samples (5%), cheese-washing waters (9.5%), cheese surfaces (5%), and edible cheese parts (1% of 2,609). In the United States, 11% (27/246) factory samples (crates, drains, and floors) and 6% (7/111) of fresh cheeses from unpasteurized milk grew *L. monocytogenes*.

Outbreaks Mexican-style cheese apparently made from raw milk caused outbreaks in Los Angeles County in 1985 (142 cases, including 93 pregnant women and 48 deaths [20 fetuses, 10 neonates, and 18 nonpregnant adults]), and in North Carolina in 2000 (13 cases in Hispanic women, including 11 pregnant women, resulting in five stillbirths, three premature deliveries, and three infected newborns). In Japan in 2001, *L. monocytogenes* 1/2b was isolated from 1 of 123 domestic cheeses, the factory, and consumers; of 86 infected consumers, 38 reported gastroenteritis or common cold. In Switzerland in 1983–1987, soft cheese was implicated in an outbreak with 65 pregnancy-related cases and 57 nonpregnant adults.

Salmonella. Pasteurization destroys *Salmonella* in milk, but contamination after processing is a hazard. Cheese is a reported vehicle for many serovars, including *Salmonella enterica* serovars Berta, Dublin, Entertidis, Heidelberg, Javiana, Paratyphi, Stourbridge, and Typhimurium.

Outbreaks Numerous outbreaks are on record.
- North America. In Canada in 1998, serovar Enteritidis in prepackaged lunch packs containing pasteurized cheddar cheese affected some 700 persons (6135). In Canada in 1994, serovar Berta in unpasteurized soft cheese produced on a farm and sold at local markets caused 82 cases (2181). In Canada in 1984, serovar Typhimurium phage-type 10 in Cheddar cheese caused 1,500–2,000 cases. Concentration in cheese was 0.4–9/100 g. The serovar Typhimurium survived refrigerated storage for up to 8 months (1701). In the United States in 1997, serovar Typhimurium DT104 (resistant to five antibiotics) in Mexican-style cheese made from raw milk caused 164 infections (1494, 7831). In the United States in 1989, mozzarella cheese contaminated with serovar Javiana at production caused 136 infections; the concentration in cheese was 0.4–4 bacteria/100 g (3221). In 1976 in Colorado, serovar Heidelberg in cheddar cheese caused 28,000–36,000 cases; embargo of 2,087 kg of cheese may have prevented a further 25,000 infections (2451).
- West Europe. In France in 2001, serovar Enteritidis phage type 8 in fresh (matured for <2 months) cheese made with raw milk from one dairy farm caused an outbreak with 190 cases (3055). In France in 1997, serovar Typhimurium in unpasteurized soft cheese caused an outbreak with 130 cases; cheese from the refrigerators of two patients, and a symptom-free neighbor grew the same epidemic strain (1843). In France in 1993, serovar Paratyphi in unpasteurized goat milk cheese caused 273 infections (1892). In the United Kingdom in 1989, serovar Dublin in an imported, unpasteurized, soft cheese caused 42 cases, mainly in adults (4642). In 2005, serovar Stourbridge from unpasteurized goat cheese from France caused an international outbreak, with 16 cases in France, 6 in Sweden, 3 in the United Kingdom, 2 in Switzerland, and at least one each in Austria and Germany (7680)

Shigella. In Spain in 1995–1996, fresh, pasteurized milk cheese was the vehicle implicated in an *S. sonnei* outbreak with >200 cases (2626).

***Streptococcus* (1138, 4379).** Cheese was implicated in an outbreak of GAS tonsillopharyngitis; a food handler, absent at the time of the outbreak, tested positive for GAS. GCS in homemade cheese caused an outbreak with 14 cases of invasive GCS disease and 2 (14%) deaths.

***Y. enterocolitica* (2879, 3364, 7242).** *Y. enterocolitica* is recovered from cheese and cream, and cheese is a suspected vehicle of sporadic yersiniosis.

Fungi
Air and surfaces of cheese factories and ripening rooms and spoiled cheese have yielded yeasts, e.g., *Candida*, and molds, e.g., *Aspergillus versicolor* and *Penicillium roqueforti* (3365, 4151). There is no indication, however, that

commercial, quality cheese is a source of fungal infections in immune-competent humans.

CREAM, ICE CREAM, YOGURT, AND BUTTER

Cream is the fat-rich top part of milk that is left standing or centrifuged, while skimmed milk is the fat-poor bottom part. Butter is churned and hardened cream. Curd is the semisolid part from coagulated milk, while whey is the watery part. Cheese is processed curd. Yogurt is semisolid bacteria-fermented (*Lactobacillus bulgaricus* and *Streptococcus thermophilus*) and coagulated milk. Kefir is a brew of fermented milk (originally from camel milk). Ice cream, sorbets, and other frozen, sweet desserts are based on water, cream, or milk powder, sugar or sweetener, flavoring substances, and possibly chocolate, fruits, cream cheeses (e.g., mascarpone), or eggs.

Exposure. In the United States, the consumption of cream per person per year was 1.5 liters in 1980, 2.7 liters in 2000, and 3 liters in 2001. For yogurt, the corresponding figures were 1 liter, 2.8 liters, and 3 liters. Ice cream consumption per person per year was 8 kg in 1980, 7.5 kg in 2000, and 7.4 kg in 2001 (http://www.census.gov/prod/2004pubs/03statab/health.pdf).

Infections (1963, 3259, 4126, 4547). Agents in sweet dairy products can result from tainted source materials, poor manufacturing, or improper handling (at the factory, in the kitchen, or on the street). Yogurt frequently grows harmless commensals. Ice cream from street vendors can be hazardous. Outbreaks due to homemade desserts may be underreported but are limited geographically. Outbreaks due to commercial products are rare but may be widespread.

Viruses

An amazing knowledge gap exists concerning viruses from ice cream.

Bacteria

The most frequent agent from sweet dairy products is *Salmonella*, the most serious is *Clostridium botulinum*. Ice cream may be an underrated source of *L. monocytogenes*. Agents demonstrated in ice cream, cream, or yogurt but infrequently implicated in outbreaks include *Aeromonas hydrophila* (8300), *B. cereus* (7016), *Campylobacter* (2116), *E. coli* (5191, 6105), *S. aureus* (4126), *S. pyogenes* (GAS tonsillopharyngitis) (4379), and *Y. enterocolitica* (2165).

***C. botulinum* (341, 2491, 3364, 7016, 7075, 7534).** In general, dairy products account for <1% of cases of foodborne botulism. However, in Italy in 1992–1996, 4% (7/192) of botulism cases from 112 outbreaks were due to dairy products, including cream cheese, cheese sauce, commercial, artisanal, and locally prepared cheese, sour milk, and yogurt.

In Georgia, in 1993, 8 of 22 patrons at a delicatessen contracted botulism, and one died. On 1 October, all of the ill, but none of the 14 well patrons, had consumed potato stuffed with meat and cheese sauce. An open can of commercial cheese sauce contained type A toxin and grew *C. botulinum*. It was concluded that cans of cheese sauce became contaminated by spores when opened, and the spores germinated and grew toxin when left at room temperature. In the United Kingdom in 1989, *C. botulinum* type B in commercial hazelnut yogurt from one producer caused 27 cases, including one death.

In Italy in 1996, commercial "mascarpone" served as dessert (tiramisù) caused an outbreak of type A botulism with 8 patients 6–23 years of age, including one death; a break in the cold chain at retail likely caused spores to germinate and produce toxin. The concentration of botulinum toxin A was 2,495 50% lethal doses (LD_{50})/g in unopened mascarpone, and 125 LD_{50}/g in leftover tiramisù. An international alert was issued, and the mascarpone was recalled. Of the retail mascarpone, 32.5% (331/1,017) tested positive for *C. botulinum* spores; of mascarpone from the outbreak plant, 0.8% (7/878) yielded toxin A, and of 260 other dairy products, 2.7% tested positive for spores.

***L. monocytogenes* (4592, 8214).** Ice cream and butter can be vehicles of *L. monocytogenes*. In Costa Rica, *L. monocytogenes* was isolated from homemade but not from commercial ice cream. In Finland in 1998–1999, serotype 3a in packaged dairy butter caused an outbreak with 25 cases; in most butter samples, levels of *L. monocytogenes* 3a were low (5–60 CFU/g), except one sample that contained 11,000 CFU/g. Although no error in operation was identified, the outbreak strain was isolated in 4 of 430 samples from the butter plant, including conveyor of the butter wagon, the likely source.

***Salmonella*.** In the United States in 1966–1976, homemade ice cream caused 22 outbreaks with 292 salmonellosis cases; *S. enterica* serovar Typhimurium accounted for 45% of outbreaks (3005). In the United States in 1994, serovar Enteritidis in a brand of ice cream caused ~224,000 cases nationwide; a tanker trailer that had transported unpasteurized liquid eggs had cross-contaminated pasteurized ice cream premix (3259). The infective serovar Enteritidis dose in finished products was estimated to 28 agents per sundae cone (73 g) (7877). In the United Kingdom, serovar Enteritidis in homemade ice cream affected 30 (81%) of 37 attendees at a birthday party (1963).

In low-income countries, *Salmonella* is recovered from street-sold ice creams, including serovar Typhimurium

(4126, 6145). In Pakistan in 1994, eating ice cream or food from street vendors was a risk for acquiring serovar Typhi (4547).

S. aureus. Cream-filled pastries are notorious for staphylococcal food poisoning (see section 8.1).

Protozoa
In tropical countries, ice cream is a suspected vehicle of enteric protozoa, although good evidence is missing. Among U.S. travelers who contracted giardiasis in Madeira, ice cream was an epidemiologically implicated vehicle (4510).

MILK CHOCOLATE
Milk chocolate is solid chocolate that includes milk (chocolate milk is milk flavored with chocolate).

Infections. The main agent from milk chocolate is *Salmonella*. Other potential hazards include *E. sakazakii*, which was isolated from the environment of a chocolate factory (3807), and *Y. enterocolitica* from an ingredient-contaminated chocolate milk, causing an outbreak (680).

Salmonella **(1627, 3815, 3820, 6312, 6328, 8052).** *Salmonella* survives in chocolate for years. In leftovers from outbreaks, chocolate yielded 2–90 *Salmonella* serovars/100 g. The infectious dose from chocolates is ~5–40 *Salmonella* serovars/25 g, perhaps because fats in chocolate protect *Salmonella* from gastric acid.

In North America in 1973–1974, *S. enterica* serovar Eastbourne in Christmas-wrapped chocolate balls caused an outbreak with 119 cases in 23 U.S. states and 7 Canadian provinces. In 2001–2002, serovar Oranienburg in a brand of chocolate caused 373 infections in Germany, 16 in Denmark, 4 in The Netherlands, and 2 in Sweden, and contaminated chocolate was recovered and withdrawn in Canada. In Norway and Finland in 1987, serovar Typhimurium in chocolate bars from Norway apparently contaminated by avian wildlife caused several thousand infections, including 349 culture-confirmed cases, predominantly among children, many of whom developed bloody diarrhea. Retail samples grew the outbreak strain, mostly at low concentrations (in 90% ≤10 agents/100 g). In the United Kingdom in 1982, serovar Napoli in chocolate bars from Italy caused 202 primary and 43 secondary cases; leftovers yielded counts of 2–23 serovar Napoli/100 g. In 1970 in Sweden, serovar Durham in chocolate caused an outbreak with 110 cases.

7.2 EGGS AND EGG PRODUCTS
Hen's eggs are purchased as dated shell eggs and are consumed as boiled, fried (sunny side up), or scrambled eggs or mixed in salads or sandwiches.

Exposure. In the United States, the number of eggs consumed per person per year was 271 in 1980, 250 in 2000, and 251 in 2001. Of this amount, shell eggs were 236 (87%) in 1980, 177 (71%) in 2000, and 179 (71%) in 2001 (http://www.census.gov/prod/2004pubs/03statab/health.pdf).

Infections. Shell eggs do not keep at room temperature. Even after boiling for 9 min, shell eggs can become contaminated from the outside and do not keep for more than a few weeks. Cracked or outdated eggs should be discarded. Hands and utensils should be washed after work with raw eggs. Eggs should be boiled or fried well, until yolk and white are hardened.

In high-income countries, eggs and egg products have been on average implicated in 15% (997/6,819) of reported food-borne outbreaks (6356). In Australia in 1995–2000, eggs accounted for 4% of food-borne outbreaks and 10% of cases of food-borne disease (1721).

Exposure history (Box III.1). In the exposure history, inquire about the consumption of raw eggs, "running" eggs, the use of raw yolk or white in recipes, and where eggs were purchased (grocery store or farm).

SHELL EGGS
Infections. The main concern about shell eggs is bacteria, while viruses, protozoa, or helminths have not been reported. Among bacteria, the principal agent from raw or undercooked eggs is *S. enterica*, mainly serovar Enteritidis. Less frequent agents include *E. coli* (ETEC) and *S. pyogenes* (GAS pharyngitis), the latter mainly from boiled or creamed eggs, egg salads, and mousse. *S. maltophilia* has been cultured from eggs, but the epidemiological significance of this finding is unclear.

Salmonella **(382, 582, 2253, 3258, 3457, 3875, 5128).** Eggs are typical vehicles, particularly *S. enteria* serovar Enteritidis. In hens, *Salmonella* can cause silent bacteremia and infect ovaries and eggs hematogenously. *Salmonella* can also access eggs through the shell, for instance, in the nest. Serovar Enteritidis is cultured from 1 per 10,000–20,000 commercial eggs. Risks for sporadic *Salmonella* infections include consumption of raw or "runny" eggs, fried eggs sunny side up, scrambled eggs, or any kind of eggs outside the home.

Outbreaks *(490, 1194, 5112)* In the 1960s–1990s, serovar Enteritidis emerged as a major egg-borne agent, causing a protracted epidemic in North America and western Europe. Epidemic occurrence is ongoing, however, as recent egg-borne serovar Enteritidis outbreaks in Canada and the United States demonstrate.

- North America (1194, 3875, 5082, 5763). In the United States in 1985–2001, serovar Enteritidis outbreaks occurred at a rate of 54–56/year, for an average load of 34–35 cases per outbreak, and a lethality of 0.1–0.4%. Of outbreaks with confirmed vehicles, 78–82% were associated with eggs and egg products, including raw eggs in salad dressing, egg batter, egg rolls, and eggnog. The serovar Enteritidis disease rate peaked in 1995, with 3.9 cases/10^5. In South Carolina correctional facilities in 2001, eggs in tuna salad caused a serovar Enteritidis outbreak with 688 infirmary visits among 2,317 inmates, for an attack rate of 30%.

    Eggs are also vehicles for other salmonellae. In Oregon in 2003, egg salad made from commercial kits that included hard-boiled, chopped egg yolk, and mayonnaise dressing sealed in plastic pouches caused an outbreak of serovar Typhimurium with 18 infections.

- West Europe (582). In France during many years of food-borne infection surveillance, *Salmonella* has been implicated in >90% of egg and egg-product-related outbreaks. In Austria in the summer of 2002, serovar Enteritidis phage type 5 caused a regional outbreak with several hundred cases, and 70 confirmed infections were traced to flocks of a local egg producer.

EGG PRODUCTS

Many recipes are based on egg yolk or white. Egg products include mayonnaise, mousse, omelet, pancake, and quiche. Mayonnaise is a creamy emulsion made from vegetable oil, egg yolk, and vinegar or lemon juice.

Infections. Products based on raw yolk or white carry a risk of *Salmonella*, in particular, *S. enterica* serovar Enteritidis. Other agents from egg products include *B. cereus* (mayonnaise) (2669), *C. botulinum* (gravy) (1081), EHEC (mayonnaise) (5349), and *Shigella* (dressings) (6253).

Salmonella **(443, 2267, 2961, 5128, 5763, 7327, 7498).** Reported vehicles for *S. enterica* serovars Enteritidis and Typhimurium include salad dressings, hollandaise sauce (from butter, egg yolk, and lemon juice), mayonnaise, chile rellenos, lasagne, omelet, pancake, French toast (egg-coated, "fully heated"), creams, custards, ice cream, tiramisú (from cream cheese), cream pie, and meringue (sugary, stiffly beaten egg white baked at a low temperature).

Outbreaks Outbreaks are well documented.
- Australasia (115, 5041, 7498, 7651). In Australia in 2002, serovar Typhimurium U290 affected 10 customers of a popular bakery that served >3,000 customers over one weekend; cream- and custard-filled products were the vehicle implicated, and cross-contamination was suspected, both by food handlers (3 of 37 admitted to diarrhea) and equipment (egg pulper, cream whipper, and cloth piping bags). In Australia in 2001, serovar Typhimurium U290 was isolated in nine cases; implicated vehicles were a pastry-filled custard tart and a jelly glaze prepared at a cake shop. In New South Wales in 2002, serovar Potsdam in mayonnaise caused an outbreak with 17 cases. In Saudi Arabia in 1996, serovar Enteritidis from mayonnaise was implicated in an outbreak with 124 cases.

- Europe (443, 2267). In the United Kingdom, in 1992, two serovar Enteritidis PT4 outbreaks were traced to one bakery: the first was due to custard slices, and the second to fresh cream cakes. Cross-contamination and inadequate cleaning of nozzles for piping cream were implicated. Also in the United Kingdom, a serovar Enteritidis PT4 outbreak with 17 patients was traced to custard from one bakery that had changed its recipe to fresh shell eggs 2 weeks earlier.

7.3 POULTRY

White meat includes chicken (including fillet, drums, and wings), duck, goose, and turkey. For flocks, see section 3.7.

Exposure. In the United States, consumption of poultry (boneless and trimmed) per person per year was 18.5 kg in 1980, 30 kg in 2000, and 30 kg in 2001. Chicken accounted for 80% of total poultry in 1980, 80% in 2000, and 79% in 2001 (http://www.census.gov/prod/2004pubs/03statab/health.pdf). In Australia, ~80% of the population consumes poultry at least once per week (2961).

Infections. The focus is on poultry-borne bacteria, while knowledge about viruses, microsporidia, protozoa, and helminths is scarce.

At the abattoir, carcasses can be contaminated from the inside via evisceration, or from the outside via excreta and defeathering. Immersion chilling can reduce but not eliminate surface load. In high-income countries, poultry on average is implicated in 4% (282/6,819) of reported food-borne outbreaks (6356). In Australia in 1995–2000, poultry accounted for 13% of food-borne outbreaks and 11% of cases (1721). In U.S. schools in 1973–1997, poultry accounted for 19% of 218 food-borne outbreaks with a single, known vehicle (1738). In the United Kingdom in 1992–1999, 20% of 1,426 food-borne diarrhea outbreaks were linked to poultry, mainly chicken (in nearly 75%) followed by turkey (in >20%) and duck (in 2%) (3904).

Exposure history (Box III.1). Inquire about the consumption of barbecued or "red" chicken and other poultry (turkey and duck) and with whom meals were prepared or shared.

Viruses

Although humans can acquire avian influenzaviruses from handling chicken or poultry (4056), food-borne transmission is unlikely and has not been reported.

Bacteria

Poultry-borne outbreaks are mainly attributed to *Salmonella* (in 30–55%), *Clostridium perfringens* (in up to 20%), *S. aureus* enterotoxin (in up to 20%, including cold chicken), and *Campylobacter* (in ~5%) (1613, 3052, 3904).

Other agents include *B. cereus* (6957), *C. botulinum* (1081), *Enterococcus*, *E. coli* (EHEC, ETEC) (1722), *Listeria*, *Streptococcus* group G (GGS pharyngitis, from chicken salad), and *Y. enterocolitica* (7242).

Campylobacter (157, 168, 1880, 2263, 2541, 3839, 6360, 6991, 7168, 8200).
Undercooked poultry is a well-documented vehicle, including barbecued or home-fried chicken and chicken from restaurants.

By the producer and test method, *Campylobacter* prevalence in commercial poultry is 30–90%. In the United States, 69% (229/330) of raw broilers from local supermarkets yielded *C. jejuni*, with highs (87–97%) in May–October, and lows (7–33%) in December–January. In the United Kingdom in 1995–2000, 47–81% (overall 57% or 632/1,127) of raw retail chickens grew *Campylobacter*; seasonal trends were not seen. In Iceland in 1999, 62% (1,309/2,099) of broiler chicken carcasses grew *Campylobacter*.

Chicken and turkey are a reservoir and can be the vehicle of fluoroquinolone-resistant *Campylobacter*. In Minnesota in 1997, 80 (88%) of 91 retail chickens yielded *Campylobacter*, and 18 (23%) isolates were ciprofloxacin resistant (13 *C. jejuni* and 5 *C. coli*).

Food-borne *Campylobacter* outbreaks are infrequent. Of *Campylobacter* outbreaks with a known or suspected food as vehicle, however, up to 20–35% have been attributable to poultry.

Enterococcus (2627, 4886, 5716).
The focus is on cross-resistance, mainly between veterinary avoparcin and human vancomycin (VRE), and between veterinary virginiamycin and quinupristin-dalfopristin, a last-resort therapy for VRE. In Italy, 18 months after the European Union had banned avoparcin in 1997, the percentage of poultry that yielded VRE fell from 15% (49/334) to 8% (22/271). In the United States in 1998–1999, quinupristin-dalfopristin-resistant *Enterococcus faecium* was isolated from 237 (58%) of 407 whole broiler chickens purchased in 26 retail stores. It is feared that VRE and quinupristin-dalfopristin-resistant *E. faecium* might become enzootic in poultry and the food industry at large.

L. monocytogenes (2548, 6354).
Reported prevalence is 10–65% in retail poultry, 10–20% in turkey, and 15–65% in broiler, frozen, and precooked chicken. Defeathering, chilling, recycled water, and hands of workers are sources of cross-contamination. In California in 2001, *L. monocytogenes* serotype 1/2a from catered, precooked, sliced turkey affected 16 (36%) of 44 birthday party attendees; leftover turkey yielded 1,600 million CFU/g.

Salmonella (2253, 3457, 3948, 7745, 8200).
(http://www.fsis.usda.gov/OPHS/haccp/salm4year.htm) Poultry is a major vehicle of *Salmonella*, including for *S. enterica* serovars Enteritidis and Typhimurium.

Of broiler carcasses, 10–70% (typically 50%) grow *Salmonella*. In the United States in 1998–2001, 9–12% of 31,439 raw broiler samples, ~16% of 997 raw ground chicken, and ~29% of 3,712 ground turkey grew *Salmonella*. In the United Kingdom in 1995–2000, by producer, 0–44% (overall 11% or 123/1,127) of raw retail chicken grew *Salmonella*. Frequently isolated were serovars Bredeney (20%), Enteritidis (18%), and Kentucky (13%). In The Netherlands, serovar Java yields from poultry of several regions, seasons, and sales points increased from 0.8% ($n = 1,359$) in 1995 to 8% ($n = 1,196$) in 2002, and its share among *Salmonella* isolates increased from 2% to 60%. This increase was not paralleled by an increase in infections in humans.

Outbreaks A risk for sporadic serovar Enteritidis infection is eating chicken away from home. Poultry-borne outbreaks are documented in North America and West Europe.

- North America. In the United States in 1985–1999, 5% (20/371) of serovar Enteritidis outbreaks with confirmed vehicle were due to poultry (5763). In Canada in 1996, cooked chicken was the vehicle for a serovar Typhimurium outbreak (5112).
- West Europe. In the United Kingdom in 1986, serovar Typhimurium in chicken caused an outbreak that affected 195 (46%) of 427 attendees of a medical conference; delegates eating ≥2 chicken pieces had an incubation period of 17 h, compared with 21 h for delegates who ate only 1 piece (2782). In Spain in July–August 2005, serovar Hadar in a single brand of precooked, vacuum-packed roast chicken caused >2,100 cases of gastroenteritis in 17 of 19 regions, mainly Andalucia, Castilla La Mancha, Murcia, and Valencia (4342).

Protozoa

Cryptosporidium parvum (3).
Chicken salad was implicated in an outbreak that affected 15 of 26 attendees of a social event.

T. gondii (6465, 7217). Undercooked poultry and raw eggs are largely unexplored as vehicles. In Switzerland, 192 seroreactive pregnant women reported significantly more frequently that they ate chicken more than once per week than 196 seronegative control women. In Costa Rica by bioassay, *T. gondii* was recovered from 27 (54%) of 50 "criollo" farm chicken.

7.4 MEAT AND MEAT PRODUCTS

Red meat includes muscle (and bone, fat . . .) from cattle (beef), pigs (pork), sheep (lamb and mutton), goats, horses, rabbits, hunted deer (venison), and hunted other animals (game). In meat products, muscle texture is no longer visible. Products include sausage, deli (cold and sliced meats), and minced meat.

Exposure. Global meat consumption (7647) (http://www.wri.org/wr2000) is 38 kg per person per year (3–12 kg in low-income countries and 42–122 kg in high-income countries). In the United States, consumption of red meat (boneless and trimmed) per person per year was 57 kg in 1980, 52 kg in 2000, and 51 kg in 2001. During this period, shares of beef (57%) and pork (42%) remained constant (http://www.census.gov/prod/2004pubs/03statab/health.pdf).

Infections (1721, 1738, 6356, 6977, 8138) (Box 7.2). Inspected meat that is chilled and maturated for ≥24 h is generally considered safe.

In high-income countries, meat and meat products are on average implicated in ~8% of reported food-borne outbreaks. In U.S. schools in 1973–1997, beef was implicated in 6% of 218 food-borne outbreaks with a single, known vehicle. In Australia in 1995–2000, beef accounted for 4% of food-borne outbreaks (and 4% of outbreak cases), pork for 2% (2%), and lamb for 1% (0.1%). In the United Kingdom in 1992–1999, 16% of 1,426 food-borne diarrhea outbreaks were linked to meat; in meat-borne outbreaks, beef was implicated in 34%, pork in 32%, and lamb in 11%.

Exposure history (Box III.1). Inquire about the consumption of raw (tartar) beef, "red" hamburgers, sausages, or other products from friends or travel (souvenir meat), and game. Where was the product purchased? With whom were the products prepared and shared?

BEEF MEAT

The focus is on beef-borne bacteria, while knowledge about prions, viruses, and microsporidia is scarce.

Prions

Variant Creutzfeldt-Jakob disease (CJD) has been associated with the consumption of meat products tainted with high-risk materials from cattle incubating BSE (7359). As the epizootic is fading, the rate of variant CJD is expected to decrease, with a lag time of more than 10 years.

When the United Kingdom BSE epizootic dampened meat consumption, meat-borne disease outbreaks decreased at the same time.

Viruses

Handling of raw meat in enzootic areas is a likely risk for contracting Crimean-Congo hemorrhagic fever virus (CCHFV).

Bacteria

Major beef-borne bacteria are *C. perfringens* and *E. coli* (Box 7.2).

C. perfringens (1146, 6302). Beef is a significant vehicle of *C. perfringens*, including roast beef, ground beef, corned beef, and beef stew.

E. coli (1335, 3655, 3838, 5998, 6105, 7597, 7685). Beef and beef products are major vehicles for enterohemorrhagic *E. coli* O157 (EHEC), in particular, in the United States, including steak, sirloin tips, grilled beef, beef from private slaughter, beef tacos, roast beef, and beef products (see "Ground Beef, Hamburgers, and Corned Beef" and "Sausages, Deli, and Ham" below). By place, operation (meat factory, butcher, market, and retail store), and test, 1–35% (typically <5%) of raw beef grows EHEC. In Auvergne, France, in 1997–1998, EHEC was isolated from 4% (16/411) of beef samples purchased from retail stores, and the Shiga toxin gene was amplified in 11% (47/411), but a majority of EHEC isolates were not considered pathogenic. Points of cross-contamination via hands, utensils, and surfaces include shops and home kitchens. Raw- and cooked-meat operations should be separated.

Box 7.2 Agents from meat and products, by cluster

For livestock, see section 2.3; for work, see sections 12.4 and 12.5. Typical vehicles are shown in parentheses.

Feces-food	*C. botulinum*, *C. perfringens* (meats, winter peak), *E. coli* O157 (beef, mutton, and products), *Listeria* (cold meats and sausages), *Salmonella* (meats, summer peak); *Y. enterocolitica* (pork); *Toxoplasma* (pork, mutton, and meat products); *Trichinella* (pork products, horse, and game), *T. saginata* (beef), *T. solium* (pork and fecally polluted foods)
Zoonotic	BSE prions (brain); CCHFV (mutton); *B. anthracis* (private butchering), *Francisella* (rabbit and game)
Skin-blood	*S. aureus* (handled ham)

In 350 outbreaks of *E. coli* O157 reported in the United States in 1982–2002, beef was implicated in 86 (25%), mostly ground beef (87% or 75/86), infrequently (13% or 11/86) other beef meats (6105). Contaminated meat grinders at two retail supermarkets were implicated in two EHEC outbreaks in Bethel, Conn., in 1994, with 19 primary and 2 secondary cases, for an attack rate of ~0.1% (418). In Scotland in 1997, an *E. coli* O157 epidemic with 512 cases, including 17 (3%) deaths, was traced to a butcher shop, where ready-to-eat food was cross-contaminated by raw meat; ironically, this shop had been awarded "best Scottish beef butcher" shortly before the epidemic (1611, 1629). In the United Kingdom in 2001, cross-contamination at a butcher franchise in a supermarket caused an *E. coli* O157 outbreak with 30 confirmed cases (6085).

Beef-borne bacteria. Minor beef-borne bacteria include the following. *Bacillus anthracis* (1168, 4143). Beef from privately butchered, infected cattle or water buffalo (*Bubalus bubalus*) is an occasional source of foodborne anthrax, typically in clusters or outbreaks. *Brucella* (1305, 6808). In enzootic areas, meat from infected livestock is a source of sporadic brucellosis. *Campylobacter* (2541, 6680). In the United Kingdom in 1995–1999, meat or meat products were implicated in 3 (6%) of 50 reported *Campylobacter* outbreaks. On the other hand, in the United States in 1982–1983, none of 520 beef samples from distributors in a midwestern city grew *C. jejuni*. *C. botulinum* (1081, 7014). Beef dishes can be vehicle of botulism, including beef chilli, roast beef, and hamburger. *L. monocytogenes* (3673). In Switzerland in 1992–2000, 3% of 132 cured-and-dried meat samples, 6% of 255 cooked-and-cured meat samples, and 15% of 142 fermented sausages grew the agent. *Salmonella.* About 1–2% of beef carcasses grow *Salmonella*. In the United States in 1985–1999, beef was implicated in 8 (2%) of 371 *S. enterica* serovar Enteritidis outbreaks with a known vehicle (5763). In Texas, in 1995, surveillance identified an unusual number (18) of serovar Agona isolates. The source was air-dried raw beef shredded in a kitchen blender and served as "machacado" in a Mexican food restaurant (7369). In Canada in 1997, roast beef was the vehicle for an outbreak of serovar Thompson (5112). In the United Kingdom in 1964, serovar Typhi in canned beef caused an outbreak with 507 cases (403 culture confirmed and three deaths) (7917).

Protozoa
Sarcocystis hominis. Undercooked beef is a vehicle of intestinal sarcocystosis in humans.

T. gondii. Although debated (2048), beef was infective in bioassay (3756, 8266), 1–6% of beef samples tested positive by PCR (320, 8286), and tasting or eating undercooked beef was a risk in epidemiological studies (1554, 7217). Part of the issue may be beef adulterated or cross-contaminated with pork.

Helminths
Undercooked beef is an established source of ***Taenia** saginata* (3593, 6951). Risks include lack of meat inspection and the habit of eating beef raw. Modeling suggests that importing infested beef can be hazardous even if the imported quantity is small (≤3% of all beef).

Toxocara **(2234).** Meat that contains viable (parathenic) larvae is a rare, but confirmed vehicle.

Trichinella **(5994, 6916, 7952).** In People's Republic of China, 1 (0.2%) of 548 *Trichinella* outbreaks recorded in 1964–1999 was due to beef, and larvae were identified in beef. In the United States, before trichinellosis was controlled in commercial swine, beef adulterated or cross-contaminated with pork caused outbreaks.

PORK MEAT
The focus is on pork-borne bacteria, protozoa, and helminths (Box 7.2), while knowledge about viruses and microsporidia is scarce.

Viruses
Food-borne HEV appears to be an emerging risk (426, 8333). In Hokkaido in 2001–2002, 9 of 10 patients with acute, sporadic HE reported consumption of grilled or undercooked pig liver 2–8 weeks before disease onset; 7 (2%) of 363 packages of raw pig liver sold in grocery stores amplified HEV by NAT.

Bacteria
Major pork-borne bacteria are *Salmonella* and *Yersinia* (Box 7.2).

Salmonella **(489, 2253, 3077, 5263, 5966, 5999).** Although in Switzerland none of 865 raw retail pork samples grew *Salmonella* in 2002, pork and pork products are documented sources of *Salmonella* outbreaks. A serotype typical for pork is *S. enterica* serovar Typhimurium. In Japan in 1993, serovar Typhimurium in roasted pork caused an outbreak with 105 cases. In a village on the French Riviera in 1997, pork served at a festival was implicated epidemiologically in a serovar Typhi outbreak with 13 confirmed typhoid fever cases.

Y. enterocolitica **(489, 3364, 5651, 7242, 7802).** In Switzerland in 2002, 15% (133/865) of raw retail pork samples grew *Y. enterocolitica*. Pork is frequently implicated in sporadic cases in humans, in particular, due to serogroups O:3, O:8, and O.9. Eating raw or undercooked pork is a risk. In Norway, eating pork or sausages was a risk among 67 cases compared with 132 age- and sex-matched controls, and the patients tended to report a preference for rare meat.

Pork-borne bacteria. Minor pork-borne bacteria include the following. ***B. cereus* (4545).** A pork barbecue at a university excursion caused an outbreak of *B. cereus* disease, for an attack rate of 22% (139/643). ***Campylobacter* (157, 168, 3819).** Although the prevalence in retail pork seems low (≤0.2%), eating barbecued pork or sausages is a reported risk. ***C. perfringens* (6186, 7355).** Pork is a vehicle. Precooked, vacuum-sealed pork caused an outbreak affecting 17 (39%) of 44 exposed hospital patients. ***E. coli* (6161, 6565).** By sampling and location, reported prevalences of *E. coli* O157 in pork are ~1–10%, in retail pork typically 1–2%. ***Erysipelothrix rhusiopathiae* (7946).** *E. rhusiopathiae* is prevalent in the abattoir environment, including in pig carcasses. Although most infections are occupational, a potential for transmission exists via undercooked pork. ***Vibrio parahaemolyticus* (2808).** *V. parahaemolyticus* has been recovered from roast pork, roast lean pork, and meat roll.

Protozoa
Sarcocystis. Pork is a vehicle of *S. suihominis.*

Toxoplasma. Eating raw or undercooked pork is a risk (3816). Pork is the main vehicle for food-borne toxoplasmosis (2047). By bioassay, 3–10% of pork samples are infective (3756, 6423). By PCR, 19 (33%) of 57 commercial pork samples tested positive in the United Kingdom (320). However, a European multicenter study did not demonstrate a risk for eating poorly cooked pork (1554). In Korea, two small outbreaks were linked to raw pork liver, one from a wild pig and one from a domestic pig (1412).

Helminths
Well-known pork-borne helminths are *Taenia* and *Trichinella*. An unusual and perhaps underdiagnosed helminth from pork in Southeast Asia and Japan is *Gnathostoma* (5446).

***Taenia* (3593).** Viable *T. solium* larvae (cysticerci) in undercooked (measly) pork, and *T. asiatica* larvae in raw pork liver cause human intestinal taeniasis. Risks include lack of meat inspection, the habit of eating pork raw, and, perhaps, preparation of measly pork with bare hands. In contrast, any foods fecally polluted by *T. solium* eggs from human carriers can be vehicles of cysticercosis.

Trichinella. Pigs and wild boars can be infected with *Trichinella britovi*, *T. pseudospiralis*, or *T. spiralis*, and species identification should be attempted from muscle biopsy or leftover pork. ***T. britovi* (5995, 7681).** In Italy in 1948–2000, 13 (76%) of 17 outbreaks with species determined were due to *T. britovi*, mostly from pig or boar meat. These 13 outbreaks caused 598 cases (46 per outbreak). In France in 2003, six persons contracted *T. britovi* after consuming boar meat which had been frozen immediately after killing. The six ate the boar lightly cooked, while a seventh attendee, who requested his serving to be reheated, escaped infection. *T. britovi* was identified from frozen meat, the estimated density was three larvae per gram. ***T. pseudospiralis* (3744, 6107).** In an outbreak in Thailand in 1994–1995 with 59 cases, raw pork from a wild pig was implicated. *T. pseudospiralis* was isolated from pork and confirmed experimentally and by molecular fingerprinting. In southeastern France in 1999, four persons contracted trichinellosis from barbecueing boar meat; *T. pseudospiralis* was detected in meat and muscle biopsies and confirmed by molecular fingerprinting. ***T. spiralis* (638, 6447, 7952).** In the United States, pork was implicated in 31% (22/72) of cases reported in 1997–2001; in a further 28% (20) of cases, a vehicle was not known. In contrast in People's Republic of China, 96% (525/548) of outbreaks in 1964–1999 were due to pork. In Henan Province, People's Republic of China, the prevalence of *T. spiralis* in retail pork and mutton was 1.6% by digestion assay. **Vehicles (1475, 3068, 6447, 7299).** Vehicles implicated in recent outbreaks have been raw pork, pork chops, roasted pork, pork jerkey, and smoked pork. In the United States, while there is almost no risk from commercially produced pork, home-raised pork remains a hazard.

MUTTON, LAMB, AND GOAT MEATS
Infections. In some low-income countries, meat from freshly slaughtered sheep or goats is preferred over chilled meats, and live animals rather than frozen carcasses are traded. Concerns from undercooked mutton, lamb, or goat include CCHFV, *E. coli*, *Salmonella*, and *Toxoplasma* (Box 7.2).

Prions
There is currently no evidence that scrapie or BSE prions can be acquired from mutton, lamb, or goat meat.

Viruses
In an outbreak in Saudi Arabia in 1991–1993, contact with fresh mutton was a risk for contracting CCHFV (2159).

Bacteria
B. anthracis-infected, privately butchered sheep is a rare source of food-borne anthrax in humans. About 2–3% of

retail lamb grows *E. coli* O157:H7 (1335, 2018). *E. rhusiopathiae* is prevalent in the abattoir environment, and it is recovered from sheep carcasses, lamb, and mutton (7946). In Calcutta, the prevalence of *Salmonella* in 200 goat meat samples was 6%.

Protozoa
***T. gondii* (320, 748, 1554, 2048, 3756, 3816, 8286).** Tasting or eating raw or undercooked mutton, lamb, or goat meat is a risk. In Brazil in 1993, 17 attendees at a party acquired acute toxoplasmosis from eating raw mutton. By sampling (carcass and retail), location, and test (bioassay and PCR) 5–65% of sheep, lamb, or mutton samples test positive.

Helminths
Trichinella from mutton (638, 5994, 7952) is unusual and has been reported only from People's Republic of China. There, 7 (1%) of 548 outbreaks recorded in 1964–1999 were due to mutton. In Henan Province, People's Republic of China, the prevalence of *T. spiralis* in marketed mutton was 0.6% by digestion assay.

HORSE MEAT
Concerns from horse meat have mainly been *Salmonella* and *Trichinella* (Box 7.2).

Salmonella. In the United States, 62 (27%) of 233 horse meat samples grew *Salmonella* at a packing plant (209). Poor slaughtering technique seemed responsible for contamination of meat surfaces.

***Trichinella* (195, 733, 5994).** In 1975–2000, horse meat caused 13 trichinellosis outbreaks with >3,200 cases. All outbreaks occurred in France and Italy, although horse meat is as popular in Belgium (consumption 1 kg per person per year) as in Italy (1 kg) or France (0.5 kg). This is attributed to the habit, in France and Italy, of eating horse meat undercooked or raw (tartar or minced). Infective horse meat had been imported into France and Italy from eastern Europe (in 8 of 13 outbreaks), the United States (in 2), and Canada and Mexico (in one each).

Particularly large outbreaks had occurred in France in 1976 (with 125 cases) and in 1993 (with >500 cases). In Italy, in six outbreaks from horsemeat in 1948–2000, *T. spiralis* was identified in three outbreaks (with 628 cases) and *T. britovi* in two (with 390 cases), while the species was not identified in one outbreak (with 13 cases).

RABBIT MEAT
E. coli and other enteric bacteria have been recovered from prepacked rabbit meat at supermarkets (6366). Undercooked meat from domestic rabbits is an unusual source of *Salmonella* (660), and a suspected source of *Francisella* (3672), *Encephalitozoon cuniculi*, and *Toxocara* (7222). In Rimini, Italy, in 1997, roasted rabbit served at a restaurant was the vehicle for 29 *S. enterica* serovar Hadar cases among patrons.

VENISON AND GAME
Venison and game (including marine mammals) can carry viruses, bacteria, protozoa, and helminths, in particular, when butchered privately and bypassing meat inspection. The main concerns are emerging agents, anthrax, botulism, tularemia, toxoplasmosis, and trichinellosis.

Viruses
HEV (7392). In Japan, seven cases of acute HE were linked to undercooked meat from wild-caught Sika deer (*Cervus nippon-nippon*).

Severe acute respiratory syndrome-coronavirus (SARS-CoV) (2975, 8402). The preference in parts of People's Republic of China for exotic foods such as palm civet (*Paguma larvata*) is assumed to have promoted the jump to humans of the virus that caused the SARS pandemic in 2003.

Bacteria
B. anthracis. Infected game is a putative source of human anthrax.

***C. botulinum* (3186).** In Canada in 1971–1984, 59% (36/61) of botulism outbreaks were due to raw, fermented, or parboiled meat from marine mammals, and 93% (113/122) cases concerned native Americans.

E. coli. Venison is an occasional vehicle, including EHEC. In Oregon, in 1995, homemade venison jerky was implicated in an outbreak with six confirmed and five presumptive EHEC cases; *E. coli* O157:H7 counts were 3–93 CFU/g in leftover jerky and 150 CFU/g in uncooked venison (3878). In the Northwestern Territories, Canada, in 1991, minced caribou meat caused an EHEC outbreak in six Inuit communities that secondarily propagated person-to-person; overall, there were 521 cases, including 22 cases of hemolytic-uremic syndrome (HUS), and two deaths (5636).

F. tularensis. Meat from hunted rabbits, hares, and other game is an unusual source of tularemia. In Memphis, Tenn., deer meat was the only explanation for an isolated case of tularemia (4294). In Germany in 2002, a father and his daughter came down with tularemia, 16 and 20 days after they had consumed a hare that the father had killed on the road with his car (6313). In France, handling of deer and boar meet was associated with sporadic tularemia cases (4270).

Protozoa

Sarcocystis. Undercooked deer meat with demonstrated cysts of *S. capreolicanis* was the likely vehicle for two cases of sarcocystosis (6713).

***T. gondii* (1554, 2048).** Many game animals can carry cysts, and eating raw or undercooked game is a risk. In arctic Quebec, Canada, in 4 months of 1987, four pregnant Inuit women seroconverted; suspected vehicles were raw caribou meat and dried seal meat (4885). In the United States in 1980, three deer hunters were diagnosed acute toxoplasmosis after eating rare venison (6509).

***T. cruzi* (1599, 8099).** Raw game meat is a likely source of infection in humans.

Helminths

Trichinella. Reported vehicles (2101, 6027, 6447, 6657, 7952) include meats (raw, roasted, and fried) and meat products (smoked, jerky, and ground) from polar bear, black bear, cougar, fox, walrus, wild boar, muntjak, and bamboo rat.

In North America (6447, 6657, 6994), *T. nativa* has been identified in meat from black bear (*Ursus americanus*) and cougar (*Felis concolor*). In the United States, game meat was implicated in 42% (30/72) of cases reported in 1997–2001. Most of the game-related cases were due to bear meat.

In 2003, a man contracted trichinellosis in New York State from bear meat obtained from a custom slaughter house, and a couple contracted trichinellosis in Tennessee from a black bear (*U. americanus*) the man had shot in Canada. The couple who cooked the bear meat on an outdoor grill for themselves and four guests ate the steaks medium rare, while four guests ate theirs well done and apparently remained well. Leftover meat from both instances yielded *T. nativa*.

In People's Republic of China (7952), 7 (1%) of 548 outbreaks recorded in 1964–1999 were due to game meat.

GROUND BEEF, HAMBURGERS, AND CORNED BEEF

Ground meat (or minced meat) should be made from beef unless declared otherwise. In the United States, >15% of ground beef is made from cull dairy cows (7573). Ground beef patties are the basis for hamburgers.

Exposure. In the United States in 2000, 18–40% (mean, 32%) of 13,113 respondents from eight states reported to have eaten hamburgers at their homes in the past 7 days.

Infections. Ground beef is a substrate for bacterial growth. It should be used fresh and not be kept. Handling with unwashed hands or utensils increases risks by working agents into bulk meat. In the United Kingdom in 1999, 8% (260/3,128) of ready-to-eat retail burgers were of poor microbiological quality, although none grew *Salmonella*, *Campylobacter*, or *E. coli* O157 (4460). Ground beef is a vehicle mainly for *E. coli* O157 and *Salmonella*, but also for other enteric bacteria such as *C. perfringens* and *L. monocytogenes*.

Bacteria

***E. coli* (1190, 3655, 3838, 5112, 5647, 5744, 6289, 7620).** Ground beef and hamburgers are major vehicles of *E. coli* O157, including raw and precooked patties, ready-to-eat burgers, and tacos. Eating undercooked (pink) hamburgers (at home or away from home) is a risk. By test and sampling, the reported prevalence of *E. coli* O157 in retail ground beef is 0.3–34% (typically ≤0.5%). However, because the production of ground beef is high (~3,600 million kg/year in the United States alone), even low frequencies have an impact on public health. As traditional measures have failed to reduce the rate of *E. coli* O157:H7 infections in the United States, a proposed alternative is irradiation of ground beef.

Outbreaks Outbreaks have mainly been reported in the United States. Hamburgers as a vehicle of *E. coli* O157:H7 were first observed in Oregon and Michigan in 1982, when ≥47 patrons of a fast-food restaurant chain contracted dysentery (6275). Between 1982 and 2002, ground beef in the United States caused 75 *E. coli* O157 outbreaks (four per year) with 1,760 cases (23 per outbreak; range, 2–732) (6105). At a junior high school in Minnesota in 1988, *E. coli* O157:H7 in preheated meat patties caused hemorrhagic colitis in 32 students, for an attack rate of 8%. Frozen patties from the implicated plant produced on the same dates as the outbreak patties grew *E. coli*, albeit not serotype O157:H7 (541).

Along the food chain, a single strain from a farm can cause a widespread outbreak. In 1992–1993, hamburgers served at restaurants of a fast-food chain caused 501 EHEC disease cases in Washington State, including 45 (9%) cases of HUS, and 3 (0.6%) deaths; this outbreak extended into California (34 cases), Idaho, and Nevada (58 cases) (531, 1455, 6830). Outbreak ground beef patties grew EHEC at a concentration of 68 per patty (7620). In 2002, EHEC in ground beef caused an outbreak with 24 cases in seven states. In response, one company recalled 8.4 million kg of beef (1190).

Few outbreaks have been reported elsewhere. In Okinawa, Japan, in 2004, frozen beef patties purchased from a U.S. military commissary caused a family outbreak of *E. coli* O157:H7 infections (1241).

***L. monocytogenes* (2876, 4915, 6354).** Carcasses are frequently contaminated with *L. monocytogens* during slaughter. Vehicles include ground beef and inadequately cooked meat products. The prevalence in ground meat and processed meat products is 10–80%. Levels are usually low, but 10–20% of samples may grow >100 CFU/g. In France, the proportion of ready-to-eat meat products that yielded *L. monocytogenes* was 13% in 1993–1994 ($n= 1,533$) and 9% in 1995–1996 ($n = 1,750$), and 1.6% and 0.7% of respective samples grew ≥100 CFU/g.

Salmonella. Ground beef and hamburgers are important vehicles. In the United States in 1998–2001, the prevalence of *Salmonella* in raw ground beef ($n = 74,758$) was 3.4%, with a peak of 6.4% in 1998, and a low of 2.8% in 2001 (http://www.fsis.usda.gov/OPHS/haccp/salm4year.htm).

Outbreaks Outbreaks have mainly been reported in the United States. Raw hamburger emerged as a source of *S. enterica* serovar Newport outbreaks in 1975 (2450). In 2002, serovar Newport in undercooked ground beef caused an outbreak with 47 cases in five states; the common source was a meat-packing plant that complied with standards of hygiene. Three isolates were resistant to amoxicillin-clavulanate and two exhibited reduced susceptibility to ceftriaxone (8377). In 1975, serovar Newport in ground beef caused >27 cases in three states; the vehicles implicated were rare hamburgers and ground beef meals supplied by one processing plant (2450). In Wisconsin during the 1994 Christmas season, 158 serovar Typhimurium infections occurred that were traced to raw ground beef from one butcher. A poorly cleaned meat grinder was the likely source (6370).

Few outbreaks have been reported elsewhere. In Aberdeen, Scotland, in 1964, corned beef was implicated in a typhoid fever outbreak with 403 culture-confirmed cases and 66 clinical cases (7917). In France in 1998–2000, refrigerated or frozen hamburgers caused three outbreaks and 69 salmonellosis cases (3050). In Germany in III–VII/2004, 115 persons contracted serovar Give from raw ground pork, with peak population rates of $1.5/10^5$ in Sachsen-Anhalt (3647).

Shigella. At a Haiti resort, rare hamburgers were implicated in an outbreak of *Shigella flexneri* (7069).

Y. enterocolitica. Y. enterocolitica has been recovered from ground beef (7242). Meatballs or stuffed vegetables made from ground meat carry a risk of cross-contamination or undercooking (7802).

Protozoa
Eating raw or undercooked ground-meat products is a risk for infection with *T. gondii* (3816). In New York in 1968, "very rare" hamburgers served at a university dormitory snack bar were the common vehicle for acute toxoplasmosis in five medical students. The butcher who provided the meat insisted "that the hamburger meat was pure beef" (3868).

Helminths
Ground pork meat was implicated in a *Trichinella* outbreak in Germany (6190).

SAUSAGES, DELI, AND HAM
Sausages are products made from ground meat (mainly pork), trimmings, and fat, to which spices and other ingredients are added and which are precooked, cured, fermented, or smoked. Varieties include "hot dog" (heated, in rolls), "Bologna" (precooked), "Mortadella" (precooked, with fat cubes), "Mettwurst" (cured and fermented, soft), "Salame" (cured and dried), and "Bratwurst" (typically fresh). Ham is meat from pig hind legs, unprocessed (fresh, needs heating) or precooked and cured (country-style, Prosciutto). Deli (charcuterie) is sliced, cold meats or meat products. Pâté is pie with meat or other filling.

Infections. Meat products have been suspected or confirmed vehicles of prions, bacteria, protozoa, and helminths. With barbecueing or pan frying there is a risk that parts remain undercooked (7802). Vacuum technology and radiation are means to reduce risks from handling and inadequate preservation (7028).

Prions
Whether prions can be borne by meat products is uncertain (927, 1224, 1526, 7359).

Before the BSE epizootic in the United Kingdom, bovine nervous tissue was often added to sausages, broths, stews, and other heated, cheap "meat" products. During the epizootic, tissue from cattle that were incubating BSE or had early signs of illness (downers) conceivably entered the human food chain. Mathematical modeling suggested 0.4–1.6 million infective cattle. Heat could not guarantee absence of prion infectivity. Although sausages that incorporated high-risk organs were putative vehicles of variant CJD in the United Kingdom, firm epidemiological or microbiological evidence for this is not available.

Viruses
Meat products are infrequently reported vehicles.

HAV (6295). In Bavaria, Germany, in 1998, a butcher with acute hepatitis A (HA) contracted on the Canary Islands infected two family members working in his butchery, which was source of contaminated sausages that caused 75 acute HA cases in institutions served by his shop.

***Norovirus* (1737).** In Texas in III/1998, deli sandwiches were implicated in a *Norovirus* outbreak with 125 cases.

Ham handled by an infective person amplified *Norovirus* by reverse transcriptase (RT)-PCR.

Bacteria

The main bacteria from sausages and cold meats are *C. botulinum*, *E. coli*, *L. monocytogenes*, *Salmonella*, and *S. aureus* (Box 7.2). Other bacteria from meat products include *Aeromonas* (2786), *Campylobacter*, *Enterococcus* (2757), and *Y. enterocolitica*. *Aeromonas* was isolated from ready-to-eat Mortadella (2786). In the United Kingdom in 2002, 0.03% (1/2,894) of ready-to-eat, cold, sliced meats grew *C. jejuni*; the single, positive item was cold beef (3457).

***C. botulinum* (1080, 3364, 5659, 7433).** For killing, bacteria need heat (60°C) for a few minutes, while spores need 110–112°C. Cold meats, sausages (botulus means sausage in Latin), and home-cured ham are significant vehicles.

Outbreaks Outbreaks are mainly reported from high-income countries.
- Africa. In Morocco in 1999, type B botulism caused 78 cases, including 20 (25%) deaths; mortadella was the vehicle implicated in the outbreak (5659).
- America. In the United States in 1990–2000, of 75 outbreaks and 132 cases with a known vehicle, two were carried by sausages, and one each by hamburger, meat balls, beef chili, roast beef, and liver pâté (7014). In Buenos Aires in 1998, 9 of 21 bus drivers developed botulism after eating meat rolls served at a bus stop (7832).
- Europe. France in 1991–2000 recorded 142 outbreaks of botulism, with 278 cases (including 5 [1.8%] deaths). Dried, crude ham was implicated in 61 (43%) outbreaks, pâté or rillettes (pork mash) in 13 (9%), other cold meats in 12 (9%), and other or unknown foods in 56 (39%) (3054). In Italy in 1992–1996, of 192 cases reported in 112 outbreaks, 23 (12%) were carried by ham or sausages (7 homemade and 16 commercial), and 12 (6%) by preserved meat or fish (7075). Portugal in 1970–1984 recorded 13 outbreaks with 50 cases; vehicles were home prepared, smoked ham in 9 (69%) outbreaks, and bacon, sausage, and mussels in 1 each (4290). In Switzerland in 1993–1994, commercial, crude, salted ham caused an outbreak with 12 cases of type B botulism (7565).

***E. coli* (187, 1335, 3261, 4603).** Beef and other meat products can be vehicles for *E. coli* O157:H7 (EHEC), including cooked and fermented sausages. Reported prevalence was 4% (3/73) in retail lamb sausages, and 4% (18/484) in lamb burgers.

Outbreaks Reported vehicles are salami and Mettwurst.
- Salami (4603, 7479, 8188). In Canada, *E. coli* O157 from salami caused outbreaks in 1998 (39 cases in Ontario) and 1999 (143 cases in British Columbia). Both outbreaks prompted a national recall of salami brands. In a United States salami-borne outbreak, the concentration of *E. coli* O157:H7 in positive samples was low (<0.3–0.4 bacteria/g), and the infective dose was estimated to 2–45 bacteria.
- Mettwurst (3261, 5756). In Australia in 1995, *E. coli* O111:H- in locally produced mettwurst caused HUS in 20 children; 18 required renal dialysis (for a median of 14 days), and 1 child died.

***L. monocytogenes* (1193, 3623, 5604, 6667, 7028).** Meat products can be contaminated from the environment after processing, and cool temperatures do not prevent growth.

Outbreaks Delis, meat pies, and other products frequently grow the agent and have been implicated in outbreaks.
- United States. In 2002, in the United States, sliceable turkey deli meat was implicated in an outbreak with 46 culture-confirmed cases, 7 deaths, and 3 miscarriages in eight states; the producer recalled 12 million kg of ready-to-eat products and suspended operations. In 2000, sliced, processed turkey from a delicatessen was implicated in an outbreak of serotype 1/2a with 30 culture-confirmed cases including four deaths (at 67, 67, 77, and 78 years of age) and three miscarriages in 11 states; the implicated producer voluntarily recalled 7 million kg of processed meat.
- Europe. In France in III–XII/1992, pork tongue in jelly and cross-contaminated delis were implicated in a *L. monocytogenes* serovar 4b outbreak with 279 cases (92 pregnancy related and 187 others).

***Salmonella*.** Traditional methods of salting, drying, and smoking do not safely eliminate *Salmonella* from meat products (5003).

Outbreaks Outbreaks have been reported, mainly in Europe.
- North America. In Canada in 1997, sausages were implicated in an outbreak of *S. enterica* serovar Hadar (5112).
- Europe. In Italy in 1995, serovar Typhimurium from salami caused 83 cases; insufficient ripening had allowed the serovar Typhimurium to survive (5966). In the United Kingdom in 1987–1988, serovar Typhimurium in salami sticks (from Germany) caused an outbreak with 101 cases; suboptimal fermentation was the likely cause (1612). Also in the United Kingdom, a community outbreak of serovar Typhimurium definitive type 124 was traced to ham and a single producer (4473). In The Netherlands in 1985, 17 patients

contracted salmonellosis from fermented pork sausage prepared by a butcher; the implicated sausage grew serovar Typhimurium (10^6 CFU/g), *C. perfringes* (10^4 CFU/g), and *S. aureus* (10^3 CFU/g) (7742). Also in The Netherlands, serovar Typhimurium in traditionally salted, smoked, and dried ham affected 38 (35%) of 109 attendees of a family party (5003). In Germany, in 2001, raw, fermented sausage was the vehicle implicated in a serovar Goldcoast outbreak with 44 cases (855). In Switzerland in 1993, serovar Braenderup in meat pies caused infectious diarrhea in 213 patients, prosthetic valve endocarditis in one, and reactive arthritis in one, for an attack rate of 7.5%. The implicated meat pies were contaminated from jelly during processing and contained >10^6 CFU/g. Ten of 24 workers at the incriminated food factory shed the epidemic strain in stool, and one worker reported gastroenteritis before the outbreak (7656).

S. aureus (1152, 6251). Ham is a frequently reported vehicle of staphylococcal food poisoning. *S. aureus* grows rapidly and produces enterotoxins best at 20–37°C. Staphylococcal enterotoxins are heat resistant. In Florida, in 1997, 18 attendees of a party acquired staphylococcal food poisoning from precooked packaged ham, for attack rates of 65% among consumers and 2% among nonconsumers. Although the food handler denied pyodermia and reported having reheated the ham at 204°C for 1.5 h before serving it cold on the following day, leftover ham tested positive for enterotoxin type A. At Rhode Island elementary schools in 1990, centrally prepared school lunches resulted in staphylococcal food poisoning, for attack rates of 18–47%; ham was implicated epidemiologically, and leftover ham yielded enterotoxin A.

Protozoa
Knowledge is limited. In a European multicenter study, eating raw sausage, salami, or dried cured pork was a risk for infections with *T. gondii* (1554).

Helminths
Pork products such as sausages, ham, and jerky can be vehicles for *Trichinella*.

T. britovi (2824). In southern Spain in 2000, *T. britovi* in sausage made from boar meat and pork caused an outbreak with 38 cases.

T. spiralis.
Outbreaks Vehicles implicated in outbreaks include pork sausages (5996, 6190, 6447), pork salami (5996), pickled pig feet (6447), and pork dumplings (jiaozi) (1673, 7299).

- North America. In Illinois in 1975, 23 of 50 Dutch-Germans contracted trichinellosis from eating raw, homemade summer sausage; a pork sample that had been officially inspected was later found to contain *T. spiralis* larvae (5987). In Iowa in December 1975–January 1976, 77 of 242 persons who ate "summer sausage" (made from pork and venison) contracted trichinellosis; 23 of 45 sausage samples yielded larvae, at counts of 1–65/100 g (1687). In July–September 1990, 90 (72%) of 125 Southeast Asian refugees in six states and Canada contracted trichinellosis from uncooked pork sausage served at a wedding in Des Moines (4865). Small outbreaks by raw pork or homemade pork products (sausages and jerky) continued to be reported in 1999 (Illinois, two cases), 2000 (Illinois, two cases), and 2001 (California, eight cases) (6447).
- Asia (1673, 7299). In People's Republic of China, pork dumplings (jiaozi, mixed with vegetables, and wrapped in dough) are popular at celebrations; when lightly boiled, the pork inside can remain infective. In Zhengzhou City, People's Republic of China, in 1996, dumplings caused an outbreak with 212 cases and 79 infections.
- Western Europe (5487, 6190, 7141). Around Trier, Germany, in 1982–1983, Mettwurst caused an outbreak with 406 cases. In Northrine-Westfalia, Germany, in 1998–1999, two outbreaks occurred, one due to ground pork (eight cases) and one due to pork Mettwurst (44 cases). Ground pork from the implicated supermarket that used pork from Germany, Belgium, and The Netherlands yielded *T. spiralis* larvae. In Germany, three patients contracted trichinellosis from smoked ham imported from the Balkan.

7.5 SEAFOOD, FISH, AND MOLLUSCS

Fish (finfish) is the class of vertebrates that inhabit marine, brackish, and fresh waters. Crustaceans is a class of arthropods that includes crabs, shrimps, and lobster. Molluscs is the phylum of animals that includes bivalves (clams and oysters), cephalopods (squids and octopuses), and marine, freshwater and terrestrial gastropods (abalone, slugs, and snails). Shellfish is a collective term for crustaceans and bivalves. Seafood is a collective term for shellfish, marine fish, and abalone. Caviar is graded, brined, and cured fish roe.

Exposure (1006, 5979) (http://apps.fao.org/faostat, www.wri.org/wr2000). By catch and culture, world fishery production is 130 billion kg/year. Fish consumption per person per year is 13–66 kg in high-income countries and 6–11 kg in low-income countries. In the United States, consumption of fish and shellfish (boneless and trimmed) per person per year was 5.6 kg in 1980, 6.9 kg in

2000, and 6.7 kg in 2001 (http://www.census.gov/prod/2004pubs/03statab/health.pdf). In the United States in 2000, 22–39% of 13,113 respondents from eight states reported consumption of fresh fish in the past 7 days, and 1–4% reported consumption of oysters (http://www.cdc.gov/foodnet/surveys/Pop_surv.htm).

Infections (1006, 1721, 2739, 6356). The estimated disease rate is ~$0.4/10^5$ servings. In high-income countries, by dietary habits and location and whether toxins are included, 7–70% (typically 10%) of food-borne disease outbreaks are attributed to fish and seafood. In the United Kingdom, the ratio fish to shellfish in seafood outbreaks is ~1. Agents naturally dwelling in seawater do not correlate with sewage influx and fecal indicator agents (2070, 4457). Sewage is a major source of seafood contamination.

Exposure history (Box III.1). Inquire about when last, where, and with whom raw fish, seafood, or snails were consumed, including: fish (raw, marinated, steamed, grilled, or dried) or fish soup; shrimps, prawns, lobster, crabs, or seafood salad; marinated, steamed, boiled, or heated clams, cockles, mussels, or oysters; abalone, terrestrial snails, or vegetable salads with visible slug traces.

FISH

Edible fish are from several orders, including Clupeiformes, e.g., anchovy (*Engraulis*), herring (*Clupea*), and sardine (*Sardina*); Gadiformes, e.g., cod (*Gadus*) and haddock (*Melanogrammus*); Perciformes, e.g., mackerel (*Scomberomorus*) and tuna (*Thunnus*); Pleuronectiformes, e.g., flounder and turbot (flat, several species); and Salmoniformes, e.g., salmons and trouts (*Salmo*, *Salvelinus*, and *Oncorhynchus*).

Infections (1006). The main agents are bacteria and helminths (Box 7.3). Knowledge about viruses (e.g., *Enterovirus*) fish is surprisingly scarce.

Bacteria

First-line agents to consider from fish are *Aeromonas*, *Clostridium*, *Listeria*, and *Vibrio*. Second-line agents include *E. coli* (EHEC in salted salmon roe caused an outbreak in Japan) (4680) and *S. pyogenes* (GAS in tuna salad caused an outbreak of tonsillopharyngitis) (4379). *S. maltophila* has been cultured from frozen fish (1886), but the epidemiological meaning of this finding is unclear.

Aeromonas **(2903).** Fish and fish eggs can be vehicle, including for *A. hydrophila* and *A. sobria*. In Japan, stools of 2% from healthy adults and of 11% from adults with diarrhea yield *Aeromonas*. In Norway, *A. hydrophila* was implicated in an outbreak of food poisoning due to raw, fermented fish.

Clostridium. C. botulinum **(1080, 1081, 1214, 3054, 3536, 7014).** *C. botulinum* is prevalent in fish and fish products, including wild and farmed, marine and freshwater fish, and seafood is a significant vehicle, typically *C. botulinum* type E. In Finland, this type was identified by PCR in 3% ($n = 123$) of air-packed fishery products and 5% ($n = 214$) of vacuum-packed products. In the United States, vehicles implicated in outbreaks included pickled herring, fermented fish, salted, uneviscerated fish, and fish eggs. In France in 1991–2000, seafood was implicated in 6 (4%) of 142 botulism outbreaks. Reported vehicles included commercial fish soup in a cardboard pack. ***C. perfringens*** **(3309).** In several outbreaks, precooked, cold salmon served as an hors d'oeuvre was implicated in *C. perfringens* food poisoning.

L. monocytogenes **(972, 2225, 2876, 3480, 3673, 5035, 6354).** Fish is a significant vehicle for *L. monocytogenes*, including raw, cold-smoked, and vacuum-packed fish.

The prevalence is 1–15% in retail fresh fish, 10% in cold smoked fish, and 10–30% in frozen seafood. Foods imported into Australia are subjected to laboratory testing. *L. monocytogenes* was isolated from 8.6% of 388 samples; smoked, vacuum-packed fish was the item that most frequently failed Australian standards.

In France, proportions of seafood and fish products that were contaminated were 10% in 1993–1994 ($n = 841$) and 10% in 1995–1996 ($n = 1,125$), and proportions of items that grew ≥100 CFU/g were 0.7% and 0.5%, respectively.

Box 7.3 Agents from fish and seafood. For fish as intermediate hosts, see section 3.9.

Any seafood:	*C. botulinum*, *L. monocytogenes*, *Salmonella*, *Vibrio*
Fish:	Also *Aeromonas*, GAS pharyngitis; *Anisakis*, *Capillaria*, *Diphyllobothrium*, *Gnathostoma*, biliary (*Clonorchis*, *Opisthorchis*), and intestinal flukes
Crustaceans:	Also *Aeromonas*, *E. coli*; *Angiostrongylus* (snails and slugs), *Gnathostoma*, *Paragonimus* (freshwater crabs and crayfish)
Bivalves (in particular raw oysters):	Also HAV, HEV, *Enterovirus*, *Norovirus*; *E. coli*, *Plesiomonas shigelloides*, *Shigella*, *Yersinia*; *Cryptosporidium*
Gastropods:	*A. cantonensis* (snails), *A. costaricensis* (slugs)

In Switzerland in 1992–2000, 12% of 471 imported hot-smoked fish samples, 14% of 814 cold-smoked fish, and 38% of 125 marinated fish grew *L. monocytogenes*.

Outbreaks In Finland, five healthy persons developed febrile gastroenteritis after consuming vacuum-packed, cold-smoked rainbow trout (*Oncorhynchus mykiss*) that grew *L. monocytogenes* serotype 1/2a indistinguishable from patient strains (5035). In Sweden, cold smoked rainbow trout made by one producer caused an outbreak with nine cases (2225).

Vibrio. V. parahaemolyticus (167, 2808, 3509, 7326). Fish, fish balls, and fish cakes are reported vehicles. At a boarding school in Thailand, food handlers and cooking utensils were the suspected source for an outbreak of *V. parahaemolyticus* in fish balls. *V. cholerae* (46, 1470, 2773, 4128, 7145). Raw fish ("ceviche" in Latin America and "sushi" in Japan), dry fish (in Africa and the Pacific), and undercooked fish are reported vehicles of toxigenic *V. cholerae* O1. In the United States in 1995–2000, of 24 reported local cholera cases, three were acquired from imported fish, three from mixed seafood, two from sushi, and 10 from other or unknown vehicles. In Tarawa, Gilbert Islands, raw fish and shellfish from the lagoon were vehicles for an explosive cholera outbreak, together with contaminated drinking water. In an outbreak in the Ukraine in 1994–1995, marinated fish (*Cluponella: Clupeidae*) was a vehicle. *V. vulnificus* (3464). Fish are reported vehicles, including cultured eels.

Fungi

Microsporida from several orders are reported in fish, including *Enterocytozoon salmonis*. However, whether fish are sources of human infections is not known.

Helminths

The main fish-borne helminths are *Anisakis*, *Clonorchis*, *Diphyllobothrium*, *Gnathostoma*, and *Opisthorchis*.

Other helminths (1648, 2884, 4624, 8356) from raw, pickled, or salted fish include *Capillaria* from freshwater or brackish fish, *Echinostoma* from freshwater loach (*Misgurnus*), *Heterophyes* from estuarine mullet (*Mugil cephalus*) and freshwater *Tilapia nilotica*, *Metagonimus* from freshwater fish, e.g., oriental trout (*Plecoglossus altivelis*), dace (*Tribolodon taczanowskii*), and perch (*Lateolabrax japonicus*), and *Metorchis* from estuarine white sucker (*Catostomus commersoni*).

Anisakis and *Pseudoterranova* (1606, 5644, 7294, 7751). Fish are significant vehicles for *Anisakis* and *Pseudoterranova*. Larvae survive cold smoking, brining, and marination. Patrons erroneously believe vinegared sushi is "safe": larvae can survive vinegar for up to 51 days. Larvae are inactivated by heat (all parts at 60°C for a few minutes), or deep freezing (below -20°C for 1–7 days). Fish must be prepared fresh and eviscerated as soon as possible. The chopping board should be washed clean after preparing raw fish.

The low number of cases in humans in North America is explained by the habit of purchasing salmon frozen and consuming it cooked. In Japan, cheap and frequently infected fish (e.g., halibut, cod, herring, mackerel, and salmon) are usually eaten at home, while sushi shops contribute few cases, as these serve expensive and infrequently infected fish (e.g., blue-fin and big-eye tuna, striped marlin, flounder, and horse mackerel). In northern Japan, infections in humans due to *Pseudoterranova decipiens* outnumber infections due to *Anisakis simplex*.

Clonorchis sinensis (1368, 1410, 4389). Vehicles in Asia are raw, pickled, dried, salted, or undercooked freshwater fish. Fish imported from enzootic areas or infested pisciculture are a risk. Over 100 fish species are listed as secondary intermediate hosts. The main hosts are Cyprinidae, particularly riverine, Eurasian stone moroko (*Pseudorasbora parva*). Unlike in snail hosts, the prevalence of infection in fish is high, in general. In Korea, by river, 30–100% of *P. parva* carried metacercariae, for an average density of 78 per g flesh.

Diphyllobothrium (1137, 1900, 2832, 3583, 6375, 6570). Eating raw, undercooked, or cold-smoked fish, and tasting during preparation are risks. "Risk recipes" include Latin American "cebiche," Japanese "sashimi" served at sushi bars, Jewish "gefillte" (stuffed) fish, and Italian and French "fish carpaccio." *D. latum* is acquired from fish that spent at least part of their life in freshwater, while *D. pacificum* is acquired from saltwater fish. In British Columbia in 1973, a "liver paste" made from salmon was likely the vehicle for an infection with *D. ursi*. In California in 1980, raw salmon served at a sushi party caused two diphyllobothriasis infections. Subsequently, an outbreak in the Pacific states and Hawaii was detected, involving 30 persons and linked to raw sockeye salmon (*Oncorhynchus nerka*) from Alaska. Apparently, an unusually large salmon run had overwhelmed the freezing and canning capacity (that destroyed plerocercoid larvae), and salmon was shipped fresh as a result. In 2004, *D. latum* appeared in consumers of sashimi in São Paulo, Brazil.

Gnathostoma (1287, 1920, 3079, 3579, 4981, 5167). Raw freshwater fish from enzootic areas is a major vehicle. Leftover fish may serve to identify *Gnathostoma* larvae.

Opisthorchis (2725, 3172, 8347). The vehicle for *Opisthorchis* is raw or inadequately cooked fish, mainly carp (Cyprinidae). In Russia, a hazardous, popular dish is slightly salted, frozen raw fish (stroganina). The infection prevalence in vector fish is high, in general. In Laos, metacercariae were found in seven species of Cyprinidae, with a prevalence range of 2–63%. The highest prevalence (63% or 17/27) was in *Cyclocheilichthys repasson* caught in ditches between paddy fields.

CRUSTACEANS

Edible crustaceans are in one of two orders: (i) Brachyura (crabs), e.g., *Cancer*, or (ii) Decapoda, including shrimps and prawns (crevettes, gambas, scampi, e.g., *Crangon* and *Penaeus*), lobsters (langouste and langoustine, e.g., *Homarus*, *Nephrops*, and *Palinurus*), crayfish (e.g., *Procambarus*), and king crabs (e.g., *Munida* and *Paralomis*).

Infections (Box 7.3). The focus is on bacteria and helminths. Although viruses are described in shrimps (e.g., white spot syndrome and yellow head viruses) and prawns (e.g., white spot bacilliform and gill-associated viruses), data on viruses infective to humans and microsporidia from crustaceans are lacking.

Bacteria

The focus is on *Listeria* and *Vibrio*.

***L. monocytogenes* (6267, 6667, 7435).** Reported vehicles for *L. monocytogenes* include shrimps and crayfish (*Procambarus*). In the United States in 2001, *L. monocytogenes* was detected in 3 (4%) of 78 raw crayfish samples and in 1 (0.6%) of 181 plant environmental samples, but in none of heat-treated, finished products. In New York City in 1989 listeriosis was diagnosed in 10 (28%) of 36 attendees of a club party; shrimps were the common vehicle implicated epidemiologically.

***Vibrio*.** Crabs, shrimps, and prawns can harbor *Vibrio* spp. ***V. alginolyticus* (501).** Crayfish is a reported vehicle of *V. alginolyticus*. ***V. cholerae* (501, 1837, 2249, 4422, 7145, 7887).** Raw or undercooked crabs and shrimps are reported vehicles of *V. cholerae* (O1 and non-O1, non-O139). In the United States in 1995–2000, of 24 reported local cholera cases, four were acquired from crabs and two from shrimps. In Mexico City, 3 of 18 shrimp cocktails from street vendors yielded *V. cholerae* non-O1, non-O139. In Brazil, *Crassostrea rhizophorae* is a suspected *V. cholerae* carrier crab. In Manila, Philippines, rice noodles with shrimps (pansit) from street vendors have been a vehicle of cholera. On a flight from Peru, crab salad was the vehicle for 75 cholera cases. ***V. mimicus* (501).** Crayfish is a reported vehicle of *V. mimicus*. ***V. parahaemolyticus* (167, 501, 1837, 4540, 4843, 5102, 8330).** Locally harvested or imported prawns, shrimps, and crabs have yielded the agent and are reported vehicles. In an outbreak in New Orleans, La., in 1986, boiled, unpeeled, and peeled shrimps grew *V. parahaemolyticus*. In Niigata Prefecture, Japan, in VIII/1996, boiled red queen crabs (*Chionoecetes japonicus*) sold at a crab shop caused an outbreak with 691 cases. ***V. vulnificus* (1958, 3464, 8330).** Chinese Giant tiger prawns (*Penaeus monodon*) and mantis shrimps (*Squilla oratoria*) from Chinese coast city markets have yielded *V. vulnificus*. Wild-caught and cultured shrimps and crabs can be vehicles.

Other agents. Other agents from crustaceans include *Aeromonas*, *C. botulinum*, *E. coli*, *Salmonella*, and *S. pyogenes*. ***Aeromonas* (1006, 3639, 6079).** *Aeromonas* has been isolated from shrimps, mainly *A. hydrophila* and *A. sobria*. In Dhaka, Bangladesh, *Aeromonas* was isolated from freshwater prawns (*Macrobrachium malcolmsonii*) sold at local fish market, at densities of 10^4–10^7 CFU/g. However, the epidemiological meaning of these findings is unclear. ***C. botulinum* (3054).** Reported vehicles include deep-frozen shrimps. ***E. coli* (1722).** In the United States in 1975–1995, shrimps and crabmeat were implicated in one each of 14 food-borne ETEC outbreaks. ***Salmonella* (2739, 5979).** Prawns are a reported vehicle. *S. enterica* serovar Typhi (7537). In northern Vietnam, eating shellfish was a risk for typhoid fever: 76% (68/90) of cases and 63% (114/180) of neighborhood controls reported to eat shellfish (from 1 time/month to 4 times/week), for an odds ratio of 1.8 (95% CI 1.1–3). ***S. pyogenes* (GAS) (4379).** Vehicles in food-borne outbreaks of GAS tonsillopharyngitis reviewed since 1941 included shrimp salad (in 1965) and prawn cocktail (in 1986).

Helminths

***Paragonimus* (104, 1408, 7522, 7631, 7793, 7818).** More than 50 species of raw or undercooked crustaceans can be vehicles of *Paragonimus*. Examples of crayfish hosts are *Cambaroides similis* and *C. dauricus*, examples of crab hosts are in Latin America *Hypolobocera emberarum* and *H. aequatorialis*, in Africa *Callinectes marginatus* and *Sudanautes africanus*, and in Asia *Eriocheir japonicus*, *E. sinensis*, *Geothelphusa dehaani*, and *Sinopotamus*. In West Africa, 5% of 176 retail *C. marginatus* carried metacercariae. The prevalence of crabs that carry metacercariae can be high, often 20–40%. In Korea, prevalence was 36–78% in the 1960s, and ~12% in 1990, with respective averages of 8–23 and two metacercariae per infected crab. In Ecuador in 1988–1991, 444 (43%) of 1,043 crabs from 45 streams yielded metacercariae (probably of *P. mexicanus*); viscera were the most frequently parasitized organs, followed by flesh.

Other helminths from crustaceans. *Angiostrongylus cantonensis* (5682, 7438).
Undercooked land crabs, freshwater prawns, and fish are alternative vehicles to snails. ***Echinostoma* (2884, 8356).** Shrimp are a reported

Echinostoma vehicle. **Gnathostoma (4981, 5167, 5470).** Putative vehicles of Gnathostoma include poorly cooked shrimp, crab, and crayfish. Two Japanese travelers contracted *G. malaysiae* from raw freshwater shrimps consumed in Myanmar.

BIVALVES

Edible bivalves (Mollusca) include clams (e.g., *Mercenaria* and *Pecten*), cockles (e.g., *Cardium*), mussels (e.g., *Mytilus*), and oysters (e.g., *Crassostrea* and *Ostrea*).

Exposure. Some 10% of American adults eat raw oysters at least once per year (167).

Infections (1006, 1007, 5979, 6852) (Box 7.3). Bivalves are "filter feeders" that accumulate microorganisms. When harvested from sewage-polluted waters, raw bivalves are hazardous. Bivalves carry mainly viruses and bacteria to humans. In the United States, the main agents of shellfish-borne diseases in 1984–1990 (14,349 cases) and 1991–1998 (2,162 cases) were *Norovirus* (3% and 52% of cases), *V. parahaemolyticus* (1% and 29%), *V. vulnificus* (1% and 8%), *S. enterica* serovar Typhi (23% and 0%), and HAV (13% and <1%).

Viruses

Infections. Oysters are well-known vehicles of viruses. In Japan, >50% of small (<20 cases) outbreaks of viral diarrhea have been attributed to oysters (3559). Molluscs can simultaneously transmit >1 viral agent (627, 782, 2560, 6579). In Japan in 2001, 22 of 57 people contracted diarrheal disease from steamed butter clam (*Saxidomus purpuratus*); initially *Norovirus* was detected by RT-PCR, and ~1 month later, four attendees developed acute HA confirmed by RT-PCR from stools. Clams were imported from People's Republic of China and tested positive for both viruses. In Valencia, Spain, in 1999, in a HAV outbreak with 184 cases, coquina (*Donax*) clams were implicated; clams were imported frozen from Peru, complied with European Union standards, but nevertheless 75% of samples tested positive for HAV by RT-PCR, and occasionally for other enteric viruses. Switzerland imports oysters at a rate of >300,000 kg/year; of 87 samples in 2001–2002, 8 (9%) amplified *Norovirus*, and 4 (5%) *Enterovirus*.

Major viruses from bivalves are HAV and *Norovirus*. Other viruses include HEV from raw clams (4034), and human adenovirus and *Enterovirus* from mussels (*Mytilus edulis* and *M. galloprovincialis*) and oysters (*Ostrea edulis* and *Crassostrea gigas*) (2464).

HAV. Seafoods are a significant vehicle, mainly oysters (1537, 2464, 6403) (initially reported in 1956 in Sweden), but also clams (2560, 6387, 6579), cockles (5538), and mussels (1398, 2464). HAV is widespread where sewers are discharged into coastal waters, and it has been amplified in oysters (*C. gigas*) and mussels (*M. galloprovincialis*) from the Atlantic Ocean and Mediterranean Sea (2464). In Spain in 1999–2001, bivalves imported from South America that amplified HAV were wedge clam (*Donax*, 1 of 6), carpet clam (*Tapes*, 2 of 6), and scallop (*Argopecten*, 1 of 5) (6387). In southern Italy in 1999–2000, 53 (18%) of 290 mussels (*M. galloprovincialis*) from markets and other sources tested positive for HAV by NAT; and 18 (6%) were positive in cell culture (1398).

Outbreaks Outbreaks are well documented. Of 46 bivalve-borne outbreaks reported worldwide in 1969–2000, 8 (17%) were due to HAV (5979).

- America. In Florida in 1988, raw oysters caused 61 acute HA cases in five states, for attack rates in patrons of seafood establishments of 2/1,000 servings (a serving consisted of 12 oysters) (1893).
- Australasia. In Shanghai in 1988, raw clams caused an epidemic with 290,000 case of acute HA, for an attack rate of 4%. Clams were the vehicle implicated in a case-control study, and HAV was cultured in clams from the Shanghai markets, and from the catch area in Jiangsu Province (3096). In Singapore, cockles and oysters repeatedly caused outbreaks of acute HA (5110). In 1983, an outbreak with 189 HA cases was linked to consumption of raw cockles (*Anadara granosa*) grown in uncontrolled conditions. In 2001, consumption of raw and inadequately cooked cockles (*A. granosa*) caused 134 cases of acute HA. In New South Wales, Australia, oysters caused an outbreak with 467 HA cases (1537).
- Europe. Around Valencia, Spain in 1999, clams from South America caused 189 serologically confirmed cases of HA (6579).

Norovirus. Clams, cockles, mussels, and raw oysters, in particular, are significant vehicles of food-borne *Norovirus* infections (627, 1006, 2009, 2017, 2560, 2952, 3004, 3565, 4031, 4273, 4317, 5657, 5727, 6852, 6903, 7099). There is growing evidence that oyster beds are contaminated by human rather than marine animal sources (4031, 6903). *Norovirus* was detected in oysters and mussels from the North Sea, Atlantic Ocean, and Mediterranean Sea (2464).

Outbreaks Outbreaks are well documented. Of 46 bivalve-borne outbreaks reported worldwide in 1969–2000, 18 (39%) were due to *Norovirus*, causing a total of 5,923 cases (~330 per outbreak) (5979).

- America. In 1993, oysters harvested from a remote oyster bed in Louisiana were implicated in a multistate outbreak with ≥73 cases, for an attack rate among patrons of 83% (2009, 4031). Again in Louisiana in XII/1996–I/1997, oysters caused a multistate outbreak with 525 cases (6852). In V/1998, *Norovirus* in oysters (*C. gigas*) from Tomales Bay 80 km north of San Francisco caused 171 cases (6852).

- Pacific. In Australia, in the winter of 1978, *Norovirus* in oysters from the Georges River in the Sydney area caused >2,000 cases of diarrhea (2952). In New Zealand, consumers of raw oysters had >5-times greater risk of *Norovirus* illness than nonconsumers (6903).
- Europe. In 2002–2003, oysters from Etang de Thau in the south of France caused *Norovirus* gastroenteritis in France (90 cases) and Italy (>200 cases). Heavy rains had caused overflow of a water purification plant and fecal pollution of the pond (Etang) (2017).

Bacteria

A. Major bacteria from bivalves are *Salmonella* and *Vibrio*. Oysters, in particular, are well-known vehicles of *Vibrio* (1006, 5979).

***Salmonella* (1006, 3237, 6100, 8201).** By location, 1–50% of seafood samples yield *Salmonella*. In the United States in 1990–1998, *Salmonella* prevalence was 1% in domestic seafood ($n = 768$), but 7% in imported seafood ($n = 11,312$). In ready-to-eat seafood, prevalence was 0.5% in domestic samples (shucked oyster and shark cartilage powder) and 2.6% in imported samples (cooked shrimp, shellfish or fish paste, smoked, salted, or dried fish, or caviar). In Northern Ireland in the 1990s, the prevalence was 8% in 433 bivalves (2% in bivalves from beds suitable for immediate consumption according to European Union standards).

Outbreaks Outbreaks are well documented. Of 46 bivalve-borne outbreaks reported worldwide in 1969–2000, 3 (7%) were due to *Salmonella* (causing a total of 98 cases) (5979).

- America. In the United States in 1986, shrimp salad polluted with *S. enterica* serovar Typhi caused 10 cases of typhoid fever (4427).
- Asia. In Japan in 1993, consumption of raw oysters caused 27 cases of paratyphoid; serovar Paratyphi A was isolated from all patients and two mud samples from the area where oysters were grown (7235). In Singapore in 1979, imported fresh oysters were implicated in a serovar Paratyphi A outbreak with 61 confirmed cases (2805).
- Europe. In the United Kingdom in 1998, serovar Enteritidis in cockles caused an outbreak with eight cases (2927). In Norway and Sweden in 2001, commercial fish gratin likely cross-contaminated from egg powder at a factory caused 60 cases of unusual serovar Livingstone infection (2982).

***Vibrio* (1006, 4540, 5731, 5979).** Oysters can concentrate *Vibrio* up to 100-fold. Some 20% of shellfish-borne bacterial illness is due to *Vibrio*. Of 46 bivalve-borne outbreaks in 1969–2000, 12 (26%) were by *Vibrio*: 5 by *V. parahaemolyticus*, 4 by *V. cholerae*, and 1 each by *V. hollisae*, *V. mimicus*, and *V. vulnificus* (for a total of 880 cases). Further vibrios from shellfish include *V. alginolyticus* and *V. damsela*. Vehicles include clams (account for ~40% of cases in the United States), cockles, mussels, oysters (account for ~50% of cases in the United States), and scallops. ***V. cholerae* (2115, 2249, 3796, 4422, 7887).** *V. cholerae* is isolated from shellfish. Reported vehicles for toxigenic *V. cholerae* O1 include undercooked or raw clams (in Italy "arselle"), mussels (in Italy "cozze"), oysters, and squid. In the Philippines mussel soup from street vendors was an outbreak vehicle; aboard an aircraft it was seafood salad. In Hong Kong in 1994, seawater tanks for holding alive bivalves, shrimps, and crabs were likely outbreak vehicles. Oysters are also vehicles for *V. cholerae* non-O1, non-O139. In Mexico city, 8 of 18 raw oysters from street vendors yielded *V. cholerae*. In southern Italy, this agent was demonstrated in mussels (*M. galloprovincialis*). ***V. parahaemolyticus* (262, 1155, 1162, 1837, 2249, 2562, 4916, 5731, 7668, 8330).** Bivalves, squids, and abalones have yielded *V. parahaemolyticus*, and the reported vehicles in outbreaks have included caught or farmed, locally consumed or imported oysters, as well as clams, cockles, mussels, squids, and in Singapore also blood cockle (*Anadara granosa* or "see hum") and mud mussel (*Glauconome rugosa* or "tua tow"). In Nigeria, 64 (58%) of 110 clams (*Mercenaria*) from the Calabar River estuary and purchased at local market grew *V. parahaemolyticus* and *V. alginolyticus*. In Mexico City, 1 of 18 raw oyster samples from street vendors yielded *V. parahaemolyticus*. In an estuary in northeastern Brazil, *V. parahaemolyticus* was isolated from 1 (0.3%) of 300 oysters (*C. rhizophorae*), while in a natural bed in southeastern Brazil, 21 (53%) of 40 mussels (*Perna perna*) grew the agent, for counts of <3 to 93/g. In southern Italy, the agent was demonstrated in 8% (39/513) of mussels (*M. galloprovincialis*), 4% (1/25) of bait mussels (*Modiola barbata*), 8% (4/49) of oysters (*Ostrea edulis*), and 14% (8/57) of hen-clams (*Tapes decussatus*). *V. parahaemolyticus* can enter the food chain also after harvesting and processing. In Calcutta, India, infections in strict vegetarians were explained by flies that contaminated foods.

In North America in 1997, 209 culture-confirmed cases were linked to eating raw oysters harvested in California, Oregon, Washington, and British Columbia. In an outbreak in New Orleans in 1986, raw and cooked oysters grew *V. parahaemolyticus*; counts in raw oysters reached 28/g. ***V. vulnificus* (770, 5731, 8330).** Oysters, mussels, and clams have yielded *V. vulnifidus*, and can be vehicles. Razor clams (*Sinonovacula constricta*) from Shanghai City markets have yielded *V. vulnificus*. In southern Italy, *V. vulnificus* was demonstrated in 3% (15/513) of mussels (*M. galloprovincialis*), 10% (5/49) of oysters (*O. edulis*), and 2% (1/57) of hen-clams (*T. decussatus*).

B. Other bacteria from bivalves include *Clostridium, Escherichia, Listeria, Plesiomonas, Shigella, Streptococcus,* and *Yersinia*.

C. botulinum. *C. botulinum* is identified in shellfish (1081). Reported vehicles include deep-frozen clams (coquilles Saint-Jacques) (3054).

E. coli. In the United States in 1975–1995, scallops were implicated in 3 (21%) of 14 food-borne ETEC outbreaks (1722). In Trinidad, 77% (154/200) of raw oysters from vendors, 45% (89/200) of condiments, and 77% (154/200) of oyster cocktails grew *E. coli* (6100). In southern Italy in 2000–2002, in 4% (27/644) of edible bivalves counts of *E. coli* exceeded 230/100 g of pulp (the European Union standard) (5731).

L. monocytogenes. Bivalves can be vehicles of *L. monocytogenes*, including smoked mussels (4915). Of 46 bivalve-borne outbreaks reported worldwide in 1969–2000, 1 (2%) was due to *L. monocytogenes* (causing four cases) (5979).

P. shigelloides. Infections in travelers suggest that oysters and other seafoods can be vehicles (6144). In an outbreak at an oyster roast in North Carolina, *P. shigelloides* was recovered from a patient and an oyster (6481). Of 46 bivalve–borne outbreaks reported worldwide in 1969–2000, 2 (4%) were attributed to *P. shigelloides* (causing 54 cases overall) (5979).

Shigella. Of 46 bivalve-borne outbreaks reported worldwide in 1969–2000, 2 (4%) were due to Shigella (one by *S. flexneri* and one by *S. sonnei*, for a total of 64 cases) (5979). In southeastern Texas, raw oysters were vehicle for an *S. sonnei* outbreak with 24 cases among patrons of eight restaurants; the source was a single carrier on an oyster boat that used pails as an on-board toilet (6180).

***S. pyogenes* (GAS).** Among food-borne GAS pharyngitis outbreaks since 1941, one (in 1984) was carried by conch salad (4379).

Y. enterocolitica. Consumption of shellfish has caused *Y. enterocolitica* infections in humans (6974).

Protozoa
Except for *Cryptosporidium* and *Giardia*, parasites are said to be poorly transmitted by shellfish (5979).

***Cryptosporidium* (2339, 4536).** *Cryptosporidium* can be carried by bivalves. Hosts include eastern oysters (*Crassostrea virginica*), freshwater clams (*Carbicula fluminea*), and mussels (*Mytilus edulis* and *M. galloprovincialis*). In the Chesapeake Bay, *C. parvum* oocysts were isolated in oysters from commercial harvesting sites by immune fluorescence microscopy. Oocysts have also been reported in Northern Ireland, in river water, treated sewage effluent, and marine mussels (*M. edulis*). *M. edulis* can filter seawater at a rate of 100 liters/24 h and accumulate oocysts.

***Giardia* (2887).** Cysts were detected in homogenized clams (*Macoma balthica* and *M. mitchelli*) from a contributory river to the Chesapeake Bay. By molecular fingerprinting, cysts belonged to a *G. lamblia* genotype infective to humans. Although *Macoma* clams are not of commercial value, they can serve as surrogate measures of water quality.

CEPHALOPODS, GASTROPODS

Edible cephalopods (Mollusca) include squid, octopus (e.g., *Sepia*), and cultivated abalone (*Haliotis*). *Edible gastropods* (Mollusca) include cultivated Burgundy snail (*Helix pomatia*) and related *H. aspersa* (Helicidae), the African giant snail (*Achatina fulica*, a "pest and pet" snail), and a few other terrestrial and freshwater snails.

Infections (Box 7.3). The focus is on helminths, mainly *A. cantonensis* (eosinophilic meningitis) and *Angiostrongylus costaricensis* (acute eosinophlic ileitis). For helminths from vegetables and salads, see section 8.2. Recovery of *V. parahaemolyticus* from abalone (*Haliotis diversicolor*) is relevant for aquaculture industries in Taiwan and Japan (4303). Snails are also major intermediate hosts for trematodes.

***A. cantonensis* (306, 3525, 5926, 7471, 7580, 7581, 7937, 7949, 8295).** Snails from enzootic areas are vehicles for *A. cantonensis* confirmed in outbreaks and by demonstration of infective larvae (L3), either by consumption or via handling. On Okinawa, likely sources for 35 cases of eosinophilic meningitis included snails in 9 (26%) cases, toads (*Bufo asiaticus*) in 3 (9%), fresh vegetables in 1 (3%), and handling of snails in 5 (14%). In Taiwan, of 82 children hospitalized for eosinophilic meningitis, 68 (83%) gave a history of contact with *Achatina fulica*, including playing and eating. Host snails include *Achatina* (Achatinidae), *Ampullaria*, and *Lanistes* (both Ampullariidae). *A. fulica* is abundant in Southeast and East Asia. In enzootic areas, 10-60% of *A. fulica* carry larvae of *A. cantonensis*, at densities of 1–441 (mean, 14) L3/snail.

Host snails are consumed for curiosity (by children), as a delicacy (by adults), or for medicinal or other purposes.

Outbreaks Food-borne outbreaks are well documented. In Egypt, three patients likely contracted *A. cantonensis* from *Lanistes carinatus* snails found at irrigation canals (919). In Jamaica in 2000, after an outbreak in tourists, *A. cantonensis* larvae were recovered from 4 (40%) of 10 *Thelidomus asper* land snails (4442). In American Samoa in 1980, Korean fishermen were sold a large basket of *A. fulica* snails; 16 of 24 fishermen who ate raw or partially cooked snails fell ill, compared with none of five who ate boiled snails, and none of three who abstained from eating snails (3992). In outbreaks in People's Republic of China, patients with eosinophilic meningoencephalitis due to *A. cantonensis* reported consumption of raw "golden apple snail" *A. canaliculatus* or related freshwater *A. gigas* (7949, 8295).

A. costaricensis (4090, 4189, 4850, 6093). Slugs are the main intermediate hosts for *A. costaricensis*, mainly of Veronicellidae (*Phyllocaulis variegatus*, *Sarasinula linguaeformis*, and *Vaginulus plebeius*), but also of Limacidae (*Deroceras laeve*). In southern Brazil, by season 7–86% of slugs were infected with metastrongylid larvae (likely *A. costaricencis*), for burdens of 1–75 larvae/slug. Small slugs can be inadvertently ingested hidden in unwashed leafy vegetables. Slugs can shed larvae with slime, and slime on unwashed garden salads and vegetables should be considered infective. In Guatemala in December 1994–August 1995, in an outbreak with 22 cases, raw mint was implicated epidemiologically.

***Anisakis* (336, 5644).** Squid is a reported vehicle for human anisakiasis in Japan where *A. simplex* was identified in flying squid (*Todarodes pacificus*).

***Echinostoma* (2884, 8356).** Raw, pickled, and inadequately cooked snails (e.g., *Gyraulus*, *Lymnaea*, *Pila*, and *Physa*), clams, and mussels (e.g., *Corbicula*, *Idiopoma*, and *Unis*) can be vehicles.

Snails as intermediate hosts. Freshwater snails participate in biological cycles of *Clonorchis*, *Echinostoma*, *Fasciola gigantica*, *Fasciolopsis*, *Heterophyes*, *Metagonimus*, *Opisthorchis*, *Schistosoma haematobium*, and *S. mansoni*. Mud-dwelling or amphibious snails support *Fasciola hepatica* and *S. japonicum*. Aquatic *and* terrestrial snails are primary intermediate hosts for *Paragonimus*.

While not infective by ingestion, the unprotected handling of host snails (*Bulinus*, *Biomphalaria*, and *Oncomelania*) at freshwater habitats exposes to *Schistosoma* cercariae in water.

8

Plant-Derived Foods

8.1 Cereals, pasta, bakery, and sweets

8.2 Vegetables, salads, fruits, and spices

8.1 CEREALS PASTA, BAKERY, AND SWEETS

Cereals (6914, 6988, 7647) (http://www.wri.org/wr2000) is the term for grain crops, mainly barley (*Hordeum*), corn (*Zea*), millet (e.g., *Panicum* and *Sorghum*), oat (*Avena*), rice (*Oryza*), rye (*Secale*), and wheat (*Triticum*, all Poaceae), and grain products such as flakes, bread, pasta, and porridge. Pasta is dried dough pressed into forms (e.g., macaroni, noodles, and spaghetti). Pastry is baked dough that is plain, filled, or sweet (e.g., biscuits, buns, cakes, cookies, croissants, doughnuts, muffins, rolls, tarts, and waffles). Bakery is bread and pastry, homemade or from bakeries and grocery stores.

Exposure. Consumption of cereals appears to range broadly, from 160–975 kg/person per year in high-income countries, and 145–250 kg/person per year in low-income countries. In the United States, consumption of flour and cereal products per person per year was 66 kg in 1980, 91 kg in 2000, and 89 kg in 2001. Wheat flour, milled rice, and corn products accounted for 81%, 6%, and 9% in 1980, 73%, 10%, and 14% in 2000, and 72%, 10%, and 15% in 2001 (http://www.census.gov/prod/2004pubs/03statab/health.pdf).

Infections (1721, 2653, 5602, 6356). The main agents are hepatitis A virus (HAV), *Norovirus*, *Salmonella*, and *Staphylococcus aureus* from handling, and *Bacillus cereus* from precooked, reheated rice. Agents recovered from baked foods but considered harmless for immune-competent hosts include *Enterobacter*, *Lactobacillus*, *Klebsiella*, and *Serratia*; *Aspergillus*, *Candida parapsilosis*, *Fusarium*, *Penicillium*, and *Rhizopus*.

In high-income countries in the 1990s, sweet bakery was implicated in ~6% (369/6,819) of food-borne outbreaks, pasta in 0.8% (53). In the United States in 1988–1997, baked foods accounted for 1% (64/5,174) of food-borne outbreaks and also 1% (1,673/163,431) of cases. In Australia in 1995–2000, grains accounted for 2% of food-borne outbreaks, desserts for 4%.

Exposure history (Box III.1). Inquire about when last and with whom pasta and baked goods were consumed, including rice, noodles, corn flakes, spaghetti, cakes, and doughnuts. Who prepared "pasta and pastry," and were dishes reheated?

PASTA AND CEREALS

The main risks are handling, cross-contamination from additives (sauces), and reheating. In the United Kingdom, the rate of disease from rice has been estimated at $1/10^5$ servings (54).

***B. cereus* (373, 883, 1145, 6480).** *B. cereus* is isolated in up to 100% from raw rice and retail noodles, and in up to 60% from boiled or fried rice. In Malasia, up to 90% of *B. cereus* isolates from dry foods are enterotoxigenic. Precooked reheated rice is the classical vehicle for outbreaks of *B. cereus* food poisoning.

***Enterobacter sakazakii* (3807).** *E. sakazakii* is an environmental contaminant. In The Netherlands, *E. sakazakii* has been isolated from 23% (6/26) of samples from a pasta factory, from 27% (4/15) in a potato flower factory, and from 4/9 in a cereals factory.

***Escherichia* (1722).** Pasta is a reported vehicle of enterotokigenic *Escherichia coli* (ETEC).

***Salmonella* (1052, 1261, 2791, 3184).** In the United States in 1998, uncommon *Salmonella enterica* serovar Agona in a brand of plain, toasted oat cereals caused an outbreak with 162 cases. In Spain, spaghetti alla carbonara was the vehicle for an outbreak of *S. enterica* serovar Enteritidis at a school with 100 cases; food handlers and undercooked eggs rather than pasta were the source. Also in Spain, hard pastry with vanilla cream (coca) caused 1,435 cases of serovar Enteritidis gastroenteritis; fresh eggs and unhygienic handling were the implicated sources. In Hesse, Germany, in 2002, tortellini and red pesto sauce were likely the vehicle for 10 infections with unusual serovar Madelia.

***Streptococcus pyogenes* (group A *Streptococcus* [GAS]) (4379).** Vehicles of food-borne GAS pharyngitis recorded in 1941–2002 included rice dressing in 1983 (from the throat of a food handler) and macaroni with cheese sauce in 1991 (from the hands of a food handler).

***Giardia lamblia* (5850).** In a food-borne outbreak the implicated vehicle of *G. lamblia* was cold noodle salad.

PASTRY AND BAKERY

Handling and utensils can contaminate baked products. Fillings (cream, and cold custard) and toppings (glaze and "frost") may be unheated, supporting the growth of *S. aureus* and other agents (6988).

Viruses
HAV (1356, 2393, 6320, 6696, 8040). Food handlers have contaminated pastry after baking by glazing or icing. In New York in 1994, an immunoglobulin M-positive baker contaminated cooked doughnuts while applying a sugar glaze, causing an outbreak with ≥64 cases. In Michigan in 1968, 61 acute hepatitis A (HA) cases were traced to a local bakery and an icteric food handler. In Glasgow, United Kingdom, in 1974–1975, 12 of 118 members of a golf club developed acute, icteric HA after attending a dinner at a hotel; the vehicle was an unbaked sherry trifle and cream prepared by an incubating food handler. In Germany in 2004, an outbreak with 64 cases was linked to confectionery and "Berliner" (filled pastry) from an incubating food worker at one bakery.

***Norovirus* (939, 4153).** In the Minneapolis-St. Paul area, Minn., in 1982, cakes from an ill food handler at one bakery who prepared cake frostings was the likely source for ~3,000 cases of *Norovirus* diarrhea. Custard slices contaminated in a large United Kingdom bakery caused 104 cases in six districts.

Bacteria
The focus is on *Salmonella* and *S. aureus* from improper handling.

***Bacillus* (6480, 6988).** From soil, *B. cereus* and *B. subtilis* get onto grains, and from grains, cells, and spores are milled into flour. In the United States, 18% of mill samples grew *B. cereus*, and 45% grew *B. subtilis*. Spores that survive baking can germinate and produce toxin. However, regular bread is an unlikely vehicle for food-borne illness, although occasional outbreaks have been reported for bread with high *B. subtilis* counts. More critical are ethnic cereal products that receive surface heat only, e.g., flat breads, crumpets, pikelets, and waffles.

***Providencia* (5264).** Cereals are a rare vehicle for *Providencia*. At two kindergartens and one high school in Japan in 1996, *P. alcalifaciens* caused diarrhea in 270 of 610 exposed children and teachers. The implicated vehicle was warmed lunch bread from a single facility.

***Salmonella* (2267, 4828, 7193, 7555).** Bakery items are significant vehicles for *Salmonella*. In British Columbia, Canada, in 2000, 47 confirmed cases of *S. enterica* serovar Enteritidis diarrhea were traced to a Chinese bakery and an egg paste made from raw shell eggs. At a school in Toyohashi City, Japan, in 2001, lunch dessert buns made from chestnut paste wrapped with jelly were vehicle for 96 serovar Enteritidis infections in children, for attack rates of 0.1–0.5%; buns were likely cross-contaminated in a jam-filling machine at factory A, via liquid eggs from factory B. In Adelaide, Australia, in 2002, 20 patients acquired serovar Typhimurium from cream-filled buns and cakes prepared in a bakery where infected food handlers worked with contaminated bakery piping bags. In the United Kingdom in 1992, a bakery practicing poor hygiene was involved in two serovar Enteritidis outbreaks, one by custard slices and one by fresh cream cakes.

Shigella **(4037).** In Texas in 1996, doughnuts and muffins intentionally inoculated with *Shigella dysenteriae* caused dysentery among 12 (27%) of 45 laboratory staff.

S. aureus **(5830, 6988, 8005).** Filled, handled bakery is a reported vehicle for *S. aureus*. While food-borne *S. aureus* outbreaks are uncommon in many high-income countries, cream-filled bakery remains a hazard where good manufacturing practice and refrigeration is not followed. Cream fillings are an excellent medium for growing *S. aureus* and formation of enterotoxin. In Brazil, a cream-filled cake caused food poisoning in 12 attendees of a birthday party; enterotoxin A was detected in the cake, and enterotoxin-producing *S. aureus* was recovered from the cake and the nose, fingernail, and healed neck infection from the food handler. At a high school in Taiwan, staphylococcal food poisoning was carried by salad bread contaminated by an infected food handler at a local bakery.

S. pyogenes **(4379).** Reported vehicles in outbreaks of food-borne GAS pharyngitis included custard in 1952 (from the throat of a food handler), custard cake in 1986 (from food handlers), and mousse in 1984.

8.2 VEGETABLES, SALADS, FRUITS, AND SPICES

Vegetables (6914) are edible (nonwoody) bulk plant parts. Salads are vegetables that are eaten raw (plain, or mixed with eggs, meat, or fish, e.g., as "Caesar," "Niçoise"). Fruits are ripened reproductive parts of vascular plants, colloquially only fleshy, sweet products, botanically also capsules, nuts, and legumes. Spices are sparingly used plant parts with a strong smell or taste.

Infections (304, 1080, 7845). Infections from vegetables, fruits, and spices are diverse (Box 8.1), originating from soil, manure, waste irrigation, hands, and utensils (e.g., in salad bars).

Food plants may yield agents that are considered innocuous when ingested by immune-competent individuals, including *Aeromonas*, *Enterobacter*, *Klebsiella*, *Providencia*, *Pseudomonas*, *Staphylococcus*, and *Serratia*; *Aspergillus* and yeasts; and free-living amebas. Vegetables should be washed well under running, clean water. Unwashed vegetables should be kept away from clean surfaces.

Exposure history. Ask when vegetables were last (salads) (Box III.1) eaten raw, without or with dips or sauces, including seed sprouts, lettuce, tomatoes, and coleslaw. Are vegetables and fruits always washed before eating? When was a salad bar visited last? When did you last eat homemade products, e.g., tofu (soy bean curd) or pickles?

VEGETABLES AND SALADS

Vegetables (6914) (roots, stalks, grean leaves, dry fruits; for sprouts, see "Seed Sprouts" below) are from about a dozen plant families, including: Alliaceae, chive and leek (*Allium*); Apiaceae, carrots (*Dacus*); Asteraceae, lettuce (*Lactuca*); Brassicaceae, broccoli and cabbage (both *Brassica*) and radish (*Raphanus*); Chenopodiaceae, spinach (*Spinacia*); Cucurbitaceae, pumpkin (*Cucurbita*), Fabaceae, beans (*Cicer*, *Glycine*, *Phaseolus*, and *Vicia*), and Solanaceae, pepperoni (*Capsicum*), potato (*Solanum*), and tomato (*Lycopersicon*).

Mixed salads include eggs, seafood, ham, poultry, or other items. Dressings and dips served with salads can confound the association with salads. Products from vegetables include potato chips and canned, frozen, pickled, and fermented vegetables (e.g., tofu).

Exposure. In the United States, the consumption of vegetables per person per year was 153 kg in 1980, 193 kg in

---

Box 8.1 Agents from vegetables, salads, fruits, and spices

For waste irrigation of crops, see section 6.1. Vehicles are shown in parentheses.

Viruses:	HAV (raw vegetables, green onions, and berries), and *Norovirus* (raw vegetables, berries, and melons)
Bacteria:	*B. cereus* (sprouts and spices), *Campylobacter* (mixed salads), *C. botulinum* (home-canned, restaurant-prepared, or commercial vegetables and spices), *C. perfringens*, *E. coli* (EHEC, ETEC; ready-to-eat produce, sprouts, dressings, marketed fruits, and spices), *Listeria*, *Salmonella* (vegetables, sprouts, peanuts, melons, dried fruits, nuts, and spices), *Shigella* (handling and dips), *S. pyogenes* (handling), *V. cholerae* (tropics: vegetables and fruits), and *Yersinia* (vegetables and salads)
Protozoa:	*Cryptosporidium* (raw vegetables), *Cyclospora* (salads, berries), *E. histolytica* (tropics: raw vegetables and handled fruits), *Giardia* (salad bars), and *Toxoplasma* (raw vegetables)
Helminths:	*Angiostrongylus* (tropics: salads), *Ascaris* (tropics: vegetables and salads), *Fasciola* (privately collected field salads), *Toxocara* (private vegetable gardens), *Trichuris* (tropics: vegetables and salads)

2000, and 188 kg in 2001. Fresh vegetables accounted for 45% in 1980, 47% in 2000, and 48% in 2001. In 2001, the top-ranking fresh vegetables were potatoes, head lettuce, onions, tomatoes, and carrots (http://www.census.gov/prod/2004pubs/03statab/health.pdf). In the United States in 2000, ~60–70% of >13,000 respondents from eight states reported to have consumed lettuce at home in the past 7 days (http://www.cdc.gov/foodnet/surveys/Pop_surv.htm).

Infections. Unwashed, raw vegetables are significant vehicles of viruses, bacteria, protozoa, and heminths (Box 8.1). Acidic dressings, in general, prevent growth of *E. coli*, *Salmonella*, *S. aureus*, and some other agents (6998). In high-income countries in the late 1990s, vegetables plus fruits were implicated in ~1.5% (99/6,819) of reported food-borne outbreaks (6356). In U.S. schools in 1973–1997, salads accounted for 6% of 218 food-borne outbreaks by a single, known vehicle (1738). In the United Kingdom in 1992–2000, ~6% (83/1,426) of food-borne diarrhea outbreaks were attributed to salad vegetables or fruits (4499). In Australia in 1995–2000, fruits accounted for <1% of food-borne outbreaks, vegetables for <1%, and salads for 6%. (1721).

United Kingdom surveillance data allow the calculation of food-borne disease rates per 10^5 servings; estimates are 0 for fruits and cooked vegetables and 0.6 for salad vegetables (54).

Viruses

HAV. Food workers have contaminated salads with HAV (2393, 4539, 5258, 5790, 6411). In Kentucky in 1988, iceberg lettuce was the implicated vehicle for 202 HA cases in patrons of three restaurants supplied by the same local fresh produce distributor. In Florida in 1989, green salad contaminated by a pantry worker caused a restaurant outbreak with 97 cases among patrons. At a camp in central Australia in 2003, mishandled coleslaw (cabbage and carrots in a mayonnaise and capsicum sauce) was the vehicle implicated in an outbreak. In Finland in 1996, two HAV outbreaks were traced to salads that contained imported items (tomato and celery) and were distributed to schools and day-care centers by a central kitchen that served 2,900 meals per day.

Green onions (*Allium fistulosum*) have emerged as a vehicle for HAV in the United States (1204, 1885). In Pennsylvania in 2003, green onions were implicated in a restaurant-associated HAV outbreak with >550 HA cases; onions were likely imported from Mexico for the preparation of "salsa" (a spicy Mexican dish). In Ohio in 1998, green onions served at a restaurant were implicated in an outbreak of 40 acute HA cases; onions likely came from Californian or Mexican farms.

***Norovirus* (200, 1310, 2668, 2870, 4499).** In the United Kingdom in 1992–2000, 17% (13/83) of diarrhea outbreaks from salad vegetables or fruits were due to *Norovirus*. Implicated vehicles in endemic or epidemic infections include "salads," potato salads, pasta salads (rotini or bow-tie), tossed salad, pumpkin (*Cucurbita*) salad, and a salad bar.

Bacteria

A. The main agents from raw vegetables in high-income countries are *Clostridium botulinum*, *E. coli*, *L. monocytogenes*, *Salmonella*, and *Shigella*.

***C. botulinum* (3054, 7014, 7075, 7433, 7774).** Vegetables are a significant vehicle of botulism. Spores survive inadequate preservation and germinate at >4°C. By location and investigation, home-canned vegetables are implicated in about 10–80% of events (high in the Republic of Georgia, low in France, mean in United States and Italy). In Italy, preservation in oil increased risks by 5 times compared with preservation without oil. In France, *C. botulinum* was demonstrated in thickening materials, including starch. Vehicles of transmission are as follows.

- Home-preserved and home-prepared vegetable vehicles (22, 6856, 7014, 7433, 7774, 8254) include asparagus, bamboo shoots, beans, beef chilli, beets, mixed vegetables, mushrooms, olives, peppers, pickles, potato salad, salsa, tofu, tomatoes, and tomato juice. Preserved asparagus (*Asparagus officinalis*) and olives (*Olea europaea*) are major vehicles in the United States and western Europe. In France in 2000, 9 of 12 people attending a family gathering contracted type B botulism from home-canned asparagus: seven were hospitalized and six needed intubation. In Thailand in 1998, home-canned bamboo (Poaceae) shoots caused 13 cases of type A botulism; the pH of unopened cans was 5.3–5.7. In China in 1958–1983, homemade soy bean (*Glycine max*) curd (tofu) was the vehicle in 74% of 986 botulism outbreaks.

- Restaurant-associated vehicles include onions, potatoes, and cheese sauce (231, 4604, 6749, 7014). At a restaurant in Illinois in 1983, fresh onions (*Allium*) served as sauté on a patty-melt sandwich caused 20 cases. In Texas in 1994, baked potatoes (*Solanum tuberosum*) held in aluminum foil at room temperature for several days and used in dips served at a Greek restaurant caused 30 cases of type A botulism (patrons were identified through meal tickets, credit card receipts, and checks). In Colorado in 1978, potato salad consumed in a restaurant caused 12 cases of type A botulism.

- Commercial vehicles are less frequent but risks of wide distribution are higher. Reported vehicles include bean dip, burrito, chopped garlic, tinned asparagus, vegetable pie, and lotus roots (5655, 5990, 7014, 7088, 7433). In

Vancouver, Canada, commercially chopped garlic (*Allium*) in soybean oil caused a protracted and widely dispersed outbreak with 36 cases of type B botulism. In Spain in 1997, commercially tinned asparagus caused an outbreak with three cases. In Fukuoka Prefecture, Japan, lotus roots (*Nelumbo nucifera*) distributed for mustard making caused 36 cases of type A botulism; the roots had been fried, vacuum packed, and sold unrefrigerated, allowing for spores to germinate.

E. coli. Fecally contaminated, raw, unwashed or washed vegetables and salads, as well as fresh produce from markets and retail stores, yield *E. coli* (2056, 4512, 6526, 7845). Of interest are vehicles for ETEC and enterohemorrhagic *E. coli* (EHEC).

- ETEC (51, 1722, 2248). Reported vehicles include salads, zucchini, potatoes, and dressings. In Mexico City, 17 (40%) of 43 street-vended chili sauces were fecally contaminated, and two (5%) yielded sufficient numbers of ETEC to cause disease. In 1998, the prevalence of *E coli* in tabletop sauces was 66% (47/71) in Mexican-style restaurants of Guadalajara, Mexico, and 40% (10/25) in Houston, Tex. In Guadalajara, of typed isolates, four were ETEC (and 14 were enteroaggregative *E. coli*).
- EHEC (42, 551, 3320, 5112, 7306). Reported vehicles include lettuce, coleslaw, potato salad, and raw potatoes. In the United States in 1996, EHEC from "mesclun lettuce" (mix of lettuce leaves) caused >50 cases (including three cases of hemolytic-uremic syndrome [HUS]); the source was contaminated fields and wash water at one producer. In the United States in 1995, EHEC from lettuce caused bloody diarrhea in >70 cases (including one case of HUS).

L. monocytogenes (6526, 6667). Many vegetables are reported vehicles, including asparagus, broccoli, cabbage, cauliflower, celery, lettuce, tomato, and various salads (bagged and ready-to-eat salads, and corn, rice, fish, and chicken salads).

In France, 5% of 1,740 ready-to-eat salads grew *L. monocytogenes* in 1993–1994, and 4% of 1,426 salads in 1995–1996, for a proportion of 0.3% with growth of ≥100 CFU/g (2876). In maritime Canada in 1980–1981, serotype 4b in coleslaw caused an outbreak with 34 perinatal and 7 adult cases (6669). In northern Italy in 1993, serotype 1/2b in rice salad caused gastroenteritis in 18 (46%) of 39 immune-competent, young, nonpregnant adults attending a private food party (6543). In northern Italy in 1997, an outbreak of febrile gastroenteritis occurred among students and staff of two primary schools served by the same caterer; of 2,189 persons interviewed, 1,566 (72%, immune-competent) reported symptoms; *L. monocytogenes* serotype 4b was isolated from 1 of 40 blood cultures, 123 (87%) of 141 stool cultures, and one specimen of cold corn and tuna salad implicated epidemiologically, and 3 of 45 catering plant environmental samples (a work surface and two sink drains) (342).

***Salmonella* (4499, 4512, 4924, 6526, 7303, 7845).** In the United Kingdom in 1992–2000, 34 (41%) of 83 vegetable-borne diarrhea outbreaks were due to *Salmonella*. By production, provenance, processing, and test, the prevalence on vegetables is 0–20%, in high-income countries typically <1%. Vegetables can be vehicles of resistant salmonellae and occasionally of *S. enterica* serovar Typhi.

Outbreaks

- Non-Typhi salmonella outbreaks from salad vegetables include the following. **Lettuce (7100).** In Queensland, Australia, in 2001, 32 cases of serovar Bovismorbificans enteritis were associated with 1 of 15 outlets of a fast-food chain around the state; though a food item could not be implicated epidemiologically, residues from the lettuce shredder of the salad manufacturer grew the same isolate and phage type. **Tomatoes (569, 1676, 3220).** In the United States, tomatoes were vehicles for several outbreaks: in 1993 with 100 cases due to serovar Montevideo, in 1990 with 176 infections due to serovar Javiana, and in 1998–1999 with 86 confirmed cases (including 16 hospitalizations and three deaths) and an estimated 3,300 cases due to rare serovar Baildon in several states. Case-control studies implicated domestic raw tomatoes from >12 restaurants, fast-food outlets, and nursing homes; scattered exposure suggested contamination during harvesting, processing, or packing. In Australia in 1998–1999, fresh, unprocessed garlic was initially implicated in an outbreak of serovar Virchow that affected 32 persons. Subsequently, however, serovar Virchow was isolated from oven-dried tomatoes, to which garlic had been added. **Other salads (2331, 6526, 7514, 7958).** In Oregon in 1984, intentionally contaminated salad bars caused 751 serovar Typhimurium infections. At a canteen in Italy in 1994, serovar Hadar in meat salad caused 448 cases. In the United Kingdom in 2001, 0.2% (6/3,852) of ready-to-eat, bagged salad vegetables were of unacceptable quality, growing *Salmonella* (serovars Durban, Neport, and Umbillo) or *Listeria*. In the United Kingdom in 2001, serovar Newport was isolated from prepacked, ready-to-eat salad distributed by a major supermarket retailer.
- Serovar Typhi from salads (5029, 7116, 7681). In West Africa in 2001, 24 French army personnel contracted typhoid fever from cucumber salad polluted by carrier kitchen workers. In France in 2003, salad polluted by a food handler was vehicle for seven typhoid fever cases. On Kos, Greece, in 1983, 20% (59/289) of visitors from

nine European countries acquired typhoid fever at one hotel, from salad handled by kitchen workers who were carriers.
- Salmonellae from salad sauces (1172). At a hotel restaurant in Nevada in 1997, hollandaise sauce served with broccoli was implicated in an serovar Enteritidis outbreak with 91 cases.

Shigella (1163, 1767, 2075, 2542, 3818, 3946, 4499). Many vegetables are reported vehicles, including lettuce (*S. sonnei*), fresh parsley (*S. sonnei*), green onions (*S. flexneri*), uncooked maize and tossed salads (*S. flexneri* and *S. sonnei*), and potato salad (*S. flexneri*).

In Texas in 1986, *S. sonnei* in shredded lettuce served at fast-food restaurants caused 347 culture-confirmed cases. In North America in 1998, *S. sonnei* in fresh parsley caused seven outbreaks that were linked by common patterns in pulsed-field gel electrophoresis; likely sources were a farm in Baja California and four farms in California.

In the United States in 2000, *S. sonnei* in a commercial bean dip distributed nationwide through a grocery chain caused diarrhea in 406 patients from 10 states; over 40% reported bloody diarrhea. The dip consisted of five layers (beans, salsa, guacamole, nacho cheese, and sour cream) that were assembled manually; an ill food handler and a cheese mill were implicated epidemiologically. In the United Kingdom in 1992–2000, 1% (1/83) of diarrhea outbreaks reported for salad vegetables or fruits was due to *Shigella* (*S. sonnei*).

B. Many other bacteria have been demonstrated in or carried by raw salads and vegetables.

Acinetobacter (590). DNA was amplified from 17% (30/177) of vegetable samples, and raw vegetables are a suspected source of *A. baumannii* in hospitals.

Bacillus (6480). Vegetables frequently yield *B. cereus*.

Campylobacter (2263, 6371, 6399). Vegetables and salads are suspected vehicles of sporadic and epidemic infections. In Cardiff, United Kingdom, in 2001, 75% (159/213) of sporadic cases reported to have eaten salads, compared with 56% (635/1,144) of controls, for an odds ratio of 2 (95% confidence interval [95% CI] 1.7–3). At a congregational school in Brussels, Belgium, in 1995, *C. coli* diarrhea was diagnosed in 24 persons; salad mixed with ham and feta cheese was implicated. In a Wisconsin summer camp in 1995, tuna salad was the suspected vehicle for an outbreak with 79 cases, for an attack rate of 13%. The tuna salad likely became cross-contaminated through the hands of a food handler or a work surface.

Clostridium perfringens (5093, 6321). Spinach boiled with fried bean curd and legumes in a minestrone soup are reported vehicles of *C. perfringens* food poisoning.

Plesiomonas (1156). In New York, salad washed with tap water that contained *P. shigelloides* was implicated in an outbreak that affected 56 attendees of a party, for an attack rate of 57%.

Stenotrophomonas (6059). In the United Kingdom, *S. maltophilia* was cultured from 78% (14/18) of ready-to-eat salads from supermarkets, at concentrations of 150–196,000 CFU/g. Washing in chlorinated water before sale was insufficient, or prepacked salads were contaminated after washing. Immune-impaired patients could become colonized from foods.

S. pyogenes (1468, 4379). Vegetable vehicles for foodborne GAS pharyngitis included potato salad in 1973 and 1985, and cabbage salad in 1990 and 1991. In the cabbage outbreaks, food handlers were confirmed to carry GAS.

Vibrio. V. cholerae (4049, 6359, 6931, 7089, 8085). Reported vehicles of *V. cholerae* are unwashed vegetables and vegetables washed with unsafe water, as well as groundnut sauce, chick peas, millet gruel, and leftover rice. Acidic foods (pH 4.5–5) such as sauces based on lime or tomato reduce risks, while neutral or alkaline foods tolerate growth. **V. parahaemolyticus (2808)** *V. parahaemolyticus* was recovered from raw celery, spring onion, cucumber, and coriander leaves, sold at market.

Yersinia. Y. enterocolitica (1898, 7287). Green, cucumber, and carrot salads and ready-to-eat, cooked, and processed vegetables (Chinese cabbage, onion, potatoes, spinach, and tofu) yielded *Y. enterocolitica*. In Washington State in 1981–1982, tofu was implicated in an outbreak with 50 cases. **Y. pseudotuberculosis (5509).** In Finland in 1998, serotype O:3 caused a nationwide outbreak with 47 cases (of age 2–77 years, median 19 years); one sepsis patient died, and five patients had appendectomies. The vehicle was iceberg lettuce served in four lunch cafeterias and produced on local farms.

Protozoa

In high-income countries, locally produced or imported vegetables have yielded *Cyclospora*, *Cryptosporidium*, and *Giardia*, including lettuce, sprouts, and herbs (4507, 6334).

Cryptosporidium (1153, 5639, 6446, 7303). Vegetables can be vehicles. Curiously, raw vegetables have also been reported to be protective. In the United States in

1997, unwashed green onions (*A. fistulosum*) served at a Spokane restaurant caused cryptosporidiosis in 54 (87%) of 62 patrons (the high attack rate made it difficult to establish an association with a particular food). In Brazil, 1% of 172 commercial vegetable samples yielded *Cryptosporidium*; in Peru, 19% of 172 samples from 28 small markets, including basil, cabbage, green onions, leeks, lettuce, and parsley yielded the same.

***Cyclospora* (1232, 1969, 3285, 4507, 5639).** Salads and leafy vegetables yielded *Cyclospora* by microscopy or PCR. In Lima, Peru, in 1995–1996, *Cyclospora* was identified in 3 (2%) of 172 vegetables, including lettuce and herbs, from 28 small markets. Salads and vegetables are reported vehicles, mainly in North America, occasionally in western Europe. In Pennsylvania in 2004, *C. cayetanensis* was identified in 40 (19%) of 215 persons exposed at a residential facility, and 56 (26%) were probable cases; raw snow peas imported from Guatemala and served in pasta salad were the vehicle implicated. In Germany in 2000, *Cyclospora* on salad served for luncheons at a restaurant caused illness in 34 (85%) of patrons; the implicated salads were imported from France (butterhead lettuce) and Italy (mixed lettuce).

***Entamoeba* (560, 7303, 7785).** In Brazil, 25% of 172 commercial vegetable samples yielded *Entamoeba*. In Mexico City, cysts were isolated in 1% (2/212) of carrots obtained from a supply center. Raw, unwashed vegetables and salads from endemic areas, and unsafe water for washing are hazards for the acquisition of *E. histolytica*/*E. dispar*.

***Giardia* (4510, 5071, 7213, 7303).** In Brazil, *Giardia* was identified in 4 (2%) of 172 commercial vegetable samples. Vegetables are a reported vehicle. Among U.S. travelers returning from Madeira with giardiasis, raw vegetables were implicated epidemiologically. In the United Kingdom in 1998–1999, eating lettuce was a significant risk in 192 cases compared with 492 age-, sex-, and location-matched community controls. In the United States in 1990, an outbreak at an insurance company cafeteria caused 18 confirmed and 9 suspected cases; sliced raw vegetables from the salad bar were implicated, and an employee who prepared the food was found to be infected.

***Toxoplasma* (3816).** Eating unwashed, raw salads, vegetables, or fruits is a risk, presumably by contamination with oocysts from cat feces.

Helminths

The global health impact of food-borne helminths contrasts with limited evidence for the presence of helminth eggs and larvae on vegetables.

***Angiostrongylus*.** Unwashed vegetables, salads, and fruits with infective (L3) larvae are vehicles, either from inadvertently swallowed small slugs, or from snail or slug slime (8375). For snails as foods, see section 7.5. ***A. cantonensis* (306, 6963).** In 2000, 12 (52%) of 23 U.S. tourists to Jamaica developed eosinophilic meningitis, likely from Romaine lettuce served in Caesar salad. In an outbreak in Okinawa in 2000 with seven patients, ingestion of fresh lettuce or cabbage was the likely vehicle. ***A. costaricensis* (4090, 8375).** In Guatemala in 1994–1995, in an outbreak of abdominal angiostrongyliasis with 22 cases, raw mint ("hierba buena," *Mentha*, Lamiaceae) was the implicated vehicle, eaten alone, or as an ingredient with "ceviche." Salt and vinegar do not eliminate risks. The proportion of L3 that remained viable in bioassay was 1.8% after incubation in saturated NaCl for 12 h, and 2.4% after incubation in vinegar.

***Ascaris lumbricoides*.** Vegetables yield *A. lumbricoides* eggs (4301, 7303, 7785). In Brazil, eggs were identified in 2% (3/172) of commercial vegetable samples. In Mexico City, 2% (4/212) of carrots from a supply center yielded eggs, as well as 3% (2/76) of potatoes, 6% (4/66) of spinach bundles, 7% (2/29) of coriander bundles, and 20% (4/20) of sweet potatoes. On Seoul markets, eggs were found on the inside, leafy parts of 2% of Chinese cabbage and 12% of lettuce.

Unwashed raw vegetables and salads are vehicles of human infections, even sugar cane (*Saccharum officinarum*, Poaceae) (3383, 3441, 6083). In 732 children from Laos, rarely washing vegetables or never washing hands before eating were significant risks. In Finland in the winter of 1982–1983, imported vegetables were implicated in an outbreak of *A. lumbricoides* that affected 12 persons.

***Echinococcus*.** Surprisingly, data on eggs of *E. multilocularis* or *E. granulosus* on vegetables, mushrooms, berries, fallen fruits, or cider seem unavailable. In Uruguay, having a fenced fruit or vegetable garden was a risk for *E. granulosus* infection (1086). In contrast in Spain, consumption of raw green vegetables was not a risk in a case-control study (1051).

***Fasciola hepatica* (351, 676, 1459, 1591, 1723, 4793, 5044).** Metacercariae on plants are infective. Sticky metacercariae from raw water and on kitchen utensils can cross-contaminate foods. Habitats for infective plants include pastures, brooks, and home gardens, rarely commercial production beds. By provenance and dietary habits, reported vehicles include common (*Nasturtium officinale*) and wild (*Rorippa amphibia*) watercress (both Brassicaceae), dandelion (*Taraxacum officinale*, Asteraceae), lamb's lettuce (*Valerianella locusta*, Valerianaceae), spearmint (*Mentha spicata*, Lamiaceae), in the Andes also rushes (*Juncus*, Juncaceae), in Africa also *Oxalis pescaprae* (Oxalidaceae), *Portulaca oleracea*

(Portulacaceae), and *Rumex tingitanus* (Polygonaceae). On markets in Peru and Uzbekistan, 1–10% of lettuces and green vegetables yielded metacercariae.

In Europe, watercress is a major vehicle of infections and family clusters. In Bolivia in 1991, in an outbreak with 30 suspected cases, "kjosco" (a water plant, botany not specified) was the putative vehicle.

Fasciolopsis buskii (1818, 2747, 2885, 4275, 8356).
Metacercariae on water plants are infective. Typically plants are eaten raw or undercooked, including stalks or fruits, or hulls are peeled with the teeth. Reported vehicles include lotus (*Nelumbo nucifera*), water caltrop (*Trapa natans*), water chestnut (*Eliocharis tuberosa* or *Trapa natana*), water hyacinth (*Eichornia crassipes*), water lily (*Nymphaea*), water bamboo (*Zizania aquatica*), and water spinach (*Ipomoea reptans*).

Hookworm (7303).
In Brazil, hookworm eggs were isolated in 27 (16%) of 172 commercial vegetable samples. If food-borne transmission is possible, this mode is underrated. Alternatively, the findings could merely reflect fecal contamination.

Toxocara (4640, 7303, 7785).
In Brazil, *Toxocara* eggs were identified in 1 (0.6%) of 172 commercial vegetable samples. In Mexico City, eggs of *T. canis* were found in 2% (4/212) of carrots from a supply center and in 7% (2/31) of radishes. Of all eggs, two thirds were unembryonated, and one third was embryonated (infective). Vegetables as a vehicle seem underrated. In France, 20 of 25 *Toxocara*-infected respondents reported to regularly consume "pissenlits" (*Taraxacum officinale*) and other field salads.

Trichuris (3383).
Unwashed or raw vegetables and salads are putative vehicles. In 732 children from Laos, rarely washing vegetables or never washing hands before eating were significant risks.

SEED SPROUTS
Edible sprouts include alfalfa (or lucerne, *Medicago*), clover (*Melilotus* and *Trifolium*), soy bean (*Glycine*), and mung bean (*Phaseolus*) from Fabaceae, and mustard (*Brassica*), radish (*Raphanus*), and cress (*Lepidium*) from Brassicaceae. In eight states in 2000, ~5% of >13,000 respondents reported to have consumed alfalfa sprouts at home in the past 7 days (http://www.cdc.gov/foodnet/surveys/Pop_surv.htm).

Infections (904, 5121, 7333) (Box 8.1).
Worldwide in 1973–1998, seed sprouts carried 14 outbreaks with ~8,140 culture-confirmed cases (4 to 6,000 per outbreak). A major hazard from sprouts is *Salmonella*. Soaking seeds in calcium hypochlorite ($CaOCl_2$) reduces but does not eliminate risks. Irradiation may be best for the delivery of safe sprouts.

Bacteria
B. cereus (7333).
Of 14 sprout-associated outbreaks worldwide in 1973–1998, one was due to *B. cereus*, causing four culture-confirmed cases in the United States.

E. coli.
Vehicles for EHEC are radish sprouts (5031, 7306, 7968), alfalfa sprouts (868, 2357, 5121), and clover sprouts (7333).

Outbreaks Outbreaks are well documented (868, 2357, 5031, 7306, 7333, 7968). Of 14 sprout-associated outbreaks worldwide in 1973–1998, four were due to *E. coli* O157, two each in the United States and in Japan.

- United States. In 1997, an outbreak of *E. coli* O157:H7 with 64 cases in Michigan and 32 cases in Virginia was traced to alfala sprouts harvested in Idaho; possible sources of sprout contamination included water, cattle manure, and deer feces. In Minnesota and Colorado in 2003, 20 EHEC cases were traced to alfalfa sprouts from the same seed distributor.
- Japan. In Sakai City in July to August of 1996, contaminated white radish sprouts (kaiware-daikon) from a single farm and distributed with school lunches through a central kitchen were the vehicle for an EHEC epidemic with >7,400 cases among school children. In Kyoto (~50 km away from Sakai) in July 1996, radish sprout salad caused an EHEC outbreak at a factory, with 47 (1.5%) of 3,155 employees meeting the case definition.

Salmonella.
Reported vehicles include alfalfa and mung bean sprouts. Outbreaks have been well documented (3412, 4657, 5112, 7333, 7704). Of 14 sprout-associated outbreaks worldwide in 1973–1998, nine in North America and West Europe were due to *Salmonella*, with a total of >1,900 culture-confirmed cases. In North America in 1995, *S. enterica* serovars Newport and Stanley in alfalfa sprouts caused ~20,000 infections. Contaminated seed lots were traced to The Netherlands from where they had been distributed to growers in Europe and America. In Canada, alfalfa sprouts were vehicles for outbreaks by serovars Newport in 1996, Meleagridis in 1997, and Paratyphi B in 1999, the last episode with 52 cases. In Canada in 2001, mung bean sprouts imported from People's Republic of China and distributed by an Edmonton supplier to ethnic (Vietnamese, Chinese, and Japanese style restaurants) caused 84 cases of serovar Enteritidis of a particular phage type.

Protozoa
In Norway in 1999–2001, mung bean sprouts tested positive for *Cryptosporidium* and *Giardia*, and radish sprouts also for *Giardia* (6334). However, sprout-borne infections or outbreaks do not seem to have been observed.

FRUITS

A botanical definition (ripened reproductive vascular plant parts) of fruits would include nuts (see "Nuts" below), legumes (e.g., peas and lentils), olives, and tomatoes (see "Vegetables and Salads" above). Here, fruits in the colloquial sense are sweet and juicy reproductive plant parts. Examples are Anacardiaceae, mango (*Mangifera*); Arecaceae, date (*Phoenix*); Bromeliaceae, pineapple (*Ananas*); Cucurbitaceae, cantaloupe and melon (both *Cucumis*) and watermelon (*Citrullus*); Ericaceae, blueberry (*Vaccinium*); Musaceae, banana (*Musa*); Rosaceae, apple (*Malus*), apricot, plum, peach (all *Prunus*), blackberry and raspberry (*Rubus*), and strawberry (*Fragaria*); Rutaceae, grapefruit, orange (both *Citrus*); and Vitaceae, grape (*Vitis*).

Exposure. In the United States, consumption of fruits per person per year was 123 kg in 1980, 127 kg in 2000, and 125 kg in 2001. Fresh fruits accounted for 39% in 1980, 45% in 2000, and 46% in 2001. In 2001, the top-ranking fresh fruits were bananas, apples, watermelons, oranges, and cantaloupes (http://www.census.gov/prod/2004pubs/03statab/health.pdf).

Infections. Fresh fruits can transmit viruses, bacteria, and protozoa (Box 8.1). Peeling fruits with dirty hands can contaminate edible parts. Washing fruits with clean hands and clean water reduces but does not eliminate risks (11). Dried fruits such as apricots and raisins are potential vehicles of enteric agents (8234). For handled fruits such as dates surprisingly little information exists on enteric bacteria. Dried fruits should be included in the exposure history (Box III.1).

Viruses

HAV. Reported vehicles of HAV include blueberries, strawberries, and raspberries.

- Blueberries (1033). In New Zealand in 2002, blueberries carried an HAV outbreak with 43 cases. During 2–7 weeks before onset of illness, the patients consumed raw blueberries significantly more often (56% or 19/39) than random telephone controls (14% or 10/71), for an odds ratio of 8 (95% CI 3–22). Blueberries were traced to a single commercial orchard and amplified HAV DNA by PCR. Audit of the orchard revealed opportunities for fecal contaminaton of blueberries by pickers.
- Strawberries (3522, 5447). In the United States in 1990, frozen strawberries processed at a single plant in California caused two outbreaks. The first outbreak at a school in Georgia was carried by strawberry cakes and caused 15 cases among 827 students and 60 teachers, for an attack rate of 10%. The second outbreak at an institution in Montana was carried by a strawberry dessert and caused 13 cases among 174 residents and 467 staff members, for an attack rate of 8%. Frozen strawberries again caused an outbreak in 1997, with 213 cases from 23 schools in Michigan (median attack rate, 2%) and 29 cases from 13 schools in Maine (median attack rate, 0.3%). The implicated strawberries had been grown in Mexico, processed in a California plant, and distributed through a national school lunch program.
- Raspberries (6102, 6192). In Scotland in 1988, a raspberry pavlova dessert caused five cases of HA; the raspberries had been purchased frozen from a fruit farm where at least one picker was diagnosed with confirmed, clinical HA. Also in Scotland, an outbreak of 24 HA cases was traced to a city hotel, and raspberry mousse prepared from frozen raspberries was the implicated vehicle.

Norovirus. Reported vehicles of *Norovirus* include melons and raspberries.

- Melons (3600) were implicated in an outbreak at a banquet that caused gastroenteritis in 206 (86%) of 239 attendees.
- Raspberries (2671, 4274, 5964). In Helsinki, Finland, in 1998, an outbreak with >100 diarrhea cases was traced to frozen raspberries. In southern Sweden in 2001, cakes with cream topping from frozen, whole raspberries caused an outbreak with 30 gastroenteritis cases; *Norovirus* was amplified by nucleic acid amplification test (NAT) from stools of five patients and from raspberries. In the Quebec area, Canada, in 1997, raspberries from Bosnia were epidemiologically and virologically implicated in gastroenteritis outbreaks with >200 cases.

Bacteria

Raw, unwashed strawberries, cherries, peaches, apples, and other fruits have been reported to yield *Citrobacter*, *Enterobacter*, *Escherichia*, *Klebsiella*, *Proteus*, *Pseudomonas*, *Salmonella*, *Staphylococcus*, and other bacteria (11). Dried fruits have yielded *Bacillus*, *Clostridium*, *Salmonella*, and *S. aureus* (8234). Some agents are innocuous when ingested, while *E. coli*, *Salmonella*, and *S. aureus* are of concern.

***E. coli* (11, 2056, 3498).** Oranges, cantaloupes, and other fruits have yielded *E. coli*. Unwashed fruits are likely sources of ETEC and diarrhea in travelers (11). In Australia in 2002, compared with randomly selected population controls, eating berries in the 10 days before illness was a significant risk for sporadic dysentery due to EHEC, for an odds ratio of 11 (95% CI 1.3–96). Reported vehicles included strawberries, blueberries, and blackberries.

Salmonella. Reported vehicles of *Salmonella* include melons and tropical fruits.

- Melons (1140, 1191, 2056) grow *Salmonella* at a rate of ~1%; washed cantaloupes have also yielded *Salmonella*. In the United States, cantaloupes have been the vehicles for several outbreaks. The first outbreak in 1990 by *S. enterica* serovar Chester caused 245 infections. A second outbreak in 1991 by serovar Poona caused 400 infections. Again in 2000–2002, serovar Poona on cantaloupes caused three outbreaks with 155 cases. Cantaloupes were imported from Mexico and suspected to be contaminated by waste irrigation, unsafe water for cleaning or cooling, or packing by food workers.
- Mango (6941). In the United States in 1999, an increase of serovar Newport in nationwide surveillance suggested a common source outbreak that was traced to mangoes imported from a farm in Brazil. Hot-water treatment to prevent importation of a fruit fly was the possible source of contamination.
- Mamey (*Manilkara zapota*, Sapotaceae) (3846). In Florida in 1998–1999, contaminated mamey fruits used for preparing fruit shakes caused 16 cases of typhoid fever (mamey tree is a historical source of chewing gum).
- Cocoa (*Theobroma*, Sterculiaceae) (2658) was the vehicle for an outbreak of serovar Durham.

In South Africa, batches of high-moisture, dried prunes and raisins grew *Salmonella*, at concentrations of 10–40 CFU/g (8234).

Shigella. Imported watermelon was implicated in an *S. sonnei* outbreak (2512).

S. aureus (8234). In South Africa, batches of high-moisture, dried raisins grew *S. aureus* at concentrations of 20 CFU/g (the permitted level is 10 CFU/g).

V. cholerae (5242, 7145). Eating unwashed fruits is a risk for contracting *V. cholerae*. In the United States in 1996, two persons acquired cholera from sliced cantaloupe prepared by an asymptomatic food handler.

Fungi
Peanuts, date fruits, almonds, and other nut fruits may yield *Aspergillus flavus* and *A. parasiticus* that produce aflatoxins, as well as *A. niger*, *Fusarium*, and *Penicillium* that do not produce aflatoxins.

Protozoa
By location, sample size, and test method, locally produced or imported fruits may yield *Cyclospora*, *Cryptosporidium*, and *Giardia* (3354, 6334).

Cyclospora (3285, 3354). Fruits are reported vehicles of *C. cayetanensis*, mainly raspberries. Outbreaks are well documented in North America (2432, 3287, 3288, 3354, 4076). In Florida in 1995, following a laboratory report of six infections, a study of 24 cases and 69 matched controls identified fresh raspberries as a significant risk. At a restaurant in Boston in May 1996, 57 (61%) of 94 attendees at a wedding reception contracted enteric illness, including 12 with confirmed *Cyclospora*; a dessert that contained raspberries, strawberries, blackberries, and blueberries was implicated. In North America in 1996, in a widespread outbreak with 1,465 cases (67% confirmed), imported raspberries were implicated, for attack rates of 24–100%. *Cyclospora* on raspberries recurred in 1997 with 762 cases (25% confirmed) from 15 states or provinces. Again raspberries from Guatemala were implicated, and the mode of contamination remained unknown. In Philadelphia in 2000, *C. cayetanensis* detected by PCR in a wedding cake filling that included raspberries caused diarrhea in 54 (68%) of 79 interviewed guests. The catering company had imported raspberries from a farm in Guatemala implicated in a previous outbreak; raspberries were served fresh and frozen.

G. lamblia (5971, 6334). In an outbreak, the implicated vehicle of *G. lamblia* was a home-prepared fruit salad. In Norway, *G. lamblia* was demonstrated on strawberries.

Helminths
Angiostrongylus (919). In Egypt in 1994, eosinophilic meningitis in three children of aged 10–12 years was traced to date fruits that the children had picked from irrigation canals in which snails yielded *A. cantonensis* larvae.

Toxocara (1019, 5175). Eggs of *T. pteropodis* from fruit bats (*Pteropus alecto*) are suspected to have contaminated mango fruits and to have caused hepatitis-like illness among 148 residents of Palm Island off Townsville, Australia, in 1979.

NUTS
Nuts botanically are dry, indehiscent fruits whose hard walls surround a single seed. Colloquially, nuts include almond (*Prunus*, Rosaceae), coconut (*Cocos*, Arecaceae), hazelnut (*Corylus*, Betulaceae), peanut (*Arachis*, Fabaceae), pinyon (*Pinus edulis*, Pinaceae), pistachio (*Pistacia*, Anacardiaceae), pumpkin seeds (*Cucurbita*, Cucurbitaceae), and walnut (*Juglans*, Juglandaceae).

Exposure. In the United States, consumption of peanuts (shelled) per person per year was 2.2 kg in 1980 and 2.6 kg in 2000. Tree nut consumption was 0.8 kg in 1980 and

1.1 kg in 2000 (http://www.census.gov/prod/2004pubs/03statab/health.pdf).

Infections. Reported agents include *C. botulinum*, *Salmonella*, and *V. cholerae*. Although *Aspergillus* is recovered from peanuts, except aflatoxins, there is little evidence for peanuts as vehicles.

***C. botulinum* (1418, 1636, 5537).** In Taiwan in 1986, peanuts canned in a small, family-owned business caused seven cases of type A botulism. Because workers of a printing factory were affected, intoxication by a solvent was initially suspected. In the United Kingdom in 1989, hazelnut purée added to yogurt caused 27 cases of type B botulism including one death; product processing was inadequate to kill spores.

Salmonella. Reported vehicles for *Salmonella* include almonds and peanuts.

- Almonds (1304, 3867). In Canada in 2000–2001, isolates of an unusual *S. enterica* serovar Enteritidis phagetype prompted an investigation that identified natural, raw, whole almonds as the vehicle. Almonds were sold by one chain of stores that was supplied by a firm in the United States. Based on a study of 15 cases and 15 controls matched for age and neighborhood, whole almonds and almond-containing snacks were recalled and removed from retail stores of the implicated chain. In North America in 2003–2004, raw almonds were the vehicle implicated in an outbreak of serovar Enteritidis with 29 patients from 12 U.S. states and Canada. As in the first outbreak, almonds originated from California that produces ~80% of the world supply, exporting to America, Europe, and Asia. Given the shelf life of >1 year, the producer announced a nationwide and international recall, although the majority of recalled almonds likely had been consumed months previously.
- Peanuts (3957, 6654). In South Australia in 1996, serovar Mbandaka in retail peanut butter caused an outbreak with 15 cases; the likely source was a producer from another Australian state. The agent was isolated in opened jars of peanut butter from case households and in unopened jars from retail outlets. In 2001, serovars Stanley and Newport in peanuts caused an international outbreak with cases in Australia (55), Canada (44), and the United Kingdom (10), mainly of Asian ethnicity; flavored or roasted peanuts of one brand grew serovars Newport and Stanley and other salmonellae. The source could not be identified, but products were recalled in the three countries.

***V. cholerae* (7368).** In Maryland in 1991, coconut milk imported from Thailand caused cholera in four of six consumers who attended a private picnic; toxigenic *V. cholerae* O1 was recovered from patients and unopened brand.

SPICES

Spices (6914) (http://www.cdc.gov/foodnet/surveys/Pop_surv.htm) are strongly aromatic plant parts or mixtures (e.g., curry), e.g., Apiaceae, cilantro (*Coriandrum*) and parsley (*Petroselinum*); Lamiaceae, basil (*Ocimum*) and oregano (*Origanum*); Lauraceae, cinnamon (*Cinnamomum*); Myristicaceae, clove (*Syzygium*) and nutmeg (*Myristica*); Myrtaceae, allspice (*Pimenta*); Solanaceae, chilli and paprika (both *Capsicum*); Piperaceae, pepper (*Piper*); Iridaceae, saffron (*Crocus*); Orchidaceae, vanilla (*Vanilla*); Pedaliaceae, sesame (*Sesamum*); and Zingiberaceae, cardamom (*Elettaria*).

Americans consume ~1 kg per person per year of herbs and spices. In the United States in 2000, of >13,000 respondents from eight states, 6–16% reported consumption of parsley in the week before the survey, and 4–23% (9%) reported cilantro.

Infections (5648). Agents from spices include bacteria and protozoa (Box 8.1). Small quantities per servings are offset by frequency of consumption and raw usage. Spores in spices may resist heating. Irradiation is a proposed method to reduce health risks from spices.

Bacteria
***Bacillus* (238, 2624, 4461, 6480, 6988).** Spices and spiced ready-to-eat foods frequently yield cells or spores of *B. cereus* and *B. thuringiensis*. Levels >10^5 spores per g can be associated with production of *B. cereus* toxin. In Nigeria, *B. cereus* was cultured from a majority of 230 unprocessed, marketed spices, including red and black pepper and curry powder. In Mexico, *B. cereus* was present in 32 of 304 samples of spices (garlic powder, cumin seeds, black pepper, oregano, and bay leaves), mostly packed in polyethylene bags.

***E. coli* (2250).** In Mexico City in 2000, 43% (44/103) of taco dressings (chili sauce and raw coriander) sold by street vendors on open markets ready-to-eat grew *E. coli*.

***C. botulinum* (439, 3794, 7409).** Spices can be vehicles. In the United States in 1973, commercially canned pepper in oil caused seven cases of type B botulism; the brand had been distributed to ~1,300 market consignees and ~93% could be recalled. In the United States in 1978, home-canned jalapeño peppers consumed as hot sauce or in "nachos" at one Mexican restaurant caused 59 cases of type B botulism, for an attack rate of 4% among all patrons. In Texas in 2001, 15 (40%) of 38 attendees of a church supper contracted botulism type A; the vehicle was a brand of frozen chili (*Capsicum annuum* and *C. frutescens*) likely spoiled during storage at a "salvage" (second hand) food store. Toxin A was recovered from stools, leftover chili, an opened chili container, and an unopened container at a concentration of 160 ng/g.

***Salmonella* (2250, 4324).** In Mexico City in 2000, 5% (5/103) of taco dressings (chili sauce and raw coriander) sold by street vendors on open markets ready-to-eat grew *S. enterica* serovars Agona and Enteritidis and group B salmonellae. In Germany in 1993, a nationwide outbreak with ~1,000 salmonellosis cases was traced to potato chips to which contaminated paprika (*C. annuum*) powder had been added, for an attack rate of $10/10^5$ exposed persons. Serovars Saintpaul, Rubislaw, and Javiana were isolated from patients, chips (0.04–45 organisms per g), and paprika powder. The infective dose was ~4-45 organisms.

Protozoa
Information is limited to *Cyclospora* (3359, 4507). In Missouri in 1999, cyclosporiasis affected 62 attendees at two events; chicken pasta salad served at one and tomato basil salad served at the other were most strongly associated with illness, and the vehicle implicated was fresh basil (*Ocimum basilicum*, Lamiaceae), grown in Mexico or the United States. In British Columbia, Canada, in May 2001, basil of "Siam Queen" variety imported from the United States and used raw in Vietnamese cuisine to garnish noodle soups, salads, and been sprouts, was implicated in an outbreak with 17 cases.

HONEY
Honey (7006) is plant nectar and pollen modified by honey bees. Main constituents are fructose (38%), glucose (30%), and water (17%).

Infections (7006). Bacteria do not replicate in honey. The main agents recovered from honey are yeasts and spore-forming bacteria (*Bacillus* and *Clostridium*). Postharvest, honey can become contaminated via dust, utensils, and handling.

***C. botulinum* (343, 5389, 6695, 7332, 7433).** Honey is a major vehicle of infant botulism. In infants spores can germinate and form toxin in vivo. Since recognition of the condition in the late 1970s, >1,000 cases have been reported in the United States until 2000. In western Europe, honey-borne sporadic cases of infant botulism were reported in Denmark (in 1995) and Germany (in 1998). By test method (PCR and bioassay) and provenance, *C. botulinum* spores are detected in 6–16% of retail honey (Europe, 6–7%; America, 7–10%; imported honey 16%). Spore counts range broadly, from 2 to 8,000/100 g. Honey should not be given to infants <12 months old.

MUSHROOMS
Edible mushrooms (Table 20.1, plants for practical purposes) include Basidiomycetes, e.g., champignon (*Agaricus pisporus*), pepper mushroom (*Cantharellus cibarius*), and stone mushroom (*Boletus edulis*), and Ascomycetes, e.g., morel (*Morchella esculenta*) and truffle (*Tuber melanosporum*).

Exposure. In the United States, consumption mushrooms per person per year was 0.5 kg in 1980, 1.2 kg in 2000, and 1.2 kg in 2001 (http:www.census.gov/prod/2004pubs/03statab/health.pdf).

***C. botulinum* (3434, 4292, 5877), (7014, 7433).** Fresh mushrooms commonly carry spores of *C. botulinum*, typically at a concentration of ~40/100 g. Mushrooms are a vehicle of botulism.

In the United States, plastic wraps for fresh mushrooms were introduced in 1967. Wrapped mushrooms quickly metabolized oxygen, creating an anaerobic environment that was favorable for *C. botulinum* and cases of botulism. Punching holes in plastic wrap remedied the problem. In New York City in 1974, home-bottled mushrooms in olive oil caused three cases of type B botulism in a family of 10. Mushrooms were eaten cold by the three ill members only. The first patient died after a 10-day illness without botulism being suspected, the second patient died after cardiorespiratory arrest and after botulism was diagnosed, the third patient suffered from dysphagia only.

In Italy in 1997, commercially canned truffle cream and commercially roasted mushrooms in oil each caused one case. In the United Kingdom, home-preserved mushrooms bottled in oil caused two cases of type B botulism among a family who had received a batch from Italy.

***L. monocytogenes* (3772).** In Finland, an 80-year-old man developed septicemia one day after consuming homemade, salted *Lactarius rufus*. Serotype 4b was isolated from blood and mushrooms (10^6 CFU/g) which were stored in cold for 5 months and had an NaCl concentration of 7.5%.

***S. aureus* (4376).** In the United States in 1989, canned mushrooms imported from People's Republic of China caused 99 cases of food poisoning, at two cafeterias, one pizzeria, and one restaurant; enterotoxin A was identified in mushrooms.

***A. lumbricoides* (7785).** In Mexico City, eggs were isolated from 9% (2/22) of mushrooms obtained at a supply center.

9

Finished Foods

9.1 Snacks and sandwiches
9.2 Menus and ethnic foods

Finished foods include ready-to-eat foods, snacks, and meals. Ready-to-eat food is immediately consumable, without a need for peeling, washing, or heating. Ready-to-eat foods are typically wrapped in plastic (tear-open), e.g., potato chips or bagged salads. Snacks are light, fast foods. Snacks are typically eaten "on-the-go," from paper or boxes, e.g., sandwiches, French fries, hot dogs, or pizza. Meals are menues served at table, e.g., of Chinese, French, or Italian cuisines.

Infections (1721, 4461). Street venders, outlets, and snack bars have the advantage of short circuits but the disadvantage of food handling at inadequately equipped places. In Australia in 1995–2000, sandwiches accounted for 5% (11/214) of food-borne outbreaks and 16% (1,321/8,124) of cases. In contrast, for centralized kitchens and home delivery services, thermal food history is critical, including cold storage over weekends and hot delivery time to clients. Tear-open foods of international brands are generally considered safe.

9.1 SNACKS AND SANDWICHES
VIRUSES
Sandwiches are reported vehicles of hepatitis A virus (HAV), *Norovirus*, and *Rotavirus*. In contrast, popular French fries have virtually never been implicated in outbreaks.

HAV (1402, 2393, 3591, 5018). In the United States in 1968–2001, in seven outbreaks with 500 acute hepatitis A (HA) cases (71 per outbreak) sandwiches were implicated that had been served at restaurants or cafeterias and prepared by infected food handlers. At a U.S. hospital in 1973, cafeteria-made sandwiches were implicated epidemiologically in an outbreak with 44 clinical and 22 subclinical acute HA cases among employees, and ≥7 community cases; sandwiches had been prepared by incubating food handlers. In Colorado 7 of 11 persons developed symptoms of HA 2.5–5 weeks after attending a picnic. Tuna salad sandwiches prepared by the index case were implicated, and the number of sandwiches consumed was inversely related to the incubation period. In Bari, Italy, in 2002, sandwiches prepared in a delicatessen were the vehicle for 26 cases of acute HA.

Norovirus (1737, 4478, 5725). Vehicles reported in outbreaks included turkey and tuna salad sandwiches and deli ham sandwiches. I could locate a single outbreak at a school cafeteria likely due to *Norovirus* from an ill food handler in which French fries were an implicated vehicle, besides hamburgers (2987).

Rotavirus (2438). In the United States, deli sandwiches served at a campus dining hall were implicated epidemiologically in an outbreak with 85 cases that met the case definition, for an attack rate of 5%.

BACTERIA

Sandwiches are reported vehicles of *Escherichia coli*, *Listeria monocytogenes*, *Salmonella*, *Shigella*, *Staphylococcus aureus*, and *Streptococcus pyogenes*. A promising method to increase the safety of ready-to-eat products is postmanufacturing irradiation.

E. coli (741, 1099, 5744). In Canada in 1985, ham, turkey, and cheese sandwiches were implicated in an outbreak of enterohemorrhagic *E. coli* (EHEC) in a nursing home. In Canada in 2002, salads or sandwiches prepared in a psychiatric hospital kitchen were implicated in an outbreak of *E. coli* O157:H7. In the United Kingdom in 1994–1996, a case-control study identified sliced meat in sandwiches from caterers as a vehicle of EHEC.

L. monocytogenes (1164, 2890, 8199). In 1998–1999, hot dogs (and delis) were implicated in a multistate outbreak by serotype 4b that caused 101 cases, including 21 deaths. In Northern Ireland, 5 (0.7%) of 725 prepacked sandwiches purchased from retail supermarkets, cafés, gas stations, and other premises grew *L. monocytogenes* at concentrations ≥100 CFU/g; the five infective samples were one chicken sandwich, one egg plus bacon sandwich, one ham plus tomato sandwich, and two chicken plus salad sandwiches. In the United Kingdom, sandwiches sold at a hospital shop caused four cases of hospital-acquired listeriosis over a 2-month period.

Salmonella (3752, 3931, 4324, 4800, 5112). Snacks and sandwiches have been reported vehicles. In the United Kingdom, Israel, Canada, and the United States in 1994–1995, *Salmonella* enterica serovar Agona in a peanut-flavored, ready-to-eat "kosher" snack manufactured in Israel caused ≥85 cases. In Canada in 1998, sandwiches were implicated in an outbreak of *S. enterica* serovar Heidelberg, and prepackaged lunch was implicated in an outbreak of serovar Enteritidis. In the United Kingdom in 1989, 47 cases of unusual serovar Manchester were traced to savory corn snacks and back to yeast powder and flavorings. In Germany in 1993, serovars Javiana, Rubislaw, and Saintpaul in paprika-powdered potato chips caused a nationwide outbreak with ~1,000 cases. Snacks contained 0.04–0.45 agents per g, and the estimated infective dose was ~4–45 agents. In the United Kingdom in 2000, egg mayonnaise sandwiches were implicated in a hospital outbreak of serovar Indiana with 17 cases among staff, relatives, and patients.

Shigella (3222). Cold sandwiches were implicated in a *S. sonnei* outbreak aboard aircrafts.

S. aureus (6251). In Rhode Island in 1990, centrally prepared lunches were vehicles for an outbreak of staphylococcal food poisoning in five elementary schools, for attack rates of 18–47%.

S. pyogenes (group A *Streptococcus* [GAS]) (1468, 4379). Vehicles in outbreaks of GAS pharyngitis included egg salad sandwiches. In Sweden in 1990, sliced-egg sandwiches caused an outbreak of GAS pharyngitis that affected 72% (122/169) attendees of a church party.

PROTOZOA
Giardia (8074). Sandwiches were implicated in a nursing home outbreak of *G. lamblia*.

9.2 MENUS AND ETHNIC FOODS
International cuisines are standard menus that are widely available, including Chinese, French, Italian, and Mexican recipes and dishes, from French fries, to noodle soups, pizzas, and tacos. Ethnic cuisines are customary, locally or seasonally relished dishes.

Infections. Hazards from ethnic foods derive from raw ingredients (for milk, see section 7.1; for egg, see section 7.2; for meats, see section 7.4; for seafoods, see section 7.5; viscera), prions in high-risk organs (brain, marrow, and eyes from bovines), home-preserved foods, and privately butchered, noninspected meats. In Australia in 1995–2000, specialty or ethnic foods accounted for 2% (5/214) of food-borne outbreaks and 0.6% (46/8,124) of cases (1721).

INTERNATIONAL CUISINE
Epidemiologists and microbiologists rightly aim to identify and report specific food vehicles. From this, a bias toward underreporting of mixed foods (menus) may result. Reported vehicles include cheesecakes, lasagnes, quiches, soups, and tacos. In U.S. schools in 1973–1997, Mexican-style foods accounted for 6% of 218 food-borne outbreaks with a single known vehicle (1738). In the United Kingdom, 6% (157/2,354) of ready-to-eat quiche were of unsatisfactory (high aerobic colony counts) quality and two were unacceptable for *E. coli* concentrations >10^4 CFU/g (2740).

Norovirus. In Australia in 2004, pizza from a nationally franchised fast-food chain was the likely the vehicle for an outbreak with seven cases (2962). Clear soup (consommé) with vermicelli (tiny pasta) contaminated by a chef was implicated in an outbreak at a banquet that caused 57 (74%) cases among 77 attendees (3600).

Clostridium. Reported vehicles of *C. botulinum* include soups, dips, and sauces (7014). In Australia in 2004, meat pizza from a nationally franchised fast-food chain was the microbiologically confirmed vehicle for an outbreak of *C. perfringens* with six cases (2962).

***E. coli* (3655).** Beef tacos from a Mexican-style fast-food restaurant chain were implicated in the United States in 1999, in an outbreak of *E. coli* O157:H7 that caused 13 cases in three states.

Salmonella.

Outbreaks A typical vehicle in outbreaks are dishes that include eggs or cheese.

- North America (818, 1172). At a Chinese restaurant in El Paso, Tex. in 1993, *S. enterica* serovar Enteritidis in egg rolls caused two outbreaks with 19 cases. In California in 1997, cheesecake privately prepared from raw egg whites was implicated in a serovar Enteritidis outbreak that affected 13 of 17 exposed persons; on the farm that supplied the eggs, serovar Enteritidis was isolated from 4% (21/476) of environmental (manure, feed, and water) samples, and from 0.5% (1/200) of pooled egg samples. In the District of Columbia in 1997, serovar Enteritidis in commercial lasagne caused an outbreak that affected 43 of 75 exposed persons; ingredients included a mixture of raw shell eggs, cheeses, and spices. Traceback led to a farm where environmental samples from 5 of 13 poultry houses yielded serovar Enteritidis. In Arizona in 1998, serovar Enteritidis in chile rellenos served at four Mexican restaurants affected 58 persons; the rellenos consisted of raw egg white batter on roasted green chile peppers stuffed with cheese and were commercially prepared, cooked, packed, and frozen in Mexico.
- West Europe (2610, 5523). In Switzerland in 1986, spring rolls were a vehicle for serovar Typhimurium with 126 cases. In 1996, lasagne was implicated in an outbreak of serovar Enteritidis that affected 19 British guests at a tourist resort hotel; the lasagne had been made with fresh egg pasta.

***S. aureus* (6988, 8265).** Handling can inoculate *S. aureus* into tortillas, lasagne, and similar foods. Although heat kills *S. aureus*, enterotoxin is heat-resistant. At a pasta manufacturer in Italy, mishandled lasagne caused an international outbreak of staphylococcal food poisoning with 47 cases reported in the United Kingdom, and high levels of *S. aureus* in dried lasagne imported into France, Italy, Luxembourg, and the United Kingdom.

AFRICAN CUISINES

Street foods (2635, 4986, 6145). Popular street foods include "ful" in Egypt (fava beans, *Vicia faba*, in pocket bread), and "fufu" in Ghana (pounded cassava, *Manihot esculenta*, with plantain, *Musa paradisiaca*, yam, *Dioscorea* or cocoyam, *Colocasia esculenta*). Street-sold ice cream is a health hazard. In Accra, Ghana, street-prepared "fufu" was microbiologically unacceptable.

Fish (1141, 7993). In Egypt in 1991, "faseikh" (uneviscerated, salted, mullet of Mugilidae) caused 91 cases of type E botulism, including 18 (20%) deaths. Concentration of toxin titrated in two samples was 16,000 and 64,000 mouse lethal doses per g (a concentration of ~7,000/g is lethal for humans) (7993). Immigrants may retain traditional diets in arrival countries. In New Jersey in 1992, "moloha" (uneviscerated, salt-cured fish) caused four cases of type E botulism.

Exotic foods (4005, 5612). An odd vehicle for *C. botulinum* reported from Kenya are white ants (termites). In Benue state, Nigeria, meat from *Rattus norvegicus* "*is a delicacy*" and a reported vehicle of *Toxoplasma gondii*; the seroprevalence in this community is 57% (557/978).

AMERICAN CUISINES

Street and catered foods (2249, 2635, 3450, 7370, 7832). Popular street foods include "ceviche" (raw, marinated fish), "tortillas" (unleavened bread from corn, *Zea maïs*), and "empanadas" (beef-stuffed pastry). Street-sold ice cream in Latin America is a health hazard. In Huancayo, Peru, in 1988, "salchipapas" (fried potatoes, hot dogs, and eggs dressed with mayonnaise) served at a local restaurant caused 12 cases of type B botulism, including two (16%) deaths. In Buenos Aires, Argentina, in 1998, "matambre" (meat rolls sealed in heat-shrinked plastic wrap and stored in poorly working refrigerators) was the vehicle for type A botulism in 9 (41%) of 21 bus drivers. In San Antonio, Tex., in 1981, "barbacoa" (steamed bovine heads, with lips, ears, tongue, and eyes) served at a Mexican-style outlet caused 80 cases of typhoid fever; *S. enterica* serovar Typhi was isolated from the stool of 1 of 31 employees.

Meats (1174, 1214, 1305, 1776, 4885, 6027). Traditional diets of Arctic Natives (Inuit and Indians) include uncooked caribou meat that is a reported vehicle of *Brucella* and *Toxoplasma*, fermented walrus meat ("igunaq") that is a vehicle of *Trichinella nativa*, fermented skin with blubber ("muktuk"), and other fermented products that are vehicles of *C. botulinum* type E. In 1950–2000, Alaska recorded 226 cases of botulism, all in Alaska Natives and all from fermented foods. In 2001, fermented beaver tail and paw caused botulism in 7 of 14 consumers. In 2002, 8 of 14 persons who ate muktuk from a beached beluga whale contracted type E botulism.

Fish (1920, 2249, 2860, 4178, 4981, 5167, 7887). "Ceviche" (raw fish marinated in lemon or lime juice) and "callos" (pieces of raw fish fillet) are popular in much of Latin America. Ceviche is a reported vehicle of *Vibrio cholerae* (O1 and non-O1, non-O13), *Anisakis-Pseudoterranova*, and *Gnathostoma*.

Exotic foods (10, 4296). "Chitterlings" (raw sausages from pig intestines) that are traditionally prepared by some African-Americans for Thanksgiving and Christmas are a reported vehicle of *Yersinia enterocolitica*.

ASIAN CUISINES
Street and catered foods. Popular street foods include in Southwest Asia "falafel" (a snack from chick peas, *Cicer arietinum*) and "döner" (vertically grilled mutton) often in pita (flat bread), in Southcentral Asia "samosa" (pea-stuffed, fried, triangular pastry), and in Japan "yakitori" (grilled chicken on sticks).

Street-sold ice cream is a general health hazard (2635). In the Philippines, "pansit" (rice noodles with shrimp, meat, and vegetables) sold by street vendors is a vehicle for *V. cholerae* (4422). Similarly in Singapore, "sambal sotong" (cooked squid) is a vehicle for *V. cholerae* (2809). When including raw fish or seafood, sushi, a Japanese snack from vinegared cold rice, fresh fish or seafood, and algae or vegetables, can transmit viruses, bacteria, and helminths. In Queensland, Australia, in 2004, 12 patrons contracted *S. enterica* serovar Singapore from sushi outlets (451). In the United Kingdom in 1995, "kebab" and yoghurt relish were vehicles of a serovar Typhimurium outbreak with 22 cases (2265). In the United Kingdom in 1997, stir-fried food served at a "Hawaiian theme" restaurant was implicated in a *Campylobacter jejuni* outbreak that affected 12 (41%) of 29 customers. Inadequate cooking time of large chicken pieces were the suspected cause (2261).

Meats (1721, 1834, 3068, 7274). Raw meats are risky. In Lebanon, "kibbi" (a dish that may include raw meat) is a suspected vehicle of *Toxoplasma*. Also in Lebanon, raw pork served for "kubeniye" at Christmas or New Year is a vehicle of *Trichinella*. In 1995, ~200 inhabitants of a village (one fourth to one fifth of the population) were suspected to have contracted trichinellosis at kubeniye. Larvae of *T. spiralis* were identified in pork supplied by a local butcher. In Thailand "laembo" (raw pork) is a vehicle for *V. cholerae*. In People's Republic of China, "shengpi" and "oru" (raw pork) are vehicles of *Trichinella*. In Victoria, Australia, in 1997, Asian-style pork rolls that include eggs, chicken liver pâté, and pork caused an outbreak of serovar Typhimurium with 862 cases.

Fish and seafood. Raw products are popular in Asia.

- Southwest Asia. In Israel and the United States in 1987, "kapchunka" or "ribbetz" (uneviscerated, salted air-dried whitefish) caused eight cases of type E botulism; fish viscera appeared to provide a low-salt anaerobic environment suitable for *C. botulinum* (6958, 7400).

- Southeast Asia. In Thailand, raw fish is an ingredient of many traditional dishes, including "pla som," "lab pla," "yum," and "koi-pla" (groundup raw fish, occasionally given to babies). Contrary to common belief, salt or vinegar do not eliminate risks of trematode infections from raw fish (8236). In Singapore, "ikan bilis" (dried anchovies in porridge) was the vehicle for 33 cases of multiresistant *S. enterica* serovar Typhimurium infections, mainly in small children (4447). Chinese in Singapore relish raw or partially cooked cockles, as such ("see-hum") or ingredients to "satay bee hon" or "laksa"; shellfish-borne HA attack rates are higher in Chinese than Malays and Indians who do not have this preference (5110). In the Philippines "bagsit" (small *Hypseleotris bipartite* fish eaten raw in a single bite) is a vehicle of *Capillaria philippensis* (1648), and "kilawen" (raw fish, shrimps, and molluscs in vinegar, salt, and spices) is a vehicle for *Echinostoma* (2884).

- East Asia (336, 1368, 1408, 3583, 6570). In Korea, "marcgulee" (sliced raw freshwater fish coated with hot bean paste) is customary in rural areas and implicated in *Clonorchis sinensis* transmission. Preference for marcgulee by males explains higher infection rates in males than females. "Kejang" (freshwater crabs soaked in soybean sauce) are a traditional dish and an implicated vehicle for *Paragonimus*. In Japan, "sashimi" (raw fish or seafood) served at sushi bars or at homes, carries risks of raw seafood, including diphyllobothriasis and acute anisakiasis. Recently, *Diphyllobothrium latum* infections acquired from sashimi were detected in São Paulo, Brazil.

- Pacific. In Hawaii, "lomi-lomi" (raw salmon) is a traditional Polynesian dish.

Dairy (126). In Yemen, "laban" (buttermilk) carries a significant risk of brucellosis.

Exotic foods. In some Islamic countries, raw or lightly heated liver dishes (marra or umfitfit) are customary and reported vehicles of *Bacillus anthracis* (613) and *Brucella* (564, 4690, 5119). In Turkey in 1988, two families contracted giardiasis from sheep tripe in a soup (3823). Many paratenic hosts can harbor larvae of *Toxocara* in viscera and tissues, and raw giblets from chicken (5310), lamb (6548), and pig (7351) are reported sources of toxocariasis.

Dog meat is a vehicle for *Trichinella* in People's Republic of China (1672, 2082, 7952). In People's Republic of China, 8 (1.5%) of 548 trichinellosis outbreaks in 1964–1999 were due to dog meat. Raw, scalded, roasted, or semicooked dog meat caused nine outbreaks with 59 cases (6–7 per outbreak), mainly in northeast People's Republic of China. In Kunming City, Yunnan Province, four (4%) of dog meat samples sold at markets yielded *Trichinella* larvae.

In East Asia, traditional medicines or sources of foods include snakes, frogs (legs and raw liver), and toads. Consumed raw, amphibians, and reptiles can be vehicles of *Angiostrongylus cantonensis* (6626) and *Gnathostoma* (2860, 5353, 5553).

In Australia, in a *Toxoplasma* outbreak that involved 12 acute infections in adults and one congenital infection, the implicated vehicle were "rare kangaroo medaillons" (6345).

EUROPEAN CUISINES

Street and catered foods. Popular street foods include in Germany "Bratwurst" and in Greece gyros (grilled meat). At a ceremony in Sweden, "landgång" (a "smorgasbord" that contains shrimps with mayonnaise, liver pâté, ham, sausage, and legume salad) was vehicle for an outbreak of *Aeromonas* food poisoning that affected 24 of 27 attendees (4118).

Meats. Raw beef in strips ("carpaccio," from Venezian painter V. Carpaccio, 1450–1525) is a potential vehicle of *E. coli* (EHEC). Raw, fermented pork sausage ("Mettwurst") in Germany (6190) and raw or lightly heated horse meat in France and Italy have caused trichinellosis outbreaks.

Fish and seafoods. In Spain, "boquerones en vinagre" (pickled raw anchovies) are a vehicle of *Anisakis* (336, 6226). In northern Europe, raw, smoked, or marinated herring ("green" or "soused" herring, "gravlax," "kipper," "maatje") is a historical or extant vehicle of *Anisakis* (336, 7751). Smoked eel is a reported vehicle of *Salmonella*. In an outbreak of unusual *S. enterica* serovar Blockley in Germany in 1998, 75% (9/12) of cases but only 10% (2/21) of controls gave a history of eating smoked eel, for an odds ratio of 29 (95% CI 4–235); the eel was traced to fish farms in Italy (2353).

Exotic foods. In France, "rillettes" (pâté-like, ready-to-eat pork) and pork tongue in jelly are vehicles of *L. monocytogenes*, having caused outbreaks in 1992 with 279 cases (including 92 pregnancy related) (3623), in 1993 with 38 cases (31 maternoneonatal, 7 nonpregnant adults) (2877), and in 1999–2000 with a total of 42 cases (1844). Other exotic dishes include "andouillettes" (sausages from pig trip and mesentery) in France and kidney pie in the United Kingdom.

10
Drinking Water and Other Beverages

10.1 Bottled waters and ice
10.2 Municipal high-income tap water
10.3 Private and low-income water supplies

Drinking water is water from taps, fountains, or other sources that is purified or naturally safe for drinking. Supplies can be municipal (public, piped, delivered year-round, for >1,000 customers) or private. In high-income countries, most (>90%) customers are connected to municipal supplies. Beverages include bottled water, soft drinks, fruit and vegetable juices, and ice. Technically, drinking water and beverages are foods.

Exposure (468, 3503, 4286, 6542, 7851, 8273). A minimum quantity for domestic needs is 15 liters per person per day. A traditional indicator of drinking water quality is *Escherichia coli* that should not be found in 100-ml samples. However, viruses and protozoa have been detected in drinking water free of *E. coli*. Wildlife, domestic animals, and runoff can fecally pollute sources and reservoirs, and leaks, failed sewer pumps, and negative pipe pressure can pollute water in pipes. Biofilms in dead-end pipes support *Legionella* and environmental mycobacteria that are resistant to standard dose disinfectants.

Infections (682, 2774, 3164, 4286, 7851, 8117). Drinking water and other beverages can carry viruses, bacteria, protozoa, and helminths (Box 10.1 and Table 10.1). Concentrations are typically low and correspond to low infective doses: 1–10 viruses, 1–100 protozoa, or a few hundred bacteria.

In Devon in the 1840s–1870s, W. Budd (1811–1880) discovered that typhoid fever was due to a contagious matter discharged with feces and that lemonade water polluted by a leaking cesspool was responsible for a hotel outbreak. In London in the 1850s, J. Snow (1813–1858) concluded that cholera spread via drinking water.

Preventive measures include source protection (well and groundwater), water purification (sedimentation, filtration, and chemical), pipe mainenance, clean storage and home use, and a rolling boil to inactivate viruses, for 1 min (at sea level) to 3 min (at elevations >2,000 m).

Exposure history (Box III.1). Inquire about the type of water supply (municipal or private), failure (no flow, foul odor, and brown color), and habitual use, such as tap water for drinking, mineral water for brushing teeth, fresh juices from street vendors, ice cubes, and canned soft drinks. An agent that causes malodorous drinking water is *Pseudomonas aeruginosa*. Technically unexplained

> **Box 10.1** Agents from drinking water
>
> High-income municipal supplies
>
> - Main agents from temporary failure: HAV, *Norovirus*; *Campylobacter*, *E. coli*, *Salmonella*, *Shigella*; *Cryptosporidium*, *Giardia*
> - Unusual hazards, mainly for groups at risk (children and immune-impaired patients): *Enterovirus*; *Acinetobacter*, *Legionella*, environmental mycobacteria, nontoxigenic *V. cholerae* O1, *Y. enterocolitica*, *P. aeruginosa*; microsporidia; *Cyclospora*, *Naegleria*, *Toxoplasma*
>
> Untreated private and low-income supplies: seasonal or endemic risk from all above, plus
>
> - Enteric adenovirus, HEV, human astroviruses, poliovirus (endemic areas), *Rotavirus*
> - *Aeromonas*, *B. pseudomallei*, *Francisella*, *Helicobacter*, *Leptospira*, *Plesiomonas*, *S. enterica* serovar Typhi, *Streptobacillus*, toxigenic *V. cholerae* O1
> - *Balantidium coli*, *E. histolytica*
> - *Dracunculus*, *Fasciola*

outbreaks or unusual agents should be the alert for intentional release and bioterror.

10.1 BOTTLED WATERS AND ICE
BOTTLED AND MINERAL WATERS

Mineral water is groundwater that contains sodium, calcium, magnesium, and other minerals. Bottled water is water intended for drinking and filled in sealed bottles. For milk drinks, see section 7.1.

Exposure. In the United States, consumption of bottled water per person per year was 9 liters in 1980 and 67 liters in 1999. For coffee, the figures were 101 liters (1980), 100 liters (2000), and 92 liters (2001) (http://www.census.gov/prod/2004pubs/03statab/health.pdf). In eight U.S. states in 2000, 12–27% (mean, 20%) of 13,113 respondents in a representative sample reported commercial, bottled water as their primary source of drinking water (http://www.cdc.gov/foodnet/surveys/Pop_surv.htm).

Infections (5824, 7578). Bottled, branded, carbonated, and unopened water is mostly safe. Commensals in bottled water could indicate fecal pollution. In Taiwan, 74 (54%) of 136 of bottled, uncarbonated mineral water samples did not meet standards for heterotrophic counts. In the United Kingdom in 2001, a supplier of bottled mineral water had to withdraw products after fecal indicators were isolated from stored samples. Rarely have outbreaks been associated with bottled water. An emerging potential risk is enteric viruses in bottled water.

Viruses
Hepatitis A virus (HAV) (7207). In Italy in 1988–1989, in an outbreak with 47 acute hepatitis A (HA) cases, raw mussels or a single brand of mineral water was implicated.

***Norovirus* (628).** In Switzerland, *Norovirus* was amplified from 11 European brands of mineral waters by reverse transcriptase-PCR. Minerals, carbonic acid, and pH did not correlate with viral RNA. Samples from three noncarbonated brands were monitored weekly for 1 year, and 33% (53/159) samples tested positive for RNA at least once. Levels were estimated at 10–100 genomic

Table 10.1 Outbreaks from drinking water by known infectious disease agents in high-income countries[a]

Organism	United States, 1990–2002[b] No. of outbreaks	United States, 1990–2002[b] No. of cases	United Kingdom, 1970–2000 No. of outbreaks	Sweden, 1986–1996 No. of outbreaks
Giardia	31	2,892	1	4
Norovirus	12	3,335		4
Cryptosporidium	11	5,269	33	1
Escherichia coli	11	504	1	
Shigella	8	605		
Campylobacter	7	1,134	17	8
Legionella	6	80		
Hepatitis A virus	5	90		1
Salmonella	3	833	1	
Other infectious agents[c]	7	106		2

[a]From references 682, 2375, and 6532 and previous issues.
[b]Excludes outbreaks from recreational waters and the 1993 Milwaukee *Cryptosporidium* outbreak (403,000 cases).
[c]*Aeromonas*, *Plesiomonas*, *Vibro cholerae* non-O1, *Yersinia enterocolitica*, microsporidia, and *Entamoeba histolytica*.

equivalents per liter. When stored in darkness at room temperature, RNA persisted in 10/10 positive samples for 6 months and in 9/10 samples for 12 months.

Bacteria

Bottled waters may yield agents that are considered innocuous for oral uptake by immune-competent individuals, e.g., *Acinetobacter, Aeromonas, Alcaligenes, P. aeruginosa,* and *Stenotrophomonas.* However, noncarbonated bottled water may be a source of resistant *Stenotrophomonas maltophilia* in immune-impaired hosts (8175).

Campylobacter **(2263, 2742).** In the United Kingdom, epidemiological studies have suggested a risk from bottled water. In 2001, 114 (54%) of 213 sporadic cases reported drinking bottled water compared with 420 (37%) of 1,144 controls, for an odds ratio of 2 (95% confidence interval [95% CI] 1.5–2.7). Also, 64% (150/272) of *C. coli* cases reported drinking bottled water compared with 54% (1,646/3,489) of *C. jejuni* cases, for an odds ratio of 1.5 (95% CI 1.1–2). The associations seemed plausible because raw water has yielded *C. coli.*

Salmonella enterica. **Non-Typhi serovars (4310).** In a multistate outbreak of serovar Bareilly in the United States in 2000, water from private wells as well as water bottled by one facility were implicated. **Serovar Typhi (1092, 2840).** In the capital city and several states of Mexico in 1972–1973, a typhoid epidemic caused 13,578 reported cases; contaminated water bottled by one company was the suspected source. In this outbreak, chloramphenicol-resistant serovar Typhi was detected.

Vibrio cholerae **(688).** During a cholera epidemic in Portugal in 1974, *V. cholerae* was isolated from two springs that supplied mineral water to a commercial bottling plant; significantly more cases than controls were found to have consumed bottled, noncarbonated water.

Protozoa

Cryptosporidium **(2494, 5416).** By molecular methods, oocysts can be detected in mineral waters. In commercial brands of mineral water in São Paulo, Brazil, detected concentrations were 0.2–0.5 per liter.

Amebas (5824). Because free-living amebas have been reported from bottled water, the routine use of bottled water for rinsing contact lenses is not advised.

ICE CUBES

Infections (96, 3952, 4049). The quality of ice is a result of the quality of source water, manufacturing, and handling. Ice-producing machines need regular maintenance. Ice from street vendors is a health hazard. Demonstration of ice as a vehicle for infections can be confounded by contaminated beverages. Ice has been implicated in outbreaks of *Enterovirus, Norovirus, E. coli* (enterotoxigenic *E. coli* [ETEC]), and *S. enterica* serovar Typhi.

Viruses

Enterovirus **(3548).** In 1991, an outbreak of coxsackievirus B1 pleurodynia among football players was linked to eating ice cubes from the team's ice chest and to drinking cooler water.

Norovirus **(716, 1059, 2431, 3912, 5793).** Ice cubes were implicated in several outbreaks, and drinks with ice were established as a significant risk. In Andorra in 2002, the diarrhea attack rate among ski holidaymakers from Ireland was 39% in 136 consumers of drinks with ice cubes compared with 21% in 79 ice nonconsumers, for a relative risk of 1.9 (95% CI 1.2–3). Ice produced in Pennsylvania and served in Delaware (at a fund-raiser) and Philadelphia (a football game) was implicated in 191 diarrhea cases, for an overall attack rate of 31% (191/614). In New York state in 1986, ice was implicated in two *Norovirus* outbreaks, one at a restaurant that affected 50% of ~700 patrons, and one at a graduation party that affected 26 (30%) of 87 attendees.

Bacteria

Ice has potential for transmitting all waterborne agents, including *Salmonella* and *Vibrio.*

E. coli **(1739, 2289, 5415).** Enteroaggregative *E. coli* has been identified from commercial ice samples. In the United Kingdom, 1% of ice samples used to cool drinks at retail and catering premises grew *E. coli.* Ice cubes from bunkered water were implicated in three ETEC outbreaks aboard cruise ships, with a total of 1,349 diarrhea cases.

Mycobacterium **(2684, 4170).** Ice machines can be a source of environmental mycobacteria such as *M. fortuitum.*

S. enterica **serovar Typhi (679, 2652).** In Semarang, Indonesia, in 1992–1994, consuming ice or purchasing ice from street venders was a significant risk in 75 culture-confirmed typhoid cases compared with 75 randomly selected, age- and sex-matched neighbor controls. In Chile in 1980–1981, purchased, flavored ice was a significant risk for 81 culture-confirmed typhoid cases in individuals 3–14 years of age who were compared with an equal number of age- and sex-matched neighbor controls.

V. cholerae **(4049, 6269).** Risks for *V. cholerae* include ice-containing beverages and flavored ices (helados) offered by street venders in cholera-endemic areas.

Protozoa

In Denmark, an incontinent and psychotic *Cryptosporidium* carrier caused a nosocomial outbreak by picking ice from a machine (6148).

In Washington State in 1990, circumstantial evidence suggested ice as the vehicle in a giardiasis outbreak; the employee who had served ice to ill attendees had a diapered child who shed *Giardia* (6051).

JUICES

Fruit and vegetable juices are cold, nonalcoholic, fresh, pasteurized, or preserved plant fluids, e.g., from apple, grape, grapefruit, lemon, lime, orange, pineapple, or tomato. Cider is freshly pressed apple juice that may or may not be fermented.

Consumption. In the United States, consumption of fruit juices per person per year was 30 liters in 1980, 33 liters in 2000, and 32 liters in 2001. The corresponding figures for vegetable juices remained constant at about 1 liter per person per year (http://www.census.gov/prod/2004pubs/03statab/health.pdf). In eight U.S. states in 2000, 8–19% (mean, 13%) of 13,113 respondents reported consumption of unpasteurized orange juice within 7 days, and 3–5% reported consumption of apple juice or cider (http://www.cdc.gov/foodnet/surveys/Pop_surv.htm).

Infections. Nonpasteurized fruit juices have been reported vehicles of HAV, *Bacillus cereus*, *E. coli*, *Salmonella*, *Shigella*, *V. cholerae*, and *Cryptosporidium*.

Viruses

HAV (2499). At a resort in Hurghada, Egypt, in 2004, in an outbreak with 351 acute HA cases in tourists from nine countries of western Europe, fruit juice from the breakfast buffet was a significant vehicle consumed by 82% of cases and 64% of controls, for an odds ratio of 2.6 (95% CI 1.1–7). Cases drank orange juice on significantly more days than controls. A non-significant association was found for grapefruit juice. Fruit juices were not heat treated, and supplier hygiene was deficient.

Bacteria

***B. cereus* (7314).** At at French police school, orange juice concentrate was the vehicle for an outbreak with 43 cases.

***E. coli* (618, 1495, 3321, 5112).** Fresh or unpasteurized cider has been a reported vehicle of *E. coli* O157 (enterohemorrhagic *E. coli*). In the United States in 1996, *E. coli* O157:H7 in unpasteurized apple juice caused 70 infections; of these, 25 (36%) patients were hospitalized, 14 (20%) developed hemolytic-uremic syndrome, and 1 (1%) died (1495).

***Francisella tularensis* (1272).** At a geriatric home in Czechia in 1978, juice from fallen, rodent-contaminated apples caused an outbreak with 103 tularemia cases in 3 weeks.

***S. enterica*. Non-Typhi serovars (715, 1557, 4096, 5112).** In 1999, *S. enterica* serovar Muenchen in unpasteurized orange juice caused 207 confirmed infections in 15 of the U.S. states and 2 provinces of Canada. In 1995, serovar Hartford in unpasteurized orange juice served at an Orlando, Fla., theme park caused 62 infections in 21 of the U.S. states. In Florida in 1999, commercial orange juice was implicated in an outbreak of serovar Anatum with several cases. Juice from the production line grew coliforms and tested positive for *Salmonella* antigen. ***S. enterica* serovar Typhi (657, 3846).** At a New York hotel in 1989, a carrier preparing orange juice caused an outbreak with 43 confirmed and 24 probable typhoid fever cases, for attack rates of 31% (26/85) among juice consumers and 5% (1/20) among nonconsumers. In Florida in 1998–1999, a contaminated fruit shake caused one probable and 15 confirmed typhoid cases; the vehicle was frozen mamey (*Manilkara zapota*, Sapotecaceae) fruit imported from Central America.

***Shigella* (7474).** An outbreak of *Shigella flexneri* from fresh orange juice has been reported among visitors to a game reserve in South Africa.

***V. cholerae* (5242, 7368).** In the United States in 1991, four of six persons attending a picnic contracted toxigenic *V. cholerae* O1 from commercially sold fresh coconut milk imported from Thailand. In Peru, an acidic (pH 4.1) drink made from "toronja" (a citrus fruit) was protective; protection increased with increasing quantity of toronja consumed.

Protozoa

***Cryptosporidium* (5046).** In Maine in 1998, fresh cider served at an agricultural fair caused illness in 160 of 759 attendees, for an attack rate of 21%. Oocysts were identified in cider, cider press, and stool of a calf on the farm that supplied apples.

***Trypanosoma cruzi* (1599).** The light at palm presses operated at night can attract triatomine bugs. Bug feces are an unusual but plausible source of *T. cruzi* in palm juice and its consumers.

Helminths

In Taiwan in 2001, five of a family of 10 contracted eosinophilic meningitis due to *Angiostrongylus cantonensis* from daily drinking raw vegetable juice for constipation and health (7579).

SOFT DRINKS

Soft drinks are cold, flavored, carbonated, nonalcoholic beverages such as lemonades. In the United States, consumption of soft drinks per person per year was 133 liters in 1980 (2.5 liters per week) and 187 liters (3.5 liters per week) in 2000 (http://www.census.gov/prod/2004pubs/03statab/health.pdf).

Carbonated, canned, or bottled soft drinks are safe. A rare outbreak was reported at an army facility in Texas in 1998, where soda water from a dispenser was implicated in a *Norovirus* outbreak with 99 infections among trainees (283). In contrast, mass complaints at five Belgian schools in 1999 ascribed to a soft drink were likely "sociogenic" (2590).

In contrast, open street beverages are a health hazard in low-income countries (4049, 6269, 6591). In Guatemala in 1993, in 26 hospitalized, urban cholera cases and 52 age-, sex-, and neighborhood-matched controls, consumption of street-vended, noncarbonated beverages was a significant risk. In Puebla, Mexico, 7 (26%) of 27 street fruit drinks tested positive for *Entamoeba histolytica/dispar*, 1 (4%) for *Giardia lamblia*, 13 (48%) for *Trichuris trichiura*, and 4 (15%) for *Ascaris lumbricoides*.

10.2 MUNICIPAL HIGH-INCOME TAP WATER

Municipal supplies (468, 682, 6532, 8117) in high-income countries are safe most of the time. Temporary breakdowns can cause outbreaks. In Europe in 11 years (1986–1996), 17 countries reported 710 waterborne disease outbreaks (four per country per year), with an average number of 220 cases per outbreak (range, 2–3,500). By area and diagnostic workup, major agents are *Norovirus*, *Cryptosporidium*, *E. coli*, and *Campylobacter* (Table 10.1). In the United States in 1990-2002, numbers/outbreak were largest for *Cryptosporidium* (479, excluding the 403,000 Milwaukee cases), *Norovirus*, and *Salmonella* (~280, each).

VIRUSES

Highly sensitive tests are becoming available that should improve detection of waterborne viruses (626, 6234, 7851) (Box 10.1). By adsorption, precipitation, and nested PCR, human adenoviruses have been detected in 5% (10/188) treated drinking water samples in South Africa (7732).

HAV (468, 2375, 4180, 6851).
HAV from human feces can pollute defective municipal supplies. Outbreaks of HAV from high-income municipal drinking water supplies have become rare (Table10.1). In Europe in 1986–1996, several waterborne disease outbreaks were attributed to HAV, including in Croatia, Czechia, Estonia, Latvia, Malta, Romania, Slovakia, Slovenia, but mainly in Spain. Among French military recruits in 1992–1993, drinking tap water was a risk.

Norovirus (2375, 5144).
Norovirus in small amounts of human feces can pollute defective municipal supplies over long distances. The agent can pass through simple filters and resists regular chlorination.

Outbreaks *Norovirus* is a significant cause of waterborne disease outbreaks (Table 10.1). Because of diagnostic difficulties, *Norovirus* is underrepresented in the statistics of the 1990s (in Europe in 1986–1996, only Sweden reported *Norovirus* outbreaks). Municipal waterborne outbreaks have been reported recently.

- United States (682). At a golf course in Arizona in July 2002, 71 cases (probably facilitated by poorly maintained water dispensers and ice machines) were reported.
- Europe (716, 939, 1097, 4136, 4849). At a tourist resort in southern Italy there were 275 cases among guests (attack rate, 9–11%) and 69 among staff (attack rate, 38%). In a Swiss township there were 1,600 cases among 3,360 inhabitants, in a United Kingdom bakery there were 30 cases among employees (attack rate, 23%), in a Finnish township there were 1,700–3,000 cases per 4,860 inhabitants, and in a Swedish ski resort there were ~500 cases.

Rotavirus (3420).
Outbreaks by municipal waters appear to be rare in high-income countries. In a township in Colorado, a waterborne outbreak caused 41 cases among 128 residents for an attack rate of 32%.

BACTERIA

Water standards and purification technologies have greatly reduced bacterial risks from drinking water, keeping municipal supplies clean most of the time (468, 8117) (Box 10.1). Increasing maintenance costs and biofilms that support growth of environmental mycobacteria and of *Legionella* in hot-water systems are emerging threats, however. Also, immune-impaired hosts may be susceptible to opportunistic bacteria.

Although *Legionella* has been recovered from drinking water supplies, infections result from aerosols or aspiration rather than drinking (for buildings, see section 6.2). Similarly, *Pseudomonas aeruginosa* infections in immunecompetent individuals result from contact rather than ingestion.

Acinetobacter baumannii (8117).
A. baumannii has been demonstrated in 5–90% of tap-water samples at low

concentrations (about 8/100 ml). Oral uptake of this agent by immune-competent persons is considered innocuous.

***B. cereus* (8117).** *B. cereus* is readily demonstrated in water, but "waterborne food poisoning" has not been documented.

***Campylobacter* (157, 168, 2208, 5519).** Sources of fecal pollution by *Campylobacter* include livestock grazing on water-capture land, birds using reservoirs, and, for humans, leaks in pipes and repair work. *Campylobacter* has been isolated from water in outbreaks. In Sweden, long water pipes and dense ruminants paralleled increased infection rates. Drinking untreated water is a risk.

Outbreaks Of all waterborne outbreaks in high-income countries with a known agent, 2–10% were attributed to *Campylobacter* (468, 682, 2541).

- United States (6510, 7858). In Vermont in 1978, municipal water caused an outbreak with 3,000 cases, for an attack rate of 19%. In Florida in 1983, municipal water caused an outbreak with ~865 cases; attack rates increased with the increasing amount of water consumed, from 9% to 56%.
- New Zealand (7137). In 1990, an outbreak at a modern convention center caused 44 cases, for an attack rate of 44%.
- Europe (2208, 2541, 4162, 4967, 4968). In Norway, in summer of 1984, 680 of 1,000 inhabitants of a town contracted *C. jejuni* from polluted tap water. In northern Norway in 1988, at latitude 70°N, an outbreak caused 330 (15%) cases among 2,200 exposed inhabitants. In Denmark in the winter of 1995–1996, *C. jejuni* in the water caused ~2,400 cases, for attack rates of 50–88%. In the United Kingdom in 1995–1999, *Campylobacter* caused four waterborne outbreaks. In a municipality in northern Finland in August 1998, 442 inhabitants contracted *C. jejuni* enteritis from drinking unboiled tap water, for an attack rate of 19% among consumers; repair work at the mains was the likely source of contamination.

***Escherichia* (1514, 5475).** *E. coli* in drinking water is an indicator of fecal pollution. Irregularities of water supply may herald risk.

Outbreaks Waterborne outbreaks have been reported, including for enterohemorrhagic and enteroinvasive *E. coli* and ETEC.

- United States (1161, 5603, 6408, 7281). At Crater Lake National Park in Oregon in 1975, waterborne ETEC caused >2,200 cases. In a township in rural Missouri in 1989–1990, *E. coli* in unchlorinated water caused 243 cases, including 86 with dysentery and 2 with hemolytic-uremic syndrome. In 1998, *E. coli* O157:H7 from unchlorinated municipal water in Alpine, Wyo., caused 157 cases in 15 states, including four with hemolytic-uremic syndrome, for attack rates of 23% in residents and 50% in visitors. At a fair near Albany, N. Y., in 1999, attended by >100,000 persons, at least 10 children contracted *E. coli* O157:H7 diarrhea, probably from contaminated well water.
- Europe (3731). In Fife, Scotland, fecally polluted water supply caused an outbreak of *Campylobacter* and *E. coli* O157 with 633 cases.

Klebsiella pneumoniae. *K. pneumoniae* naturally inhabits nutrient-rich waters. The agent is considered innocuous when taken up orally by immune-competent individuals.

***Mycobacterium* (1610, 1715, 2297, 7490, 7511, 7869, 8393).** Piped water is a reservoir for environmental mycobacteria that form biofilms on pipe walls and silicone tubings. Isolates from drinking water include *Mycobacterium avium* complex, *M. avium paratuberculosis*, *M. chelonae*, *M. fortuitum*, *M. kansasii*, *M. malmoense*, *M. marinum*, *M. mucogenicum* (*chelonae*-like), *M. scrofulaceum*, and *M. xenopi*. By test (culture and nucleic acid amplification test [NAT]), mycobacteria have been identified in 30–35% of samples from public drinking-water supplies and in 54% of ice samples. *M. avium* complex resists conventional chlorine treatment. Environmental mycobacteria are of concern for immune-impaired hosts who are advised to boil tap water for drinking, e.g., as tea. At a hospital in Atlanta, Ga., *M. avium* complex disease correlated well with isolates from hospital hot water.

***Salmonella* (232, 682, 4310, 6532).** In high-income countries, *S. enterica* serovar non-Typhi accounts for 0–4% of waterborne disease outbreaks (Table 10.2). In a Missouri township in 1993, *S. enterica* serovar Typhimurium in unchlorinated municipal water caused an outbreak with 650 cases; the town water reservoir was found to be accessible to birds.

After C. J. Eberth (1835–1926) reported serovar Typhi in 1880, waterborne typhoid hit Chicago in 1891, causing nearly 2,000 deaths. "There is no excitement among the inhabitants of the city on the score of typhoid fever" wrote an observer in 1892. The situation has changed, and in the twenty-first century, most typhoid fever cases in high-income countries are imported.

Outbreaks Waterborne outbreaks have been reported in North America and Europe.

- North America (880, 2350, 5355). Reports of *Salmonella* outbreaks include Monark Springs, Mo., in 1956, with 34 cases and an attack rate of 6%; Audrain, Mo., in 1968 with 25 cases and an attack rate of 23%; a

migrant worker camp in Florida in 1973, with 201 culture-confirmed and 29 probable cases, for an attack rate of 13%; and a tourist resort in Quebec province, Canada, in 1976 with 137 cases.
- Europe (468, 602). In Zermatt, Switzerland, in 1963, a waterborne outbreak of *Salmonella* caused 437 international cases and 3 (0.7%) deaths. In 1986–1996, 45 presumably waterborne outbreaks of typhoid fever were reported, mainly from Albania and Spain.

***Shigella* (130, 468, 469, 4849)**. Temporary failures of municipal supplies have caused waterborne outbreaks of *Shigella* in the United States and Europe. In Europe in 1986–1996, 191 waterborne outbreaks were reported to be due to "bacterial dysentery," mainly in Albania, Croatia, Estonia, Hungary, Romania, Slovakia, Slovenia, and Spain.

***Tsukamurella* (8117)**. *T. paurometabola* is an occasional spillover from sedimentation tanks and activated sludge. This agent is a cause of invasive disease in immune-impaired hosts.

***Vibrio* (468, 4091, 8117)**. Waterborne *V. cholerae* O1 is largely controlled in high-income countries. In Europe in 1986–1996, several waterborne outbreaks were attributed to cholera, mainly in Romania in 1991–1993 (286 cases), Albania in 1994 (626 cases), and Ukraine in 1994–1995 (1,370 cases). Implicated sources included sewage spill and contaminated surface water. In the twenty-first century, however, most cholera in high-income countries is imported. In contrast, nontoxigenic *V. cholerae* O1 can be isolated from surface and coastal waters in temperate climates, occasionally also from tap water.

***Yersinia enterocolitica* (682, 5651, 8117)**. Fecally polluted drinking water is a likely source of human infections. In Bavaria, *Y. enterocolitica* was isolated from 82 (5%) of 1,650 municipal water samples, including serogroup O3 pathogenic to humans.

FUNGI
Microsporidia (1596, 2008, 2480). *Encephalitozoon intestinalis*, *Enterocytozoon bieneusi*, and other microsporidia have been amplified from surface water, groundwater, sludge, and municipal water in Guatemala. Drinking water is a suspected vehicle. In France, in the summer of 1995, water was implicated in a microsporidiosis outbreak among human immunodeficiency virus-infected persons, for an attack rate of 1%. Although the outbreak did not meet all criteria for waterborne spread, water was the only common vehicle.

PROTOZOA
Cysts and oocysts may resist ordinary treatments. *Cryptosporidium* and *Giardia* are significant agents of high-income municipal water outbreaks.

***Cyclospora* (2008, 3285, 3469)**. *C. cayetanensis* has been isolated in municipal water in Guatemala, and drinking water is a suspected vehicle. At a hospital dormitory in Chicago in 1990, stagnant water from a tank was the suspected source of *C. cayetanensis* for an outbreak among staff with 21 cases.

***Cryptosporidium* (468, 621, 3164, 5416)**. Human and animal feces are sources of *Cryptosporidium* oocysts in drinking water. Oocysts can be detected in municipal water by screening large volumes (100–1,000 liters) with sensitive, molecular methods. Typical densities are 4,000 oocysts per 100 liters of untreated water, and 0.1/100 liters of filtered water. Oocysts resist ordinary chlorination, and combination methods (coagulation, sedimentation, and filtration) are necessary for their removal.

Drinking tap water is a confirmed risk (251, 2813, 3505), in particular, for AIDS patients. In the United Kingdom, the risk of sporadic cryptosporidiosis increased with glasses of tap water consumed at home each day.

Outbreaks (468, 682, 1631, 2559, 3447, 4600, 6532) (Table 10.1) Since the mid-1980s, >80 waterborne outbreaks have been reported. By location, 5–75% of waterborne outbreaks from a known agent are due to *Cryptosporidium*. In the United States in 2002–2002, 1 (5%) of 19 waterborne outbreaks by infectious agents was due to *Cryptosporidium*. In the United Kingdom in 1970–2000, public water supplies recorded 33 *Cryptosporidium* outbreaks. In a county town in 2000, 58 inhabitants contracted disease from drinking unboiled main tap water, for an attack rate of 0.3%. Stools from patients yielded *C. parvum* genotype 2, and water reservoir and tap water yielded oocysts, at concentrations of 8–90/100 liters. Spain in 1995–2003 reported 11 *Cryptosporidium* outbreaks, with a total of 1,455 cases (132 per outbreak). For six outbreaks, a vehicle was reported: contaminated municipal water in three, water from a hotel swimming pool in two, and untreated water from a well in a cattle-breeding area in one. Perhaps the largest epidemic was observed in Milwaukee, Wis., in spring 1993, where the temporarily polluted city supply caused ~403,000 cases. By setting, attack rates can reach 40–70%.

***E. histolytica* (468, 977, 4115)**. In Chicago, Ill., in 1933, a cross-connection at a hotel that linked waste with tap water caused an amebiasis outbreak with ≥800 cases. Waterborne amebiasis has become rare in high-income countries. In Europe in 1986–1996, seven outbreaks of amebic dysentery were reported, five in Albania, and one each in Slovenia and Sweden, but only Slovenia reported cases from contaminated drinking water.

***G. lamblia* (621, 3164, 3570, 6101, 7922)**. Human and animal feces can contaminate supplies with *G. lamblia* at source, reservoir, or in pipes. Water roof tanks for a block of flats were suspected to have been deliberately contaminated in Edinburgh, United Kingdom, in 1990. Cysts can be detected in routine and outbreak drinking-water samples by screening large (100–1,000 liters) volumes with sensitive methods (filtration and molecular). Reported densities are 0.3–100 cysts per 100 liters of untreated water, and <0.1 cyst per 100 liters of treated water. A proposed level that should trigger action is three to five cysts per 100 liters. Cysts resist ordinary chlorination and are best removed by a combination of methods (coagulation, sedimentation, and filtration).

Outbreak and sporadic cases can be waterborne. Water from taps or wells is a risk (1884, 2508, 7213). In Dunedin, New Zealand, in the 1980s, laboratory-confirmed disease rates per 10^5 person-years were 33 in the sector that received unfiltered (microstrained) water and 10 in the sector that received water filtered with two media (anthracite and silica sand), for a relative risk of 3 (95% CI 1.1–10).

Outbreaks   Waterborne outbreaks have been well documented (Table 10.1). By location and definition of supply, 2–15% of waterborne outbreaks with a known infectious agent can be due to *G. lamblia*.

- North America (682, 3570, 3896, 5174, 6824, 8048). In Penticton, British Columbia, in 1986, the town water supply caused 362 confirmed cases, for an attack rate of 1.4%. In Creston, British Columbia, two waterborne outbreaks occurred within 5 years, one with 83 and one with 124 confirmed cases; an infected beaver was suspected to have contaminated the water supply. Residents infected in the first outbreak were less likely to be infected in the second outbreak than nonprimed individuals. In Rome, N.Y., in 1974–1975, 350 residents contracted giardiasis from city water, for an attack rate of 11%. In Red Lodge, Mont., in 1980, contaminated city water caused ~780 cases. In Pittsfield, Mass., in 1985–1986, chlorinated but unfiltered tap water caused ~3,800 cases; attack rates were 1.4% in residents served by the defective reservoir, and 0.7% in residents served otherwise. In the latest U.S. surveillance period (2001–2002), three waterborne giardiasis outbreaks were reported, one in Colorado from community water, with six cases; one in Florida from a well, with six cases; and one at a New York trailer park, also with six cases.
- West Europe (468, 2864, 3689, 4470, 5381, 6532). In Mjövik, Sweden, in 1982, polluted municipal water caused 56 cases (and 557 cases by an unidentified other agent, in retrospect, likely *Norovirus*). In Bristol, United Kingdom, in 1985, contaminated municipal water caused 108 confirmed cases. At a Swedish ski resort in 1986, sewage overflow into drinking water caused an outbreak with >1,400 confirmed cases. At a community in Rheinland-Pfalz, Germany, in 2000, eight cases were confirmed waterborne by cyst recovery from supplies.

Toxoplasma **(255, 814, 1554).** Drinking tap water is a risk for *T. gondii*. In Europe, 27% (53/194) of infected pregnant women reported drinking untreated water, compared with 18% (123/697) of uninfected control women. In greater Victoria, British Columbia, in 1995, unfiltered, chlorinated municipal water was implicated in an outbreak that caused 2,900–7,700 infections, including 74 manifest cases.

10.3 PRIVATE AND LOW-INCOME WATER SUPPLIES

Private supplies in high-income countries are typically small (for single houses, hamlets, and camps), using untreated water from boreholes, wells, or rain tanks. Low-income supplies are unimproved supplies in low-income countries, using untreated water from unprotected wells or springs, surfaces (canals, rivers, and ponds), or vendors. A minimum quantity is 20 liters per person per day for drinking, body hygiene, and laundry. Access should be easy and not exceed a distance of 1 km or a roundtrip time of 30 min.

Exposure (235, 6532, 7650, 8117, 8273). In high-income countries, 0–10% of water supplies are private. In low-income countries in 2002, about 20% of the population depended on unimproved supplies, 5–20% in urban areas and 15–60% in rural areas. Unlike municipal high-income supplies, hazards from private or unimproved supplies tend to persist (endemically or perennially) or to recur.

Infections (4067, 5938, 8117, 8273). Hazards span collection, transportation, storage, and retrieval of water in households. Untreated waters can transmit a broad agent spectrum, including viruses, bacteria, and protozoa of high-income supplies (Box 10.1). Unsafe water is a major vehicle of infectious diarrhea in low-income countries (see section 14.7). Untreated tap water should be considered unsafe and boiled for drinking.

VIRUSES

Confirmed to be spread by ingestion of water (8117) are enteric adenoviruses, *Enterovirus*, HAV, hepatitis E virus (HEV), *Norovirus*, and *Rotavirus*. All can persist in water at 20°C for >1 month, and all are moderately resistant to conventional chlorine treatment.

Adenovirus (4309). Enteric adenoviruses have been detected in urban tap water, including types 40 and 41.

***Enterovirus* (190, 4309, 6234, 7851).** *Enterovirus* has been detected in tap water, including coxsackievirus, echovirus, and vaccine poliovirus, including from urban tap water. In the city of Vitebsk, Belarus, in 2001, waterborne *Enterovirus* (mainly coxsackie B4) caused an outbreak.

HAV (468, 1600, 3753, 4180). HAV has been detected in tap water. In low-income countries, HAV is typically acquired at an early age when many infections are inapparent. Likely endemic sources include untreated drinking water. Drinking unboiled water from taps is a risk. Nonimmune residents living in endemic areas are susceptible. In Djibouti in 1993, 37 acute, waterborne HA cases occurred, mainly in French residents.

In high-income countries, outbreaks from private supplies have been reported (704, 1830, 1944). In Georgia State in 1982, 16 of 18 susceptible residents of a trailer park contracted acute HA after using water from a private well. During an outbreak in Canada in 1995, HAV was recovered by NAT from patients, well water (that did not grow coliforms), and a cesspool. In a college in Rome, Italy, in 1987, six acute cases and seven infections were traced to a well from which HAV had been isolated.

HEV (1582, 1584, 3753, 5316, 6063, 6752). HEV has been detected in municipal water in low-income countries. Unlike HAV, a significant fraction of HEV infections has been in adults and is manifest. Risks include water from rivers for drinking, cooking, and bathing, inadequately treated municipal water, and defecation into rivers. In Islamabad, Pakistan, attack rates during an outbreak were high (16%) in sectors supplied exclusively by a failing water plant, intermediate (5–12%) in sectors with mixed supply, and low (2%) in sectors not served by that plant.

Outbreaks Waterborne outbreaks of acute HE have been well documented in low-income countries.
- Africa. Outbreaks were reported in Algeria in 1980–1981 (788 cases in 4 months) (527, 7708), in Namibia in 1983 (hundreds of cases among refugees from Angola, confirmed retrospectively in 1998) (3573), in Chad in 1983–1984 (7708), in Ethiopia in 1988–1989 (7589), in Somalia in 1988–1989 (11,413 cases, attack rate 4.6%, lethality 3%) (644), in Djibouti in 1993 (43 cases) (1600), and in Morocco in 1994 (566).
- Latin America. Outbreaks were reported south of Mexico City in 1986, first by water at the start of the rainy season with 94 cases and an attack rate of 5% (94/1,757), then in another village likely by person-to-person spread with 129 cases and an attack rate of 6% (129/2,194) (7791).
- Asia. Outbreaks were reported in Kashmir, India, in 1978 (famous first outbreak, 52,000 cases, confirmed retrospectively) (3923), in Xinjiang, People's Republic of China, in 1986–1988 (~120,000 cases) (354), in Yangon, Myanmar, in 1989 (111 cases in an army camp of 600) (7629), in Kalimantan, Indonesia, in 1991 (>2,500 cases) (1582), in Kanpur, India, in 1990–1991 (79,091 cases, attack rate 3.8%) (5316), in Islamabad, Pakistan, in 1993–1994 (3,827 cases, attack rate 10%) (6063), in Vietnam in 1994 (anti-HEV immunoglobulin [Ig] G demonstrated in 76% of 50 patients and 38% of 100 community controls) (1584), in Nepal in 1995 (32 cases in 8 weeks, in a army camp of 692) (1478), and in rural Java, Indonesia, in 1998 (615 cases, attack rate 19%) (6752).

***Norovirus* (535, 682, 4261, 5520, 5727).** Outbreaks have been associated with tap and well waters, including private supplies in high-income countries. In the United States in 2001–2002, private well water caused *Norovirus* outbreaks in Wyoming at a snowmobile lodge (230 cases) and at a bar (83 cases), in Connecticut at a camp (142), and in New Hampshire at a camp (201 cases). At a new resort in Arizona, a contaminated deep-water well caused ~900 cases. At a restaurant and bus stop in Alaska, a contaminated well caused 18 (69%) cases among 26 employees, and 108 (39%) cases among 274 bus passengers. In western Norway in 2002, water from a camp caused an outbreak with 134 cases, for an attack rate of 65%.

Poliovirus (3942). In the remaining endemic areas such as Nigeria and India, infections are typically inapparent and acquired at an early age. In Taiwan in 1982, type 1 virus caused 1,031 paralytic polio cases; a significant risk was water from a non-municipal source.

***Rotavirus* (3059, 3501, 7263).** *Rotavirus* is a significant cause of waterborne diarrhea in low-income countries. At a private school in Rio de Janeiro a waterborne outbreak had an attack rate of 75% (including a concurrent *Shigella sonnei* outbreak). In northeastern People's Republic of China in 1982–1983, explosive rotavirus B epidemics led to >12,000 cases of diarrhea in adults, for attack rates of 13–14%. In the first phase, fecally polluted drinking water was implicated, and in a later phase there was person-to-person spread.

BACTERIA

Confirmed to be spread by ingestion of water (8117) are *Burkholderia pseudomallei*, *Campylobacter*, *E. coli*, environmental mycobacteria, *S. enterica* serovar Typhi and non-Typhi, *Shigella*, *V. cholerae*, and *Y. enterocolitica*. All of these agents are sensitive to chlorine, except environmental mycobacteria that are resilient and multiply in water supplies.

***Aeromonas* (766, 4794).** Untreated well water is an infrequent source of infection in humans. In India,

5 (28%) of 18 municipal supplies and 24 (51%) of 47 private supplies (wells and sources) yielded *Aeromonas* ≥10^3/ml, mostly *A. hydrophila*.

***Burkholderia* (1686, 3556).** In Australia, high water temperatures in tanks and pipes support spread of *B. pseudomallei* by drinking water. In a township of 300 in western Australia in 1997, *B. pseudomallei* caused five melioidosis cases in 5 weeks; 1 year later, an identical *B. pseudomallei* strain was isolated from a water-storage tank. In an township that recorded nine melioidosis cases in 28 months, a water storage tank yielded *B. pseudomallei*.

***Campylobacter* (682, 2116, 2541, 4999, 6532, 8117).** *Campylobacter* is detectable in impacted river waters (at concentrations up to 90–2,500 per liter), lakes and reservoirs (up to 20–500 per liter), pristine rivers (0–1,100 per liter), and groundwater (0–10 per liter). Private supplies are a hazard, including in Australia and New Zealand where rainwater is saved for domestic use. At an island resort in Queensland, Australia, in 1997, rainwater from tanks feeding water dispensers was implicated in an outbreak with 23 cases. In the United States in 2001–2002, private well water caused outbreaks in Alaska among cannery workers at a bunkhouse (six cases) and in Wisconsin at a household (13 cases). In the United Kingdom in 1970–2000, *Campylobacter* was implicated in one half (13/25) of the outbreaks from private supplies; 758 persons were affected (58/outbreak), for a mean attack rate of 42%.

***E. coli* (682, 5680, 6532).** In the United States in 2001–2002, *E. coli* O157:H7 was implicated in 1 (5%) of 19 outbreaks by known infectious agents. In the United Kingdom in 1970–2000, *E. coli* O157 was implicated in 1 (4%) of 25 outbreaks from private supplies. In southern India in 1996, water from two open wells was the likely source of an outbreak with 20 cases due to enteroggregative *E. coli*, for an attack rate of 15%.

***Francisella* (2920, 3249, 5037, 6202).** Water is a suspected vehicle of *F. tularensis*. In the Kosovo, during the Balkan conflict in 1999–2000, an outbreak caused >900 suspected cases; water from wells accessible to rodents was implicated. Around Bursa, Turkey, in 1988–1997, oropharyngeal lesions in most (83%) of 205 cases and the frequent involvement of young women who used water from aqueducts suggested waterborne spread. In Tuscany, Italy, in 1982, unchlorinated town water was implicated in 49 cases. In a village in the Appenines in 1988, water was likely the vehicle for nine tularemia cases and 11 infections.

***Helicobacter* (395, 924, 979, 2849, 3830, 4122, 5511, 6621).** *H. pylori* is endemic in low-income countries, and spread via untreated drinking water is likely. *H. pylori* has been detected in water from various sources, including water-storage pots, and use of unsafe drinking water in rural and urban areas has been correlated with increased prevalence of infection. Similar evidence is accumulating in high-income water supplies. In Japan, *H. pylori* was amplified from cow feces, soil, stream water, and drinking water. *H. pylori* DNA was also identified from well water in Germany. The presence of *H. pylori* DNA in water correlated with colonization or infection identified by breath test or anti-*H. pylori* IgG.

***Leptospira* (247, 1022, 4369).** Water is a natural reservoir for *Leptospira*. So far, *Leptospira* does not seem to have been detected in drinking water. Nevertheless, outbreaks suggest such a mode. In 4 (14%) of 28 leptospirosis outbreaks reported in 1930–2000, drinking water was implicated: in Portugal in 1931 (126 cases from a fountain polluted by rat urine), in Greece in 1931 (31 cases from coffee polluted by rat urine), in Russia in 1954 (62 cases from a well contaminated by pigs), and in Italy in 1984 (33 cases from a reservoir that had trapped a hedgehog). In the Tottori area of Japan in 2000, a man contracted leptospirosis by drinking water from a well muddied by an earthquake.

***Plesiomonas* (1156, 7598).** Water is a natural reservoir, but *P. shigelloides* seems to be inactivated by water treatment. In New York in 1996, water from a well was implicated in 56 (30%) cases of *P. shigelloides* diarrhea among 189 party attendees. In Japan, *P. shigelloides* was implicated in two waterborne diarrhea outbreaks.

***S. enterica* serovar Typhi (353, 2945, 7275, 7537).** *S. enterica* serovar Typhi is endemic in low-income countries. Drinking untreated water is a risk for contracting typhoid fever. In communities that rely on untreated water from streams, springs, and ditches waterborne outbreaks are a continuous threat.

Outbreaks A summary of reports follows.
- Africa (2137, 6169). In Alger, Algeria, in 1990–1992, a waterborne outbreak caused 34 hospitalized cases.
- Southwest Asia (124). In Haifa, Israel, in 1985, a fecally polluted periurban well was the vehicle for 77 cases. In Tabuk in northeast Saudi Arabia, in 1992, breakdown of a water desalinization plant led to an outbreak with 81 culture-confirmed and 104 suspected cases, for attack rates of 0.1–1/1,000.
- Southcentral and northcentral Asia (3801, 4393, 6623, 7342). In Sangli, Maharashtra, India, in 1975–1976, polluted city water caused a massive outbreak with 9,000 typhoid fever cases. In Kashmir, India, in 1988, waterborne multidrug-resistant serovar Typhi caused

46 culture-confirmed and 184 suspected cases. In Tajikistan in 1996, a waterborne epidemic followed by interhuman spread caused >24,000 cases. In Bharatpur (population, 92,000), Nepal, in 2002, the municipal water supply caused 5,963 confirmed or suspected typhoid fever cases in 7 weeks, for a crude attack rate of 6.5% (the true size of the epidemic could be 2,085–59,830 cases).

- Southeast and East Asia (3951, 5410). In 1983, an outbreak in Taiwan caused 52 confirmed cases; drinking tap water was a risk. In southern Vietnam in 1993, a waterborne outbreak and secondary interhuman spread caused 3,049 cases.

Untreated water is an occasional source of *S. enterica* serovar Typhi in high-income countries. Near Barcelona, Spain, in 1994, water from a drinking fountain likely contaminated by a nearby broken sewer pipe led to nine cases of typhoid fever (7661).

Shigella **(2138, 6568, 7593).** *Shigella* is endemic in low-income countries, and outbreaks from untreated waters are a risk. In Israel in 1985, polluted municipal water caused an outbreak of *S. sonnei* with >8,000 cases and borehole water in Zimbabwe was a vehicle of infection.

Untreated private waters can be sources of shigellosis in high-income countries as well. On Crete, Greece, village springs were implicated in an outbreak with 35 culture-confirmed *S. sonnei* cases.

Streptobacillus moniliformis **(4895, 6532).** At a boarding school in the United Kingdom in 1983, an outbreak affected 304 (47%) of 700 students; water from a spring inhabited by rats was implicated.

Vibrio **(659, 1470, 6814).** Untreated water is a risk for *Vibrio*, including from lakes, streams, municipal supplies, large water vessels (into which household members can put dirty hands), and during droughts when water is scarce. Widespread and explosive outbreaks point to water as a vehicle.

Outbreaks A summary of reports follows.
- Latin America (7280). During an outbreak in Trujillo, Peru, in 1991, 3 (6%) of 50 municipal water samples yielded *V. cholerae* O1.
- The Pacific (505, 4128). In the Marshall Islands in 2000–2001, cholera was associated with the transportation (from Kwajalein to Ebeye Island), handling (scooping), and storage (buckets and jugs) of chlorinated drinking water. Boiled or bottled water and use of water coolers with a spout for water outlet were protective. On Tarawa, Gilbert Islands, the main water supply was implicated in an explosive cholera epidemic; lagoon water and shellfish were also found to be contaminated with *V. cholerae*.

PROTOZOA

Confirmed to be spread by the ingestion of water (8117) are *C. parvum*, *C. cayetanensis*, *E. histolytica*, *G. lamblia*, *Naegleria fowleri*, and *Toxoplasma gondii*. All resist conventional chlorine treatment. Most are able to persist in water at 20°C for >1 month. These agents are typically endemic in rural and urban areas of many tropical countries (7216).

Amebas (682, 1998, 6841, 7603). Free-living amebas have been recovered in drinking water. In India, an infant contracted fatal primary amebic meningoencephalitis (PAM) from bathing water that yielded *N. fowleri*. In Papua New Guinea, five of six babies contracted PAM after being washed in well or lagoon water. The custom of splashing water around the face was postulated to deposit amebas to nostrils, allowing passage to the brain. In Australia in the summers of the 1960s–1970s, unchlorinated, domestic water from overland water pipelines was implicated in cases of PAM among nonswimmers. Occurrence was controlled by continuous water chlorination. In Arizona in October of 2002, two previously healthy children contracted fatal PAM from home bathtubs and swimming pools served by the community water supply; a reservoir and a house refrigerator filter tested positive for *N. fowleri*. It remained unclear if infection resulted from drinking or immersion.

C. parvum **(2495, 6170, 6532, 8117).** Oocysts have been detected in impacted river waters (at concentrations up to 480 per liter), lakes and reservoirs (up to 4–290 per liter), pristine rivers (up to 2–240 per liter), and groundwater (0–1 per liter). Endemicity extends into communities on the United States-Mexico border that lack adequate municipal water and sewage services. Drinking-water purification has been protective. In the United Kingdom in 1970–2000, *Cryptosporidium* was implicated in ~10% (3/25) of outbreaks from private supplies; 75 persons were affected (25 per outbreak); where known, attack rates were 22–57%.

C. cayetanensis **(594, 1038, 3285, 4506, 5033, 6066, 6845).** Oocysts have been detected in sewage, surface, reservoir, well, and tap water and chlorinated drinking water. Drinking untreated water is a risk for residents, expatriates, and travelers. In Guatemala in 1997, 91% (62/68) of infected persons reported drinking untreated water in 2 weeks before illness onset, compared with 73% (88/120) uninfected controls (odds ratio 4, 95% CI 1.4–11) (594). A waterborne outbreak in Nepal in 1994 caused 12 diarrhea cases (92%, six confirmed) among 14 exposed British soldiers.

Entamoeba **(471, 560, 703, 1365).** In environmental samples, cysts of *E. histolytica* should be distinguished from *E. moshkovskii* and *E. dispar* by molecular methods. Untreated tap water is a risk for *E. histolytica* infection and invasive disease (amebic liver abscess). Waterborne outbreaks have been reported. In Tbilisi, Republic of Georgia, in 1998, water caused an outbreak with 37 cases of amebic liver abscess and ~84,000–225,000 cases of enteric illness. In Taiwan in 1993, well water caused diarrhea in 730 (49%) of 1,481 students; the agents were *E. histolytica* and *S. sonnei*. None of 64 staff who was served by a different supply became infected.

Giardia **(1457, 2495, 6170, 6532, 8117).** Cysts are detectable in impacted river waters (at concentrations up to 470 per liter), lakes and reservoirs (up to 2–30 per liter), pristine rivers (up to 2 per liter), and groundwater (0–1 per liter). Near Mexico City, in an area of artificial groundwater recharge, household risks included storing water in open receptacles (buckets and tanks) and not washing hands. *G. lamblia* is endemic in communities on the United States-Mexico border that lack adequate municipal water and sewage services. In the United Kingdom in 1970–2000, *G. lamblia* was implicated in 1 (4%) of 25 outbreaks from private supplies.

Isospora **(4443).** *Isospora* oocysts are suspected to be spread by tap water.

Toxoplasma **(383, 558, 3094).** Drinking untreated water is a risk for *T. gondii*. In a township of Rio de Janeiro State, Brazil, in 1997–1999, 316 residents not connected to treated water or sewerage had a >3 times higher seroprevalence than 301 residents receiving municipal supplies. Following jungle training in Panama and consumption of water from a small stream, 35 (32%, 31 confirmed, 4 probable) of 98 U.S. soldiers came down with acute toxoplasmosis. In India, in a community of strict vegetarians (Jains) who wash vegetables and do not keep cats, acute cases pointed to drinking water as a source, as did a high seroprevalence (47% or 8/17) compared with vegetarian Hindus (28% or 24/85) and nonvegetarian Hindus (32% or 48/139).

HELMINTHS

Drinking water is the only vehicle for acquisition of *Dracunculus medinensis*. For *Fasciola*, drinking water is an alternative to water plants. *Schistosoma* is acquired from water contact rather than ingestion.

A. lumbricoides **and** *T. trichiura* **(304, 1087, 4521).** Although assumed, epidemiological evidence is unavailable to support transmission of *A. lumbricoides* and *T. trichiura* via drinking water. Instead, lack of water and sanitation are risks. In an urban area of Nigeria, *Ascaris* infection prevalence was least in children whose families had tap water and flush toilets.

D. medinensis **(1028, 8117).** *D. medinensis* is acquired by the ingestion of unfiltered surface water that contains infective copepods.

Echinococcus **(1086, 4225).** Spread of *E. granulosus* by drinking water is uncertain. In Uruguay, water from small dams (cachimba) or tanks that collect rainwater from ground or roof (aljibe) is a risk. In contrast, in a case-control study in Uruguay, having tap water provided protection from infection with *E. granulosus*.

Fasciola **(1723, 2240, 4792, 8117).** In endemic areas, up to 13% of *F. hepatica* metacercariae are free floating or sticking to floating straws or leaves. At a site in the Andean altiplano, concentration of metacercariae in water reached 7/500 ml. Drinking raw, untreated water is a risk. In an endemic area of Peru, epidemiological findings suggested acquisition from drinking irrigation canal water.

Fasciolopsis buski **(2885).** Metacercariae can float in surface water, and untreated water is a potential source.

Gnathostoma **(3671).** Accidental swallowing of water from ponds or rice fields that contains infective copepods is a possible source.

Taenia saginata **(6646).** Eggs can be carried to cattle via water. In Alberta, Canada, in 2000, during an outbreak of cysticercosis in cattle, *Taenia* eggs were identified in water sediment.

SECTION IV
Humans

- 11 Human Domiciles
- 12 Human Work
- 13 Human Leisure and Lifestyle
- 14 Human Community

Humans are significant sources of infection, including shedding carriers and incubating, reconvalescent, and relapsing patients. Exposure can take place at home, in the workplace, during leisure, and in the community.

Infection risks in populations are influenced by age structure (see section 14.2), growth rate, and density. The extremes of age are particularly vulnerable, infants who are not yet immune, and elderly with waning immune memory. Live births (~130 million/year worldwide) generate continuous cohorts of susceptible individuals. Global population density is 40/km^2, with a range of <1–2/km^2 in deserts and highlands to >500/km^2 in megacities, India, and western Europe. Of ~57 million deaths worldwide in 2002, 22% (~12.5 million) were due to infectious (and parasitic) diseases, mainly respiratory tract infections (7% of all deaths, or 4 million), AIDS (5% or 2.8 million), diarrhea (3% or 1.8 million), tuberculosis (2.7% or 1.6 million), and malaria (2% or 1.3 million) (http://www.who.int, WHO health report).

11

Human Domiciles

11.1 Regular domiciles
11.2 Substandard domiciles
11.3 Homeless persons
11.4 Refugees and relief camps
11.5 Orphans and adoptees
11.6 Adults in long-term care
11.7 Detention facilities
11.8 Hotel accomodation

Domiciles are all permanent housings (manor house to shanty town). Variable fractions of the population live in institutions (orphanages, correctional facilities, camps, and nursing homes). In the United States in 2000, 1–9% (mean, 4%) of 13,113 respondents from eight states reported to have lived on a farm in the week before the survey (http://www.cdc.gov/foodnet/surveys/Pop_surv.htm).

Exposure (2630, 4313, 5152). Agents are brought to domiciles by children (from day care or school), playmates, traveled (from abroad) or reconvalescent (from hospital) household members, promiscuous sex partners, and pet animals. Domiciliary spread is by droplets, skin contact, shared objects, sex, and foods. Hazards include crowding, lack of tap water and sanitation, rodents on the premises, and sites close to mosquito-breeding sites.

Exposure history (Box 11.1). Inquire about the type and location of domicile, sanitary installations, rooms available, number of people and pets in the household, and members or pets who are ill. A measure of crowding is the number of household members per sleeping room.

Prevention. Good housing with electricity, tap water, toilet, regular garbage removal, and insect- and rodent-proofed doors and windows can prevent many, but not all, infections. Childhood vaccines prevent droplet-borne infections. Live polio vaccine should not be given to members of households with immune-impaired individuals, because of the risk of person-to-person spread.

11.1 REGULAR DOMICILES

Regular domiciles are defined here by the presence of indoor tap water and flush toilet. Types include single-family homes, apartments, condominia, flats, and townhouses.

Infections. The focus is on intrafamilial spread by droplet-air, feces-food, and skin-blood clusters (Box 11.2).

DROPLET-AIR CLUSTER, REGULAR DOMICILES
Exposure (5149, 5429, 7187). Respiratory agents readily spread in households. Consistently higher attack rates in women than men suggest that children

> **Box 11.1 Suggested domiciliary exposure history**
>
> **Right now:**
> - In what kind of domicile (house, institution, or relief camp) do you live? Where is it located (city or rural)? What kind of utilities (tap water, flush toilet, screened openings, and number of rooms)? How many people and animals, including infants, preschool children, and adults, occupy the domicile?
> - Is there anybody in the household, who is ill, in the hospital, wearing diapers, in day care, recently returned from travel, having AIDS or suppressive chemotherapy? Have pet animals become ill or died?
>
> **In the past 3 months:**
> - Did you share utensils (e.g., tooth brush) with household members or a bed with your children?
> - Did you eat foods with your bare hands? Did you use bednets? Have you had any outdoor overnight stays or stays in cabins?
> - Did you notice rats, bugs, or ticks in or around the house? Are livestock or open waters within visual range?
>
> **In your lifetime:**
> - Have you ever been in an orphanage or prison, ever used injection drugs, or ever been tested for HIV?
> - Have you or your partner ever completed or interrupted treatments for tuberculosis, AIDS, or STI?
> - How many sex partners have you ever had?

are major sources of infections in households, including children in day care and kindergarten. Parental smoking increases the risk of respiratory tract infections in children, including from respiratory syncytial virus (RSV).

Control (5106, 5111, 6311). Important questions are (i) the presence of susceptible infants, pregnant women, and immune-impaired individuals in the household, (ii) ongoing outbreaks in day care, school, or workplace, and (iii) timely (within 24–72 h) availability of vaccines, immunoglobulins (Ig), and prophylactic antimicrobials. By national guidelines, chemoprophylaxis should be considered for susceptible household contacts of diphtheria, meningococcal meningitis, *Haemophilus influenzae* b (Hib) disease, and pertussis cases. Catch-up, booster, or full-dose postexposure or emergency vaccines should be considered for susceptible contacts or during outbreaks of diphtheria, meningococcal meningitis, pertussis, measles, or varicella. If live vaccines (measles and varicella-zoster virus [VZV]) are contraindicated, e.g., for pregnant women or immune-impaired individuals, normal human Ig should be considered instead. Adults with cough for >2 weeks should be evaluated for *Bordetella* and *Mycobacterium*.

Viruses

High coverage with vaccines against measles virus, mumps virus, and rubella virus (MMR vaccine) and VZV is assumed (for these viruses, see section 11.2 below). Vaccine nonpreventable respiratory viruses include *Enterovirus* (EV), Epstein-Barr virus (EBV), parainfluenzavirus (PIV), parvovirus B19 (PVB19), RSV, *Rhinovirus*, and coronavirus causing severe acute respiratory syndrome (SARS-CoV).

EV (1323, 5354, 7308, 7820). EV readily spreads in households. In São Paulo, Brazil, EV71 infection rates

> **Box 11.2 Agents from standard homes, by cluster**
>
> For pets, see section I; for utensils, see section 6.4; for STI, see section 14.7.
>
> | | |
> |---|---|
> | Droplet-air | If vaccine (MMR, VZV, DP, Hib) coverage is high: *Enterovirus, Influenzavirus,* PIV, PVB19, RSV; *C. pneumoniae, M. tuberculosis, M. pneumoniae, N. meningitidis, S. pneumoniae; Cryptococcus* |
> | Feces-food | • Mainly interpersonal spread: HAV, *Norovirus, Rotavirus; Helicobacter, Shigella; Cryptosporidium* |
> | | • Mainly food borne: *Campylobacter, Listeria; Fasciola, T. solium* (cysticercosis) |
> | | • By either mode: *Escherichia* (EHEC, EPEC), *Salmonella, Y. enterocolitica; Entamoeba, Giardia* |
> | | • By foods or cat feces: *Toxoplasma* |
> | Zoonotic | *B. burgdorferi* |
> | Skin-blood | CMV, GBV-C, HBV, HCV, HDV, HIV, HPV, HSV, HTLV; bacterial STI, *S. pyogenes; Enterobius* |

were 28% (11/40) in households with an EV71 index case, but 1% (4/387) in control households. In Taiwan in 2001–2002, EV71 over 7 months spread to 84% (70/83) of siblings, 83% (19/23) of cousins, 41% (72/175) of parents, 28% (10/36) of grandparents, and 26% (5/19) of uncles and aunts, for an overall secondary household infection rate of 52% (176/399). In Germany in 1996, EV secondary attack rates were 26% (28/109) in households with a sick child in day care, compared with 2% (2/119) in control households. Epidemic conjunctivitis due to EV has been reported in slum populations.

EBV (1628, 1651, 2430, 7246). EBV can spread in households. Spread has been demonstrated in 20% (7/35) of families having an index child with mononucleosis. In families with an index child case, adult shedding can be reactivated. Risks for spread include crowding, sharing a bedroom with a family member, and having a single parent. In crowded households, virtually all children are EBV-infected by school age, while under optimal living conditions, 30–50% of adolescents escape EBV infection.

***Influenzavirus* (1095, 3203, 3512, 3848, 5151, 5282).** *Influenzavirus* readily spreads in households, including subtypes A/H1N1, A/H3N2, and B. By case definition (clinical or virological) and case mix (children or adults, vaccinees, users of neuraminidase inhibitors), secondary attack rates in households with an index case are ~10–40%.

PIV (1564). PIV circulates in preschool children at a high rate (in Seattle 44/100 person-years).

PVB19 (212, 2828, 3141, 6239, 7692, 8351). PVB19 readily spreads in households. Children bring PVB19 home. In households with an index case, secondary attack rates in susceptible members reach 45–50%. Infections can be a hazard for pregnant women in the household. In Denmark, in a population study of 30,946 pregnant women, compared with having no child in the household, the odds of acute PVB19 infection were 3 (95% confidence interval [95% CI] 2–5) with one child in the household, 6 (95% CI 4–9) with two children, and 8 (95% CI 4–15) with three or more children. In pregnant women of unknown serostatus who are exposed to PVB19 at home, the risk of fetal loss is <2.5%.

RSV (971, 1564, 3089, 5429). RSV readily spreads in families. In Seattle, rates of ~20/100 person-years were observed in preschool and schoolchildren. Secondary attack rates can reach 30% in infants and 17% in adults. Crowding, older siblings, and smokers in the household increase infection and disease risks. Secretions, hands, and objects can be infective. Crowding (≥4 children per household, ≥2 persons per living room) likely explains the high rates of RSV infections and hospitalizations in Alaskan native infants.

***Rhinovirus* (2484, 3680, 5419).** *Rhinovirus* rapidly spreads in households. By family size and age of index cases, secondary attack rates in households are 25–70%, typically 50%. In the elderly, the impact of *Rhinovirus* on health is comparable to *Influenzavirus*.

SARS-CoV (2803, 3575, 4236). SARS-CoV can spread in households, although apparently not very efficiently. Reported secondary attack rates in household contacts of SARS patients are 5–15%. In the SARS epidemic in 2003, visiting patients was a risk; having a health worker in the family was not.

Bacteria

High coverage with vaccines against *Bordetella pertussis* (P vaccines), *Corynebacterium diphtheriae* (D or d vaccines), and *H. influenzae* b (Hib vaccine) is assumed (for these bacteria, see "Substandard Domiciles" below). Vaccine nonpreventable respiratory bacteria include the "pneumos": *Chlamydophila pneumoniae*, *Klebsiella pneumoniae*, *Mycoplasma pneumoniae*, and *Legionella pneumophila*. In contrast to hospitals, the household epidemiology of *K. pneumoniae* is almost not documented. *L. pneumophila* does not spread person-to-person (for buildings, see section 6.2).

***Chlamydophila* (698, 699, 2719, 5182, 8323).** *C. pneumoniae* spreads in households, and outbreaks in households have been reported, although transmission seems inefficient. In Italy in 1991, in a community of former injection drug users (IDUs) half of whom were human immunodeficiency virus (HIV)-infected, 62% (15/26) contracted *C. pneumoniae* respiratory disease (mostly pneumonia).

***Mycobacterium* (1472, 2521, 3032, 5282, 5869, 6074, 6132, 6775, 7233, 8364).** *M. tuberculosis* can spread in households, mainly by smear-positive (open) cases. Crowding is an established risk, and HIV coinfection is an emerging risk. **Infection.** By age and HIV status, the infection risk (by skin reactivity) in households with smear-positive cases is 25–60%, and after exposure for months up to 100%. Relative to age-matched community controls, the infection risk is 30–50% higher in households exposed to smear-positive pulmonary cases, but only ~5% higher from exposure to smear-negative, culture-positive cases. **Disease.** In endemic areas, by contact tracing and HIV status, the risk of active tuberculosis after household contact with a smear-positive case is 0.2–6%. Part of this variability results from uncertainty about which nonhousehold contacts to contact for diagnostic workup.

Outbreaks in households have been reported. A babysitter caused an outbreak of isoniazid (INH)-resistant tuberculosis. Good ventilation appears to reduce the infectivity in rooms.

***Mycoplasma* (1564, 1994, 2487).** *M. pneumoniae* circulates in households, including infants, schoolchildren, and adults (in Seattle, Wash., at a rate of ~10/100 person-years). In The Netherlands through 30-months of 1997–1999, PCR detected *M. pneumoniae* from nose and throat swabs in 39 (3%) of 1,172 random outpatients with acute respiratory tract infections. For 30 of them, all 79 household members could be examined (after 14–30 days), and 12 (15%) were infected, that is, 4.5-times the population rate. Of 12 infected household members, 9 (75%) were children. In Seattle, in 1963–1965, 55 (36%) of 151 members from 36 families with a pneumonia index case grew *M. pneumoniae* in throat swabs, compared with none of 390 members from 74 families with a pneumonia case negative for *M. pneumoniae*.

***Neisseria meningitidis* (397, 1104, 1559, 1846, 3171, 3366, 5282, 5819, 6904, 7936).** In households with a disease index case, carriage is increased to 20–50%. High carrier prevalence signals threatened spread of virulent clones. Crowding is a risk. In the 1940s–1980s, secondary attack rates in untreated households were ~0.5–6%, typically 2%. In the United Kingdom in the 1980s, the median interval from index to secondary case was 7 weeks. In a postal survey in the United Kingdom in 1993–1995, the secondary household attack rate in the first month of exposure was 0.2%, that is, 1,200 times higher than in the population during days 0–6, and 150 times higher than during days 7–30. Chemoprophylaxis within 24 h is advised to close contacts.

In the meningitis belt of sub-Saharan Africa, exposure to smoke from cooking fires and sharing a bedroom with a patient are risks. Slum areas such as in Nairobi, Kenya, may suffer from high rates of invasive disease.

***Streptococcus pneumoniae* (2768, 3036, 4335, 5525, 5901, 7775).** Serogroups readily spread in households. Risks for carriage and spread include children in the household and respiratory coinfections. The prevalence of nasal carriage typically builds up after age 6 months, reaches a peak at age 1½ years (~30%), and decreases in older siblings (~10% at 5–10 years of age) and parents (1%). Older children can bring new serogroups into households, including from day care centers. Carriage is not limited to the nose: in families in Papua New Guinea, 8% (2/24) of mothers and 36% (13/36) of their children grew *S. pneumoniae* from their hands.

Fungi

Occasional family clusters have been reported, likely from common exposure rather than from person-to-person spread. The main risk is immune-impaired household members. For indoor molds, see section 6.2.

***Coccidioides immitis* (6887).** In Arizona in 1959–1980, rates of disseminated disease among Native Americans per 10^5 per year decreased from 9 in the first 11 years to 4 in the second observation period, while the infection prevalence (skin reactivity) was stable (~35% on reservation land and ~17% off the reservation). This decrease was explained by housing, which changed from wickiup or adobe to regular, with less exposure to dust.

***Cryptococcus* (5750, 7282).** In metropolitan Rio de Janeiro, Brazil, 13% (20/154) of domiciliary samples (dust, soil, and avian droppings) grew *C. neoformans*, including houses with AIDS patients, houses with AIDS patients coinfected with the fungus, and houses with healthy inhabitants; the principal hazard was peridomestic birds. In Bujumbura, Burundi, *C. neoformans* was recovered in house dust from 20 of 44 AIDS patients coinfected with the fungus, 13 of 20 patients reported frequent contacts with pigeons, and, from six houses, pigeon guano grew the fungus.

***Pneumocystis jirovecii* (8239).** Infectivity in the household of persons with *Pneumocystis* pneumonia seems low.

FECES-FOOD CLUSTER, REGULAR DOMICILES
Exposure (2253, 2741, 2962, 3053, 5083, 5602). Sources of home enteric infections are colonized, incubating, or ill household members, tainted foods, and pet animals. Households are world top "caterers," and good cooking practice is essential. By surveillance and geography, private homes are sites for ~10–35% of food-borne disease outbreaks. Domiciliary clusters may escape notice. Among 57,667 enteric infections reported in Denmark in 1991–2001, links with postal codes and street numbers identified largely unrecognized outbreaks in 2–13% of households. Of 226 domiciliary outbreaks reported in the United Kingdom in 1992–99, 192 (85%) were food borne; main vehicles (in about two thirds of the outbreaks) were poultry, desserts, and egg dishes. On interviewing, most households admit to some form of food mishandling.

Prevention (2731, 6741). The advice for prevention of food-associated infections is (i) to wash raw vegetables, salads, and fruits; (ii) to consider meats as raw, even when wrapped in plastic; (iii) to wash hands, surfaces, and utensils after work with raw items, and to separate raw from heated or ready-to-eat items; (iv) to heat products throughout, and to serve them immediately (in 5–10 minutes); (v) to avoid raw seafood, milk, eggs, and their products; (vi) to cool cooked items rapidly (in <15 min) and store them in the refrigerator (at 4°C), away from insects and rodents; (vii) to respect shelf life, and discard spoiled items.

Viruses

Major viruses that circulate in regular homes are hepatitis A virus (HAV), *Norovirus*, and *Rotavirus* (Box 11.2, for poliovirus, see section 11.2 below). Poor food-handling practice in households is a risk (1849).

HAV (1652, 1894, 4853, 5072, 6431, 6525, 7096). Spread in households seems mainly person-to-person rather than by food. Risks include not washing hands before cooking or after gardening. Unrecognized infections, e.g., traveled adults or children in day care can be sources of secondary household infections. Reported secondary attack rates in high-income countries, by susceptibility and follow-up period, are 5–25% without control measures, occasionally up to 50%. In a randomized vaccine trial in Italy, secondary attack rates were 6% (12/207) in control households and 1% (2/197) in vaccinated households. The number of vaccinees needed to prevent one secondary infection was 18 persons. Vaccine should be offered to household and sex contacts of confirmed acute HA cases during days 0–7 after disease onset (d_0) in the index case, or normal human Ig during days 8–14.

***Norovirus* (448, 1849, 3305, 3822).** *Norovirus* readily spreads in households, apparently mainly person-to-person, less frequently via food. In outbreaks, reported secondary household attack rates are 19–44%.

***Rotavirus* (1849, 2372, 4054, 6784).** Some 20% infections can be acquired at home. Home spread seems mainly person-to-person, from children to household members, less frequently via food. Risks include crowding and contact with manifest cases.

Bacteria

Campylobacter and *Listeria monocytogenes* spread in households mainly by foods, *Helicobacter pylori* and *Shigella* spread mainly by contact, while *E. coli*, *Salmonella*, and *Yersinia enterocolitica* use either mode (Box 11.2).

***Campylobacter* (157, 2253, 3817, 5112).** *Campylobacter* spreads in households mainly via food and occasionally person-to-person. In Canada in 1996–1997, 42% (489/1,165) of sporadic and epidemic *Campylobacter* infections were acquired at home, compared with 39% (453) by travel or 17% (201) at restaurants. In Denmark in 1991–2001, 3% of *Campylobacter* cases were reported from household outbreaks. However, underreporting is considerable. In Denmark in 2000–2001, of 168 small household outbreaks uncovered by address-linking, only 8 (5%) had been reported.

***E. coli* (4938, 5112, 5743, 7827).** *E. coli* readily spreads at home, both via food and person-to-person. In Canada in 1996–1997, 51% (90/178) of sporadic and epidemic diarrheagenic *E. coli* infections were acquired at home, compared with 26% (47) at restaurants or 18% (32) by travel. In the United States, risks of sporadic *E. coli* O157:H7 infections included not washing hands and surfaces after handling raw ground beef, and eating home-prepared hamburgers in the week prior to illness. Enterohemorrhagic *E. coli* (EHEC) and enteropathogenic *E. coli* (EPEC) are quite infective, and reported household secondary attack rates are 4–15%. In an EPEC outbreak at a Finnish school, secondary attack rates were 5% (85/1,749) in households with ≥1 outbreak-related attendee, but only 1.5% (7/476) in households without an attendee.

***Helicobacter* (924, 1609, 2016, 4425, 6425, 7759).** Infections cluster in families. Spread appears to be person-to-person, and crowding is a risk. In rural Shandong, People's Republic of China, in 1997–1998, among 3,288 adults, *H. pylori* was significantly more prevalent if more than two persons shared a bed, or if hands were not regularly washed before meals. A further risk is children sharing beds with parents. In Germany in 1998, the prevalence of *H. pylori* in children 5–7 years of age was 10% (31/305); infections were about three times more prevalent if parents had anti-*H. pylori* IgG in saliva than if they did not. In Guatemala seroreactivity was correlated between mother and child, and between siblings. In addition, *H. pylori* DNA was amplified from buccal cavities and fingernails; hands could carry *H. pylori*, in particular, when eating from bare hands.

***Listeria* (625, 4915, 6543).** Spread at home is via food (for mother-to-child spread, see section 14.7). Kitchens yield the agent, allowing cross-contamination. In The Netherlands, *L. monocytogenes* was isolated from 45 (21%) of 213 housholds, including from refrigerated vegetables, refrigerator compartments, dishcloths, brushes, and sinks.

***Salmonella* (1864, 2253, 2731, 4029, 5112, 5763, 6741, 7860).** Domiciliary spread can be via food or via person-to-person contact. In the United States in 1985–1999, 13% (112/841) of *S. enterica* serovar Enteritidis outbreaks occurred at home. In Canada in 1996–1997, 44% (359/825) of sporadic and epidemic *Salmonella* cases were contracted at home, compared with 37% (304) from travel and 18% (150) from restaurants. In Europe, by geography and species, 5–85% of outbreaks were linked to households. In Denmark in 1991–2001, ~6% of reported serovar Typhimurium cases and ~13% of serovar Enteritidis cases were part of household outbreaks, suggesting a high tendency for home spread. In the United Kingdom in 1970–1982, 1,175 deficiencies were identified in 566 food-borne *Salmonella* outbreaks, including preparation >12 h in advance in 20% (240), inadequate cooking in 12% (139), and storage of cooked food at ambient temperature in 9% (172). A risk for sporadic salmonellosis is never or only rarely to wash hands between meat work and nonmeat items.

Risks for serovar Typhi transmission in households include not using soap for handwashing, sharing food from the same plate, and not having a toilet in the household.

Shigella (2080, 2253, 3010, 5123). Spread of *Shigella* at home seems mainly person-to-person. In households with young children, secondary attack rates can exceed 30% and reach 50%. In Denmark in 1991–2001, ~10% of reported *Shigella* cases were part of household outbreaks, suggesting a high tendency for household spread.

Yersinia (2253, 3031, 4296, 4775). Home infections by *Y. enterocolitica* can result from foods and animal or human contacts. In a family outbreak in the United States, a sick bitch and her puppies were the primary source, but secondary spread was person-to-person. In a family outbreak in Canada without an environmental source, intrafamilial spread was likely. In Denmark in 1991–2001, 2% of reported cases were part of household outbreaks.

Protozoa

In households (Box 11.2), *Cryptosporidium* spreads mainly by contact, *Entamoeba histolytica* and *Giardia lamblia* spread by food or contact, and *Toxoplasma gondii* spreads by food or cat contact.

Cryptosporidium (3230, 5046, 5399, 6331). Domiciliary spread is mainly person-to-person. Contact with a diarrhea case is a risk. Reported home secondary attack rates are ~15–20%. In a diarrhea outbreak at a child day care center in Oklahoma, 23% (6/26) of household members with an infective child tested positive for *Cryptosporidium*, compared with 2% (1/53) of unexposed members.

Entamoeba (2660, 2661, 7064, 7468, 7878). Spread at home is by foods, contact, and apparently sex, on occasion including in high-income countries. In Texas in 1974, two cousins from an extended family developed amebic liver abscess (ALA), likely by contact; 46% (74/183) of members were seroreactive, and 13% (14/111 tested) shed *E. histolytica/dispar*. In Italy in 1992, six persons contracted amebiasis, likely via food tainted by a carrier housemaid from the Philippines: two children and one friend developed diarrhea, the mother contracted dysentery, and the father and one friend were diagnosed with ALA; the friend with ALA died. Of 24 cases of ALA diagnosed in Denmark in 1987–1991, three were acquired in Denmark, through "intimate contact" with persons from endemic areas. When carriers are identified in households, screening of members may be warranted.

Giardia (1884, 3424, 5850, 5971). Spread of *G. lamblia* at home is by food and person-to-person. Risks include handling of diapers, contact with a child in day care, and contact with a manifest case. Home-prepared meals are sources of party outbreaks. Female home foodhandlers in contact with shedding infants or pet animals have been sources of outbreaks.

T. gondii (1381, 1834, 4561, 6511, 6840). Family outbreaks are food borne, including raw milk, undercooked meat, or tap water, or linked to cats that contaminate the household. Acute, isolated cases may signal a common home source and further, inapparent household infections.

Helminths

Fasciola hepatica (1459, 1591). Shared meals can cause household clusters. In Basque Country, Spain, in 1983–1992, four outbreaks occurred in families who consumed watercress, for a total of 17 cases (4 per outbreak).

Taenia solium (3492, 6652, 7046). *T. solium* carriers who work or live in affluent households are a potential source of cysticercosis by polluting foods with eggs. Because cysticercosis is a significant health hazard, screening of household employees from enzootic-endemic areas is advised.

ZOONOTIC CLUSTER, REGULAR DOMICILES

Houses can be located close to transmission foci. Pets can harbor agents or bring ectoparasites home. Tick-borne agents include tick-borne encephalitis virus (TBEV), *Borrelia*, *Rickettsia*, and *Babesia*. For insect-borne agents, see section 11.2 below.

Viruses

TBEV (4061). Domiciles close to TBEV foci are a risk, mainly for children and housewives.

Bacteria

Borrelia burgdorferi (4061, 4848, 6619). Residence in an enzootic, tick-infested area is a likely risk for *B. burgdorferi*. The nearer a domicile is to a focus, the higher are the infection risks for its residents. The larger a property, the more likely it features habitats that support ticks. Residential development in parts of the United States has created clearings enclosed by patchy woodlands that are favorable for deers, deer ticks, and *B. burgdorferi*.

Chlamydophila psittaci (3919, 4221). Pet birds have been a reported source of household outbreaks of *C. psittaci*.

Coxiella burnetii **(966, 4066).** Dogs and cats have been reported sources of household outbreaks of *C. burnetii*.

Rickettsia conorii **(6828, 8310).** Shared exposure to ticks explains household *R. conorii* case clusters. In a desert settlement in southern Israel in 1984–1986, cases of spotted fever were diagnosed in 4% (13/341) of residents; cases clustered at the settlement fringe.

Protozoa
Babesia **(3215, 6459).** Housing in enzootic, tick-infested areas is a risk for *Babesia*. In the northeastern United States periurban residential areas bring deer ticks to the backdoors of humans.

ENVIRONMENTAL CLUSTER, REGULAR DOMICILES
Clostridium tetani **(4564, 5792).** The home environment can be a source of wound tetanus in nonvaccinated household members. In Italy in 1998–2000, of 71 cases with a known mode, 5 (7%) (5) acquired *C. tetani* at home, and 4 (6%) acquired it on the street. In Finland in 1969–1985, 17 (16%) of 106 tetanus patients were housewives or service workers.

SKIN-BLOOD CLUSTER, REGULAR DOMICILES
Exposure (1180, 3711, 7449). Modes of spread include skin contacts, shared use of personal objects, and sex. Genital infections in children should be an alert for child abuse. Spread of sexually transmitted infections (STI) in households is mainly from infective uninformed and unprotected partners. In a 1997 U.S. telephone survey of ~34,000 civilian, noninstitutionalized adults 18–49 years of age, 5% (Montana) to 18% (Nevada) of sexually active respondents (11% overall) reported multiple sex partners in the past year. Similarly, in a 1999–2001 United Kingdom survey of ~10,000 adults 16–44 years of age, 9% of females and 15% of males reported more than one sex partner in the past year.

Preventive measures (1845, 6056, 7142, 7905). Preventive measures include body hygiene, disclosure of infection status, and safe sex. In the United States, 40% of 203 HIV-infected individuals refused to disclose the infection status to their partners. Consistent use of condoms reduces or prevents spread of herpes simplex virus 2 (HSV2), HIV, and other STI, and male circumcision reduces the spread of HIV.

Viruses
Spread by domiciliary sex is mainly documented in monogamous, discordant couples.

Cytomegalovirus (CMV) (76, 4468). Domiciliary spread of CMV is via breast-feeding, skin contact, and sex. Living conditions have an impact on spread. In People's Republic of China in 1986–1987, in a random sample of 1,950 households, urban housing and breast-feeding correlated with the seroprevalence in children. Children can bring CMV home from day care.

GB virus C (GBV-C, hepatitis G virus) (3811). Reactivity in sex partners of hepatitis G virus (HGV)-infected individuals suggests sexual spread.

Hepatitis B virus (HBV) (503, 3467, 4026, 4338, 5040, 5072). Domiciliary spread of HBV is mother-to-child or via skin contact, shared objects, or sex. Contacts and sex partners of household members positive for HB surface antigen (HBsAg) are at risk and should be offered vaccination. By age, length of follow up, and test (HBsAg IgM and antibody to core HBV [anti-HBc]), secondary infection rates in households with an index case are 5–25%. Carrier parents seem to spread HBV to children less efficiently than carrier siblings. In uninfected sex partners infection rates per 100 and per year were 13 (anti-HBs conversion) to 61 (HBsAg conversion). From 42 index cases in households, 23% (3/13) of susceptible sex partners but none of 68 parents or siblings acquired HBV after follow-up for ≥12 months.

Hepatitis C virus (HCV) (39, 173, 950, 1068, 4979, 5899, 7444). Domiciliary spread of HCV is via contact and likely via sex. Compared to the general population, seroreactivity is 5–10-fold higher in households with an infected member. The risk for a long-time susceptible sex partner to acquire HCV is 0–4%. In an intervention trial on heterosexual discordant partners, the HCV infection rate in the control group was 1 (95% CI 0.3–2) per 100 person-years. Among couples, females with seroreactive partners were 3.7 times as likely to be anti-HCV positive than males with seronegative partners.

Hepatitis D virus (HDV) (2567). Domiciliary HDV spread accounts for a majority of chronic HD in children.

HIV (1845, 2915, 3340, 6056, 6448). Domiciliary spread is mother-to-child or via breast milk or sex. Risks for uninfected partners to contract HIV from 100 sex acts with infected individuals are 0.03–0.14 in high-income countries and 0.1–5.6 in low-income countries. Infectivity is influenced by infection stage (with highs in early and late infections), gender, male circumcision, and use of condoms. In Zambian discordant couples in 1985–1987, infection rates per 100 per year were 8 for husbands, but 26 for wives. In Uganda, among 415 discordant couples monitored for up to 30 months, seroconversion rates per 100 person-years were 12 for male-to-female spread, and nearly the same (11.6) for female-to-male spread. None of 50 circumcised males seroconverted, compared with a rate of 17/100 person-years in 137 uncircumcised males. To their female partners, circumcised males were less efficient spreaders (rate, 5/100 person-years) than uncircumcised males (rate, 13/100). In a prospective study of 256 stable, serodiscordant couples in Europe, use of condoms with each of 15,000 sex acts fully protected from HIV (zero infection), while inconsistent use was associated with seroconversion rates of 5/100 person-years (95% CI 3–8, 12/12,000 sex acts).

Human papillomavirus (HPV) (452, 3356). Spread of HPV via domiciliary sex is likely. A majority (64% or 309/480) of male partners of females with cervical condyloma (294 cases) or intraepithelial neoplasia (186 cases) were diagnosed with condylomata acuminata or HPV genital lesions.

HSV (1575, 7905). Spread of HSV via domiciliary sex is likely. Infection risks per 100 sex acts are 0.02 for uninfected male partner, and 0.09 for uninfected female partners.

Human T-cell leukemia virus (HTLV) (1879, 4717). Family clusters of HTLV have been reported. In discordant couples, infection rates per 100 person-years are 4.9 for male-to-female spread, and 1.2 for female-to-male spread.

Bacteria
Skin flora can spread by contact. Unusual agents are rarely spread sexually, e.g., *C. burnetii*. After nine sheep shearers contracted Q fever in Spain and returned home to Poland, three of their spouses were seroreactive; because no other household members contracted the infection, and *C. burnetii* antigen was detected in the semen of two shearers, sexual spread was suspected (4125).

***Streptococcus pyogenes* (group A *Streptococcus* [GAS]) (654, 670, 1197, 1762, 2160, 4810, 5282, 6341).** *S. pyogenes* (GAS) is usually brought home by school-aged children. Crowding is a risk for colonization. The proportion of colonized household members is 10% on contact with a carrier, and 25% on contact with a GAS pharyngitis case. Although the rate of GAS disease in households with an index invasive disease case is 0.07–0.32%, that is 20–200 times the risk in the population, it is considered too low to routinely recommend chemoprophylaxis to household contacts. Furthermore in one study, even when ~90% (78/82) of index cases complied with chemoprophylaxis, spread continued in ~50% (39/82) of households.

Helminths
***Enterobius vermicularis* (47, 1325, 3488, 7253).** *E. vermicularis* spreads at home, in the same individual ano-orally, or person-to-person via eggs on hands, fingernails, and skin, and likely via inhalation of egg-ladden dust from linen and underwear. Viable eggs have been reported from hands, fingernails, bedding, clothes, furniture, and house dust. In infected households, average concentrations in dust can reach 8–13 eggs per g of dust. Risks include crowding, closed, poorly ventilated rooms, poor body hygiene, not washing hands before meals, nail biting, sucking fingers, and playing on the floor.

11.2 SUBSTANDARD DOMICILES
Substandard domiciles are defined here by the lack of indoor tap water and flush toilets. Earth floors, walls made from fortified mud or sundried bricks (adobe), tin roofs, and outdoor pit latrines are typical. Slums (colonias, favelas, and shantytowns) are precarious dwellings of insecure tenure that lack any utilities and are prone to floodings or mud slides.

Exposure (1392, 6737) (http://www.unhabitat.org.). Of currently 3 billion urban residents, about one third live in slums (few in high-income cities, 30% in Latin America, 70% in sub-Saharan Africa), for an overall slum population of about 1 billion. For urban risks, see section 6.3.

DROPLET-AIR CLUSTER
Infections (2449, 6737) (Box 11.3). The main risks include crowding, acute and chronic upper and lower respiratory tract infections, tuberculosis, bacterial meningitis, lack of water and hand, nose, and body hygiene, sharing of unclean personal objects, and low vaccine coverage.

Viruses
Droplet-spread viruses of regular domiciles circulate in substandard homes, in general, at an earlier age and higher rate (for vaccine nonpreventable viruses, see section 11.1 above). Here, the focus is on mumps virus, measles virus, rubella virus, MMR vaccine and VZV.

Measles virus (1502, 2614, 3416, 5776, 5945, 7714, 8119, 8120). Measles virus readily spreads in households. By losing maternal protection by 6–9 months of age, infants become vulnerable, in particular, in crowded situations such as slums. This "susceptibility window" can be narrowed by advancing the first vaccine dose to age groups younger than 12 months. As immunogenicity is suboptimal at this age a booster dose is needed after age 12 months. Without vaccine, secondary attack rates in susceptible household contacts younger than 15 years are ~75–85%, and by age 9 years, 90% of household members will have had measles.

Mumps virus (1564, 2295, 3416, 3941). Mumps virus readily spreads in households, typically as an inapparent

> **Box 11.3** Agents from substandard homes, by cluster
>
> For regular homes, see Box 11.2.
>
> | | |
> |---|---|
> | Droplet-air | Measles, mumps, polio, and rubella viruses, VZV; *B. pertussis*, *C. diphtheriae*, *H. influenzae*, *M. tuberculosis* |
> | Feces-food | *E. coli* (ETEC), *S. enterica* serovar Typhi, *V. cholerae*; *B. coli*; *Ascaris*, *Trichuris* |
> | Zoonotic | Arboviruses (e.g., CCHFV, DENV, JEV, RRV, WEEV, and WNV), vertebrate-borne viruses (*Hantavirus*, lymphocytic choriomeningitis virus, rabies virus); *B. duttoni*, ocular *C. trachomatis*, *R. rickettsii*, *R. typhi*, *Streptobacillus*, *Y. pestis*; *Leishmania*, *Plasmodium*, *Trypanosoma*; *E. granulosus*, *O. volvulus*; myiasis |
> | Environmental | *Leptospira*; *Sporothrix*; hookworm, *Schistosoma*, *Strongyloides*, *Toxocara* |
> | Skin-blood | HIV, HHV8; pyodermia, STI, *T. pertenue pertenue*; tinea capitis; *Hymenolepis*; *Pediculus*, *Sarcoptes* |

infection in preschool or young school children. Reported secondary attack rates in unvaccinated members of households with an index case are ~10–40% (typically 30%), and by 29 years of age, 90% of household members will have had mumps.

Rubella virus (1693). Rubella virus in low-income countries is typically acquired at 2–8 years of age; by location, the proportion of women of childbearing age that is susceptible (seronegative) ranges from <10% to >25%.

VZV (302, 1543, 3234, 3416, 4230, 6790, 8061). VZV is highly infective. An index case can rapidly and broadly contaminate the home environment. Secondary attack rates in susceptible household contacts <15 years of age are 65–85%, and by age 11 years, 90% of household members will have had varicella. In Switzerland in 1992–1995, anti-VZV IgG in adolescents increased with increasing the number of siblings, from 90% (182/202) in households with no siblings, to over 97% (1,199/1,235) with one or two siblings, and 98% (156/159) with three siblings, to 100% (47/47) with four or more siblings. Vaccination may not fully suppress the spread. VZV DNA has been amplified from the nasopharynx of immune household contacts, and vaccinated individuals with a rash could shed either wild-type (breakthrough varicella) or vaccine-type (mitigated varicella) VZV.

Bacteria

Droplet-spread bacteria of regular domiciles circulate in substandard homes, in general, at an earlier age and higher rate (for *N. meningitidis*, *S. pneumoniae*, and vaccine nonpreventable bacteria, see section 11.2). Here, the focus is on *B. pertussis* ($P_{acellular}$ or $P_{whole\ cell}$ vaccines), *C. diphtheriae* (D_{infant} or d_{adult} vaccines), *H. influenzae* b (Hib vaccine), and *M. tuberculosis* (Bacillus Calmette Guérin [BCG] vaccine).

Bordetella **(449, 664, 1832, 2179, 3098, 3235, 6015, 6104, 7567, 8223).** *B. pertussis* readily spreads in households. Infants are susceptible from the first few weeks of life. As the primary DP_a vaccine series is begun at 2–3 months of age, there is a "susceptibility window" that can be closed by chemoprophylaxis. By age, vaccination, and postexposure treatment, secondary attack rates in households are 10–70%, often 30–50%. Home index cases are sources for 70–100% of secondary household cases. Children can carry *Bordetella* home, and likewise, infected parents can be a home source for pertussis in children. Mothers are typical home sources of pertussis in infants.

Corynebacterium **(2322, 2579, 4186, 4569, 4733, 6050, 6806, 7427).** Crowding and poor living conditions are risks for *C. diphtheriae*. In an outbreak in San Antonio, Tex., in 1970, with 196 diphtheria cases, the disease rate was low ($6/10^5$) in census tracts of the upper socioeconomic quartile, intermediate ($25/10^5$) in tracts of interquartile levels, and high ($63/10^5$) in tracts of the lower quartile. In Dhaka, Bangladesh, 98% (1,292/1,372) of diphtheria cases diagnosed in 1973–1974 came from crowded housing. Index diphtheria home cases increase the risk of carriage and diphtheria in households. Some 5–25% of household contacts will test positive for toxigenic *C. diphtheriae* and in the first 30 days postexposure, the risk of diphtheria is increased ≥10-fold. The diphtheria epidemic in eastern Europe in the late 1980s was initially amplified in hospitals, military barracks, kindergartens, and schools. In the Republic of Georgia in 1995–1996, compared with 408 matched controls, risks in 218 diphtheria cases included household exposure to diphtheria, lack of vaccination, sharing of bed and cups, and infrequent bathing. In Finland in 2001, a 3-month-old nonvaccinated boy contracted diphtheria and died. Guests from Russia who had arrived 5 days before and stayed overnight were likely sources for the boy and his sister whose throat swab tested positive.

Hib (6812, 7301, 7566, 7957). Hib is spread in households. Infection risks include crowding (family size >6, or >1 person per room), having siblings, and not being vaccinated. Household contacts have secondary infection rates that decrease with age, from 6% at <1 year, to 2% at

1–3 years, and 0.5% at 4–5 years. In the prevaccine era in the United States, 9 (0.5%) of 1,687 household contacts of <6 years of age developed invasive Hib disease in the 30 days following first manifestation of an index case, compared with none of 2,624 contacts ≥6 years of age. Children of preschool age with home exposure are at >500 times greater risk of invasive Hib disease than the general population.

***M. tuberculosis* (1472, 6074, 6604, 7807).** Tuberculosis disease is correlated with crowding. In Canada, rates of reported tuberculosis among native Americans were $19/10^5$ (95% CI 13–25) in communities housing 0.4–0.6 persons per room, but $113/10^5$ (95% CI 95–131) in communities with 1–1.2 persons per room. In a slum in Peru in 1989–1993, the rate of pulmonary disease was 364 (95% CI 293–528)$/10^5$/year. In highly endemic areas, a minor fraction (~13–23%) of tuberculosis is acquired in households, while the greater portion is acquired in the community, from "social mixing." Outbreaks have been reported among employees of a chicken farm who live in a trailer park and among members of a traveling circus.

FECES-FOOD CLUSTER
Infections (337, 3135, 3491, 3805, 5060, 6557, 8321) (Box 11.3). The main risks include open sewer drains that are used as water sources, domestic animals, carriers in households, unwashed hands, polluted foods, and stored water. Viruses, bacteria, and protozoa are causes of acute diarrhea in infants; protozoa and helminths can cause chronic diarrhea and malabsorption. Multiple pathogens are carried by up to one third of slum dwellers.

In a slum in Dhaka, Bangladesh, the rate of diarrhea in 289 children 2–5 years of age was 1.8 per child-year. Agents from watery stools included *G. lamblia* in 11%, enterotoxigenic *E. coli* (ETEC) in 9%, *Cryptosporidium* in 8%, *E. histolytica* in 8%, *Rotavirus* in 5%, and *Shigella flexneri* in 4%. Agents from dysenteric stools included *S. flexneri* in 12%, *E. histolytica* in 9%, and *C. jejunii* in 6%. In slums, soil-transmitted helminths in children can reach prevalences of 50–90%. For community-acquired diarrhea, see section 14.7.

Among a religious group in Los Angeles that shared meals from a communal kitchen, ate with their hands, and washed the perineum after defecation with bare hands, of 220 members 115 (52%) tested positive for *Dientamoeba fragilis*, 50 (23%) for *G. lamblia*, 9 (4%) for *E. histolytica/dispar*, and 2 (1%) for *E. vermicularis*, and the group had experienced outbreaks of HAV, shigellosis, and staphylococcal pyodermias.

Prevention (5300, 6212, 6802). Adapted means include washing hands with soap, boiling drinking water, adding disinfectant or bleach (NaClO) to stored water, and adding quicklime (CaO) to excrements.

Viruses
All viruses of regular domiciles circulate, including HAV, enteric adenoviruses, *Norovirus*, and *Rotavirus* (3491, 6557, 8321).

HAV (160, 1783, 4276, 4338, 5181). HAV is endemic in crowded domiciles that lack sanitation. Risks include crowding (two or more persons per room), no kitchen, and open sewers in front of the house. In Texas, children from colonies along the border to Mexico had a significantly higher seroprevalence (37% or 39/105) than children from urban border areas (17% or 11/65) or metropolitan San Antonio (6% or 7/115). In Rio de Janeiro, Brazil, in 1997, seroreactivity in 3,271 randomly selected residents sharply increased after age 3 years, approaching 100% by age 30 years; the average age of primary infection was 10 years. In Madrid, Spain, in 1990, seroprevalence related to housing conditions, with 23% (12/51) in children from houses with tap water, toilets, and 1.5 persons per bedroom, 46% (25/54) in children from orphanages with tap water, toilets, and five persons per bedroom, but 63% (32/51) in Gypsy children from domiciles of which only 50% had tap water and toilets and three persons per bedroom. Vaccine is advised for children in endemic areas and for recurring epidemics.

HEV (644, 6947, 6948). Household HEV spread seems uncommon, and reported secondary attack rates have been low (<5%).

Poliovirus (2688, 3942, 6013, 7743). Poliovirus circulates in substandard domiciles, in nonvaccinated populations who lack sanitation, mainly by contact rather than by water or food. In Louisiana in 1953–1955, after exposure to wild virus, >90% (136/148) of susceptible household contacts seroconverted. In Namibia in 1993–1994, type 1 virus caused an outbreak with 27 cases; the attack rate in preschool children of Windhoek was 0.06%. Inadequate sanitation and unsafe water were thought to have fostered the outbreak. In an outbreak in Taiwan in 1982 with 1,031 cases, risks doubled in families who shared toilets with other families.

***Rotavirus* (3491).** *Rotavirus* is a frequent cause of diarrhea in the first year of life. In that age group, up to 20% of diarrhea is due to *Rotavirus*.

Bacteria
Diarrheal disease is rampant in households that lack sanitation, with rates of 4–10 episodes per child per year compared with 0.5–2 per child per year in regular domiciles (2984). Compared with the frequency in controls, the main diarrheagenic bacteria are *E. coli* (ETEC), *Shigella*, and *Vibrio* (3491).

Campylobacter **(5547, 6110).** Risks for *C. jejuni* include the lack of domestic water and the presence of animals and garbage in the cooking area. In a Peruvian shantytown, *Campylobacter* was isolated from 156 (9%) of 1,711 residents, 9 (7%) of 134 environmental samples (chicken feces and hand washings), and 682 (40%) of 1,711 free-ranging chicken. The *Campylobacter* infection rate was 0.8 per child-year, and the disease rate was 0.4 per child-year. The reported diagnostic yield in preschool children with diarrhea is ~10%.

E. coli **(3491).** ETEC and EPEC are frequent causes of diarrhea in the first 3 years of life. Spread is by foods or person-to-person. The reported diagnostic yield in preschool children with diarrhea is ~10–15%.

***Salmonella enterica* serovar Typhi (2652, 4583).** Risks include having contact with a case, living in a house without municipal tap water or with an open sewer, and not washing hands before eating.

Shigella **(3491).** *Shigella* is a frequent cause of diarrhea in children. Spread is mainly person-to-person.

Vibrio cholerae **(46, 1569, 2340, 4321, 4422).** Risks for *V. cholerae* include life in slums, crowding, contact with a case, lack of home tap water, >10 min walk to a water source, and use of unboiled water. Depending on *Vibrio* biotype, 5–25% of home contacts of a cholera case become ill, and another 20–25% become infected.

Protozoa
Major agents are *Cryptosporidium*, *E. histolytica*, and *G. lamblia*.

Balantidium **(1909, 2238).** Pigs on the premises are a risk for *Balantidium*, mainly in association with lack of sanitation.

Cryptosporidium **(597, 4277, 5397, 5399, 6557).** Risks for *Cryptosporidium* include crowding and living in slums. In Texas, children 6 months to 13 years of age from colonias along the border to Mexico have been seroreactive to *C. parvum* (89% or 93/105) more frequently than children from urban nonborder areas (46% or 50/109). In colonias, consumption of municipal water compared with bottled water was a risk. In a slum in Brazil, oocysts were found in household members, city water samples, and household animals (including in 10% of dogs). In households with an index case, the secondary transmission rate was 19%. In a periurban community of Peru, *Cryptosporidium* diarrhea was more frequent in children who defecated in a field than in children who could use a latrine or flush toilet in the house.

Entamoeba **(337, 560, 829, 980, 3134, 3135, 5077).** Risks for *E. histolytica/dispar* infection and disease include lack of domestic water and crowding. Amebiasis is endemic in slums. Fecal prevalence of *E. histolytica/dispar* in children in slums has been 2–20%. In the slums in Fortaleza, Brazil, *E. histolytica* (excluding *E. dispar*) was prevalent in 11% (60/564) of stools from inhabitants of all ages. Seroprevalence in slum dwellers of all ages can reach 20%. In a slum in Dhaka, Bangladesh, the *E. histolytica* diarrhea rate in 289 children 2-5 years of age was 0.08 per child-year, and the *E. histolytica* infection rate was 0.28 per child per year.

Giardia **(337, 2746, 4655, 5077, 5396, 6000).** Risks for *G. lamblia* include lack of toilets, domiciles with mud floors, animals in the house, open sewage nearby, and rubbish on the premises. Water containers accessible to flies and hands are a domestic source, and cysts have been detected in household drinking water. Properly stored water is protective. *G. lamblia* is endemic in slums. By age 2 years, virtually all children have gone through infections or disease episodes, or are still infected. The prevalence in children in the slums can reach 20%.

Toxoplasma **(91, 2518).** A source of *T. gondii* in low-income countries is soil contaminated by cat feces, including for children who play on the ground, and adults who cook and do other work on the ground. In Costa Rica, humans could acquire infection inside houses with cement floors, if cats defecated in the house.

Helminths
Ascaris **(304, 337, 1087, 3046, 3805, 5535, 7592, 8191).** Risks for *A. lumbricoides* include crowding, poor housing, lack of toilets and domestic water, many persons per toilet, promiscuous defecation, and an uneducated mother. In Minas Gerais, Brazil, crowding had a five times greater effect on the prevalence of *A. lumbricoides* in households when it was associated with a lack of water in the house. Worm burden is clustered, although part of the overdispersion may be due to predisposition rather than exposure. *A. lumbricoides* is endemic in slums and its prevalence in slum children can reach 50–90%.

Clonorchis sinensis **(1368, 1410).** This snail-borne trematode is maintained by the deposition of human feces into snail-infested freshwaters. Residence along rivers is an infection risk. In Korea, the infection prevalence in snails has been inversely correlated with the distance of snail habitats from houses.

T. solium **(1091, 2440, 2621, 2628, 2848, 5407).** Risks for *T. solium* infections in domestic pigs and cysticercosis in humans include open sewers, a carrier in the household that fecally pollutes foods, and crowding. Eggs can be recovered from dirt under the fingernails of carriers. In Ecuador, members of households with a neurocysticercosis case were three times more frequently seroreactive (11.6% or 20/173) than control households (3.8% or 2/53).

Trichuris (337, 3046, 3805, 7165). *T. trichiura* is endemic in slums. Prevalence in slum children can reach 65–100%. Lack of sanitation is a risk.

ZOONOTIC CLUSTER

Exposure (1946). Arthropods, birds, bats, rodents, monkeys, and other mammals can be sources of infection in residents of substandard domiciles. Slum dwellers are particularly at risk. Along the trans-Amazon highway in Brazil, risks for arboviral infections included living in straw houses and sleeping outdoors for hunting or clearing land.

Although not confirmed disease vectors, bedbugs can be prevalent in substandard houses in low-income countries.

Prevention (1691, 4446). Prevention includes maintenance, garbage collection, and mosquito barriers. Means against mosquitoes include location away from breeding sites, screened doors, windows, and ceilings, impregnated bednets, and indoor residual spraying.

Viruses: Arthropod Borne

Residents of substandard homes in enzootic areas are most heavily exposed to mosquito-borne viruses (e.g., dengue virus [DENV], Japanese encephalitis virus [JEV], Ross River virus [RRV], St. Louis encephalitis virus [SLEV], western equine encephalitis virus [WEEV], and West Nile virus [WNV]) and to tick-borne viruses (e.g., Crimean-Congo hemorrhagic fever virus [CCHFV]). Some evidence is reviewed below.

CCHFV (166, 993, 2419). CCHFV is mainly borne by ticks and blood from infected animals. However, CCHFV seems to spread among home contacts of cases, although not efficiently. In an outbreak in Pakistan in 1976, with an index case and 10 secondary cases, the father of the index case, and the wife and a sister of a secondary case contracted CCHF.

DENV (2712, 3302, 6208, 7201, 7396, 7421). Risks for DENV include living in slums, elevated homes with wooden floors, use of pit or outdoor toilets, cans and other water receptacles on premises, gutters for rainwater, and lack of waste collection. Transmission in urban areas can be intense. In inhabitants of Salvador City in northeastern Brazil, the seroprevalence was 69%, and the infection rate was 70/100 per year. Some 0.5–25% (mean, 7%) of houses had one or more sites with larvae of *Aedes aegypti*; even in areas with the lowest house index, the DENV rate reached 55/100 per year. In Iquitos, Peru, *A. aegypti* adults clustered by frequent feeding and short flight range in "key" houses. Window and door screens offer significant protection. In an outbreak in Laredo, Tex., and adjacent Nuevo Laredo, Mexico, low seroprevalence in Laredo demonstrated protection also by air conditioning.

JEV (5773). In a JEV outbreak on Saipan island, infection risks included crowding and lack of air conditioning.

RRV (7291). Living in a rural, enzootic area is a risk. During the 1990–1991 outbreak in Northern Territory, Australia, attack rates were significantly lower in urban Palmerston ($165/10^5$) and Darwin ($228/10^5$) than in the hinterland (Litchfield Shire, $866/10^5$).

SLEV (3737, 7583). In an SLEV outbreak in Texas in 1986, compared with age- and sex-matched controls, living in mosquito-accessible domiciles was a risk in 17 cases. In Louisiana in 2001, most of the 70 cases came from poor living areas, with houses run down, screens in disrepair, premises with abundant breeding sites, and mosquito pools that yielded SLEV.

WEEV (1259). Residence in a rural, enzootic area is a risk for WEEV.

WNV (3114, 6630). In a WNV outbreak in Bucharest, Romania, in 1996, the old sewer system, designed to drain rainwater, contained standing water and *Culex pipiens* larvae. The basements of some houses were flooded with a mix of drinking water and sewage, allowing for *Culex* breeding sites. Risks included having mosquitoes in the house, having a flooded basement, and time spent outdoors.

Viruses: Vertebrate Borne

Ebola virus (EBOV) (1535, 2010, 7387). EBOV can spread at home and among contacts of cases. In the Sudan in 1976, secondary attack rates were 81% among 48 relatives who treated patients, 23% among 23 relatives who slept with patients in the same room, and 13% overall (30/232 household contacts). In the Congo (formerly Zaire) in 1976, when family was defined by living in contiguous domicile and shared eating facility, secondary attack rates were 6% (62/1,103 contacts). In the Congo in 1995, secondary attack rates were 16% (28/173) in household contacts of cases and nil (0/78) in household members without physical case contact.

Hantavirus (1120, 1388, 1650, 2441, 3549, 4664, 6405, 8293). Humans contract hemorrhagic fever with renal syndrome or *Hantavirus* pulmonary syndrome (HPS) from rodent contacts or aerosols. Only for Andes virus is there evidence for person-to-person spread. In Chile, 1.9% (95% CI 0.3–6%) of 106 home contacts of patients with HPS had IgG antibodies to Andes virus, compared with 0% (0–3%) of 109 health care workers with patient contacts; domiciliary contacts included shared lodging, work in a closed room, or transportation for >1 h.

Domiciliary risks include living in enzootic areas, solitary houses close (<50 m) to the forest, bushes around the house, observing rodents on the premises, rodent-infested houses, regular work in the forest (for >16 h/month), storing of firewood around the house, cleaning out rodent-infested cellars, sleeping on the ground, and overnight stays in field huts and wilderness camps. In People's Republic of China in 1961, an outbreak caused 1,314 cases of hemorrhagic fever with renal syndrome, for an attack rate of 0.2%; risks in 351 hospitalized patients included sleeping on the ground and in field huts.

A preventive measure (2005, 3417) is proofing dwellings against rodents by sealing the openings at foundations, doors, roofs, and pipes and by repairing window and door screens. Trapping and removing deer mice from ranch buildings paradoxically can result in an increased number of mice entering the buildings, with an increased risk of mouse-to-human spread.

Lassa virus (4880, 7406). Houses are considered the most important transmission habitat. Rodent-infested houses and food contaminated via rodent urine are hazards.

Lymphocytic choriomeningitis virus (1249, 1386, 1387, 5733). Peridomestic cycles exist among (wild) house mice and (pet) hamsters. The reported population seroprevalence is 4–5%. Risks include increasing age and low household income.

Machupo virus (7177). A reported risk for Machupo virus is sleeping in rodent-infested shelters.

Marburg virus (612, 2683, 4780). In the Marburg 1967 outbreak, 1 of the 31 cases was the wife of a patient which suggested spread by contact or sex. In 1975, the companion of an Australian index case developed secondary disease. In the Congo outbreak in 1998–1999, person-to-person spread was confirmed. Sources of infections in households included patients and ritual contacts with corpses.

Bacteria

Flies carry agents mechanically feces-to-food, feces-to-face, and face-to-face, including ocular *Chlamydia trachomatis*. Fleas carry *Rickettsia typhi* and *Yersinia pestis* to humans; ticks carry *Borrelia* and *Rickettsia*. *Streptobacillus* is rodent associated; substandard housing is a risk for contracting rat bite fever (6495).

***Borrelia* and tick-borne relapsing fever (TBRF). Africa (2787, 3962, 7315).** *Ornithodoros moubata*, the vector of *Borrelia duttoni*, is well adapted to rural houses, where it dwells in cracks of walls and earthen floors. In endemic villages in Tanzania, up to 88% of houses are infested. **North America (423, 820, 1567, 2103, 2787, 4190, 5772, 7315, 7456, 7481).** In enzootic areas of the United States, typical sites for exposure to TBRF are cabins, cottages, vacation homes, and rural housings that are visited by rodents and have become tick infested. At Grand Canyon National Park, 15 visitors contracted TBRF after an overnight stay in cabins; rodent nests were found above the ceilings and below the floors of many cabins. In an outbreak in the Grand Canyon in 1973, attack rates per 100 person-nights were significantly higher in cabins at the northeast rim (0.62 in employees and 0.32 in tourists) than in all other housings (0–0.25), including cottages, dorms, and trailer parks. Prevention includes rodent proofing and habitat treatment with acaricides. Care should be taken when clearing out cabins. In Texas, a 34-year-old woman contracted TBRF several days after she cleared rats nests from underneath her country home.

***Chlamydia* (2199, 3461, 4571, 6660).** Risks for *C. trachomatis* include no tap water, no toilets, garbage or cattle on the premises, flies in the house, flies on the faces of children, crowding, and sharing a sleeping room with an individual with an active infection. Trachoma clusters in households; solitary cases are rare. Prolonged close contacts and high fly densities support intense transmission.

***R. rickettsii* (2550, 3740, 5184, 6284, 6795, 8167).** Some 4% of spotted fever cases occur in family clusters, which are explained by common exposure or intrafamilial spread. Detached dwellings in enzootic, woody, or brushy areas are a risk. In Espirito Santo, Brazil, in 1990, the wife of one of four hunters who developed spotted fever removed numerous ticks from her husband's clothing and found an embedded tick on her body 10 days before becoming ill herself.

***R. typhi* (665, 1211, 6246, 6896).** Barns, port warehouses, and substandard domiciles can attract rats and vector fleas. Rodent-infested domiciles are a risk for *R. typhi*. Cases can cluster in rodent-infested houses. In Israel, significantly higher disease rates in Arabs than Jews have been associated with higher rat and rat flea densities in bedouin houses with murine typhus cases than in neighboring Jewish houses. In Brazil, workers contracted murine typhus from naps on grain sacks in a warehouse. Rat proofing can prevent infections.

***Y. pestis* (458, 735, 1328, 1643, 2564, 6974, 8137).** Plague risks include residence in an enzootic or epizootic area, substandard or rodent-infested housing, fleas in or around the home, and a plague case at home. In outbreak areas of rural Mozambique and Ecuador, exposed people live in thatched huts, often sleeping on the floor. In Mahajanga, Madagascar, in 1995–1998, >90% (473/515) of patients with confirmed disease resided in the most densely populated city areas. Of 357 cases reporting details, 33% (117) found dead rats in the house, and another 25% (88) saw dead rats in the vicinity of their homes. Plague can spread person-to-person, typically in families, both by droplets (pneumonic plague) and the human flea (*Pulex irritans*). In Peru in 1988, an interval of 20–25 days from primary to secondary cases suggested spread by *P. irritans*, an outbreak-prone situation. Household contacts should receive chemoprophylaxis.

Protozoa

Exposure. Residents of substandard houses are exposed to *Leishmania* and *Plasmodium* (by mosquitoes), *Trypanosoma brucei gambiense* (by tsetse flies), and *Trypanosoma cruzi* (by bugs).

Prevention (502, 1269, 3268, 4520, 6755, 8099). Improving walls and roofs and residual insecticides are effective means of vector control, and impregnated curtains can protect bedrooms from triatomines. Although uncommon in well-plastered houses, however, triatomine bugs can maintain domestic cycles in high-quality houses by feeding on dogs, e.g., in Texas.

Leishmania. **Cutaneous leishmaniasis (CL) (2352, 5585, 7833, 8009, 8303).** In South America, indoor *Lutzomyia* abundance correlates with the rate of CL. In Venezuela, the indoor density of *L. ovallesi* females needed for new cases to occur was estimated at ≥800 per house per year. Infection risks include domiciles close (≤200 m) to vector-breeding sites or foci, tall trees near the house, solitary house (>15 m away from neighbor), dirt floor, roof from permeable materials, permanent openings for windows, animals in or near the house, and outdoor activities, such as fetching water, bathing, and farming. In a shack settlement without piped water, sewage, and electricity, 35 km from Rio de Janeiro, Brazil, in 1984–1986, an outbreak carried by peridomestic *L. intermedia* caused 105 cases; lesions took 3 months to develop, and *L. braziliensis* was isolated from patients, domestic dogs, and equids. **Visceral leishmaniasis (VL) (445, 596, 3696, 4791, 5179, 7423, 8426).** Infection risks include residence close to a focus, no tap water, no sewage, no electricity, houses with mud floors or walls, open garbage containers, animals (dogs and livestock) in or near the house, and living with a case in the household. In an enzootic area of Venezuela, seroreactivity was 10% (19/187) in families with an index case, but only 3% (5/169) in neighborhood controls without an index case. Bednets and good housing reduce but do not eliminate risks. In Bihar State, India, in 1997, domiciles of 938 confirmed cases were brick houses in 23%, mud houses in 68%, and grass-covered houses in 8%. Homes of 78% of the cases were situated ≤15 m from a cowshed, and to prevent theft 22% took animals into the house at night.

Plasmodium **(240, 1039, 1101, 1346, 2602, 3026, 3062, 4446, 7095, 7719).** Infection (*Plasmodium* parasitemia) and disease cluster in households. Major determinants of domiciliary exposure include proximity to breeding sites (high risk if within <100–1,000 m from ditches, canals, swamps, and lagoons), building material (high risk if built from mud, straw, palm, or makeshift), type (high risk if level to earth or camps), maintenance (high risk if cans are around), rainwater drainage (high risk if clogged gutters and stagnant ditches), mosquito proofing (high risk if thatched roof, open eaves and windows, in particular, in sleeping rooms), and nocturnal activities (bednets, high risk during visits to privy).

The principal malaria vector in Africa, *Anopheles gambiae*, enters houses preferably through overhanging roofs and open eaves. In the Amazon, outbreaks of vivax and falciparum malaria occurred in new settlements along roads where population turnover was high and housing inadequate. In Kampala, Uganda, rates of clinical malaria per person-year were 2.2 in residents close to a swamp but only 0.4 in residents >100 m away from the swamp. In Sri Lanka in 1996, compared with remote houses, the odds of clinical malaria were 6 (95% CI 4–9) in houses within 750 m from a breeding site. Similarly, compared with houses ≥1,000 m from the site, the odds were 7.6 for nearby (<250 m) houses to harbor *A. culicifacies*. In Papua, Indonesia, malaria reemerged when traditional village huts were replaced with new houses equipped with drainage ditches that served as breeding sites.

Protection (1530, 1692, 1915, 3025, 4446, 5135, 6327, 8394). Impregnated curtains at doors, windows, and eaves reduce overall mortality. Houses treated with residual insecticides protect from mosquitoes and clinical malaria for 6 months. The mean number of *A. gambiae* was 7 (95% CI 4–11) per night in a control hut, but only 1.3–1.5 per night in huts with net or plastic screen ceilings, a reduction of 78–80%. House spraying, unlike aerial spraying, by being targeted is environmentally acceptable; to abandon it will likely contribute to the reemergence of malaria. Deltamethrin works on cement, bamboo, and wood, less on mud walls. Despite their efficiency, impregnated bednets and indoor residual spraying have been underused. In Africa, median child coverage with bednets is 15%, that with insecticide-treated nets is only 2%.

Trypanosoma. Domiciliary exposure includes in Africa *T. brucei gambiense*, in Latin America *T. cruzi*. ***T. brucei gambiense*** **(1127, 8090).** In tsetse fly territory, *T. brucei gambiense* is transmitted peridomestically (by "palpalis" group *Glossina*), at water sites, shade trees, plantations, and rice fields. Exposed groups include children playing in water, women fetching water, preparing cassava, or washing clothes, and men landing boats or fishing. The dry season, in particular, congregates tsetse flies and humans at water sites. ***T. cruzi*** **(1599, 8099).** Chagas disease is the "poor man's housing disease." Triatomines adapted to (rural) houses include *Rhodnius prolixus*, *Triatoma dimidiata*, and *T. infestans*. *R. prolixus* mainly inhabits straw roofs. *T. dimidiata*, the principal domestic vector, colonizes floors, camouflaged in dust. Light can attract bugs to houses. There have been many instances of occasional incursions of triatomines into houses. Bugs might also access houses with construction material or firewood. **Risks (225, 1269, 1786, 1936, 3035, 5784, 6378, 8099, 8212, 8383).** Risks for *T. cruzi* include thatched roofs, loose walls, dirt floors, piles of firewood, indoor crop storage, and the presence of rats or other mammals. By location, house type, and control, the proportion of bug-infested houses in enzootic areas is <0.1% (Uruguay) to 10–60% (rural areas). Infection risks are considered low for house infestation indices <2%. In the domestic cycle, humans are the main reservoir. Sources of blood for peridomestic triatomines are humans (in 50–90%), dogs (45–80%), cats (0.1–9%), and chickens (5–15%).

In a town in Costa Rica in 1964–1968, 181 (35%) of 523 houses harbored 3,885 bugs, for a density of 22 bugs per house. In rural Guatemala in 1998, of 550 persons in 121 adobe (brick) houses (~25% *T. dimidiata*-infested), 9% were seroreactive, and the infection rate was ~0.5/100 per year, in contrast to 670 persons in 117 bajareque (stick-plaster) houses (~8% *R. prolixus*-infested) where 39% of residents were seroreactive, and the infection rate was ~4/100 per year. In Venezuela in 1988–1996, 34 (58%) of 59 patients with acute Chagas disease reported bugs at home. Houses of 85% (29/34) of those reporting bugs harbored *T. cruzi*-infested bugs, and 38% (13) harbored reactive or parasitemic dogs. Bugs positive for *T. cruzi* or *T. rangeli* were also recovered from palm trees (*Acrocomia*) near the houses of five of the cases. In northeastern Argentina, ~15–55% of dwellings were infested by triatomines, including *T. infestans*.

Helminths
Echinococcus **(198, 4225, 7950, 7976).** Risks for *E. granulosus* include unhygienic contacts with dogs and their feces, home slaughter, and a history of infection.

Onchocerca **(8087).** A risk for *O. volvulus* is housing close to rivers where *Simulium* can breed.

Ectoparasites
Fly larvae can cause myiasis (see section 4.6) (5459, 5694). The Congo floor maggot, *Auchmeromyia luteola* (Calliphoridae, ex *A. senegalensis*) occurs in sub-Saharan Africa. Larvae hide in cracks on the floor of dwellings; at night, they crawl to hosts, including pigs and humans. Feeding lasts 10–20 min. Sleeping on the floor or on mats is a risk. Because larvae do not climb more than a few centimeters, beds on a frame are preventive.

ENVIRONMENTAL CLUSTER
Major environmental agents from substandard homes are *Leptospira* and some helminths.

Bacteria
Leptospira **(632, 1450, 3718, 3825, 3844, 4369, 6616).** Risks range broadly and include slum and rural homes, proximity to stagnant waters or open sewers, domiciles prone to floodings, rainwater catchment, lack of sewage, lack of garbage disposal, garbage on the premises, seeing rats on the premises during the day, water-related domestic activities (e.g., washing clothes and watering plants), walking barefoot on the premises, skin wounds, and dogs or cats in the house. In Peru in 2000, seroprevalence was 28% (182/650) in residents of a slum near Iquitos built on stilts because of seasonal floods, 17% (52/316) in residents of an uphill well-drained area, and 0.7% (1/150) in a desert shantytown south of Lima. In the seasonally flooded area, seroconversion rate was ~28,800/10^5 per year. In Mumbai, India, in 2001, after heavy rainfall and floods, an outbreak among children in the slums caused 32 confirmed cases.

Sporothrix **(4591).** *S. schenckii* is a risk in endemic areas, in houses with dirt floors or raw wood ceilings.

Helminths
The main hazards are peridomestic defecation by humans and animals and contact with unsafe freshwater.

Hookworms (*Ancylostoma duodenale* and *N. americanus*) (337, 1416, 3805, 4711, 7221). *A. duodenale* and *N. americanus* are endemic in slums that force people to defecate around houses. Poorly maintained latrines can be a rich source of infections. In Thailand, 63–85% of 2,527 inhabitants from 120 villages had latrines in their homes, 20–40% regularly used them, and a similar percentage reported to have defecated outside latrines in the past month. Hookworm prevalence of 5–45% is reported in slums. Load is often uneven (overdispersed), with most individuals carrying a light burden, and a few harboring most of the community biomass. Wearing shoes is protective.

Cutaneous larva migrans (due to *A. braziliense* and *A. caninum*) is also prevalent in slums (3304).

Schistosoma **(622, 2163, 3117, 3318, 4400, 7655, 7671).** Risks for *Schistosoma* include rural domiciles in endemic areas, location near a transmission site, lack of toilets, and water-related domestic activities, such as walking through creeks and marshlands, collecting water at holes or ponds, washing clothes and kitchen utensils, growing vegetables, harvesting water grasses and reeds, fishing, boating, swimming, and playing in water. On the shores of Lake Victoria, Kenya, the prevalence of *S. mansoni* decreased with the increasing distance of homes from the lake, from 60% at 0–1 km to 22% at 3–4 km. In Minas Gerais, Brazil, 597 individuals had a mean of 118 (range, 0–504) water contacts per week.

Strongyloides **(475, 1551, 1594, 3083, 5956).** *S. stercoralis* infections in slums are aggregated (overdispersed) in some households. Possible explanations include common exposure or human-to-human spread. Risks include lack of indoor toilets, communal latrines, houses with earth floors, poor personal hygiene, and home contact with infected individuals. By human-to-human spread, the worm can be introduced into regular households. In France, the only risk found in a 23-year-old military person with strongyloidiasis was that his parents had traveled to Thailand and Mexico a few years ago. Also in France, *S. stercoralis* was isolated in two friends 4 and 5 years of age; both had never left the country and lived in the same flat, under poor hygienic conditions, and the father of one was from West Africa and had been diagnosed with massive strongyloidiasis.

Toxocara **(1458).** In northwestern Spain in 1991–1994, the seroprevalence was 3% (14/455) in middle-class children living in an urban environment, but 57% (52/91) in age- and sex-matched children of the same area living in shacks without plumbing, where dogs were common around dwellings.

SKIN-BLOOD CLUSTER
Inner-city and marginal communities and inhabitants of slums are at risk of infections by skin contact and STI. The review below is circumstantial only.

Viruses
HIV. HIV is endemic in adult slum populations. Seroprevalence >20% in pregnant women 15–24 years of age has been reported from capital cities of the following countries in southern Africa: Zimbabwe (22%), South Africa (24%), Lesotho (28%), Botswana (33%), and Swaziland (39%) (7643).

HDV (3047, 4719). Intrafamilial spread of HDV is suspected in indigenous people in Latin America who exhibit a high prevalence of HBV markers.

Human herpes virus 8 (HHV8) (5937). In rural French Guiana, a study of pairs (717 mother-child, 1,140 child-child, and 126 spouses) suggested mother-to-child and child-to-child but not husband-to-wife spread of HHV8.

Bacteria
Haemophilus ducreyi **(3110).** In Winnipeg, Manitoba, Canada, in 1975–1977, 88 (65%) of 135 patients with chancroid were Native Indians or Métis living in the inner city, in old rooming houses and hotels.

Mycobacterium leprae **(889, 1076, 1290, 1941, 3078, 3630, 3903, 7702).** *M. leprae* is spread in households, likely via droplets from nasal smear-positive individuals. Risks include poor living conditions and sharing a room or bed with a case, although spread among discordant, life-long spouses is said to be rare. Infectivity that varies with type of leprosy may confound the association. Household contacts have a relative risk of 2–4 for tuberculoid leprosy and of 8–10 for lepromatous leprosy. In Hyderabad, India, a history of contact was available for 119 (39%) of 306 children with leprosy; most (95% or 113) were exposed in families, and only 5% (6) had other contacts. In Sulawesi, Indonesia, of 101 newly diagnosed leprosy cases, sources were households in 28 (28%), neighborhood in 36 (36%), social network in 15 (15%), and unknown in 22 (22%). Early detection should focus on households and neighborhood contacts, and in low prevalence areas, postexposure prophylaxis in household members is an option.

Staphylococcus aureus **and** ***S. pyogenes*** **(GAS) (5337).** The incidence of GAS pharyngitis can be high in children in slums, in northern India up to one episode per child-year. Although likely endemic in crowded habitats, staphylococcal and streptococcal skin infections are poorly documented in slum populations.

Treponema pertenue **(3043).** Yaws is spread in households via skin contacts.

Fungi
Dermatophytes (178, 2526, 7772). Dermatophytes such as *Trichophyton tonsurans* can spread person-to-person. Crowding and lack of domestic water are risks. In 31 families with a tinea capitis index case, the prevalence of *T. tonsurans* scalp infection was 63% (20/32) in children and 14% (5/35) in adults, compared with 15% (8/53) in children and 13% (2/16) in adults from 20 control families without an index case.

Helminths
Enterobius **(47, 1325, 2745, 7253).** Risks for *Enterobius* include crowding, lack of domestic water, and poor personal hygiene.

Hymenolepis (**4804, 5077**). In India in 1996–2001, the prevalence of *Hymenolepis nana* among slum dwellers of all age groups was 10% (93/939). An urban risk is contact with an infected sibling.

Ectoparasites

In a slum in Fortaleza, Brazil, in 2001, point prevalences in a randomly selected block of 1,185 inhabitants were: cutaneous larva migrans 3% (95% CI 2–4), scabies 9% (95% Cl 7–11), tungiasis 34% (95% Cl 31–36), and pediculosis capitis 43% (95% Cl 41–46) (3304).

Pediculus (**4444**). Crowding is a risk for *P. capitis*.

Sarcoptes (**1417, 1446, 3229, 4205, 6818, 8042**). Risks for *S. scabiei* are substandard housing and crowding. Family clusters have been reported. In households with an index case, reported secondary attack rates are 27–38%. On average, an index case infects two persons.

11.3 HOMELESS PERSONS

Homeless persons (743, 4412, 6444) are people who lack a domicile (postal address) and live in temporary housing such as abandoned buildings, subway halls, parks, public shelters, and homes of friends (couch hopping and doubling up).

Exposure (912, 2458, 4451, 7816). The proportion of city populations that is homeless is ∼0.2–0.4% in the United States, 0.1% in Marseille, France, ∼0.7% in the United Kingdom, and 0.8% in Moscow (0.1 million/12 million). Unemployed adults, minorities, drug addicts, female sex workers, runaway youths, and abandoned children are overrepresented among the homeless.

Infections (270, 2449, 2458, 3900, 4412, 5278, 5557, 6115, 6443, 6444, 8419). Homeless persons are particularly susceptible to respiratory, skin, enteric, and bloodstream infections (Box 11.4). Risks are compounded by smoking, alcoholism, injection drug use (IDU), and unprotected sex for money, drugs, or shelter. In Montreal, Canada, in 1995–1996, 46% (200/437) of street youths 14–25 years of age reported IDU. In Minneapolis in 1998–1999, 15% of 201 homeless youths reported IDU, 20% were tattooed, 37% reported use of marihuana, and 68% reported HIV testing. Health care of homeless persons is difficult and fragmentary, and the morbidity and mortality for this group are above age-specific rates. In Montreal, Canada, in a cohort of 1,013 street youth monitored in 1995–2000, mortality was $921/10^5$ person-years, >11 times the rate of the city youth population.

DROPLET-AIR CLUSTER, HOMELESS

Crowded shelters expose individuals to respiratory tract infections (4634, 5528), including pneumonia and tuberculosis. Respiratory tract infections are prevalent in homeless persons. In Melbourne, Australia, in 1995–1996, 77% of 284 homeless persons were smokers, and productive, persistent cough was a common complaint (3899). Chronic bronchitis has been reported in 2–20% of homeless persons (6115). To cover the homeless with booster vaccines and observed treatments is a challenge.

Viruses

Information is scant. Influenza and other respiratory viruses are putative risks for homeless persons in shelters.

Bacteria

C. diphtheriae (**2579, 2969, 4186**). Homeless persons are at risk of respiratory and cutaneous diphtheria.

C. burnetii (**910**). In Marseilles, France, in 2000, increased seroreactivity to *C. burnetii* was reported among homeless persons in a shelter located downwind from an abandoned slaughterhouse that was used once a year for the ritual killing of sheep by Muslims.

M. tuberculosis. Homeless persons are at risk of *M. tuberculosis* infection and disease (2691, 3044, 3597, 3900, 4265, 4336). In the United States in 1994–2003, of all reported tuberculosis cases ∼6% concerned homeless persons. In New York City, 15% (16/106) of AIDS patients living in single-room-occupancy hotels had previously been diagnosed with tuberculosis, and one half (8/16) of those history positive were noncompliant with treatment.

Box 11.4 Agents and infections in homeless people, by cluster

Droplet-air	Pneumonia, tuberculosis
Feces-food	Acute and chronic diarrhea by bacteria, protozoa, or helminths
Zoonotic	*Hantavirus*; *Bartonella elisabethae*, *B. henselae*, *B. quintana*, *B. recurrentis* (LBRF), *R. prowazekii* (LBT); consider tick bites and bites from vertebrate animals (rabies)
Skin-blood	HBV, HCV, HIV; pyodermias; bloodstream infections, endocarditis; tinea pedis, onychomycosis; lice, scabies. Check "body, clothes, and blankets" for lice (can contribute to agent recovery), and blood culture-negative endocarditis for *Bartonella* and *Tropheryma*

In Melbourne, Australia, in 1995–1996, 3% of homeless persons had a history of tuberculosis. **Prevalence (2458, 3900, 4047, 6115, 8419)**. Reported infection prevalence in homeless persons (by skin test reactivity) is 9–79% (typically 20–30%), disease prevalence (by chest X ray and sputum tests) is 2–11%. **Risks (3044, 3900, 4047, 4265, 5226, 6604, 8419)**. Infection and disease risks include long duration of homelessness, domicile in crowded shelters or single-room hotels, IDU, HIV coinfection, treatment noncompliance, and a history of tuberculosis. In the United States in 1994–2003, compared with nonhomeless cases ($n = 167,148$), homeless persons with active tuberculosis ($n = 11,369$) were more often male (87% versus 61%), smear positive (53% versus 35%), HIV positive (20% versus 9%), recently incarcerated (9% versus 3%), and IDU (14% versus 2%). In San Francisco, in a cohort of 2,774 homeless persons, the tuberculosis rate was 0.27/100 per year: 0.06 in whites, 0.35 in African Americans, and 0.45 in other nonwhites. In Denver, Colo., mandatory screening and prompt treatment reduced disease rates per 100 per year from 0.5 (1995) to 0.1 (1998). In a shantytown of Lima, Peru, with 34,000 inhabitants, the tuberculosis rate by capture-recapture method was $360/10^5$ per year. **Clusters and outbreaks (937, 3029, 4336, 5226)**. Case clusters and outbreaks are common among the homeless. In the United States, three fourths or more of cases among HIV-infected, African American homeless are clustered. In the late 1980s, New York City experienced a tuberculosis epidemic, with disease rates of $170/10^5$ per year in central Harlem. In France, molecular fingerprinting identified 95 (36%) clusters among 272 strains of *M. tuberculosis* from 272 patients; clusters were strongly associated with homelessness. **Shelters (4336, 4893, 5421, 5467, 7693)**. Shelters are a source of clusters or outbreaks. In the United States in 6 weeks of 1986–1987, seven cases occurred in a shelter for males ≥50 years of age, while in the year before the outbreak, only nine cases had been reported in ~1,000 clients. In North Carolina in 1999–2000, an outbreak among 25 homeless persons was linked to a particular shelter; 24 (96%) of 25 patients were male, and 22 (88%) were African American. In Maine in 2002–2003, active pulmonary tuberculosis in six of seven homeless males was linked to shelters; prompt investigation of ~1,100 contacts prevented further spread. In Paris, in 2001–2002, a crowded shelter for migrants was venue for an outbreak with 56 cases of active tuberculosis. **Other venues (4265, 4336)**. Other venues for tuberculosis clusters include hostels for migrant workers and single-room-occupancy hotels.

S. pneumoniae (4987, 6816). In Alberta, Canada, in 2000–2002, rates of bacteremic pneumococcal pneumonia were increased in the homeless ($267/10^5$ person-years) compared with the general population ($10/10^5$ person-years). Alcoholism predisposes to pneumococcal disease. In the United States in 1988–1989, of 39 cases of pneumococcal pneumonia among homeless persons who had recently stayed in a shelter, 35 were smokers, 32 were alcoholics, and 29 had an identical *S. pneumoniae* type.

FECES-FOOD CLUSTER, HOMELESS

Information is scant. In Melbourne, Australia, in 1995–1996, 74% of 284 homeless persons were alcoholics, 28% had raised γ-glutamyltransferase, and gastroenteritis was a common complaint (3899). Poor hygiene predisposes to feco-oral spread of enteric agents. In downtown Los Angeles in 2000, 14% of 200 homeless persons were seroreactive to HEV (6983). In Rio de Janeiro, Brazil, soil-transmitted helminths were prevalent in the homeless: 9% tested positive for hookworms, 33% for *Trichuris*, and 49% for *Ascaris* (2821).

ZOONOTIC CLUSTER, HOMELESS

Poor body hygiene and outdoor overnighting predispose homeless persons to lice-, flea-, tick-, and rodent-borne zoonoses. (912). For animal bites and rabies, see section I.

Hantavirus **(6983)**. Exposure to rats is a putative risk. In downtown Los Angeles in 2000, 0.5% (1/200) of homeless persons were seroreactive to SEOV.

Bartonella **(912, 1532, 2994, 3617, 4851, 6494, 6983, 7058)**. In inner-city residents and homeless persons, reported *Bartonella* seroprevalence is 2–70%. Of 200 homeless persons from downtown Los Angeles, 12.5% were seroreactive to *B. elizabethae*, 9.5% to *B. quintana*, and 3.5% to *B. henselae*. In Paris, France, the *Bartonella* seroprevalence in the homeless was 54% (31/57; 95% CI 41–68), compared with 2% in age-, sex-, and area-matched blood donors. Risks for reactivity were age ≥40 years and homelessness for ≥3 years. Although serological cross-reactivities preclude species identification, *B. elisabethae*, *B. henselae*, and *B. quintana* have been confirmed in the homeless. In Marseille, France, 7.5% (70/930) of homeless persons were reactive to *B. quintana*, and 50 (5%) grew the agent in blood cultures. Traditional risks for *B. quintana*-associated trench fever have been lack of personal hygiene, crowding, and infestation with body lice. Today, these risks apply to homeless people. In Marseille and Moscow, *B. quintana* has been confirmed by nucleic acid amplification (NAT) in lice from the homeless.

Borrelia recurrentis **(912, 956)**. A threat exists that infected immigrants from endemic areas could reintroduce louse-borne relapsing fever (LBRF) among the homeless. In Marseille, France, in 2000–2003, 1.6% (15/930) homeless persons had anti-*B. recurrentis* IgG (cutoff dilution, 1:100), compared with none of 467 control blood donors.

Rickettsia **(376, 912, 1534).** Although outbreaks of louse-borne (epidemic) typhus (LBT) have not been reported in the homeless, a risk of reintroduction exists. In Marseille, France, in 2000–2003, 0.75% (7/930) homeless persons had anti-*R. prowazekii* IgG (cutoff dilution, 1:64), compared with none of 467 control blood donors. A sporadic case in a homeless person from Algeria was reported in that city in 1999, and an autochtonous case in a homeless person (coinfected with *B. quintana*) in 2002. In Baltimore, Md., 16% (102/631) of inner-city IDU had an anti-*R. akari* IgG, suggesting an increased risk of mite-borne rickettsial pox among this population.

The outdoor life of homeless persons also exposes them to tick bites and increased rates of rickettsial infections of the spotted fever group (*R. conorii*, *R. rickettsii*, and others).

SKIN-BLOOD CLUSTER, HOMELESS

Infections (2458, 6115). Skin diseases are prevalent in the homeless, including frostbite, infected wounds, pyodermias, tinea, and ectoparasitoses. IDU is prevalent in some communities, and correspondingly frequent are infections with HBV, HCV, and HIV.

Viruses

HBV (6115). Reported HBsAg prevalence in the homeless is 2–12%.

HCV (4784, 6443). In Montreal, Canada, in 1995–1996, 13% (95% CI 10–16) of 437 street youths 14–25 years of age tested positive for anti-HCV; 46% had a history of IDU, and use of crack cocaine and injection drugs were independent risks. In Goiânia, a city in central Brazil with 1 million inhabitants, seroprevalence in street youths was 1% (4/391) in youths with family links, and 3% (3/100) in youths without family links.

HIV (912, 1869, 4087, 6115, 8419). Reported infection prevalence in homeless persons ranges broadly, from 0.2% to 20%. In San Francisco in 1987–1998, the infection rate in 8,065 street-recruited IDU was ~1/100 person-years. Risks included an age of 20–30 years, sex with men, selling sex, and African American ethnicity. Of male Toronto street youths 14–25 years of age, 2% (15/695) were seroreactive. Infection risks were IDU, prostitution, and incarceration; 57% of youths were on their own for ≤3 years, and 60% had stayed in hostels or homeless shelters in the past 6 months.

Bacteria

Skin infections commonly result from scratching bites by ectoparasites (6115). In San Francisco, of 833 urban poor and homeless, 190 (23%) were nasal carriers of *S. aureus*, and 23 (3%) carried methicillin-resistant strains (MRSA) (1342). Risks were IDU and hospitalization in the past year (1342).

Bacteremia, sepsis, or endocarditis may result from skin or other foci. In Marseille, France, blood cultures from 930 homeless persons yielded *Staphylococcus* (coagulase-negative) in two (0.2%), *Streptococcus* in two (including one *S. bovis*), *Acinetobacter* in two, and diphtheroids in one (0.1%), compared with no isolates in 217 control blood donors (912).

Fungi

Dermatophytes (6115, 7190). Tinea pedis and onychomycosis are common in the homeless. In Boston the prevalence of tinea pedis in homeless persons was 38%, far above the prevalence in the general population.

Arthropods

Pediculus. In Marseille, France, in 2000–2003, 205 of 930 (22%) of homeless persons had skin lesions that suggested body lice; 676 body lice were collected, mostly from clothes, but one fourth (176) from the blankets in shelters (912).

Sarcoptes **(912, 6115).** Scabies is prevalent in homeless persons. The reported prevalence is 3–57%.

11.4 REFUGEES AND RELIEF CAMPS

Displaced persons have been forced to leave their home place by war, religious violence, political persecution, or natural disaster (for floods, see section 5.2). In their home country, they are "internally displaced," after crossing national borders, by legal status, they become refugees, asylum seekers, or stateless. In contrast, migrants (see section 15.6) leave homes for economic reasons. Emergencies are disaster (crisis) situations that require immediate relief. They can be spatially limited or widespread (complex), affecting one or more political subunits or countries.

Exposure (1544, 5236, 5465, 6542) (http://www.unhcr.ch). Hazards include lack of safe water or food, crowded shelters, breakdowns of infrastructure (electricity, water and sewage pipes and pumps, and roads) and health services (ambulances, hospitals, and supplies). In the 2000s, by actual political and emergency situation, estimates were of ~9–12 million refugees, ~4–25 million internally displaced persons, ~2 million stateless persons, and ~1 million asylum seekers.

Infections (1142, 2895, 2931, 4686, 4736, 6542). Displaced persons carry agents enzootic or endemic at their home places and acquired in transit. In emergency camps, acute and chronic infections coexist. Most (65-80%) infections and deaths in camps are due to respiratory tract infections, diarrheal disease, malaria, and measles (Box 11.5). In Somalia in 1992, crude mortality in camps for displaced persons was 0.4–1.7/1,000 per day. In Angola at the end of decade-long civil war, crude mortality in resettlement camps was 0.1–0.2/1,000 per day. In Darfur, Sudan, in 2004, crude mortality among displaced persons was 0.2–0.3/1,000 per day. A proposed threshold to separate limited from complex emergencies is a rate of 0.1 deaths/1,000 per day.

Prevention (444, 1142, 2992, 4736, 5236, 5465, 6542, 6769). Initial measures focus on shelter, sanitation, safe water (at least 15 liters per person per day), and food (2,100 kcal or 8.8 MJ per person per day).

Good site planning, early evaluation, entry vaccinations, and targeted surveillance can prevent outbreaks. Priority vaccines are measles (coverage of children of age 6 months to 5 years ≥90%), and meningococcal meningitis. In camps, single-dose treatments are preferred. Camps are good for limited emergencies but may be inadequate in complex emergencies.

Predeparture or arrival screening of refugees could include: tuberculin skin test and chest radiography, complete blood cell count (anemia, lymphopenia, eosinophilia), serology for HBV (HBsAg, anti-HBs, anti-HBc), HIV (anti-HIV, age >14 years), *Treponema pallidum* (rapid plasma reagin [syphilis], age >14 years), and stool microscopy for parasites.

DROPLET-AIR CLUSTER, RELIEF CAMPS

Risks (122, 951, 1544, 4736). Pneumonia, measles, and acute bacterial meningitis in camps are high-risk infectious diseases that should be made instantly reportable. In long-term refugee camps in the West Bank of Palestine, the frequency of pharyngitis, ear infection, flulike illness, and bronchitis was associated with crowding, cold, damp, and moldy housing, dust, smoke, and poor ventilation, and lack of electricity. Moderate or severe acute respiratory tract infections in camps can occur at rates of up to 0.2/100 per day.

Measles (1544, 2190, 3804, 5187, 7260, 7507). Measles, a major health problem in camps, is aggravated by outbreaks. The reported lethality in camp outbreaks is 1–33%. Recent measles outbreaks in camps include Darfur, Sudan, in 2004 (with at least 725 cases), refugees from Burundi in Tanzania in 2000–2001 (with 1,062 cases), refugees from Mozambique in Malawi in 1987–1989 (with 6,775 cases, for a peak attack rate of 2.5/100 per month), and evacuees from Pinatubo Vulcano in the Philippines in 1991 (with 18,000 cases). Early measles vaccination is important. Measles mortality can be controlled by high vaccine coverage.

***C. diphtheriae* (1399, 4104).** By age and source country, vaccine coverage can be low among refugees. In southern Italy in 1999–2000, of 1,128 Kosovar and Kurd refugees, 618 (55%) were protected by antitoxin IgG levels ≥100 IU/liter, 30% had "basic" protection (IgG 1–99 IU/liter), and 15% were susceptible (IgG <1 IU/ml). In Germany in 1985–1986, toxigenic *C. diphtheriae* was isolated from the throat or nose of 3 (0.06%) of 4,751 asylum seekers.

***M. tuberculosis* (444, 1043, 3019, 3907, 4414, 6496, 7264, 7466).** Displaced persons are at increased risk of infection, disease, and death. Lethality in crisis situations can reach 5–9%. In Guinea-Bissau in 1997–1998, lethality in a "war cohort" of 101 irregularly treated patients was 3-fold higher that in a "peace cohort" of 108 regularly treated patients. Among refugees arriving in Thailand and the Philippines from Vietnam, the prevalence of bacteriologically confirmed pulmonary tuberculosis was 0.6%, and the infection risk by skin test conversion was 2.2/100 per year. Although difficult, daily supervised treatment has given good results, even in complex emergencies.

Refugees account for a significant fraction of tuberculosis cases in high-income countries. Evaluation should include tuberculin skin test and BCG vaccination status.

Box 11.5 Measures of infection control for displaced persons and in relief camps	
Check	Immediate needs, itinerary (transit and origin), past treatments (tuberculosis and malaria)
Consider	• Shelter (tents and buildings), water (drinking and hand washing), toilets, supply (food, firewood, and soap) • Vaccines (entry, catchup): flu, measles, polio; cholera, diphtheria, meningococcal meningitis, pertussis, typhoid fever • Mosquito and malaria prevention; screening for HBV
Detect	And promptly treat HAV, HEV, diarrhea, shigellosis, amebiasis; bacterial meningitis, tuberculosis; zoonoses (dengue, LBRF, LBT, scrub typhus, trench fever, and malaria); pyodermia, ectoparasites
Monitor	Target conditions: e.g., daily diarrhea, deliveries, and deaths ("DDDD"), flulike illness

Indurations that are ≥10 mm indicate infection, indurations ≥5 mm indicate infection if the individual has had contact with an active case, has an abnormal chest X ray, or is immune compromised. Of refugees arriving in the United States, 49% had skin indurations to tuberculin ≥10 mm, the active disease rate was 0.5 (95% CI 0.4–0.6)/100 per year (~80-fold the national figure), and the sputum-positivity rate was 0.09 (95% CI 0.05–0.1)/100 per year. In Norway, 14% of BCG nonvaccinated arriving Kosovar refugees had latent infection, and the rate of active tuberculosis was 0.05%. Refugees can introduce virulent strains such as the "Beijing" genotype locally. This genotype was brought to Gran Canaria Island, Spain, in 1993, by a smear-positive refugee from West Africa. Beijing genotype accounted for zero cases in 1991–1992, 10 (5.5%) in 1993, 12 (8%) in 1994, 18 (16%) in 1995, and 35 (27%) in 1996.

Mycoplasma (7237). An outbreak of *M. pneumoniae* is reported at a refugee center in Thailand.

N. meningitidis (3056, 6606). In Uganda in 1994–1995, a *N. meningitidis* serogroup A outbreak in a camp that hosted an average of 96,860 refugees lasted >1 year, causing >290 cases and an attack rate of 0.3%. Mass vaccination can curtail outbreaks in camps caused by serogroups included in the vaccine.

FECES-FOOD CLUSTER, RELIEF CAMPS
Risks (951, 2689, 4414, 4736). Dehydrating or bloody diarrhea, jaundice, and acute flaccid paralysis are camp risks that should be made instantly reportable. Infectious diarrheal disease can reach rates of 0.25–0.35/100 per day. Enteric infections in refugees and camp inhabitants reflect endemicity of source and transit countries. Polyparasitism is prevalent among refugees.

Viruses
HAV (1400, 1401, 3784, 6607, 6769). HAV is a relief camp risk, mainly for children, as most (>90%) adults from endemic areas are immune. Two major earthquakes hit Turkey in 1999, one in August at Golyaka (a force of 7.4–7.8 on the Richter scale) with 300,000 damaged houses and 17,225 deaths, and one in November at Dücze (a force of 7.2) with 40,000 damaged houses and 845 deaths; the provision of water and sanitation was slow in Golyaka and by ~1 week faster in Dücze. HAV seroprevalence in children in postquake camps was significantly higher in Golyaka (69% or 64/93) than in Dücze (44% or 172/383). HEV seroreactivity showed the same significant trend (17% or 16/93 versus 5% or 18/383), underscoring the instant need for prompt delivery of safe water and sanitation.

HEV (1400, 2201, 2881, 3573, 6769). HEV is a relief camp risk. In Namibia in 1983, jaundice likely due to HEV affected hundreds of Angolan refugees in settlements that lacked drinking water and sanitation. Outbreaks were reported among internally displaced persons in Sudan in 2004 (5,000 cases), in war-damaged cities in Iraq in 2004 (hundreds of cases), in a refugee camp in Somalia in 1985–1986 (>2,000 cases), and in a refugee camp in Sudan in 1985–1986 (~2,000 cases). Unlike HAV, a variable proportion of adults from low-income countries (40–85%) remains susceptible to HEV.

Poliovirus (1263, 3598). By vaccination coverage, poliomyelitis is a relief camp risk. In Angola in 1999, type 3 virus caused 634 cases and 39 (6%) deaths, mainly among displaced persons. In Czechia in 1995, type 1 caused 146 cases and 6 (4%) deaths; the outbreak strain was associated with military conflict in the Caucasus.

Rotavirus (5439). In long-term refugee camps in Jordan, *Rotavirus* was detected by antigen capture in stools from 35% of children with gastroenteritis (n = 220) and 3% of age- and sex-matched control children. Risks included age <2 years, use of unboiled tap water for formula milk, and the summer season (June–August).

Bacteria
The main enteric infections in relief camps are cholera and bacterial dysentery (1544).

S. enterica serovar Typhi (742, 823, 2350). Outbreaks of serovar Typhi have been reported in war zones and in camps for refugees and migrant workers.

Shigella (2, 1142, 3542, 4736, 5722). Shigella outbreaks have been reported in relief camps in Africa and Asia. In the Kivu region of Zaire in 1994, an epidemic among Rwandan refugees caused 15,550 cases. In Rwanda in 1993–1994, in a camp with 20,000 refugees from Burundi, *S. dysenteriae* caused 6,122 cases, for an attack rate of 32%. A multiresistant strain was involved in an outbreak of *S. dysenteriae* in Somalia. In Nepal in 1992, in a camp for Bhutanese refugees, an outbreak of *S. flexneri* followed a cholera outbreak.

Vibrio (2, 659, 874, 931, 1569, 4736, 5187, 5246, 5276, 8085). Arriving refugees can seed new strains of *V. cholerae* into camps. Outbreaks have been reported under conditions of war, and in camps in Africa, and less often in Asia. Attack rates reported among refugees and in camps are ~1–5%. By time and access to oral and parenteral treatments, lethality ranges from 0–10%. In Goma, Zaire, in 1994, an explosive outbreak among Rwandan refugees resulted in 60,000–85,000 cases and 12,000 deaths. In Somalia in 1985, an outbreak among refugees from Ethiopia caused ≥2,600 cases and 700 deaths. In Sudan in 1985, an outbreak among refugees from Ethiopia caused 1,175 cases in 6 weeks and 51 deaths (13 in hospital but 38 in domiciles). The average volume of intravenous fluid was 8 liters per case, and at the height of the epidemic, usage was 1,000 liters per day. In Nepal in August–November 1992, an outbreak among ~68,500 Bhutanese refugees in camp caused 764 cases, for a crude attack rate of 1.1%, and a peak attack rate of 0.05% *per day*.

Protozoa
Risks (2633, 2689, 4414, 8059). Enteric protozoa are expected to be prevalent in camp populations that lack safe water and sanitation. By age and provenance mix, and treatments in source and transit countries, the reported arrival prevalence in refugees is 5–15% for *G. lamblia*, 3–18% for *D. fragilis*, 1–10% for *E. histolytica/dispar*, and 0–0.2% for *C. parvum*. With all of them, person-to-person spread is possible. In a camp on the Thai-Cambodian border, amebic dysentery peaked in children 12–23 months of age, for a rate of 6/100 per month.

Helminths
Risks (444, 2633, 2689, 4414, 8059). By age and provenance mix, and treatments in source and transit countries, the reported arrival prevalence of enteric helminths in refugees is 1–6% for *A. lumbricoides*, 0.4–15% for *T. trichiura*, 0–7% for *C. sinensis*, and 0–1.4% for *Taenia* sp. Some 10–20% of refugees may have enteric polyparasitism. Most infections are inapparent. Screening on arrival in high-income countries by examination of one to three stool specimens and of blood for eosinophilia may be an alternative to routine administration of anthelminthics.

ZOONOTIC CLUSTER, RELIEF CAMPS
Risks (1544, 4736). Vector-borne diseases are risks in relief camps that should be made immediately reportable, in particular, dengue, LBRF, LBT, and clinical malaria.

Viruses
Mosquitoes and rodents in camps are a hazard.

Viral hemorrhagic fevers (1544). Viral hemorrhagic fevers are a threat in complex emergencies, including by CCHFV, EBOV, Lassavirus, and yellow fever virus.

DENV (789, 8159). DENV seems to be an underreported threat. At a refugee camp in Somalia in 1985–1987, outbreaks of flulike illness were confirmed due to DENV2. In camps for displaced persons at the Thai-Kampuchean border, 4 (6%) of 67 randomly selected, febrile inmates were diagnosed with dengue.

Bacteria
Lice, fleas, mites, and rodents in camps are a hazard.

Bartonella **(6119).** Trench fever made its reappearance in Burundi after civil war began in 1993. *B. quintana* was detected in lice from refugees in camps and prisoners in jail.

Borrelia recurrentis **(932, 5089, 7252).** Crowding and poor body hygiene in slums and camps are risks for pediculosis and LBRF. Outbreaks have occurred in camps for prisoners of war and a camp for refugees. In a camp in Somalia affected by epidemic LBRF, most (86%) refugees lived under tents that measured 2 × 4 m; average occupation was five persons per tent, and the prevalence of louse infestation was ~60%.

Orientia tsutsugamushi **(8159).** In camps for displaced persons at the Thai-Kampuchean border, 6 (9%) of 67 randomly selected, febrile inmates were diagnosed with scrub typhus.

R. prowazekii **(360, 2477, 3884, 5835, 6119, 8089, 8417).** Crowding and poor body hygiene in camps for refugees and prisoners of war are risks for pediculosis and LBT. In refugee camps in Burundi and Congo, under appalling conditions, LBT returned in the 1995–1997 with >27,000 clinical cases, 20 years after an outbreak in 1975 that had caused 9,000 reported cases. *R. prowazekii* was detected from lice by NAT.

R. typhi **(2058, 8159).** In camps for displaced persons at the Thai-Kampuchean border, 39 (58%) of 67 randomly selected, febrile inmates were diagnosed with flea-borne (murine) typhus. In Thailand in 1988–1989, an outbreak in a camp for displaced Khmer refugees caused 26 cases, for monthly attack rates of 0.3% in children and 1.9% in adults.

Protozoa
Mosquitoes in camps, influx of asymptomatic carriers (adults) and nonimmune individuals (infants), and lack of mosquito nets are hazards.

Leishmania. CL and VL can be transmitted in refugee camps. **CL (901, 4036, 6441).** In Pakistan in 1997, an outbreak of anthroponotic CL occurred in a camp for Afghan refugees; 38% (304/799) of refugees surveyed had active lesions, and 17% (106) had fresh scars. From culture and PCR the agent was identified as *L. tropica*. *Phlebotomus sergenti* was captured in the camp. In 16 Afghan camps in 1998, the prevalence of active lesions was 0.3–8.8% (mean 2.7%), and the disease rate was ~0.4–0.5/100 per year. In Pakistan in 2002–2003, 2.7% of 21,046 refugees in camps had active lesions of anthroponotic CL, as had 1.7% of 7,305 village residents; the respective prevalence of scars was 4.2% and 4.9%, and the rate of anthroponotic CL in refugees was 1/100 per year. **VL (806).** In Kenya in 2000, an outbreak among Somali refugees caused 34 cases of kala azar.

***Plasmodium* (496, 798, 4409, 5486, 6439, 6442, 6797, 7067).** Malaria is a well-documented threat to refugees in camps, including resistant falciparum malaria. Under conditions of scarce resources, however, malaria can be overdiagnosed. Transmission can be at camp sites, or malaria can be introduced into camps. Gametocytemic refugees arriving in high-income countries are a potential source of introduced (locally transmitted) malaria. **Prevalence (5359, 7067).** In Quebec, Canada, in 2000–2001, 19% (98/521) of refugees arriving from Tanzania tested positive for parasitemia by smear, antigen test, or NAT, 95% (93/98) for *P. falciparum* (81 solitary and 12 mixed). In Uganda camps for internally displaced persons, the microscopic prevalence of *P. falciparum* parasitemia was 9% (61/661) in users of distributed, impregnated bed nets and 14% (70/508) in nonusers. **Risks (496, 4736, 4948, 5486).** Risks for outbreaks include mass movements and mixings of people and breakdowns of health services. In Cuba in 1991–1992, an epidemic in a camp for Haitian refugees caused 235 falciparum malaria cases, for an attack rate of 1.6/100 per 3 months. Transmission was not demonstrated in the camp, but the *P. falciparum* prevalence among asymptomatic camp residents was 1.7%. In Nepal in September 1992, the attack rate of suspected malaria among Bhutanese refugees was 5.6%; of 5,100 blood smears from suspected cases, 212 (4%) were positive for *P. falciparum*, and 265 (5%) were positive for *P. vivax*. In Thailand in 1983–1985, in camps for displaced Khmers, the infection risk was 1.2–3.6/100 per year, and transmission was year-round. Also in Thailand in 1992–1997, in camps for displaced Karen, disease rates per 100 person-years were 13–38 for falciparum malaria and 29–55 for vivax malaria. **Control (444, 798, 2891, 2892, 6439, 7067).** Control requires prompt management of cases, elimination of *Anopheles* breeding sites, and impregnated nets, bedding materials, or tents. In high-income countries, fever in refugees should prompt search for malaria by blood smear or rapid tests.

***Trypanosoma brucei* sensu lato (sl) (1544).** Conflict and the collapse of control programs in Congo in the 1960s led to a resurgence of cases of human African trypanosomiasis.

Arthropods
***Cimex* (2680).** In Freetown, Sierra Leone, virtually all (98% or 233/238) rooms in camps for internally displaced persons were infested by bedbugs, mainly adults (68% or 398/584), but also by nymphs (25% or 145) and egg clusters (7% or 41). In 3 weeks, most (86% or 196/221) inhabitants exhibited typical bite reactions (wheels).

ENVIRONMENTAL CLUSTER, RELIEF CAMPS
Bacteria
In the Sudan, an outbreak of *M. ulcerans* among internally displaced persons caused ~940 cases.

Helminths (1836, 2633, 2689, 2693, 3335, 3769, 4414, 4745, 8059, 8337)
By age and provenance mix, and treatments in source and transit countries, reported arrival prevalences in refugees are 0.5–35% for hookworms, 0–26% for *S. mansoni*, and 0.2–38% (typically 1–5%) for *S. stercoralis*. In France, the prevalence of *S. stercoralis* was ≤1% in refugees from Vietnam, 6–12% from Laos, and 8–23% from Cambodia. *S. stercoralis* can be perpetuated through autoinfection. In Australia, 2 (2%) of 87 Laotians tested positive for larvae of *S. stercoralis* 12 years after their arrival in the country.

SKIN-BLOOD CLUSTER, RELIEF CAMPS
Risks (951, 5796). Although knowledge is limited, impetigo, fungal infections, pediculosis, and scabies should be suspected and managed aggressively in refugee and camp populations. In camps and crisis situations, scabies is a proxy for scarce water, and pediculosis capitis for crowding.

Viruses
HBV (444, 1400, 1401, 4414, 6607). The prevalence of HBsAg among refugees is high, in general, by country of origin 2–19% (typically 7%). Screening refugees for HBV is recommended, for HBsAg (detects infection: current, carriage, or chronic) and anti-HBs (detects immunity: from past infection or vaccination), possibly anti-HBc (narrows window period of infectivity).

HCV (444, 1400, 1401). In Italy, the anti-HCV prevalence was 0.1% (1/1,005) in Kurd refugees and 0.3% (2/670) in Albanian refugees. In high-income countries, screening refugees for risks rather than anti-HCV is proposed.

HIV (444). Prevalences in refugees mirror endemicity and risk behavior in source and transit countries. In the United States, refugees ≥15 years of age are tested for HIV before resettlement.

Bacteria
***Treponema pallidum pallidum* (444).** In the United States, refugees ≥15 years of age are tested for syphilis before resettlement. A difficulty is serological cross-reactions with nonvenereal *Treponema*.

Parasites

Pediculus (2306, 4713, 8086, 8089). Molesting but innocuous head lice (*P. humanus capitis*) can be prevalent in refugee populations. By location and age, the reported prevalence can exceed 10–30%. Far more critical are body lice (*P. humanus corporis*) that can rapidly infest refugee populations under unhygienic conditions. Large-scale use of insecticides in camps is recommended by the World Health Organization.

Hymenolepis (2633, 2689, 3335, 4745). *H. nana* can spread person-to-person. By age and location, the reported prevalence in refugee populations is 0.6–11%.

Sarcoptes (7410). Although poorly documented, scabies is a risk among crowded refugee populations (camp itch). In Sierra Leone, in a camp for the internally displaced, the microsopically confirmed prevalence in individuals 1–15 years of age was 67% (84/125), with a peak in preschool children.

11.5 ORPHANS AND ADOPTEES

Orphans are children (to age <18 years) who have lost a mother or father, double orphans have lost both. Adoptees are children with legal but nonbiological parents. This section deals with orphans, adoptees, as well as mentally retarded children in institutions.

Exposure (www.unicef.org). In 2003, more than 16 million children worldwide (1% of all) were *double* orphans, including >7.5 million (~2%) in sub-Saharan Africa, 8 million (~0.7%) in Asia, and >0.5 million (~0.3%) in Latin America. The number of orphans living in institutions is not known. Global adoption statistics are not available. In high-income countries, ≤2% of children born to unmarried mothers are offered for adoption, and ~2% of married women adopt a child. In the United States in 2003, ~120,000 children were adopted: 100,000 domestic and 20,000 international adoptees, mainly from China, Russia, and Guatemala.

Infection risks (Box 11.6). **Orphans** (3798, 4437, 6492). HIV and AIDS have had a significant impact on numbers of orphans in sub-Saharan Africa and on infant survival. Orphans may be cared for by extended families. Health of surviving orphans is comparable to nonorphans in the same community, including episodes of diarrhea, respiratory tract infections, and *Plasmodium* parasitemia. In crowded, poorly resourced orphanages, respiratory and intestinal infections are likely risks similar to day care (see section 14.3). **Adoptees** (3438, 3714, 6708). Health conditions in international adoptees observed on arrival range broadly, likely by variable preselection procedure and nationality mix. Vaccinations are found to be incomplete on arrival in ~15–35% of adoptees. Documented vaccinations do not guarantee protection. Of 98 children entering The Netherlands from People's Republic of China for adoption, 15 (15%) had nonprotective diphtheria antitoxin titers (≤0.01 IU/ml) compared with 5% (8/157) of Dutch control children. For tetanus antitoxin, proportions of susceptible children were 13% and 0%, respectively. Adoptees can be victims *and* vectors of infections, including measles, HBV, respiratory and enteric agents that are transmissible in households.

DROPLET-AIR CLUSTER

Risks. In orphanages in high-income countries vaccine coverage is presumably high. Reports from low-income countries are scant, but droplet-borne infections are a likely hazard for susceptible children in crowded orphanages. By age, vaccinations, and source country mix, arriving international adoptees may present with acute upper respiratory tract infections, otitis media, mumps, rubeola, and varicella (3674).

Viruses

Outbreaks among children in homes and orphanages have been reported for *Enterovirus* (1291), measles virus (4354), PIV4 (4239), RSV (2388), and VZV (2695).

Measles virus. In 2001, an unusual number of measles cases was reported among adoptees arriving in the United

---

Box 11.6 Agents and infections in orphans, adoptees, and children in institutions, by cluster

Droplet-air	*Enterovirus*, measles, RSV, VZV; invasive Hib disease, pertussis, tuberculosis; *Pneumocystis* pneumonia
Feces-food	Diarrhea, mainly by *Shigella*, microsporidia, *Cryptosporidium*, *E. histolytica*, *Giardia*, *Ascaris*, *Trichuris*
Environmental	Hookworm, *Strongyloides*
Skin-blood	HBV, HCV, HIV; *T. pallidum*; *Enterobius*, *Hymenolepis*; scabies

Notes
- Document source institution, itinerary, medical history, and vaccination status
- Screen physically (scabies and BCG scars), tuberculin skin test, stools (for parasites), and serologically (for HBV, HIV, *T. pallidum*, possibly antitoxin titers of *C. diphtheriae* and *C. tetani*)
- Complete vaccines: HAV, HBV, MMR, polio, VZV; DTP$_a$, Hib; in sickle-cell anemia *N. meningitidis*, *S. pneumoniae*

States (1189). An orphanage in People's Republic of China was the presumed source for 13 cases. Again in 2004, nine adoptees imported measles into the United States, and one nonvaccinated student contracted measles on contact with an ill child (1268).

PIV. At an institution for disabled children in Hong Kong in the fall of 2004, 38 children and 3 staff contracted PIV4 in 3 weeks, for approximate attack rates of 19% and 2.5%, respectively (4239).

Bacteria
Bordetella **(1196, 2417, 7155).** In a home for the neurologically impaired, 44 (67%) of 66 residents were diagnosed with recent *B. pertussis* infections and 12 (27%) developed clinical pertussis; 7 (11%) residents were seronegative but culture positive. In a facility for the developmentally disabled, 149 residents had evidence of *B. pertussis* infection, including 130 with respiratory illness, for infection rates of 6–91% by affected wards. Most infected residents were adolescents and adults who had received a full vaccine course. Culture-confirmed pertussis was diagnosed in North Carolina, in an infant 10 months of age who had been adopted from Russia.

H. influenzae **(6156).** In an orphanage in France in 1996, the average monthly carriage of non-b serotypes in 53 Hib-vaccinated children 0–24 months of age was 45%. For a closed community, this prevalence was not considered unusual.

M. tuberculosis. **Orphans (1921, 2695).** In an orphanage in Jamaica in 2001–2002, 4 of 24 HIV-infected children contracted tuberculosis, and two of the four not receiving antiretroviral therapy died; all staff were tuberculin skin test negative. In Havana, Cuba, in 1995–1998, molecular fingerprinting in a clinic for the mentally handicapped identified a cluster of 12 infections. **International adoptees (3438, 3714, 6534, 7090).** The reported prevalence of tuberculin skin reactivity (induration ≥10 mm) is 3–19%. Internationally adopted children should be screened by skin test.

Mycoplasma **(6553).** An outbreak of *M. pneumoniae* has been reported in a home for boys.

Fungi
P. jirovecii **(2097, 2776, 6171).** In Shiraz, Iran, in 1961–1968, a protracted outbreak of *Pneumocystis* pneumonia claimed the lives of 68 orphans 3 days to 3 years of age. Diarrhea and malnutrition preceded *Pneumocystis* pneumonia. In the United States in the 1970s, *Pneumocystis* pneumonia was diagnosed in malnourished children adopted from Vietnam (operation babylift).

FECES-FOOD CLUSTER
Risks (3577, 3644, 4676, 7090, 8341). Crowding and poor hygiene expose children in institutions to enteric viral, bacterial, and parasitic infections. Screening for enteric parasites is recommended from three fecal samples collected 2–3 days apart.

Viruses
HAV, *Norovirus*, and *Rotavirus* are likely to circulate in orphanages and adoptees, but information is scant.

HAV (228, 7090, 7285). In high-income countries, HAV is a rare hazard for children in institutions. Testing for anti-HAV and vaccination may be an option for international adoptees >2 years of age.

Bacteria
Enteropathogenic bacteria are likely to circulate in orphanages and adoptees, but information is scant.

Salmonella **(5263).** In Japan in 1993, in a home for mentally handicapped students, *S. enterica* serovar Typhimurium caused an outbreak with attack rates of 83% (89/107) among students and 48% (16/33) among staff.

Shigella **(2203).** *Shigella* is a risk for institutionalized children, mainly because of poor body hygiene and person-to-person spread. In Proisy, France, in 1998–1999, in an institution for neuropsychiatrically handicapped children, 45 *S. sonnei* cases were diagnosed (29 confirmed, 6 probable, and 10 possible), for attack rates of 33% (35/106) in children and 6% (10/164) in staff.

Fungi
Microsporidia **(5256).** In well-nourished, HIV-negative, nondiarrheic Thai orphans, the prevalence of microsporidia was 6% (13/221).

Protozoa
Enteric protozoa are prevalent and comparatively well documented in orphans (2996, 5256, 6937) and adopted children (3714).

Blastocystis **(409, 1462, 2996, 3714, 5256, 7158).** Living in an institution is a hazard for infection by *B. hominis*. The reported prevalence in institutionalized children is 0.5–44%. Of 61 children from Romania seen at U.S. adoption clinics, 2 (3%) were shedding the agent.

Cryptosporidium **(2996, 3644, 5256).** The prevalence of *Cryptosporidium* in institutionalized children is 4–10%.

Dientamoeba. Living in institutions is a risk (8327) for *D. fragilis*.

Entamoeba **(3714, 4676, 6197, 6937).** *E. histolytica/ dispar* has been identified in the feces of 7–9% of institutionalized children in endemic areas. In the United Kingdom in 1983, in a hostel for educationally subnormal children, 5 of 10 residents were shedding *E. histolytica/ dispar* cysts. Of 61 children from Romania seen at U.S. adoption clinics, 3 (5%) were shedders.

Giardia **(2996, 3438, 3644, 3714, 4676, 5256, 6534, 6937).** The reported prevalence of *G. lamblia* is 8–23% in institutionalized children and 9–19% in international adoptees.

Isospora **(6937).** In mentally handicapped children and adults living in institutions in Thailand, the fecal prevalence of *I. belli* was 0.1% (1/993).

Helminths
Enteric helminths are prevalent in orphans in low-income countries (409, 6937) and international adoptees (3674, 3714).

Ascaris **(409, 2996, 3714, 5256, 6937).** The reported prevalence of *A. lumbricoides* is 0.5–36% in children living in institutions in endemic areas and 8% in international adoptees.

Trichuris **(154, 409, 2996, 3714, 6937).** The reported prevalence of *T. trichiura* is 2–45% in children living in institutions in endemic areas and 3% in international adoptees. In the United Kingdom, an outbreak on a ward for the mentally handicapped affected 22 of 29 residents. Under conditions of poor body hygiene, *T. trichiura* seems able to persist in institutionalized children. Because eggs of *T. trichiura* need to embryonate to become infective, modes of spread in institutions are unclear.

ENVIRONMENTAL CLUSTER
Hookworm (409, 6937). In children living in institutions in endemic areas, the reported prevalence of hookworms is 5–7%.

Strongyloides **(2996, 3714, 6937).** *S. stercoralis* is transmissible person-to-person. The reported fecal prevalence is 2–3% in institutionalized children in endemic areas, and 5% in international adoptees.

Tunga **(1749, 2343).** Tungiasis has been diagnosed in international adoptees.

SKIN-BLOOD CLUSTER
Parents and staff should be aware of the increased prevalence of HBV, HCV, and HIV in international adoptees and orphans.

Viruses
CMV (6534). CMV was recovered in the urine from ~45% of international adoptees, and adoptees were diagnosed with CMV disease.

HBV (645, 2525, 3180, 3438, 3714, 4210, 5274, 6534, 7090). HBV is a hazard for children in institutions. HBV can be prevalent in low-income orphanages. In Somalia, by location, the prevalence of HBV markers (HBsAg, anti-HBc, anti-HBs) in children in institutions was 20–75%, and susceptible children acquired HBV at rates of 10–50/100 per year. In Romania, 85% (183/215) of orphans had markers of HBV and 18% (38) were carriers of HBsAg. Many adoptees are from areas where HBV is endemic. The marker prevalence in these children is ~20–50%, and 3–7% can be carriers of HBsAg. However, markers in infants could be confounded by maternal antibody and HBV vaccination. International adoptees from countries where HBV is endemic should be screened for HBsAg, anti-HBc, and anti-HBs; if they are susceptible, they should be vaccinated; if they are carriers, the host households should be vaccinated, because there is a risk of adoptee-to-family spread.

HCV (3180, 6534, 7090). Knowledge of HCV is scant. Reported seroprevalence is 4% (9/215) in orphans in Romania and 0.8% (4/496) in international adoptees. Screening could be considered for adoptees from endemic areas with a history of blood transfusion, or a mother who is an IDU.

HIV (3281, 3798, 4437, 6492, 7090) (http://www.unicef.org). In 2003, 0.6–0.7 million children <15 years of age contracted HIV, and 1.9–2.5 million were living with HIV or AIDS. In sub-Saharan Africa, on average >25% of children have been orphaned because of AIDS. In Uganda, of 518 children, 10% had lost one or both parents (6% fathers only, 3% mothers only, and 1% both). On follow-up over 3 years, 83 parents died, leaving 169 new orphans. In Kinshasa, Zaire, children of HIV1-positive mothers became orphans at a rate of 8/100 women-years. In Romania by 1990, 95% (1,094/1,168) of reported AIDS cases were in children; two thirds of whom (683/1,094) were abandoned, living in orphanages. International adoptees should be tested for HIV on arrival, and again after 6 months, if recent infection is suspected.

Bacteria
T. pallidum **(3714, 7090).** Congenital syphilis is reported in international adoptees. Syphilis testing is recommended on arrival.

Helminths
E. vermicularis **(1443, 2996, 3935).** The prevalence in institutionalized children can be unusually high, 43–74%.

Hymenolepis (2996, 3714, 4676, 6937, 6938). Intrapersonal spread of *H. nana* is possible. Reported prevalence is 2–13% in institutionalized and 10% in international adoptees.

Arthropods
Sarcoptes (2695, 3674, 4766). Scabies is prevalent in international adoptees. Outbreaks have occurred among children in homes and institutions.

Pediculus (3674). Pediculosis has been diagnosed in international adoptees.

11.6 ADULTS IN LONG-TERM CARE

Long-term care is health and custodial care given to persons with chronic conditions living in institutions, including rehabilitation centers, mental and psychiatric hospitals, and geriatric and nursing homes (for children, see "Orphans and Adoptees" above).

Exposure. In the United States in 2000, 35 million (12% of the population) were ≥65 years of age (~50,000 were ≥100 years of age). In high-income countries, ratios of acute-to-chronic care patients have shifted from 2:1 in the 1970s to 1 in the 2000s. In the United States in 2000, 4.5% of the population ≥65 years of age was living in nursing homes, with a steep gradient by age, from 1.1% at age 65–74 years, to 4.7% at age 75–84 years, and 18.2% at ≥85 years. Reported crude mortality in nursing homes is ~20–30/100 residents per year (2026, 2186).

Infections (Box 11.7). Infections can be acute, exacerbating, relapsing, chronic, and multiple. Major sources of infections in long-term care are endogenous flora of residents, caregivers, and visitors, and the nosocomial environment (see section VI). Staff of chronic care facilities should be offered the same prevention program as for acute-care workers (see section 12.6).

DROPLET-AIR CLUSTER, LONG-TERM CARE
Risks (2301, 5237, 5297, 5427, 7801). At anyone point in time, respiratory tract infections are prevalent in 0.5–3% of residents. Reported rates of acquisition are up to 2/1,000 resident-days. The reported rate of nursing home-acquired pneumonia (NAP) is 1/1,000 resident-days. Lethality of NAP is high, 7–19% with inhouse treatment and 13–41% with referal treatment.

Oubreaks (2371, 4484, 7192) of respiratory tract illness in nursing homes can occur throughout the year, with a peak in winter. In Toronto, Canada, surveillance over 3 years detected 16 respiratory tract disease outbreaks in nursing homes, for an average of 30 cases per outbreak, attack rates of 2–25%, an incidence density of 0.4/1,000 resident-days, and a crude lethality of 8%.

Viruses
Risks (2301, 4484, 5237). Nearly 10% of NAP is attributed to viruses, mainly PIV, influenza A and B viruses, and RSV. Droplet- and aerosol-borne viruses that leave life-long immunity are not diagnosed in long-term care.

Adenovirus (AdV) (6589, 6770). AdV is infrequent in long-term care. Crowding and unhygienic behaviors are risks. At a United States chronic-care facility in 1995, an outbreak of AdV35 caused 53 pneumonia cases, for attack rates of 26% (14/53) among residents and 2% (4/200) among staff. At a nursing home in Spain in 2001–2002, an outbreak of AdV8 keratoconjunctivitis caused 102 cases, for attack rates of 36% among residents and 13% among staff; spread was likely interpersonal.

Influenzavirus (2027, 2028, 2186, 2371, 4484, 5153, 5759, 6460, 6663). Outbreaks of *Influenzavirus*-

---

Box 11.7 Agents in long-term care facilites, by cluster

Risks and remarks are in parentheses.

Droplet-air	*Influenzavirus*, PIV, *Rhinovirus*, RSV; *B. pertussis* (cough for >2 weeks), *Chlamydophila* (poorly ventilated rooms), *H. influenzae*, *Legionella* (aspiration), *Mycoplasma* (from visitors), *N. meningitidis* (following viral infection), *M. tuberculosis* (cough for >2 weeks), *Pseudomonas*, *S. pneumoniae* (epidemic pneumonia)
Feces-food	*Norovirus* (interhuman), *Rotavirus* (interhuman); *Enterococcus* (colonization), *E. coli* (foods, interhuman, ESβL), *C. difficile* (colonization and antibiotics), *C. perfringens* (foods), *Klebsiella* (endogenous, ESβL), *Salmonella* (foods, interhuman), *Shigella* (interhuman); *E. histolytica* (local pockets), *Giardia*
Environmental	*Strongyloides*, *Toxocara*
Skin-blood	HBV, HCV, HIV; *S. aureus* (flora, MRSA); *Candida* (flora); *Enterobius*, *Hymenolepis*; *S. scabiei*

Note: Consider the reason for entry (old age or disability), comorbidities (organ failure, devices, and medications), epidemiological hazards (hygiene, crowding, and season), and vaccines (*Influenzavirus*, *B. pertussis*, and *S. pneumoniae*).

associated illness are common in nursing homes. Risks include large numbers of residents, low vaccine coverage (<50–80%), high season (December to January), double-room occupancy, advanced age, and comorbidities. Occasional offseason (summer) outbreaks have been reported. By season, vaccination coverage, rapidity of detection, and use of antivirals (neuraminidase inhibitors), reported attack rates range broadly from nil to 60%. Up to 25% of patients with manifest illness can develop life-threatening complications or die. Outbreaks typically last for 12 weeks and can occur despite high (90%) vaccination coverage.

PIV (4484, 7192, 7491). PIV is a frequent cause of outbreaks in homes and of epidemic NAP. Reported attack rates are 20–30%, and lethality can reach 16%.

RSV (2186, 2301, 4484, 7043, 7192, 7823). RSV is a cause of exacerbating chronic obstructive pulmonary disease and of NAP in the elderly and nursing home residents. Risks resemble *Influenzavirus*, but the RSV season starts earlier (in mid-September to November) and lasts longer (typically 26 weeks). Outbreaks of RSV-associated illness are common in nursing homes. The endemic disease rate is ~4–8/100 per year. In 1975–2000, at least seven outbreaks were reported in nursing homes in North America and Europe, for attack rates up to 40–50%. Reported lethality is 2–20%.

Rhinovirus (4525, 7909). *Rhinovirus* can cause outbreaks and clinically relevant respiratory tract illness in long-term care residents. In the United States in 1993, in a 685-bed, long-term-care facility, 33 (49%) of 67 ill residents grew *Rhinovirus*, including five (15%) on steroids or bronchodilators, one (3%) with pneumonia, and one (3%) who died of respiratory failure.

VZV. VZV can become reactivated as zoster in nursing home populations.

Bacteria
Risks (4484, 5237, 5297). Most NAP has a bacterial etiology. The main agents include *S. pneumoniae* (0–40%), *S. aureus* (0–35%), non-typeable *H. influenzae* (0–20%), *P. aeruginosa*, and other gram-positive rods (0–55%). Significant epidemic agents of NAP are *C. pneumoniae* and *L. pneumophila*.

Bordetella (64, 2371). Residents with waned immunity constitute an inapparent infection reservoir. In Wisconsin in 1985, 38 (36%) of 105 nursing home residents were seroreactive, and 4 (4%) grew *B. pertussis*. Clustering in one wing, and a high infection rate suggested spread in the home. Staff can be infected as well. Cough for >2 weeks should prompt evaluation for *B. pertussis*.

Chlamydophila (4484, 7192, 7322, 7574). Outbreaks are well documented in nursing homes. Reported attack rates are ~40–70%, for a lethality of 2–3%. Staff can be affected as well, with attack rates of 22–34%. In outbreaks in Canadian nursing homes, a smoke room was suspected to have facilitated airborne spread of *C. pneumoniae*.

Haemophilus (2799, 5237). *H. influenzae* is a cause of NAP. At a nursing home in California in the fall of 1991, eight residents in an outbreak grew identical, nontypeable strains; person-to-person spread was assumed.

Legionella (4485, 5068, 5372). *Legionella* outbreaks have been documented in rehabilitation centers and nursing homes. Aspiration and aerosols from indoor water supplies are likely modes of spread, although in an outbreak of *L. sainthelensi* in Ontario, Canada, in 1994, eating pureed food was a significant risk.

M. tuberculosis (3545, 7192). In the United States, disease rates per 10^5 per year are ~40 in nursing home residents compared with ~20 in the elderly in the community. Outbreaks in nursing homes have been reported. Reactivated tuberculosis may go unrecognized for weeks and sustain spread in the home and into the community. In rural Arkansas, an outbreak in a nursing home was detected from an increase in tuberculin skin test conversion among employees. Cough for >2 weeks should prompt evaluation for *M. tuberculosis*.

Mycoplasma (1143, 3984). Visitors are a suspected source of *M. pneumoniae*. Outbreaks among institutionalized persons have been documented, with primary attack rates of 7–25%, and secondary attack rates of 12%. Staff can also be affected.

Neisseria (2044, 3567). Outbreaks of *N. meningitidis* have been documented in chronic care facilities. Carriage seems infrequent, and chemoprophylaxis could be limited to patients and staff in close contact with a case. Viral and *Mycoplasma* coinfections may predispose to invasive disease.

S. pneumoniae (861, 3000, 5508, 6052, 7192). Carriage in a nursing home was 23%, compared with ≤10% in adults from the community. Outbreaks in nursing homes seem to reemerge; since 1990, ≥10 outbreaks have been reported, for attack rates of 10–13% and lethality of 14–27%. In outbreaks, vaccination has been offered to residents and staff, and chemoprophylaxis to residents.

FECES-FOOD CLUSTER, LONG-TERM CARE
Risk (4940, 7192). Bowel, urinary devices, and skin ulcers are likely reservoirs of resistant agents, including of

Enterococcus (vancomycin-resistant *Enterococcus* [VRE]), *E. coli* that produces extended-spectrum β-lactamase (ESβL), *K. pneumonia* (can produce ESβL), and *Salmonella* (fluoroquinolone resistant). Susceptibility (antibiotic treatment and achlorhydria) and hygiene problems (mental disability and incontinence) facilitate spread and outbreaks. In the United Kingdom in 1992–2000, of 739 infectious diarrhea outbreaks in hospitals with known wards, 64% (470) occurred on geriatric wards and 8% (56) on psychiatric wards. For food-borne agents, see section III.

Viruses

Astrovirus (2914, 4940). Astrovirus is rarely (<1%) reported in epidemic diarrhea in chronic care. An outbreak of infectious diarrhea in a home for the elderly affected 80% (34/42) of residents and 44% (13/29) of the staff.

HAV (1384). Circulation in chronic care seems rare. In a nursing home in Missouri, the seroprevalence was 80%.

HEV. HEV does not seem to have been reported in nursing homes.

***Norovirus* (2313, 2922, 3226, 3646, 4940, 6400, 7956).** *Norovirus* is a major, well-documented cause of diarrhea in institutionalized adults. Spread is via close contact (in ≥25% of outbreaks), by inhalation of vomit-generated droplets or aerosols, or from the contaminated environments. In an outbreak in Rotterdam, feeding residents was a risk for staff. The spread of *Norovirus* through homes can be rapid.

Outbreaks **(2313, 2922, 3226, 3646, 4163, 4786, 5889, 6400)** Of all *Norovirus* outbreaks, from ~25% (United States in 1997–2000, 59/217; Sweden in 1994–1998, 106/407) to 39% (United Kingdom in 1992–2000, 724/1,877) have occurred in institutions for elderly, such as nursing homes, retirement centers, and residential care homes. During outbreaks, >50% of symptomatic residents may test positive for *Norovirus* as the only enteric pathogen. Typical case loads are ~40–45 per outbreak, with a range of ~5 to >200 per outbreak. Attack rates are ~5–60%, often 25–30%. Staff can also be affected, with attack rates comparable to residents (~30–55%). A common source or vehicle can be difficult to identify.

***Rotavirus* (2937, 3101, 4198, 4756, 4940).** *Rotavirus* in institutions seems to spread human-to-human. Outbreaks in long-term care facilities have been documented. In the United Kingdom, ~2% of epidemic diarrhea in geriatric or psychiatric hospitals is due to *Rotavirus*. Reported attack rates are 27–56% in residents and 17% in staff. Reported lethality in residents is 0.4%.

Bacteria

Sporadic and epidemic diarrhea is frequent in nursing homes.

Urinary tract infections (5427, 7801, 7964, 7970). The prevalence of urinary tract infections in residents is 1–3%, and the disease rate is 0.5–4/1,000 patient-days. Bladder catheters are a risk. Common agents of urinary tract infections in nursing homes are *Enterococcus*, *Escherichia*, *Pseudomonas*, *Proteus*, and *Providencia*.

***Aeromonas* (7192).** *Aeromonas* outbreaks in nursing homes are documented but unusual.

***Bacillus* (5822, 7192).** Outbreaks of *B. cereus* have been reported. At a nursing home in Spain, the attack rate was 18% (77/425).

***Campylobacter* (4940, 7192).** *Campylobacter* outbreaks in nursing homes have been documented but are unusual (<1% of all outbreaks).

***Clostridium*.** Both *C. difficile* and *C. perfringens* can occur in nursing homes. **ic. difficile* (549, 4228, 4940, 7192).** Of residents, 4–30% can be colonized. *C. difficile* is a significant cause of antibiotics-associated diarrhea and of outbreaks in nursing homes. In the United Kingdom, ~9% of epidemic diarrhea in geriatric or psychiatric care is due to *C. difficile*. In Baltimore, Md., lethality in an outbreak was 38% (19/49). **C. perfringens* (656, 4377, 4940, 5093, 6302, 7192, 7319).** Food-borne outbreaks have been reported in homes. In the United States in 1975–1987, 496 residents were affected in six outbreaks (83 per outbreak), with two (0.4%) deaths. At a home for the elderly in Germany in 1998, *C. perfringens* food poisoning affected 21 (10%) of 208 residents, and 2 (10%) died; precooked and repeatedly reheated beef heart ragout was the vehicle implicated epidemiologically and microbiologically.

***Enterococcus* (1275, 1403, 2175, 7558, 8391).** Residents are a reservoir for VRE. Risks for colonization or infection include: being bedridden, having a bladder catheter or decubitus ulcer, or prior or current use of antibiotics. In long-term care facilities, 4–45% of residents carry *Enterococcus*, including VRE. Reported VRE point prevalence ranges similarly, by body site and type of care from 3.5 to 45%. Interfacility transfers increase the risk of spread.

***E. coli* (741, 1099, 4940, 5777, 7192, 7558, 8154).** Spread of *E. coli* in institutions is human-to-human or via foods. Nursing home residents are a reservoir of *E. coli* that produces ESβL. Outbreaks in nursing homes have been documented, including *E. coli* O157 (EHEC). At a psychiatric hospital in Canada in 2002, salads or sandwiches prepared at a hospital kitchen were vehicles for an

E. coli O157:H7 outbreak that affected 74 staff and 35 patients; 20 (18%) cases had bloody diarrhea. Ground beef was the vehicle for *E. coli* O157:H7 outbreaks in two U.S. institutions for persons with retardation. Reported attack rates are 33% in residents and 13–19% in staff. Hemolytic-uremic syndrome complicates 0–40% of cases in residents. Reported lethality is 2–35%.

***Helicobacter* (732, 923).** Risks for *H. pylori* include living in an institution, a long stay, and regurgitation of food.

***Klebsiella* (652, 2760, 7558, 8154).** Patients in geriatric units and nursing homes are reservoirs of *K. pneumoniae*, including of strains that produce ESβL. Colonization risks include immobility, dependence on daily care, and frequent hospital admissions. At a skilled-care unit, the point prevalence of *K. pneumoniae* producing ESβL by cultures from rectal, nasal, wound, and axillary specimens from residents was 18% (21/117). After an outbreak at a Scottish hospital, 38 patients colonized with ESβL-*K. pneumoniae* (74% in urinary tract, 58% in bowel, 29% in respiratory tract, and 11% in wounds) were discharged to 22 nursing or residential homes; there was no evidence of spread after a mean observation period of 298 days.

***Salmonella* (4377, 4940, 5599, 5763, 7109, 7192).** *Salmonella* is a significant cause of epidemic diarrhea in institutionalized adults. Food seems to be the main vehicle, but human-to-human spread is possible as well. In the United States in 1975–1987, *Salmonella* accounted for 20% (27/115) of food-borne outbreaks in nursing homes, causing 1,004 cases (37 per outbreak), and in 1985–1999, 89 (11%) of 841 *S. enterica* serovar Enteritidis outbreaks concerned nursing homes or hospitals. In the United Kingdom, ~26% of epidemic diarrhea in geriatric or psychiatric hospitals is due to *Salmonella*. Lethality of fluoroquinolone-resistant serovar Schwarzengrund in nursing homes is 27% (3/11).

***Shigella* (4658, 4870, 4940).** Spread of *Shigella* is predominantly person-to-person. Outbreaks of *S. sonnei* have been documented in chronic care. At an institution for the disabled in New Orleans, La., in 1990, *S. sonnei* affected 101 residents (95% >19 years of age), for attack rates of 2–63% (mean, 33%). Staff and community members can acquire shigellosis during nursing home outbreaks.

***S. aureus* (4377, 4940, 7192).** Food-borne *S. aureus* outbreaks have been reported in chronic care. In the United States in 1975–1987, *S. aureus* accounted for 10% (12/115) of food-borne outbreaks in nursing homes, with 517 cases (43 per outbreak). In the United Kingdom, <1% of epidemic diarrhea in geriatric or psychiatric hospitals is due to *S. aureus*.

***Vibrio* (2810).** In Singapore in 1984, an outbreak of *V. cholerae* in an institution for the aged caused 21 cholera cases and 75 inapparent infections. Food contaminated by two kitchen helpers was implicated.

Protozoa
When looked for, enteric protozoa are surprisingly prevalent in institutionalized adults.

***Blastocystis* (1462).** In Italy in 1994–1997, prevalence of *B. hominis* was 6% (6/105) in controls, 14% (15/110) in elderly living in an residential center, and 32% (76/238) in psychiatric inpatients.

***Cryptosporidium* (7192).** Although reported, outbreaks of *C. parvum* in nursing homes seem unusual.

***Entamoeba* (15, 1373, 2384, 3495, 5311, 6146, 6643).** Risks for carriage, infection, or invasive disease by *E. histolytica* (colitis and ALA) include living in an institution, unhygienic behavior (geophagia and coprophagia), and sex among men. The reported fecal prevalence of *E. histolytica/dispar* in institutionalized adults is 1–15%. In Japan, in an institution for persons with mental retardation, the fecal prevalence was 13% (78/620); most zymodemes were pathogenic, and a seroprevalence of 27% (164/620) suggested past invasive disease. In Pavia, Italy, in 1979–1989, 16 (30%) of 53 cases of ALA were diagnosed in institutions for persons with mental retardation.

***Outbreaks* (15, 7192, 7420)** Outbreaks have been documented in nursing homes and institutions for persons with mental retardation. Epidemic infection rates can reach 28–30%. Also spread patient-to-staff seems negligible; attack rates in staff can reach 5%.

***Giardia* (3495, 7192, 7420, 8074).** Spread of *G. lamblia* in institutions can be human-to-human or via foods. In an Israeli government home for adults with mental retardation, the fecal prevalence was 2% (2/106).

Outbreaks Outbreaks have been documented in nursing homes. At a home in Minnesota in 1986, *G. lamblia* in 6 weeks affected 35 residents, 38 staff (including kitchen and child care), and 15 children in day care at the home. At a dormitory for persons with mental retardation in Washington, D.C., in 1977, an outbreak affected 15% (15/98) of residents and 5% of staff.

ENVIRONMENTAL CLUSTER, LONG-TERM CARE
***Strongyloides* (840, 2693, 3495, 5956, 6022).** Fecal incontinence and uncontrolled behavior facilitate human-to-human spread. In institutionalized adults, reported prevalences range from 1% to 15% or higher. In Victoria, British Columbia, in 1984–1985, *S. stercoralis* was

identified in stools of seven residents with severe disabilities, but up to 10 stool specimens were needed for parasitological diagnosis. *S. stercoralis* larvae have been recovered from soiled linen.

***Toxocara* (3495).** In an Israeli government home for adults with mental retardation, the seroprevalence was 9% (9/106). Most of the reactive residents shared apartments and used to play with dogs.

SKIN-BLOOD CLUSTER, LONG-TERM CARE

Risks (5427, 7192, 7801). Infected ulcers and other soft tissue infections are prevalent in 1–6% of residents, for a rate of 0.1–2/1,000 patient-days. Outbreaks of skin infections have been reported in chronic care. Hand hygiene and precautions apply to caregivers in long-term care in the same way as for health workers in acute care hospitals (see section 12.6).

Viruses

Invasive procedures are health hazards for residents. Although sexually inactive, residents in homes may be infective and vectors of HBV, HCV, and HIV in caregivers.

HBV (1255, 1384, 1828, 6409, 7725). Of adults in institutions, 23–62% test positive for markers of HBV. Infection risks include shared finger-stick devices for blood sampling or monitoring of glucose levels and shared personal objects (razor blades and objects of podiatric care). Outbreaks of acute HB have occurred in long-term care facilities in North America and Europe.

HCV (410, 1384, 6409). The reported anti-HCV prevalence in residents is 5–20%. Infection risks include a history of blood transfusion and end-stage renal disease.

HIV (544, 6409). Patients in nursing care facilities may include drug-dependent and AIDS patients. In four of the U.S. states, 3% of 931 persons with mental illness were HIV infected (eight times the population estimate). A healthcare worker has been reported to have contracted HIV and HCV from a nursing home resident.

Bacteria

***S. aureus* (1632, 2026, 2269, 2797, 4929, 5098, 7558).** *S. aureus* can be endemic in nursing homes. The reported point prevalence is ∼10–35%. From 4 to 7% of staff may also carry methicillin-resistant *S. aureus* (MRSA), including on the skin of hands and in the nose. Of all *S. aureus* isolates from residents, 30–80% are MRSA and the remaining are methicillin-sensitive (MSSA). Mainly nostrils, chronic wounds, and the urinary tracts of residents are colonized by MRSA. Risks of colonization include recent use of antibiotics and multiple interfacility transfers. MRSA can be acquired at rates of ∼1–15/100 per year. Colonization may clear spontaneously. Carriers of MRSA are at increased risk of infection: *S. aureus* infection rates per 100 per year were 25 in MRSA carriers, but only four in MSSA carriers and five in noncarriers. However, MRSA colonization in long-term care patients seems to progress less often to infection than in acute care. The value of an admission screen for MRSA is controversial.

***S. pyogenes* (GAS) (338, 3143, 8428).** In metropolitan Atlanta in 1994–1995, rates of invasive GAS disease per 10^5 per year were 5 in the general population, 9 in community-living elderly (≥65 years of age), but 74 in nursing home residents. Occasional outbreaks have been reported in long-term care facilities.

Fungi

***Candida* (2311).** Elderly are an infection reservoir. *Candida* commonly colonizes the buccal cavity (in 10–65%, without or with denture, mainly *Candida albicans*, also *C. glabrata*), skin (wet sites and nails), and urogenital tract of residents in long-term care. Elderly are also at increased risk of invasive *Candida* disease (Fig. 20.3).

Helminths

Both *E. vermicularis* and *H. nana* can spread human-to-human.

***E. vermicularis* (3495, 4492).** Prevalence of *E. vermicularis* in institutionalized adults can be high, up to 3–26%.

***H. nana* (3495).** In an Israeli government home for adults with mental retardation, the fecal prevalence was 1% (1/106).

Arthropods

***S. scabiei* (197, 994, 1417, 2001, 3405, 4855).** Scabies can be a problem in long-term care, in particular, when misdiagnosed as eczema or senile pruritus. In Ontario, Canada, 20% of 130 long-term care institutions reported problems with scabies. Outbreaks are frequently reported in long-term care. In a nursing home in Ontario, Canada, an index case was the source for scabies in 42 (74%) of 57 residents and 15 (30%) of 50 staff. An outbreak was also reported at a workshop for the handicapped.

11.7 DETENTION FACILITIES

Detention, correction, and incarceration facilities are penitentiary holding places (behind bars) for legally arrested or sentenced juveniles and adults. Jails are communally-operated, short-term facilities (with annual turnover that clearly exceeds total holding capacity), while prisons are state- or federally operated, long-term facilities (with low annual turnover).

Exposure (744, 1540, 6198, 8011). The point prevalence of people in detention is ~0.2% (10 million/6 billion) worldwide, with a range of 0.08% in Switzerland to 0.7% in the United States (2 million/282 million) and 0.8% in Russia.

Infections (2059, 6198, 6427, 6573, 7118, 8011) (Box 11.8). Hazards in penitentiary facilities include IDU, unsafe sex (STI), prolonged time in prison, and high numbers of prisoners per m^2. Detainees can enter the facility infected or become infected in the facility. Many detainees do not know their infection status.

Prisoner of war and "volunteer" prisoners were participants of infamous trials (285, 6219, 6407) in Manchuria (with botulinum toxin, by Japanese occupants) and in the United States (with *Plasmodium* and *Giardia*).

Prevention. Inquire about IDU and past detentions and treatments for tuberculosis, STI, and AIDS. Review detention conditions (sanitation and number of mates per room) and HBV, HCV, and HIV infection status. The entry screen should focus on infectivity and could include a verbal screen for scabies (itch) and STI (ulcer and purulent discharge), tuberculin skin test, and seroscreen for HBV, HCV, HIV, and *T. pallidum*. Entry HBV vaccination could be offered, as HAV-HBV combination, if HAV risk in prison is considered high (3620). Detainees should be given advice on shared invasive materials (injections, tattooing, and shaving) and condoms.

DROPLET-AIR CLUSTER, PRISONS

Hazards in "closed communities" include crowding, comorbidities, and restricted access to health services.

Viruses

Influenzavirus **(350, 8350).** Outbreaks in prisons have been reported. At a prison in Australia in January 2003 (Southern Hemisphere summer), A/H3N2 caused an outbreak with 37 clinical cases; virus was detected in 50% (11/22) of respiratory specimens.

Measles virus (2734). In young, detained populations, measles outbreaks are a threat. Prevention is by catch-up vaccination on entry into the facility (as MMR), with special consideration for HIV-infected detainees.

Rubella virus (1404, 2734, 6176). In the United States in 1990–1999, 14 (22%) of 65 outbreaks occurred in detention facilities. In the United States in 1985, three prison outbreaks caused 93 cases; postexposure vaccinations were given to 7,239 inmates and 1,404 staff.

VZV (4380). Spread in prison is a risk, and outbreaks in prison have been reported. In Australia, four cases and 23 contacts were linked to an index case during transport from prison to court and the court holding cell. In the outbreak, >300 inmates were exposed, including an HIV-infected inmate who developed shingles despite serologically confirmed immunity.

Bacteria

N. meningitidis **(3616, 7334).** Detention increases the risk of carriage and disease. In Los Angeles jails in 1993, pharyngeal carriage was significantly more frequent in men entering jail (17% of 162) or leaving jail (19% of 379), than in jail staff (3% of 121) or community residents (1% or 214). Meningococcal disease in the community was strongly associated with exposure to jail inmates or workers. Disease outbreaks have been reported in correction facilities.

M. tuberculosis **(537, 1539, 1540, 2032, 3741, 4919, 6008, 7695).** Prisons are reservoirs of *M. tuberculosis* infection. Tuberculosis in prisons is a problem that is compounded by crowding, HIV coinfection, incarceration for >2 years, late detection, poor compliance with treatment, and previous incarceration. Visitors and infected prison staff can carry *M. tuberculosis* from the facility into the community. In the United States in 1995–1999, an outbreak in an urban jail was followed by circulation of agent strains in the nearby community that were indistinguishable by molecular fingerprinting from jail strains. **Impact.** Impact varies by location, type of facility, inmate mix (IDU and HIV), and multidrug-resistant (MDR) isolates. **Infection (71, 1073, 2032, 4611, 4776).** Infection is diagnosed by skin testing. The reported infection prevalence is 18–56%, while the rate (conversion) is 6/100 person-years.

Box 11.8 Agents and infections in prisons, by cluster	
Droplet-air	Vaccine-preventable viruses (MMR, *Influenzavirus*, VZV) and bacteria (DP$_a$, *M. tuberculosis* including MDR, *N. meningitidis* mainly C, and *S. pneumoniae*)
Feces-food	HAV, *Norovirus*; food poisoning, *Salmonella*
Skin-blood	Agents from skin, sex, invasive procedures, in particular: HBV, HCV, HIV; genital *C. trachomatis*, *N. gonorrhoeae* (can be inapparent), syphilis, *S. aureus* (including MRSA); *Trichomonas*; ectoparasites

Disease (71, 537, 1359, 1540, 2033, 2034, 4364, 5865, 6577, 7695). Disease is diagnosed from symptoms (cough for >2 weeks and night sweats), chest X ray, and culture. Reported prevalence is ~0.5–2.5%, while the rate (newly active tuberculosis) in prisons is 0.1–7 (often 2)/100 per year. In detention facilities in Madrid, Spain, in 1993–1994, the rate of culture-proven new disease was 2/100 per year (216/6,308 inmates), and ~84% of recently infected prisoners were HIV coinfected. In prisons in Russia and Central Asia, rates are higher. In Russia, >50% of new tuberculosis cases are estimated to arise in prisons. **MDR tuberculosis (1359, 2033, 5865, 7695).** Since the 1990s, sporadic and epidemic MDR tuberculosis has increasingly been reported in prisons. In New York City in 1990–1991, 32% of prison isolates were MDR. In Azerbaijan in 1995, this proportion was 52% (34/65). In Samara Oblast, Russia, in 2001–2002, 26% (55/211) non-Beijing strains but 62% (216/349) of Beijing strains were MDR, mainly from prisons.

Outbreaks (4919, 5766, 7696) Outbreaks in prisons are well documented. In North Carolina in 1999, an HIV-positive source patient not detected for 2 months caused skin conversions in 75 (66%) of 114 inmates in a sector that housed only HIV-infected men, while within 6 months of recognition of the source patient, 30 additional inmates and 1 health worker contracted active tuberculosis.

S. pneumoniae (3380, 6816). In Alberta, Canada, in 2000–2002, rates of bacteremic pneumococcal pneumonia in persons in prison were higher (52/10^5 person-years) than those in the general population (10/10^5 person-years). An outbreak occurred in an inadequately ventilated and crowded jail, housing nearly double its planned capacity.

Fungi
Systemic fungal infections seem rare in prison and are confined to endemic areas. A case of blastomycosis has been reported in an inmate (6221). In a New York prison in 1978–1981, *Histoplasma capsulatum* infected 10 staff, 3 inmates, and 2 community members; the source was the cleaning of bird-dropping sites.

FECES-FOOD CLUSTER, PRISONS
Enteric viruses and bacteria can enter prisons via foods and tap water. Endogenous flora can spread human-to-human, in particular, in crowded, unsanitary prisons in low-income countries.

Viruses
Information seems largely limited to HAV and *Norovirus*.

HAV (174, 1639, 3620, 5557, 6946, 7872, 8011). By age and inmate mix, reported seroprevalence of HAV in inmates is ~10–45% in high-income prisons, and up to >95% in low-income countries. A majority (>60–70%) of inmates in high-income countries remain susceptible. Infection risks include past detention and IDU (presumably through poor hygiene). Outbreaks in prisons of high-income countries seem rare, although a risk exists that incubating individuals such as IDU could seed and spread HAV in prison. For facilities with high prevalence of susceptible inmates, during community outbreaks, or when expected or past HAV infection rates in prison exceed population rates by ≥2 times, vaccination is recommended, preferably in combination with HBV.

Norovirus **(1213).** An outbreak occurred in a Washington State county jail.

Bacteria
Common enteric bacteria should be expected in detainees, including *Salmonella* and *Shigella*, although evidence is circumstantial. Food hazards include long distribution paths from the central kitchen and uneducated kitchen staff.

C. jejuni **(2361).** *C. jejuni* seems infrequent in detainees. In Madrid, Spain, in 1991–1993, *C. jejuni* was isolated in 28 detainees coinfected with HIV, 27 (96%) were males and 25 (90%) were IDU. Of isolates, 48% were resistant to fluoroquinolones.

C. perfringens **(3881, 7355).** In Nice, France in 1998, roast turkey from a jail kitchen caused 93 cases of food poisoning by *C. perfringens*, for an attack rate of 16%. In a Florida correctional facility in 1984, roast beef caused food poisoning in 74 (27%) of 276 inmates, 8 days later, ham caused a second outbreak with 100 (36%) cases.

E. coli **(5103).** *E. coli* seems infrequent in detainees. Outbreaks of *E. coli* O157 have been documented in prisons in the United Kingdom.

Salmonella **(5405, 5763).** In the United States in 1985–1999, 20 (2%) of 841 *S. enterica* serovar Enteritidis outbreaks occurred in prisons. At an institution in Singapore in 1995, serovar Enteritidis from canned luncheon pork was implicated in an outbreak with 188 cases. The last report of a typhoid fever outbreak in a prison dates back to the early 1960s.

Shigella **(2079).** Traditionally, inmates have been considered at risk for *Shigella*. Although likely spread human-to-human in crowded prisons, recent information seems unavailable.

S. aureus **(4947).** Food poisoning with *S. aureus* has been reported in prison.

S. pyogenes **(GAS) (4379).** In New South Wales, Australia, in 1999, curried egg salad sandwiches were the likely vehicle for GAS tonsillopharyngitis in 72 (28%) of 256 inmates. The presumed source was a food handler with infected hand wounds.

Parasites
By location and inmate mix, intestinal protozoa and helminths can be prevalent (~10–30%) in detainees in or from endemic areas (164, 800). Reported parasites include *Giardia*, *Cryptosporidium*, *Ascaris*, and *Trichuris*.

ENVIRONMENTAL CLUSTER, PRISONS
Hookworm and *Strongyloides* have been documented in detainees in or from endemic areas (164, 800).

SKIN-BLOOD CLUSTER, PRISONS
Risks. Crowding and poor hygiene foster pyoderma, tinea, and ectoparasitic infections (386, 2896, 4349). Some 2–30% of detainees are believed to engage in sex, including among men and with staff (8011). In Malawi in 2000–2001, 4% (178/4,229) of inmates were diagnosed with STI, mainly (46%, 83) urethral discharge and (34%, 60) genital ulcer disease; 20% (35) had epididymoorchitis. The rate of prison-acquired STI was ~1.2/100 inmates per year (8363). Little is known about rape in prison.

Some 25–55% of entering prisoners have a history of IDU and continue while in prison (1641, 2059, 3242, 4498, 6198, 6427).

Viruses
IDU, sharp instruments, and shared personal objects predispose to blood-borne infections. For human bites see section 13.5; for invasive procedures see section 18.1.

CMV (2568). Information about CMV is scant. In Virginia, 64% of 459 entering female prisoners were seroreactive. Reactivity was associated with age, ethnicity, and a history of gonorrhea.

GBV-C (194). In Greece, 46% of 106 incarcerated IDUs were seroreactive to GBV-C.

HBV (174, 1641, 4498, 4542, 5557, 6426, 8011). HBV is a major prison hazard. By age, inmate mix (IDU and HIV), and location, ~5–45% of inmates test positive for HBV markers (anti-HBc, HBsAg, anti-HBs) that indicate past or current infection. In high-income countries, reported anti-HBc prevalence ranges from 6% (Ireland) to 33% (Australia). In Australia, 2.5% of entering 3,627 prisoners tested positive for HBsAg. In correctional facilities in the United States, 1–4% of inmates, typically ~2% are diagnosed with chronic HBV infections, a prevalence that is 2–6 times higher than in the general adult population. HBV infections can be acquired in prison at rates of 13/100 person-years (Australia) to 22/100 per year (China).

Outbreaks (1175, 3518, 3620) Outbreaks of acute HB in prison have been documented. In the United States, 8% of dormitory mates of a chronically infected prisoner had evidence of acute HBV infection. In Scotland in 1993, needle sharing among inmates caused seven HBV infections. Screening and vaccination are recommended at least for inmates with high-risk behavior who enter or reside in long-term detention facilities.

HCV (174, 194, 1641, 3242, 3406, 4498, 4808, 5278, 5557, 6198, 6952, 8011). HCV is a major prison hazard. Risks include IDU, no use of condoms, past detention, past hepatitis, tattooing, or piercing, and in youths a history of STI. By age, past inprisonment, inmate mix (IDU), and location, ~5–75% (typically 20–60%) of detainees test positive for anti-HCV; a high of 77% is reported in prisoners in Greece who are IDU. In Washington State in 1999–2001, 2% (6/305) of incarcerated youths 9–21 years of age tested positive for anti-HCV. In Melbourne, Australia, in 1996, 21% of 90 male adolescents 15–18 years of age residing in juvenile detention tested positive for anti-HCV; all reactive youths injected heroin for more than one year.

By seroconversion, new acquisition rates per 100 person-years in prisons are 1–27 (1301, 1641, 6198), with a low of 1 in the United States, an intermediate rate of 18 in Australia, and variable rates of 1–27 in Europe. In a Scottish prison in 1999–2000, rates per 100 person-years in adult males were 1 in never injection drug users, 12 in ever injection drug users, 19 in current injection drug users, and 27 in current injection drug users sharing equipment.

In North America, ~15% of inmates are considered chronically infected (2459, 6198, 6952, 8011).

HIV (174, 744, 958, 1641, 4498, 4808, 6427, 6504). HIV is a major hazard in detainees. IDU can acquire HIV before, during, or after detention, mainly from needle sharing. Other risks are sex among men and tattooing. By age, inmate mix, and location, the reported infection prevalence in detainees is ~0.1–19% (typically 1–4%). In a nationwide survey in the United States in 1992–1998, the prevalence was 3% (16,797/459,155), and self-reported previous tests suggested that 56% of infections were newly detected. In São Paulo, Brazil, in 1993–1994, in a prison with ~4,700 inmates, the prevalence in 631 randomly selected prisoners was 16% (95% CI 13–19%). In Europe, seroprevalence in prisoners ranged from 0.03% (Hungary) to 12% (Switzerland).

The rate of seroconversion in Maryland state prisons in 1985–1987 was 0.4/100 prison-years (871). An outbreak with eight prison-acquired infections occurred in a Scottish prison (7357).

HTLV (2980). In Tijuana, Mexico, 7% (29/410) of inmates in the state penitentiary tested positive for HTLV, with comparable prevalence in women (9%, 3/34) and men (7%, 26/376), but higher prevalence in IDU (25%, 21/85) than in non-IDU (3%, 8/325).

Bacteria
C. trachomatis, **genital (545, 3138, 5005).** In U.S. detention facilities, the reported prevalence by age, specimen (urine or swab), test (culture or NAT), and screen (entry or resident) is 6–22% in women and 15–16% in men.

N. gonorrhoeae **(545, 2177, 3138, 5005).** In U.S. detention facilities, the reported prevalence by age, specimen (urine or swab), test (culture or NAT), and screen (entry or resident) is 3–9% in women and 1–3% in men. Most (>90%) culture-positive entering men had inapparent urethral infections.

S. aureus **(386, 1177, 1675, 5704).** Skin infections by methicillin-resistant strains (MRSA) and nasal carriage of MRSA in prison seem to have increased in the 1990s-2000s. Risks include crowding, poor hygiene, and immune impairments from HIV, IDU, diabetes, and end-stage liver or renal disease. In a Mississippi state prison in 2000, 86 (5%) of 1,757 inmates were nasal carriers of MRSA. Women carried MRSA (6% or 73/1,241) more frequently than men (2.5% or 13/516). In Texas in 1999–2001, MRSA infections were acquired in prison at a rate of 1/100 person-years. In California jails in 1997–2002, the proportion of MRSA among all *S. aureus* increased from 23% to a plateau at about 74%. Outbreaks of MRSA have been reported in prisons. In one, MRSA caused skin infections in 59 inmates, mostly (78%) women.

T. pallidum **(3783, 4808, 6242, 7781, 8240).** *T. pallidum* can be a prison hazard. In Louisiana in 1994–1998, 1% (494/38,573) of screened detainees were diagnosed with untreated syphilis. Estimates for the year-prevalence of early syphilis were 0.8–0.3% in detainees and 0.2–0.03% in the East Baton Rouge community, for a decreasing time trend in both settings. In Rhode Island, 1.4% (86/6,249) entering female detainees were seroreactive, and 29 (0.5%) were diagnosed with primary or secondary syphilis, that is 49% of the state total. In Alabama prisons for men in 1999, undetected and untreated, infective inmates, by transfers and multiple partnerships, caused syphilis outbreaks. Syphilis seroprevalence was 8% in 1,284 inmates in Mozambique, and 18% (95% CI 15–21%) in 631 randomly selected prisoners in São Paulo. Entry screen and treatment of infective cases seems warranted.

Fungi
Tinea pedis and tinea cruris can be prevalent in crowded prisons, including causative dermatophytes such as *C. albicans*, *Trichophyton mentagrophytes*, and *T. rubrum*. However, recent information is scant.

Protozoa
Trichomonas vaginalis **(2617, 3983, 7040).** By age, ethnicity, and location, reported prevalence of *T. vaginalis* in incarcerated female youths and adults is ~30–45%. Sex work is an infection risk. *T. vaginalis* seems to be a marker for *T. pallidum* and perhaps other STIs. Infections appear to be imported into prison rather than acquired there, and outbreak risks in jail are considered low.

Helminths
Enterobius appears not to have been documented in detainees.

Arthropods
Scabies (3710, 4349). Scabies is a problem in crowded jails. Outbreaks have been reported, with crusted or unrecognized and untreated cases as major sources.

Body lice (662, 2477, 6119). Body lice can transmit LBT (by *R. prowazekii*), LBRF (by *B. recurrentis*), and trench fever (by *B. quintana*). LBT has reemerged in prisons in East Africa. In a Burundi prison in 1995–1997, 45,558 epidemic cases were diagnosed clinically. In Rwanda in 2001, *R. prowazekii* was detected by NAT in 7% of body lice removed from jail inmates.

11.8 HOTEL ACCOMMODATION
Hotels, motels, lodges, conference centers, resort complexes, country inns, dude ranches, and bed and breakfast hostels are all establishments for short-term lodging. Beds may range from one to hundreds. U.S. cities with large numbers of hotel rooms include Las Vegas (147,000), Orlando (118,000), and Chicago (98,000).

Exposure. Most nations collect statistics of overnight accomodations that are part of the global travel industry (see chapter 15). However, compared with international travel, less information is available on hotel accomodations. Major international chains are Cendant (>6,400 hotels, e.g., Days Inn, Ramada Inn, Super 8, and Travelodge), Choice (>4,900, e.g., Comfort Inn, Econolodge, and Quality Inn), Best Western (>4,100), Accord (>3,800, e.g., Motel 6, Novotel, and Sofitel), and Intercontinental (>3,500, e.g., Crowne Plaza and Holiday Inn).

Box 11.9 Agents from hotels, by cluster	
Droplet-air	*Influenzavirus*, SARS-CoV; *Legionella, N. meningitidis; Histoplasma*
Feces-food	HAV, *Norovirus; Campylobacter, Salmonella* (including serovar Typhi), *Shigella, V. parahaemolyticus; Giardia*
Environmental	*Schistosoma*
Skin-blood	STI

Infections (Box 11.9). Presumed risks include poorly maintained pools, spas, and sanitary installations; crowded conference rooms; contaminated foods; the presence of mosquitoes, ticks, and rodents; and casual sex with bar and massage staff. Hotel-based outbreaks with worldwide media attention include legionellosis and SARS. For dormitories, see section 14.4; for military barracks, see section 12.3; for food-borne disease, see section III; for hotel work, see section 12.7; and for buildings, see section 6.2.

DROPLET-AIR CLUSTER, HOTELS

Given the volume of accomodations, hotel-associated incidences are infrequent. Low risks from short contact periods may be outweighed by poorly ventilated rooms and rooms shared with cough patients. Hotels have been used to trace or quarantine exposed travelers.

Viruses

Published evidence centers on vaccine-preventable *Influenzavirus* and vaccine nonpreventable SARS-CoV.

***Influenzavirus* (3489, 3999, 6516, 7595).** Several infections mimic flulike illness, notably Pontiac fever. The risk of flulike illness is increased when sleeping facilities are shared. An influenza outbreak was reported at an international medical conference. Barracks of an air squadron were venue for an *Influenzavirus* A/H1N1 outbreak.

SARS-CoV (5406, 6072, 8051, 8164, 8354). At a hotel in Hong Kong in II/2003, an index case (superspreader) from Guangdong, People's Republic of China, infected 13 hotel guests, including seven on the same floor. From there, incubating guests imported SARS into North America, Asia (Singapore and Vietnam), and West Europe (Germany and Ireland). Later on in Hong Kong, in March–April 2003, SARS hit a private housing complex, with 321 cases among residents. The seeder was a patient with chronic renal disease who incubated SARS and visited his brother in the estate. Suggested routes of spread included sewage droplets sucked back into bathrooms through fans, carriage by black rats, and aerosols in a plume of warm air.

Bacteria

There is evidence for vaccine-preventable *N. meningitidis* and vaccine nonpreventable *Legionella* in hotels.

***Legionella* (562, 1049, 2379, 2598, 2872, 3751, 4345, 5241).** Travel-related legionellosis is overwhelmingly linked to hotels. In France in 1998–2001, of 1,015 cases of legionnaires' disease or *Legionella* pneumonia with exposure known, 225 (22%) were hotel associated. Species of *Legionella* recovered from hotel water samples include *L. pneumophila*, *L. micdadei*, and *L. bozenanii*. Sources are aerosols from hot and cold tap-water supplies, thermal spas, whirlpools, swimming pools, shower nozzles, faucets, decorative fountains, storage tanks, and air conditioners.

Outbreaks Outbreaks are well documented in hotels, including at popular tourist destinations, conference and training centers, and leisure complexes. Hotels in Philadelphia, Pa., and Benidorm, Spain, have become notorious for legionellosis.

- North America (562, 1248, 2354, 2507, 3489). In Philadelphia in 1976, 182 (4%) of 3,683 attendees (legionnaires) of the American Legion convention contracted a new form of pneumonia from airborne exposure at a hotel lobby, and 29 died, for a lethality of 16%. At a California hotel in 1988, *L. anisa* caused 34 cases of Pontiac fever among conference attendees, for an attack rate of 82%; the agent was isolated from a decorative fountain in the hotel lobby. In 1999, an outbreak at a Georgia hotel caused two cases of legionnaires' disease and 22 cases of Pontiac fever; *L. pneumophila* serogroup 6 was isolated from the index patient and the hotel whirlpool spa. Attack rates were 38% (10/26) in guests exposed to the spa and 7% (2/29) in guests exposed to the pool area only. At an Illinois hotel in 2002, ≥50 guests contracted Pontiac fever, likely due to *L. micdadei* from the swimming pool and whirlpool spa area. At a hotel in Ocean City, Md., in 2003–2004, eight guests contracted legionnaire's disease. All had showered or bathed in their rooms, six reported exposure in the swimming pool and whirlpool spa area, and *L. penumophila* serogroup 1 was recovered from multiple environmental sites.
- Latin America (1615, 6668). At a resort in St. Croix, U.S. Virgin Islands, Legionnaire's disease cases occurred among tourists in 1981–1982 (27, including 6 from Denmark), 1998, and again in 2002 (three cases, all Danes). In the first outbreak, 41% of hotel employees were found seroreactive. The continued source for all outbreaks was showers with water that yielded *L. pneumophila* in 1981–1982 and again in 2002–2003.
- Australasia (533, 4396, 8299). At a training center in Tokyo, Japan, in 1994, *L. pneumophila* caused Pontiac

fever in 43 trainees and 2 staff members; a cylindrical, open cooling tower on top of the building was the implicated source. In Australia in 10 years (1991–2000), 5 of 22 *Legionella* outbreaks occurred at accommodation facilities: one at a Sydney hotel with four cases, one at a Sydney hotel car park with four cases, one at a Queensland holiday apartment with three cases, one at a tourist resort on Kangaroo Island with four cases, and one at a Victoria hostel with two cases. A hotel in Sydney, Australia, reported four cases; on investigation, 28 (18%) of 152 responding attendees of a seminar reported symptoms compatible with legionellosis, and 33 (22%) had raised antibody titers ($\geq$1:128) to *L. pneumophila* serogroup 1 in immunofluorescence assay. A site implicated epidemiologically was the hotel car park. Case clusters were also reported from hotels in Bangkok, Thailand, and Beijing, People's Republic of China.

- West Europe (427, 2814, 2872). On the west coast of Scotland over Christmas and New Year of 1987–1988, Pontiac fever affected 170 persons who visited a leisure complex, for an attack rate of 91%; *L. micdadei* was isolated from the whirlpool spa, which was the implicated source. In Tyrol, Austria, in 1989–1990, *Legionella* was cultured from the cold-water system of 11 (31%) of 35 hotels and from the hot- or mixed-water system of 9 (26%); water pipes were main site for growth and dissemination of the agent. In hot- and cold-water systems, first-flush samples yielded higher counts than samples taken after flushing for 5–10 min, which suggested that biofilm formation was significant. In northern Sweden in 1999, an outbreak affected 29 hotel guests, for attack rates of 54% in visitors of the whirlpool area, and of 1% in non-pool using guests.

N. meningitidis (2044). Hotels as venues for outbreaks are unusual. In Florida in 1995, *N. meningitidis* B invasive disease was diagnosed in five cases from two overcrowded hotels hosting 730 guests and staff, for an attack rate of 0.3%; chemoprophylaxis was offered to 480 guests and staff on site (66% of target). In Mallorca, Spain, infections in three United Kingdom and one German child were linked to a leisure hotel complex that catered for >2,000 guests.

Fungi

Dust from construction sites and from soil in plant pots are putative sources of hotel-associated fungal infections.

Histoplasma (1184, 5193). In 2001, an *Histoplasma* outbreak among college students traveling to Acapulco, Mexico, was associated with a stay at a beach hotel. Of 757 travelers who stayed at that hotel, 262 (36%) met the case definition for a febrile respiratory tract illness, and sera of 148 (54%) from 273 persons tested positive. In a telephone survey, the risk of infection was 10.5 times (95% CI 4–31) higher in frequent users than nonusers of hotel stairways on which construction work was ongoing.

FECES-FOOD CLUSTER, HOTELS

Risks (1954, 2259, 3139, 4889, 6762, 7069). All common food-borne agents are to be expected at hotel and resort accomodations. Recognition of a causative agent can be confounded by recovery of more than one genus, species, or strain of enteric pathogens from guests and foods. For instance, among 224 travelers returning from Greece to the United Kingdom with past or current diarrhea, 70 (31%) yielded one or more agents, including *G. lamblia* in 58 (83%), *C. parvum* in 11 (16%), *Campylobacter* in 4 (6%), *Salmonella* in 3 (4%), *E. histolytica/dispar* in 2 (3%), and *Rotavirus* in 1 (1%).

In the United Kingdom in the 1990s, 13% (128/983) of food-borne disease outbreaks occurred in hotels. Risks include cold buffets, fresh juices, and meals from raw eggs. Person-to-person spread is also reported in hotels. Secluded resorts have infection control problems that resemble cruise ships, with large numbers of short-stay visitors, diversity of foods served, and food handlers who maintain chains of infections among departing and arriving visitors.

Viruses

HAV (704, 1645, 6306). In Georgia in 1982, an outbreak at a trailer park served by a private well caused 16 cases. An increased risk of HAV infection was reported in homosexual men who visited a large sex resort in the southern United States. At a holiday resort in Ibiza, Spain, in 2000, 13 German tourists contracted acute HA, in the wake of a community outbreak that affected a kitchen worker.

Norovirus. *Norovirus* is a significant cause of hotel-associated diarrhea.

Outbreaks Outbreaks have been reported in North America and West Europe.

- North America (201, 1938, 4534, 6762). At a Winnipeg, Canada, hotel, guests contracted *Norovirus* gastroenteritis, likely from food prepared by a shedding kitchen employee recovering from diarrhea. In Virginia in 2000, an outbreak in an well-run hotel caused gastroenteritis in three arriving cohorts, for attack rates of 28–49% among guests and 29% among staff: 17% (1/6) in dishwashers, 19% (13/67) in food workers, 41% (9/22) in housekeepers, and 78% (7/9) in front desk workers. Food consumed outside the hotel was the vehicle implicated epidemiologically, but person-to-person and environment-to-person spread were suspected as well. At a hotel in Colorado in 2000, 52% (69/133) of attendees of a professional meeting and 8 staff complained of illness, and *Norovirus* was detected in three stool specimens. An outbreak vehicle was not implicated, but there was evidence for improper food handling. In Wyoming in 2001, an outbreak at a snowmobile lodge caused illness among 35 (43%) of 81 guests. Illness was associated with drinking water, and attack rates increased with the number of glasses of water consumed, from 21% (6/29) with zero glasses, 43% (6/14) with one to three glasses, 83% (5/6) with four to five glasses, and 100% (3/3) with more than five glasses.

- West Europe (716, 1097, 1362, 5889). In the United Kingdom in 1992–2000, 8% (147/1,877) of confirmed *Norovirus* outbreaks had hotels as venues. In the United Kingdom in 1996, environmental contamination was detected in a hotel outbreak that extended from January to May. At a tourist resort in southern Italy in 2000, 275 guests and 69 staff contracted *Norovirus* gastroenteritis, likely from contaminated drinking water. In Sweden in 2002, a waterborne outbreak at a winter holiday resort caused ~500 cases among guests and residents, for attack rates of ~40%.

Rotavirus **(3139).** *Rotavirus* was isolated in travelers returning from resorts.

Bacteria

Campylobacter **(4999, 6139).** In Australia in 2001, 10 (34%) of 29 delegates at an international academic meeting contracted diarrhea, and two grew *C. jejuni* from stools; a vehicle was not identified. At an island resort in Queensland, Australia, 23 guests contracted *Campylobacter* diarrhea, likely from tank water. An outbreak was also reported at a resort in Ontario, Canada.

E. coli **(6984).** In the United Kingdom in 1994, enteroaggregative *E. coli* caused diarrheal disease outbreaks at a conference center (with 51 cases) and a hotel (with 53 cases).

Salmonella **(657, 2930, 5696, 5914).** At a New York hotel in 1989, orange juice served for breakfast and prepared by an unrecognized *S. enterica* serovar Typhi carrier caused 44 confirmed and 24 probable typhoid fever cases. At a national convention in a Montreal hotel in 1995, 69 attendees from across Canada contracted diarrheal disease due to serovar Enteritidis, likely from a soufflé made with raw eggs and served for lunch. In Victoria, Australia, in 2001, 19 persons contracted serovar Typhimurium from a hotel buffet, likely from lamb's fry and bacon in an onion gravy. At a medical conference in the United Kingdom, chicken pieces were the vehicle for an outbreak of serovar Typhimurium DT9 that affected ≥196 delegates.

Shigella **(138, 7069).** At a resort club in Haiti in 1984, a *Shigella* outbreak affected 339 tourists and expatriate staff among ~1,900 exposed persons, for a crude attack rate of ~18%. Eating rare hamburgers and having an ill roommate were significant risks. At a hotel in La Gomera, Canary Islands, 14 of 28 tourists contracted *S. sonnei* gastroenteritis. Although a common source was suggested by epidemiological and microbiological investigations, a single vehicle was not confirmed.

V. parahaemolyticus **(485, 7085).** At a hotel in Bangkok in 1978–1979, in an outbreak that lasted for 12 months, 150 (0.07%) of 209,901 guests and 116 (15%) of 800 staff developed diarrhea; from 45 (31%) of 146 guests and 17 (15%) of 116 staff, *V. parahaemolyticus* was isolated, and seafood was the likely vehicle. In an Australian island resort in 1968–1969, 131 guests and staff contracted *V. parahaemolyticus* diarrhea, likely from frozen, precooked prawns, crabs, and lobsters that were thawed in contaminated bore water.

Protozoa

Cryptosporidium **(4620).** For a *Cryptosporidium* outbreak at a resort in Wisconsin in 1993, with 51 cases, swimming in the hotel pool was a significant risk.

Entamoeba **(3139, 4510, 5674).** *E. histolytica/dispar* was isolated in travelers returning to Europe and North America with diarrhea. At a hotel in Punta Cana, Dominican Republic, in 2002, some 76–216 Spanish tourists contracted gastroenteritis, likely due to *E. histolytica*, from tap water, ice, or meals served at the buffet.

Giardia **(3139) (4510).** *G. lamblia* was the likely cause of diarrhea in travelers returning from the Mediterranean to the United States and the United Kingdom. In Madeira, Portugal, in 1976, 323 (39%) of 859 responding U.S. travelers reported diarrhea; 27 (47%) of 58 stool samples contained *G. lamblia*, and (5%) *E. histolytica/dispar*, while 3 (9%) of 35 stools grew *Shigella*, and 1 (3%) grew *Salmonella*. Vehicles implicated epidemiologically included tap water, ice cream, and raw vegetables.

Outbreaks Giardiasis outbreaks have been reported at winter and summer resorts, and a trailer park.
- North America (655, 3590). At a trailer park in Vermont, 37 (30%) of 122 residents contracted giardiasis. At a Colorado ski resort in 1981, waterborne giardiasis

caused an outbreak with peak attack rates (42%) in persons who drank ≥6 glasses of water per day.
- West Europe (4470). At a Swedish ski resort, >1,400 persons contracted confirmed giardiasis from sewage that spilled into the drinking-water system.

ZOONOTIC CLUSTER, HOTELS

Ponds, vases, and freshwater bodies on hotel premises can be significant breeding sites for mosquito larvae, with a risk of arboviral infections and malaria. Gametocytemic guests are an unusual source of "hotel malaria." In 2000, a German couple contracted *P. vivax* malaria after staying at a hotel in northern Greece. Hotel malaria was assumed after excluding alternative routes of acquisition, and when an American who on return from Mozambique stayed at the same hotel came down with malaria. The season made transmission by local mosquitoes likely (8032).

Infrequently used or abandoned cabins can be rodent or tick infested, with a risk of acquisition of *Hantavirus* or *Borrelia*. In Idaho, three cases of TBRF were associated with lakeside cabins (7480). For substandard housing, see section 11.2 above.

ENVIRONMENTAL CLUSTER, HOTELS

At a holiday resort in metropolitan Belo Horizonte, Minas Gerais, Brazil in 2002, 17 patrons contracted acute schistosomiasis from the resort swimming pool (2214). Patrons reported the pool to be clean and free of snails. Investigations established *Biomphalaria glabrata* that shed *S. mansoni* cercariae in a nearby pond and in a water tank that served the pool, and *S. mansoni* infections in five of seven resort residents. Rural tourism with accommodation in farm hotels (hotel-fazenda) or boarding houses can put noninformed persons at risk of unusual infections.

SKIN-BLOOD CLUSTER, HOTELS

Bar and other hotel workers are likely to mirror locally endemic infections, including STI. For hotel-based sex work, see section 13.6.

12
Human Work

12.1 Construction and mining
12.2 Manufacture and maintenance
12.3 Military, police, and guards
12.4 Field, forest, herd, and abattoir
12.5 Catering
12.6 Health and laboratory work
12.7 Cleaning and waste work
12.8 Transportation work
12.9 Clerk, class, and sales work

To be is to do (Sartre), *To do is to be* (Camus), *Do be do be do* (Sinatra)
From a graffito

Work is the multitude of human activities (Table 12.1) intended to sustain us through life. A job is a particular piece of work. Employment is contracted and salaried work.

Infections (Table 12.1). Occupational infections are acquired at the workplace or during work time. A link with work is supported by (i) compatible exposure (type and intensity), (ii) compatible incubation period and manifestations, (iii) infections significantly more prevalent in workers than controls or populations of corresponding age, and (iv) recovery of identical agent strains from humans and the workplace. Modes of acquisition include contact (environment, animals, and patients), ingestion (foods and hands), inhalation (animal droplets and dust), and inoculation (cuts and sharps). In the United Kingdom in 1996–1997, 1,037 occupational infections were reported, including 921 (89%) cases of diarrhea (mainly health workers and mainly *Campylobacter* and *Salmonella*), 71 (6%) cases of scabies (mainly staff in long-term care facilities), 18 (2%) cases of legionellosis, 8 (1%) cases of pulmonary tuberculosis, and 19 (2%) other cases (6418). While the focus in the following chapter is on workers as victims, workers can also be vectors of infection, for instance, food handlers of *Shigella* (2626), miners of *Plasmodium* (6092, 7787) and human immunodeficiency virus (HIV) (5691, 5925), and truck drivers of HIV (450, 6098) and *Treponema pallidum* (1558).

Exposure history (Box 12.1). Exposure history should include current and lifetime workplaces; hazards on the job, including from outdoor and indoor activities and contacts with animals, plants, foods, and people; absenteeism; and preventive measures.

Prevention. Vaccination and exposure prevention can reduce occupational infection risks. Examples include influenza (vaccination), legionellosis (ventilation), tuberculosis (rapid case finding), diarrhea (hand hygiene), pyoderma (showers), HIV (education), and malaria (mosquito proofing and chemoprophylaxis).

Table 12.1 Occupational groups and examples of work-related infections

Section	Occupation	Examples of agents or infections
12.1	Construction, mining	Tuberculosis, malaria, arboviroses, leptospirosis
12.2	Manufacture, maintenance	Influenza, *Legionella*, mycobacteria, *Coxiella*, anthrax
12.3	Military, police, guard	Meningococcal meningitis, diarrhea, STI, malaria, VHF
12.4	Farm, forest, herd, abattoir	Brucellosis, erysipeloid, ornithosis, tickborne agents, tularemia
12.5	Cooking, catering	Food poisoning, infectious diarrhea
12.6	Health, laboratory	HBV, HCV, HIV, SARS, tuberculosis, scabies
12.7	Cleaning, garbage, waste	Tuberculosis, HAV, HBV, typhoid
12.8	Classroom, clerk, store	Respiratory infections
12.9	Transportation	STI (HBV, HIV, gonorrhea, syphilis)

12.1 CONSTRUCTION AND MINING

"Orange casque" work includes construction, renovation, and demolition work, at buildings, on roads, and in tunnels, prospecting, surveying, and archeological digging.

Infections (1572, 2066) (http://www.cdc.gov/malaria/history). Special climate conditions underground that resemble caves and precarious sanitation put workers at risk of respiratory tract and enteric infections. Migration and social disruption increase the risks of sexually transmitted infection (STI). Outdoor life exposes workers to arboviruses, malaria, and rodent-borne infections. When Americans built the Panama Canal in 1904–1914, W. C. Gorgas (1854–1920) was in charge of vector control. By clearing jungle, draining marshes, and larviciding ponds, he controlled yellow fever and malaria, reducing malaria deaths in workers from 1.2/100 in 1906 to 0.1/100 in 1909. For dust, see section 5.5; and for dams, see section 6.1.

DROPLET-AIR CLUSTER
Bacteria
***Bacillus anthracis* (7616).** In Australia in 1997, a severe epizootic caused >180 bovine cases; for control, >78,000 cattle from >450 herds were vaccinated. While neither winds, feeds, animal carcasses, arthropods, or movement of personnel could explain the epizootic, extensive earth work in the 1980s that had stirred up anthrax "graves" and warmer-than-usual soil temperatures were suspected to be conducive conditions.

Box 12.1 Suggested occupational exposure history

Right now:
- Does your work mainly involve natural materials (rock, roads, mines, or soil), plants or animals (field, farm, zoo, or abattoir), people or human materials (security, education, rescue, health, and laboratory), foods (packing, cooking, and vending), or installations (maintenance, manufacture, and cleaning), or are you jobless, retired, or in training?
- Describe your current workplace, work schedule, and job responsibilities.
- Are you aware of any colleagues from your shift, team, or workplace who are ill like you?

In the past 1–4 weeks:
- Have you had any injury from a sharp object, splash into the eye, or "accident" (laboratory or animal bite)?
- Have you had any contacts with patients (vomit, diarrhea, fever, or rash), diapered children, or the elderly? Any international travel?

In the past 1–6 months:
- Did you perform any work with patients, human materials, biomaterials, waste, soil, water, animals, animal products, plants, plant products, or foods? Have you had any training sessions outdoors, at field camps, or stations? Have you had any foods from canteens?
- How many days have you been sick off work? Did the condition aggravate before, during, or after work?

In your lifetime:
- Have you ever had chickenpox, jaundice (acute hepatitis A, B, or C), typhoid fever, or tuberculosis, or have you ever passed or been treated for tapeworms (carrier)?
- Name all job titles that you have had. Have you ever switched jobs for health reasons?

Mycobacterium. *M. tuberculosis* **(2789, 7033).** Gold miners in South Africa are at risk of infection and disease. Spread is mainly among miners. In four South African gold mines in 1995 (HIV seroprevalence of ~21%), the disease prevalence was 1.6%, and ≥50% of the 419 cases detected were acquired in the mining community. Among a cohort of 326 South African mine workers observed for ~1–3 years, 65 (20%) had recurring disease, for a rate of 10/100 person-years; of 39 patients molecularly fingerprinted, only 25 (64%) had relapses while 14 (36%) had evidence for reinfection. **Environmental mycobacteria (1409).** In black-coal-mining areas of Moravia and Silesia, Czechia, in the 1970s–1990s, miners were at increased risk of *M. kansasii* infection, likely from industrial and drinking water. A likely hazard was industrially polluted air. In endemic areas, average disease rates per 10^5 per year were 20 in males, 6 in females, and 12 overall.

***Neisseria meningitidis* (7034).** New, young miners seem at high risk. In the gold mines in South Africa, meningococcal disease outbreaks have occurred at intervals.

Fungi

Dust is a hazard for fungal pulmonary infections in orange casque workers. For renovation work in hospitals, see section 17.7.

***Aspergillus* (286, 5841).** A likely risk for *Aspergillus* is demolition and repair of moldy buildings.

***Coccidioides* (5851, 8055).** In California in 1970, 61 of 103 students excavating Indian ruins contracted coccidioidomycosis. At Dinosaur National Monument, Utah, in 2001, 10 of a team of 8 students and 10 archeologists contracted coccidioidomycosis from sifting dirt through screens.

***Cryptococcus* (1572).** In HIV-infected South African gold miners, *C. neoformans* accounted for an unusual proportion (44%) of deaths.

***Histoplasma* (1233, 7375).** *Histoplasma* is a hazard for orange casque workers, including construction workers, miners, caveguides, and archeologists. Histoplasmin skin reactivity in occupationally exposed groups is greater in males than females. Safety equipment for high-risk activities, e.g., disturbing soil with bird droppings, should include disposable coveralls, rubber boots, and respirator.

Outbreaks Occupational outbreaks have been reported since the 1950s, virtually only from the United States, at demolition, repair, and construction sites, from buildings, factories, bridges, subways, and golf courses. Earth movements and dust from cleaning bat guano or bird droppings from buildings and bridges are major sources. In 1962 in Mason City, Iowa, bulldozing work in a park stirred up spores and caused some 8,400 infections, for an attack rate of 25% (1698). In Indianapolis in 1978–1979, a first outbreak caused 435 documented cases and ~100,000 infections; construction of a tennis complex was the likely source (8066). A second epidemic of similar magnitude occurred in 1980; construction of a swimming pool was the likely source (6670, 8065). In 1980, an outbreak in a limestone quarry in Michigan caused 138 cases; the source was a pulley stored in a gull-nesting area (7913). In Kentucky in 1995, five members of a demolition crew fell ill after work at an abandoned city hall in which bats had lived; of 55 exposed workers or residents, 19 had clinical or serological evidence of acute infection (4356). In 2001, archeological work at Dinosaur National Monument in Utah caused 10 acute cases among workers and archeologists; in contrast, among 397,800 visitors to the park in 2000, no cases became known (4735). In Nebraska in 2003, 25 of 724 workers acquired confirmed histoplasmosis disease from soil carefully excavated and deposited for repair of an underground pipe (1233).

***Sporothrix* (2385, 7842).** Infections are a hazard for construction and brick factory workers and farmers. Outbreaks occurred in South African gold mines in 1914, 1941, and later. The 1941 outbreak caused >2,400 cases among miners. Timbers used to support underground mines were the likely source.

FECES-FOOD CLUSTER

Information is scant. Adequate sanitation is a problem in underground mines. Camp kitchens carry a risk of foodborne infections.

Bacteria

At a worker camp in Saudi Arabia, 168 of 419 Filipino workers who ate from a single kitchen developed acute *Salmonella enterica* serovar Minnesota gastroenteritis; 1 of 27 cooks tested positive for the agent (118). In 1973, likely waterborne serovar Typhi was reported in a migrant camp in Florida with 225 probable or confirmed typhoid fever cases (2350). In Singapore in 1982, 37 foreign construction workers acquired *Vibrio cholerae* O1 from seafood served at the construction canteen (2809).

Protozoa

Of 154 pan miners in Pará State, Brazil, the feces of 14% tested positive for *Entamoeba histolytica/dispar* and of 5% for *Giardia lamblia* (6611). In the United States, soil-related occupations are a hazard for infections with *Toxoplasma gondii* (3734).

Helminths

Of 154 pan miners in Pará State, Brazil, the feces of 47% tested positive for *Ascaris lumbricoides* and of 3% for *Trichuris trichiura* (6611).

ZOONOTIC CLUSTER

Information is scant. In enzootic areas, protected housing, impregnated clothes, and repellents against mosquitoes, flies, and ticks should be considered for workers (1105).

Viruses
Dengue virus (DENV) (5771). At a construction site in Pakistan in 1995, an outbreak of febrile illness was confirmed due to DENV2.

Ebola virus (EBOV) (612). In northeastern Gabon, antibodies to EBOV were prevalent in gold-panning villages.

Marburg virus (MARV) (491, 612). Working in Congo (formerly Zaire) gold mines was a risk for MARV infection, by as yet unidentified sources. Index cases for an outbreak in Congo in 1998–1999 were miners who were thought to have acquired MARV from animal contact, perhaps bats.

Protozoa
Leishmania **(6151).** Occupational hazards are mainly forest-related (see section 5.4). In rural Guyana, mining and military service are confirmed risks for cutaneous leishmaniasis.

Plasmodium **(2043, 6721, 7289, 7787).** *Anopheles* breeding sites in industrial complexes include drains, water tanks, sluice-valve chambers, and water reservoirs.

Infection risks include construction work in endemic areas, open day mines, prospecting, outdoor night shifts, migrant work, and sleeping outdoors. Open mining operations, in particular, foster mosquito breeding and enhance transmission, including drug-resistant *P. falciparum*, e.g., in the Amazon, and rain forest areas of West Africa, Southcentral and Southeast Asia, and the Southwest Pacific.

In Brazil, gold miners (garimpeiros) are at particular risk ("gold fever") (1604, 1784, 2045, 6611, 7787). Of 186 pan miners in Pará State, Brazil, 65 (35%) were infected; a majority (34 or 52%) of parasitemias was inapparent, although close to 100% of miners reported ≥1 malaria episode in the past decade.

In Orissa, India, miners of iron and other ores, and mining settlements, were at particular risk; parasitemia prevalences in mining settlements were 14–24% (~three fourths due to *P. falciparum*) (8302). In a gem-mining area in dry central Sri Lanka, entomological inoculation rates from main vectors (endophagic *Anopheles culicifacies* and *A. subpictus*, exophagic *A. varuna*) were ~6–7 infective bites per person per year. Crude disease rates/1,000 person-years were 123 for *P. vivax* and 26 for *P. falciparum*, with significantly higher rates in men than women (8331). In jungle areas of Cambodia, gem miners remote from medical services were at particular risk, and reported falciparum malaria lethality reached 10–15% (5870).

Large mines provide opportunities for malaria control and prevention as well (1604, 6002, 6721). At a security camp in the forest of Assam, northeast India, in 1998–2001, chemoprophylaxis, mosquito nets, and repellents reduced the disease rate in workers from 6.7 to 0.06/1,000 person-nights.

Trypanosoma cruzi **(1919).** In Minas Gerais, Brazil, ~12% of 301 construction workers were seroreactive, and 31% of seroreactive workers had electrocardiographic anomalies, compared with 7% of seronegative workers.

Helminths
Mansonella. Bites by midges are a hazard for orange casque workers. In South America, the hazards are living in forest mining camps and panning for gold (5178).

Onchocerca. Bites by black flies are a hazard. In South America, daytime outdoor work such as gold mining is a risk (4662).

ENVIRONMENTAL CLUSTER
Water and soil contacts frequently expose orange casque workers.

Bacteria
Clostridium tetani **(4564, 4565).** Occupational tetanus is poorly documented. In Finland in 1969–1985, 9 (9%) of 106 tetanus patients were construction workers.

Leptospira **(611, 4369, 5622, 5894).** At risk are road, construction, and oil exploration workers, storm drain cleaners, gold panners, and miners. Tunnels and shafts can become wet and rat infested. In Nigeria in 1990–1991, seroprevalence was 46% (41/248) in coal miners, and 4.5% (4/62) in hospital laboratory workers. In Gabon in 1996, seroprevalence was 14% (19/132) in gold panners, 8% (3/36) in traders, and 15% (5/33) in housewives.

Mycobacterium **(1573, 4751, 8427).** Miners are at risk of infection with environmental mycobacteria, in particular, workers with a history of tuberculosis or pneumoconiosis. Of 32 miners with pulmonary disease from environmental mycobacteria, 23 grew *M. kansasii*, 7 grew *M. scrofulaceum*, and 1 each grew *M. avium* and *M. abscessus*.

Helminths
Hookworm (5799, 6611). Risks are soil related. In 1880, numerous workers contracted hookworm anemia from working in the Gotthard Tunnel across the Swiss Alps.

Lack of sanitation and tunnel temperatures of 36–38°C were favorable for local transmission of *Ancylostoma duodenale*. In Pará State, Brazil, 61% (94/154) pan miners tested positive for hookworms.

Schistosoma (5958, 7053, 8399). Risks are water related and include mining and dam building, e.g., Diama Dam (on the Senegal River) and Manantali Dam (on the Bafing River) in West Africa for *S. haematobium* and *S. mansoni*, and Three Gorge Dam (on the Yangtze River) in People's Republic of China for *S. japonicum*. In Zaire, tin mining requires large amounts of water to wash out deposits and veins. Construction of canals and reservoirs creates man-made foci of infection.

Strongyloides (1594, 1798, 6611, 7894). Risks are soil related. Mines with favorable microclimates that lack sanitation support transmission. Infections have been reported in coal and pan miners.

SKIN-BLOOD CLUSTER
Viruses
Migrant construction workers and miners are at increased risk of hepatitis B virus (HBV) and HIV infections.

HBV (6611). Of 185 pan miners in Pará State, Brazil, 157 (85%) had positive markers of HBV, and 11 (6%) were carriers of hepatitis B surface antigen (HBsAg).

HIV (1572, 5691, 8179). In a mining community in South Africa, in 1998, HIV prevalence was 20% in men in the community, 29% in gold miners, 37% in women in the community, and 69% in mine sex workers. In South Africa, compared with 2,970 HIV-negative miners, 1,792 HIV-infected miners were at greater risk of hospitalization for tuberculosis, bacterial pneumonia, and cryptococcosis. In a remote gold-mining camp in Guyana, 6.5% (14/216) of the workforce was HIV-infected.

Bacteria
In the 1940s, yaws affected 67 workers of the springs mines at Witwatersrand; transmission was shown to occur at ~2,100 m below surface, where temperatures were tropical and miners worked with frequent skin contacts (3043). Of 185 pan miners in Pará State, Brazil, 77 (42%) were reactive in a *T. pallidum* (syphilis) microhemagglutination test (6611).

Fungi
Coal miners in the United Kingdom seemed at high risk of tinea pedis (3198). Besides the usual agents of tinea, *Trichophyton rubrum* and *T. mentagrophytes* were observed in Nigerian coal miners (2991).

Helminths
Enterobius vermicularis was isolated in pan miners in Pará State, Brazil (6611).

12.2 MANUFACTURE AND MAINTENANCE
"Blue collar" work includes manufacturing and assembling of machines, automotive and electronic parts, the chemical, plastic, and print industries, supplies of electricity, gas, and oil, and the maintenance and repair of cars, water and sanitation systems, and heating and air conditioning installations. For work with animal products, see section 12.4.

Infections. Because substrates (e.g., metals, oils, and chemicals) are noninfective, in general, the main risks are respiratory tract infections in crowded, poorly ventilated rooms, e.g., assembly halls and workshops, and pyodermias and dermatophytes from tight professional gowns. Confounders include smoking, inhalational allergens, toxic chemicals (hypersensitivity pneumonitis, oil akne), and infections from home or leisure habitats. How chemicals and infectious agents interact is inadequately known (3460).

DROPLET-AIR CLUSTER
In workers well covered by routine vaccines, the main risks are Legionnaires' disease and tuberculosis.

Viruses
Adenovirus (AdV) (5124, 7073). Respiratory AdV can circulate in blue-collar workers, and outbreaks of AdV keratoconjunctivitis have been reported in industrial settings.

Influenzavirus (878, 3724). In the placebo arm of a randomized vaccine trial, the rate of laboratory-confirmed influenza disease in healthy adult workers was 4% (6/137) in the 1997–1998 season, and 10% (14/137) in the 1998–1999 season. On an oilrig in Darwin Harbor, Australia, in December 1996, an off-season *Influenzavirus* B outbreak affected 56% of workers. Consistent with a general pattern, influenza in the tropical part of Australia can be transmitted throughout the year. Anticipated outbreaks can be prevented by annual vaccination of the workforce.

Bacteria
B. anthracis (411, 5864). Organic dust can be a source of anthrax, including in textile mills and felt factories (see "Field, Forest, Herd, and Abattoir" below). However, organic material can be inconspicuous, e.g., pipe insulation material from goat hair.

***Bordetella pertussis* (1216).** Occupational infections in blue-collar workers are rare. In Illinois in 2002, an outbreak at an oil refinery caused 15 cases among workers, for an attack rate of 10%. The source was an ill superviser. Active surveillance identified 24 outbreak-related cases, of whom 21 (88%) were of age ≥20 years.

Chlamydophila pneumoniae. In South Africa, seroreactivity was significantly more prevalent in mine workers (66%) than in factory workers (22%), and 17% of miners observed for 6 months seroconverted (461).

***Legionella* (151, 1049, 2544, 3295, 5536).** Industrial settings that produce water aerosols are reported sources of sporadic and epidemic cases of Legionnaires' disease, Pontiac fever, or *Legionella* pneumonia. In France, ~4% of reported cases of Legionnaires' disease are occupational. *L. pneumophila* was suggested to be associated with sick-building syndrome.

- Plumbers and air-conditioning maintenance workers (965, 2762, 2817). Legionellosis should be a hazard, but the evidence is limited and equivocal. By antibodies and history of pneumonia, risks were comparable in 21 "high-risk" workers (cleaning and servicing cooling towers and evaporative condensers) and 27 "low-risk" workers (not involved in service work). At a power-generating plant with a contaminated cooling tower that yielded *L. pneumophila* serotype 6, seroreactivity was nil in workers with low cooling-tower exposure, 4.6% in workers with intermediate exposure, and 7.6% in workers with high exposure.
- Other work (461, 3255). A risk for construction workers is suggested in Singapore where in 1986–1996, 53% of foreign construction workers were found to be seroreactive, compared with 10–22% in the general population. In South Africa, seroreactivity was significantly more prevalent in mine workers (36%) than in factory workers (10%), and 18% of miners monitored for 6 months seroconverted.

Outbreaks Outbreaks among blue-collar workers have been reported mainly in North America and Australia. At an Ontario, Canada, automobile assembly plant in 1981, coolant caused 317 cases of Pontiac fever among workers, for attack rates of 0–100%, depending on work location (3295). In the United States in 1988, three cases of Legionnaires' disease were linked to a factory that used water to cool molded plastics (5262). In an Ohio car factory in 2001, an outbreak caused 4 cofirmed and 13 possible cases among ~2,500 employees; compared with 86 controls, cases were more likely to be exposed to aerosols from the cleaning work line (odds ratio 3; 95% confidence interval [95% CI] 1.1–9) (151, 2544). At a sugarbeet processing plant in Minnesota in 2000, 14 workers contracted Pontiac fever from high-pressure water cleaning work; water yielded *L. pneumophila* at concentrations of 10^5 CFU/ml (1123). In Sydney, Australia, in 2001, three infections were linked to a cooling tower in the workplace (921).

***Mycobacterium. M. tuberculosis* (2035, 6074).** Undetected smear-positive cases expose blue-collar coworkers in the same, confined spaces, e.g., manufacturing halls. Tuberculosis outbreaks in factories have been reported. **Environmental mycobacteria (2298).** In automobile manufacturing, "hypersensitivity pneumonitis" has been attributed to aerosols from metal-working fluid that contains *M. avium* or *M. intracellulare*. Similarly, granulomatous pneumonitis in life guards (lifeguard lung) at indoor swimming pools with waterfalls and sprays was suggested to be due to mycobacteria-containing aerosols.

Fungi
A histoplasmosis outbreak at a paper factory with 16 (30%) cases among 53 workers was traced to sweeping bird guano from a roof on a windy day (7178).

FECES-FOOD CLUSTER
In Kyoto, Japan, in 1996, radish sprout salad served at a factory cafeteria caused an outbreak of enterohemorrhagic *Escherichia coli* among workers (7968). In a Zimbabwe textile factory in 1994, *Shigella sonnei* and *S. boydii* affected 38 workers who had drunk contaminated water from boreholes, for an attack rate of 51% (7593).

ZOONOTIC CLUSTER
Indoor exposure of blue-collar workers to arthropods seems negligible. The main zoonotic risk is from dust.

***Coxiella* (4755, 7755).** *C. burnetii* is a risk for blue-collar workers. In Wales, United Kingdom, in 2002, renovation work at a cardboard-manufacturing plant was followed by a Q fever outbreak with 95 acute cases, for an attack rate of 38% among 253 tested employees; the likely source was holes drilled into straw board ceiling. In a truck-repair plant, *C. burnetii* infected 16 of 32 employees; a suspected source was dust from clothing of an employee who owned an infected cat.

***Erysipelothrix* (5969).** In a shoe factory, raw material that grew *E. rhusiopathiae* was vehicle for an outbreak among workers.

***Francisella* (1272, 2972).** *F. tularensis* is a risk for factory workers. In a sugar factory in Vienna, Austria, in 1959–1960, 795 (77%) of 1,028 workers contracted tularemia, mainly through inhalation of aerosolized cleaning water from sugar beets inadvertently milled with mice carcasses. Similar, smaller outbreaks occurred in Moravia, Czechia, in the 1960s, with a total of 87 tularemia cases in sugar factory workers.

ENVIRONMENTAL CLUSTER

Burkholderia (2577). In Australia, two mechanics of a remote town garage in the melioidosis belt developed skin lesions that grew an identical strain of *B. pseudomallei*; both worked mainly on muddy off-road vehicles. A container with commercial hand wash from which mechanics dispensed detergent by means of a garden hose readily grew *B. pseudomallei* strains that differed from clinical strains.

Leptospira (222). In France, canal workers and locks workers who reported water contacts were at risk of inapparent *Leptospira* infections.

12.3 MILITARY, POLICE, AND GUARDS

"Uniformed" work includes military (army, navy, and air force) personnel, police and security forces, customs officers, coast guards, fireworkers, and rescue teams. In 2000 worldwide, armies counted ~22 million personnel (0.3–0.4% of the world population).

Exposure (6973) results from crowded barracks and dormitories, inadequate sanitation in field camps, mosquito and tick bites during deployment, large movements of troops, unsafe leisure behavior, and periods of war. At high risk are "unseasoned" recruits. Some 2,000 wars and warlike events were recorded in 4 millenia (350 since World War II). Countries with large armies include People's Republic of China (2.6 million, 0.2% of its population), United States (1.5 million, 0.5%), Russia (1.3 million, 0.9%), India (1.3 million, 0.1%), and North Korea (1.1 million, 5%).

Infections (Box 12.2). **Military personnel (1655, 1987, 2654, 2925, 3529, 5550).** Risks vary by time (availability of antimicrobials), services (training and war), and location (temperate or tropical). The main infectious diseases in World War I (1914–1918) were influenza and trench fever, and in World War II (1939–1945) they were viral hepatitis, louse-borne typhus, typhoid fever, and malaria. In the Vietnam War (1964–1973), dengue, Japanese encephalitis, plague, and malaria were reported, but apparently not schistosomiasis. During the Persian Gulf War in 1991, respiratory tract and enteric infections were common, and tropical infections and STIs were unusual; only 12 cases of visceral leishmaniasis were reported among ~0.7 million U.S. troops. **Police personnel (5675, 7029).** In police officers, reported rates of exposure to human blood from needlestick or bite are 0.4% (New York) to 0.7% (Amsterdam). Uniformed service personnel and institutions have contributed to the advancement of diagnostics, vaccines, and antimicrobials. Uniformed workers can be victims *and* vectors (61, 392, 3991) of infections. For the latter, examples are rubella (with a risk for nonimmune females in households), pertussis (misdiagnosed, of high infectivity), meningococcal meningitis, tuberculosis, and STI (including HIV). For carriers in the population, see secton 14.1. **Prevention.** Vaccines to consider on entry into services for periodic updating and predeployment could include (i) commercial vaccines routinely recommended for civilian populations, i.e., hepatitis A virus (HAV), HBV, influenza, measles-mumps-rubella (MMR) vaccine, polio, varicella-zoster virus (VZV), Bacillus Calmette Guérin (BCG), diphtheria, tetanus, pertussis$_{acellular}$ vaccines dTp$_a$), *N. meningitidis*, and *Streptococcus pneumoniae*, and (ii) vaccines targeted by risk and availability (can be investigational) (6473), i.e., AdV, arboviral encephalitis (eastern equine encephalitis virus [EEEV], Japanese encephalitis virus [JEV], tick-borne encephalitis virus [TBEV], Venezuelan equine encephalitis virus [VEEV], and western equine encephalitis virus [WEEV]), rabies virus, viral hemorrhagic fevers (Rift Valley fever virus

---

Box 12.2 Agents and infections from uniformed work, by cluster

Droplet-air	• Vaccine preventable: *Influenzavirus*, MMR, VZV; diphtheria, pertussis, *S. pneumoniae*, tuberculosis • Vaccine nonpreventable: AdV, *Chlamydophila, Coxiella, Mycoplasma, N. meningitis* group B
Feces-food	HAV, HEV, *Norovirus; Campylobacter, E. coli* (mainly ETEC), *Salmonella* (*S. enterica* serovars non-Typhi and Typhi), *Shigella* (*S. flexneri* and *S. sonnei*); *Cryptopsoridium, E. histolytica* (endemic areas)
Zoonotic	• Viral hemorrhagic fevers (DENV and HFRS), viral encephalitis (JEV, rabies, TBEV) • Anthrax, borrelioses (mainly Lyme), *Coxiella, F. tularensis*, rickettsiae (*Orientia* and *Rickettsia*), *Y. pestis* • *Leishmania* (cutaneous and visceral), *Plasmodium* (*P. falciparum* and *P. vivax*); lymphatic filariasis
Environmental	• *Acinetobacter* (wound infection), melioidosis, leptospirosis • Hookworm (enteric and cutaneous), *Strongyloides, Schistosoma* (urinary and enteric)
Skin-blood	HBV, HCV, HIV; *C. trachomatis* (genital), *N. gonorrhoeae, S. aureus, S. pyogenes, T. pallidum*

[RVFV], Junin virus [JUNV], and yellow fever virus [YFV]), variola virus, *B. anthracis, Clostridium botulinum, C. burnetii, F. tularensis, S. enterica* serovar Typhi, *V. cholerae*, and *Yersinia pestis* (manufacture was discontinued in 1999).

DROPLET-AIR CLUSTER, UNIFORMED SERVICES

Risks (947, 2911). Respiratory tract infections are a significant cause of illness and hospitalization in the uniformed services. Hazards include crowded quarters (on land, ships, and submarines) and low coverage with vaccines (police and customs). In the United States in the 1990s, army recruits were hospitalized for acute respiratory illnesses at a rate of ~0.15/100 per year compared with ~0.05/100 per year in young adult civilians.

Viruses: Vaccine Preventable

Influenzavirus **(2911, 3831).** Despite annual use of vaccine, laboratory surveillance is critical, as risks persist in crowded quarters. Outbreaks are well documented in the uniformed services (2109, 3999, 4127, 4683). In 1918, during the 1917–1918 pandemic, A/H1N1 affected 106,897 (19%) of 569,470 U.S. Navy personnel, for a lethality of 4.5%. In 1996, A/H3N2 affected 42% of the personnel aboard a U.S. Navy ship, despite 95% had been covered by vaccine. At an air force training center in Greece in 1996, recent influenza B infections were documented serologically in 27% (15/55) of randomly selected recruits (in parallel, there was an outbreak of meningococcal disease).

Measles virus (1699, 2681, 2781). While vaccine coverage of ≥85% with a single dose is inadequate, coverage with two doses that approaches 100% will prevent outbreaks in the uniformed services. In Italy in 1986–1997, reported disease rates/10^5 per year tended to be higher in military personnel (100–1,300) than civilian males of corresponding age (≤200).

Mumps virus (268, 1504, 1699). In the prevaccine era, mumps caused considerable morbidity in the uniformed services. In Italy in 1986–1997, reported mumps rates/10^5 per year were higher in military personnel (25–65) than civilian males of corresponding age (15–45). Wild-virus mumps was diagnosed in the United Kingdom, in 4 (2%) of 180 Gurkha army recruits 16 days after receiving measles, mumps, rubella (MMR) vaccine in Nepal.

Rubella virus (61, 1621, 1699, 4839, 7164). The main risk is exposure of pregnant women from male personnel. High vaccine coverage is required to control circulation. In Italy in 1986–1997, reported disease rates/10^5 per year were higher in army personnel (~250–2,300) than in civilian males of corresponding age (≤200). In Switzerland in 1986, 9% (595/6,877) of recruits were seronegative on entry into the service, and of 475 recruits monitored for 3 months, 113 (24%) seroconverted.

Outbreaks were reported in the 1950s–1980s, and less frequently in the 1990s. In North Carolina in 1995, in an outbreak among visiting German soldiers, 6 of 10 nonimmune individuals contracted clinical rubella while four other nonimmunes received immunoglobulin (Ig) in ≤12 h after recognition of the index case. In Bosnia in 1996, four male British soldiers contracted rubella, and one pregnant soldier was repatriated to minimize the risk of intrauterine infection. In Australia in 1991, an outbreak affected 32 naval apprentices and 3 air force members at a nearby base; 2 of the 35 cases reported contacts with pregnant women.

VZV (1699, 3266, 4500). Pockets of nonimmune personnel persist, including in conscripts from some tropical areas. In Italy in 1986–1997, reported varicella rates/10^5 per year were higher in army personnel (600–1,900) than civilian males of corresponding age (≤200). Among Puerto Rican recruits deployed to Texas for training in 1986–1987, 42% were susceptible and two outbreaks ensued, for attack rates of 30% and 70%, respectively, and a total of 105 cases. A varicella outbreak was reported during the Gulf war.

Viruses: Vaccine Nonpreventable

AdV (453, 1782, 2342, 2912, 3317, 3534, 4038, 6490, 6581). AdV is a well-documented hazard in the uniformed services. In the 1950s, recruits were hospitalized for AdV infections at rates reaching ~10%. In the United States in 1996–1998, ~50% of >3,000 throat cultures from symptomatic trainees yielded AdV, mostly types 4, 7, and 3. Of 678 military recruits monitored for 8 weeks, 626 (92%, 1.2/100 person-weeks) developed respiratory symptoms, 115 (17%, 0.2/100 person-weeks) were hospitalized, and 79 (69%) of those hospitalized yielded AdV (type 4 in 70, type 3 in 7, and type 21 in 2). Of 249 recruits providing paired sera, 49% (82/166) treated as outpatients and 83% (69/83) of those hospitalized seroconverted to AdV type 4.

Outbreaks have been well recognized in the uniformed services. With no vaccine currently available, 100s to 1,000s of personnel can be affected, in particular, at training centers, for attack rates in affected units up to 10% per week. Outbreaks of AdV keratoconjunctivitis have also been reported in the uniformed services.

EBV (3095). Infections in recruits have been reported. However, rare secondary infections in roommates of index cases suggest low contagiousness in the uniformed services.

Bacteria: Vaccine Preventable

B. pertussis (1436, 2911, 3991). Pertussis risks include personnel and dependent families. In 1989, 18% of U.S. Marine trainees who reported ≥7 days of cough were diagnosed with acute *B. pertussis* infections. In a pertussis outbreak in Israel in winter 2001, attack rates in an infantry regiment were 21% (cough for ≥30 days) or 9.5% (cases confirmed by PCR or anti-*Bordetella* IgA or IgM). *B. pertussis* was detected by PCR well into reconvalescence in a high proportion (20%) of patients.

Corynebacterium (1943, 2579, 6965, 8068). Diphtheria is a risk for nonimmune personnel. In 1940–1941, when Halifax, Canada, was a World War II winter port, crew of a Norwegian tanker ignited a diphtheria outbreak with 649 cases. In the 1990s, 100,000 demobilized Russian troops not routinely vaccinated carried the agent home from Afghanistan, contributing to a massive epidemic. Nontoxigenic *C. diphtheriae* has also been reported in military personnel.

M. tuberculosis (2032, 6759). Groups at risk of infection include armed forces recruits, police cadets, and prison guards. **Infections (1562, 1646, 6978).** Infections can be prevalent in the uniformed services. Of 44,128 U.S. Navy recruits tuberculin-tested in 1997–1998, 1,531 (3.5%, 95% CI 3.3–3.7) were considered latently infected: 1% (9) had indurations of 5–9 mm and scars on chest X ray or a history of exposure, 21% (327) had indurations of 5–9 mm and a history of disease, 27% (419) had indurations of 10–14 mm, and 51% (776) had indurations of ≥15 mm (in the 1980s, infection prevalences were ~1%). In New South Wales, Australia, in 1987–1990, of 4,704 police cadets skin tested, 7% of those who had never received BCG were reactive to tuberculin. **Disease (804, 1699).** In Italy in 1986–1997, rates of reported pulmonary tuberculosis per 10^5 per year were higher in army personnel (8–13) than in civilians of corresponding age (4–5.5). In Greece, disease rates were also higher in military than in civilian individuals, although rates per 10^5 per year fell in 1965–1993, from 60 to 18 in army personnel, 50 to 25 in navy personnel, and 38 to 15 in air force personnel.

Outbreaks (3894, 4196, 7853) Outbreaks have been reported on an amphibious ship and in military units.

N. meningitidis (199, 2960, 3730, 5376, 6280). Classical investigations have demonstrated the spread of *N. meningitidis* by crowding, and reduced risks of carriage and disease by spacing beds >1 m apart (droplet distance). Strains resistant to rifampicin (MIC >256 mg/liter) have been isolated in military settings. **Infection (199).** In closed rooms with smokers, the proportion of carriers can reach 40–50%. The risk of carriage and disease in uniformed personnel is particularly high in the first 0–12 weeks of contact. In Denmark, on entrance into the service at different seasons, 39–47% of 1,969 military recruits were pharyngeal carriers; after 3 months, one third had changed carrier state at least once. **Disease (663, 1699, 2960, 4675).** In Finland in 1974, although the entrance prevalence was low (1–5%), serogroup A disease rate in unvaccinated recruits reached $71/10^5$ in 9 months. In Italy in 1986–1997, disease rates per 10^5 per year were 0.5–6.5 in army personnel compared with 0.5–1.5 in civilians of corresponding age. Serogroup C peaked in Italy in 1985–1986, for a disease rate of 11 per 10^5; by vaccination, rates in 1988–1989 reached a low of 0.2 per 10^5. In the Israeli armed forces, most (~80%) bacterial meningitis is due to *N. meningitidis*, and typically there is a winter peak. In the 1990s, three fourths of meningococcal meningitis was due to serogroup C.

Outbreaks (1952, 4683) Outbreaks occurred in troops in World War I. Meningococcal meningitis by vaccine nonpreventable serogroup B remains a threat, even for vaccinated employees. In Norway in 1967–1988, a protracted serogroup B outbreak caused 188 cases, for rates per 10^5 per year of 40 in military personnel, and 10 in civilians of the same age. At an air force training center in Greece in 1996, an outbreak of *N. meningitidis* group C caused 10 cases; concomitant was an influenza outbreak.

S. pneumoniae (2911, 3481, 5283, 6583). Outbreaks of pneumococcal pneumonia occurred in the armed services before and after penicillin was introduced during World War II. In Illinois in 1918, *S. pneumoniae* in a military camp put 2,349 into the hospital, for a lethality of 50%. After a period of silence in the 1960s–1980s, pneumococcal pneumonia reemerged. At a marine training camp in California in the winter of 1989–1990, an outbreak caused 128 such cases. In the winter of 1998–1999, 30 (13%) of 239 ranger trainees contracted pneumococcal pneumonia; *S. pneumoniae* was cultured from 61% (11/18) hospitalized cases and from throat swabs of 14% (30/221) other trainees. The outbreak was controlled by azithromycin chemoprophylaxis.

Of 157 invasive strains obtained from U.S. military hospitals in 1997–1999, 30% (50/157) exhibited intermediate or high-level resistance to penicillin, and 15% were multiresistant. The most common serotypes were 14 (23%), 9V (12%), 4 and 6B (12% each), and 19F (10%).

S. pneumoniae is a cause of epidemic conjunctivitis among military trainees (1656).

Bacteria: Vaccine Nonpreventable

Chlamydophila (579, 1665, 2153, 3986). Cases of *C. pneumoniae* (sore throat and mild pneumonia) and outbreaks should be expected in military personnel at all seasons. Because of diagnostic difficulties and because symptoms overlap with *Mycoplasma* and AdV, *C. pneumonia* may be underdiagnosed. Outbreaks in Finland lasted ~6 months, with attack rates of 6–8%. In a Norwegian military camp in 1990, 35 (7%) of 500 conscripts and officers became ill, and another 49% seroconverted.

Mycoplasma (2342, 2911). *M. pneumoniae* infection rates can be high in the uniformed services, and outbreaks have been reported. In the 1960s–1990s, up to 56% of pneumonias in recruits were *M. pneumoniae* (2911). At a U.S. military training academy in 1996, 317 (54%) of 586 trainees were diagnosed with mycoplasmal respiratory illness; *M. pneumoniae* was confirmed by PCR from oropharyngeal swabs in 28 of 42 tested trainees. Risks included residence in a particular building, having an ill roommate, and more than three visits to the campus health clinic.

Fungi
The main risk is inhalation of dust in endemic areas.

Coccidioides (1659, 7110). Desert training is a risk. Reported infection rates are ~6–32/100 per year. In an endemic area of California in 2001, 10 (45%) of 22 navy personnel acquired *C. immitis* disease from training that included camping and digging holes. Similarly, after training in California, 8 of 27 (30%) marines were found to be infected.

Histoplasma (759, 7577). Infections and acute disease have been diagnosed in military personnel. Of 232 French legionnaires screened by chest radiography on returning from 2-year assignments in French Guiana, two legionnaires had lung nodules due to *H. capsulatum*, and six had probable histoplasmosis.

FECES-FOOD CLUSTER, UNIFORMED SERVICES
Risk (3527, 3529, 3728, 6598). Diarrheal disease is a significant risk for troops deployed to low-income countries (troopers' diarrhea). Reported attack rates are 10–50%, or 1.3 per person-year. Causative agents resemble "travelers' diarrhea" (see section 15.4) and by geography include *E. coli* (enterotoxigenic *E. coli* [ETEC] and enteroaggregative *E. coli* [EAEC]), *Campylobacter*, and *Shigella*, *Norovirus* and *Rotavirus*, and *Cryptosporidium*.

Viruses
Astrovirus (538). Astrovirus was recovered from French military recruits with diarrhea.

HAV (976, 1699, 2493, 2744, 3196, 3343, 4823). HAV is a risk for nonimmune military populations deployed to endemic areas. Vaccination has changed the epidemiology. In the 1980s–1990s, anti-HAV prevalence in active-duty personnel from high-income countries ranged from 10% (United States) to 25% (Italy). Reported infection rates are ~1/100 per year, while disease rates range from ~3 to $50/10^5$ per year. Prevaccination screening is not considered cost-effective for personnel with seroprevalences <20%.

Outbreaks (557, 1600, 1987, 2493, 6451) Outbreaks were recorded in World Wars I and II. Outbreaks were also reported in service personnel in the 1970s–1990s by contaminated water, food, or interpersonal spread; one at a military post in Anchorage, Alaska, caused 116 clinical cases.

Hepatitis E virus (HEV) (953, 969, 1478, 2605, 7589, 7629, 7708). Acute hepatitis E (HE) seems to be an emerging hazard for peace-keeping forces and military personnel deployed to or residing in endemic areas. In Chad in 1983–1984, an outbreak among French soldiers caused ≥38 cases, confirmed retrospectively. In Ethiopia in 1988–1989, waterborne HEV caused 423 icteric cases in military camps. In Haiti in 1995, four members of the Bangladeshi peace-keeping force contracted acute HE; a survey demonstrated seroprevalence of 2–6% in American forces (United States, 2/109; Guatemala, 6/111; Honduras, 6/109) and of 27–62% in Asia forces (Bangladesh, 28/105; India, 40/107; Nepal, 42/114; and Pakistan 68/109). At a remote training camp in Nepal in 1995, an outbreak caused 32 cases among 692 soldiers. In Yangon, Myanmar, in 1989, an outbreak at an army camp caused 111 hospitalized cases among 600 recruits. In Pakistan in 1988, fecal contamination of the water supply was the likely vehicle for an outbreak at an urban military academy with 107 hospitalized hepatitis patients for an attack rate of 13%.

Norovirus (283, 917, 3529, 4872, 6598). *Norovirus* is a common cause of diarrhea in military personnel. Outbreaks have been documented at home base, aboard vessels, and during deployment. In Texas in 1998, an outbreak among 835 army trainees caused 99 cases of diarrhea for an attack rate of 24%, and a hospitalization rate of 12%. In Afghanistan in 2002, 29 British soldiers and staff of a field hospital contracted *Norovirus* illness; manifestations included diarrhea, headache, and stiff neck.

Rotavirus (6598). *Rotavirus* was recovered from U.S. military personnel deployed to Egypt.

Bacteria
Campylobacter (95, 2541, 4158, 6597). *C. jejuni* is a common cause of diarrhea in the uniformed services,

both at home base and during deployment abroad. In the United Kingdom in 1995–1999, 8% (4/50) of reported *Campylobacter* outbreaks occurred in military venues. In Finland, following outdoors infantry drill, 75 of 88 conscripts contracted *C. jejuni* enteritis; the outbreak was associated with consumption of untreated surface water from which *C. jejuni* was isolated. In Thailand, most strains from military personnel were quinolone resistant.

E. coli **(3483, 3527, 3529, 5634, 5665, 6598, 8195).** *E. coli* is a major cause of troopers' diarrhea, that is, in military units assigned to low-income countries. Mainly ETEC is involved, but EAEC and enteroinvasive *E. coli* (EIEC) have been implicated as well. In outbreaks among field units, ETEC and EIEC have been implicated. During Operation Desert Shield in Saudi Arabia in 1990, ETEC was recovered from 29% (125/432) of diarrhea cases.

Helicobacter **(3108, 3530).** Army personnel seem at increased risk of *Helicobacter pylori* infection, either by crowding or by assignments to low-income countries. Among 1,000 personnel deployed abroad for 5–6 months, the seroconversion rate was 1.9 per person-year. Seroprevalence was 19% in 74 German air force members, 21% in 186 French infantrymen, and 38% in 63 German submarine crews of similar age.

Providencia **(1406).** At a Czech army field hospital in Turkey in 1999, food-borne *P. alcalifaciens* was implicated in 27 diarrhea cases and 11 infections among 65 personnel.

Salmonella **(1699, 5029, 6598, 6973, 7327).** *S. enterica* serovar Non-Typhi diarrhea and typhoid fever are risks for troops living in poor sanitary conditions. In Turkey, an outbreak of serovar Enteritidis affected 60 (36%) of 168 soldiers; three food workers grew the agent, and the suspected vehicle was omelet. In the Spanish-American war (1898), >150,000 recruits were gathered in camps in the United States, when typhoid fever caused ~24,000 cases and 2,000 deaths. In Italy in 1986–1997, typhoid fever rates per 10^5 per year were lower in military personnel (0.5–3) than in civilians of corresponding age (1.5–9), pointing to protection of the military by typhoid vaccine. In Côte d'Ivoire in 2001, 24 typhoid fever cases (14 confirmed and 10 probable) occurred in a French camp with 94 army personnel; the likely vehicle was cucumber salad contaminated by carrier food workers, for an attack rate among consumers of 40% (18/45).

Shigella **(1507, 3527, 3728, 6598).** Military personnel are at risk of diarrhea due to *S. flexneri* or *S. sonnei*. Diagnostic yield from diarrhea cases among U.S. troops deployed to Egypt (in 2001) and Saudi Arabia (in 1990) ranged from 2% (*S. flexneri*) to 27% (*S. sonnei*). Disease rates ranged broadly as well, from 1.3–7.8/100 per year in Israeli recruits undergoing field training (*S. sonnei* and *S. flexneri*, peak in summer) to 0.3 per person-year in Peruvian recruits undergoing combat training in the Amazon (mainly *S. flexneri*).

Streptococcus. *S. pyogenes* **(group A** *Streptococcus* **[GAS]) (4379).** A fraction of respiratory GAS illness is food-borne. Of 35 outbreaks of food-borne GAS tonsillopharyngitis reviewed in 1941–1997, 12 (1/3) occurred in military settings. **Group G** *Streptococcus* **(GGS) (1505).** At a military camp in Israel in 1983, food-borne GGS caused an outbreak with 37 cases of sore throat, fever, or tonsillitis; 8 of 29 contacts and 6 of 28 food-handlers grew GGS.

Vibrio. *V. cholerae* **(6587).** Cholera is a risk for troops operating in endemic or epidemic areas. In the placebo arm of a vaccine trial among recruits in Peru, rates per 1,000 person-weeks were 0.6 for *V. cholerae* infections and 1 for cholera disease. *V. parahaemolyticus* **(521, 4337).** Outbreaks have been reported among military personnel. In Var department, France, in 1997, an outbreak affected 44 military personnel; seafood (moules or crevettes) was the likely vehicle.

Protozoa

Enteric protozoa are less well characterized agents of troopers' diarrhea than viruses and bacteria.

Cryptosporidium **(5227, 6598).** Among U.S. army personnel deployed to Egypt in 2001, 7% (9/129) of diarrhea cases were diagnosed as *Cryptosporidium*. On a U.S. coast guard cutter in 1993, within 3 weeks of filling tanks with Milwaukee city water, 40 of 52 crew contracted *Cryptosporidium* diarrhea, and two had asymptomatic infections.

Cyclospora **(6066).** At a military station in Pokhara, Nepal, in 1994, a waterborne *Cyclospora* outbreak affected 12 of 14 British soldiers.

E. histolytica/dispar **(6598).** Among U.S. Army personnel deployed to Egypt in 2001, 2% (2/129) of diarrhea cases were diagnosed as *E. histolytica*.

Sarcocystis **(282).** In a remote area of Malaysia in 1993, 7 of 15 U.S. military personnel contracted muscular sarcocystosis from an unidentified source.

T. gondii **(558).** Drinking stream water during jungle training caused an outbreak of acute toxoplasmosis in a U.S. military unit.

ZOONOTIC CLUSTER, UNIFORMED SERVICES

Risks (494, 1437, 1655, 3385). By location and prevention, bites from arthropods, dust, and contacts with infective mammals are the main outdoor risks for uniformed services. Preventive measures include showers and soap against lice, impregnated uniforms and bednets, residual spray against mosquitoes, vaccines, chemoprophylaxis, and targeted surveillance.

Some of the agents discussed below are considered suitable for weaponizing. For laboratory safety, see section 12.6.

Viruses: Vector Borne

Crimean-Congo hemorrhagic fever virus (CCHFV). During World War II, ~200 Soviet military personnel contracted the disease in Crimea (8075).

DENV (577, 3330, 3971, 5021, 5829, 6823, 7564). Infections with DENV have been reported in Canadian, Australian, and Italian peace-keeping forces in East Timor and in U.S. troops in Somalia and Haiti. In East Timor in 1999–2000, 16 (3%) of 595 soldiers of the Italian peace-keeping contingent had serological evidence of inapparent infection (3, 20%), mild dengue (3, 20%), or classical dengue (10, 60%). Duties away from the base camp increased risks; regular use of bednets was protective. Among ~2,500 Australian forces returning from East Timor, nine had viremic dengue; education, surveillance, and vector control prevented local spread in Queensland. In Vanuatu in 1989, DENV3 spilled from the population into a military camp, causing 40 cases, for an attack rate of 8.6%. Dengue has also been observed in French troops deployed to the Caribbean and French Polynesia.

EEEV (3385). Natural exposure risks of EEEV are considered low for U.S. troops.

JEV (2663, 3385, 3906, 6536, 6942). During the Korean War in 1950–1953, 300 epidemic cases of JEV occurred in U.S. troops. During the Vietnam War in 1964–1973, a few cases of JEV were reported in Australian troops, but observed seroconversion rates in 2,000 personnel reached 20.9%. Among U.S. troops in Vietnam, >10,000 became infected, and >50 contracted encephalitis. In 1991, after >16 years of silence, three nonvaccinated U.S. marines contracted encephalitis on Okinawa Island.

RVFV (2088, 2089, 5435, 8031). In Chad in 2001, RVFV was isolated from 2 of 50 febrile French soldiers; one had stayed in N'Djamena, while the other had visited a nomad camp and was offered milk to drink. In 1978–1979, in the wake of the Egyptian epidemic, seroconversions were demonstrated in 8 (5%) of 170 Swedish peace-keeping forces stationed in Egypt and the Sinai Peninsula.

Ross River virus (RRV) (2489, 3484). During a joint Australia-U.S. military exercise in 1997, four infections were diagnosed in 6 weeks. In 1998–2000, RRV was amplified by reverse transcriptose-PCR from pools of mosquitoes captured at a military training area in Queensland, Australia.

Sandfly fever virus (2148, 5433). Sandfly fever was reported in peace-keeping troops stationed in the Mediterranean basin. In 1985, 4% (11/298) of Swedish soldiers seroconverted after 6 months of deplyoment in Cyprus.

TBEV (1622, 3385, 4001). At risk for TBEV are border guards in enzootic areas. Personnel who work with dogs may be at particular risk. For U.S. troops, the exposure risk was considered low (1%). In unvaccinated soldiers deployed to Bosnia in 1996, 0.4% (4/959) seroconverted in 6–9 months. Vaccine was offered to personnel at high risk on a voluntary basis.

VEEV (2500, 6586, 7980, 7981). VEEV is a risk in enzootic areas in Latin America. U.S. soldiers contracted VEE during jungle training in Panama in 1967 (seven cases) and again in 1981 (five cases). Inapparent infections and disease cases were documented in nonimmune troops stationed in the Peruvian Amazon.

WEEV (3385). Natural exposure risks for WEEV are considered low for U.S. troops.

West Nile virus (WNV) (3847, 5510). At a military camp in the Negev Desert, Israel, in 1980, 32 soldiers contracted West Nile fever. In Congo (formerly Zaire) in 1998, a WNV outbreak at a military camp caused 23 confirmed cases.

YFV (1617, 6175). In the Spanish-American War in 1898, hundreds of U.S. soldiers died of yellow fever on Cuba. Deaths prompted investigations and human experiments by a Yellow Fever Commission under W. Reed (1851–1902) that confirmed transmission by *Aedes aegypti* proposed by C. J. Finlay (1833–1915). Cases have not been reported in vaccinated personnel.

Viruses: Vertebrate Borne

Hantavirus **(1481, 1947, 3494, 4299, 5434, 5963).** Outbreaks of hemorrhagic fever with renal syndrome (HFRS) have been reported in military settings, including by Hantaan virus (HTNV), Puumala virus (PUUV), and Seoul virus (SEOV). In the 1930s, ~12,000 of the 1 million Japanese troops who occupied Manchuria contracted HFRS. The Korean War (1950–1953) claimed thousands of cases, including ~3,200 cases among peace-keeping forces in the demilitarized zone, for a lethality of 10–15%. Compared with 295 controls, risks in 196 Korean military included staying in a hut, mice on the premises, and exposure to dust; repellents were protective. In 1986, 14 of 3,754 U.S. Marines on training in Korea developed HFRS and 2 (14%) died. During the Bosnian-Herzegovinian War (1992–1995), at least two cases of HFRS were reported among multinational forces. During military maneuvers in Germany, 16 cases were reported among U.S. troops. In Sweden, seroconversion rates per 10^5 per year were 360–1,110 in military personnel, compared with 3–14 in civilians from the same area.

Lassa virus (6256, 7405, 8131). Personnel deployed to enzootic-endemic areas in West Africa can be at risk. Lassa fever cases have been reported among United Nations peace-keeping forces.

Nipah virus (147). In Malaysia in 1998–1999, to curb an epizootic in pigs and epidemic in farmers, >1,600 military personnel assisted in culling ~1 million pigs; of 1,412 personnel examined, 6 (0.4%) had antibodies to Nipah virus, suggesting low transmissibility.

Rabies virus (1870, 2682, 3385). Cases were reported during the Vietnam War. At a U.S. Navy base in the Philippines in 1984, 315 of ,55,000 military and civilian residents reported for exposure evaluation: 285 (91%) for bites, 29 (9%) for scratches, and 1 (0.3%) for saliva splash; postexposure prophylaxis (PEP) was completed by 79 (25%) of 315 consultees. Military active-duty personnel reported the highest number of exposures and the highest proportion of completed PEP. In Israel, despite a succesful population vaccination program, a soldier contracted rabies, likely from a rat or mouse bite; because these rodents were considered nonvectors, PEP was not given. Border guards and police force impounding stray animals are likely at risk, but evidence is not available. For animal bites, see chapter 1.

Bacteria: Vector Borne

"Lousy wars"

***Anaplasma phagocytophilum* and human granulocytic ehrlichiosis (HGE) (494, 8238).** Work in tick-infested, enzootic areas (North America and Europe) is a risk for *A. phagocytophilum* and HGE. In German parachutists monitored for 10 months, the infection rate was 6/100 per year.

***Bartonella quintana* (1437).** Trench fever was significant in times of trench warfare, in particular, World War I. For the homeless, see section 11.3.

***Borrelia*. *B. burgdorferi* and Lyme disease (438, 5512, 6689, 7874).** In Tyrol, Austria, 4% (2/50) of recruits developed erythema migrans in 8 weeks, and 20% (11/50) had increased antibody titers. In Dutch military personnel engaging in outdoor work and wearing protective clothes (long sleeves and long trousers closed at the ankles) the seroconversion rate (~2/100 per year) was comparable to indoor military work (~1/100 per year). In northern Italy in 1987–1991, 3% (9/299) of soldiers were seroreactive. Similarly, low seroprevalence (0.1%) and seroconversion rates (2/10^5 person-years) have been reported for U.S. military personnel. **Relapsing *Borrelia* and louse-borne relapsing fever (LBRF) (775, 2664, 7252).** Notorious from World War II, LBRF remains a risk in civil and military conflicts. In Ethiopia in 1991–1992, returning soldiers sparked an outbreak with ≥289 cases.

***Ehrlichia chaffeensis* and human monocytic ehrlichiosis (HME) (494, 3884, 5853, 8336).** Work in tick-infested, enzootic areas (the Americas, Europe, and Southeast Asia) is a risk. *E. chaffeensis* was isolated following infections at Fort Chaffee, Ark. in 1989–1990. In New Jersey in 1987, 9 (12%) of 74 army reservists with arthralgia in retrospect were diagnosed with HME from seroconversion to *E. canis* antigen. In Arkansas in 1990, 1% (15/1,194) of exposed military personnel seroconverted (10 of 15 converters did not report symptoms).

***Orientia tsutsugamushi* and scrub typhus (494, 1587, 2490, 3700, 3884, 4868, 7267).** There were >36,000 cases of *O. tsutsugamushi* infection among Japanese and allied forces in World War II, and only sporadic cases in the Korean War. In Vietnam War, 20–30% of fevers of unknown origin were attributed to scrub typhus. Work in mite-infested, enzootic areas (Central, East, and Southeast Asia) continues to be a significant risk. In Thailand, by location, function, and test, seroprevalence in military personnel was 0–30% (typically 5–10%), and the seroconversion rate was 2.7/100 per year. Among Indonesian peace-keeping forces deployed to Cambodia in 1992–1993, 8% (19/241) were initially reactive to *O. tsutsugamushi*, and one individual seroconverted, for a rate of 0.8/100 per year. Outbreaks have been well documented among camped troops. Attack rates ranged from 1% (Camp Fuji, Japan, 2000–2001) to 22% (Thailand, 1965). In Queensland, Australia, outbreaks in troops caused 17 cases in 1996 and 11 cases in 1997.

***Rickettsia*. *R. prowazekii* and louse borne (epidemic) typhus (LBT) (494, 3884, 6119).** Estimates are of millions of LBT cases during and shortly after World War I, of 1/4 million in World War II, and of 32,000 in the Korean War (1950–1953, with 6,000 deaths, mainly in Korean military and civilian populations). No cases of LBT were reported in the Vietnam War (1964–1973), but LBT flared up in Central Africa in the 1990s, and focally in Central and

South America. ***R. typhi* and flea-borne (murine, endemic) typhus (FBT) (494, 1587)**. Few (<1,000) cases of LBT were reported in U.S. troops in World War II, and none in the Korean War. In the Vietnam War, however, 15–30% of fevers of unknown origin were attributed to FBT. In Cambodia in 1992–1993, 37% (91/248) of peacekeeping-forces from Indonesia were reactive to *R. typhi* predeployment, and 1% (3) seroconverted, for a rate of 2 (95% CI 1–5)/100 per year. **Spotted fever rickettsiae.** Spotted fever rickettsiae are significant for troops stationed in enzootic areas, notably in sub-Saharan Africa (*R. africae*), the Mediterranean and Asia (*R. conorii*), and the Americas (*R. rickettsii*) (494, 3683, 6582, 6999, 8336). In Botswana in 1992, 23% (39/169) of U.S. soldiers contracted African tick bite fever from field training that lasted 10 days; many patients recalled "insect" bites, but a recovered tick failed to amplify *R. africae* DNA. In Arkansas and Virginia, 1–2.5% of exposed personnel seroconverted to *R. rickettsii* group antigen. Conversions were associated with a history of tick attachment. The majority of infections was inapparent.

***Y. pestis* (1437)**. In World War II, plague cases were not reported in allied troops from enzootic areas in Asia. In the Vietnam War, when deployed U.S. troops were vaccinated, only eight cases were reported, a rate far lower than in Vietnamese troops.

Bacteria: Vertebrate Borne

***B. anthracis* (1949, 3554)**. In Manchuria in the 1940s, Japanese army personnel apparently used *B. anthracis* spores in biowarfare. Bioterrorism was attempted in Japan in 1995 (by the infamous aum-shin-rikyo group), and in the United States in 2001 (anonymously).

***Brucella* (1437)**. Brucellosis is a reported but poorly quantified health risk for troops in enzootic areas. *Brucella* is a potential biowarfare agent.

***Coxiella* (202, 1437, 4633, 7071) (6393, 8325)**. Outbreaks of *C. burnetii* were reported among troops during and since World War II. In 1941–2002, at least 16 outbreaks were recorded among troops stationed in North Africa and Europe, with 10–1,700 (median, 127) cases per outbreak. In Cyprus in 1975–1976, 4% (20/534) of Swedish peace-keeping forces were seroreactive; because part of the batallion had tested negative before departure, and 1,390 domestic Swedes were all seronegative, locally acquired infections were assumed. In Spain in 1992, Q fever hit a military detachment that camped at an abandoned farm, for an attack rate of 43% (48/105); straw and wool were likely sources. In Bosnia and Herzegovina in 1997, an outbreak among Czech peacekeeping forces caused 14 cases and 12 infections, for a rate of 4.6%. Helicopters were suspected to have stirred up dust from a nearby lambing sheep farm. In Iraq in 2003, >60 pneumonia cases were diagnosed in U.S. troops; the patients reported contact with domestic mammals (dogs, cats, sheep, goats, and camels), tick bites, and consumption of raw sheep's milk.

***F. tularensis* (1437, 6202)**. In World War II, tens of thousands of tularemia cases occurred in German and Soviet troops along the Don and Volga rivers. At Stalingrad in 1942–1943, case numbers could have reached 100,000; intentional release was neither confirmed nor rejected. Shortly after the war in Kosovo in 1999–2000, >300 cases were reported, mainly due to rodent-polluted foods and water.

Protozoa

***Leishmania*.** *Leishmania* is a risk for uniformed services (armed and peace-keeping forces, and police) in enzootic-endemic areas. **Cutaneous leishmaniasis (CL) (293, 1203, 1655, 1820, 8010) (4415, 5020)**. CL is a risk in warm climates.

- Africa (2546). In a multinational force in the Sinai, Egypt, *L. major* disease rates, by location and nationality, were 0–2/100 per year in 1989–1991, and 15/100 and 6 months in 1983–1985.

- Asia (2654, 3529, 3764, 8010). During World War II, 500–750 soldiers contracted CL in Iran, for a rate of 0.2/100 in 3 months. During the Persian Gulf War in 1990–1991, 20 CL cases (due to *L. major*) were reported among ~0.7 million troops. In Jordan in 1995 for 5.5 months, zoonotic CL affected 36 (45%) of 80 members of a Jordanian army unit. In 2002–2003, >600 U.S. soldiers contracted CL, mainly in Iraq, rarely in Afghanistan or Kuwait. Most lesions were multiple (up to >40 per person), and lesions grew *L. major*. In contrast, *Phlebotomus* females amplified *L. infantum* by PCR.

- South America (1820, 4415, 5020). Exposure has typically been in forested areas. At an air command in Manaus, Brazil, in XI/1994, an outbreak caused 48 CL cases. In French Guyana in 1998–1999, French troops were hit by an outbreak with 326 cases, for an attack rate of ~3/100 person-years. Soldiers consistently using mosquito nets and repellents had significantly fewer skin lesions than noncomplying soldiers.

- Central America (3267, 6584, 7295). In Panama in 1977, the rate of CL in deployed U.S. soldiers was 0–5 (typically 2)/100 per 6 months. In Belize in 1978–1990, among a British garrison holding ~1,500 troops, 306 CL cases were reported. Lesion counts were 1 in 71%, 2 in 16%, 3 in 8%, and 4 in 4%. Of 117 culture-positive cases, 66% grew *L. braziliensis* sensu lato (sl), 25% grew

L. mexicana sl, and in 9% the species was not identified. In Panama, the CL attack rate in Puerto Rican national guard undergoing jungle training was 22% (14/64).

Visceral leishmaniasis (VL) (2654, 3529, 4638, 5294, 8411). During the Persian Gulf War in 1990–1991, 12 VL cases were reported among ~0.7 million troops. Visceral specimens yielded *L. tropica* rather than *L. donovani*. In 2001–2003, two U.S. military personnel contracted VL in Afghanistan; recognition was delayed in one by initially microscopy-negative bone-marrow and liver-biopsy specimens.

Plasmodium. Malaria has a heavy impact on peace-keeping forces and troops operating in malarious areas. Risks (4073, 5746, 5931, 6580, 7920) include nocturnal activities, noncompliance with exposure prevention and chemoprophylaxis, drug resistance, and lack of resources.

Outbreaks Examples of disease rates and outbreaks in the uniformed services are summarized below.
- West Africa (5036, 7602). In Sierra Leone in 1996 (close to 100 cases) and again in 2000, British army personnel were hit by outbreaks of falciparum malaria. In Côte d'Ivoir in 2002, French troops were exposed to two to three infective mosquito bites per week, and observed rates of falciparum malaria were 0.2–3.6/100 person-months.
- Central and East Africa (5402, 5423, 5746, 6580, 7920). In Somalia in 1992–1993, U.S. army and marine personnel were exposed to falciparum and vivax malaria, mainly in the first few weeks of deployment; about one third of the cases occurred in the country, and two thirds after return home. In French troops in Gabon in 1994–1996, the rate of falciparum malaria was 3/100 per month, largely because of noncompliance with chemoprophylaxis and the use of an ineffective chloroquine-proguanil combination; newly arriving reinforcement troops were mainly affected. In Angola in 1995–1996, an outbreak of falciparum malaria among Brazilian troops largely due to chemoprophylaxis noncompliance caused an attack rate of 18% (78/439) and a lethality of 3.8% (3/78).
- Central Asia (4073, 6779). From Afghanistan in 1981–1983, 7,683 Russian soldiers returned home with vivax malaria. Also from Afghanistan in VI–IX/2002, 38 U.S. troops returned home with vivax malaria, for a disease rate of 52/1,000; 52% of the troops were compliant with weekly chemoprophylaxis.
- Southeast Asia (2108, 3422, 3972, 5828, 7256). In the Vietnam War, U.S. troops counted >21,000 malaria cases. In peninsular Malaysia in 1967–1985, the disease rate in army personnel receiving chemoprophylaxis was 0.5–3/100 per year. In Cambodia in 1992–1993, Dutch marines contracted falciparum and vivax malaria (ratio of 2:1) at breakthrough rates of 0.05–0.6/100 person-weeks; all vivax malaria was manifest after return home. In Thai troops stationed in the malarious northeast of their own country the disease rate was 41/100 in 6 months, despite chemoprophylaxis and use of bednets. In East Timor in 1999–2000, multinational (mainly Australian) troops contracted falciparum and vivax malaria despite chemoprophylaxis, and in the wet season; attack rates reached 13.5%.
- East Asia (4302, 5732). In 1993, vivax malaria reemerged in the demilitarized zone of Korea. In 2000, vivax malaria was reported in military personnel (5,577 cases, 40% of reports), veterans (discharged since <2 years, 3,641 cases, 26%), and civilians (4,685 cases, 34%).
- Pacific (3755). During World War II on Guadalcanal in 1942, when atabrine was not yet available, the disease rate in the U.S. Navy reached 150/100 per year.

Trypanosoma. T. cruzi. Although of concern in enzootic areas, reports about *T. cruzi* are not available from troops. Because treatment is difficult, exposure prevention is important. *T. brucei* sl and human African trypanosomiasis (HAT) (2061, 5148). Military personnel is at risk of HAT. Two French parachutists contracted *T. brucei rhodesiense* from deployment in Rwanda.

Helminths
Lymphatic filariae (1655, 2592, 7549). In World War II, 14,000–16,000 soldiers were diagnosed with lymphatic filariasis, mainly from the South Pacific. In Algeria in 1951, *Brugia malayi* was diagnosed in ~150 servicemen returning from North Vietnam, 31% were French and 69% were North Africans.

ENVIRONMENTAL CLUSTER, UNIFORMED SERVICES
Exposure to freshwater and mud are major risks, including during training, maneuvers, and deployments.

Bacteria
***Acinetobacter* (1769).** *A. calcoaceticus-baumannii* is an emerging cause of war wound infections (e.g., shrapnel) and osteomyelitis (e.g., open fractures). Sources in combatants are unclear but might be nosocomial rather than environmental.

***Burkholderia* (4420, 4623, 4879, 7436).** Soil contact in endemic areas is a risk. During the Vietnam War, acute and reactivated melioidosis was reported in U.S. soldiers. Reported seroprevalence ranged from 0.2% in the armed forces in Singapore to 1–7% in U.S. soldiers in Vietnam, and 2% (18/905) in troops from the United Kingdom, Australia, and New Zealand that were stationed in Malaysia, at a camp where *B. pseudomallei* was isolated from surface water.

Leptospira **(1437, 4369, 5894, 6475).** Risks for *Leptospira* include contact with mud and freshwater (trench training). During the Vietnam War, up to 20% of fevers of unknown origin in soldiers were attributed to *Leptospira*. Outbreaks were reported among military personnel in Panama (7296), Peru (6475), Hawaii (3845), and Okinawa (1583). During jungle training in Panama in 1981–1982, U.S. soldiers contracted leptospirosis, for attack rates of 2–8%. In Peru in 1999, 78 (40%) of 193 Peruvian military recruits contracted leptospirosis from exposure in a ravine that drained farm animal feces. On Okinawa island in 1987, an outbreak affected military personnel, for attack rates of 5% (7/15) among recreational swimmers and of 18% (15/82) among combat trainees. The likely mode of spread was the swallowing of water rather than immersion only.

Helminths
Hookworm. Intestinal (3883). Hookworm was reported in veterans returning from deployment in endemic areas. The prevalence in conscripts should reflect local endemicity, but information is amazingly scant. During the U.S. military operation in Grenada in 1983, ≥200 (~20%) of 1,040 exposed troops acquired *Necator americanus* in the first 5–7 weeks of deployment, mainly from soil near quarters. **Cutaneous (larva migrans) (2921).** In Belize in 1999, cutaneous larva migrans was diagnosed in 13 (87%) of 15 British military personnel undergoing jungle training, despite "*full protective clothing at all times*" was worn; possibly, because of heavy exposure to mud, larvae were able to penetrate through textiles.

Strongyloides **(1594, 2693, 2733, 2963, 5818, 6021).** A major risk of *S. stercoralis* is contact with soil during training or deployment in endemic areas. Recycling (auto-reinfection) maintains the worm for decades. In the United Kingdom in 1946, strongyloidiasis was diagnosed in ex-prisoners of war from the "bridge over the river Kwai" camp. Subsequently, strongyloidiasis was confirmed in veterans and ex-prisoners of World War II in Canada (in 0.6% or 4/694), the United States (37% or 52/142), Australia (28% or 44/160), and the United Kingdom (15% or 88/602), up to 30–37 years after exposure.

Schistosoma **(1655, 2925, 4253, 4741).** Water contact in endemic areas is a risk for *Schistosoma*. In World War II, >1,500 allied troops contracted schistosomiasis in Nigeria, and hundreds contracted it on Leyte in the Philippines. Apparently no infections were reported in the Vietnam War. From surgery for diverticulitis, a veteran who had not left the continental United States since World War II was diagnosed with active *S. japonicum* infection 30 years after exposure in the Philippines. Following a French military operation in Chad in 1973–1974, 181 (23%) of 790 soldiers became infected during deployments that lasted 3–6 months, 148 (82%) with *S. mansoni* alone, 14 (8%) with *S. mansoni* plus *S. haematobium* or *S. intercalatum*, and 19 (10%) with unidentified species.

SKIN-BLOOD CLUSTER, UNIFORMED SERVICES
Risks (419, 4910, 5675, 7029). On entry into uniformed services, recruits typically represent the local civilian population of corresponding age, and STI and blood-borne infections are likely to be equally prevalent in both collectives. Exposures during service include injury, shared objects, contact (skin, sweat, and saliva), and unprotected sex. In New York City in 1992–1993, police reported needlestick injury and human bites at a rate of 0.4/100, with equal rates in males and females. In Amsterdam, The Netherlands in 2000–2003, police reported exposure to viruses at a rate of 0.7/100 per year; most (79% or 89) exposing sources could be tested, and 4% were positive for HBV, 4% for HIV, and 18% for hepatitic C virus (HCV). Without preventive measures, accumulated infection risks in veterans and reservists may substantially differ from risks in the population. During conflicts with mass casualties, safe blood supply can be critical.

Viruses
HBV (153, 420, 1699, 6744). Risks of HBV for the uniformed services include deployment in hyperendemic areas, work (customs, police, and prisons) with high-risk clients, and a history of injection drug use (IDU) or STI. HBV infections were a particular risk for U.S. troops engaged in the Korean and Vietnam Wars. In Texas in 1973–1975, a protracted outbreak with 792 hospitalized military cases was largely due to IDU, shared needles, and close contacts. In Italy in 1986–1997, the acute HB rate per 10^5 per year was similar in army personnel (7–33) and civilians (7–20) of corresponding age. In 2001, the anti-HBs (immunity) prevalence in a random sample of 2,400 U.S. recruits was 31.5% (95% CI, 30–33). Vaccine is recommended on entrance into armed forces, and for public safety workers at risk of occupational exposure to blood.

HCV (3528). In 1997, the overall anti-HCV prevalence in 10,000 U.S. military personnel was 0.5%, with a low of 0.1% among recruits and a high of 3% among active-duty troops and reservists ≥40 years of age. From sequential samples, the infection rate was estimated at $20/10^5$ per year. Lower risks in military than in civilian populations of comparable age were attributed to the dissuasion of IDU in armed forces by testing for illicit drugs.

HIV. Police (392, 3377, 6489). In Denver, Colo., in 1989–1991, police officers reported 137 exposures to blood or saliva, for a low rate of 0.03/100 person-months. Of 42 hazardous exposures to blood (no time for protective gloves and deep needle stick), 32 (76%) sources could be tested, of which 5 (16%) were HIV positive. In Dar es Salaam, Tanzania, in 1994–1998, 14% (378/2,733) of police officers tested positive for HIV1 (males, 13% or 323/2,427; females 18% or 55/306); on follow-up, seroconversion rates were 20/1,000 person-years (20 in males, 22 in females). Incident evaluation, counseling, and documentation should be offered to police officers who have been exposed. In Cambodia in 1996, 12.5% of 322 male police and military personnel were HIV-infected. **Army (5394, 6127, 6622, 7347).** Armies may or may not screen and exclude HIV-infected individuals. Unrecognized infections are a risk for the individual (progression, use of contraindicated live vaccines) and the unit (spread). However, 10 HIV-infected unrecognized soldiers tolerated unintentional exposure to smallpox vaccine (three primary and seven repeat vaccinations) surprisingly well. In the United States, 0.08% of 5.34 million applicants to the armed services (army, navy, air force) in 1985–2000 tested positive for HIV1 (0.3% in 1985, 0.04% in 2000), and seroconversion rates per 1,000 person-years decreased from 0.3–0.7 (in the 1980s) to 0.08 (current). In army personnel in sub-Saharan Africa, the HIV prevalence can exceed a staggering 40%. Army preventive programs include education, promotion of condoms, and early recognition and treatment of STI.

Bacteria

***Chlamydia trachomatis.* Genital (serovars D–K) (891, 1270, 2677, 4910).** By test and sample, reported infection prevalence is 3–9%. In South Carolina in 1998–1999, the infection prevalence in male recruits was 5% (119/2,245) by nucleic acid amplification test (NAT) from urine; only 14% (17/119) of infections were symptomatic. In female recruits from all 50 of the United States in 1996–1997, the prevalence by the same method was 9% (1,215/13,204). **Systemic (serovars L1–3) (6649).** During the Vietnam War, the rate of lymphogranuloma venereum in U.S. military personnel reached 1.4/100 per year.

***Klebsiella granulomatis* (5480).** A case of granuloma inguinale (donovanosis) was reported in a soldier returning from deployment in Djibouti for 6 months.

***Neisseria gonorrhoeae* (891, 1270, 4910, 6127).** By test and sampling, the reported infection prevalence is 0–5%. In South Carolina in 1998–1999, the infection prevalence by NAT from urine was 0.6% (5/884) in male recruits; only 40% (2/5) of infections were symptomatic. Among 400 male soldiers with urethritis, *N. gonorrhoeae* was detected by Gram stain or culture in 94 (24%). In the Korean and Vietnam Wars, gonorrhea rates in U.S. troops per 1,000 person-years reached 300–500, while in troops at home rates remained at 26. In the 2000s, military rates (∼5) were comparable to civilians of the same age.

***S. aureus* (1047).** *S. aureus* readily spreads in military settings. In San Diego, Cal., in 2002, methicillin-resistant *S. aureus* (MRSA) from the community caused skin infections in 22 military trainees, for a rate of ∼1/100 person-weeks.

***S. pyogenes* (GAS) (947, 1653, 1658, 2911).** Colonization and GAS pharyngitis are frequent in military personnel. In the United States in 1985–1994, 18% (10,789/59,818) of pharyngeal cultures from army trainees grew GAS. GAS can spread well in military settings. In the late 1970s, an outbreak of streptococcal pyodermia at a military institution affected >1,300 persons in 18 months. At a U.S. military training center in 2002, despite entry chemoprophylaxis with parenteral penicillin or oral erythromycin, GAS caused 29 cases of pneumonia and 2 cases of toxic shock syndrome among ∼4,500 recruits in 7 weeks, for an attack rate of 0.7%.

***T. pallidum* (392, 1471, 4909, 6127, 6489).** In World War II, the reported prevalence of syphilis in U.S. draftees was 4.5%, with a low of 1% in the New England states, and a high of 11% in southern Atlantic states. At Fort Braggs, N.C., in 1985–1993, the incidence of primary and secondary syphilis in the military (and surrounding civilian communities) reached epidemic levels, with a military peak of 123/10^5 per year. In Dar es Salaam, Tanzania, in 1994–1998, the prevalence of active syphilis in police officers was 3% (88/2,850), and on follow-up, the rate of new syphilis was 8.6/1,000 person-years. In Cambodia in 1996, 12.5% of 322 male police and military personnel were seroreactive. Seroscreening uniformed services populations for syphilis on entry into services seems warranted and cost effective.

***Ureaplasma* (4910).** In 400 male soldiers with urethritis, *U. urealyticum* was detected in 52 (13%).

Fungi

Dermatophytes (890, 3557). In southern Italy in 2002, the prevalence of superficial, mycologically confirmed fungal infections in navy cadets was 3% (33/1,024); only 2 (6%) of 33 were aware they had tinea. Tinea pedis was suspected in 12% (126) and confirmed in 2.9% (30 cases,

23 or 77% by *T. mentagrophytes* var. *interdigitale*). Onychomycosis was suspected in 6% (64) and confirmed in 0.2% (2 cases, 1 each by *T. mentagrophytes* var. *interdigitale* and *T. mentagrophytes* var. *mentagrophytes*). Tinea cruris (of groin) was suspected in 2.7% (28) and confirmed in 0.1% (one case due to *Epidermophyton floccosum*). Other fungi (*Aspergillus*, *Fusarium*, *Paecilomyces*, and *Penicillium*) were isolated from 5% (48) but were considered nonpathogenic in this context.

The main dermatophyte is tinea pedis. By sampling and setting, reported prevalence of confirmed infections in the uniformed services is 2–30% (typically 10%). Of 73 Danish soldiers deployed to ex-Yugoslavia, 16% (12) had predeparture diagnoses of tinea pedis or onychomycosis, mainly by *T. mentagrophytes* or *T. rubrum*. After six months of deployment, prevalence was 32% (24), and the main cause was *Candida albicans*.

Ectoparasites
Epidemic waves of infestation by head lice (*Pediculus humanus capitis*) were reported in Israeli soldiers (5066). Scabies was reported in army personnel (5065).

12.4 FIELD, FOREST, HERD, AND ABATTOIR

"Crop-and-herd" work (Table 12.1) is work with plants, animals, and animal products, in fields, orchards, green houses, forests, farms, corrals, and abattoirs, including horticulture, lumbering, breeding and rearing of livestock, pisciculture, and bone, hide, leather, wool, and textile industries, and as rancher, herdsman, game warden, fisher, hunter, butcher, veterinarian, pest controller, and pet shop worker.

Exposure. About one fourth (36 million/136 million km^2, without Antarctica and Greenland) of the terrestrial surface is under agriculture. Agriculture accounts for 4% of the global Gross Domestic Product (1–4% in high-income countries and 6–60% in low-income countries).

Infections (1904, 4419, 6418, 8172) (Box 12.3). Modes of acquisition include contact, ingestion, inhalation, and inoculation. Because leisure exposure (to animals and plants) is a confounding factor, high seroprevalence in groups at risk alone does not constitute proof of occupational acquisition. Infections in crop-and-herd workers are not usually notifiable, and statistics are fragmentary. In meat workers, reported rates were 0.4–4/1,000 per year for diarrhea, and 0.65/1,000 person-days for skin infections. Female U.S. veterinarians in the United States have reported needlestick injuries at a rate of ~9/100 practice-years; hazardous materials included vaccines, antibiotics, and animal blood.

Prevention. Prevention includes education, employment entry screen, vaccinations, and storage of null serum; good practice when dealing with plants (ploughing, harvest, and milling), animals (feeding, milking, delivery, and shearing), and their products (factory air); and protective gear (for manure, dairy products, sick animals, and animal tissues).

DROPLET-AIR CLUSTER, CROP-AND-HERD WORK
Hay and decaying plants can release spores. Sneezing, urinating, and defecating animals can release droplets or generate aerosols.

Viruses
Influenzavirus. A concern is the spread of *Influenzavirus* to humans, mainly to crop-and-herd workers. **Avian viruses (877, 4056, 5813).** In Hong Kong in 1997, after an epizootic in poultry, virulent avian A/H5N1 virus caused disease in 18 humans (it was lethal in 6 or 33%), and infection (two-step testing) in ~10% of 1,525 poultry

Box 12.3 Main agents and infections from crop-and-herd work, by cluster	
Risks are listed in parentheses. For bites, see chapter 1.	
Droplet-air	Influenza (human, avian, and swine); *M. tuberculosis* (migrant workers); *Coccidioides* (endemic areas), *Histoplasma* (bird sites)
Feces-food	HEV (pigs); *Campylobacter*, *E. coli*, *Salmonella* (MDR), *Y. enterocolitica*; *Toxoplasma*
Zoonotic	Rabies, encephalitis (JEV, LCMV, and TBEV), hemorrhagic fevers (CCHFV, EBOV, GUAV, *Hantavirus*, JUNV, RVFV, and YFV), simian retroviruses, WNV; anthrax, *Bartonella*, *Borrelia* (Lyme, relapsing), *Brucella*, *C. psittaci*, *Coxiella*, *Erysipelothrix*, *Francisella*, *Pasteurella*, rat-bite fever, rickettsiae (*Anplasma*, *Ehrlichia*, *Orientia*, and *Rickettsia*), *S. suis*, *Vibrio* (parenteral), *Y. pestis*; *Leishmania*, malaria, trypanosomiasis (African, Chagas); *Echinococcus*, filariae
Environmental	*Aeromonas* (fishermen), environmental mycobacteria (fishermen and farmers), *Leptospira*, melioidosis (farmers), *C. tetani* (nonvaccinated farm families); chromomycosis, mycetoma, *Sporothrix*; hookworm, *Schistosoma*, *Strongyloides*, *Toxocara*; myiasis
Skin-blood	Dermatophytes; myiasis

workers and 3% (9/293) of workers assisting in poultry culling. Infection risks included butchering and working with flocks with high (>10%) mortality; feeding flocks was not a risk. Avian A/H5N1 reemerged in People's Republic of China in 2003, in a family of 5 who returned from a visit to Fujian Province. This threat is extending into 2006. In Dutch poultry farms in 2003, an epizootic of virulent avian A/H7N7 spread to poultry workers and 3 (4%) of 83 household contacts. A/H7 was recovered from conjunctival samples of 24% (83/349) of workers reporting conjunctivitis, and 8% (7/90) of workers with flulike illness. **Porcine viruses (357, 5492, 5595).** In Wisconsin in 1996–1997, 23% (17/74) of swine farmers, but only 1% (1/114) of urban controls, were seroreactive to swine A/H1N1 virus; seropositivity was associated with being a farm owner or farm family member, living on a farm, or entering a swine barn ≥4 days/week. In southern Mexico in 2000, 2% (2/115) of inhabitants practicing "backyard" (combined pig and poultry) farming were reactive to classical swine A/H1N1 virus. In Austria in 1994–1995, anti-A/H1N1 seroprevalence was ~25% in fattening pigs and 9% (12/137) in veterinarians (significantly higher in practitioners than in swine-nonexposed veterinarians).

Rubella virus (1743, 6176). Humans are the only source of rubella virus. In the United States in 1990–1999, 13 (20%) of 65 rubella outbreaks occurred at work places, including meat-processing plants. In Nebraska in 1999, confirmed rubella was isolated in 52 mostly Hispanic meat packers and their home contacts (attack rate, 1.4%), 16 children in day care and their parents (attack rate, 8.8%); and 15 residents living in crowded census tracts.

Severe acute respiratory syndrome coronavirus (SARS-CoV) (8353). In Guangdong Province, People's Republic of China, in 2003, the prevalence of IgG antibodies to SARS-CoV was 1% (1/84) in healthy adults, 3% (4/137) in hospital workers, but 13% (66/508) in inapparent workers at live animal markets, which suggested a zoonotic origin of the virus. By traded animal, reactivity was 73% (16/22) in traders of masked palm civets, 57% (16/28) of wild boar, 56% (9/16) of muntjac deer, 46% (6/13) of hares, 33% (3/9) of pheasants, 19% (8/43) of cats, 12% (3/25) of fowls, and 9% (23/250) of snakes.

Bacteria
Legionella. *Legionella* is unusual in crop-and-herd workers (for potting earth, see section 5.3). At a floral trade show in The Netherlands in 1999, where a whirlpool spa caused a large Legionnaires' disease outbreak, 742 exhibitors had higher mean antibody levels than the general population (785).

***M. tuberculosis* (4891, 5559).** Migrant farm workers are at increased risk of tuberculosis, likely from human sources. At a freezing works in New Zealand's North Island in 2002, late detection of an index case, recirculated unfiltered air, and a virulent strain of *M. tuberculosis* caused an outbreak with 10 (3%) cases and 29 (9%) infections in workers (n = 342), and 9 (16%) cases and 11 (20%) infections in household and social contacts (n = 55). Zoo workers exposed to infected mammals were latently infected. For *M. bovis*, see "Zoonotic Cluster, Crop-and-Herd Work," below.

Fungi
Hay, crops, barns, and feathers are sources of fungal spores, but occupational risks have been documented.

Blastomyces. Occupational exposure to *Blastomyces dermatitidis* seems unusual.

***Coccidioides* (2686, 3723).** Farmers stirring up dust in endemic areas are at risk of infection with *C. immitis*. Infections were reported in cotton mill workers.

Cryptococcus. Occupational contact with birds is a putative risk of *Cryptococcus*.

***Histoplasma* (4941, 7227, 7375).** Reported hazardous jobs include clearing cane in which birds have roosted, cleaning out chicken houses, removing bird roosts, gamecock handling, spreading chicken droppings, and cleaning bat guano from structures. In Cuba, poultry workers were significantly more frequently skin-reactive to histoplasmin (29% of 392) than non-poultry-exposed workers (13% of 285). Contact with chicken manure, and length on poultry jobs increased infection risks.

***Paracoccidioides* (707, 5076).** Farm workers and woodcutters in endemic cases appear to be at risk of *Paracoccidioides*. In a large series, 46% of 422 cases were farm workers.

FECES-FOOD CLUSTER, CROP-AND-HERD WORK
Crop-and-herd workers can be victims of zoonotic infections or sources of fecal contamination of foods.

Viruses
HAV (3329). Humans are reservoir, and plant or animal work is not usually a risk. Outbreaks were reported in chimpanzee handlers.

HEV (2031, 4985, 8145). Human-infective strains likely circulate in pigs. Putative risks include raising pigs, cleaning barns, and assisting parturient sows. In 8 U.S. states, the prevalence of anti-HEV IgG in 295 swine veterinarians was ~25% or ~1.5 times that in blood donors of the same states. In Bali, Indonesia, where pork is commonly consumed, 20% (54/276) of residents were seroreactive, compared with 4% (17/446) in Lombok and 0.5% (2/393) in Java, two mainly Muslim areas (in contrast, anti-HAV prevalence was 95% in Bali, 90% in Lombok, and 89% in Java). In Moldavia in 1997–1998, swine farmers were significantly more often seroreactive (51% or 135/264) than controls (25% or 63/255).

Bacteria

Campylobacter. Work with animals is a likely risk, including for farmers, abattoir workers, poultry processors, and butchers (1011, 2116, 3297, 7451). In Ontario, Canada, in 1978–1985, rates of sporadic campylobacteriosis per 10^5 per year were 350–400 in farm residents, 65–85 in rural nonfarm residents, and 80–90 in urban residents. However, risk estimates in farm residents were confounded by frequent consumption of raw milk. At a pheasant farm in Wyoming, in 2000, an outbreak of *C. jejuni* affected 53% (8/15) of workers, mainly first-time and fecally exposed workers. Long-term exposure of poultry abattoir workers has been suggested to lead to partial immunity.

E. coli **(119, 6900, 7161, 7554, 7685, 8202).** Farm, poultry, and meat workers are at likely risk of infection, including verotoxin-producing (enterohemorrhagic *E. coli* [EHEC]) and antibiotics-resistant *E. coli*, likely from contact with animals or manure. In Canada, stools of 6% (21/335) of farmers and their families and 46% of cattle tested positive for EHEC, and 0.3% grew *E. coli* O157:H7. Also in Canada, human EHEC cases (1,276 in 1996–1998, mostly *E. coli* O157:H7) correlated with the ratio of beef cattle to residents and the practice of spreading solid or liquid manure onto farm land. In Italy, EHEC was isolated from 1% (4/350) of farm workers on 276 dairy farms. In Switzerland, stools from 3.5% of healthy meat industry workers tested positive for EHEC by PCR.

Listeria **(4915).** Animals may shed *L. monocytogenes* from feces, milk, and birth secretions. At least 17 cases of animal-to-human spread have been reported in farmers or veterinarians from contact with congenitally infected calves.

Salmonella **(209, 620, 1547, 1993, 2281, 2448, 3077).** The intestinal tract of domestic and wild vertebrates is a major reservoir. The enteric prevalence in intensive animal husbandry is high. Animals can shed large numbers of salmonellae for many months. Antibiotic resistance and typing (e.g., *S. enterica* serovar Typhimurium definite type 104) help to trace spread. Modes of spread include contaminated feeds, and interanimal (among and across species) and animal-to-human contacts.

In the United States, compared with infections by other serotypes, humans infected with *S. enterica* serovar Typhimurium DT104 resided in areas with higher cattle farm densities and more frequently reported contact with livestock. In Canada, living on a livestock farm was a risk for sporadic serovar Typhimurium DT104 infections. In the United Kingdom, direct contact with farm animals was associated with sporadic serovar Typhimurium DT104 and family outbreaks.

Infected animals carry agents to abattoirs and practices. In the United States, stools of 1% (2/158) of horsemeat plant packing workers grew salmonellae. In pig abattoirs in Europe, hands of 3.7% of 874 workers and 2.8% of knives grew salmonellae. At a U.S. veterinary clinic in 1999, cats caused multiresistant serovar Typhimurium infections in clients and staff. In the United Kingdom in 1982, 1.6% (26/1,625) of veterinary professionals self-reported salmonellosis, for a rate of 0.1/100 person-years.

Shigella **(1163, 3889).** Humans are a reservoir, and animal-to-human spread is not a risk, except where animals acquired *Shigella* from humans. At a primate research unit, *S. flexneri* was isolated in technical assistants who had regular contact with infected macaques. However, farm and food workers are a potential source of *Shigella* in foods.

Yersinia **(793, 2879, 4990).** *Y. enterocolitica* is an occupational risk for butchers, in particular, work with swine throats and intestines. Putative further groups at risk include cattle breeders, hunters, and animal workers.

Fungi

Information is scant. In Slovakia, 5% (5/98) of slaughterhouse workers were seroreactive to *Encephalitozoon*, compared with none of 92 forestry workers, 22 dog breeders, and 150 blood donors (1464)

Protozoa

Cryptosporidium **(4341).** Occupation is a putative risk. In Wisconsin, dairy farmers were more likely to be seroreactive than non-dairy farmers; hazards included feeding and milking cows.

Cyclospora **(594).** Infected farm workers are putative sources of contaminated foods. In Guatemala in 1997, the stools of 2% (4/176) of raspberry farm workers tested positive for *Cyclospora*; three of four shedders were asymptomatic.

T. gondii **(1554, 1903, 3734, 3756, 3766, 5492, 7112, 7217, 8311).** Oocysts in the soil from infective kittens seem more important sources than oocysts on the fur of animals, or cysts in raw viscera. In a representative U.S. sample, 37% (95% CI 32–44%) of 1,041 persons with occupational soil contact were seroreactive, compared with 25% (95% CI 24–27%) of 13,487 persons with jobs not involving soil contact. Occupational groups at risk include gardeners, floriculturists, farmers, cat breeders, zoo workers, veterinarians, hunters, abattoir workers, butchers, and meat workers. Occupational risks can be confounded by animal ownership and dietary habits.

Helminths

Wastewater irrigation (see section 6.2) of root and leaf vegetables, and the use of raw feces for fertilizer are hazards. As foods are the main vehicles, evidence of occupational risks is circumstantial.

Ascaris. Pig farming is a putative risk of *A. lumbricoides*. For *A. suum*, see section 2.4.

***Capillaria* (3767).** Handling rodents infected with *C. hepatica* is a risk, e.g., for zoo workers.

***Fasciolopsis* (2885).** *F. buski* can be maintained in fish ponds by feces from pigs and humans that are used as fish fodder.

***Opisthorchis* (7039).** *O. viverrini* is prevalent in farmers in Southeast Asia, presumably in association with water development projects.

***Taenia solium* (2620).** Risks of intestinal and tissue infections include raising and butchering pigs, and processing and selling pork. In Latin America, mainly small-scale producers of local, pork-containing foods are affected. Carriers should not work in the food industry.

***Trichinella* (638).** In Henan Province, People's Republic of China, larvae of *T. spiralis* were recovered from the washing meat slop in abattoirs.

***Trichuris* (3441).** Vegetable gardening is a putative occupational risk of infection with *T. trichiura*.

ZOONOTIC CLUSTER, CROP-AND-HERD WORK

Occupational exposure to zoonotic agents spans domestic, pet, laboratory, zoo, and wild mammals, other vertebrates, and invertebrates, in particular, attached ectoparasites.

Prions

Risks for workers to acquire sporadic Creutzfeldt-Jakob disease (CJD) from work seem negligible, except, perhaps, for butchers (1492).

Viruses: Arthropod Borne

By diurnal and nocturnal activities, farmers, herdsmen, and forest workers can be at risk of arthropod-borne viral infections, including encephalitis and hemorrhagic fever. Fragmentary evidence for this follows below.

***Bunyaviridae* (1046).** In California in the 1960s–1980s, 10% of rangers and other employees with outdoor work in remote areas were reactive to Jamestown Canyon virus. **CCHFV (2159, 2419, 3168, 8189).** CCHFV risks include exposure to tick-infested mammals, viremic blood, or infective tissues, through sheep shearing, and in abattoirs and butcher shops. In Saudi Arabia, ~1% (3/354) of farm and quarantine station workers and 13% (16/122) of abattoir workers were seroreactive. In Oman, 30% (73/241) of non-Omani animal workers and 2% (1/41) of Omani animal workers were seroreactive.

Outbreaks Outbreaks among workers have been well documented.
- Southwest Asia. In Mecca, Saudi Arabia in 1989–1990, 40 abattoir workers contracted confirmed or suspected CCHFV infection, and 12 (30%) died (2159). In the United Arab Emirates in 1994, an outbreak caused 35 cases; 16 of 28 cases with occupation known were livestock market workers, abattoir workers, or skin processors, and of all workers, 4% (12/291) were seroreactive (3911).
- South Africa (7277, 8138). During an epizootic in 1984, five persons contracted CCHF from butchering and cow carcasses. In 1996, an outbreak at an ostrich abattoir affected 16 workers involved in defeathering, skinning, stunning, and evisceration. Ostriches were heavily infested by *Hyalomma* ticks; their abundance was attributed to high rainfall.

RVFV (1157, 4487, 6563, 8209, 8263). Hazardous activities include milking, sheltering of animals in domiciles, camel breeding, assisting livestock at birth or abortion, treating sick animals, slaughtering, handling carcasses, and being near herds during epizootics. During an epizootic in Kenya in 1989, 40% (12/30) of herdsmen were seroreactive.

Flaviviridae. **JEV (5339).** Rice farming is a putative risk of JEV. In rural Uttar Pradesh, India, in 1988, in an encephalitis epidemic that affected 4,544 inhabitants and 2,770 villages, the observed female-to-male ratio of 1:1.8 was explained by increased outdoor exposure by men. **St. Louis encephalitis virus (SLEV) (7582).** Farming communities appear to be at increased risk of infection by SLEV. **TBEV (1460, 1463, 4061, 6025, 7497).** Groups at potential occupational risk of TBEV include woodcutters, forest rangers, hunters, game wardens, farmers, road constructors, and surveyors. By area, occupational group, and vaccination status, reported risks have been low. In Italy in 2002, only 0.6% (11/174) of nonvaccinated forest rangers were seroreactive in two-step procedure (screening by enzyme-linked immunosorbent assay [ELISA], confirmation by neutralization assay). Vaccination should be limited to workers frequently exposed in foci. **WNV (648, 2771).** Occupational risks of WNV are emerging. In Wisconsin, when febrile cases were reported at a turkey-breeding farm in 2002, 42% (8/19) of exposed workers had anti-WNV IgM, compared with 5% (2/38) of other farm workers, and none of 14 non-turkey-exposed residents at or near the outbreak farm. The findings suggested the possibility of transmission by contact. Turkey workers were advised about hand hygiene, to wear protective gear, and to use mosquito repellents. In Israel in 1998, following an epizootic at goose farms, the seroprevalence in people who had close contact with sick geese reached 86%. **YFV (1796, 6335, 8136).** At risk of YFV are nonimmune individuals with outdoor jobs in enzootic areas, including farm, plantation, and forest work, harvesting of latex, hunting, and working for oil companies. In South America, ~80% of YF cases are in occupationally exposed male adults.

Togaviridae. **WEEV (1259).** Farm work in enzootic areas is a reported risk for WEEV.

Viruses: Vertebrate Borne

The significance of inapparent infections (seroreactivity and seroconversion) is often uncertain (harmless versus longterm effects). For the professional handling of animals, standard precautions (see section 12.6) are nevertheless advised.

Arenaviridae. **Guanarito virus (GUAV) (1815).** In enzootic areas, Venezuelan hemorrhagic fever is a risk for farm workers throughout the year, with a peak in November to January, when crops (corn, sorghum, cotton, rice, sunflowers, sugarcane, melons, and beans) are harvested, soil is tilled, and the dry season sets in. **JUNV (455, 4669, 8029).** In enzootic areas, Argentine hemorrhagic fever is a risk for rural residents and farm workers. Cases in humans peak in parallel with rodent populations in April to June when corn and sorghum are harvested. **Lymphocytic choriomeningitis virus (LCMV) (2167, 2536, 3766).** Occupational contacts with mice are a LCMV risk. Of persons occupationally exposed to rodents, 1.2% (1/72) had anti-LCMV IgG. In The Netherlands in 1993, none of 102 veterinarians, but 2.6% of 191 pig farmers were seroreactive. At the Vienna Zoo in Austria, 13% of 60 employees were seroreactive.

Coronaviridae. **Avian infectious bronchitis virus (AIBV) (5795).** Higher levels of anti-AIBV were reported in individuals exposed to poultry than in nonexposed individuals.

Filoviridae. **EBOV (2462, 5057, 5074, 5075, 6384).** Work with captured monkeys is a risk for EBOV. At Reston, in 1989, during an epizootic among captive cynomolgus monkeys (*Macaca fascicularis*), four animal handlers were seroreactive, none had signs of disease; at the monkey provider facility in the Philippines, 12 (6%) of 186 workers were seroreactive. During a second epizootic in the United States in 1996, when quarantine procedures were rigidly followed, none of the staff seroconverted; at the provider facility in the Philippines, 1 of 246 animal workers was reactive and none reported symptoms of disease. In the Taï forest of Côte d'Ivoire in 1994, a Swiss research worker contracted EBOV disease from necropsy of a chimpanzee. **MARV (4781).** In Marburg in 1967, 25 of 31 epidemic cases were exposed to green monkeys (*Cercopithecus aethiops*), their blood, or cells.

Bunyaviridae. The *Hantavirus* SEOV is a cosmopolitan risk from wild rats (see section 3.3). Other hantaviruses are regionally enzootic.

- Far East (4299). HTNV circulates, mainly affecting farmers.
- Northern Europe (6405, 6876, 7764). PUUV circulates, mainly affecting farm and forest workers. In Finland in 1989–1994, from 5,132 PUUV infections, risks were significant for farmers, for a risk ratio of 1.7 (95% CI 1.5–1.8) relative to the population. In high-risk age groups (20–29 years) and areas, the infection rate in farmers reached 0.07/100 per year.
- Western and central Europe (1903, 1904, 2167, 3766, 4769, 5512, 6876, 7112). Dobravavirus (DOBV), HTNV, PUUV, Tulavirus (TULV), and likely further species circulate. At likely risk are farm and forest workers, hunters, and zoo workers. Reported seroprevalence is 0% in veterinarians, 1–4% in farmers, 6–7% in forest workers, and up to 10% in hunters and game wardens.
- North America (2467, 2536, 7847, 8381). Sin Nombre virus (SNV) and avirulent species (e.g., Prospect Hill virus) circulate. Occupational risks are uncertain. Reactivity to SNV was not found in any of 84 forest and park rangers mainly working outdoors nor in 72 persons occupationally intensely exposed to rodents. In contrast in the 1980s, reactivity to HTNV or Prospect Hill virus in immunofluorescence assay (IFA) was reported for forest workers from Mississippi (1% or 1/85), Virginia (1% or 1/79), and Alaska (2.5% or 9/360).
- Latin America (1119, 5922). Andes (ANDV) and other viruses circulate. Likely risks are rural work or residency, and rodent contacts. In an enzootic area of northern Argentina, 10% (20/201) of rural workers (farms and sawmills) were reactive, compared with 1% (1/97) of urban workers (employees, health, and students).

Paramyxoviridae. **Newcastle disease virus (NDV) (1069, 1547, 1904, 5795).** At risk of infection by NDV or disease are chicken workers, hunters, and veterinarians, including in laboratories. In the United Kingdom in 1982, 81 (5%) of 1,625 veterinary professionals self-reported Newcastle disease, for a rate of 0.3/100 person-years. People exposed to poultry had higher levels of anti-NDV than nonexposed individuals. In Austria, 4% of hunters were reactive to NDV in an indirect hemagglutination test, compared with none of 50 urban controls. Half of reactive hunters had a history of rearing pheasants or quails. **Nipah virus (1440, 5757, 6529).** In Singapore and Malaysia in 1998–1999, an epizootic in pigs resulted in 265 cases in humans, mainly in small-scale pig farmers. Dominance of males among patients suggested spread by contact or secretions rather than by mosquitoes. Subsequently, in Singapore, pigs from Malaysia set off an outbreak among abattoir workers in 1999. Of abattoir workers who slaughtered pigs, 1.6% (7/435) were seroreactive compared with none of 233 workers who slaughtered ruminants.

Picornaviridae. **Encephalomyocarditis virus (1903).** Hemagglutination inhibition antibodies were more frequent among hunters (15%) than urban residents (8%), abattoir workers (8%), farmers (7%), and veterinarians (5%).

Poxviridae. **Cowpox virus (3766, 5817).** At a Finnish veterinary meeting in 2001, antibodies to *Orthopoxvirus* in IFA among participants increased with age, from 10% (2/19) at ≤25 years, to 50% (50/101) at 26–50 years, and 100% (18/18) at ≥51 years. Orthopox (cowpox) antibodies were also demonstrated in Vienna Zoo workers. **Orf virus (6340, 7674).** In New Zealand, 231 employees from 18 sheep slaughterhouses contracted orf virus infections over 1 year, for attack rates of 1.4% among all employees, and 4% among slaughter board workers. Most (95%) lesions were on the hands. In Turkey in 2003–2004, six housewives and three teachers contracted Orf of the hands from nonskilled slaugther of goats or sheep for a Muslim feast. **Pseudocowpox virus (8053).** Pseudocowpox virus is an occasional cause of milker's nodules in persons in contact with infected cattle.

Retroviridae. **Feline retroviruses (1003).** Risks for feline retroviruses appear small. At a veterinary conference, none of 204 attendees tested positive for feline immunodeficiency virus (FIV), feline foamy virus (FeFV), or feline leukemia virus (FeLV), despite long (mean, 17 years) and intense (yearly traumas) work with cats. **Simian retroviruses (1151, 2292, 3253, 6601).** Viruses that may infect captive primates for life include simian immunodeficiency virus (SIV), simian foamy viruses (SFV), simian T-lymphotrophic viruses (STLV), and simian D retroviruses. Vehicles may include blood, breastmilk, and genital secretions, as well as organs and cells. Infections were documented for SIV by serology in 0.6% (3/427) of primate workers, and for SFV by serology, NAT, or culture in 2% (4/231) workers. Furthermore, in North America, 3% (4/133) zoo workers were seroreactive to SFV. Infections can persist in exposed humans and may or may not be associated with disease or interhuman spread.

Rhabdoviridae. **Rabies virus (2454, 2898, 7341).** Rabies case reports suggest occupational risks for ranchers, bat fanciers, workers at animal shelters, quarantine and impound stations, veterinary clinics, and wildlife rehabilitation centers. Preexposure vaccination should be considered for occupational contacts with nonvaccinated animals in or from areas with enzootic bat or terrestrial rabies. **Vesicular stomatitis virus (VSV) (6195).** During an epizootic in the United States in 1982–1983, 13% (17/133) of occupationally exposed individuals (veterinarians, research workers, and students) and 6% (3/52) of unexposed controls had neutralizing antibodies to VSV. Risks included examining the mouths of animals, animals that sneezed into the face of examiners, saliva splash into unprotected eyes, and skin lesion on hands or arms.

Bacteria: Arthropod Borne

Serosurveys are likely plagued by cross-reactivity. Latent infections need confirmation by a second highly specific serotest or by NAT.

Borrelia. **Tick-borne relapsing fever (TBRF) (820, 2426, 6258).** Relapsing borreliae circulate in the Old and New Worlds, although apparently not simultaneously with *B. burgdorferi*. In North America, a risk was reported for park rangers sleeping in rustic cabins. In the U.S. Virgin islands, a park ranger who cleared out rodent-infested sheds and trapped mongooses contracted TBRF. **Lyme disease (5896).** Although farm and forest workers appear at risk, the published evidence is of variable quality and likely confounded by leisure activities.

- Farmers (1407, 5512, 7112, 7445, 8054). Reported seroprevalence is 0.2–14%. In the United Kingdom, however, when a two-step procedure (screening by ELISA and confirmation by Western blot) was used, only 0.2% (1/518) of randomly selected farm workers tested positive. Where controls were included, seroprevalence was significantly increased in Polish but not in Swedish farmers. In Sweden in 1994, 8% (19/253) of farm and forest workers were seroreactive, marginally more than clerks (5%, 13/249).

- Forest workers and rangers (984, 1407, 1460, 3188, 3459, 4135, 5307, 5512, 7497, 8401). The same caveats apply as with farmers, but controlled studies have supported a true risk. Reported seroprevalence is 7–35%. Compared with controls (4–5%), seroprevalence was significantly increased in forestry workers in France, Germany, Italy, The Netherlands, and Switzerland, as well as in Croatia, Poland, and Romania. In Italian and Dutch forest workers, seroconversion rates were 5–10/100 per year, but clinical manifestations were not seen. In Switzerland, seroreactivity in workers increased with increasing years on the job.

- Hunters (1904, 5512). Reported seroprevalence is 8–42%. In Austria, 42% of 147 hunters, but none of 50 control urban residents had IgG to *B. burgdorferi* sl in ELISA.
- Other occupational groups (3766, 5512, 6728). In New Jersey in 1987, of employees in the department of environmental protection with outdoor jobs, 6% (624/381) were seroreactive in the parks and forestry division, 5% (8/156) in the fish, game, and wildlife division, and 5% (3/64) in the coastal resources division. In Italy in 1987–1991, 17% (5/30) of fishermen were seroreactive. Of 60 Vienna Zoo employees, 10% were seroreactive.

Rickettsiales. *A. phagocytophilum* **(1460, 2389, 2949, 5513, 7445).** Farm and forest workers seem at risk, although some surveys have reported antibody prevalence of up to 2% in apparently unexposed (likely cross-reactive) controls. By test and location, reported seroprevalence in West Europe was 0.6–14% in forest workers or rangers, 1.5% in farm workers, and 6% in hunters. True infection prevalence is likely <2%. In Italy in 2002, while 16 (8.8%) of 181 of forest rangers tested positive in IFA, only one infection was confirmed by Western blot, for an adjusted prevalence of 0.6%. Cases of granulocytic ehrlichiosis (HGE) do not appear to be reported in crop- and-herd workers in Europe. *E. chaffeensis* **(1904, 7445).** In the United Kingdom in 1991–1995, 0.2% (1/518) of farm workers were seroreactive. In Austria, 15% (23/147) of hunters but none of 50 urban controls had IgG in indirect IFA, and 3% (4) had IgM. However, cases of monocytic ehrlichiosis (HME) do not appear to be reported in crop-and-herd workers in Europe. *O. tsutsugamushi* **(920, 6891, 7202, 7390, 7978).** Groups at risk of infection and disease (scrub typhus) in Southeast and East Asia include rice farmers, orchid farm workers, oil palm workers, and rubber plantation workers. Reported seroprevalence is 1–10% in control groups and 7-57% in occupational groups at risk.

Rickettsia. *R. africae* **(3683).** Mainly hunters, but also film crews seem at risk for *R. africae*. *R. conorii* **(1735, 6468, 7884).** Groups at risk for *R. conorii* in South Europe and Southwest Asia include farmers, livestock breeders, shepherds, and hunters. Reported seroprevalence is 4% in control groups and 10–13% in occupational risk groups. *R. helvetica* **(2476).** Forest workers seem at risk for *R. helvetica*. In France, 9% (35/379) of forest workers were seroreactive. *R. typhi* **(1735, 7202, 7390).** By location and test, compared with controls (0.8–7% seroreactive), groups reported at risk for *R. typhi* in South Europe and Southeast Asia included farmers and livestock breeders (3%), rubber estate workers (3% reactive initially, 14% after 4 months of follow-up), and orchards and orchid farm workers (13%).

Y. pestis **(2569, 8093, 8109, 8405).** Work with infected mammals is a risk for *Y. pestis*, including the slaughtering and butchering of camels, the skinning and cutting of marmots, and the handling of flea-infested rodents. Groups at risk include hunters, trappers, veterinarians, and field biologists. Noncommercial vaccine should be considered for workers regularly exposed to wild rodents or their fleas in plague enzootic or epizootic areas.

Bacteria: Vertebrate Borne

Bacillus anthracis **(411, 1807, 2697, 5864, 5873, 5882, 6865, 6975, 7682).** Anthrax is an unusual but well established occupational risk. Furthermore, spores in effluents from tanneries and hide workshops have been suspected to pollute nearby soils. Occupational groups at risk include farmers, herdsmen, and shepherds; veterinarians and other animal health providers; abattoir workers, skinners, and butchers; meat transporters, handlers, and inspectors; leather, wool, and textile workers; hair, hide, bone, and gelatine workers; machinists handling contaminated fodder sacks; and gardeners handling bone meal fertilizer.

Of 38 anthrax investigations in the United States in 1950–2001, about one third were for textile mills, close to two thirds concerned farms and livestock, and five were for contaminated products. Of 27 cases in textile mills, 21 (78%) were cutaneous, and 6 (22%) were inhalational. On farms, there were >3,600 cases in animals (in cows, sheep, pigs, and horses), and 13 cases in humans (all cutaneous, most in ranchers and farm hands). In the United Kingdom in 1961–1980, most (84% or 122/145) reported cases were occupational and in males (93% or 113/122). Also in the United Kingdom in 1981–2000, 14 suspected cases were reported; of these 10 (71%) were occupational. In France in 1980–2000, >200 cases were identified, all but three were related to animal contacts. **Rates (821, 1547).** Anthrax has become a rare disease. In U.S. mills that processed raw goat hair in the 1950s, the anthrax rate reached 1/100 workers per year. In the United Kingdom in 1982, 0.4% (6/1,625) veterinary professionals self-reported anthrax, for a rate of $16/10^5$ person-years.

Outbreaks (411, 1807, 5290, 5864, 5944, 7822) Outbreaks are unusual in high-income countries, although *B. anthracis* may persist in wild herds or contaminated soils (for anthrax in livestock, see section 2.3). Noncommercial vaccines are manufactured for groups at high risk only.

- North America. Natural epizootics are reported in bison herds. In 1957, an outbreak at a goat-hair-processing plant caused four cutaneous cases (all recovered) and five inhalational cases (four died).
- West Europe. In Italy in 1991, 3 of a farm family of 11 contracted anthrax from assisting in delivery of a cryptically infected cow. In Switzerland in 1978–1981, an outbreak in a textile factory caused 24 cutaneous cases and 1 inhalational case; the source was goat hair imported from Pakistan.
- Africa. Natural epizootics are reported in wild and domestic herd animals. Outbreaks have resulted from the butchering of sick animals and the consumption of meat from sick animals.
- Asia. Natural epizootics have been reported in livestock. In Kazakhstan in 1998, ≥53 humans contracted anthrax, largely from slaughtering or butchering; most cases were cutaneous. In Tamil Nadu, India, in 1998–2001, cutaneous anthrax was diagnosed in 15 children and 8 adults, mainly from cattle or goats dying at home or in the neighborhood, or from handling meat.

Bartonella. B. henselae **(1903, 3766, 5452, 5492).** Occupational risks for *B. henselae* are inadequately known. High seroreactivities have been reported in veterinarians (7–51%) and zoo workers (65%). At a veterinary conference in Ohio, 25 (7%) of 351 veterinarians and related professionals were reactive. Similarly, at a meeting in Styria, Austria, 70 (51%) of 137 veterinarians were reactive. Unsolved problems include confounding by private cat ownership, specificity of serological tests, uncertain modes of spread, and lack of clinical correlates. ***B. vinsonii*** **(8034).** *B. vinsonii* has been isolated from a febrile cattle rancher.

Brucella **(2167, 3851, 5080, 5615, 6223, 6808, 7921, 8135, 8348).** *Brucella* is an occupational hazard, mainly from aborting and parturient livestock. Manure and pastures can yield viable agents for several months. Use of clippers, cleavers, or other sharp implements on animals or their products increases the risks. Contaminated farm machinery can be a source of infection. In U.S. abattoirs, attack rates correlated with airflow, and negative air pressure in kill halls reduced risks in other work areas, findings that suggested airborne transmission. For foodborne brucellosis, see section III.

Occupational groups at risk include farm workers, cattle ranchers, sheep shearers, dairy farmers, veterinarians, and abattoir, pork-processing, and meat workers. Hunters have contracted *Brucella suis* from dressing feral swine carcasses. **Seroprevalence (1903, 2167, 5615, 6223, 6808, 7424).** By location, work safety, and test, reported seroprevalence in occupational groups in enzootic areas is 0.5–38%. In enzootic provinces of People's Republic of China, 18–38% of slaughterhouse, carcass, and packing-house workers were reactive, and with students as baseline, seroprevalence was elevated in farmers (11-fold), veterinarians (27-fold), herdsmen (46-fold), and coat and leatherworkers (48-fold). In The Netherlands in 1993, 4.5% of 102 veterinarians but none of 191 pig farmers were seroreactive to *Brucella abortus* antigen. In contrast in Germany, none of 137 veterinarians, 152 farmers, or 147 abattoir workers tested positive for *B. abortus* (complement binding) or *B. suis* (microagglutinaton). **Infection rates (1547).** Infection rates have been poorly documented. In the United Kingdom in 1982, 11% (186/1,625) of veterinary professionals (563 veterinarians and 1,062 support and laboratory staff) self-reported brucellosis, for a rate of 0.8/100 person-years.

Outbreaks Occupational brucellosis outbreaks are well documented.

- United States (3502, 7571, 7921). At a pork-processing plant in the United States in 1992, an outbreak affected 18 workers. In a follow-up survey, 19% (30/154) kill-floor workers had evidence of infection. In Argentina, an epizootic among goats was followed by 33 brucellosis cases among farm workers, including 14 confirmed by culture due to *Brucella melitensis*.
- Asia (1775, 3636, 4203, 5080). At a meat-packing plant in Israel in 1994, ~2–4 months after 800 infected cattle had to be killed, nine workers contracted chronic brucellosis. During a *B. mellitensis* outbreak at a kibbutz in Israel, infection risks included working in a cowshed, assisting parturient calves, and consumption of unpasteurized milk. At an abattoir in Australia in 1979–1980, an outbreak caused 22 acute cases (abattoir fever). The epidemic agent, *B. abortus* biovar 2, was unusual; it was explained by aerosol transmission from infected pregnant cattle.
- Europe (5099, 6364). In Zaragoza, Spain, in 1998–1999, a *B. mellitensis* biotype 1 outbreak affected 28 slaughterhouse workers; by work area, attack rates were 11–33%. In Germany in 1983, when a sheepshearer contracted *B. melitensis* through a work injury, an investigation detected 15 further cases, including 7 with contacts to infected sheep herds, 4 with contacts to infected cattle herds, and 4 without herd contacts.

Chlamydophila **(1166, 1327, 1903, 2866, 3339, 3766, 6723, 7112).** Occupational groups at risk for *C. psittaci* include poultry farmers and abattoir workers, wildlife rangers, hunters, quarantine station workers, veterinarians, bird fanciers, zoo workers, pet shop employees, and taxidermists. For laboratory work, see section 12.6.

By sampling and test, endemic seroprevalence in occupational groups at risk is 1–21%. In Northern Ireland, the seroprevalence among randomly selected farmers was 11%. In Styria, Austria, in 1995, 21% (29/137) veterinarians were seroreactive to *C. psittaci* in a complement fixation assay.

Infection rates (1547, 5393) have been poorly documented. In the United Kingdom in 1982, 0.1% (2/1,625) of veterinary professionals self-reported ornithosis, for a risk of $9/10^5$ person-years.

Outbreaks Occupational outbreaks have been documented. For workers at risk, proposed preventive measures include gloves and facial masks.

- North America (3224). In Minnesota in 1986, an epidemic caused 186 cases (122 confirmed and 64 suspected) among workers at a turkey processing plant and farm, for an attack rate of 10%. In the outbreak year, Minnesota produced nearly 35 million turkeys raised in flocks of 10–20,000 birds.
- Asia (3339, 8183). During an outbreak at a duck farm and processing plant in Victoria, Australia, in 1989, 76% of workers were seroreactive. Also in Victoria, an outbreak by *C. psittaci* (or possibly *C. pneumoniae*) affected 15 men and 1 woman; compared with neighborhood controls, the only risk in cases was to spent more time in gardens and to mow lawns in the 3 weeks before illness onset.
- West Europe (4293, 5393, 5693, 6723). At a duck-processing plant in the United Kingdom in 1985, ornithosis affected 16% (13/80) of workers, with a peak in the production line. Of 37 new employees, 18 (49%) were diagnosed with recent infection in the first 3 months of employment, and 5 (14%) also had clinical evidence of ornithosis. Also in the United Kingdom, 15 (44%) of 34 veterinary surgeons contracted ornithosis from a training visit to a duck-processing plant. Exposure to duck feathers was associated with 1.7 times higher attack rates. In France, three or more outbreaks occurred in abattoirs for ducks, turkeys, and chickens: in 1998 with 6 cases in humans, 1997 with 15 cases, and in 1990 with 18 cases and an attack rate of 32%. At a poultry farm and processing plant in Germany, ornithosis was diagnosed in 8 (9%) of 87 workers of whom two died. On follow-up, 70% (57/82) of outbreak plant workers were seroreactive, compared with 19% (16/83) of workers at a chicken slaughterhouse, and 27% (22/82) of age- and sex-matched controls. Discussed modes of spread included inhalation of dried excretions or aerosols and hand-to-mouth uptake.

Coxiella **(17, 3176, 4672, 4852, 4932, 6294, 6468, 7140, 7228, 7446, 8018).** *C. burnetii* is an occupational hazard, mainly from aborting and parturient livestock, birth products, manure, wool, and dust. Even farmed birds are a reported source. For raw milk, see section 7.1; for ticks, see section 4.1, and for professional clothes, see section 6.4.

Occupational groups at risk for *C. burnetii* include farmers, stock breeders, animal transporters, abattoir and animal product workers, and veterinarians. In South Australia in 1986–1990, of 130 confirmed cases notified, 90% (118) were males of working age, 55% (71) were meatworkers, 20% (26) were farm, dairy, or wool workers, and 9% (12) were animal transporters. To prevent spread, animals should be separated from herds for delivery, and birth assistants are advised to wear face mask and gloves. Placenta, carcasses, and other infective materials should be collected in closed containers for safe disposal. **Seroprevalence (17, 5492, 7112, 7228, 7446).** Reported seroprevalence ranges broadly by herd infection, type and length of job, and test. In Japan in 1997–2000, veterinarians were ~3 times more frequently reactive (14% or 36/267) than health care workers (5% or 18/352) or blood donors (4% or 73/2,003). In a serosurvey in Spain, 52% (100/194) of farm workers were reactive, significantly more than other workers (31% or 65/212). In the United Kingdom, seroprevalence was 27% (105/385) in farm workers compared with 11% (43/395) in police and emergency service workers. Full-time workers were >4 times more likely to be reactive than part-time workers, and cumulative exposure seemed more important than exposure to a particular animal. In Northern Ireland, the seroprevalence among randomly selected farmers was 28%. In Austria in 1995, 13 (10%) of 137 veterinarians were reactive in a complement fixation test; veterinarians who reported handling placenta with their bare hands were reactive significantly more often than veterinarians who reported use of gloves. **Infection rates (45, 1547, 4672, 4912, 7446).** In a 2-year vaccine study among abattoir workers in Australia, the rate of Q fever in the placebo arm was 2/100 and year (55/1,365). In a retrospective 10-year study at an abattoir in Australia that slaughtered and boned cattle, sheep, and swine and manufactured ham and corned beef, the overall disease rate in 9 interepidemic years was 1/100 per year, compared with 8/100 per year in 1 epidemic year. In West Australia, employment in the farm animal industry increased infection risks 25-fold. In the United Kingdom, infection (seroconversion) rates in farm workers were 0.8/100 per year (95% CI 0.1–2). In the United Kingdom in 1982, 0.5% (8/1,625) of veterinary professionals self-reported Q fever, for a rate of 0.03/100 person-years.

Outbreaks Outbreaks of Q fever among professionals have been documented in North America, Australia, and Europe.

- North America (3176, 4511). At a meat-packing plant in California, after five cases of *Coxiella*-hepatitis had occurred, 12 (29%) of 42 employees had evidence of recent infection, and 19 (45%) had evidence of past infection. In an outbreak in Canada, 37% (66/179) of goat farmers had evidence of recent *C. burnetii* infection.
- Australia (961). At an abattoir that usually slaughtered cattle and sheep, an outbreak with 70 cases occurred in 1979, when the abattoir began to slaughter goats.
- Europe (6294, 6694, 7627). At a breeding, teaching, and research farm in Hessen, Germany, in 1997, infected sheep caused an outbreak with 47 cases, for attack rates of 8% (5/59) among staff and 44% (26/59) among students (further cases occurred among visitors). In addition, 21 inapparent, recent infections were diagnosed. In Berlin, Germany, in spring 1992, sheep brought to an animal clinic caused an outbreak with 80 cases in humans. In Poland in 1992, an outbreak at a tannery caused 18 cases among workers in contact with imported skins of wild animals.

E. rhusiopathiae (4635). Case reports suggest occupational risks for abattoir workers, butchers, fish handlers, farm workers, and veterinarians, mainly via inoculation or microtrauma.

F. tularensis. The main occupational risks are hunting and farm work. An emerging risk seems to be landscaping. On Martha's Vineyard, Mass., infection risks were reported for tree workers, property managers, lot clearers, and professional gardeners (2349). Of landscapers, 9% (9/132) were seroreactive in a microagglutination test, compared with 0.3% (1/3010) of resident and physician visit controls. Landscapers using power blowers were at particular risk. In contrast in Austria, none of 137 veterinarians, 152 farmers, and 147 abattoir workers were seroreactive (1903).

- Hunters (1272, 1883, 2838, 2972, 3205, 4270, 4367, 5257, 5561, 5562). At risk are hunters, trappers, fur traders, venison dressers, and cooks, mainly from handling hares, rabbits (lagomorphs), muskrats, or beavers (rodents), including carcasses and furs. In Québec, Canada, in 1992–1993, 2.4% (4/165) of trappers but only 0.6% (1/165) of age-, sex-, and area-matched controls were seroreactive. Unlike arthropod-borne tularemia that peaks in summer and fall, vertebrate-borne tularemia in hunters peaks in fall and winter coinciding with the hunt. In France; 80–85% of reported cases (375 in 1988–1993) resulted from hunters or cooks handling hares. In Spain and Czechia, too, handling of hunted, tularemic hares has been the principal source. In Switzerland, in 1967, five butchers contracted tularemia from work with 2,100 hares trapped in Austria in the previous year and imported deeply frozen. An infrequent source is hamsters. In Hungary in 1970–1976, 45 of 50 of reported cases concerned hamster hunters.
- Farmers (1714, 2172, 7283). In enzootic or epizootic areas, farmers are at risk. Tularemia on farms can be acquired via inhalation of dust from hay cutters, handling of hay or straw, cleaning of grain bins, or threshing grain that was inhabited by rodents. In northern Sweden in the fall of 1966, an airborne epidemic caused 676 cases. In an outbreak in northern Finland in 1982, 50 of 53 patients contracted respiratory tularemia while farming. In this outbreak, suspected sources besides dust included picking potatoes, repairing the tractor in the barn, and poking at a dead rabbit.

Mycobacterium bovis (1589, 5540). Livestock keepers, herdsmen, farmers, and slaughterhouse workers exposed to infected cattle or captive deer seem at increased risk of *M. bovis* infection or zoonotic tuberculosis.

Pasteurella. P. multocida (1419, 1979). Work with infected pigs or cattle can result in oropharyngeal colonization or inapparent infection. For bites, see chapter 1. **P. aerogenes (2149).** Work with or bites from pigs has caused occasional infections in workers.

Streptobacillus moniliformis (3060, 6875). *S. moniliformis* infections are a risk of rodent handlers, pet shop workers, and farmers. From a minor finger wound at a contaminated rat cage, a 24-year-old U.S. pet shop employee developed fatal rat bite fever.

Streptococcus suis (2167, 4057, 5798, 6332, 7188, 7343, 7825). Case reports and surveys corroborate a risk of *S. suis* for farm and abattoir workers, butchers, hunters, and meat workers. In Spain *S. suis* was recovered from two adults with meningitis, a butcher, and an abattoir worker. In Germany, 7 (5%) of 132 workers in pig-slaughtering and -processing industries carried *S. suis* in the pharynx. Compared with veterinary students, increased seroreactivities were reported in veterinarians, pig and dairy farmers, and meat inspectors.

Vibrio (1719, 3351). By the handling of fish and seafood, fishermen, dockworkers, and oyster shuckers are at risk of percutaneous infections with *V. parahaemolyticus* and *V. vulnificus*. Eviscerating European eel (*Anguilla anguilla*) seems a particularly hazardous activity. These predominantly male jobs explain the preponderance of males with *Vibrio* wound infections.

Protozoa
Well-conducted studies of occupational risks are scarce.

***Babesia* (3979).** Case reports and some serosurveys suggest a risk of *Babesia* for crop-and-herd workers.

***Leishmania*. Cutaneous leishmaniasis (CL) (220, 6151, 8303).** Reported risk groups comprise persons participating in outdoor (nocturnal) activities in enzootic or endemic areas, mainly farming, harvesting, and entering forests for lumbering, hunting, and collecting of firewood or gum (chicleros). **Visceral leishmaniasis (VL) (724, 7423, 8411).** Reported risk groups are farmers, livestock workers, shepherds, poultry workers, and game wardens.

***Plasmodium* (1039, 2224, 6081).** Nonimmune migrant workers are at high risk, including in the Amazon and Southeast Asian forests, in logging, newly colonized, or plantation areas. Migrants often sleep in the forest, without mosquito protection. In Vietnam, attack rates in migrants reached 0.2 per person-year for all types of malaria, and 0.1 per person-year for falciparum malaria. In peninsular Malaysia, workers exposed to falciparum malaria include rattan collectors.

***Trypanosoma*. *T. brucei gambiense* (1127, 2919).** With *T. brucei gambiense*, "tsetse flies go to hosts." In West Africa, peridomestic, daytime activities are a major risk for women, men, and children, including bathing, washing clothes, gathering firewood, and fishing. In Cameroon, hunting is a significant risk. ***T. brucei rhodesiense*.** With *T.brucei rhodesiense*, "hosts go to tsetse flies" (4863, 8281). In East Africa, daytime activities in tsetse territory are a major risk, including hunting, fishing, and honey gathering. ***T. cruzi* (1599, 7395).** Although the main risk is nocturnal and domestic, activities in forests and forest fringes in enzootic areas are likely additional risks, including hunting, woodcutting, and the collection of latex and palm fronds. However, little recent evidence is available, except for palm fronds (e.g., piassaba *Attalea funifera*) that host infective sylvatic triatomines (e.g., *Rhodnius brethesi*) that may attack collectors, including by flight.

Helminths
***Echinococcus*. *E. granulosus* (1620, 1903, 4225, 6043, 7976).** Putative groups at risk of *E. granulosus* include farmers, herdsmen, hunters, fur farmers, and abattoir workers. However, many serosurveys are plagued by cross-reactivity and lack confirmation by imaging on follow-up. In low-income countries, home slaughter of infected livestock and feeding of raw offal to dogs is a better established risk for exposed workers to contract infection or (cystic) disease. In Rio Negro province, Argentina, having a father who slaughtered sheep at the workplace was an infection risk for children. ***E. multilocularis* (2758, 3901, 5488, 6142).** In enzootic areas of Europe, farmers are at risk of infection and (alveolar) disease. Of 210 cases reported in Europe, 22% reported exposure from farming. In southern Germany, the odds of infection in farmers compared with the population were 9–15 to 1. Putative other groups at risk include abattoir workers and veterinarians. In Alaska, dogs rather than wild carnivores are the principal source of *E. multilocularis*.

Filariae. *B. malayi* (4674). In Malaysia, subperiodic *B. malayi* has been reported in rubber estate workers, including tappers, weeders, and latex factory hands. ***Loa loa* (7955).** Occupational risks for *L. loa* have been poorly documented. Farm and forest workers seem at risk. ***Onchocerca volvulus* (111, 5628, 7782, 8267).** Daytime outdoor work in endemic areas is a hazard, including fishing, farming, timber cutting, hunting, and coffee plantation work.

ENVIRONMENTAL CLUSTER, CROP-AND-HERD WORK
Bacteria
***Aeromonas* (3639, 4292, 6766, 7876).** Fish, mollusks, and crustaceans raised in tanks, estuaries, and bays, by crowding and overfeeding create favorable conditions for *Aeromonas* spp., including *A. hydrophila*. Abrasions from handling fish, molluscs, or crustaceans can result in *Aeromonas* skin infections.

***B. pseudomallei* (1421, 7257).** In Southeast Asia, a majority of melioidosis is diagnosed in (rice) farmers, in particular, diabetic farmers. In Australia, melioidosis affects crop-and-herd workers.

***C. tetani* (3388, 4565, 5792, 6472, 7690).** High densities of spores are to be expected in soils grazed by farm animals. Although vaccine-preventable, tetanus is a risk on farms. In Louisiana in 1998, only 54% (352/657) of farm women were current with tetanus boosters. In Italy in 1998–2000, for 56% (40/71) of cases with a known source tetanus resulted from farm work, and in 25% (18) it resulted from gardening. In central Italy in 1996–1999, of 32 cases, the mean age was 75 years, 91% (29) were females, 84% (27) were farm workers, and 16% (5) were housewives. In Finland in 1969–1985, of 106 cases, 26% (28) were occupational, including 15% (16) in farm and forest workers, and the rate of occupational tetanus was $\sim 1/10^5$ accidents. Most infective injuries were minor, and 61% were at the hand. In the United Kingdom in

1984–2000, only 13 (10%) of 133 tetanus cases with a known source reported work-related injuries: six from farms, three from outdoor engineering, three from manual work, and one from small animals.

Environmental mycobacteria. *M. marinum* (229, 6855). Fishermen and fish dealers are at increased risk of infection. *M. ulcerans* (1959, 4768). Reported infection risks are irrigation and wetland farming, and long walks to farmlands.

***Leptospira* (2286, 4152, 8049).** Sources include the urine of rodents and of inapparently infected cattle, pigs, sheep, and goats, mud in yards and stables, and freshwaters. In Germany, a retired forest warden contracted leptospirosis from gathering walnuts in muddy ground close to a creek. In wet farming areas (southern People's Republic of China, southern India, and northeastern Italy), leptospirosis can be enzootic and endemic. **Occupational risk groups (632, 1044, 1903, 3387, 3766, 4369, 5348, 5894, 7325, 7411, 7463).** Occupational risk groups are diverse and include rice and irrigation farming, sugar cane and banana plantation work, rice mill work, potato picking, forest work, logging, dairy farming, swine herding, game keeping, rodent trapping, hunting, abattoir work, carcass dressing, offal handling, butchering, meat inspection, animal health work, fishing, fish and prawn raising, zoo work, and animal health and research work, including small and large mammals. Occupational risks vary locally. In Thailand, most infections are in rice farmers, and plowing wet fields, applying fertilizer, and pulling rice sprouts are significant risks. In Australia, groups at risk are meat workers, dairy workers, wool workers, and animal transporters. In Denmark in 1970–1996, 41% of 118 confirmed cases were fish farmers, and 28% were farmers. **Seroprevalence.** A range of occupational groups were seroscreened on all continents for inapparent infection:

- Africa (3382, 5622). Reported seroprevalence is 20–44% in bush, farm, and plantation workers, ~20% in abattoir workers and butchers, and 4–6% in laboratory workers and blood donors.
- America (206, 4367). In Québec, Canada, in 1992–1993, 9% (15/165) of trappers and 5% (8/165) of age-, sex-, and area-matched controls were reactive. In Hawaii, seroprevalence in sugar cane workers and other high-risk occupational groups was 12–82%.
- Asia (685, 686, 5348). At rodent-infested rice mills in Tamil Nadu, India, 68% of workers were reactive, significantly more than other occupational groups. In New Zealand, 44% of dairy farm workers, 25% of pig farmers, and 8% of sheep and beef farmers were seroreactive, as were 10% of 1,215 meat inspectors and 6% of 1,248 meat workers. The main serovars in dairy farmers of Australia and New Zealand are Hardjo and Pomona.
- Europe (1903, 2167, 5512, 7112). Reported seroprevalence is 0.5–12% in farm and forest workers, <1% in fish farmers, and 0–3% in veterinarians.

Rates (1547, 2737, 7463). In the United Kingdom in 1961–1981, disease rates per 10^5 person-years were 33 in fish farmers but 0.1 in the population. In the United Kingdom in 1982, 0.2% (4/1,625) of veterinary professionals self-reported leptospirosis, for a rate of $17/10^5$ person-years. In New Zealand in 1990–1998, disease rates per 10^5 per year were 164 in meat workers, 92 in livestock workers, and 24 in forestry workers.

Outbreaks (1044, 4367, 7411, 7447) In Missouri in 1998, nine pig workers contracted leptospirosis; smoking or drinking beverages at work were risks, and washing hands after work was protective. On a dairy farm in New Zealand in 1992–1993, four cases occurred in 1 month; of 19 randomly selected cows from the nonvaccinated dairy herd, 79% were reactive in the microagglutination test. At an abattoir in New South Wales, Australia, in 1998, eight meat workers contracted leptospirosis in 2 months; a source was not found, but all cases reported exposure to large volumes of animal urine.

In Canada, only 69 (42%) of 165 trappers reported wearing gloves when handling animals. Preventive measures include vaccination of livestock and protective clothes for milk, livestock, and abattoir work.

Fungi
Chromomycosis (5070, 6817, 6894, 6895). Most chromomycosis cases concern males. Farmers and woodcutters are at risk, mainly through injury or walking barefoot. In Maranhao state, Brazil, 2 of 30 patients had chronic lesions at the buttocks (an atypical site); both worked as palm tree cutters and seemed to have contracted *Fonsecaea pedrosoi* from sitting on palm shells (the babaçu palm *Attalea phalerata* is a source of charcoal that is used to smoke rubber).

Mycetoma (4666). Walking barefoot is a hazard for both actinomycetoma and eumycetoma.

***Sporothrix* (1522, 1538, 1811, 1945, 1988, 2718, 3070, 3850, 4502, 7842).** Plants are a major source of *S. schenckii*, in particular, moss, moldy hay, and rotting wood. A less frequent source is fish. Occupational risks include farming, horticulture, gardening, flower work, forest work, tree nursing, Christmas tree farming, topiary production, hay baling, and masonry work. In the United States in 1988, the vehicle for an outbreak with 84 cases in 15 states was sphagnum moss; 8 of 102 sphagnum and other environmental samples grew *S. schenckii* (and 56 grew other *Sporothrix* spp). In an outbreak in Queensland, Australia, all of 16 cases had contact with moldy hay.

Helminths
Hookworms (2578, 3496, 7633). Unprotected skin exposes farmers and gardeners in endemic areas to hookworm larvae from soil, including of *N. americanus*, *A. duodenale* (ancylostomiasis), and zoonotic *A. braziliense* (cutaneous larva migrans). In North Vietnam, women who reported using fresh human feces as fertilizer had significantly higher hookworm egg counts than women who used treated feces or nonusing women. Surprisingly, in the Niger delta in Nigeria, ancylostomiasis was more prevalent in fishermen than farmers, and water was a postulated additional source. In Naples, Italy, in 2001, fecally polluted plant material (flowers, bark, and ears of corn) dried in a barn for a flower basket was the source for six cases of cutaneous larva migrans.

Schistosoma. Risks of *Schistosoma* are domestic and occupational water-related activities in endemic-enzootic areas, including farming, sugar cane cutting, ploughing wet fields, loading and repairing boats, herding, fishing, and hunting (32, 430, 1705, 2163, 3318, 4398, 4400, 5358, 5947). Exposure can be intense. In endemic parts of Egypt, farmers are exposed to canal or irrigation water, for ~4 h/week (*S. haematobium*) (5947) to ~8 h/week (*S. mansoni*) (32). Impact can be heavy. In a fishing boat community on Lake Dongting, People's Republic of China, in 2001, 58% (61/106) of members tested positive for *S. japonicum* by stool microscopy, 64% (68) by miracidium hatching test, and 37% (39) had evidence of liver fibrosis by ultrasound (4398). The economic consequences can be significant. On a sugar cane estate in Pernambuco state, Brazil, in 1978, loss of productivity due to intestinal schistosomiasis in cane cutters was estimated to ~9% (430).

Strongyloides **(6361, 6390, 6642).** The main occupational source of *S. stercoralis* is soil. A major group at risk is farmers in endemic areas. Around Valencia, Spain, 18% of the working population is engaged in farming and *S. stercoralis* is endemic in farm workers, for a prevalence of 12% (31/250, 95% CI 8–16). While housing was adequate, 3% of workers admitted to defecating in fields. In a case-control study in the same area, the only significant occupational risk was work in rice fields. In an endemic area of northeastern Italy, 104 (69%) of 150 patients reported farm or garden work.

Toxocara **(574, 1483, 1903).** Except in the United States, occupational risks of *Toxocara* are likely, although serosurveys are not proof of risk. In New Zealand, seroprevalence was 27% (52/192) in hydatid disease control officers, 14% (11/79) in dog breeders or exhibitors, 6% (1/18) in veterinarians, 7% (13/187) in rural blood donors, and 3% (9/318) in urban blood donors. In the United Kingdom, 6–16% of dog handlers, breeders, or exhibitors and 11% of small animal veterinary surgeons were seroreactive, compared with 3% of 922 healthy controls. In Austria, 48% of farmers, 27–34% of veterinarians, 25% of abattoir workers, 21% of zoo workers, and 17% of hunters were seroreactive (ELISA and Western blot), compared with 2% of urban controls. Eosinophilia in dog breeders and kennel workers should prompt evaluation for visceral, ocular or cutaneous larva migrans or inapparent infection by *T. canis*, *T. cati*, or related species.

SKIN-BLOOD CLUSTER, CROP-AND-HERD WORK
Prions (1492)
Several studies failed to detect occupational risks. A possible exception is butchers who are suspected to be at increased risk of sporadic CJD.

Bacteria (277)
Pig farmers seem to be at increased risk of nasal colonization with *S. aureus* of porcine origin. The feet of rice farmers are vulnerable to skin infections.

Fungi
Dermatophytes (1547, 4701). In Italy, floor samples of 50 private veterinary clinics yielded *Microsporum canis*, *M. gypseum*, *T. mentagrophytes*, *Trichophyton terrestre*, and other fungi. Materials from pets are suspected to enhance spread of zoophilic dermatophytes in veterinary clinics. In the United Kingdom in 1982, 17% (280/1,625) veterinary professionals self-reported animal ringworm, for a rate of 1.2/100 person-years.

Arthropods (19, 1284, 1688, 4806)
Case reports have suggested a risk of myiasis for farm managers, cattle workers, shepherds, goat farmers, woodcutters, and hunters. Implicated fly larvae include *Chrysomya*, *Dermatobia*, *Hypoderma*, and *Oestrus*.

12.5 CATERING
"Pot-and-pan" work includes cooking and catering, from preparation to serving, including bakers, barmen, cooks, food industry workers, kitchen aids, street vendors, and waiters at canteens, outlets, restaurants, and grocery stores. Although households are the "world's top caterers" (see section 11.1), the focus here is on salaried catering.

Exposure. Large, international chains include McDonald's (>31,000 restaurants in >100 countries), Kentucky Fried

Chicken (>13,000 in >90), Pizza Hut (>12,000 in >80), and Burger King (>11,200 in >60). Food work is an integral part of the exposure history (Box 12.1). For foods, see section III; for restaurants, see section 13.2; for infected livestock, see section 2.3.

Infections. Pot-and-pan workers can be victims or sources (Box 12.4). **Victims.** Pot-and-pan workers can contract infections at the workplace, from ingestion (e.g., tasting raw foods), contact (e.g., unwashed hands), inoculation (e.g., microtrauma), or inhalation (e.g., droplets from colleagues). Causative agents reflect hygiene at the workplace, susceptibility of the worker, and local endemicity. **Sources (vectors) (2250, 3300, 4986, 7859).** Ill or shedding food handlers can spread infections; for carriage, see section 14.1. Some countries require the exclusion of carriers of enteric agents from food work. In Germany in 1994–1996, 0.6% of 13,434 food workers carried enteric pathogens, mostly *Salmonella*. Because of low prevalence, a change of legislation was proposed. Uneducated migrant workers in high-income countries and nonregulated street vendors in low-income countries are important sources of food-borne infections. Street hazards include cooking on the ground or well in advance of consumption, fecally polluted water for washing hands, foods, or dishes, or production of ice cubes, reuse of water from buckets, lack of toilets or knowledge of hygiene, dirty hands, and flies.

Preventive measures. Preventive measures include good manufacturing and retailing practices, continued education of workers, sanitary installations, hand hygiene, protective clothes, audit of premises, and surveillance. Workers should report target illnesses to a responsible person before starting food work. In some situations, screening may be warranted, e.g., for HAV, *S. enterica* serovar Typhi, and *M. tuberculosis*. By type and job experience, vaccinations, endemicity (e.g., HEV and *V. cholerae*), and legal requirements, workers may need to be temporarily excluded from work (consult Table 14.1 for outpatients).

DROPLET-AIR CLUSTER, CATERING

Workers contract acute respiratory infections and tuberculosis at rates comparable to the community. At a hospital kitchen in Jerusalem, Israel, in 1999, Q fever affected 16 (39%) of 41 kitchen staff; the source of *C. burnetii* remained unknown (7148).

Pot-and-pan workers with ill household members, in particular, children in day care, are a potential food safety hazard. Sneezing and coughing workers could potentially contaminate unwrapped foods with adenovirus, *Rhinovirus*, SARS-CoV, and vaccine-preventable *C. diphtheriae* and *M. tuberculosis*. Workers should report cough illness, sore throat, coryza, and eye infections to management.

FECES-FOOD CLUSTER, CATERING

Workers contract acute diarrhea (6418) and hepatitis A (2493) at rates comparable to the community. In the United Kingdom in 1996–1997, rates of occupational diarrhea per 1,000 workers per year were 0.1 in bakers and 0.2 in cooks (6418).

Carriers, migrants, workers returning from visits to tropical countries, and workers with diapered children at home risk fecally contaminating unwrapped foods. In Jakarta, Indonesia, enteric agents shed by 128 street food vendors included *S. enterica* serovar Typhi (0.8%), *G. lamblia* (1.5%), *E. histolytica/dispar* (1.5%), and *S. enterica* serovar non-Typhi (3%) (7859). Vaccine-preventable food-borne agents include HAV, serovar Typhi, and *V. cholerae*. Workers should report vomiting, diarrhea, and jaundice to management.

Viruses
HAV (2393, 3411, 7096, 7462). Incubating food workers are a source of food-borne HAV and outbreaks.

Box 12.4 Agents and infections in and from pot-and-pan workers, by cluster

Risks are listed in parentheses.

Droplet-air
- Victim: respiratory tract infections
- Source: AdV; *M. tuberculosis*

Feces-food
- Victim: acute diarrhea
- Source: HAV, *Norovirus*; *E. coli* (EHEC, after recovery), *Campylobacter* (low-income vendors), *S. enterica* serovar non-Typhi (after recovery), serovar Typhi (carriers), *Shigella* (after recovery), *V. cholerae* (low-income vendors), *V. parahaemolyticus* (in endemic areas); *Cryptosporidium*, *E. histolytica* (carrier in or from endemic area), *Giardia*; *T. solium* (carrier in or from endemic area)

Skin-blood
- Victim: injury
- Source: *S. aureus* food poisoning (carrier and skin lesion), *S. pyogenes* epidemic pharyngitis (carrier, skin lesion)

Source and vehicle are often suspected too late, when leftover foods are no longer available, and PEP with Ig is no longer recommended. In Spokane County, Wash., in 1997–1998, a community epidemic caused 527 acute HA cases, including 107 (20%) in IDU, and 30 (6%) in food workers; none of the infected workers was the source for food-borne secondary cases, but IgG was administered for PEP to >3,000 patrons, and >9,000 food workers were vaccinated over 15 months. A model case was a deli meat and cheese worker at a grocery store in Alberta, Canada, in 2001, who promply reported jaundice and was excluded from work for 2 weeks during which acute HA was confirmed. The public was informed, potentially contaminated ready-to-eat foods were recalled, Ig was administered to ~5,400 potentially exposed customers, and secondary cases did not occur.

Outbreaks Outbreaks of acute HA from foods handled by infective workers are well-documented in high-income countries. Some have argued that such outbreaks are not frequent enough in high-income countries to justify routine immunization of food workers (1652).

- North America (2393, 4218, 4539, 4811, 8040). In the United States in 1968–2001, 17 outbreaks were linked to infected food handlers: 8 at restaurants, 5 at cafeterias, and 2 each at bakeries, and caterers; there were 1,114 acute cases or 11–228 (mean, 66) per outbreak. Implicated vehicles included salads, sandwiches, pastry icing, and glazed bakery. At a restaurant in Massachusetts in 2001, a food worker was the suspected source for 21 HA cases. At a Kentucky catering company in 1994, a food worker (who adhered to good hygiene practice) was source for 91 HA cases, for an attack rate of 7% among 1,318 patrons. At a bakery in Rochester, N.Y. in 1994, sugar glaze contaminated by an infected worker was vehicle for 64 HA cases. At a Florida restaurant in 1989, cold food handled by infected pantry workers, waitresses, or a bartender carried an outbreak with 97 cases among patrons.
- Europe (1402, 6295). At a delicatessen in Bari, Italy, in 2002, sandwiches handled by an incubating worker were vehicle for 26 HA cases. At a butcher shop in Bavaria, Germany, in 1998, sausages were the vehicle for 75 cases; the master butcher had contracted acute HA on a visit to Teneriffa, Spain, where he had consumed molluscs.

HEV. As adults can contract acute HE, food work is a potential risk.

Norovirus (2668, 3600, 5577, 5725, 5727). Foodhandlers are a significant source of food contamination and outbreaks. Because the infectious dose is low, and virus in stool is concentrated, already spotty contamination has an impact. Infectivity begins in the incubation period (before d_0, the first day of symptoms). By test, virus is demonstrated in stool for up to 14 days. However, infectivity may last longer: in the United Kingdom in 1985, a chef was the suspected source in two outbreaks that were separated by 24 days. Exclusion from work for 3 days after recovery may be inadequate to prevent spread.

Outbreaks Outbreaks are well-documented in high-income countries.

- North America (1310, 1737, 3837, 4153, 5725). At a Christmas dinner banquet in Ohio, tossed salad was implicated in an outbreak of gastroenteritis that affected 93 (68%) of 137 attendees; a food handler at a local caterer was the suspected source. At a restaurant in Ohio, a food handler who delivered sandwiches caused ≥50 diarrhea cases among 325 patrons. At a university cafeteria and deli bar in Texas, ham contaminated by a food handler was vehicle for 125 cases among student patrons. At a company luncheon in Alaska, potato salad contaminated by a food handler caused 191 cases among 343 patrons. At a bakery in Minneapolis, cake frosting contaminated by a worker caused ~3,000 diarrhea cases.
- Asia (4016). In Japan, a food handler and a school lunch from a particular caterer were likely sources in a gastroenteritis outbreak that affected 3,236 (42%) of 7,801 schoolchildren at nine elementary schools, and 117 (39%) of 297 teachers.
- West Europe (2870, 4478). In the United Kingdom, turkey and tuna salad sandwiches contaminated by a food handler and served in four hospitals caused 195 diarrhea cases among patients and staff. In Sweden in 1999, the same *Norovirus* genotype was recovered from epidemic cases of 30 day care centers served by the same caterer, and from two food handlers (one ill and one asymptomatic).

***Rotavirus* (2438).** Information is limited. At a college in the District of Columbia in 2000, 85 students contracted *Rotavirus* diarrhea presumably from sandwiches, for an attack rate of 5%; two cooks with diarrhea amplified *Rotavirus* by NAT.

Bacteria

For a majority of enteric bacteria, food animals rather than humans are the principal source, and contamination at farm or slaughter is the main hazard.

***Campylobacter* (5600, 7524).** The main hazard is contamination by *Campylobacter* at farm or slaughter. Food workers are a rare source. In southern Brazil, the *Campylobacter* point prevalence in 177 kitchen workers is 6%. At a school luncheon in Kansas in 1998, a cafeteria worker and mishandled food were implicated in an outbreak of *C. jejuni* that affected 27 (17%) of 161 attendees.

***E. coli* (1352, 3827, 5637, 6085).** Although animal feces *and* shedding workers are potential sources, few reports address EHEC, EIEC, and ETEC in food workers. After an illness episode, children and adults can shed EHEC for days, weeks, or up to 4–5 months. In the United Kingdom, a butcher's counter was implicated in an outbreak with 30 confirmed cases of *E. coli* O157. In India, 3% of food workers with diarrhea yielded EHEC.

***Providencia* (1406).** In Turkey in 1999, in an outbreak among Czech peace-keeping forces with 27 diarrhea cases and 11 asymptomatic infections, an ill cook was the implicated source of *P. alcalifaciens*, and pork schnitzel with potato salad was the implicated vehicle.

***Salmonella.* *S. enterica* non-Typhi serovars.** (123, 959, 3300, 5263, 6420, 7859, 8316). The main hazard is contamination with serovar non-Typhi at the farm or slaughter. Acutely ill workers are an alternative source; carriage by healthy workers is rare ($\leq 0.6\%$) in high-income countries. In Tokyo, Japan, in 1961–1997, stools of only 0.07% of healthy food handlers grew *Salmonella*. In contrast in low-income countries, food vendors are a relevant source. In Jordan, 6% of 283 food handlers yielded *Salmonella*. In a review of 32 studies and 2,814 patients, median shedding periods were 7 weeks in preschool children, and 3–4 weeks in persons ≥ 5 years of age. After 12 weeks, 45% of preschool children (219/486), and 6% (83/1,489) of older persons were still shedding. Antibiotics are widely considered not to reduce or even enhance shedding.

Outbreaks Some outbreak reports follow.
- North America (3223). At a fast-food restaurant in Minnesota, *S. enterica* serovar Enteritidis in curly-fried potatoes and ice from a food worker caused 37 diarrhea cases.
- Asia (3497). At a Korean-style restaurant in Adelaide, Australia, *S. enterica* serovar Typhimurium in mango pudding dessert from a food worker caused 28 diarrhea cases among ~240 patrons, for an attack rate of ~12%.
- Europe (1052, 2492). At a fish-and-chip shop in the United Kingdom, food handlers caused an outbreak of *S. enterica* serovar Paratyphi B. In Spain in 2002, infected food handlers and fresh eggs contributed to an outbreak of serovar Enteritidis with 1,435 cases.

***S. enterica* serovar Typhi (3925, 4202, 4748, 7681, 7859).** Humans are the only reservoir, and carriers are a major source of food-borne typhoid fever. At the turn of the nineteenth to the twentieth century, "Typhoid Mary" Mallon, an Irish immigrant to the United States was a cook and carrier and was associated with nine typhoid outbreaks and 54 cases. Meanwhile, carriage has become rare in high-income countries, where most current infections are imported or diagnosed in foreign born individuals. In low-income countries, the reported prevalence of carriers among food handlers or vendors is 0.2-0.8%.

Outbreaks Typhoid fever outbreaks have become unusual in high-income countries.
- North America (657, 4427, 7370, 7429, 8343). At a restaurant in New York in 2000, seven cases were traced to an immigrant worker. At a family gathering in 1990, food prepared by a carrier infected 6% (17/293) of attendees. At a hotel in New York in 1989, orange juice prepared by a carrier caused 67 infections. At a fast-food restaurant in Maryland in 1986, shrimp salad prepared by a carrier caused 10 cases. At a takeout food service in San Antonio, Tex., in 1981, a carrier caused 80 cases.
- Europe (7660, 7681, 8288). At a restaurant in France in 2003, salad was the vehicle implicated in seven cases; no breaks in hygiene were found, and none of the seven food workers had a history of typhoid fever, but one had visited an endemic country a year before, and the fourth of six stool samples grew serovar Typhi. He was freed of serovar Typhi by quinolone treatment for 4 weeks followed by a cholecystectomy (for stones) and a second course of quinolones. In northern Spain in 1988–1994, a casual food handler and carrier caused 70 infections. At a public school in Madrid, Spain, in 1991, salad or custard prepared by a carrier caused cases in 54 students.

Shigella. Humans are reservoirs, and infected food workers can contaminate ready-to-eat food. In high-income countries, *Shigella* is rarely recovered from stool samples of healthy food workers. In Tokyo, Japan, yield in food workers has decreased from 0.3% in 1961 to almost zero since the mid-1970s (8316). In Jordan, 1.4% of 283 food handlers shed *Shigella* (123). Many point-source outbreaks have been reported (123, 1767, 2075, 2626, 3222, 4386, 7551).

***Vibrio. V. cholerae* (2809, 4049, 4422, 7145).** Street food vendors, food handlers, and kitchen helpers can be sources of *V. cholerae* O1. In the United States, cantaloupe sliced by an asymptomatic food handler caused two *V. cholerae* O1 infections. In Guatemala in 1993, in a study of 26 patients hospitalized with urban cholera and 52 age-, sex-, and neighborhood-matched controls, consumption of street-vended food items was a significant risk. At a construction canteen in Singapore, seafood handled by two food workers (one symptomatic, one inapparent) caused an outbreak with 37 confirmed *V. cholerae* O1 infections. **V. parahaemolyticus (2808, 7326, 8387).** In Singapore in 1977–1980, 2% (38/2,036) of food handlers shed *V. parahaemolyticus*. In Tokyo, Japan, in 1962, 7% (14/200) of sushi cooks and 82% (107/130) of kitchen utensils grew *V. parahaemolyticus*. At a Thai boarding school in 1998, fish balls implicated in an outbreak were likely contaminated by kitchen utensils and food handlers, one of whom grew *V. parahaemolyticus*.

Y. enterocolitica **(5215).** Food workers have rarely been implicated. At a camp in New York State in 1981, infected kitchen workers were the likely source in a food-borne outbreak of *Y. enterocolitica*.

Protozoa
Cryptosporidium **(6058).** In high-income countries, the main hazard is contamination at farm or slaughter. Few reports address *C. parvum* in food workers; oocysts are infective when shed. At a university cafeteria in the United States in 1998, an infected food handler was implicated in an outbreak with 92 diarrhea cases.

Cyclospora. In high-income countries, the main hazard is imported food that is contaminated with *C. cayetanensis* at the farm. Oocysts from workers are not immediately infective when shed.

Entamoeba **(123, 7859).** In low-income countries, 1–10% of food handlers or vendors shed *E. histolytica/dispar* with feces. Cysts are infective when shed. Unlike *Cyclospora*, imported food is not a reported epidemic vehicle.

Giardia **(123, 5071, 6051, 7859, 8074).** In low-income countries, ~0.5-5% of food handlers or vendors shed *G. lamblia* with feces. Cysts are infective when shed. Food handlers are a source of outbreaks, including in high-income countries. At the cafeteria of a large insurance company in the United States in 1990, an infected food handler caused 27 cases (18 confirmed and 9 suspected), likely by preparing raw vegetables, cold meats, and cheeses for the salad bar (5071). At a nursing home in Minnesota in 1986, spread by food and person-to-person contact caused 88 cases in residents, staff, and children in day care; the index ill food handler had an infected toddler in day care.

Helminths
Food vendors in low-income countries can harbor *Ascaris* and *Trichuris* (7859). Eggs are not infective when shed, however.

T. solium **(2440, 3492, 6578, 6617, 6652).** Enteric *T. solium* is prevalent in ~0.2-2% of people in low-income countries where pork is consumed. Street vendors, food handlers, and household aids in or from endemic areas, by shedding eggs, are a potential source of cysticercosis for customers and household members.

SKIN-BLOOD CLUSTER, CATERING
Pot-and-pan workers seem to be at risk of injury and contact dermatitis. Skin infections in workers can be sources of food poisoning in clients. Workers should report wound and skin infections and flulike illness to management.

S. aureus **(303, 1613, 3364).** Pot-and-pan workers with staphylococcal skin infections or nasal carriage are the main sources of enterotoxigenic *S. aureus*. About one third to one half of *S. aureus* from carriers (see section 14.1) are enterotoxigenic. Alternative sources include cross-contamination and contamination at the farm. For toxin production and food poisoning, contaminated foods typically need mishandling during preparation (temperature and time abuses).

Outbreaks Although outbreaks are frequent, food workers are infrequently confirmed as sources, likely because many small outbreaks (e.g., in households) are not reported.
- United States (1957, 5830, 6251). In Rhode Island in 1990, an infected food handler who prepared ham for school lunches was the source for food poisoning at several elementary schools, for attack rates of 18–47%. At a church gathering in Minas Gerais, ~4,000 of 8,000 attendees contracted staphylococcal food poisoning from a menu of chicken, beef, rice, and beans that was pre-prepared by eight food handlers who all tested postive for enterotoxigenic *S. aureus*. At a birthday party in Brazil, a food handler who grew enterotoxigenic *S. aureus* from nose, fingernails, and a healing neck infection, was source for 12 cases of food poisoning, and a cake cream filling was the confirmed vehicle.
- Asia (8005). At a high school in Taiwan, *S. aureus* from the hand wound of a food worker caused 10 cases of food poisoning among 356 students, for an attack rate of 3%.

S. pyogenes (GAS) **(3849).** Workers with GAS in the throat (carriers and sore throat) or in hand lesions are a source of epidemic pharyngitis from handled, typically cold foods such as egg salads.

Outbreaks
- North America (4878). At a picnic in Arizona, 45% (63/139) of attendees contracted culture-confirmed pharyngitis from potato salad that was implicated epidemiologically and confirmed microbiologically.

- Asia (4832). At a company sports meeting in Japan in 1996, 192 of 255 employees contracted pharyngitis (90%) or food poisong (10%) from a lunch meal that yielded GAS; however, all 10 food workers tested negative for GAS after 1 month.
- Europe (1468, 2706). At a church party in Sweden in 1990, sandwiches prepared in a crowded, hot kitchen, by persons who grew erythrogenic, exotoxin-producing GAS, were likely the vehicle for 122 (72%) GAS disease cases among 169 attendees. At a naval school in France in 1992, eggs (oeufs mimosa) prepared by a GAS throat carrier were likely the vehicle for streptococcal pharyngitis in 212 clients, for an attack rate of 7.5% (212/2,800).

12.6 HEALTH AND LABORATORY WORK

Handwashing is the single most effective hygiene practice for minimizing health care associated infections.
Ministry of Health (5115)

Health work includes work by physicians, surgeons, anesthetists, dentists, medical students, nurses, midwives, phlebotomists, physiotherapists, and rescue workers, and, in a broader sense, laboratory technicians, clinical microbiologists, and pathologists. For cleaning and waste work, see section 12.7; for nosocomial infections, see section VI.

Exposure (4032, 6791). The health care industry is huge. In the United States, the health sector employs ~9 million workers, including ~0.5 million in dental health (dentists, hygienists, and technicians) and ~0.5 million in laboratories. Median numbers of health workers per 10^5 population in high- (and low-) income countries are: physicians, 200–500 (100); dentists, 40–70 (20); and nurses, 600–900 (80–200).

Health workers are exposed to care-seeking persons, clinical materials (secretions, excreta, organs, and tissues), objects (e.g., syringes, sharp instruments, clothes, and beddings), and procedures (e.g., venipuncture and recapping of needles), in a variety of settings, including medical, dental, podiatric, and alternative care offices, ambulances, emergency rooms, and laboratories (Box 12.1).

Accidental injury (1523, 2842, 3286, 5109, 5401) (http://www.osha-slc.gov/SLTC/needlestick/index.html). At the highest risk of percutaneous injury are nurses, surgeons, and midwives. By setting, reported injury rates are ~10/100 workers per year, ~30/100 occupied beds per year, and ~2 per worker-year.

Laboratory hazards include aerosols and mucosal splash, e.g., from sonication, centrifugation, or opening of cultures with concentrated or sporulating agents, sharp objects, oral pipetting, and smoking or eating at the workplace. Reported laboratory accident rates are ~8/100 person-years.

Infections (Box 12.5). Health workers are among the best-studied occupational groups. Agents are reviewed in the following sections.

- Trauma (543, 2701, 5109, 6909). From an infective source in high-income countries, susceptible workers acquired infections at rates per 100 injuries of 0.3 (HIV) to 0.5–2 (HCV), and 1–40 (HBV, 1–5 from HBe-negative, but 20–40 from HBe-positive source). In low-income countries, corresponding risk estimates are of 0.2–0.5 (HIV), 6 (HCV), and 20–40 (HBV).
- Laboratory (2944, 5910, 7812, 7915). By mail survey among United States laboratory workers, the rate of infections from the laboratory was estimated at 0.15–0.35 per 100 per year. In the United Kingdom, clinical laboratories self-reported work-acquired infections at rates per 100 person-years of 0.04–0.1 (1980s) to <0.02 (1990s). Of ~3,900 laboratory infections gathered in 1949–1974, 27% were viral, 60% were bacterial, and 9% were fungal.

Sources. Health workers are victims and sources (vectors) of infection. Unwashed hands can spread nosocomial

Box 12.5 Main agents and infections from health work, including laboratory, by cluster	
Droplet-air	• Vaccine preventable: *Influenzavirus*, MMR, VZV; *B. pertussis*, *C. diphtheriae*, *M. tuberculosis*, *N. meningitidis* • Vaccine nonpreventable: AdV, EBV, *Enterovirus*, PIV, RSV, SARS-CoV; *Legionella*; *Pneumocystis*; cultured fungi
Feces-food	HAV, *Norovirus*; *H. pylori*, *Shigella* (pediatrics), VRE; endemic areas: *S. enterica* serovar Typhi, *V. cholerae*
Zoonotic	Viral encephalitis, VHF from Arenaviridae, Bunyaviridae, Filoviridae, Flaviviridae, Rhabdoviridae, Togaviridae; *B. anthracis*, *Borrelia*, *Brucella*, *Coxiella*, *Francisella*, Rickettsiales, *Streptobacillus*, *Y. pestis*; *Leishmania*, *Plasmodium*, *Trypanosoma*
Environmental	Laboratories: *Burkholderia*, *Leptospira*; *Strongyloides*
Skin-blood	Prions; CMV, HBV, HCV, HIV and related retroviruses, HSV1; *S. aureus* (MRSA), *S. pyogenes*; *Candida*, *Trichophyton*; *S. scabiei*

agents, in particular, MRSA and *Enterobacteriaceae*, but also respiratory viruses. Breaks in standard procedures can also transmit blood-borne agents such as plasmodia.

Likewise, laboratories can be sources of viable viruses and bacteria (1246, 2217), perhaps fungi.

- In 2003–2004, SARS-CoV was reported to have escaped on three occasions from laboratories in Asia. In 2004, exposure to EBOV was reported in a United States and a Russian laboratory.
- In March 2005, Canadian health authorities detected Influenzavirus A/H2N2 (subtype of the 1957–1958 pandemic) in a test sample from a U.S. reference laboratory that in October 2004–February 2005 had erroneously sent such samples (instead of A/H3N2 and A/H1N1 that circulated at the time) to >3,500 laboratories in 16 countries. However, all samples were destroyed, and virus did not escape.
- Variola virus survives frozen at laboratories in Georgia (United States), Novosibirsk (Russia), and perhaps elsewhere.
- A supplier in the United States in 2004 shipped living instead of inactivated *B. anthracis* from Maryland to California for research.

Cross-contamination and mislabeling of specimens (1765, 6632, 6901) are further laboratory hazards. In a United Kingdom laboratory, working stocks of "*Rhinovirus*" turned out to contain poliovirus type 1. Blood culture bottles improperly vented by a technician with impetigo of the hand led to a pseudo-outbreak with 10 bacteremias due to *S. pyogenes* and *S. aureus*.

Prevention. Preventive measures include education, vaccinations, precautions, PEP, good laboratory practice, good waste disposal practice, and building technology (e.g., airflow and isolation rooms). **Vaccines (747, 1278, 1523, 5115, 6473)** (Table 12.2). The vaccine status of health workers should be reviewed on entry into service and periodically during service, and updated when indicated. By national guidelines and epidemic risks, vaccines to consider for health workers include HAV, HBV, *Influenzavirus*, MMR, polio, rabies, and VZV, as well as BCG, dT (possibly p_a), meningococci, *S. enterica* serovar Typhi, and *V. cholerae*. Health and laboratory workers, like uniformed services (see section 12.3), may benefit from targeted (noncommercial) vaccines in addition to routine vaccines, that protect from particular biohazards and potential weaponized agents, e.g., arboviral encephalitis, viral hemorrhagic fever, and variola. **Standard precautions (817, 3296, 4032, 5101, 5109, 5115).** Standard precautions are "good practices" in health work, mainly hand hygiene, consistent and appropriate use of protective gear (gloves and gown, and eventually face mask and eye shield) for any exposure to blood (e.g., venipuncture), solutions (e.g., breaking of ampouls), and secretions (e.g., suction), asepsis, safe disposal of one-time-use sharp objects in containers with device autodestruction, and proper decontamination or autoclavation of reuse material. For contact and droplet precautions, see section 14.1. **Hand hygiene.** Hand hygiene is crucial. Hands can be washed under running water with soapy solutions, or hands can be rubbed waterless, with gel or liquid disinfectant carried by workers all the time. Indications for hand hygiene include (i) before and after patient contacts, e.g., taking blood pressure and wound inspection; (ii) before and after procedures, e.g., venipuncture and insertion of a urinary catheter; (iii) before donning sterile gloves and after having removed gloves; and (iv) whenever hands are dirty, before leaving the toilet, before eating, or when having touched likely infective objects. **PEP (747, 5115, 5714).** Consider PEP, including for prions (wash immediately); cytomegalovirus (CMV, possibly CMV-Ig), HAV (vaccine, Ig), HBV (vaccine and HBV-Ig), HCV (possibly antivirals), HIV (antiretroviral combinations), measles (vaccine, Ig), rabies (wash immediately, vaccine, rabies-Ig), VZV (VZV-Ig); *C. tetani* (vaccine, tetanus-Ig), *C. diphtheriae* (benzathin-penicillin), *N. meningitidis* (vaccine, rifampin). **Clinical material.** Clinical material should be considered infective, including of human, animal, or environmental origin, and for assembling, packaging, transporting, opening, and processing. For shipping (8140), international regulations may apply, including three-layered packaging: a core (labeled) receptacle, a middle (absorbing) layer, and an outer (durable) case; the envelope must show a biohazard logo. **Biosafety levels (BSL) (1159, 1523, 3286, 5502)** (http://www.cdc.gov/od/ohs/biosfty/, http://www4.od.nih/oba/, and http://www2.niaid.nih.gov/biodefense/bandc_priority.htm) (Table 12.3). BSL were developed to minimize infections from work with agents in office, hospital, and reference laboratories. Levels are cumulative, that is, BSL3 includes measures from BSL1 and BSL2. For research, the National Institutes of Health proposed similar risk groups (RG1–4). Agents with high weaponizing potential require BSL4: *Arenaviridae*, *Filoviridae*, *Poxviridae*, *Hantavirus*, DENV, RVFV; *B. anthracis*, *F. tularensis*, *C. botulinum*, and *Y. pestis*.

DROPLET-AIR CLUSTER, HEALTH WORK

Patients, workers, and visitors continuously move in and out of acute-care hospitals. Such fluctuations, concomitant community outbreaks, and season confound the intramural (within hospitals and laboratories) spread of infections.

Table 12.2 Measures to consider for health workers on entry and after exposure, by agent or infection[a]

Agent or infection	Suggested measures[b]
Bordetella pertussis	On entry: review vaccine, boost ($p_{acellular}$) if laboratory work with *Bordetella*.
	Exposure: if asymptomatic, recommend chemoprophylaxis; if ill, exclude from work until 5 days from start of antibiotic therapy.
Corynebacterium diphtheriae	On entry: review vaccine; boost if necessary (dT).
Clostridium tetani	On entry: review vaccine; boost if necessary (dT).
CMV	On entry: discuss risks for neonates, transplant recipients, and immune compromised patients.
Enterovirus	Shedding: exclude from neonates and immune compromised patients until recovered.
HAV	On entry: review vaccine; vaccinate if fecal peril, e.g., infants, incontinent patients, in laboratory.
	Exposure: evaluate need for vaccine and standard Ig; if ill, exclude from food and patient work until 7 days from onset of jaundice.
HBV	On entry: review markers, vaccinations; boost if parenteral or mucosal peril; retest for anti-HBs.
	Carrier (HBsAg positive): counsel or exclude from work with parenteral or mucosal peril.
	Exposure: evaluate need for tests, vaccine, and hyperimmune Ig.
HCV	On entry: review markers; archive serum.
	Exposure or infected (anti-HCV): offer tests; evaluate periodically. If ill, no restrictions apply.
HSV	Oral herpes: evaluate need to exclude from high-risk patients. Hand herpes: exclude from clinical work until recovered. Genital herpes: no restrictions apply.
HIV	On entry: review status; archive serum.
	Infected (HIV positive): refer for treatment. If pregnant, consider CMV reactivation and shedding.
	Exposure: evaluate need for testing and PEP (antiretrovirals).
Influenzavirus	For each flu season: offer vaccine according to national policy or for work with high-risk patients.
Measles virus	On entry: vaccinate (MMR), if no proof of two age-adequate doses or laboratory tests of immunity.
	Exposure: if susceptible, vaccinate (days 0-3 from e_0) or give standard Ig (days 4-7 from e_0) and exclude from work (days 5-19 from e_0). If ill, exclude from work (days 0-7 from start of rash).
Mumps virus	On entry: review vaccine, vaccinate (MMR) if age is <45 years.
	Exposure: if susceptible, exclude from work (days 10-24 from e_0).
	Parotitis: exclude for 9 days.
Neisseria meningitidis	On entry: vaccinate if laboratory work with *N. meningitidis*.
	Exposure (contact, e.g., resuscitation): give PEP (chemoprophylaxis); consider vaccine (A, C).
	Infected: give antibiotics and exclude from work for ≥24 h.
Prion	On entry: counsel on precautions with high-risk patients and tissues.
Rubella virus	On entry: vaccinate (MMR), if no proof of two age-adequate doses, or laboratory test of immunity.
	Exposure: if susceptible, test and exclude from work (days 7-21 from e_0), If pregnant, consider standard Ig. If ill, exclude from work (days 0-7 from start of rash).
SARS-CoV	On entry: counsel on precautions; archive serum.
	Exposure: monitor (symptoms, temperature twice a day).
Staphylococcus aureus	Carrier: if not linked to spread, no restrictions apply; if MRSA, hand hygiene is essential.
	Skin lesions: exclude from food and patient work until recovered.
Streptococcus pyogenes	Infected: exclude from food and patient work until treated for ≥24 h.
Mycobacterium tuberculosis	On entry and periodically: skin test; if converter, evaluate for disease (clinically, chest X ray).
	Active disease: exclude from work until clinically and microbiologically considered noninfectious.
VZV	On entry: vaccinate and test response if history is blank for varicella and worker is seronegative.
	Exposure: if susceptible, exclude from work (days 8-22 from e_0) or allow work with face mask. If pregnant, give hyperimmune (or standard) Ig (days 0-4 from e_0).
	Varicella: exclude from work until lesions are dry. Localized zoster: cover lesions and exclude from high-risk patients until lesions are dry.
Conjunctivitis	Exclude from patient work until discharge ceases.
Diarrhea	Exclude from food and patient work until recovered; if *Norovirus*, negative stool tests desirable.
Pediculosis	Head lice: exclude from patient work until treated and confirmed cured.

[a] From references 747, 4032, 5109, and 5115.
[b] e_0 day of first exposure; Ig, immunoglobulin.

Table 12.3 Biosafety levels (BSL) for work in laboratories

BSL	Risk and agents	Task and precautions	Laboratory requirements
1	Oral; commensal or low-virulent agents readily treated or prevented, e.g., *Escherichia coli*	Office laboratory. Universal precautions (gloves), no eating or drinking in laboratory.	Sink for hand washing, water-impermeable work bench
2	Percutaneous; agents for which vaccines or antimicrobials are available, e.g., HBV, measles virus, *Salmonella*, *Toxoplasma*	Hospital, public, or commercial laboratory. Staff is regularly trained and proficient. Sharps precaution, hand (gloves) and face (mask)protection, gown, null sera archive, vaccines updated.	Lockable doors, biohazard signs, safety cabinets, autoclaves
3	Aerosols (e.g., from culture); life-threatening agents difficult to treat, e.g., JEV, *Mycobacterium tuberculosis*, fungi	Reference or production laboratory. Staff wears respiratory protection and gowns are decontaminated for laundry.	Isolation zone, entry from double doors, controlled (inward) air flow
4	Highly infective or lethal viruses (VHF), e.g., CCHFV, EBOV, Lassa fever virus	Dedicated, national security laboratory. Entrance clothing and exit showers.	Separate building, one-way locks, self-contained utilities

Viruses: Vaccine Preventable

These include *Influenzavirus*, measles, mumps, and rubella viruses (MMR), and VZV. Incubation periods that exceed length of stay in hospitals obscure the recognition of nosocomial spread or of outbreaks.

***Influenzavirus* (2168, 5669).** Flulike illness, confirmed influenza, and inapparent shedders should be distinguished. Nosocomial outbreaks have been documented. In a large (1,156 bed) hospital, A/H3N2 infected 118 workers and 49 patients, and nosocomial spread was assumed. In four hospitals in Glasgow, United Kingdom, in a preepidemic (October) to postepidemic (January) period of 1993–1994, 23% (120/518) of health workers seroconverted, including 59% (71/120) who did not report influenza. In contrast, 31% (161/518) workers reported influenza, including 70% (112/161) who remained seronegative. Altogether 8% (42/518) of staff seroconverted *and* took leave for influenza (for a median of 4 days).

- Workers as victims (591, 875). Evidence is limited. During the A/H5N1 (bird flu) epidemic in 1997, patient-to-staff spread was suggested by higher seroreactivity rates in staff exposed to patients with A/H5N1 infection (4% or 8/217) compared with nonexposed staff (1% or 2/309). A vaccinated woman hospitalized for influenza complications shed A/H3N2 virus for ≥4 days from admission, passing influenza to her attending, vaccinated physician, but to none of 28 exposed, nonvaccinated workers.
- Workers as sources (2260, 4685, 5109, 6460). Evidence is circumstantial. Of 17 influenza outbreaks in U.S. hospitals in 1959–1994, staff-to-patient spread was implicated in 5, with 1–49 (mean, 14) cases per outbreak. Vaccination of patients and caregivers is thought to reduce morbidity of patients in long-stay facilities.
- Vaccination (1083, 5109, 5986, 6639, 8160). At geriatric facilities, vaccination of workers rather than patients has seemed to reduce patient mortality. Reduced patient mortality by vaccination of workers was confirmed in a randomized, controlled trial, although confirmed infections were similarly frequent in the vaccine (5.4%) and nonvaccine (6.7%) groups. A randomized trial at Baltimore teaching hospitals failed to show the impact of vaccination among young, healthy workers; while 2% (3/180) of vaccinees but 13% (24/179) of controls had serological evidence of infection, both groups reported comparable numbers of febrile respiratory illness days (29 versus 41/100), and absence days (10 versus 21/100). Another randomized, controlled trial demonstrated that vaccination of workers reduced absenteeism from respiratory tract infections by 28%. Despite these limitations, yearly vaccination of health workers is recommended.
- Recommended BSL is 2 (human strains) to 3 (avian strains). A few laboratory infections have been reported.

Measles virus (4767, 5328, 6062, 6106). Measles virus can circulate in health care settings. Nosocomial outbreaks are well documented. Besides noncompliance with vaccines, high infectivity in the prerash period and delayed recognition of cases are major threats. During a community outbreak in Florida in 1985, hospitals were sites of frequent transmission. However, at a hospital that complied with strict respiratory isolation, secondary spread among in-patients did not occur.

- Workers as victims (305, 1771, 5109, 5583, 8409). By age and vaccine coverage, 0–7% of health workers in high-income countries are nonimmune. Patient-to-staff spread seems more important than staff-to-patient. In the United States in the 1980s, health workers were two to eight times more likely to contract measles than the general population, and 4% of measles were acquired nosocomially (2% in outpatient settings and 2% in hospital). On entry into services, workers should present records, and two vaccine doses (preferably MMR) should be completed. Exposed staff vaccinated once should receive a second dose within 72 h from e_0 (first exposure day). Exposed nonvaccinated staff should be vaccinated and excluded from work, at least for days 5–19 from e_0.

- Unrecognized patients (e.g., travelers, migrants, or children from endemic areas) bring measles to hospitals, including by short, overnight stays for observation.
- Recommended BSL is 2.

Mumps virus (2409, 5109, 8063). Nosocomial spread is infrequent, but a risk for workers and patients exists, and nosocomial outbreaks have been reported. In a pediatric hospital in the United States, a child patient, a physiotherapist, and a nurse contracted mumps from an immigrant with mumps.

- Workers as victims (305, 5109, 5583, 8063). About 3–17% of health workers in high-income countries are nonimmune. Although most mumps in workers is community acquired, mumps from nosocomial exposure has been reported. On entry into services, workers should present vaccine records, and two doses (preferably as MMR) should be completed. Exposed, susceptible workers should be excluded from work for days 10–24 from e_0.
- Patients have occasionally acquired mumps in hospitals, mainly from visitors during community outbreaks (8063).
- Recommended BSL is 2.

Rubella virus (3298, 5960, 7189). In a metropolitan hospital in California, nosocomial rubella occurred among 3,900 workers in departments who had been offered voluntary vaccination, but not among 1,400 workers of the gynecological and pediatric units who had received mandatory vaccine. Nosocomial spread is a particular hazard for pregnant patients, pregnant staff, and pregnant visitors.

- Workers as victims (305, 5109) (5583). About 2–15% of health workers in high-income countries are likely to be nonimmune. As PEP cannot fully prevent congenital infections even when Ig is administered within 48 h from e_0, emphasis is on vaccination before exposure. Because neither a history of rubella nor a history of rubella vaccination reliably predicts immunity, new workers should submit proof of immunity or be vaccinated (preferably as MMR). Infected workers should be excluded from work for days 0–7 from rash onset.
- A dietary worker was the likely source for a hospital outbreak with 47 cases among workers (5960).
- Recommended BSL is 2.

VZV (2317, 3760, 5109). Droplets and aerosols from patients with varicella are highly infectious, and less so, skin lesions from patients with zoster. Patients should be placed in air isolation, on wards remote from wards with neonates or pregnant or immune-impaired patients. Hospital outbreaks have been recorded. In a metropolitan hospital in Australia, after a community outbreak, 20 adult varicella cases were observed, including 13 cases determined to be nosocomial (nine secondary and four tertiary).

- Workers as victims (305, 1780, 4351, 5109, 5583). Most (>90%) workers in high-income countries are latently infected (seroreactive), and only ~3–4% are likely to be susceptible. As a history of varicella validly predicts past infection (predictive positive value >99%), seroscreening can be limited to workers whose history is blank (~15–25% of female workers). New, seronegative workers should be offered vaccine on employment. Exposed and susceptible workers should be excluded from work for days 8–22 from e_0; if not pregnant, they also should receive vaccine for PEP within 3 days; if pregnant, they should also receive VZV-specific Ig within 4 days.
- Nosocomial spread from staff to patients has been reported (5109).
- Recommended BSL is 2.

Viruses: Vaccine Nonpreventable

Droplets and hands from patients admitted for nonrespiratory illness and from incubating or shedding visitors and staff are the main vehicles of nosocomial spread. Groups at main risk are immune-impaired children. Staff is presumed at lower risk because of partial protection from past natural infection.

AdV (3694, 5109, 5318, 6365). Ocular and respiratory AdV can spread nosocomially.

- Epidemic keratoconjunctivitis is a nosocomial risk, including from eyes and unwashed hands of patients and workers. In an ophthalmology clinic, AdV was cultured from the hands of physicians with epidemic keratoconjunctivitis, even after they had washed hands.
- Rhinopharyngitis and pneumonia due to AdV can be acquired in hospitals. Mainly at risk are immune-impaired patients, but also nursing staff. Immune-

impaired children can shed respiratory AdV with feces for ≥3 weeks.

- A few laboratory-acquired AdV infections are also reported. Recommended BSL is 2.

Epstein-Barr virus (EBV) (2752, 5109). Patient-to-staff spread has occasionally been reported, but the risk seems small. In an obstetric and gynecology clinic over 4 weeks, 9 (31%) of 29 health workers contracted EBV infection, presumedly from poorly washed coffee cups. Recommended BSL is 2.

Enterovirus **(387, 1523, 7302).** Given recurrent seasonal outbreaks, spread in hospitals and laboratories seems infrequent and concentrated to neonatal units. At a Tokyo clinic in 1996, four neonates contracted echovirus type 7 nosocomially, but none of nursing staff. Recommended BSL is 2.

Parainfluenza virus (PIV) (5125, 5417, 6926). Hospital outbreaks have been recorded. During an outbreak among neonates in an intensive care unit (ICU), 2 of 52 workers yielded PIV from the nasopharynx. Patients, visitors, staff, and surfaces can be sources, and PIV can spread patient-to-patient and staff-to-patient. Immune-impaired patients are at risk, including at hospital outpatient departments. Control may need air isolation or cohorting. Recommended BSL is 2.

Parvovirus B19 (PVB19) (2011, 4491, 4563, 5094, 5109, 6155, 6772). In high-income countries, ~50% of workers may be immune to PVB19, including pregnant women. PVB19 appears to spread mainly staff-to-staff and patient-to-patient, infrequently patient-to-staff. Hospital outbreaks have been reported. By setting, reported attack rates in exposed staff are ~3-45%. For PVB19 in pregnancy, see section 14.7. Laboratory infections have been reported. Recommended BSL is 2.

Respiratory syncytial virus (RSV) (99, 678, 3085). During epidemic waves, 15–20% of staff can shed RSV inapparently. RSV can survive on the skin for up to 20 min. Hands of staff can transmit RSV in hospitals. Hand washing is a powerful means of transmission prevention. RSV was detectable in air by NAT up to 7 m away from patients. Recommended BSL is 2.

SARS-CoV (2803, 2853, 4237, 4238, 4483, 6644). Care for patients with SARS emerged as a hazard in the 2003 epidemic, when in Asia ~20–50% of suspected, probable, or confirmed cases were health workers. At 16 Hong Kong hospitals in 2003, attack rates were 0–2% (mean, 0.3%) in medicotechnical staff, 0–5% (1%) in nurses, and 0–13% (3%) in support staff. High-risk care activities included suction of the airway and intubation of patients, other contacts with mucous membranes or respiratory secretions, and even manipulation of oxygen masks. In Toronto, Canada, in 2003, 7 (10%) of 69 intensive-care staff contracted SARS from exposure that had lasted from 11 min to 22 h. Health workers who comply with preventive measures (hands, N95 masks, goggles, caps, gloves, and gowns) can protect themselves and prevent nosocomial spread.

Laboratory (4421, 4535). A laboratory infection has been documented in Singapore, through work with a WNV culture heavily contaminated with SARS-CoV. Laboratories can be potential sources of SARS-CoV. Recommended BSL is 3.

Bacteria: Vaccine Preventable

***B. pertussis* (478, 1250, 1432).** Nonrecognized and nonisolated cases of *B. pertussis* are major sources of nosocomial spread and outbreaks. Modes of spread include worker-to-patient, patient-to-worker, and worker-to-worker. For patient-to-patient spread, average periods in the hospital may be too short.

- Workers as victims (99, 478, 1250, 1432, 1803, 1832, 5109, 8274). By location and service, up to 50% of health workers may be susceptible to *B. pertussis*. Health workers may or may not be at greater risk of pertussis than the population. Inapparent infections have been documented in workers, for reported seroconversion rates of ~1 (range, 0–4)/100 per year. At the children's hospital of Cincinnati, during a pertussis community outbreak, 84 workers were clinically diagnosed with pertussis, and ~17% (>620 of >3,760) of all employees were given antibiotics for PEP. Exposed and susceptible workers should receive PEP, preferrably macrolides. Exposure is defined by close (within 1 m) contact with a pertussis patient for >1 h, or sharing the room with a patient (*B. pertussis* DNA was detected in the air up to 4 m away from patients).

- Workers as sources (478, 4454). Workers >50 years of age with cough for >2 weeks should be suspected sources. Immune-impaired patients are at increased risk of pertussis. An outbreak among eight pediatricians and five nurses resulted in six pertussis cases in neonates.

- Laboratory infections from inhalation have been reported (1523). Recommended BSL is 2.

***C. diphtheriae* (3169, 5109).** Diphtheria has become rare in high-income countries, but health workers should be prepared to deal with cases, e.g., from endemic areas. Corynebacteria other than *C. diphtheriae* isolated in nosocomial venues include *C. jeikeium* or *C. striatum*.

- Workers as victims (4229, 4568, 5109). From antitoxin titer <0.01/ml, 10–50% of health workers are expected to be nonimmune, in particular, the 20–50-year age group. Although patient-to-worker spread has been reported, the risk is considered small. Throat and nasopharyngeal cultures from 328 Swedish workers who nursed patients with diphtheria or carriers were all negative, as were cultures from 67 Finnish health workers in contact with three cases. Health workers should complete a primary vaccine series (3 doses, preferably in combination with tetanus), and a booster every 10 years (at least one at age 50 years).
- Cutaneous and throat diphtheria from the laboratory have been reported (1523, 2687, 3169). At an advanced training course in Germany in 1996, an experienced technician acquired diphtheria likely from improperly handling pure cultures; none of 25 other participants became infected. Recommended BSL is 2.

H. influenzae. Presumed risks are patient-to-patient spread, of Hib on pediatric wards and of nontypeable *H. influenzae* on respiratory or geriatric wards. In contrast, occupational infections in health and laboratory workers seem unusual. Recommended BSL is 2.

M. tuberculosis. Hospital outbreaks are well documented (844, 1238, 3127). Spread, including of multidrug-resistant (MDR) strains, can occur patient-to-patient, patient-to-worker, and, rarely, worker-to-patient.
- Workers as victims (414, 758, 844, 3081, 3524, 4822, 5713, 5788, 6759, 8047). Patient-to-worker spread is significant, in particular, in areas where tuberculosis is endemic. Risks include transportation and nursing of tuberculosis patients, nursing of HIV-infected patients and IDU, respiratory therapy and physiotherapy, and emergency care. Patients with suspected or confirmed tuberculosis should be air isolated and nursed on wards remote from immune-impaired patients. On nonisolation wards with MDR tuberculosis patients, workers were more likely to skin convert (34% or 11/32) than workers on other wards (2% or 1/47). In particular, HIV-infected patients can be a source of MDR tuberculosis in workers. In the United States in 1983, an intubated patient with cavitary pulmonary tuberculosis spending 4 h in the emergency room infected 16 (14%) of 112 health workers of whom five developed active tuberculosis. Also in the United States, a patient with a tuberculous hip abscess was source for nine secondary cases and 59 skin test conversions.
- Rates (711, 758, 5713, 8047). In New York and Boston health care facilities in 1994–1995, 2,117 (40%) of 5,232 health workers were skin reactive to tuberculin, and 30 (1.5%) of 1,960 negative workers converted, for rates/100 person-years of 1 in United States-born workers, 3.6 in foreign-born workers, and 1.6 overall. This difference suggested some nonoccupational exposure in foreign born workers. In Lima, Peru, 40 of 98 hospital physicians tested negative to tuberculin; after 1 year, 14% (5/35) of those retested converted and 5% (2/40) developed active tuberculosis, for a disease rate of 2/100 per year. Measures can reduce conversion rates to <1/100 per year or interrupt spread.
- Workers are rare sources of tuberculosis for patients (3315). At an outpatient renal dialysis center in Nevada in 2003, a hemodialysis technician with pulmonary tuberculosis exposed >400 persons and infected 29 patients and 13 staff.
- Laboratory (1523, 2944, 5804, 6759, 7664, 7915). Although difficult to define, occupational tuberculosis is a risk, including for microbiologists, laboratory technicians, pathologists, coroners, and employees of funeral homes. In the United Kingdom in 1980–1989, clinical pathologists self-reported 30 work-acquired cases, for rates of 0.02–0.04/100 person-years. Recommended BSL is 2 (acif-fast staining of smears) to 3 (culture).

***N. meningitidis* (2749, 5109, 5885).** Although reported, direct patient-to-staff spread is unusual, e.g., from mucosal splash. In contrast, the risk of carriage and invasive disease is increased in exposed workers. In the United Kingdom, by retrospective analysis, the disease attack rate in health workers was estimated at $1/10^5$, which was 25 times the population rate. Spread is prevented by wearing face masks and eye protection when close (≤1 m) to suspected or confirmed patients. Workers exposed to respiratory secretions from patients that did not complete 24 h of antibiotics should receive antibiotic PEP and vaccine, if the causative strain is vaccine preventable.

Laboratory (2995, 4486). *N. meningitidis* is an uncommon, but serious hazard. Reported disease rates in laboratories are $\sim 10/10^5$ per year, compared with $0.2/10^5$ per year in the community of similar age. PEP is advised for laboratory exposure as above. Recommended BSL is 2 (or 3, if aerosols are likely).

Vaccine Nonpreventable Bacteria
C. pneumoniae. Most *C. pneumoniae* infections are acquired in the community. Putative hazards are aerosols and contaminated surfaces. Recommended BSL is 2.

***K. pneumoniae* (3277).** *K. pneumoniae* can remain on unwashed hands of workers, so prevention is by hand hygiene. Recommended BSL is 2.

***Legionella* (778, 4557, 6200, 6349).** *Legionella* is a hazard for immune-impaired inpatients and health workers exposed to aerosols such as spa workers, physiotherapists, and dentists. At a French hot spring spa, 11% of 230 therapists had *Legionella* antibodies, and titers were significantly higher than in 904 control blood donors. In Portugal, 7% (3/42) of therapists working at one spa were reactive to one or more of five *Legionella* antigens, compared with 3% (5/172) of patients frequenting the spa and 1% (7/503) of blood donors. Mean antibody levels were highest in therapists. In North America and Europe, *Legionella* antibodies are more prevalent among dentists and dental assistants than healthy controls. However, infection seems more important in dental personnel than disease. Recommended BSL is 2 (or 3 for procedures that generate aerosols).

M. pneumoniae. Most infections are aquired in the community. Nosocomial spread seems unusual. Recommended BSL is 2.

Fungi
Major hazards are inhalation of spores in the laboratory and immune-impaired health workers.

***Blastomyces* (116, 6791).** Cultures of *B. dermatitidis* can form infectious conidia. Laboratory hazards include inhalation and injury. Laboratory infections are known from inhalation and injury. Recommended BSL is 3.

***Coccidioides* (6791).** Cultures of *C. immitis* can form infectious arthroconidia. Inhalation is a laboratory hazard. In the United States in 1969–1989, 202 laboratory infections were reported. Recommended BSL is 3.

***Cryptococcus* (1523, 2770).** Needle sticks with fungemic blood caused *C. neoformans* infections in laboratories and in a health worker. Recommended BSL is 2.

***Histoplasma* (6791).** Cultures can form infectious arthroconidia. Inhalation is a laboratory hazard. In 1969–1989, 152 laboratory infections were reported, largely from U.S. laboratories. Recommended BSL is 3.

Paracoccidioides brasiliensis. Recommended BSL is 3.

***Pneumocystis* (4331, 6065, 7770).** The concept of reactivation and animal reservoirs have hampered understanding of *Pneumocystis* for a long time. Higher antibody titers in 24 health workers exposed to AIDS patients than in 24 control health workers suggested AIDS patients as a source. Case reports and clusters and molecular epidemiology confirmed interpersonal spread of *P. jirovecii*. Patient-to-worker spread may result in colonization rather than infection. Recommended BSL is 2 (nonculture diagnostic procedures).

FECES-FOOD CLUSTER, HEALTH WORK
Unwashed hands of patients and workers can spread enteric viruses and bacteria, mainly patient-to-patient and patient-to-worker. Alternative sources of occupational diarrhea in workers include foods and drinking water. In the United Kingdom in 1996–1997, the risk of work-acquired infectious diarrhea per 100 per year was 0.03 in nurses and 0.07 in care assistants (6418).

Viruses
HAV (363, 2493, 3874, 4338, 5109, 6412). Incubating or patients with unrecognized acute HA are a source of HAV in health workers, including in ICU, nursing homes, day care centers, institutions for disabled persons and for nurses, therapists, physicians, dentists, laundry workers, and relief workers. Nosocomial outbreaks have been reported. In a neonatal ICU, 13 (20%) infants, 22 (24%) nurses, 8 other nursing staff, and 4 household contacts contracted HAV; risks included care for a patient with HAV and drinking beverages in the unit. Another outbreak in an ICU involved 15 nurses, 2 premature babies, and 1 mother. Although standard precautions can reduce risks, in high-income countries where >50% of health workers are expected to be susceptible, vaccination is recommended for work potentially exposing the worker to feces (e.g., babies, incontinent patients, and health care in camps), possibly in combination with HBV vaccine. **HAV in laboratories (1652, 1926).** In the 1950s–1970s, acute cases were reported in laboratories and in persons handling chimpanzees. Vaccination is recommended for work with HAV. Recommended BSL is 2.

***Norovirus* (3917, 4589, 8414).** *Norovirus* readily spreads person-to-person, via hands, feces, and aerosols from vomiting. Foods and surfaces are additional vehicles. Outbreaks have been reported in acute and long-stay facilities (see section 11.6). Reported attack rates in nosocomial outbreaks are 14–57% in patients and 18–41% in workers. Outbreaks can last for >2 weeks and can disrupt services, with a need to close wards for 6–11 days. Control requires hand hygiene by workers, patients, and visitors and containment of infective persons to wards remote from high-risk hospital areas. Recommended BSL is 2.

***Rotavirus* (6365, 8388).** Patients shed large amounts of virus with feces. *Rotavirus* is resilient, surviving well on hands and surfaces. Hands are a major vehicle for patient-to-patient and patient-to-worker-to-patient spread. About 2–30% of hospitalized children can acquire RoV nosocomially (>72 h after admission). At the children's hospital in Seattle, Wash., in 2001–2004, promotion of hand hygiene decreased rates of hospital-associated *Rotavirus* episodes per 1,000 discharges from ~6 to ~2.

Poliomyelitis virus. Laboratory infections with poliovirus are rare. Recommended BSL is 2.

Bacteria

In high-income hospitals, enteric bacteria, in general, pose low risks to workers.

Campylobacter. Given the frequency of tests, laboratory *Campylobacter* infections are rare. Recommended BSL is 2.

Clostridium (271, 3842). Bowel, hands, and clothes of health workers can become colonized with *C. difficile*. In Japan, 4% (12/284) of health workers were shedding *C. difficile*, compared with 9% (53/627) of ground force employees and 11% (25/234) of students. Disease is rarely reported in workers, the main risk being use of antibiotics. Recommended BSL is 2 for *C. difficile* and *C. botulinum*.

Enterobacter (3136, 8357). Hands of health workers can spread *E. cloacae*. Recommended BSL is 2.

Enterococcus (344, 760, 1275, 5109). *Enterococcus* is part of the skin and enteric flora. The agent can spread via skin and hand contacts, including vancomycin-resistant strains (VRE). Although patients with open wounds and decubitus ulcers can be colonized with VRE, the risk for health workers to become colonized with VRE is small. Infectivity of VRE is considered moderate (R_0 is estimated at 3–4). Hand hygiene is the most effective means of infection control. Recommended BSL is 2.

E. coli (7915). *E. coli* seems a rare occupational hazard. Hands of workers could spread the agent, including EHEC, ETEC, producers of extended-spectrum β-lactamase, and quinolon-resistant strains. Given the frequency of tests, laboratory infections are rare. Recommended BSL is 2 (3 for EHEC).

H. pylori (732, 3322, 4431, 8180). There is evidence for patient-to-staff spread. At a Dutch institution, longstanding employees having intense contacts with disabled persons were at increased risk of infection. In Switzerland in 1989–1998, 54 gastroenterologists who universally used gloves for endoscopy acquired *H. pylori* infections at a rate of 2.6/100 per year, compared with 0.14/100 per year in 103 age- and ethnicity-matched controls. In Germany, the seroconversion rate in 165 nursing trainees was 2.3/100 per year, clearly higher than the expected population rate. In contrast, dentists were not at increased risk. Recommended BSL is 2.

Salmonella (355). Food-borne outbreaks in hospitals have been reported. A hazard is not to wash hands, including after patient contacts and the handling of specimens. Nosocomial transmission of *S. enterica* serovar non-Typhi as well as serovar Typhi seems infrequent in high-income countries. An Asian pregnant woman with undiagnosed typhoid fever who delivered within 10 min of admission was the source of confirmed serovar Typhi for her baby and 13 secondary cases, despite isolation immediately after delivery and room disinfection. Vaccination is an option for health workers in endemic areas. Health workers who carry serovar Typhi can continue to work if they comply with hand and personal hygiene. **Laboratory (2944, 6791, 7144).** Of 6,962 laboratory infections reported internationally in 1969–1989, 2% (114) were attributed to serovar non-Typhi and 8% (551) to serovar Typhi. Of 1,393 confirmed typhoid cases reported in the United States in 1994–1999, 9 (0.6%) involved laboratory workers and their households. In the United Kingdom in 1980–1989, clinical pathologists self-reported three laboratory cases of typhoid fever. Recommended BSL is 2.

Shigella (1226, 7915). *Shigella* can spread patient-to-staff, in particular, in day care centers (see section 14.3), pediatric care units, and laboratories. A major hazard is not to wash hands. **Laboratories (2944, 6791).** In 1969–1989, 2% (138) of 6,962 internationally reported laboratory infections were due to *Shigella*. In the United Kingdom in 1980–1989, clinical pathologists self-reported 35 infections, for a rate of 0.03/100 person-years. Recommended BSL is 2.

V. cholerae (1484, 1523, 2812). Outbreaks of *V. cholerae* in hospitals have been reported, mainly in pediatric or psychiatric units, via hand or close contacts. Standard precautions can prevent spread. Laboratory infections are unusual; perhaps the first occurred in 1886, in Robert Koch's laboratory in Berlin. Recommended BSL is 2.

Fungi

Microsporidia (5256, 7731). Evidence is scant. In a Bangkok, Thailand, orphanage, the prevalence of asymptomatic, intestinal microsporidiasis in child health workers was 2% (2/105). A laboratory worker contracted *Encephalitozoon cuniculi* keratoconjunctivitis 3 weeks after concentrated culture supernatant splashed into his eyes; one year later, one cornea remained opaque. Recommended BSL is 2.

Protozoa

Health workers seem to rarely acquire *C. parvum*, *C. cayetanensis*, *E. histolytica*, *G. lamblia*, *Isospora belli*, and *T. gondii* from work (935, 3286, 6791). A main risk is inadvertent ingestion in the laboratory. For *T. gondii*, the risk of infection from U.S. laboratories is estimated at 4/100 person-years; mainly research workers seem at risk. Recommended BSL for these protozoa is 2.

Helminths
A hazard is ingestion from handling of stool or tissues that contain infective ova or larvae (3286). Recommended BSL is 2 (*Ascaris*, *Trichuris*, *Taenia*, and *Trichinella*).

ZOONOTIC CLUSTER, HEALTH WORK
Risks (6473, 7338). Most BSL 3–4 agents are in this cluster. Major hazards are injury and inhalation. Sources include viremic patients, infective tissues, and laboratory animals (rodents and monkeys). Exposed workers should be aware of risks. Accidents should be reported by a PEP plan. At a U.S. Army research laboratory in 1989–2002, in workers fully vaccinated and treated prophylactically, 5 (2%) of 234 exposures to bioterror agents resulted in disease, one case each of chikungunya fever, vaccinia, glanders, Q fever, and suspected VEEV infection. Note that none of the workers contracted anthrax or plague.

The focus in the following section is on laboratory infections. For viral hemorrhagic fevers, see section 17.8.

Viruses
Arenaviridae **(1159, 1523).** Infections in laboratories have been reported. Except LCMV, recommended BSL is 4, including for GUAV, JUNV, Lassa virus, Machupo virus, and Sabia virus. **JUNV (8028).** In Argentina in 20 years, 35 of ~280 people working with the virus developed clinical illness, three died. Seroconversions and mild illnesses were also documented. **LCMV (41, 2107, 3337, 7763).** Recommended BSL is 3. Over a dozen laboratory infections have occurred, including from exposure to Syrian hamsters (*Mesocricetus auratus*), hamster cells, and mice (*Mus musculus*). Outbreaks have occurred in laboratories in the United States and Germany.

Bunyaviridae **(1159, 1523).** Infections have been reported in laboratories and hospitals. Recommended BSL is 3 for *Hantavirus*, Oropouche virus, and RVFV, and 4 for CCHFV. **CCHFV (166, 1347, 2418, 2419, 5717).** Although by 1999 at least eight laboratory infections were recorded and including one death, the risk is greater for health workers who are exposed to secretions and blood from CCHF patients. Recommended BSL is 4. **Hantavirus.** In research laboratory workers in the 1970s–1980s, infections with cosmopolitan, rat-associated SEOV were reported in the United Kingdom, Belgium, Russia, Sinagpore, and Japan (1897, 4475, 7641, 8253). Old World viruses (e.g., DOBV, HTNV, PUUV) seem a minor laboratory hazard, except perhaps HTNV. New World viruses (e.g., ANDV and SNV) (1120, 5504, 5673, 7512, 7846, 8038). Although hantavirus pulmonary syndrome has been diagnosed in health workers, and family clusters in Latin America suggested person-to-person spread, nosocomial acquisition of ANDV is unlikely, and cases or seroconversions in health workers have not been documented. **RVFV.** By 1999, 47 laboratory infections had been documented, including one death.

Filoviridae **(1159, 1523, 2462).** *Filoviridae* infections have been reported in laboratories and hospitals. Recommended BSL is 4.

Flaviviridae **(1159, 1347, 1523).** *Flaviviridae* infections in laboratories or hospitals have been reported. Major risks are summarized below. Recommended BSL is 2 for routine laboratory diagnosis of DENV, 3 for JEV, Murray Valley encephalitis virus (MVEV), Powassan virus (POWV), SLEV, TBEV, WNV, and YFV, and 4 for Kyasanur Forest disease virus (KFDV) and Omsk hemorrhagic fever virus (OHFV). **DENV (1847, 5378, 7896).** Health workers have contracted dengue by needlestick injury from viremic travelers. At least 10 laboratory infections have been recorded. **JEV.** More than 20 JEV laboratory infections have been recorded. **TBEV (7898).** At least eight TBEV laboratory infections have been recorded. In Finland, a series of laboratory infections was controlled by vaccination and improved biosafety. **WNV (1045, 2798).** At least 20 WNV laboratory infections have been recorded. Because BSL3 could hamper routine diagnostic capacities, BSL2 with modest modifications has been proposed. **YFV (1555).** In the prevaccine era, laboratory infections were a risk; >30 laboratory infections are recorded. Of note, microbiologist H. Noguchi (1876–1928), who claimed *Leptospira* to be the cause of yellow fever, died in Ghana of yellow fever that he acquired from work with icteric sera.

Paramyxoviridae. Recommended BSL is 4 for NDV. **NDV (1523).** Several laboratory infections with NDV have been reported. A technician acquired culture-confirmed NDV in Malaysia, from grinding chicken in the laboratory and droplets that came into his eyes.

Reoviridae. Recommended BSL is 2 for Colorado tick fever virus (CTFV). **CTFV (3981).** At least 16 laboratory infections with CTFV have been recorded from work with viremic blood.

Rhabdoviridae. Recommended BSL is 2 (routine tests) or 3 (production and research) for rabies virus and VSV. **Rabies virus (7482, 8218).** Some laboratory infections with rabies virus have been reported. In New York in 1977, a technician who had received a primary vaccine series and annual boosters developed rabies, 5 months after the last booster. **VSV (1523).** Of 46 VSV laboratory infections, 31 were reported from a single institution.

***Togaviridae* (1159)**. Recommended BSL is 3 for Chikungunya virus (CHIKV), EEEV, Mayaro virus (MAYV), O'nyong-nyong virus (ONNV), SFV, VEEV, and WEEV. **CHIKV (6473).** By 1999, 39 CHIKU laboratory infections had been reported. **MAYV (3771).** Several laboratory infections with MAYU have been recorded. A worker became infected 6 days after preparing antigen, probably through inhalation. **VEEV (6473).** Inhalation of VEEV is a laboratory hazard. By 1999, 150 laboratory infections had been reported, including one death.

Bacteria

***A. phagocytophilum* (909).** The recommended BSL for culture of *A. phagocytophilum* is 3.

***B. anthracis* (1246, 1523, 4621).** The recommended BSL for *B. anthracis* by procedure is 2 or 3. The main laboratory hazards are inhalation or injury. Over 100 cases have been documented in research, production, and diagnostic laboratories. In California in 2004, a laboratory unknowingly received a suspension of viable rather than inactivated agents from another laboratory for research; the suspension was centrifuged on an open bench and 12 workers were potentially exposed, but no infections resulted.

***Borrelia* (1523).** The main hazard for *Borrelia* is injury. Recommended BSL is 2. *B. recurrentis* laboratory infections have been reported.

***Brucella*.** *Brucella* is a significant agent in hospitals and more so in laboratories. **Hospital (3927).** In a tertiary hospital in Saudi Arabia, nine expatriates (from the United States and the United Kingdom) contracted brucellosis: a nurse, an obstetrician, and seven bacteriology technologists. **Laboratories (1523, 2944, 2968, 5490, 6791, 8307).** Brucellosis is a one of the most frequently diagnosed laboratory-acquired infections, and 2% of all cases may result in laboratories. In 1969–1989, 10% (717/6,962) of international laboratory infections were due to *Brucella*. In laboratories in enzootic areas, the disease rate can reach 8 per 100 worker-years. Modes of acquisition include ingestion, mucosal splash, or trauma, e.g., from handling blood cultures, but the main mode is inhalation, e.g., from viable agents on an open bench or from sniffing plates. *B. melitensis* is particularly infectious in laboratories. Clinicians should alert laboratories when submitting specimens. Recommended BSL for culture is 3.

Outbreaks   Outbreaks are documented in high-income laboratories.

- North America (7121). At a microbiology laboratory in 1988, eight workers developed acute brucellosis (five grew *B. melitensis* from blood) in 5 months, for an attack rate of 31%. Spread was presumed airborne as 6 weeks before the outbreak, a frozen isolate was thawed and subcultured without use of a safety cabinet, and epidemic isolates were indistinguishable from the stocked *B. melitensis* isolate.
- Asia (8309). At a hospital laboratory in Israel that frequently isolated *B. melitensis* from blood cultures, seven infections occurred in workers, although breaches in safety practices were not found.
- Europe (2397, 5588). At a university laboratory in Italy, a broken centrifuge tube caused 12 *B. abortus* infections among workers, for an attack rate of 31%. At a vaccine production laboratory in Spain, defective ventilation caused 22 *B. melitensis* cases and 6 infections among workers, for an attack rate of 17%.

***Chlamydophila psittaci* (6791).** Aerosols are a laboratory hazard. In 1969–1989, 3% (190/6,962) internationally reported laboratory infections concerned *C. psittaci*. Recommended BSL is 3.

***C. burnetii* (4852, 6473, 6791).** The main *C. burnetii* hazard is inhalation of aerosols, mainly in settings that use sheep or goats for research or training. **Hospitals (4961).** At a university campus in Colorado, where sheep were used in education, 41 persons with sheep contact and 96 without contact became infected; attack rates were highest in animal care (75%, 15/20) and perinatal units (60%, 15/25). The clothes of patients can be an unusual source of *C. burnetii*. **Laboratories (3090, 3243, 6791, 6912).** In 1969–1989, 7% (462/6,962) of internationally reported laboratory infections concerned *C. burnetii*. In Germany in 1947–1999, the venue for two of 40 Q fever outbreaks was laboratories (one each in 1947 and 1948). Surgery experiments on sheep at a university laboratory in the United Kingdom caused an outbreak with 11 Q fever cases and 4 infections. In Toronto, Canada, 18% of 331 animal research workers were seroreactive, a 30 times higher prevalence than in blood donors. Recommended BSL is 3.

***F. tularensis* (827, 909, 6791, 6811).** Hazards for *F. tularensis* are inhalation or inoculation. *F. tularensis* has a reputation of laboratory infections. A prominent victim was E. Francis (1872–1957), for whom the agent was named. In 1969–1989, 5% (354/6,962) of internationally reported laboratory infections were due to *F. tularensis*. Laboratory infections continue to be reported. In Massachusetts in 2000, 11 workers required doxycycline for laboratory and autopsy exposure to a man with fatal pulmonary tularemia that was not initially suspected. Recommended BSL is 3 (serology and culture).

P. multocida. Recommended BSL for *P. multocida* is 3.

***Rickettsia* (909, 5837, 6119, 6791, 7339, 8373).** Aerosols, accidents, and bites by arthropods are hazards. Health workers in endemic areas are at risk for LBT due to *R. prowazekii*. In 1995, a Red Cross nurse working with inmates in a Burundi prison contracted LBT.

In 1969–1989, 3% (206/6,962) of internationally reported laboratory infections concerned typhus. In Sicily, a technician contracted boutonneuse fever due to *R. conorii* from accidental inoculation in the laboratory. Recommended BSL is 3 for culture. Note that both H. T. Ricketts (1871–1910) and S. von Prowazek (1875–1915) died of laboratory-acquired typhus.

S. moniliformis. Recommended BSL for *S. moniliformis* is 2. Laboratory workers handling rodents are at risk of rat bite fever (211).

***Y. pestis* (1206, 1523, 2569).** Inhalation or inoculation are hazards for *Y. pestis* in laboratories (blood culture) and hospitals (pneumonia and bacteremia). Ideally, facilities are notified about possible plague risks. Plague vaccine is recommended for laboratory workers who routinely perform procedures that involve viable *Y. pestis*. Recommended BSL is 3.

Protozoa
Risks include accidental inoculation (infective blood and vector pools) and laboratory-reared vectors (mosquitoes and ticks) or reservoir rodents (3286). Recommended BSL is 2 for *Babesia*, *Leishmania*, *Plasmodium*, and *Trypanosoma*.

Leishmania. At least a dozen laboratory infections have been reported, including by *L. donovani*, *L. braziliensis*, and *L. tropica* (1865, 6791). At a research laboratory, a technician injected her left thumb while inoculating a hamster with a macerate that contained ~2,000 *L. braziliensis* amastigotes per μl; after 18 weeks, the infection was confirmed parasitologically and treated.

***Plasmodium* (176, 5202).** Health workers can be victims and sources. For instance, at a hospital in Massachusetts, falciparum malaria was transmitted from a patient to a nurse via injury, and from the nurse to another patient via nonstandard injection. Plasmodia can also spread patient-to-patient and in the laboratory. In Italy, a blood glucose meter was the vehicle for patient-to-patient spread of falciparum malaria.

- Workers as victims (176, 1090, 5876, 6075, 7338). Instances have been well documented. Health workers have contracted malaria from needlestick injury, or blood that spilled on unprotected, chapped hands. An English woman traveling in Namibia, Botswana, and Zimbabwe became unwell when returning home, stopping in Sicily; there, the attending Italian doctor sustained a needlestick injury and contracted fatal falciparum malaria (the patient was able to travel to United Kingdom where she was diagnosed with falciparum malaria and made a full recovery.
- Workers as sources (176, 5202). Health workers have transmitted *P. falciparum* to patients by invasive nonstandard procedures.
- Laboratory malaria (2040, 3286, 4142, 4402, 5229, 6791, 8184). At least 34 laboratory infections are on record, mainly (15 or 44%) *P. falciparum*, but also *P. vivax* and monkey plasmodia (*P. cynomolgi* and *P. knowlesi*). A technician contracted falciparum malaria from infective, laboratory-reared mosquitoes. In Germany, a technician intentionally inoculated herself 13 times in 2 years with *P. falciparum* that she obtained from patients.

***Trypanosoma. T. cruzi* (3286, 3376, 8099).** Over 70 infections have been documented in laboratory technicians, physicians, and research workers, from human and animal blood, culture, and triatomine bug feces. In Brazil, the risk of *T. cruzi* infection in exposed personnel was estimated at 2/100 person-years. ***T. brucei* sl (2198, 3286).** Four *T. brucei gambiense* and two *T. brucei rhodesiense* laboratory infections are on record. In Nigeria in 1988, a research laboratory technician contracted *T. brucei gambiense* from scratching his forearm with an infected needle.

Helminths
Echinococcus. A putative hazard for *Echinococcus* is the handling of infectious dogs, cats, or foxes and their feces. Recommended BSL is 2.

ENVIRONMENTAL CLUSTER, HEALTH WORK
Bacteria
***Leptospira* (1313, 6791).** Injury with leptospiremic blood is a hazard in hospitals and laboratories. In India, *Leptospira* was detected by microscopy in the blood of reconvalescent patients for up to 43 days. Recommended BSL is 2.

Burkholderia. Laboratory infections have been reported for *B. mallei* and *B. pseudomallei* (1523, 6791). Recommended BSL is 3. ***B. mallei* (6473).** Exposure to *B. mallei* in the laboratory resulted in human glanders. ***B. pseudomallei* (311, 1684).** Hazards for *B. pseudomallei* include inoculation and inhalation, but risks for workers are considered low. At a Los Angeles diagnostic laboratory in 2003, *B. pseudomallei* was isolated in a man with diabetes mellitus who had traveled in El Salvador and died of fulminant sepsis. Of 17 exposed laboratory workers, 13 reported high-risk activities such as sniffing culture plates for odor, picking colonies, and subculturing. All 17 workers were offered PEP with cotrimoxazole within 48 h and for 3 weeks. None of the workers contracted melioidosis.

Fungi
Sporothrix (1523). Inoculation or mucosal splash with *Sporothrix* is a rare hazard. Recommended BSL is 2.

Protozoa
Environmental amebas (e.g., *Acanthamoeba* and *Naegleria*) (3286). Mucosal splash with environmental amebas is a potential hazard. Recommended BSL is 2.

Helminths
Schistosoma (3286, 7730). At least eight *Schistosoma* infections have been documented, principally in research laboratories (eggs in stool samples are not infective). In Belgium, *S. mansoni* was isolated in a laboratory assistant who tested molluscicides in *Biomphalaria pfeifferi* from Senegal. Recommended BSL is 2.

Strongyloides (3286, 6369). Handling samples that contain viable *Strongyloides* larvae is a risk. Laboratory infections are reported from handling human and horse feces. Recommended BSL is 2

SKIN-BLOOD CLUSTER, HEALTH WORK
Risks include injury with sharp objects, mucosal splash, and contact with unprotected skin and unwashed hands. Blood is hazardous during viremia, bacteremia, fungemia, or parasitemia ("agentemia") with viable agents.

Prions
CJD (581, 1492, 2862, 4032, 5090, 6244). Health workers are at potential risk of CJD, mainly from handling clinical or autopsy materials. High-risk organs and tissues (Table 14.2) are brain and spinal cord, for variant CJD, also lymphatic tissues (spleen, tonsils, and appendix) and blood. Though patient-to-worker transmission is unlikely, about two dozen sporadic CJD cases have been reported in health workers, including a physician, neurosurgeon, and pathologist. Prions are not identified in dental pulp of patients with sporadic CJD. Technicians, pathologists, and histopathologists should follow guidelines for diagnostic or research procedures. Recommended BSL is 3.

Viruses
Flaviviridae. HCV (152, 1344, 7245). Risks vary with portal (intact or broken skin and mucous membrane), inoculum (volume and viremia), host (susceptibility), and HCV endemicity in the area served. Spread can be patient-to-worker, worker-to-patient, in the laboratory, and (rarely and by modes not fully understood) patient-to-patient, e.g., in hematology and dialysis units.

- Workers as victims (173, 543, 1344, 2933, 3435, 3563, 8334). Groups at risk include nurses, phlebotomists, students, surgeons, anesthetists, workers in emergency rooms and ICUs, and dentists. From comparison with population prevalence, risks for health workers appear to be moderate and include venipuncture and high viral load in source blood (>1 million copies per ml). Following injury with HCV-infected patients or blood, 0–10% (typically 2–3%) of workers seroconvert. In Swiss health workers in 1997–2000, 12% (317/2,685) of sources of percutaneous or mucosal exposure were positive for anti-HCV, and five instances of patient-to-worker spread were detected, for a rate of 1.6%. Currently, PEP is limited largely to the early detection of chronic liver disease. However, PEP with antivirals has potential to substantially lower risks.

- Workers as sources (783, 1496, 2242, 6305, 6419, 6722). Spread from workers to patients has been reported in hospitals in North America and West Europe, mainly by infected surgeons, gynecologists, and anesthesists. Reported rates of transmission from infected workers are 0.04–0.8/100 exposed patients. In Spain in 1988–1994, a cardiothoracic surgeon infected 5 of 643 operated patients, for a risk of 0.8/100. In Germany in 1999, a woman contracted acute HC from a cesarean operation by an HCV-positive gynecologist; follow-up of 2,285 operated women in 1993–2000 identified seven HCV infections, all distinct from the genotype of the gynecologist, for an overall risk of 0.04/100 exposed patients. Workers confirmed by NAT to be HCV-infected should be counseled.

- Laboratory (2944, 7915). Sporadic infections have been reported. Recommended BSL is 2.

Hepadnaviridae. HBV (543). HBV is a risk in hospitals and laboratories. From blood, HBV concentration is higher and the percentage of empty envelopes is lower than in other body fluids (saliva, semen, and breastmilk), and infectivity is higher in the former than the latter. The disease risk is 1–6% from exposure to single-positive (HBsAg+/HBeAg negative) blood, but 20–30% from double-positive (HBsAg+/HBeAg+) blood.

- Workers as victims (543, 750, 2807, 2933, 4338, 5109, 5115, 6967). Dentists in Singapore were significantly more frequently carriers of HBsAg (11% or 13/114) than the population (4% or 19/454). HBV infection rates per 100 health workers per year were 0.07 in northern Europe, 0.5 in western Europe, and 1.5 in southern Europe. In 4% (100/2,685) of percutaneous or mucosal exposures reported by health workers in Switzerland in 1997–2000, the source was HBsAg-positive; because 94% of workers were vaccinated, not a single transmission event occurred. Workers should be offered vaccine on employment, including care of IDU and disabled individuals in institutions. PEP should be planned in advance. For vaccinated health workers who are known responders, no further steps are needed.

- Workers as sources (101, 2946, 4424, 5587, 7927). Workers who are carriers are a potential risk for patients. In the United Kingdom, a tattoo artist was implicated in 31 acute HB cases, and another HBeAg-positive acupuncturist over 3.5 years caused five confirmed acute HB cases, for a rate of 1.7/100 clients. In Switzerland, 41 HBV infections were linked to a family doctor with chronic HB. In the United Kingdom in 1975–1990, 12 instances of worker-to-patient spread were documented; follow-up detected 95 HBV infections. In 11 of the 12 incidents, surgeons were implicated, 10 were HBeAg-positive (in one, status was unknown). In the United Kingdom in 1994–1995, 6 of ~8,000 hospital physicians (including 3 surgeons) were HBeAg-positive, for a rate of confirmed HBV transmission of 0.2/100 patients (95% CI 0.004–1.1). Published transmission rates from infected workers to patients were 3% in orthopedic surgery and dentistry, 8% in cardiac and dental surgery, and 10% in obstetrics and gynecology.
- Laboratories (1523, 2944, 6791). Hazards are percutaneous and mucosal exposure to blood and body fluids. Infection risks in laboratory workers are about three times higher than in other health workers and ~10 times higher than in the population. In the United Kingdom, reported HBV infections in laboratories per 100 person-years were ~0.2 in the 1970s and 0.01–0.03 in the 1980s. Recommended BSL is 2.

Herpesviridae. **CMV (407, 412, 5109).** Although saliva and urine of patients with primary infection can be infectious for weeks or months, the risk of patient-to-worker spread seems small. In the United States in 1984–1988, two thirds (783/1,250) of health workers were seroreactive on enrollment; in 300 seronegative workers, the conversion rate was 2/100 per year, and risk activities were not recorded. Over 5 years, seroconversions were comparable in transplant and hemodialysis nurses (n = 263), neonatal ICU nurses (n = 204), student nurses (n = 225), and control blood donors (n = 251), for an overall rate of 1.8/100 per year. Recommended BSL is 2. **HSV (2004, 5109).** HSV1 can spread patient-to-worker and worker-to-patient. Sources include hand lesions (herpetic whitlow), but also orolabial and ocular lesions and respiratory secretions from latently infected patients. In high-income countries at age >20 years, 70% of the population is expected to be latently HSV1 infected.

- Workers as victims. Groups at risk include nurses, anesthesiologists, respiratory therapists, and dentists. Latex gloves are protective. For PEP, antivirals (e.g., famciclovir and valaciclovir) are an option.
- Workers as sources. Workers with lesions that cannot be covered with dressing should be restricted from work with patients, in particular, neonates, burn patients, and immune-impaired patients. Recommended BSL is 2.

Human herpes virus 8 (HHV8) (2648). A risk for HHV8 may exist. In a German hospital, 7% (5/72) of health workers who nursed patients with HHV8 risks had anti-HHV8 IgG, compared with 0.7% (1/152) of workers nursing nonrisk patients. Recommended BSL is 2 or 3.

Poxviridae. **Monkeypox virus (MPXV).** Recommended BSL for MPXV is 3 or 4. **Vaccinia virus (VACV) (1523, 6473, 8237).** VACV laboratory infections have been reported. A nonvaccinated, previously healthy laboratory technician contracted generalized vaccinia confirmed by electron microscopy and culture from a cut at the finger by a cover slip while working with VACV. **Variola virus (VPXV) (1523).** Smallpox has been eradicated, but VPXV is stockpiled at biodefense (or bioterror) laboratories. In London, United Kingdom, in 1973, three persons contracted smallpox: a visitor to a laboratory (who survived), and two contacts of the visitor (both died). In Birmingham, United Kingdom, in 1978, a person contracted smallpox in a building that housed a smallpox laboratory. Recommended BSL is 4.

Retroviridae. **HIV (3189, 4387).** Blood, semen, vaginal secretions, breastmilk, and unfixed tissues from HIV-infected individuals can be infective (Table 13.2). In contrast, urine, feces, vomitus, and blood-free saliva are highly unlikely sources of HIV. Expected population prevalence varies by location; in emergency rooms, 4% (95% CI 2–6) of patients tested positive for HIV.

- Workers as victims (543, 1075, 1298, 2258, 2933, 3562, 5714, 6038, 6310). HIV infections in health workers mainly result from nonoccupational exposure. Worldwide, ~300 occupational HIV infections (100 confirmed and 200 possible) have been reported in health workers, >90% in high-income countries. Risk groups include nurses and midwives (account for ~40% of infections), clinical laboratory workers (~15%), physicians, medical students, and resuscitation workers. The bulk (~80%) of exposure is percutaneous, from needle sticks. The risk increases with increasing volume of blood inoculated and high viral load. Compared with 665 exposed but uninfected workers, significant risks in 33 seroconverting workers included deep injury, large-gauge needle, visible blood on device, intravascular procedure, and a source with terminal AIDS. The risk of HIV infection from percutaneous exposure to HIV-infected blood is 0.01–0.6% (typically 0.2%). The risk is similar or lower from mucosal exposure. In Swiss health workers in 1997–2000, 9% (244/2,685) of percutaneous or mucosal exposures had a HIV-positive source, but not a single HIV transmission was detected.

PEP should be planned in advace. When given within hours, antiretrovirals reduce infection risks. For minimal trauma from blood of low viremia (<1,500 RNA copies per ml), a combination with two antiretrovirals is considered adequate. For trauma with large-bore needle or deep puncture, and from highly viremic or symptomatic source (florid AIDS), ≥3 antiretrovirals are recommended. Start of PEP >72 h after e_0 is discouraged.

- Workers are rarely sources of HIV (1451, 4524). In Florida in 1984–1989, five HIV infections were epidemiologically and virologically linked to invasive procedures by a dentist. An orthopedic surgeon who developed AIDS in retrospect was the likely source for one infection in 983 patients, a woman without HIV risks who had tested negative before total hip replacement by this surgeon. By molecular fingerprinting, her HIV strain was closely related to the surgeon's.
- Laboratory (6791). Infections seem infrequent. In the United States, 25% (25/101) of occupational HIV infections have been in laboratory technicians. Recommended BSL is 2 (diagnostic) to 3 (research and production).

HTLV (4387, 5271). By age and location, 1–10% or more of patients are expected to be infected by HTLV, and 3% of resuscitation procedures expose workers to infected blood. Recommended BSL is 2 (diagnostic) to 3 (research). **SiFV (3253).** In the United States, 2% (4/231) workers at primate research facilities had evidence of latent SiFV infection. Recommended BSL is 2. **Simian herpes virus (SHV, includes cercopithecine herpesvirus 1) (1510, 1755, 3398, 5690).** SHV is an occupational hazard from primates. Three men who worked at an animal research facility contracted SHV from macaques. Manifestations varied from self-limited aseptic meningitis to fulminant encephalomyelitis and death. Of 24 cases reported in humans in 1932–1972, 18 (75%) were fatal. The risk of secondary spread seems low. At a research facility in Florida in 1987, three workers contracted SHV from monkeys; contact tracing identified 159 exposed persons (21 at the facility and 138 others) but no further cases. Recommended BSL is 4. **Simian retrovirus D (SRV) (4350).** In the United States, 0.9% (2/231) research facility workers were reactive in Western blot. One worker had been exposed to a variety of monkeys for 23 years; the other was exposed for 5 years. Recommended BSL is 3.

Bacteria

***C. trachomatis* (6791).** Sporadic laboratory *C. trachomatis* infections have been reported. Recommended BSL is 2.

S. aureus. Health workers can be victims or sources of methicillin-sensitive *S. aureus* (MSSA) and MRSA.

- Workers as victim (5109, 8025). *S. aureus* can spread patient-to-worker. In Canada in 1995–1996, 17 patients with invasive *S. aureus* disease were monitored for spread; of workers who spent ≥24 h/week with these patients, 27% (13/48) yielded identical serotypes, while workers who spent less time with source patients, only 2% (1/54) were colonized. Patients with respiratory *S. aureus* infections and purulent *S. aureus* lesions are the most frequent sources of hospital outbreaks.
- Workers as source (5109). Sites colonized in health workers are anus, vagina, and nose. Nosocomial outbreaks from nasal carriers are uncommon. However, *S. aureus* is readily transferred from nose to hands that are a major vehicle. Health workers with *S. aureus* hand infection should be excluded from work until the lesions are resolved.

  MRSA (144, 1498, 1618, 2270, 4956, 5109, 6164, 7191). In Canada, the proportion of MRSA among all *S. aureus* strains steadily increased, from 0.9% (1995) to 1.7% (1996), 2.6% (1997), and 3.9% (1998). Unlike MSSA, *nasal* carriage of MRSA is increased in hospital workers, for typical prevalence of 4–8%. At a teaching hospital in Paris, France, the prevalence of MRSA in health workers by nasal swab in a nonepidemic period was 6% (60/965, 95% CI 5–8). Households of 10 workers were investigated, and identical MRSA was found in four households. Nosocomial spread is mainly via hands of workers who are nasal MRSA carriers, although patients are further sources. Workers and patients can shuttle MRSA hospital-to-hospital, acute-to-chronic care facility, hospital-to-household, and community-to-chronic care facility. Universal and contact precautions apply. MRSA colonized or infected workers should be referred to a hospital infectiologist for counseling. Masks are an option for workers caring for carrier patients.
- Recommended BSL is 2.

***S. pyogenes* (GAS) (1523, 5109).** Workers who carry epidemic strains have been implicated in nosocomial outbreaks of invasive GAS disease, including after surgery and delivery. Invasive GAS disease should be reported to the hospital infectiologist. Diagnosis of a single case should prompt enhanced surveillance, diagnosis of ≥ 2 cases should prompt an epidemiological investigation.

Few laboratory infections have been reported. Recommended BSL is 2.

Treponema. Accidental inoculation with *Treponema* is rare (1523, 6791). Recommended BSL is 2.

Fungi
***Candida* (754, 2311, 3504).** Health workers and patients are frequently colonized (overall, $>50\%$), including by *C. albicans* and *C. parapsilosis*. Strains of *C. albicans* from hands of ICU workers were found to match strains from patients, suggesting exogenous sources. Recommended BSL is 2.

***T. tonsurans* (1523, 8257).** A nosocomial outbreak of *T. tonsurans* has been reported on a long-stay ward. Inoculation is a laboratory hazard. At least 160 laboratory infections have been reported. Recommended BSL is 2.

Ectoparasites
***P. humanus* (5109).** The risk of nosocomial spread of head, body, and pubic lice is considered low.

***Sarcoptes scabiei* (197, 3405, 3705, 5545, 6344).** Outbreaks have been well documented in hospitals and nursing homes. Scabies is a significant hazard for health workers, in particular, from patients with unrecognized scabies, or "crusted" scabies in immune-impaired patients. In the United States, a patient with unrecognized crusted scabies was source for 112 cases over 12 months, with high attack rates among roommates (78% or 11/14) and nursing staff (49% or 27/55).

12.7 CLEANING AND WASTE WORK
"Brown collar" work includes cleaning of buildings, hotels, and streets, garbage collection and incineration, sewerage maintenance, sewage purification and sludge production, and work with corpses, including at funerals, at mortuaries, and in disasters. For abattoir work, see section 12.4; for agents from liquid waste, see section 6.2.

Exposure (2967, 3975). In high-income countries, domestic waste production per person per day amounts to 0.5–2 kg of solid waste and of up to 500 liters of liquid waste. Solid waste is recycled, incinerated, or dumped. Liquid waste is discharged into the environment or purified at plants. Air inside waste plants can be loaded with bacteria (e.g., *Klebsiella* and *Pseudomonas*, $>10,000$ CFU/m^3) and fungi (e.g., *Aspergillus*, $>100,000$ CFU/m^3). Annual accrual is 57 million corpses worldwide and billions of animal carcasses.

Infections (Box 12.6). Evidence is scant, and significant knowledge gaps exist for refuse collectors and street cleaners. Infections in brown collar workers can result from inhalation (e.g., *M. tuberculosis*), inoculation (e.g., prions, HBV, *N. meningitidis*), ingestion (e.g., HAV), or contact (e.g., EBOV, *V. cholerae*, or *P. humanus* from corpses). Evaluation of occupational risks is confounded by past infections, domiciliary risks (e.g., crowding), leisure activities (e.g., travel), exposure prevention, vaccines, and years on the job.

Prevention (400, 3214, 3975). Prevention includes education, good practice, and vaccines. Protective equipment, changing of clothes at the workplace, and hand hygiene are part of good practice. In addition for work with corpses, bags are recommended, and face masks if death was due to respiratory tract infection.

DROPLET-AIR CLUSTER
Bacteria such as *Acinetobacter*, *Klebsiella*, *Pseudomonas*, and *Serratia*, and fungi such as *Acremonium*, *Aspergillus*, *Cladosporium*, *Fusarium*, and *Penicillium* have been identified in air at waste facilities (3975). Similarly, garbage collectors are exposed to seasonally variable amounts of dust, bioaerosols, and cell wall components such as endotoxins that can cause nausea and diarrhea (3599, 8326).

Box 12.6 Agents or infections from cleaning and waste work, by cluster

Risks are given in parentheses.

Droplet-air	*Legionella* (waste), *M. tuberculosis* (autopsy), *N. meningitidis* (injury)
Feces-food	HAV (waste); *Salmonella* (laundry), *V. cholerae* (funeral), *E. histolytica* (waste)
Zoonotic	EBOV (funeral), FMDV (carcass), Hantavirus (cleaning); *E. granulosus* (carcass)
Environmental	*C. tetani* (waste), *Leptospira* (waste), *Schistosoma* (endemic areas), *Strongyloides* (waste, garbage)
Skin-blood	Prions; HBV, HIV; bacteremia (corpses); ectoparasites

Unfortunately, risks in brown collar workers are poorly documented.

***Legionella* (2928).** *Legionella* seems to be a hazard for brown collar workers. In Denmark, five workers at a wastewater plant contracted Legionnaires' disease after repair work near an aerosol-generating decanter.

M. tuberculosis. *M.tuberculosis* is a reported hazard for hotel workers, medical waste workers, and those who work with corpses.

- Hotels (2882). At a resort outside New York City the sudden death from tuberculosis of a dishwasher prompted an investigation among workers who shared the poorly ventilated dishwashing station with the deceased worker. Of 52 initially skin test-negative, exposed individuals, 8 (15%) converted on follow-up.
- Medical waste (3716). In Washington State in 1997, three waste workers contracted pulmonary tuberculosis. Strains were different by DNA fingerprints, and disposal practice suggested a work-related source. Waste delivered from hospitals, laboratories, and medical and dental offices in containers was emptied manually into chutes for shredding, blowing, compacting, and electrothermal decontamination, to be deposited at a landfill.
- Corpses (2944, 7167, 7401, 7664). Coroners, pathologists, and embalmers are at risk of infection and disease. After autopsy of a corpse with unsuspected tuberculosis, all five tuberculin-negative attendees' skin-tests converted, and two became sputum-culture positive. In the United Kingdom in 1980–1989, 30 cases of occupational tuberculosis were reported, including 14 in postmortem workers, pathologists, and mortuary technicians.

FECES-FOOD CLUSTER
Exposure to fecal matter is a putative hazard for waste plant and canalization workers. Corpses from floods or other natural disasters can be a source of enteric agents.

Viruses
HAV (299, 2493). Potential HAV hazards include aerosols from liquid waste, splash into the face, and skin contact with sludge. Wastewater workers and hospital laundry workers seem at risk of infection. Vaccine prevents outbreaks and is likely beneficial where the proportion of naturally immune individuals is low (say <20%).

- Wastewater workers in North America (1831, 7572, 7873, 8035). In Columbus, Ohio, in 1998–1999, 26% (42/163) wastewater workers and 12% (17/139) control workers were reactive; after adjustment for age, past HA, and ethnicity, there was no significant difference. In a convenience sample in Texas in 1996–1997, the anti-HAV prevalence was 28% in wastewater workers ($n = 359$) and 24% in drinking-water workers ($n = 89$), for an odds ratio of 2 (95% CI 1.0–4) after adjustment for age, education, and ethnicity. In Quebec City, Canada, seroprevalence was similar in municipal sewer workers (54%, $n = 76$) and age- and sex-matched controls (49%, $n = 152$). In contrast, an outbreak in Florida in 1988–1989, with 18 primary HA cases that followed stormwater and sewage overflow, underscored potential risks.
- Wastewater workers in West Europe (299, 938, 1024, 6949). In Greece, compared with controls, the odds of HAV infection for wastewater workers was 3.5, and vaccine was recommended for susceptible workers. At a water and sewerage company in the United Kingdom, 50 workers frequently exposed to raw sewage were at significant risk of HAV infection compared with 191 other workers, for an odds ratio of 3.7. In France, sewage workers were more frequently seroreactive (60% or 93/155) than water workers (47% or 33/70); reactive workers were longer on the job (by ~3 years) than seronegative workers. In Copenhagen, Denmark, seroprevalence in males matched for age and duration of employment were 80.5% in wastewater workers ($n = 77$), 60.5% in gardeners ($n = 81$), and 48% in clerks ($n = 79$).
- Hospital laundry workers (771). Exposure to infected linen seems a risk. In a Malta hospital, 55% of laundry personnel ($n = 22$) but 14% of age-matched health workers ($n = 37$) were seroreactive to HAV; reactivity was higher in workers who handled dirty laundry than in workers who handled clean laundry.

HEV (3659). Clinical HE was not more frequent in 349 Swiss waste workers than 429 municipal control workers, and anti-HEV IgG was comparably prevalent in exposed (3%) and control (4%) workers.

Bacteria
Enterobacter, *E. coli*, and *Yersinia* have been isolated in air at waste plants (3975), pointing to the inhalational risks of fecal bacteria. However, no clinical correlates for these findings exist.

***H. pylori* (2535, 3659).** From serology, infection risks were not discernible in sewage workers in Sweden. Likewise in Switzerland, peptic ulcer disease was as frequent in waste workers ($n = 349$) as in municipal control workers ($n = 429$), and anti-*H. pylori* IgG was prevalent in both groups (34% versus 50%).

***Salmonella* (6787, 7109).** Hospital laundry workers rather than wastewater plant workers appear at risk for *Salmonella* At a nursing home in Tennessee, *S. enterica* serovar Hadar affected 32 (mostly incontinent) residents and eight workers. Spread among residents was food borne. Laundry workers, however, who did not eat food from the home's kitchen and had no contact with residents contracted salmonellosis, likely from heavily soiled linen, not wearing gloves consistently, and eating in the laundry room.

V. cholerae **(3007).** Washing and transporting corpses with cholera as a cause of death is a hazard. The recommended procedure is disinfection (e.g., bleach: 2% NaOCl) and burial within 24 h.

Protozoa
Giardia **(3216, 4007, 6676).** In France, the prevalence of *G. lamblia* is 4% (17/480) in wastewater workers but 1% (5/363) in food handlers. Giardiasis has been observed in sewage workers in Germany and the United Kingdom. In Norwich district in 1991, three workers were diagnosed with giardiasis: one at high-pressure water hoses, one at a sewage treatment plant, and one a pump engineer.

E. histolytica **(3111, 4007, 4008).** Wastewater workers seem at risk of both intestinal amebiasis and invasive disease. In Hamburg, Germany, in 1980, a sewer worker contracted amebic liver abscess, 14 weeks after falling into the clearing basin of the city purification plant.

Helminths
In France, the fecal prevalence of *T. trichiura* was similar in wastewater workers (0.6%, 3/480) and food handlers (0.6%, 2/363) (6676).

ZOONOTIC CLUSTER
Garbage collectors and street cleaners are likely exposed outdoors to animals such as dogs, rodents, and mosquitoes, with a putative risk of zoonoses such as rabies and arboviral infections. People in slums who search refuse for goods are at similar, putative risks. In return, collection of cans, bottles, and tires removes breeding opportunities for mosquitoes

EBOV (2698). EBOV seems to remain viable in corpses (for days or a few weeks) and in secretions on corpses. Funerals have been venues for the spread of EBOV. When handling such corpses, protective clothes should be used.

Foot-and-mouth-disease virus (FMDV) (1805, 6747). Animal carcasses are considered highly infective with FMDV. In the United Kingdom in 2001, for control of a massive epidemic, >4 million animals were killed. Culling and rendering capacities were overwhelmed, calling for alternatives such as mass burial at engineered sites.

Hantavirus **(2537).** Cleaning rodent-infested buildings and sheds is a risk for aquiring New World hantavirus cardiopulmonary syndrome or Old World HFRS.

E. granulosus **(1086).** Handling infected animal carcases is a risk for *E. granulosus* infection. In Florida, Uruguay, the prevalence by ultrasound and serology was higher in persons who fed, buried, or burned slaughter offal (2.8–3.2%) than in persons who used other means of waste disposal (0.8–1.5%).

ENVIRONMENTAL CLUSTER
C. tetani. Nonvaccinated sewerage workers, garbage collectors, and street cleaners are at putative risk of tetanus.

Leptospira **(1831, 2275, 3387, 4279, 4369, 4496, 5894).** Garbage collectors, wastewater workers, septic tank cleaners, and sanitation workers are at risk of *Leptospira*. In Denmark in 1970–1996, sewage was the source in 7% of 118 laboratory-confirmed cases. In Quebec City, Canada, seroprevalence was 12% in municipal sewer workers ($n = 76$) but 2% in age- and sex-matched controls ($n = 152$). Risks include abundance of *Leptospira* in waste and unprotected contact of broken skin with wastewater or sludge.

Free-living amebas (7844). Free-living amebas have been identified in sewage.

Schistosoma **(3826, 4400, 5958).** Washing cars with water from transmission foci is a risk of *Schistosoma*. At Lake Victoria, Kenya, the risk of *S. mansoni* infection increased with the number of cars washed per week.

Strongyloides **(1594, 5956).** Risks of *S. stecoralis* include unprotected contacts with sludge, sewage, or garbage, including for plumbers, swimming pool maintenance workers, and garbage collectors. In France, strongyloidiasis was diagnosed in a garbage collector who had never left the country but without wearing gloves cleaned camping sites frequented by immigrants.

SKIN-BLOOD CLUSTER
Injection materials from home treatments or street injection drug use can expose nonprotected garbage collectors and street cleaners to sharp injury. In Taiwan, 37% of municipal refuse collectors ($n = 533$) reported injuries from sharps compared with 12% of control municipal employees ($n = 320$), for an odds ratio of 3.5 (95% CI 2–5) (8326).

Corpses (3214, 5195) can be a source of prions, viruses (HBV, HCV, and HIV), and bacteria (*N. meningitidis, S. aureus,* and *S. pyogenes*). Percutaneous injury can result in sepsis. Funeral workers and embalmers have acquired *P. humanus* or *S. scabiei* from handling infested corpses.

HBV (299, 2006, 7619). In Boston, 13% of 133 embalmers were positive for HBV markers, that is twice the prevalence in blood donors. Risks were being on the job for >10 years and not wearing gloves routinely. HBV is quite stable in the environment. In a suburb of Piraeus, Greece, in 1999–2001, the prevalence of HBsAg in municipal solid waste workers was 11% (8/71) compared with 4.5% (4/88) in employees not exposed to waste. Differences were significant for anti-HBc (24% or 17/71 versus 8% or 7/88). Also in Greece, 32% (35/108) of wastewater workers were positive for anti-HBc compared with 6% (5/86) of control residents; vaccination was recommended for susceptible workers.

HIV (246, 393, 512, 3189, 6126). In the United States, 3% (15/539) of morticians reported percutaneous exposure to blood from a decedent with AIDS. HIV RNA was amplified from 4% (3/80) of syringes discarded by health workers after intramuscular or subcutaneous injection of HIV-infected patients. HIV is susceptible to drying. Injury is a putative hazard for garbage collectors, but data are not available.

Female and male hotel service and bar workers in low-income countries seem at risk of HIV infections. In Dar-es-Salaam in 1990–1998, of a cohort of hotel workers with no access to antiretroviral therapy, 10% (196/1,887) were reactive to HIV1 on enrollment and 8% (133/1,691) sero-converted during a median follow-up period of 41 months.

12.8 TRANSPORTATION WORK

"Buckled-up" work includes bus, truck, and taxi drivers, railway and subway conductors, sailors, ship crew and captains, dock and warehouse workers, flight cabin crew and pilots, and astronauts. For infections in passengers, see section V; for military, see section 12.3; for transported animals, see section 16.1.

Exposure. Global transportation statistics are not publicly available. Numbers of truck drivers are >3 million in the United States, and probably >0.5 million in Canada.

Infections. Infections overall have been poorly documented in buckled-up workers. Putative or confirmed risks include droplets in congested, poorly ventilated compartments, unsafe foods, bites by transported mammals (see section I), exposure to arthropods, and STI in socially disrupted long-distance truck drivers. Besides being victims, buckled-up workers are sources and vectors of infections along major transportation routes.

DROPLET-AIR CLUSTER

SARS has heightened awareness of respiratory risks in buckled-up workers. In a questionnaire survey, 62% (158/256) of flight crew members self-reported upper respiratory tract infections in 6 months (7649), and 10% of female flight attendants self-reported five or more episodes of cold or flu in the past year (8069).

Crowding is likely to expose nonvaccinated crews to respiratory tract infections, including *Influenzavirus*, measles virus, mumps virus, *Rhinovirus*, and rubella virus. In 1997, rubella outbreaks affected crew members of two commercial cruise lines (1262).

Stress-induced inapparent reactivation of VZV was demonstrated in astronauts by analysis of saliva before, during, and after space flight (4953)

FECES-FOOD CLUSTER

Snacks from street vendors, truck stops, or galleys are potential sources of diarrheal disease in buckled-up workers.

HAV (3024, 6881). Risks of HAV appear to vary with age, country of origin, and destination. In Norway, seroprevalence was comparable to the population in seamen born after 1945 (5%, 10/209), but elevated 33% (54/154) in older seamen. In Switzerland, nonimmune air crew members with destinations to low-income countries seem at risk for an infection rate of 0.15/100 year. Rates were three times higher in male flight attendants than in female attendants or pilots.

H. pylori. Crowding and limited sanitation aboard submarines seem to facilitate spread among crew members (3108).

V. cholerae. Dock workers can be exposed to seawater in polluted harbors.

Entamoeba (7992). Pathogenic zymodemes were identified in 4 of 99 Lufthansa flight staff who shed *E. histolytica/dispar*.

ZOONOTIC CLUSTER

Unprotected outdoor diurnal and nocturnal activities expose buckled-up workers to bites by invertebrate vectors, in particular, during overnight stays.

R. typhi (7540). A historical risk in dock workers has been murine typhus, in port cities of the Atlantic, Indian, and Pacific oceans, and the Australian, Chinese, Caspian, and Mediterranean seas.

S. suis (5442, 7188). Pig bites commonly occur during capture, transport, or slaughter. A truck driver who transported pigs was diagnosed with *S. suis* septic shock.

Plasmodium (1018, 5868, 6867). Malaria is a risk for buckled-up workers, including seamen (for centuries), long-distance truck drivers, and air crews. In Japan in the 1990s, seafarers accounted for ~5% of all imported malaria. On a humanitarian transport through the Sahara, four French truck drivers contracted *P. falciparum* in Mauritania, probably from sleeping outdoors as none of eight companions who slept inside trucks were affected. In air crews from the United Kingdom to sub-Saharan Africa who were provided air conditioning at airports and hotels and during ground transport, the rate of falciparum malaria was $1.6/10^5$ nights (95% CI 0.5–3.7).

ENVIRONMENTAL CLUSTER

The scarcity of reports on environmental infections in buckled-up workers contrasts with road conditions during rainy seasons in tropical countries that offer ample opportunities for soil and water contacts.

Leptospira **(8018).** Leptospira infections in animal transporters have been reported.

Schistosoma **(1336).** During a weekend in Ghana, 10 of 14 British air crew swam in the freshwater estuary of the Volta River; 8 of 10 exposed crew members developed acute schistosomiasis (after 2–5 weeks), one developed swimmer itch, and one remained symptom-free. *S. mansoni* eggs were identified in stool or rectal biopsy in 5 individuals.

SKIN-BLOOD CLUSTER

Risks in buckled-up workers include HBV, HCV, HIV, gonorrhea, and syphilis. In Chad in 1989, 45% (41/92) of truck drivers admitted to sexual contacts during displacements, 88% (81) never used preservatives, and 13% (12) reported urethral discharge in the past 4 months (7546).

CMV. Inapparent reactivation of CMV was demonstrated in astronauts by analysis of urine before, during, and after space flight (4954).

HBV (2675, 3628, 4714, 6881). The infection prevalence of HBV in buckled-up workers has increased. In Iran, HBsAg carriage among 1,113 truck drivers randomly selected at 51 police stations along roads of 17 provinces was 6% (95% CI 4.5–7%), compared with ~1.7% in the population. In Norway, HBV markers (HBsAg, anti-HBs, and anti-HBc) were significantly more prevalent (9%, 49/523) in merchant seamen than the population, and in seamen who reported frequent casual sex abroad (15%) than in seamen with few or no sex contacts abroad (6.5%).

HCV (4605). Of trawlers departing from Australia, 27% of crew (n = 45) had anti-HCV, of IDU among the crew (n = 20) even 55%.

HIV (1012, 2675, 4173, 4714, 6098). HIV risks in drivers include long-distance drives, border crossings, stops for sex, sex with female or male prostitutes, a history of urethritis or genital ulcer disease, and reactivity to *T. pallidum*. The reported prevalence in drivers is 1% in Brazil, 1–16% in India, and 27% in East Africa (on the Mombasa-Nairobi Highway); even higher prevalence has been reported in drivers in southern Africa.

N. gonorrhoeae **(2675, 5728).** Increased gonorrhoea prevalence has been reported in motorcycle taxi drivers in Peru and long-distance truck drivers in India.

T. pallidum **(2675, 4173, 4714, 5243).** Reported seroprevalence (by VDRL or other test) in long-distance drivers are 8–13% in Brazil and 21–22% in India. The diary of a *T. pallidum* infected sex worker revealed sex with 168 long-distance truck drivers.

12.9 CLERK, CLASS, AND SALES WORK

"Neck-tie" work includes work in classrooms, offices, stores, and studios. It aggregates many of the jobs from groups 1–5 of the International Standard Classification of Occupations (ISCO-88, http://www.ilo.org), including administrators, bankers, clerks, managers, office assistants, receptionists, secretaries, politicians, salespersons, supervisors, and teachers.

Infections (5292, 8069) (Box 12.7). Overall, of all occupational groups, infection risks are lowest in neck-tie workers. Agents such as *Influenzavirus* and *Rhinovirus*, and flulike illness can be risks for neck-tie workers in poorly ventilated, crowded rooms. Teachers are instrumental in student health education. For hazards from buildings, see section 6.2; for infections in schools, see section 14.4.

DROPLET-AIR CLUSTER

Flulike illness is a cause of absenteeism in neck-tie workers; per flu season, 2–10% of workers may take sick leave for 1–5 days (106, 1752, 1931, 5180, 5413, 5596).

Box 12.7 Agents from clerk, class, and sales work, by cluster	
Droplet-air	Vaccine-preventable viruses (MMR) and bacteria (dp_a), PVB19; *Legionella*, *M. tuberculosis*
Zoonotic	*B. anthracis* (from intentional release)

Influenzavirus **(106, 1752, 1931, 5180, 5413, 5596).** A variable proportion (about one third to one fourth) of flu-like illness is attributable to *Influenzavirus* and can be prevented by vaccine that is well matched to circulating virus.

Mumps virus (3814). In Chicago, Ill., in 1987, mumps affected 119 persons, mostly nonvaccinated bankers and their household contacts; 21 (18%) patients had complications, and 9 (8%) were hospitalized.

PVB19 (212, 2729, 2743, 7692). Nursery and elementary school teachers and the staff of child care centers are at risk of PVB19. In Denmark, in a population study of 30,946 pregnant women, nursery school teachers had a three-times higher risk of acute PVB19 infection than other pregnant women. During community or institutional outbreaks, the infection rate is greater in primary school teachers and child care staff (10–30%) than in the population (10–15%).

Rubella virus (149, 2533). At a bank in Manhattan, N.Y., in 1983, 86 clinical cases were reported, including 72 in office workers in one of three affected buildings, for an attack rate of 1.6% (72/4,594). In 1984, the financial district of lower Manhattan reported 60 clinical cases, including 11 in bankers and brokers; subsequently, 1,639 workers (about one third of the workforce) were vaccinated.

B. pertussis **(1832).** Neck-tie workers can contract pertussis at the workplace. In particular, teachers seem at greater risk of pertussis than the population.

L. pneumophila. *L. pneumophila* is a risk in buildings by aerosols from faucets and air-conditioning systems (see section 6.2).

M. tuberculosis **(4193, 4613).** Undetected, infective cases of *M. tuberculosis* at the workplace are a risk. In a London office, an index case infected three of seven colleagues. In Australia, two office workers were sources for infection in ≥24% of 210 employees.

N. meningitidis **(8259).** In Cheshire, United Kingdom, in 1997–99, teachers and school administrators were at higher risk of invasive disease ($41/10^5$ per year) than resident adults ($8/10^5$ per year), for a risk ratio of 6 (95% CI 3–13). Preventive policies for schools should consider teachers for inclusion.

ZOONOTIC CLUSTER

B. anthracis **(8021).** For intentional release in the United States in 2001, spores were sent in letters by regular mail, causing infections and anthrax in postal workers and office workers.

Coxiella **(6308, 8219).** In Germany in 2001, among a movie team of 25 working in a hay barn in artificial wind for 10 h, 9 (36%) contracted Q fever. In the United Kingdom in 1983, an outbreak at a post-sorting office caused 13 cases; a source was not identified, but dust was a likely vehicle.

SKIN-BLOOD CLUSTER

For kindergarten teachers, CMV seems to be an occupational risk. In Belgium, 16–34% female kindergarten workers were reactive, but having children was a significant confounder (3963).

Sexually transmitted infections. Adult film workers in the United States are at increased risk of STI (1245). **HIV.** In 2004, a previously test-negative worker contracted HIV in Brazil; on return to California, he participated in film productions, in which he engaged in unprotected sex with 13 females, infecting three previously test-negative workers, for an attack rate of 23%. ***C. trachomatis.*** Compared with a national sample of similar age, the prevalence in male (5.5% versus 3.7%) and female (7.7% versus 4.7%) heterosexual film workers was increased. ***N. gonorrhoeae.*** Again compared with the national sample, the prevalence was increased in males (2% versus 0.4%) and females (2% versus 0.4%).

13

Human Leisure and Lifestyle

13.1 Fairs and mass gatherings
13.2 Catered events and restaurants
13.3 Swimming pools and spas
13.4 Outdoor sports and hobbies
13.5 Indoor sports and hobbies
13.6 Female prostitution
13.7 Sex among men
13.8 Injection drug use

Another result of the (AIDS) epidemic is that physicians now know how crucial it is to discuss sexual behavior with their patients.

M. S. Gottlieb (2868)

Leisure is free time that is spent indoors or outdoors, at home or away from home, alone or with others, during day or night. For travel, see section V; for hotel accommodations, see section 11.8.

Exposure. Minimal risk activities include reading, listening to radio, or watching television alone. Human contacts include playing cards and board games with others, singing in choirs, and visits to libraries, cinemas, clubs, gyms, discos, and night clubs. Outdoor hobbies and sports include visits to playgrounds, parks, and zoos, as well as jogging, boating, and going to the beach. Depending on age, leisure time may exceed 5 h/day. The exposure history should address current and past leisure activities (Box 13.1).

Infections (6675). Infections can result from exposure to the environment (see section II), equipment, animals, and humans.

13.1 FAIRS AND MASS GATHERINGS

Fairs are places where people meet for buying, selling, exhibiting, and viewing goods, animals, and performing humans. Included here are bazaars, carnivals, churches, cinemas, concerts, exhibitions, festivals, funerals, markets, mosques, museums, shopping malls, temples, and theme parks. Mass gatherings (399, 2897, 3022, 4946, 5340, 5710, 5768, 6836, 7450, 8023) attract large numbers of people (say >10,000–100,000). Examples include car rallies, football games, Olympic games, open-air concerts, political and religious unions, youth days, and world championships. For catered events, see section 13.2; for pilgrimage, see section 15.4; for food-borne infections, see section III.

Exposure. Amusement and theme parks attract hundreds of million visitors per year, and sportive, religious, or music events attract hundreds of thousands or millions of participants. At Olympic games, athletes and visitors from ~200 countries participate.

Box 13.1 Suggested leisure exposure history
Latest leisure activity inside or outdoors, during day or nighttime: • Visits, e.g., playground, zoo, festival, friend, party, and bar • Sports, e.g., gym hall, swimming pool, and hiking • Other leisure activities, e.g., card play and gardening **In past 1–4 weeks:** • Did you attend any catered event, including garden party, restaurant salad bar, or private dinner? • Did you sustain any bite, scratch, or other injury, e.g., from an insect, dog, or equipment? • Did you share towels, clothes, equipment, combs, or other belongings with your team? **In your lifetime:** • Name all your hobbies and sportive activities. • Ever diagnosed with an STI? Your sexual preference? Number of sex partners? Ever practiced oral or anal sex? • Ever used injection drugs? Which substances, how were they administered? Any hospital stays because of injection drug use?

Infections (Box 13.2). Infections vary with the location, season, and current global infectious disease situation.

- Mass gatherings (399, 3750, 5254, 6836, 8060). Conditions that trigger health visits include heat, injury, and respiratory and gastrointestinal symptoms. During the 2002 winter Olympics in Salt Lake City, of >59,000 chief complaints recorded, 25–50% were respiratory, 2–4% were gastrointestinal, 2–3% were rash, and 0.01–1% were neurological. At the 1984 summer Olympics in Los Angeles, there were 0.2 visit/100 attendees, and 29% of visits ($n = 5,516$) required physician evaluation. At football games in South Carolina in 1995, with a mean number of 69,400 spectators per game, nurses, paramedics, and physicians provided care at rates of 0.07–0.15/100 spectators, and 4% of patients needed transfer to a hospital. At the 1996 summer Olympics in Atlanta, physician visits per 100 accredited persons were 16 for athletes, 9 for officials, 5 for media staff, 2 for volunteers, and 4 overall. During the 2000 summer Olympics in Sydney, emergency department visits increased by 5% over baseline.
- Animal fairs (552). There is a risk of zoonoses. More than two dozen such incidents have been documented.

Prevention (532, 2897, 3131, 3750). Prevention includes planning for instant multilingual communication, sanitation, expected infections (Box 13.2), surveillance (outbreaks, and bioterrorism) at ports, stations, hotels, and emergency rooms, and response capacity. Planning of surveillance for the 2000 Olympics in Sydney took nearly 3 years. Lessons can be learned from mass gatherings, pandemics, and most recently from severe acute respiratory syndrome (SARS).

Prevention has been promoted at health fairs and in cinemas, and screening has been offered at fairs.

DROPLET-AIR CLUSTER, FAIRS

Because fairs are short and participant turnover is high, spread is difficult to document. At regional, crowded indoor fairs, locally prevalent respiratory viral and bacterial agents are likely to circulate. At international fairs a broad agent spectrum must be assumed, including intentionally released, weaponized agents.

Viruses

Influenzavirus. Humans and animals are potential sources at fairs.

- Humans (413, 2154, 6060). Substantial risks are documented among pilgrims to and in Mecca (hajj). Flu-like illness on the hajj was reported in ~30–35% of influenza-vaccinated pilgrims and in ~40–60% of nonvaccinated pilgrims.
- Animals (7563, 7996, 8036). Live bird markets can be sources of low-virulent and high-virulent avian influenza viruses (for birds, see section 3.7). Animal venues can also be sources of swine influenza. In Wisconsin in 1988, a pregnant women died of pneumonia 8 days after a visit to an farm fair; the only agent detected was an influenza virus antigenically related to swine influenza virus. Swine exhibited at that fair had flulike illness, and

Box 13.2 Agents or infections at mass gatherings, by cluster	
Droplet-air	Vaccine preventable: mainly influenza, measles, rubella; *M. tuberculosis*, *N. meningitidis* Vaccine nonpreventable: SARS-CoV; *Legionella*
Feces-food	HAV, *Norovirus*; *Campylobacter*, *E. coli*, *Salmonella*, *Shigella*, staphylococcal food poisoning, *V. cholerae* (endemic areas); *Cryptosporidium*
Zoonotic	Agents from invertebrate vectors, agents from sacrificed livestock

76% (19/25) of swine exhibitors were seroreactive to *Influenzavirus*, compared with none of 25 swine exhibitors from a neighboring county.

Measles virus (2139, 2378, 2631). Fairs can be transmission sites. In Adelaide, Australia, in 2003, a worker returning from New Zealand and a coworker of the same supermarket set off an outbreak with four secondary cases at the supermarket, and seven secondary and four tertiary cases at a concert hall in a hotel that one index case had attended. At the 1991 International Special Olympics in Minneapolis, a track and field athlete from Argentina with measles caused an outbreak with 16 primary and 9 secondary cases; transmission occurred at the opening ceremony in a domed stadium, or at track and field events. In rural Senegal in 1983–1986, 7% (30/402) of primary measles cases were acquired at gatherings.

Rubella virus (8396). In an outbreak in People's Republic of China in 1989–1990 with an attack rate of 37%, all 196 first-generation rubella cases reported visiting a particular cinema.

SARS-coronavirus (CoV) (5658). Humans are confirmed sources, while living mammals offered on Asian markets are a suspected source. To curb the SARS epidemic in Beijing, People's Republic of China, in 2003, ~30,000 residents were quarantined for 14 days, at home or at dedicated sites. Exposure was defined by contact with a SARS patient for ≥30 min, at home, the workplace, school, public transport, or the hospital. Quarantine was evaluated in one district. SARS attack rates were ~3% (95% confidence interval [95% CI] 2–4) in 5,186 quarantined persons and 0% (0–3%) in persons not meeting quarantine requirements. Although quarantine was effective, efficiency could have been increased by limiting it to SARS patient contacts, because attack rates peaked among quarantined persons (~4%, 3–6%) in the contact group.

Bacteria
***Legionella* (1579, 2625, 3645, 5887).** *L. pneumophila* is a risk at fairs that feature aerosol-generating devices. For buildings, see section 6.2. In an outbreak in Murcia, Spain, walking within a 200-m radius from the source was a significant risk. For risk reduction, aerosol-producing devices were proposed to be banned from fairs.

Outbreaks Venues for outbreaks include fairs, grocery stores, shopping centers, open concerts, and the centers of cities.
- North America (4661, 6167). At a grocery store in Bogalusa, La., in 1989, an ultrasonic mist machine to mist vegetables was source for 33 cases of Legionnaires' disease among shoppers. In a rural county of Maryland in 1986, 75% (12/16) of residents developed legionellosis within 2 weeks after visiting a retail store compared with 14% (4/28) sex- and age-matched community controls; adjacent to the store, excavation and construction work was ongoing, which was the suggested outbreak source.
- Australia (4396). In 10 years (1991–2000), 3 (of 22) outbreaks occurred in shopping centers, in Sydney in fall 1992 (26 cases), in Sydney in summer 1995 (11 cases), and in Victoria in winter 1998 (4 cases). In all three outbreaks, cooling towers were the likely source.
- West Europe (1827, 1876, 4362, 5797) About 30–45% of cases are community acquired. At an annual flower show in The Netherlands in 1999, two whirlpool spas were sources for ≥188 cases among 77,061 visitors and exhibitors. At a commercial fair in Belgium in 1999, 93 of ~50,000 visitors contracted *L. pneumophila* serogroup 1 disease, likely from an aerosol-producing whirlpool.

***Mycobacterium tuberculosis* (179, 6074, 7697).** Unrecognized infective cases are a plausible source. Pulmonary tuberculosis was a cause for hospitalization of hajj pilgrims. Venues for outbreaks have included concert rooms, singing choirs, Christmas parties, a church gathering, and a traveling circus. Two unrecognized infective musicians of a Dutch rock band were sources for 40 tuberculosis cases in small concert rooms and probably hundreds of infections. In rural Kentucky and Tennessee in 1995, 68% (224/328) contacts of an unrecognized infective case were reactive to tuberculin, compared with a community infection prevalence of 3% (4/149). Reactivity was 100% (28/28) among close (family) contacts, 71% (165/231) among contacts at the clothing factory where the index case worked, and 46% (31/68) among social contacts described as "hanging out at the local gasoline station at night."

***Neisseria meningitidis* (7749).** At an international football tournament in Belgium in 1997, serogroup C disease caused an outbreak with cases in Germany (1), Denmark (2), and The Netherlands (2 primary and 4 secondary at the team's home village).

FECES-FOOD CLUSTER, FAIRS
Hazards (2894, 8064) are unauthorized food vendors, inadequate sanitation (particularly at open-air fairs), and exhibited animals. For foods, see section III.

Viruses
Hepatitis A virus (HAV) (2894). In the United States in 2003, 25 attendees contracted acute hepatitis A (HA) at outdoor camping and concert events.

***Norovirus* (2262).** At a metropolitan concert hall (capacity, 2,000) in the United Kingdom in 1999, *Norovirus* gastroenteritis affected >300 attendees in 5 days; the outbreak was triggered by a patient who vomited in the auditorium and adjacent toilet. Disinfection was inadequate; maintenance workers likely acquired virus from aerosols, attendees from walking on soiled carpet or from using soiled toilets. The overall attack rate was 21%, with a range of 0.6–75%, and a high in attendees seated in the same tier as the index case.

Bacteria
***Campylobacter* (1161, 5190).** At a festival in the United Kingdom, 72 attendees contracted *Campylobacter* likely from unpasteurized milk sold at the event. Well water was a likely source for *C. jejuni* enteritis at a fair near Albany, N.Y.

Escherichia coli.

Outbreaks Venues for outbreaks include fairs and pet zoos and farms (for the latter, see section 13.4).
- North America (2094) (1161, 7773). At a fair in Texas in 2003, 25 livestock exhibitors and visitors contracted *E. coli* O157:H7 likely from animal contact. Patients ranged in age from 1½ to 67 years, 88% (22) were female, and four developed hemolytic uremic syndrome (HUS). The outbreak strain was cultured from seven cases and environmental samples. At a fair in Ohio in 2001, 111 attendees reported diarrhea, including 23 who met a definition for *E. coli* O157 infection. Risks included visits to a building on the fairgrounds, attending a dance inside the building, and handling sawdust; as waterborne and food-borne spread was unlikely, and sawdust and rafters grew identical *E. coli* O157 strains, airborne spread was assumed. At a fair in New York in 1999, with ~108,000 attendees, unchlorinated water from a shallow well used by food vendors for beverages and ice was implicated in an outbreak with 921 diarrhea cases, 11 HUS cases, and 2 deaths.
- West Europe (1624). At an open-air festival in the United Kingdom in 1997, 8 of ~80,000 attendees had evidence of enterohemorrhagic *E. coli* (EHEC) infection at widely dispersed camp sites; dairy cows that had grazed on the site shortly before the festival were the most likely source.

***Salmonella* (1052).** In Catalonia, Spain, "coca" pastry is popular at the Eve of Saint John festival in June. In 2002, coca de crema (with vanilla cream) from one bakery caused 1,435 cases of *Salmonella enterica* serovar Enteritidis gastroenteritis among 6,500–7,500 estimated consumers, for an attack rate of ~22%.

***Shigella* (4304, 8064).** *Shigella* is a risk at fairs, including from foods and human contact. At an outdoor music festival in Michigan, in 1988, >3,150 of 6,400 participants contracted *S. sonnei* gastroenteritis; uncooked tofu salad prepared by >2,000 volunteer food handlers was the likely vehicle. At a camp gathering in a national forest, poor sanitation was implicated in an *S. sonnei* outbreak that affected >50% of the >12,000 attendees.

***Staphylococcus*, enterotoxigenic (1957).** In Minas Gerais, Brazil, in 1998, of ~8,000 catered attendees, ~4,000 (50%) contracted staphylococcal food poisoning within 4 h, ~2000 (25%) sought medical care; in the ensuing chaos, 396 (5%) were hospitalized, 81 (1%) were admitted to intensive care units (ICU) (for dehydration), and 16 (0.2%) died (of shock and multiorgan failure).

***Vibrio* (4064, 4540).** At a scientific conference in New Orleans, La., in 1986, 12% (160/1,380) of questioned participants reported diarrhea, and of 479 submitted stool samples, 51 (11%) grew *Vibrio*, including *V. parahaemolyticus* (35), *V. cholerae* non-O1 (13), and *V. vulnificus* (3). Raw and cooked oysters were the vehicle confirmed epidemiologically and microbiologically. In Papua, Indonesia, attending a funeral during an El Tor cholera outbreak was a risk for contracting cholera.

Protozoa
***Cryptosporidium* (309, 5046).** In Tasmania, Australia, in 2001, an outbreak with 48 cases was traced to an agricultural show; of 19 first-wave (within one incubation period) cases, 14 had visited an animal nursery, and most had touched exhibited animals (goats, lambs, calves, puppies, rabbits, pet rats, and chickens). At an agricultural outdoor fair in Maine in 1993, about one fourth of >700 attendees contracted *Cryptosporidium* diarrhea from fresh-pressed apple cider.

ZOONOTIC CLUSTER, FAIRS
Hazards include day-active vectors, sacrificial animals, and refuse from markets that attract scavengers and flies.

Dengue virus (DENV) (3170, 6890, 7201). At the 2002 carnival in Rio de Janeiro, an extreme clustering of dengue cases was observed. In Thailand, foci of dengue transmission included a school and a Buddhist temple.

Crimean-Congo hemorrhagic fever virus (CCHFV) (3637). In Pakistan, in 2000, livestock from enzootic, rural areas moved into Karachi for a Muslim festival were likely the source of acute CCHF in at least six residents who had not left the city in the preceding few weeks.

***Echinococcus* (198).** On markets in enzootic areas of Africa, where livestock, infective viscera from slaughter, dogs, and people congregate, conditions are favorable for transmission of *E. granulosus*.

Arthropods (624). At a shopping mall in Austin, Tex., in 1981, decorative wheat infested by the straw itch mite (*Pyemotes ventricosus*) was the source for an outbreak of dermatitis.

SKIN-BLOOD CLUSTER, FAIRS

At crowded places, skin contacts are a putative hazard.

Variola (3418). Preeradication, funerals were sites for smallpox outbreaks in West Africa.

***Mycobacterium leprae* (6111).** In some urban areas in India, the point prevalence of leprosy among beggars can reach 30%, and 17% can be smear positive. Open cases among destitute persons are considered a potential source of infection for relatives and the public at crowded places such as bus stops.

13.2 CATERED EVENTS AND RESTAURANTS

Catered events include commercial venues that sell ready-to-eat foods, e.g., cafeterias, canteens, deli shops, drive-through outlets, ice cream parlors, restaurants, salad bars, street stalls, and vending machines, as well as noncommercial invitations and parties, e.g., for birthday, Christmas, New Year, and Thanksgiving celebrations.

Exposure (1524) (http://www.cdc.gov/foodnet/surveys/Pop_surv.htm). In 2000, visits in the preceding week reported by a representative sample ($n = 13,113$) from eight of the U.S. states included community events by 1–2%, food takeouts by 6–19%, cafeterias by 10–18%, restaurants by 22–44%, fast-food chains by 22–45%, and salad bars by 30–45%. Of 2,000 shoppers surveyed in the United States in 1996, >10% purchased ready-to-eat, take-out food at least once per week. However, consumer attitudes and habits are continuously changing. For the exposure history (Boxes III.1 and 13.1), consider local events and the celebration calendar, in particular, when two or more food-borne diarrhea cases are diagnosed within hours or days.

Infections (500, 1954, 2259, 2961, 3052, 3223, 5602, 6275, 6830, 7100) (Box 13.3). In high-income countries, restaurants or catered events are venues for ~35–55% of food-borne outbreaks. In Australia in 2004, restaurants were the most frequent site for food-borne outbreaks implicated in 36% (42/118) of outbreaks. In North America, fast-food chains have been implicated in outbreaks of *E. coli* O157:H7 and *Salmonella*. In France, about one third of food-borne outbreaks occur at private parties. Although most food-borne infections are enteric, respiratory agents can be acquired from foods (or at parties).

DROPLET-AIR CLUSTER, CATERING

Poorly ventilated rooms and smoke are a hazard for respiratory tract infections from restaurants and bars.

***Legionella* (3739).** In Tennessee in 2002, Pontiac fever was diagnosed in 117 patrons of a restaurant; common foods were not identified, but 58% of ill patrons and only 18% of well clients sat near a large fountain that grew *L. anisa*, and 11 of 22 ill patrons had a $\geq$4-fold increase in titer of antibody to the outbreak strain of *L. anisa*.

***M. tuberculosis* (3994, 5324).** Bars are reported transmission sites for *M. tuberculosis*.

***N. meningitidis* (3551).** A campus bar was the site for an outbreak with nine cases of *N. meningitidis* serogroup C disease in patrons.

FECES-FOOD CLUSTER, CATERING

All viruses, bacteria, protozoa, and helminths in this cluster could be acquired from catered foods.

Viruses

Food handlers are the principal source of HAV and *Norovirus* in foods.

HAV (1204, 1885, 4218, 4539). Restaurant-associated outbreaks of HAV have been well documented. Sources can be food handlers or food polluted during harvest or processing. At a restaurant in Pennsylvania in 2003, 13 food workers and >540 patrons were diagnosed with acute HA, and three persons died; the implicated vehicle was green onions. At a restaurant in Ohio in 1998, green onions caused an outbreak with 40 acute HA cases.

Box 13.3 Agents and infections from catered events, by agent cluster	
Droplet-air	Legionellosis, meningococcal disease, tuberculosis
Feces-food	HAV, *Norovirus*; botulism, food poisoning (*B. cereus*, *C. perfringens*, and staphylococcal), enteritis by *Campylobacter*, *E. coli* (EHEC, ETEC), *Salmonella* (serovar Typhi, non-Typhi serovars), *Shigella*, *V. cholerae* (endemic areas), *V. parahaemolyticus*
Skin-blood	Food-borne streptococcal pharyngitis

***Norovirus* (4744).** Although primarily food borne, *Norovirus* can be aerosolized from vomiting, and it can spread person-to-person at restaurants.

Outbreaks Outbreaks are well documented.
- North America (200, 2313, 5727). Restaurants and catered events were sites for 39% of *Norovirus* outbreaks reported in the United States in 1996–2000; in 217 outbreaks, 5–800 (median, 33) persons were affected. In 2000, after a New York-based car dealership supplied banquet meals to 52 dealers nationwide, 13 states reported 333 (44%) diarrhea cases among 753 attendees, and the virus was detected by reverse transcriptase-PCR in 32 of 59 stool samples from eight states. A subcontracter to the Ohio-based caterer was the likely source, and salads were the implicated vehicle.
- Australasia (3342, 4765). In Nagasaki, Japan, in 2 days of 2003, *Norovirus* gastroenteritis was diagnosed in 44% (660/1,492) of tourists who ate lunch in one restaurant; the same genogroup virus was amplified from cases, workers, and the kitchen table. At a Mediterranean-style restaurant in suburban Victoria, Australia in 1998–1999, sources for three sequential *Norovirus* outbreaks appeared to be guests who typically ate food with their fingers from a common platter.
- West Europe (3407, 5889). In the United Kingdom in 1992–2000, only 6% (105/1,877) of laboratory-confirmed *Norovirus* outbreaks occurred in restaurants. At a restaurant in the United Kingdom, 49 patrons contracted diarrhea, and the virus was identified in six cases and one chef who had prepared the salad that was implicated epidemiologically. Interestingly, the chef had been symptom free for 48 h before returning to work.

Bacteria
Restaurant-associated outbreaks are typically limited to local guests. In contrast, restaurants catering to tourists and fast-food chains may reach an international clientele.

***Bacillus cereus* (2669, 6957).** *B. cereus* Food poisoning at catered events has been reported. At a food party in Canada, 25 (70%) of 36 attendees contracted food poisoning, likely from mayonnaise served in potato salad (2669).

***Campylobacter* (155, 2541).** In the United Kingdom in 1995–1999, 32 (64%) of 50 reported *Campylobacter* outbreaks occurred at catered venues: restaurants (50% or 16), hotels (31% or 10), bars (13% or 4), a hall (3% or 1), and a canteen (3% or 1). At a private party in Germany, five of six attendees from Austria, Germany, and Liechtenstein contracted *C. jejuni* enteritis from barbecued chicken; the outbreak strain was traced to a food shop in Tyrol and further to an abattoir and a farm in Carinthia.

Clostridium. C. botulinum* (3794, 7014).** Restaurant botulism has mainly been reported in North America. In the United States in 1990–2000, two outbreaks occurred at restaurants, one in Texas in 1993 by "skordalia" (potato-based dip) with 17 cases, and one in Georgia in 1993 by cheese sauce with eight cases. At a church supper in Texas in 2001, frozen chili was an outbreak vehicle. ***C. perfringens. Food poisoning is well documented at catered events, as are outbreaks.

Outbreaks
- North America (2958, 5852). At a factory banquet in Connecticut in 1985, gravy was the suspected vehicle for an attack rate of ~44% among 1,362 attending employees.
- Australia (7403). At a wedding reception at a hotel in Brisbane, Australia, in 1993, chicken vol-au-vent was vehicle for 53 cases, for an attack rate of 62%.
- West Europe (267, 6612). At a restaurant in Bari, Italy, in 1997, "pasta al ragu" was vehicle for 25 cases. At a restaurant in Spain, ravioli and cheese sauce were vehicle for 17 cases, for an attack rate of 71%.

***E. coli* (3838).** Eating at restaurants is a risk for infection with with *E. coli* O157:H7 (EHEC) and enterotoxigenic *E. coli* (ETEC).

Outbreaks Outbreaks have been documented in North America and Asia.
- North America (531, 3614, 3655, 5317). In 1999, an EHEC outbreak with cases in Arizona, California, and Nevada was traced to beef tacos from a fast-food Mexican-style restaurant chain. In Minnesota in 1998, chopped parsley was implicated in two restaurant-associated ETEC outbreaks. In the Pacific Northwest in 1993, salads from bars were implicated in EHEC outbreaks at four chain restaurants. In 1992–1993, a multistate EHEC outbreak with >500 cases (including 45 HUS cases and 3 deaths) was traced to hamburgers from a fast-food chain.
- Asia. In Japan in 2002, grilled beef served by a 63-branch restaurant chain was the vehicle for an EHEC outbreak with 43 cases (1–77 years of age) from 19 restaurants located in Hyogo, Kyoto, Nara, Wakayama, and Okayama (7597).

Salmonella. Both *S. enterica* serovar Typhi (5601, 7687, 8343) and non-Typhi *S. enterica* (379, 2252, 4928, 5041, 7514) can be restaurant associated. For serovar Typhi, sources are carrier food workers; for non-Typhi serovars, sources are foods or ill workers. In Oregon in 1984, serovar Typhimurium was intentionally released in restaurants. **Non-Typhi serovars.** Numerous restaurant outbreaks underpin these agents as a major hazard.

Outbreaks
- North America (5763, 6813). In the United States in 1985–1999, 62% (522/841) of serovar Enteritidis outbreaks occurred at commercial food establishments (restaurants, caterers, delicatessens, bakeries, and cafeterias). At a restaurant in Sioux Falls, S.D., in 1996, 52 patrons, attendees at three luncheons, and workers were diagnosed with serovar Thompson infections, and roast beef was the implicated vehicle.
- Australasia (115, 7651). At a restaurant in southwestern Saudi Arabia in 1996, 124 patrons contracted serovar Enteritidis enteritis (91 culture confirmed), likely from mayonnaise served with fried chicken. At a restaurant in New South Wales, Australia, in 2002, 17 cases of serovar Potsdam enteritis were traced to Caesar salad dressing and a mayonnaise bottle that grew the agent.
- West Europe (379, 660, 2252). At a restaurant in Denmark in 2003, a buffet prepared by an assistant chef was implicated in >70–390 serovar Typhimurium enteritis cases (67 laboratory confirmed) among Danish, Swedish, Norwegian, and German patrons, for an overall attack rate of ~7%. At a Chinese restaurant in the United Kingdom in 2002, egg-fried rice left at room temperature for 7 h before use caused an serovar Enteritidis outbreak with 38 cases. At a restaurant in Rimini, Italy, in 1997, 29 patrons contracted serovar Hadar enteritis from well-roasted rabbit; handling and poor storage contributed to the outbreak.

Serovar Typhi (5601, 7687, 8343). In New York City in 2000, seven typhoid fever cases were linked to a restaurant in Queens, likely from an immigrant employee. In Nauru, in the South Pacific, in 1998–1999, 50 patrons contracted typhoid fever (19 culture confirmed) from two restaurants that employed carrier workers. At a floating restaurant in France in 1998, 27 guests (15 culture confirmed) contracted typhoid fever; a source could not be identified.

***Shigella* (5317, 6253, 7069, 7551).** Outbreaks of *Shigella* at catered events have been reported, including fast-food restaurants catering centrally prepared foods. Sources of *Shigella* are food workers or imported fresh produce. In Canada and the United States in 1998, *S. sonnei* from imported, cut parsley caused restaurant-associated outbreaks. At a wedding anniversary banquet in Alberta, Canada, in 1982, an outbreak caused 115 cases, for an attack rate of 71%; home-prepared turkey dressing and person-to-person spread were implicated.

***Vibrio. V. cholerae* (5907, 6814, 7089).** Raw oysters, a significant vehicle, are frequently eaten at street food stands. Restaurant-associated non-O1 *V. cholerae* infections have been documented in Italy. Attending funeral feasts for persons deceased from cholera is a risk. At a funeral in Guinea in 1986, a cholera outbreak was linked to women who cleaned the body and bed of a cholera victim and subsequently helped to prepare foods for the funeral. ***V. parahaemolyticus* (2961, 3487, 5102).** Restaurant-associated *V. parahaemolyticus* outbreaks have been reported. In Shiga Prefecture, Japan, in 1998, catered meals caused an outbreak with 1,167 cases.

Protozoa
Catered events seem infrequent sources.

***Cryptosporidium* (1153).** At a dinner banquet in a Spokane, Wash., restaurant, in 1997, an *Cryptosporidium* outbreak caused an attack rate of 87%.

***Giardia* (5971, 6051).** Reported outbreak venues are a restaurant and a party. At a restaurant in Washington State in 1990, 75% (27/36) of attendees of a meeting became ill compared with 3% (1/31) nonattending employees; no vehicle could be implicated.

Helminths
***Angiostrongylus* (8295).** At a restaurant in Wenzhou, People's Republic of China, in 1997, 45% (47/105) of consumers of undercooked snails (*Ampullaria gigas*) contracted eosinophilic meningitis, compared with none (0/77) of snail nonconsuming patrons. Attack rates in consumers were higher (86%, 25/29) in those who ate four or more pieces than in those (20%, 22/76) who ate one to three pieces. Larvae (L3) of *A. cantonensis* were recovered from *A. gigas* taken from the locality, and adult worms were recovered from local rats.

***Anisakis* (3476, 5644, 7294).** In France, two anisakiasis cases resulted from fish consumption at Japanese restaurants. In Japan and parts of the Americas (California, Hawaii, and Brazil) sushi is popular and prepared at bars or supermarkets. Sushi bars are considered infrequent sources of anisakiasis.

***Trichinella* (4865).** At a wedding party among 250 mostly Laotian refugees in North America in 1990, uncooked sausages homemade from commercial pork caused 90 trichinellosis cases, for an attack rate of 36%.

SKIN-SEX CLUSTER, CATERING
***Staphylococcus aureus* (114, 4376, 5602).** Nasal carriers (see section 14.1) of enterotoxin-producing strains are

potential sources of *S. aureus*. Restaurant-associated outbreaks seem rare, however. In the United States in 1993–1997, *S. aureus* food poisoning accounted for only 1.5% of reported food-borne outbreaks, and cafeterias, delicatessens, or restaurants were venues for only 17% (7/42) of *S. aureus* outbreaks. Mushrooms served at a restaurant, a pizzeria, a university cafeteria, and a hospital cafeteria were the vehicle for staphylococcal food poisoning in 99 patrons; canned mushrooms imported from China yielded staphylococcal enterotoxin A.

Box 13.4 Agents and infections from pools and other treated recreational waters, by agent cluster

Droplet-air	Enterovirus; *Legionella*
Feces-food	HAV, Norovirus; *E. coli*, *Shigella*; *Cryptosporidium*, *Giardia*
Environmental	*Pseudomonas* (dermatitis), mycobacteria (granuloma)
Skin-blood	Warts, molluscum contagiosum; tinea pedis

***Streptococcus pyogenes* (group A *Streptococcus* [GAS]) (2597, 4379).** GAS from the throats of workers can be sources of food-borne pharyngitis. Of 35 food-borne outbreaks of GAS pharyngitis in 1941–1997, four occurred at church or charity lunches, three at private or picnic parties, two at banquets, and two at conferences, including a microbiology conference in Oregon in 1981. At a restaurant in Italy in 1986, GAS pharyngitis was diagnosed in 63 attendees of wedding banquets; prawn hors-d'oeuvre and custard cakes were suspected vehicles. Six staff, five of whom were in the restaurant manager's family, were colonized with the outbreak strain.

13.3 SWIMMING POOLS AND SPAS

Pools and spas are treated, recreational, public or private water habitats, including indoor and outdoor swimming pools, wading pools, hot tubs, spas, water fountains, whirlpools, and water parks.

Exposure (1461, 3872, 7814). Swimming is a popular recreational activity. In high-income countries, 6–8% of people reported pool visits in the preceding 7 days. In the United States alone, there are 360–400 million pool visits per year, and ~5 million hot tubs, whirlpools, and spas are in use. In the United States, of 5,385 pools inspected in 2002, 18% of wading pools violated codes, as did 14% of therapy pools, and 14% of motel pools. Of 4,533 spas inspected in 2002, 11% were closed immediately, mainly for violated water chemistry or filtration, and most often at campgrounds, hotels-motels, clubs-gyms, and apartments-condominiums.

The exposure history (Box 13.1) should address the dates and types of pools visited, the numbers and ages of users, the appearance of the pool water (clear, cloudy, or irritating), and maintenance (staff and records).

Infections (469, 4310, 8340) (Box 13.4). Sources of contaminated pool water are people (feet, skin, urine, and feces), animals, and runoff water. Diapered infants in wading pools are a fecal peril. Infections are acquired from ingestion (swallow), inhalation (aerosol), or contact. In the United States in 1990–2002, 141 pool-related outbreaks with a known infectious agent were reported (Table 13.1). Warm water promotes growth of bacteria. In temperate climates, recreational water disease outbreaks peak in the summer (Fig. 13.1).

Preventive measures (1234, 3872, 5250, 7901). Preventive measures include user education (shower and hygiene), maintenance (cleaning and filter and tube checks), water management (weekly to monthly renewal

Table 13.1 Outbreaks from treated recreational waters (swimming pools and spas) by known infectious disease agents: United States 1990–2002[a]

Illness	Agent	No. of outbreaks	No. of cases	No. of cases/outbreak
Respiratory	*Legionella*	7	177	25
Diarrhea	*Cryptosporidium*	44	12,483	284
	Giardia lamblia	5	187	37
	Norovirus	5	115	23
	Shigella	5	131	26
	Escherichia coli O157:H7	4	60	15
	Other enteric bacteria (e.g., *Salmonella* and *Campylobacter*)	2	9	
Dermatitis	*Pseudomonas aeruginosa*	67	1,142	17
	Other skin bacteria (e.g., *Bacillus* and *Staphylococcus*)	2	23	

[a]From references 469, 4310, and 8340 and previous issues.

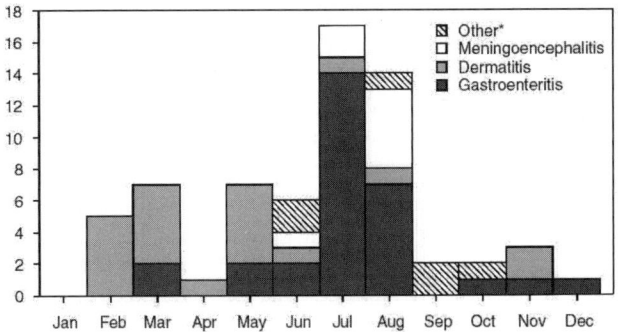

Figure 13.1 Recreational water-related disease outbreaks, United States 2001–2002. The number of outbreaks (y axis, n = 65) is given by month (x axis) and syndromes: gastroenteritis (black), dermatitis (light gray), meningoencephalitis (white), and others, e.g., respiratory or chemical (hatched). From reference 8340.

and chlorination), and surveillance (temperature, pH, free chlorine, and microorganisms). Water quality should be monitored weekly for *E. coli* and enterococci. European Union limits for *E. coli* in bathing waters are 200 CFU/100ml.

DROPLET-AIR CLUSTER, POOLS

Indoor pools and spas are more likely habitats for respiratory tract infections than outdoor pools.

Viruses
Adenovirus (3145, 5719). Adenovirus is a cause of pharyngoconjunctivitis in swimmers.

***Enterovirus* (1595, 3873, 7901).** *Enterovirus* has been identified in pools and recreational waters. *Enterovirus* has caused pool outbreaks, including of aseptic meningitis by echovirus. When an outdoor swimming pool was opened at a seaside village in Northern Ireland in 1992, the index attendee with confirmed echovirus 30 infection vomited into the pool, and subsequently 33 other bathers fell ill with vomiting, diarrhea, and headache.

Bacteria
***Legionella*.** Warm, nutrient-rich waters support growth of *Legionella* spp., including in pools and spas.

- Pools (4347). In Bologna, Italy, 2 of 48 pool water samples, and 27 of 48 pool hot-water showers grew *Legionella* (10–19,250 CFU/liter), including *L. micdadei*, *L. bozemanii*, and *L. pneumophila*.
- Spas (thermal, therapeutic, and whirl) (778, 1049, 6349). *Legionella* concentrations in hot-spring spas can reach 1,000–100,000 CFU/liter. In Portugal during the spa season (spring to fall), on repeat sampling of 10 sites, 6 *Legionella* spp. were isolated, mainly *L. pneumophila* and *L. londiniensis*. Spas seem to readily generate aerosols. In France in 1998–2001, of 1,015 legionellosis cases with exposure known, 26 (3%) were associated with thermal cures.

Outbreaks Venues for outbreaks include whirlpools at hotels and exhibitions.

- North America (562, 567, 2379, 8340). At least seven recreational outbreaks were reported in 1990–2002, for a mean of 25 cases per outbreak (Table 13.1). At an Illinois motel in 2002, a spa was the source for 68 cases of Pontiac fever. From a whirlpool at a hotel in Georgia in 1999, 24 persons from three states contracted Pontiac fever or Legionnaires' disease. At a Wisconsin hotel in 1998, guests who used the whirlpool spa contracted Pontiac fever at a rate of 71% (35/49); *L. micdadei* was recovered from the spa water. At a home-improvement store in Virginia in 1996, a display whirlpool spa caused an outbreak with 23 confirmed cases of Legionnaires' disease; walking by was sufficient for exposure.
- Asia (5322). In Ishioka City, Japan, in 2000, 34 persons contracted Legionnaires' disease (20 confirmed and 14 probable) from communal bath water that failed circulation and filtration.
- West Europe (1876, 2872, 4894). At a Swedish hotel in 1999, Pontiac fever attack rates were 71% (27/38) in guests who visited a whirlpool, but 1% (3/323) in non-visiting guests. In The Netherlands in 1999, whirlpool spas and sprinklers in halls of a flower show were the source for 188 cases in visitors. In the United Kingdom a spa pool on display at a retail outlet was the source for three seemingly unlinked, sporadic cases.

***N. meningitidis* (1053).** In Spain, cases of meningococcal disease were linked to a swimming club and indoor swimming pool.

FECES-FOOD CLUSTER, POOLS
Viruses
HAV (4659, 7318). Few outbreaks of HAV have been reported. At a campground in Louisiana in 1989, 20 (2%) of 822 residents contracted acute HA; all cases reported swimming in one of the public pools, and cases were more likely than controls to swim for >1 h, and to submerge their heads. In suburban Melbourne, Australia, in 1997, seven young males contracted acute HA from using a spa pool that included "spitting whales" (that spit mouthfuls of spa water).

***Norovirus*.** Small children are presumed sources. *Norovirus* is a cause of recreational diarrhea outbreaks reported in high-income countries.

Outbreaks
- North America (1234, 3822, 8340). At a Vermont swimming club in 2004, a kink in the chlorine feeder

tube and presumed fecal contamination from an infant pool user caused an outbreak with 53 cases, for an attack rate of 28%. At a motel in Wisconsin in 2002, a pool was the source for 15 cases. In Ohio, a contaminated pool at an elementary school caused an outbreak with 103 cases among students and staff.
- Europe (3367, 4847). In The Netherlands, on a hot summer day, *Norovirus* caused gastroenteritis in ≥90 school children playing at a recreational water fountain, for an attack rate of 54% (90/167); identical strains were recovered from children and fountain water samples. In Helsinki, Finland, in 2001, bathing in an outdoor wading pool resulted in a gastroenteritis outbreak with 242 cases, mostly children (age: median, 9 years; range, $^3/_4$–73 years); *Norovirus* was amplified from patients and pool bottom water (in addition to astrovirus from patients).

Bacteria

Shallow or poorly maintained pools are a hazard, principally for *Escherichia* and *Shigella*, rarely *Campylobacter* or *Salmonella* (Table 13.1).

***E. coli* (873, 2531, 3877).** Near Portland, Oreg., in 1991, swimming at a lakeside park caused 21 *E. coli* O157:H7 infections in children, including bloody diarrhea and HUS. In the United States, a party at a trailer park pool was followed by 10 diarrhea cases (*E. coli* O157:H7 isolated in one) among 51 attendees and residents; swimming in the pool was the only significant risk. In the United Kingdom in 1992, a paddling pool for children was implicated in an EHEC outbreak with five cases and one infection.

***Shigella* (1181, 3877).** In the United States in 2001, a wading pool in a large city park caused 45 primary cases (within 3 days of exposure) and 24 secondary cases (within 3 days of a household index case); 26 stool samples yielded *S. sonnei*. Near Portland, Oreg., in 1991, swimming at a lakeside park caused 38 *S. sonnei* infections, mostly in children.

Protozoa

***Cryptosporidium* (2479, 6331, 6662, 7098).** *Cryptosporidium* oocysts have been identified in pool water or filter samples. Recreational infections are a risk. In Australia, swimming in pools has been a significant risk for epidemic *and* sporadic cases.

Outbreaks Outbreaks are well documented.
- North America (1877, 4526, 4820, 4864, 7041, 7814, 8340). Over 40 recreational outbreaks of *Cryptosporidium* were reported in 1990–2002, for a mean of 284 cases per outbreak (Table 13.1). In British Columbia in 2003, 14 confirmed cases contracted *C. parvum* from a recreational pool; oocysts were detected in pool water at a density of 14 per 100 liters. In Ohio in 2000, a club pool was the source for 601 suspected plus 144 confirmed cases; swimming was a significant risk, and *C. parvum* human and bovine genotypes were identified from humans and the pool filter. At a sport club in Massachusetts in 2002, a pool was the source for 767 cases. At a Minnesota zoo in 1997, a water sprinkler fountain in which children were playing was the likely source for 369 cases (333 of age ≤10 years). At an indoor water park in Oregon in 1992, waves generated by heated pools were implicated in 55 cases; free chlorine pool levels which were documented at least twice daily exceeded the recommended minimum of 0.8 mg/liter on 99% of readings. At a private pool in Los Angeles County in 1988, 44 (73%) of 60 pool users contracted cryptosporidiasis, including a water polo team, a scuba class, a swimmer group, and lifeguard staff; attack rates increased with increasing hours in water.
- Australia (6032). In New South Wales in 1998, an outbreak caused ~1,020 cases in 5 months; compared with 200 controls, 100 cases were more likely to report swimming at a public pool (odds ratio, 2.7; 95% CI 1.4–5) or in natural freshwaters (odds ratio, 4.8; 95% CI 1.1–20).
- West Europe (1631, 3560, 3706). In the United Kingdom in 1988, a swimming-pool-related outbreak caused 67 cases; oocysts were detected in pool water. In Spain in 1995–2003, two *Cryptosporidium* outbreaks were reported from hotel swimming pools. In Sweden in late summer of 2002, swimming in a public outdoor pool was implicated in an outbreak with ~800–1,000 cases, for primary attack rates of 40–50% and secondary attack rates among household pool nonusing contacts of 8–10%.

***Giardia lamblia* (2479, 4310, 5972, 6662, 8340).** *G. lamblia* cysts have been detected in pool water or filter samples. Recreational infections are a risk. Outbreaks have mainly been reported in North America. Mean case loads in five recreational outbreaks were 37 (Table 13.1). At an indoor pool in New Jersey in 1985, *Giardia* affected nine swimmers (all females, two children, seven adults); attack rates were highest (39% or 5/13) in the adult lap group exposed on a day when a handicapped child had a fecal accident in the pool. Pool records showed that no chlorine levels were taken on that day, and that chlorine level was zero on the following day. Including the child with the accident, 9 (45%) of 20 handicapped swimmers tested positive for *G. lamblia*.

Fungi

Microsporidia have been identified in pool water by PCR (2479). Swimming in pools appears to be a risk (3521).

ENVIRONMENTAL CLUSTER, POOLS

Skin manifestations from exposure to artificial recreational water include dermatitis (by *Pseudomonas* and *Schistosoma*), granuloma (by environmental mycobacteria), external otitis, and keratitis (by free-living amebas).

Bacteria
Environmental mycobacteria (2298, 3544, 4346). Environmental mycobacteria have been detected in water from pools, whirlpools, and hot tubs. In Finland, five of seven indoor pools grew mycobacteria, including *M. kansasii* and *M. fortuitum* sensu lato (sl); counts were highest in a small pool with high temperature, low pH, and low content of free chlorine. **M. marinum (2412, 4363).** *M. marinum* has occasionally caused "swimming pool granuloma," which is considered an occupational hazard for lifeguards. **M. avium complex (1804, 2197, 2236, 4709).** *M. avium* complex infections have been reported after exposure in hot tubs. In Colorado in 1998, indistinguishable isolates of *M. avium* complex were obtained from hot-tub water and from three of five members of a family who used the tub; *M. fortuitum* was also isolated, from water and a fourth family member.

***Pseudomonas* (3394, 5169, 7348).** *P. aeruginosa* has been isolated from recreational water samples, including pools, and from equipment such as swimming pool inflatables. In Northern Ireland 3,510 water samples from 132 amenities were tested over 2 years, 31% (4/13) of hydrotherapy pools, 38% (26/68) of swimming pools, and 73% (37/51) of jacuzzis and spas grew *P. aeruginosa* at least once.

P. aeruginosa is a significant cause of recreational dermatitis that typically affects skin not covered by swimming suits. Dermatitis has resulted from whirlpools, hot tubs, swimming pools, saunas, and water slides and from contact with equipment.

Outbreaks Outbreaks have been well documented.
- North America (2398, 4310, 6133, 8340) (Table 13.1). Typical venues are whirlpools, hot tubs, and spas. A motel pool and spa in Alaska in 2002 was source for 110 *P. aeruginosa* dermatitis cases. In Newfoundland, 26 (72%) of 36 guests who used the hotel whirlpool developed *P. aeruginosa* folliculitis. Also in Canada, a wading pool was source for 40 *P. aeruginosa* infections in children; the manifestation was painful, erythematous nodules of the feet (hot-foot syndrome).
- West Europe (2268, 7348). From outdoor games in the United Kingdom in 2001 that included a water slide, 151 (26%) of 593 children from 24 junior schools contracted a papulopustular rash located predominantly over the lower trunk and buttocks; *P. aeruginosa* was isolated from water samples. Also in the United Kingdom, *P. aeruginosa* from brands of swimming pool inflatables caused 35 cases of folliculitis, mainly of the trunk, buttocks, arms, and legs.

Fungi
In Berlin, Germany, in 1981, *Sporothrix schenckii* was isolated from the floor near a shower of an indoor swimming pool.

Protozoa
Free-living amebas (4133, 4156, 4911). Free-living amebas such as *Acanthamoeba*, *Hartmannella*, and *Naegleria* have been detected in water from swimming pools, whirlpools, and hot-spring spas, including in water that grew *Legionella*, and in minimally chlorinated water. In Germany in 1982, 34 of 100 indoor swimming pool water samples yielded *Acanthamoeba*; on follow-up in 1983, most of contaminated pools had reverted to negative. *Acanthamoeba* was more frequent in pools with many visitors than in pools with <50 visitors per day. Amebic keratitis is a putative risk from swimming, diving, or wrestling under water.

Helminths
***Schistosoma* (2214).** Poorly maintained swimming pools (that harbor vector snails) and ablution basins are reported transmission sites. At a resort in Belo Horizonte, Brazil, 17 guests contracted acute intestinal schistosomiasis from swimming in the resort pool. For dermatitis from lakes, see section 5.2.

***Strongyloides* (614).** Leisure activities that include contact with muddy soil or water are a hazard in endemic areas. In Geneva, Switzerland (a nonendemic area), the only risk in a patient with presumed locally contracted *S. stercoralis* was frequent visits to swimming pools.

SKIN-BLOOD CLUSTER, POOLS
Human papillomavirus (HPV) (3717, 7871). Although plausible, there is limited evidence for the acquisition of warts and HPV from swimming pools and public showers.

***Molluscipoxvirus* (838, 5432, 8022).** Swimming in pools is a risk for acquiring molluscum contagiosum. In kindergarten and elementary school children in Japan, the rate of molluscum contagiosum in swimmers was double that in nonswimmers. In Denmark, an outdoor public swimming pool was associated with 125 cases.

***Chlamydia trachomatis*, ocular.** In adolescents and adults in high-income countries, putative sources of inclusion conjunctivitis include water from swimming pools and autoinfection from genital secretions.

Dermatophytes (177, 331, 1595, 2979, 3557, 3800, 4094). *Candida albicans, Epidermophyton floccosum, Trichophyton mentagrophytes*, and *T. verrucosum* have been recovered from the floors of showers, dressing rooms, and around pools, and *C. albicans, T. mentagrophytes*, and *T. verrucosum* have also been recovered from pool water. In some settings, tinea pedis and onychomycoses are associated with visits to public pools. In Montreal, Canada, the feet of 15% (22/150) of regular swimmers grew *T. mentagrophytes* or *T. rubrum*; 64% (14/22) of infections were manifest (athlete's foot), while the remaining were subclinical. In Japan, *T. mengagrophytes* was cultured from 72% (101/140) of students in swimming classes. In Iceland, swimmers had a three times higher prevalence of onychomycoses than the general population.

Trichomonas (4109, 5387). Acquisition of *T. vaginalis* from pool water is unlikely. Wet surfaces and objects in dressing rooms are unconfirmed, theoretical sources of *T. vaginalis*.

13.4 OUTDOOR SPORTS AND HOBBIES

Outdoor sports can be performed on earth or rock, in water, air, or caves, or on snow, either alone (e.g., jogging, hiking, and swimming [see section 13.3]) or in teams (e.g., badminton, football, and tennis) and with equipment (e.g., archery, biking, boating, camping, car racing, canoeing, climbing, diving, golfing, parachute gliding, rowing, skiing, and surfing), or with animals (e.g., horses, dogs, pigeons, fishing, and hunting).

Outdoor leisure activities are diverse and include bird watching, gardening, mushroom collecting, nature photography, and visiting zoos, farms, and wildlife centers.

Exposure (985, 1179, 5992) (http://www.cdc.gov/foodnet/surveys/). Volume and intensity of leisure exposure are poorly known. In a national U.S. sample (n = 5,238), 67% of respondents reported gardening or yard work in the preceding 30 days and 20% reported outdoor bicycle riding. In other U.S. surveys, 2–5% of respondents reported visits to zoos or animal farms in the preceding week. At a festival in Idaho, 63–68% of attendees (n = 320, mainly American Indian) reported fishing (for 13–37 days/year), 60–84% reported camping (7–24 days), 53–70% reported hiking (21–47 days), and 39–68% reported hunting (2–49 days).

Infections (Box 13.5). Infections are acquired from contact with water, soil, or plants (see section II); from bites by animals (for mammals, see section I; for arthropods, see chapter 4); by inhalation (for dust, see section 5.5); or by ingestion of beverages and foods, e.g., at camps (for foods, see section III).

Prevention. Prevention is based on exposure avoidance and vaccines. Wild large mammals, rodent burrows, and shelter in abandoned (rodent-infested) cabins should be avoided. Clothes should be checked for ticks. Washing hands should be routine after touching animals and defecation, and for barbecuing. Water should be boiled for drinking.

DROPLET-AIR CLUSTER, OUTDOOR LEISURE

Crowded camps seem a risk. In contrast, outdoors, droplets from humans or animals are likely to dissipate rapidly below the infective dose. Leisure activities that stir up soil have a potential for aerosolization of soil-dwelling agents.

Viruses

***Enterovirus* (4918, 6094, 7901).** *Enterovirus* was recovered from lake water. Outbreaks were reported at camps. In Connecticut in August of 2003, echovirus 9 caused 12 cases of aseptic meningitis and 24 cases of echoviral illness among 201 campers, for a meningitis attack rate of 6%. The likely source was a crowded campground pool; attack rates increased with increasing density of campers per site and provided evidence of secondary spread. At a remote children's camp in Alaska in 2001, echovirus 18 caused 29 meningitis cases among 113 attendees, for an attack rate of 26%; implicated risks included crowding and a fecally polluted surface water source. At a scout

Box 13.5 Agents and infections from outdoor leisure, by agent cluster	
Droplet-air	From camps, road dust: *Enterovirus; Mycoplasma, N. meningitidis; Histoplasma*
Feces-food	From camps, farms: HAV, HEV, *Norovirus; Campylobacter, C. perfringens, E. coli, Salmonella, Shigella; Cryptosporidium, Giardia, Toxoplasma*
Zoonotic	From camps, hiking, biking: *Hantavirus*, rabies virus, arthropod-borne viruses; *B. burgdorferi* sl, *Francisella*, Rickettsiales; *Babesia, Plasmodium; E. multilocularis*
Environmental	From beach, camps, lakes, parks: *Aeromonas, Burkholderia, Leptospira, Pseudomonas; Rhinosporidium, Sporothrix;* free-living amebas; hookworm, *Schistosoma, Strongyloides, Toxocara*
Skin-blood	From discarded syringes in parks: HBV

summer camp in Switzerland in 2000, coxsackie B5 virus caused 10 meningitis cases among 32 attendees; person-to-person spread was implicated, and a source was not found.

Influenzavirus **(4593).** At a crowded ski resort hostel in Austria in 1997, influenza (likely A/H3N2 virus) affected 49% of 81 ski school students; two students were hospitalized and one died.

Bacteria
Chlamydophila **(3349).** In Sweden in 1992–1993, after myocarditis caused unexpected deaths among Swedish orienteer runners, athletes were seroscreened for *C. pneumoniae*, but seroprevalences were comparable in runners (53%, 947/1,790) and control blood donors (57%, 183/319).

Mycoplasma **(908).** Outbreaks of *M. pneumoniae* were reported in summer camps, in Vermont in 1968 and in Wisconsin in 1978.

M. tuberculosis **(5559).** Infections and outbreaks of *M. tuberculosis* have occurred in circus and zoo animals (e.g., primates, elephants, and rhinos), but apparently not in visitors.

N. meningitidis **(6217).** At a campsite on the Costa Brava in Spain in 2000, a Dutch and a Polish girl contracted serogroup C invasive disease. In 1998, holiday camps were sources for serogroup C disease for two campers in France and two others in Scotland.

Fungi
Histoplasma **(5936).** Dust is a putative hazard, including from off-road vehicles. Cutting and gathering firewood in endemic areas has been associated with outbreaks of acute pulmonary histoplasmosis.

FECES-FOOD CLUSTER, OUTDOOR LEISURE
Fecal perils exist in camps, including from poor hand and kitchen hygiene, unsafe drinking water, lack of latrines, and animal manure on campgrounds. Compared with camps, lower risks are reported for gardening, and the "garden variety" bug better be called "camp variety." For army camps, see section 12.3; for mining camps, see section 12.1; for refugee camps, see section 11.4.

Bathing in polluted freshwater is a further risk. Of 827 triathlon swimmers and 773 control athletes monitored for two summers, 0.4–5% of swimmers but only 0.1–2% of controls developed gastroenteritis in the week after exposure, for an odds ratio of 1.6–2.3 (7700). Rates in swimmers were significantly increased when mean water levels of *E. coli* exceeded 355 counts per 100 ml.

Viruses
HAV (2609, 5258). In the prevaccine era, outbreaks occurred in camps, from contaminated foods or water and interpersonal spread. At a campground in Australia in 2003, 21 attendees of a 5-day youth camp contracted acute HA, for an attack rate of 9%; food (coleslaw) was the implicated vehicle. Seroreactivity was 14% (16/117) in surfers exposed to marine water, 5% (6/117) in wind surfers exposed to freshwater, and 5% (6/119) in nonexposed army personnel.

Hepatitis E virus (HEV) (294). In India, after a 2-day trekking trip, 17 of 20 school children developed HEV infection, including 10 with jaundice.

Norovirus **(1213, 1361, 1541, 5520).** Outbreaks of *Norovirus* have been reported in camps. At a youth camp in Virginia in 2001 with ~40,000 attendees, an outbreak affected 23% (56/244) of people in three subcamps. Further spread was halted by limiting contacts between ill and well persons, dedicating latrines and washing facilities, and supply of drinking water. At a religious summer camp in Norway in 2002, 134 participants reported illness, for an attack rate of 65%; virus was detected in patients, but not from fecally contaminated, untreated water supply, although drinking water and taking showers at the camp were significant epidemiological risks.

Bacteria
Campylobacter. Risks from *Campylobacter* include food and water from camps and visits to dairy farms (from drinking raw milk).

Outbreaks Outbreaks are reported from these venues.

- North America (6371, 6992, 8258). Of 20 milk-borne *Campylobacter* outbreaks in 1981–1990, 15 were associated with school field trips to dairy farms where children were offered raw milk. In Minnesota in 2000–2001, diarrhea outbreaks occurred at a farm day camp at which *Campylobacter* was isolated from eight attendees (four *C. jejuni*, three *C. coli*, and one *C. lari*) and from four calves (all *C. jejuni*).
- Europe (2264, 5888, 6301). In Germany in 2000, during educational visits to farms, 28 (74%) of 38 students and three of four adults who drunk raw milk contracted *C. jejuni* enteritis; leftover milk was not available, but milk from cows of that farm grew *C. jejuni*. In the United Kingdom in 1994, after a school trip to a dairy farm, 20 (53%) of 38 children and 3 (28%) of 13 adults had *C. jejuni* enteritis; illness was significantly associated with drinking raw milk, for a relative risk of 5 (95% CI 1.4–20), and attack rates increased with increasing quantity consumed.

***Clostridium* (3415).** At a youth camp in New Zealand in 1994, chicken was implicated in an outbreak of *C. perfringens* food poisoning that affected 241 (42%) of 574 participants.

***E. coli* (903, 1454, 1514, 3838, 6992).** *E. coli* is a hazard at fairs (see section 13.1), farms, pet zoos, and camps, but also from gardening and playing in manured gardens. At pet farms and zoos, visitors can touch animals and consume food at the same time. Few laboratories screen for non-O157 EHEC that are easily overlooked.

- Farms (1179, 1663, 5064, 5527, 6992, 7554). Risks have been well documented. In Minnesota in 2000–2001, diarrhea outbreaks occurred at a farm day camp at which *E. coli* O157:H7 was isolated from children and calves. In the United States in 2000, among 51 confirmed or suspected EHEC infections that followed farm visits, contact with cattle was a significant risk, and 13% (28/216) of cattle on the farms shed *E. coli* O157:H7 indistinguishable from patient strains; washing hands before eating was protective. In the United Kingdom in 1994–1997, of 69 reported EHEC cases, 23 (33%, visitors, farm workers, and farm families) reported contact with farm animals, and in seven, human isolates matched animal isolates. In the United Kingdom in 1996–1997, 13% (62/511) of community controls but 24% (87/369) of sporadic EHEC cases reported farm contacts in 5 days before illness onset, for an odds ratio of 2.5 (95% CI 1.5–4, adjusted for season, age, and sex). Reasons for farm visits were recreational (day visit or holiday) or occupational (delivery and maintenance) but not for farm work.
- Pet zoos (2961, 3308). The risks are similar to those on farms. In The Netherlands, a child with HUS grew *E. coli* O157 that was indistinguishable from goat and sheep strains from a pet farm the child had visited. In South Australia in 2000, EHEC affected six persons or their contacts who had visited a petting zoo; a pig at the zoo grew a strain that was indistinguishable from the clinical strain.
- Camps (903, 1148, 3449, 6005, 6408). Outbreaks at camps have been well documented. At a youth camp in Texas in 1999, 55 (11%) of 521 participants fell ill, and 2 (18%) of 11 grew *E. coli* O111:H8; illness was associated with various foods, including salad and ice. At a summer camp in Virginia in 1994, rare ground beef cooked over the campfire was implicated in an EHEC outbreak with 20 cases (including one HUS), for attack rates of 13% among campers and 10% among counselors. At Crater Lake National Park in 1975, contaminated park water caused an ETEC outbreak with >2,200 cases. In the United Kingdom, private water supplies on rural campsites have been associated with *E. coli* outbreaks. At an agricultural showground in Scotland in 2000, *E. coli* O157 was implicated in an outbreak that affected 6% (20/337) campers likely taken up from the pasture via hands or foods.

***Salmonella* (940, 1868, 2835, 6005).** Food from camps is a risk, and outbreaks have been reported. In Wales, *S. enterica* serovar Enteritidis PT 6B caused illness in 46 of 49 campers; the implicated vehicle was a lemon meringue pie prepared and transported at ambient temperature. Egg products should be cooked well, and cold boxes should be used for transport and storage of perishable foods.

***Shigella* (4681, 6297, 8064).** Risks for *Shigella* include camping and swimming in freshwater. At a poorly developed campsite in a U.S. national forest in 1987, *S. sonnei* attacked ~50% of the estimated 12,700 attendees, likely by spread from food, water, and contact. Attendees dispersed the agent nationwide, and outbreaks in three states were linked to the campsite. In Germany in 1998, *S. sonnei* affected 18 (30%) of 60 participants of a scout tent camp; poor hygiene was the most likely explanation.

***Y. enterocolitica* (5215, 6827).** Foods from camps have been a reported risk. In New York State in 1981, an outbreak affected 39% (129/327) of campers, 24% (29/117) of staff, and 9% (1/11) of kitchen staff. Vehicles were powdered milk and turkey chow mien that were prepared at the camp and yielded *Y. enterocolitica*.

Protozoa

***Cryptosporidium* (1777, 4902, 5046, 6992).** Farms and wildlife centers are reported sources of *C. parvum* in visitors, mainly from petting of calves, lambs, or other animals. In Minnesota in 2000–2001, diarrhea outbreaks occurred at a farm day camp at which *C. parvum* was isolated from 17 attendees and 25 calves. In 1998, apple cider from an agricultural fair in Maine caused *Cryptosporidium* enteritis in 160 (21%) of 759 attendants. In Scotland in 2005, 62 visitors contracted *C. parvum* from petting animals at a wildlife center.

***Giardia*.** Outbreaks have been reported in camps and at picnics.

- Picnic (5850). In rural Connecticut, 13 (81%) of 16 adult picnic attendees contracted illness from cold salad.
- Camps (432, 3421). In Colorado in 1983, geology students and faculty camped for field studies in two sequential groups: the first group who used untreated stream water for drinking had an infection rate of 74% (31/42), while the second group who was discouraged from using stream water had a rate of 0/36. In Utah in 1974, mountain stream water was the putative source

for an outbreak among university students who hiked and camped in the Uinta Mountains, for an attack rate of 64% (34/53). Neither stream water, nor feces of beaver, muskrat, and sheep from the area tested positive for *Giardia*.

***Toxoplasma* (4063).** Frequent gardening is a *T. gondii* infection risk.

Helminths
***Ascaris* (7717).** Vegetable gardening is a risk for *Ascaris* infection in endemic areas.

***Spirometra* (5699).** In Italy, a freshwater sports fisherman contracted subcutaneous sparganosis, likely from drinking copepod-contaminated surface water.

ZOONOTIC CLUSTER, OUTDOOR LEISURE
Hazards include bites by mammals (see chapter 1) and invertebrate vectors (see chapter 4), mainly ticks and mosquitoes. Inadvertent ingestion of animal feces, e.g., via gathering berries, is a poorly substantiated putative hazard.

Viruses
Bunyaviridae. **CCHFV (1333).** Sleeping outdoors is a risk for CCHFV, presumably from increased exposure to ticks. **Hantavirus (281, 1650, 4615, 7179, 8349).** Exposure in 112 of the first 200 cases of hantavirus pulmonary syndrome (HPS) that followed the 1993 outbreak of sin nombre virus (SNV) in the southwestern United States included peridomestic rodents in 86 (77%), work (farming and trapping) in 16 (14%), and leisure (camping and hiking) in 10 (9%). Rodent-infested dwellings, cleaning out abandoned cabins, and dust from rodent feces are risks in enzootic areas, both in the United States (for HPS) and Europe (for hemorrhagic fever with renal syndrome or epidemic nephropathy due to Puumala virus). A German tourist was diagnosed with Puumala virus infection and acute renal failure 3 weeks after a visit to Sweden where he had stayed in a mouse-infested vacation home. To reduce risks, first air out cabins, then remove all garbage and cover foods and utensils before cleaning. An emerging risk seems to be all-terrain vehicles. In Utah, their heavy use is believed to enhance Sin Nombre virus infection of deer mice (*Peromyscus maniculatus*) and woodrats (*Neotoma lepida*) by producing open spaces that restrict rodents to crowded microhabitats. **La Crosse encephalitis virus (2230).** In the United States in 2000, 15 children with confirmed La Crosse encephalitis virus infections spent significantly more time outdoors (6 h) than febrile control children (4 h); in contrast, no differences were observed for clothing, use of insect repellents, or home window screens.

Flaviviridae. **DENV (4588).** During a community-assistance program in the British Virgin Islands, in 1995, 69% (22/32) of participants contracted dengue; 15 cases were confirmed by anti-DENV immunoglobulin M (IgM). None of the participants had used effective mosquito repellents, and only two (6%) had used bednets. **Powassan virus.** Stays in rural vacation homes and camping on untended properties that provide habitats for ticks are a hazard for Powassan virus. **Tick-borne encephalitis virus (3021, 7261, 8284).** Outdoor sports (e.g, hiking and jogging) or hobbies (e.g., gathering mushrooms or berries, fishing, and hunting) in enzootic areas may expose to tick-borne encephalitis virus, but the evidence is inadequate. At an orienteer race in Sweden in 1990, after excluding vaccinees, seroprevalence was 1% (5/334) among orienteers and 0–5% among various controls ($n = 652$).

Rhabdoviridae. **Rabies virus (2446, 6919).** Injury from stray animals and wildlife, including bats, is a hazard. An interesting observation has been reported from Alaska, where 1 (4%) of 26 trappers had naturally acquired neutralizing lyssavirus antibodies, of a titer (2 IU/ml) clearly above protective threshold (0.5 IU/ml). The reactive individual had never been vaccinated and had trapped and skinned Arctic foxes (*Alopex lagopus*) for >45 years, an observation that suggests the occurrence of inapparent rabies virus infections.

Bacteria
***Anaplasma phagocytophilum* (7726).** In The Netherlands in the fall of 1998, a frequent camper contracted human granulocytic ehrlichiosis.

***Bartonella* (4899).** In Sweden in 1992–1993, 30% (355/1,136) of orienteers but only 7% (22/322) of time-matched blood donors had antibodies to *Bartonella*; nearly 90% (312/355) of reactivity was to *B. elisabethae*.

Borrelia. ***B. burgdorferi* (1429, 2285, 3021, 4206, 6619).** Outdoor leisure activities in enzootic areas are a risk for *B. burgdorferi*. At a summer camp in Maryland in 1995, of 537 campers 200 found ticks on skin or clothing, and six contracted Lyme disease in camp, for a rate of 3/1,000 campers in 10–14 days of exposure. Of 230 ticks, 44 (19%) were *Ixodes scapularis*: 37 (84%) nymphs and 7 (16%) larvae; of nymphs, 4 (11%) tested positive for *B. burgdorferi*. Heavily used hiking trails and picnic areas near San Francisco, Calif., were sampled biweekly for one year. While picnic areas yielded few ticks, 1,911 adult ticks were collected from hiking trails, mostly (64%) *Dermacentor occidentalis* and (26%) *Ixodes pacificus*, rarely (0.2%) *Dermacentor variabilis*. Microscopic *B. burgdorferi* prevalence in adult ticks was 0% (0/861) in *D. occidentalis*, 1.6% (2/126) in *D. variabilis*, and 0.2% (1/609) in *I. pacificus*. At an orienteer race in Sweden in October 1990, seroprevalence was 9% (31/362) in orienteers and 1–9% in various controls ($n = 652$). In Switzerland, orienteers were significantly more frequently seroreactive than controls; however, when monitored, rates of Lyme disease in orienteers (0.8/100 per year) were not different from the popoulation. In France, of 170 hunters ~15% were seroreactive, significantly more than blood donors. **Relapsing Borrelia and tick-borne relapsing fever (2255, 6726, 7456).** Cleaning out or staying in rodent- and tick-infested cabins in enzootic areas is a risk. In Montana, in an island habitat covered with ponderosa pine, Douglas fir, grassland, and rocks, five persons contracted tick-borne relapsing fever after staying in a cabin infested with *Ornithodoros hermsi* ticks. In Washington State, in 1968, 11 (26%) of 42 boy scouts and scoutmasters who camped out contracted TBRF.

***Coxiella* (4596).** In a Q fever outbreak in Germany, visits to sheep farms or walking near sheep pastures were risks for *C. burnetii* infections.

***Ehrlichia chaffeensis* (7108).** At a golf-oriented, densely wooded retirement community in Tennessee that bordered a wildlife management area, 10 cases of monocytic ehrlichiosis were observed, and seroprevalence of community members was 12.5% compared with 3.9% in a retirement community 30 km away.

***Francisella* (196, 2348, 4876).** Mowing the lawn or clearing brush are disease risks. On Martha's Vineyard, Mass., in 2000, 15 tularemia cases occurred among residents and visitors; mowing the lawn or cutting brush were risks, and one patient reported exposure to a rabbit while cutting brush. In central Spain in 1998, 11 men and 8 women contracted ulceroglandular tularemia (biovar B) from fishing and handling crayfish (*Procambarus clarkii*); it was concluded that river water and mud at the fishing site were contaminated with *F. tularensis*.

***Orientia tsutsugamushi* (1681, 5551).** In a rain forest (Litchfield) park 140 km south of Darwin, Australia, five visitors contracted scrub typhus in 1990–1993. More cases have been reported since in visitors to Litchfield Park.

***Rickettsia* (3683, 6429).** In Delaware in 1996, 4 of 223 attendees of a summer camp contracted Rocky Mountain spotted fever (due to *R. rickettsii*) for an attack rate of 1.8%; risks included camping and hiking off trails. At risk of *R. africae* are safari tourists, backpackers, hunters, sports competitors, and film crew members.

Protozoa
***Babesia* (3292, 3979).** The risks of outdoor leisure have been poorly documented; putative hazards include hiking and camping in enzootic areas.

***Plasmodium* (6820, 7255).** Nocturnal outdoor activities and sleeping in the open in malarious areas are plausible risk behaviors. In Michigan in 1995, a campground in a swampy area, close to a racetrack frequented by international travelers, was a site for presumed nighttime local transmission of vivax malaria.

Helminths
***Echinococcus multilocularis* (3901).** In Europe, 46% of 210 patients reported outdoor activities, including on vocational farms and in gardens and forests.

ENVIRONMENTAL CLUSTER, OUTDOOR LEISURE
Water, soil, and plant contacts are potential hazards, including from gardening and hiking. In a national U.S. sample of respondents reporting gardening or yard work, 1.6% (3,514/5,230; 95% CI 1–2) sustained an injury from that activity in the preceding 30 days, compared with 0.9% (1,035/5,236; 95% CI 0.3–1.4) of outdoor bicycle riders (5992). In Washington State, following mud wrestling (in a building), 21 wrestlers contracted folliculitis; topsoil that had been purchased from a gardening supplier grew *Enterobacter*, *Klebsiella*, and *Pseudomonas* (73). For agents in soil, see section 5.3.

Bacteria
***Aeromonas* (7694).** In Australia, on a warm summer day in 2002, ≥26 participants at a rugby competition that involved body and mud contact on a wet playing field acquired *A. hydrophila* disease, for an attack rate of ~40%. Besides skin infections, 22 of 26 patients had rash, malaise, or fever. *A. hydrophila* was isolated from patients and a nearby river from which the playing field had been irrigated days before the game, and in which players washed after the game.

***Burkholderia* (4458, 5811).** Children with cystic fibrosis in educational summer camps have acquired *B. cepacia* from person-to-person spread.

***Clostridium tetani* (6472).** Any leisure injury in a nonvaccinated individual is a risk, including from walking barefoot. In the United Kingdom in 1984–2000, 61% (81/133) of tetanus cases with known exposure sustained the injury in the garden or at home, and 10% (14) sustained it on the road.

***Leptospira* (740, 1450, 3038, 3844, 4369, 5192, 5341, 7159, 7325).** Leisure exposure to natural waters is a well-established risk, including from stagnant and running fresh waters. In high-income countries, recreational exposure is increasing at the expense of occupational exposure. Heavy rains and floods increase recreational risks. Reported exposing activities include wading, bathing, swimming, triathlon, canoeing, kayaking, rafting, fishing, duck hunting, and even caving.

- Swimming (3613, 4369). Of 28 outbreaks reported worldwide in 1930–2000, 22 were associated with swimming in natural waters such as creeks, rivers, ponds, lakes, or canals, for 2–114 (median, 16) cases per outbreak. In rural Illinois in 1991, 5 of 18 (28%) boys contracted leptospirosis from swimming in a small hole; *L. interrogans* serovar Grippotyphosa was isolated from the urine of two boys and pond water, and 29% (4/14) of nearby cattle were reactive to that serovar.
- Canoeing (740). At a white-water canoeing event in Dublin, Ireland, in 2001, 6 (9%) of 65 participants contracted leptospirosis (serogroup Icterohaemorrhagiae). Compared with only 5% (3/56) of controls, 50% (3/6) of cases ingested more than one swallow of river water.
- Rafting (6203, 7159). In October 1996, after whitewater rafting in Costa Rica, 9 (35%) of 26 rafters were diagnosed with leptospirosis in the United States; risks were having ingested river water and being submerged after falling into the river. In Germany, ~18 days after a boat-rafting tour during which the boat capsized in a high flood river, all three participants came down with clinically manifest leptospirosis.
- Athletism (3038, 3064, 5192, 6761, 7393). In 2000, following an "eco-challenge" in Malaysia that involved jungle trekking, caving, outrigger sailing, canoeing, scuba diving, mountain biking, and a 12-km swim in jungle rivers, 80 (42%) of 189 athletes met a clinical case definition for leptospirosis, and 26 (68%) of 38 tested athletes were seroreactive. At a contest in Illinois in 1998, following heavy rains, 98 (12%) of 834 triathletes reported illness, and 52 (11%) of 474 tested athletes were seroreactive; swallowing lake water was a risk. In Germany, a participant at an iron man contest in the Philippines that involved running through a dense rain forest for 40 km and canoeing in rough seas for 7 km was diagnosed with leptospirosis.
- Hunt (4102). In the greater Darwin region, Australia, in 2000, two men who hunted duck barefoot and three women who hunted turtle barefoot contracted leptospirosis.
- Fruit gathering (8049). After collecting nuts under a walnut tree (*Juglans regia*) close to a creek where rats lived, a retired forest worker developed leptospirosis.

***Pseudomonas* (3500).** Children with cystic fibrosis in summer camps have acquired *P. aeruginosa* via cross-infection (person-to-person spread).

Fungi

***Rhinosporidium* (6871, 7882).** Bathing or swimming in stagnant waters is a risk for *R. seeberi*.

***Sporothrix* (4502).** Outdoor rural leisure activities such as fishing and hunting are a risk for *S. schenckii*.

Protozoa

Free-living amebas (929, 4777). Splash into the face and submerging in water are risks for amebic keratitis, acute primary amebic meningoencephalitis, and subacute granulomatous amebic encephalitis. Hazardous sports include swimming, fishing, and water skiing.

HELMINTHS

***Ancylostoma duodenale, A. braziliense,* and *A. caninum* (5503).** Potential transmission sites are public places in endemic areas that are accessible to defecating humans or dogs. At public elementary school playgrounds in São Paulo, Brazil, of sandboxes, 0.6% (3/535) yielded eggs of *Ancylostoma*, and of schools, 36% (10/28) in summer and 46% (13/28) in winter yielded hookworm larvae.

***Strongyloides* (475, 1594, 3769, 5956, 7074).** Leisure activities that are associated with soil contact in endemic areas are a risk. Camping is a risk, including outside endemic areas, at sites that receive visitors from endemic areas but lack sanitation. In Nottingham, United Kingdom, a 17-year-old girl contracted *S. stercoralis* locally, seemingly by regularly walking barefoot in parks and at home.

***Schistosoma* (667, 2257, 2616, 3924, 4809, 5980, 6078, 7843).** Transmission is from contacts with snail-inhabited freshwaters in endemic areas, such as lakes, river banks, ponds, natural pools, and even "*crystal clear and cold water*" (8424). By age and sex, exposing leisure activities include fording a creek, playing in water, swimming, standing under a waterfall, freshwater scuba diving, water skiing, river rafting, and panning for gem stones in brooks. Water contacts that last a few to 30 min are sufficient for transmission. In South Africa, three scuba divers contracted Katayama fever and *S. mansoni* while recovering a boat engine from the shallows of a dam.

***Toxocara* (1121, 2415, 6861).** Sandy soils from public places that are accessible to dogs and cats are well-known sources of *Toxocara* infection. Uptake is via hands or geophagia. Eggs (*T. canis* and *T. cati*) were isolated in up to 35–85% of samples from sandpits in kindergartens, playgrounds, and public parks. Of dog feces collected in squares and parks, 14% tested positive for *T. canis* eggs. Eggs of *T. cati* have been recovered from 1–66% of soil samples from parks or playgrounds.

SKIN-BLOOD CLUSTER, OUTDOOR LEISURE
Discarded syringes (5521). The risk of blood-borne infections from discarded syringes in city parks and public places is unclear and debated. In South London, of 106 discarded syringes collected from four parks over 4 months, five (5%) tested positive for hepatitis C virus (HCV), and also five (5%) for HBV. **HBV (5521).** In the United Kingdom in 1988–1991, accidental exposures and postexposure prophylaxis (PEP) for HBV were reviewed retrospectively. Over 50% (1,805/3,535) of exposures occurred in the community. Of needle-stick injuries 16% (289/1,805) occurred in the street, 12% (217) from contact with rubbish, 6% (108) in the park, and 4% (72) on the beach. Better education of injection drug users (IDU) about safe disposal of needles has been suggested. **Human immunodeficiency virus (HIV) (693, 3189).** The risk for children to percutaneously contract HIV from discarded syringes is considered close to zero. The HIV transmission rate from discarded injection material at public places of <0.3/100 accidents was considered too low to routinely recommend PEP, unless syringes are visibly blood stained or from a source known to be HIV-positive.

For sports injuries see section 13.5.

13.5 INDOOR SPORTS AND HOBBIES

Disco fever

S. T. Cookson et al. (1561)

Indoor sports can be performed singly (e.g., aerobics, billiards, bowling, gymnastics, shooting, and weight lifting), with an opponent (e.g., boxing, judo, fencing, karate, squash, table tennis, and wrestling), or in teams (e.g., basketball and handball).

Indoor hobbies are diverse and include indoor plants and pet animals (aquarium fish, terrarium reptiles, caged birds, and rodents), culture (e.g., opera, reading, and theater), collection (e.g., art, stamps, and rocks), relaxation (e.g., listening to music, massage, sauna, and solving puzzles), and entertainment (e.g., board and card plays, going to discos, movies, or nightclubs, and watching television).

Exposure (2867). In the United States each year, ~30 million children and adolescents participate in organized sports.

Infections (5379) (Box 13.6). Sports apart, infections from indoor leisure activities are poorly documented or rare. For pet animals, see chapter 2; for plants, see section 6.3; for beauty parlors, see section 18.1.

Human bites (2935, 7311, 7857). Human bites result from fights, sports or leisure (love bites). Bites can transmit oral flora (e.g., CMV, *Fusobacterium*, *Eikenella*, and *Candida*). Some 10–50% of human bite wounds become infected, typically at the hand, and, in particular, bites into a clenched fist.

- Viruses (6, 3189) reported to be transmissible through bites include HBV, HCV, HIV, HSV1, and HSV2. Children in day care who are carriers of HBV are a risk for susceptible victims, for whom PEP is recommended (vaccine and specific Ig). The risk of HIV transmission via bites is considered low.
- Bacteria (2429, 2935, 7311). Over 50% of bite wounds grow a mixture (up to 20) of bacteria, ~40% grow only aerobes, and 2% grow only anaerobes. Frequent aerobes are *S. aureus* and CoNS (in >50%), and *Streptococcus anginosus*, *S. oralis*, and *S. pyogenes* (in >80%). *Eikenella corrodens* is recovered in ~25% of indolent, chronic infections from clenched-fist bites. Infrequent aerobes are *Corynebacterium*, *Gemella*, *Haemophilus*, *M. tuberculosis*, *Neisseria*, and *Treponema pallidum pallidum*. Frequent anaerobes are *Fusobacterum nucleatum* and *Prevotella melaninogenica*. Infrequent anaerobes are *Actinomyces*, *Bacteroides*, *Clostridium*, and *Peptostreptococcus*. Tetanus results from secondary wound infection rather than from human bites.

Prevention (204, 205, 536, 5379). Prevention of sports infections includes education, vaccines, and maintenance (installations and equipment). Vaccines recommended for indoor team athletes include HBV, *Influenzavirus*, measles-mumps-rubella, tetanus (as dT), and *N. meningi-*

Box 13.6 Main agents or infections from indoor leisure activities, by agent cluster

Droplet-air	From indoor sports, games, parties, bars: • vaccine preventable: *Influenzavirus*, MMR, varicella; *M. tuberculosis*, *N. meningitidis* • vaccine nonpreventable: *Enterovirus*; *Coxiella*, *Legionella*
Feces-food	From indoor sports teams, parties: HAV, enteric bacteria
Skin-blood	By contact: HBV, HPV, HSV1 (herpes gladiatorum); pyoderma (*S. aureus* and *S. pyogenes*); dermatophytes

tidis A/C. By risk and athlete (elite), further vaccines to consider include HAV, rabies, tick-borne encephalitis virus, varicella-zoster virus, and *S. pneumoniae*. Clothes, towels, and mats should be cleaned regularly, and towels and utensils should not be shared. Athletes should report skin infections and bleeding trauma for treatment, possible exclusion from training or game, and PEP in contacts.

DROPLET-AIR CLUSTER, INDOOR LEISURE

Crowded and poorly ventilated rooms are a hazard. Members of sports teams and visitors of parties, discos, bars, and night clubs are potential victims *and* sources of respiratory tract infections.

Viruses

***Enterovirus* (140, 447, 3548, 5170, 5379).** Sports teams have experienced outbreaks. In the United States in 1978–1980, seven outbreaks affected teams of football players, for attack rates of 20–70%. At a high school in Alabama in 1989, coxsackievirus B2 and aseptic meningitis affected 25% (81/319) of students and staff, with a peak attack rate (53%) among the football team. *Enterovirus* can spread by contact or shared bottles or other utensils. At a school in upstate New York in 1991, 20% (17/87) of football players were diagnosed with coxsackievirus B1 pleurodynia; the most likely vehicles were water from a cooler or ice from an ice chest.

***Influenzavirus* (5379).** Clusters of cases have been reported in sports teams.

***Measles virus* (1149, 1772, 5379).** Clusters and outbreaks of measles have been reported at sports events and in sports teams. In an outbreak in Alaska, 11% (7/63) of cases acquired measles at indoor soccer games.

***Rubella virus* (4743).** A rubella outbreak in Hawaii in 1977 affected mainly women 20–24 years of age, for an attack rate of 0.2%; a case-control study identified a disco and a singing piano player as the likely source. For PEP, vaccine was given to 6,523 women.

***Varicella* (5379).** Case clusters of varicella have been reported in sports teams.

Bacteria

***Coxiella* (4213, 5923).** Parturient cats inside rooms were likely sources of *C. burnetii* in 12 members of a poker-playing group and in 11 of 15 family members attending a family reunion.

***Legionella* (1875, 4052, 4396).** *Legionella* is spread environment-to-person, not person-to-person. In a bar in Missouri in 1996, when floodwater was pumped out, aerosols by a leaky pump caused disease in one of five staff, and 1 (1.4%) of 70 customers. In Australia in 1991–2000, 1 of 22 outbreaks involved a football club, with four cases likely resulting from the club spa pool and shower. In Haarlem, The Netherlands, in 1991–1996, Legionnaires' disease was diagnosed in six regular visitors of a particular sauna; patient strains matched a strain isolated from the sauna footbath. The sauna hot-water installations had to be remodeled and the stagnant parts were removed.

***M. tuberculosis* (6074).** Outbreaks of *M. tuberculosis* have been reported in sports clubs (volleyball and rowing), bars, night clubs, and a sauna.

- Bars (3994, 5324, 6074). Risks include poor ventilation and delayed diagnosis in patrons or bartenders. In Minneapolis, Minn., in 1992, an infective, regular homeless patron of a bar caused infections in 41 (42%) of 97 contacts (4 bartenders and 93 patrons), including 14 cases of active tuberculosis. In the city in that year, bar-related cases accounted for 35% (17/49) of all active tuberculosis, occurring in a perimeter of 3.2 km around the bar. In Nagasaki, Japan, pulmonary tuberculosis in four alcoholic patients was linked epidemiologically and by fingerprinting to a bar visited by all four patients.
- Night clubs (717, 3690, 4641). In Wichita, Kans., in 1994–2000, DNA fingerprints linked 18 tuberculosis cases among entertainment (exotic) dancers and other persons; 12 of the cases reported use of cocaine or amphetamines, and 10 had been incarcerated. Of 302 contacts evaluated, 25% had latent infection. In Georgia in 1996, an outbreak occurred among three participants of an illegal card game. The index case identified family contacts but did not disclose the game, nightclub work, and a liaison with a woman of whom his wife was unaware. Initially, 61 contacts were named (of whom 31 or 51% were reactive to tuberculin), only 19 months later, 282 additional contacts were named (of whom 53 or 19% were reactive).
- Sauna (5327). In an office, shopping, and amusement sector of Tokyo, molecular fingerprinting and overnight stays in public saunas linked three clusters of pulmonary tuberculosis.

***N. meningitidis*.** Many indoor leisure habitats dispose participants to increased carriage or disease.

- Sports clubs (1053, 4028, 5635, 7749). Contacts among or with members are a risk. In Northern Ireland, 4–5 days after a rugby match, four spectators developed invasive serogroup C disease of the same serotype; two died. In a United Kingdom town in 1995, six of seven cases were rugby players or linked to the local rugby club.

- Campus (5369). Risks for carriage among university students include smoking, visits to bars or night clubs, and intimate kissing. Risks for invasive disease among students include catered hall accomodations.
- Parties (2391, 2424). In Maryland, three serogroup C cases occurred among attendees of a party at which many smoked tobacco or marijuana or drank alcohol. In a school outbreak in Wales, United Kingdom, carriage was associated with attending an informal party.
- Discos (1561, 1757, 3183). In the city of Corrientes in northeastern Argentina in 1996, eight serogroup C cases occurred among attendees of a disco ("disco fever"); cases were 15–45 (median, 19) years of age. In Wales, United Kingdom, regular attendance at a disco was associated with an increased proportion of carriers among contacts of outbreak cases. In an outbreak during carnival in Germany in 1998, visits to local discos linked five serogroup C cases.
- Bars (3551, 6432). In the United States in 1991–1992, eight university students and one college student contracted serogroup C disease. Screening of 1,528 throat cultures yielded five identical further strains; two of these were from workers of a campus bar that the case students had visited. Smoking and crowding at peak hours were suspected to facilitate transmission. At a campus in the United Kingdom, carriage (19% or 88/454) was associated with patronage of the campus bar; in 2 weeks before the outbreak, 41 carriers spent an average of six evenings in the bar, compared with four evenings by 48 controls.
- Nightclubs (2748, 3660). At a university campus in 1997, of five cases of serogroup C disease who did not know each other, three had attended the same nightclub the evening before their illness. In Sydney, Australia, in 1996, 7 of 10 young adults had a direct or indirect link with a local night club, and 10 of 11 systemic *N. meningitidis* isolates were of the same C serotype 2a:P1.5.

FECES-FOOD CLUSTER, INDOOR LEISURE

The bulk of infections is acquired from nonleisure exposure. Travel to sports events in areas with poor hygiene and foods served at clubs and parties are hazards (233).

HAV (2529, 4316, 5217). An outbreak by contaminated drinking water was reported in a college football team, for an attack rate of 34%. Saunas are meeting places for homosexual men in some areas. In Amsterdam, The Netherlands, compared with controls, significant risks in acute HA cases were visits to gay saunas and darkrooms.

***C. jejuni* (7104).** An outbreak was reported at an orienteer rally in Switzerland in 1981, at which participants were offered raw milk drinks. Over 500 participants contracted enteritis, for an attack rate of >75%; the source was traced to a cow from a single dairy farm.

***S. sonnei* (3222).** *S. sonnei* in cold sandwiches served aboard a U.S. aircraft affected 21 (32%) of 65 football team members.

ENVIRONMENTAL CLUSTER, INDOOR LEISURE

The indoor environment is a rare source for leisure infections. For flower potting soil, see section 5.3.

Chromomycosis (6041). In Finland, cases of this essentially tropical fungal infection were attributed to traditional saunas, which are wooden huts with an earth floor and in which heat and water were considered conductive for growth of causative fungi.

SKIN-BLOOD CLUSTER, INDOOR LEISURE

Risks (6, 57, 233, 925, 5379). Although the bulk of infections is acquired from nonsports exposure, body contact and trauma from contact and collision sports can result in human-to-human spread of skin or blood-borne agents. Infrequently, training rooms, equipments, or personal items (e.g., nail clippers) are vehicles. In professional U.S. football, bleeding trauma occurs at a rate of 3–4 per team and game; most (~90%) injuries are abrasions, ~10% are lacerations.

Because transmission risks are low, athletes with known HBV, HCV, or HIV infection should not be excluded from competitive sports, and tests should not be required. Instead, infected athletes should be counseled on reporting bleeding trauma and on protective play.

VIRUSES

> ...staff of athletic programs aggressively should promote HBV immunization among all athletes and among coaches, athletic trainers, equipment handlers, laundry personnel...
> — American Academy of Pediatrics (6)

HBV (3834, 7488). Spread of HBV via sports trauma has been reported. In a university football team in Japan, 5 of 65 members were diagnosed with acute HB, and six were diagnosed with HBV infection over 19 months, for a rate of 17%. At a high school club in Japan, 5 of 10 sumo wrestlers were diagnosed with HB.

HCV (233, 5379). Risks from sports trauma seem minimal but are poorly known.

HIV (233, 925, 5379, 7515). HIV has occasionally been spread via sports trauma. Transmission of HIV is less frequent than that of HBV. From rates of bleeding, rates in health care, and HIV prevalence in college men, the risk of HIV player-to-player spread was estimated at <1 per 85 million game contacts.

HPV (3717, 5379, 6697). Contact sports and barefoot use of public places are risks for skin and plantar warts. Among 146 adolescents 10–18 years of age, plantar warts were much less prevalent (1%) in adolescents from a public school who did not use public showers regularly than in adolescents from a swimming club (27%) who regularly used communal showers.

HSV1 (205, 540, 5379). "Herpes gladiatorum" is a risk for contact sports. Lesions are typically located at contact (lock-up position) sites, mainly head, neck, shoulders, and extremities. Outbreaks are reported among wrestlers. During the Minnesota high school league wrestling season of 1999, 61 wrestlers and 3 coaches were affected. In the United States in 1989, skin-to-skin transmitted HSV1 infection was diagnosed in 60 (34%) of 175 high school wrestlers attending a four-week training camp; attack rates were 25% in the lightweights group, and 1–67% in the heavyweights group.

Molluscipox virus (5379). Spread of molluscum contagiosum via contact seems to occur.

Bacteria
***S. aureus* (520, 2615, 4439, 7094).** Skin infections and outbreaks have been reported among athletic teams, including wrestling, rugby, and football teams, and basketball players. Risks include body contact, abrasions from artificial grass (turf burns), body shaving, and shared objects such as bath towels, lubricants, and equipment. By equipment, infections can spread to athletes with little skin-to-skin contact, e.g., fencers (via sensor wire), and household members. Community-acquired methicillin resistant *S. aureus* strains should be suspected in skin infections that do not respond to standard antibiotics.

- Wrestling (2615, 4439). In Vermont in 1993–1994, 6 of 32 members of a high school wrestling team contracted MRSA skin infections, and one member became colonized.
- Football (520, 2615, 3864, 5409). In Missouri in 2003, 5 (9%) of 58 professional players contracted MRSA skin infections at turf-abrasion sites; the same epidemic strain was isolated from a competing team and from clusters in the community. In Los Angeles in VIII–IX/2003, 10% (11/107) of players of a team developed boils and other skin lesions, and 8% (8/99) grew MRSA from nasal cultures. In camp, four players shared a dormitory, and preexisting skin lesions and sharing soap bars were risks. In Connecticut in 2003, 10 of 100 players of a college football team contracted cellulitis or skin abscess; six wounds grew methicillin-resistant *S. aureus*.
- Basketball (7048). At Kentucky high school in 1986–1987, an outbreak of furuncles affected 25% (31/124) of male athletes. Significant risks included frequent abrasions, cuts that required bandaging, friends with a furuncle, and being member of varsity football or basketball teams.

***S. pyogenes* (GAS) (2290, 4560).** GAS spread among attendees of an indoor football tournament. In the United Kingdom in 1984, 7 rugby players and 2 girl friends contracted nephritogenic GAS that caused impetigo and glomerulonephritis.

***T. pallidum* (825).** In Melbourne, Australia, of volunteers from a sauna club for homosexual men 18% (114/623) were seroreactive, and 2.7% (17) were diagnosed with new (primary) syphilis.

Fungi
Risks are stronger for tinea corporis that is infrequent, and weaker for tinea pedis that is frequent.

Tinea corporis (gladiatorum) (58, 536, 2155, 3458, 5379). Contact sports (e.g., wrestling) increase the risk for infection with anthropophilic *Trichophyton tonsurans*. Outbreaks among wrestlers have been reported in North America and Europe. In Sweden in 1993, visiting wrestlers from the United States were the likely source of *T. tonsurans* for 19 Swedish patients.

Tinea pedis (340, 1070, 3800). *T. rubrum* has been recovered from athletes, training mats, and shower rooms. The main isolates in skin culture are *T. rubrum* and *T. mengagrophytes*.

About one half to three fourths of tinea pedis in athletes is inapparent. Sports increase infection risks moderately (1.3- to 3-fold), but independent from age or comorbidity (e.g., diabetes).

Risks extend beyond swimmers, to athletes who wear tight shoes. In marathon runners in Canada, the prevalence of athlete's foot was 22% (89/405), with a high in men (24%) and a low in women (6%). In Japan, the prevalence of athlete's foot was 23% (32/137) in control students, but 72% (101/140) in swimming students, and overall 43% (122/282) in other athletes, including judokas (prevalence, 23% or 5/22), kendokas (33% or 12/36), basketball players (39% or 24/61), soccer players (44% or 35/79), water polo players (53% or 9/17), swimmers (55% or 17/31), and long-distance runners (56% or 20/36).

13.6 FEMALE PROSTITUTION
Prostitutes are women who trade sex for money or drugs, including in bars, massage salons, commercial brothels,

and the street. Sexual violence in females is manifest by prostitution of adolescents, trafficking and sexual abuse of girls, female circumcision, and rape. Lesbians (2534) are women who have sex with women. In the United States, 20–30% of female IDU are reported to be lesbians. For STI in the population, see section 14.7; for infections in IDU, see "Injection Drug Use" below; for carriers in the community, see section 14.1.

Exposure (4963, 5069, 7797, 7979, 8194). Global statistics are not available. Estimates are of 0.2% (2 million/1 billion) for prostitutes in brothels in India, and of 3% of prostitutes in Nha Trang City, Vietnam (by the capture-recapture method). About 13% of women report having been sexually assaulted in their life. Annually, ~0.7–2 million women are trafficked, mainly in eastern Europe, Asia, and Latin America, and ~1 million children are forced into prostitution.

STIs (757, 2173, 4752, 5095, 5383, 7127, 7657) (Box 13.7). Age, country (law and religion), area (urban or rural), work (street or brothel), clients (tourists, IDU, or demand for oral sex), and prevention influence the prevailing STI. Where neither condoms nor screening are promoted, 25–85% of prostitutes have curable STI at any one time, including *C. trachomatis* (5–15%), *N. gonorrhoeae* (10–30%), and *T. pallidum* (10–30%). In massage parlors in Bangkok, Thailand, rates of STI/100 woman-months ($n = 163$) were 43 for genital *C. trachomatis*, 32 for gonorrhea, two for trichomoniasis, and 77 overall. In contrast, where condoms are used and workers are treated, the prevalence can be low (<2% for *N. gonorrhoeae* and <0.1% for HIV).

Multiple STIs can coexist. Nearly half of STI may be inapparent. Lesions at atypical sites may indicate acquisition from oral or anal sex. However, agents from the feces-food cluster are less frequently reported from prostitutes than homosexual men (Box 13.7), and the focus below is on the skin-blood cluster. Prostitutes can be victims and sources of STI. The same is true for clients for which knowledge is limited. In Atlanta in 1990–1991, of 69 clients 2.9% were seroreactive to HIV, 10% to *T. pallidum*, and 25% to markers of HBV. Bacterial vaginosis seems an emerging STI in lesbians.

Preventive measures (3118, 7127). Preventive measures include promotion of condoms and access to care, periodic screening, and prompt treatment of infected sex workers. In Thailand, public campaigns raised the proportion of condom users among prostitutes from 14% in 1989 to 94% in 1993; at the same time, the proportion of males with one or more of five major STI declined by 79%.

SKIN-BLOOD CLUSTER, PROSTITUTES
Genitoanal Discharge

Manifestations include vaginal or anal discharge, itch, frequent urination, and dysuria. The main agents of vaginitis, cervicitis, and urethritis are *Chlamydia*, *Neisseria*, and *Trichomonas*. In addition, *Mycoplasma genitalium* (5826, 7600) has been identified by nucleic acid amplificaion test (NAT) in cervical swabs from prostitutes, for prevalences of 13% (Japan, $n = 174$) to 26% (West Africa, $n = 826$).

C. trachomatis **(522, 3852, 5383, 6080, 7127, 7224, 7600, 7657).** *C. trachomatis* is endemic in prostitutes worldwide. By sampling and test, reported infection prevalences are 5–25% in Africa, 10–30% in Latin America, and 10–45% (often, 30%) in Asia. In Dhaka, Bangladesh, in 2002, 44% (174/400, 95% CI 39–48) of hotel prostitutes tested positive by NAT from endocervical swab. In Kenya, the infection rate by NAT from urine in the placebo arm of a chemoprophylaxis trial was 14.5/100 women-years; 84% of infections were asymptomatic.

N. gonorrhoeae **(522, 3852, 5383, 6080, 7127, 7600, 7657, 8084).** *N. gonorrhoeae* is endemic in prostitutes worldwide. By sampling and test, reported infection prevalence is 5–50% (often 15%) in Africa, 2–25% (often 10%) in Latin America, and 0–60% (often 20%) in Asia. These figures are roughly in line with reports from the 1980s, suggesting little change. In Dhaka, Bangladesh, in 2002, 36% (143/400, 95% CI 31–41) of hotel prostitutes tested positive by culture from endocervical swab. In Kenya, the infection rate by NAT from urine in the placebo arm of a prophylaxis trial was 13/100 women-years; 73% of infections were asymptomatic.

Box 13.7 Sexually transmitted agents and infections in prostitutes and homosexual men, by cluster

Droplet-air   Males: *N. meningitidis*; *P. jirovecii*
Feces-food   Males: HAV; *Campylobacter, Salmonella, Shigella*; microsporidia; *Cryptosporidium, Giardia*
Skin-blood   Females and males: • discharge: *C. trachomatis, N. gonorrhoeae*; *T. vaginalis*; • ulcer: HSV2; *H. ducreyi* (mainly male), *T. pallidum pallidum*; • warts: HPV; • other manifestations: CMV, HBV, HIV, HTLV1; *C. trachomatis* (lymphogranuloma venereum, mainly male); ectoparasites (pediculosis, scabies)

***T. vaginalis* (253, 522, 3852, 5383, 6080, 7127, 7330).** *T. vaginalis* is prevalent in prostitutes worldwide. By sampling and test (wet mount and culture), reported infection prevalence is 8–60% (often 25%) in Africa, 10–20% in Latin America, and 4–45% (often 7%) in Asia. In Dhaka, Bangladesh, in 2002, 4% (17/400) of hotel prostitutes tested positive by microscopy of wet mount from a vaginal swab. In Manila, Philippines, the prevalence in "waitresses" or "hostesses" was 15%, that is ~5 times the prevalence in control women. In a prophylaxis trial among prostitutes in Kenya, the infection rate in the placebo arm was 20/100 women-years by culture; 80% of infections were inapparent.

Genitoanal Ulcers

Regional adenopathy may or may not accompany the presence of one or more genital or proctoanal ulcers. The prevalence of genitoanal ulcer disease in prostitutes is 0.1–20% (typically 10%) (7127). Main considerations are HSV2, *Haemophilus ducreyi*, and *T. pallidum pallidum*.

HSV2 (3163, 5383, 6080, 7127, 7654, 7657). HSV2 is endemic in prostitutes worldwide. Reported seroprevalence is 65–85% in Latin America and 35–80% in Asia. In Dhaka, Bangladesh, in 2002, 35% (138/400, 95% CI 30–39) of hotel prostitutes were reactive in enzyme-linked immunosorbent assay (ELISA). Primary or reactivated lesions are considerably less prevalent. In Fukuoka, Japan, in 1985–1986, 5% (13/284) of prostitutes presented with HSV2 florid genital lesions.

***H. ducreyi* (683, 3110, 5946, 7126).** Chancroid is associated with prostitution and endemicity of HIV. It is more readily diagnosed in men than women. In Nairobi, Kenya, in 1981–1982, sources of chancroid reported by 300 men with culture-confirmed infection were prostitutes (in 57%), casual (anonymous) sex partners (in 36%), regular (known by name) sex partners (in 4%), and spouses (in 3%). At that time, the infection prevalence in Nairobi prostitutes was 0.8% (10/1,222). In high-income countries, chancroid is uncommon. In Los Angeles in 1981–1983, an outbreak caused 271 confirmed cases, 254 (94%) in Hispanic men, mainly migrant workers who had sex with prostitutes. In Winnipeg, Canada, in 1975–1977, in an outbreak with 135 cases, risks included unstable partnerships, and domicile in the core city.

***T. pallidum pallidum* (522, 3028, 3852, 5383, 5566, 6080, 6968, 7127, 7476, 7657, 8296).** The primary manifestation is often an ulcer, although later stages are disseminated. By sampling and test, reported seroprevalence in prostitutes is 1.5–40% (often 10%) in Africa, 2.5–15% (often 5–9%) in Latin America, 0.5–35% (often 10%) in Asia, and 3% in Madrid, Spain. In Madagascar in 1998, 18% (58/316) of registered prostitutes were reactive in rapid plasma reagin (RPR) test; their age was 15–42 (median, 23) years, the age at first sex was 11–22 (median, 17) years, and one fourth served foreign clients. Risks included multiple clients per week and, paradoxically, regular use of condoms. In Dhaka, Bangladesh, in 2002, 9% (34/400, 95% CI 6–12%) of hotel prostitutes were seroreactive in RPR and *T. pallidum* hemagglutination (TPHA) tests, including 4% (17) who were diagnosed with active syphilis. In a prophylaxis trial among prostitutes in Kenya, the seroconversion rate by RPR in the placebo arm was 3.8/100 women-years. An epidemic of syphilis seems to have emerged in Russia that in the 1990s reached western Europe with prostitutes from eastern Europe.

Genitoanal Papules

The main consideration is HPV. For donovanosis and lymphogranuloma venereum, see section 14.7; for ectoparasites (pediculosis or scabies), see section 4.6.

HPV (7443, 7727). HPV is associated with genital warts (condylomata acuminata), inapparent cervical infection, and cervical neoplasia. Genital warts (and HIV) increase the risks of cervical infection.

- Prostitutes (2364, 2764, 4106, 7533, 7727) are at increased risk of HPV infection and are considered a reservoir of oncogenic HPV. In Vienna, Austria, however, prevalence by DNA in situ hybridization were comparable in registered prostitutes ($n = 978$) and women attending STI clinics ($n = 5,493$). By sampling, HIV coinfection, and test (pap smear or NAT) reported infection prevalence in prostitutes are 24–37% in Africa, 18–57% in Latin America, and 7–32% in Europe.
- Lesbians (385, 4753). HPV seems to be transmitted among Lesbian women, who should be offered cervical smears like other women.

STI From Microtrauma

GB virus C (GBV-C, "hepatitis G virus") (6634, 8275). Sexual transmisison seems possible. In Japan by NAT or serology, prevalence was 25% (58/234) in non-IDU prostitutes, but 9% (7/71) in matched controls. In Taiwan by NAT, prevalence was 21% (30/140) in prostitutes, but 5% (2/40) in control women; infections were significantly associated with the monthly number of paying sex partners.

HBV (203, 2802, 3028, 3372, 3578, 5566, 7657). HBV infection risks include sex work and being the customer of an infected prostitute. Reported HBsAg prevalences in prostitutes are 0.3% (Mexico City), 0.6% (Tokyo), 1.3% (southern Mexico), 3.5% (Madrid, Spain), and 9% (Cambodia). In Europe and Australia, HBV marker prevalence can be 2–4 times higher in migrant than local prostitutes. HBV vaccine is recommended for susceptible prostitutes, but difficult access limits program success.

HCV (3028, 3578, 4979, 5331). Whether HCV is transmitted sexually (prostitute-to-client or client-to-prostitute) remains unresolved. Injection drug use is a confounding risk. Reported seroprevalence in prostitutes is 0.8–12%. In Madrid, Spain, in 1998–2003, 0.8% of migrant prostitutes ($n = 762$) were seroreactive.

HIV (3578, 5886, 7127, 7643, 7644). By sampling, prevention, and test, reported seroprevalences in prostitutes are 10–80% (often 40%) in Africa, 0.5–50% in Latin America, and 0–45% (often 1%) in Asia. Prostitutes are driving HIV epidemics in parts of Africa, the Caribbean, and Southeast and East Asia.

- Africa (2888, 3852, 6358). In Djibouti in 1991–1992, the HIV-1 seroprevalence was 12% (64/540) in "bar hostesses," and 38% (153/408) in street prostitutes. In a randomized, double-blind trial among prostitutes in Kenya, azithromycin prophylaxis for 2 years reduced the rates of *N. gonorrhoeae* and *C. trachomatis* infections but not of HIV1 infections that remained at 3–4/100 women-years. Locally, HIV2 can surpass the prevalence of HIV1 in prostitutes.
- Latin America (7047, 7657). In Chiapas State, Mexico, 0.6% of 484 bar-based prostitutes were infected. In contrast in IDU prostitutes in Argentina, the HIV1 seroprevalence was 44–50%.
- Asia (1509, 5566, 7797, 8194). In India, 85% of HIV infections are acquired heterosexually and few prostitutes use condoms. Their promotion reduced HIV infections in prostitutes, in Thailand from 28% to ~12%, and in Cambodia from 40–55% to ~30%. Of children forced into prostitution in Southeast Asia, ~50–90% are estimated to be HIV infected.
- Europe (546, 3028). In Madrid, Spain, in 1998–2003, 5% of migrant prostitutes ($n = 762$) were seroreactive to HIV1. In six large cities in Spain in 2000–2001, the HIV seroprevalence in prostitutes attending STI clinics was 0.7% (21/3,149). Among a small subset of IDU prostitutes, the prevalence was 16% (3/19).

Abuse (3189). In the United States in 1981–1997, of 9,136 HIV-infected children, 26 (0.3%) were suspected to have resulted from sexual abuse.

HHV8 (1058, 4254). Sexual transmission is believed to occur in the milieu, in particular, from high-risk (oral and anal) sex.

HTLV1 (546, 3028, 7244, 7575, 7799, 8429). Prostitutes are at increased risk. HTLV1 seroprevalence is 4- to 7-fold higher in prostitutes than in women from the population. Risks include advancing age, IDU, history of STI, and intercourse during menstruation. By age and IDU, reported HTLV1 seroprevalence in prostitues is 7% in Africa, 4–14% in Latin America, and 0.2–16% in Europe. In Madrid, Spain, in 1998–2003, 0.2% of 762 migrant prostitutes had antibodies to HTLV1. In Spain in 2000–2001, 0.3% of prostitutes ($n = 3,149$) were reactive to HTLV1 (0.2% to HTLV2). Of the few IDU sex workers, 16% (3/19) were reactive to HTLV1.

13.7 SEX AMONG MEN

Homosexual men have sex with men (MSM). Bisexual men have sex with men and women. Transvestites are biologically male but emotionally female. Male prostitutes trade sex for money or drugs. Male prostitutes may have wives or girlfriends and may perceive their male clients as heterosexual (5216). Male prostitutes can bridge populations of various strata and risks. Sexual violence in males is manifest by prostitution and sexual abuse of boys and by forced sex of men in prison.

Exposure (2845, 3711, 4963, 8392). About 0.5–2.5% of men in People's Republic of China and 2–5% of men in Europe report to have ever had sex with men in their life. About 3% of men worldwide report to have ever been sexually assaulted. Of adolescent male high school students in the United States ($n = 3,267$), 8% of heterosexual men, 21% of homosexual men, and 59% of bisexual men reported to have been forced into sex. MSM can also be injection drug users (IDU, see section 13.8). An "unfortunate quartet" are HIV-positive MSM who are IDU and practice sex. For STI in the population, see section 14.7; for carriers in the community, see section 14.1.

Infections (1800, 2173, 2845, 5676, 6461) (Box 13.7). Risks include unprotected anal, insertive, or receptive sex, orogenital sex, fisting, having multiple (casual) sex partners, and IDU.

Promotion of safe sex among MSM was successful in the early 1990s, but rates of HIV, *C. trachomatis*, and other STI in MSM have rebounded. Of >20,000 MSM in San Francisco, 58% (95% CI 56–59) reported anal sex in 1994, but 61% (95% CI 60–63) in 1997; concurrently, regular use of condoms for anal sex dropped from 70% (95% CI 68–71%) to 61% (95% CI 59–63).

MSM can be victims and sources of STI. Little is known about clients of male prostitutes. In Atlanta in 1990–1991, 16% of clients ($n = 82$) were reactive to *T. pallidum pallidum*, 37% to HIV, and 58% to markers of HBV.

Prevention (2064, 3893, 6461, 8268). Prevention is based on education, promotion of safe sex, vaccines (HAV and

HBV), and periodic (annual) or opportunistic (visit based) screening. Agents to consider for screening are HAV and HBV (in nonvaccinees); HCV and HIV; *T. pallidum pallidum*; urethral, rectal (in MSM reporting anal sex), and pharyngeal (oral sex in the past 2 weeks) *N. gonorrhoeae*; and urethral and rectal *C. trachomatis*. In Amsterdam, The Netherlands, safer sex among 532 young MSM brought a decline of herpes seroreactivity, for HSV2 from 51% in 1984–1985 to 19% in 1995–1997, and for HSV1 from 81% to 59%.

DROPLET-AIR CLUSTER, MSM
In HIV-infected MSM, AIDS-defining opportunistic respiratory tract infections comprise the expected spectrum, including mycobacteria (*M. avium* complex and *M. tuberculosis*) and fungi (*Pneumocystis* pneumonia, disseminated histoplasmosis, and extrapulmonary cryptococcosis) (3732).

N. meningitidis (7585). In Toronto, Canada, in 2001, six MSM linked via bathhouses in 10 weeks contracted a unique *N. meningitidis* serogroup C strain; two patients died. In oral swabs from MSM, *N. meningitidis* must be differentiated from *N. gonorrhoeae*.

FECES-FOOD CLUSTER, MSM
Enteric infections (1678, 3937, 4241, 4742, 6055, 6213). Enteric infections in MSM can result from unprotected anogenital, orogenital, or oroanal sex. Agents of proctitis or diarrhea in MSM (gay bowel) include HSV2, *Campylobacter*, *N. gonorrhoeae*, *Shigella*, and *G. lamblia*. In HIV-infected MSM, AIDS-defining infections span the expected spectrum; in addition to the agents given above, enteric AdV, CMV, *Rotavirus*, *C. difficile*, *V. parahaemolyticus*, *Cryptosporidium*, *Isospora*, and *Toxoplasma* can also cause infections.

Viruses
HAV (1501, 1576, 1602, 2493, 3074, 6201). By endemicity, vaccination, and condom use, HAV is a moderate to substantial risk for MSM, including from gay venues (e.g., saunas and bar darkrooms), casual sex, multiple anonymous sex partners, group sex, and oroanal or anogenital sex. In the pre-HIV era, reported rates of acute HA among MSM were 7–22/100 per year, and 20–50% of MSM had antibodies to HAV.

Outbreaks of acute HA among MSM have reemerged in North America (38, 1597, 3260), Australia (7180), and West Europe (1862, 4860, 6201, 6314, 7250). In Europe, recent outbreaks have been reported in cities such as Copenhagen, London, Munich, Paris, Oslo (Norway), and Rotterdam (The Netherlands).

Vaccine (38, 1597, 2493) is recommended for MS, at least for subgroups who engage in high-risk sex. For young adults, prevaccination antibody testing is not necessary.

Bacteria
***C. jejuni* (2666, 6055).** Sexual spread of *C. jejuni* among MSM has been reported, including strains that are resistant to fluoroquinolones.

***Salmonella* (6213).** Sexual spread of *Salmonella* among MSM is likely. In the United States in 2000, two cases of typhoid fever and seven serovar Typhi infections were diagnosed among MSM who had sex with a culture-confirmed carrier.

***Shigella*.** Sexual spread of *S. flexneri* or *S. sonnei* among MSM is a significant risk, mainly from genitoanal, oroanal, and orogenital sex. Sources are men who are reconvalescent or prolonged shedders.

Outbreaks Since the 1970s, outbreaks have been reported among MSM in high-income countries.
- North America (375, 1254, 3982). Cities with outbreaks include Chicago, Quebec, San Francisco, and Seattle. In San Francisco in 2000, of 199 culture-confirmed *S. sonnei* cases, 121 (61%) were self-reported MSM, for a rate of $259/10^5$ per year, compared with $16/10^5$ per year in the population.
- Australia (5542). In Sydney in 2000, *S. sonnei* biotype G caused an outbreak with 123 infections, of which 98 (80%) were in MSM. Visiting a sex venue in 2 weeks before illness onset was the only risk. In Australia, sex venues are commercial establishments that require an entry fee and provide rooms and showers.
- West Europe (4732). In Berlin in 2001, an outbreak of *Shigella* caused ≥15 cases.

Fungi
Microsporidia (3521, 5631, 7856). Intestinal microsporidiosis is a hazard for MSM with AIDS. Modes of spread are not well established but might include sex and swallowing pool water. In Italy in 1992–1995, all 19 patients with intestinal microspiridiasis were HIV positive, and one half (10/19) were MSM. *Enterocytozoon bieneusi* was isolated by electron microscopy in 20 (30%) of 67 MSM with AIDS and chronic diarrhea. Jejunal biopsies were more often positive (44% or 16/36) than duodenal biopsies (17% or 6/35), and release of spores into the bowel lumen was seen.

Protozoa
***Cryptosporidium hominis* (3241, 3937, 7044).** Sexually transmitted *Cryptosporidium* has been reported in MSM. Risks include having changed sex partners, attending sex venues, and insertive anal sex. In Los Angeles in 1983–1992, cryptosporidiosis was reported in 3.8% (638/16,953) of AIDS patients, significantly more often in

sexually (3.9%) than nonsexually (2.6%) acquired AIDS; in gay and bisexual males, prevalence decreased with age.

Entamoeba. Past reports of the high (15–40%) prevalence of inapparent *Entamoeba histolytica* infections in urban MSM could in retrospect be explained by confounding with *E. dispar* (4463, 5565, 6146, 7114, 8016). Although at a much reduced rate, however, sexual spread of *E. histolytica* has been confirmed in MSM, including invasive disease. In Japan in 2000–2001, ~90% (53/58) of invasive amebiasis cases (colitis and liver abscess) were acquired locally (in Tokyo, Yokohama, and Osaka), and >50% (31/55) of male patients were MSM.

***Giardia* (640, 3074, 3869, 4742, 5685)**. Sexual spread of *G. lamblia* in MSM is likely. Reported prevalence in urban MSM communities is 3–18%.

SKIN-BLOOD CLUSTER, MSM

In HIV-infected MSM, AIDS-defining opportunistic infections cover the expected pattern, including CMV retinitis, HSV disease, and esophageal candidiasis (3732).

Genitoanal Discharge

Symptoms include purulent urethral discharge (drip), tenesmus, and purulent bowel movement. The main agents are *C. trachomatis* and *N. gonorrhoeae*.

***C. trachomatis* (1948, 3893, 6461)**. MSM are frequently infected, and infection enhances the risk of HIV. In San Francisco in 2003, >6,400 MSM were tested for *C. trachomatis* by NAT. Positive were 5.2% of urethral, 7.9% of rectal (after receptive sex), and 1.4% of pharyngeal (after oral sex) tests. The majority (53%) of infections was extraurethral. About 42% of urethral but 85% of rectal infections were inapparent. Diagnostic yield was higher in manifest than inapparent MSM, from urethral (15.1% versus 2.7%) and rectal (20.7 versus 7.6%) sites. In Europe, ~2% of asymptomatic MSM had urethral infection by NAT or culture, and of all infections in MSM, ~50% were inapparent.

***N. gonorrhoeae* (1983, 2485, 3893, 7335)**. MSM are frequently infected, and infection enhances the risk of HIV. In United States cities, the proportion of gonorrhea attributed to MSM increased from 5% (219/4,858 diagnoses) in 1992 to 13% (591/4,465) in 1999. Sites for gonococcal infections in MSM include urethra (40–80%), rectum (10–30%), and pharynx (5–20%). In San Francisco in 2003, >6,400 MSM were tested for *N. gonorrhoeae* by NAT. Positive were 6.0% of urethral, 6.9% of rectal (after receptive sex), and 9.2% of pharyngeal (after oral sex) tests. The majority (64%) of infections was extraurethral. About 10% of urethral but 85% or rectal infections were inapparent. Diagnostic yield was higher in manifest than inapparent MSM, from urethral (26.9% versus 0.8%) and rectal (19.8 versus 6.1%) sites. Outbreaks among MSM have been reported.

T. vaginalis. The prevalence of *T. vaginalis* in MSM seems comparable to the male general population.

Genitoanal Ulcers

Regional adenopathy (bubo) may or may not accompany the presence of one or more genital or anorectal ulcers. Main considerations are herpes simplex virus (HSV), *H. ducreyi*, and *T. pallidum pallidum*.

HSV (2064, 3163, 4117, 6224). Both HIV1 and HIV2 can infect MSM. MSM shed HSV2 mainly perianally and inapparently, and HSV1 mainly orally. Reported seroprevalence is high: 20–55% for HSV2, and up to 60–80% for HSV1. Of latently HSV2–infected MSM, 15% reported reactivated herpes in the preceding year. Infection with HSV2 increases the risk of subsequent infection with HIV, probably because both viruses are spread by the same risk behaviors.

***H. ducreyi* (1922, 5007)**. Although a major cause of male genital ulcer disease, knowledge for MSM is limited. In an outbreak of genital ulcer disease in Mississippi with 56 confirmed chancroid cases, risks in men included sex with a cocaine user, sex for money or drugs, and multiple sex partners.

***T. pallidum pallidum* (1218, 1236, 1965, 2765, 3028, 3228)**. *T. pallidum pallidum* circulates among MSM. In the United States, increasing rates of primary and secondary syphilis in 2001–2002, and an increasing male-to-female rate ratio underscore a recently enhanced spread among MSM. In Chicago, Ill., MSM accounted for an increasing proportion of primary and secondary syphilis in the city: 15% in 1998–2000, but close to 60% in 2001–2002. In the United Kingdom in 2000, 48% of syphilis in males was attributed to MSM. Oral sex is a significant mode of acquisition. In Chicago in 1998–2002, oral sex as exclusive exposure was reported by 7% (10/145) of heterosexual females, 6% (10/157) of heterosexual males, but 20% (66/325) of MSM. Highly infectious primary (ulcer) and secondary (patchy) lesions at lips, tongue, and buccal mucosa are well known. Transvestites seem at unusually high risk. In Madrid, Spain, 16% (21/128) of immigrant transvestite male prostitutes had "active" syphilis. Syphilis outbreaks are well documented among urban MSM communities.

Genitoanal Papules Or Granulomas

The main considerations are HPV and *C. trachomatis* serovars L1–3 (lymphogranuloma venereum). For donovanosis, see section 14.7; for ectoparasites, see section 4.6.

HPV (186, 847, 1391, 2528, 5689, 7862). Condylomata acuminata can be inconspicuous, and penile infections can be inapparent. HPV is endemic in MSM. HPV was detected by PCR in 93% of HIV-infected ($n = 346$) and 61% of HIV-negative ($n = 262$) MSM. Among HIV-negative MSM from four U.S. cities (Boston, Denver, New York, and San Francisco) in 2001–2002, 57% (692/1,218) amplified HPV from the anal canal. MSM appear at increased risk of intraepithelial neoplasia from genital and anal warts, and anal cancer due to HPV. HPV was also detected in oral brushings by PCR in 7% ($n = 57$) of HIV-infected individuals.

C. trachomatis L1–3 (492, 2871, 7710). Risks include HIV infection and unprotected anal sex. Lymphogranuloma venereum reemerged among MSM in The Netherlands in 2003. While in The Netherlands typically <5 cases per year were diagnosed, reported cases in 2003–2005 rose to >140. Most patients presented with bloody proctitis rather than genital lesions and bubo. Confirmation was by proctoscopy, PCR from rectal swabs, and serum antibodies. From Amsterdam and Rotterdam, the epidemic L2 serovar spread to other cities in Europe and North America, with >120 cases in Paris and Bordeaux and >30 in London.

STI From Microtrauma
CMV (186, 3074, 6322). CMV is a hazard for MSM. In Göteborg, Sweden, in the 1980s, anti-CMV IgG or IgM were detected in 88% (113/129) of inapparent MSM but only 59% (61/104) of heterosexual men. In one third of IgM-reactive men, CMV was isolated from urine or semen. CMV was also detected in oral brushings by PCR in 3.5% ($n = 57$) of HIV-infected individuals. In France in 184 HIV-positive but CMV-negative individuals, the CMV seroconversion rate was 9/100 person-years (95% CI 7–12), with a high rate among MSM. In consistent users of condoms, risks were significantly reduced.

HBV (416, 1501, 2820, 3074, 4255, 7284). HBV is a hazard for MSM, including male prostitutes. The excess risk for MSM has been estimated at 40–50%. In high-income countries, 10–15% of notified acute HB cases have been attributed to MSM. In western Europe in the 1980s, 50–80% of MSM tested positive for HBV markers, including 4–7% for HBsAg. Vaccine should be offered to susceptible MSM, preferrable pre-HIV, as HIV infection may increase HBV infectivity and reduce vaccine efficacy in MSM.

HCV (2608, 4979, 6137). HCV is a hazard for MSM, mainly from IDU, less from sex. A review of 21 studies concluded that "sexual transmission of HCV occurs, but infrequently" (4979). Reported seroprevalence in MSM is 0–33% (up to 90% in MSM who are IDU). A majority of infections (about two thirds) are silent for years. In a Swiss cohort study, the seroconversion rate was 0.6/100 person-years (7 in IDU).

HHV8 (1058, 2065, 5645). HHV8 appears to spread sexually among MSM. Risks include preexisting HIV infection and insertive or receptive orogenital sex with multiple partners. In MSM from high-income countries, reported seroprevalence is high (20–25%). In a cohort of 1,458 Dutch MSM monitored in 1984–1996, 215 participants seroconverted, for a rate of 3.6/100 person-years.

HIV (1176, 1244, 1813, 7643, 7988). HIV is a hazard for MSM. Risk factors include previous STI, irregular condom use, casual sex partners, HIV-positive sex partners, sex work, and IDU. In the United States in 2001, of 35,602 HIV infections, 22% (7,674) were attributed to MSM, 2% (641) to MSM who were IDU; risks were not reported for 54% (19,137). Also in the United States in 2004–2005, 25% (450/1,767) of MSM from five cities tested positive for HIV (range, 18–40%), and 48% of the infected (217/450) said to be unaware of the infection, although most (84% or 184) of the infected individuals had been tested previously for HIV. MSM are driving HIV epidemics in parts of East Asia, North and Latin America, Australia, New Zealand, and West Europe.

- By sampling, reported infection prevalence is: in the Americas (1813, 5216, 6478, 7988), 1–7% in Canada ($n = 635$ MSM, 126 male prostitutes), 17.5% in New Orleans (211 male prostitutes), 14% (95% CI 11–17) in Buenos Aires ($n = 694$ MSM from nightclubs, porno cinemas, or streets), and 22% in Montevideo ($n = 200$ transvestite prostitutes); in Asia (1411), 3% (95% CI 2–5) in Beijing; and in Europe (3028, 3105), median 14% in 13 studies (low 2% in Belgium and high 26% in London), and 11% in Madrid ($n = 128$ immigrant male transvestite prostitutes from Ecuador).
- Transmission (Table 13.2) risks vary by source and mode of spread, with a rate of 5–30 per 1,000 unprotected receptive anal sex acts.
- Risks (159, 3105, 6727, 6981). In San Francisco in 1989–1998, by sampling and test, the infection rate in MSM was 1.6–6.6/100 and year. Reported rates in MSM in Europe are 1.1–4.7/100 person-years. Indications for (nonoccupational) PEP include unprotected receptive anal sex and needle sharing with a known HIV-infected source; in contrast, PEP is controversial for these exposures, if the source is a "high-risk partner" or its HIV status is unknown.

HTLV (459, 8429). HTLV is a hazard for MSM. Risks include a history of gonorrhea, HIV coinfection, long

Table 13.2. Risk of HIV acquisition from exposure to HIV-positive sources

Event	Vehicle	Infections per 1,000 events
Transfusion	Blood	900–1,000
IDU, shared needles	Blood	7
Work-related injury	Blood	2–4
Childbirth	Perinatal fluids	130–450
Nursing	Breast milk	0.01–0.04
Unprotected receptive sex		
Anal	Semen, secretions	5–30
Vaginal	Semen, secretions	0.5–1.5
Oral	Semen, secretions	<0.5
Unprotected insertive sex		
Anal	Semen, secretions	0.7–1
Vaginal	Semen, secretions	0.5–1
Oral	Semen, saliva	0.05

homosexual activity, and multiple sex partners. In Trinidad, seroreactivity to HTLV1 was higher in MSM (15%) than in the population (2%). In Peru, seroreactivity was three times higher in MSM (6%, 3/48) than in healthy pregnant women (2%, 5/211).

13.8 INJECTION DRUG USE

IDUs depend on parenteral administration of illicit drugs, mainly heroin and cocaine (both drugs can be snorted or inhaled as well). IDUs are notorious for being difficult to reach and for poor treatment compliance such as tuberculosis treatment (837).

Exposure (36, 1266, 2039, 6389) (http://www.census.gov/prod/2004pubs/04statab/health.pdf). In the 2002 national household survey on drug use and health in the United States, 46% of respondents ≥12 years of age ($n = 72,000$) reported to have ever used any illicit drug in life and 8% reported current (in the past month) use. Current users mentioned, among others, marijuana and hashish (6%), cocaine (0.9%), methamphetamine (0.3%), heroin (0.1%), and, for comparison, alcohol (51%). Worldwide, IDUs are estimated to 13–15 million, for a prevalence of 0.3% among adults. In 2003, median population prevalence was estimated at 0.6–0.7% in North America, 0.4–0.8% in Australia, Japan, and New Zealand, and 0.4% in West Europe.

Infections (507, 2243) (Box 13.8). Acute, recurrent, and chronic infectious diseases are one of several major burdens in IDUs. In Madrid, Spain, in 1995–1996, of 304 female IDUs, 18% reported tuberculosis in the past 5 years, 21% reported sex for income, 23% were homeless, 31% reported STI in the past 5 years, and 32% had been in prison at least once since first drug use. Frequent infections in IDUs include skin, respiratory, and bloodstream infections. *S. aureus* is the single most important bacterial agent in IDUs. Causes of excess mortality in IDUs include AIDS and endocarditis. For prostitution, see section 13.6; for homelessness, see section 11.3; for STI in the community, see section 14.7; for infections in prison, see section 11.7; and for sex among men, see "Sex among Men" above.

DROPLET-AIR CLUSTER
In HIV-infected IDUs, AIDS-defining opportunistic respiratory tract infections comprise the expected spectrum, including mycobacterial disease (*M. avium* complex and *M. tuberculosis*), recurrent bacterial pneumonia, and *Pneumocystis* pneumonia (3732). In a cohort of HIV-infected IDUs ($n = 197$), the rate of bacterial pneumonia in 1988–1992 was 2/100 person-years (1025).

IDUs might profit from MMR, VZV, *C. diphtheriae* (as dT), and *S. pneumoniae* vaccines.

***C. pneumoniae* (698).** In 1991, an outbreak in a community of 26 ex-IDUs (13 HIV-infected) affected 15 (58%) members (11 with pneumonia, 2 with pharyngitis, and 2 with flulike illness).

***C. diphtheriae* (2556, 2969, 2978).** IDUs are at risk of colonization and infection with nontoxigenic strains. In Switzerland in 1990–1996, 38 (58%) of 65 nontoxigenic strains of *C. diphtheriae* were obtained from IDUs or their contacts (20 or 31% other strains were from imported skin infections). In Zürich in 1991–1992, nontoxigenic *C. diphtheriae* was isolated from the throat of 5 (4%) of 117 homeless IDUs, and from 5 (18%) of 28 skin ulcers. The 10 strains belonged to a single clone. During the same period no strain was isolated from 200 controls.

***M. tuberculosis* (837, 1173, 3882, 4146, 6046).** Infection and disease are endemic in IDUs. By age and comorbidity, 15–40% of IDUs are skin reactive (latently

> **Box 13.8** Main agents or infections in injection drug users (IDUs), by agent cluster
>
> | | |
> |---|---|
> | Droplet-air | *C. diphtheriae*, mycobacteria (*M. avium* and *M. tuberculosis*), recurrent bacterial pneumonia, *Pneumocystis* pneumonia |
> | Feces-food | HAV; chronic diarrhea and wasting, microsporidia, *Cryptosporidium* |
> | Zoonotic | *Bartonella*, *R. akari*; *Plasmodium* |
> | Environmental | *B. cereus*, *C. botulinum* (wound botulism), *C. tetani*, and clostridia that form gas and gangrene |
> | Skin-blood | HBV, HCV, HDV, HHV8, HIV1, HTLV1 and 2; *S. aureus* (abscess and infective endocarditis), *S. pyogenes* bacteremia; STI (homosexual IDUs) |

infected). In Italy, the prevalence of latent infection among non-Bacillus Calmette Guerin (BCG)-vaccinated IDUs was 11% (27/237) by induration of ≥10 mm in tuberculin skin test, and 26% (61) by induration ≥5 mm. In Montreal, Canada, of 246 IDUs, 22% had skin test indurations ≥5 mm: 5% of HIV-infected (likely anergic) IDUs, but 28% of HIV-negative IDUs. Reactivity increases with years of injection drug use. A history of a positive skin test is unreliable as nearly one third of IDUs actually test negative, likely from anergy.

In the United States, the risk of active tuberculosis in skin-test-positive IDUs is 1–7.6/100 person-years, which is 1–6 times the risk in the population within 1 year from skin-test conversion. In The Netherlands in 1986–1996, the rate of culture-confirmed tuberculosis per 100 person-years was 0.6 (95% CI 0.4–0.9) in drug users overall, with a high of 1.5 (0.9–2) in HIV-infected users and a low of 0.2 (0.1–0.4) in HIV noninfected users.

FECES-FOOD CLUSTER

In HIV-infected IDUs, AIDS-defining opportunistic enteric agents to be expected include microsporidia and *Cryptosporidium* (3732). Accordingly, HIV-infected IDUs may suffer from chronic diarrhea and wasting (>10% loss of body weight). For wound botulism from *C. botulinum*, see "Environmental Cluster" below.

HAV (38, 2493, 5530, 7060, 7462). Major infection risks are poor personal hygiene and contact with individuals with jaundice. Parenteral mode of spread is uncertain. In high-income countries, 10–30% of reported acute HA cases are in IDUs. Outbreaks in IDUs have been described. In Italy in 2002, acute HA affected 47 persons of whom 35 were IDUs. At a resort on the English coast in 1998–1999, 14 IDUs contracted acute HA, and 11 further cases were connected to injection drug use. Vaccination is recommended for IDUs, in adolescents without prevaccine testing.

ZOONOTIC CLUSTER

By life in parks, streets, and city cores, IDUs are exposed to rodents and arthropods. Shared needles may replace arthropods as infection vectors.

***Bartonella* (1531, 1532).** IDUs are at risk of *Bartonella* infections. In Baltimore in 1988–1989, 37% of 630 inner-city IDUs were seroreactive to either *B. elisabethae*, *B. henselae*, or *B. quintana*. In New York City in 1997–98, 46% of 204 IDUs were reactive to *B. elisabethae*; lower reactivities to *B. henselae* and *B. quintana* were interpreted as cross-reactions.

***Borrelia* (4515).** TBRF is reported in IDUs.

***Rickettsia akari* (1531, 1534).** In the United States, from 9% of IDUs in New York City to 16% in inner-city Baltimore (95% African Americans) were seroreactive.

***Plasmodium* (481, 1355, 4477).** Needle sharing is a risk for falciparum and vivax malaria in IDUs. Small amounts of blood may be sufficient for transmission. An invisible inoculum of 0.05 ml from a donor carrying 5,000 parasites per µl, is estimated to correspond to 24 succesful sporozoites that develop to 24 hepatic schizonts, 480,000 merozoites, and 240,00 invaded red blood cells. Of IDUs with malaria, about 45–80% are coinfected with HIV.

Outbreaks Needle sharing has caused outbreaks of falciparum and vivax malaria, mainly in cities outside malarious areas (481, 2834, 5186).

- America (481, 6825). In the United States in 1970–1972, in the wake of the Vietnam War, 55 malaria cases were reported in IDUs. In São Paulo, Brazil, in 1988–1990, three vivax malaria outbreaks affected 2, 9, and 119 IDUs, respectively.
- Asia (1355). In Ho Chi Minh City (Saigon), Vietnam, where malaria is not endemic, 32 IDUs contracted falciparum malaria in 1991–1996 from shared needles, for a lethality of 20%.
- Europe (2834, 5186). In Madrid, Spain, in 1984, five young (age 17–18 years) male white IDUs contracted vivax malaria from shared injection material. In Milano, Italy, in 1981, falciparum malaria was diagnosed in 16 IDUs.

ENVIRONMENTAL CLUSTER

In nondebrided wounds and necrotic tissues, spores of *C. botulinum* or *C. tetani* can germinate and produce toxin, with a risk of wound botulism, tetanus, or severe bacterial infection. Spore-forming bacteria in IDUs are endogenous (skin and pharynx), or injected into skin or muscle (popping) with "street-drugs" or dirty injection material (863). IDUs should be offered tetanus vaccine (as dT) updates according to national policy at any occasion.

***Bacillus* (1732).** Aspirate from an IDU with crepitant (gas) cellulitis at the forearm and a sample of his own heroin both grew *B. cereus*.

***Clostridium*.** Spores survive heat from "cooking up" of heroin. Besides *C. botulinum* and *C. tetani*, unusual clostridia may be recovered from IDUs. ***C. botulinum* (842, 863, 1223, 4997, 8056).** Wound botulism is manifest like food-borne botulism. Wound botulism is a risk for IDUs. In California in 1994–1998, "black tar" heroin was vehicle for 93 cases of wound botulism among poppers; only 12 small (<0.5 g) samples of black tar could be obtained, and all tested negative for botulinum toxin. In the United Kingdom in 2000–2004, >55 cases of wound botulism were diagnosed in IDUs (most due to type A and a few by type B). ***C. histolyticum* (842).** This rare agent was diagnosed in the United Kingdom in 2003–2004 in 12 poppers. ***C. novyi* (93, 1431).** *C. novyi* is an emerging agent in IDUs. In Scotland in 2000, life-threatening disease was diagnosed in 108 long-standing IDUs who injected heroin; 13 grew *C. novyi*, together with other clostridia and *Bacillus*. ***C. sordellii* (3947).** Black tar heroin was the vehicle for necrotizing fasciitis in IDUs, and of a toxic shock-like syndrome, for a lethality of 44% (4/9). ***C. tetani* (27, 863, 1158, 7475).** Tetanus is a risk for IDUs. In California in 1987–1997, 27 (40%) of 67 reported tetanus cases were in IDUs; all were poppers. Injection abscesses were seen in 67% (18/27) of patients. In Vietnam in 1993–2002, 4.4% of 2,422 tetanus cases were due to injections, mainly self-administered injections in IDUs. In the United Kingdom in 2003, seven tetanus cases (four men, three women) were diagnosed in IDUs; two cases were unvaccinated, and one case had received one vaccine dose (9 years previously). In 2003–2004, case numbers in IDUs increased to 20.

SKIN-BLOOD CLUSTER

In HIV-infected IDUs, AIDS-defining opportunistic infections to be expected include HSV disease and esophageal candidiasis (3732).

Viruses

HBV, HCV, and HIV frequently coinfect IDUs. Screening should include at least these three viruses. A convenient material is saliva collected on filter paper (3758).

GBV-C (1050, 5456, 7561). Reported prevalences in IDUs by serology or NAT are 35–50% in Europe and 43% in Japan.

HBV (416, 1423, 2820, 6573). Risks include sharing injection material, e.g., with sex partners and mates in prison, and years on drugs. In high-income countries, ~15–20% of reported acute HB is attributed to injection drug use. Outbreaks among IDUs may escape ordinary surveillance, being detected only by molecular fingerprinting at central laboratories.

- Prevalence (328, 1890, 2243, 2647, 6573, 7135, 8027). In urban IDUs, reported HBV marker prevalence is ~25–75%.
- Rates (1890, 7135). In New York City in 1997–1999, the infection rate in 630 IDUs (all on heroin, 50–80% on cocaine) 18–30 years of age was 20/100 person-years (95% CI 14–29). In Switzerland, of susceptible IDUs in a prevention program ($n = 854$), seroconversion rates were 8/100 in the first year, and 4/100 in the second year.
- Preventive measures (4338, 6045, 6047, 6967). Preventive measures include education, clean injection material, screening, and vaccine for susceptible IDUs. However, only a fraction of IDUs may participate in vaccination programs, e.g., in Italy in 2001, only 32% (308/965) of IDUs were vaccinated compared with 42% (54/130) of noninjecting drug users. Response in IDUs to standard vaccine schedule may be suboptimal. Reasons for nonresponse include HIV or HCV coinfection and older age.

HCV (173, 1890, 4979, 6389, 6430, 6573, 6585, 7467). Since blood banks have introduced sensitive screening tests in the 1990s, IDUs in high-income countries account for >50% of newly detected HCV infections. Modes of spread include sharing injection materials (e.g., syringes, cookers, and filters) with friends, strangers, and for sex, reusing materials, "splitting drugs wet," and "shooting in gallery." Risks are increasing with older age, years on drugs, unsafe sex, sex work, and a history of incarceration. It would seem that a "silent" HCV epidemic is ongoing in IDUs of comparable proportion to HIV; unlike HIV, HCV gets little public attention.

- Prevalence (328, 1640, 1890, 2647, 3758, 6045, 8027). Documentation abounds. By age, place, and years on drugs, from 4% (London, United Kingdom) to virtually 100% (typically 70%) of IDUs test positive for anti-HCV. Viral RNA is detected by NAT in nearly 50% of IDUs in Australia and in ~25–90% in Europe.
- Rates (1640, 1890, 2647, 3758, 4952, 6445, 7135, 7467). Seroconversion rates per 100 person-years reported in IDUs are ~10–20 in North America, 38 (95% CI 28–

49) in People's Republic of China, 20 in Australia, and 4–24 in Europe.
- Prevention. As vaccines are not available, prevention is based on harm reduction by education, clean injections, safe sex, and periodic testing.

Hepatitis D virus (HDV) (7430). HDV is parasitic on HBV. In Thailand, of 55 HBsAg-positive IDUs, 12 (22%) tested positive for anti-HDV, and 8 (15%) amplified HDV-RNA by reverse transcriptase-PCR.

HHV8 (328, 1058). HHV8 infections seem associated with IDUs. In San Francisco in 1998–2000, 11% (218/1,905) of IDUs were seroreactive, including 10% (53/556) of female heterosexual IDUs, 10% (103/1,074) of male heterosexual IDUs, and 23% (62/275) of homosexual IDUs.

HIV (1176, 7643). Risks in IDUs are the same as with HBV and HCV infections in IDUs. In the United States in 2001, of 35,602 new HIV infections, 8% (2,941) were in IDUs, and an additional 2% were in homosexual IDUs (641); for 54% (19,137) risks were not reported. IDUs are driving HIV epidemics in parts of North Africa, North and Latin America, India, Southeast and East Asia, Australia, and Europe.
- Prevalence (328, 1890, 2243, 2647, 3105, 6045, 7047, 8027). By age, location, and sexual orientation, reported infection prevalences in IDUs are ~0.5–25% in North America, ~30–80% in Argentina, 17% in southern People's Republic of China, and ~1–60% (often 5–15%) in Europe, with highs typically in urban homosexual IDUs.
- Rate in IDUs (1890, 2647, 3758, 3968, 7118, 7135). Reported HIV1 seroconversion rates per 100 person-years are 0.4 (95% CI 0–2.5) in New York City, 11–57 in Thailand (0.2–5 in drug smokers or inhalers), 7 (95% CI 5–10) in People's Republic of China, 1 in Switzerland, 3 (95% CI 1.8–6.6) in London, United Kingdom, and 6 in Berlin, Germany.
- Prevention is based on education, clean injection materials, periodic testing, and early highly active antiretroviral treatment (HAART).

HTLV (7037, 7244, 8027). IDU is a risk. In Buenos Aires, Argentina, of street-recruited IDU, 2% (4/174) tested positive for HTLV1, and 14% (25/174) for HTLV2. In Italy, the HTLV seroprevalence in IDU was 3.5–6%. In Spain, 95% (107/113) of individuals reactive for HTLV2 were IDU.

Bacteria

Syringe abscess (477, 650, 842, 3262). Unclean subcutaneous or intramuscular (popping) or intravenous injections are risks. Among a San Francisco community sample of 169 IDUs, 54 (32%) had abscesses, cellulitis, or both. Common abscess locations include arms and groin. Self-treatment is common; in San Francisco, 27% of IDUs lanced abscesses, and 16% purchased antibiotics on the street. Despite self-treatment, skin infections are a main reason for hospitalization of IDUs. For evaluation, wound and blood cultures are recommended. **Microbiology (586, 842, 3262, 7018, 7247).** Skin abscesses of IDUs on average yield three to four agents. Oral flora can be prominent, perhaps from licking hypodermic needles for injection. Main isolates are *S. aureus*, *S. pyogenes* (GAS), oral streptococci, and anaerobes, e.g., *Actinomyces*, *Bacteroides*, *Fusobacterium*, *Peptostreptococcus*, and *Prevotella*, occasionally *Clostridium* (see "Environmental Cluster" above). **Outbreak (731).** In Switzerland in 1997, a GAS clone caused an outbreak among IDU, with 19 cases (16 subcutaneous needle abscesses, 2 erysipelas, 1 osteomyelitis).

Bloodstream infection (BSI). Skin abscesses and intravenous injections are sources of bacteremia, BSI, sepsis, and endocarditis in IDU. *S. aureus* **(4541, 5078).** *S. aureus* is the main agent, causing subcutaneous abscesses, osteomyelitis, and life-threatening infective endocarditis in IDUs, including of intact valves. Endocarditis in IDUs is an emergency that requires immediate hospitalization and treatment. Infection risks appear to be increased in HIV-infected IDUs, perhaps because of a greater need for invasive procedures. Colonization is a risk for subsequent infection. *S. pyogenes* **(GAS).** *S. pyogenes* is a cause of bacteremia in IDUs.

STI in IDUs. *C. trachomatis* L1–3 (493). An outbreak of lymphogranuloma venereum has been described among crack cocaine users. *T. pallidum pallidum* (3313, 6045). Sex for drugs is a risk in IDUs. In the Veneto area of Italy in 2001, 16 (1.7%) of 965 IDUs were reactive in *T. pallidum* hemagglutination test compared with none of 130 noninjecting drug users.

14

Human Community

14.1 Colonization, carriage, and contact

14.2 Age

14.3 Day care

14.4 Schools and training

14.5 Minorities

14.6 Latency, reactivation, and immune impairment

14.7 Community-acquired syndromes

There is no such thing as society. There are individual men and women, and there are families.

M.Thatcher (1925-)

"Community-acquired" is often used to describe all infections acquired outside hospitals. This broad sense aggregates community habitats such as homes, workplaces, and leisure venues. Here, the term is used more restrictively, for day care and schools, public places, and the "general" population.

Exposure. Determinants of endemicity in communities include municipal utilities (tap water, sanitation, and garbage), age of primoinfection, carrier prevalence, and herd (collective) immunity. Poorly integrated or reached minorities can be significant community infection reservoirs. In the history, address type of neighborhood and selective life-time exposures (Box 14.1).

Infection. Infection is acquired from carriers in the community, inhalation (utility-generated aerosols, see section 6.2), ingestion (catered events), or inoculation (e.g., sharps at public places, see section 13.4). Control and preventive measures should involve community members, e.g., participation in programs for safe water, sanitation, vaccination, and elimination of breeding sites. For cities, see section 6.2.

14.1 COLONIZATION, CARRIAGE, AND CONTACT

"Normally sterile sites" are sheltered body parts that do not grow agents in healthy persons, e.g., blood, pleura, and cerebrospinal fluid. Colonized sites (401, 661, 726, 1717) are surfaces (skin and mucosa) inhabited by commensals or opportunists (normal flora). Assignment to "normal flora" can be arbitrary. An opportunist may be flora (harmless) at one site (e.g., skin) but not at another (e.g., blood), or in one host (immune competent, outpatient) but not in another (e.g., antimicrobials, devices, and intensive care). Flora is lost and reacquired, and it competes for niches.

In general, flora is considered to protect the body from virulent agents (e.g., *Lactobacillus* in the vagina). In the pharynx, *Streptococcus pneumoniae* seems to

> **Box 14.1** Suggested history of community exposure
>
> **Right now:**
> - What is your address, type of domicile, and neighborhood (e.g., industrial, ethnic). How long have you been at this address?
> - What is the total number of people in your household? Are there any children in day care? Any children in school?
> - Has anybody been ill (with . . .) in the neighborhood, in day care, at school, at work, or among friends? Have you heard rumors of an outbreak?
>
> **In past 1–4 weeks:**
> - Has there been any municipal service breakdown (malodorous tap water, sewerage overflow, garbage heaps, and dust clouds)?
> - Have you had any snacks or meals from school kitchens, outlets, or street stalls?
> - Have you made any visits to malls, theaters, zoos, saunas, or discos or stayed at camps, dormitories, or friends' homes?
> - Have you encountered any dust or "mist" (from an industrial plant, or in an office) or unusual weather condition?
> - Have you missed any school or work days or visited a doctor or hospital?
> - Have you received any antimicrobials (prescribed or self-administered) or vaccines?
>
> **In the past 1–12 months:**
> - Has there been any international travel?
>
> **In your lifetime:**
> - Have you ever had chickenpox, jaundice, tuberculosis, typhoid fever, or an STI?
> - Name and document all vaccines ever received (including respiratory and enteric)
> - Have you ever been bitten by a vertebrate animal, tick, or other living thing?
> - Have you ever been HIV tested or injected drugs or had sex with same sex or anal sex? What is your number of sex partners and pregnancies?

prevent *Staphylococcus aureus* carriage. In contrast, *Rhinovirus* seems to promote nasal coagulase-negative *Staphylococcus* (CoNS), and *S. pneumoniae* and *Haemophilus influenzae* seem to synergize *Neisseria meningitidis*.

Contact (6, 2641, 5282, 6252) is physical, via hands, skin touch, kissing, or "bridging," via droplets that fall on hands, skin, or mucosa (within 1–3 m) or are inhaled in closed rooms (shared with others for hours). Typical venues for contacts are households, day care centers, classrooms, dormitories, aircrafts, and hospitals.

Shedding is determined in outbreaks, follow-up studies, and volunteers. Similarly, infectivity is determined from secondary attack rates in contacts. A reference point is disease onset (d_0), the day when vomit, diarrhea, skin eruption, fever, or malaise are first noticed. Shedding and infectivity typically straddle d_0, from late incubation to the early recovery. Pre-d_0 shedding usually cannot be prevented, except in outbreaks or when the exposure date (e_0) is known, e.g., from travel or an injection.

Carriage is the prolonged, silent presence of an unwanted, typically acquired agent (opportunist or pathogen) at a site. Carriage often follows disease, although acquisition can be silent or mitigated by vaccines or antimicrobials. Carriage and reinfection can reliably be separated only by molecular study. Carriage in blood ("agentemia") is nonshedding. Shedding is via droplets, saliva, sputum, tears, skin scales and eruptions, fistules, vomit, feces, urine, urethral and vaginal discharge, menstrual blood, lochia, semen, and breast milk (Box 14.2). Only viable and developed agents are immediately infective. How vaccines modify carriage is a neglected area of research, e.g., via systemic and mucosal immune responses.

Prevention (6, 2641, 5101, 5115, 6252). Spread can be prevented by health education, precautions, postexposure prophylaxis (PEP) (antibiotics, vaccines, immunoglobulin [Ig]), contact tracing, and possibly exclusion from school or work, and quarantine. Precautions (Table 14.1) include:

- Standard precautions by hand hygiene and protective equipment, e.g., gloves (see section 12.6).
- Airborne precaution (air isolation) is for highly infective patients, including aerosols from viral hemorrhagic fevers (see section 17.8), measles, severe acute respiratory syndrome (SARS), varicella, zoster (disseminated, or immune-impaired patient), and infective (sputum-positive) tuberculosis. Room is air tight, ventilated separately, ideally under negative air pressure, or with a high-efficiency particulate air filter.
- Droplet precaution is for patients likely shedding agents from respiratory secretions, e.g., adenovirus (AdV),

> **Box 14.2** Agents from carriers and contacts, by site
>
> Prevalence in high-income countries shown in parentheses.
>
> **Nose, mouth, and throat**
> - AdV, CMV, EBV, *Enterovirus*, HAV, HBV, HCV, HHV8, HIV, HSV1, *Influenzavirus*, MMR, PIV, PVB19, rabies virus, RSV, VZV
> - *B. pertussis*, *C. pneumoniae*, *C. diphtheriae* (<0.3%), *H. influenzae* (all strains, 10–75%), *K. kingae* (children up to 10%), *K. pneumoniae*, *M. pneumoniae*, *N. meningitidis* (1–25%), *P. aeruginosa* (0–3%), *S. aureus* (MSSA, 10–35%), *S. pneumoniae* (1–50%), *S. pyogenes* (GAS, 1–70%), viridans streptococci
> - *Candida* (20–70%, mainly hospital), *Pneumocystis*
>
> **Bowel**
> - AdV, ASTV, HAV, HEV, *Norovirus* (0.3–1%), *Rotavirus* (10%)
> - *C. difficile* (1–10%), *C. perfringens* (2–60%), *Enterococcus* (50%), *E. coli* (EHEC, 0–1%; EPEC, 0–20%), *H. pylori* (25–50%), *K. pneumoniae* (5–40%), *L. monocytogenes* (0.8%), *P. aeruginosa* (3–25%), *S. enterica* serovar Typhi (0.04–0.7%), *Shigella*, *Staphylococcus* (MSSA), *Streptococcus* (GBS, *S. bovis*, viridans)
> - *Candida* (30–50%)
> - *Cryptosporidium*, *Entamoeba*, *Giardia*
> - *Enterobius*, *Hymenolepis*, *Strongyloides*, *T. solium*
>
> **Skin and urogenital tract**
> - CMV (genital and colostrum), HAV (skin), HIV (genital), HPV (skin, genital: 5–25% of adults), HSV (HSV1 skin, HSV2 genital), polyomavirus (urine)
> - *Acinetobacter* (skin, 1–40%), *C. trachomatis* (ocular, genital: 0.5–13% of adults), *C. difficile* (vagina, 8–18%), *Enterococcus* (skin and genital), *M. genitalium* and *M. hominis* (genital: 1–50% of adults), *N. gonorrhoeae* (genitoanal: 0.1–0.4% of adults), *P. aeruginosa* (wet skin), *S. epidermidis* (skin), *Streptococcus* (GBS, vagina: 1–40%), *T. pallidum pallidum* (genital and skin), *U. urealyticum* (genital: 15–80% of adults)
> - *Candida* (15–20%), dermatophytes
> - *Trichomonas* (genital)

Influenzavirus, mumps virus, parvovirus B19 (PVB19), respiratory syncytial virus (RSV), rubella virus; *Bordetella pertussis* (cough disease), *Corynebacterium diphtheriae*, *H. influenzae* b, *N. meningitidis* (invasive disease), and *Streptococcus pyogenes* (group A Streptococcus [GAS]: pharyngitis, pneumonia, and scarlet fever). Patients are moved to access-restricted rooms. Patients, visitors, and workers can enter and leave only by appointment. Workers and visitors need face masks when close (1 m) to patents. Hands must be washed before and after patient contact.

- Contact precaution is for patients likely shedding agents from skin lesions, vomit, or feces. These include diarrhea agents (mainly in infants and incontinent adults): hepatitis A virus (HAV), *Enterovirus*, *Norovirus*, *Rotavirus*; *Clostridium difficile*, vancomycin-resistant *Enterococcus* (VRE), *Escherichia coli*, *Shigella*; *Giardia*; skin agents: herpes simplex virus (HSV) (neonates and mucocutaneous); methicillin-resistant *S. aureus* (MRSA), *Treponema pallidum* (skin lesions), *S. aureus* (impetigo), *S. pyogenes* (impetigo), varicella-zoster virus (VZV), (localized or disseminated); *Pediculus*, *Sarcoptes*; finally, object-born agents such as RSV. Movement restrictions and hand hygiene are the same as for droplet precaution. Instead of masks, emphasis is on gloves and gowns that are donned on entry into the patient's room. Gowns and equipment are dedicated, and left in the room. Excretions are disinfected for disposal.

In hospitals, precautions in addition to outpatient settings may apply (Table 14.1).

Cohorting (1565). Patients with the same illness are nursed together, in a designated area (room, ward section, or ward: patient cohorting) or by designated staff (nurse cohorting). Cohorting can be used to control spread of MRSA and to meet emergency demands, e.g., influenza outbreaks.

Quarantine (4307) (see glossary). SARS has provided the opportunity to evaluate quarantine. In Taiwan in 2003, of 131,132 persons quarantined, 133 (0.1%) were subsequently diagnosed with SARS. Reasons for quarantine (SARS attack rates) were: health work (0.3%, 6/1,751), patient home care (0.3%, 22/6,663), being close (≤3 m) to a patient (0.1%, 6/4,351), classmate and teacher in the same room with patient for ≥1 h (0.1%, 9/14,919), aircraft passenger close (≤3 rows) to patient (0.4%, 5/1,380), travel to area reporting SARS (0.03%, 21/80,813), passenger on bus or train carrying patient for ≥1 h and other likely exposures (0.3%, 64/21,255). Attack

Table 14.1 Infectivity for selected agents and precautions in ambulatory and hospitalized patients (HP), by site

Agent (type of infection)	Shedding	Secondary attack	Precautions[a]
Agents from respiratory secretions			
Adenovirus (pharyngeal)	While ill	Up to 55%	None. **HP:** Droplet and contact (children).
Bordetella pertussis	Weeks	10–70%	No school to $t_0 + 5$ days, consider vaccine and chemoprophylaxis. **HP:** Droplet
Cytomegalovirus	Weeks to years		None
Corynebacterium diphtheriae (pharyngeal)	Days to weeks		Refer. **HP:** Droplet, to two negative cultures
EBV (mononucleosis)	Months		None
Enterovirus	Up to 1 week	25–50%	None. **HP:** Contact
Haemophilus influenzae (invasive)	Days to weeks	0.5%	No school to $t_0 + 2$ days. **HP:** Droplet, to day $t_0 + 1$ day
Influenzavirus	Around illness	10–40%	No work to $d_0 + 2$ days. **HP:** Droplet or cohort
Measles virus	5–7 days	85%	No school to $d_0 + 5$ days. **HP:** Air isolation
Mumps virus	Up to 2 weeks	10–40%	No school to $d_0 + 5$ days. **HP:** Droplet, to $d_0 + 9$ days
Mycobacterium tuberculosis (infective)	Months	0.2–6%	Refer. **HP:** Air isolation, to clinical recovery or 3 negative cultures
Mycoplasma (pneumonia)	While ill	15–35%	None. **HP:** Droplet
Neisseria meningitidis (invasive)	Months	0.5–6%	Refer, chemoprophylaxis, consider vaccine if serogroups match. **HP:** Droplet
PIV (pseuocroup)	Weeks		None. **HP:** Children: droplet and contact
PVB19 (acute, chronic)	Days to years	45–50%	None. **HP:** Children: droplet, to $d_0 + 7$ days
RSV (bronchiolitis)	Days to weeks	15–30%	None. **HP:** Children: droplet and contact
Rubella virus	Up to 3 weeks		No health work to $d_0 + 7$ days. **HP:** Droplet, to $d_0 + 7$ days congenital rubella: contact, for 1 year
Pneumocystis (pneumonia)	Months		None
SARS-CoV (SARS)	Probably days	Up to 15%	Quarantine. **HP:** Droplet
Streptococcus pneumoniae	At least 1 month		None
Yersinia pestis (pulmonary)	While ill		Refer. **HP:** Droplet, to $t_0 + 3$ days
Agents from bowel			
Campylobacter (diarrhea)	Weeks	Low	Educate (handling of food and diapers)
Clostridium difficile (diarrhea)	Weeks to months		None. **HP:** Contact
Cryptosporidium (diarrhea)	Weeks to months	15–20%	Educate (handling of food and diapers)
Entamoeba histolytica (colitis)	Days to years	15–50%	Educate (food and sex)
Enterococcus	Lifelong	Unknown	None. **HP:** Contact, to negative culture
Escherichia coli (diarrhea)	EHEC: weeks	5–15%	Educate (handling of food and diapers). **HP:** Contact
Giardia (diarrhea)	Weeks to months		Educate (handling of food and diapers). **HP:** Contact
HAV (hepatitis A)	Weeks (months)	5–50%	Educate (handling of food and diapers); consider vaccine. **HP:** Contact
HEV (hepatitis E)	Probably weeks	<5%	None. **HP:** Contact
Norovirus	Days to 2 months	20–40%	Educate (handling of food and diapers). **HP:** Contact
Rotavirus	Weeks		Educate (handling of food and diapers). **HP:** Contact
Salmonella			
non-Typhi	Weeks		Educate (handling of food and diapers)
Typhi	Mostly weeks		Refer. **HP:** Contact to $t_0 + 2$ days
Shigella	Weeks to months	Up to 50%	Educate (handling of food and diapers). **HP:** Contact
Vibrio cholerae	Days		Educate (handling of food and diapers)
Yersinia enterocolitica	While ill	Low	Educate (handling of food and diapers). **HP:** Contact
Agents from the skin and urogenital tract			
Candida (mucosal, invasive)	Months		None
HIV (latent, AIDS)	Lifelong		None. **HP:** By opportunists, co-infections

(continued)

Table 14.1 (continued)

Agent (type of infection)	Shedding	Secondary attack	Precautions[a]
HPV (genital herpes)	Weeks to years		None
HSV (herpes, invasive)	Days to months	Low to 35%	None. **HP:** Contact
Pediculus (pediculosis)	Lifelong		None. **HP:** Contact, to $t_0 + 1$ day
Sarcoptes scabiei (scabies)	Years	Up to ~40%	No skin contact, to $t_0 + 1$ day. **HP:** same
Staphylococcus aureus (pyodermia)	Days		No skin contact, to $t_0 + 1$ day. **HP:** same
Streptococcus pyogenes			
(pyodermia)	Days		No skin contact to $t_0 + 1$ day
(pharyngitis)	Months		None. **HP:** Droplet to $t_0 + 1$ day
VZV			
(varicella)	Days -4 to $+5$	60–85%	No school, to crusts. **HP:** Air isolation
(zoster)	While lesions		No skin contact, to recovery. **HP:** If immune impaired: air isolation.

[a] *In addition* to standard precautions. HP, precautions for hospital patients; e_0, d_0, and t_0, first day of exposure, disease, or treatment, respectively.

rates were low among quarantined persons, and SARS-coronavirus (CoV) was detected by PCR in pharyngeal swabs from only 5 (7%) of 68 quarantined patients subsequently suspected of infection with SARS.

AGENTS FROM NOSE, MOUTH, AND THROAT

Flora (726, 5525). Over 40 bacterial species constitute oral flora, for densities up to 10^9/ml. Agents can be shed with droplets and saliva from the naso- and oropharynx. Saliva is of diagnostic interest, for demonstrating viruses by the nucleic acid amplification test (NAT) in infants or outbreaks and for genotyping. Nasopharyngeal washings are less reliable but easier to collect than swabs that need insertion through a nostril of the tilted head and guidance to the nasopharyngeal wall.

Viruses

Viruses demonstrated in saliva include cytomegalovirus (CMV), Epstein-Barr virus (EBV), hepatitis B virus (HBV), hepatitis C virus (HCV), human herpes virus 8 (HHV8), human immunodeficiency virus (HIV), herpes simplex virus 1 (HSV1), measles, mumps, and rubella viruses (MMR), VZV, as well as HAV and rabies virus.

Load and shedding over time suggest infectivity that is confirmed epidemiologically, e.g., by infections from kissing or spitting or from community or experimental studies. In viruses such as HAV and measles virus that induce long-lasting protective immunity (circulating and secretory Ig and cellular), shedding is typically limited to the acute phase of the disease, from late incubation to early reconvalescence.

AdV. AdV is shed from respiratory secretions (pharyngitis) or tears (conjunctivitis). Infectivity peaks around the first few days of acute illness.

CMV (77, 3835, 4554, 5109). Saliva is a significant source of CMV. Shedding can last weeks to many months in immune-competent individuals, and months to many years in untreated infected neonates or HIV-infected individuals. Children who acquired CMV in day care were shedding CMV in urine or saliva for ½–3½ (mean, 1½) years.

EBV (186, 3541). Saliva is a significant source of EBV. Inflammation of salivary glands or gingiva may reactivate or enhance shedding. EBV has been detected in oral brushings by PCR in 42% (24/57) of HIV-infected individuals, 65% (26/40) of renal transplant recipients, and 17% (5/30) of age-matched healthy controls. Persistent or intermittent shedding can go on for many months.

HBV (3490, 7716). HBV can be shed with saliva. In 27 patients with chronic HB, median HBV loads (RNA equivalents per milliliter) were 210,000 in serum and 22,700 in saliva. Bites by carriers and mucosal exposure can transmit HBV.

HCV (7271, 8156). Viremia in patients with chronic HC can persist for 25 years. A few infected individuals (<1%) seem able to carry the virus for the same period of time. HCV can be shed with saliva. In 26 anti-HCV-positive individuals, mean loads (RNA copies per milliliter) were 510,000 in serum, 31,000 in gingival fluid, and 19,000 in saliva. Aerosols from dental procedures at the gingiva (e.g., for periodontitis) are a potential source.

HHV8 (4554, 7376). HHV8 can be shed with saliva from immune-impaired persons. In Sweden, none of 15 controls, but 11% (5/44) of HIV-infected individuals excreted HHV8 in saliva. In prostitutes in Mombasa, Kenya, HHV8 was detected in 28% of oral swabs and 4% of cervical swabs, with higher yields in HIV1-positive (44% and 10%) than HIV1-negative (24% and 2%) individuals.

HIV (6874). HIV can be shed with saliva. In <10% of HIV-infected individuals, the load in saliva is higher than in blood. In these individuals, the buccal cavity is a possible site for HIV sequestration. Bites by latently infected individuals could transmit HIV.

HSV1 (7349). HSV1 is shed from primary and recurrent skin lesions and from saliva, including from inapparently infected individuals. Shedding is typically for a few weeks but can go on intermittently or persist. At an oral and maxillofacial surgery department in Japan, 4.7% of 1,000 outpatients were shedding HSV1 by PCR.

Influenzavirus. *Influenzavirus* is shed from respiratory secretions. Virus has been demonstrated in nasal secretions (usually for 7 days, longer in infants and immune-impaired patients). Infectivity peaks in the 24 h before onset of symptoms (d_0).

Measles virus (1382). Measles virus is shed from respiratory secretions. Virus has been demonstrated in saliva for at least 1 week. Patients are infective from 4 (typically 1–2) days before the onset of the rash (d_0) up to 4 days after d_0.

Mumps virus (5574). Mumps virus is shed from respiratory secretions. Virus can be demonstrated in saliva for a few days to ~2 weeks. Patients are infective from 7 (typically 1–2) days before the onset of parotitis (d_0) up to 4–5 days after d_0.

Enterovirus. *Enterovirus* can be shed from respiratory secretions. Infectivity is believed to last <7 days.

Parainfluenzavirus (PIV). PIV is shed from respiratory secretions. Children shed PIV from 1 week before d_0 to several weeks after d_0.

PVB19. PVB19 is shed from respiratory secretions. Patients with acute disease are infective before disease onset (d_0) and 0 (infectious erythema) to 7 (aplastic crisis) days after d_0. Immune-impaired patients with chronic infections can shed PVB19 for years.

RSV. RSV is shed from respiratory secretions, usually for 3–8 days, in infants for up to 4 weeks.

Rubella virus. Rubella virus is shed from respiratory secretions. Postnatal patients are believed to be infective from 13 (typically ≤7) days before onset of the rash (d_0) to up to 7 (typically 2) days after d_0.

VZV (1543, 7919, 8362). VZV is detected in skin lesions (typically for ~3 days), saliva (ophthalmic zoster, for up to 34 days), and the nasopharynx of immune but exposed persons. Immune-competent patients with varicella are infective from 4 (typically 1–2) days before onset of rash (d_0), to crusting of all lesions, that is ~7 days after d_0. Immune-impaired patients can be infective as long as florid lesions persist.

Bacteria

Respiratory secretions frequently grow commensals such as *Lactobacillus* and anaerobes. Opportunists in the nose, mouth, or throat include *Actinomyces* (in dental plaques, the "grass-in-the-mouth" source is obsolete) (6033), *Haemophilus parainfluenzae* (in the nasopharynx of 4% of children) (359), *Kingella kingae* (in the oropharynx of 10% of preschool children) (2332, 8306), *Klebsiella pneumoniae* (in the nasopharynx of 1–6% of people) (5948), *Moraxella catarrhalis* (in the pharynx of 30–70% of children and 1–10% of adults) (5803, 6785, 7775), and viridans streptococci (in the oropharynx).

***B. pertussis* (6666, 7087).** *B. pertussis* is shed with aerosolized droplets. By age, vaccine status, and antimicrobial treatment, patients shed the agent and can be infective from 2 weeks before the onset of cough (d_0), to 2–6 weeks after d_0. Waning immunity permits nasopharyngeal colonization, including during outbreaks.

***Chlamydophila pneumoniae* (699, 5481, 6684).** By test, reported population point prevalence of *C. pneumoniae* in the throat is 2–6% up to 23%.

***C. diphtheriae* (2322, 4104, 4982, 5968, 8196).** *C. diphtheriae* is shed from throat and skin lesions and from colonized individuals. By vaccine status and antimicrobial treatment, shedding is for <4 days to 6 weeks. *C. diphtheriae* is grown from the throat or nasopharynx of ≤0.06% to 0.3% of the population, in endemic pockets from up to 4%. At a sexual health clinic in the United Kingdom, 0.06% (1/1,696) of heterosexual attendees, and 0.3% (2/578) of homosexual men grew nontoxigenic *C. diphtheriae* from the throat. In urban Italy, none of 515 healthy adults yielded *C. diphtheriae* from the nasopharynx. In Germany in 1985–1986, *C. diphtheriae* was isolated from the throat or nasopharynx of 0.07% (2/3,993, both isolates nontoxigenic) of students and adults, but from 1% (46/4,751, 3 or 0.06% isolates toxigenic) asylum seekers.

***H. influenzae* (359, 794, 5803, 6112, 6156, 6785, 6812, 7775).** Carriage of *H. influenzae* is for weeks or months. Risks for carriage include young age, closed rooms (e.g., classroom), and an index case in the household. By age, vaccine status, and setting, point prevalence is 10–75% for all strains, and 0.5–10% for serogroup b (Hib) strains.

- America (2822). By age and vaccine status, 1–80% of children grow nonencapsulated strains, and <1–8% yield Hib. In the Dominican Republic, 8% (76/983) of periurban children had Hib in the nasopharynx: 1.5% at age 0–5 months, 12.5% at 6–11 months, 6% at 12–23 months, 8% at 24–35 months, and 10% at 36–47 months.
- Asia (359). In urban Turkey, 17% (51/300) of randomly selected children 7–12 years of age yielded *H. influenzae* from the nasopharynx, and 3% (9) yielded Hib.
- Europe (794, 5803, 6156). In The Netherlands in 1999, the nasopharynx of 37% (96/259) of children in day care, but 11% (30/276) of other children, was colonized by any strain, and 1.5% (4) and 0.4% (1), respectively, carried Hib (all five Hib carriers were vaccinated). In a French orphanage, the prevalence of non-b *H. influenzae* was 45%. In Catalonia, Spain, in 1996, the pharyngx of 26% (95% confidence interval [95% CI] 24–28%) of 1,212 school children (95% not vaccinated) grew *H. influenzae*; 25% of strains were nontypeable, 0.4% were Hib, and the remaining strains were e (0.5%), f (0.4%), and c (0.08%).

Person-to-person spread has not been well documented. Shedding is with respiratory secretions. Antimicrobials shorten shedding to 1–2 days.

Mycobacterium leprae (629, 3177). Patients with lepromatous leprosy can shed the agent with nasal secretions. In endemic areas, *M. leprae* is identified by NAT in nasal scrapings from 3–8% of healthy individuals.

Mycoplasma pneumoniae (3532). *M. pneumoniae* is spread by droplets, mainly during the incubation period. After recovery, the throat can remain colonized for several months. After an outbreak, oropharyngeal point prevalence in adults was 7–13%.

N. meningitidis (643, 5885, 6037, 7115). *N. meningitidis* is shed with respiratory secretions. Antimicrobials shorten shedding to 1–2 days. *N. meningitidis* colonizes the nasopharynx, on average for 9 months. About 3% of reconvalescent patients are carriers on leaving the hospital without chemoprophylaxis.

Besides invasive disease, risks for carriage include young age, large households (more than three members), and outbreaks. Pharyngeal, cutaneous, *and* conjunctival carriers of epidemic strains are infective. **Carriage prevalence (401, 1974, 5761, 5885, 6415).** By age and habitat, reported nasopharyngeal prevalence is 1–2% (preschool children) to 15–25% (adolescents), in endemic periods typically 10%. In British Columbia, Canada, in 2001, after a serogroup C outbreak, *N. meningitidis* was present in the pharynx of 8% (153/2,004; 95% CI 7–9) of vaccinees; only 4% (6/153) of the strains were C. In Turkey, 1% (17/1,382) healthy children 0–10 years of age carried *N. meningitidis*, including serogroups Y (53%, 9), B (29%, 5), and 6% (1) each A, D, and W-135.

S. aureus. *S. aureus* can be sensitive (MSSA) or resistant (MRSA) to methicillin.

- MSSA (18, 114, 726, 728, 1342, 1374, 1733, 2966, 3294, 4410, 6602, 7021, 8370) colonizes the nares and nasopharynx, temporarily also healthy skin (hands, axilla, umbilicus, groin, and perineum), irritated skin (>90% of patients with atopic dermatitis), wounds, exit sites (intravascular and bladder catheters), and stomata (tracheostoma). About 10–35% of the population are persistent carriers who almost always grow the agent, 20–75% are intermittent carriers, and 5–50% are refractory, almost never testing positive. In stable carriers, the elimination half-life is ~40 months. Colonization peaks at 10–11 years of age. Epidemiologically, particularly important adult carriers include farm workers, butchers, bakers, health workers, and the urban poor. In Kuwait, 27% of restaurant workers ($n = 500$) are nasal carriers, and 87% of *S. aureus* strains tested positive for enterotoxins. After outbreaks of staphylococcal scalded-skin syndrome in a maternity unit, 500 pregnant women attending an antenatal clinic were screened, and 164 (33%) carried *S aureus*: 100 (61%) in the nose, 41 (25%) at the perineum, 3 (2%) at the axillae, and 20 (12%) at multiple sites.
- MRSA (1374, 1770, 2966, 4410, 5323, 6521, 6549, 8370) accounts for a fraction of all *S. aureus*. In the population, 0.1–3% carry MRSA. In the United States in 1998–1999, 19% (54/291) healthy urban preschool children carried *S. aureus* in the nasopharynx, and 2% (5) carried MRSA. In central Italy in 2000–2001, 0.1% (1/812) of school children and routinely examined women carried MRSA in the nose. Household members who are hospital workers increase nasal community prevalence. Removing them in a metaanalysis reduced the carriage prevalence in the community from 1.3% to 0.2%. In hospitals, risks for MRSA colonization include advanced age, severe illness, interhospital transfer, extended length of stay, central venous catheters, and use of cephalosporins. In the United Kingdom, among a random sample of persons ≥65 years of age living in long-term stay facilities, 27% (257/962, 95% CI 24–30) were carriers of MSSA, and 0.8% (8/962, 95% CI 0.3–1.4) were carriers of MRSA. MRSA carriage was considered uncommon and mainly attributed to an ongoing hospital epidemic.

Streptococcus. **S. pneumoniae (726, 728, 1374, 4335, 4729, 4973, 5525, 5803, 5857).** *S. pneumoniae* is part of the nasopharyngeal flora. Colonization is established in the first month of life and may temporarily reach 100%. Risks include young age, belonging to a minority group, households with more than three members, older siblings, children in day care, or smokers, and a history (in the preceding 1–3 months) of acute otitis media, sinusitis, or antibiotics. A serotype is typically carried for ∼1 month and on occasion for 6–9 months. Carriage lasts longer in preschool children (∼2 months) than in schoolchildren and adults (2–3 weeks). More than one serotype can be carried at a time. Invasive disease seems most likely soon after a new serotype has been acquired and less likely in persistent carriers. By age and location, 10–50% of children and 1–20% of adults are carriers. In the United States in 1998–1999, 16% (47/291) of healthy, urban preschool children carried *S. pneumoniae* in the nasopharynx, and 6% (3) grew strains with intermediate sensitivity to penicillin. In 13 Italian cities in 2000, 9% (242/2,799) of healthy children in day care or elementary school carried *S. pneumoniae* in the nasopharyngx; frequent serotypes were 3 (12%), 19F (11%), 23F (11%), 19A (11%), 6B (10%), and 14 (7%). **S. pyogenes (GAS) (3652, 3813, 4773, 7171).** GAS colonizes the throat of healthy persons. By age and season, point prevalence is 1–70%, with a high (45–70%) in crowded children in winter, and a low (1–20%) in adults. In schoolchildren monitored for 4 years, the carriage prevalence was 4–26% (mean, 16%), and carriage of a particular type lasted 6 months to >2 years. Likewise, patients with GAS pharyngitis or scarlet fever can shed the agent for 1–12 (typically 2–3) months. Antimicrobials abolish shedding in 1–4 days.

FUNGI
Candida **(30, 2311, 2942, 4797, 5908, 7120, 7784).** Species of *Candida* colonize the oropharynx of immune-competent hosts, including *C. albicans* and *C. glabrata*. Colonization of the oropharynx by *C. albicans* builds up in the first month of life. By age (neonates and elderly) and test (culture and PCR), reported oral prevalence is 20–70% (extremes, 5–95%). In hospitals, the risk of person-to-person spread exists. Risks for nosocomial colonization and spread are mainly immune impairments (HIV infection, devices, extremes of age, diabetes, and neutropenia), but also interhospital transfer and dentures. Immune-impaired and colonized hosts are at risk of invasive disease.

Pneumocystis **(4082, 4798, 4945, 5206, 7298, 7527, 7904).** Before recognition of *P. jirovecii* as the species that infects humans and the main agent of *Pneumocystis* pneumonia (PCP), reports were confounded by zoonotic *P. carinii*, and human-to-human spread was uncertain. There is growing evidence that *P. jirovecii* is shed with respiratory secretions. Initially, HIV-infected individuals were shown to carry *P. jiroveci* inapparently for up to 9.5 months after PCP. Then, *P. jiroveci* DNA was amplified in oropharyngeal samples from healthy adults for up to 6 months. Now, by age, clinical material, and HIV status, *P. jirovecii* is detected by NAT in respiratory samples from 5 to 70% (often 20%) of individuals. However, as viability cannot be demonstrated by NAT, a reservation about human-to-human spread remains, in particular, for immune-competent individuals.

Protozoa
Free-living amebas (26, 436, 1393, 2837, 5030, 5129, 6902, 7844). Apparently 1–9% of healthy children and adults can carry free-living amebas such as *Hartmannella*, *Naegleria*, and *Acanthamoeba* in the naso- or oropharynx. A difficulty is to distinguish virulent from commensal species. Risks include previous water contact and granulomatous sinusitis.

AGENTS FROM THE BOWEL
Bacteria, yeast, and protozoa constitute the bulk of bowel biomass. Bacteria reach concentrations of up to 10^9/ml in the ileum and 10^{12}/g in the colon. Infective agents are mainly shed with vomit or watery or loose stools. For shedding food workers, see section 12.5.

Viruses
AdV (109, 7747). Enteric AdV is shed with feces. Children shed AdV for 1–14 (often 4) days, from 7 (mean, 3) days before d_0 to 11 (mean, 5) days after recovery. Infectivity seems to peak at about d_0.

Astrovirus (ASTV) (109, 1669, 5086). Immune-competent children with or without diarrhea can shed ASTV for 1–35 (often 4–8) days. Immune-impaired children can shed virus for many months.

HAV (4622, 4723). HAV is typically shed in the feces for less than 2 weeks, but it can be detected by NAT for 3 weeks to 3 months, in particular, in infants or outbreaks. HAV can also be demonstrated in saliva. Infectivity is greatest 1–2 weeks before illness onset (d_0) and is minimal by 1 week after d_0. In hospitals, standard precautions apply; for diapered infants and incontinent patients, contact precautions also apply.

Hepatitis E virus (HEV) (1476). HEV can be shed with feces for 2 weeks.

Norovirus **(109, 1848, 2594, 4764).** Carriers in the community exist, but their prevalence seems low, ∼0.3–1%. During a hospital outbreak, 26% of asymptomatic staff and 33% of asymptomatic patients tested positive by NAT (for a nonepidemic *Norovirus* strain). Virus is shed with vomit and stool, in stool typically for 1–56 (often 7–14) days. Patients are infective for at least 2–3 days after recovery. Related *Sapovirus* is shed for 1–15 days.

***Rotavirus* (208, 1302, 3059, 5196, 5902, 6138, 7091, 7959).** Disease caused by *Rotavirus* mainly affects children 6 months to 2 years of age. Immune-competent individuals typically shed virus in stools for ~1–10 days, with a range from 3–5 days before d_0 to 1–21 days after d_0. Impaired systemic or mucosal immune response can prolong shedding, up to at least 5 weeks. Children shed 10^{10}–10^{11} particles per g of feces, adults 10-to-100-fold less. Inapparent infections are reported in neonates, repeatedly infected children, and adults, for an approximate point prevalence of 10% in high-income countries and up to 15–35% in outbreaks and low-income countries. Carriage is not commonly discussed, but likely to occur, including in adults.

Bacteria

A bowel commensal is *Lactobacillus*. Bowel opportunists include *Bacteroides*, *Clostridium perfringens* (shed by ~2–60% of healthy persons) (7790), *Fusobacterium*, *K. pneumoniae* (in ~5–40% of samples) (5948), *Pseudomonas aeruginosa*, and *Streptococcus bovis* (in up to 12% of samples) (3990). Bowel opportunists can cause acute appendicitis, cholecystitis, bacterial liver abscess, and other endogenous infections.

Campylobacter. Human-to-human spread of *C. jejuni* is unusual. Untreated patients can shed the agent for 2–3 weeks from d_0.

***C. difficile* (435, 462, 2346, 5301, 6521, 6859, 7605).** *C. difficile* colonizes the intestinal tract of 5–70% of healthy neonates, 1–10% of healthy adults, and 10–30% of hospitalized adults. Risks for nosocomial colonization include advanced age, comorbidities, interhospital transfer, extended length of stay, use of antimicrobials (clindamycin and β-lactams), tube feeding, and gastrointestinal surgery. Colonization does not seem to increase risks of *C. difficile*-associated diarrhea (CDAD). Although neonates carry *C. difficile* more frequently than adults, neonates less frequently develop CDAD, perhaps because toxins cannot attach to neonatal mucosa, or because neonates are protected by maternal antibodies. In Sweden, breast-fed infants were less often colonized than bottle-fed infants: 21% versus 47% at age 6 weeks, and 19% versus 39% at age 6 months.

***Enterococcus* (374, 1986, 2604, 4185, 6521, 6898, 7712, 8178).** Molecular epidemiology confirms person-to-person, vehicle-to-person, and animal-to-person spread of *Enterococcus* in the community, hospitals, and nursing homes. By use of antimicrobials and hospitalizations, ~50% of people carry *Enterococcus*, and 2–10% carry vancomycin-resistant *E. faecalis* or *E. faecium* (VRE). Hospital patients, nursing home residents, and healthy persons, even livestock can carry VRE. Risks for nosocomial colonization with VRE include advanced age, comorbidities, interhospital transfer, extended length of stay, and treatment with fluoroquinolones. Carriage can last months or years. During a prolonged outbreak in Massachusetts in 1993–1995, 253 patients were colonized or infected with VRE; of 49 patients monitored, 34 (70%) continued to yield VRE for 19–303 days.

***E. coli* (4359, 4799, 5493, 5529, 6900).** *E. coli* is part of the bowel flora and a reservoir of antimicrobial resistance. From birth, the prevalence of "residential" *E. coli* builds up to virtually 100%. However, most diarrheagenic *E. coli* seems acquired rather than endogenous. Among randomly selected long-term care residents, 51% (25/49) shed fluoroquinolone-resisant *E. coli*; of colonized residents, 73% (16/22) shed resistant agents for 2–20 (median, 5) months, and of noncolonized residents, 30% (7/23) acquired resistant agents after 1–8 (median, 6) months. Enterohemorrhagic *E. coli* (EHEC) and enteropathogenic *E. coli* (EPEC) readily spread person-to-person. Although carriage of EHEC is unusual, children and patients with diarrhea can shed EHEC for a few days to 14 weeks, typically for 2–3 weeks. Shedding of enterotoxigenic *E. coli* (ETEC) is shorter, typically <1 week. Patients can be infective for the entire period of shedding.

***Helicobacter* (697, 923, 1609, 2073, 4684).** Some 50% of the world population are *H. pylori* carriers, 70–90% of adults in low-income countries and 25–50% of adults in high-income countries. Carriage persists for years or life, but infections can be cleared (by treatment or spontaneously) at a rate of 0.1–1.8/100 per year.

***Listeria* (3803, 5249).** Of 2,000 fecal samples from healthy persons, 0.8% grew *L. monocytogenes*, and 2% grew *L. innocua*. Carriage is unusual, but two colonized healthy adults shed *L. monocytogenes* in stools for 1.5 to >2 years.

***Pseudomonas* (690, 2685, 4871, 7948).** *P. aeruginosa* is part of mucosal flora. Of healthy adults and patients on hospital admission, 0–3% grow *P. aeruginosa* from nasal mucosa and 3–24% grow from feces. Of 628 hospitalized patients, 7.6% were colonized on admission, and 1.7% of 580 initially uninfected patients acquired the agent nosocomially on follow-up. Of patients with cystic fibrosis, up to 50–80% can be carriers (persistently colonized).

Salmonella. Non-Typhi *Salmonella enterica* (959). Non-Typhi serovars are typically shed for ≤4–12 weeks. However, 45% of infants and 5% of children and adults still shed 3 months from d_0, and 1% shed after 1 year. Antimicrobials prolong rather than shorten carriage. Patients are likely infective during the entire period of shedding. ***Salmonella enterica* serovar Typhi** (3430, 4372, 4748, 5220, 7681). Patients with typhoid fever can shed *S. enterica* serovar Typhi from ~2 weeks before d_0 (poorly defined), to ~4 weeks after d_0. Some 2–4% of typhoid patients shed serovar Typhi for >3 months, eventually for life. Well-known shedders and sources of typhoid are "typhoid Mary," and "milker N." In endemic areas, the population prevalence of serovar Typhi carriers is 0.04–0.7%.

Shigella (3437, 4373, 6538). *Shigella* carriage for >1 year is rare but exists. Carrier prevalence reported for low-income countries is 0.8–6.4%. Without treatment, patients shed *Shigella* for 1 day to 2–3 months, often 4 weeks. Patients are infective during the entire period of shedding.

Vibrio. V. cholerae (2340, 7667, 8088). By age and season, the fecal point prevalence of *V. cholerae* in endemic areas is 0.02–20% (typically <1%). Carriage is uncommon, except for HIV-infected adults who can shed the *V. cholerae* for months, and carriers can bring the agent to uninfected areas. Cholera patients shed *V. cholerae* for 5–7 or more days. ***V. parahaemolyticus*** (2808, 8387). In Japan in 1962, 16 (0.8%) of 2,000 healthy hotel employees shed *V. parahaemolyticus*. Carriage does not seem to occur, however. In Singapore in 1977–1980, 23 (79%) of 29 persons cleared their infection in a few days, and 6 (21%) cleared it in 10–21 days.

Yersinia (5650, 6009). For both *Y. enterocolitica* and *Y. pseudotuberculosis*, shedding beyond reconvalescence appears to be rare.

Fungi
Candida (2134, 2311, 2456, 4101). *Candida* can colonize the bowel of healthy children and adults, for a point prevalence of up to 30–50%. Risks in children include use of antimicrobials and coinfection with enteric pathogens, but there is neither evidence for *Candida* overgrowth from antibiotics nor of *Candida*-associated diarrhea.

Protozoa
Enteric protozoa shed with feces include *Cryptosporidium*, *Cyclospora*, *Dientamoeba*, *Entamoeba*, and *Giardia*, infrequently (in <1%) also *Balantidium*, *Isospora*, and *Sarcocystis*. Infectivity upon shedding is largely limited to *Cryptosporidium*, *Entamoeba*, and *Giardia*.

Cryptosporidium (7136). Children can shed *C. hominis* oocysts for 1–7 weeks or longer. HIV-infected individuals can shed oocysts for months.

Entamoeba (702, 2661, 6147). For evaluation of infectivity, differentiation of *E. histolytica/dispar* is crucial, in particular, in food and health workers. Humans can carry *E. histolytica* cysts for at least 1 year. In Vietnam, the shedding half-life in 43 carriers of *E. histolytica* monitored by PCR was 10–16 months. In endemic areas, continued exposure and reinfection often outweigh the benefits of treatment. In high-income countries, confirmed carriers are recommended treatment to prevent spread and subsequent invasive disease.

Giardia (4655, 5904). Patients with chronic diarrhea or malabsorption can shed *G. lamblia* for weeks or months. Inapparent infections seem to persist for 3–12 or more months.

Helminths
Worm eggs, larvae, proglottids, or juveniles can appear in feces, including of the nematodes *Ascaris*, *Ancylostoma*, *Enterobius*, *Strongyloides*, and *Trichuris*, the cestodes *Hymenolepis* and *Taenia*, and the trematodes *Clonorchis*, *Fasciola*, and *Schistosoma*. However, immediate infectivity upon shedding is limited to *Enterobius vermicularis* (typical prevalence, 5–20%), *Hymenolepis nana* (typical prevalence, 0.5–3%), and *Strongyloides stercoralis* (typical prevalence, 2–10%). Untreated, all three worms are often maintained by reinfection (see chapter 20).

Taenia solium (1091, 2440, 2621, 4737, 5407, 5474, 6003, 6086, 7938). Unlike *T. saginata*, eggs of *T. solium* from carriers are the source for cysticercosis in 5–40% of carriers themselves (through regurgitation or external autoinfection), as well as in their environment (households and catering facilities). The prevalence of *T. solium* carriage in enzootic areas is 0.1–38%, typically 1%. Untreated, carriage can continue for 10 or more years.

AGENTS FROM SKIN
Flora. Skin harbors residential (propagating) and temporary (nonpropagating) flora transferred from hands, skin and surface contacts, and droplets. Healthy residential flora antagonizes temporary flora. Skin grows bacteria at densities up to 10^3–10^5/cm^2. Skin flora is a potential source of skin (pyoderma), wound, and surgical site infection (SSI) and of contaminated blood cultures. Skin sheds agents from squames, lesions (e.g., vesicles), fistules, and draining wounds.

Viruses
Infective skin lesions include warts for human papillomavirus (HPV) and vesicles for labial herpes (HSV1) and

varicella-zoster virus (VZV). Infective anogenital lesions include genital herpes (for HSV2), and genital warts (for HPV).

Transient viruses on skin and mucosa include HAV, RSV, PIV, and VZV, resident viruses include HPV, HSV1, and HSV2. Transmission from lesions or inapparent skin is by skin or sexual contacts. For sexually transmitted infection (STI) in the community, see section 14.7; for prostitutes, see section 13.6; for homosexual men, see section 13.7.

Bacteria
Residential bacteria on the skin include *Corynebacterium minutissimum* (moist skin), *Micrococcus*, *Propionibacterium*, and coagulase-negative staphylococci (CoNS, *S. epidermidis*). Acidic pH promotes residential bacteria and prevents colonization by temporary bacteria.

Temporary bacteria on skin include *Acinetobacter* (in 1–40% of people, for days to weeks) (589, 7740), *Pseudomonas* (in moist interdigital spaces), and *S. aureus*.

C. diphtheriae **(1789, 4053).** Cutaneous diphtheria is infective and contributes to the bacterial reservoir. In the rural United States, two patients with impetigo-like lesions that grew *C. diphtheriae* were the source for 10 (19%) pharyngeal colonizations in 52 classroom contacts.

S. aureus. *S. aureus* can temporarily colonize the hands of nasal, vaginal, or rectal carriers. Colonized hands are of concern in health care (see section 17.1), and for the spread of staphylococcal impetigo. Contact precaution may apply for 24 h after treatment onset (t_0), unless lesions can be covered.

***S. pyogenes* (GAS).** *S. pyogenes* (GAS) on the skin is usually associated with disease such as cellulitis, erysipelas, or fasciitis. Contact precaution may apply for 24 h after t_0, unless lesions can be covered.

Fungi
Residential fungi of the skin include *Candida*, dermatophytes, and *Malassezia* (in close to 100% of adults) (6733).

Candida **(29, 1914, 4637).** *C. albicans*, *C. tropicalis*, and other species can colonize skin, nails, and hair, in Egypt in 13% of children. Risks for colonization include corticosteroids, diabetes, HIV infection, and perhaps use of antimicrobials. Human-to-human spread seems to occur at least occasionally.

Dermatophytes. Humans can be carriers of anthropophilic dermatophytes. Human-to-human spread is by contact with hair or skin.

- Tinea capitis (148, 585, 1670, 2526, 4637). Main agents are *Trichophyton* and *Microsporum*. By location and test (culture from hair brush), reported carrier prevalence is 0.2–2.5% in South America, Southwest Asia, and Europe, 3–4% in North Africa, and up to 50% in southern Africa where *T. violaceum* is endemic.
- Tinea pedis, onychomycosis (3557). In Italy, the prevalence of culture-confirmed carriage in adults is ~3%.

Protozoa
Although *Leishmania* skin lesions are not directly infective, humans constitute the only vertebrate reservoir for anthroponotic cutaneous leishmaniasis (CL), principally through mild, untreated, persistent infections. Also, for zoonotic CL, an infection that persisted for decades has been reported (2988).

Ectoparasites
Patients with pediculosis and scabies are infectious from the incubation period and indefinitely after d_0 (see section 4.6). Standard and contact precautions apply until 24 h after t_0. For *Pediculus humanus capitis*, treatment covers scalp hair, combs and brushes, head covers (hat or turban), scarfs, pillow linen, and close contacts. For *Pediculus humanus corporis*, treatment covers clothes, blankets, linen, and close contacts.

AGENTS FROM THE UROGENITAL TRACT
Usual bacterial counts are 10^2–10^4/ml in first-void, midstream urine, and 10^5–10^9/ml in vaginal secretions. Residential commensal flora is protective; residential opportunistic flora and temporary flora can lead to endogenous infections, including pelvic inflammatory disease, and prostatitis. Agents can be shed with urine, urethral and vaginal discharge, menstrual blood, lochia, and semen. In particular, HBV and HCV are demonstrated in vaginal secretions. For STI in the community, see section 14.7; for prostitutes, see section 13.6; for homosexual men, see section 13.7.

Viruses
EBV (1628, 3586, 6943, 7701). EBV has been detected in urethral discharge of men and cervical secretions of women, and there is evidence for sexual spread, including among homosexual men. In The Netherlands, 95% (81/85) of HIV-positive men who have sex with men (MSM), 80% (90/113) of HIV-negative MSM, and 82% (93/114) of HIV-negative heterosexual men amplified EBV from blood lymphocytes, and 67%, 39%, and 6% in the respective groups were seroreactive.

CMV (1918, 5109, 6839). Following primary infection, CMV can be shed with urine for weeks or months. In women in Taiwan, shedding increased during pregnancy, in cervical swab by PCR from 13% to 40% and in urine from 1% to 13%. In Taiwan in 1992–1993, of 63 immunologically competent kindergarten children monitored for 1 year; none of 33 seronegative but 27 of 30 reactive children were shedding CMV, either continuously (13) or intermittently (14). CMV is also shed with semen and breast milk.

GB virus C (GBV-C, "hepatitis G virus") (2522). Evidence exists for sexual spread of GBV-C.

HCV (1982, 7444). There is evidence for occasional sexual spread of HCV. Risks increase with the number of lifetime sex partners, HIV, or *Trichomonas* coinfection, and sex among men.

HIV (2396, 3709, 4081, 6056, 7804). HIV1 is shed in the genital tract. RNA load in plasma can predict genital shedding; transmission seems infrequent if plasma yields <1,500 copies/ml, although genital shedding has been demonstrated in women with <500 copies/ml in plasma.

HPV (1122, 5222, 5684, 5997, 6863, 8166, 8260). Latently infected adults (males and females) can shed HPV genitally. By sexual activity, location, and test, latent genital infections and shedding are detected in 5–25% of adults. Low-risk and oncogenic types are amplified in genital samples from shedding adults. Reported infection rates in sexually active young adult females are 13–17/100 per year. Condoms are likely to protect from genital warts and are recommended for nonmonogamous sex.

HSV (3163, 3194, 5748, 5974, 6512, 6650, 7907). Latently infected adults can shed HSV2 intermittently for months or years. In the placebo arm of a controlled trial, 38 (66%) of 58 infected females shed HSV at least once in 112 days. Men with a history of genital herpes ($n = 68$) or without a history but seroreactive ($n = 11$) self-obtained daily cultures; HSV2 was shed during 343 (5%) of 6,806 culture-days, in 210 (61%) days with recurrent genital herpes, and in 133 (39%) inapparent days. Of note, HIV-infected men and women could shed HSV2 not only genitally but also anally.

Reported seroprevalence varies considerably. In Japan, 2% of male blood donors ($n = 41$) and 14% of pregnant women ($n = 290$) were reactive. In Bangladesh, 6% (8/134) of married nonpregnant women 15–50 years of age and 6% (10/178) of men of the same age were reactive. In Italy, the HSV2 seroprevalence in a national sample of 1,169 healthy men was 0.1%.

***Polyomavirus* (2189, 5962).** Children and adults shed BK polyomavirus (BKV) and JC polyomavirus (JCV) from urine. A reported point prevalence for JCV shedding is 5%.

Bacteria

A commensal is *Lactobacillus*, which is supported by acidic pH. Likely opportunists include *Bacteroides fragilis* (carried by 7% of pregnant women) (4360), *C. difficile* (in 8–18% of women) (7286), *C. perfringens* (in 1–10% of women) (3100), mycoplasms, and ureaplasms.

***Chlamydia trachomatis*.** **Lymphogranuloma (serovars L1–3).** A carrier state is not reported. **Genital (serovars D–K) (5827, 5991, 6735, 7529).** By age, material (urine, cervix), test (NAT and antigen), sex, and location (low or high income), reported genital prevalence is 0.5–13%.

- High-income countries (1981, 2133, 2355, 5004, 7617, 7753). In representative samples and with sensitive tests, genital carriage prevalence of 1–7% among males and 1–5% among females was found. In a 1997–1998 Baltimore probability sample of 579 persons 18–35 years of age, the prevalence of untreated genital infection by NAT from urine was 1.6% in males and 4.3% in females. In a 1999–2001 United Kingdom survey, the prevalence by NAT from urine was 2.2% (95% CI 1.5–3.2) in males ($n = 1,474$) and 1.5% (95% CI 1.1–2.1) in females ($n = 2,055$). In The Netherlands, by NAT from home-obtained urine mailed to the family physician, 2% (42/1,809) of asymptomatic men and 3% (79/2,751) of asymptomatic women tested positive. In Sweden in 1985–1995, of 103,870 cervical samples from women 15–39 years of age, 5.4% (5,648) tested positive.

- Low-income countries (2423, 2699, 3194, 4802, 5764, 7983, 8174). Reported carriage prevalence is 0.5–4% (median, 2%) in males, and 0.5–13 % (median, 4%) in females. High prevalence was reported in South Africa among pregnant women (13%, $n = 6,948$) and in Haiti among women attending antenatal services (11%, $n = 476$). In contrast, prevalence by NAT from urine was low in rural Bangladesh, 0.5% (4/753) in nonpregnant women 15–50 years of age and 0.5% (3/607) in men (married or unmarried) of the same age.

***Haemophilus ducreyi* (3195, 4145).** Inapparent *H. ducreyi* infections have been documented by NAT in prostitutes in West Africa, but seem very rare in men.

***Klebsiella* (ex-*Calymmatobacterium*) *granulomatis*.** Although humans are the only reservoir for *K. granulomatis* carriage has not been reported.

Mycoplasms. Mycoplasms can colonize the genital tract of males and females. By material, test, and gender, the reported carriage prevalence is:

- 1–20% for *M. genitalium* (1113, 3870, 4168, 4980, 5827, 7529, 7600)
- 5–50% for *M. hominis* (2193, 3870, 7381)

- 15–80% for *Ureaplasma urealyticum* (1972, 3870, 4450, 5827, 5991).

Neisseria gonorrhoeae. Carriage exists.

- High-income countries (2699, 6735, 7617). The reported carriage prevalence at reproductive age is ∼0.4% in females and ∼0.1% in males. In Baltimore, Md. in 1997–1998, in a probability sample of 579 persons 18–35 years of age, the weighted infection prevalence by ligase chain reaction (LCR) from urine was 6.7% in females and 3.8% in males. In Birmingham, Ala., in 2001, the prevalence by LCR in asymptomatic males attending an STI clinic was 3% (5/145).

- Low-income countries (2423, 2699, 3194, 4950, 5764, 5827, 6489, 7983, 8174). Reported carrier prevalence ranges broadly, with medians of 0.4% in females and 0.1% in males. In women attending antenatal or family-planning services, prevalence is typically 1–8%. In men in West Africa and Southeast Asia, reported carriage prevalence is ∼5%.

***Streptococcus agalactiae* (group B *Streptococcus* [GBS]) (5019, 6702).** The prevalence of vaginal or rectal carriage is 30–40% in sexually active women, and 10–30% in pregnant women at about the time of delivery. GBS carriage can be transient, intermittent, or chronic.

***T. pallidum pallidum* (2423, 2699, 4950, 6489, 6917, 7983, 8174).** Primary, secondary, and early latent syphilis stages are infective, mainly via sex. Shedding has been poorly documented. In high-income countries, the seroprevalence in adults is ∼0.5%. In low-income countries, where nonvenereal *Treponema* interferes with syphilis serology, overall seroprevalence in adults are perhaps 0.5–0.6%, although in the 1980s and 1990s, an average seroprevalence of 7–12% was reported in healthy men and women.

Fungi
***Candida* (2780, 4797, 4819, 6682, 7895).** *C. albicans*, *C. glabrata*, *C. tropicalis*, and other species can colonize the vagina. A suspected, but unconfirmed risk is antibiotic treatment. By age and sample, the reported vaginal prevalence is 15–20%. In pregnancy, the risk of vulvovaginitis is 8% in noncolonized women, but 25% in colonized. Mother-to-child spread can occur.

Protozoa
***Trichomonas vaginalis* (4110).** Untreated infections in men can persist inapparently for ≥4 months. Men clear about one third of newly acquired infections spontaneously. For STI in the community see section 14.7.

14.2 AGE

Age groups are preschool children (0–4.9 years, with neonates of 0–4 weeks and infants of 1–11.9 months), school children (5–14 years), adults (15–64 years; adolescents, 15–19 years; and reproductive age, 15–50 years), and elderly (≥65 years).

Of the world population, ∼10% are preschool age, 20% are school age, 63% are adults, and 7% are elderly. The world population was 6 billion in 2000, growing to 6.3 billion in 2004, for annual growth rates of 1% (73 million), from annual birth rates of ∼2% (130 million live births) minus annual death rates of ∼1% (57 million).

Infections (Box 14.3). Although confounded by age-characteristic exposures, age significantly modifies susceptibility and disease expression (e.g., HBV and *Rotavirus*). By exposure and immunity, infection or disease rates can peak in one or more age groups. **Peak in one age group.** Unimodal peaks are explained by primary infections that leave life-long protection and cause protective immune

Box 14.3 Age peaks of agents or infections in well-vaccinated communities, by agent cluster

	Preschool age	School age	Adults	Elderly
Droplet-air	AdV, influenza, PIV, RSV, N. meningitidis, S. pneumoniae	PVB19, M. pneumoniae	AdV, EBV, rubella virus, N. meningitidis, M. tuberculosis	Influenza, B. pertussis, Legionella, M. tuberculosis, S. pneumoniae
Feces-food	HAV, enteric bacteria, infant botulism	Ascaris, Trichuris	HAV	C. difficile, Listeria, S. stercoralis
Zoonotic	Plasmodium		Arboviruses, Coxiella, Plasmodium	
Environmental			Leptospira, hookworm	C. tetani
Skin-blood	CMV, HBV, molluscum, S. aureus bacteremia, Candida, Enterobius	GAS pharyngitis, tinea capitis	CMV, HBV, HCV, HIV, bacterial STI, tinea pedis, Sarcoptes	Classical CJD, zoster, S. aureus bacteremia, onychomycosis, Candida, Pediculus

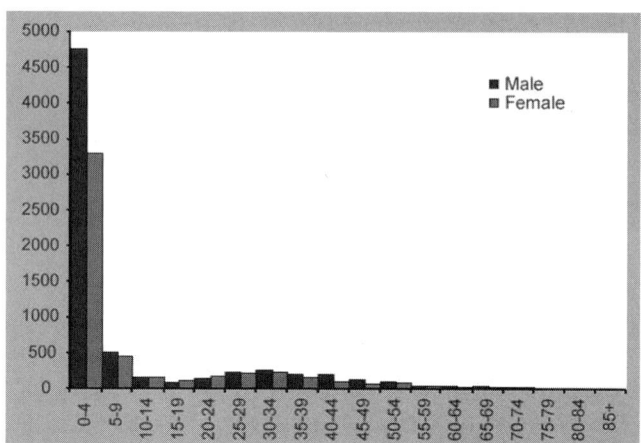

Figure 14.1 Laboratory reports of adenovirus infections, Australia 1991–2000 ($n = 13,924$). Reports (y axis) are given by age groups (x axis, in years) and sex (females, light; males, dark). From reference 6350. Copyright by Commonwealth of Australia. Reproduced with permission.

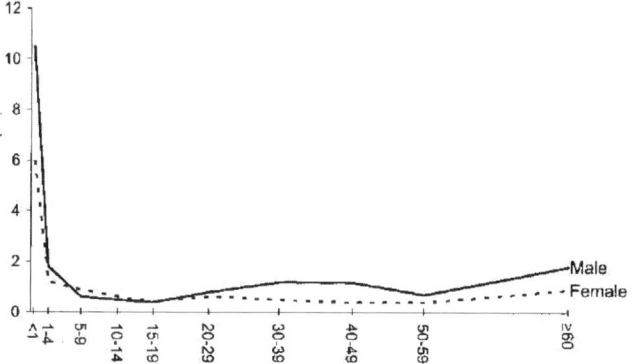

Figure 14.2 Invasive *Salmonella* disease reported by FoodNet, United States, 1996–1999, ($n = 540$, mainly serovar Typhimurium). Rate is given per 10^5 (y axis), by age group (x axis, in years), and sex (males, line; females, dots). From reference 7881.

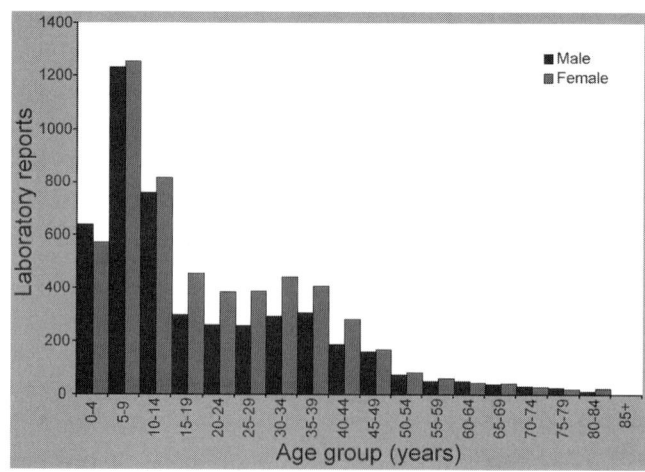

Figure 14.3 Laboratory reports of *Mycoplasma pneumoniae*, Australia 1991–2000 ($n = 10,620$). Reports (y axis) are given by age groups (x axis, in years) and sex (females, light; males, dark). From reference 6350. Copyright by Commonwealth of Australia. Reproduced with permission.

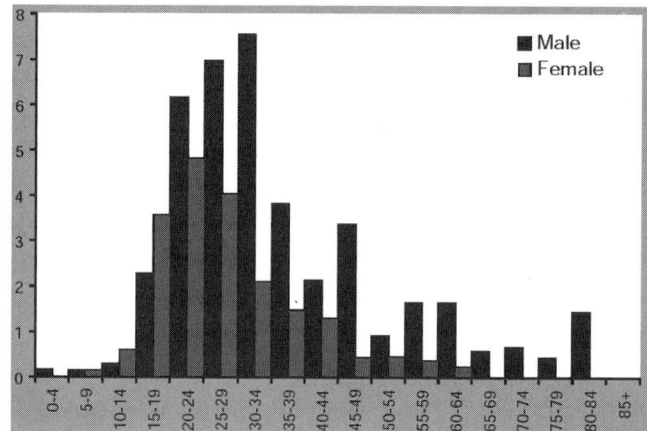

Figure 14.4 Incident hepatitis B reports, Australia, 2002 ($n = 400$). Rate per 10^5 (y axis, overall 2) is given by age groups (x axis, in years) and sex (females, light; males, dark). From reference 8342. Copyright by Commonwealth of Australia. Reproduced with permission.

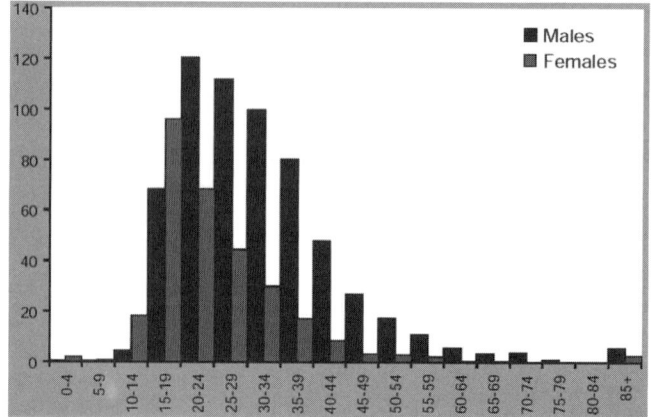

Figure 14.5 Gonococcal infection reports, Australia, 2002 ($n = 6,247$). Rate per 10^5 (y axis, overall 32) is given by age groups (x axis, in years) and sex (females, light; males, dark). From reference 8342. Copyright by Commonwealth of Australia. Reproduced with permission.

responses (e.g., neutralizing antibodies) to accumalate with age. The time of primary infection depends on exposure at home, school, or work or leisure places.

- Peak at preschool age. Examples are congenital infections and some vaccine-preventable infections, e.g., measles (peak at age 6–9 months in low-income settings) (3804, 6042), poliomyelitis, HAV infections, and invasive Hib disease. Other examples are RSV infections, AdV infections (Fig. 14.1), and invasive *Salmonella* disease (Fig. 14.2).
- Peak at school age. By exposure and endemicity, examples are mumps, varicella, rubella (1781), diphtheria, *M. pneumoniae* (Fig. 14.3), and enteric helminths.
- Peak in adolescents. Again, by exposure and endemicity, examples are acute HB (Fig. 14.4), HCV infections (injection drug users [IDU]), STI such as primary genital HPV infection and gonorrhea (Fig. 14.5), and rubella (Fig. 14.6).

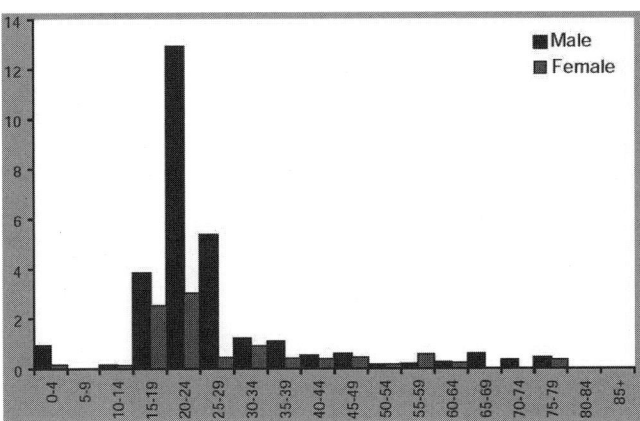

Figure 14.6 Rubella reports, Australia, 2002 ($n = 254$). Rate per 10^5 (y axis, overall 1.3) is given by age groups (x axis, in years) and sex (females, light; males, dark). Reports included 56 cases in women of child-bearing age (15–49 years). From reference 8342. Copyright by Commonwealth of Australia. Reproduced with permission.

- Peak in elderly. Examples are *Legionella* pneumonia (Figure 14.7) (8342) and neuroinvasive West Nile virus disease (Fig. 20.2) (3206). Some peaks in the elderly are explained by waining immune memory and vigor. Rates of human granulocytic ehrlichiosis (HGE, by *Anaplasma phagocytophilum*) and human monocytic ehrlichiosis (HME, by *Ehrlichia chaffeensis*) increase with age, with peaks at 60–69 years or ≥70 years, respectively (1872). **Peaks in two age groups.** Explanations for bimodal age peaks include continued exposure, reinfection because immunity is short-lived or nonprotective, latent infection that is reactivated (see section 14.6), and cohorts (transmission or susceptibility that changes from one generation or birth year to another).

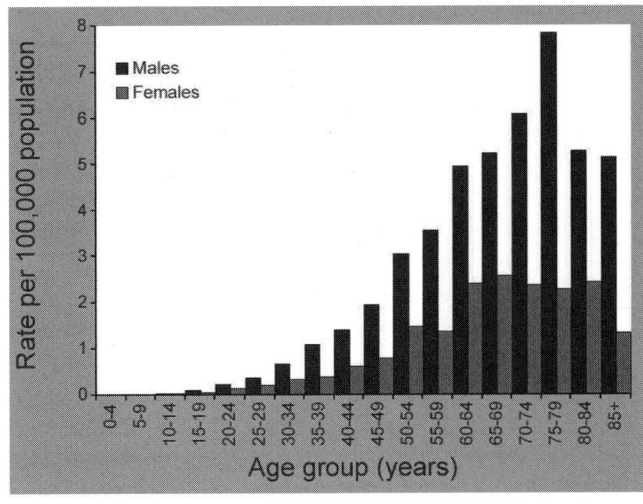

Figure 14.7 *Legionella* infection reports, Australia, 2002 ($n = 318$). Rate per 10^5 (y axis, overall 1.6) is given by age groups (x axis, in years) and sex (females, light; males, dark). From reference 8342. Copyright by Commonwealth of Australia. Reproduced with permission.

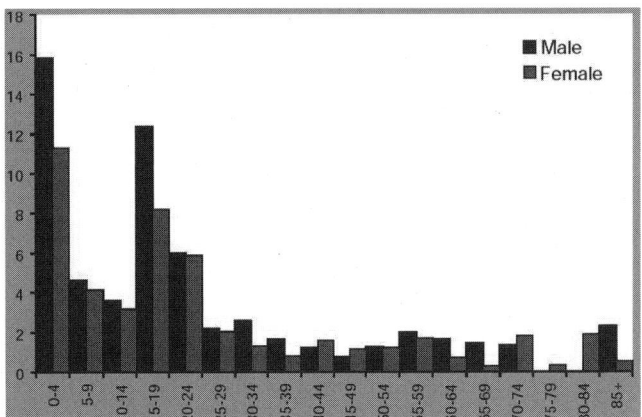

Figure 14.8 Invasive meningococcal disease reports, Australia, 2002 ($n = 684$, 53% B, 39% C). Rate per 10^5 (y axis, overall 3.5) is given by age groups (x axis, in years) and sex (females, light; males, dark). Age-specific rates were highest at age 0–4 years ($13.6/10^5$) and 15–19 years ($10.3/10^5$). From reference 8342. Copyright by Commonwealth of Australia. Reproduced with permission.

- First peak at preschool age that is followed by a second peak: either in adolescents, e.g., invasive meningococcal disease (Fig. 14.8), in adults, e.g., CMV infection (Fig. 14.9) and *G. lamblia* infection (3423), or in elderly, e.g., influenza (Fig. 14.10), invasive pneumococcal disease (Fig. 14.11), and some nosocomial infections such as candidemia (Fig. 20.1) (5892).
- First peak in adults that is followed by a second peak in elderly. The classical example is active and reactivated tuberculosis (Fig. 14.12).

PRESCHOOL AGE (0–4.9 YEARS)

Exposure (726, 5493) begins during pregnancy, extends to birth, and continues for life. Colonization of skin and

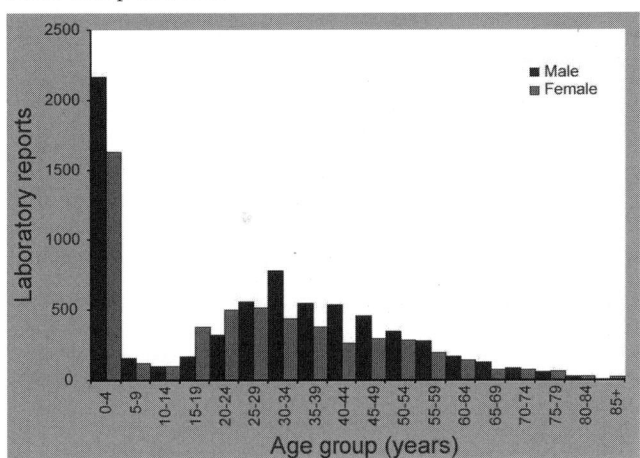

Figure 14.9 Laboratory reports of cytomegalovirus infections, Australia 1991–2000 ($n = 13,928$). Reports (y axis) are given by age groups (x axis, in years) and sex (females, light; males, dark). From reference 6350. Copyright by Commonwealth of Australia. Reproduced with permission.

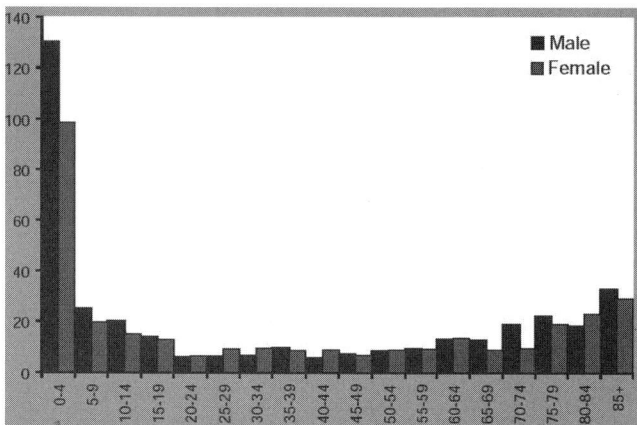

Figure 14.10 Laboratory confirmed influenza reports, Australia, 2002 ($n = 3{,}665$, 99% A/H3N2). Rate per 10^5 (y axis, overall 18.6) is given by age groups (x axis, in years) and sex (females, light; males, dark). From reference 8342. Copyright by Commonwealth of Australia. Reproduced with permission.

mucosa with "normal" flora begins at birth and is established in the first month to year of life. Maternal antibodies in cord blood and breast milk contribute to protect neonates from invasive diseases. Once weaned, and when Ig is washed out, infants are susceptible to exposure from foods, siblings, animals, and the environment. High infectious disease rates in preschool children point to ongoing disease transmission. Timely vaccines help to close a "window of vulnerability" that is open at age 3–24 months.

Impact (955, 4256). Of the world population, >10% (>600 million) are preschool children, for a low of 5% in Europe and a high of 16% in Africa. About 10–11 million preschool children die each year, including 4 million

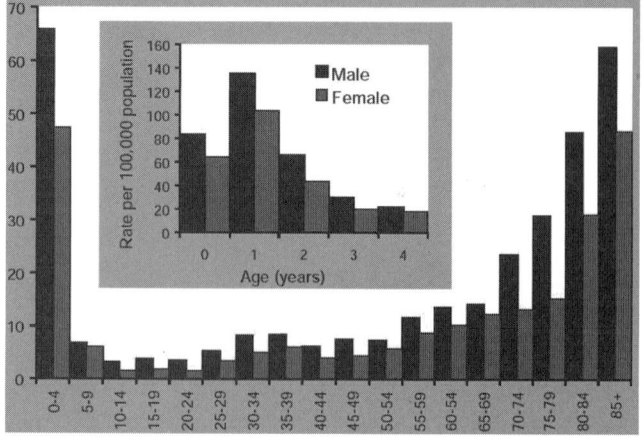

Figure 14.11 Invasive pneumococcal disease reports, Australia, 2002 ($n = 2{,}271$). Rate per 10^5 (y axis, overall 11.5) is given by age groups (x axis, in years) and sex (females, light; males, dark). Age-specific rates were highest at age 0–4 years (insert, $57/10^5$) and >85 years ($52/10^5$). From reference 8342. Copyright by Commonwealth of Australia. Reproduced with permission.

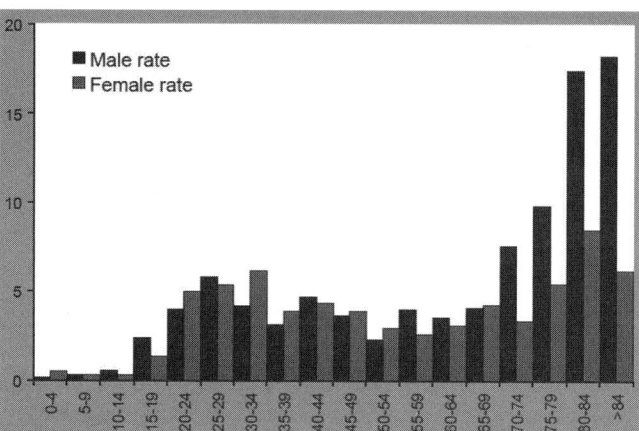

Figure 14.12 Bacteriologically confirmed tuberculosis reports, Australia, 2001 ($n = 771$). Rate per 10^5 (y axis, overall 4.0) is given by age groups (x axis, in years) and sex (females, dark; males, light). From reference 4567. Copyright by Commonwealth of Australia. Reproduced with permission.

(38%) neonates. Main infectious causes of death in preschool children are neonatal sepsis and tetanus, pneumonia, diarrhea, malaria, measles, and HIV.

Droplet-Air Cluster

Respiratory illness (4643, 5149, 5252, 6351, 7640, 8078, 8342) peaks in preschool children, for rates of 7–8/year, compared with 4/year in adults. Agents that circulate widely in preschool children include AdV, *Enterovirus*, PIV (croup), RSV (bronchiolitis), *N. meningitidis* (Fig. 14.8), and *S. pneumoniae*, and where vaccine coverage is low *Influenzavirus* (Fig. 14.10), measles virus, VZV, *B. pertussis*, and Hib.

In the United Kingdom, *Enterovirus* isolation rates/10^5 and year are ~4 in the population but 140 in infants. Invasive *S. pneumoniae* disease has a first peak at age <2 years (Fig. 14.11). In San Jose, Costa Rica, in 1995–2001, 56% of 135 episodes of invasive pneumococcal disease in children were diagnosed at age <2 years, and 73% at age <5 years.

Feces-Food Cluster

Infectious diarrhea typically affects preschool children. Although viruses such as HAV induce immunity for life, most enteric bacteria and protozoa do not, allowing for reinfections.

Agents (343, 1516, 2632, 4684, 7881, 8342) that circulate at high rate in preschool children, predominantly in low-income countries, include HAV; *Campylobacter*, *Clostridium botulinum* (infant botulism from intestinal toxin production, at age 0–6 months), *E. coli* (EHEC, EPEC, ETEC), *H. pylori*, *Salmonella*, *Shigella*; *Cryptosporidium parvum*, and *G. lamblia*. Hemolytic-uremic syndrome (HUS) from EHEC infections typically affects preschool children. In the United States, rates of invasive salmonellosis (mainly by *S. enterica* serovar Typhimurium)/10^5 per year were 7.8 in infants, ≤0.8 in adolescents and adults, and 1.3 at age >60 years (Fig. 14.2). In Louisiana in 1975–1996, rates of seroconversion to *H. pylori* in 224 children peaked at age 4–5 years (2/100 per year).

Zoonotic Cluster
By crawling and walking, infants become exposed to pet mammals and bites by arthropods. In endemic areas, malaria is a severe disease in preschool children. *Wuchereria bancrofti* can also be acquired at this age (8231).

Environmental Cluster
From filthy faces and flies, children acquire ocular *C. trachomatis*. From sand boxes and through geophagia, children acquire *Toxocara* and visceral larva migrans.

Skin-Blood Cluster
The main hazards are infective mothers and siblings. Skin-, blood-, and secretion-borne agents and infections that exhibit peaks at age 0–4.9 years include congenital viral infections, CMV infection (Fig. 14.9), invasive *S. aureus* disease, *S. agalactiae* (GBS) invasive disease, and *Candida* fungemia (Fig. 20.1).

SCHOOL AGE (5–14 YEARS)
Of the world population, ~20% (~1,200 million) are children of school age (27% in Africa and 12% in Europe). In high-income countries, infection risks are typically low at this age, with rates exhibiting a trough. Venues for exposure include class rooms, sports teams, excursions to zoos and farms, and holiday camps.

Droplet-Air Cluster
Infections (699, 1974, 4733, 6350) that peak at school age include PVB19, *C. pneumoniae*, and *M. pneumoniae*; in children who have missed vaccines because of parental objection, absenteeism, or other reason, measles virus, *B. pertussis*, and *C. diphtheriae* are also seen. In some settings, carriage of *N. meningitidis* peaks in school children.

Feces-Food Cluster
Food-borne worms (5157, 7165). Both prevalence and intensity of *Ascaris lumbricoides* and *Trichuris trichiura* infections typically peak at school age, then level off or decline in adolescents and adults. This pattern is explained by intense exposure followed by acquired partial immunity.

Zoonotic Cluster
Although arthropod-borne infections typically peak in adults, some notable exceptions exist. Dengue and dengue hemorrhagic fever predominantly affect school children in low-income countries (2977). The incidence of *Rickettsia conorii* disease (boutonneuse fever) in western Europe (86) and of *R. rickettsii* disease (spotted fever) in the Americas (5584, 6794) peaks in school children. Possible explanations include exposure to ticks on the way to school, from pet animals or in backyards.

Environmental Cluster
In endemic areas, *Schistosoma* (3776, 7225) infections (*S. haematobium*, *S. japonicum*, and *S. mansoni*) peak in older children and adolescents; prevalence and intensity can level off or decline in adults.

Skin-Blood Cluster
Infections (726, 838, 1908, 6329, 8042). Infections that peak at school age include molluscum contagiosum, nasal *S. aureus* (peak of ~50% at age 10 years), streptococcal pharyngitis, tinea capitis (by anthropophilic *Trichophyton*), enterobiasis (mainly kindergarten and elementary school children), pediculosis capitis, and scabies.

ADULT AGE (15–64 YEARS)
Of the world population, 63% (~3,825 million) are in this age group (54% in Africa and 68% in Europe). Typical exposing activities include work, travel, reproduction, unsafe sex, and injection drug use (IDU). Annually, ~0.5 million mothers die from pregnancy-related causes (4256).

Droplet-Air Cluster
The majority of adults are immune to vaccine-preventable agents, from vaccination or natural infection. However, to interrupt transmission, the proportion of susceptible individuals in the community should be below 5–10%.

Agents (1603, 4567, 6350, 8342) that circulate in adults at high rates include AdV (Fig. 14.1), EBV (Fig. 14.13),

Figure 14.13 Laboratory reports of Epstein-Barr virus infections, Australia, 1991–2000 ($n = 18,219$). Reports (*y* axis) are given by age groups (*x* axis, in years) and sex (females, light; males, dark). From reference 6350. Copyright by Commonwealth of Australia. Reproduced with permission.

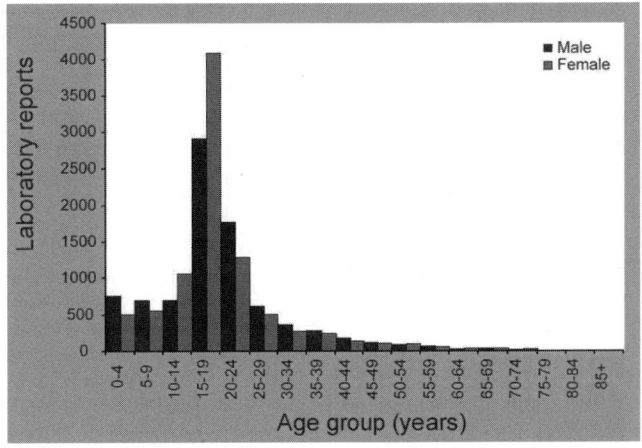

PVB19 (second peak in adults), *M. tuberculosis* (first peak in young adults; Fig. 14.12), and *Neisseria meningitidis* (second invasive peak in adolescents; Fig. 14.8).

Mononucleosis has a typical peak at age 15–19 years ("first kiss disease"). In North America, West Europe, and Australia, the first peak of incident, active tuberculosis is largely due to foreign-born, adolescent and young adult immigrants.

Feces-Food Cluster
In high-income countries, sanitation and spacious housing have shifted enteric infections from preschool to adult age. Consequently, international travelers are likely to be susceptible to HAV and poliovirus and should be offered vaccines.

Infections (2580, 7881, 8342) for which peaks (first or minor second) are apparent in adults in high-income countries include *Campylobacter*, *Salmonella* (non-Typhi serovars and serovar Typhi), *Shigella*, and *Cryptosporidium*.

Zoonotic Cluster
Outdoor activities expose adults to vertebrate- and arthropod-borne agents.

Agents (40, 946, 6350, 8342), that reach peak rates in adults include Ross River virus (RRV), sindbis virus (SINV), yellow fever virus (YFV); *Coxiella burnetii*, *Chlamydia psittaci* (ornithosis), and imported *Plasmodium*. In Australia, *Coxiella burnetii* typically infects male adults, for a male:female ratio of 5:1. In contrast, tick-borne encephalitis (TBE) cases in western Europe have been diagnosed in a wide age range, from 1 to >80 years.

Environmental Cluster
Outdoors activities expose adults to surface water, soil, and dust. Agents (3440, 7463) that are typical for this group include *Leptospira* and hookworms (intestinal and cutaneous larva migrans).

Skin-Blood Cluster
Unsafe sex and IDU are major risks. A common condition in young women is vaginitis due to *Gardnerella*, *Candida*, or *Trichomonas*.

Agents (1425, 4503, 6350, 6679, 8056, 8342) that circulate at high rates in young adults include CMV (second peak, Fig. 14.9), HBV, HCV, and HIV, HSV2, genital *C. trachomatis* (Fig. 14.14) and *N. gonorrhoeae*. In contrast, rates of syphilis (combined primary, secondary, and latent stages) are spread more widely over adult age groups. Tinea pedis, which is uncommon in children, becomes prevalent after puberty. Wound botulism is closely associated with IDU (popping).

ELDERLY (≥65 YEARS)
Of the world population, ~7% (440 million) are elderly (low of 3% in Africa and high of 16% in Europe). Their

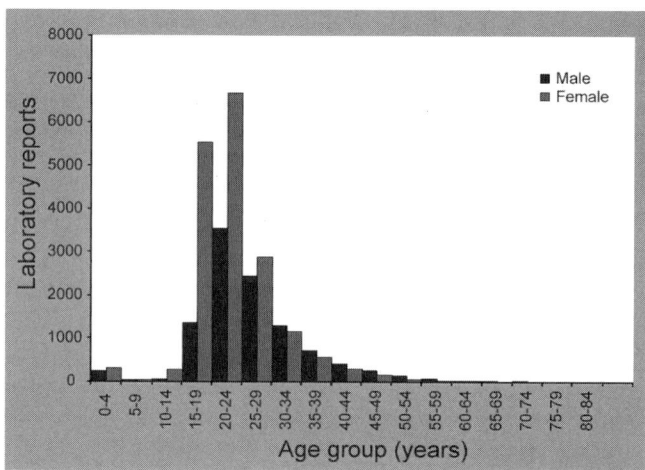

Figure 14.14 Laboratory reports of genital *Chlamydia trachomatis* infections, Australia, 1991–2000 ($n \sim 30,000$). Reports (y axis) are given by age groups (x axis, in years) and sex (females, light; males, dark). 57% of reports were for age group 15–24 years. From reference 6350. Copyright by Commonwealth of Australia. Reproduced with permission.

share is projected to increase to 12% by 2030 (to 4% in Africa and 24% in Europe) (2875). Decreasing immune memory and function, increasing utilization of care, and increasing comorbidities make elderly vulnerable to infections, including nosocomial and reactivated infections.

Droplet-Air Cluster
Agents (4567, 6351, 6706, 6908, 8342) that affect the elderly, in particular, include *Influenzavirus* (second peak [Fig. 14.10], accounts for 1–95% of excess deaths in the population), *B. pertussis* (second peak), *L. pneumophila* (elderly account for up to three fourths of all cases; Fig. 14.7), *M. tuberculosis* (second peak in nationals; Fig. 14.12), and *S. pneumoniae* (second peak of invasive disease [Fig. 14.11], for a lethality of ~20%).

Feces-Food Cluster
Agents (7440, 8342) that cause peak disease rates with advancing age include *C. difficile*, *L. monocytogenes* (Fig. 14.15), and some nosocomial Enterobacteriaceae. Reactivations to consider in the elderly include *S. enterica* serovar Typhi and *E. histolytica*.

Zoonotic Cluster
West Nile virus (WNV) neuroinvasive disease exhibits a curious peak in the elderly (Fig. 20.2) (3206).

Environmental Cluster
Elderly are at increased risk of *Clostridium tetani* and *P. aeruginosa* (243, 2704, 5747, 5792). Reactivated agents to consider in the elderly include *Strongyloides* and *Schistosoma*. In the United States in 1998–2000, reported

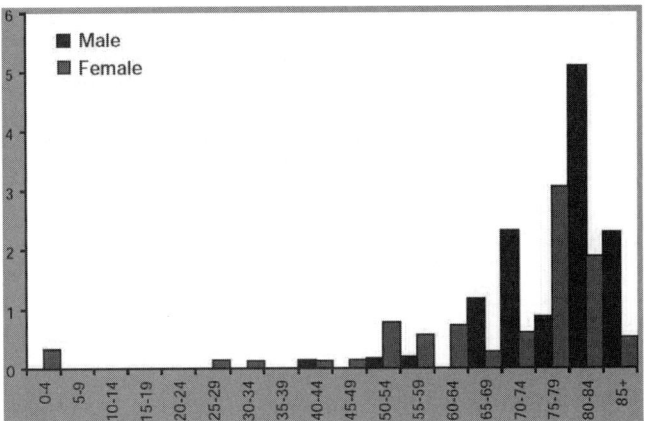

Figure 14.15 Listeriosis reports, Australia, 2002 ($n = 59$). Rate per 10^5 (y axis, overall 0.3), by age groups (x axis, in years) and sex (females, light; males, dark). From reference 8342. Copyright by Commonwealth of Australia. Reproduced with permission.

age groups of 130 tetanus cases were <20 years in 9% (12), 20–59 years in 55% (71), and ≥60 years in 36% (47) (Fig. 14.16). Tetanus risks peak in the elderly, for rates/10^5 per year of ~0.03 in North America and 0.3–0.8 in West Europe. High rates in the elderly coincide with lost protection. In a U.S. population sample in 1988–1991, 70% had protective (>0.15 IU/ml) antitoxin levels, with a high (>80%) in children and young adults, and a low (28%) at age ≥70 years.

Skin-Blood Cluster

Infections (1975, 2125, 5892, 5905) typical for the elderly include sporadic Creutzfeldt-Jakob disease (CJD), zoster, *S. aureus* bacteremia, candidemia, tinea pedis, and onychomycosis. Zoster rates increase with advancing age. In the United States, the zoster rate is ~0.2/100 person-years, and only ~5% of cases younger than 15 years. In the United Kingdom, rates of first zoster per 100 person-years are 0.1–0.2 in children but >1 at age ≥85 years.

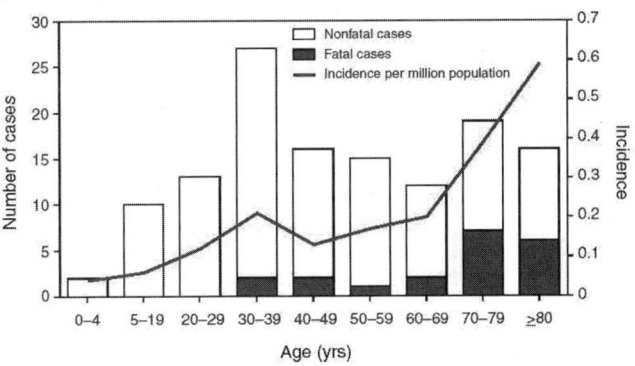

Figure 14.16 Reported tetanus cases, United States, 1998–2000. Number (left y axis, $n = 130$), rates/million/year (line, right y axis, overall 0.16) is given by age groups (x axis, in years) and lethality (dark, fatal). From reference 5747.

Candidemia rates are U-shaped, with highs/10^5 per year of 9–11 in infants and 4–10 in elderly (Fig. 20.1).

14.3 DAY CARE

Children in day care centers may be a global reservoir of worldwide prevalent strains of drug-resistant pneumococci.

R. Sa-Leao et al. (6497)

Day care means care of preschool children during the day and away from home at private or communal centers. Families may share care by rotation. Included here are playgroups and day facilities for children with handicaps. For orphanages, see section 11.5.

Exposure (77, 2370) (http://www.cdc.gov/foodnet/surveys/Pop_surv.htm). In the United States in 2000, of respondents representing eight states ($n = 13,113$), 6–10% reported to have ≥1 child in day care. The proportion of preschool children attending child care is ~37% in Australia, and ~50% in the United States.

Infections (2370, 2443, 3748, 6125, 7639, 7908) (Box 14.4). Risks in day care include crowding, poor hygiene by small children and untrained staff, and inadequate facilites. Compared with home care, children in day care are at increased risk of days ill, antibiotic prescriptions, and infections, in particular, otitis media. In Sydney in 1992, 80% (74/92) of day care centers reported ≥1 outbreak, mainly diarrhea, conjunctivitis, and pediculosis.

Preventive measures (6, 2370, 6252). Preventive measures include staff education (hand hygiene and cleanliness), sanitary installations (e.g., diaper-change areas and wash basins), vaccines for children and staff, and a policy for ill children and staff.

Vaccines for children recommended by many national programs (and usual age for first dose) include HBV (at birth), diphtheria, tetanus, pertussis$_\text{acellular}$ (DTP$_\text{a}$), Hib, polio, *S. pneumoniae* (all at 2 months), MMR, and VZV

Box 14.4 Agents and infections in or from day care, by agent cluster

Droplet-air	Otitis media; AdV, *Enterovirus, Influenzavirus, Rhinovirus*, VZV; *B. pertussis, C. pneumoniae, H. influenzae, K. kingae, M. catarrhalis, M. tuberculosis, N. meningitidis* (B, C), *S. pneumoniae*
Feces-food	Diarrhea; enteric AdV, ASTV, HAV, *Norovirus, Rotavirus*; *E. coli, Shigella*; *Cryptosporidium, Giardia*
Skin-blood	CMV, HBV; *Enterobius*

(at 1 year). Vaccines for workers should consider the same vaccines recommended for health and laboratory workers (see section 12.6). Likely infective children should be excluded from day care, e.g., febrile rash, bloody diarrhea, difficult breathing, or purulent conjunctivitis. However, when substantial shedding is suspected to occur before the disease is manifest (d_0), exclusion is ineffective and not indicated. For infectivity and shedding, see section 14.1 and Table 14.1; for schools, see section 14.4.

DROPLET-AIR CLUSTER, DAY CARE
Risks (6, 5803, 6252, 7056). Pharyngeal carriage of respiratory agents is 2–5 times more frequent in children in day care than in control children. In Brazil, the rate of respiratory illness in children in day care was 10/100 child-days.

Children with febrile rash should be excluded until the cause is confirmed noninfective. Further reasons for exclusion include difficult breathing, purulent conjunctivitis, measles (for 5 days from rash onset), mumps (for 5 days from parotitis onset), diphtheria, Hib-invasive disease (for 2 days from treatment onset or t_0), pertussis (for 5 days from t_0), varicella (for 5 days from rash onset, may not be effective), or infective tuberculosis (rare, for 2 weeks from t_0).

Viruses: Vaccine Preventable
Risks (1743, 6486, 7056). The main viruses that circulate in day care centers include *Influenzavirus* and VZV, while high vaccine coverage has significantly reduced rates of measles, mumps, rubella, and polio in high-income countries.

Influenzavirus **(3513, 7056).** Influenza is a day care hazard, including complications such as otitis media. In Brazil, A and B viruses accounted for 6% (8/129) of respiratory viruses in day care. In a vaccine trial in winter of 1996–1997, the rate of influenza A/H3N2 or B in unvaccinated control children in day care was 51% (26/51) in 14 weeks. Annual vaccination is recommended for children ≥6 months of age at risk of influenza complications.

VZV (2584, 3608, 3748, 4351). Varicella outbreaks in day care centers have been reported. Reported attack rates in susceptible (nonvaccinated) children sharing rooms with an index case are 86–88%. In Sydney, Australia, in 1992, one third (24/72) of outbreaks in day care were due to varicella, and these outbreaks had the highest caseload (9–10/outbreak), and lasted longest (for 4 weeks on average). Most (>90%) day care workers can be expected to be seroreactive.

Viruses: Vaccine Nonpreventable
Risk (7056). Agents that frequently circulate in day care children include AdV, EV, PIV, and *Rhinovirus*. In children in day care in Brazil, the rate of acute viral respiratory infections was 0.8/100 child-days.

AdV (4926, 5670, 7056). Respiratory AdV infections and epidemic conjunctivitis have been reported in day care. In Brazil, AdV accounted for 12% (16/129) of respiratory viruses in day care.

Enterovirus **(EV) (1307, 1322, 3239, 5122, 7056, 7521, 7820).** EV is a significant risk in day care centers and nursery schools. Spread is via droplets, hand and surface contacts, and feces. Changing diapers is a risk; handwashing is protective. Syndromes are variable and can be due to coxsackievirus, echovirus, or EV proper. In Brazil, EV accounted for 15% (19/129) of respiratory viruses from day care.

Hand-foot-and-mouth disease outbreaks have been reported in Asia and Europe, from coxsackievirus A and EV71. Also, outbreaks of EV30 have been reported in day care centers in the United States and Europe, for attack rates of ~40–75% among children and 5–15% among staff. Children can carry EV from centers to homes and become a source for siblings and other household members, for secondary attack rates of ~15–60%.

Rhinovirus **(7056).** *Rhinovirus* circulates in day care. In Brazil, the virus accounted for 52% (67/129) of respiratory viruses in day care.

Roseolovirus **(human herpesvirus 6) (2517).** Human herpesvirus 6 (HHV6) can circulate in day care, causing rashes or febrile illness. In outbreaks at 8 day care centers in Belém, Brazil, in 1997, two thirds (256/401) of children had evidence by enzyme-linked immunosorbent assay (ELISA) and NAT of recent HHV6 infection.

PVB19 (4020, 4779, 5108, 6252). PVB19 caused outbreaks of erythema infectiosum (slapped cheek disease) in preschool and school children, for attack rates of 11–67%. Index children do not seem to present significant risks for pregnant staff or household members. Exclusion from day care is ineffective and not recommended.

PIV (7056). PIV circulates in day care. In Brazil, PIV2 and 3 accounted for 11% (14/129) of respiratory viruses in day care.

Reovirus (7208). Reovirus has been reported in day care.

RSV (7056). Although important in infants and preschool children, RSV has been poorly documented in day care. In Brazil, RSV accounted for 4% (5/129) of respiratory viruses in day care.

Bacteria: Vaccine Preventable
B. pertussis **(3210, 7087).** Although vaccines reduce pertussis risks, cases can occur, even in centers with high vaccine coverage. That vaccinated children can be a source is perhaps explained by good systemic (antitoxin)

response but inadequate mucosal response to whole-cell vaccine.

C. diphtheriae. Diphtheria has become very unusual in day care since the vaccine era, at least in high-income countries; in low-income countries with endemic diphtheria, day care is not popular.

H. influenzae. Day care is a significant risk for infection and for invasive disease by capsulated serotype b (Hib).

- Carriage (1426, 1706, 2071, 2460, 2753, 5803). Compared with home care, day care significantly increases carriage. By age, vaccine use, tested site (oro- or nasopharynx), and endemicity, 1–40% of children in day care carry any *H. influenzae* in the pharynx, and 0–1% carry capsulated strains, including Hib. Strain turnover may be rapid, or carriage could last up to 9–12 months. Whether nontypeable (noncapsulated) strains are beneficial by preventing colonization with Hib or epidemic strains is uncertain.
- Outbreaks (217, 2753, 4935, 6812, 7569) have been reported, including invasive Hib disease and conjunctivitis by a nontypeable strain. Infectivity in centers appears to extend for up to 60 days. Among children of age <2 years sharing day care rooms with an index case, reported secondary infection rates are 0–2.7%.
- Prevention (6, 2460, 4935). Vaccine prevents disease and reduces carriage. Although chemoprophylaxis in day care is not universally accepted, outbreaks of invasive Hib disease in day care may be an indication for rifampin prophylaxis in contacts.

M. tuberculosis (102, 2029). *M. tuberculosis* can circulate in day care. At a Greek day care center, a 24-year-old trainee teacher with tuberculous pleuritis and positive sputum by direct smear was the source for 24 (89%) infections among 27 children 1.5–6 years of age attending day care who were not vaccinated with bacillus Calmette Guérin (BCG); 5 (21%) infected children had symptoms suggestive of active tuberculosis. The high transmission rate was explained by intense exposure (for 6 h/day, 5 days/week) and high virulence rather than delay of treatment. Contacts of index cases must be evaluated for infection.

N. meningitidis (6, 1774, 1846, 2932, 5531). Day care does not seem to increase carriage. Invasive disease in preschool settings has been reported. Compared with the population, the risk of secondary cases in the month after a primary case is up to 40-fold, for attack rates of 70–80/10^5 among preschool contacts, and up to 685/10^5 among household contacts. Serogroups B and C case clusters and outbreaks have been reported in day care. Chemoprophylaxis for contacts is recommended, and tetravalent vaccine (A, C, W135, Y) should be considered.

S. pneumoniae (727, 1710, 2071, 2768). *S. pneumoniae* circulates widely in day care. Day care increases risks for carriage, infection, and invasive disease, mainly in children of age <2 years. Children in day care can carry *S. pneumoniae* home to siblings.

- Carriage (727, 2071, 2767, 5438, 5803). By age and setting, ~35–60% of children in day care carry *S. pneumoniae* in the nasopharynx. Risks include young age, crowding, and use of antibiotics. Carriage may or may not include strains that are resistant to penicillin. In The Netherlands in 1999, penicillin-resistant strains were not isolated from children in day care ($n = 259$) or control children ($n = 276$); prevalent serotypes were 19F, 6B, and 6A. In a 4-km perimeter around a day care center in Israel, marked strain differences were observed in eight day care centers.
- Outbreaks (1265, 1376, 1710) seem infrequent in day care. In 1994, three of six children in family day care contracted pneumococcal bacteremia.
- Prevention (6, 1711). Vaccine reduces respiratory morbidity and antibiotic use in children in day care. By age and risks, conjugate or polysaccharide vaccines are recommended.

Bacteria: Vaccine Nonpreventable
Chlamydophila (5481). In Sweden by NAT, 23% (103/453) of children in day care and 23% (33/142) of staff carried *C. pneumoniae* the agent in the pharynx; carriage did not correlate with respiratory symptoms.

Kingella (6964). *K. kingae* seems to readily spread among children in day care.

Moraxella (4730, 5803). Some 5–80% of preschool children carry *M. catarrhalis* in the nasopharynx, and children in day care are at increased risk of carriage.

Mycoplasma (5067). *M. pneumoniae* seems unusual in day care. An outbreak has been reported in a nursery school in Japan.

FECES-FOOD CLUSTER, DAY CARE
Risks (6, 6252). Poor hygiene and close contact enhance child-to-child spread of enteric viruses (e.g., HAV and *Norovirus*), bacteria (e.g., *E. coli* and *Shigella*), and protozoa (*Cryptosporidium* and *Giardia*). Reasons for exclusion from day care include vomiting (more than once), acute purulent or bloody diarrhea (for 24 h after recovery), acute HA (for 5 days from d_0), EHEC (until two cultures are negative), *Salmonella*, and *Shigella* (until stool culture is negative). For diapers, see section 6.4.

Viruses

Risks (109, 7373). AdV, ASTV, *Norovirus*, and *Rotavirus* are frequently isolated in day care in children with *and without* diarrhea.

AdV (109, 4385, 7373, 7747). Enteric AdV circulates in day care. About half of all infections are inapparent. AdV can accout for 15–40% of diarrhea in day care. At some centers, children with diarrhea shed AdV about as frequently as children without diarrhea (2%). Outbreaks in day care have been reported. In Texas in 1986–1991, AdV was detected in 10 (1%) of 96 diarrhea outbreaks in day care, and in 38 % (94/249) of children in these outbreaks.

ASTV (109, 4385, 5086, 6893, 7373). ASTV circulates in day care. ASTV can account for 15% of diarrhea in day care. At some centers, children with diarrhea shed ASTV significantly more often (4%) than children without diarrhea (0.7%). Outbreaks in day care have been reported. During an outbreak at a day care center that lasted 11 weeks, 32% of 368 stool samples from 36 children amplified ASTV by NAT; median shedding was 4 days.

HAV (6, 261, 752, 2493, 3048, 3123). HAV can circulate sporadically or epidemically in day care. Centers are sources of HAV in workers, households, and the community. Risks may vary for new or well-trained workers. Risks for outbreaks include large centers (>50 children), non-toilet-trained attending children, and children or parents returned from travel to endemic areas. Vaccine should be considered routinely for children from endemic communities of high-income countries, all new staff, and in outbreaks for contacts whether the source has acute HA or is infected inapparently.

Outbreaks Outbreaks have been well documented in day care centers. Immigrant children are an emerging source of outbreaks in day care.

- North America (1894, 3048, 7805). In Florida in 1988–1989, of 311 cases in three urban areas (attack rates, 0.4–6/10^5), 37% were linked to day care centers. An outbreak at a center in Oklahoma in 1979 caused acute HA cases among 15% (4/27) of workers and 17% (19/115) of households with a child in the center; altogether 41 cases occurred, all in adults.
- Australia (3123). Of 114 first HA cases in day care, 18 (16%) heralded outbreaks. The 18 outbreaks resulted in 105 acute HA cases, and administration of Ig to 928 children and 105 staff.
- West Europe (261, 751, 1553, 6788). At a center in Spain in 2002–2003, HAV affected children (attack rate, 9%), 2 staff (11%), and 13 household contacts. At a nursery school in Italy in 1996, an outbreak caused 11 cases in children (primary attack rate, 27%) and 10 cases in household contacts (secondary attack rate, 9%). At a center in France in 1994, an outbreak caused 11 cases in children (of age 2–3 years, primary attack rate 56%), 2 in staff, and 4 in households (secondary attack rate 28%). At a kindergarten in Switzerland in 1990, an outbreak caused 20 cases (11 in children and 9 in adults), and 5 subclinical infections, for an attack rate of 15% (20/136 susceptible); spread was human-to-human, and the source was a traveler to Mexico who on return home shared a bottle of beer with the father of a child in the affected kindergarten.

Norovirus (109, 2593, 2870). *Norovirus* can accout for 15% of diarrhea in day care. Outbreaks with *Norovirus* and related *Sapovirus* have been reported in day care. In Sweden in 1999, *Norovirus* gastroenteritis affected 30 day care centres served by one caterer. Food (pumpkin salad) was the likely vehicle for early cases (primary attack rate, 27%), but human-to-human spread was more likely for later cases (secondary attack rate, 14%).

Rotavirus (1792, 2372, 2565, 3121, 5902, 5903, 6231, 7373). *Rotavirus* can circulate in day care, including groups A and C. A major source of *Rotavirus* seem to be children who are incubating diarrhea. Children in day care can carry *Rotavirus* to households and the community, for reported secondary attack rates of 15%. Outbreaks in day care are well documented.

Bacteria

Risks (6, 1145, 5546). Person-to-person spread is the main risk. Agents that are mainly food borne are infrequently reported in day care, including *Bacillus cereus*, *C. jejuni*, and non-Typhi *S. enterica* serovars, although preschool children can be *Salmonella* carriers, as were 6.7% of children in a center in Mexico.

E. coli (542, 5349, 5529, 6193, 7279). Enteroaggregative *E. coli* (EAEC), EHEC, EPEC, and ETEC can circulate at centers, causing diarrhea and outbreaks. EHEC readily spreads person-to-person. In Minnesota in 1988–1989, at centers with an index child, the number of all EHEC infections was 2–18 (median, 2). In EHEC outbreaks, reported primary attack rates are 3–38% (typically 20%) among children, and 20% among workers; secondary attack rates can reach 20%. While sources of outbreaks are often not identified, in an outbreak at a center in Germany in 1992, deep-frozen stuffed cabbage rolls and turkey scallops in batter were implicated microbiologically. Handwashing is recommended before eating (including snacks) and after changing diaper or toileting.

Shigella (2692, 3010, 5123, 5903, 6807). Children in day care are sources of shigellosis in workers, households, and communities. By age of the index child, reported secondary attack rates are 26–49%. Risks include diapered infants, volunteer workers, poorly trained workers, handwashing facilities that are inaccessible to children, and poorly disposed diapers.

Outbreaks Outbreaks are well documented in centers in high-income countries.
- United States (1226, 5123, 6807, 7526). In 2001–2003, several *S. sonnei* community outbreaks had their origin in day care. Cases in the community diluted the proportion of cases attributed to day care to 50–20% or less. In an outbreak in Cincinnati, Ohio, in 2001, with 1,642 *S. sonnei* cases, attack rates were 1–33% (median, 10%) in children in day care, and 0–17% (median, 6%) in staff. In Kentucky in 1991, 14 licensed centers were involved in an outbreak.
- Australasia (2692, 8317). At a center in Melbourne, Australia, in 2000, an outbreak affected 47% of children and 37% of staff. At a center in Tokyo in 1998, *S. sonnei* caused 20 cases among kindergarten children 13 cases among their families, and 3 inapparent infections.

Protozoa
Blastocystis **(4079, 5058, 7158).** *Blastocystis* has been reported from day care. In Montreal, Canada, in 2000, *B. hominis* was identified in 5% (4/78) of children and 30% (3/10) of staff; a source was not identified. In low-income countries, ~15–30% of children in day care may shed *Blastocystis* in stools.

Cryptosporidium **(3126, 5058, 6367, 7136, 7181, 7324).** *C. hominis* is a hazard in day care, mainly from spread person-to-person. Risks include young age (<36 months), diapered children, and non-toilet-trained children. The reported prevalence in day care is 3–10% in high-income countries and up to 89% in children low-income countries. With good hygiene, the risk of spread seems low, including from HIV-infected children.

Outbreaks at centers have been well documented. In an outbreak in Georgia, infection rates were 49% (39/79) in children, and 13% (2/23) in staff. In an outbreak at a day nursery in the United Kingdom, the infection rate in children was 18% (13/74).

Entamoeba **(5058, 7181).** Children from endemic areas can be carriers of *E. histolytica/dispar*. For instance in Trujillo, Venezuela, 1% of 301 children in day care were shedding *E. histolytica/dispar*. With good hygiene, the risk of spread is low.

Giardia **(65, 227, 767, 2083, 2667, 5058, 5904, 6367, 7154, 7181).** *G. lamblia* is a day care hazard, mainly from person-to-person spread. Risks include poor practice with diapers and dirty linen, poor handwashing, toddlers at the center, and children who attend for >3 months. Good hygiene can reduce risks. By age, setting, and number of stool samples examined, the reported point prevalence in day care is 1–35% in high-income countries and 20–70% in low-income countries. Infections have also been reported in 1–20% of (female) workers and 7–23% of household members (siblings) of attending children.

Outbreaks at centers are well documented. In Wisconsin in 1983–1985, three outbreaks occurred in one center, for attack rates of 17–47% in children, 9–35% in staff, and 5–17% in household contacts.

Helminths
In low-income countries, 10–20% of children in day care may shed eggs of *A. lumbricoides* and *T. trichiura* in stools. However, eggs are not transmissible person-to-person when shed.

ENVIRONMENTAL CLUSTER
Risks (5058). Play grounds are potential sources of *Strongyloides* (from contact with soil) and *Toxocara* (from taking soil into the mouth). In Venezuela, the point prevalence of *S. stercoralis* in 301 children in day care was 0.3%.

Surfaces and objects soiled with fresh droplets, saliva, hands, vomit, or feces are potential sources or vehicles of respiratory (e.g., PIV, *Rhinovirus*, and RSV), enteric (e.g., HAV, *Norovirus*), and other agents (e.g., CMV), and of "horizontal" spread of infections. For toothbrushes, see section 6.4.

SKIN-BLOOD CLUSTER
Risks (6, 6252). In day care, spread from skin contact and saliva (licking and drooling) is likely. For agents from respiratory secretions, see section 14.1. Reasons for excluding children from day care include impetigo (to recovery t_0 plus 24 h), streptococcal pharyngitis, scarlet fever (to t_0 plus 5 days), herpetic gingivostomatitis with drooling, and scabies (to t_0 plus 24 h).

Viruses
Risks (6). Nose bleeding and bleeding wounds are potential sources of viruses, mainly HBV. Transmission of HCV or HIV has not been documented in day care, and risks from infected children are considered small. Entry screen for HBV, HCV, or HIV should not be required. HBV vaccine is recommended for all children in day care. Standard precautions apply for all children who are bleeding. For human bites, see section 13.5.

CMV (6, 75, 77, 1956, 3523, 3835, 4468, 6839). Preschool children in day care and in centers for the handicapped frequently acquire inapparent CMV infection. In day care or kindergarten, ~20–70% of children may acquire CMV, and 20–40% may shed CMV with urine or saliva (for months or years). Shedding children are a risk for susceptible (seronegative) female workers, play mates, and mothers. However, screening children for shedding and isolation are ineffective means of control. In contrast, hand hygiene is protective for seronegative, pregnant women who are exposed to a shedding child.

HBV (893, 2422, 4904). HBV transmission is reported in day care, in particular, in centers with children in or from highly endemic communities. In Denmark, the anti-HBc prevalence was low (<1%) by screening of saliva from children in day care, even at centers with a high proportion (>50%) of immigrant children.

HSV (2369, 6685). Transmission of HSV1 has been documented in day care. Labial lesions or saliva rather than gingivostomatitis are potential sources. At a center in Sydney, Australia, in 1993, 5 (26%) of 19 children <2 years of age, and two older siblings contracted HSV1.

Bacteria
Bacterial skin infections in child care are poorly documented. Impetigo is a putative risk.

S. aureus (7509). Nasal carriage of MSSA and MRSA strains has been reported from children in day care without known risks.

S. pyogenes (GAS) (1426, 3404, 3465, 7483, 8308). By age and setting, 2–8% of children in day care may carry GAS in the nasopharynx. Outbreaks have been reported in day care, including of pharyngotonsillitis, and scarlet fever. Reported infection rates are 42–49% in children, 0–8% in workers, and 23–36% in household members.

Fungi
An outbreak of culture-confirmed *Microsporum audouinii* at a Danish kindergarten affected 12 (12%) of 98 exposed persons, 8 contracted tinea capitis, and 4 had tinea corporis (3049). For *Candida*-associated diaper dermatitis, see section 6.4.

Helminths
Enterobius, *Hymenolepis*, and *Strongyloides* can be spread person-to-person.

Enterobius (2667, 5505, 7030). *E. vermicularis* can be endemic in day care. Reported prevalence is 0–30%. At day nurseries in Schwerin, Germany, in 1997, the prevalence was 3% (35/1,174) in children (age 1–7 years) and 0.7% in staff (1/137). In Havana, Cuba, infection rates per 100 per year in children in day care ($n = 469$) were lower before treatment (10–11) than after treatment (20–23), likely because of reinfection from significant home reservoirs.

Hymenolepis (2999, 5058). *H. nana* is a hazard mainly in low-income countries where the point prevalence in children in day care is 1–9%.

Arthropods
Sarcoptes scabiei and *P. humanus capitis* readily spread by contact, *P. humanus capitis* also spreads by hair brushes.

S. scabiei (6615). A scabies outbreak was reported in a day care center, for an attack rate of 22%.

P. humanus capitis (773). By setting and time period, head lice can be absent or prevalent in children in day care. In Minas Gerais, Brazil, of 884 children from various institutions of 0–15 years of age, 35% had evidence of *P. humanus capitis* infestation.

14.4 SCHOOLS AND TRAINING
Educational habitats include elementary or primary school (primary, for age groups ~6–11 years), secondary or junior high school (secondary, for age groups ~12–17 years), vocational schools, gymnasiums, colleges, universities, and private and adult learning institutions. For day care, see section 14.3 above.

Exposure. Almost 100% of children of school age in high-income countries and 50–95% in low-income countries are likely to attend school, at least part-time. The history (Box 14.1) should address the number of children attending school, school food programs and excursions, school days missed, ill class mates, and the size and type of classes.

Infections (Box 14.5). School-associated infections can be acquired from inhalation (e.g., classrooms and dormitories), ingestion (e.g., catered lunch, campus cafeterias, and boarding), inoculation (e.g., sports, piercing, and IDU), or contact (e.g., skin and sex).

Prevention (6, 2641, 3093, 5632, 6252). Schools provide excellent opportunities for the promotion of healthy lifestyle and vaccines, and for screening for infections such as tuberculosis and schistosomiasis. Schools may opt for health services by nurses or physicians.

By endemicity and national policy, vaccines to consider for school children include HAV, HBV, *Influenzavirus*, MMR, polio, VZV, and YFV; DTP_a, and meningococci. A legal requirement for vaccination before admission to schools has been shown to increase vaccine coverage.

Box 14.5	Main agents or infections in or from schools, by agent cluster
Droplet-air	High-income countries with high coverage of routine vaccines: AdV, EBV, *Enterovirus*, *Influenzavirus*, PVB19; *C. pneumoniae*, *M. pneumoniae*, *N. meningitidis*, *M. tuberculosis*, *S. pneumoniae*
Feces-food	ASTV, HAV, *Norovirus*, *Rotavirus*; *Campylobacter*, *C. perfringens*, *E. coli* (EAEC, EHEC, and EPEC), *Salmonella*, *Shigella*, staphylococcal food poisoning
Zoonotic	Low-income countries: DENV; *Plasmodium*
Environmental	Low-income countries: hookworms, *Schistosoma*, *Strongyloides*, *Toxocara*
Skin-blood	HBV, HSV; *S. pyogenes* (GAS); tinea capitis; *Enterobius*; pediculosis, scabies

Students considered infectious should be excluded from school. For infections with substantial spread before the first day of disease manifestation (d_0), e.g., influenza or mononucleosis, however, exclusion is ineffective and not recommended.

DROPLET-AIR CLUSTER, SCHOOLS

Risks (6, 6252). Risks include crowded, poorly ventilated rooms, and the number of susceptible and colonized students in class. In winter, respiratory and flulike illnesses can cause significant absenteeism.

Reasons for exclusion from school include suspected rubella (from d_0 for 5 days), meningococcal meningitis (from t_0 for 24 h), and pertussis (from t_0 for 5 days), possibly outbreak cases of *Enterovirus* aseptic meningitis.

Viruses: Vaccine Preventable

***Influenzavirus* (1741, 4262, 5965).** Although students are at low risk, influenza outbreaks are documented at schools (by A/H3N2) and universities (by A/H1N1). Reported attack rates among nonvaccinated students are 10–70%.

Measles virus (1229, 5391, 5776, 6274). Nonimmune students are at risk for measles. In the United States in 1980–1985, college-related measles cases accounted for 5% (1,113/24,186) of national case reports. Risks include poorly ventilated class rooms, deficient ventilation, living in campus dormitories, overdue secondary vaccine dose, and recent travel to an endemic area.

Outbreaks Outbreaks are well documented in educational settings, in particular, where vaccine coverage is low (<80–90%).

- North America (1229, 3280, 4204, 4826, 5391, 6274, 6336). In Pennsylvania in 2003, an index patient with measles from Beirut, Lebanon, caused 10 confirmed cases, including 8 at a boarding school; of 663 students, 8 (1%) had never received vaccine, 26 (4%) had received one dose, and 629 (95%) had received two doses. In Arkansas in 1986, 284 measles cases were confirmed in 18 counties, 32 schools, and 1 university, for attack rates of 0%, 1%, 5%, or 10%, when a vaccine dose dated back 0–4, 5–9, 10–14, or 15–19 years, respectively.

- West Europe (5228, 5776, 7714). In a municipality in Finland in 1989, an index case infected 22 schoolmates in one day, probably during an assembly in a poorly ventilated hallway.

Mumps virus (3279). Nonimmune students are at risk. In Kansas in 1988–1989, 77% (208/269) of mumps cases were students (98% or 203 with documented vaccination), for attack rates of 0.7% at elementary school, 2% at high school, and 8% at junior high school.

Outbreaks Outbreaks are well-documented in schools.

- North America (887, 1360, 3279, 3941, 8062). By vaccination and case definition, attack rates were ~5–50%. Venues for outbreaks included school classes and rallies. At a high school in Tennessee in 1991, 68 students developed mumps in 7 months. At a high school in Texas in 1990, 54 students contracted mumps, 77% 12–20 days after a schoolwide pep rally. During a countywide outbreak in Nashville, Tenn., a public high school recorded 332 mumps cases; the suspected source was a pep rally 17 days before the outbreak peak. At a middle school in Ohio in 1982, an outbreak caused 110 cases, for attack rates (by case definition) of 25–49% among unvaccinated students.

- West Europe (8002). At a secondary school in the United Kingdom in 1996, mumps virus affected 34 (32%, 30 clinical and 4 inapparent) of 106 teenaged students, and 14 individuals in the community; 13% (4/30) of student patients reported severe headache and stiff neck.

Rubella virus (738, 6176). Nonimmune adolescent students are at risk for rubella virus. Risks include poorly ventilated rooms, overdue vaccine, and travel to endemic areas. In the United States in 1990–1999, rubella rates/10^5 per year decreased from 0.6 to 0.06 at age <15 years but increased from 0.1 to 0.2 at age 15–44 years, with an increased risk of congenital rubella syndrome, in particular, in infants born to Hispanic mothers.

Outbreaks Outbreaks have been well-documented in educational settings, in high-income countries mainly at high schools.

- North America (738, 1422, 6176). In Newfoundland, Canada, in 1986, an outbreak at a high school affected 64 unvaccinated students; confinement of students to classrooms for a large portion of the day was suspected to have facilitated the outbreak.
- Europe (7172)
- Low-income countries (4724). At a crowded school in St. Vincent, Caribbean, in 1983, an outbreak caused 143 cases: 133 (43%) among 312 students 5–12 years of age, 4 (33%) among 12 teachers, 5 among mothers of index students, and 1 in a nurse.

VZV (2102, 3093, 4297, 5165, 7604). Nonimmune students are at risk of varicella. Vaccine protects well from moderate or severe varicella, but breakthroughs are possible in students whose vaccination dates back >5 years. As VZV can spread before d_0, outbreak control by exclusion from school when the rash sets in is likely ineffective. In contrast, vaccine may shorten varicella outbreaks.

Elementary schools have been venues for outbreaks. At a primary school in Oregon in 2001, an outbreak caused 21 cases in 9 of 16 classes, for attack rates of 12% (18/152) in vaccinated students, and 43% (3/7) in nonvaccinated students (194 students had had varicella); attack rates were low (3% or 3/87) in recently (preceding 1–5 years) vaccinated students, but high (23% or 15/65) in students vaccinated >5 years previously.

Viruses: Vaccine Nonpreventable

Droplet-borne viruses that may circulate in educational settings include AdV, EBV, EV, human metapneumovirus, PIV, PVB19, and RSV. Viruses that primarily affect preschool children (see section 14.3) and have protective immunity are infrequent in school children, being largely limited to children with comorbidities (e.g., obstructive airway disease).

AdV (3145, 5783). Pharyngoconjunctival fever from AdV has been reported in schools.

EBV (1729, 5170). EBV can circulate in boarding and high schools. In Hong Kong in 1988, nearly 95% (968/1,039) of university freshmen were seroreactive; after 1 year, 25% (16/62) of seronegative freshmen had seroconverted.

EV (140, 3548, 3949, 5170). Outbreaks have been reported in schools, including among sports teams. Various syndromes have caused outbreaks in schools, including aseptic meningitis (from coxsackievirus, echovirus, and EV), conjunctivitis (from EV), and pleurodynia (from coxsackievirus); for hand-foot-mouth disease, see section 14.3.

PVB19 (213, 2940, 3369, 5108, 6239). PVB19 can circulate in kindergarten, elementary schools, and boarding schools, and outbreaks have occurred in these settings, for reported attack rates of 3–67%. At a London primary school in 1994, attack rates were 3% (3/32 susceptibles) in nursery children, 31% (32/103) in students, and 47% (7/15) in staff. At a primary school in The Netherlands in 2001, PVB19 affected 33 (14%) of 230 schoolchildren; none of 12 staff were pregnant or had symptoms. As shedding begins pre-d_0, exclusion from school is ineffective and not recommended.

Bacteria: Vaccine Preventable

B. pertussis (857, 1434, 3596, 3920). Infectivity is high, and 50–80% of class mates of an index case can become infected. Risks include overdue vaccine and nonvaccinated school mates and friends. Schools are frequent venues for outbreaks. For instance in Massachusetts in 1996, 18 of 20 pertussis outbreaks occurred at schools. An outbreak at a primary school in the United States caused 36 student (primary) cases, for an attack rate of 17%, and 16 other (secondary) cases among contacts (households, neighbors, and friends). The earlier the infection is detected, the more effective exclusion will be; cough illness with dyspnea or vomiting should raise suspicion and prompt exclusion until pertussis is rejected or confirmed (for 5 days from t_0). Chemoprophylaxis is recommended for household contacts.

C. diphtheriae (2322, 5051). Vaccine coverage is typically high in high-income countries. After exposure at school, carriage prevalence is 0–5%, exceptionally 30%. School outbreaks were reported in high-income countries in the prevaccine era. At a primary school in Texas in 1967, an outbreak caused 15 culture-confirmed cases and 89 carriers among students and staff, for an overall attack rate of 5% (15/306).

H. influenzae (794, 964, 3589). Nontypeable strains circulate in schools; Hib circulates infrequently, depending on vaccination. In Spain, 316 (26%) of 1,212 randomly selected school children carried H. influenzae in the pharynx: 5 (0.4%) carried Hib, 12 (1%) carried types c, e, or f, and 299 (25%) carried nontypeable strains. The risk of invasive Hib disease in students is low, but carrier students can be a source of Hib for younger siblings. A school and community outbreak of Haemophilus-conjunctivitis was observed in Georgia, United States, in 1981.

N. meningitidis. N. meningitidis can circulate in various educational habitats. Facilities are recommended to develop plans of action for sporadic invasive disease cases and for outbreaks, particularly by types B or C.

- Schools (1974, 3612, 5367). By endemicity, the reported carrier prevalence in schools is 5–10%. Risks for carriage include the high number of students in class, crowded rooms, and particular classes, e.g., school band. Carriage can be reduced by vaccine (~3.5–fold, for 6 months), and chemoprophylaxis with rifampin (also ~3.5–fold, for perhaps 1 month).

Outbreaks   Outbreaks (647, 1774, 3171, 3612, 6705, 8374) in primary and secondary schools in high-income countries are dominated by serogroups B and C. The number of primary cases is often small (2–4), and most (about three fourths) secondary cases occur within 7–14 days of a primary case. By age, setting, and control measures, risks for school and household contacts are increased several fold compared with the population, for rates of 2.5–295/10^5. In the United States in 1994–2002, venues for meningococcal disease outbreaks were primary or secondary schools in 25% (19/76) and colleges in a further 17% (13). Close contacts (e.g., kissing and food halls) should receive chemoprophylaxis, and tetravalent vaccines (A, C, W135, and Y) should be considered.

- High schools and universities (647, 936, 2748, 3157, 5368, 5369, 6432). Carriers rapidly increase in the first week after campus reopens, from 7% (on the first day), to 11% (on the second), 19% (on the third) and 24% (on the fourth). Infection networks, case clusters, and outbreaks have been reported on campus. In the wake of a campus outbreak, carriage in undergraduate students was 25% (147/587), which is an expected range. Risks for invasive disease include freshmen who stay in campus dormitories, and eat in halls. By type of student, reported disease rates on campus are 2–13/10^5 and year, that is several times the rate in populations of the same age. In the United States, tetravalent conjugate vaccine is recommended for freshmen before entry into high school.
- Training centers (3616). At a residential corps training center in the United States, an outbreak caused nine cases.

M. tuberculosis **(219, 1032, 1690, 2279, 5351, 5869, 6074, 6265, 6508, 7535).** Risk of *M. tuberculosis* include delayed diagnosis of sources among students or staff and poorly ventilated classrooms. Infectious cases are a risk that increases with dose shed (smear-positive and cavitation) and exposure time (months undetected). By history of exposure, skin test conversion, or comparison with controls, untreated cases cause latent infections in contacts, at school in 10–65%, on school buses in 30%, and in households in 40–75%, as well as pulmonary or extrapulmonary disease, at school in 0.5–6% of contacts, on buses in 1–2%, and in households in up to 60%. To detect all active disease cases, follow-up may be necessary for up to 2 years after e_0.

Outbreaks   School outbreaks from undetected cases are well-documented in high-income countries; a review in 1965–95 computed ≥34 school outbreaks. At a California high school in 1993, a student infectious for 29 months caused tuberculin skin conversions in 94 (10%) of 928 initially negative students. At a Missouri high school, a 15-year-old student infectious for 6 months was source for five of five household members (three ill and two infected) and 7 (19%) of 67 bus riders (one ill and six infected); in addition, 58 (10%) of 559 school mates were skin reactive.

In Japan, a school teacher infectious for 3 months caused latent infections in 47% (72/153) of students and 5% (3/63) of teachers; despite chemoprophylaxis, four students and two teachers contracted active disease.

S. pneumoniae **(761, 4508, 6264).** The pharynx of ~3.5–35% of school children may yield pneumococci. By place and time, ~3–65% of carried strains are penicillin resistant. Putative risks for carriage include having younger siblings in the household, use of antibiotics, and recent hospitalization.

Outbreaks   Outbreaks of pneumococcal conjunctivitis (4332, 4774, 7611) have been reported at U.S. schools. In New Hampshire in 2002, nontypeable *S. pneumoniae* caused 574 (81 confirmed and 493 probable) cases of conjunctivitis among 5,060 college students, for an attack rate of 11%. Similarly, in Maine in 2002, nontypeable *S. pneumoniae* caused conjunctivitis among 101 (28%) of 361 kindergarten and primary and secondary grade students.

Bacteria: Vaccine Nonpreventable
Chlamydophila **(3238, 5854, 6684).** Colonization and carriage for weeks have been reported in ~6% of schoolchildren. *C. pneumoniae* is a significant cause of community-acquired pneumonia (CAP) in children of school age, for a rate of 0.2/100 per year. School outbreaks have been reported. Reexamination of an outbreak at a boarding school in the United Kingdom in 1980 suggested *C. pneumoniae* as the causative agent; 20 boys, 2 teachers, 1 kitchen worker, and 1 investigator were affected, and person-to-person spread was suspected from a continued single source.

Moraxella **(4730, 6729).** *M. catarrhalis* can circulate in primary and boarding schools. An outbreak of follicular conjunctivitis due to *Moraxella* has been reported.

Mycoplasma **(908, 3238, 3806).** *M. pneumoniae* is a significant cause of CAP in children of school age, for a rate of 0.5/100 per year. School outbreaks have been reported. At a summer camp in Wisconsin in 1978, 71% (139/196) of attendees had evidence of *M. pneumoniae* infection; attack rates decreased with increasing age.

Fungi
Histoplasma. Outbreaks of *H. capsulatum* have been documented in U.S. schools (465, 1296). At a high school

in Indiana in 2001, 77% (523/678) of tested students and staff had serological evidence of infection, and 29% (355/1,207) of exposed individuals were diagnosed acute histoplasmosis; the outbreak source was soil in the school courtyard rototilled after trees had been felled on which birds had roosted. Samples from soil and air filter adjacent to the tilled area grew *H. capsulatum*. In Illinois, in 1980, four workers disturbed piles of bat droppings in the attic of a 100–year-old school building that was inhabited by big brown bats (*Eptesicus fuscus*); 7–10 days later, all four workers, and 16 of 73 visitors of the building contracted acute pulmonary histoplasmosis.

FECES-FOOD CLUSTER, SCHOOLS

Risks (500, 1738, 1954, 2259, 3052, 5602, 6252). School foods are a major risk. In the United States in 2000, >27 million children were served catered school lunches daily. Schools are venues for ~4% (United States and United Kingdom) to ~15% (France) of food-borne outbreaks reported in high-income countries. U.S. schools in 1973–1997 reported 604 food-borne outbreaks (9–44/year; median, 25) with nearly 50,000 cases (1–1,000/outbreak; median, 42). Frequently implicated vehicles were poultry (15% or 50/333 outbreaks) and salads (13% or 42 included poultry, fish, eggs, and potatoes).

Person-to-person spread is unusual in schools. A risk is poor hygiene. Reasons to exclude students from school include acute diarrhea (to recovery plus 24 h), *Norovirus* infection (to recovery plus 3 days), and typhoid fever (to recovery and negative stool culture).

Viruses

ASTV (5569). ASTV can be food borne. In Osaka, Japan, in 1991, epidemic diarrhea affected >4,700 students and teachers at several schools, and food-borne ASTV was implicated.

HAV (38, 752, 1738, 7830). In high-income countries, student-to-student spread is uncommon. Rather, outbreaks at schools have a common source in the community. In U.S. schools in 1973–1997, HAV accounted for 1.5% (9/604) of food-borne outbreaks and 0.5% (232/49,963) of HA cases. In contrast, at a public school in Rio de Janeiro, Brazil, in 1999, in an outbreak with 25 acute HA cases, ~50% of students were susceptible, and spread was person-to-person. In Florence, Italy, in 2002, older siblings of children attending day care were carrying HAV to secondary school, causing an outbreak with 11 student cases and 6 parent cases. Rapid vaccination of school and household contacts can shorten outbreaks. In some settings, routine HBV-HAV combined vaccine programs may be cost-effective.

HEV (3564). HEV can be a hazard in schools in low-income countries. At a college in Pakistan in 1987, a waterborne outbreak caused 133 clinical cases, for an attack rate of ~20%.

Norovirus (1738, 2313, 3929, 4407, 5657, 5889). In U.S. schools in 1973–1997, *Norovirus* accounted for 0.8% (5/604) of food-borne outbreaks and 1.6% (804/49,963) of cases. Given diagnostic difficulties in that period, these figures likely underestimate the *Norovirus* impact. Indeed in the United States in 1997–2000, 13% (31/217) of *Norovirus* outbreaks occurred at schools or day care centers (6–200 cases per outbreak; median, 56); food was implicated in 45% (14/31) of outbreaks. Settings included a college cafeteria in Florida (attack rates of 40% in students and 15% in staff), and a university freshman dining hall in Cambridge, Mass. (attack rate 52%). There is, however, considerable geographic variation. In Kyushu, Japan, schools were venues for 12 (67%) of 18 diarrhea outbreaks by "small round structured viruses." In contrast in the United Kingdom in 1992–2000, only 4% (73/1,877) of laboratory-confirmed *Norovirus* outbreaks occurred at schools.

Rotavirus (2438, 4831, 5039). *Rotavirus* outbreaks have been reported from educational settings. At a university in Washington, D.C., in 2000, in an outbreak with 85 (1.6%) cases among 5,453 students, sandwiches from the campus dining hall were implicated. In Japan in 1988, an outbreak at primary schools caused 675 (22%) cases among 3,102 students. Symptoms were mild, and the outbreak subsided within 2 days; though food was the suspected vehicle, no particular item was implicated. In contrast, in Japan in 2001, 42% (45/107) school children contracted *Rotavirus* diarrhea during a 3-day school trip, likely by person-to-person spread from an index pupil.

Bacteria

Major risks for school-based food-borne outbreaks are transportation, improper holding temperature, and improper handling. Later eating shifts may be associated with an increased risk of food-borne infectious diarrhea. Commercial products such as ice cream are infrequently implicated.

Bacillus (883, 1738, 4545, 7314). Reported settings for *B. cereus* include schools, a university, and a police academy. Free meals served at an excursion were the implicated vehicle in a university outbreak, for an attack rate of 22% (139/643). In U.S. schools in 1973–1997, *B. cereus* accounted for 1% (6/604) of food-borne outbreaks and 0.8% (390/49,963) of cases. In a further 19 (3%) outbreaks, *B. cereus* emetic toxin or staphylococcal enterotoxin was suspected because of the short (≤6 h) incubation period and frequent (≥80%) vomiting.

Clostridium (1738). At a conference for cake decorators in Michigan in 1990, minestrone soup caused *C. perfringens* food poisoning among 76% (32/42) of attendees (6321). In United States schools in 1973–1997, *C. perfringens* accounted for 4% (25/604) of food-borne outbreaks and 4% (2,165/49,963) of cases.

***Campylobacter* (1738, 2541, 8258).** Outbreaks of *Campylobacter* have been well documented in educational settings. Reported vehicles included contaminated school tap water, free school milk and raw milk from school field trips, and school lunches. In U.S. schools in 1973–1997, *Campylobacter* accounted for 1.3% (8/604) of food-borne outbreaks and 0.6% (279/49,963) of cases. In the United Kingdom in 1995–1999, schools were venues for 12% (6/50) of reported *Campylobacter* outbreaks.

***E. coli* (551, 903, 1738, 3595, 7306, 7827).** EAEC, EHEC, and EPEC have been implicated in school outbreaks. Vehicles have included school lunches (e.g., coleslaw and radish sprouts), meals at school camps (e.g., salad and dinner rolls), ice from barrels, and dairy cow feces from visited farms. In U.S. schools in 1973–1997, EHEC (*E. coli* O157:H7) accounted for 0.8% (5/604) of food-borne outbreaks and 0.3% (156/49,963) of cases. In Japan in 1993, an EAEC epidemic caused 2,697 diarrhea cases among primary and junior high school students. In Sakai City, Japan, in 1996, food-borne EHEC caused an epidemic with >5,700 cases among school children. In Finland in 1987, EPEC caused an epidemic at a school that affected 611 students and 39 adults, for an overall attack rate of 72%; although a specific item was not identified, the likely vehicle was food served at the school.

***Salmonella* (1738, 4453, 4828, 5763, 7660).** In U.S. schools in 1973–1997, *Salmonella* accounted for 14% (87/604) of food-borne outbreaks and 15% (7,529/49,963) of cases; implicated serotypes included serovars Enteritidis (44% or 38 of 87 *Salmonella* outbreaks), Typhimurium (24% or 21/87), and Heidelberg (7% or 6/87). Of all *S. enterica* serovar Enteritidis outbreaks reported in the United States in 1985–1999, schools or churches were the venue in 7% (55/841). For serovar Enteritidis frequent vehicles in schools are eggs, poultry, and egg-based desserts such as buns and chocolate mousse. Visually displayed menus were used successfully to overcome recall bias in case-control investigation.

At a school in Madrid, Spain, in 1991, salad prepared by an serovar Typhi carrier was vehicle for 54 typhoid fever cases.

***Shigella* (1365, 1738, 4644).** *Shigella* outbreaks are well documented at schools, from foods or by person-to-person spread. In U.S. schools in 1973–1997, *Shigella* accounted for 1.5% (9/604) of food-borne outbreaks and 2% (1,040/49,963) of cases. In Taiwan, *S. sonnei* affected 730 students (along with *E. histolytica*); the implicated vehicle was contaminated drinking water. At a primary school in the United Kingdom in 1993, canteen food and person-to-person spread of *S. sonnei* were implicated in an outbreak that affected 42% of 327 students and staff.

***V. parahaemolyticus* (1738, 7326).** *V. parahaemolyticus* is an occasional hazard in schools. In U.S. schools in 1973–1997, *V. parahaemolyticus* was identified in 1 of 604 of food-borne outbreaks with eight cases. In Thailand in 1998, fish balls served at a boarding school caused 132 cases, for attack rates of 16% (127/810) among students and 10% (4/41) among teachers.

***Yersinia* (1738, 3632, 7412).** *Yersinia* is an occasional school hazard. In U.S. schools in 1973–1997, *Y. enterocolitica* was identified in 1 of 604 of food-borne outbreaks with 286 cases of whom 50 (17%) were hospitalized. At a primary school in Finland in 1987, 50 infections with *Y. pseudotuberculosis* (34 confirmed and 16 suspected) were diagnosed among 246 children; a vehicle was not identified. In Finland in 2001, a school linked 89 cases (39 culture confirmed) scattered in a northern municipality; iceberg lettuce and eating outside the home were risks implicated epidemiologically.

Protozoa

Enteric protozoa in endemic areas are likely contacted at home and at a preschool age. Conversely in high-income countries, infections likely result from travel to endemic areas during school holidays, or from foods served at home.

***Cryptosporidium* (6058).** At a university in Washington, D.C., in 1998, raw produce served at campus cafeterias was implicated in 92 cases of *C. parvum* diarrhea.

***Giardia* (1738).** In U.S. schools in 1973–1997, *G. lamblia* was implicated in 2 (0.3%) of 604 food-borne outbreaks with altogether 71 cases.

Helminths
Food-borne helminths (900, 1271, 6738). *Ascaris* and *Trichuris* are prevalent in school children in low-income countries. In Sivas City in central Turkey, *Taenia* spp. were detected by the cellophane tape test in 1.6% (32/2,029) of students from six primary schools.

ZOONOTIC CLUSTER, SCHOOLS

Dust, animals at school, and day-active mosquitoes are potential hazards.

In the United Kingdom in 1987, at a school that kept goats and poultry, *C. burnetii* caused an outbreak with five Q fever cases and inapparent further infections (3749). In rural Thailand, dengue transmission was concentrated at two villages and one school (7201). By level of endemicity, from <10% to >50% of students (Table

20.3) can carry *Plasmodium*. Clinical malaria is a cause of absenteeism from school. Transmission in school has not been reported, perhaps because of the nocturnal feeding habits of *Anopheles*.

ENVIRONMENTAL CLUSTER, SCHOOLS

Contaminated school yards and ponds near schools are potential hazards.

Soil. Enteric nematodes (900, 3390, 6738). In tropical countries, hookworms (*Ancylostoma duodenale* and *Necator americanus*) and *S. stercoralis* can be prevalent in school children. **Zoonotic hookworms (259).** At a school in Brazil, cutaneous larva migrans due to *Ancylostoma* affected 6 (38%) of 16 students (37.5%) who were exposed at two playgrounds. ***Toxocara* (967, 3391, 6514).** Seroreactivity has been reported in school children from high- and low-income countries of all continents.

Water (900, 3776). Many surveys from endemic areas show the prevalence of *Schistosoma haematobium*, *S. mansoni*, and *S. japonicum* in school children in endemic areas. Mass treatments have been conducted at schools. Water sites near schools can become foci of transmission, if vector snails are available and students use sites for defecation, urination, and recreational purposes.

SKIN-BLOOD CLUSTER, SCHOOLS

Fungal infections of the skin and hair can be spread person-to-person.

Concordant with first sexual experiences by adolescents, there is a marked increase of STI in the community (see section 14.7). School curricula should include education of safe sex and prevention of IDU. Epistaxis, sports injuries, and fights are potential sources of HBV, HCV, or HIV infection (see section 13.5). However, risks from bleeding trauma are considered small, and much lower than parenteral risks (piercing and IDU) and risks from unsafe sex (6). By national policy, HBV or HAV-HBV vaccines are routinely offered to students. Medical and dental students should be offered prevention as for health workers (see section 12.6).

Viruses

HBV (6, 866, 4429, 6556). In New York City public schools in 1978–1982, staff and students exposed to carriers with mental retardation in class were at increased risk of HBV infection, for seroconversion rates per 100 per year of 0.7 in students and 1.3 in staff. In general, however, transmission risks in schools are considered low. Routine vaccination of neonates or adolescents has contributed to significantly reduce HBV infections in newly admitted students.

HSV (25, 2726). Both HSV1 and HSV2 infect students. **HSV1.** HSV1 infections of the mouth and skin are common in students. In the United States in 1979–1983, 26% of 623 freshmen and 28% of 449 fourth-year students had a history of "cold" (herpetic) sores, and the corresponding anti-HSV1 prevalence was 37% and 46%. **HSV2.** In the same study, none of freshmen and only 1% of fourth-year students gave a history of genital herpes, and the respective anti-HSV2 prevalence was 0.4% and 4.3%. Predictors of HSV2 reactivity were previous STIs, duration of sexual activity, and African-American ethnicity. In Mexico, of 898 students from 92 schools in Morelos State 11–24 years of age, ~6% (51/898) were reactive to HSV2. Females were twice as likely to be infected than males, and unlike other reports, females in junior high school were significantly more often reactive (9.6%) than female university students (3.3%), a difference that was explained by early first intercourse and low use of condoms by junior high students.

Bacteria

***S. aureus* (6, 1738).** MSSA and MRSA strains can colonize the nares, rectum, and vagina of students (see section 14.1), and temporarily also the skin. Infections in students include pyoderma, abscess, and cellulitis. To prevent spread, students with lesions that cannot be safely covered should be excluded from school until lesions are healed. Treatment of MRSA may need expert advice. Enterotoxigenic *S. aureus* has caused outbreaks of food poisoning in schools. In U.S. schools in 1973–1997, *S. aureus* accounted for 10% (60/604) of food-borne outbreaks and 13% (6,591/49,963) of cases of which 319 (5%) needed hospitalization. In most (>80%) outbreaks, handled meat or poultry was the vehicle implicated.

***S. pyogenes* (GAS) (6, 1928, 3652, 4416).** GAS can colonize or infect students. Spread is via droplets, contact, and occasionally droplets on foods. Some 18–28% of school children are pharyngeal carriers. Risks for colonization include crowding and poor home hygiene. GAS pyodermias are managed in the same way as staphylococcal pyodermias.

Outbreaks (1493, 1738, 3368, 4772, 6471). GAS has caused outbreaks of impetigo, pharyngotonsillitis, and scarlet fever in schools. In U.S. schools in 1973–1997, 2 (0.3%) of 604 food-borne outbreaks with 337 cases were attributed to GAS. In The Netherlands, a GAS outbreak affected 21 (72%) of 29 elementary school children within 1 month: five had impetigo, eight had pharyngitis, and eight had scarlet fever; outside of the affected class, a further six children had impetigo, pharyngitis, or scarlet fever. Contacts should be evaluated for GAS and treated if GAS is identified.

Fungi
Tinea capitis (6, 352, 3199). Risks for tinea capitis are crowding and poor hygiene. In London schools, the presence of two or more carriers of *Trichophyton tonsurans* in class was correlated with tinea capitis in students, suggesting person-to-person spread. At a primary school in Kenya, ~40% (68/164) of children had clinically diagnosed tinea capitis, and 30% (50/164) grew *T. tonsurans*. *T. tonsurans* remains viable on combs, hair brushes, and fabrics.

Helminths
***E. vermicularis* (1271, 1325, 5444).** Although primarily prevalent in preschool children (see section 14.3), prevalence in school children can reach 10–40%. Crowding in class increases the risk of person-to-person spread.

Ectoparasites
For pediculosis and scabies, students should be excluded from school until treated (to t_0 plus 24 h) (6).

***Pediculus* (807, 963, 1445, 5374).** Spread of *P. humanus capitis* is person-to-person. Pediculosis is a frequent problem among students of both high-income and low-income countries. For reasons not understood, *P. humanus capitis* may heavily infect some classes and others not at all.

Sarcoptes. Spread of *S. scabiei* is person-to-person, rarely via bedding or clothes.

14.5 MINORITIES
Minorities are small, neglected, or opposing groups who live separately from main populations by religious, linguistic, social, or other barriers.

Magnitude. Worldwide, there are hundreds of ethnic groups ("from Aceh to Yanomami"). Examples of minorities are Pygmies and San, in Africa; American Indian, Amish, and Inuit in America; Aborigines, Hmong, Maori, and Orang Asli in Australasia; and Roma in Europe. In the U.S. 2000 census, one of every four residents reported themselves as a minority. For refugees, see section 11.4; for migrant workers, see Table 15.6; for island populations, see section 5.4; and for adopted children, see section 11.5.

Infections (67, 3324, 3396, 4325, 5581, 6658, 6738, 6832, 7337, 8041, 8425) (Box 14.6). Infection hazards include substandard housing (see section 11.2), proximity to livestock (see section 2.3), invasive rites (see section 18.1), and irregular access to care.

Nomads by their lifestyle evade soil-transmitted helminths and crowding, but run risks of low vaccine coverage and infections from herds and lack of water. Infections typical for nomads include trachoma, tuberculosis, brucellosis, Q fever, and nonvenereal treponematoses. Chronic infections overrepresented in other minorities include pyodermias, scabies, otitis media, tuberculosis, STI, and infections from IDU. At a juvenile correctional facility in Spain in 1993–2000, of delinquent Roma 13–17 years of age ($n = 222$), 22% had incomplete vaccinations, 36% admitted to unsafe sex, 7.6% were seroreactive to HCV, 6.3% to HBV, 2.7% to HIV, and 0.4% to *T. pallidum*.

Community size is critical for the maintenance of human-infective agents. For island populations, see section 5.4. Circulation arrests, if herd immunity is high (and $R_0 < 1$). Conversely, agents persist in susceptible (nonvaccinated) minorities (pockets). Recognition of innate susceptibility or resistance can be confounded by behavior and living conditions. Epidemiological, twin, molecular, and experimental studies suggest, however, that genetic make-up indeed modulates susceptibility, e.g., to prions, HIV, *M. tuberculosis*, and *Plasmodium*. Former markers (blood groups and histocompatibility antigens) are now being replaced by specific descriptions of receptors and metabolic pathways.

DROPLET-AIR CLUSTER: MINORITIES
Minorities that object to vaccines for fundamental reasons can maintain pockets of endemicity and jeopardize control efforts. An unresolved issue is how far communities committed to disease eradication tolerate minority claims of civil liberties, thereby, risking program failure.

Viruses
Viruses likely to circulate in remote minority communities include vaccine-preventable viruses (*Influenzavirus* and MMR), also on contact or during epidemics AdV, PIV, PVB19, *Rhinovirus*, and RSV.

***Influenzavirus* (5414).** In the United Kingdom in 2001–2002, influenza A/H3N2 affected 43% (151/350) of a highly vaccinated religious community. Unusual time (at the end of the season), age group (mainly ≤2 years and few elderly), and communal living (semienclosed) were suggested to have reduced efficacy of the vaccine that was well matched to circulating strains.

Measles virus (1482, 2414, 5042, 5881, 7265, 7714, 7750). Although humans are the only reservoir for measles virus, carriers are not known. This means that susceptible birth cohorts must maintain the virus: ≥15,000 births per year from an estimated minimum population of 0.2–0.5 million people. Probably >95% of people need to be covered with two doses of vaccine to interrupt transmission. Measles outbreaks have occurred

> **Box 14.6** Main agents and infections among minorities, by agent cluster
>
> | | |
> |---|---|
> | Droplet-air | Vaccine-preventable: MMR, *Influenzavirus*, poliovirus; *B. pertussis*, Hib, *M. tuberculosis*, *N. meningitidis*, and *S. pneumoniae*; from outbreaks: AdV, PIV, PVB19, and RSV; *B. dermatitidis* |
> | Feces-food | HAV, *Rotavirus*; *C. botulinum*, *Shigella*; *Cryptosporidium*, *Giardia*, *Toxoplasma*; *Ascaris*, *Trichuris* |
> | Zoonotic | *Plasmodium*; *E. granulosus* |
> | Environmental | *C. tetani*; hookworm, *Strongyloides*, *Toxocara* |
> | Skin-blood | HBV, HCV, retroviruses; pyodermias, bacterial STI (*H. ducreyi*, genital chlamydia, *K. granulomatis*, and *N. gonorrhoea*), nonvenereal *Treponema* (*T. pallidum endemicum*, *T. pallidum pertenue*), *M. leprae*; dermatophytes (*T. tonsurans*); *Hymenolepis*; scabies |

among minorities in North America and West Europe that object to vaccination. In The Netherlands in 1999, an outbreak among a religious minority caused ~3,000 cases, including 3 deaths (0.1%) in children. In the United Kingdom in 1997, an outbreak among an anthroposophic community caused 293 cases in 9 months.

Mumps virus (5867, 7713). Like measles, fresh numbers of susceptibles at high density are needed to maintain the mumps virus in the community. Probably >90% of people need to be covered with two doses of vaccine to interrupt transmission. Nonimmune minorities are vulnerable to outbreaks. On St. Lawrence Island, Alaska, mumps was not known until 1956, when a boy from Fairbanks introduced it, causing an epidemic with 363 cases among indigenous Inuit. In 1997–1999, mumps in an undervaccinated, tight-knit, networking, religious community caused outbreaks in New York, Israel, Russia, and London, United Kingdom, with 144 cases (51 confirmed from antibody in saliva).

PVB19 (1797). Isolated communities may escape PVB19 infection. In Brazil, 43% (231/542) of Belem residents were seroreactive, compared with only 5–11% of 461 American Indian tribe members.

RSV (971). From surveillance data, Alaskan native infants have the highest RSV hospitalization rate recorded worldwide (15.6/100 per year).

Poliomyelitis virus (2141, 4148, 5627, 5758, 6191, 7197). Recent outbreaks of polio among minorities include Jordan in 1991–1992 (37 cases) where vaccine coverage with three doses was 96% overall, but low among children of Bedouins (63%), Pakistani (21%), and Roma (9%); Romania in 1990–1992 (13 cases) mainly among Roma; The Netherlands in 1992–1993 (71 cases and 2 deaths) among a religious group; Bulgaria in 2001 (three cases and two infections) among Roma; Nigeria in 2003 (>350 cases) among fundamentalists; and the United States in 2005 (four infections) among the Amish in Minnesota. From Nigeria in 2003, polio subsequently spread to countries in Africa and Asia. To be 95% sure that local transmission has ceased, ≥0.2 million inhabitants must be free from cases for >3 years.

Rubella virus (3066, 3610, 4974, 6176). In the United States in 1990–1999, 22% (14/65) of outbreaks occurred among religious minorities. In Ohio, Amish often claim exemption from vaccination; in 1990–1991, an outbreak among Amish caused 276 rubella cases (99% in the state). As a result, the rate of congenital rubella rose to 2/100 live births. In The Netherlands in 2004–2005, a rubella outbreak among unvaccinated members of a reformed church caused 309 confirmed cases, including 23 in pregnant women (nine in the first trimester). From ties with a community in Canada, the outbreak spilled into southwest Ontario, with 214 confirmed cases (five in pregnant women).

Bacteria

***B. pertussis* (664, 2254, 6754).** In the United States, pertussis rates are significantly higher (1.7-fold, 95% CI 1.4–2) among Hispanic infants ($60/10^5$) than other infants ($36/10^5$). Outbreaks in unvaccinated minorities have been reported in North America (in Massachusetts) and Europe (among Roma).

***H. influenzae* (2543, 2899, 6414).** African Americans, American Indians (Apache and Navajo), and Alaskan natives seem disproportionately susceptible to invasive Hib disease, perhaps because of deprived living conditions. In Pennsylvania, where Amish were reluctant to accept Hib vaccine, Amish children were at increased risk of *H. influenzae* carriage and invasive Hib disease.

***Mycobacterium*.** Tuberculosis is a risk for minorities, but how much exposure, malnutrition, and innate susceptibility contribute to this risk is uncertain.

- North America (1472, 3741, 4413, 7123). Skin testing confirms minorities (African Americans and American Indians) to be at severalfold increased risk of latent infection. The same is true for active tuberculosis disease. In Canada, the rate of notified tuberculosis was severalfold higher in American Indians on reserves than in the population.

- Australasia (5052, 6352, 8041). Minorities in Taiwan have a severalfold higher tuberculosis mortality than the population. In Australia for 10 years, Aborigines have been at increased risk of disease; in 2001, rates of new cases/10^5 were 10 in indigenous Australians and 1 in Australia-born Caucasians.

***N. meningitidis* (396, 5787, 6904, 8211).** In New Zealand, carriage of *N. meningitidis* was more prevalent in Maoris and Pacific islanders (22–37%) than Caucasians and other ethnicities (11%), and the risk of invasive disease was 2.5–4.5 times higher in the former than the latter. Similarly in Australia, indigenous Australians are at increased risk of invasive disease.

***S. pneumoniae* (67, 571, 726, 850, 4905, 5526, 5821, 6351, 8078).** Increased risks are reported for African Americans, American Indians (Apache and Navajo), Alaskan Natives, indigenous Australians, and Maoris, for both nasopharyngeal carriage and invasive disease. In preschool children, reported rates of invasive disease per 100 per year are 0.1–2.4 in minorities but 0.05 in the (Australian) population. In the United States in 2002, rates of invasive, drug-resistant *S. pneumoniae* disease per 10^5 were 1.5 in African Americans but 0.7 in Caucasians, for a rate ratio of 2.1. Whether these differences are attributable mainly to innate susceptibility or to lifestyle is uncertain. Also, innate mechanisms may not be uniform; rather, local conditions may have selected for ethnicity-specific genetic mechanisms.

Fungi
In the United States, African Americans are reported at increased risk of *B. dermatitidis* (1061) but not *Coccidioides immitis* (67) infections. In Missouri, blastomycosis rates per 10^5 per year were 2.8 in African Americans but 0.6 in Caucasians.

FECES-FOOD CLUSTER: MINORITIES
Prions
Kuru (2576, 2816) was endemic among the Fore ethnicity in the highlands of Papua New Guinea. Spread likely involved ritual cannibalism, but genetic predisposition might have contributed to endemicity.

Viruses
HAV (67, 325, 637, 5000, 5778). In the 1980s, religious communities in the United States experienced HAV outbreaks, including in Indiana (69 cases, attack rate 1.5%) and at the Utah-Arizona border (204 cases, attack rate 5.8%). Up to the 1990s, acute HA was 3–10 times more frequent in American Indians and Alaska Natives than Caucasians; vaccination diminished this gradient. In 2002, reported rates of acute HA per 10^5 were ~4 in American Indians, 2 in African Americans, and ~1 in Caucasians. Similar increased risks are reported for indigenous Australians.

***Rotavirus* (2469, 4449, 6357).** *Rotavirus* among isolated communities was characterized by a sequence of introduction, epidemic spread, abrupt disappearance, and long silence. Outbreaks have affected isolated communities in the Amazon and the Pacific.

Bacteria
Clostridium. C. botulinum. Botulism is an increasing hazard in Alaska, largely because traditional fermentation of foods in barrels (outside the house, below ground, for weeks to months) has been replaced by fast fermentation in plastic containers (inside the house). Of food-borne botulism cases in the United States, more than one fourth is reported in Alaska. In 1950–2000, Alaska recorded 114 outbreaks with 226 cases. ***C. perfringens*** **(4260, 5280).** Necrotizing enteritis due to *C. perfringens* (pigbel) is curiously limited to the highlands of Papua New Guinea.

***H. pylori* (6342).** *H. pylori* is highly endemic in indigenous communities in South America, perhaps from intense transmission within households.

***Shigella* (67, 6410, 7013).** In 1994–1996, *S. sonnei* outbreaks occurred in eight traditional Jewish communities in the United States and Canada, with >1,000 culture-confirmed cases; intercommunity travel was the suspected mode of spread.

American Indians are at increased risk of shigellosis; in Manitoba, Canada, in 1980–1994, rates per 10^5 person-years were 219 in American Indians but 8 in the population. In the United States in 2002, rates of shigellosis reports per 10^5 were ~20 in American Indians and Alaska natives, 17 in African Americans, and 4 in Caucasians. These gradients are explained by poor sanitation and personal hygiene rather than susceptibility. This explanation is supported by rather uniform *Salmonella* reports in the United States (in 2002, rates per 10^5 were ~17 in American Indians and Alaska natives, 11 in African Americans, and 11 in Caucasians).

Protozoa
***Cryptosporidium* (2506).** *Cryptosporidium* can be prevalent in minorities. In Bedouin children in Israel, the prevalence is 2% and the peak rate is 3/100 person-months.

***Giardia* (475, 2506, 7337, 7453).** *G. lamblia* can be prevalent in up to 25% of minorities, e.g., Wichí Aboriginals in northern Argentina, Bedouin children in

Israel, indigenous Australians, and free-camping Roma in France.

***Toxoplasma* (4355, 7015).** By lifestyle and dietary habits, *T. gondii* infections may be absent or hyperendemic in remote minorities. In central Brazil reported seroprevalences in American Indians are 40–100%, and >50% of preschool children can be reactive.

Helminths
Food-borne helminths (5478, 6738, 8425) can be highly prevalent in minorities, e.g., Orang Asli in Malaysia and Queimada in Brasil. The reported prevalence in children is 40–60% for *Ascaris* and 30–90% for *Trichuris*. Likely reasons are poor living conditions, including homes without indoor toilets or tap water.

ZOONOTIC CLUSTER: MINORITIES
Tropical forest people can be exposed to wild mammals and invertebrates, and nomadic pastoralists can be exposed to infected herds and their ectoparasites. Both groups can "bridge" habitats when meeting people on roads, at market places, and in villages.

Viruses
Humans are the only vertebrate reservoir for dengue virus (DENV). The minimum community size needed for this reservoir function is estimated at 0.15–1 million (4147). During the 1981 epidemic in Cuba, African Americans were found to be less susceptible to dengue hemorrhagic fever than Caucasians (841). In the United States in 2002, comparable rates per 10^5 were reported for WNV encephalitis in American Indians (0.2), African Americans (1.1), and Caucasians (0.8) (67).

Bacteria (67, 6524, 6658)
In Chad, 4% of 860 nomadic pastoralists were seroreactive to *Brucella*, and 1% of 368 were reactive to *C. burnetii*. In minority communities, rickettsial infections can be endemic. In Sarawak, Malaysia, *Orientia tsutsugamushi* and *Rickettsia typhi* were endemic in forest communities. In the United States in 2002, comparable rates per 10^5 were reported for Rocky Mountain spotted fever in American Indians (1), African Americans (0.2), and Caucasians (0.4). In contrast, rates of Lyme disease were clearly higher in Caucasians (7.8) than in American Indians (2.1) or African Americans (0.7).

Protozoa
***Trypanosoma cruzi* (1515, 6377, 7337).** Remote American Indian communities may reflect presettlement transmission. High seroprevalence has been reported for forest-dwelling Wichí (18%) in northern Argentina and for hunter-gatherers (12%) in the Paraguayan Chaco, where noninfective *Triatoma sordida* and *T. infestans* were isolated in temporary dwellings and from a bag for carrying belongings. In contrast, none of 168 Xavénte American Indians from reservations in Mato Grosso, central Brazil, tested positive.

Plasmodium. Genetic, nutritional, and immunological mechanisms of resistance to *P. falciparum* and *P. vivax* have been described. In the field, these are difficult to separate from exposure.

Helminths
***Echinococcus* (997, 3891, 4629, 6043, 6803, 7510, 7950).** *E. granulosus* is enzootic-endemic among nomads in Africa, the Middle East, and central Asia. In central Asia, dogs of nomads, traditionally fed viscera, are more likely infected than dogs of sedentary farmers. In New Zealand, traditional fragmented Maori farms and the feeding of raw offal to working dogs in the past maintained infections at a high level.

Filariae (4662, 7817, 7850). Some species seem well adapted to indigenous people. In the Colombian Amazon, *Dirofilaria immitis* is transmitted among Tikuma American Indians and their dogs. Tikuma live in a single house, together with their domestic animals. *Onchocerca volvulus* has been well studied among Yanomami American Indians. Their open houses and scanty clothing favor continued exposure to the vector.

ENVIRONMENTAL CLUSTER: MINORITIES
Bacteria (6698, 7635)
Tetanus. Rites that include tattooing, scarification, or piercing, and male and female circumcision carry a risk of tetanus in unvaccinated persons. The same is true for some traditional methods of umbilical stump treatment.

Helminths
Hookworms and *Strongyloides* (475, 5478, 5701, 6019, 6738, 7337, 7453, 8337, 8425). Hookworms and *Strongyloides* can be prevalent in minorities such as Pygmies in central Africa, Wichí in northern Argentina, Queimada in Paraná, Brazil, Orang Asli in Malaysia, and indigenous Australians. By ethnicity and endemicity, the reported prevalence is 5% to >95% for hookworms and 0–50% for *Strongyloides* (mostly *S. stercoralis*, in central Africa also *S. fuelleborni*). Risks include houses with earth floors and lack of toilets. In France in 1993, *S. stercoralis* was isolated in 18% (8/45) of Roma from seven families who lived in an informal camp in scrub vegetation (garrigue) without sanitation.

***Toxocara* (7337).** A surprisingly high seroprevalence of *Toxocara* of 22% was reported from Wichí Aboriginals in northern Argentina.

SKIN-BLOOD CLUSTER: MINORITIES
Viruses
Viruses likely to circulate in remote minority communities include CMV, EBV, HBV, HCV, HSV, VZV, *Retroviridae* (e.g., HIV, human T-lymphotropic virus [HTLV], and SiFV), and *Polyomaviridae* (e.g., BK virus).

HBV. HBV can be hyperendemic in many ethnicities.

- Tropical Africa (4083, 5286). Hepatitis B surface antigen (HbsAg) prevalence of 6–12% is reported for Manos in Liberia, Bantu and Pygmy in Cameroon, Korekore in Zimbabwe, and Turkana in Kenya.
- United States (67, 362, 1165, 3150). High-risk minorities include American Indians of North and South America, African Americans, Alaskan natives, Pacific islanders, and children in households of immigrants from endemic countries. In central Brazil, the HBsAg prevalence among American Indians is 4.5%. In the prevaccine era, 13% (189/1,479) of Alaskan natives tested positive for HBsAg. In 2002, reported rates of acute HB/10^5 were 5.6 in American Indians and Alaska natives, 3.9 in African Americans, 2.2 in Pacific islanders, and 1.5 in Caucasians.
- Australasia (2736, 5268). As an example, HBsAg prevalence of 12–36% is reported from tribes of the Andaman and Nicobar islands and Karen. HBV is also hyperendemic among indigenous Australians. In schoolchildren from western Australia in 1986, the HBV marker prevalence was 28% (78/275) in Aboriginals and nil (0/300) in Caucasians.

HCV (4083, 4528). Risks of HCV seem to resemble those of HBV. Anti-HCV prevalence of 13–19% has been reported from forest people in southern Cameroon.

Retroviruses. HIV (2055). By lifestyle (traditional or not) and remoteness (economic pressure, war, and access to preventive services), minorities may escape HIV infection or be at increased risk. In the United States, mortality from AIDS is disproportionately high in African Americans. **HTLV (2055, 3347, 4846, 4943).** HTLV2 is endemic among Pygmy in central Africa and American Indians in North and Latin America. **Simian foamy virus (SiFV) (5805, 8243).** Infections have been reported from hunter and gatherer communities in sub-Saharan Africa. Road construction, migration, and sex work favor the escape of SiFV and related viruses from remote forest populations to villages, market places, and larger settlements.

Bacteria
Bacteria likely to circulate in remote minority communities include *C. trachomatis*, *H. ducreyi*, *Klebsiella granulomatis* (donovanosis, e.g., among Australian natives) (5244), *Neisseria gonorrhoeae*, and *Treponema pallidum pallidum*. Disparities of STI risks seem largely to result from high-risk behavior and poor case management of minorities rather than innate susceptibilities.

Trachoma, non-venereal *Treponema*, and *M. leprae* are endemic in some minority communities in low-income countries.

STI. *C. trachomatis* (67, 5059). In a representative sample of U.S. adults 18–26 years of age, genital infection by NAT from first-void urine was more prevalent in African Americans than in Caucasians, both in females (14%: 95% CI 11–17, versus 2.5%: 95% CI 2–3.5) and males (11%: 95% CI 9–14, versus 1.5%: 95% CI 1–2). In 2002, reported rates of genital *C. trachomatis* per 10^5 were 806 in African Americans, 512 in American Indians, 108 in Pacific islanders, and 90 in Caucasians. **H. ducreyi (2442, 3110).** In the United States, a high proportion of chancroid is diagnosed in African Americans. In an outbreak in Winnipeg, Canada, in 1975–1977, mainly American Indians and Métis who lived in a deprived inner-city area were affected. **N. gonorrhoeae (67, 1823, 5059).** High gonorrhea rates have been reported among some minorities, in particular, in North America and less in Australia. In a representative sample of U.S. adults 18–26 years of age, the prevalence of genital infection by ligase chain reaction from first-void urine was ~20-times higher in African American males and females (2%, 95% CI 1.5–3) than in Caucasian males and females (0.1%, 95% CI 0.03–0.3). In 2002, reported rates of gonorrhea per 10^5 were 570 in African Americans, 96 in American Indians, 18 in Pacific islanders, and 24 in Caucasians. In northern Alberta, Canada, an outbreak in 1999–2001 affected 81 individuals 15–60 years of age from eight neighboring communities. Cases were associated with visits at a public bar, multiple sex partners, and mostly (96%) among American Indians. **T. pallidum pallidum (67, 3511, 4671, 4673).** Syphilis can be endemic among minorities. In the United States in 2002, reported rates of primary and secondary syphilis per 10^5 were 9.4 in African Americans, 2.3 in American Indians, 0.8 in Pacific islanders, and 1.1 in Caucasians. In the far north of western Australia, syphilis rates were >700/10^5 in 1986 and ~200/10^5 in 1998. In the Kimberley in 2000–2002, 74 cases of early syphilis (32% primary, 39% secondary, 28% latent, and 1% congenital) were reported among residents; except for one, all were Aborigines. In the United Kingdom in 1994–1997, of women treated for syphilis in pregnancy, more than three fourths (106) were of Black (African and Caribbean), Asian (Indian and Chinese), other, or unknown ethnicity; less than one fourth (33/139) were Caucasians.

Nonvenereal infections. *C. trachomatis* (2278, 6833). Trachoma is a disease of poor living conditions. It can be hyperendemic in remote communities. An example is

Australian Aborigines. Obstacles to control include continued poor housing, mobility within and between communities, and poor treatment compliance. **M. leprae (402, 4527, 4578).** *M. leprae* can persist in minorities. On small islands off Sulawesi, Indonesia, in 2000, 96 cases (85 new and 11 known) were detected among 4,140 inhabitants, for a prevalence of 2%. Leprosy was clustered on islands and in households. In Australia in 1951, an outbreak affected Aborigines in the Northern Territory, for an attack rate of 0.3%. In 1922–1950, leprosy hit the island of Rapa 1,100 km southeast of Tahiti, with 230–408 inhabitants on 22 km^2. New cases peaked in 1935–1939, for a rate of 1/100/year, while disease prevalence peaked in 1959, with 6.8%. **S. pyogenes (GAS) (764, 2359, 2846, 6833, 7198).** GAS skin infections can be prevalent among minorities such as Australian natives. Probably by crowding and from GAS on skin, Aborigines are at increased risk of rheumatic fever and glomerulonephritis. In the United States, acute rheumatic fever has mainly been a disease of underprivileged children living in inner cities.

Treponema. Nonvenereal treponematoses can confound serological tests for syphilis in minorities. **T. pertenue (237, 1817, 3284, 6739).** Yaws can persist in tropical forest communities in central Africa, the Amazon, and the southwestern Pacific, including Vanuatu and Papua New Guinea. ***T. pallidum endemicum* (1667, 5142).** Bejel persists in a few nomad communities in arid areas with scarce water for body hygiene. In West Africa, 3–84% of roaming or sedentary nomads are seroreactive, and active lesions confirm that transmission is ongoing. For highly infected sedentary nomads, the only water supply was ~10 km away. Public waterskins contaminated by customers with buccal lesions are a putative source of bejel. In Saudi Arabia in 1976–1980, 276 (17%) of 1,620 nomads were seroreactive.

Fungi
Candida **(1593).** Oral and vaginal colonization by *Candida* are likely increased in communities endemic for HIV infection. In the United States, African American women have been reported at increased risk of vaginal carriage during pregnancy.

Tinea capitis (4479, 7772). In North America, for reasons poorly understood, *T. tonsurans* is endemic in African American children but sporadic in Caucasians. In California in 1993, griseofulvin prescriptions as a surrogate for tinea capitis provided attack rates of 2.5% in African American children and of 0.2% in Caucasian or Hispanic children.

Helminths
Hymenolepis **(475, 7453).** Maintained by person-to-person spread, *H. nana* can be endemic in minorities, e.g., Australian Aborigines and free-camping Roma in France.

Ectoparasites
Sarcoptes **(1072, 8251).** Scabies is endemic in Australian natives, as are pyodermias associated with scabies.

14.6 LATENCY, REACTIVATION, AND IMMUNE IMPAIRMENT

There is only a thin veneer protecting humankind from potentially devastating infectious disease epidemics.

J. Lederberg et al. (4292)

Latency is the silent presence of agents (dormant metabolism, slow propagation, and low gene expression) in cells (preferrably long-lived) or tissues. It follows manifest, mild, or inapparent primary infection. Latency lasts months, years, or decades. Month- or year-long incubation periods can mimick latency (e.g., CJD and tuberculosis). Unlike carriage (see section 14.1) or reactivation, latently infected individuals are not usually infective.

Relapse is the rebounding manifestation of disease during treatment or antimicrobial washout, indicating clinical treatment failure. Reactivation (Box 14.7) is the revival of an agent from latency, either manifest by new symptoms (e.g., vivax malaria) or silent by resumed shedding (e.g., HSV). Because primary and reactivated agents are identical, molecular fingerprinting helps to separate reactivation from reinfection. Triggers of reactivation include intercurrent infections and invasive interventions.

Resistance is the set of mechanisms that prevents agents from accessing or infecting hosts. Innate (natural) resistance relies on intact barriers, instantaneous activity of complement and leukocytes, and nonexpression of receptors. Acquired (adaptive) resistance is antigen driven and relies on the time-consuming recruitment of immune-competent cells and production of local and circulating Ig. Immune impairment (Box 14.8) is the clinically relevant malfunctioning of innate or acquired resistance.

Box 14.7 Triggers of shedding or manifest reactivation	
Constitution	Age (preterm, >80 years), pregnancy, innate immune impairment, end-stage organ disease
Susceptibility	Past infections (e.g., HIV, varicella, and tuberculosis), vaccines, known antibodies, minority groups
Lifestyle	Injection drug use, alcoholism, smoking, homelessness, and malnutrition
Medical	Devices, transfusions, transplants, implants, suppressive treatments (malignancy, neutropenia)

> **Box 14.8** History pointing to innate or acquired immune impairment
>
> **Risky lifestyle**
> - Have you ever taken illicit drugs? If so, which? Have you ever injected drugs? If so, was it by "popping" or into vein? Have you ever shared injections?
> - Have you ever had an HIV test? If so, what was the result? Were you ever told you had AIDS or were HIV infected?
> - What is the number of sex partners you have had in your life? Have you ever had sex with a member of the same sex?
>
> **Poor defense**
> - Were you ever told you did not respond to skin antigens (e.g., tuberculin), vaccines (e.g., HBV), or antimicrobials?
> - Have you had any infections last for over 2 weeks (e.g., fever, cough, or diarrhea) or recur over 1–3 months (e.g., herpes)?
> - Were you ever told you carried or shed an agent (e.g., HBV, *S. enterica* serovar Typhi, fungi, and worms)?
>
> **Poor healing**
> - Have you had any wound that did not heal in 2 weeks? Have you had any wound infections? Any gingivitis? Umbilical stump festering?
>
> **Treatments**
> - Have you taken any antimicrobial in the preceding 3 months? If so, which and when? Have you had any syringe abscess or device infection (e.g., catheter)?
> - Have you ever been hospitalized for an infection? If so, what kind and when? Have you ever had a life-threatening infection (e.g., sepsis)?

Acquired causes include malnutrition, injection drug use, lymphotropic (anergy-inducing) agents such as HIV, measles, *Mycobacterium*, and *Leishmania*, comorbidity (e.g., diabetes and end-stage organ disease), medications that induce neutropenia (neutrophils <1,000/µl, even <500–100/µl), and barrier-disruptive devices.

Exposure (Boxes 14.7 and 14.8). The longer the incubation period, the less likely is the recall of exposure. Examples of diseases with long incubation periods and typically a blank exposure history include CJD, leprosy, and echinococcosis. In patients with nonrevealing exposure history, endogenous or reactivated agents should be considered (Boxes 14.7 and 14.9). The history may provide clues that point to immune impairment. (Box 14.8).

Infections (Box 14.9). Latent infections are recognized in asymptomatic individuals by sensitive skin, blood, or other screening tests, in pregnant women from intrauterine infections or perinatal transmission (see section 14.7), and in donors of blood, tissues, or organs from transfusion- and transplant-associated infections in recipients (see sections 18.4 and 18.5). Latent infections may have serious consequences, including oncogenesis.

Immune-impaired hosts (Box 14.10). A review of infections in immune-impaired hosts (56, 573, 1992, 2142, 2381, 3315, 5821, 5900, 6519, 6719, 6781, 7653, 8229) in general, and in AIDS patients in particular is beyond the scope of this book. A few noteworthy points follow.

> **Box 14.9** Latent agents that can be reactivated or have long-term effects, by agent cluster
>
> *Oncogenic agents.
>
> | | |
> |---|---|
> | Droplet-air | PVB19, VZV; *M. tuberculosis*; *Histoplasma*, *Pneumocystis* |
> | Feces-food | *H. pylori* (*gastric adenocarcinoma); *E. histolytica*, *Toxoplasma*; *C. sinensis* (*cholangiocarcinoma) |
> | Zoonotic | Rabies virus; *Bartonella*, *Borrelia*, *Brucella*, *R. prowazekii*; *Leishmania*, *P. malariae*, *P. vivax*, *T. cruzi*; *E. granulosus*, filiariae, *T. solium*-cysticercosis |
> | Environmental | *B. pseudomallei*; *Strongyloides*, *Schistosoma* (**S. haematobium*: bladder carcinoma), *Toxocara* |
> | Skin-blood | Variant CJD, CMV, EBV (*lymphoma, nasopharyngeal carcinoma), HBV (*liver carcinoma), HCV (*liver carcinoma), HHV8 (*sarcoma), HIV, HSV, HPV, HTLV1 (*T-cell leukemia), polyomavirus; *Treponema* |

> **Box 14.10** Agents and infections in immune-impaired hosts, by cluster
>
> Risks are shown in parentheses. *AIDS-defining conditions.
>
> Droplet-air PVB19 (sickle cell disease), VZV; *H. influenzae* (asplenia, Ig-deficiency), *M. tuberculosis* (malnourished, suppressive treatment, *if manifest), *N. meningitidis* (asplenia, Ig-deficiency), *S. pneumoniae* (suppressive treatment, sickle cell disease, asplenia, Ig-deficiency), *Cryptococcus* (*if extrapulmonary), *Histoplasma* (*if disseminated), *Pneumocystis* (*if pneumonia), other respiratory fungi (neutropenia, suppressive treatment)
>
> Feces-food *C. difficile* (necrotizing colitis: neutropenia), *Enterococcus* (suppressive treatment), *Listeria* (suppressive treatment), *Salmonella* (suppressive treatment, *if sepsis), *Y. enterocolitica* (β-thalassemia); *Encephalitozoon*; *Cryptosporidium* (*if chronic diarrhea), *Cyclospora*, *Toxoplasma* (suppressive treatment, *if encephalitis)
>
> Zoonotic *Babesia* (asplenia), *Leishmania* (HIV), *Plasmodium* (malnourished, possibly HIV coinfection)
>
> Environment (All neutropenia): *Alcaligenes*, *Capnocytophaga*, environmental mycobacteria (* if disease), *Fusobacterium*, *Lactobacillus*, *Leuconostoc*, *Pseudomonas*-ecthyma, *Rhodococcus*, *Stenotrophomonas*, *Stomatococcus*; *Scedosporium*, *Trichosporon*; *Strongyloides* (corticosteroids, transplant)
>
> Skin-blood CMV (*if retinitis), HHV8 (*if sarcoma), HIV (*if encephalopathy), HPV (*if squamous cell carcinoma), HSV (*if chronic); *C. jeikeium* (neutropenia), *Staphylococcus* (*S. aureus*, CoNS: suppressive treatment); *Candida* (*if esophagitis).
>
> **Syndromes**
>
> Recurrent respiratory tract infections (neutropenia, Ig-deficiency, *if bacterial pneumonia), chronic UTI (neutropenia, malnourished), BSI (neutropenia, malignancy), anergy (HIV, measles, end-stage organ disease, malnourished), gingivitis (neutropenia), and reactivation (suppressive treatment)

- Cystic fibrosis patients are susceptible to bacterial infections of the airway, including the "wet agents" *Burkholderia cepacia*, *Pseudomonas aeruginosa*, *Ralstonia pickettii*, and *Stenotrophomonas maltophilia*.
- Of neutropenic patients with fever (axillary temperature, ≥37.5°C, oral temperature ≥38°C), ≥50% will have an infection. Bacteremia and fungemia are particular risks for neutropenic patients. Of febrile patients with ≤100/μl neutrophils, ≥20% are bacteremic.
- AIDS patients (701, 1992, 2105, 3626, 5096, 5117, 5453, 6487, 6638). Infections include diarrhea (*Cryptosporidium* and microsporidia), pneumonia (recurrent bacterial, mycobacterial, and PCP), fever (sepsis), and encephalitis (viral, *Cryptococcus*, and *Toxoplasma*).

General features that distinguish infections in immune-impaired from immune-competent hosts include broad agent spectrum, multiple and unusual infection sites, tissue invasion and dissemination, minimal inflammatory response, inadequate treatment response, and shedding of larger quantities of viable agents, over longer periods (months rather than days) and from more sites.

Preventive measures. Preventive measures include promoting awareness, testing and counseling, vaccines, early treatment, partner information, safe lifestyle (e.g., sex, injection materials), and planned PEP.

Vaccines. Vaccines should be offered pretransplant and pretreatment, at a time when an adequate immune response is still likely. Patients with surgical or functional asplenia benefit from vaccines against encapsulated bacteria (Hib, *N. meningitidis*, and *S. pneumoniae*). Live vaccines, in general, are contraindicated in hosts with advanced immune dysfunction. In stem cell recipients, immune restoration takes ≥2 years from donation. Postvaccinal antibody testing is advisable when immune vigor is in doubt.

Screening (20). A basic screen for any immune impairment could include tuberculin skin test, leukocyte count, and total Ig. For HIV screening (ELISA), proposed indications are: client demand, member of a risk group (IDU, sex with a HIV-infected person, sex among men, sex for drugs, and more than one sex partner), suggestive illness (suspected acute AIDS, tuberculosis, and AIDS-defining opportunists), pregnancy, or occupational exposure. For HIV infection that is confirmed by Western blot, basic tests might include: viral load, complete blood count including CD4 cells, tuberculin skin test, serology for CMV, HBV (HBsAg, anti-HBs), HCV, *T. pallidum*, and *T. gondii*, and urine by NAT for *C. trachomatis* and *N. gonorrhoeae*.

Treatment (5096). Highly active antiretroviral therapy has changed opportunistic infections in AIDS patients. In Europe, the rate of AIDS-defining illnesses per 100 person-years was reduced from 30 (95% CI 28–33) in 1994 to 3 (95% CI 2–3) in 1998.

LATENT PRIONS

CJD (3323, 3331, 5107, 5794, 6091) (Table 14.2). Diagnostic tests for incubating CJD are sorely missed. Before invasive procedures, and for processing instru-

Table 14.2 Risks from patients with CJD or their organs

Level of risk	Type of individual	Organs or tissues
High	Patients with unclear progressive neurosyndromes (e.g., ataxia, paresthesia, or dementia) suspected of CJD	Brain, spinal cord, dura mater, pituitary gland, eye (retina, nerve), all[a]
Moderate	Persons with a suspected history: growth hormone, dura mater, prion diseases in family, residence in the United Kingdom in 1986–2000	Cerebrospinal fluid,[a] lymph nodes,[a] spleen, liver, lung, kidney, placenta. For variant CJD, also tonsils,[a] appendix, blood
Low or none	Healthy population	Saliva, urine, feces, skin, muscle, bone marrow

[a] Instruments in contact with these organs or tissues should be considered high risk.

ments, risks from patients with suspected CJD or their organs should be evaluated. Risk evaluation is advised before endoscopy (in particular, with biopsy), ear-nose-throat surgery (in particular, tonsillectomy), donation of blood and organs, and autopsy.

LATENT VIRUSES

Many systemic viral infections cause viremia that lasts hours to days. Latent viruses with eventual reactivation (one or intermittent episodes) include *Herpesviridae* (CMV perhaps in leucoid progenitor cells, EBV in B lymphocytes, and HSV and VZV in neuronal cells), *Retroviridae* (HIV and HTLV both in T lymphocytes), HBV and HCV (both in hepatocytes), HPV (in epithelia), polyomaviruses, PVB19 (in erythroid progenitor cells), and rabies virus (in neuronal cells). NAT and antigen tests can detect inapparent reactivation that is significant for transmission.

Herpesviridae. **CMV (2038, 4955, 5198, 7382, 8382).** While immune-competent individuals tend to suppress viremia, infections can persist in immune-compromised patients. Triggers of reactivation include breast-feeding, transplantation, and immune-suppressive treatments. By type and follow-up, triggers typically reactivate 30–65% of latent infections (with extremes of ~5–100%). Reactivation during pregnancy is not usually associated with intrauterine transmission. **EBV (3609, 7086, 7477).** Following primary infection, EBV can persist in peripheral lymphocytes of immune-competent individuals. Reactivation can be demonstrated in oropharyngeal lymphoid tissues, or in blood by NAT. Kidney transplants appear to trigger early reactivation, that is in the first week of immune-suppressive treatment. **HSV (5974, 6650).** Triggers of reactivation include febrile illness, coinfection with HIV, suppressive treatments, and invasive interventions, including transplantation. Manifestations of reactivation include labial, buccal, and genitoanal lesions, Stevens-Johnson syndrome, pneumonia, encephalitis, and disseminated disease. Silent and manifest HSV2 reactivations are particularly frequent in HIV-infected adults. By antiretroviral treatment, HIV-infected men may shed HSV2 on 10% to >25% of all days, compared with <5% of all days in HIV-negative homosexual men. HIV-infected men reported genitoanal lesions on 3–11% of all days. **HHV8 (1128, 3686).** From primary infection HHV8 persists for life. Seroprevalence cumulates with age, to reach 20–60% in endemic areas of the Mediterranean and Africa. HHV8 is associated with Kaposi's sarcoma. Reactivation goes along with shedding from saliva. **VZV (301, 2561, 4953, 6790, 7458).** Relapsing varicella is rare. Decreasing protection from vaccination can result in mitigated, clinical varicella. Acute-type immune responses and NAT confirm the occurrence of inapparent reactivations or reinfections in immune-compromised and -competent hosts. In general, symptomatic reactivations are manifest as zoster. However unusual manifestations are reported, e.g., in children and immune-impaired individuals, including facial paralysis, Guillain-Barré syndrome, pneumonia, or dissemination. Triggers of reactivation include transplantation, suppressive treatment, surgery, intercurrent infections, e.g., with EBV, HIV, or *Plasmodium*, and stress.

Other latent viruses. HBV (749, 2676, 3605, 4088). HBV can become latent and oncogenic. Some 80% of cases of primary liver cancer are attributable to chronic HBV. Therefore, even low HBsAg prevalence is undesirable, calling for prevention by vaccine. In the 1990s, the reported HBsAg prevalence was ~0.5% in Canada, 1–2% in Italy, Spain, and Portugal, ~0.7% in Germany, 0.4% in the United Kingdom, and 0.05% in Scandinavia. **Polyomaviruses (BKV, JCV, Simian virus 40[SV40]) (3344, 4164, 5962, 7826).** Polyomaviruses have low virulence and long latency in humans. BKV and JCV are aquired in childhood, and latent infections persist for life. Immune impairment can trigger reactivation. Serious complications associated with reactivation include nephropathy (BKV), progressive multifocal leukoencephalopathy (JCV), and mesothelioma (SV40), but causation is uncertain. Reactivation in healthy individuals results in inapparent excretion of BKV and JCV. **PVB19 (2444, 5295, 8351).** While immune-competent patients clear viremia,

PVB19 can persist in immune-compromised hosts for years. **Rabies virus (1239, 1267).** The incubation period for rabies virus can exceed 1 year. In the United States and Germany, organs from a donor incubating unrecognized rabies caused fatal rabies in recipients. Donors from areas where rabies is enzootic in terrestrial animals or bats should be considered for screening.

Latent Bacteria

Bacteria that can become latent include intracellular *Bartonella*, *Brucella*, *Chlamydia*, *Helicobacter*, *Mycobacterium*, and *Rickettsia*, as well as extracellular *Borrelia*, *Burkholderia*, and *Treponema*.

Bartonella quintana **(2471).** Trench or "quintan" fever was characterized by fever for a few days that recurred at intervals of 4–6 days.

Borrelia. **Lyme borreliosis (*B. burgdorferi* sl) (4488, 7111, 7128).** Lyme borreliosis infections that escape early recognition and treatment can cause joint, neurological, or cardiac complications, typically weeks or months after primary infection, occasionally after years. **Louse-borne (LBRF, *B. recurrentis*) and tick-borne (TBRF, *B. duttonii* and other borreliae) relapsing fevers (7111).** Characteristic are fevers that relapse, typically after afebrile intervals of 3–30 days.

Brucella **(7346, 8135).** *Brucella* can cause latent or chronic infections manifest for ≥6 months by vague, flulike symptoms, night sweats, and lassitude. In Turkey, of 119 confirmed cases, 15% (18) were classified as relapses.

Burkholderia **(4623, 4859, 5842, 6035).** *B. pseudomallei* is a "retarded tropical bomb" (5842) that can be latent for years or decades, to become manifest by febrile or tuberculosis-like illness (melioidosis).

H. pylori **(7636, 7759).** After years of latency, *H. pylori* can cause peptic ulcer disease. Untreated *H. pylori* can be oncogenic, with a lifetime risk of gastric neoplasia of ~0.1% to 3%.

M. tuberculosis **(1173, 4199, 7033).** Latent *M. tuberculosis* infections can progress to active tuberculosis months to decades after the primary infection. The risk of progression per 100 person-years is greatest in the first year after e_0 (~1.3), decreasing in the next 6 years (to ~0.2). Risks are 0.2–1.4 in persons with residues on chest radiography and 3.5–16 in HIV-infected persons. Concepts of progression and reactivation were challenged by molecular fingerprinting that uncovered reinfection in postprimary tuberculosis. Of South African miners with culture-confirmed tuberculosis monitored for 1–3 years, 36% (14/39) had reinfections, and 64% (25) had reactivations; risks of reinfection per 100 person-years were much greater in HIV-infected miners (11) than in HIV-negative miners (0.4). To prevent progression, latent infections should be detected (contact tracing and targeted screening) and treated.

Rickettsia prowazekii **(4580, 6494, 7138, 7339, 7610).** *R. prowazekii* can be latent for years or decades. Amazingly, cases of reactivation (Brill-Zinsser disease) continue to be reported in the 1990s, both in North America and Europe.

Treponema. T. pallidum pallidum **(5836, 6917).** About 10–15% of untreated infections result in tertiary syphilis, after year-long latency (or incubation, if primary and secondary phases are bypassed). Reported latency periods are 1–46 years for "late benign syphilis" (manifest by gummas), 5–20 years for "neurosyphilis" (manifest by dorsal tabes and progressive paralysis), and 10–30 years in "cardiovascular syphilis" (manifest by aortitis and aneurysm). *T. pallidum pertenue* **(3043).** Reactivations were reported in the 1940s in South African mines.

LATENT FUNGI

Latent and reactivated fungi include the opportunists *Blastomyces*, *Coccidioides*, *Histoplasma*, *Paracoccidioides*, and *Pneumocystis*. Except *Pneumocystis*, skin test reactivity can demonstrate latent infection.

Blastomyces **(2054).** Reactivations of *B. dermatitidis* have been reported in expatriates up to 30 years after exposure in endemic areas.

Cryptococcus **(3514, 5088).** Latent *C. neoformans* infections have been suggested by fingerprinting, serosurveys, and routine autopsy findings.

Histoplasma **(135, 2989, 5335).** From skin test surveys, >95% of sporadic primary *H. capsulatum* infections are inapparent. Latent infections can be reactivated by immune-suppressive treatments, transplantation, or intercurrent HIV infection. Reactivations can occur 5–10 years after exposure in endemic areas. Reactivated histoplasmosis can manifest as pulmonary, ocular, or disseminated disease.

P. jirovecii **(4720, 5313, 7904, 8239).** As with tuberculosis, the concept of PCP from reactivation needs revision because some cases likely result from reinfection. Arguments in favor of reinfection include clusters from common exposure, molecular identity of clustered strains, and high turnover of strains in carriers of *P. jirovecii*. From 2% to 21% of PCP is estimated to be newly acquired from human sources.

Paracoccidioides **(103, 944, 4718, 5390).** Reactivations of *P. brasiliensis* have been reported in expatriates from months to 60 years after exposure in endemic areas.

LATENT PROTOZOA

Latent and reactivated protozoa include tissue-dwelling *Babesia, Entamoeba, Leishmania, Plasmodium, Toxoplasma,* and *Trypanosoma*. Unlike reactivated viruses, reactivated protozoa are potential sources of intrauterine infection.

Babesia **(2859, 3410, 4099, 4329, 6715, 8006).** Inapparent *Babesia* infections are documented in humans and well-known in animals. Of 18 blood donors monitored for 2 years, 10 (56%) had inapparent parasitemia by PCR and/or hamster inoculation. In the eastern United States, *B. microti* DNA was amplified from the blood of untreated persons for up to 24 months. However, reactivation has not been reported. Predisposing to disease manifestation are advanced age, coinfections, and splenectomy (mainly *B. divergens* in Europe).

Entamoeba **(3375, 6146).** *E. histolytica* can be latent for 10–30 years before disease becomes manifest. In particular, amebic liver abscess (ALA) can develop months, years, or decades after exposure, although in travelers returning from endemic areas, 95% of ALA is stated to occur within 5 months.

Leishmania. **Visceral leishmaniasis (VL) (724, 4271).** For anthroponotic VL, humans are the only vertebrate reservoir, mainly primary infections in children with a long incubation period, inapparent infections, and post-kala azar dermal leishmaniasis. For zoonotic VL, humans are incidental hosts. However, *L. infantum* can circulate in the blood of healthy, seroreactive individuals at low density. Latent VL can be reactivated by triggers such as intercurrent HIV infection. **Cutaneous leishmaniasis (CL) (1695, 6614, 8008).** In Colombia, of 77 cases with active cutaneous lesions, one third (24) represented new infections, while two thirds had scars suggestive of reactivations (or reinfections). Also in Colombia, from fingerprinting of *L. braziliensis*, 12 of 24 patients had reactivations, and 12 had reinfections. Median times from primary to secondary lesions was 1–28 (typically 5.5) months in reactivations but 6–60 (19.5) months in reinfections, and the proportion of secondary lesions within 0–5 cm of primary lesions was 75% (9/12) in reactivations, but only 17% (2/12) in reinfections. Reported triggers of reactivation include suppressive treatments, HIV infection, and surgery. An elderly man developed cutaneous leishmaniasis after surgery for a basalioma of the face; the man had not left the United Kingdom for 20 years, and likely exposure dated back 50 years.

Plasmodium **(1702, 2090, 2801, 4059, 7495, 7839).** Latent liver infections (hypnozoites) resistant to "noncausal" antimalarials are characteristic for *P. vivax* and *P. ovale* that cause relapsing malaria. Vivax malaria relapses occur after 1–4 months (tropical strains) to 6–12 months, occasionally after 1–4 years (temperate or "hibernans" strains). In contrast, untreated *P. malariae* remains subpatent (perhaps in red blood cells) to be reactivated after years or decades ("quartan" malaria). *P. falciparum* does not develop hypnozoites, nor is it latent for more than about 1 year. In partially immune residents of endemic areas, all four plasmodia infective to humans can cause patent, inapparent parasitemia. By age, season, and test (microscopy and PCR), typical parasitemia prevalence is 15–30% in sub-Saharan Africa (>90% by *P. falciparum*), 10% in the Amazon (5–75% by *P. falciparum*), 1–25% in Southcentral Asia (15–75% by *P. falciparum*), and 0–25% in Southeast Asia (up to 60–80% *P. falciparum*).

T. gondii **(21, 3133, 3392, 3756, 4058, 4854, 7923).** Congenital toxoplasmosis can take months to years to become manifest. After primary infection, *T. gondii* "bradyzoites" persist for life, inside cysts located in the brain, eye, or virtually any other organ or tissue. After months, years, or decades, infections can reactivate, releasing "tachyzoites" into the bloodstream. Disease manifestations of reactivated toxoplasmosis include uveitis, in immune-compromised hosts encephalitis and congenital infection.

T. cruzi **(1785, 3955, 4248, 8099).** Resolution of acute Chagas disease is followed by latency in muscle and neuronal cells. Latency can be accompanied by subpatent parasitemia detectable by xenodiagnosis. After years, even decades, chronic disease can become manifest. Immune suppression in transplant recipients can reactivate Chagas disease.

LATENT HELMINTHS

Both intestinal and tissue helminths can be latent for months or years, in particular, light infections in travelers. Helminths with potentially serious long-term health effects (Box 14.9) include *Clonorchis, Echinococcus, Schistosoma, Strongyloides, T. solium* cysticercosis, *Toxocara, Trichinella,* and *Wuchereria*. Screening is performed on stool samples for *Clonorchis, S. japonicum, S. mansoni,* and *Strongyloides*, on urine for *S. haematobium*, on night blood for *W. bancrofti* (microfilariae), and by serology for *Echinococcus*, tissular *T. solium, Toxocara,* and *Trichinella*. In contrast, most *O. volvulus* infections are symptomatic, with pruritus as an early symptom.

Clonorchis sinensis **(4570, 6873).** Light *O. sinensis* infections (<100 worms) can be mildly symptomatic or latent for years, occasionally up to 25 years. Heavy infections are rare in travelers. Long-term consequences of heavy clonorchiasis include recurrent cholangitis, bile duct fibrosis, and cholangiocarcinoma.

***Echinococcus* (1620, 2758)**. *E. multilocularis* and *E. granulosus* can be latent for 5–20 years before being manifest by space-occupying lesion or other signs.

***Schistosoma* (1279, 1556, 3155, 4741)**. *Schistosoma* infection or disease has been reported in expatriates and migrants years or decades after exposure in endemic areas, *S. haematobium* after >20 years, *S. mansoni* after >30 years, and *S. japonicum* after >30–40 years. A long-term consequence of hepatobiliary schistosomiasis is fibrosis of the liver. A consequence of urinary schistosomiasis is bladder carcinoma.

S. stercoralis (1836, 2732, 2878, 4334, 4587, 5818, 6021). Self reinfection maintains infections outside endemic areas for years or decades, including among immigrants in Australia, Canada, and France, and among expatriates or World War II veterans in Australia, Canada, the United States, the United Kingdom, and France. Suspected record highs have been latencies of 57 years (2732) and 65 years (4334).

Corticosteroid treatments and transplantations are associated with a risk of reactivated, massive, or disseminated disease (1798, 2964, 5688, 5985, 6879).

***T. solium* (1620, 8004)**. Cysticercosis can be latent for years, occasionally up to 20–30 years, before becoming manifest by space-occupying lesions (neurocysticercosis) or other signs.

***W. bancrofti* (1940, 2025)**. *W. bancrofti* infections can be latent as: (i) occult form with adults demonstrated by ultrasound, (ii) subpatent microfilaremia with antigenemia, and (iii) patent and persistent microfilaremia. Although patent microfilaremia seems to infrequently progress to manifest disease, latent infection can result in filarial fevers and lymphatic obstruction.

14.7 COMMUNITY-ACQUIRED SYNDROMES

Major community-acquired diseases include respiratory tract infection (RTI), diarrhea, and STI. Mother-to-child transmitted infections are included because agents can be acquired in the community and because of the potential for lifelong disability. A comprehensive description of community-acquired syndromes is beyond the scope of this book, however.

COMMUNITY-ACQUIRED PNEUMONIA

Cold wars

C. B. Hall (3085)

Upper RTIs are manifest by abrupt onset of coryza, cough, sore throat, pain on swallowing, frontal headache, or earache, and include pharyngitis, sinusitis, and otitis media. Lower RTIs are manifest by worsenend cough, newly purulent sputum, difficult breathing, tachypnoea, wheeze, chest pain, and fever, and include bronchitis, bronchiolitis, and pneumonia. Community-acquired pneumonia (CAP) is suspected from lower RTI, and confirmed by infiltration on chest radiograph. Unlike nosocomial pneumonia, CAP is not usually confirmed culturally, but NAT from naso- or oropharyngeal swabs or washings may expand diagnostic tools in the near future.

Exposure (Box 14.1). The history should address season, crowding, ill friends, and air quality (heating and dust) at home, in class, and at work, current respiratory vaccines (*Influenzavirus*, MMR, DP_a, Hib, and pneumococci), and use of antimicrobials.

Risks (1546, 2434, 3039, 3097, 3202, 4612, 4704, 5149, 6456, 6593, 7715)

Acute respiratory infections are the most common illnesses experienced by people of all ages worldwide

B. G. van den Hoogen et al. (7715)

Reported rates of RTI per person per year are 5–8 for children and 2–4 for adults. Physicians may be consulted for acute RTI at rates of 0.1–0.6/100 visits per week.

By age and diagnostic criteria, rates of CAP per 100 persons per year are 1–5.5 in high-income countries and up to 28 in low-income countries (with high rates at extremes of age). CAP hospitalization rates are typically 0.3–3/100 persons per year. By location and case mix, lethality is 5–35%, often 15%. In low-income countries, CAP accounts for ~18% of all deaths in preschool children.

Predisposing for CAP are extremes of age, season, crowding, and comorbidities. In favor of outpatient management are: (i) age <50 years, (ii) none of five comorbidities (cardiac, cerebral, renal, hepatic, and neoplastic), and (iii) five good vital signs (alert, respiration <30/min, pulse <125/ min, temperature of 35–39.9°C, and systolic blood pressure >90 mm Hg).

Etiology (463, 670, 2302, 2382, 2425, 4319, 4328, 5252, 5626, 5862, 6593, 7157) (Box 14.11). More than 100 agents have been implicated in CAP. By age, case mix, season, vaccinations, use of antimicrobials, specimen (saliva, pharyngeal washings, sputum, broncheal lavage, blood, and urine), and test (culture and NAT), a causative agent of CAP is identified in 5–40% (up to 50–80% in studies of CAP). Of causative agents, 20–80% are viruses, and 30–60% are bacteria. CAP can be polymicrobial, a virus can be followed by a bacterium, or hosts can be coinfected.

In neonates, agents from the birth canal prevail, typically *S. agalactiae* (GBS), *E. coli*, and *C. trachomatis*. In children, the main agents include RSV, *H. influenzae*, and

> **Box 14.11 Main agents of community-acquired RTI, by type**
>
> Relative frequencies are shown in parentheses.
>
> **Pharyngitis**
> Viruses*: 40–80%; *S. pyogenes* (children, 15–30%; adults, 5–10%); infrequent (<1–5%): *C. pneumoniae, C. diphtheriae, M. pneumoniae, N. gonorrhoeae*
>
> **Sinusitis**
> Viruses*: dominate; *S. pneumoniae* (children up to 35%, adults ~5%), *H. influenzae* (5–30%, non-b), *M. catarrhalis* (children 20%, adults 2–10%); infrequent: anaerobes, *Acinetobacter, Enterobacter, Escherichia, Klebsiella, Pseudomonas, S. aureus*, free-living amebas
>
> **Otitis media**
> Viruses*: 45–75%; *H. influenzae* (15–45%, non-b, can produce β-lactamase), *M. catarrhalis* (children 1–35%, often 7%), *S. pneumoniae* (children 20–70%, often 40%, can be penicillin-resistant); infrequent (<5%): GAS, *Pseudomonas, S. aureus*
>
> **CAP**
> Viruses*: 20–80%; *S. pneumoniae* (children 15–40%, adults 5–50%), "atypical" (1–30%, *C. pneumoniae, C. burnetii, L. pneumophila, Mycoplasma*), *H. influenzae* (0–13%, non-b); infrequent in adults (≤5%): mycobacteria, *S. aureus*, fungi
>
> *In well-vaccinated populations: AdV, *Enterovirus*, HuCoV, HuMPV, *Influenzavirus*, PIV, *Rhinovirus*, RSV

S. pneumoniae. In the elderly, main agents are *Influenzavirus*, RSV, and *S. pneumoniae*.

Viruses

Viruses frequently (in >5%) implicated in lower RTI or CAP are *Influenzavirus*, PIV, and RSV. Less frequently or regionally implicated are viruses such as AdV, *Hantavirus* (pulmonary syndrome), human coronavirus (HuCoV, in 6–9%), human metapneumovirus (HuMPV, in 6% of test-negative preschool children), measles virus (low vaccine coverage), PIV (in <1% of hospitalized preschool children), *Rhinovirus*, and SARS-associated coronavirus (SARS-CoV, epidemic).

Influenzavirus **(737, 1413, 4319, 5626, 6350).** *Influenzavirus* contributes seasonally to lower RTIs and CAP. By season, case mix, and test, diagnostic yield was low in infants in the United Kingdom in winter 1997–1998, but ~10–20% in cold seasons in Australia, The Netherlands, and Canada. Sources in the community are rarely reported, except A virus contracted from work with birds. Avian subtype H5N1 can cause severe pneumonia and acute respiratory distress.

Measles virus (1149, 2631). Measles virus is rarely listed as an agent of CAP, perhaps because pneumonia is considered secondary and bacterial. Measles virus is truly community acquired. In Senegal, sources for 402 index cases were at hamlets (62%), schools (12%), dispensaries (6%), gatherings (6%), and buses or travel (14%); for 908 secondary cases, sources were households (96%) and visitors (4%). In Juneau, Alaska, sources for 63 epidemic cases were schools (49%), homes (22%), indoor soccer games (11%), and others (18%).

PIV (737, 4319, 5252, 6350). PIV contributes seasonally to CAP. By season, age, case mix, and test, diagnostic yield for types 1–3 is ~1–13% (6% in Australia in 1991–2000, or 2,255/36,320 specimens). In contrast in the United Kingdom, only 0.3% (434/97,783) of lower RTIs in hospitalized preschool children were attributed to PIV.

RSV (737, 4319, 5252, 6350, 7994). RSV contributes seasonally to CAP. Diagnostic yield is ~25–50% (45% in Australia in 1991–2000, or 16,349/36,320 specimens). Indeed, of lower RTIs in hospitalized preschool children 18% (United Kingdom in 1995–1998, 22,229/97,783) to 19% (Gambia in 1994–1996, $n = 4,799$) were attributed to RSV.

Bacteria

Bacteria frequently implicated in CAP are *S. pneumoniae*, *H. influenzae*, and *S. aureus*. Agents of "atypical" CAP (mild infiltration) are *C. pneumoniae, C. burnetii, Legionella pneumophila*, and *M. pneumoniae*. Exposure is of diagnostic value for atypical agents.

Bacteria (2382, 6173, 7150) infrequently (in <5%) implicated are anaerobes (aspiration), *Acinetobacter, Bacillus anthracis* (biowarfare), *B. pertussis* (cough illness for >2 weeks), *B. pseudomallei* (regional in up to 15% of adults), *C. psittaci, Klebsiella* (comorbidities, antimicrobials), *M. catarrhalis, M. tuberculosis* (low-income countries, AIDS patients, and the homeless), and *P. aeruginosa* (comorbidities and antimicrobials).

***Chlamydophila* (699, 1048, 2382, 2383, 2386, 2916, 7150).** *C. pneumoniae* accounts for 1–15% (often 5–8%) of CAP. Reported rates of *C. pneumoniae* CAP are 3–17/10^5 per year.

***Coxiella* (2382, 2386, 6571, 7150).** *C. burnetii* accounts for 0.5–2% of CAP, locally or in outbreak up to 19%.

***Haemophilus* (35, 2382, 2386, 4074, 5862, 7150, 7951, 8346).** *H. influenzae* accounts for 0–13% of CAP (2.5% in a meta-analysis of 33,148 cases). Similiar proportions have been reported for adults in low-income countries. While mainly non-b strains are implicated, Hib has a role in CAP that is evident from vaccination.

***Legionella* (634, 2382, 2383, 3751, 4754, 7150, 7185).** By age, season, and test (urine), *Legionella* accounts for 0–15% of CAP, in adults typically 5%. Cases can be sporadic or epidemic. In Europe in 2000–2002, 20% (38/189) of outbreaks had sources in the community (mean case load, 28 per outbreak). Sources included cooling towers, hot- and cold-water systems, and whirlpool spas. Reported rates of *Legionella* CAP are 4–6/10^5 per year.

***M. tuberculosis* (2382, 4754, 7150).** *M. tuberculosis* is an infrequent cause of CAP in high-income countries, including patients who are hospitalized for CAP. In contrast, its share in low-income countries can reach 10%. Acute caseous pneumonia can mimic lobar pneumonia, and staining of sputum smear should be part of the emergency case management. Sources include crowded shelters and jails. Environmental mycobacteria may account for ~1% of CAP.

***Mycoplasma* (1309, 1330, 2382, 2383, 3109, 3594, 5022, 5252, 5308, 6350, 7951).** By age, test (NAT and serology), and setting, *M. pneumoniae* accounts for 0.5–30% of CAP, often for 2–10% in adults and for 0.5–8% in children. In Australia in 1991–2000, diagnostic yield from lower RTI specimens was 10% (3750/36,320). Reported rates of *M. pneumoniae* CAP have been 6–38/10^5 per year. In an outbreak in Colorado in 2000, the community attack rate was 0.7%.

***S. aureus* (2382, 2386, 7150).** *S. aureus* may account for 0.5–5% of CAP in adults.

***S. pneumoniae* (2382, 2386, 2727, 4074, 4704, 4754, 5252, 5626, 5862, 7951, 8346).** Confirmation of *S. pneumoniae* is difficult, requiring cultures from blood and sputum, and Gram stain of sputum smear. This may change, when new tests from urine (antigen capture) or pharyngeal swab (NAT) have been validated. By diagnostic criteria and workup, pneumococci account for 5–50% of CAP in adults and 15–40% in children, in hospitalized CAP typically for 15%. Crowding is suggestive of epidemiological evidence.

Fungi
Unlike nosocomial pneumonia, fungi are infrequently implicated universally, except *Pneumocystis*. PCP (2382, 4754, 7150) is diagnosed in 0–8% (often 1–2%) of CAP, mainly where the case mix includes a high proportion of HIV-infected patients.

Fungi of regional importance include *Blastocystis*, *Coccidioides*, *Histoplasma*, and *Paracoccidioides*.

COMMUNITY-ACQUIRED ACUTE DIARRHEA
Diarrhea is defined by three or more watery stools every 24 h (enteritis), plus one or more of these symptoms: cramps, nausea or vomiting (gastritis, for food poisoning, see section III), dehydration ("secretory" diarrhea), fever ("invasive" diarrhea), or visibly purulent or bloody stools ("dysentery"). Acute diarrhea should last <7 days. In contrast, chronic diarrhea lasts >14 days and goes along with flatulence (gas) and foul-smelling stools.

Risks (1474, 1848, 2961, 2984, 3135, 4067, 4546, 4670, 6645). Acute diarrhea in high-income countries occurs at a rate of ~0.5–2 per person per year. In any 1 month, 10% of the population has had an acute diarrhea episode. Only 15–30% of patients consult a physician. In low-income countries, rates in preschool children are 2–3 up to 24 per child per year. In any 2 weeks, 5–25% of preschool children have had a diarrhea episode. Attributable diarrhea mortality in preschool children is 0.5/100 per year, for 2 million deaths per year worldwide.

Etiology (1848, 2984, 4161, 6645, 7504, 8067) (Box 14.12). Workup should focus on agents that need treatment or public health attention. Proposed targets for laboratory workup include: dehydrating diarrhea in children (focus on *Rotavirus*, *E. coli*, and possibly *V. cholerae*), invasive diarrhea or repeated vomiting (focus on *Campylobacter*, *Salmonella*, *Shigella*, and enterotoxins), international travel in the preceding 12 months (focus on *V. cholerae*, and *S. enterica* serovar Typhi), hospital stay in the preceding 4 weeks (focus on *C. difficile*), or suspected outbreak (more than one case with a common source). In high-income countries, only 2–8% of diarrhea is examined microbiologically.

Preventive measures. Preventive measures include avoiding unsafe foods and beverages, promotion of hand-washing, safe storage of water, simple home water filtration, and provision of tap water and sanitation. Contaminated weaning foods are a major risk for diarrhea in young children. Oral rehydration corrects dehydration and saves lives but does not prevent diarrhea.

> **Box 14.12** Agents of community-acquired enteric infections, by syndrome
>
> Diagnostic yield and remarks appear in parentheses.
>
> **Acute diarrhea**
> **Viruses (10–30%):** HAV (rare), *Norovirus* (5–10%), *Rotavirus* (3–8%, higher in children)
> **Bacteria (5–40%):** mainly *C. jejuni* (1.5–12%), *C. perfringens* (0.5–3.5% enterotoxin), *E. coli* (0.5–5%), *Salmonella* (0.5–5%), *Shigella* (0–1%), infrequent: *Aeromonas*, *B. cereus* (toxins), *C. difficile* (up to 10% of outpatients), *Listeria*, *Plesiomonas*, *Vibrio*, *Yersinia*
> **Parasites (<1%):** *Cyclospora*, *Cryptosporidium*, *Giardia*, *Entamoeba*; *Trichinella*
>
> **Acute abdomen: upper or lower quadrants**
> Parasites (infrequent in high-income countries): *Cryptosporidium* (lower), *Entamoeba* (lower: colitis, upper: amebic liver abscess), *A. costaricensis* (upper), *Anisakis* (upper), *Ascaris* (ileus, upper by aberrant migration), *Strongyloides* (upper)
> **Chronic diarrhea (for >2 weeks)**
> *Salmonella*, *Shigella*, *M. tuberculosis*
> **Impaired immunity (by HIV, unless noted)**
> CMV; *Campylobacter*, *M. avium*; *Candida*, microsporidia; *C. hominis*, *C. cayetanensis*, *E. histolytica* (corticoids), *I. belli*; *S. stercoralis* (corticoids)
> **Malabsorption**
> *Giardia*, *D. fragilis*; *Ascaris*, *Capillaria philippensis*, *Strongyloides*

Viruses

Etiology (1385, 1848, 1881, 2938, 6350, 6690, 7504). By season, setting, and age, ~10–30% of acute community-acquired diarrhea is viral. Frequent viruses are *Norovirus* and *Rotavirus*, in endemic areas likely also HAV. Infrequent (≤5%) viral causes of acute diarrhea are enteric AdV (in 3–5.5%, diagnostic yield can exceed 10%), ASTV (in 0–9%), and *Enterovirus* (infrequent, diagnostic yield can reach 8%). For food poisoning, see section III; for travel, see section 15.4; for nosocomial diarrhea, see section 17.7.

***Norovirus* (and related Sapporo virus) (1385, 1848, 2314, 5332, 5727, 7504).** *Norovirus* is a major agent, accounting for 5–10% of acute, community-acquired diarrhea in high-income countries. In outbreaks in the United States in 1996–2000 ($n = 348$), implicated sources were foods in 39%, humans in 12%, water in 3%, and unknown in 46%.

HAV (6967). HAV circulates in children in endemic areas; sources include foods, tap water, and humans with infections.

***Rotavirus* (1848, 1881, 5332, 5411, 7504).** *Rotavirus* is a major agent, accounting for 3–8% of acute, community-acquired diarrhea in high-income countries, in children up to 30–45%. *Rotavirus* diarrhea is commonly associated with *E. coli* or *Shigella* coinfections.

Bacteria

Overview (801, 1848, 2938, 2984, 6129, 7504, 7880). By season, setting, and age, ~5–40% of community-acquired acute diarrhea is due to bacteria. In high-income countries frequent (by reporting rate $>1/10^5$ per year in the United States, or diagnostic yield >1% in most regions or groups) are *Campylobacter*, *E. coli*, *C. perfringens*, *Salmonella*, and *Shigella*. Infrequent in high-income countries are *Aeromonas*, *B. cereus*, *C. difficile*, *L. monocytogenes* (rate, $0.1–0.5/10^5$ per year), *Plesiomonas* (diagnostic yield regionally up to 4%), and *Yersinia* (rate, $0.1–0.6/10^5$ per year).

***Aeromonas* (2938, 3639, 4794, 4841).** Diagnostic yield of *Aeromonas* in endemic areas is 1–9%. However, enteropathogenicity of species such as *A. caviae*, *A. hydrophilia*, or *A. sobria* is controversial.

***Campylobacter*.** Diagnostic yield of *Campylobacter* is ~1.5–12%. In the United States, the reporting rate is 6–32 (overall 13)/10^5 per year.

***C. difficile* (3345, 6277).** *C. difficile* is mainly but not exclusively acquired in hospitals. By recent antibiotic use and test (culture, toxin), the diagnostic yield in outpatients can be 3–11%.

***E. coli* (6338).** By age, setting, and test, the overall diagnostic yield is 0–15% (often 0.5–5%). The frequency of pathotypes in diarrheic stool samples is variable. EPEC (atypical and typical) is identified in 3–13% of stools, EAEC in 3–6.5%, ETEC in 0.3–13%, enteroinvasive *E. coli* (EIEC) in 0–2%, and EHEC (O157) in 0–0.6%. In the United States, the reporting rate for *E. coli* O157 is 0.5–5 (overall 1.7) per 10^5 per year.

Salmonella. By age and setting, diagnostic yield for *Salmonella* is 0.5–5% in high-income countries, but 1–12% in low-income countries. In the United States, the reporting rate is 10–21 (overall 16) per 10^5 per year. The two most frequent community-acquired serotypes are *S. enterica* serovar Typhimurium (25% of isolates) and serovar Enteritidis (15%). Outbreaks are typically traced to foods (see section III).

Shigella (4072, 7229). By age and setting, diagnostic yield of *Shigella* is 0–1% in high-income countries, but 5–15% in low-income countries. In the United States, the reporting rate is 2–22 (overall 10) per 10^5 per year. Most (85%) isolates are *S. sonnei*.

Community outbreaks (1395, 3507, 4687, 5123, 6807, 7013) are documented in the Americas, Africa, and Asia. In Rwanda in 1981–1982, the population attack rate was ~5%. In Zaire in 1980–1982, there were ≥0.1 million cases, for an attack rate of ~6%; the "epidemic front" advanced 1,000 km in 1 year. By person-to-person spread, community outbreaks can go on for weeks or months.

Vibrio (V. cholerae O1, O139, other serogroups). Diagnostic yield of *Vibrio* in endemic areas is 0.1–1%. In the United States, the reporting rate for *Vibrio* spp. is 0.1–0.4/10^5 per year. Although person-to-person spread is important, endemicity depends on environmental reservoirs.

Protozoa
Overview (184, 1074, 2938, 2984, 3821, 7880).
Diagnostic yield varies with age, season, case mix (children, travelers, and disease duration), and test (fresh or preserved stool samples, number of specimens). Causality assessment may be confounded by carriers intercurrently infected with known viral or bacterial enteropathogens and self-treatments.

Protozoa are more often associated with chronic than acute diarrhea. In nontraveled residents of high-income countries with acute diarrhea diagnostic yield is typically <1%, including for *Balantidium coli*, *C. hominis*, *Cyclospora cayetanensis* (yield 0.4–0.5%, reporting rate 0.1/10^5 per year), *Dientamoeba fragilis* (yield 0.4–0.5%), *E. histolytica*, *G. lamblia*, and *Isospora belli* (yield <0.1%).

Colonic protozoa occasionally associated with acute appendicitis include *B. coli*, *C. hominis*, and *E. histolytica*.

Enteropathogenicity of *B. hominis* is controversial. In the United States, its diagnostic yield is 3–23%.

Protozoa frequently associated with chronic diarrhea in AIDS patients include *Cryptosporidium* and *G. lamblia*.

C. hominis (1369). Diagnostic yield is 0.2–7% in high-income countries but 6–12% in low-income countries, even up to 20% in AIDS patients with chronic diarrhea. In the United States, the reporting rate is 1.4/10^5 per year.

E. histolytica/dispar. Diagnostic yield is <1% in high-income countries (in the United States in 1987, it was 0.01% or 1,841/216,275 specimens) but >10% in low-income countries. In Bangladeshi preschool children with diarrhea, *E. histolytica* was isolated in 8% (69/893), *E. dispar* in 12% (107).

G. lamblia. A significant decrease over time is reported in the United States, with diagnostic yields of 7.2% in 1987 (15,497/216,275 specimens) (3821) but 0.3% in 2000 (19/5,792 specimens) (184). In high-income countries, diagnostic yield can exceed 10%, including children and AIDS patients with chronic diarrhea.

Fungi
Microsporidia are important causes of persisting diarrhea in immune-compromised patients.

Helminths
Overview (1961, 3821).
Except for acute trichinellosis in high-income countries, and dysentery from heavy enteric *Schistosoma* and *Trichuris* infections in tropical countries, helminths rarely cause acute diarrhea.

Acute abdomen is a feature of abdominal angiostrongyliasis, anisakiasis, and ascariasis. Colonic helminths occasionally associated with acute appendicitis include *E. vermicularis*, *S. mansoni*, *S. stercoralis*, and *T. trichiura*.

Helminths that may or may not be associated with chronic diarrhea include *Ascaris*, intestinal flukes, *S. mansoni*, *Taenia* spp., and *Trichuris*. In the United States in 1987 diagnostic yield from 216,275 specimens was 1.5% for hookworm, 1.2% for *Trichuris*, 0.8% for *Ascaris*, 0.6% for *Clonorchis-Opisthorchis*, 0.4% for *Strongyloides*, and <0.1% each for *Fasciola*, *Schistosoma*, and *Taenia*.

SEXUALLY TRANSMITTED INFECTIONS
STIs are infections that are *mainly* but not exclusively transmitted by sex. Manifestations can be genitoanal (discharge and ulcer), or extragenital (e.g., post-primary syphilitic skin eruptions, gonococcal arthritis, and chlamydial pelvic inflammatory disease).

Agents (1630, 1982, 3859, 5024, 8084) (Box 14.13). Arbitrarily included are CMV, HBV, HIV, HSV, HHV8,

> **Box 14.13** Agents of STI, by syndrome
>
> Relative frequency is listed in parentheses.
>
> | | |
> |---|---|
> | Discharge disease | *C. trachomatis*, mycoplasms, *N. gonorrhoeae*, and *T. vaginalis* |
> | Ulcer disease | HSV (~15–50%), *H. ducreyi* (1–40%), *T. pallidum pallidum* (3–12%), and no agent (15–40%) |
> | Granuloma disease | *C. trachomatis* (lymphogranuloma venereum) and *K. granulomatis* (donovanosis) |
> | By microtrauma | CMV, HBV, HIV, and HHV8 |

HPV; chlamydiae (*C. trachomatis* A–K and L1–3), *H. ducreyi* (chancroid), mycoplasms (*M. genitalium* and *U. urealyticum*), *N. gonorrhoeae*, *K. granulomatis* (donovanosis), *T. pallidum pallidum* (syphilis); *T. vaginalis*; *P. pubis*, and *S. scabiei*.

About 10–40% of patients have multiple STIs, including HIV and agents of discharge disease (*N. gonorrhoeae, C. trachomatis*, and *T. vaginalis*), or HIV and agents of ulcer disease (*H. ducreyi* and *T. pallidum pallidum*). Inapparent STIs escape treatment and reporting.

While data from STI clinics are useful, self-selection among clinic patients is likely to introduce bias.

Risks (1180, 2356, 3333, 5730, 8143). Worldwide, four readily treatable agents (*C. trachomatis, N. gonorrhoeae, T. pallidum pallidum*, and *T. vaginalis*) cause 340 million infections per year, for a global rate of 9/100 sexually active adults per year. Rates peak in young adults. Infection risks include casual (anonymous) sex, multiple sex partners, female sex work (see section 13.6), sex among men (see section 13.7), unprotected sex, receptive oral or anal sex, and life-years of sexual activity. In a United States survey in 1997, 11% of 33,913 respondents admitted to multiple sex partners. In a stratified probability sample of 11,161 men and women in the United Kingdom, median numbers of lifetime partners were four in women (ethnic range, 1–5) and six in men (ethnic range, 1–9); 9–22% of women and 23–44% of men reported one or more new heterosexual partners in the preceding year, and 0–1% of women and 0.1–2% of men reported one or more new homosexual partner. Lifetime STI risks in the United Kingdom are 11% in men, and 13% in women.

Victims of STI can also be sources of STI. Infected individuals have an obligation to disclose their infection status to sex partners. STI in children are suspicious of sexual abuse.

Preventive measures. Preventive measures include promotion of stable (monogamous) partnerships, safe sex, and condoms, as well as contact tracing and vaccines (HAV and HBV). **Condoms (210, 1982, 3401, 7905, 7961, 8268).** Although inadequately documented, consistent use of quality condoms is likely to considerably reduce the acquisition and spread of STIs, including HPV (genital warts), *C. trachomatis* (by 25% in prostitutes), HIV (by 35–95%), *N. gonorrhoeae* (by 60% in prostitutes), and HSV2 (by up to 90% in females). However, the preventive potential of condoms has not been fully exploited. In the United States in 1996–2000, only 20% (95% CI 18–21) of sexually active adults reported use of condoms at the last sexual intercourse. **Contacts (1575, 1982, 5006, 8268).** Contacts are indicated by patients and traced by teams, for early treatment, screening, prevention of spread, and risk alert. Contact tracing and treatment is a priority for "classic" agents (*C. trachomatis, H. ducreyi, N. gonorrhoeae*, and *T. pallidum*) and genital ulcer disease (to reduce spread of HIV). Screening for inapparent infections should be cost-effective. New tests are simplifying screening (Table 14.3). Sites for gonococcal screening could be selected according to the history of oral or anal sex. Pregnant women should be screened on first antenatal visit for HBV, HIV, *T. pallidum*, and *C. trachomatis*, by risks also for HCV and *N. gonorrhoeae*.

Genitoanal Discharge: Community

Overview (53, 2623, 2766, 8084). Conditions associated with discharge include urethritis, vaginitis, cervicitis, and anoproctitis. Outpatients commonly report complaints (itch and discharge) indicative of urethritis or

Table 14.3 Screening of inapparent women and men for STI[a]

Agent	Test	Specimen
HIV	Anti-HIV	Blood
HBV	Anti-HBc, anti-HBs, or anti-HBsAg	Blood
HPV	Microscopy (pap smear)	Swab (cervical)
Chlamydia	NAT	First-void urine, tampon, or swab (cervix, urethra, or rectum)
Neisseria	NAT or culture	First-void urine or swab (cervix, urethra, rectum, or pharynx)
Treponema	Anti-*Treponema*: RPR and TPHA	Blood
Trichomonas	Microscopy (wet or pap smear) or culture	Swab (vagina or urethra)

[a] From reference 811 and 4963.

vaginitis (30% in Italy in 1991–1996, or 13,459/44,438). Discharge disease can be highly infectious, requiring prompt evaluation and treatment. Frequent agents are *C. trachomatis*, *N. gonorrhoeae*, and *T. vaginalis*. In females, additional agents include *Candida*, *Gardnerella vaginalis*, and mycoplasms. *Candida* (53) is an agent of vulvovaginitis that is not considered an STI. By age and sample, the genital infection prevalence in females is ~0.5–20%, and the disease prevalence is 4–5%. *G. vaginalis* is associated with vaginosis, perhaps vaginitis. Its reported prevalence in female outpatients is 15–20%.

C. trachomatis (1225, 1982, 5991, 6054, 6735, 7105, 7529, 8043).

C. trachomatis is a main agent of vaginitis and nongonococcal urethritis (NGU). Worldwide, >9 million adults are infected, for a minimum prevalence of 2%. Spread seems equally efficient male to female and female to male. Diagnostic yield by gender, test (NAT and culture), and diagnosis (urethritis, NGO, and postgonococcal urethritis) is 10–80%. Although in the United States screening is recommended for sexually active women <26 years of age and for all pregnant women, <40% of target women are actually screened.

- Prevalence (1225, 2293, 2355, 2623, 3333, 4908, 5059, 5677, 5730, 6735, 7617). By age, ethnicity, sampling (random and STI clinics), material (urine and swab), and test, genital infection prevalence in high-income countries is 1–17% in females and 2–14% in males, with highs in young adults. For instance in Sweden, the prevalence of *C. trachomatis* by NAT from first void urine and cervical sample was 10% (45/465) in women attending an STI clinic (32% symptomatic), compared with 2% (1/59) in young women in a cancer-screening program. In the United States, prevalence is highest in African-American young women. In females, up to 70% of infections are inapparent. In low-income countries, the reported prevalence is similar, ~2–10% in females and 2–13% in males.
- Incidence (2956, 3486, 8342). In high-income countries, genital infection rates reported for both sexes are 50–300/10^5 per year, with peaks (up to 1,000/10^5) in young adults.

Mycoplasms. M. genitalium (1113, 1982, 2293, 3580, 4576, 4980, 5827, 7529).

M. genitalium is an emerging agent of genital discharge disease. NAT detects the agent in ~5–45% of females and 10–25% of males attending STI clinics. In contrast, 0–15% (typically 6–7%) of asymptomatic men test positive by NAT or culture. In Sweden, the prevalence of *M. genitalium* by NAT from first void urine and cervical sample was 6% (26/461) in women attending an STI clinic (23% symptomatic), compared with nil (0/59) in young women in a cancer-screening program. *M. genitalium* is a consideration in males with recurrent, persistent, or nongonococcal, nonchlamydial urethritis. **M. hominis (2193)** *M. hominis* is considered a commensal, although in Sweden, colonized women consulting for family planning more often reported casual sex and sex with more than one partner in the preceding 6 months than did noncolonized women. **U. urealyticum (1972, 5827, 5991).** *U. urealyticum* is a likely cause of NGU in men. However, yield is comparable in men with urethritis and in asymptomatic men. By NAT, prevalences are 25–30% in men with urethral discharge, and >40% in females visiting for family planning.

N. gonorrhoeae (1824, 1982, 5827, 8043).

N. gonorrhoeae is a major cause of vaginitis and purulent urethritis. Gonorrhea is more often diagnosed in male than female. Worldwide, there are >60 million infections, for a prevalence of 1.6% in adults. Diagnostic yield (NAT and culture) in symptomatic males at STI clinics is ~20–60%. A high proportion (≥50%) of strains is penicillinase producing. Simple infection chains are being replaced by "networks." In Alberta, Canada, in 1999, an outbreak with 107 index cases revealed sexual networks that were centered around a motel bar, with 2–39 individuals per network.

- Prevalence (5059, 5991, 7617). In high-income countries, untreated infection prevalence in adults is 0.03–3%, often 0.3–0.6%.
- Incidence (2924, 2956, 3486, 7077, 8342). In high-income countries, gonorrhea rates increased in the 1950s–1960s, plummeted to a low in the 1980s, and resurged in the 1990s. In the 2000s, rates in North America, Australia, and West Europe are ~10–130/10^5 per year, with peaks (up to >200/10^5) in young adults.

T. vaginalis (53, 1982, 2623, 3194, 3859, 4011, 5024, 6735, 7040, 7983, 8043, 8174).

T. vaginalis is a major cause of vaginitis, and a cause of NGU. Worldwide, there are >170 million infections, for a prevalence of ~5% in adults. By sample (from STI clinics and contacts) and test (microscopy, culture, and NAT), prevalence in high-income countries is 5–35% (females) to 0.5–20% (males). Prevalence in females in low-income countries ranges broadly, from 1–60%. In Brazil, the prevalence from 20,356 pap smears for cancer screening was 5–10%. In Uganda, the prevalence by culture from self-collected vaginal smear in the control arm of a randomized community intervention trial ranged from 14% (261/1,815) to 24% (785/3,270) over time; in the intervention group, home mass treatment with a single dose of metronidazole reduced the prevalence from 24% (797/3,323) to 9% (182/1,968). In South Africa, prevalence was ~40% in pregnant women ($n = 6,948$), and ~60% in nonpregnant women ($n \sim 49,000$). In males, the reported prevalence is 0.6–14%, with a high in symptomatic men.

Genitoanal Ulcers: Community

Overview (523, 729, 943, 1441, 4695, 5007, 8084). Genital ulcer disease (GUD) includes indolent or painful ulcers of the genital, perianal, or proctal areas, without or with regional adenopathy. Ulcers are highly infectious, requiring prompt evaluation, treatment, and reporting. Main agents are HSV (genital herpes), *T. pallidum pallidum* (primary syphilis), and *H. ducreyi* (chancroid). Their relative proportions may change over time. In ~15–40% of patients, an agent is not detected.

HSV. Both HSV1 (primarily oral) and HSV2 (primarily genital) can cause GUD. **HSV1 (943, 1982, 3944, 6745).** World infection (sero)prevalence in adults is 25–90%. Risks for genital HSV1 infections include orogenital sex, being female, and age <25 years. In the United States, HSV1 accounts for 20% of genital herpes. In Scotland in 1986–2000, HSV was identified in 3,181 (30%) of 10,547 genital swabs, HSV1 accounted for 49% (1,530) and HSV2 for 51% (1,596) of infections typed. Among 372 GUD patients at an STI clinic in Amsterdam, The Netherlands, culture detected HSV1 in 5.6% and PCR in 7.8% of attendees. **HSV2 (943, 1982, 2766, 3486, 3944, 4695, 5315, 7230).** By age and setting, infection (sero)prevalence in adults is ~10–40%. Of infected individuals, only ~20–45% give a history of herpes. Predictive of infection are age, sexual preference, years of sexual activity, number of lifetime sex partners, and past STIs. In high-income countries, infection prevalence in homosexual men, heterosexual men, and heterosexual women gradually increases with numbers of lifetime sex partners, from 0–7% with one partner, to 70–90% with >50 partners. By gender, endemicity, and test, ~15–50% of all GUD is attributable to HSV. In Italy, genital herpes was diagnosed in 8% (3,435/44,438) of outpatients. In the United Kingdom in 1990–1999, rates of first genital herpes were 25–40/10^5 per year.

***H. ducreyi* (943, 1922, 4695, 5007, 7126).** Risks of *H. ducreyi* include sex with prostitutes, sex for drugs, and sex with drug users. The prevalence of IgG that should reflect past infection can reach 5%. By age, case mix (screened for syphilis), and test (culture and PCR), the proportion of GUD (females and males) attributable to *H. ducreyi* is 1–40% in high-income countries and 7–95% (often 30%) in low-income countries.

***T. pallidum pallidum* (522, 943, 1965, 1982, 2423, 2623, 2956, 3194, 4695, 8342).** Only the primary stage is manifest as GUD. Risks are the same for syphilis as for other STIs. Worldwide, there are 12 million infections, for a prevalence of 0.3% in adults. By setting, gender, and test (serology and NAT), the proportion of GUD attributable to *T. pallidum pallidum* is 3–12% in high-income countries and 16–24% in low-income countries. Reported community seroprevalence in low-income countries is ~0.5–0.7%, in females it is up to 7%. In North America, Australia, and Europe, rates of primary and secondary syphilis reports are ~0.2–10/10^5 per year (high in Australian males and low in English females).

Genitoanal Granulomas: Community

Agents include HPV, *K. granulomatis* (donovanosis), and *C. trachomatis* (serovars L1–L3 that cause lymphogranuloma venereum) (8084). For HPV, see section 13.6 and 13.7; for lymphogranuloma, see section 13.7.

***K. granulomatis* (473, 6757, 8285, 8342).** Donovanosis is infrequently diagnosed in patients with granulomatous or ulcerous lesions of the genitals. In Australia, the disease affects indigenous communities, for <40 case reports per year. Donovanosis was targeted for elimination by 2005. In India, donovanosis accounts for 0.3–6.3% of all STIs. In South Africa, 42% (14/33) of women with donovanosis had coinfections with *T. pallidum*.

STI From Microtrauma: Community

For agents shed from the urogenital tract, see section 14.1.

CMV (1982, 2024, 6838). CMV can spread sexually. In Taiwan, cervical infections were detected by PCR in 25% (17/70) of women at a gynecological clinic, in 35% (65/187) of women consulting for STI, and in 40% (76/195) of licensed prostitutes.

HBV (416, 1982, 3231, 4338, 6967). HBV can spread homosexually and heterosexually. In the United Kingdom, in 13% (1,140/8,956) of reported acute HB cases sex was the attributed mode of spread. Risks include sex with a carrier, sex with multiple partners, and a history of STI. Vaccine is recommended for groups at risk.

HIV (1176, 1205, 6679, 6727, 6981, 7644). In sub-Saharan Africa, the main mode of spread is heterosexual. In ~40 countries of that region in the 1990s, the median infection prevalence in men attending STI clinics in urban areas was 16%. In high-income countries, there is a mix of homosexual and heterosexual spread, and of spread in IDUs. In the United States in 2001, of 35,602 new HIV infections, 13% (4,537) were attributed to heterosexual spread while modes were not reported for 54% (19,137). Relative to other modes, heterosexual mode is increasing in high-income countries. Unlike other STIs, lesions do not signal new infection, for which the only way of detection is by testing. In the United States in 2001, ~30–65% of the adult civil population reported HIV tests. At an STI clinic in San Francisco in 1989–1998, among 34,866 of 117,272 attendees tested, the overall seroprevalence was 9.5% (males, 12%; females, 1%). PEP can be beneficial if given in ≤72 h from e_0.

HHV8 (6236). HHV8 seems to spread sexually in areas where Kaposi's sarcoma is endemic.

MOTHER-TO-CHILD TRANSMITTED INFECTIONS

Mother-to-child transmitted infections are infections of the embryo, fetus, or neonate that result from intrauterine (congenital and transplacental), peripartal, or nursing (postpartal) transfer of maternal agents. Intrauterine infections result from exposure in pregnancy. Peripartal infections result from exposure during delivery. Nursing infections result from exposure during nursing.

Infections (Box 14.14). Sources are agents from maternal blood ("agentemia": viremia, bacteremia, and parasitemia), the colonized birth canal, breast milk, hands, and the environment.

Prevention (6, 1428, 3862, 6214). Prevention is based on vaccines, exposure avoidance, screening, and, in tropical countries, intermittent treatments of *Plasmodium falciparum* parasitemia and intestinal helminths.

Routine prepregnancy vaccines include HBV, MMR, and dT. Attenuated live vaccines are contraindicated in pregnancy.

Exposure avoidance includes foods (raw, exotic, and unwashed), home (sick older children, unsafe sex, pet animals, and shoes), and work (domestic animals, soil, and infective patients and materials).

Screening on first antenatal visit could include clinically for STI, microbiologically (birth canal) for *C. trachomatis* and *N. gonorrhoeae*, and serologically for HBV, HIV, rubella virus, *T. gondii*, and *T. pallidum pallidum*, in endemic areas also by test for *M. tuberculosis*, *Plasmodium*, and *T. cruzi*. Confirmed infections should be treated provided safe drugs are available. Screening should be repeated before delivery, with a focus on STI (see section above) and *S. agalactiae* (GBS).

Box 14.14 Agents transmitted mother-to-child, by period and impact

Transmission rates and remarks appear in parentheses.

Prepartal: during pregnancy, from "agentemia"
Mainly:
- CMV (~50%), HIV (5–45%), PVB19 (30–50%), rubella (by gestational week <10% to 90%)
- *Listeria* (80–95%), *T. pallidum* (10–100%, by disease stage)
- *Plasmodium* (~0.5–90%, by parasite density), *Toxoplasma* (1–80%, by treatment and trimester), *T. cruzi* (1–10%)

Others:
- DENV, *Enterovirus*, HHV6, HSV, JRV, LMCV, measles virus, WNV, VZV
- *Anaplasma*, *Borrelia*, *Brucella* (~50%), *Chlamydophila*, *C. trachomatis*, *Coxiella*, *Gardnerella*, *M. tuberculosis*, *M. pneumoniae*
- *Pneumocystis*
- *Babesia*, *Leishmania*, *T. brucei*

Peripartal: during labor and delivery, from birth secretions or via umbilical cord
Mainly:
- HBV (10–90%, by HBsAg and HBeAg satus), HCV (2–12%, by viremia), HIV (~13–18%), HSV (1–50%, by reactivation or new acquisition)
- *C. trachomatis* (36%), *E. coli*, *Klebsiella*, GBS (1–20%), *N. gonorrhoeae* (30–50%)

Others:
- CMV
- *Campylobacter*, *Enterobacter*, GAS, *L. monocytogenes*, mycoplasms, *Pseudomonas*, *Serratia*, *S. aureus*, *T. pallidum*
- *Candida*; *Trichomonas*

Postpartal: during nursing, from breast milk or environment
Mainly:
- CMV (10–40%), HIV (5–20%)

Others:
- EBV, *Enterovirus*, HBV, HSV, HTLV (15–30%), *Rotavirus*, WNV; *Burkholderia*, GBS *Leptospira*, *Listeria*, *M. tuberculosis*, *Salmonella*

Intrauterine Infections

Acquired or reactivated (see section 14.6) infections in pregnancy can cause intrauterine infection, principally from viremia, bacteremia, or parasitemia. Possible pregnancy outcomes include abortion and congenital manifest or inapparent infection. As acquired immunity increases with increasing age of mothers, the age at which women are pregnant influences the risk of mother-to-child transmission, tending to be lower at advanced age.

Useful steps in the evaluation of infection risks in pregnant woman include: (i) If a pregnant woman is seronegative (susceptible), what is her risk for a first-time infection in pregnancy? If she is seroreactive (latently infected), what is her risk for reactivation? (ii) If maternal "agentemia" is detected, what is the risk for transmission and infection for the fetus? (iii) Seroreactivity in the newborn, is it maternal (pseudo-infection) or self-produced (congenital infection)? (iv) Confirmed congenital infection, is it inapparent at birth or becoming manifest on follow-up (for perhaps 1 year)?

Intrauterine Viral Infections

Viremia is a poorly documented, apparently infrequent pregnancy hazard. Main viruses associated with intrauterine infections include CMV, HIV, PVB19, and rubella virus.

Because of rare exposure, low maternal susceptibility, or low virulence, viruses infrequently implicated in intrauterine infections include DENV (6935), *Enterovirus* (7210), GBV-C (viremia transmission rate ~75%, inapparent viremia persists in about one half of infected infants for 12 months) (4428, 8033), HSV, Japanese encephalitis virus (JEV) (1353), lymphocytic choriomeningitis virus (LCMV) (467), measles virus (a suspected cause of abortion, low birth weight, and viremia in neonates) (5333), *Roseolovirus* (HHV6), and WNV (2798).

CMV (77, 87, 1822, 2482, 2702, 7102).

- Maternal infections. In high-income countries, by age and lifestyle, 10–65% of women of child-bearing age are susceptible to CMV. Reported primary infection rates are 2–4/100 women. Many primary infections are inapparent or not recognized. Furthermore, latent infections can be reactivated, and seroreactive women can become reinfected.
- Mother-to-child transmission (77, 2702) is highest in primary infections, for rates of ~50%.
- Impact (87, 142, 2481, 2482, 2702, 5270, 5385). By maternal risks, the rate of congenital infection is 0.1–2/100 live births. In Brazil, filter-paper blood-screening from 15,873 neonates identified 16 congenital infections, for 0.1/100 live births; 69% (11/16) of infections remained inapparent for up to 2 years. Of 125 infants with congenital infection from primary maternal infection (primary group), and 64 congenital infections from maternal reactivations (secondary group), only infants from the primary group (18%) were symptomatic at birth. After follow-up for nearly 5 years, 25% from the primary group, and 8% of the secondary group had developed symptoms, including mental impairment and hearing loss.

HCV (4965).
For the prevention of rhesus incompatibility, 2,533 women were inadvertently exposed to HCV-contaminated anti-D Ig in Germany in 1978–1979. Of children from 74 women with self-limited HCV infection and from 86 women with chronic HC monitored for 10–15 years, 1% (3/231) had seroconverted. Chronic HC was not diagnosed in seroconverted children, and the risk of intrauterine, perinatal (see below), or postnatal intrafamilial spread was considered low.

HHV6 (3086, 5749).
Almost 100% of women of childbearing age are seroreactive, but reactivation in pregnancy can cause intrauterine infections. The risk of congenital infection is ~1/100 live births, which is comparable to CMV. However, unlike CMV, congenital HHV6 infection seems innocuous.

HIV.
Roughly one third of HIV infection in infants is intrauterine (974, 4077, 5364).

- Maternal infection (6385, 7644). In the 1990s, the median prevalence in women in antenatal care was 4% in sub-Saharan Africa, 0.2% in Latin America, 0.4% in People's Republic of China, and 0.06% in western Europe. In South Africa in 2000, the prevalence in rural mothers was 28% (365/1,303).
- Mother-to-child transmission (974, 4703, 4192, 5158, 5364, 6385, 7290, 7388). By viral load and CD4 count, untreated rates range from ~5–45%, with a high in sub-Saharan Africa. Antiretrovirals (short course or single dose) in late pregnancy, during labor, and in neonates can reduce transmission and infection risks for neonates.
- Impact (1176, 1607). In Paris, France, in 1990–1991, of 43 HIV-positive women with pregnancy outcome known, 2 (5%) had ectopic pregnancies, 21 (49%) had abortions (2 spontaneous, 5 therapeutic, and 14 elective), and 20 (46%) delivered babies. In the United States in 2001, 543 (1.5%) of 35,602 new HIV infections were reported in children. Untreated, HIV infection in infants is almost always fatal.

PVB19. Maternal infection (2729, 3141, 7692).
In high-income countries, 35–50% of pregnant women are susceptible. Rates of seroconversions during pregnancy are 0.2–2/100 susceptible women, during outbreaks 10–

20/100. **Mother-to-child transmission (4021, 5049, 5507, 5875).** The risk is 30–50%. Whether transmission is largely limited to the first half of pregnancy or spans the whole gestation period is contentious. **Impact (2729, 3141, 4384, 5049, 5507, 5875).** Infections in pregnancy are associated with a 7–10% increased risk of fetal loss. The majority of neonatal infections is asymptomatic. In the United Kingdom, of 186 infected mothers who elected to go to term, 156 (84%) delivered healthy babies, and on follow-up to age 1 year, no abnormalities were detected.

Rubella virus. Ophthalmologist N. M. Gregg (1892–1966) reported congenital rubella disease in 1941 (2929).

- Maternal infection (5942, 5943). By endemicity, and without routine vaccination, at least 5–15% of women are susceptible, including in low-income urban areas.
- Mother-to-child transmission (417, 5048, 5942). By week of gestation, the risk of congenital rubella syndrome (CRS) from confirmed rubella in pregnancy is 50–90% during weeks 1–8, 20–50% during weeks 9–16; and small ($\leq$10%) after week 16.
- Impact (417, 706, 1693, 4214, 4215, 5385, 5943, 8096, 8413). In the prevaccine era, the rate of CRS was 0.1–0.2/1,000 live births in endemic years, to 0.5–4/1,000 in outbreak years, with few differences between high- and low-income countries. In countries with low vaccine coverage, CRS persists at rates of 0.1–0.9/1,000 live births. Due to vaccination, CRS has become rare in high-income countries. Pockets of endemicity remain, however. In the United States, CRS disproportionally affects Hispanic women. In El Paso, Tex., CRS rates/1,000 live births were 0.3 compared to U.S. rates of 0.001–0.008, and all CRS cases were of Hispanic origin. In Brazil, screening of 15,873 neonates identified 11 infections (69/10^5 neonates); 55% (6/11) were inapparent until age 2 years. Outbreaks of CRS were reported in Brazil, in Acre state in 2000 (five cases, 0.6/1,000 live births), and Pernambuco State in 1998–2000 (31 cases, 0.9/1,000).

VZV (2205, 3142, 5751). In high-income countries, >90% of pregnant women are immune. After primary maternal varicella or zoster, the mother-to-child transmission risk is low (<1–2%). Congenital varicella syndrome is rare, but eventually severe.

Intrauterine Bacterial Infections

Putative sources of intrauterine infections are bacteremia and ascending genital infection. The main bacteria associated with intrauterine infections are *Brucella*, *Listeria*, and *Treponema*.

Because of rare exposure, low maternal susceptibility, or low virulence, infrequently implicated in intrauterine infections are *A. phagocytophilum* (from tick bite) (3432), *B. burgdorferi* (from tick bite) (2178), *Borrelia* that cause TBRF (from tick bite; abortion, preterm labor, and stillbirth) (2873), *Chlamydophila abortus* (from aborting ruminants) (4959), *C. psittaci* (from sick birds) (3531), *Chlamydia trachomatis* (miscarriage) (5543), *Coxiella* (fetal and neonatal deaths) (7139), *G. vaginalis* (miscarriage) (5543), *M. tuberculosis* (from untreated disease in pregnancy, ~300 congenital cases reported) (4305), and *M. pneumoniae* (7659).

***Brucella* (3916, 4978).** Untreated brucellosis in early pregnancy is a pregnancy hazard. In Saudi Arabia in 1983–1995, 92 pregnant women were diagnosed with acute brucellosis, for an incidence of 1.3/1,000 deliveries; of infected women, 43% aborted in the first to second trimesters, and 2% lost fetuses in the third trimester. Prepartal antimicrobial therapy protected from abortion.

***L. monocytogenes* (4609, 6884).** Of all reported listeriosis, 34–43% of cases are pregnancy related. Both intrauterine and peripartal modes are plausible.

- Maternal infection (2511, 4915, 6303, 6897). Pregnant women are particularly susceptible. Rates in pregnancy can be >10/10^5 compared to population rates of <1/10^5 per year. Infections in pregnancy can be flulike. Although mild, such infections can result in bacteremia and intrauterine infection. Antimicrobial treatment can reduce or prevent neonatal infection.
- Mother-to-child transmission (4609, 4915, 6303, 6884, 6897). *L. monocytogenes* has a predilection for placenta. Concentration in amniotic fluid can be high (10^8 CFU/ml). Including spontaneous abortions, untreated transmission rates are likely 80–95%.
- Outcome (2511, 4915, 6303, 6884, 6897). By treatment in pregnancy, 0–20% of intrauterine infections result in abortion, 15–45% in fetal death or stillbirth, and 55–65% in preterm or term delivery. Of live births, >80% will become manifest as early (days 0–6) or late congenital listeriosis syndrome that is characterized by sepsis, meningitis, or the formation of microabscesses (granulomatosis infantiseptica). Lethality of neonatal listeriosis is 5–50%.

***T. pallidum pallidum* (6561, 7916).** Worldwide, syphilis affects 1 million pregnancies per year, for 0.46 million abortions or stillbirths, 0.27 million low-birth-weight babies, and 0.27 million congenital infections. Most maternal and neonatal morbidity can be prevented by screening and treating pregnant women.

- Maternal infection (525, 5802, 6561, 6917, 7054, 7916, 7975, 8187). Most infections in pregnancy are inapparent and detected only by seroscreening. In high-income countries, seroprevalence in pregnant women is generally low (0.02%), except in pockets of endemicity such as in inner cities where the prevalence can reach 4.5%. In low-income countries, the reported seroprevalence in pregnant women is 1–18%. Reactivity should alert for congenital syphilis.

- Mother-to-child transmission (587, 3511, 5802, 6561, 6917, 7054). Risks include no antenatal care, no testing, and no treatment. In Bolivia in 1996, of 1,368 delivering women, 1,043 (76%) had received antenatal care, but only 227 (17%) had been tested for syphilis. By stage, untreated transmission rates are 70–100% in primary syphilis, 30–60% in early-latent syphilis, and 10% in late-latent syphilis.
- Outcome (6561, 6917, 7054, 7916, 7975, 8187). Untreated syphilis in pregnancy can result in abortion, fetal death, prematurity, low birth weight, and latent or manifest congenital syphilis. More than half of congenital infections are inapparent at birth. Lethality of congenital disease is 6–38%. Early (0–2 years) manifestations include radiographic bone anomalies (in 75–100%), skin rash (in 40%), hepatomegaly (in 33–100%), and low birth weight (in 10–40%). Late (2–15 years) manifestations include hearing loss and teeth and bone deformities. In the United States, the incidence of congenital syphilis per 10^5 live births was 107 in 1991, 14 in 2000, 21 in 2001, and 11 in 2002. During an outbreak in inner-city Baltimore that erupted in 1994, the incidence of congenital syphilis reached 270/10^5 live births.

Intrauterine Fungal Infections

Intrauterine transmission of *Pneumocystis* is rare but confirmed (4130, 5219). In Moravia in the 1950s, PCP in neonates 16 days of age strongly suggested intrauterine acquisition.

Intrauterine Protozoal Infections

Parasitemia in pregnancy is well documented for *Plasmodium*. The main protozoa associated with intrauterine infections include *Plasmodium*, *Toxoplasma*, and *T. cruzi*. Cases of congenital infections have also been reported for *Babesia* (6), *Leishmania*, and *Trypanosoma brucei* (8262).

***Leishmania* (730, 4964, 7666).** Congenital visceral leishmaniasis has been reported both in and outside endemic areas, including western Europe. Mothers can be manifestly ill or infected inapparently. Treatment in the second trimester has been attempted.

***Plasmodium* (52, 1702, 1951, 5366, 6454, 7153, 7489).** Immunity (partial in resident women, absent in traveling women; Table 20.3) modifies the effects of parasitemia and clinical malaria in pregnancy that range from anemia to cerebral malaria. PCR can detect subpatent parasitemias in partially immune mothers and neonates protected from maternal antibodies. Serology can separate partially immune resident mothers from nonimmune traveling mothers. Microscopy of placenta can establish parasite sequestration.

- Maternal infection (1951, 2408, 5366, 5591, 5729, 7489). In sub-Saharan Africa, 5–55% of pregnant women can be parasitemic (mainly by *P. falciparum*), and some more women have placental infection without patent parasitaemia.
- Mother-to-child transmission (6168) is influenced by maternal age, parity, season, and use of antimalarials. In rural Malawi in 1987–1990, 36% (111/311) of neonates from mothers with *P. falciparum* parasitemia, and 35% of neonates (134/388) from mothers with infected placentas had umbilical cord blood parasitemia. When parasites were not detected in maternal blood or placenta, the parasitemia prevalence in umbilical cord was 1.6% (29/1,769) and 0.4% (6/1,692), respectively. When parasite densities were $\geq 10,000/\mu l$ in maternal blood or placenta, cord blood parasitemia rates were 89% (25/28) and 63% (32/51), respectively.
- Impact (52, 404, 1702, 1951, 2408, 4312, 5366, 5591, 5729, 6454, 7153). By immunity, effects of clinical malaria or parasitemia in pregnancy include fetal loss, intrauterine growth retardation, low birth weight, neonatal parasitemia, and clinical congenital malaria, and neonatal death. Congenital infection is diagnosed from parasitemia on days 0–7 postpartum that matches maternal *Plasmodium* species. Most congenital infections are due to *P. falciparum*, but *P. vivax* and *P. malariae* have been reported as well. Congenital infections (in neonates from partially immune mothers) are often self-limited. By location and test, their reported prevalence is 0–40% (often 5–10%). In contrast, manifest congenital malaria (in neonates from nonimmune mothers) carries a lethality of 25%. Congenital clinical malaria may account for 0–30% of congenital infections.

***T. gondii* (2518).** As with other congenital infections, determinants of risks include the proportion of pregnant women who are susceptible (seronegative), the rate of new (parasitemic) infections in pregnancy, the rate of transplacental transmission, and the manifestation index in neonates.

- Maternal infection (1107, 2273, 3624, 3735, 3756, 4282). From numerous studies in high-income countries, ~45–85% of pregnant women can be expected to be susceptible. This proportion may be similar to or somewhat lower in low-income countries. Maternal

Table 14.4 Pregnancy outcome of new *T. gondii* infection in pregnancy, by trimester[a]

Outcome	% with maternal infection in		
	First trimester	Second trimester	Third trimester
Subclinical infection	1–10	10–30	60
Stillbirth	5	2	0
Congenital disease	78	16	10

[a]From reference 5155.

infections are often inapparent or mild, for rates of 1–5/1,000 susceptible pregnant women.

- Mother-to-child transmission (1709, 2518, 4069, 4282, 5155, 7926) (Table 14.4, from [5155]). Transmission risks vary with type of treatment and trimester, for rates of 1–10% in the first trimester to 30–80% (typically 60%) in the third trimester. In contrast, congenital disease shows an opposite trend, with a high manifestation index (~80%) in the first trimester, and low index (10%) in the third trimester.
- Impact (649, 1107, 1709, 2273, 3649, 3756, 4058, 4282, 4504, 4854, 5386, 7217, 7923, 7926, 8198). By prenatal treatment and completeness of initial evaluation (eye and imaging), ~60–100% of infections are inapparent at birth. By postnatal treatment and length of follow-up (1–20 years), a variable, additional fraction of infants becomes manifest, mainly by ocular lesions (~18–24%). However, >70% will remain free from lesions. By location, maternal management, and follow-up, reported overall rates of congenital infections are 0.07–1 (typically 0.3–0.8) per 1,000 live births. For congenital *T. gondii* chorioretinitis rates per 100 person-months of 0–2.8 at age 0–12 months and of 0–1.2 at age 2–13 years were reported.

***T. cruzi* (3016).** Intrauterine infections are a significant hazard in enzootic areas. In Argentina in 1994–2001, 1,136 congenital infections were reported (~15% of the estimated true number). In Argentina, congenital infections outnumbered vector-borne acute cases by a factor of 10.

- Maternal infection (8099) varies by age and exposure in enzootic area. For transplacentel transmission, parasitemia during pregnancy is required, rather than current residence in an enzootic area.
- Mother-to-child transmission (672, 6479, 7520, 8099, 8367). Reported risk in (latently) infected pregnant women, by test and length of follow-up is ~1–10%.
- Impact (672, 3016, 7520, 8367). Most infections are inapparent at birth but can evolve to serious disease. Manifestations include stillbirth, preterm delivery, low birth weight, and jaundice. Lethality of neonatal Chagas disease is 2–14%.

Peripartal Infections of Neonates

Peripartum is the time from rupture of the membranes to cutting the umbilical cord. Neonatal is the period of the first month of life. "Early-onset" neonatal disease begins in the first 3–6 days of life, reflecting intrauterine or peripartal exposure. "Late-onset" disease begins on days 4–7 postpartum, reflecting intrauterine, peripartal, *or* environmental sources (for the latter, see "Postpartal Infections of Neonates" below).

Infections (1013, 6930). Peripartal neonatal infections result from contact (ascending maternal infection and amnionitis), ingestion (aspiration) of secretions or excretions during delivery, or inoculation (umbilical cord, microtrauma).

In the United States in 1990–1998, 4% (559/13,324) of neonates (age 0–30 days) were diagnosed with infections, ~30% in inpatients and 70% in outpatients. Attack rates per 100 inpatients (outpatients) were 0.4 (0.04) for pneumonia, 0.02 (1.8) for other respiratory tract infections, 0.4 (0.03) for bloodstream infections (BSI), 0.02 (0.06) for meningitis, and 0.01 (0.11) for urinary tract infections (UTI). In Utah in 1999–2002, of 1,298 febrile neonates and infants (temperature ≥38°C, age 1–90 days), 8% (105) had serious bacterial infections (growth from normally sterile site, pathogen in stool, or significant growth in urine); diagnoses included UTI (in 67%), bacteremia (in 27%), and meningitis (in 4%). Most (98%) infections were community acquired.

Peripartal Viral Infections of Neonates

Agents from peripartal secretions or blood are CMV, HBV, HCV, HIV, and HSV.

CMV (142, 6006, 6533). Peripartal (from secretions) and nursing (from breast milk) neonatal CMV infections seem more frequent than intrauterine infections. Most peripartal and nursing neonatal CMV infections are inapparent, few are severe and manifest as pneumonia or deafness.

HBV (171, 2256, 6962). HBV is a major delivery hazard in areas where antenatal screen and vaccines are not routine, and HBsAg prevalence is high (>8%).

- Maternal infection. HBsAg prevalence varies by location and risks. In the United States, the overall HBsAg prevalence in pregnant women is 0.6% (95% CI 0.2–1), with lows of 0.1% (95% CI 0.02–0.5) in Hispanic and of 0.6% (95% CI 0.3–1) in Caucasian women, and highs of 1% (95% CI 0.5–1.5) in African American and of 6% (95% CI 4.5–7) in Asian women.

- Mother-to-child transmission. Perinatal transmission is efficient. For HBsAg-positive, HBeAg-negative mothers, the transmission risk is 10–40%. For HBsAg-positive, HBeAg-positive mothers, the risk is 70–90%.
- Impact. Administration of HB-Ig and vaccine, starting at birth, reduces transmission risks to <10%. HBV infection acquired from birth persists in 20–70% of neonates (from HBsAg-positive, HBeAg-negative mothers) to 70–90% of neonates (from HBsAg-positive, HBeAg-positive mothers). About 25% of persisting infections progress to chronic HB, cirrhosis, or primary liver carcinoma.

HCV (173, 1344, 3506, 4965, 7151). The main risk of HCV is maternal virema (detected by NAT). Although breast milk can test positive for HCV, breast-feeding (and type of delivery) do not seem to influence transmission.

- Maternal infection (3506). Infection prevalence varies by location and risks. In the United States, 2–5% of women of childbearing age are infected.
- Mother-to-child transmission (173, 1344, 1549, 2721, 3506, 7151, 8033). Transmission is rare if mothers are negative by NAT, but more likely if NAT detects maternal viremia of $>10^6$ copies/ml. Coinfection with HIV seems to enhance risks. Overall transmission risks are 2–12% (often 4–7%). (2900, 4862, 5567, 6228, 7331).
- Impact (3506). Infection in infants is confirmed by NAT at age >1 month, and by antibody that persists beyond age 18 months. Some 1.5%-80% of infected infants progress to chronic infection with potential liver damage.

HIV (6, 974, 3709, 4077, 5364, 7214). Roughly one third of pediatric HIV infections are perinatal. By viral maternal load and CD4 cell count, peripartal bleeding, and duration of labor, risks of peripartal transmission are ~13–18%. Cesarean section reduces risks, vaginal delivery increases risks, in particular, episiotomy, vacuum extraction, or other invasive delivery procedures that are not performed routinely.

HSV (8076). Peripartal transmission accounts for most (85%) of neonatal HSV infections. Sources are reactivated or primary infections of the birth canal.

- Maternal infections (1575, 4537, 8076). In high-income countries, 20–60% of women of childbearing age are seroreactive to HSV2, that is, latently infected, and in 0.5–3% of pregnant women, genital HSV2 infection is demonstrated. Of acquired infections, ~20% are inapparent.
- Mother-to-child transmission (6, 933, 1575). The risk is <1–5% from reactivated infection, but 15–50%, if a seronegative women acquires HSV2 in the third trimester of pregnancy.
- Impact (3027, 3943, 8076). Most neonatal infections are manifest. Without treatment, lethality is high (up to 60%). Even with treatment, lethality ranges from 4% (CNS disease) to 29% (disseminated disease), and neurological sequelae can remain. Reported rates of neonatal HSV infections are 0.1–0.4 per 1,000 deliveries.

Peripartal Bacterial Infections of Neonates

Maternal sources of peripartal neonatal infections include (i) endogenous or transient flora in the birth canal (e.g., *S. aureus*, *S. agalactiae*, and *S. pyogenes*) through ascension after early rupture of membranes, (ii) agents of STI (e.g., *Chlamydia*, gonococci, mycoplasms, and *Treponema*), (iii) the bowel (e.g., *Enterobacter*, *Escherichia*, *Klebsiella*, *Pseudomonas*, *Listeria*, and *Serratia*), and (iv) peripartal bacteremia (e.g., *Campylobacter fetus*).

A neonatal source for neonatal infections is the umbilical stump (e.g., for sepsis agents, *C. tetani*). Agents of invasive neonatal disease (1013, 3218) are *Enterobacter*, *E. coli* (in 25–60% of cases), *K. pneumoniae* (8%), *P. aeruginosa*, *L. monocytogenes*, *Staphylococcus*, GBS, and *S. marcescens*.

C. trachomatis (1753, 6648). *C. trachomatis* is a significant cause of conjunctivitis, ophthalmia, and pneumonia in neonates. Of 131 colonized women, 36% gave birth to infected neonates.

C. tetani (2844, 3350, 7756). Maternal and neonatal tetanus are acquired from dirty environments. Birth attendants who wash hands and use clean instruments reduce tetanus risks. Vaccination during pregnancy eliminates risks for mothers and neonates (by antibody transfer). Yet worldwide, there are ~200,000 deaths per year from neonatal tetanus, and ~30,000 cases per year of maternal tetanus. In Montana in 1998, tetanus was diagnosed in a neonate. The mother had refused vaccine for "philosophical" reasons, instead, she applied "beauty clay powder" for home umbilical cord care from a "direct-entry midwife."

- Maternal infection (674). Hazards include home delivery by untrained women, criminal abortion, and female circumcision.

- Outcome (570, 1286, 3350, 6049, 6698, 7544, 7635). Hazards include home delivery, unhygienic delivery, traditional birth attendance, and traditional umbilical cord care. Reported hazardous procedures include the application of coconut oil into the vagina for delivery, delivery on soil, delivery close to domestic animals, application of butter (ghee) to neonates, application of cow dung to the umbilicus, and wrapping neonates in sheepskin. In the prevaccine era, rates of neonatal tetanus in rural areas were 5–8/100 live births.

L. monocytogenes **(2215, 2511, 6884, 6897).** Delivering mothers can shed *L. monocytogenes* with feces, urine, birth canal secretions, and lochia. Peripartal infections of neonates from aspiration are plausible. The rate of neonatal listeriosis is 0–40 (typically 5) per 10^5 live births.

Mycoplasms (4168, 5377). Febrile postpartal or postabortal women grow *M. hominis* (~1%) or *U. urealyticum* (~2%) from blood. Blood cultures from febrile pregnant women should include these agents. Low-birth-weight babies with respiratory failure born to febrile mothers were reported to grow *M. hominis* or *U. urealyticum* from blood or respiratory fluid. In contrast, maternal *M. genitalium* does not seem to affect pregnancy outcome.

N. gonorrhoeae **(3720, 4179).** In general, infection prevalence in pregnant women is <1% in high-income countries but 3–15% in low-income countries. The risk of mother-to-child transmission during delivery is 30–50%. A manifestation of neonatal infection is conjunctivitis (gonococcal ophthalmia), which can cause blindness. In low-income countries, the risk of neonatal gonococcal infection is ~3/100 live births.

Staphylococcus **(1013, 4175, 5377).** *S. aureus* is a cause of maternal and neonatal illness. In Bordeaux, France, in 1988–1990, 0.3% (2/620) of febrile postpartal or postabortal women grew *S. aureus* in blood culture. *S. aureus* can be transmitted peripartally, from vaginal flora, but postnatal cross-infection is more frequent. In Utah, *S. aureus* was recovered from 8% (8/105) of infants with serious bacterial infections. A neonatal disease is staphylococcal scalded-skin syndrome (SSSS).

S. agalactiae **(GBS) (1761, 2730, 3314, 6702, 6707).** Around delivery, GBS colonizes the birth canal of 10–30% of pregnant women (high in North America, low in Asia). Risks include young age, intrauterine devices, tampons, and African-American ethnicity. GBS is a cause of maternal bacteriuria, amnionitis, and puerperal sepsis. Prepartal screening for vaginal and rectal carriage is recommended in the United States. Intrapartal antimicrobial treatment targeted to colonized women seems beneficial for neonatal health.

- Mother-to-child transmission (2730, 3314). By screening and intrapartum treatment, rates of transmission from colonized mothers are 1–20%.
- Outcome (1013, 2730, 3217, 3533, 4559, 4594, 6702, 6703, 6882). Neonatal invasive GBS disease includes sepsis and meningitis. GBS is recovered in 6% of infants with serious bacterial infections, and it accounts for 40–50% of neonatal meningitis. Lethality is 5–10%. Risks for neonatal invasive GBS disease include maternal colonization, early rupture of membranes, intrapartum fever ($\geq 38°C$), preterm delivery, and a history of an infant with invasive GBS disease. The well-documented rate of neonatal invasive GBS disease ranges broadly, from 0.2 to 6/1,000 live births. Rates per 1,000 live births of early-onset disease are 0.2–0.6 in North America and 0.5 in Europe; rates of late-onset disease are 0.4 in North America and 0.2 in Europe.

S. pyogenes **(GAS) (7205).** To prevent spread of GAS and puerperal fever, I. Semmelweis (1818–1865) pioneered hand hygiene. Today, in general, GAS is isolated in <3% of postpartum infections. An outbreak has been reported on an obstetric ward.

Peripartal Other Infections of Neonates

C. albicans **(6, 6677, 7895).** *C. albicans* colonizes the vagina, and vulvovaginal infections are frequent in pregnant women. Mild mucocutaneous infection is also frequent in healthy infants, while disease is rare.

T. vaginalis **(125).** Some *T. vaginalis* infections have been reported in female neonates.

Postpartal Infections of Neonates

Sources of postpartal infections in neonates include breast milk and nursing and home environment (Box 14.14).

Protection from breast milk (33, 415, 971, 3729, 3989, 4655, 5493, 5938, 6424, 6438, 6522, 6557). Breast milk protects neonates from infection. However, although plausible, protection is difficult to confirm, for reasons that include poor compliance (partial breast-feeding, early abandoning), assessment of outcome, and confounding by innate resistance, transplacentally transferred IgG, and vaccines. Despite these caveats, there is evidence for protection, by continuous breast-feeding for 3–6 months, from otitis media, lower RTI, diarrhea, and infections by RSV; Hib, *H. pylori*, *Salmonella*, *Shigella*; *Giardia*, *Cryptosporidium*, and *P. falciparum*. In Gabon, Central Africa, rates of parasitemia (2/1,000 person-months) and clinical falciparum malaria (1/1,000 person-months) were >100–fold lower in infants <3 months of age than in older infants.

Viruses from breast milk (975, 2551, 3112, 3709, 5213, 6214, 6462, 7214, 8332). There is evidence for transmammary transmission of CMV, EBV, HBV, HIV, HSV, HTLV, and WNV. **CMV (3112, 4795, 4955, 7103, 8332).** Breast milk is the main source of postnatal CMV infection. By NAT, CMV is detected in milk from ~15–70% of breast-feeding mothers, and in ~40–95% of seroreactive mothers (likely from reactivation), with a peak viral load at ~4 weeks after delivery. By birth weight and length of follow-up, rates of postnatal transmission from infected mothers to infant are ~10–40%. Of neonatal infections, 0–50% are inapparent. **HIV.** Maternal lethality (4883, 5365). Lethality of HIV-infected nursing mothers is high in sub-Saharan Africa: 3–4% have died within 1 year of delivery, and 11% within 2 years.

- Mother-to-child transmission (975, 1605, 5213, 6160). The risk is 5–20%, ~10% after 1 month of breast-feeding, and ~15% after 18 months. In high-income countries, replacing breast-feeding with formula milk can prevent postnatal HIV1 transmission. In low-income countries, this choice is difficult, given the benefits of breast-feeding, and the cost of formula feeding.
- Impact (974, 4077, 5213, 5364, 6160). There is firm evidence for HIV1 transmission through breast-feeding. By NAT, HIV1 is demonstrated in 30–60% of milk samples from infected mothers. Roughly one third of HIV infections in infants result from breast-feeding.

HTLV (2551, 3833, 4159, 6462). The main transmission risk is postnatal. Both HTLV1 and HTLV2 can be transmitted through breast milk.

- Maternal infection (3833, 4159, 4610). In Okinawa, Japan, an endemic area, maternal seroprevalence decreased from ~20% in the 1980s to ~6% in the 2000s, apparently by shortened or abandoned breast-feeding. In other areas such as Spain, maternal seroprevalence of HTLV1 and HTLV2 is low, not warranting antenatal screening.
- Mother-to-child transmission (4159, 4717). The reported rate is 15–30%.
- Impact (4610). The impact on neonatal health has been poorly documented. HTLV seems nonpathogenic for infants.

WNV (2798, 5558). Transmission through breast-milk is reported. A 40-year-old woman received red blood cells from a WNV-positive donor 24 h after delivery of a healthy baby. The mother developed WNV encephalitis 12 days posttransfusion, and her baby whom she breast-fed up to 16 days postpartum tested positive for WNV at age 25 days.

Bacteria from breast milk (185, 431, 5649, 5686, 6061, 6087). Agents grown from breast milk include skin flora, *Bacteroides*, *B. pseudomallei* (6087), *E. coli*, *S. aureus*, CoNS, *S. agalactiae* (GBS), and *S. pyogenes* (GAS). There is evidence for transmammary transmission of *Brucella*, *B. pseudomallei*, *Leptospira*, *Listeria*, *M. tuberculosis*, *Salmonella*, and GBS.

Parasites from breast milk. Hookworm infections in neonates (5518) and recovery of larvae from colostrum (6783) suggest transmammary transmission of *A. duodenale* but not of *N. americanus* (1642).

Agents from the environment. Sources of postpartal infections in neonates include hands and skin of mothers, diapers (see section 6.4), and formula feeding. Whereas reports of infections in neonatal intensive care units (ICU, see section VI) abound, few reports address community-acquired neonatal infections. Bottle-fed infants are at increased risk of otitis media, lower RTI, and diarrhea, including in high-income countries (415, 4227). Formula-associated diarrhea in infants likely results from unhygienic preparation or handling. **EV (7798).** EV is acquired seasonally and can be acquired early in life. Sources include maternal droplets and feces, surfaces, and objects. In Utrecht, The Netherlands, in 2000–2001, PCR identified EV in blood, cerebrospinal fluid, or feces from 11 (58%) of 19 infants (≤60 days old) admitted from home. In the same area in 1993–1995, the rate of EV disease in neonates (≤30 days old) was 0.3/1,000 live births. **Rotavirus (669, 4448, 6784).** A prospective study of breast-fed and bottle-fed infants found no evidence for protection. Hands and the nursing environment are likely sources. In a matched case-control study, bottle feeding was a risk. In Melbourne, Australia, the rate of *Rotavirus* diarrhea was 1.5% (22/1,464) in babies roomed with their mothers, 14% (36/251) in babies in a special care nursery, and 17% (54/326) in a routine, communal nursery. **Citrobacter (2793).** *Citrobacter* is an agent of invasive disease in neonates indicative of acquisition from nosocomial or home environments.

SECTION V
Travel and Transport

15 Human Travel

16 Transported Animals and Goods

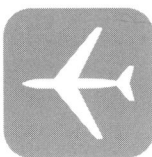

Droplets around the world in less than 80 days.

Previous sections dealt with autochthonous (indigenous) agents and infections. Here, displaced agents and infections are discussed. Travel is the act of going to places, including border crossing and overnight stay. Transport is the movement of people, animal, or goods by vehicle, train, boat, or aircraft. In imported infections, place of acquisition and place of domicile and diagnosis are clearly separated, for instance, by at least a domestic if not a national border. In introduced infections, import results in local spread.

Trade routes are traditional corridors of dissemination of agents and infections. "Epidemiological portals of entry" are bus and railway stations, seaports, and airports. Depending on presymptomatic shedding (see section 14.1) and sensitivity of procedures, screening of arriving passengers or animals may or may not be effective to prevent spread. In the 2003 severe acute respiratory syndrome (SARS) pandemic, health declarations by 45 million travelers at international borders detected only four SARS cases, and thermal scanning of >35 million international travelers for fever did not detect a single case (532). Quarantine is an ultimate measure to control spread.

Infections that advanced along land and sea routes included plague, cholera, and human immunodeficiency virus (4181, 4930). Highways such as the trans-Saharan and trans-Amazon affect agent spread as corridors but also by altering settlement (1946). Ship's ballast, bilge, and sewage water transported *Vibrio cholerae* shore-to-shore (4874). International flights take less time than many incubation periods, with a risk for incubating passengers to arrive and spread agents before disease is manifest. In Gran Canaria, Spain, a tourist from mainland Europe was the likely source for an outbreak of echovirus 13 meningitis that affected 152 children and adolescents (5832). At a campground in Queensland, Australia, in 2002, a 29-year-old man with *Plasmodium vivax* infection acquired in Asia in 1998 introduced vivax malaria to 10 adults camping nearby; at the time of outbreak, *Anopheles farauti* sensu lato was abundant at the campground (3124).

> **Box V.1 Suggested travel exposure history**
>
> **Commuting**
> - Describe your way to work, school, or shopping.
>
> **Last international travel**
> - Give departure and return dates of last international travel, with stopover places and names of countries visited.
> - Give the reason for that travel, how you traveled, and type of overnight accomodations.
> - List any use of antimalarials, bednets, or repellents. Have you had any water (e.g., hands), soil (e.g., beach), or casual sex contacts?
>
> **Travel in past 12 months**
> - List all places you visited within your country further than 100 km away from home.
> - Have you had any overnight stays with friends, in camps, cabins, or tents, or in the open air?
> - Did you book any flight, cruise, or package tour? Any border crossing by car, ferryboat, or train?
> - Have you taken home any souvenirs, including food, animals (living and carapace), or goods (e.g., leatherwear and textiles)?
> - Have you been bitten by a dog, cat, bat, tick, insect, or other animal?
>
> **Lifetime travel**
> - List all continents visited ever, with years and duration of visit

Exposure history (Box V.1) should include international and domestic travel. Examples of domestically imported infections include in the United States Colorado tick fever (5032), tick-borne relapsing fever (2255), and plague (1968) that are acquired in the West and diagnosed in the East, and in Europe *Dirofilaria immitis* that is acquired in Corsica and diagnosed in mainland France (6069).

The history should also address international stopovers and single-night accommodations as these may suffice to contract infections, for instance, malaria, or Mayaro fever from dining outdoors (7517). For hotel accommodation (see section 11.8). The latest information is available at http://www.who.int/ith and http://www.cdc.gov/travel/index.htm.

15 Human Travel

15.1 Local travel
15.2 Ships and seaports
15.3 Aircraft and airports
15.4 International short-term travel
15.5 Expatriates
15.6 Immigrants and migrants

15.1 LOCAL TRAVEL

Local travel is all regular travel for work, school, shopping, and leisure, in a perimeter of a about a 2-h drive (100 km) from home. Means include walking, bicycle, taxi, bus, tram, rail, subway, and ferryboat (see section 15.2). Of emerging importance are transports by ambulances between facilities of care.

Exposure. Although significant, international statistics are unavailable. Car density is 0.1–0.5 per person in high-income countries, and 0.005–0.02 per person in low-income countries. Cities with large subway systems (billion rides per year) include Moscow (3.2), Tokyo (2.6), Mexico City (~1.4), Seoul (~1.4), and New York City (1.4).

Infections (2710, 4181, 5646) (Box 15.1). "Commuting infections" have been poorly documented. Rural residents visiting cities are at risk of respiratory tract infections and sexually transmitted infections (STI). Urban residents visiting the countryside are at risk of vector-borne or environmental infections. In Quidbo, northwestern Colombia, travel out of the city in the preceding 8–14 days increased falciparum or vivax malaria risks in city residents.

DROPLET-AIR CLUSTER

Sources include crowded buses, subways, rails, even taxis, incubating visitors and migrants, and patient transports. As exposure time is short, shedding with droplets from incubating or ill passengers must be massive for effective spread.

Viruses

Influenzavirus **(1154, 2715, 3973, 7996).** Transportation of troops by railway contributed to the spread of the 1918 "Spanish flu." In the 1957–1958 pandemic, A/H2N2 was carried from People's Republic of China into Russia on the trans-Siberia Railway. Crowded public transports may trigger local outbreaks. In summer of 1998, acute respiratory tract infections were reported in travelers to Alaska and the Yukon Territory, in particular, among groups of 40–50 passengers who shared common transportation; A/H3N2 virus was implicated in the outbreak. On living animal (wet) markets in Asia, where chicken, ducks, pet

> **Box 15.1** Agents or infections from local travel, by agent cluster
>
> | | |
> |---|---|
> | Droplet-air | Influenza, measles, SARS; *Klebsiella* (ESβL by patient transport), *Legionella, M. tuberculosis*, and *N. meningitidis* |
> | Feces-food | HAV; *C. botulinum, C. difficile* (by patient transport), *Enterococcus* (VRE by patient transport), *E. coli* (ESβL by patient transport), *Salmonella*, and *V. cholerae* |
> | Zoonotic | FMDV, YFV; *C. burnetii; Plasmodium*, and *Leishmania* |
> | Environmental | *Serratia* (by patient transport); *Sporothrix* |
> | Skin-blood | HIV; *S. aureus* (MRSA by patient transport), *T. pallidum pallidum*; and *Candida* (by patient transport) |

birds, dogs, and other animals are traded under crowded conditions, species jump of A virus subtypes is greatly facilitated.

Measles virus (2631, 3240). In the United States in 1994, one index case and 10 immunoglobulin M (IgM)-positive measles infections were diagnosed among 94 college students, faculty, and relatives who traveled on two buses in the southwest for 3 days, seven infections were from the bus with the index case, and three were from the other bus. In rural Senegal in 1983–1986, 14% (57/402) of primary measles cases were acquired on buses or during local travel.

Poliomyelitis virus (8121). By 2003, circulation of wild poliovirus had been contained to three countries each in Africa (Egypt, Niger, and Nigeria) and Asia (Afghanistan, India, and Pakistan). By 2004, virus had been seeded into eight previously polio-free countries in West and Central Africa, resulting in 63 cases. Of eight index cases, two reported travel, and six reported residence in commercial centers with much regional traffic. Furthermore, analysis of virus types (1 and 3) suggested repeated crossings of the Niger-Nigeria border.

Severe acute respiratory syndrome-coronavirus (SARS-CoV) (8276). In Beijing, People's Republic of China, during the 2003 SARS epidemic, taking a taxi more than once per week was an infection risk, for an odds ratio of ~3 (95% confidence interval [95% CI] 1.3–8) compared with persons not taking taxis. Risks from taking a bus (odds ratio, 1.7; 95% CI 0.9–3) or subway (odds ratio, 2.5; 95% CI 1–7) more than once per week were approaching significance.

Bacteria

***Legionella* (4105, 6298).** Person-to-person spread of *Legionella* has not been documented. Management of air temperature in public transport systems is a putative source, however. In Germany in 1999, a 55-year-old healthy man contracted *Legionella* pneumonia 2 days after returning from a bus tour through Austria and Italy; no other cases were identified. In Switzerland in 1977, a 66-year-old man contracted *Legionella* pneumonia 2 days after exposure on the train to a group of coughing and febrile American tourists.

***Mycobacterium tuberculosis*.** Not recognized, symptomatic cases are a risk for passengers on buses and trains, in particular, on long trips and in poorly ventilated buses. Because school busing is typical for North America, most instances are reported from this region.

- Buses in North America (5869, 6074, 6508, 8359). In Nova Scotia, Canada, one bus driver and two nuns escorted 48 girls (including one open index case) on a 10-h bus trip; bus windows were closed because of the cold. Both nuns and all girls converted to tuberculin (98% or 50/51), as did 41% (234/574) of class mates, and 35 cases were diagnosed. In Missouri, a high school student with untreated cavernous tuberculosis was the likely source for seven infections in bus riders, including one with active disease. In upstate New York, a school bus driver was undiagnosed and symptomatic for several months; compared with an infection prevalence of ~2% in the community, 32% (85/266) of children riding the bus regularly were skin-test positive, and 19% (51) developed disease. The reactivity prevalence increased from 22% if the time spent on the bus was <10 min, to 30% for exposure for 10–39 minutes, and to 57% for exposure for ≥40 minutes.

- Buses in West Europe (2280). At a school in Spain in 1992, 81 infections and 12 new cases were diagnosed among 232 students and 127 teachers, including 21 infections and 5 cases among participants of a bus trip from Malaga to the Sierra Nevada. Compared with nonparticipants, the odds ratio for infection among bus riders was 3.4, and most infected bus riders were sitting close to an index case.

- Trains (5172). In 1996, smear- and culture-positive tuberculosis was diagnosed in a 22-year-old African

American who had traveled on two U.S. passenger trains for 29 hours, and on a bus for 5.5 hours; 240 passengers and crew were screened by tuberculin skin test, and 4 (2%) converted. For two of them, no risks were identified other than exposure to the index passenger.

Klebsiella **(1560, 3360, 4283, 5143, 6521, 8154).** Interfacility patient transfer and transport of extended-spectrum β-lactamse (ESβL)-producing *K. pneumoniae* is a hazard that has emerged in North America and Europe. Nursing home patients are a significant source of ESβL strains. Ways of spread include home-to-hospital and hospital-to-hospital. International spread among facilities has also been reported. A multiresistant *K. pneumoniae* strain has been carried from Bahrain to London, and from there to Oxford.

Neisseria meningitidis **(3156, 3616).** Of 21 *N. meningitidis* serogroup C outbreaks reported in the United States in 1980–1993, venue for one outbreak with five cases was a school bus jointly used by elementary and junior high school students; spread was limited to the bus, for an attack rate of 7% (5/72).

Fungi
Histoplasma **(3023).** In Tennessee in 1980, 81% (69/85) of participants of an overland wagon train contracted *Histoplasma* infection from a former blackbird roost, soil samples of which grew *H. capsulatum*.

FECES-FOOD CLUSTER
Sources include snacks and foods consumed while commuting, agents from locally transported foods, and patient transfers.

Viruses
Hepatitis A virus (HAV) (8014). Border crossing can be a risk. In San Diego County, California, in 1998–2000, 67% (89/132) of Hispanic children (age <18 years) with acute HA reported travel to Mexico (mostly nearby Tijuana) in the 2–6 weeks preceding illness onset, compared with 25% (88/354) of susceptible, healthy Hispanic control children matched for age and exposure period, for an odds ratio of 6 (95% CI 4–10). Foods from street vendors and eating salads or vegetables were significant travel risks.

Bacteria
Clostridium. C. botulinum **(7832).** Food stalls have been a reported source of botulism for bus drivers in Buenos Aires, Argentina, who ate meat rolls along bus itineraries. *C. difficile* **(6521).** Interfacility transfer of colonized patients is a hazard for nosocomial spread of *C. difficile*.

Enterococcus. Residents of nursing homes are an important source of vancomycin-resistant *Enterococcus* (VRE) (2175). Of travelers repatriated to Germany (2402) and The Netherlands (3787), 2–4% were found to carry VRE. Interfacility transfer of colonized patients has been associated with an increased risk of nosocomial VRE acquisition (7556).

Escherichia coli **(8154).** Nursing home patients are a significant source of ESβL-producing strains of *E. coli*, and interfacility transfer of colonized patients is a nosocomial hazard.

Salmonella **(3259).** Trucks can disperse *Salmonella* with raw foods. In the United States in 1994, nondisinfected tanker trailers first used to transport liquid egg that grew *Salmonella enterica* serovar Enteritidis, then pasteurized ice cream premix, were vehicles for ~224,000 salmonellosis cases nationwide, through cross-contamination of the premix.

Vibrio cholerae **(8085).** *V. cholerae* can spread along transportation routes by carriers who walk to marketplaces and gatherings, truck drivers, and boatmen.

Helminths
Fasciola hepatica **(4793).** In Bolivia, vegetables are transported from enzootic-endemic areas in the altiplano to uncontrolled markets in La Paz, for a risk of urban fascioliasis.

ZOONOTIC CLUSTER
Sources (2483, 4530, 7032, 7035). Sources of zoonotic infections include local herds, birds, commuting cars and trains that carry arthropods or parasitemic passengers, and tick foci in the area. *Rattus norvegicus* and *Mus musculus* were recovered from trains arriving at Chinese ports. *Aedes* mosquitoes were found in cars, trucks, and trains. For long-distance dispersal, see sections 16.1, 16.2, and 16.3.

Viruses
Foot-and-mouth disease virus (FMDV) (2722). In the FMDV epidemic in the United Kingdom in 2001, likely modes of dispersion in 1,849 reported animal cases included milk tankers in 11 (1%), motor vehicles in 28 (2%), and "local" means (within 3 km of a infected premise) in 1,454 (79%).

Yellow fever virus (YFV) (8083). In Brazil in 1985, three truck drivers on the road from São Paulo to Mato Grosso states were diagnosed with yellow fever in the town of Presidente Prudente; viremic drivers are feared to carry YFV into cities along highways that are receptive by the presence of *Aedes aegypti*.

Bacteria

Coxiella burnetii **(6558).** In a periurban area in the United Kingdom, an outbreak of Q fever with 29 cases was linked to farm vehicles that had brought contaminated straw, manure, or dust into the city.

Borrelia **(2255).** After visiting a remote, uninhabited cabin in New Mexico in 2002, 11 (28%) of a party of 40 had laboratory evidence of *B. hermsii* infection (an agent of tick-borne relapsing fever).

Protozoa

Plasmodium **(2092, 2483, 3574, 3974, 6404).** *Anopheles* or gametocytemic travelers can conceivably introduce malaria to receptive areas along trade corridors such as the trans-Saharan (oases) and pan-American (colonias) highways. At the Djibouti-Ethiopia border station, trains were examined for *Anopheles* and human carriers; *Anopheles* was not found, but humans with *P. falciparum* parasitemia were identified, and it was concluded that the railway could potentially spread malaria. In South Africa, two women living 140 km away from malarious areas, but 80 m from a taxi rank serving commuters to and from malarious areas, contracted falciparum malaria in the same month of 1995; spread of vectors by taxi was suspected. In Cambodia in 2000, local spread by traders and mobile laborers seemed plausible as 2% (16/666, 94% *P. vivax*) were parasitemic. In Italy, carriage of infective *Anopheles* by car was suspected in a woman with falciparum malaria who lived 5 km from a local airport (with occasional arrivals from tropical countries), but 25 km from an international airport (Fiumiciono near Rome). Last, drivers are at risk while driving through malarious areas (see section 12.8).

Leishmania **(3928).** In Tadjikistan cutaneous leishmaniasis was carried by sandflies imported by car and by helicopter from neighboring Afghanistan.

ENVIRONMENTAL CLUSTER

On fragile lands, offroad and sports utility vehicles can compact and erode soil, and stir up infective dust and aerosols (see section 5.5). Further sources include patient transports and accidents.

Serratia marcescens **(3273, 3727, 6521).** Patient transfers are a hazard for the nosocomial spread of *S. marcescens*.

Sporothrix. Motor vehicle accidents that cause soil to be inoculated into skin and soft tissues have been associated with sporotrichosis (3850).

SKIN-BLOOD CLUSTER

Sources include sex contacts along trade corridors, patient transports, and accidents.

Human immunodeficiency virus (HIV) (3325, 4181, 7982). In rural West Africa, seroprevalence was higher in women reporting casual sex in a city than in women not reporting such exposure. Among adults from Uganda ($n = 1,292$), seroprevalence was high (26% in men, 47% in women) at trading centers along main roads, intermediate (22% in men, 29% in women) in villages along minor roads, and low (8% in men, 9% in women) in farm villages. For spread of HIV by truck drivers, see section 12.8. A 32-year-old American was reported to have acquired HIV from a motor vehicle accident in Rwanda, in which he sustained lacerations that were contaminated with blood from similarly injured passengers.

Staphylococcus aureus **(691, 2402, 3787, 6521).** Patient transfers are a hazard for the nosocomial spread of methicillin-resistant *S. aureus* (MRSA). Of travelers repatriated to Germany or The Netherlands, 2–4% were found to carry MRSA. Interfacility transfers of colonized or infected patients may increase risks of subsequent nosocomial acquisition up to 7-fold. From hospitals and nursing homes, patients, residents, and health workers have carried MRSA to their home communities where strains become established.

Treponema pallidum pallidum **(1558).** In North Carolina in 1985–1994, mean syphilis rates per 10^5 per year were 37 in five urban counties, 38 in counties along highways, but significantly lower (16) in the remaining 84 counties.

Candida **(6521).** Patient transfers are a hazard for the nosocomial spread of *Candida*. Interfacility transfers of colonized or infected patients may increase risks of subsequent nosocomial acquisition up to 21-fold.

15.2 SHIPS AND SEAPORTS

"Ship" here includes any sea-going vessel, from "fishing and ferry boat to container and cruise ship," including submarines, tankers, and yachts.

Exposure (66, 4257). International statistics of travel by ferries and cruise boats are not available. In the United States in 1975–1985, captains reported 22,767 cruises that docked at ports; typical cruises lasted 7 days and carried 600–700 passengers. By volume of passengers, the major cruise ports are Miami and Ft. Lauderdale/Port Everglades, both in Florida.

Infections (2977, 4930, 5233, 5816) (Box 15.2). Seaports have been portals of plague in the past. At the end of the nineteenth century, steamboats carried infected rats and their fleas port-to-port, contributing to the spread the third plague pandemic. Today, ports remain portals for

> **Box 15.2 Agents or infections on ships and at seaports, by cluster**
>
> Droplet-air   Mainly influenza. Also: rubella; *C. diphtheriae, Legionella, M. tuberculosis,* and *N. meningitidis*
> Feces-food   Mainly: *Norovirus; E. coli* (ETEC), *Shigella, V. parahaemolyticus*. Also: *Salmonella, V. cholerae, Y. enterocolitica; Giardia;* and *Trichinella*
> Zoonotic   DENV, WNV; *Plasmodium*

mosquitoes, arboviruses such as dengue virus (DENV), and *Plasmodium* ("boat malaria" or "port malaria").

DROPLET-AIR CLUSTER

Incubating passengers and crew and stops at ports are sources of respiratory agents on ships. By type of passengers, season, crowding, and epidemiological situation, captains of commercial and navy ships might consider recommending predeparture vaccines for passengers and crew, e.g., *Influenzavirus* and measles-mumps-rubella (MMR).

Viruses

***Influenzavirus* (3973).** During the 1957–1958 pandemic, A/H2N2 virus was carried from Hong Kong to Singapore and Japan by sea. Spread across oceans, of A/H2N2 in 1957–1958, and of A/H3N2 in the 1968–1969 pandemic, took several months.

Outbreaks   Outbreaks have been well documented on ships mainly in the Northern Hemisphere, both in winter and summer (1424, 2109, 2368, 4932).

- Northern Hemisphere (1424, 2109, 4127, 5050). On a cruise on the Baltic Sea in June–July 2000, B virus caused an outbreak. On a cruise from New York to Montreal in August–September 1997, 3% (39/1,445) of passengers and 0.5% (3/631) of crew reported flulike illness; on the return cruise from Montreal to New York with the same crew, 1% (19/1,448) of new passengers and 3% (17/631) of crew had flulike illness; A/H3N2 virus was implicated in both outbreaks. On a U.S. Navy ship in December 1977 to January 1978, A/H1N1 virus caused ≥57 cases and inapparent infections in 3 (16%) of 19 personnel. On a U.S. Navy ship in waters off southern California in February 1996, A/H3N2 virus caused 232 cases among a crew of 548, for an attack rate of 42%; although 95% of the crew were vaccinated, the vaccine virus was ill fitted to circulating wild virus.
- Southern Hemisphere (4932). On a cruise from Sydney to Noumea in September 2000, 310 (28%) of 1,119 passengers reported flulike illness; attack and hospitalization rates were not different among vaccinated and nonvaccinated passengers.

Rubella virus (3373, 8407). Outbreaks of rubella virus on ships have been reported. In May–June 1996, a German navy ship experienced an outbreak with 18 cases and 2 infections, for an attack rate of 57%.

Bacteria

***Corynebacterium diphtheriae* (2131).** In 1997, a non-vaccinated, 71-year-old woman developed a sore throat while on a 12-day cruise on the Baltic Sea that included visits to Oslo, Copenhagen, St. Petersburg, Tallinn, Stockholm, and Amsterdam; on return to the United Kingdom, her tonsils grew toxigenic *C. diphtheriae* indistinguishable from epidemic strains circulating in Russia at the time.

***Legionella* (1116, 3692, 6436).** Water or air management systems rather than patients are the sources of *Legionella* on ships, including the water supply and whirlpool spas. Whirlpool spas on cruise ships increase the odds of disease by 16 (95% CI 3–352). With every hour spent in spa water, the risk of disease increases by 64% (95% CI 12–140). Sporadic cases or outbreaks have been reported from ferryboat, fish trawler, cargo ship, cruise ship, sail training ship, river cruiser, and missile cruiser. Because many ferryboat trips are short, it has been proposed to limit ferry-related cases to people who used cabins.

***M. tuberculosis* (3140, 3444, 4196, 6074, 7270).** Long contact and recirculated air are risks aboard ships. In particular, in submarines, closed air circulation is conducive for transmission. On a U.S. Navy cruiser, two crew members were diagnosed with disease, and 209 (46%) of 456 crew members skin-test converted. On another U.S. ship, 46% (139/308) of crew members became infected, and 5% (7/139) of skin converters developed disease. On a U.S. amphibious ship, a marine had cavitary pulmonary tuberculosis for 3 months before being diagnosed and treated; of 3,338 crew skin-tested, 712 (21%) had new, latent infections, and 21 had active tuberculosis.

***N. meningitidis* (2324).** Meningococcal meningitis was suspected in a young sailor onboard an aircraft carrier at sea in 2003. Chemoprophylaxis was given to 99 close contacts, and authorities of a port were contacted where the case had spent time days before illness onset.

FECES-FOOD CLUSTER

Sources (4050, 6401, 6402). Sources include raw, underheated, and handled foods, beverages, and ice from aboard ships and stops at ports, as well as polluted water taken aboard from ports, improper loading and storage of water, and lack of water treatment.

Risks (66, 3576, 4050, 4257, 6401, 6402). In the 1970s–1980s, diarrhea outbreaks affected 0.6% (98/17,322) of cruises from U.S. ports that typically lasted 3–15 days. A government inspection program was instituted that is ongoing (scores available at http://www2a.cdc.gov/nceh/vsp/vspmain.asp). Currently, ~0.4% of cruises report outbreaks (defined by attack rates >3%). A review of passenger ships for 1970–2003 identified 20 waterborne outbreaks (~0.5 per year) with 5,858 cases (293 per outbreak), and 50 food-borne outbreaks (1–2 per year) with 9,861 cases (197 per outbreak).

Prevention (4050). Over 50% of outbreaks could be prevented by cooking seafoods well, using pasteurized eggs, excluding ill food handlers from work, and not allowing onshore catering for offship excursions.

Viruses

Norovirus. Norovirus is a major agent of diarrhea on ships. Numerous outbreaks (66, 1586, 1623, 3006, 3576, 4050, 4872, 5664, 6401, 7465, 7840) have been documented on ships. Some examples follow. On one ship from Florida to the Caribbean in 2002, *Norovirus* outbreaks occurred on six consecutive 7-day cruises, despite aggressive sanitization after the second cruise. On cruise 1, 4% (84/2,318) of passengers had gastroenteritis. On cruise 3, 8% (192/2,456) of passengers and 2% (23/999) of crew had gastroenteritis. Several strains of *Norovirus* were recovered from five of the six cruises, for an overall yield of 45% (25/55) and confirming several introductions aboard. Dinners from two restaurants, breakfast from one restaurant, and person-to-person spread among cabin mates were all implicated. On a U.S. naval aircraft carrier in 1997, *Norovirus* caused ~1,800 diarrhea cases, for attack rates up to 44% in 2 weeks. A vehicle was not identified. Similarly in 1999, *Norovirus* caused outbreaks aboard two U.S. Navy ships, with attack rates of 6–9%, and no apparent source. In Southeast Asia in 1996, 7% (49/721) of troops aboard a U.S. ship contracted diarrhea in 3 months; 45% (21/47) of cases but none (0/38) of controls tested positive for *Norovirus*.

Bacteria

Main agents are *E. coli*, *Shigella*, and *Vibrio parahaemolyticus*. *Campylobacter*, *Salmonella* non-Typhi, *Salmonella enterica* serovar Typhi ("typhoid at sea") (1764), and *Yersinia* have also been reported aboard ships.

***E. coli* (1739, 5664, 6401, 6402, 7007).** Enterotoxigenic *E. coli* (ETEC) is a major agent of diarrhea on cruise and naval ships. Potato salad and cold buffet were implicated in an outbreak of invasive *E. coli* diarrhea on a cruise ship with ≥47 cases. Three ETEC outbreaks on cruise ships with 1,349 diarrhea cases altogether were associated with beverages served with ice cubes aboard ships; water bunkered at ports was the implicated source.

***Shigella* (66, 1147, 4386, 5001, 6402).** *Shigella* is a major agent on cruise and other ships, in particular, *S. flexneri*. Outbreaks have been well documented. Reported vehicles included handled foods such as potato salad and ice cubes. On a cruise from California to Mexico in 1994, 37% (586/1,589) of passengers and 4% (24/594) of crew reported diarrhea, and *S. flexneri* was isolated from ill passengers.

***Vibrio. V. cholerae* (819).** On a cruise ship from Hong Kong to Thailand in 1994, 62 (10%) of 630 passengers developed diarrhea, including 15 (2%) with suggestive cholera antitoxin titers, 6 (1%) with clinical cholera, and 2 (0.3%) with confirmed *V. cholerae* O139; yellow rice from an on-shore buffet in Bangkok was implicated. ***V. parahaemolyticus* (66, 4258, 4916, 5664).** *V. parahaemolyticus* is a major agent on cruise and naval ships. On cruises in the Caribbean in 1974–1975, seafood cocktails contaminated with seawater were implicated in two outbreaks, one with 36% (252/703) of passengers and none of 321 crew ill, the other with 61% (445/734) of passengers and 5% (27/570) of crew ill. In Alaska in 2004, locally farmed, raw oysters were the vehicle for 22 (17%) cases among 132 interviewed cruise passengers and ≥48 cases in the community. Patients, oysters, and water from oyster farms all yielded the epidemic strain.

***Yersinia enterocolitica* (366).** On an oil tanker from Croatia to Italy in 2002, 18% (22/120) of crew contracted diarrhea due to *Y. enterocolitica* 0:3; food could not be implicated, and person-to-person spread was suspected.

Protozoa

***Giardia* (7455).** Foods and drinking water are likely vehicles. In 1973, after a cruise in the Mediterranean, 70% (95/136) of children and teachers tested positive for *G. lamblia*, and 40% (52) had suggestive symptoms; the implicated vehicle was drinking water.

An unlikely zoonotic source is ship rats infected with *G. muris*.

Helminths

***Trichinella* (6916).** On a luxury liner from California to Alaska in 1974, beef was implicated in a trichinellosis outbreak that affected 2% (13/693) of passengers.

ZOONOTIC CLUSTER

West Nile virus (WNV) (2021). An outbreak affected crew of a cargo ship on passing the Suez Canal, from Romania to Yokohama, Japan.

Plasmodium. Malaria can be contracted on ships (ship malaria) (5436, 6867, 7500, 8408). For centuries, sailors have been considered at risk when sailing along malarious coasts. In Croatia in 1990–1993, port health authorities recorded 23 malaria cases aboard ships: 19 in sailors, and 4 in tourists, for an attack rate of 0.3% (23/8,379). In Japan, ~5% of imported malaria cases concerned seafarers. For a German couple who contracted falciparum malaria on a diving cruise in New Ireland, Solomon Islands, anchoring ~100 m off the malarious shore and leaving the cabin door open for the night was the only identified exposure.

Malaria can also be contracted in port cities (seaport malaria) (1867, 5816). In Ghent, Belgium, a ship docking at the fruit port terminal was suspected to have carried infective *Anopheles* and to have caused a case of falciparum malaria. In Marseille, France, in the summer of 1993 when the temperature was continuously >18°C and relative humidity >60%, two residents without travel or other risks contracted falciparum malaria; since vessels from West Africa could arrive at Marseille port within 6–8 days, the most likely source was infected *Anopheles* carried by a container ship.

SKIN-BLOOD CLUSTER
For STI in truck drivers, sailors, and air crew, see section 12.8.

15.3 AIRCRAFT AND AIRPORTS
Aircraft denotes conveyance through air, including by long-range commercial jet, propeller airplane, helicopter, air ambulance, and military aircraft (even hot-air balloon).

Exposure. Worldwide in 2003, >13,000 airports had paved runways, and >850 (many in high-income countries) had long (>3 km) runways for jets. Worldwide, airlines transport >1.5 billion passengers per year. Long-distance range and passenger capacity are increasing, while stopovers seem to decline. Of 59 million United Kingdom residents who departed in 2002, 76% (45 million) traveled by air, only 17% (10 million) by sea, and 7% (4 million) by tunnel.

Infections (2013, 4708, 8130) (Box 15.3). In general, the risk for infection to spread on aircraft is considered low. The rate of in-flight health problems is ~0.1/1,000 passengers. Most (70%) events are managed by cabin crew. Abdominal symptoms (diarrhea and vomiting) rank 1 and account for >25% of health problems; infections rank 7.

Prevention (1580). By destination, clients, and epidemiological situation, vaccines to consider for air ambulances and commercial aircraft crew include hepatitis B virus

---

Box 15.3 Agents or infections on aircraft or at airports, by cluster

Droplet-air	Mainly: influenza; *M. tuberculosis*, *N. meningitidis*. Also: measles, SARS
Feces-food	Mainly: *Norovirus*. Also: botulism, food poisoning (*B. cereus*, *C. perfringens*, and *S. aureus*), *Salmonella*, *Shigella*, *V. cholerae*, and *V. parahaemolyticus*
Zoonotic	DENV, some viral hemorrhagic fevers; *Coxiella*; *Plasmodium*

(HBV), MMR, and diphtheria-tetanus, possibly HAV, *Influenzavirus*, polio, varicella-zoster virus (VZV), YFV, and *N. meningitidis*. Malaria prophylaxis (continuous and emergency self-treatment) should also be considered for flights to malarious areas.

Passengers with measles or varicella should not be admitted to commercial flights. Passengers falling ill on the flight should report to the crew. SARS or viral hemorrhagic fever (VHF) has been suspected from abrupt and persisting fever (>38°C), exposure in hospitals, hotels, or outbreaks, or visits to infected areas in the preceding 3 weeks. Crew should consult with experts via phone before arrival, including for suspected bioterror, and alert responsible airline and airport staff.

DROPLET-AIR CLUSTER
Risk (4708, 8130, 8146). Cabin air quality is generally well maintained. There is a residual risk, however, for passengers to carry, spread, and acquire respiratory agents on board.

Viruses
Viruses with confirmed or likely onboard transmission are *Influenzavirus*, measles virus, and SARS-CoV.

***Influenzavirus* (3999, 4762, 5223, 6625).** Although difficult to confirm, transmission on aircraft seems to occur. An aircraft with an index A/H3N2 case and 54 passengers was grounded for 3 h without ventilation; within 72 h, 72% of passengers had developed flulike illness. At a naval air station in Florida in October–November 1986, A/H1N1 virus caused 60 clinical cases, including 41 (68%) from a squadron that had returned from Puerto Rico; transmission seemed to occur in barracks in Florida and Puerto Rico, and on two aircraft. At the quarantine station of Nagoya Airport, Japan, in 1996–1999, 6% (30/504) of gargle solutions from passengers with respiratory symptoms yielded *Influenzavirus*: 28 A/H3N2 virus and 2 B virus. Molecular and epidemiological evidence suggested that travelers contributed to the 1997–1998 and 1998–1999 domestic seasonal waves.

Measles virus (188, 1139, 2378). Risks on aircraft vary by duration of flight, air management, seating, and passenger age mix, but appear low overall. On a 7-h flight from Japan to Hawaii with a measles case onboard, none of 276 passengers monitored (from 336 exposed) developed febrile rash illness. A naval officer was the source for seven measles cases, six (five at Seattle airport and one office manager) on his flight from San Diego to Seattle, and one (a passenger) on his return flight.

SARS-CoV. Aircraft (1978, 8164) transporting incubating patients were the most likely mode by which SARS in 2002–2003 spread to 28 countries. In II–V/2003, six SARS cases were imported into Singapore before arrival screening was implemented. Only the first imported case caused secondary cases; of 442,973 air passengers screened, 136 were sent to a designated hospital for further evaluation and none was diagnosed with SARS.

Spread on a flight (532, 869, 4535, 5598, 8165) seems possible but unusual, and concentrated to the second week of illness (Table 15.1). In-flight transmission was documented only on one of three flights to Singapore with SARS patients on board, for an attack rate of ~0.6% (1/156). In Taiwan in 2003, 9 of the 11 first SARS patients had traveled in affected areas; three flights were investigated. Flight 1 from Hong Kong to Taipei (1.5 h) with one incubating SARS case on board did not result in secondary cases among 314 passengers and crew. Neither did flight 3 from Hong Kong to Taipei with four manifest SARS cases on board among 245 passengers and crew. In contrast, flight 2 from Hong Kong to Beijing (3 h) with one manifest index case resulted in 22 secondary cases among 119 passengers and crew, for an attack rate of 19%. A confirmed SARS passenger on a flight from Hong Kong to Frankfurt (12.5 h) did not cause secondary cases, nor did cases on other flights that lasted for 2–10 h.

Bacteria
Bacteria with confirmed onboard transmission are *M. tuberculosis* and *N. meningitidis*.

M. tuberculosis (2030, 3898, 5053, 5736, 7779, 8077). Because one third of the world population is latently infected, it is likely that infectious passengers will be onboard aircraft. In 1992, over 5 months, a flight attendant was source for two skin-test conversions in 212 crew and possibly four conversions in 59 frequent flyers; risks increased with hours exposed. In 1994, a passenger with open, multidrug-resistant (MDR) tuberculosis traveled back and forth Honolulu-Baltimore-Chicago. On the longest flight lasting 8.75 h, 6 of 15 tuberculin-positive contacts had no other risks than exposure to the index case, and all six were seated in the same section with him; four of the six were skin-test convertors. In 1998, a Thai passenger on a Bangkok-Athens-Zürich flight was hospitalized in Switzerland with abundant acid-fast rods in spontaneous sputum; Greek authorities made 600 phone calls and sent 190 letters to contact 144 passengers and crew and to obtain three baseline tuberculin skin-test results, a meager yield that was not considered worth the effort.

Spread on aircraft seems rare, however, requiring a highly infectious source, long exposure (cumulative >8 h), and proximity to the source, for an overall estimated rate of about one secondary case per 1,000 flights with a source case onboard. Nevertheless, accurate passenger lists when kept for 3 months would facilitate contact tracing.

N. meningitidis (647, 4263). Association of meningococcal disease with flights has been defined by its occurrence within 14 days from a flight that lasted ≥8 h. The risk of secondary spread on aircraft seems low. In the United States in 2000, of eight reports of flight-related disease, no secondary cases among contacts were reported. Despite this, airlines may need to provide complete passenger lists for contact tracing. Chemoprophylaxis should be considered for passengers who have been exposed to respiratory secretions from a primary case, or for anyone seated next to an index case on a flight lasting >8 h.

FECES-FOOD CLUSTER
Risks (4708, 5874) (http://www.epa.gov/airlinewater/). In the 1970s–1980s, food samples from International Airports (Bangkok and London-Heathrow) had yielded *E. coli* (in ~20–50%), *Bacillus cereus* (in 3%), *V. parahaemolyticus* (in 3%), *Salmonella* (in 0.4–9%), *S. aureus* (in 0.2–2%), and *Clostridium perfringens* (in 0.2%). In

Table 15.1 Risk of SARS transmission during commercial flight

Flight	Duration (h)	Index case	Rate (%) (no. infected/no. on plane)	Reference
Hong Kong-Singapore	Short	1, manifest	0 (0/47)	8165
Hong Kong-Taipei	1½	1, incubating	0 (0/315)	5598
Hong Kong-Taipei	1½	4, manifest	0 (0/246)	5598
Hong Kong-Beijing	3	1, manifest	19 (22/120)	5598
Hong Kong-Frankfurt	12½	1	0	869
New York-Singapore	Long	1, manifest	0.6 (1/156)	8165

1947–1999, 41 in-flight food-borne outbreaks were documented, including 15 *Salmonella* outbreaks (with nearly 4,000 infections and 7 deaths) and 8 *S. aureus* outbreaks. Since the 1990s, foods onboard aircraft have generally met high standards of hygiene. A residual risk remains from hazardous foods (see section III). An emerging risk is fecal contamination of the onboard environment. Also, tap water on aircraft should be considered unfit for drinking.

Viruses
***Norovirus* (8148).** On an 8-h flight from London to Philadelphia, 5 (5%) of 93 passengers and 8 (57%) of 14 crew members reported vomiting or diarrhea, and *Norovirus* was recovered from stools. Passenger cases used board toilets significantly more often than noncases; a likely scenario was environmental contamination by vomit, although attack rates were low, and no passenger noticed soiled toilets.

Bacteria
***C. botulinum* (5100).** In 1987, a kosher meal from Switzerland for a flight from Nice, France, to London, United Kingdom, caused a severe case of botulism. Rice and vegetable salad, which the patient described as smelling offensive, was implicated; he tasted a small amount and discarded the bulk.

***Salmonella* (7354).** Of 23 food-borne outbreaks reported on aircrafts in 1947–1984, 7 (30%) were attributed to *Salmonella*. In the United States in 1984, *S. enterica* serovar Enteritidis was implicated in 186 cases on 29 flights.

***Shigella* (3222).** In the United States in 1988, *S. sonnei* in cold sandwiches hand-prepared on board caused 30 culture-confirmed cases among 725 (4%) passengers on 13 flights.

***S. aureus* (2146, 7354).** Of 23 food-borne outbreaks reported on aircrafts in 1947–1984, 5 (22%) were attributed to *S. aureus*. Aboard a commercial flight in 1975, 196 (57%) of 344 passengers and 1 steward contracted *S. aureus* food poisoning from a ham handled by a cook with lesions on his fingers. Attack rates were 86% in the consumers of handled ham and 0% in other passengers.

***Vibrio* (7354).** Of 23 food-borne outbreaks reported on aircrafts in 1947–1984, 5 (22%) were attributed to *Vibrio*. ***V. cholerae* (2115, 7266).** In 1992, cold seafood was the vehicle for cholera on a flight from South America to Los Angeles; 100 (30%) of 336 passengers had laboratory evidence of *V. cholerae* O1 infection, 75 (22%) had cholera, 10 (3%) were hospitalized, and 1 (0.3%) died. In 1972, cold hors d'oevres prepared at Bahrain and Singapore were the vehicle for cholera on a flight from London to Sydney: while none of 26 first-class passengers were affected, 47 (14%) of 331 economy passengers grew *V. cholerae* El Tor, 25 (8%) had cholera, and 1 (0.3%) died. ***V. parahaemolyticus* (5807).** In 1972, on a flight from Thailand to London, nine passengers and three of six cabin crew developed diarrhea, including three with dehydration and shock; cooked white crab meat in hors d'oevres was the vehicle implicated.

ZOONOTIC CLUSTER
Risks (2997, 3828, 4708, 8130). International health regulations aim to reduce international spread by surveillance, prescribed vaccines (cholera and yellow fever), and aircraft disinsection (preboarding residual or postboarding knockdown). Disinsection is inconsistently performed, however. At Paris International Airport, ~20% (85/400) of inbound airlines did not comply with disinsection, mainly of cabins and cargo holds. At this airport in 2000, two live *Anopheles gambiae* were detected in 42 examined aircrafts from tropical Africa, one unengorged and one engorged female, which had likely fed on a passenger or crew member. Animals must not be allowed in cabins. For dispersal of mosquitoes by aircraft, see section 16.2.

Transit (1545, 3574, 3662, 5953, 6300). Time spent in transit at airports in enzootic or endemic areas can be sufficient for passengers or crew to contract arthropod-borne infections. Airport transmission was suspected in a German couple returning from Hawaii with acute dengue. Stopovers at malarious airports (even of ≤1 h) on flights between nonmalarious countries were reported sites for the acquisition of *Plasmodium* and malaria (transit malaria).

VHF (339, 1438, 7134). VHFs that require special precaution include Crimean-Congo hemorrhagic fever (CCHF), filoviruses (*Ebolavirus* and *Marburgvirus*), Latin American arenaviruses (Guanarito virus [GUAV], Junin virus [JUNV], Machupo virus [MACV], and Sabiá virus), and orthopoxviruses (monkeypox virus and variola virus).

In contrast, infectivity of Old World Lassa virus on aircraft is low. In 15 years, ≥12 patients with Lassa fever traveled on international aircrafts without causing secondary infections. After a 4-month stay in West Africa, a 38-year-old businessman died of Lassa fever shortly after returning to the United States; none of five high-risk (body fluid) contacts, nor any of 183 low-risk contacts (139 health workers, 16 laboratory workers, 9 relatives, and 19 passengers on the London-Newark flight seated close to him) contracted Lassa fever.

For emergency repatriation, special teams are on call at some large airports. Preventive measures include exposure avoidance (blood and other body fluids), transportation in an air-sealed container, and protective equipment for health workers (clothes, respirator, and filters removing particles of 0.03–3.0 μm).

Q fever (278, 7071). Dust generated by helicopters near farms, herds, or slaughterhouses has been implicated in outbreaks of Q fever, for instance in southern France and among Czech forces in Bosnia and Herzegovina.

Plasmodium **(1668, 2997, 3572, 3675, 3828, 6404).** Live, infective *Anopheles* females on aircraft have caused airport malaria cases in a perimeter of ~25 km from international airports that receive long-distance flights from malarious areas. For airport malaria, perimeter residents should have a blank history of travel and other malaria risks for the incubation period of the causative *Plasmodium* species, and weather conditions should be favorable for *Anopheles* survival. Most airport malaria originated in sub-Saharan Africa and was reported in West Europe, for 78 cases in 1977–2000, most by *P. falciparum* and a few by *P. ovale*. In airport perimeters of Madrid, Spain, the estimated rate of airport malaria was ~$3/10^5$ per year. A case of airport malaria due to *P. vivax* was also reported in Cairns, Australia, in October 1996.

15.4 INTERNATIONAL SHORT-TERM TRAVEL

The traveler can be seen as an interactive biological unit who picks up, processes, carries and drops off microbial genetic material.

M. E. Wilson (8207)

International is travel that crosses national borders, oceans (overseas), or continents (intercontinental). Typical means are aircraft, ferryboat, train, car, and truck. Here, short-term means a duration of ≤4 weeks (~60–85% of international travel is short-term).

Exposure (3104, 7508, 7733, 8163). Worldwide, there were 25 million international arrivals in 1950 but 715 million in 2002. In the United States in 2000, 1–2.5% of >13,000 respondents in a representative sample from eight states reported international travel in the preceding 7 days. Popular destinations include the Mediterranean (southern Europe and North Africa), the Caribbean, North America, Southeast and East Asia, and Australia. Tropical countries receive ~80 million visitors per year. Purposes include holiday (40–70%, "backpacking to beach"), work (10–40%, "aid to business"), visits (10–40%, "families to friends"), and pilgrimage. Rome in Italy and Mecca in Saudia Arabia receive masses of pilgrims each year. For mass gatherings, see section 13.1; for hotel accommodation, see section 11.8.

Infections (241, 2081, 3147, 3326, 3362, 6372, 7070, 7130) (Box 15.4). Frequent complaints by travelers to tropical countries are diarrhea, fever, skin conditions (pyoderma, tinea, cutaneous larva migrans, bites from arthropods or vertebrates, and itch), and STI.

Prevention (369, 3456, 3909, 6372, 7132) (http://www.cdc.gov/travel/diseases.htm and http://www.who.int/ith/). By destination, length of stay, mode of travel (e.g., package, adventure), season, and epidemiological situation, prevention is based on exposure avoidance, vaccines, and malaria chemoprophylaxis. Exposure avoidance includes avoiding hazardous foods and beverages, using repellents, bednets, and condoms, and avoiding water, soil, and animal contacts.

International vaccines include universal HAV, MMR, polio, and diphtheria tetanus (dT), and targeted HBV, *Influenzavirus*, Japanese encephalitis virus (JEV), rabies

---

Box 15.4 Agents and infections in international travelers from high-income countries, by cluster

*Agents or infections for which imported cases account for >25% of reported cases.

Droplet-air	Influenza, measles,* rubella, SARS; diphtheria,* legionellosis, meningococcal meningitis, pertussis, tuberculosis; coccidioidomycosis,* histoplasmosis
Feces-food	HAV,* HEV*; *Rotavirus*, *C. jejuni* (quinolone-resistant*), *H. pylori*, *Plesiomonas*, *S. enterica* non-Typhi serovars, serovar Typhi (multiresistant*), *Shigella*, *V. cholerae*;* microsporidia; *Cryptosporidium*, *E. histolytica*,* *Giardia*;* acute tissue helminthiases, e.g., trichinellosis*
Zoonotic	Rabies virus, DENV,* JEV,* RRV, WNV, YFV,* viral hemorrhagic fevers;* *Brucella*, relapsing borreliae,* rickettsiae (e.g., *R. africae**), *Y. pestis*; leishmaniasis,* malaria,* trypanosomiasis*
Environmental	*Burkholderia*, *Leptospira*, environmental mycobacteria; *Penicillium*; cutaneous larva migrans,* *Schistosoma**; myiasis* (*Dermatobia* from Latin America and *Cordylobia* from Africa)
Skin-blood	CMV, HBV, HIV, HPV; cutaneous diphtheria, *S. aureus*; STI: chancroid,* genital *Chlamydia*,* lymphogranuloma venereum,* *N. gonorrhoeae*, *T. pallidum pallidum*; *Hymenolepis**

virus, tick-borne encephalitis virus (TBEV), YFV; *N. meningitidis*, *S. enterica* serovar Typhi, and *V. cholerae*.

DROPLET-AIR CLUSTER

Overview (236, 2266, 3362). Risks of acute upper and lower respiratory tract infections (RTI) have been poorly documented in tourists. RTI are a reason for physician visits during or after travel. While up to 8% of tourist may report RTI, rates of physician-confirmed RTI are lower, probably <1%. Among international travelers with pneumonia, a broad spectrum of community-acquired agents should be considered (see section 14.7).

Travelers are not only victims but also vectors of RTI. Emerging examples are measles and resistance to antimicrobials.

Viruses

Influenzavirus. **Human viruses (5223, 5846, 7673).** Outbreaks have been reported among tourists. In Alaska (United States) and Yukon Territory (Canada) in the summer (May–September) of 1998, A/H3N2 caused a protracted outbreak among tourists and tourism workers from 37 countries; cases of acute respiratory illness were estimated at >33,000, for attack rates of 1–1.5/100 per week at the height of the epidemic. In 1999, flulike illness rates among tourists returning to the United States from Ireland were 45% (10/22) in age groups <65 years but 100% (8/8) in age groups ≥65 years. Vaccine should be considered for travelers ≥65 years of age to destinations expecting a seasonal influenza wave. **Avian viruses (5450).** The avian A/H5N1 virus emerged in East and Southeast Asia in 2003, causing an epizootic that is ongoing. Travelers are advised to avoid contact with live poultry in markets and farms and with surfaces contaminated by bird droppings. Poultry and eggs are safe for consumption if heated well (>70°C) throughout. No vaccine is currently available against avian viruses.

Measles virus. Travelers can be victims and vectors of measles virus. The latter role was detected after measles transmission had been interrupted in the Americas. Introduction of measles by (nonvaccinated) travelers has now been confirmed in high-income countries.

- America (1202, 1779, 7883). The bulk of measles in the United States is now travel related. Of 2,632 reported measles cases in 1993–2001, 39% (1,023) were travel related (17% imports, 15% foreign genotypes, and 7% linked). Of 215 cases reported in 2001–2003, 80% (173) were travel related (45% imports, 27% linked, and 8% foreign genotypes). In 2001–2003, returning U.S. residents and visitors generated 42 secondary chains that lasted up to 2 months. In 2001–2002, a traveler returning from Europe introduced measles into Venezuela, causing an epidemic with 2,501 cases in Venezuela and 140 cases in Colombia.

- Australia (4200). In 1999, an woman returning from Bali brought introduced measles into Melbourne; through her work at a cinema complex, she was the source for an infection chain with 40 cases.

- Europe (3103). In 2001, a child returning from the Philippines introduced measles in Jutland, Denmark, causing 19 secondary cases (despite a nearly 100% vaccine coverage in the population).

Vaccine should be recommended to travelers according to national policy.

Rubella virus (6176). Travelers can be victims and vectors of rubella virus. In the United States in 1997–1999, 7% (55/817) of reported cases were considered imported, mainly from Mexico (17 cases), Russia (7 cases), and Japan (6 cases). Molecular typing suggested that single imported sources seeded at least two outbreaks.

SARS-CoV (1222, 7272, 8111). The 2003 epidemic demonstrated how international travel could disperse infections around the globe in a matter of days or weeks. From a hotel in Hong Kong, 12 incubating travelers carried SARS-CoV to their home countries, triggering infection chains that led to >8,000 cases in >30 countries, with nearly 800 deaths. In Toronto, Canada, 222 (99%) of 225 residents who met the SARS case definition were linked to a single index patient from Hong Kong.

Bacteria

Reported etiologies of pneumonia in international travelers include *C. burnetti*, *Legionella pneumophila*, *M. tuberculosis*, *Mycoplasma pneumoniae*, and *Streptococcus pneumoniae* (236). Other droplet-borne agents in travelers include *Bordetella pertussis*, *C. diphtheriae*, and *N. meningitidis*.

***B. pertussis* (8161).** *B. pertussis* is not usually reported in short-term travelers. In 2002, of 358 pilgrims from Singapore to Mecca, five by cough for >1 week and seroconversion acquired pertussis in 1 month, for an attack rate among nonimmune persons of 8% (3/40). Pertussis vaccination ($p_{acellular}$) should be considered (8161).

***C. diphtheriae* (398, 1943, 2131, 2322, 2579, 2978, 3169, 4568, 4569, 4577).** Sporadic diphtheria of the throat and skin has been well documented in susceptible travelers from North America and western Europe. In Finland, the risk has been estimated at 0.1 case per 10^5 travelers. In Germany in 1994–1999, 14 (78%) of 18 diphtheria cases were travel related (imports and links). Imported toxigenic strains occasionally spread locally, causing outbreaks.

- North America (2131, 2322, 4577). After a 1-week trip to rural Haiti where diphtheria is endemic, a previously healthy, unvaccinated 63-year-old resident from Pennsylvania fell ill with laryngeal diphtheria and died; throat swab and pseudomembrane were culture-negative, but PCR-positive for C. diphtheriae toxin genes. Close contacts (travel companions, wife, and health workers) tested negative for C. diphtheriae but were given chemoprophylaxis and offered vaccine. In 1994, two travelers from the United States contracted diphtheria while staying in outbreak areas in eastern Europe. In 1990, visitors to Haiti were suspected to have imported diphtheria into Florida, with death of an nonvaccinated child and colonization of 23 contacts.

- Australasia (398). In New Zealand in 1998, a nonvaccinated child developed toxigenic diphtheria after parents had returned from a visit to Bali.
- West Europe (1943, 2131, 2579, 2978, 4568, 5878). In 1993–1997, 12 cases of toxigenic diphtheria were imported into the United Kingdom, including six cutaneous cases. In Switzerland, 20 (31%, all cutaneous) of 65 nontoxigenic cases were imported. In the 1990s, troops returning from Afghanistan seeded toxigenic strains in East Europe, initially in cities such as Moscow, St. Petersburg, and Kiev. In subsequent epidemics, diphtheria spread along traffic corridors. By 1994, it had reached all 15 newly independent states. In 1992–2000, cases from travel to East Europe emerged in Belgium (3), Finland (10), Germany (8), Greece (1), Mongolia (triggering an outbreak), Poland (19), and the United Kingdom (1).

Legionella (1049, 2598, 3751, 4366, 6262, 8094).
Legionella surveillance is well developed in Europe. The reported rate in travelers is ~0.3–3/10^5 per year. Lethality was 6% (38/632) in 2003. In 2000–2002, 10–20% of sporadic cases but 60% of outbreaks (113/189) were travel related. Outbreaks caused 315 cases (3 per outbreak). Most cases were reported from Spain, Italy, and France. However, when related to volume of visitors (available for the United Kingdom in 1999–2001), rates per 10^5 visitors were highest from travel to Mexico (2–3), Turkey (1–1.5), and Italy (0.3–0.4). While about two thirds of outbreak sites were international, about one third were domestic. Of 107 accommodation sites investigated, 22 caused a notice on the internet. Mostly (~85–90%) hotels (see section 11.8) were implicated and rarely (5–15%) other accommodations such as campsites, caravans, or private homes.

M. tuberculosis (619, 2956, 6266).
In the United States in the 2000s, >25% of reported cases were in foreign-born individuals. Risks in travelers are considered small, not warranting bacillus-Calmette-Gúerin (BCG) vaccination. However, frequently crossing borders (hopping) between low-risk and high-risk countries is considered a risk. Examples are borders between Mexico and the United States, and between Morocco and Spain.

N. meningitidis (84, 3065, 5173, 7478, 8162).
At risk of invasive disease are nonvaccinated travelers to outbreak areas and pilgrims. For aircrafts, see section 15.3.

In 1987, an outbreak that originated in Mecca, Saudi Arabia, caused 735 international cases among nearly 1 million pilgrims for a rate of 77/10^5. In 2000, serogroup W135 affected pilgrims and their contacts, with cases reported in the United States (3), the United Kingdom (20 pilgrims and 22 contacts), France (9 pilgrims and 15 contacts), Germany (8), six other European countries (16), Oman (3 pilgrims and 9 contacts), Saudi Arabia (30), and other Asian countries (10), for overall rates of 25/10^5 among pilgrims and of 18/10^5 among household contacts. After the 2001 pilgrimage, again 33 cases of W135 meningitis were observed in the United Kingdom (6 in pilgrims, 16 in contacts, and 11 unlinked), for a lethality of 27% (9/33), compared with 16% (8/51) in 2000.

S. pneumoniae (5261, 7011).
Travelers are likely means of "clonal expansion" and international spread of penicillin-resistant strains of S. pneumoniae. There is evidence from the late 1980s for the spread of clones from Spain to the United States and from Spain to Iceland.

Fungi
A network of travel and tropical medicine clinics in 1998–2003 reported 32 cases of respiratory mycoses among travelers. Diagnoses included histoplasmosis (in 23 or 73%), coccidioidomycosis (in 3 or 9%), cyptococcosis (in 3 or 9%), blastomycosis (in 2 or 6%), or paracoccidioidomycosis (in 1 or 3%) (5706). Risks include dust (see section 5.5) from winds and off-road driving, and visits to caves (see section 5.4).

Coccidioides (390, 1029, 1354, 5425, 5706).
Travelers from nonendemic areas of the United States, Australia, and Europe have become infected while visiting endemic areas in the southwestern United States and Mexico. In New York in 1989–1997, of 49 culture-confirmed cases, 26 (53%) had traveled to endemic areas. Of 126 members of a church group from Washington State that traveled to Tecate, Mexico, for construction work, 21 (17%) contracted coccidioidomycosis; C. immitis was isolated from soil at the construction site. On return from holiday in Mexico, an Australian was diagnosed with erythema nodosum and pulmonary coccidioidomycosis by histology and culture. A United Kingdom resident who attended a championship for model airplane flying in Kern County, California, developed acute coccidioidomycosis 1 week after returning home.

Histoplasma (236, 1184, 5193, 5347, 5706, 7686, 8015, 8244). *H. capsulatum* pneumonia has been diagnosed in international travelers. Disease risks include adventure travel, ecotourism, spelunking, and any visit to endemic areas. In 2001, students contracted acute histoplasmosis from a visit to Acapulco, Mexico; the subsequent investigation identified >260 cases from one hotel that underwent construction. Also in 2001, an outbreak affected 14 of 15 adventure travelers returning from Nicaragua; all 14 who visited a small, bat-infested cave for ~10 min had serologically confirmed infection, and 12 (86%) had fever, cough, or other symptoms. The only traveler who did not enter the cave remained well and tested negative in serum and urine. Visits to bat-inhabited caves are a well-known source of acute histoplasmosis and of outbreaks among visitors.

Paracoccidioides. *Paracoccidioides* has occasionally been isolated in travelers (5390, 5706). By serology and skin test, paracoccidioidomycosis was diagnosed in three German adventure travelers who spent 4 weeks in Brazil; accomodations included shacks, and foods included hunted monkeys and birds.

FECES-FOOD CLUSTER

Risks. Feces-food-transmitted infections in travelers include diarrhea (for definition, see section 14.7), acute hepatitis A (HA), and typhoid fever.

Diarrhea (797, 1105, 2081, 3701, 7133, 7870). By destination and risk behavior, rates of self-reported diarrhea in short-term travelers from high-income countries are ~2–6% in other high-income destinations, but 15–55% (often 30%) in low-income destinations. Some 0.1–0.2% of patients are hospitalized. Among 280 backpackers hiking the Appalachian Trail in 1997, drinking untreated surface water was a risk, while water treatment, washing hands after urination and defecation, and cleaning utensils with warm soapy water reduced risks. In ~50% of cases, no agent can be implicated, and in ~15%, stool analysis detects more than one agent.

Viruses
Overview (3701, 6013). In the prevaccine era, travelers were affected by and contributed to the spread of wild polioviruses and HAV. Vaccine has greatly reduced these risks. A main viral agent of diarrhea in international travelers is *Rotavirus*. Enteric adenoviruses are detected in ≤3% of cases.

HAV (1448, 1652, 2493, 3147, 6967, 7394, 8014, 8057). In susceptible (nonvaccinated) international travelers, by destination and behavior, reported infection risks are 0.03–0.3/100 per month. Risks include adventure travel, travel to tropical countries, the Mediterranean, or eastern Europe, outbreak situations, and traveling children of immigrants, for instance, from California to Mexico. In high-income countries, ~30% of acute HA may now be travel related. At travel and tropical medicine clinics, HAV infections are diagnosed in 0.2–5% of attending travelers. Outbreaks (2499, 6314) are still reported in travelers. In 2000, an outbreak affected German travelers to Ibiza. At Hurghada resort on the Red Sea, Egypt, in 2004, an outbreak caused 357 HAV infections among tourists, 284 from Germany (271 primary and 13 secondary), and 73 from eight other European countries (60 primary and 13 secondary). By national policy, vaccine should be offered to groups at risk or all susceptible short-term travelers.

Hepatitis E virus (HEV) (1616, 3546, 4034, 5623, 6314, 6731). Infections and sporadic, acute hepatitis E (HE) cases are increasingly recognized in international travelers. Of the comparatively small numbers of reported cases in high-income countries, up to 90% are travel related. In travelers from Louisiana, the anti-HEV prevalence before departure was 2% (9/384), and 6 months after travel, 2% (4/236) of susceptible travelers had seroconverted. From imported cases, high-risk countries include the Indian subcontinent (Bangladesh, India, Nepal, and Pakistan), People's Republic of China, and Southeast Asia.

Norovirus **(3701, 3905).** *Norovirus* is curiously absent from many studies of travelers' diarrhea. Possible explanations include diagnostic difficulties and a preference for cold season, whereas international travel "goes for the sun." Outbreaks have been reported (2520, 5793, 5812). On the Appalachian Trail in Virginia in 1999, 45 (64%) of 70 hikers contracted *Norovirus* diarrhea; tap water from a general store was the implicated source, but person-to-person spread was not excluded. In 2002, 71 (30%) of 234 Irish ski holidaymakers visiting Andorra contracted *Norovirus* diarrhea; ice cubes were the implicated source. At Lourdes, France, in 2002, 33 (28%) of 119 pilgrims representing 29 institutions from Switzerland and 36 accompanying personnel contracted *Norovirus*; on returning home, 11 (38%) institutions reported ≥380 secondary cases, including one death.

Rotavirus **(3362, 3701, 7070, 7361).** *Rotavirus* is a significant cause of diarrhea in international travelers. By destination, diagnostic yield is ~1–10% and at least an equal proportion of cases is attributable to this agent.

Bacteria
Overview (3072, 3701). Main bacterial agents of diarrhea in international travelers are *Campylobacter* (can be quinolone resistant), *E. coli* (ETEC, enteroaggregative

[EAEC]), *Salmonella*, and *Shigella*. Travelers are suspected vectors of antimicrobial resistance.

Aeromonas **(3701, 7824, 8315).** The pathogenicity of *Aeromonas* is debated. Diagnostic yield in travelers is 2–6%. In Barcelona, Spain, of 18 isolates from 863 overseas travelers in 1999–2001, nine were *A. veronii*, seven were *A. caviae*, and one each was *A. hydrophila* and *A. jandaei*.

Campylobacter **(1516, 2116, 2150, 2589, 3147, 3701, 6360, 6597, 6699).** International travel is a risk of *C. jejuni*, including to low-income countries. By destination, yield in travelers with diarrhea is ~0.5–10% (often 1–2%). In northern Europe, >50–60% of reported infections have been imported. In travelers returned to Sweden after an overnight stay abroad, rates per 10^5 were highest from the Indian subcontinent (~1,250), intermediate from Africa (~50–75), and low (3) from northern Europe. Above-average risks have also been reported for travelers to Southeast Asia. **Resistance (3072, 6991).** Travelers seem to contribute to spreading quinolone-resistant strains. In 1996–1997, 75% (96/130) of Minnesota residents with quinolone-resistant *C. jejuni* isolates had a history of foreign travel in the 7 days preceding illness onset, compared with 23% (59/260) of controls with quinolone-sensitive isolates matched for age, residence, and date of specimen collection. In Finland in 1995–2000, isolates from international travelers resistant to fluoroquinolones increased from 40% (82/205) in 1995–1997 to 60% (90/149) in 1998–2000.

E. coli **(49, 1293, 3362, 3701, 5349, 5552, 5666, 7070, 7769, 8092).** *E. coli* is a significant cause of diarrhea in international travelers. EAEC, enterohemorrhagic *E. coli* (EHEC), enteroinvasive *E. coli* (EIEC), enteropathogenic *E. coli* (EPEC), and ETEC all have been implicated. Overall, ETEC and EAEC are the most frequent types. By destination and age, ETEC accounts for 5–35% of all diarrhea in international travelers, EAEC for 1–25%, EPEC for 3–4%, EIEC for 2–3%, and EHEC for 1%. Of U.S. travelers to Mexico, 11% (4/37) contracted ETEC infections in the first 2 weeks abroad, and 22% (8/37) contracted EAEC. In Wales in 1990–1998, 9% (37/415) of EHEC cases reported foreign travel in the week preceding illness onset. Few outbreaks have been reported (5789). In 1997, EHEC caused an international outbreak among tourists to the Canary Islands, Spain, with cases in the United Kingdom (8), Finland (5), Denmark (1), and Sweden (1).

Helicobacter **(5983).** Risks are considered low but are perhaps underrated or mitigated by concomitant antimalarials (mefloquine seems active in vitro against *H. pylori*). Of 104 backpackers traveling to Africa, Latin America, or Asia for 3–16 (mean, 6) months, 36 (35%) were seroreactive before travel, 4 (4%) seroconverted after travel, and 10 (10%) reverted to negative, for an infection rate of 6/100 per year.

Plesiomonas **(3701, 4002, 6144, 6854, 8315).** *P. shigelloides* seems to have emerged as an agent of diarrhea in international travelers. Reported yields have been 0.02% in general travelers (989/5,648,066 travelers in transit in Japan) and ~3–5.5% in travelers with diarrhea.

***Salmonella*.** **Non-Typhi (2151, 3147, 3701, 5128, 8315).** Travel is a risk for non-Typhi *S. enterica* serovars. By destination, *Salmonella* accounts for 0.5–7.5% of diarrhea in travelers. In Sweden in 1997–2003, 24,803 cases were reported in international travelers. Rates per 10^5 were lowest (1.7) for destinations in northern Euope and highest for the Indian subcontinent (474, 95% CI 330–681), East Africa (471, 95% CI 294–755), West Africa (279, 95% CI 180–432), and East Asia (270, 95% CI 247–295). In Europe, a significant fraction of non-Typhi salmonellae are now acquired abroad. In Denmark in 1997–1999, 25% (115/455) of patients with sporadic *S. enterica* serovar Enteritidis infections had a history of travel compared with 8% (40/507) of population controls matched for gender, age, and municipality. **Resistance (175, 3073).** Travelers seem to contribute to the spread of resistant salmonellae. In Norway in 2000, 50% (75/151) of multiresistant *S. enterica* serovar Typhimurium was imported. In travelers from Finland, the proportion of isolates with reduced susceptibility to ciprofloxacin (MIC $\geq$0.125 µg/ml; overall, 66/629) increased from 4% in 1995 to 24% in 1999; the increase was particularly high in isolates from Thailand (6% in 1995 and 50% in 1999). ***S. enterica* serovar Typhi (43, 1130, 1488, 3362, 3668, 4996, 6317, 7144, 7469).** Travel to endemic areas is a risk for serovar Typhi. About 50% of travelers develop symptoms while abroad, whereas the other 50% become symptomatic 1–26 days (often 10 days) after returning home. By destination, risks, vaccine, and surveillance, reported rates range broadly from 0.1 to 1,000 per 10^5 travelers. From package tours to Indonesia in 3 months of 1994–1995, 4% (6/156) of Dutch participants in four groups contracted typhoid fever; isolates from patients represented different clones. In high-income countries, 75–95% of typhoid cases are now imported. In the United States, major source countries (>75% of imports) are Mexico, Haiti, the Indian subcontinent, and the Philippines. In Europe, the major source countries (>50% of imports) are the Indian subcontinent and Turkey. **Resistance (7469).** In the United Kingdom in 1999, 23% of isolates (mainly from travelers to India and Pakistan) had reduced susceptibility to ciprofloxacin (MIC 0.25–1.0 mg/liter), and >50% were resistant to chloramphenicol, ampicillin, and trimethoprim.

***Shigella* (3147, 3362, 3701, 6317, 7069, 7070).** By destination, *Shigella* accounts for 0–14% (often 1%) of diarrhea in internatinal travelers. In Germany, 65–85% of cases are imported, mainly from North Africa, the Indian subcontinent, and Turkey. *S. sonnei* accounts for 80% of isolates, *S. flexneri* for 15%, *S. boydii* for 3%, and *S. dysenteriae* for 2%. An outbreak at a Caribbean resort in 1984 affected >60% of 1,893 tourists likely from handled food and person-to-person spread. **Resistance (421, 7353).** Resistance to co-trimoxazole (in 3–20%) and ampicillin (30%) was reported for *Shigella* isolates from international travelers.

***Vibrio* (3701).** By destination and food preference, yield in international travelers with diarrhea is 0–3%. ***V. parahaemolyticus* (4829, 7085).** *V. parahaemolyticus* is a cause of diarrhea in travelers, in particular, those from Japan to Southeast Asia. ***V. cholerae* (315, 4656, 7085, 7145, 8088, 8235).** Sporadic cases of cholera have been documented in international travelers. Aboard a return flight from the Philippines, a United States traveler developed cholera that required emergency landing in Anchorage. At a London, United Kingdom, hospital emergency room, a man with a distended abdomen was suspected to have diabetes when evacuating 500 ml of fluids that, because of language problems were mistaken for urine, only on the ward did severe dehydration and cholera become obvious.

Risks include low gastric acidity (e.g., by antacids) and consumption of raw seafood, but they are low overall, for rates of 0.01–0.5/10^5 travelers. Given the low risk, vaccine is not usually recommended for healthy travelers to nonepidemic areas.

***Y. enterocolitica* (3147).** Diagnostic yield of *Y. enterocolitica* in overseas travelers with diarrhea is low (0–0.4%).

Fungi

Microsporidia (4517, 5248) are an emerging cause of diarrhea in international travelers. In Germany, stool samples of 6% (9/148) of returned travelers tested positive by PCR for *Enterocytozoon* or *Encephalitozoon*.

Protozoa

Overview. The main protozoal agents of diarrhea in international travelers are *Cyclospora* and *Giardia*. *Isospora belli* (3770, 7045) and *Toxoplasma gondii* (1554) are infrequently implicated in travelers. Pathogenicity of *Blastocystis* and *Dientamoeba* is debated.

***Blastocystis* (1462, 3147, 3428, 3669).** The reported prevalences of *B. hominis* in travelers is ~5–15%. In Italy travelers having visited tropical countries had a lower prevalence (3%, 12/409) than resident controls (6%, 6/105). In contrast in Germany, *B. hominis* was detected in 15% (69/469) of tourists with diarrhea but only 6% (21/326) of asymptomatic control travelers; in 51 of the 69 symptomatic travelers, *B. cystis* was the only enteric agent detected.

***Cryptosporidium* (3147, 3505, 3664, 3701, 3725, 6446).** *Cryptosporidium* is a risk for international travelers. Originally, the agent was reported in travelers to St. Petersburg (Leningrad), Russia. By destination and behavior, 0–3% (often ≤1%) of diarrhea in travelers is attributable to *Cryptosporidium* (likely *C. hominis*). Of reported cases in high-income countries, about 10% were imported.

***Cyclospora* (2649, 2650, 3147, 3287, 3456, 3664).** *C. cayetanensis* is a risk for international travelers. By destination, 1–4% of diarrhea in travelers is attributable to this agent. In North America, most sporadic cases seem related to international travel. In the United Kingdom, ~50% of all cases were imported (308/598 in 1994–2002). In Europe, major source destinations are the Indian subcontinent (India and Nepal), Southeast Asia (Indonesia), and Latin America.

***Dientamoeba* (3147, 5476).** People acquire *D. fragilis* from international travel. In 2000, 1% (7/662) of German overseas travelers with diarrhea excreted *D. fragilis*.

***Entamoeba* (3456).** In high-income countries, *E. histolytica* is an imported infection. While cysts could be confounded with *E. dispar*, amebic liver abscess (ALA) and other forms of invasive disease are characteristic for *E. histolytica*.

- Noninvasive infection (3147, 3362, 3701, 7070, 7912, 8016). *E. histolytica* is considered "a very uncommon cause of diarrhea in short-term travelers," as it usually takes >1 month of exposure to become infected (6146). By destination and case mix, *E. histolytica/dispar* is isolated in 0–5% of feces from returned travelers. In infected German travelers (n = 60) returning from tropical or subtropical countries, *E. dispar* to *E. histolytica* ratios varied by length of exposure, from 6 to 1 in foreign residents, 3 to 1 in long-term travelers, and 1 to 2.5 in short-term travelers. Also in Germany, only 5 (8%) of 61 *E. histolytica/dispar* isolates from travelers represented pathogenic zymodems.
- Invasive disease (1808, 2121, 2384, 3001, 7468). In Pavia, Italy, in 1979–1989, 70% (37/53) of ALA occurred in travelers returned from endemic areas. At a luxury hotel in Phuket, Thailand, in 1988, 16 of 160 Italian tourists contracted invasive disease (seven colitis and nine ALA), probably from raw vegetables, salads, fruits, or ice. A

Dutch family acquired *E. histolytica* from a summer holiday visit in southern Italy: the father developed ALA, the mother contracted amebic dysentery, and one of their three children passed cysts; the three isolates were indistinguishable by molecular fingerprinting.

Giardia **(892, 3045, 3139, 3147, 3362, 3670, 3701, 3726, 7070).** *G. lamblia* is a significant cause of diarrhea in travelers, initially recognized in the 1960s–1970s, in travelers to eastern Europe. In 1969–1971, 6% (91/1,419) of U.S. tourists to Russia tested positive for *G. lamblia*, and clinical attack rates by destination were 20–40%. Modes of acquisition are often not determined; potential sources include tap water, ice cream, other foods, and person-to-person spread. By destination and case mix, yield in travelers with diarrhea is 0–12%; in short-term travelers it is often 1–3%. Of 662 overseas travelers returning to Germany with diarrhea, 46 (7%) excreted *G. lamblia* in the feces. Also in Germany, *G. lamblia* was isolated as the sole enteric pathogen in 352 (3%) of 13,566 traveled outpatients. A major source country is the Indian subcontinent.

Helminths

Overview. Acute, manifest, food-borne tissue helminths are recognized in short-term international travelers rather than persistent, inapparent, enteric helminths such as *Ascaris* and *Trichuris*, which are more characteristic for expatriates (see "Expatriates" below). Helminths causing acute syndromes include *Angiostrongylus*, *Anisakis*, *Fasciola*, *Gnathostoma*, and *Trichinella*. These are infrequent, but common-source outbreaks are possible. Rare food-borne worms in travelers are *Capillaria* (1383), *Echinostoma* (1007), and *Heterophyes* (480).

Angiostrongylus **(4476, 6963, 7438).** Food-borne eosinophilic meningitis due to *A. cantonensis* has been reported in travelers returning from the Pacific and the Caribbean. In 2000, 12 (52%) of 23 U.S. tourists who visited Jamaica for 1 week developed eosinophilic meningitis within 6–31 days after returning home.

Anisakis **(651, 7803).** A 26-year-old woman from Switzerland with recurrent urticaria was diagnosed with *A. simplex* infection that she had contracted from eating fish in Portugal. A 62-year-old man from Belgium contracted suspected acute anisakiasis from eating fish either in Chile or on his flight from Chile to Brazil.

Fasciola **(4217, 4533, 5012, 7220).** Acute cases of *F. hepatica* have been reported in travelers. Risks are consumption of salads from wild water plants or from homegrown plants in enzootic areas.

Gnathostoma **(1858, 2196, 2860, 3079, 3456, 3671, 4981, 5167, 5470).** Cases of *Gnathostoma* have been reported in international short-term travelers. The main source is raw fish. In the United States and South Africa in 1998, a father and a son were diagnosed with gnathostomiasis 12–14 days after they had fished in Zambia and eaten raw fish marinated in lemon juice. In France in 1991–2000, five cutaneous cases were reported in travelers returning from Southeast Asia, after average stays of 34 days. In the United Kingdom in 2000–2001, 16 cases were reported in travelers returning from Africa, Asia, or America.

Trichinella **(1475, 4866, 5487, 5917).** Travel-related *Trichinella* cases have been documented. In the United States in 1975–1989, 26 cases were reported, including (rates per 10^5 travelers) 10 from Central America (0.01), 5 from Africa (0.4), 7 from Asia (0.04), and 3 from Europe (0.003). A couple from Denmark contracted *Trichinella* from pork consumed in Serbia. Of a Dutch family, parents developed symptoms 2 days after consuming pork in Montenegro, and two of the three daughters had serological evidence of recent infection. In Germany, three patients contracted trichinellosis from smoked ham brought home from the former Yugoslavia.

ZOONOTIC CLUSTER

Modes of acquisition include bites by arthropods and bites by vertebrates (see section I).

Fever (241, 3147, 3362, 6687, 8057). By destination, behavior (diurnal or nocturnal exposure and bednets), chemoprophylaxis, and vaccines (YFV), main zoonotic causes of fever in short-term travelers are malaria (in 0–14% of cases) and arboviruses (dengue in 0–2%). Perhaps because of lifestyles that are different from local people, VHFs are rare in short-term international travelers.

Arthralgia (3656). In travelers returning from the tropics with persistent arthralgia, causative alphaviruses include Chikungunya virus (CHIKV) from Africa or Asia, O'nyong-nyong virus (ONNV) from Africa, Mayarovirus (MAYV) from South America, and Barmah forest virus (BFV) and Ross River virus (RRV) from Australia.

Viruses

Priority zoonotic viruses in travelers are vaccine-preventable rabiesvirus (see section 1.1), JEV, and YFV, and vaccine-nonpreventable DENV and RRV. Other zoonotic viruses suspected or confirmed in short-term international travelers include CHIKV (5114, 5911), Colorado tick fever virus (CTFV) (5032), Lassavirus, MAYV (7517), ONNV (8261), Rift valley fever virus (RVFV) (7752), sandfly fever virus (5114, 6734), simian herpes virus (SHV, enzootic among macaques in temples in Bali, Indonesia) (3485), TBEV (8368), and WNV.

DENV (1487, 2498, 5982, 6317, 7254). By destination, reported infection rates range from 0.6/100 travelers per month to 3 (95% CI 2–5) per 100 person-months, and disease rates are ~4–28/10^5 travelers (with high rates in Thailand and Brazil). Although a majority (up to three fourths) of infections in travelers is inapparent, classical dengue and on occasion dengue hemorrhagic fever (DHF) have been diagnosed in travelers returning to high-income countries.

- America (1182, 2735, 6149, 6270, 6760). In the United States in 1986–1994, 937 imported cases were reported clinically, and 204 (22%) were confirmed serologically or virologically. The southern United States is receptive to DENV reintroduction, and local spread has been reported in Florida and Texas. This risk is nontrivial given the volume of border crossings. Between Laredo in Texas (DENV-free), and Nuevo Laredo in Mexico (DENV-endemic), there are ~2 million border crossings per month. A similar situation exists on the southern cone. In Argentina, with 1.6 million arrivals per year from DENV-endemic areas, DENV was reintroduced in 1998, after a break of 72 years.
- Australasia (5982, 6287, 7254, 8314). In Japan in 1996–1999, 74 imported cases were reported. North Queensland, Australia, is receptive for DENV. In 1994–2002, North Queensland reported importation of 69 viremic travelers (all four serotypes). Outbreaks have been recorded since the late nineteenth century, recently in 1992 around Townsville, which has an international airport, and in 1997–1999 around Cairns, Port Douglas, and Mossman, in which viremic travelers were suspected to seed foci, including at backpacker hostels.
- Europe (377, 1487, 2130, 2498, 3665, 4436). For decades, only imported cases have been recorded. In Europe in 3 years, 294 imported cases were reported, including 212 (72%) confirmed by DENV isolation or ≥4-fold rise of neutralizing antibody titer, and 5 (2%) with signs of hemorrhagia (petechiae and low platelet counts). Of German travelers returning from DENV-endemic areas in 1996–2004, 4.7% (51/1,091) presenting for fever were seroreactive, as were 1.1% (13/1,168) of travelers without recent fever.

JEV (982, 1126, 3165, 6866, 8233). Transmission of JEV is perennial in tropical Asia and seasonal (summer epidemics) in temperate East Asia. Only 0.1–0.4% of infections are believed to be manifest. Estimated rates in nonvaccinated travelers per 10^5 per month are 20 for the infection and 0.1 for the disease (JE). At risk are travelers who plan to stay in villages close to rice fields or domestic animals, either in the summer in temperate Asia or any time in tropical Asia, including short-term backpackers and bikers. In 1978–1992, ≥24 cases were recorded in travelers from high-income countries. A 22-year-old nonvaccinated woman from the United States contracted JEV from traveling in Thailand for 1 month; her accomodations included sleeping in a mosquito nonproof dormitory. Although debated for safety, vaccine should be considered for travelers at risk.

Lassa virus (3008, 3341, 3399, 8158, 8430). Imported sporadic Lassa fever cases have been reported in North America, Asia, and Europe. Secondary cases have not occurred. For instance in 1976, of 552 contacts with a peace corps worker returned to the United States with Lassa fever, none contracted the disease. Low contagiosity in travelers contrasts with high contagiosity in hospitals.

RRV (3886, 4617, 4646, 5114, 8430). RRV is enzootic in parts of Australia and the Pacific. Cases in international travelers have been documented in Australia, New Zealand, and Europe. In Queensland, Australia, the rate of clinically diagnosed epidemic polyarthritis among visitors who are exposed on average for 6–10 days is ~5/10^5 (88/1,818,179). Of 183 travelers having visited Pacific islands during the 1979–1980 epidemic, 79 (43%) became seroreactive, and many developed illness compatible with epidemic polyarthritis. Besides being victims, travelers are suspected vectors. The 1979–1980 epidemic in the Pacific was likely seeded by a viremic traveler from Australia.

WNV (1343, 3378, 6316). In 2002 (one case), 2003 (two cases), and 2004 (one case) manifest cases were reported in tourists from France and Germany who had visited infected areas in the United States. Previously, infections had been reported in Irish travelers to the Algarve in Portugal, a German traveler to Kenya, and Austrian travelers to tropical countries. However, not all of earlier infections had been confirmed by neutralization assay or paired sera, leaving open the possibility of cross-reactions.

YFV (380, 1188, 1520, 1930, 5139, 6299). YFV is enzootic in parts of Africa and South America. In infected areas, tourist arrivals are 9 million per year. In sub-Saharan Africa, disease risks per 1,000 per month for nonvaccinated travelers are about one in enzootic areas and 7.5 during outbreaks, while in Latin America risks are 10 times lower. In 1950–2004, at least 14 imported cases were reported in North America and Europe, principally in nonvaccinated travelers. Of 15 participants of a 6–day fishing tour to the Rio Negro in the Amazon of Brazil in 2002, seven were not vaccinated, and one nonvaccinated participant died of yellow fever. In Senegal in 1979, three travelers contracted yellow fever; the only common exposure was a stay at a tourist resort for ≤24 h. Vaccine is recommended for travelers who plan to visit infected areas. Last-minute changes of travel schedules should be considered when planning predeparture vaccines. Besides being victims, viremic travelers are potential vectors and a hazard for urban areas infested by *A. aegypti*.

Bacteria

Priority bacteria in febrile international short-term travelers are Rickettsiales (*Orientia* and *Rickettsia*). Macular rash and eschar are useful clinical signs (4761). Other zoonotic bacteria reported in short-term travelers include *Bartonella bacilliformis* (Oroya fever and verruga peruana) (4837), *Brucella*, *Coxiella*, relapsing *Borrelia* (louse-borne relapsing fever [LBRF] and tick-borne relapsing fever [TBRF]), *Spirillum*, and *Yersinia pestis*.

Brucella **(292, 1415, 4585, 6317, 7594, 8348).** Dairy products consumed during travel or purchased locally and brought home are vehicles for brucellosis in travelers and persons residing outside enzootic areas. The finding of *B. melitensis* in a U.S. high school student triggered an investigation that identified five unrecognized cases in classmates; the source implicated was cheese consumed during travel to Spain. In Germany, about two thirds of reported cases are imported.

Coxiella **(3456, 3550, 5981, 6064).** Travel-related Q fever is infrequent. In the United Kingdom in 1990–2002, only 3% (49/1,459) of reported infections were related to recent travel, mainly the Mediterranean. Risks include inhalation of animal dust, visits to and stay in animal shelters, and touching mammals. During a 1-week safari in Masai-Mara reserve in Kenya, 4 (8%) of 50 travelers contracted *C. burnetii* (two overt and two inapparent), probably from inhalation of dust when entering a shack made of cattle hides and straw.

Orientia **(2078, 2401, 2950, 3456, 3966, 4761, 6073, 6891).** *O. tsutsugamushi* is said to "readily infect visitors to areas where disease transmission occurs" (7977). Scrub typhus accounts for 2–14% of rickettsial infections in travelers. At risk are campers and trekkers in enzootic areas. Reported source countries include Thailand, Korea (mainly for travelers from Japan), and Malaysia, Papua New Guinea, and the Philippines (mainly for travelers from Europe). A German woman contracted scrub typhus during 10 days in Thailand where she trekked in the forest barefooted, camped in a tent, and ate with indigenous people.

Relapsing borreliae. LBRF (6304, 6317). Imported cases have been reported sporadically, for instance, in Germany: 2 in 2000, 1 in 2002, and 0 in 2003. Of the two cases reported in 2000, both had stayed with families in West Africa, had blood films to exclude malaria, and one had skin lesions suggestive of lice bites. *B. recurrentis* was identified in blood smears. **TBRF (1350, 1519, 1768, 2103, 6131, 6304).** Cases have been reported in travelers in North America and Europe. Risks include sleeping outdoors, staying in rodent-infested cabins, spelunking, and adventure traveling. A 13-year-old Caucasian boy from Hawaii contracted TBRF in Texas, after staying in a summer camp and visiting a cave. Two Belgian women contracted TBRF in Senegal from sleeping outdoors. A German woman contracted TBRF in the U.S. Rocky Mountains from visits to parks.

Rickettsia **(3456, 3684, 4761, 6073).** The main imported agents are *R. africae* (African tick bite fever [ATBF]), *R. conorii* (boutonneuse fever), and *R. typhi* (murine typhus). Infrequently reported are *R. akari* (rickettsial pox) (230), *R. australis* (Queensland tick typhus) (6330), *R. prowazekii* (louse-borne typhus [LBT]), and *R. sibirica* (North Asian tick typhus); the term "spotted fevers" is used for cases in whom an agent is not identified. Countries in Europe have reported 0–10 cases per year (e.g., Germany, 22 cases in 5 years; Switzerland, 60 cases in 6 years; and the United Kingdom, 66 cases in 12 years). ***R. africae*** **(1106, 2478, 3684, 3685, 5370, 6116, 6792).** *R. africae* has been increasingly recognized in travelers. Risks include game hunting and travel in the winter months (XI–IV). Of travelers to rural sub-Saharan Africa 4% (38/940) were diagnosed with ATBF (27 confirmed and 11 probable). Among travelers with flulike illness, this proportion increased to 27%. A major source country is South Africa. Of 119 patients with ATBF, 71 (60%) had traveled to there. At an adventure race in South Africa in 1997 that lasted 2 weeks, ≥13 of 450 participants acquired ATBF, for a minimum attack rate of 3%. In V/1999, six Italian tourists contracted ATBF in Mkaya National Park, Swaziland. At a development project in Swaziland in 1998 that lasted 3 weeks, 2 of 34 participants contracted confirmed ATBF and in seven other participants ATBF was suspected clinically, for attack rates of 5–23%. ***R. conorii*** **(3663, 4761, 5687, 5737).** Boutonneuse fever has been diagnosed in travelers to the Mediterranean, Africa, and Asia. Some cases from Africa may in retrospect represent cases of ATBF misdiagnosed as Boutonneuse fever. ***R. typhi*** **(2015, 2950, 3456, 4176, 4761, 5740, 5880, 6073, 6960, 7720).** Murine typhus has been documented in travelers. Reported source countries include Botswana, Ethiopia, Indonesia, and Thailand. A 62-year-old man returned ill to the United Kingdom from a nine-day bird-watching safari in Ethiopia; VHF was initially suspected, but he was later diagnosed with murine typhus; except for one night in a "dilapidated caravan," exposure was unrevealing. In Bali, an Australian woman who attended a conference and stayed in a five-star hotel contracted murine typhus; no risks were identified except an episode of walking barefoot through damp grass. During a 3-week holiday in Thailand, an Austrian contracted murine typhus while staying in simple guest houses; the history was blank for flea bites or rat contacts. ***R. prowazekii*** **(3456, 5412, 6317).** Cases of LBT (epidemic typhus) have been reported in travelers. In Marseille in 1998, LBT was diagnosed serologically and microbiologically in an Algerian who lived in France (5412). In Germany, imported cases were reported from Ethiopia (one, 2003), Gabon (one, 2001), and Thailand (one, 2001). **R. sibirica.** In Mongolia in 2001–2002, 4 (31%) of 13 paleontologists camping in arid and riparian areas of the Gobi Desert contracted typhus; two of four patients recalled tick bites (4388).

Spirillum **(6889).** A traveler contracted spirillary rat-bite fever (sodoku) in Saigon, Vietnam, from strolling in sandals and being bitten on the toe by an urban rat.

Y. pestis **(1968, 8241).** Few plague cases have been reported in travelers. A mammologist in Bolivia collecting and dissecting small mammals in an plague-enzootic area for 4 weeks returned to the United States with fever and lymphadenopathy; culture-confirmed plague was diagnosed and successfully treated. A resident of Arizona contracted *Y. pestis* from a cat in Colorado and died of primary pneumonic plague at home; a mouse flea (*Aetheca wagneri*) collected by burrow swabbing at the exposure site tested positive for *Y. pestis*.

Protozoa

Priority in international short-term travelers is for *Leishmania* and *Plasmodium*. Other protozoa reported in travelers include *Babesia* and *Trypanosoma*.

Babesia **(4532, 5458).** Cases in travelers are rare. *B. microti* imported from the United States was reported in Czechia. After a hiking trip in Wales, a 72-year-old man was diagnosed with *B. divergens* infection in Switzerland.

Leishmania. **Cutaneous leishmaniasis (CL) (3148, 3293).** Travelers from North America and Europe have contracted CL abroad. Risks include visits to forests or parks, ecotourism, and field research. Exposure of ≤1 week (in about one fourth of cases) or ≤48 h (in 10%) can be adequate for transmission. In the United States in 1985–1990, 129 cases were reported in civilian travelers; 53% (69) acquired CL in Latin America. Among travelers to Latin America, estimated rates per 10^5 ranged from <0.1 in Mexio to 100 in Suriname. In Germany, 30 cases in tourists were reported in 2 years, 11 (37%) from Latin America (mainly Brazil), 10 (33%) from Europe (mainly Spain and Malta), 6 (20%) from Asia (Syria and Turkey), and 3 (10%) from Africa. Diagnosis is often made late. In the United States, patients consulted 1–7 (mean, 2) physicians before the diagnosis was made. In Germany, the time to diagnosis was 3 weeks to 2 years (median, 4 months). **Visceral leishmaniasis (VL) (3148, 3657).** Travelers, mainly from Europe, are at risk. In Germany, 18 cases in tourists were reported in 2 years, 5 in children (8 months to 11 years of age) and 13 in adults (31–70 years of age). Source countries were Italy (mainland, Ischia, and Sicily), Spain (mainland and Ibiza), Greece (Korfu), France, Malta, Tunisia, and People's Republic of China. In France in 1986–1987, 70 (79%) of 89 reported cases were autochthonous, 19 (21%) were imported, and 5 were preschool children. Source countries included Greece, Italy, Spain, and India. Time to diagnosis can be considerable; in Germany it was 1–16 (median, 4) months.

Plasmodium **(318, 826, 1668, 2081, 3785, 6502, 6665, 6801).** In high-income countries, most cases are imported by civilians and army personnel. Entomological inoculation rates in travelers are projected to be comparable to or lower than in local residents. By accommodation and prevention, estimated disease rates per 100 travelers per month are 0.3–3 in sub-Saharan Africa (mostly *P. falciparum*), 0.001–0.2 in Latin America (virtually nil in capital cities) and Asia, and up to 6 in the southwestern Pacific, with highs if no prophylaxis is taken. Prevention includes mosquito avoidance by clothes, repellents, and bednets, chemoprophylaxis, and self-treatment in an emergency.

Of malaria in travelers, 10–15% is manifest abroad and 85–90% after returning home. By 1 month after return, 80% of falciparum malaria has become manifest, by 2 months, 20–40% of vivax malaria, and by 12 months 99% of all malaria. Disease in travelers, despite compliance with chemoprophylaxis (breakthrough malaria) or treatment failures, may herald drug resistance. Destination determines the proportion of falciparum disease and hence lethality. Nonimmune travelers are rarely sources of introduced malaria, unlike partially immune immigrants (see section 15.6) or refugees (see section 11.4) who can be carriers of gametocytes.

- North America (1132, 2171, 6801). In 1990–2003, the United States reported 17,583 malaria cases (∼1,255 per year), most (60–70%) from Africa, and 45–53% due to *P. falciparum*. Overall lethality was 0.4–0.6%. In 2003, of cases with date of onset known, 12% were manifest before arrival in the United States, and 0.8% >1 year after arrival. A few cases have been acquired locally each year, congenitally, from transfusion or needle-stick, or "cryptically."
- Australasia (4108, 6343, 8342). Australia in 1999–2003 reported 3,451 imported cases (on average, 690/year), mainly from Papua New Guinea and Southeast Asia, and 20–43% were due to *P. falciparum*. In 1980–1992, New Zealand imported on average 67 cases/year, mainly from Papua New Guinea, Solomon Islands, and Vanuatu, and 23% were due to *P. falciparum*; lethality was 0.3%. Australia has been malaria-free since 1983, although *A. farauti* is present north of latitude 17–18°S. Malaria

was introduced by gametocytemic individuals in north Queensland in 1986 with seven local vivax cases, and again in 2002 with ten local vivax cases.

- Europe (3456, 4291, 6317, 6502, 7734, 8032). On average, imported cases reported per year were 1,500–2,000 in the 1970s, 7,000 in the mid 1980s–1990s, but ~13,000 in 1999; corrected for underreporting, the true number is likely two to three times higher. About 70–80% of cases are acquired in Africa, 60–80% are due to *P. falciparum*, and lethality is 0.3–2%. At a hotel in Chalkidiki, Greece, in 2000, a German couple and an American tourist contracted vivax malaria in a seemingly malaria-free area.

Trypanosoma. T. cruzi **(888).** Cases in travelers are rare. In Colombia, after overnight stays in a thatched hut for 11 days, a French woman contracted culture-confirmed, acute Chagas disease complicated by pancarditis. ***T. brucei*** **sl (2061, 4523, 4688, 4698, 5298).** Human African trypanosomiasis (HAT) has been imported sporadically into the United States and Europe. Of 109 cases reported in 1904–1965, 90% (98) were males, 10% (11) were females. The rate in travelers is low, probably ~$0.3/10^5$.

- Subacute *T. brucei gambiense* (1728, 4523) was diagnosed in a student, a geologist, a construction worker, and expatriates. Acquisition near cities and after a "brief" stay is possible (7677).
- For acute *T. brucei rhodesiense* (3661, 4523, 4688, 5164, 5298, 6929), risks include safaris in game parks, hunt, and field research. In 2001, nine or more cases were reported in travelers to game parks in East Africa. For savanna, see section 5.4.

Helminths

In general, exposure is too short for short-term travelers to acquire vector-borne helminths. Occasional infections in tourists have been reported for *D. immitis* (6069), *D. repens* (5700), *Mansonella ozzardi* (5516), *M. perstans* (3926), and *Onchocerca volvulus* (6030). In the United Kingdom in 1990, onchocerciasis was diagnosed in 22 (26%) of 85 travelers who had visited Cameroon in 1988 for 27 days to 15 months (mean, 3 months).

ENVIRONMENTAL CLUSTER
Bacteria
Burkholderia pseudomallei **(1731, 3676, 7841).** Cases of melioidosis have been reported in travelers, including from India, Malaysia, Thailand, and Australia. Putative risks are water or mud contacts. An English photographer on assignment in Malaysia during a massage sustained a rib fracture that was treated locally; after 10 days, *B. pseudomallei* was isolated from a skin abscess in the United Kingdom.

Leptospira **(3038, 3387, 5145, 7707, 7735, 8171).** Cases of *Leptospira* have been reported in travelers to Africa, Asia, and Latin America. In 1987–1991, 32 cases were reported in Dutch travelers, mostly from Southeast Asia; in 31, exposure to surface waters was the source implicated. In Denmark in 1970–1996, 8% of 118 laboratory-confirmed cases were related to international travel. Risks include river crossing; swallowing river water, in particular, after floods that may flush out bank rodents; trekking; and other adventure travel.

Mycobacterium **(6768).** A Canadian journalist presented with a painless, furuncle-like, persisting lesion of the calf after travel in Africa for 8 months in 1993–1994; the lesion eventually grew *M. ulcerans*.

Fungi
Penicillium marneffei **(5706).** In 1988–1994, penicilliosis disease (tuberculosis-like) was diagnosed in 14 HIV-infected travelers from the United States, Australia, and Europe.

Sporothrix schenckii. Although conceivable, sporotrichosis does not appear to have been reported in travelers.

Helminths
The main hazards are schistosomiasis from freshwater contacts, and cutaneous larva migrans (CLM) from soil contact. Unlike expatriates, enteric hookworms and *Strongyloides* seem infrequent in international short-term travelers.

CLM (687, 858, 2578, 2921, 3147, 3304, 5326, 5765, 7547, 7794). CLM is an infection of the skin by zoonotic nematode larvae, mainly hookworm (*A. braziliense* and *A. caninum*), occasionally *Gnathostoma*.

Acquisition is through the skin from soil polluted by dog or cat feces. Risks include barefoot walking in countries with warm climates, unprotected skin contact with beach sand, wearing sand-filled sandals or muddy clothes (larvae can penetrate textiles, including uniform cloth), and handling soil.

The incubation period is 1 day to 4–16 (typically 2) weeks. Manifestation is a creeping, serpiginous, itchy eruption, typically at the feet or buttocks. Diagnosis is clinical. CLM resolves spontaneously in 1 week to 12 (typically 2) months. Treatment options include topical thiabendazole, or oral albendazole or ivermectin.

By case mix, CLM has been diagnosed in 0–3% of international travelers, mainly from the Caribbean, Africa, and Southeast Asia. Autochthonous cases have been reported in Texas and Florida as well as parts of Europe (Italy, France, Germany, and United Kingdom). In favelas in Fortaleza, Brazil, the point prevalence was 3% (95% CI 2–4). In residents on Montserrat, Caribbean, the rate was $64/10^5$ per year. Outbreaks have been reported among travelers, pupils, and military personnel. At a resort in Barbados, Caribbean, 32 (25%) of 126 Canadian holidaymakers contracted CLM.

***Schistosoma* (2948, 3147, 5893, 6078, 6347, 8082).** All infections in high-income countries have been imported. Risks in travelers include swimming in rivers, snorkeling, diving, boat trips, and rafting.

A first, often inapparent stage within hours from exposure is cercarial dermatitis (see section 5.2). A second, acute stage (Katayama fever) associated with juvenile worms may ensue in weeks after exposure. Katayama fever has been well documented in travelers, including from outbreaks. *S. mansoni* has most often been implicated; infrequently, *S. haematobium*. Established visceral infection has been confirmed by the demonstration of eggs in urine (*S. haematobium*) or feces (*S. mansoni* and *S. japonicum*) after completion of the prepatent period (see chapter 20).

Travelers account for 20–60% of imported cases in Europe, immigrants for 80–40%. Infections in travelers, because of short exposure, are typically light, difficult to detect, inapparent (in 20–70%), and uncomplicated, unlike immigrants who may have been exposed for years. By area visited, *S. mansoni* accounts for 10–80% of imported infections, *S. haematobium* for 5–70%, and *S. intercalatum* for 0–8%; 10% of infections are mixed, and in 10–30%, a species is not determined. Of 662 overseas travelers returning to Germany with diarrhea in 2000, 6 (1%) excreted eggs of *S. mansoni* in the feces. If screening is targeted to travelers from Africa with a history of water exposure, expected diagnostic yield is increased to 18%. Sources for most (90–95%) travelers from Europe are countries in sub-Saharan Africa, in particular, the Niger, Sambesi, and Volta rivers, and Lake Malawi.

Arthropods
Cases of Myiasis (see section 4.6) and tungiasis (see section 4.6) have been reported in travelers.

SKIN-BLOOD CLUSTER
Exposure. Hazards include accidents that require emergency transfusion of unsafe blood and travel for casual sex (sex tourism).

Sex tourism (300, 1102, 3193, 4734, 4836, 4969, 5245, 6372). Destinations popular with sex tourists include Caribbean (Dominican Republic) and Southeast Asia (Thailand). By age and sex, 5–65% of tourists plan or have sex with new, casual partners abroad. Of 4,680 Danes 18–59 years of age who traveled to Greenland, sex with partners at risk of HIV infection (IDUs, prostitutes, homosexual men, and residents from sub-Saharan Africa) was reported by 5% of first-time and 10% of repeat female visitors, and 16% of first-time and 34% of repeat male visitors. At STI clinics in Glasgow, United Kingdom, in 1993–1994, patients reported new sexual encounters at rates of 0.1 per week (before travel) and 0.25 per week (abroad). Of international travelers attending a London outpatient department, 19% (141/757) reported new sex partners on the most recent travel abroad; nearly two thirds of those who had sex abroad did not use condoms consistently, and 6% (43) contracted STI. Risk behavior may not be limited to travel, but in the United Kingdom, ~10% of gonorrhea and ~20% of acute, infectious syphilis is travel related.

Viruses
Cytomegalovirus (CMV) (2651). CMV is a cause of fatigue syndrome in travelers that has been discussed.

HBV (6967, 7129). Travel to high-endemicity areas is a hazard. In the prevaccine era, the rate of acute hepatitis B in travelers was ~20–60/10^5 per month.

HIV (5843, 7848). Risk behavior and excess seroprevalence in sex tourists and epidemiological studies suggest that HIV infection can be acquired during travel. Travelers can also be vectors of HIV. "Travelers contribute to the spread of HIV-1 genetic diversity worldwide." (5843).

Human papillomavirus (4734). At Swedish family-planning and youth clinics, the prevalence of cervical HPV was significantly higher (11%) in 276 women admitting casual travel sex than in 720 control women (0.7%) who negated casual travel sex.

Bacteria
Skin infections (1129). Skin infections from international travel include impetigo and infected insect bites. Of 269 travelers (three fourths tourists) presenting in Paris, France, for skin problems from tropical countries, 18% had pyodermia, and 10% had arthropod-reactive dermatitis. Infrequent but important for differential diagnosis are cutaneous diphtheria and leprosy. ***C. diphtheriae* (1789).** Cutaneous diphtheria is rare in high-income countries but endemic in pockets in some tropical countries. In the United Kingdom in 1995–2002, all of 17 confirmed cases were imported (12 from Asia and 5 from Africa). Of 15 presenting documents, six patients had received four vaccine doses (a full primary series), two had received three doses, and seven (47%) were nonvaccinated. Cutaneous diphtheria can be the source for respiratory carriage or laryngeal diphtheria, and it should be managed accordingly. ***Mycobacterium leprae* (2376).** *M. leprae* is rarely confirmed in travelers. An Italian male, after visits that lasted 20–30 days each to Sri Lanka in 1980 and 1981, India in 1987, and Cuba in 1988, presented with paresthesias in 1989 that led to a diagnosis of leprosy in 1992.

S. aureus (3787, 6388). Travelers and repatriated patients can be vectors of MRSA strains. In 1993, a patient returning from India introduced MRSA into British Columbia, Canada, which subsequently spread to several hospitals, covering >1,600 km within 6 weeks and causing 12 cases of disease (including 11 deaths) and 14 colonizations.

STI (2140). STI from international travel include genital *Chlamydia trachomatis* (serovars D–K), gonorrhea, and syphilis. Infrequent but predominantly imported STI include chancroid (*Haemophilus ducreyii*), donovanosis (*Klebsiella granulomatis*), and lymphgranuloma venereum (*C. trachomatis* serovars L1–3). For STI among homosexual men, see section 13.7. **Genital *C. trachomatis* (495, 3334, 4734).** Although casual sex abroad is a risk, most infections are acquired domestically, in Finland 89–97%. *N. gonorrhoeae* (1829, 2918, 3334, 3362, 6372, 6458). *N. gonorrhoeae* is a major, travel-related STI. Travelers can be victims and vectors. The latter is exemplified by penicillinase-producing strains (PPNG) that emerged in 1976. Within 5 years, PPNG from epicenters in Southeast Asia and Africa spread to Europe and North America, largely carried by travelers. In some high-income countries, up to 30–60% of gonorrhea cases can be imported. *T. pallidum pallidum* (1829, 3362, 6372, 6847). Syphilis can be acquired during travel. In high-income countries, up to 30% of new cases can be imported. In the wake of syphilis resurgence in Russia in the 1990s, syphilis was diagnosed in travelers returning from outbreak areas.

Helminths

Hymenolepis **(3456).** In the United Kingdom in 1990–2003, 185 (42%) of 445 laboratory reports concerning *H. nana* provided information about travel; in 62% (115/185) of these reports, immigrants were mentioned and travel was also noted, mainly to the Indian subcontinent and sub-Saharan Africa.

15.5 EXPATRIATES

Expatriates in this book are people from high-income countries living in low-income countries for months or years while keeping their original citizenship. Examples are aid and construction workers, missionaries, and delegates of diplomatic missions. Included here are long-term travelers who are abroad for ≥1 month, often on more than one continent. For migrant workers, see section 15.6; for peacekeeping forces, see section 12.3.

Exposure can result from ingestion (drinking water and foods), inhalation (droplets from people and dust), inoculation (unsafe injections, tattooing, and injection drug use), or contact (unsafe sex, freshwater, and rodent-infested domiciles). "Seasoned" expatriates will assimilate local "flora" and acquire partial immunity to latent infections. Difficulties with recall can bias the history of expatriates, e.g., exposure to foods and animals.

Infections (601, 3361, 4365, 4403, 5380, 7131, 7218). With increasing duration of exposure and assimilation of local lifestyles, clinical profiles in expatriates shift from short-term travelers (acute or light-inapparent infections) toward immigrants (chronic infections manifested by complications). On home leave, a Swiss missionary working in Gabon for 12 years was diagnosed with six parasitologically confirmed infections: *Loa*, *Mansonella*, *Onchocerca*, and *Wuchereria* tissue infections and *Strongyloides* and *Trichuris* enteric infections.

For illness, expatriates mainly consult local health services. As a consequence, expatriates are less well studied than tourists. Frequent infections in expatriates (and approximate rates per 100 person-years) include diarrhea (50/100), RTI (~35), presumptive malaria (8), STI (8), and ectoparasites (6), in Africa also schistosomiasis (6).

Prevention (3361, 8081). Measures resemble short-term travelers (see section 15.4), but malaria chemoprophylaxis should be adapted to local risks. Employers may plan emergency repatriation by air and postemployment medical visits. Evaluation should consider exposure history and physical examination, tuberculin skin test, complete blood count (anemia and eosinophilia) and smear for *Plasmodium* and microfilariae, serology for HBV, HCV, HIV, syphilis, *Schistosoma*, and *Strongyloides*, stool samples for cysts (*E. histolytica* and *G. lamblia*), eggs (*S. mansoni* and *Ascaris*), and larvae (*Strongyloides* and hookworm), and urine for sediment, hematuria, *C. trachomatis*, *N. gonorrhoeae*, and eggs of *S. haematobium*.

DROPLET-AIR CLUSTER

Evidence is limited. Respiratory viruses, bacteria, and fungi likely reflect endemicity in resident communities. The focus is on chronic or reactivated conditions such as tuberculosis and systemic fungal infections.

Bacillus anthracis **(5774).** An African resident in France presented with inhalational anthrax 3 days after a 3-month trip in West Africa.

M. tuberculosis **(1489, 3897).** Work (e.g., health, aid) and location (countries with infection risks ≥1/100 per year) are risks for infection and disease in expatriates. In The Netherlands in 1994–1996, of immune-competent long-term travelers to high-risk countries, 1.8% (12/656) skin converted to tuberculin, for an infection rate of 4/100 person-years, and 0.3% (2) developed active tuberculosis, for a disease rate of 0.7/100 person-years. At a

U.S. government office in Botswana in 1998, 15% (3/22) of United States-born employees converted to tuberculin.

Blastomyces. *B. dermatitidis* is endemic in North America, Africa, and Asia. A 3-years-old child who had been born and lived in the United States was diagnosed with pulmonary and cutaneous blastomycosis (7792).

***Paracoccidioides* (103, 3433, 4718).** At least 42 cases of paracoccidioides in expatriates have been reported in Europe and North America. Culture-confirmed paracoccidioidomycosis was diagnosed in a Canadian expatriate who had lived in Brazil in 1958–1964 and in Argentina in 1979–1981, and in a German legionnaire who had worked in Brazil for many years.

FECES-FOOD CLUSTER
Evidence is limited. Enteric viruses, bacteria, and parasites likely reflect endemicity in resident communities. The focus is on chronic conditions such as carriage of enteric helminths, persisting diarrhea due to enteric protozoa, and eosinophilia due to tissue helminths.

Viruses
HAV (5560, 5906, 5957, 6971). By length of stay, work, and vaccination status, expatriates are at variable risk of infection and acute hepatitis A, including from contact with infective family members and local children. In the prevaccine era, infection rates in expatriates were 0.8/100 person-years, and disease rates ranged from 0.2/100 person-years to 4/100 per year.

HEV (3642, 6971). By geography, reported seroprevalence in adult expatriates ranges from ~2% (Southwest Asia) to ~7% (sub-Saharan Africa, Southeast Asia, and Latin America) and 10% (Indian subcontinent). Of 328 North American missionaries, none was initially reactive, and none seroconverted after a mean exposure period of 7 years. Most infections in expatriates seem inapparent or mild.

Bacteria
Enteric bacteria (516, 1856, 3668, 7362) reported in inapparent or symptomatic expatriates include *Campylobacter* (in 0.7%), *H. pylori*, *S. enterica* non-Typhi serovars (in 0.2–0.7%), serovar Typhi, *Shigella* (in 0.5%), and *V. cholerae*. For serovar Typhi and *V. cholerae*, vaccines are commercially available. ***H. pylori* (516).** *H. pylori* is a consideration in expatriates with gastrointestinal disease. Among 312 American missionaries working in low-income countries on an average for 7 years, the rate of *H. pylori* infection was 1.9/100 per year. **Serovar Typhi (3668).** Likely risks include domicile in remote area, poor sanitation, and poor food and water hygiene. The rate of typhoid fever in expatriates is estimated to 0.5/100 per year. ***V. cholerae* (2809, 7362).** By geography and epidemiological situation, cholera can be a risk. In Lima, Peru, during the 1991–1993 cholera epidemic, 5 (1.6%) of 317 Americans working at the U.S. embassy were diagnosed with confirmed cholera; three of the five attributed their illness to food served on the beach. In Singapore in 1982, 22 foreign construction workers contracted cholera, and a further 15 had *V. cholerae* O1 infection; the implicated vehicle was seafood from a canteen.

Protozoa
Enteric protozoa (2545, 3289, 3381) reported in inapparent or symptomatic expatriates include *B. hominis* (in 15–20%), *Cryptosporidium* (in 1%), *C. cayetanensis* (in 1–12%), *E. histolytica/dispar* (in 1–7%), *G. lamblia* (in 1–8%), and *Isospora* (in 0.5–1%). Expatriates with diarrhea should be evaluated for these agents.

Helminths
Enteric helminths (1856, 2545, 3147, 3456, 7119) reported in inapparent or symptomatic expatriates include *Ascaris* (in ~0.5–5%) and *Trichuris* (in ~0.5–10%), and sporadically *F. hepatica* and *Taenia*. Most *Ascaris* and *Trichuris* infections diagnosed in high-income countries are imported, typically from sub-Saharan Africa and the Indian subcontinent.

***Taenia. T. saginata* (3456, 8071).** In the United Kingdom in 1990–2003, for 185 of 475 *T. saginata* laboratory reports foreign travel was the mentioned source, in 52% (97/185) this was sub-Saharan Africa, in particular, (43%, 42/97) Ethiopia. *T. saginata* was isolated in an Ethiopia-born student in Texas, after a visit to Mexico where she ate uncooked beef. ***T. solium* (1351, 3456, 7046).** Both enteric (taeniasis) and tissue (cysticercosis) infections seem infrequent in short-term travelers and expatriates. However, in California in 1988–1990, 7% (9/138) of reported cysticercosis cases concerned United States-born travelers to Mexico.

ZOONOTIC CLUSTER
Risks include domiciles in remote areas and adventurous travel. The focus is on chronic conditions such as persisting arthralgia due to arboviruses, relapsing fever from *P. vivax*, and persisting pruritis due to *Onchocerca*.

Viruses
Expatriates can be exposed to the full spectrum of zoonotic and vector-borne viruses, including CHIKV, DENV, JEV (7068), rabies virus, RRV, YFV, and agents of VHF. Febrile expatriates should be evaluated for dengue, and expatriates with neurological symptoms should be

evaluated for rabies. Vaccines are commercially available for JEV, rabies virus, TBEV, and YFV. Avoidance of mosquito, tick, and vertebrate bites is generally advised.

CHIKV (2147). Infection and disease are reported in expatriates. Of German aid workers, on average exposed for 38 months, 1% (9/670) had immunoglobulin G (IgG) antibodies to CHIKV.

DENV (2147, 3618, 3643, 4436, 4588). DENV infections and disease have been reported in adventurous travelers, e.g., campers, and expatriates, e.g., aid workers. By destination and test, ~4–6% of expatriates have been confirmed seroreactive. In German aid workers, the seroconversion rate was ~2/100 per year. Risks seem to increase with increasing length of stay. Travelers from Sweden with dengue ($n = 74$) had spent 11–496 (median, 30) days abroad; 61% (45/74) of the travelers had been abroad for ≥25 days compared with 15% (44/292) of randomly selected control travelers without dengue, for an odds ratio of 9 (95% CI 5–16). Concurrent with cumulating exposure time, risks of dengue hemorrhagic fever (DHF) or shock syndrome (DSS) seem to increase. In the United Kingdom, a Malaysian woman and a Pakistani man developed DHF after visits to their homelands. Exposure avoidance is advised for expatriates in endemic areas.

Rabies virus (677, 3179). In 296 Norwegian missionaries and foreign aid workers living in areas with enzootic rabies, the cumulative risk of exposure in 4–5 years was ~7/100 expatriates. In Swiss and German expatriates, dogs were the source in 69% of 72 potential exposures.

Bacteria

Expatriates can be exposed to the full spectrum of zoonotic bacteria, including *Bartonella*, *Borrelia*, *Brucella*, Rickettsiales (*Anaplasma*, *Ehrlichia*, *Orientia*, and *Rickettsia*), and *Y. pestis*. Febrile expatriates with compatible exposure histories should be evaluated for the respective agents (3361)

Protozoa

Expatriates can be exposed to the full spectrum of vector-borne protozoa. Screening inapparent expatriates by blood smear and serology for *Leishmania*, *Plasmodium*, *Trypanosoma*, and invasive *Entamoeba* can be inefficient, for an expected yield <1% (1856). Use of sensitive tests (e.g., nucleic acid amplification test) may change the efficiency. Febrile expatriates with compatible exposure histories should be evaluated for the respective agents (3361).

Leishmania **(641, 3361).** Expatriates are at risk of visceral (febrile) and cutaneous (nonfebrile) leishmaniasis. In Saudi Arabia in 1977, European expatriates not familiar with CL frequently exposed themselves at dusk, when gathering around swimming pools. Of 87 persons surveyed, 47 had active lesions (1–28 per patient; median, 4), mainly shallow ulcers.

Plasmodium **(601, 2219, 3361, 7131, 8081).** Expatriates are at risk of malaria disease. Hyperreactive splenomegaly, blackwater fever, and cerebral malaria have all affected expatriates. Partial immunity may take many years to develop and cannot reliably protect them from malaria. Of expatriates and their families in Abidjan, Cote d'Ivoire, by 15 years in the country, 50% had had one or more clinical malaria episodes. Risks include being an expatriate child, domicile in rural areas, and noncompliance with prevention. In Africa in 1987, the incidence of falciparum malaria in peace corps volunteers complying or not with chloroquine chemoprophylaxis was 8/100 per year. In 1989–1990, 4% (316/7,114) of the United Nations assistance group in Namibia consulted for suspected malaria and in 60% (191/316) of these, malaria was slide confirmed.

Trypanosoma. Infections in expatriates are infrequent but severe. ***T. brucei* sl (2061, 3538, 4698).** In 1904–1965, of 86 HAT expatriate cases with occupation known, 15 (17%) were missionaries, 15 (17%) were military personnel, 10 (12%) were outdoor workers (farm, forest, and hunt), 8 (9%) were miners or engineers, 8 (9%) were traders, 8 (9%) were health workers, 8 (9%) were administrators, 6 (7%) were boatmen, and 8 (9%) had other professions. While *T. brucei rhodesiense* does not seem to have been reported in expatriates (perhaps because fulminant infections were treated locally), cases of *T. brucei gambiense* have been reported in expatriates living or working in rural or remote areas. ***T. cruzi.*** Acute Chagas disease has not been reported in expatriates. Seroreactions in blood banks have been explained by infected immigrants rather than infected expatriates.

Helminths

Filariae diagnosed in expatriates include *Loa* (in 0–0.1%), *Mansonella perstans* (in 0–1.5%), *Onchocerca* (in 0–1.5%), and *Wuchereria* (in 0–0.05%) (1856). In general, acquisition results from exposure for months or years. In 64 expatriates with filariases, mean time spent abroad was 5½ years (7218).

Loa **(802, 1447, 3997, 5515).** *L. loa* is a cause of migrating soft-tissue edema and inflammation in expatriates. Many cases of loasis have been reported in expatriates from Africa, typically after stays of 1–3 years. Among 20 Peace Corps volunteers working in Gabon for 2 years and not taking diethylcarbamazine for prophylaxis, rates per 100 per year were 25 for infection and 15 for disease.

***Onchocerca* (2204, 2788, 3768, 7218).** *O. volvulus* is a cause of corneal opacity, persistent pruritus, subcutaneous nodules, and adenopathy in expatriates. Imported cases have been reported in North America and West Europe.

***Wuchereria* (2947, 7218).** *W. bancrofti* is a rare cause of adenopathy and edema in expatriates. Sporadic infections have been confirmed by antigen test or microfilaremia in long-term travelers and expatriates.

ENVIRONMENTAL CLUSTER

Expatriates can be exposed to the full spectrum of environmental agents, including bacteria (e.g., *B. pseudomallei*, *Clostridium tetani*, *Leptospira*, and environmental mycobacteria), fungi (e.g., lobomycosis by *Lacazia*, rhinosporidiosis by *Rhinosporidium*, and sporotrichosis by *Sporothrix*), environmental amebae (*Acanthamoeba* and *Naegleria*), helminths (from soil and water), and sandfleas (*Tunga*). The focus, however, is on persisting infections by hookworms, *Schistosoma*, and *Strongyloides*.

Hookworms (3456). Most cases of hookworms in high-income countries are imported, mainly by immigrants or expatriates, rarely by travelers. By geography and self-treatment, 0.5–2% of expatriates harbor *Ancylostoma duodenale* or *Necator americanus*.

***Schistosoma* (601, 1277, 1856, 2948, 3666, 5893, 8081).** All schistosomiasis in high-income countries is imported, ~15% by expatriates and 85% by immigrants. Risks include contact with water in river banks, lake shores, and ponds, for instance, by washing hands, swimming, or wind surfing. By geography and tests, 0–0.3% of expatriates harbor *S. haematobium*, and 0.2–1.3% harbor *S. mansoni*. When stratified by exposure ($n = 387$), 5% of expatriates reporting no water contact tested positive (eggs and serology), compared with 13% reporting occasional freshwater contact and 19% with frequent contact. At the time of diagnosis, ~60% of infections in expatriates are inapparent. In 440 expatriates with exposure at Lake Malawi, seroprevalence increased with increasing time abroad, from 11% for stays of 1 year to 48% for stays of ≥4 years. In 1987, infections in Peace Corps volunteers occurred at a rate of <1/100 per year.

***Strongyloides* (1856, 3147, 3456, 3769, 7231).** Most *S. stercoralis* infections in high-income countries have been imported, mainly by immigrants or expatriates, rarely by travelers. By geography, self-treatment, and test, 0.1–0.4% of expatriates have tested positive for *S. stercoralis*. In 2000, of 662 overseas travelers returning to Germany with diarrhea, one (0.2%) excreted larvae in feces.

SKIN-BLOOD CLUSTER

Some 30% of male and female expatriates have reported casual sex with local partners, but only two thirds of these consistently used condoms (1799). The focus is on persisting infections, mainly HBV, HCV, HIV, and syphilis.

Viruses

Priority is for HBV, HCV, and HIV.

HBV (1490, 5560, 5957, 6971, 7211). By age and geography, the HBV marker prevalence is 8–12%, figures that are generally higher than in comparable domestic populations. Risks include adopting children into the household, health work, invasive procedures (ritual, dental, and injections), and sex with local residents. Without vaccine, reported rates were 1.7–2.8/1,000 person-months for seroconversions, and 0.6–1.1/100 per year for acute hepatitis B. Vaccine reduced the disease rate to 0.05/100 per year. Susceptible expatriates should be offered vaccine.

HCV (6971, 7211). Main risks are unsafe procedures and blood products and injection drug use. Seroprevalence in expatriates seems comparable to domestic populations, for <1% by second-generation immunoblot assay. The reported infection (seroconvesion) rate is 0.4 per 100 person-years.

HIV (1799, 5430, 5589). Reported infection prevalence in expatriates is 0.3–2.7%. Risks include unsafe sex with infected partners, unsafe procedures (venipuncture and intramuscular injection), unsafe blood products, and injection drug use.

Bacteria

M. leprae has been diagnosed in ≤0.1% of expatriates (1856).

STI in expatriates reflect patterns of short-term travelers. However, serodiagnosis of syphilis may be confounded by nonvenereal *Treponema* infections in expatriates, including *T. carateum* (pinta), recognized in an Austrian expatriate returning from Cuba (8247), *T. pallidum endemicum* (endemic syphilis) recognized in an expatriate girl returning from Mali (7675), and *T. pallidum pertenue* (yaws) recognized in a girl from Ghana visiting The Netherlands (2210).

Helminths

By case mix, 0.1–0.2% of expatriates test positive for *Enterobius vermicularis*, and 0.2–0.4% test positive for *H. nana* (1856).

Ectoparasites

The expected prevalence of scabies in expatriates is 0.5% (1856).

15.6 IMMIGRANTS AND MIGRANTS

Migrants are people who leave their home place for economic reasons, typically for seasonal work. Transmigrants settle in their home countries. Immigrants cross borders (documented or nondocumented) and enter host high-income contries with plans to settle permanently. There are ~160–175 million (im)migrants worldwide (9% in Africa, 27% in America, 32% each in Australasia and Europe) (7642). For refugees, see section 11.4.

Exposure. Typical jobs for immigrants include kitchen, farm, harvest, cleaning, waste, abattoir, and sex work (see section 13.6). Access to care can be difficult, utilization of care can be below or above average, and housing is typically below standard.

Infections (1372, 2019, 3535, 4516) (Box 15.5). Infections in immigrants mirror enzootic and endemic occurrence in source and transit countries. In Spain in 1989–1999, the main symptoms in 988 immigrants were fever (29%), pruritus (29%), abdominal pain (14%), and cough (13%); main findings were eosinophilia (23%), visceromegaly (16%), and anemia (15%). Immigrants can be victims *and* vectors of infection if host countries are receptive for agents carried or shed by immigrants.

Prevention (1517, 5240). Screening could follow suggestions for expatriates (see section 15.5). Screening for tuberculosis and HIV is debated, in particular, mandatory screening for HIV. By likely pretest prevalence, presumptive treatment for enteric parasites can be more cost-effective than screening.

DROPLET-AIR CLUSTER

Overview (2019, 4516). RTI have been documented inadequately in immigrants. By origin, ~10–20% of immigrants may report cough. Agents in immigrants may mirror endemicity in source, transit, or host countries (see section 14.7). Compared with the remaining United States, influx counties within 100 km from the Mexican border have had increased rates of mumps (1.3-fold), measles (1.2-4-fold), rubella (2-fold), and diphtheria (2-3-fold). Vaccine coverage may be low in immigrants.

The focus in immigrant children and adults is on vaccine-preventable and reactivated latent respiratory infections.

Viruses

Immigrants seem at increased risk of vaccine-preventable viruses, including measles, rubella, and varicella (8073). Review of reliable vaccination records may help to guide laboratory identification of agents.

Rubella virus (3535, 5943, 8413). Immigrants and their contacts are at increased risk of infection and disease. In the United States, congenital rubella syndrome is a health problem largely limited to pregnant Hispanic immigrant women.

Poliovirus (4129). Up to the 1970s and 1980s, immigrants and their families contributed ~60% of polio cases imported into high-income countries.

Bacteria

Diphtheria, invasive *Haemophilus influenzae* b disease, pertussis, and tuberculosis are vaccine preventable. Tuberculosis can be reactivated or newly acquired. Review of reliable vaccination and tuberculin skin test records could be helpful.

***C. diphtheriae* (4104, 7427).** In Germany, the proportion of carriers of toxigenic strains was higher in immigrants than the local population. In Thailand in 1996, migrants from Laos and northern Thailand (Hmong) were suspected sources of diphtheria outbreaks in Nan (5 cases) and Saburi (18 cases) provinces.

***M. tuberculosis* (1295, 1518, 1925, 2161, 3915, 4417, 5711, 5753, 6564, 7806).** Migrants, immigrants, and asylum seekers account for a significant fraction of all tuberculosis infection and disease in high-income countries. By national policy, screening (history, skin test, or

---

Box 15.5 Main agents and infections in immigrants, by cluster

*Potential for introductions.

Droplet-air	Vaccine-preventable viruses and bacteria, *C. diphtheriae* (carriage and diphtheria*), *M. tuberculosis* (latent or active*); reactivated fungi (e.g., *H. capsulatum*)
Feces-food	HAV,* HEV; ETEC, serovar Typhi (carriage, typhoid*), shigellosis*, *V. cholerae*; *C. parvum*, *E. histolytica* (carriage and invasive disease), *G. lamblia*; • *Ascaris, Clonorchis, T. saginata, T. solium* (carriage*), *Trichuris*
Zoonotic	Rabies virus, DENV, other arboviruses; *Brucella*; *Leishmania, Plasmodium* (gametocytemic* and acute), *Trypanosoma* (latent*); *Echinococcus*, filariae
Environmental	Hookworm, *S. haematobium, S. mansoni, Strongyloides*
Skin-blood	HBV* (carrier, acute, and chronic), HCV (chronic), HIV* (AIDS and coinfections); *M. leprae, Treponema** (latent); tinea capitis*; pediculosis,* scabies*

chest radiograph) should be considered for immigrants (i) from high-risk countries, (ii) with cough illness, or (iii) from transit relief camps. Screening has been questioned, however, because of cost ineffectiveness and increased risks that continued for years after arrival.

- Migrants (1452, 2514, 3597, 3871, 6710, 6834, 7973) (http://www.eurotb.org). Migrants are at increased risk of infection and disease. Disease endemicity in country of birth predicts ~85% of tuberculosis risk in migrants; additional predictors include hindered access to care, full compliance with treatment for 6 months, and unemployment. In Florida in 1992, 38% (118/310) of migrants from 14 camps were skin test positive, and 33% (18/55) of reactive migrants monitored were given chemoprophylaxis, while 2% (1) had active disease.

  By source country and ethnicity mix, disease prevalence in migrants is 0.5–9%. Disease in migrants may be different from cases in low-risk countries, including by more frequent extrapulmonary sites (e.g., spine, meninges, and abdomen).

- Immigrants (1712, 2161, 4417, 4516, 5052, 5753, 6564, 7316, 8342) (http://www.eurotb.org). Immigrants from high-risk countries significantly contribute to disease (up to 50–80% of cases) in North America, Australia, and West Europe, including MDR tuberculosis. Of 743 Vietnamese immigrants to the United States in 1991–1999, 45–53% were latently infected. In Spain in 1989–1999, 44% (200/453) of immigrants had latent infection, and 6% (57/988) had active disease. In Italy, 0.7% (8/1,232) nonregistered immigrants had active tuberculosis. In Australia for many years, reported disease rates were much higher in overseas-born than Australia-born (19 versus $1/10^5$ in 2001). Among overseas-born in Australia, disease rates mirror endemicity in home countries, with highs in 2001 among immigrants from Somalia ($592/10^5$) and Afghanistan ($159/10^5$). Bimodal cross-sectional rates in high-income countries (Fig. 14.12) are largely explained by cohorts of overseas-born young adults with active disease. In Denmark, unexpectedly, the disease rate among Somali immigrants did not decline rapidly after arrival, rather, it took 7 years to fall from 2,000 to $700/10^5$ per year.

- Asylum seekers (1925). In Hamburg, Germany, in 1997–2002, of 12,176 asylum seekers screened, 62% (7,549) were skin test positive, and 0.3% (31) had active tuberculosis. Only 29% (31/108) disease cases were detected on entry screen; while 71% (77) became manifest after a mean latency of 2½ years.

Fungi
The focus is on reactivated systemic fungi such as *Blastomyces*, *Coccidioides*, *Cryptococcus*, *Histoplasma*, and *Paracoccidioides*. As these are endemic in Latin America, Hispanic immigrants are at particular but nonexclusive risk (8073). In France in 1970–1994, *H. capsulatum duboisii* was isolated in 23 migrants from Africa, and *H. capsulatum capsulatum* was isolated in 94 other migrants, including in 54 (57%) from Latin America (7962).

FECES-FOOD CLUSTER
Overview (2019, 4516, 6857, 7945). By country of origin, 15–25% of immigrants may report abdominal pain, 10–25% are found to harbor enteric parasites, and 5–25% may have eosinophilia. About 30% can be coinfected, harboring more than one enteric parasite. Symptoms may not correlate with enteric parasite load.

Immigrants may also be at increased risk of enteric bacterial infections. Compared with the rest of the United States, influx counties within 100 km from the Mexican border have increased rates of typhoid fever (1.2-fold), shigellosis (1.2-2-fold), acute hepatitis A (1.5-4-fold), cholera (2.5-fold), and food-borne botulism (5-7-fold).

Viruses
Migrant and immigrant children seem at increased risk of HAV infection or acute hepatitis A (2019, 8073). Among immigrants from eastern Europe to Israel in 1990–1991, the prevalence of anti-HAV antibodies at 17–19 years of age was 37% (161).

In Spain, of asymptomatic immigrants mainly from sub-Saharan Africa, 6% (5/90) exhibited antibodies to HEV compared with 3% (25/863) of blood donors (7344).

Bacteria
Migrant and immigrant children seem at increased risk of typhoid fever, shigellosis, ETEC diarrhea, and cholera (2019, 8073). In immigrants, carriage of *S. enterica* serovar Typhi is probably increased. In New York City in 2000, an immigrant working at a restaurant in Queens was the likely source for an outbreak of typhoid fever with seven cases (8343).

Fungi
In Madrid, Spain, in 1989–1999, *Enterozytozoon bieneusi* was detected in 0.1% (1/671) of immigrants (4516).

Protozoa
Overview (1372, 1453, 3482, 4516). By age and country of origin, 10–15% of immigrants may shed enteric pathogenic or potentially pathogenic protozoa, including *B. hominis* (in 0.5–3%), *Cryptosporidium parvum* (in 0.1–2%), *E. histolytica/dispar* (in 0.8–7%), *G. lamblia* (in 1–10%), and *Isospora* (in 0–3%).

***E. histolytica* (2660, 4516, 4697, 5855, 8073, 8079).** Migrants and immigrants seem at increased risk of invasive amebiasis including ALA. In the United States, immigrants account for virtually all ALA cases. Migrants can also introduce virulent strains in nonendemic areas. In Italy in 1992, a housemaid from the Philippines was source for a family outbreak of six amebiasis cases. Near Cape Town, South Africa, introduction by migrants from an endemic area resulted in an outbreak on five farms, with nine hospitalized patients with invasive disease.

Helminths
Overview (517, 1372, 1453, 3482, 4516). By age and country of origin, 15–40% of untreated (im)migrants may harbor enteric helminths, including *Ascaris* (0–25%, often 5%), *Clonorchis-Opisthorchis* (0–5%), *Taenia* (0–0.4%), *Trichuris* (0–25%, often 15%), and *Trichostrongylus* (0–5.5%, often 1.5%).

***Clonorchis-Opisthorchis* (1372, 4389, 7122).** In Taiwan in 1992–1996, 5% (557/11,403) of migrant workers harbored *O. viverrini-C. sinensis*. In North America, these biliary trematodes have been isolated in immigrants from Southeast Asia, East Asia, or Russia, often years after arrival, and with eosinophilia as a pointer.

***Taenia* (4516).** In Spain, 0.3% (2/671) of immigrants harbored *T. saginata*, and 0.1% (1) harbored enteric *T. solium*.

Tissue *T. solium* infection (cysticercosis) (1857, 4516, 5619, 7046) has been diagnosed in immigrants in North America, Australia, and Europe. In the United States in 1996–1998, of 1,801 patients with 1,833 emergency visits for seizures and neuroimaging, 2% (38) were diagnosed with neurocysticercosis. Most (78%) patients were of Hispanic ethnicity, for a relative risk of 17 (95% CI 8–37).

Other helminths reported in (im)migrants include *A. cantonensis* (7580), *Dracunculus medinensis* (1085, 4440), *Fasciola* (5494), *Fasciolopsis* (1372), *Gnathostoma* (2707, 3781), *Paragonimus* (5544), and *Toxocara* (4516).

Introductions. Immigrant food workers carrying *T. solium* can shed cysticercosis in households (see section 11.1). For most other helminths, immigrants are unlikely sources. Prehistoric settlers migrating over the Bering land bridge, or post-Columbian European immigrants are believed to have introduced *Diphyllobothrium latum* into North America (1923). Refugees from Bihar or Assam in India are believed to have introduced *F. buski* into Bangladesh after World War II (2747).

ZOONOTIC CLUSTER
Immigrants are at increased risk of chronic or reactivated infections such as malaria, leishmaniasis, and Chagas disease (8073). Compared with the rest of the United States, migrant influx counties within 100 km from the Mexican border are also at increased risks of human rabies (4-fold), brucellosis (8-fold), and plague (~3-fold) (2019).

Viruses
After malaria, arboviruses are an acute cause of fever in immigrants, but considering incubation periods and lack of latency, imported arboviruses can be excluded in immigrants who become febrile >3 weeks after arrival in nonendemic host countries. In contrast, long incubation periods should be considered for rabies virus.

CHIKV (4194). Cases of CHIKV were unknown in Malaysia until 1998–1999, when migrant workers were suspected to have introduced an outbreak.

DENV (4516, 8073). Acute dengue has been reported in immigrants.

WNV. An outbreak of WNV was reported among migrants in Kisangani, Congo, in 1998 (5510).

Rabies virus (2019, 6985, 6989). Immigrants are at increased risk of rabies. Because of protracted incubation, (im)migrants may have been exposed in their home countries, months or even years before arrival. In three immigrants who died of rabies in the United States, epidemiological and molecular evidence suggested incubation periods of 11 months, 4 years, and 6 years, respectively. In the United Kingdom in 1946–2000, 20 cases were imported by people exposed in enzootic areas abroad. Alternative sources were imported, nonvaccinated puppies and other incubating animals (see chapter 1).

Bacteria
***Brucella* (1062, 2019, 8073, 8157).** Hispanic immigrants are at increased risk of brucellosis. Cases have been diagnosed in migrants from enzootic areas. Vehicles frequently implicated in migrants are raw milk and homemade dairy products.

***C. burnetii* (4125).** Nine Polish sheep shearers contracted Q fever while working in Spain.

Protozoa
***Leishmania* (2893).** Immigrants are at risk of CL and VL. Immigrants could also introduce new strains to receptive areas, an event that is difficult to detect in enzootic or endemic areas such as in the south of Italy. **CL (137, 5118, 6233, 7609).** In Bolivia, transmigrants from the Andean highlands to lowland Amazon where CL is enzootic were at increased risk of CL for several years. In Kabul, Afghanistan, an outbreak of anthroponotic CL was likely sustained by influx of susceptible migrants. In Saudi Arabia, *L. tropica* was isolated from a nasal nodule of an Egyptian laborer, underscoring the potential for migrants

to spread anthroponotic CL to nonendemic areas. In France in 1986–1987, 94% (60/64) of reported cases were imported, mainly from North Africa. **VL (3657, 7609).** VL is reported less frequently in (im)migrants. Of 95 VL cases recorded in France in 1986–1987, most were acquired locally, by residents or tourists, but 7% (7) were imported by immigrants from North Africa.

Plasmodium. Farm and forest projects attract transmigrants to potentially malarious areas. Transmigrants from nonmalarious to malarious areas within Africa, Latin America, and Asia are at high risk of infection and disease. Settlements and camps can be places where nonimmune and partially immune individuals meet. Gametocytemic, partially immune immigrants to nonmalarious areas are potential sources of introduced malaria and drug-resistant *P. falciparum*.

- Africa (4, 2973). In Ethiopia, transmigrants from the cold highlands to warm, moist, fertile, and hyperendemic lowlands are at risk of malaria. On the coast of Kenya, mathematical modeling suggested that <1% of infected immigrants would be enough to hinder malaria control by mosquito avoidance and case management.
- North America (4602, 5359, 5780, 8423). In North Carolina in 1992, of refugees arriving from Southeast Asia, 58% (187/322) were infected. All four species that infect humans were isolated. Most infections were inapparent, and many were mixed. Seasonal migrants and refugees have been sources of introduced falciparum or vivax malaria in Canada and the United States.
- South America (1542, 2046, 5870, 6092, 7787). In Brazil, clinical malaria frequently affects nonimmune transmigrants to the Amazon, including laborers, cattle hands, and miners, and outbreaks have occurred. In Leonislândia, Mato Grosso, where >60% of transmigrants originate from low-risk areas, parasitemia prevalence by season was 0.3–4%, and infection rates per 100 person-months were 3.9 for *P. vivax*, 1 for *P. falciparum*, and 4.5 overall. In Amapá, creation of a duty-free zone and population increase were paralleled by appearance of an unusual vector (*Anopheles marajoara*) and an increase of parasitemia prevalence from 4% to 15% in 9 years. Migrant miners are thought to have carried malaria to Yanomami American Indians on remote Brazil-Venezuela border, and chloroquine-resistant *P. falciparum* from south to north Guyana.
- Asia (389, 1744, 2547, 4111, 4287, 6084, 6779, 8291). Immigrants have been sources of introduced malaria in the United Arab Emirates and Central Asia. In the United Arab Emirates in 1988–1991, 5–10% of migrant workers had asexual parasitemia. On Rameswaram Island between Sri Lanka and Tamil Nadu, pilgrims from India and Nepal meet with local fishermen at seasonal camps along the coast that can become hot spots for resistant *P. falciparum* to spread to receptive people. In Indonesia, transmigrants from low-risk Java to malarious Kalimantan or Papua (formerly Irian Jaya) were at increased risk of malaria. Infections (45% *P. falciparum* and 55% *P. vivax*) in transmigrants occurred at rates per person-year of ~3 in the first two years after arrival, and of ~1 in the third year. In Yunnan, workers arriving from other provinces of People's Republic of China, Myanmar, Vietnam, and Laos are at high risk of clinical malaria; in 10 years, arrival screening reduced rates from 2 to 1/1,000, despite increased mobility and drug resistance.
- West Europe (671, 1118, 1668, 3482, 4516, 6664). Malaria is increasingly diagnosed in immigrants returning from visits to family and friends. Many are inadequately informed about prevention. Their itineraries may influence risks and parasite spectrum. For instance, Chinese immigrants passed through Africa for 3–9 months before presenting in Italy with falciparum malaria. Spain, because of proximity to Africa and the influx of parasitemic migrants, is vulnerable to local transmission. In Spain, >95% of immigrant malaria is in immigrants from Africa. In 1989–1999, 15% (149/988) of immigrants tested positive for *P. falciparum*, *P. vivax*, *P. ovale*, or *P. malariae*, ~90% of infections were manifest, more often in children than adults. Of 125 immigrant children from sub-Saharan Africa, 7 (6%) were parasitemic carriers, and 49 (39%) developed symptomatic malaria, mainly due to *P. falciparum*, after a mean period of 2 months.

Trypanosoma. ***T. brucei*** sl **(4516, 4863).** HAT is occasionally diagnosed in immigrants. Migrants may have initiated an outbreak of *T. brucei rhodesiense* in Uganda that in 1939–1945 claimed ~2,500 cases. **T. cruzi (1913, 3956, 4330, 4408, 4516).** *T. cruzi* infection prevalence in Hispanic migrants mirrors endemicity in their home countries. In the United States, by location, from 7 to 14% of blood donors report birth in or visits to enzootic areas, and 0.003–0.01% of blood donations are confirmed seroreactive. In Houston, Tex., 0.4% (9/2,107) of Hispanic pregnant women were seroreactive, compared with 0.1% (2/1,658) non-Hispanic pregnant women. In immigrants from Nicaragua and El Salvador living in Washington, D.C., the seroprevalence was 5% (10/205), and three of six reactive migrants tested positive in xenodiagnosis. The frequency of seroreactions contrasts with the paucity of Chagas disease reports in immigrants from Latin America, at least in Europe.

Helminths

Chronic tissue helminthiases in (im)migrants include cystic echinococcosis and filariasis.

Echinococcus granulosus. In California in 1981–1990, 25 (89%) of 28 cases reported were foreign born; of these, 19 (76%) had immigrated from Southwest Asia, 4 (16%) from southern Europe, and 1 each (8%) from Peru and People's Republic of China (1984).

Filariae. In Spain in 1989–1999, 25% (245/988) of immigrants were diagnosed with filariae, including ~18% with multiple species (4516). ***Loa*** **(1447, 3482, 4516).** Loasis can be diagnosed in immigrants from Africa. By geography and age, reported prevalence is 0–3%. ***Mansonella*** **(3482, 4084, 4516, 8329).** *M. ozzardi* circulates in Latin America. Reported prevalence in settlers and refugees is 1–3%. *M. perstans* circulates in Africa and Latin America. Reported prevalence in immigrants is 9–19%. *M. streptocerca* circulates in Africa. The reported prevalence in immigrants is 0.7%. ***Onchocerca*** **(780, 3482, 4516, 4662, 6247, 7782).** *O. volvulus* circulates in Africa, Latin America, and Yemen. *O. volvulus* is believed to have been introduced in America by slaves from Africa. Migrant workers from Guatemala are suspected to have established foci in Chiapas, Mexico, in the nineteenth century. In Brazil, migrant miners (garimpeiros) are thought to have brought the worm from the Amazon to Goiás and a gold mine near the Paraná River. By geography and age, prevalence in immigrants is up to 24%. ***Wuchereria*** **(4246, 4516, 5614, 7562, 8329).** *W. bancrofti* circulates in tropical Africa, America, and Asia. From forests in Southeast Asia, sea-faring people are believed to have carried the worm to islands in the Pacific and Indian oceans. Once adapted to *Culex*, spread into towns became possible. Microfilaremic migrants risk establishing new foci, including in urban, receptive Thailand. By geography, age, and test (night blood and diurnal antigenemia), reported microfilaremia prevalence in (im)migrants is 0.1–10%.

ENVIRONMENTAL CLUSTER
Bacteria
B. pseudomallei **(1731, 5752).** Melioidosis has been reported in immigrants.

C. tetani **(2019).** Nonvaccinated immigrants are at risk of tetanus. Compared with the rest of the United States, migrant influx counties within 100 km from the Mexican border had a 1.4–fold increased rate of tetanus.

Leptospira **(8073).** Leptospirosis is a differential diagnosis in immigrants.

Fungi
Deep-seated mycoses have been reported in immigrants, including mycetoma from *Actinomadura* (1802, 3200).

Helminths
Hookworm (*A. duodenale* and *N. americanus*) (1372, 1453, 3482, 4516, 6348). By age, country of origin, and deworming history, the infection prevalence reported in (im)migrants is 0.6–58% (often 15%). At a university hospital in Spain in 1984–1999, 285 infections were diagnosed among African immigrants, 52% of infected individuals had peripheral eosinophilia, and 28% had iron deficiency indicative of hookworm disease.

Schistosoma **(1312, 1657, 2272, 2948, 5893, 6347, 6422, 6552, 8232).** *Schistosoma* is well documented in (im)migrants. In Spain, overall prevalence in immigrants from Africa is 15% (200/1,321). Species mix varies with country of origin: *S. haematobium* is mainly and *S. intercalatum* is exclusively imported from Africa, *S. mansoni* is mainly from Africa and South America, *S. mekongi* is from Laos, and *S. japonicum* is from the Philippines and People's Republic of China.

In Europe, immigrants account for up to 95% of imported schistosomiasis. *S. haematobium* alone accounts for ~70–90% of infections, *S. mansoni* alone for ~10%, and both together for ~5–10%. *S. intercalatum*, *S. japonicum*, and *S. mekongi* are rarely diagnosed in immigrants in Europe.

By the presence of suitable snail hosts, countries may or may not be receptive. In Malaysia, introduction has not occurred, although schistosomiasis was imported from the Philippines, People's Republic of China, and Egypt. On the contrary in Jordan that receives thousands of infected migrants from Egypt, local *S. haematobium* transmission was confirmed at an irrigation pool inhabited by *Bulinus truncatus* snails.

S. stercoralis **(1372, 1453, 3769, 4516, 7231).** By country of origin, test, and deworming history, infection prevalence reported in (im)migrants is 0–6% (often 2%). Prevalence can be higher (17–29%), if multiple specimens are submitted from clinically suspected immigrants.

Ectoparasites
Tunga penetrans has been reported in immigrants (4796). Past corridors of spread are being debated; a scenario is from Latin America to West Africa.

SKIN-BLOOD CLUSTER
Overview (4516). In Spain in 1989–1999, STIs were diagnosed in 7% (74/988) of immigrants, superficial mycosis in 4% (39), and ectoparasites in 2% (21).

Viruses
HBV (161, 2019, 4516, 5114, 5753). By age and country of origin, reported prevalence in immigrants is 3–14% for

hepatitis B surface antigen (HBsAg) and 10–55% for anti-HBc and anti-HBs. Antenatal screening should identify HBsAg-positive pregnant women and children at risk, but programs may fail to reach immigrant mothers. Furthermore, children from HBsAg-negative immigrant mothers are still at increased risk of HBV infection from carriers in the family or neighborhood. Compared with the rest of the United States, migrant influx counties within 100 km from the Mexican border had a 1.4-fold increased rate of acute hepatitis B. In the United Kingdom, 10–20% of HBV infections appear to be acquired abroad, including by immigrants.

HCV (161, 4516). By age and country of origin, reported anti-HCV prevalence in immigrants is 1–9%.

HIV (1517, 4516, 6588, 6736, 6972). By risk group and country of origin, ~0.5–15% of (im)migrants can test positive for HIV. Expected infection prevalence in Mexican migrants to the United States is 0.03–0.3% for low-risk groups (pregnant women, farm workers, and blood donors), 0.1–0.5% for female sex workers, 6–12% for IDU, and ~15% for homosexual men. By country of origin and risk behavior, frequent coinfections in HIV-infected immigrants include HBV, HCV, *M. tuberculosis* (latent or active), *M. avium*, *Pneumocystis*, *T. gondii*, and STI. HIV-infected immigrants are victims and sources of HIV. In the United Kingdom, 46% (944/2,046) of individuals notified to have acquired HIV domestically were thought to have a source that originated from outside Europe. HIV2 was likely introduced in Portugal and France from the heartlands in sub-Saharan Africa, via corridors established during the colonial era.

Human T-lymphotropic virus (3355, 7596). Higher seroprevalence in immigrant than in host populations was reported for immigrants from Japan to Hawaii and for immigrants from Latin America.

Bacteria
Skin. *M. leprae* (1577, 2019, 4815, 5617, 5624, 7379, 7706, 8073, 8378). Immigrants are at increased risk of leprosy. Compared with the rest of the United States, migrant influx counties within 100 km from the Mexican border had a 5-fold increased rate of leprosy. In high-income countries, close to 100% of cases (in "registers") have been imported by (im)migrants and asylum seekers. Because of the long incubation period, signs on arrival may be missing. Screening was not found useful in a model that incorporated migrants from high ($\geq 10/10^5$), intermediate ($5–9/10^5$), or low ($1–4/10^5$) prevalence countries. The risk of secondary spread to the local population is considered minimal.

STI. *C. trachomatis* (4516, 6588, 6736). By country of origin, sex, and test, the reported prevalence of genital *C. trachomatis* infection in immigrants is ~2–10%. Lymphgranuloma venereum has occasionally been diagnosed in migrants. *H. ducreyi* (683). In California in 1981–1983, a chancroid outbreak mainly affected Hispanic laborers; 69% (98/142) of culture-confirmed patients reported sex with prostitutes who solicited house-to-house. *K. granulomatis* (499). Occasional donovanosis cases have been reported in immigrants. *N. gonorrhoeae* (4516, 6588). Reported prevalence of gonococcal urethritis in immigrants is 0.3–1%. *T. pallidum* (4516, 6588). Reported prevalence of latent syphilis in immigrants is 0.3–3%.

Fungi
Dermatophytes (1671, 2170, 2496). In the past 50 years, *Trichophyton tonsurans* has replaced *Microsporum audouinii* as the predominant cause of tinea capitis in North America and West Europe. A proposed mechanism for this shift is introduction by immigrants from areas where *T. tonsurans* is endemic. Tinea capitis and *T. tonsurans* are prevalent in immigrants, in particular, in children. Immigrants may account for >50% of reported domestic cases.

Protozoa
In Spain, *T. vaginalis* was detected in 5 (0.5%) of 988 immigrants (4516).

Helminths
Reported prevalence in (im)migrants (from stool analysis) is 0.4% for *E. vermicularis* and 0–8% (typically 1%) for *H. nana* (1453, 4516). Because stool is a suboptimal material, the prevalence of *E. vermicularis* is likely underestimated.

Arthropods
In Spain, 2% (21/988) immigrants were diagnosed with ectoparasites (4516). In immigrant children from sub-Saharan Africa to Spain ($n = 125$), pediculosis was diagnosed in 0.8% and scabies in 6% (3482).

16

16.1 Migrating and transported vertebrates

16.2 Transported invertebrates

16.3 Transported goods

Transported Animals and Goods

16.1 MIGRATING AND TRANSPORTED VERTEBRATES

Bioinvasion (882) is the establishment of displaced organisms in an ecosystem. Industries (e.g., food and logging), trade (e.g., pets and plants), transport, and travel contribute to bioinvasion. By displacing autochthonous organisms, introduced organisms contribute to loss of species (global estimated loss, 11 per day).

Biocontrol (4988, 5092) makes use of viruses, larvicidal *Bacillus* spp., larvivorous fish, and sterile males. Australia attempted to biocontrol rabbits (*Oryctolagus cuniculus*): by myxomavirus in the 1950s, by a rabbit flea (*Spilopsyllus cuniculi*) that spred myxovirus in the 1960s, and by another flea (*Xenopsylla cunicularis*) as vector of rabbit calicivirus in the 1990s. Although wild rabbit populations have been reduced, they remain a pest in parts of Australia.

Displaced infections (Box 16.1). Anthroponotic agents are dispersed by traveling humans (see sections 15.4–15.6), and zoonotic agents are dispersed by moving or transported vertebrates or invertebrates (see section 16.2). Although fish, birds, small mammals, research primates, and livestock have contributed to dispersing agents infective to humans, information is fragmentary.

Fish. Except anadromous fish such as salmon, information about the impact of fish migration on the dispersal of agents infective to humans is limited. Fish are traded internationally for food and aquarium pets.

Birds (4692, 4977, 6123) (http://www.npwrc.usgs.gov/resource/othrdata/migratio/routes.htm.). Infected and parasitized birds can carry agents and ectoparasites locally and long-distance. There is a poorly characterized risk for attached, infected ticks or viremic birds to introduce agents, e.g., West Nile virus (WNV) in North America or avian influenza virus in Europe. Arguments in favor of the spread of agents by birds include foci along known migration corridors, seasonal introductions over long distances, and latent infection (prolonged viremia) in migratory rather than sedentary birds.

In general, birds migrate in north–south corridors, between breeding and wintering sites. The scarlet tanager (*Piranga olivacea*) migrates from eastern Canada and the United States over Central America to forests in Colombia, Ecuador, and Peru. The stork (*Ciconia ciconia*) migrates from Europe over

> **Box 16.1** Agents displaced by vertebrates, by cluster
>
> The suspected carrier is listed in parentheses.
>
> Droplet-air   *Influenzavirus* (birds)
> Feces-food   *Salmonella* (birds and fish); *A. cantonensis* (rats and snails), *Capillaria* (fish and birds), *Gnathostoma* (fish)
>   *T. solium* (pigs and humans)
> Zoonotic   CCHFV (livestock), FMDV (livestock), *Lyssavirus* (bats, skunks, and foxes), MPXV (rodents), OHFV (rodents),
>   RVFV (livestock); *Anaplasma* (livestock), *B. anthracis* (livestock), *Brucella* (livestock), *Chlamydophila psittaci*
>   (birds); *Francisella* (rodents), *M. bovis* (livestock and wildlife), *Rickettsia* (livestock), *Y. pestis* (rodents);
>   *T. brucei rhodesiense* (cattle), *T. evansi* (bats); *E. granulosus* (birds), *E. alveolaris* (rodents, foxes)
> Environmental *B. pseudomallei* (livestock)

Southwest Asia to Africa. Fewer birds migrate between Eurasia and North America, e.g., the Eurasian wigeon (*Anas penelope*). Displaced by storms, birds from West Africa occasionally reach North America,

There is international trade in poultry and in caged pet birds, mainly of psittacines (parrots, cockatoos, and budgerigars) that probably exceeds 1 million per year.

Small terrestrial mammals (7032). Migrating lemmings apart, small terrestrial mammals are mostly displaced inadvertently. At Shanwei Seaport in People's Republic of China in 1990–1998, import and export inspection detected rodents aboard 270 (25%) of 1,093 arriving ships, as well as on trains and aircraft. Rodents arriving in People's Republic of China by aircraft included *Rattus flavipectus* (one from Japan in 1984), *Rattus norvegicus* (one from Russia in 1990 and one from Hong Kong in 1995), and *Rattus* (one from Saudi Arabia in 1990). Rodents arriving in People's Republic of China by train included *R. norvegicus* (three from Mongolia in 1989), and *Mus musculus* (ten from Russia in 1994).

There is a significant international trade in pet reptiles, including tortoises, turtles, lizards, and snakes.

Bats. Migration of bats is less well studied than migration of birds. Bats also migrate from summer roosts to hibernation sites, mainly from dusk to midnight and close to the tree canopy. Examples are long-nose bats (*Leptonycteris curasoae* and *L. nivalis*) that migrate from the United States to Mexico, the noctule bat (*Nyctalus noctula*) that migrates up to 2,000 km from northeastern to southwestern Europe, and the grey-headed flying fox (*Pteropus poliocephalus*) that migrates on the east coast of Australia.

Large terrestrial mammals (1662, 3738). Gone are the days when large herds of bison roamed the North American prairie. Migrating herds are limited to parts of Africa and Asia. Dwindling numbers of nomads still drive herds to pastures and water holes, and in the Alps, livestock is moved from lowlands to alpine summer pastures.

In contrast, livestock is increasingly trucked across borders, horses are brought to races, and wildlife is transported to zoos. New Zealand, which lacks native terrestrial mammals, is an example of bioinvasion: sheep, other exotic fauna, and manure-introduced zoonotic agents, including *Bacillus anthracis*, *Brucella*, *Leptospira*, and *Echinococcus*.

Research primates have been sources of Ebolavirus in North America.

DROPLET-AIR CLUSTER
Influenzavirus **(4977, 5482, 6869).** Migratory, aquatic birds are suspected to have introduced influenza A virus A/H5N1 in poultry farms in Hong Kong and to have triggered the 1997 epizootic. On the contrary, the A/H5N1 epizootic that began in 2003–2004 was likely initiated by living chickens transported over 1,500 km, from Gansu Province, People's Republic of China, to Lhasa, Tibet. In response to the epizootic that spilled into Southeast Asia, poultry herds were culled, and Europe banned the import of live pet birds, poultry meat, eggs, and unprocessed feathers from infected countries. Nonetheless, A/H5N1 arrived in Romania in fall of 2005, perhaps carried by migrating birds, and killed 1,800 turkeys.

FECES-FOOD CLUSTER
Salmonella **(2670, 5592).** On South Georgia in the Antarctic in 1995–1996, 1 of 30 penguins (*Pygoscelis papua*) grew *S. enterica* serovar Enteritidis. Migratory birds, human carriers, or sewage from ships are suspected to have introduced the agent in this remote habitat.

Tropical aquarium fish are transported from wholesalers to pet shops and customers in plastic bags and water from the original tanks. Water in bags and aquaria and transported fish are suitable reservoirs for *Salmonella* and hazardous for dealers and customers. Of seven humans infected with *S. enterica* serovar Paratyphi B, all reported exposure to aquarium water, aquarium fish, or fish food; serovar Paratyphi B was isolated from home aquarium water and one fish food sample (likely contaminated by an ill individual).

Angiostrongylus (3934, 3993, 6017, 6020, 6070). Likely infected rats or possibly giant African land snails (*Achatina fulica*) carried the nematode *A. cantonensis* from East Asia to Southeast Asia, Australia, and the Pacific in the 1940s–1950s, to North (Egypt), West (Cote d'Ivoire), and East Africa (Madagascar and Reunion) in the 1960s–1970s, and to Central America (Cuba and Puerto Rico) in the 1970s–1980s. By 1990, *A. cantonensis* had reached the Bahamas and New Orleans, by 1992 the Dominican Republic, and by 2002 Jamaica and Haiti. Spread by rats could explain the nematode's appearance in the port city of New Orleans and its expansion into Louisiana wildlife.

Capillaria (1648, 3809). Increasing pisciculture and new foci of human intestinal capillariasis suggest the possibility of importation of *C. philippensis* through captive fish or fish-eating migratory birds.

Gnathostoma (5352, 5353). Fish (loach, *Misgurnus anguillicaudatus*) imported live from People's Republic of China, Korea, or Taiwan into Japan was the suspected source for >50 *G. hispidum* infections in humans.

Taenia (2574, 7938). In the 1970s, transmigrants from Bali and their pigs introduced *T. solium* and cysticercosis in Papua (formerly Irian Jaya), Indonesia. Initial foci expanded, and there is a risk that the cestode could spread into Papua New Guinea.

ZOONOTIC CLUSTER
Zoonotic agents recovered out of season from unexpected hosts, or from unusual habitats, should alert for weaponized agents.

Viruses
Crimean-Congo hemorrhagic fever virus (CCHFV) (2159). Viremic sheep and their ticks arriving at Jeddah Seaport in the late 1980s were suspected to have carried CCHFV to Saudi Arabia. Subsequently, CCHFV became enzootic in West Province.

Foot-and-mouth disease virus (FMDV) (486, 2587, 2722, 6764). FMDV can spread with migrating herds, transported animal products, and fomites, including shoes from infected premises, but most likely with illegally imported, viremic livestock. The United Kingdom 2001 epizootic was enhanced by bringing infected sheep to market. Quarantine of farms reduced the spread by animals and detered people from visiting affected farms.

Inkoo virus (7932). Inkoo virus circulates in Eurasia in reindeer (*Rangifer tarandus sibiricus*) and *Aedes* mosquitoes. Viremic reindeer imported from Siberia are suspected to have introduced the virus in Alaska in the 1890s.

Lyssavirus (1548, 4103, 8134). Migrating mammals such as skunks and foxes can advance enzootic rabies "fronts" in North America and Europe. Nonvaccinated pet puppies or kittens from enzootic countries can be sources of rabies in humans in rabies-free areas. Pet dogs and cats should not be brought unrestricted into countries free of terrestrial rabies. By country, restrictions may include identification, documentation of vaccination, seroscreening, and quarantine.

By geography, bats are vectors of rabies virus, Australian bat *Lyssavirus*, and European bat *Lyssavirus*, among bats, to livestock, and humans. Natural, accidental, and intentional translocations of bats within and between continents have been recorded. Bats migrate, land or roost on ships, enter aircrafts, are transported to zoos, or are released. There is a threat for bats to expand European bat *Lyssavirus* in western Europe.

Monkeypox virus (MPXV) (1209, 1221). In the United States in 2003, Gambian giant rats (*Cricetomys*) imported from Ghana, West Africa, along with squirrels (*Funisciurus* and *Heliosciurus*), mice (*Graphiurus* and *Hybomys*), and porcupines (*Atherurus*) were implicated sources of an infection chain that began with pet vendors and distributors, included pet prairie dogs (*Cynomys*), and ultimately caused ≥87 cases in humans.

Omsk hemorrhagic fever virus (OHFV) (4586). OHFV appeared in Siberia, after muskrats (*Ondatra zibethica*) had been introduced from Canada for hunting purposes.

Rift Valley fever virus (RVFV) (298, 2566, 3754). Sheep moved from enzootic holding areas in Sudan to live markets in Egypt are believed to have introduced RVFV in Egypt in 1976, causing an epizootic in 1977–1978. Travel time was <5 days, fitting with the incubation period of RVFV in sheep. In 1993, cases in animals along the Nile again suggested introduction from the Sudan to Egypt, resulting in an epizootic in 1993. New roads seem to facilitate spread along trade routes. In contrast, traditional nomads have tended to leave areas where mosquitoes are abundant or losses among livestock are high.

Tick-borne encephalitis virus (TBEV) (1435, 3403). While rodents are rather sedentary, larger mammals and birds can carry ticks over distances. For the establishment of new TBEV foci, however, this mechanism is considered insignificant.

Bacteria
***Anaplasma* (2794).** Cattle and their ticks likely brought *A. bovis* to Nantucket Island, Mass., in the 1800s, and sports clubs introduced cottontail rabbits (*Sylvilagus*

floridanus) in the 1920s–1930s. *A. bovis* is now ezootic on the island, circulating in cottontails and *Haemaphysalis leporispalustris* ticks.

***B. anthracis* (1662, 4143).** Livestock transported and sold across borders can escape meat inspection and become a source of anthrax in humans. An example is the Myanmar-Thailand border. Livestock can also introduce *B. anthrax* in virgin territory. An example is New Zealand.

***Brucella* (1662, 3247).** Ill cattle shipped from Queensland, Australia, to the Solomon Islands were suspected the source of brucellosis in Melanesian cattle workers. *Brucella* was brought with livestock to New Zealand.

***Chlamydophila psittaci* (6296, 7162, 8271).** In 1929–1930, exotic birds shipped from Argentina carried virulent strains to North America and western Europe, causing outbreaks with ~800 cases in humans. In the United Kingdom in 1982–1986, cases in humans paralleled importation of psittacine birds that counted 10,000–40,000 per year. In Germany in 1998, traded ducklings caused eight or more disseminated cases in humans.

***Francisella tularensis* (5849).** In 2002, prairie dogs (*Cynomys ludovicianus*) cross-infected with *F. tularensis* at a pet trade shop in Texas, were shipped from the United States to Czechia, where 1 of 100 animals grew the same, holoarctic (B) strain as animals from Texas.

***Mycobacterium bovis* (1590, 1812).** Cattle imported in the colonial era likely introduced tuberculosis in Africa where it has become enzootic in wildlife. Roaming infective wildlife is a source of *M. bovis* in domestic animals, e.g., deer in the United States, and deer, boar, and badger in Europe.

***Rickettsia africae* (5738).** Cattle transported from Africa to the Caribbean in the eighteenth and nineteenth centuries, are suspected to have brought *Amblyomma variegatum* ticks and *R. africae* to Guadeloupe.

***Yersinia pestis* (4530, 4930).** In the 1890s, *Y. pestis* emerged at seaports worldwide, probably carried by ship rats and their fleas. An epidemic in San Francisco in 1899–1900 was likely portal of entry for *Y. pestis* in North America; disseminated by ground squirrels, the agent became enzootic in the western United States.

Protozoa
***Trypanosoma. T. brucei rhodesiense* (2373, 3517).** Cattle can carry *T. brucei rhodesiense* and establish new foci. In the outbreak in Soroti district, Uganda, in 1998, >50% of cattle traded at a main market originated from areas in which trypanosomiasis is enzootic. ***T. evansi* (1548).** Bats are a vector of *T. evansi* to horses and cattle; migrating bats could expand the enzootic areas. ***T. vivax* (3742).** Probably in the nineteenth century *T. vivax* was brought to Latin America by unregulated cattle transports from Africa. Meanwhile, the protozon has become enzootic in Latin America. This example is of interest, as tsetse flies are absent from America and replaced by acyclic, hematophagous tabanids (stable flies).

Helminths
***Echinococcus. E. granulosus* (198, 1662).** The cestode came to New Zealand with introduced sheep. Birds were suspected to have brought *E. granulosus* eggs to St. Kilda, an uninhabited archipelago in northern Scotland, ~60 km away from the nearest dog. On St. Kilda, sheep were estimated to ingest *E. granulosus* eggs at a rate of 2–3 eggs per sheep per year. ***E. multilocularis* (3265).** The appearance of *E. multilocularis* on Svalbard (Spitzbergen) in the Norwegian Arctic was explained by the arrival of intermediate host voles (*Microtus rossiaemeridionalis*) inadvertently imported with animal feed for Russian mining operations and by natural migration of the Arctic fox (*Alopex lagopus*, final host) from Siberia.

ENVIRONMENTAL CLUSTER
Soil on hooves and in fur is a putative mode of dispersal of environmental agents by vertebrates.

***Burkholderia pseudomallei* (1683, 5842).** Transportation of latently infected or sick animals can carry *B. pseudomallei* to melioidosis-free areas. An epizootic at Jardin des Plantes in Paris in 1975 was attributed to the arrival of sick Prejwalski horses from Iran or of an infected panda from People's Republic of China.

16.2 TRANSPORTED INVERTEBRATES

San Francisco Bay is ecological chaos.

C. Bright (882)

Microorganisms, arthropods, and other invertebrates can be dispersed passively (Box 16.2), by storm, truck, train, ship (bilge water, containers, and tires), and aircraft (cabin and cargo). For windblown mosquitoes, see section 5.5.

MICROORGANISMS FROM SHIPS
Ships (882, 1082, 6466, 7032) have carried prokaryotes and invertebrates around the world. The United States is estimated to receive nearly 80 million tons of ballast water from overseas annually. In Oregon, ballast water released by Japanese ships contained 367 plankton taxa. Marine life in San Francisco Bay has become "international," with

> **Box 16.2** Microbes and vectors internationally disseminated via aircraft, ship, or other vehicle
>
> Vehicles are listed in parentheses.
>
> **Microbes:** *Norovirus* (ship), *V. choleae* (ship), *V. parahaemolyticus* (ship)
>
> **Vectors**
> - *Aedes* (ship and aircraft): DENV, YFV; *Anopheles* (aircraft, ship, and bags): *Plasmodium*; *Culex* (aircraft): WNV
> - *Glossina* (car and boat): *Trypanosoma*; *Simulium* (wind): *Onchocerca*
> - Bedbugs (bags)
> - Fleas (ship, train, on rats): *Y. pestis*
> - Ticks (vertebrates)

taxa from around the world imported by container ships. The proportion of ships that discharges bildge water, ballast water, or even raw sewage into the sea is not known.

Viruses

Norovirus (4031, 6903). After an oyster-borne *Norovirus* outbreak in Louisiana, crew from 22 of 26 boats harvesting oysters in the Gulf admitted to disposing sewage overboard. In New Zealand, sewage effluent from recreational boats was the most likely source for the pollution of farmed oysters that were the vehicle for an outbreak with 86 cases.

Bacteria

***Clostridium botulinum* (3364).** In Australia, 1 of 281 ballast samples from a ship docked in Queensland yielded botulinum toxin type C, demonstrating the potential for ships to introduce the agent into port waters.

***Vibrio. V. cholerae* (2220, 4874, 4875, 6466, 7236).** Toxigenic *V. cholerae* O1 was recovered from nonpotable (ballast, bilge, and sewage) water of ships docked at Caribbean and United States Gulf ports, and from ships arriving in the Chesapeake Bay. Departure ports included cholera-endemic as well as noninfected countries. In Mobile Bay, Ala., in 1991, routine sampling identified toxigenic *V. cholerae* O1 distinct from the local strain, in seafood from closed oyster beds; 3 of 14 cargo ships docking at Gulf ports grew the same strain from samples of ballast water, bilge water, marine sanitation devices, and sewage-holding tanks. Effluents from ships were the suspected source of *V. cholerae* O1 that hit the Nicobar Islands in 2002. ***V. parahaemolyticus* (4216, 4678, 4829, 8142).** A "sessile" stage of the agent can attach to the bottom of boats. Boats are suspected to have contributed to the intercontinental spread of serovar O3:K6 observed since 1995.

ARTHROPODS FROM SHIPS AND AIRCRAFT

Modes of dispersal include wind (see section 5.5), local traffic (see section 15.1), baggage, ships, and aircraft.

Ships (4147, 4530, 4998, 5233, 5816, 7032). Living mosquitoes, flies, fleas (*Ctenocephalides felis*), and cockroaches have been recovered from aboard ships. Adult mosquito can be transported in cargo or containers, larvae can be transported in water collections, while eggs resist desiccation on goods such as plants and in freight. Adult mosquitoes could even reproduce aboard ships.

Aircraft (2811, 2997, 3857, 5233, 6476, 7032). Mosquitoes (*Aedes*, *Anopheles*, and *Culex*), flies (midges, *Simulium*, and others), and cockroaches (*Blatella germanica*) have been identified in aircrafts. At Dalian Airport, Liaoning province, northeastern People's Republic of China, in 1993, 20% (96/487) of arriving aircraft were infested with mosquitoes and/or flies. At Changi Airport, Singapore, in 1983–1984, 12% (39/330) of aircraft were found to harbor mosquitoes and other insects; of 100 mosquitoes caught, 62 were from the first class cabin, and 30 were from economy class.

Mosquitoes

Under favorable weather conditions, dispersed infective vector mosquitoes can infect people residing at destination seaports, airports, or train stations. Dispersed mosquitoes could also replace indigenous fauna. On Hawaii, all five species of biting mosquitoes, including *Aedes aegypti*, *A. albopictus*, and *Culex quinquefasciatus*, are nonindigenous, having been introduced from East Africa, the Caribbean, or the Pacific, mainly with bromeliads (4530).

Aedes* (2977).** Airports are potential portals of entry for Dengue virus (DENV) and yellow fever virus (YFV). ***A. aegypti* (4147, 4530, 5233).** *A. aegypti* is vector of YFV and DENV. In the fifteenth to seventeenth centuries, ships are believed to have carried *A. aegypti* from West Africa to the New World. Nearly eliminated in the Americas in the 1950s–1960s, populations recovered and have become widespread again. *A. aegypti* was identified in aircraft arriving in DENV-free French Polynesia. ***A. albopictus

(2453, 2998, 3857, 4530, 5163, 5233, 6397). *A. albopictus* is a "polyvalent" vector. Around 1985, larvae were shipped from Asia to the United States with water that remained in used tires. Quite efficiently, *A. albopictus* invaded 15 states. Then, *A. albopictus* was shipped from the United States to Europe, again with old tires. In parallel, *A. albopictus* was brought to islands in the Indian Ocean (Madagascar, Mauritius, and Seychelles) and the Pacific (Bonin, Hawaii, Mariana, and Solomon). In Africa, *A. albopictus* is expanding its range from South Africa to Central and West Africa. **Other species (4530).** Other species that have been transported by tires include *Aedes bahamensis* and *A. japonicus*.

Anopheles. For seaport malaria, see section 15.2; for airport malaria, see section 15.3; for baggage malaria, see section 16.3. *A. gambiae* **(4375, 4530, 5233).** In 1930, shipment of *A. gambiae* sensu lato (sl) was recorded from Dakar, West Africa, to Natal, northeastern Brazil. In 1930–1941, the vector covered territory by "habitat-hopping" and "hitch-hiking" on cars and trains. The result was a devastating malaria epidemic, with tens of thousands of deaths. An eradication campaign was launched that included poisoning of larval habitats with Paris green. The campaign ended the epidemic and eliminated *A. gambiae* from Brazil in 1941. Similarly, steamboats carried *A. gambiae* from Madagascar to Mauritius and Reunion, resulting in malaria outbreaks.

***Culex* (1201, 7032).** At Shanghai Seaport in 1996, live *Culex pipiens quinquefasciatus* was recovered from aboard container ships. Transportation of *Culex* by aircraft is a possible mode of introduction of WNV into New York City in 1999. In Los Angeles County in 2002, an isolated case of WN fever in humans in the absence of bird cases corroborated the hypothesis of long-distance transportation by aircraft.

Flies
***Cochliomyia* (6777).** Screwworm can be dispersed by infested livestock, adult flies perhaps also by winds. In 1988, *C. hominivorax* appeared in Tripoli, Libya. From Tripoli, it invaded a perimeter of 200 km. Invasion was controlled by a large-scale campaign.

***Glossina* (4530, 8090).** *Glossina* can be dispersed by motor vehicles and drifting vegetation. The West African island of Principe was freed of *Glossina* for 40 years, until *Glossina* was reintroduced by boat or plane from the island of Fernando Póo situated 200 km to the north.

***Simulium* (4530, 5233).** *Simulium* can travel 150–200 km without human assistance. On Galapagos Islands, construction of an airport was followed by introduction of *S. bipunctatum* from the mainland.

Fleas
***Y. pestis* (4530).** Outbreaks of plague in port cities have been related to rats and their fleas disembarking from sailing ships or freight vessels.

Tunga. *T. penetrans* is believed to have been shipped in sandbags or with slaves from Africa to Latin America.

Bedbugs
***Cimex* (4898, 5769).** *C. lectularius* can be transported in luggage and (second hand) furniture; four such instances were reported in the United Kingdom in 1999. Starved, inactive (daytime) bedbugs resemble lentils and are easily overlooked in baggage. Bedbugs have been reported to be imported from Italy to the United Kingdom hidden in the seams of a backpack.

Ticks
Dogs, cats, livestock, migratory birds, or traded reptiles can disperse ticks over short or long range.

Ticks on birds (675). Every spring about 100 million birds migrate through Sweden. From an *Ixodes ricinus* prevalence of ~2% among migrating birds and an *Anaplasma phagocytophilum* prevalence of ~5.5% in ticks, it was estimated that migrating birds would import into Sweden >0.5 million *Ehrlichia*-infected ticks each spring and export >0.1 million infected ticks each fall.

Ticks on reptiles (996). *Amblyomma sparsum* (a putative vector of *Cowdria ruminantium* = *Ehrlichia chaffeensis* in cattle) was introduced in Florida from imported reptiles.

Ticks on livestock (454, 5739, 5808). In the eighteenth to nineteenth centuries, cattle from West Africa likely brought *Amblyomma variegatum* to the Caribbean. In the 1960s–1980s, this tick invaded several Caribbean islands, likely carried by arriving migratory egrets (*Bubulcus ibis*). Although the tick was eradicated on some islands, new cattle were suspected to have brought *Rickettsia africae* to the Caribbean.

16.3 TRANSPORTED GOODS
Transported goods include foods, baggage, mail, and laboratory specimens. Outbreaks demonstrate hazards from regionally, nationally, and internationally transported foods and from privately carried food gifts and souvenirs. Transported agents and transport media are remarkably diverse (Box 16.3).

> **Box 16.3** Agents internationally disseminated via goods, by cluster
>
> Vehicles are listed in parentheses.
>
> | | |
> |---|---|
> | Droplet-air | *Cryptococcus* (seeds, wood) |
> | Feces-food | HAV (seafood), *Norovirus* (seafood); *Clostridium botulinum* (vacuum-packed and home-canned foods), *Escherichia coli* (beef), *Salmonella* (foods), *Shigella* (foods), *Vibrio cholerae* (seafood), *V. parahaemolyticus* (seafood); *Cyclospora cayetanensis* (berries); *Diphyllobothrium* (fish), *F. hepatica* (salad), *Trichinella* (pork) |
> | Zoonotic | BSE (fodder); *B. anthracis* (fertilizer, wool, textiles, leather, souvenirs, and mail); *Anopheles-Plasmodium* (baggage) |
> | Environmental | *B. pseudomallei* (manure) |
> | Skin-blood | HIV (blood products) |

DROPLET-AIR CLUSTER

***Cryptococcus neoformans* (2183, 7282).** Seeds of river red gum (*Eucalyptus camaldulensis*) are suspected to have exported *C. neoformans* var. *gattii* from Australia. In Kinshasa, Congo (formerly Zaire), *C. neoformans* var. *neoformans* was recovered from wood in a carpenter shop and a log in a living room, suggesting that exported tropical woods could disseminate the agent.

FECES-FOOD CLUSTER

In many high-income countries, imported foods are sampled for inspection and testing for food-borne pathogens (972, 8397). However, nonsampled foods remain vehicles of food-borne infections and outbreaks. Examples of imported foods that failed to pass tests in Australia in 1995–1999 (failure rate) included smoked fish (8.6%, $n = 388$) or soft cheese (1.1%, $n = 1,440$) by growth of *Listeria monocytogenes*, paprika (4.5%, $n = 369$), pepper (1.6%, $n = 1,440$), or coconut (0.8%, $n = 524$) by growth of *Salmonella*, and molluscs (2.5%, $n = 2,440$) by toxins or growth of *Escherichia coli* ($>2.5/g$) or *V. cholerae*.

Viruses

Hepatitis A virus (HAV) (6387). In Valencia, Spain, in 1999, wedge clams (*Donax*) imported from Peru caused 188 acute hepatitis A cases. Subsequently, 4 (24%) of 17 wedge clam and other imported mollusc samples amplified HAV/RNA.

***Norovirus* (628, 2961).** *Norovirus* was demonstrated in mineral water imported into Switzerland. In Australia in 2002, oyster meat imported from Japan was the implicated vehicle in a *Norovirus* outbreak at a conference; for an attack rate of 23% among >1,000 attendees. At the same time, oyster meat imported from Korea caused three *Norovirus* outbreaks in New Zealand.

Bacteria

***C. botulinum* (5877, 6292).** In Germany in 1997, a couple fell ill with botulism, after having consumed vacuum-packed smoked fish bought in Germany; the fish was caught in Canada, and smoked and packed in Finland. Home-bottled mushrooms from Italy, given to visiting family members, caused two cases (one fatal and one survived) of type B botulism in the United Kingdom.

***E. coli* (1241).** In 2004, ground beef produced in the United States, exported to Okinawa, Japan, and sold by a military commissary on the island as frozen beef patties caused three *E. coli* O157:H7 infections in a Japanese family.

***Salmonella* (8397).** Transport has been implicated in national and international outbreaks. Identification of vehicles and sources often requires international cooperation and molecular epidemiology. Of concern is dispersal of antimicrobial resistance. In the United States in 2000, Federal Drug Administration field laboratories isolated 187 *Salmonella* strains from 4,072 imported foods, including 15 (8%) that were resistant to one or more of 17 test antimicrobials, and 5 (3%) that were resistant to three or more antimicrobials.

- Sprouts and legumes (2961, 4657, 7704). *S. enterica* serovars Newport or Stanley in seed lots of alfalfa sprouts distributed from The Netherlands to growers in Europe and North America were implicated in infections in sprout consumers. In Australia in 2002, serovar Montevideo in chick peas (tahini) and sesame seeds (hommus) from Egypt caused an outbreak with 47 cases that prompted recall from consumers and trade and an international alert.
- Fruits (3846). In 1998–1999, frozen mamey (*Manilkara zapota*) fruits from Guatemala and Honduras were implicated in 16 cases of typhoid fever (3846).
- Almonds and peanuts (308, 1304). In Canada, a multiprovincial outbreak of serovar Enteritidis was traced to raw almonds imported from the United States. In Australia in 2000, serovar Stanley in dried peanuts from People's Republic of China caused a nationwide outbreak with 27 cases.

- Animal-derived foods (918, 7745) (5695). In The Netherlands in 1995–2002, serovar Java was increasingly detected in poultry but not in humans. However, in Scotland, serovar Java isolates from humans increased from 0.9% (14/1,571) in 2001 to 1.2% (14/1,127) in 2002; by pulsed-field gel electrophoresis, 10 of 28 poultry isolates, all from The Netherlands, and 10 of 29 isolates from humans fell into one cluster, strongly implying Dutch poultry as the source. Serovar Agona with fishmeal from Peru was introduced into the United Kingdom in 1970. Soon thereafter, infections were detected in pigs, chicken, and humans, and by 1971, chicken products had established an animal food cycle independent from importation.
- Ready-to-eat foods (308, 3931). In 1994–1995, serovar Agona in a kosher savory snack from Israel caused an outbreak with cases in Canada, Israel, the United Kingdom, and the United States. In 2000, serovar Typhimurium DT104 in sweets ("helva", with pine nuts, semolina, and sugar as ingredients) from Turkey caused an outbreak with 23 cases in Australia (20 in Victoria) and further cases in Norway and Sweden.

Shigella. Mainly handled and transported foods are potential vehicles of *Shigella*.
- Salads (3818). In 1994, iceberg lettuce from Spain was implicated in *S. sonnei* infections in Sweden and the United Kingdom, and in an outbreak in Norway with 110 cases linked to a salad bar.
- Fruits (2512). A Swedish woman living in Morocco took her two children and a watermelon on a home visit; she served the melon to 15 guests 3 days later, and within 24 h, 14 guests fell ill, while she and her two children stayed well. *S. sonnei* was isolated from 14 ill and 1 asymptomatic guest but not on repeat testing from any of the three host family members. Subsequently, one infected guest gave birth to a healthy baby who also grew *S. sonnei*. Although no longer available for culture, the watermelon was the implicated vehicle.

Staphylococcus aureus (4376). In 1989, canned mushrooms from People's Republic of China (Anhui, Fujian, and Sichuan provinces) were implicated in outbreaks of staphylococcal food poisoning in the United States.

Vibrio. *V. cholerae* (1133, 2387, 7368). In New Jersey in 1991, eight residents developed severe diarrhea due to *V. cholerae* O1 El Tor, after eating crabmeat brought by a traveler from Ecuador. In Maryland in 1991, frozen coconut milk from Thailand caused an outbreak among attendees of a picnic: in four of six who consumed coconut milk, and in one of six product bags, toxigenic *V. cholerae* O1 El Tor was isolated. In Italy in 1998, cholera was diagnosed in a resident who had never traveled to cholera-endemic areas; the seafood salad implicated was made from ready-to-eat shrimps, scallops, mussels, hen clams, cuttlefish, and squid, cooked and frozen in various countries of origin that were difficult to track but included cholera-endemic countries in East Asia. *V. parahaemolyticus* (2808, 5038). Clams from France were implicated in a case of *V. parahaemolyticus* diarrhea in a consumer in Germany. In Singapore in 1975–1980, 78% (158/202) of imported seafood grew *V. parahaemolyticus*, including bivalves (oysters), cephalopods (squids), and crustaceans (crabs, prawns, and crayfish).

Protozoa
***Cyclospora cayetanensis* (3285, 3287).** Raspberries and blackberries from Latin America have repeatedly been implicated in outbreaks in Canada and the United States. The 1996 outbreak was remarkable for its size (1,465 cases) and because raspberries from the implicated source country (Guatemala) accounted for only 4–20% of fresh raspberries shipped to the United States during the outbreak months.

Helminths
***Diphyllobothrium* (1394).** In the United States in 1980, sockeye salmon from Alaska caused a multistate outbreak with >30 people with infections.

***Fasciola hepatica* (1964).** In the United Kingdom, khat (*Catha edulis*, *Celastraceae*) leaves from the horn of Africa were implicated in an infection of a Yemeni woman; khat leaves are wrapped into banana leaves to keep them damp during transportation, and are chewed fresh, as a stimulant.

***Opisthorchis felineus* (8347).** In Israel, a family of four and a friend contracted the trematode from eating raw, smoked carp brought from Siberia.

***Trichinella* (195, 5996).** In France in 1993, horse meat from Canada that authorities had certified free of *Trichinella*, caused an outbreak with 538 cases in the Paris area. Workers from eastern Europe increased demand for pork in western Europe; outbreaks from uninspected pork brought as a souvenir or sent as a gift were reported in Germany (smoked boar meat from Romania), Italy (smoked pork sausages from Romania and Croatia), and the United Kingdom (pork salami from Serbia). Feeding infective food scraps to pigs risks opening new domestic cycles in countries that have achieved control of porcine trichinellosis.

ZOONOTIC CLUSTER
Prions
Bovine spongiform encephalopathy (BSE) (6995). In the wake of the 1986–2000 BSE epizootic in the United Kingdom, outbreaks in cattle in other European countries were likely seeded by exports of contaminated "meat-and-bone meal" fodder, which continued despite ban, or by illegally exported incubating cattle from the United Kingdom.

Bacteria
***B. anthracis* (1136, 1662, 5864).** Anthrax was introduced in New Zealand in the mid-1890s, with unsterilized bone dust fertilizer from India; the last local case was reported in 1954. In 1974, a Florida resident acquired anthrax from a contaminated goatskin drumhead imported from Haiti. Subsequently, in 1974–1981, 12% (26/218) of goatskins and 78% (59/76) of rugs imported from Haiti grew *B. anthracis*. Goat hair from Pakistan caused an anthrax outbreak at a textile plant in Switzerland, with 25 cases among workers. In the United States, spores were sent by mail for attempted bioterrorism (see section 6.2).

Protozoa
***Plasmodium* (1117, 3574, 4722, 4789, 6001, 6290).** Carried by baggage, bags, and suitcases, infective *Anopheles* females can cause introduced malaria (baggage malaria) in nonmalarious areas. At locations ≥30 km away from international airports or refugee camps, when weather is calm and cold, and in households with returned travelers, *Anopheles* from baggage is the most likely source of "cryptic" malaria in individuals with a blank history of recent travel, transfusion, or injection.

ENVIRONMENTAL CLUSTER
***B. pseudomallei* (2586, 5842).** In France, horse manure and compost are believed to have disseminated *B. pseudomallei* to horse clubs and French mushroom (champinion) factories.

SKIN-BLOOD CLUSTER

Complete evidence of risk does not have to exist before measures are taken to protect against the risk.
K. Wilson and M. N. Ricketts,
on the precautionary principle (8204)

Variant Creutzfeldt-Jakob disease (CJD). As a precautionary measure, some countries (such as the United States) deferred blood donors who had stayed for >3–6 months in countries reporting cases of BSE or variant CJD. Years later evidence accumulated that indeed variant CJD was transfusion transmissible (see section 18.4).

Human immunodeficiency virus (5489). In Doha, Qatar, in the 1980s, blood from commercial suppliers in Florida was the implicated source for HIV infections in children with thalassemia at 3–13 years of age who had received on average 64 blood transfusions.

SECTION VI
Nosocomial Infections

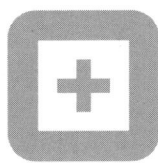

17 Noninvasive Procedures

18 Invasive Procedures

Procedures are health-related interventions. Noninvasive procedures leave natural barriers intact. Examples are medications, tape electrodes, speculum examination, and endoscopy without biopsy. Agents are spread via contact or ingestion. Invasive procedures break through skin or mucosal surfaces. Examples are injections, dental or cervical scrapings, biopsy, and surgery. Agent spread is mainly via inoculation. Devices are objects for preventive, diagnostic, or therapeutic use, be it temporary (removable) or permanent (nonremovable: implants).

Nosocomial here means procedure related. This definition includes ritual, cosmetic, and alternative procedures. Nosocomial infections can result from endogenous (activated) flora or from acquired (introduced) agents. In outpatients, sources of nosocomial infections include injection materials (e.g., in injection drug users [IDU]) and instruments (e.g., for tattooing). In hospitals, sources include hands, machinery, surfaces, and solutions.

Arguments for nosocomial acquisition include history of a procedure (Box VI.1), carriage of a device, site-typical manifestation, a compatible incubation period, recovery of an indicator agent (Box VI.2), and identical strains from patient and suspected source. For transmission within hospitals, a requirement is manifestation >48 h after admission. Acute care is defined by hospital stays for 1–59 days. For long-term care, see section 11.6. Iatrogenic infections are associated with procedures prescribed or performed by physicians. For infections in workers, see section 12.6.

Infections in inpatients (988, 6521, 8050). In the United States each year, ~35 million patients are admitted to ~7,000 hospitals, for an average stay of ~5 days. Colonization can be a precursor of infection. Of *Candida* colonizations, up to 38% go on to become infections. Characteristics of nosocomial infections include site, acquisition, agent spectrum, and impact.

Sites (988, 1230, 6637, 8019). About 80% of nosocomial infections are either urinary tract (related to bladder catheters), bloodstream (BSI, related to vascular access), or surgical-site infections, or pneumonias (ventilator associated).

Modes of acquisition (2757, 4652, 6521, 6913, 7000).
Factors that "reactivate" endogenous flora or transmit exogenous agents include recent antimicrobial therapy, recent hospitalization, facility transfer, large-volume aspiration, intubation, assisted ventilation, vascular access, bladder catheter, and need for stay in intensive care unit (ICU). These modes can be addressed in the exposure history (Box VI.1).

Rates of acquisition (988, 1230, 8019). By hospital size, unit, and inpatient days, nosocomial infection rates in high-income countries are overall 1–10/100 admissions or 1/100 patient-days. In ICU, nosocomial infection rates per 100 intervention days are 0.3–0.7 for urinary catheters, 0.3–0.7 for central lines, and 0.3–1.5 for ventilators. About 5–10% of hospitalized patients acquire one or more infections; in ICU one fourth patients acquire one or more infections.

Agents (1230, 1770, 5485, 5934, 6309) (Box VI.2). The single most important nosocomial agent is *Staphylococcus aureus*. In U.S. acute-care hospitals *S. aureus* is reported in 0.8% of discharge diagnoses. At a tertiary-care military hospital in San Antonio, Tex., the nares of 21% (95% confidence interval [95% CI] 18–24%) of 667 patients grew methicillin-sensitive *S. aureus* (MSSA) on admission, and 3% (2-5%) grew methicillin-resistant (MRSA) strains. After 1–96 (median 3) days of follow-up, 2% of initially noncolonized patients, 1.5% of initially MSSA-colonized patients, and 19% (5/26) of initially MRSA-colonized patients had infections by MRSA. Hand hygiene at Geneva hospitals reduced new MRSA infections per 100 admissions from 0.5–0.6 in 1993–1994 to 0.2–0.3 in 1997–1998. MRSA has now escaped into communities and is no longer indicative of hospital transmission. Other agents frequently acquired in ICU, burn, and other hospital units include *Acinetobacter baumanni*, *Burkholderia cepacia*, *Citrobacter*, *Enterobacter*, *Stenotrophomonas maltophilia*, *Klebsiella*, *Pseudomonas*, *Serratia*, and vancomycin-resistant *Enterococcus* (VRE).

Impact (1230, 2657, 5485, 5934, 6637, 7837, 8019). On any given day, 3–30% (often 10%) of hospitalized patients have one or more nosocomial infections. In Swiss acute-care hospitals in 2003, the point prevalence was 8% (657/8,429): 5% in small (<200 beds) hospitals, 7% in

---

Box VI.1 Suggested nosocomial exposure history

Right now:
- If an outpatient: are you wearing any device (e.g., for dialysis) or implant (e.g., of hip)? Have you received any injection (e.g., ritual or shared)?
- If hospitalized: in which hospital and unit are you in? Since when? Have you been transferred from another unit? Why? While in the hospital, was there any endoscopy, bladder catheter, infusion from a venous line, intubation for assisted ventilation, or other intervention? Name all persons who have visited you in the hospital.

In the past 4 weeks:
- Have you taken any self-administered or prescribed antimicrobial, e.g., for sore throat, fever, diarrhea, human immunodeficiency virus, or vaginitis?
- Have you had any wound from injury, tattooing, or injection (e.g., acupuncture and drug), endoscopy, or other (invasive) procedure?
- Have you had any inhalation therapy or any contact with patients or health workers, e.g., for wound dressing or physiotherapy?
- Have you been in a hospital or been readmitted for a relapse? Were you on assisted ventilation? Have you had any surgery or catheterization?

In the past 12 months:
- Have you made any visit to an herbalist, dentist, ophthalmologist, gynecologist, physician, or other health or cosmetic facility?
- Have you had any stay in an emergency room, acute-care hospital, long-term care, or other facility? For how many days?

In your lifetime:
- Do you have any piercing or tattooing? Have you ever been incarcerated? Ever used injection drugs? Any pedicure or leg shaving? Circumcision?
- Have you ever had a transfusion, transplantation, device, or implant? Have you had any intubation, general anesthesia, stay in the ICU?
- What was your last injection or venipuncture? What were the dates of your last visits to an acupuncturist, dentist, gynecologist, family doctor and/or other physician?

> **Box VI.2** Agents or infections indicative of nosocomial acquisition or spread
>
> Units or sites are listed in parentheses.
>
> **Each clinical case**
> - Epidemic conjunctivitis, severe acute respiratory syndrome
> - *Enterobacter* (burn, neonatal ICU), *Enterococcus* (burn, surgery, ICU), *Klebsiella* (ICU), *Legionella, Pseudomonas aeruginosa* (burn, ICU), *S. aureus* (burn, ICU, obstetrics), *Staphylococcus epidermidis* (ICU), *Streptococcus pyogenes, Streptococcus agalactiae* (neonatal ICU)
> - *Aspergillus* (invasive) *Candida* (ICU, invasive)
> - Scabies
>
> **Cluster of two or more cases**
> - Unexpected, unusual, or surveillance-targeted cases or agents
> - Acute hepatitis B, herpes simplex virus (pediatrics)
> - *Clostridium difficile*-associated diarrhea, MRSA, *Streptococcus pneumoniae*, VRE
> - *Candida* (BSI)
>
> **Each clinical isolate**
> - *Acinetobacter baumanni* (usually sterile, respiratory tract infection, burn, adult ICU), *Burkholderia cepacia, Citrobacter* (BSI), *Enterobacter* (BSI), *Enterococcus* (BSI), *Klebsiella* (BSI), *Serratia* (BSI), *Stenotrophomonas maltophilia*, VRE

middle-sized (200–500 beds), and 10% (340/3,289) in large (>500 beds) hospitals. Prevalence was highest (~25%) in ICU, intermediate (~8%) in medical and surgical units, and lowest (2%) in obstetrics. Nosocomial infections are often severe, prolonging stays by 1–10 days. Reported lethality is 10–35%. Numerous nosocomial outbreaks have been reported. In 63% of 1,022 hospital outbreaks analyzed, a source was identified, mainly patients in 26%, equipment or devices in 12%, the environment in 12%, and staff in 11%. The main outbreak syndromes were BSI in 37%, gastrointestinal in 29%, and pneumonia in 23%. Much clinical and microbiological research is devoted to hospital infectiology in high-income countries, although greater numbers of patients with infectious disease are treated in resource-limited hospitals of low-income countries.

Infections in outpatients (1955, 2850, 3296, 4699). Forced by economy and supported by new technologies, much of past inpatient care has now moved to outpatient and home care, broadening the scope of nosocomial infections. In the United States in 1996, ~8 million people received home medical care. Of patients in home care, ~10% carried one or more devices. Sources of nosocomial infections in outpatients include incubating patients in crowded waiting rooms, unsafe injections, improper care of exit sites, and the handling of cappings and connecting tubes. Unfortunately, nosocomial infections in outpatients are not usually monitored. In 1961–1990, of 53 transmission events in oupatient habitats, 55% (29) resulted from common sources (mainly syringes), 26% (14) from person-to-person spread, and 19% (10) from spread by droplets.

Prevention (3296, 5101, 5115). Preventive measures include education of workers *and* patients and visitors, standard precautions that apply to hospitals and outpatient habitats and include hand hygiene, gloves for venipuncture and the breaking of ampouls (see sections 14.1 and 12.6 and Table 14.1), and infection-control programs that cover disinfection, waste management, and surveillance.

17 Noninvasive Procedures

17.1 Hands
17.2 Materials and machines
17.3 Endoscopy
17.4 Bladder catheters and UTI
17.5 Intubation and nosocomial pneumonia
17.6 Drugs, bioproducts, and nosocomial diarrhea
17.7 Hospital air, water, and surfaces
17.8 Viral hemorrhagic fevers in hospitals

In 1895, W. K. Röntgen (1845–1923) discovered X rays, and W. E. Einthoven (1860–1927) developed electrocardiography. Today, an array of diagnostic, monitoring, therapeutic, and preventive technologies are available, including assisted spontaneous breathing, computer tomography, extracorporeal shock-wave lithotripsy, magnetic resonance imaging, and positron emission tomography.

17.1 HANDS

Agents on hands (817). Agents can permanently (resident flora) or temporarily (transient flora) colonize the hands of health care workers (see section 12.6) and patients; little is known about visitors who likely mirror community carriage (see section 14.1). Sources of agents on hands include own skin, nails, hairs, nose, pharynx, vagina, and anus, hands of other people, respiratory droplets, blood, wound secretions, excretions, soiled linen, objects (e.g., stethoscopes), surfaces, and solutions (e.g., liquid soap). Unwashed hands are significant mechanical vectors of nosocomial agents and infections (Box 17.1).

Prevention (550, 817, 5934). Nosocomial infections can be prevented by hand hygiene. At general hospitals in Vienna in 1844–1847, I. Semmelweis (1818–1865) investigated transmissibility of puerperal fever by the hands of staff, from boils and corpses to women in labor. He discovered that lethality could be significantly reduced (from 15–30% to ~1%) by disinfecting hands in a bowl of "chlorina liquida" before examining pregnant women. Today, disinfectants are available that are effective against enveloped viruses (e.g., hepatitis B virus [HBV], human immunodeficiency virus [HIV], herpes simplex virus [HSV], *Influenzavirus*, and respiratory syncytial virus [RSV]), nonenveloped viruses (e.g., adenovirus [AdV], *Enterovirus*, hepatitis A virus [HAV], *Rhinovirus*, and *Rotavirus*), and bacterial and fungal vegetative cells and spores.

DROPLET-AIR CLUSTER
Viruses (101, 817, 3694)
Viruses transmissible by hands include AdV, HSV1, *Enterovirus*, *Influenzavirus*, *Rhinovirus*, RSV, severe acute respiratory syndrome coronavirus [SARS-CoV], and varicella-zoster virus [VZV]. Labial herpes and herpetic lesions of the

> **Box 17.1** Hand-transmissible agents, by agent cluster
>
> *Residual flora.
>
> | | |
> |---|---|
> | Droplet-air | AdV, HSV1, *Enterovirus, Influenzavirus, Rhinovirus*, RSV, SARS-CoV, VZV; diphtheroids (e.g., *C. jeikeium*),* *Klebsiella* |
> | Feces-food | HAV, HEV, *Norovirus, Rotavirus*; *C. difficile, Enterobacter, Enterococcus* (including VRE), *E. coli, Proteus mirabilis, S. enterica* serovar Typhi, *Shigella, V. cholerae, Y. enterocolitica* |
> | Environmental | *Acinetobacter,** *Fusobacterium*, "wet bacteria" such as *B. cepacia, Pseudomonas, Serratia, Stenotrophomonas*; fungi such as *Paecilomyces* and *Rhizopus* |
> | Skin-blood | HBV, HCV (dialysis units), CMV; *Peptostreptococcus,** *S. epidermidis* (CoNS),* *S. aureus** (MRSA), *S. pyogenes* (GAS); *Candida*, dermatophytes; *Sarcoptes* |

hands are sources of HSV1. In respiratory secretions RSV can survive on unwashed hands for at least 20 min. In eye care units, AdV was spread via instruments or hands, worker-to-patient or patient-to-worker, causing outbreaks of epidemic conjunctivitis.

Bacteria (817, 6053, 7398)

Bacteria transmissible by hands include *Chlamydophila pneumoniae*, diphtheroids (e.g., *Corynebacterium jeikeium*), *Klebsiella*, and *Mycobacterium tuberculosis*. Diphtheroids are part of the skin flora. *C. jeikeium* survives in hospital air, on surfaces, and on hands of workers, and nosocomial outbreaks have been reported. *Klebsiella* frequently colonizes hands of workers transiently. Hand hygiene reduces the nosocomial spread.

Fungi

Fungal spores transmissible by hands include *Aspergillus, Cryptococcus neoformans*, and *Histoplasma capsulatum*. Transmissibility of *Pneumocystis jirovecii* by hands is uncertain.

FECES-FOOD CLUSTER
Viruses (817, 6346, 6412)

Viruses transmissible by hands include HAV, hepatitis E virus [HEV], *Norovirus*, and *Rotavirus*. Incubating or incontinent patients can spread HAV patient-to-patient, or patient-to-worker, in particular, in neonatal units. HEV appears able to spread through contact. In South Africa, 6 weeks after exposure to blood, cerberospinal fluid (CSF), and stool from a patient with acute hepatitis E, one physician and two nurses contracted acute hepatitis E. Outbreaks in care facilities have demonstrated person-to-person spread of *Norovirus*.

Bacteria

Bacteria transmissible by hands include *Clostridium difficile, Enterobacter, Enterococcus, Escherichia coli, Proteus, Providencia, Salmonella enterica* serovar Typhi, *Shigella, Vibrio cholerae*, and *Yersinia enterocolitica*.

C. difficile **(435, 462, 2703, 3722, 4897, 7440).** About 5% of patients are colonized on entry into hospital, and 5–30% acquire *C. difficile* in the hospital. Although patients are the major reservoir, *C. difficile* can be recovered from hands of workers. In Seattle, of workers caring for infected patients, 59% grew *C. difficile* from their hands. The hands of patients or workers can transfer *C. difficile*, although workers rarely contract intestinal infection from patients. Several classes of antimicrobials can promote overgrowth of *C. difficile*, but notably clindamycin. In a hospital in Perth, Australia, *C. difficile*-associated diarrhea (CDAD) decreased from 2–3 to 1/1,000 per discharges in parallel with decreased use of third generation cephalosporins.

Large hospital outbreaks have been reported (1103, 3722, 8170). During outbreaks in U.S. hospitals, rates of CDAD reached 16–20/1,000 discharges or admissions.

Enterococcus **(631, 817, 1275, 2604, 5247).** *Enterococcus* is readily transmissible by hands and skin contacts, including vancomycin-resistant strains (vancomycin-resistant *Enterococcus* [VRE]). Hands of workers can yield VRE from contact with patients *and* surfaces near infected patients. By its ease of spread and environmental hardiness, *Enterococcus* is a problem in hospitals. Hand hygiene can significantly reduce the nosocomial spread of VRE.

V. cholerae **(5025, 7276).** Cholera outbreaks have been documented in low-income hospitals. Spread can be person-to-person or by foods. A liquid tube-fed diet was a vehicle implicated in an outbreak. Cohorting and barrier nursing are advised.

Y. enterocolitica **(1056, 3964, 6134, 6974).** Nosocomial *Y. enterocolitica* infections and outbreaks have been reported. At Cincinnati University Hospital in 1987–1990, 5 (28%) of 18 infections were considered nosocomial. Suspected modes included patient-to-patient and worker-to-patient spread.

ENVIRONMENTAL CLUSTER

Agents (1821, 3569, 3985, 6618). Spores and vegetative cells of environmental agents that can contaminate hands of workers include *Acinetobacter*, *Fusobacterium*, "wet bacteria" such as *Burkholderia cepacia*, environmental mycobacteria, *Pseudomonas*, *Serratia*, and *Stenotrophomonas maltophila*, and fungi such as *Paecilomyces* and *Rhizopus*.

Sources (3985, 6618). Sources for hand contamination include sinks, other wet surfaces, solutions, and poorly serviced dispensers. After washing hands with *Serratia marcescens*-contaminated liquid soap from dispensers, hands of workers were >50 times more likely to be colonized than after washing hands with agent-free soap.

SKIN-BLOOD CLUSTER

Sources for hand contamination include endogenous flora, blood-tainted surfaces, and patients.

Viruses (143, 1874)

Viruses transmissible by hands include HBV, hepatitis C virus (HCV) (in dialysis units), and cytomegalovirus (CMV). CMV has been isolated from hands of patients and workers, and patient-to-patient and patient-to-worker spread has been documented.

Bacteria

Bacteria transmissible by hands include *Staphylococcus aureus* (methicillin-sensitive *S. aureus* [MSSA] and methicillin-resistant *S. aureus* [MRSA]), *Staphylococcus epidermidis* (coagulase-negative *Streptococcus* [CoNS]), (6815), and *Streptococcus pyogenes* (group A *Streptococcus* [GAS]).

S. aureus (631, 817, 1498, 5934, 7021). Colonized patients and workers, and infected wounds are major sources of *S. aureus* in hospitals. Modes of spread include unwashed hands and transfers of infected patients. Spread is by worker-to-patient and patient-to-patient contact while breathing and talking are insignificant. Hand hygiene reduces spread of MRSA, and combined with other measures it can achieve elimination of MRSA. A hand hygiene program at hospitals in Geneva, Switzerland, reduced MRSA transmission rates per 1,000 patient-days from 0.2 in 1994 to 0.1 in 1998.

Fungi

Fungi transmissible by hands include *Candida* and dermatophytes.

Candida albicans (2311). Nosocomial and person-to-person spread of *C. albicans* has been demonstrated by genotyping strains from throat, urine, and stools of 69 elderly patients who were monitored for 2 months.

Dermatophytes. Outbreaks of dermatophytes have demonstrated nosocomial spread (289, 4395, 7003). At a nursery in the United States, six neonates contracted *Microsporum canis* and tinea capitis from an infected nurse. At a rehabilitation facility, four workers contracted *Trichophyton tonsurans* and tinea corporis from a patient, for attack rates of 30% for intense exposure, 17% for moderate exposure, and nil for minor exposure. On a pediatric ward, 10 workers contracted *T. tonsurans* and tinea corporis from a corticosteroid-treated patient who was undiagnosed for 5 weeks, for an attack rate of 30%.

Ectoparasites

Scabies (4226, 5545, 6344, 7754). Scabies is a significant nosocomial hazard. In 1976–1996, 44 nosocomial scabies outbreaks were reported. In the United States, a patient with unrecognized scabies admitted to the AIDS unit of an acute-care hospital exposed 773 workers and 204 patients. At a hospital in Spain, a 90-year-old patient from a nursing home infected 14 workers and 13 patients. At another hospital in Spain, an outbreak affected 4% (6/140) of bedridden patients, 8% (1/11) of physicians, 21% (6/29) of nurses, 17% (3/18) of stretcher bearers, 1 ambulance driver, and 1 wife of a worker.

17.2 MATERIALS AND MACHINES

Disposable material (e.g., tongue blades), instruments (e.g., thermometers), devices (e.g., tubes), and machines (e.g., nebulizers) have been sources or vehicles of nosocomial infections, in particular, in immune-impaired patients (Box 17.2).

DISPOSABLE MATERIALS

Millions of noninvasive procedures are being performed in hospitals and outpatient settings without harm. The colonizations or infections that result from materials that are summarized here underscore diversity rather than magnitude of exposure. Risks of cross-infection (material-to-patient spread) likely originate from reusing, handling, or storing materials rather than from producing or transporting bulk material.

In pedicure salons, *Trichophyton* was recovered from mats, floors, instruments, and waste (7813). Tinea capitis of two healthy elderly women who both had visited the same hairdresser grew *M. canis* (7310).

Acinetobacter baumannii was grown from patient charts (583). Contaminated adhesive band was the vehicle for *Rhizopus* wound infections (1135, 4937). In a burn unit in Belgium in 2004, a new brand of nonsterile elastoplast bandages was the vehicle for *Absidia corymbifera* skin colonization in two patients and infections in five (confirmed by biopsy), for an attack rate of 26% (1427). In Spain, wooden tongue blades contaminated with

> **Box 17.2** Nosoinfections from materials, instruments, and machines, by cluster
>
> Sources are listed in parentheses.
>
> Droplet-air AdV (pneumotonometer), *Klebsiella* (instruments, milk pumps, respiratory machines, and dialyzer), and *Legionella* (tubes, probes, nebulizers, incubators, respirators, tap water)
>
> Feces-food *C. difficile* (thermometers), *Enterobacter* (thermometers, blood gas analyzer, and dialyzer), *Enterococcus* (thermometers and dialyzer), *Entamoeba* (colonic tubes), and *Salmonella* (thermometers)
>
> Environmental Wet bacteria, e.g., *Acinetobacter* (mattresses, respiratory machines, and dialyzer), *B. cereus* (tubes), *B. cepacia* (probes, respiratory machines, dialyzer, and blood gas analyzers), environmental mycobacteria (instruments, electrodes, and tap water), *Pseudomonas* (tubes, clamps, urine collectors, milk bottles, respiratory machines, dialyzer, and blood gas analyzers), *Serratia* (linen, probes, urine collectors, milk pumps and bottles, respiratory machines, and infusion equipment), *Stenotrophomonas* (dialyzer), and *Rhizopus* (adhesive band and tongue blades)
>
> Skin-blood Prions (instruments from CJD patients), HBV (liquid nitrogen freezer), HSV (electrodes), skin abscess (electrodes), *S. aureus* (electrodes and dialyzer), and CoNS (electrodes and dialyzer)

Rhizopus microsporus were used to prepare oral medications that caused gastric infections in five adults in the intensive care unit (ICU); patients and used and unused blades yielded identical strains while other batches from the same supplier and samples from another supplier tested negative (4728). Wooden tongue blades used to splint intravascular access sites in preterm infants caused nosocomial *Rhizopus* infections (5087). Wooden blades should not be used in ICU or immune-compromised patients. On rubber gloves, RSV can survive for at least 90 min (3088). In Turkey, contaminated theater linen was the vehicle implicated in an outbreak of *S. marcescens* (2233). In a burn unit, wet mattresses served as a reservoir for *Acinetobacter calcoaceticus* (6846).

Suctioning and tubing. Quivers on which suction tubes (3763) had been stored after use on ventilated patients in ICU were implicated in an outbreak of *Pseudomonas aeruginosa* infections; disinfection and daily changes of quivers halted the outbreak. Ventilator reusable tubes (2913) and mechanical bags (7723) are reported sources of *Bacillus cereus* colonizations, infections, and invasive disease in neonates. Nebulizer mouthpieces (1486) caused *P. aeruginosa* pulmonary infections in 21 patients with chronic obstructive airway disease; the outbreak ceased when nebulizer mouthpieces were changed every 24 h and sterilized between uses in patients. Nasogastric tubes (NGTs) are reported vehicles of *C. difficile* (435), *Helicobacter pylori* (from former gastric intubation for study of hypochlorhydria) (7360), *Legionella pneumophila* (perhaps from microaspiration) (7185), *P. aeruginosa* (in tube-fed elderly) (4327), and *S. marcescens* (in tube-fed neonates) (608). Colonic tubes were reported vehicles of *Entamoeba histolytica* (3592). In Colorado in 1978–1980, a chiropractor transmitted *E. histolytica* to ≥36 patients by colonic irrigation; six died of invasive disease.

Nursery equipment (1985, 2427, 2901, 2905, 3727). Equipment such as breastmilk pumps, tubings, and milk bottles have been reported as a source of wet agents such as *Klebsiella pneumoniae*, *P. aeruginosa*, and *S. marcescens*. Contaminated milk and milk bottles were vehicles for the colonization of babies in neonatal ICU with *S. marcescens*. A milk bank pasteurizer and bottle warmer was implicated in an outbreak of *P. aeruginosa* in an ICU which caused 31 infections, including four deaths. Reused umbilical clamps are a reported source of *Pseudomonas* infection in neonates (6810).

Electrodes. Electrocardiography leads are a reported source of VRE (2294). Transducers of internal tocographs are a reported source of *S. marcescens* in neonates and delivering mothers (608). Fetal scalp electrodes are reported sources of HSV (3860) and of polymicrobial scalp abscesses (5573) in neonates. **Probes.** Transesophageal echocardiography probes were implicated in three cases of *Legionella* pneumonia; strains from patients and water from rinsing probes were indistinguishable by pulsed-field gel electrophoresis (4382). Electronic temperature probes used with servo-controlled humidifiers were implicated in sputum findings of *B. cepacia* in 117 patients (7997). **Calibrators.** Calibrating equipment for intravascular line pressure monitoring is a reported source of *Serratia liquefaciens* in ICUs (3149).

Urine bags (4758, 5146, 6848, 7226). In high-income countries that use sterile equipment, aseptic catheterization, and closed drainage, agents of nosocomial urinary tract infections (UTI) are typically endogenous. However, most sites such as urine bags and bottles, urinals, and urometers are reported sources of outbreaks of nosocomial UTI, including by *P. aeruginosa* and *S. marcescens*. For bladder catheters and nosocomial UTIs, see section 17.4.

INSTRUMENTS
There is a risk of cross-infection (instrument-to-patient spread) from serially reused instruments that are not regularly disinfected, e.g., sphygmomanometers or stethoscopes. For endoscopes, see section 17.3.

Stethoscopes (1508, 2656, 3736, 4739, 5506). Diaphragms of stethoscopes yield *S. epidermidis* (in 70–100%), *S. aureus* (in 5–45%), MRSA (in 0–7%), *Streptococcus viridans* (in ~3%), but also *Acinetobacter*, *Bacillus*, *Corynebacterium*, *K. pneumoniae*, and *Enterobacter*. In respiratory secretions, RSV can survive on stethoscopes for up to 6 h. Diaphragms can be cleaned with alcoholic solutions. Cleaning diaphragms before auscultation appears important in patients with burns or surgical wounds.

Sphygmomanometers (5293). Blood pressure cuffs have yielded *A. baumannii*. In a special care nursery, a blood pressure cuff was associated with an increased infection rate in neonates.

Thermometers. Thermometers are reported vehicles of *C. difficile*, *Enterobacter cloacae*, *Enterococcus faecium* (VRE), *K. pneumoniae* (including extended-spectrum β-lactamase [ESβL] producing), and *Salmonella*. *C. difficile* (905, 2703, 3695). Spores can persist in the environment for months. Thermometers were suspected to contribute to nosocomial spread. In a New York hospital, 21% of electronic rectal thermometer handles yielded *C. difficile*. Replacement by disposable thermometers decreased the rate of CDAD from 2.7 to 1.8/1,000 patient-days. A randomized crossover study confirmed significantly lower CDAD rates per 1,000 patient-days with disposable thermometers (0.2) than with electronic thermometer use (0.4). *E. cloacae* (7711, 7724). In The Netherlands, rectal thermometers were implicated in outbreaks among neonates in ICU. In one outbreak, 15 (37%) of 41 exposed patients were colonized; the outbreak slowly subsided when disposable thermometer covers were introduced.

Dental instruments. Dentists and orthodontists in high-income countries typically steam autoclave or dry-heat sterilize reusable instruments, and dental laboratories disinfect materials such as dental impressions and dentures. The situation may be different in low-income countries frequented by high-income country patients for low cost.

Otorhinolaryngological instruments (1508, 3727, 4538). Otoscope handles from clinic pediatricians yielded *S. aureus* (in 38%) including MRSA in 10% (4/42). Instruments cleaned in an ultrasonic bath of nonsterile tap water were vehicles for 13 cases of otitis media due to *Mycobacterium chelonae*. Laryngoscopes are a reported source of *S. marcescens*.

Ophthalmological instruments (1529, 3694, 7691, 7914). Poorly disinfected tonometers have been vehicles of AdV and epidemic keratoconjunctivitis in outpatient and clinic settings. At an ophthalmology clinic, compared with 200 controls, risks in 58 keratoconjunctivitis cases included pneumotonometry, for an odds ratio of 10.5 (95% confidence interval [95% CI] 4–28), multiple clinic visits, for an odds ratio of 6 (95% CL 3–11), and contact with an infected physician, for an odds ratio of 3 (1.2–9). Poorly disinfected instruments were implicated in a *Mycobacterium fortuitum* infection after a sclerocorneal incision for cataract.

Although risks of prions from tonometers are negligibly low, ophthalmologists and optometrists should follow guidelines for disinfection or autoclaving, particularly when dealing with suspected CJD patients.

MACHINES
There is a risk of cross-infection (machine-to-patient) from poorly maintained and disinfected machines. Disposable mouth pieces and connecting tubes should be used whenever possible. For reuse, pieces should be easy to clean (with sterile water) and be disinfected frequently (1486, 4529).

Respiratory Ventilators, Spirometers, and Nebulizers
Machines. Machines include respiratory ventilators, medication nebulizers, spirometers, and humidifiers. Sources of contamination include tap water, cleaning water, and hands of service or health workers. For ventilator-associated pneumonia, see section 17.5.

Agents. Agents are typically "wet agents" that survive in water collections, tanks, or biofilms, including multiresistant strains. Agents from respiratory machines having caused colonizations, infections, or outbreaks through aerosolization or microaspiration include *Acinetobacter* (*A. baumannii* and *A. calcoaceticus*) (604, 3569, 5915), *B. cepacia* (4529, 5575, 5809), *Klebsiella* (*K. oxytoca* and *K. pneumoniae*) (2863, 3688), *L. pneumophila* (287, 4814), *P. aeruginosa*, *S. marcescens* (261, 7297), and *S. maltophilia* (6373).

Dialyzers
Machines (288, 604, 3789). Serviced hemofiltration machines, dialyzer fluids and distribution systems, blood from dialyzed patients, and hands of workers can be sources of contamination of dialyzer systems. For dialysis, see section 18.7.

Agents (288, 593). Agents from contaminated systems that have caused colonizations, infections, and outbreaks in hemodialysis patients include *Acinetobacter, B. cepacia, Enterobacter, Enterococcus, Klebsiella, Pseudomonas, S. aureus,* CoNS, and *Stenotrophomonas.*

Blood Gas Analyzers
Contaminated blood gas analyzers or their probes are reported sources of colonizations, infections, or outbreaks by *B. cepacia* (2908), *E. cloacae* (4174), and *P. aeruginosa* (2639). Neonatal ICUs appear at high risk. At a neonatal ICU in Australia, a blood gas analyzer was the reservoir for a *P. aeruginosa* outbreak in a neonatal ICU with 2 pseudobacteremias, 6 colonizations, and 16 infections, mainly sepsis and pneumonia, for lethality of 38% (6/16).

Incubators
Sources of agents in incubators are the hands or gloves of workers, spores in the air, and tap water, e.g., for *Legionella* (4556). On an incubator ward, *Rotavirus* caused a diarrhea outbreak in neonates; although a vehicle was not identified, the outbreak was controlled by cleaning and disinfection (8151).

Freezers
Sources of agents in freezers are leaking cryopreservation bags, spores in the air, and thermoisolating gloves. Liquid nitrogen has yielded HBV, environmental bacteria, and fungi such as *Aspergillus*. Freezers and cryopreservation tanks are suspected to have contaminated biogoods such as hematopoietic stem cells (2473, 7389) and semen.

17.3 ENDOSCOPY

Endoscopy (3296, 7991). Endoscopy is a procedure for the inspection and sampling of internal surfaces. Noninvasive examples are bronchoscopy, colonoscopy, cystoscopy, gastroscopy, and kolposcopy. Invasive examples are cardiac catheterization (through blood vessels [see section 18.2]) and arthroscopy (through synovia [see section 18.3]). By biopsy, all endoscopy becomes invasive. Endoscopy is performed routinely. In the United States, there are ~11 million gastrocolonoscopies per year and ~0.5 million bronchoscopies per year.

Infections (987, 4562, 6661, 7059) (Box 17.3). Theoretical hazards include colonizing agents, nonsterile instruments (prions), and bleeding from biopsy. By procedure and surveillance, infection rates range from clearly <1% (bronchoscopy or gastrocolonoscopy, from retrospective studies) up to ~8% (bacteriuria from cystoscopy, from prospective studies). Postendoscopic infections

---

Box 17.3 Endoscopy-associated agents, by procedure

Particular risks are listed in parentheses.

Bronchoscopy
Prions (theoretical, from incubating CJD), environmental mycobacteria, *M. tuberculosis* (defective or poorly decontaminated instrument), *P. aeruginosa*

Gastrocolonoscopy
Prions (theoretical, from incubating CJD), HBV (biopsy), HCV (biopsy), *C. difficile, H. pylori, P. aeruginosa, Salmonella, Cryptosporidium, Strongyloides*

Cystoscopy
Uropathogenic bacteria such as *Enterococcus* and *E. coli*

---

include UTI, pneumonia, and bloodstream infection (BSI). There is no conclusive evidence for transmission of prions or HIV via endoscopy.

Prevention. Prevention is based on appropriate indications and standardized reprocessing of instruments.

- Indications (3566, 6103, 6307, 7892). As bronchoscopy can induce coughing and generation of aerosols, infection risks should be considered before endoscopy in carriers and incubating, ill, or recovering patients, mainly for prions, HBV, HCV, HIV, and *M. tuberculosis*. Because tonsils and appendix of patients with variant Creutzfeld-Jakob disease (CJD) can be infective, and infectivity likely begins during the incubation period, preendoscopic risk evaluation is recommended (Table 14.2).

- Reprocessing (1614, 6103, 6307, 6482, 7084, 7931, 7991). Flexible endoscopes are sensitive, multichanneled instruments, that do not support high temperatures (134°C is required to inactivate prions) or corrosive disinfectants. Prions (see section 18.1), bacterial endospores, and *M. tuberculosis* are particulary resilient. Reprocessing should follow national or manufacturers' guidelines, including soaking in cleaning solution, brushing, disinfection, flushing with alcohol, and drying with pressurized air.

BRONCHOSCOPY
Bronchoscopy-associated agents include mycobacteria, *P. aeruginosa*, and *S. marcescens* (3959). Contaminated bronchoscopes have been sources of *Trichosporon mucoides* pseudoinfections (6921).

Mycobacteria. *M. tuberculosis* (82, 6103, 7991). True nosocomial infections with *M. tuberculosis*, through defective or inadequately decontaminated bronchoscopes, have been reported. However, magnitude is obscured by pseudo-infections from contaminated specimens and false-positive cultures in patients without symptoms or signs of disease. **Environmental mycobacteria (7940).** The same dilemma is exemplified by a study from Taiwan where in 1992, bronchial washings of 21 of 76 patients demonstrated acid-fast rods, and 18 grew *M. chelonae*. Bronchoscopes had been reprocessed by standard protocol. The source of this pseudo-outbreak was found in suction channels of four different bronchoscopes. ***P. aeruginosa*** **(689, 3959, 6307, 6655, 7038, 7084).** Bronchoscopy-transmitted outbreaks of *P. aeruginosa* have been documented. At a tertiary-care facility in Baltimore, Md., in 2001, among 414 patients who underwent bronchoscopy, 32 *P. aeruginosa* infections (28 pneumonia and 4 BSI) were diagnosed, for an attack rate of 8%. At a community hospital in Texas in 2001, *P. aeruginosa* was recovered from 20 of 60 patients and three of four new bronchoscopes that featured a loose biopsy-port cap. As a consequence, ~4,700 bronchoscopes were recalled nationwide.

GASTROCOLONOSCOPY

Reported gastrocolonoscopy-associated agents include HBV, HCV; environmental mycobacteria (*M. avium* complex), *H. pylori*, *Pseudomonas*, *Salmonella*; *Cryptosporidium*, and *Strongyloides* (3296, 6307, 7059, 7866). Bleeding is likely to increase the risks of HBV and HCV transmission.

HCV (894, 4972, 5660, 6307). After colonoscopy with biopsy of a HCV-infected patient, two other individuals examined subsequently contracted HCV infection. In France, three cases of acute hepatitis C were reported: one after retrograde cholangiography, and two after colonoscopy; in all three, decontamination of instruments was found to be insufficient. In Italy in 1994–1999, relative to acute hepatitis A ($n = 7,158$), endoscopy and/or biopsy was a significant risk for acute hepatitis C ($n = 1,023$); in contrast, no risk was discernible for acute hepatitis B ($n = 3,120$). Some blood banks exclude donors for 12 months after endoscopy.

H. pylori **(2316, 4211, 5935, 7628, 7990, 8180).** *H. pylori* can contaminate gastroscopes. Although there is a 60% chance for an infected patient to contaminate a gastroscope, standardized decontamination is highly effective. By endemicity and decontamination, reported rates of nosocomial transmission are 0.4–1.1/100 gastroscopies. Gastroscopy is a potential source of *H. pylori* in gastroenterologists, as is instrumentation of the airway for anesthetists.

Salmonella **(518, 2106, 6307, 6674).** Association with endoscopy was documented in the 1970s–1980s, including of *S. enterica* serovar Typhimurium with gastroscopy and of *S. enterica* serovar Newport with colonoscopy.

CYSTOSCOPY

By patient mix and diagnostic criteria, reported rates are ~1–3% for UTI (158, 987) and ~5–8% for bacteriuria (158, 4562). The most frequent cystoscopy-associated agent is *E. coli* (in 50%). Other agents include *Enterococcus* and *Proteus*.

17.4 BLADDER CATHETERS AND UTI

Bacteriuria (792, 7893). Bacteriuria is defined by significant amounts of bacteria ($\geq 10^5$ CFU/ml) in properly collected, transported, and processed urine from an asymptomatic individual. **UTI (5302, 6248, 6250, 7836).** UTI is defined by bacteriuria or pyuria (≥ 3 leukocytes/high-power field of unspun urine) plus compatible symptoms such as burning, urgency, and frequency ("lower UTI" or cystitis). In association with lumbar tenderness or fever ($\geq 38°C$), pyelonephritis (upper UTI) should be suspected. Nosocomial UTI is diagnosed when UTI develops ≥ 48 h after hospitalization, or when associated with a bladder catheter, cystoscopy, or surgical intervention. Some 80% of nosocomial UTI is associated with bladder catheters, in ICU up to 95%.

Risk (792, 809, 1230, 1264, 4992, 5302, 5451, 6637, 7836, 7893). In Swiss acute-care facilities in 2003, at a given day, ~25% of inpatients carried urinary catheters (in surgery 35%, in ICU even 70%). The overall point prevalence of nosocomial UTI is ~2.5–3%. By age, case mix, and hospital unit, reported rates of nosocomial UTI are 3–13/100 catheterized patients or 0.1–2.5/100 catheter-days. Nosocomial UTI accounts for 10–60% (typically 40%) of nosocomial infections.

Agents (792, 808, 6848, 7226, 8210) (Box 17.4). Bacteria are the main causative agents. Evaluation of nosocomial UTI should include urine culture. In 228 hospitals in western Europe in 1999, urine was cultured from about one third (2.4 million/7.5 million) of inpatients. About one fourth of specimens grew at least one significant agent.

More species cause nosocomial UTI than community-acquired UTI, and *E. coli* is less dominant. At least two thirds of agents are endogenous, while up to one third is acquired; nosocomial acquisition is increasingly recognized. In Taiwan in 1996, *S. marcescens* from urinals caused an outbreak of UTI with 17 cases. In Taiwan in 1998, *S. marcescens* from urine bottles caused a prolonged outbreak of UTI on a neurology ward in which this agent reached a relative proportion of 60%.

> **Box 17.4** Agents of nosocomial and community-acquired UTI
>
> Relative frequency and remarks appear in parentheses.
>
> **Viruria**
> Nosocomial: CMV, polyomaviruses BK and JC.
> Community: CMV, *Hantavirus*
>
> **Bacteriuria**
> Nosocomial and community: *E. coli* (noso, 25–45%; community, 60–90%), *Enterococcus* (noso, 15–25%; community, 0.5-12%; at risk, elderly), *Klebsiella* (noso, 5-15%; community, 0.5-12%; at risk, diabetics), *P. aeruginosa* (noso, 5–15%; community, 0–4%)
> Community: *Staphylococcus saprophyticus* (5–15%; at risk, elderly), *Proteus* (0.5–9%; can induce stones; at risk, spinal cord injury), *Citrobacter* (0.5–5%), *Enterobacter* (0.5–5%), CoNS (0–8%), *Morganella* (0–4%), *S. agalactiae* (0–2%; at risk: diabetics), *S. aureus* (0–2%), *M. tuberculosis* (0–0.6%), *Serratia* (at risk, spinal cord injury)
>
> **Funguria**
> Nosocomial and community: *C. albicans* (10%)
>
> **Helminthuria**
> Community (Africa): *Schistosoma haematobium*

Prevention (792). Prevention is based on appropriate indications, aseptic insertion and drainage techniques, and removal as soon as possible.

VIRUSES

CMV and polyomavirus BK as causes of nosocomial UTI seem relevant mainly in immune-impaired patients.

Bacteria

Frequent agents of nosocomial UTI (808, 4818, 5302, 7893). Frequent agents of nosocomial UTI are *E. coli* (20–45%, uropathogenic), *Enterococcus* (15–25%, can include VRE), *Klebsiella* (5–15%), *P. aeruginosa* (5–15%), *Proteus* (5–10%), and CoNS (2–14%). **Klebsiella.** Of 166 strains from urine, 83% (138) were *K. pneumoniae*, 13% (21) were *K. oxytoca*, and 4% (7) were other *Klebsiella* spp. Up to 40% of *K. pneumoniae* from urine can produce ESβL. **P. aeruginosa.** *P. aeruginosa* is typically of low virulence, and about one fourth of infections can be treated with catheter removal.

Infrequent agents of UTI. Infrequent agents of UTI (relative proportion ≤5%) include *Enterobacter* (3–6%), *S. aureus* (2–4%), *S. pyogenes* (2%), *Acinetobacter* (~2%), *Citrobacter* (1–4%), and *Serratia*. Urinary *Enterobacter* and *Staphylococcus* usually have low virulence, and ~60% of infections can be treated with catheter removal.

FUNGI

C. albicans (808, 6248). *C. albicans* is frequently recovered from urine of patients in ICU (in up to ~30%), but this finding often represents colonization (funguria) rather than infection. In Europe, *Candida* is considered a relevant isolate in ~10% of nosocomial UTIs.

17.5 INTUBATION AND NOSOCOMIAL PNEUMONIA

For diagnosis of pneumonia, see section 14.7. Nosocomial pneumonia is further characterized by exposure (Box VI.1) to aerosols from machines or showers, intubation with microaspiration, or assisted ventilation, and by additional signs such as increased need for suctioning or worsened gas exchange. Signs of severity include rapid progression, multilobar or multiorgan involvement, concomitant BSI, and need for ventilation and intensive care (4890). Ventilator-associated pneumonia (VAP) is nosocomial pneumonia that develops >48 h after endotracheal intubation (or tracheostomy) and mechanical ventilation.

Nosocomial pneumonia should be confirmed radiologically *and* microbiologically, including by cultures of blood and lower airway specimens (e.g., bronchoalveolar lavage) and by antigen tests of urine.

Risk (578, 1230, 2135, 2195, 4890, 6248, 6250, 7836). By age and unit (ICU wards), reported rates of nosocomial pneumonia are 0.1–1/100 patient-days or up to 1/100 hospitalized patients. A variable proportion of nosocomial pneumonias is VAP, in ICU 75–85%. Risks for VAP include endotracheal intubation with deflated cuffs that permit microaspiration, and ventilation for >24 h. By age and unit, reported VAP rates are 0.1–2.5 (often 0.5–1) per 100 ventilator-days. Of ventilated patients, 5% (children) to 20–45% (adults) develop VAP. Lethality of nosocomial pneumonia is 30–70%; one third to one half of overall lethality is due to VAP.

Agents (1592, 2195, 3922, 4705, 5237) (Table 17.1). Causative agents can be endogenous or acquired, including from procedures (e.g., suction), machines (e.g., VAP), respiratory droplets (from workers, patients, and visitors), aerosols, or dust. Acquired agents are mainly bacteria, less frequently viruses, rarely fungi.

Prevention (7836). Prevention is difficult, with a focus on education (standards of care), sterile equipments (standards of maintenance), and surveillance (early detection of clusters).

VIRUSES

Viral nosopneumonias (1754, 3679, 8007). Nosocomial acquisition and causality can be difficult to demonstrate, in particular, when viruses are associated with bacteria. Confirmed or suspected agents include vaccine-preventable viruses such as measles virus, *Influenzavirus*, and VZV, as well as vaccine nonpreventable viruses such as AdV, *Enterovirus*, HSV1, human metapneumovirus, parainfluenzavirus (PIV), RSV, *Rhinovirus*, and SARS-CoV.

BACTERIA

Colonization should be distinguished from infection, and hospitalized community-acquired pneumonia (CAP, onset in first 48 h from admission) from nosocomial pneumonia in acute care and long-term care (Table 17.1).

Frequent agents of nosopneumonia (1592, 2195, 2640, 4705, 5237, 6207, 7570). Frequent agents of nosopneumonia (approximate relative frequency) are *S. aureus* (15–30%, often 25%), *P. aeruginosa* (10–20%), *A. baumannii* (8–28%), and *K. pneumoniae* (5–14%). ***A. baumannii.*** *A. baumannii* is an emerging agent of late-onset pneumonia in critically ill patients. Lethality of VAP by *A. baumannii* is 35–45%. ***S. aureus.*** *S. aureus* nosopneumonia typically develops after stays that last >1 week. By geography and unit, up to 50–70% of *S. aureus* nosopneumonias can be due to MRSA. Lethality of VAP by MRSA is ~40%. ***P. aeruginosa.*** *P. aeruginosa* is overrepresented in nursing-home-acquired pneumonia, in which it can account for up to 50% of isolates. Lethality of VAP by *P. aeruginosa* is up to 40%.

Infrequent agents (2195, 5237). Infrequent agents (relative proportion ≤10%) are diverse and include *Enterobacter* (6–9% in VAP), *E. coli* (3–10% in VAP), *S. marcescens* (3–5%), *S. maltophilia* (3% in VAP), *C. pneumoniae* (0–6%), *Legionella* (0–6%), *M. pneumoniae* (0–1%), *B. cereus* (from machines), and *Enterococcus*. Vaccine-preventable bacteria of nosopneumonia (cases may reflect CAP) include *Bordetella pertussis*, *Haemophilus influenzae*, *M. tuberculosis*, and *Streptococcus pneumoniae*. ***Enterococcus (760, 1592, 2604).*** Although frequently colonizing patients in ICU, causality in nosopneumonia is uncertain. In Chicago, Ill., in 1995, 24% (9/38) of ventilated patients were colonized with VRE on admission to ICU, and 41% (12) acquired VRE after 3–8 (median, 5) days. In France in 1997, the prevalence of patients in ICU colonized by VRE was 37% (26/70) compared with 12% (20/169) in controls from an agricultural community. ***M. tuberculosis (509, 1989, 6286, 8047).*** Nosocomial spread is documented. In HIV-infected patients, there is an increased risk for the transmission of multidrug-resistant strains to patients and workers.

FUNGI

Fungi are significant endogenous or acquired agents of nosopneumonia. By case mix, unit, and diagnostic criteria, reported relative shares are: *Candida* (1592, 2195) 3–9%, *Aspergillus* (1592) 1%, and *Pneumocystis* rare on most wards, except wards with HIV-infected persons.

17.6 DRUGS, BIOPRODUCTS, AND NOSOCOMIAL DIARRHEA

Drugs are substances intended for preventive, curative, or stimulating use in humans, including illicit drugs, herbs

Table 17.1 Agents of nosocomial pneumonia[a]

Agent	Acute care		Nursing homes, elderly
	Children	Adults	
Viruses	10 (up to 25%)	10 (up to 25%)	10 (up to 25%)
Staphylococcus aureus	12	15–30	0–33
Pseudomonas aeruginosa	30	10–20	5–50
Klebsiella pneumoniae	15	5–14	5–40
Haemophilus influenzae	9	6	0–20
Streptococcus pneumoniae	6	1	0–40
Other or unknown agents	20	30	25–80

[a]Numbers are approximate relative frequencies (in percent). Column totals can exceed 100%, as etiology is polymicrobial in up to 30% of cases.

> **Box 17.5** Agents and infections from drugs, by agent cluster
>
> Vehicles are listed in parentheses. Abbreviations used: alternative drugs (ALT), bioproducts (BIO), and multidose vials (MDV).
>
> Droplet-air   *Klebsiella* (cosmetic, solution, and disinfectant); *A. fumigatus* (experimental)
> Feces-food   HEV (ALT); *B. cereus* (solution and disinfectant), *Enterobacter* (solution, MDV, and feed), *Salmonella* (illicit, ALT, and feed); *Anisakis* (ALT)
> Zoonotic   SHV (cosmetics), SV40 (experimentals and bioproducts); *Brucella* (cosmetics), *M. bovis* (experimental and BIO); malaria (treatment failure from fakes)
> Environmental
> - Wet agents: *B. cepacia* (cosmetic, solution, MDV, disinfectant, and feed), mycobacteria (ALT, solution, vial, and disinfectant), *Pseudomonas* (ALT, disinfectant, and feed), *Ralstonia* (solution), *Serratia* (solution, MDV, citrated tube, disinfectant, and feed)
> - Other agents: avian and simian retroviruses (BIO?), *Acinetobacter* (feed), *C. tetani* (illicit, ALT, and BIO), clostridia (illicit), *Streptomyces* (ALT); *Malassezia* (feed), *Paecilomyces* (cosmetic), *Wangiella* (cosmetic); *Toxocara* (ALT)
> Skin-blood   Prions (BIO?), HBV (MDV and BIO), HCV (experimental, fluid, MDV, and BIO), GBV-C (BIO); injection abscess, *S. aureus* (MDV), *S. pyogenes* (BIO); *Candida* (feed)

and other alternative remedies, apothecaries, pharmaceuticals, and bioproducts. Included here are cosmetic and nutritional products.

Many countries regulate medications (pharmaceuticals and bioproducts) stringently, by requiring guaranteed composition, proof and quantification of quality, effects, and risks, and continued postmarketing surveillance. Herbalists, pharmacists, physicians, and manufacturers have a duty to report adverse events to authorities. What follows is a summary of case reports rather than a systematic analysis of infection risks (Box 17.5).

ILLICIT DRUGS

Quality (381, 6285). Illicit drugs are not standardized. Street heroin ($n = 101$) and cocaine ($n = 120$) samples were analyzed for contaminants in Switzerland in 1995–1996. Heroin accounted for 32–62% of material, while impurities (e.g., papaverine), decay metabolites (e.g., monoacetylmorphine), and adulterants (e.g., caffeine) accounted for 68–38%. Similarly, cocaine accounted for 43–88% of material, while the remaining material contained impurities (e.g., cinnamoylcocaine) and adulterants (e.g., anesthetics). In Austria in 1987–1995, of heroin seized (25.6 kg) in the street, 25% (95/386) of samples contained caffeine, and 1% each contained paracetamol and metaqualon. Heroin-related deaths and quality of heroin were found to be unrelated. Black tar heroin is reportedly particularly impure.

Agents. Illicit drugs are reported vehicles of bacteria. **Spore-forming bacteria (862, 1223, 1732, 3947).** Through production and handling, street illicit drug can become contaminated with spore-forming *B. cereus* and *Clostridium* spp. (e.g., *C. botulinum* and *C. tetani*). Heating heroin for sniffing does not inactivate spores. For *Clostridium* infections in injection drug users (IDUs), (see section 13.8). **Salmonella (7363).** In the United States in 1981, marijuana likely imported from Colombia or Jamaica was vehicle for 85 *S. enterica* serovar Muenchen infections. Potential sources of contamination were fertilizer or manure from growing plants or adulteration of street drugs.

FAKE DRUGS

Fakes can be harmful by lack of efficacy duped "murder by fake drugs" (5404) or by unwanted additives. Counterfeits reported in infectiology include fake antiretrovirals, antibiotics, antimalarials, and false vaccine documents.

Antimalarials (1977, 5403). Fake antimalarials are well documented. In Southeast Asia in 1999–2000, 29% (30/104) of blister packs labeled "artesunate" did not contain any artesunate. Likewise, 38% (39/104) of samples bought from pharmacies and shops were fakes and did not contain artesunate: 11% in Thailand, 25% in Cambodia, 38% in Laos, 40% in Myanmar, and 64% in Vietnam. By 2002–2003, the proportion of fake blisters that did not contain artesunate rose to 53% (99/188). To separate pseudoresistance (by fakes) from pharmacological resistance (by vera), leftover drugs should be secured and drug blood levels determined.

Vaccines (6708, 6936, 7090). In Kenya, fake yellow fever vaccine certificates appear to be available at bookshops and travel agencies. Among children for adoption from People's Republic of China, ~30% were not adequately protected, despite complete diphtheria-tetanus (DT) and polio vaccination records. Adoptees should be revaccinated or to have antibody levels verified.

HERBAL AND OTHER ALTERNATIVE DRUGS

Herbal (phytotherapy) and other alternative remedies can cause harm through contaminants, inefficacy, and drug interactions (e.g., St. John's wort [*Hypericum*] with the antiretroviral indinavir) (5929). Formulations may include solutions, powders, organ extracts, and fetal cells (may be illegal in some countries). Alternative drugs are reported vehicles of viruses, bacteria, and helminths. For acupuncture, see section 18.1.

Viruses
***HEV* (3581).** Exposure interval and molecular study suggested that a 46-year-old Japanese man had contracted acute HE from Chinese herbal medicine.

Bacteria
***C. tetani* (2844, 8287).** In Montana, local "direct-entry" midwives used "health and beauty clay" powder to accelerate umbilical cord drying until 1998 when a case of neonatal tetanus occurred. The powder was bentonite clay from California's Death Valley manufactured without sterilization and sold as a cosmetic. In Buenos Aires, Argentina, in 1996, intramuscular injections of fetal sheep cells for alternative treatment of rheumatism caused tetanus in 12 nonvaccinated elderly women, seven (58%) of which were fatal. The index case presented with muscle rigidity at face and legs initially considered contractures.

***Mycobacterium* (2585).** In 30 of the United States in 1995–1996, an unlicensed injectable adrenal cortex extract sold and used as alternative medicine caused injection abscesses by *M. abscessus* in 87 persons.

***Pseudomonas* (6620).** A herbal concoction (gripe water) containing seed oils from dill, fennel, anise, mint, and ginger is a folk medicine for abdominal distress in babies. In the United States, an infant contracted *P. aeruginosa* septic shock from being given gripe water from India that grew *P. aeruginosa*.

***Salmonella* (4018).** In Germany in 2003, an outbreak of *S. enterica* serovar Agona affected 42 infants ≤13 months of age. Vehicles were brands of herbal teas sold to alleviate flatulence and spasms of infants. Outbreak brands contained aniseed (*Pimpinella anisum*, Apiaceae) that yielded serovar Agona. Source was a bulk aniseed producer in Turkey that used manure for cultivation of aniseed. Of note, two thirds of parents of case infants had concocted teas with boiling water (although some had cooled teas by adding cold water).

***Streptomyces* (1078).** In the United States, a 49-year-old woman with metastatic breast cancer received infusions of a compound (NeyTumorin) reportedly consisting of peptides from fetal or young pigs or cows; she subsequently developed an invasive *Streptomyces* infection.

Helminths
***Anisakis* (3476).** In France, three individuals contracted acute anisakiasis from the consumption of raw fish for medicinal purposes.

***Paragonimus* (1674, 3933, 4630).** Freshwater crabs steeped in rice wine, brine, or vinegar in People's Republic of China, crab juice in Japan, and crayfish juice in Korea are traditional medicines (in Korea for measles) and suspected vehicles for *Paragonimus*.

***Taenia* (4636).** In South Africa, self-trained healers are reported to have used segments of *T. solium* against enteric tapeworms (similia similibus) or, added to beer, to punish unfaithful husbands or lovers, a practice that puts clients at risk of cysticercosis.

***Toxocara* (508, 6394).** Raw snails used in folk medicine against ulcers are a suspected vehicle of *Toxocara* infections. Before vitamin B12 became available, raw liver against pernicious anemia was a suspected cause of hypereosinophilia and toxocariasis.

COSMETIC PRODUCTS
Cosmetic products are applied directly to the body. Cosmetics can be difficult to distinguish from medications. Examples of cosmetics (medications) include soap, skin lotion (with sunblock), shampoo (with antidandruff), make up, eye mascara, shaving lotion, lipstick (with antibiotic), toothpaste (with fluoride), and deodorant (with antiperspirant).

Storage and multiple-use containers are likely weak points. Cosmetics are reported vehicles of viruses, bacteria, and fungi. For surgical site infections, see section 18.3; for personal objects, see section 6.4.

Viruses
Simian herpes virus (SHV) (3398). In Florida in 1987, SHV in a nonprescription skin cream caused SHV infection in a user.

Bacteria
***Brucella* (2906).** At a beauty parlor in The Netherlands in 1981–1982, 4 of 15 people treated with contaminated cosmetic bovine cell suspension fell ill with brucellosis (likely due to *B. melitensis*), and two others were seroreactive.

***Burkholderia* (4824).** At two hospitals in Arizona in 1996–1998, *B. cepacia* in intrinsically contaminated mouthwash for oral care of intubated patients caused a pseudo-outbreak with 69 culture-positive respiratory samples.

***Klebsiella* (2571).** At a hospital in Paris, France, in 1993, *K. pneumoniae* in ultrasonography-coupling gel cross-contaminated six women and two neonates.

Fungi

Curvularia (3786). Saline-filled silicone breast implants became contaminated with *Curvularia* from saline bottles stored in a room with a water-damaged ceiling. The result was black sediment in removed implants.

Exophiala (1187). In North Carolina in 2002, *Exophiala* meningitis was diagnosed in five patients 27–152 days after they had received epidural injections of contaminated methylprednisolone formulated by a pharmacy for pain treatment.

Paecilomyces (5640). In a bone marrow transplant unit of a hospital in Switzerland in 1993, *P. lilacinus* in a contaminated skin lotion caused 25 infections.

EXPERIMENTAL DRUGS

Experimental formulation and reconstitution are likely weak points. Experimental drugs are reported vehicles of viruses, bacteria, and fungi.

VIRUSES

HCV (4222). In Italy in 1995, 15 of 29 volunteers who participated in two pharmacokinetics studies of oral drugs acquired acute HC from a common source, presumably on entry blood screen.

Simian virus 40 (SV40) (6798). Live SV40 contaminated an experimental RSV vaccine; after intranasal administration of the compound, 60% of volunteers developed neutralizing antibody.

Bacteria

M. bovis (7875). A bacillus Calmette Guérin (BCG)-based anticancer preparation became contaminated with *M. bovis* during reconstitution in the biosafety cabinet of a Dutch hospital pharmacy where *M. bovis* DNA was later amplified from petri discs and dust. As a result, three immune-compromised patients developed disseminated infection.

Fungi

Aspergillus (290). An experimental solution for the infusion of killer cells to cancer patients transmitted *A. fumigatus* to two patients.

SOLUTIONS, DISINFECTANTS, AND MULTIDOSE VIALS

Good practice is essential when preparing solutions for injection, infusion, or inhalation. Multidose vials (MDV) (1220) are readily contaminated and a well-documented source of nosocomial infections and outbreaks. If use is unavoidable, follow good practice: keep vials according to the manufacturer's instructions; use in a medication area; date the first opening; always disinfect and change needle for each entry; use content for a single patient if possible; discard when sterility is compromised; do not combine leftovers for later use. Good practice can reduce contamination risks. Of 1,223 weekly samples from 863 MDV cultured over 3 months, none grew bacteria. The duration of use was 1–402 days, with 13% of vials in use for more than 30 days.

Solutions and MDV are reported vehicles of viruses and bacteria.

Viruses

HBV. Bottle reuse (7995). At an alternative medicine clinic in the United Kingdom, saline from a reused bottle for autohemotherapy was the likely vehicle for HBV infections in 16% (57/356) of exposed clients and staff, and a client was the likely source. **MDV (1220).** At a private office in New York, N.Y., in 2001, poor practice that included drawing several substances from multidose vials into one syringe was the source for 21 acute HBV infections. Of 1,042 clients tested, 3.6% (38) tested positive for HBV infection. The physician was ordered to stop injections (he opted to retire).

HCV. Syringe reuse (1220). At a hematology-oncology clinic in Nebraska in 2002, a health worker routinely used the same syringe to draw blood from central venous catheters and from catheter-flushing saline bags that were used for multiple patients. In all, 85 (69%) HCV infections were detected among 139 patients with central venous catheters. **MDV (941, 1220).** At an emergency room in Spain in 2000, 9 (13%) of 70 patients visiting in 1 day contracted acute hepatitis C. All nine had intravenous catheters flushed with heparin from a multidose solution compared with only 1 (4%) of 23 HCV-negative day- and age-matched controls. At a private office in New York, N.Y., in 2001, 12 acute HCV infections were traced to multidose anesthetics vials; a carrier was the likely source of vial contamination. Among 1,315 clients available for testing since opening of the office, 19 (1%) HCV infections were detected.

Bacteria

Bacillus (2645, 3466). Contaminated ethanol bulk supply for the preparation of 70% ethanol skin disinfectant caused a *B. cereus* pseudo-outbreak. In Brazil in 1996, *B. cereus* in intravenous fluids caused sepsis and death of 36 neonates. Fluids did not yield the agent, but endotoxin was elevated (1.2–3.3 U/ml) in glucose and distilled water for injection. Fluids from the same manufacturer had been implicated in a previous *Bacillus* outbreak that involved 39 patients on an oncology ward.

Burkholderia. Both *B. cepacia* and *B. pseudomallei* survive well in moist habitats. **B. cepacia.** Risks include aspiration and flushing procedures and the preparation of solutions and disinfectants.

- Aspiration and flushing (5810, 7739). On a cardiology ward in 3 days, eight patients developed *B. cepacia* sepsis; the source was a dextrose solution bag that was aspirated to dilute heparin for injection. On an oncology ward 14 patients developed *B. cepacia* bacteremia; patients had central venous catheters flushed with heparin solution prepared by using a contaminated intravenous fluid bag.
- Solutions (2907, 6165). In an ICU, extrinsically contaminated albuterol nebulizer solution caused 44 colonizations or infections. In an ICU, indigo-carmine dye for tinting enteral tube feeding was the vehicle implicated in an outbreak.
- Multidose vials (3106, 4071) were sources of *B. cepacia* infections in Canada (intra-articular methylprednisolone) and the United States (nebulized albuterol).
- Disinfectants (3789, 5346, 5712, 7486). Hardy *B. cepacia* survives in ad hoc prepared or commercial disinfectants. Contaminated benzalkonium was implicated in four or more nosocomial *B. cepacia* outbreaks. On a dialysis unit in Texas, intrinsically contaminated povidone-iodine caused three cases of peritonitis and three pseudoinfections (by wiping tops of blood culture bottles). At the university hospital in Beirut, Lebanon, in 7 years, *B. cepacia* caused 411 BSIs in 361 patients; disinfectant alcohol diluted with tap water was implicated epidemiologically and molecularly. The outbreak abated when once-use alcohol swabs were introduced. In Thailand, nine hemodialysis patients contracted *B. cepacia* bacteremia from contaminated chlorhexidine-cetrimide in which forceps were disinfected for picking up cotton balls and gauze to dress subclavian catheters.
- Parenteral nutrition (1966). In Paris, France, in 2001–2002, *B. cepacia* was isolated from the blood of 11 patients (mainly premature infants with sepsis) on three different wards. The agent was grown from condensation droplets between plastic caps and rubber stoppers of bottles that contained lipid emulsion for parenteral nutrition. The final source was residual water inside an autoclave provided by the manufacturer of the emulsion.

B. pseudomallei (2577, 6035). In a hospital in Thailand, 16% (18/110) of chlorhexidine-cetrimide samples from wards occupied by melioidosis patients grew *B. pseudomallei*, likely from suction tubes used for respiratory care. In Australia, commercial handwashing detergent grew *B. pseudomallei*, likely from inserting a garden hose for dispensing.

Enterobacter (2889, 3136, 4825, 8357). A phlebotomist contaminated blood culture specimens with *E. cloacae* by occasionally using a contaminated thrombin solution on her finger. In Taiwan, contaminated saline for the preparation of heparin solution was the vehicle for an *E. cloacae* outbreak. In Greece, *E. cloacae* and *E. agglomerans* in intravenous fluid caused 63 sepsis cases in infants and children. The source was screwcaps on bottles from a single manufacturer. Fluids became contaminated when line-sets were inserted into bottle rubbers. At a university hospital in Switzerland, multidose vials were likely source for four *E. cloacae* infections and four colonizations of neonates in ICU.

Klebsiella (2003, 4191, 6207). *K. oxytoca* in disinfectant solution was the implicated source of sepsis in 28 infants. The disinfectant (formaldehyde, glutaral, and glyoxal) was prepared daily. It was kept in plastic containers and was used on surfaces, laminar air systems, and infusion pumps. It maintained infections on the unit for 2.5 years. In a burn unit, environmental sampling for outbreak investigation incidentally detected *K. oxytoca* in opened but not unopened detergent bottles. Dextrose solution for intravenous use was the source implicated in an outbreak of *K. pneumoniae* sepsis in a neonatal nursery.

Mycobacterium. Environmental mycobacteria are widespread in tap water and may survive in disinfectants.

- Solutions (4000, 6523). In 1985, eight patients submitting to cosmetic surgery developed *M. chelonae* wound infection; the vehicle implicated was a contaminated solution of gentian violet used for skin marking. In New Jersey in 2002–2003, four *M. chelonae* infections (three confirmed and one suspected) followed outpatient cosmetic surgery by one surgeon; *M. chelonae* was recovered from methylene blue solutions used by the surgeon to mark incisions.
- Vials (8400). In a factory hospital in People's Republic of China in 1997–1998, injectable penicillin vials stored on humid ground and contaminated with *M. chelonae* from soil caused an outbreak of 86 injection-site infections, for an attack rate of 10%.
- Disinfectants (5395, 7486, 8045). Benzalkonium (quaternary ammonium) is ineffective against mycobacteria; diluted benzalkonium contaminated with *M. abscessus* and *M. chelonae* (presumably from tap water) caused outbreaks of injection-site infections. Eight *M. chelonae* infections were linked by a podiatrist who used jet injection for lidocain administration; the agent was recovered in water for mixing disinfectant in which the injector was dipped. In Georgia in 1980, a contaminated disinfectant or topical anesthetic was implicated in three cases of *M. chelonae* keratitis.

P. aeruginosa (215, 245, 3876, 5741). Disinfecting solutions were reported sources of infections or outbreaks, including povidone iodine, chlorhexidine, and an unidentified disinfectant used for piercing at a jewelry kiosk. Although probably contaminated during preparation, intrinsic contamination (by poor manufacturing) of iodophor has been reported as well.

Ralstonia (4167). In the United States in 1998, saline solution for endotracheal suctioning caused colonization of 33 patients from four hospitals. The solution was produced by one manufacturer, and unopened vials grew *R. pickettii* genotypically related to patient isolates. The same manufacturer had been implicated in a previous outbreak.

Serratia. *S. marcecens* thrives in moist habitats. Manipulation of solutions is a risk. Reported vehicles include anesthetic solutions, liquid soap, disinfectants, blood tubes, multidose vials (MDV), solvents for antibiotics (6751), fluids for inhalation therapy (7721) and in nebulizer tanks (7297), theophylline from multiuse bottles instilled into gastric tubes (2427), and liquid waste from an electrolyte apparatus (7744).

- Anesthetics (3263, 5652, 6751). A postoperative outbreak of *S. marcescens* was traced to a single anesthetist and the anesthetic propofol; patients were >40 times more likely to have had this anesthetist and 22 times more likely to have received propofol than were controls, although samples neither from the anesthetist nor from the environment grew *S. marcescens*. In the United States in 1998–1999, a respiratory therapist manipulating and probably self-administering solutions of the opioid fentanyl was implicated in 26 cases of *S. marcescens* bacteremia on a surgical ICU. In anesthesia, a hazard is to use the same vial for >6 h and on more than one patient and to simultaneously prepare all syringes needed for the day.
- Liquid soap (264, 6618, 7297). In the United States, bottles of chlorxylenol soap carried by health workers or left standing inverted in sinks contributed to colonizations or infections of 32 neonates in ICU. In Japan, 71 colonizations or infections (including three primary BSIs) were traced to fluid tanks of three nebulizers and a liquid soap dispenser. In France, extrinsically contaminated nonmedicated liquid soap was the source for colonized hands of health workers and nosocomial *S. marcescens* infections.
- Disinfectants (786, 5330, 7486, 7821). Contaminated benzalkonium was implicated in three or more nosocomial *S. marcescens* outbreaks. Cotton balls soaked in disinfectant were the source for 10 cases of *S. marcescens* arthritis. *S. marcescens* in diluted hexetidine mouth wash caused an outbreak in an ICU. Chlorhexidine was the vehicle implicated in a hospital outbreak.
- Citrated tubes (1276). In France in 1983, contaminated, mishandled tubes for blood coagulation tests were source for 15 sepsis cases and 43 pseudobacteremias.
- MDV (2953, 3263, 7323). At an outpatient hemodialysis center, to save costs, epoetin single-use vials were punctured multiple times and residual epoetin from multiple vials was pooled. This practice caused 10 *S. liquefaciens* infections. In Japan, heparin from multidose vials contributed to an outbreak with 12 BSI.

S. aureus (3960, 8139). In Tennessee in 2001, lidocain injections from contaminated MDV caused *S. aureus* joint and soft-tissue infections in 5 (29%) of 17 injected outpatients. In Azerbaijan in 1995, measles vaccine from MDV transported house-to-house without cold chain was the source of *S. aureus* infections in five children resulting in four deaths.

PARENTERAL NUTRITION AND FORMULA FEED

Contaminated enteric feeds (given via nasogastric tube) and parenteral nutrition solutions (for infusion) are reported vehicles of infections.

Bacteria
Enteric feeds (608, 4834, 5568). Agents reported from enteric feeds include *Acinetobacter*, *Enterobacter*, *Pseudomonas*, *Salmonella*, and *Serratia*. Reused feeding bags and infusion tubes were likely sourses of *A. calcoaceticus* and *P. aeruginosa*. A likely source of contamination was bags and tubes that could not be washed and dried for reuse. In an outbreak of *S. enterica* serovar Enteritidis, lyophilized egg albumin in enteric dry feed was the implicated source.

Parenteral nutrition (2827, 7550). *E. cloacae* has been transmitted through parenteral nutrition solution. In one outbreak with nine bacteremia cases, the solution was considered intrinsically contaminated. In another outbreak with 10 cases of neonatal sepsis, the solution was believed to be contaminated during preparation. In this outbreak, *E. cloacae* DNA profiles from refrigerated solution, in-use solution, and blood of infected newborns were indistinguishable.

Infant formulas. Infant formulas are substitutes for human milk available as liquids or powders; for breastfeeding, see section 14.7. Agents from infant formulas include *C. botulinum* (864), *Enterobacter*, and *Salmonella* (7470). *Enterobacter sakazakii* (1185, 5356, 7698). Extrinsically and intrinsically contaminated dried infant formula has been implicated in cases and outbreaks of *E. sakazakii* disease in infants, including necrotizing enteritis and meningitis that are fatal in 15% to 40–80% of cases.

Fungi

***Candida* (5201, 7026).** In 1987, 8 of 27 surgical patients receiving parenteral nutrition developed systemic *C. albicans* disease, but none of 108 control patients. The implicated vehicle was nutrition bags to which an experienced nurse who carried *C albicans* in the throat had added lipids. In 3 months in 1981, five hospitalized patients were diagnosed with fungemia or vascular device colonization by *C. parapsilosis*; all five, but none of 34 controls were on parenteral nutrition. A vacuum pump used to compound solutions grew *C. parapsilosis* from multiple sites.

***Malassezia* (1742).** Neonates receiving lipids through central venous catheters have developed *Malassezia* fungemia.

BIOPRODUCTS

Bioproducts include heparin, hormones, immunoglobulins (Ig), vaccines, blood and derivatives (see section 18.4), and organs, tissues, and cells for transplantation (see section 18.5). Vaccine adverse events include infection from attenuated agents (mimicked natural infection), contaminating agents (production and handling), aberrant agents (wrong route and veterinary vaccine), and replacing agents (types not covered by vaccine).

Means to minimize risks from contaminants include donor selection and manufacturing technologies that are continuously adapted to the latest technologies, and post-marketing surveillance.

Prions

Mammal-derived bioproducts. A theoretical hazard exists for prions to get into bioproducts manufactured from bovine source materials.

- Heparin (mammalian mucopolysaccharides) and absorbable surgical sutures (cat gut). (59, 1644, 4240). Manufacturers have switched to porcine or ovine source materials.
- Vaccines (658, 1112) (http://www.fda.gov/cber/BSE/BSE.htm). Starting in 1989, manufacturers were asked to use cell lines from bovine spongiform encephalopathy (BSE)-free herds. Most manufacturers have followed this recommendation or have switched production to human cell lines. In human substrate cells, spontaneous emergence of prion could be prevented by knocking-out the prion gene.

Human-derived bioproducts (646, 836, 928, 2488, 2724, 2874, 4019, 8155). Pituitary human growth hormone (HGH) obtained from cadaveric brain was used to treat growth failure in the 1960s–1980s. HGH was first reported as a iatrogenic form of CJD in 1985. Iatrogenic CJD is rare (for dura mater, see section 18.5). To date, about 140 cases of CJD due to HGH have been documented (>80 in France, >35 in the United Kingdom, and >20 in the United States). The lifetime risk of recipients to develop CJD is 0–4%. In the United States, seven CJD cases were reported among 6,284 HGH recipients, for a cumulative risk of 0.1/100 recipients. No cases were detected in series of recipients in The Netherlands ($n = 564$) or France ($n = 1,620$). By the start or end of HGH treatment, estimated incubation periods are 4–20 years.

Viruses

Immunoglobulin. In the 1970s–1990s, due to less advanced screening and manufacturing technologies, batches of Ig were contaminated by HBV or HCV. **HBV (5189).** In Brazil in 1974, six contaminated Ig (γ-globulin) batches caused 17 acute HBV infections, for a reported attack rate of 2.5%. **HCV.** Tests for HCV became available only in the 1990s.

- Intravenous Ig for primary immune deficiencies (580, 860, 2326, 6692). Before manufacturing was modified in the 1990s, HCV could survive in some batches and infect recipients. In the United States in 1993–1994, of 341 recipients, 278 could be evaluated (mean age, 9 years) and 11% (23/210) of recipients of a particular brand were seroreactive, compared with none (0/52) of recipients of other brands.
- Intravenous anti-D against rhesus incompatibility (3892, 4965, 6979). In Ireland in 1994, batches used in 1977–1978 were in retrospect found to have been contaminated by a HCV-infected donor. All anti-D recipients of 1970–1994 were screened and 1% (704/62,667 women) had evidence of past or current HCV infection. By nucleic acid amplification test (NAT), 55% (390/704) of reactive women (likely <1% of all women) tested positive. Of NAT-positive women, 376 were evaluated ~17 years after exposure: 81% had symptoms (mainly fatigue), 47% (176/371) had transaminitis, and 2% (7/363) had cirrhosis in liver biopsy. Batches of anti-D again became HCV contaminated in Ireland in 1991–1994. This time, 0.6% (44) of exposed women tested positive for HCV by NAT, and 0.3% (19) had a genotype related to that from the single implicated donor. Similarly in Germany in 1978–1979, 2,533 women had been exposed to HCV-contaminated anti-D; after 10-15 years, at least 86 (3%) women had chronic hepatitis C.

GBV-C (580, 1635, 5495). RNA of GBV-C was amplified from Ig for intramuscular and intravenous use, and seroconversion was documented in at least one recipient. However, transmission of virus particles has not been demonstrated, and the clinical significance of apparently innocuous GBV-C RNA is uncertain.

Vaccines. Attenuated viruses can mimick natural disease, e.g., measles virus (mild febrile rash), mumps virus (mild parotitis), and poliovirus (very rarely flaccid paralysis). While being infective, mimicked disease is mostly mitigated and clears spontaneously. Rare complications include aseptic meningitis (mumps virus) and aseptic arthritis (rubella virus). In immune-impaired patients, attenuated agents can cause disseminated disease and are contraindicated.

Remote hazards of viral vaccines include errors in administration, incomplete or reversed attenuation, and contamination at production.

- Errors (588, 2829). Rabies virus veterinary vaccines for baiting wildlife are feared to be taken up inadvertently by immune-impaired children. A 58-year-old man was inadvertently injected with oral polio vaccine intramuscularly; no adverse events were observed.
- Incomplete attenuation (5723, 7934, 7986) is very rare. In Fortaleza, Brazil, in 1960, incompletely inactivated rabies vaccine caused fatal illness in 18 people, 4–13 days after the first vaccine dose. Vaccine virus was isolated from brains of victims and faulty vaccine batch. In South America in the 1960s, epidemiological and molecular evidence suggested that locally produced and inadequately inactivated *equine* vaccine for Venezuelan equine encephalitis virus had caused cases in horses and had spread to humans.
- Reversed attenuation (3908) is a very rare event reported for poliovirus vaccine.
- Comtaminants at production. Avian cell lines can introduce viruses from vertebrates, e.g., avian leukosis virus (ALV), filoviruses (5848), and SV40, and from humans, e.g., AdV, CMV, and HBV.

Avian retroviruses. ALV, endogenous avian retrovirus (EAV) (3515, 5782, 7586, 7971, 8141). In World War II, ALV likely contaminated yellow fever vaccine produced on chick embryos. Modern molecular methods detected viral genomes in brands of vaccines (including mumps virus, measles virus). However, ALV from avian cell lines was noninfectious, recipients tested negative for EAV, and neither replication nor harmful effects were demonstrated in recipients. **HBV.** In 1942, from pooled human sera used as stabilizer, lots of yellow fever vaccines became contaminated; ~50,000 of ~330,000 military recipients of contaminated lots were hospitalized with jaundice (5479). **SV40 (1001, 2212, 6386, 6798, 6886, 7200).** SV40 was discovered in 1960. In 1955–1963, simian cells were the source for SV40 in inactivated, commercial poliovaccine and a parenteral AdV vaccine; millions of recipients were potentially exposed to SV40. The concern was that SV40 could cause malignancies in recipients. However, virological evidence and large cohort and case-control studies did not support this assumption.

Bacteria

Ig. *C. tetani* (6230). In Hungary in 1950, a batch of pertussis immune serum became contaminated with tetanus toxin. According to official information released in 1997, 22 recipients contracted tetanus, and 11 died.

Vaccines. Errors of administration and bacterial contamination from handling or administration are hazards.

- Errors. Erroneous routes, doses, and vaccines have been reported. ***Bordetella* (588).** At a veterinary clinic, a child contracted *Bordetella bronchiseptica* infection from inadvertent exposure to a live aerosol veterinary vaccine (for "kennel cough") by an unrestful dog. ***Brucella* (312, 588).** In 1998–1999, 26 human exposures to live veterinary *Brucella* vaccine were reported, mainly through needle sticks, occasionally through mucosal splash. Antibiotics for postexposure prophytax is (PEP) curbed infections. ***C. diphtheriae* (6982).** In the United Kingdom in 1995, 102 school leavers received DT vaccine (high antigen dose for children), rather than dT vaccine (low dose for adults), an error that resulted in 20% excess absenteeism from school. ***M. tuberculosis* (297, 1228).** For tuberculin skin testing in the United States, ~100 patients erroneously received tetanus vaccine that mimicked positive skin reaction. Conversely, tuberculin was injected intramuscularly, as an erroneous substitute for vaccines. In a city in Iran, a nurse had the habit of administering HBV and BCG vaccines intramuscularly to newborns by the same syringe. As a result, 153 infants contracted *M. bovis* cold abscesses. BCG is an attenuated vaccine that in immune-impaired hosts could cause disseminated disease.
- Contamination from handling or delivery. Multidose vials, reused syringes, and skin flora are vehicles of agents, injection-site abscesses, and postvaccination BSI.
- Contaminants at production (774, 1377, 7169). Rare incidences include *Mycobacterium chelonae* in a lot of DTP-Polio vaccine and *S. pyogenes* in a lot of DTP vaccine in multidose vials. R. P. Strong, a graduate of Yale University with a medical degree from Johns Hopkins University, as head of Philippine Biological Laboratory in 1906 inoculated 24 inmates of Manila Central Prison with an experimental cholera vaccine contaminated by *Y. pestis*. All recipients fell ill and 13 died from plague. Strong did not publish the incident, continued to use prisoners in experiments, and despite investigations, in 1913 with the support of F. C. Shattuck was appointed head of the new department of tropical medicine at Harvard Medical School. Strong's story reminds us of the advancements manufacturing and ethics have made in the past century.

ANTIMICROBIALS AND NOSOCOMIAL DIARRHEA

Antimicrobials are substances used in vivo against multiplying viruses, bacteria, fungi, and protozoa, e.g., antiretrovirals, macrolides, β-lactams, tuberculostatics, and antimalarials. Disinfectants (550, 817, 4888) are substances with in vitro activity against microbes (cells, spores, and cysts) and for use on surfaces (skin and floors) and objects (instruments and machines), e.g., chlorine, ethanol, or iodine-tincture. No substances are available against prions.

Resistance is the persistence or multiplication of infectious agents despite adequate tissue concentration of an antimicrobial. Mechanisms can be innate (dormancy, capsule, thick cell wall, or biofilm) or acquired (mutation or gene transfer). Resistance is assayed in vitro and confirmed in vivo (pharmacokinetically and clinically).

Antimicrobial resistance (1230, 3115, 4553, 6521, 6637, 7836). A review is beyond the scope here. In brief, risks include recent exposure to antimicrobials, prolonged hospital stay, and stay in an ICU, and interfacility patient transfers. In Swiss acute-care hospitals in 2003, at a given day, nearly 25% of inpatients received antibiotics. Resistant agents can spread within and between institutions, and into the community.

Consequences of infections by resistant agents include "overgrowth" (flora imbalance) and diarrheal disease, nonresponsiveness and treatment failure, and overwhelming infection leading to death.

Unlike inpatients (Box 17.6 and Fig. 17.1) with difficult-to-treat MRSA, VRE, and multi-drug resistant (MDR) agents, the main concerns in outpatients are resistance to antiretrovirals (HIV), macrolides (*S. pneumoniae*), quinolones (*Campylobacter*, *N. gonorrhoeae*, *S. enterica* serovar Typhi), tuberculostatics (MDR *M. tuberculosis*), and antimalarials (*Plasmodium falciparum*). Judicious indications, revolving chemical classes, targeted admission screening, isolation of colonized or infected individuals, and surveillance can help to curb resistance.

Nosocomial diarrhea (101, 4212, 4519, 4940, 7990). Hospital-acquired diarrhea is defined by onset >48 h after admission. It ranks after UTI, SSI, BSI, and pneumonia as a frequent nosocomial infection. Reported attack rates per 100 hospital-days are 0.05–0.2 in patients and 0.05 in workers. Sources include overgrowing endogenous flora, roomed-in patients, and visitors. Vehicles include tap water, beverages, and foods from hospital kitchens or visitors. In large hospitals, maintaining foods at growth-inhibiting temperatures through long catering chains can be difficult. By facility, season, and age mix, reported major agents of nosocomial diarrhea are *Norovirus* (in ~50–60%), *Rotavirus* (in 1.5–18%), *C. difficile* (in 12–32%), and *Salmonella* (in 4–12%). In as much as 25% of outbreaks, a causative agent is not found. Long-stay facilities are several times more frequently venues for outbreaks than acute-care hospitals.

Antimicrobials (435, 462, 1716, 8230) are one cause of nosocomial diarrhea. By antimicrobial and underlying disease, 1–18% of patients develop treatment-attributable diarrhea. Virtually all classes of oral antibiotics have been incriminated. Diarrhea can be due to antimicrobial intolerance or to bacterial overgrowth. The implicated antibiotics should be discontinued at once, and stool samples should be tested for *C. difficile* and its toxins.

C. difficile **(435, 462, 801, 4212, 5477, 6521, 6859, 8230).** About 10–25% of CDAD is acquired, mainly from the hands of workers or patients (see section 17.1). However, a majority of CDAD results from antimicrobial pressure. In Sweden, the risk of CDAD was 1,300-fold higher in the hospital than in the community within the

---

Box 17.6 Antimicrobial resistance, by agent cluster

Prevalence is shown in parentheses. *Resistance in outpatients.

Droplet-air	*H. influenzae** (10–40% to amoxicillin), *Klebsiella* (10–40% ESβL), *M. tuberculosis** (1–13 MDR)
Feces-food	*Campylobacter** (10–30% to quinolones), *Enterobacter* (10–30% ESβL), *Enterococcus* (<1–40% VRE), *E. coli* (<1–6% ESβL), *P. mirabilis* (up to 16% ESβL), *Providencia stuartii* (up to 28% ESβL), *Salmonella** (20% to ampicillin, 0–10% to quinolones), *S. enterica* serovar Typhi* (20–35% to quinolones), *Shigella** (50–95% to co-trimoxazole)
Zoonotic	*P. falciparum** (30–80% to chloroquine, resistance to antifols and mefloquine increasing)
Environmental	*Acinetobacter*, *Pseudomonas* (20–30% ESβL)
Skin-blood	HIV*; *N. gonorrhoeae** (10–50% to quinolones), *S. aureus* (0.5–70% MRSA, emerging to vancomycin), *S. aureus** (0.5–3% MRSA), CoNS (40–90% to methicillin), *S. pneumoniae* (10–50% to penicillin, 10–30% to erythromycin); *Candida** (10% to azoles)

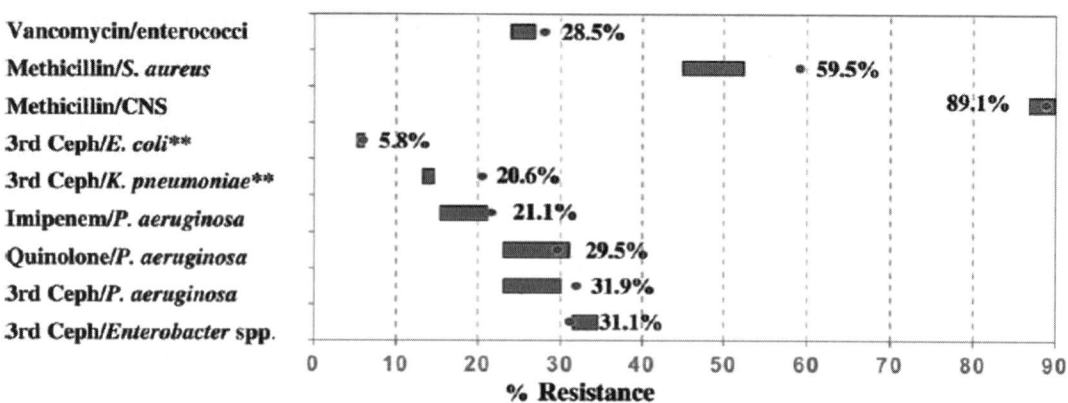

Figure 17.1 Nosocomial agents from ICU patients: resistance prevalence, United States, 1998–2003. Boxes represent standard deviations (1998–2002) and dots show 1-year prevalences (January to November 2003, >1,000 isolates /series). 3rd Ceph, expanded-spectrum cephalosporins. From reference 1230.

hospital catchment area. Concurrently, inpatients consumed 37 times more defined daily antibiotic doses than community members. Antibiotics frequently implicated in CDAD are β-lactam/anti-β-lactamase combinations, multiple antibiotics, cephalosporins (for a relative risk of 1.4–29 compared with no antibiotics), and in particular, clindamycin (for a relative risk of 16–42). Colonization may or may not predispose to CDAD. On follow-up for 1-3 weeks, 1% (2/192) of colonized patients and 4% (22/618) of noncolonized patients developed CDAD. Strains from carriers may or may not be toxigenic. Adults and children can contract CDAD.

17.7 HOSPITAL AIR, WATER, AND SURFACES

Nosocomial environments (6758) (Box 17.7). Air, water, wet cells, and surfaces are inanimate potential sources of nosocomial infections. Building maintenance, engineering of water supply, airflow, indoor climate, and managed cleaning and waste disposal are measures to minimize risks. For buildings, see section 6.2.

AIR IN NOSOHABITATS

Overview (101, 4406, 6758). Patients, workers, and visitors are animate sources of infectious droplets, secretions, or aerosols (Box 17.7). Unlike other nosocomial infections, spread of nosocomial respiratory agents is seasonal, reflecting circulation in the community. Air movements through doors, corridors, and elevator shafts can disperse aerosols and spores. Air quality and flow are of particular concern in crowded waiting rooms, operating rooms for clean surgery (low counts of airborne bacteria were shown to correlate with low sepsis rates in patients with prosthetic devices), negative-air-pressure rooms for respiratory isolation (e.g., VHF and tuberculosis), units for immune-impaired patients (hematology, oncology, dialysis, and transplantation), and reconstruction areas.

Viruses

Overview (101). In well-vaccinated communities, nosocomial spread of vaccine-preventable respiratory viruses (*Influenzavirus*, measles, mumps, and rubella [MMR], and VZV) is rare. Nosocomial spread is documented for AdV (keratoconjunctivitis and lower respiratory tract infection [RTI]) (5697), Epstein-Barr virus (EBV), *Influenzavirus*, PIV, parovirus 19 (PVB19), *Rhinovirus*, RSV (pediatric, oncology, and transplant units, via droplets or objects), measles virus, rubella virus, SARS-CoV, and VZV (by droplets or aerosols).

Influenzavirus **(101, 4696, 6550).** Spread of *Influenzavirus* is by droplets, hands, and perhaps aerosols. At least 17 hospital outbreaks were reported in 1959–1994, including acute-care hospitals (general, pediatric, and hematology units) and long-stay facilities. Rapid diagnosis by bedside antigen tests of community-acquired influenza in hospitalized children and adults is essential for the prevention of nosocomial spread. Neuraminidase inhibitors have an underevaluated potential for PEP in nosohabitats. High vaccine coverage among workers seems to reduce nosocomial spread among workers and patients.

Measles virus (1771, 1840, 4767, 8101). Measles can be acquired in hospitals, waiting rooms, and practice offices. In the United States in the 1980s, ~0.5–3% of measles cases were acquired nosocomially (about three fourths by patients or visitor and one fourth by workers). In The Netherlands in 1997, a girl from Indonesia with unrecognized measles later confirmed by virus isolation

> **Box 17.7** Agents from nosocomial droplets or aerosols (*) generated by subjects, currents, or wet sites
>
> **From air**
> - Viruses: vaccine preventable: *Influenzavirus*, measles,* rubella, smallpox (historical),* varicella;* vaccine nonpreventable: AdV, PIV, PVB19, *Rhinovirus*, RSV, and SARS-CoV
> - Bacteria: vaccine preventable: *B. pertussis, C. diphtheriae, H. influenzae* b, *M. tuberculosis**; vaccine nonpreventable: *M. catarrhalis, M. pneumoniae, Staphylococcus* (CoNS, MRSA), *S. pneumoniae*
> - Fungi: *Aspergillus,* Cladosporium,* Paecilomyces,* Penicillium*; Pneumocystis,* Rhodotorula,* Scedosporium**;
>
> **From wet sites**
> - Bacteria: *Acinetobacter,* Alcaligenes,* Aeromonas,* Burkholderia,** environmental mycobacteria,* *Legionella,* Nocardia,* Pseudomonas,* Serratia,* Stenotrophomonas**
> - Fungi: *Acremonium,* Aspergillus,* Exophiala,* Fusarium**
> - Protozoa: environmental amebas

was the source for measles in one worker and unequivocal, subclinical infection in one other worker. At a pediatric hospital in Johannesburg, South Africa, in 1999, a nosocomial outbreak affected 14 children. In Sfax, Tunisia, in 2002, despite high (>90%) vaccine coverage, an outbreak in the city hospital involved staff of several departments.

PVB19 (534, 4563). Chronically infected, immune-impaired patients are a source of PVB19. At a pediatric hospital in Philadelphia in 1988, two adolescents with sickle cell disease and aplastic crisis were sources for two nosocomial outbreaks of fifth disease among nursing staff, for attack rates of 36–38% among susceptible contacts.

Rubella virus (2439, 2769, 2917). Outbreaks have been reported in outpatient settings. At a large prenatal and family-planning clinic, an obstetrician and two other workers exposed 56 susceptible pregnant women.

SARS-CoV (2853, 7272). SARS-CoV can spread rapidly within and between hospitals. In Toronto, Canada, in 2003, the SARS outbreak was mainly nosocomial, with transmission in 58% (11) of acute-care hospitals. Of 23,103 contacts, most (70%, 16,149) required quarantine for exposure at hospitals, less (21%, 4,804) for community exposure (household, school, and work), and few (9%, 2,150) for exposure in practices. Timely and appropriate measures can control spread. Timely means detection and management of a source or outbreak within ≤1 incubation period, before secondary spread. Appropriate means isolating patients, quarantining exposed workers and visitors, and closing unaffected wards. If management is delayed, whole hospitals need to be closed, and complete lists of alls SARS contacts need to be generated in ≤48 h. In the Singapore 2003 outbreak, visitor records helped to identify individuals at risk of carrying SARS-CoV into the community.

Bacteria

Overview. In well-vaccinated communities, nosocomial spread of vaccine-preventable respiratory bacteria is rare. Nosocomial spread is documented for *B. pertussis, C. diphtheriae* (4568), *H. influenzae* (b, non-b) (7703), *L. pneumophila* (via aerosols; an air conditioner at an outpatient clinic was source for 103 cases) (5539), *Moraxella catarrhalis* (5194), *M. tuberculosis*, (via droplets or aerosols), *M. pneumoniae, Nocardia* (via dust aerosols) (6530, 8046), and *S. pneumoniae* (5724, 8026).

***B. pertussis* (478, 1433).** Spread is via droplets. Children and adults can be nosocomial sources. In a pediatric hospital in Cincinnati, measures to prevent introduction from the community included: triage of patients at the emergency unit, respiratory isolation of suspect cases, exclusion of some visitors (respiratory symptoms, children, to selected units), restricted in-hospital child care, PEP (macrolides) for exposed workers, and exclusion from work of exposed workers with cough illness.

***K. pneumoniae* (2656).** Although nosocomial clusters and outbreaks are well documented, mainly on neonatal ICUs and by strains that produce ESβL, respiratory spread is not confirmed.

M. tuberculosis. *M. tuberculosis* is a hazard to plan for in hospital *and* outpatient habitats.

- Outpatient habitats (718, 1034, 1598, 3296, 5171, 6997). Outbreaks that can last days to months and expose dozens of persons underscore the ease of spread in such settings. Index outpatients can infect workers and patients in waiting areas, including immune-impaired patients. Worker-to-patient spread is uncommon. Reported index workers include a dentist and a pediatrician. A smear- and culture-positive pediatrician had exposed 1,416 pediatric patients; follow-up identified 7 (0.5%) likely infected children but

no active cases. Facilities should have guidelines for lung function tests, sputum induction, and nebulizer treatment.
- Hospital habitats (1238, 2123, 8193). Hospital outbreaks have been reported, including of MDR strains among AIDS patients. At a U.S. community hospital in 2002, an index case was unrecognized for 3 weeks, and five secondary cases triggered tracing of 668 (two thirds of 1,045) contacts. On tracing, 23% (39/173) of contacts were skin test reactive (induration ≥5 mm), as were 32% (21/65) of workers nursing patients, 23% (6/26) of ward workers, and 7% (29/404) of other hospital workers. At a general hospital in Lima, Peru, tuberculosis disease prevalence was 13%. Among 40 sputum- and culture-positive inpatients, tuberculosis was not initially suspected in 13 (33%), although five (39%) of them had cough for 2 weeks or more, six (46%) were sputum smear-positive, and six (46%) grew MDR strains. Of the 27 initially suspect cases, 20 (74%) had chronic cough, 20 (74%) were smear positive, and 2 (7%) grew MDR strains.

***Mycoplasma* (1143, 3532).** Hospital outbreaks of *M. pneumoniae* have been documented. At a U.S. psychiatry hospital in V–X/1999, pneumonia due to *M. pneumoniae* affected 23% (60/257) of residents and 22% (82/372) of workers. PEP (azithromycin) reduced the disease rate but not oropharyngeal carriage rate. In Texas in 1993, 12% (215/4,500) of workers at a tertiary-care hospital contracted *M. pneumoniae* illness.

***Staphylococcus* (6711, 7391).** Although unusual, airborne spread of CoNS and MRSA seems possible. CoNS from 15 of 27 cardiac surgery patents and from air in the operating room were indistinguishable by pulsed-field gel electrophoresis and antibiotic resistance, suggesting an environmental source. At a head-and-neck surgery unit of a hospital in Amsterdam, The Netherlands, a single clone of MRSA caused 17 colonizations or infections; despite strict isolation, the outbreak continued for 7 months until filters of ultrasonic nebulizers were identified as the source. Environmental decontamination in addition to hand hygiene and isolation may be needed for outbreak control.

Fungi
Overview (2985, 3233, 4315, 4582, 5920, 7758).
Sources of fungal spores in hospital air include poorly filtered outside air, moist building materials, repair work, dust in air ducts and filters, and vacuum cleaning. On a hematology ward in Florence, Italy, fungal densities were 50 CFU/m^3 of air in rooms with neutropenia patients, 147 in hospital corridors, and 572 outside the building. Barriers (closed doors, barred windows, and no flower pots), air filters, and engineered flow are means to reduce spore density in hospital rooms.

Fungi identified in hospital air and air filters include *Pneumocystis*, yeast-like *Rhodotorula*, and molds such as *Aspergillus*, *Cladosporium*, *Paecilomyces*, *Penicillium*, and *Scedosporium*.

***Aspergillus* (3233, 4315, 7437).** Typical environmental sources are dust, moist structures, and construction work. However, at Rotterdam University Hospital, infected patients were an epidemiologically suspected source of conidia. **Air (291, 1882, 3436, 4315, 5920).** There apparently is little or no seasonal variation in density in air. Reported conidia concentrations in hospital air range broadly, from <1 to 2,000/m^3. In a new hospital in Chicago, mean concentrations of *A. flavus* and *A. fumigatus* in monthly air samplings increased in the 1980s, to reach 1 CFU/m^3 in 1987. In the same year the aspergillosis disease rate in immune-impaired patients reached 1.2%. Removal of contaminated air filters and improved maintenance in 1988–1990 reduced conidia concentration in air to 0.01 CFU/m^3 and disease rate to 0.3%. In Florence, Italy, in 1999–2000, *A. fumigatus* and *A. flavus* average densities were 6 CFU/m^3 from biweekly air samples outside and 1–4 CFU/m^3 inside the hospital.

Outbreaks Hospital outbreaks by *A. fumigatus* or *A. flavus* have been documented in North America, Asia, and West Europe.
- North America (286, 291, 4582, 7437). At a Texas tertiary hospital in X/2000 to II/2001, a contaminated operating room air system caused six *Aspergillus* infections. At a university hospital in Baltimore, pressure gradients, airflow into rooms, and close location to a stairwell door were hazards identified in an outbreak with 21 disease cases. Heavy growth on air filters were the source for the Chicago hospital outbreak mentioned earlier. On a renal transplant ward, a cluster of cases resulted from repair work on the next-higher floor that caused dust to filter down to the ward below.
- West Europe (3233, 4315). At a Belgium hospital, following an outbreak of *Aspergillus* disease in nine cardiac surgery patients, investigations suggested as source a restroom where stuffing and wood were moistened by water leakage; spores were likely dispersed along a lift shaft.

***Pneumocystis* (464, 5610).** DNA has been amplified from hospital air. In the United States, DNA suggestive of *P. carinii* was amplified in air samples from 55% (16/29) of hospital rooms occupied by patients with *Pneumocystis* pneumonia (PCP), 29% (4/14) of empty hospital rooms, 22% (2/9) of patients home bedrooms, and none (0/12) of office or storage rooms. In Sweden and France, air samples from five of seven rooms occupied by patients with PCP, two of four adjacent corridors, and 3 (19%) of 16 infectious disease wards amplified *P. jirovecii* DNA. Genotyping suggested person-to-person spread.

PCP outbreaks (1379, 3257) occurred on hospital units for children with malignancies, and transplantation units.

***Scedosporium* (2985).** Six inpatients with leukemia contracted fatal invasive *S. prolificans* disease from contaminated air in isolation rooms.

Protozoa

In Manchester, United Kingdom, *Acanthamoeba* was recovered from air inside of a hospital, at a concentration of 10–20 cysts/m^3 (436). *A. castellanii* is able to host *Legionella*.

HOSPITAL WATER AND WET HABITATS

It is exceptional for a water supply to be entirely free of aquatic organisms.

A. M. Emmerson (2202)

Overview (192, 2202, 7076). Sinks, drains, rarely used faucets or shower heads, dead-end tubes, and storage tanks can grow biofilms and become reservoirs for wet agents (Boxes 17.1 and 17.7) such as *B. cepacia*, *Legionella*, mycobacteria, *Pseudomonas*, *Serratia*, and *Stenotrophomonas*. Viruses, algae, and protozoa have also been detected in hospital water. Warm water temperatures enhance growth of algae.

Patients may consume hospital tap water. Humidifiers, nebulizers, and ventilators can disperse wet agents. Rinsing with tap water can contaminate instruments with waterborne agents. Water for physiotherapy is a source of *Pseudomonas* in burn patients. Infection risks from water delivery and neonatal baths are poorly known. Wet agents are a particular hazard for immune-impaired individuals.

Viruses

Viruses confirmed or suspected to be spread by hospital tap water include *Enterovirus*, HAV, HEV, *Norovirus*, and perhaps *Rotavirus* (101).

Bacteria

Ingestion of hospital water (4994, 6143). (For drinking water, see section 10.2.) Bacteria confirmed or suspected to be ingested from hospital tap water are *Campylobacter* and *Shigella*. At a hospital in Finland in 1986, 32 patients and 33 staff contracted *C. jejuni* diarrhea from the hospital's own water supply contaminated at an airing well. At a hospital laboratory in Rhode Island in 1996, a contaminated faucet handle was implicated in an *Shigella sonnei* outbreak that affected 6 (32%) of 19 technologists.

Droplets, aerosols, or contact with hospital water. Wet agents from inhalation or contact include *Burkholderia*, *Legionella*, environmental mycobacteria, *Pseudomonas*, *Serratia*, and *Stenotrophomonas*.

***Acinetobacter* (583, 2785, 3439, 7943).** *A. baumannii* is isolated from sinks, surfaces, and hospital air. A suspected mode of spread to patients is via droplets. Outbreaks demonstrated its potential for spread. Although colonized hands are a major vehicle, wet environments are a suspected alternative source.

***Burkholderia* (5346, 8371).** Both *B. cepacia* and *B. pseudomallei* have been cultured from drinking water. ***B. pseudomallei* (310, 3446).** *B. pseudomallei* resists usual levels of free chlorine, but nosocomial spread seems unusual. ***B. cepacia* (983, 6831, 6880).** *B. cepacia* has a niche in wet hospital environments. Although nosocomial outbreaks are well recorded, sources often remain obscure. In an ICU in 1997–1999, *B. cepacia* was isolated from 31 adults without cystic fibrosis, and from 3% (6/200) of environmental samples; a common source was not identified, and patient-to-patient spread was suspected. Confirmed vehicles include nebulizer solution and mouthwash (see section 17.6).

***Clostridium* (2703).** Spores of *C. difficile* can persist in the environment, and contaminated bath tubs are a suspected nosocomial source.

***Klebsiella* (5948).** Although *Klebsiella* can be recovered from wet environments, and numerous nosocomial outbreaks have been studied microbiologically, sources are infrequently investigated, and knowledge of modes of spread is inadequate.

***Legionella*.** Although duped a hospital agent, *Legionella* is widespread in outpatient habitats.

- Outpatient waters (329, 427, 1292, 4558, 8372). About 25–60% of water samples from outpatient departments yield *Legionella*. In dental offices, *L. pneumophila* and other *Legionella* spp. have been identified in water from taps, oral rinsing cups, and dental equipment, e.g., ultrasonic scaler, and turbine.
- Hospital waters (610, 765, 1747, 2202, 2394, 3751, 4006, 4051, 5839, 7149). Hot tap water ("comfort" temperature is 25–40°C) and stagnant waters in dead-end pipes are major sources of *Legionella* and nosocomial outbreaks, before cooling towers. By sampling and test, 10–85% of hospital waters yield *Legionella* spp., including *L. pneumophila* (e.g., serogroups 1, 5, and 6). In the United States, allowable water temperatures in hospitals are typically regulated at 37–55°C,

but *L. pneumophila* can be isolated from tap water at temperatures that range from 40 to 67° C. An outbreak in a Swedish hospital was ended, and *L. pneumophila* was eliminated from more than three fourths of wards when hot-water temperature was raised from 45°C to 65°C and kept at ≥60°C. Ideally, water should not be allowed to stagnate, should circulate at <20°C or >60°C, and storage tanks and calorifiers should be inspected regularly.

- Spread (427, 700, 849, 1747, 7076, 7149). Likely modes of nosocomial spread are inhalation *and* aspiration. Modes could be obscured by the better health of patients who shower than of bedridden patients who cannot shower but are prone to aspiration. Respirators, ventilators, humidifiers, ice machines, tap-water faucets, and shower heads are all potential sources of wet aerosols in hospitals. In an outbreak at a Swedish hospital in 1990–1991 with 31 pneumonia cases, 17 of 20 hot-water supplies grew *L. pneumophila* serogroup 1, and aerosols from shower nozzles were the suspected source.
- Impact (1049, 3129, 3751, 4006, 4051, 4348, 5630, 8094). Urine tests have markedly increased the recognition of nosocomial *L. pneumophila* serogroup 1 cases. By setting, endemicity, and time, 3–24% of nosocomial pneumonias are attributable to *Legionella*, and 10–35% of legionellosis cases are nosocomial. In New York hospitals, the legionellosis case rate was 1/100 discharges. Among patients at risk (solid organ or hematopoietic stem cell recipients), attack rates can reach 17–32%.
- Outbreaks (765, 1747, 3129, 3751, 4006, 5630, 6024) are well-documented in hospitals, including medical departments, ICU, and transplantation units (4370). In Europe in 2000–2002, of 189 reported *Legionella* outbreaks, 19% (36) were nosocomial, with an average of six cases per outbreak.

Mycobacteria (2042, 3853, 7076, 7868). Hospital tap water and shower heads, in particular, hot water, can yield rapid growers (*M. abscessus*, *M. chelonae*, and *M. fortuitum*) and slow growers (e.g., *M. avium*, *M. gordonae*, *M. intracellulare*, *M. kansasii*, and *M. scrofulaceum*).

- *M. fortuitum* (995, 2684, 3853, 4170, 4250). During an outbreak of *M. fortuitum* in 1989–1990, 16 patients on a rehabilitation ward became colonized; epidemiological and microbiological evidence suggested a ward shower as the source. Showerheads were the implicated source in disseminated *M. fortuitum* disease in a leukemia patient. In U.S. hospitals, ice machines were implicated in three outbreaks with 19, 30, and 47 colonized individuals, respectively; in one outbreak, cases and machine grew indistinguishable *M. fortuitum* strains.
- *M. avium* complex (MAC) (2042, 7490, 7868). MAC disease in HIV-infected patients has been linked to the hot-water supply in hospitals. At a Boston hospital, 14 (41%) of 34 water taps yielded MAC, including 11 of 16 hot-water taps with average water temperatures of 55°C and concentrations of up to 500 CFU/100 ml. Test-positive sites included heated nebulizer reservoirs, ice machines, hot and cold drinking-water faucets, sprays from toilets and utility room sinks, bedside drinking-water carafes, and water fountains.
- Impact (323, 572, 5016, 7002). Environmental mycobacteria have been associated with sporadic cases, outbreaks, and pseudooutbreaks, from instruments or containers that were in contact with contaminated tap water

***Pseudomonas* (2965, 3439, 5211).** *P. aeruginosa* grows well in faucets, shower heads, sinks, drains, flower vases, nebulizers, dental water-conducting systems, and other moist nosocomial habitats. Faucets are a reservoir. In a neonatal ICU, tap water from several faucets repeatedly grew *P. aeruginosa*, while faucets on adjacent wards supplied by the same water system grew different genotypes, and samples from the main supply tested negative.

- Sources (607, 1008, 2367, 2685, 3439, 5160, 5289). As *P. aeruginosa* is part of flora, how the environment contributes to nosocomial spread can be difficult to determine. *P. aeruginosa* in cystic fibrosis patients is suspected to almost always have environmental sources. Several reports have implicated tap water as a source of *P. aeruginosa* hospital outbreaks. Water bath to warm fresh frozen plasma and human albumin for infusion was the source for four colonized or infected neonates. A potential confounder are hands of health workers contaminated from tap or bath water. During an outbreak in a neonatal ICU, *P. aeruginosa* was indeed isolated from the hands of 3/104 health workers.
- Prevention (2685). Means to limit nosocomial spread include isolation of infected patients, hand hygiene, equipment maintenance, and hygienic disposal of sputum.

***Serratia* (264, 1016, 3273, 7226, 7297, 7863).** Sinks, urine bottles, and other moist habitats are reported inanimate sources of *S. marcescens* in hospitals.

- Living sources (1016, 1852, 6618, 7721) Patients are a significant source, and hands of patients and workers are major means of spread. *S. marcesens* can be recovered from inpatients: in 2–60% from the throat, in 0–40% from feces, and in 0–20% from urine. Readmission of carriers is a suspected source of epidemic strains.
- Outbreaks (786, 1852, 3149, 3263, 3273, 4010, 7226, 7297, 7821). Many hospital outbreaks are documented,

including on general wards, ICU, neurology, oncology, and transplantation units. Agents were *S. marcescens* and *S. liquefaciens*. Implicated sources or vehicles included colonized patients and workers, and contaminated equipment and medications.

Stenotrophomonas (1821, 1859, 6373, 6539, 7076, 7811, 8225). *S. maltophilia* is an opportunist that exploits wet niches, including water faucets, faucet aerators, sinks, suction catheters, spirometers, serviceable parts of ventilators, and plastic surfaces of intravascular and other devices. Contaminated rinsing water can cross-contaminate instruments or machines. In Australia in 1973–1974, *S. maltophilia* in deionized water used for diluting disinfectant concentrate (savlon, a mixture of chlorhexidine, and cetrimide) caused 7 infections and 56 colonizations. *S. maltophilia* in tap water used to wash preterm infants led to respiratory colonization in four, and sepsis and death in one infant. For removal of vernix and blood from delivery, preterm babies better be washed than bathed.

Fungi
Fungi that can occupy moist niches in hospital environments include the filamentous fungi *Acremonium*, *Aspergillus*, *Exophiala*, and *Fusarium*.

Acremonium (7928). *Acremonium* colonized humidifier water in an office in which cases of endophthalmitis occurred.

Aspergillus (291, 4231, 7758, 7967). Potential wet sources include aerosolized hospital water, soil in flower pots, and moistened dust. At the university hospital in Oslo, Norway, genotypes of *A. fumigatus* from water, air, and patients suggested that water was a source of spores in addition to air.

Exophiala (5496). In Rio de Janeiro in 1996–1997, 19 cases of fungemia due to *E. jeanselmei* were traced to contaminated, deionized pharmacy water used to prepare antiseptic solution; the fungus was also cultured from a water tank and a sink.

Fusarium (191). In a U.S. university hospital, *Fusarium* was recovered from 57% (162/283) of water-system samples; 88% (72/92) of sink drains yielded *F. solani*, 16% (12/71) sink faucet aerators and 8% (2/26) shower heads yielded *F. oxysporum*. Aerosolization was documented after running the showers. Of 20 cancer patients infected with *F. solani*, two had isolates that matched environmental isolates, and four had isolates that matched other patient isolates; curiously, matching pairs were recovered at intervals of five months to 5.5 years.

Protozoa
Free-living amebas (2202, 4155, 5028, 7844). Free-living amebas such as *Acanthamoeba*, *Hartmannella*, and *Naegleria* thrive in stagnant waters at ambient temperatures. Free-living amebas have been recovered from tap water in a new hospital, from water in dental and dialysis units, and from gastrointestinal washings. Because free-living amebas can harbor *Legionella*, mycobacteria, and *P. aeruginosa*, they are suspected to maintain intracellular bacteria in wet habitats.

HOSPITAL SURFACES
Nosocomial agents can be detected on linen, mattresses, bedrails, gowns, clothes, floors, walls, and hospital kitchen surfaces. However, presence of nosocomial agents proves neither persistence nor source function. From surfaces, agents can contaminate hands or become aerosolized, e.g., from walking or mopping.

Viruses
Surfaces (171, 1362, 3439, 4744, 7194) can hold several viruses (survival period), including HBV from blood, HPV from skin, *Norovirus* (up to 12 days on carpets) and *Rotavirus* from stools, and *Influenzavirus* (24–48 h), PIV (6–10 h on clothes), RSV (6 h on objects), SARS-CoV (24–72 h on objects) from droplets. In STI clinics, and at a leisure and fitness center for hospital workers, HPV was amplified by NAT from patient beds, colposcope handle, examination lamp, toilet flush handle, door handle, and light switch.

Bacteria
Bacteria (3439) get to surfaces from excretions, secretions, hands, and dust. *A. baumannii* has been isolated from beds, mattresses, and the linen of colonized patients, sinks, paper towel dispensers, cupboards, door handles, room humidifiers, and floors. Similarly, *P. aeruginosa* has been isolated from beds, mattresses, and towel racks. MRSA survives on plastic surfaces for 2 days. Although it is widespread in some hospital areas, e.g., burn units, however, the epidemiological significance of MRSA on surfaces is questionable, and spread from surfaces to patients has not been confirmed. Evidence for surfaces as bacterial reservoirs is good for *C. difficile* and VRE.

C. difficile (4856, 4897). Spores are durable and widespread in nosohabitats. Hospital floors can remain contaminated for up to 5 months. A likely infection chain is from surface to hands of workers and further to patients. In Seattle, Wash., hospital rooms occupied by patients with CDAD more often yielded *C. difficile* (49%) than rooms occupied by carriers (8%). In St. Louis, Mo., disinfecting rooms with hypochlorite (NaOC) instead of quaternary ammonium decreased rates of CDAD in hematopoietic stem cell recipients from 0.9 to 0.3/100 patient-days. By reverting to quaternary ammonium, rates returned to 0.8/100 patient-days.

VRE (6152, 8044). VRE is widespread in nosocomial habitats, in particular, in the surroundings of colonized patients who are incontinent or have diarrhea, e.g., on bed linen. VRE survives well on surfaces under dry conditions for 1 week to 4 months. *Enterococcus* survival seems independent from species (*E. faecalis* or *E. faecium*), source (patient or environment), or susceptibility to vancomycin (sensitive or resistant). On contact, VRE is readily transferred from surfaces to (gloved) hands. Spread environment-to-patient, environment-to-worker, and worker-to-patient are all likely.

Fungi

Fungi can contaminate surfaces through spores in air.

Candida **(3439) (7539, 7783).** Evidence shows that surfaces are a reservoir. *C. albicans* survives on glass for 3 days, on cotton for 14 days. *C. parapsilosis* survives on both surfaces for 14 days. By experimental deposit, *C. albicans* survives on human skin for ≤1 h. Object-to-patient spread is suspected for *C. glabrata*.

17.8 VIRAL HEMORRHAGIC FEVERS IN HOSPITALS

Hemorrhagic fevers (101, 1260, 1649, 2037) (Table 17.2). Hemorrhagic fevers are febrile illnesses with signs of spontaneous bleeding, including into skin (petechiae and purpura), epistaxis, melaena, and (micro)hematuria. Causative bacteria include mainly *N. meningitidis* but also invasive or vasculotropic bacteria such as rickettsiae, *S. enterica* serovar Typhi, and *Y. pestis*.

Here, the focus is on viruses (viral hemorrhagic fevers [VHF]). Causative viruses are from four families: *Arenaviridae*, *Bunyaviridae*, *Filoviridae*, and *Flaviviridae*. VHFs are suspected in malaria-negative patients returning within ≤21 days from visits to infected areas. An exposure history of contact with inpatients or their secretions, or of encounters with wild mammals, mainly rodents, monkeys or bats is supportive. In the latter case, rabies should also be considered (see section 1.1). VHF are confirmed by NAT, culture, and serology from throat washings, urine, blood, and CSF. Tests must be performed in biosafety level 3–4 laboratories (see section 12.6).

Spread (101, 776, 1649, 6299, 7321, 8224) (Table 17.2). Person-to-person spread is confirmed for *Arenaviridae*, *Filoviridae*, and *Nairovirus* (Crimean-Congo hemorrhagic fever virus [CCHFV]) of *Bunyaviridae*. Among remaining *Bunyaviridae*, interpersonal spread is suspected for *Hantavirus* and uncertain for *Phlebovirus* (Rift Valley fever virus [RVFV]). Exposure includes inhalation (droplets or aerosols from patients or women in labor), inoculation (injury with viremic blood or mucosal splash), and ingestion (unprotected hands in physical contact with patients, beddings, excretions, and corpses).

Prevention (327, 1649, 5361, 8224). Referral hospitals should have plans for confirmation, isolation, and management of VHF cases. Suspected patients should be repatriated by dedicated rescue aircraft, admitted to a high-security referral hospital isolation rooms by direct-circuit (bypassing emergency rooms), and nursed by trained, specially assigned workers. Recommendations for patient care (barrier nursing) include standard precautions (see section 12.6) and close-fitting filter mask, water-tight apron, and goggles for personal protection. For funeral and burial, close contact with bodies should be avoided. Contacts and caregivers should be traced to interrupt infection chains and identify infective sources.

ARENAVIRIDAE

Arenaviridae that cause VHF are Lassa virus in the Old World (perhaps the best known), and in the New World Guanarito virus (GUAV, agent of Venezuelan VHF), Junin virus (JUNV, agent of Argentinian VHF), Machupo virus (MACV, agent of Bolivian VHF), and Sabiá virus (agent of Brazilian VHF).

Lassa virus (339, 2420, 3248, 5136). Lassa fever emerged in 1969–1972, in hospitals in West Africa. The first cases known were nurses and physicians. Of 114 cases reported in 1969–1975, more than one third were acquired in hospitals from person-to-person spread. In two outbreaks in Nigeria that caused 34 cases and 22 (65%) deaths, included were six nurses, two surgeons, and one physician. Nosocomial spread was supported by lack of material and knowledge, sharing of syringes, and little protection during emergency surgery and nursing. High-risk exposures include percutaneous injury, mucosal splash from secretions or blood, and unprotected physical contact with patients. Low-risk exposures include protected work (patient care and cleaning), sharing a room with a patient, or sitting within coughing distance (1–2 m) from patients. High infectivity in hospitals contrasts with low infectivity in the community. Indeed, standard precautions and barrier nursing are considered adequate means to prevent nosocomial spread.

BUNYAVIRIDAE

Viruses from *Hantavirus* (Hantaan virus [HTNV], Seoul virus [SEOV], and Puumala virus [PUUV]), *Nairovirus*

Table 17.2 Nosocomial transmission of viral hemorrhagic fevers[a]

Family	Genus or species	Modes of spread			PEP[b]
		Human to human	Droplet	Other	
Arenaviridae	Guaranito, Junin, Machupo, and Sabiá viruses	Yes		Injury,[c] aerosol, contact, rodents in buildings	Ribavirin
	Lassa virus	Yes	Yes	Injury, aerosol, contact, rodents in buildings	Ribavirin
Bunyaviridae	CCHFV	Yes	(Likely)	Injury, (aerosol), contact, (ticks on patients)	(Ribavirin)
	Hantavirus	Yes	(Likely)	Injury, (aerosol), contact, rodents in buildings	Ribavirin
	RVFV	Yes	?	Injury, (aerosol, contact), mosquitoes in buildings	(Ribavirin)
Filoviridae	*Ebolavirus, Marburgvirus*	Yes	Yes	Injury, aerosol, contact	
Flaviviridae	Dengue virus	Mostly no	No	Injury, mosquitoes in buildings	
	Omsk hemorrhagic fever virus	Mostly no	No	Injury, (ticks on patients)	
	Kyasanur Forest disease virus	Mostly no	No	Injury, (ticks on patients)	
	Yellow fever virus	Mostly no	No	Injury, mosquitoes in buildings	

[a]Parentheses indicate that the evidence is unconfirmed.
[b]PEP, postexposure prophylaxis.
[c]Injury, contact of broken skin with viremic blood.

(CCHFV, agent of Congo-Crimean hemorrhagic fever), and *Phlebovirus* (RVFV, agent of Rift Valley fever) can all cause VHF. HTNV and SEOV are associated with hemorrhagic fever with renal syndrome. PUUV is the agent of epidemic nephropathy, causing (micro)hematuria. In contrast, New World hantaviruses such as Sin Nombre virus (SNV) are associated with cardiopulmonary rather than hemorrhagic manifestations. Of all *Bunyaviridae*, CCHFV has the greatest potential for nosocomial spread.

CCHFV (166, 327, 2419). Nosocomial transmission seems largely limited to infective blood; data are insufficient to support spread by aerosols. The following instances illustrate variability of nosocomial exposure. In Pakistan in 2002, a nurse acquired fatal CCHF after mouth-to-mouth resuscitation of a patient, and contact with his blood and vomit. A physician who performed gastric lavage on the same patient, without wearing face or eye protection, also contracted CCHF, but recovered with ribavirin therapy. In Pakistan in 1994, none of 50 health workers exposed to CCHF patients seroconverted, including four whose skin was exposed to secretions, and 16 who had skin-skin contacts. In South Africa in 1986, 2% (1/61, a laboratory technician) exposed workers were seroreactive, compared with none (0/67) of control health workers.

Outbreaks (128, 166, 327, 993, 6976, 6843, 7243). Nosocomial outbreaks occurred in Asia and Africa, in Pakistan in 2002 (three cases, one primary, two secondary), in 2000, in 1994 (three cases), and in 1976 (ten cases), in Dubai in 1979 (five cases), in Iraq in 1979 (two cases), and in South Africa in 1984 (seven cases).

FILOVIRIDAE

Both Old World filoviruses, *Ebolavirus* (EBOV) and *Marburgvirus* (MARV), are well-publicized causes of VHF.

***Ebolavirus* (3913, 5288, 8115).** Nosocomial spread of EBOV is a risk in hospitals that do not implement isolation and barrier nursing. Exposure includes blood and secretions, suctioning and mucosal splash, invasive procedures such as placing intravenous lines, even contact with soiled clothes and linen. Control measures include rapid identification and isolation of patients, barrier nursing for health workers and family members who nurse patients, and rapid burial of corpses by trained teams.

Outbreaks (8098). In outbreaks in Sudan in 1976 and Congo (ex-Zaire) in 1995, overall attack rates were 25–44%, and 33–50% of cases were health workers or caregivers. Nosocomial cases were also reported in later outbreaks in Uganda in 2000–2001 and in Gabon in 2001–2002.

***Marburgvirus* (2683, 4780, 5361, 8384).** In Marburg, Germany, in the 1967 outbreak, 16% (5/31) of cases were health workers. Nosocomial cases were also reported in outbreaks in South Africa (in 1975), Kenya (in 1980 and 1987), and Congo (ex-Zaire, in 1999–2000), for an overall occupational risk of 4% (5/130). The outbreak in Angola in 2005 with >270 cases was sparked in a pediatric ward of a provincial hospital.

FLAVIVIRIDAE

Cosmopolitan denguevirus (DENV) has the greatest impact of all VHF, by causing dengue hemorrhagic fever (DHF) and dengue shock syndrome (DSS). Other flaviviridae that cause VHF include Kyasanur Forest disease virus (KFDV), Omsk hemorrhagic fever virus (OHFV), and yellow fever virus (YFV).

Because *Flaviviridae* are arthropod-borne (see chapter 4), there is no risk for person-to-person spread by contact. However, accidental exposures and experimental infections have shown that percutaneous or transmucosal transmission can occur (without vectors) (1366). Health workers should wear gloves when removing potentially infective ticks or ectoparasites from patients. Hospitals located in transmission areas should be mosquito proofed.

RHABDOVIRIDAE

Rabies virus (101, 6216). Infective saliva from patients with unrecognized rabies (e.g., encephalitis) could expose health workers to the virus. High-risk exposure should prompt evaluation for PEP, e.g., coughed-up saliva from confirmed rabies patients in ICU or from cultured virus for production of vaccine.

18 Invasive Procedures

18.1 Instantly invasive procedures
18.2 Intravascular devices and bloodstream infections
18.3 Surgical site and wound infections
18.4 Transfusions
18.5 Transplants
18.6 Implants
18.7 Dialysis
18.8 Intensive care

18.1 INSTANTLY INVASIVE PROCEDURES

Instantly invasive are procedures that break through natural barriers for moments only, e.g., piercing, injection, and venipuncture.

Exposure (Box VI.1). Instantly invasive procedures are widely performed in nosocomial settings. The history should address injection drug use, rituals (e.g., piercing, tattooing, and circumcision), cosmetic procedures (e.g., shaving and pedicure), alternative care (e.g., acupuncture), outpatient care (e.g., dental, preventive, and medical), and hospital care.

Infections (1220, 2039, 5113, 5115) (Box 18.1). Agents from instantly invasive procedures range broadly and include skin and enteric flora and blood-borne agents.

Prevention (1220, 2039, 5113, 5115). A universal goal is to minimize risks, including from prions, hepatitis B virus (HBV), hepatitis C virus (HCV), human immunodeficiency virus (HIV), and nosocomial agents. Measures to achieve this include judicious indications and exposure avoidance, education of the public and health workers, clean working spaces, sustained and affordable supply and use of disposable materials, standard precautions (see section 12.6), proper collection of materials and instruments for safe disposal, decontamination or incineration, and surveillance.

For prion prevention, high risks should be considered *before* intervention (Table 14.1). Decontaminating instruments from prions requires three steps: cleansing (mechanical and manual), immersion (in NaOH or NaOCl for 1 h) and rinsing, then heat (best 134°C for 1 h).

INFECTIONS FROM RITUAL AND COSMETIC PROCEDURES

Tattooing is a procedure to apply color particles under the skin. Piercing is a procedure to penetrate body parts and place metallic ornaments.

Exposure (4682, 5278, 6443, 6573, 7623). By sex, group, and geography, tattoos and piercings are prevalent in 1–80% of adults, with highs in military personnel, street youths, injection drug users (IDUs), and inmates of prisons. Of 437 street youths in Montreal, Canada, in 1995–1996, 57% had tattoos and 78%

> **Box 18.1** Agents and infections from monmentous invasions, by agent cluster
>
> Risks are shown in parentheses.
>
> Feces-food   Anaerobes (injection, cosmetic), *Proteus* (podiatry)
> Zoonotic   Viral hemorrhagic fevers (injection)
> Environmental   Environmental mycobacteria (cosmetic, acupuncture, injection, and subcutaneous infusion), *Pseudomonas* (cosmetic and acupuncture), *Serratia* (cosmetic), tetanus (ritual, cosmetic, acupuncture, and injection); *Sporothrix* (cosmetic)
> Skin-blood   HBV, HCV, HIV, HPV (cosmetic), molluscum contagiosum (cosmetic); abscess (cosmetic, acupuncture, and injection), endocarditis (cosmetic, acupuncture, and dental); *Mycobacterium leprae* (tattoo), *S. aureus*, *S. pyogenes*

had piercings. In Washington State in 1999–2001, of 305 incarcerated youths, 33% had tattoos and 53% had piercings. Of 774 of IDUs in New Mexico, in 1995–1997, 75% had tattoos; of tattoos, about one half were self-made or made by friends and about one third were made in jail. In Australia in 1998, in a random sample of 10,000 persons ≥14 years of age, the lifetime prevalence was 10% for tattoo, 7% for pierced body, and 32% for pierced ears.

Viruses

HBV. HBV infections are a hazard of ritual and cosmetic procedures. **Ritual risks (832, 4970, 5443, 6573, 7623).** Ritual risks include piercing and tattooing. In Italy in 1985–1993, ear piercing and tattooing were significant risks in 6,395 reported hepatitis B cases when compared with 4,789 acute hepatitis A cases. Infection prevalence is significantly higher in tattooed than tattoo-free individuals, and HBV marker prevalence increases with increasing numbers of tattoos. By case mix, up to 10–20% of tattooed persons can be hepatitis B surface antigen (HBsAg)-positive. **Cosmetic risks (3715, 4970, 6829) (cosmetic hepatitis).** Poor practices at cosmetic parlors put clients and workers at risk. In Italy in 1985–1993, HBV risks included visits to podiatrists (foot care), manicurists (nail care), or barbers (for shaving). In a city of Hubei Province, People's Republic of China, in 1986, the HBsAg prevalence was 17% (53/316) in healthy barbers compared with 9% (29/316) in control department store workers. In urban Canada, manicurists and pedicure technicians of 72 randomly selected parlors were interviewed; most reported reusing instruments and not adhering to standard precautions; 40% (29/72) reported to be vaccinated against HBV.

HCV (3082, 3242, 4015, 5278, 5443, 6573, 7249). Tattooing and body and ear piercing are infection risks identified in a majority of epidemiological studies. Like HBV, HCV infection prevalence is significantly higher in tattooed than tattoo-free individuals, and seroreactivity increases with increasing numbers of tattoos. By case mix, 20–65% of tattooed persons can be seroreactive. In Victoria, Australia, in 2001, 35% (62/177) of inmates not having a tattoo tested positive for anti-HCV, compared with 67% (294/439) of inmates with tattooes, for an odds ratio of 3.8 (95% confidence interval [95% CI] 2.6–5.5). Inmates tattooed while in prison were more often (81%) reactive than inmates tattooed outside of prison (50%), for an odds ratio of 4.4 (95% CI 2.6–6.8). In People's Republic of China, three women 21–26 years of age contracted acute hepatitis C 45–60 days after fashionable tattooing of their eyebrows and eyelids. The reported practice in beauty parlors was use of nondisposable needles disinfected with 70% alcohol.

HIV (832, 5443, 7623). HIV infection is a suspected complication of piercing or tattooing. In Brazil in 1998–2000, 16% (28/182) tattooed persons were HIV positive.

Human papillomavirus (HPV) (833, 5858). Cosmetic removal of hairs by electrolysis has been reported to spread skin warts in a client. A man was reported to develop multiple skin warts, which were confined to a tattoo 2.5 years after tattooing by a professional. The area had been wart-free but was irritated by sunburn.

Molluscum contagiosum virus (6241). Cosmetic removal of hairs by electrolysis (thermolysis) was reported to disseminate the agent on skin, causing ~200 papules at thighs, genital, and abdomen.

Bacteria

Risks from nonsterile ritual or cosmetic invasive procedures include soft-tissue infections (107) (2447), abscesses, endocarditis, and syphilis (5443). The incidence of earlobe infection from piercing can reach 11–24%. Causative agents include skin flora and wet agents.

Soft-tissue infections. Mycobacteria. Environmental mycobacteria are a risk for ritual and cosmetic procedures.

- Tattoo (2717). In India in 16 years, 31 individuals developed leprosy over tattoo marks.
- Podiatry (8045, 8220). At a California nail salon in 2000, 110 customers developed furunculosis after whirlpool footbaths and shaving of the legs with a razor before pedicure; cultures from 32 patients and 10 footbaths grew *M. fortuitum*. In 1988, *M. chelonae* foot infections were diagnosed in eight persons who underwent invasive procedures at a podiatry office; the source was distilled water in a reusable, nonsterilized container for holding a lidocain jet injector.
- Cosmetic surgery (2246) (524, 4000, 5016). In the United States in 2004, *M. abscessus* infections were reported in 12 individuals who had undergone liposuction and abdominoplasty (tummy tuck) in the Dominican Republic. *M. fortuitum* and *M. chelonae* had previously been reported from liposuction or other cosmetic surgery. Of 82 patients who had liposuction by a single practitioner, 34 (41%) contracted cutaneous abscesses, and 12 (15%) grew *M. chelonae*. The likely vehicle was rinsed surgical equipment, and *M. chelonae* was isolated in biofilm from the office tap-water system.

***Proteus* (6484).** An outbreak of *P. mirabilis* infections from ambulatory podiatric surgery was traced to a contaminated bone drill. ***Pseudomonas* (3876).** In Oregon in 2000, ear piercing at a jewelry kiosk was associated with an outbreak of auricular *P. aeruginosa* chondritis. Of 118 individuals with 186 piercings, 18 (15%) had signs of infection (drainage of pus or blood for ≥14 days), and 7 (6%) grew *P. aeruginosa*. Upper ear (cartilage) piercing was more likely to result in infection than ear lobe piercing. The vehicle was a refilled atomizer bottle that grew *P. aeruginosa* and from which ears were misted with disinfectant before applying a piercing gun. ***Serratia* (8168).** Nondisposable instruments can be a source. At a cardiac surgery unit, 10 males contracted *S. marcescens* surgical-site infections; the source was preoperative shaving by a team of barbers. ***Staphylococcus aureus* (520, 6457).** Instruments can be a vehicle of *S. aureus*, including methicillin-resistant *S. aureus* (MRSA). Cosmetic body shaving increased the risk of MRSA-infected abrasions in football players. At a hospital hairdresser's, an epidemic MRSA strain was recovered from the equipment, a finding that suggested spread by unclean instruments.

Endocarditis (107, 5549, 6089, 7568, 8013). Endocarditis is a serious complication of nonsterile procedures. Endocarditis has been reported from piercing of nose, tongue, nipple, and naval. Recovered agents have included flora of skin or mucous membranes, and unusual *Haemophilus aphrophilus* from tongue piercing.

Fungi
In Detroit, Mich., hair removal by electrolysis spread *Sporothrix schenckii* on the skin of a patient with sporotrichosis (1942).

INFECTIONS FROM ALTERNATIVE CARE
Acupuncture involves the insertion of needles at particular sites. Autohemotherapy involves the injection of one's own blood, after mixing with saline. Reported complications of acupuncture include pneumothorax and spinal cord injury (8322).

Viruses
HBV. Acupuncture (3895, 4017, 7212, 7927, 8322). Infection clusters or outbreaks from acupuncture have been reported in North America, West Europe, and Japan. In Rhode Island in 1984, an acupuncturist by reusing needles caused 35 HBV infections among 316 clients, for a rate of 11%. **Autohemotherapy (7995).** At an alternative-medicine clinic in London in 1997–1998, 53 HBV infections had autohemotherapy as the common source, likely from contaminated saline. HBV marker rates increased with increasing visits, from 11% (21/194 exposed patients) for 1–4 visits, to 20% (17/84) for 5–9 visits, and 41% (15/37) for ≥10 visits.

HCV. Acupuncture is a risk borne out in several studies (950, 3977, 6585, 6862). In Peru, a history of acupuncture doubled the risk of HCV seropositivity. In Japan, of 262 HCV infections, 87 (33%) were attributed to past transfusions and 106 (40%) were attributed to past acupuncture. Also in Japan, besides acupuncture, vacuum therapy (folk medicine for relief of myocongestion) was a risk.

HIV (7849). Acute HIV infection following acupuncture has been reported.

Bacteria
Risks from nonsterile, alternative care invasive procedures include soft-tissue infections, tetanus, and bacteremia or endocarditis by agents such as *Propionibacterium*, *P. aeruginosa*, and *S. aureus* (2228, 6799).

***Clostridium tetani* (5792).** In Italy in 1998–2000, for 94 tetanus cases, known sources were in three fourths (72) injuries (lacerations, bruises, and cuts), and in an amazing one fourth (22) acupuncture.

Mycobacteria (8255). Three months after acupuncture for osteoarthritis, a woman developed chronic *M. chelonae* infection at the injection site.

INFECTIONS FROM DENTAL CARE

Oral flora is rich (see section 14.1), including viruses, commensal bacteria, *Streptococcus pneumoniae* (in up to 25% of people), *S. pyogenes* (in 5–10%), and *Candida albicans*. Oral flora is relevant for the interpretation of laboratory results, infections from human bites, aspiration pneumonia, and bacteremia from dental procedures. Acidic metabolites from oral streptococci by dissolving enamel and dentin may enhance the transit of oral bacteria into the bloodstream (6826). For risks from oral infections for dentists (see section 12.6).

HBV (1465, 2850, 4371). Dentists have rarely been implicated in the spread of HBV infection. Of 13 nosocomial transmission events recorded in dental offices in 1961–1990, 9 concerned HBV. Among 970 residents of Chihuahua, Mexico, a history of dental procedures doubled the risk of HBV infection.

HCV (6585). Among blood donors and hospitalized patients in Peru, a history of dental procedures in the preceding year was a significant hazard.

HIV (1451). Transmission dentist-to-patient is rare. In Florida, a dentist diagnosed HIV infection in 1986 and AIDS in 1987 during 1987–1989 was source for 5 of his clients. Transmission patient-to-worker has also been documented.

Endocarditis. Antibiotic prophylaxis is recommended for high-risk patients scheduled for high-risk dental work. High-risk patients include carriers of prosthetic heart valves, and a history of endocarditis. High risk dental procedures include periodontal probing and surgery, and tooth extraction (6826).

INFECTIONS FROM BLOOD SAMPLINGS

Risks are minimal, if blood is taken professionally and disposable equipment is used (5392) (1574, 2582, 7614). Complications from venipuncture include cellulitis and phlebitis, for a rate of $<1–2/10^5$ acts. For risks from blood for health workers, see section 12.6.

HBV (1255, 1828, 2007, 5959). Outbreaks of acute hepatitis B have been well documented from devices for capillary blood sampling. In long-stay facilities in the United States in 2003–2004, outbreaks were attributed to shared devices for blood glucose monitoring and breaks in infection control, for acute hepatitis B attack rates among residents of 6%, 9%, and 36% in three states.

HCV (1891). At a long-stay facility for children with mucoviscidosis or diabetes in France in 1995, the HCV seroprevalence was unusually high (40% or 86/215); the investigation implicated a self-administered capillary blood-sampling device for blood glucose determination.

INFECTIONS FROM INJECTIONS AND OTHER INSTANT PROCEDURES

Injections. Injections are a means for the parenteral administration of drugs, including into muscle, joints (intra-articular), or other sites. Syringes were introduced in the 1840s; disposable syringes were introduced in the 1950s (2039).

Exposure (3519, 6679, 6909). In low-income countries, injections are administered at estimated rates of 2–11 (typically 3) per person per year. For $\geq 80\%$ of these injections, indications can be questioned. The proportion of injections that is unsafe because of reused material or poor hygiene is 1–75% (often 50%).

Infections (365, 1694, 3519, 4543, 4906, 6679, 8282) (Box 18.1). By method and site, complications from unsafe injections include local infections (e.g., abscess and septic arthritis), systemic infections (e.g., endocarditis), systemic response to local infection (e.g., tetanus), and aggravation or reactivation of a latent infection (e.g., poliomyelitis). By frequency rather than efficiency, injections cause more blood-borne infections than blood transfusions.

Prions

For surgery-associated Creutzfeldt-Jakob disease, see section 18.3.

Viruses

Injection equipment from viremic patients is a risk for the transmisison of many viruses when reused on other patients. Major risks are HBV, HCV, HIV, and agents of viral hemorrhagic fever (VHF) (see section 17.8).

HBV (1220, 1536, 2946, 3151, 3182, 3808, 6909). Unsafe injections are estimated to cause 10–20 million new HBV infections per year, or >20–30% of the world total. Sources of HBV include reused injection equipment contaminated by patient blood or latently infected, unrecognized workers. In an Oklahoma pain clinic in 2002, a nurse anesthetist who reused syringes to sequentially administer sedation medication transmitted HBV to 4% (31/793) of clients. In the United States in 1992, an infected thoracic surgeon infected 13% (19/144) of his susceptible patients. In Switzerland in 1973–1977, a physician infected 41 patients before he died from hepatic cirrhosis.

HCV (950, 1220, 1536, 3182, 3808, 4548, 4608, 6585, 6909). Unsafe injections have been estimated to cause 2–5 million new HCV infections per year, or 40% of the world total. As with HBV, sources of HCV include other patients or infected workers. The more frequent the injections, the higher the risk. In a case-control study in

Pakistan, the odds of HCV infection increased with increasing number of injections received in the preceding 10 years. In an Oklahoma pain clinic in 2002, a nurse anesthetist who reused syringes to sequentially administer sedation medication transmitted HCV to 9% (71/795) of clients. The clinic was closed and was assessed a $99,000 fine. At a hematology-oncology clinic in Nebraska in 2000–2001, 99 patients acquired HCV infection from the practice of flushing venous catheters with saline contaminated by reuse of syringes.

HIV (3182, 3281, 3808, 6679, 6909). Unsafe injections are estimated to cause 0.1–0.3 million new HIV infections per year, or 2.5–5% of the world total. In Romania, by the end of 1990, ~600 children had contracted HIV from unsafe injections.

Bacteria
Soft tissue infections (895, 896). Pyogenic agents from subcutaneous or intramuscular injections include *S. aureus*, *S. pyogenes* (group A *Streptococcus* [GAS]), and anaerobes such as *Peptostreptococcus* and *Clostridium*. Anaerobes in abscesses of the buccal or abdominal cavities include gram-negative enteric rods, *Bacteroides*, *Fusobacterium*, *Prevotella*, and *Porphyromonas* that typically invade from colonized, adjacent sites.

***C. tetani* (6698, 7475).** Unclean injections are a cause of iatrogenic tetanus, in particular, in low-income countries. Mainly intramuscular injections are associated with tetanus, including antibiotics, vitamins, and irritating substances such as quinine.

Mycobacteria (1971, 3561, 5312, 5468, 7528). Injections have been associated with infections by *M. fortuitum* and *M. kansasii*. *M. fortuitum* infections have also been reported for subcutaneous infusions, and reused, disinfected and rinsed electromyographic needle-electrodes.

Protozoa
Injection equipment from parasitemic patients is a risk for the transmission of tissue protozoa when reused on other patients. The main risk is for *Plasmodium*. *Plasmodium* (176, 3631), including *P. falciparum*, has been transmitted by needle-stick injury, shared syringes, improper use of saline flush syringes, multidose heparin vials, and other instantaneous invasive procedures.

18.2 INTRAVASCULAR DEVICES AND BLOODSTREAM INFECTIONS
Intravascular devices are devices that remain in blood vessels for hours to weeks, for monitoring, diagnostic, or therapeutic purposes, including needles (e.g., "butterflies"), cannulas, peripheral and central (CVC) venous catheters (lines), and surgically implanted devices (subcutaneous port catheters). For hemodialysis, see section 18.7.

Exposure (2638, 4381, 6637). Vascular access is a hallmark of hospital care. In the United States, >150 million catheters and >5 million CVC are sold per year. Acute-care hospitals in the United States in 2000 performed 1.2 million cardiac catheterizations ($440/10^5$ population) and ~1 million procedures for obstructed coronary arteries ($370/10^5$). In Swiss acute-care hospitals at a given day in 2003, 2% (obstetrics) to 64% (intensive care units [ICU]) of patients had a CVC (median, 14%).

Infections (234, 1637, 1726, 2136, 2502, 2638, 4177, 4381, 4901, 4993, 5451, 6883) (http://www.esgni.org). Risks vary by device (type, insertion site, and dwelling time), hospital unit (ICU, special unit, and ward), and patient (age, critically ill, or burn). In the 1990s, 2–3% of CVC in adults became infected, and 6% of CVC in children in ICUs needed removal for suspected sepsis. In the 2000s, improved technologies and site care have reduced overall infection rates to 0.2–2/100 catheter-days. Infections from cardiac catheterization or arterial angiography are rare, occurring in <0.25% of patients.

In the 1870s–1880s, microbiologists such as L. Pasteur (1822–1895), C. A. T. Billroth (1826–1894), E. Klebs (1834–1913), R. Koch (1843–1910), and A. Ogston (1844–1929) investigated wound infection and "pyemia." We now distinguish local (site) infections, systemic infections, and rare metastatic infections (e.g., septic coxarthritis from angiography). A summary of systemic syndromes follows. **Systemic inflammatory response syndrome (SIRS).** SIRS is diagnosed clinically, from hypothermia (<35–36°C) or hyperthermia (>38–38.5°C), tachycardia (>90/min), poor breathing (rate >20–30/min, P_aCO_2 <32 mm Hg, or need for ventilation), and leukopenia (<4,000/μl) or leukocytosis (>12,000/μl). Biochemical parameters may support the diagnosis of systemic inflammation, e.g., procalcitonin or C-reactive protein levels. **Sepsis.** Sepsis is the clinical diagnosis of SIRS plus systemic infection suspected from susceptibility (e.g., impaired immunity), exposure (e.g., device), clinical signs (e.g., hypoperfusion), or focus (e.g., urinary tract infection [UTI]). Although desirable, the diagnosis of sepsis is independent of microbiological confirmation. Septic shock is characterized by unexplained systolic hypotension (<90 mm Hg) that persists despite volume replacement. **Bacteremia.** Bacteremia is a microbiological diagnosis, from agents identified in blood by culture, smear (Gram stain), or nucleic acid amplification test (NAT). In hospitals in Europe, blood cultures are obtained at a rates of ~20–25/100 inpatients. Contamination is diagnosed from ≥1 commensal in ≥1 blood culture. Typical contaminants are skin flora such as diphtheroids, *Micrococcus*, and *Propionibacterium*. Bacteremia is considered significant if a single pathogen is isolated in two or more blood cultures, if only one but the same commensal is isolated in two or more blood cultures, or if any bacterium is isolated from a highly susceptible (e.g., neutropenia), highly exposed (invasive procedure), or critically ill (e.g., rigor) patient. For fungemia, viremia, and parasitemia, comparable criteria do not exist, but density of agents in blood helps to recognize significant findings. By focus, bacteremia is primary (no focus) or secondary (from known focus). Bacteremia is nosocomial if diagnosed >48 hours after admission or within 7 days from hospital discharge (Table 18.1). **Bloodstream infection (BSI).** BSI is a clinical diagnosis (SIRS or sepsis) that is confirmed microbiologically (significant bacteremia, fungemia, viremia, or parasitemia).

LOCAL VASCULAR DEVICE INFECTIONS

Colonization (6272). Catheters can become colonized by biofilm-forming agents, mainly coagulase-negative *Staphylococcus* (CoNS), *S. aureus*, and *Candida*. For CVC, reported colonization rates are ~10–50 (often 20–30)/1,000 catheter-days, or ~5–25% (often 10%) of catheters.

Site infections (3166, 4993). Manifestations include circumscribed inflammation and purulent discharge: around (2 cm) the exit site, of the port-pocket or tunnel (surgically implanted devices, e.g., Port-a-Cath or Hickman catheter), or along peripheral parts of catheters (phlebitis). Causative bacteria correspond to agents from biofilms or BSI (see below). Cultures from removed catheter tips correlate with agents of BSI.

Management options include catheter removal or "watchful waiting."

NOSOCOMIAL BACTEREMIA, FUNGEMIA, AND PARASITEMIA

Overview (510, 2002, 3654, 4627, 5707) (http://www .esgni.org). About one fourth to one half of bacteremias diagnosed in hospitals are nosocomial, while the majority is community-acquired. Reported overall lethality is ~20–30% (bacteremia) to ~30–45% (candidemia). Lethality attributable to nosocomial bacteremia is 12–17%.

Risks. Nosocomial bacteremia (5890, 6883). The risks of nosocomial bacteremia include invasive procedures and devices. Main sources are central and peripheral venous catheters (in 15–35%) and bladder catheters (in close to 10%). Of vascular catheter-associated bacteremias, 66–80% are attributable to CVC, 19% to peripheral catheters, 0–14% to tunneled catheters, and 0–1% to arterial catheters. **Nosocomial candidemia (510, 4627, 6254).** Risks include CVC, systemic antimicrobials, total parenteral nutrition, and neoplasm. In France, 50% of candidemia patients have neoplasms. Sources are cryptic (primary) in two thirds of the cases, urinary tract (in 9%), and other known sites (in nearly one-fourth).

Rates. Bacteremia (2002, 3654, 5707, 5890, 8227). Reported bacteremia rates are ~0.06/100 patient-days, or 0.3–1.7% of admissions. Rates are highest in ICU and hematology, nephrology, and oncology units. **Candidemia (319, 3452, 4627, 5952, 6254).** By geography and case mix, reported rates are 0.03–0.05/1,000 patient-days, 0.1–0.8/1,000 hospital discharges, or 1–5/10^5 population year.

Agents (319, 2122, 5884, 5890, 5892, 7646, 7836). More than 100 agent genera have been identified in nosocomial agentemias. About one half to two thirds are gram-positive bacteria (mainly *Staphylococcus*), one fourth to one half are gram-negatives (mainly *Enterococcus*, *Escherichia coli*, *Klebsiella*, and *Pseudomonas*), ~8% are polymicrobial, and 7–12% are fungi. Relative frequencies and absolute risks of fungemias have substantially increased in the past two decades.

Bacteria

Frequent isolates (>1%) in nosocomial bacteremia (1264, 2122, 3451, 3454, 5884, 5890, 7969) (http://www .esgni.org) (Table 18.1). Frequent isolates in nosocomial bacteremia are *Acinetobacter*, *Citrobacter*, *Enterobacter*, *Enterococcus*, *Klebsiella*, *Proteus*, *Pseudomonas*, *Serratia*, *Staphylococcus*, and *Streptococcus*. **Acinetobacter (511).** Most isolates are *A. baumannii* and a few are *A. calcoaceticus*. Sources include peripheral venous and pulmonary arterial catheters. **Enterococcus (3453, 4677).** Most *Enterococcus* bacteremias are nosocomial. The main sources are the urinary tract, intravascular devices, intraabdominal infections, surgical wounds, and burn wounds. In the United Kingdom, of >6,000 nosocomial bacteremia isolates in 2003, a majority were *E. faecalis* (2% vancomycin-resistant *Enterococcus* [VRE]), a minority were *E. faecium* (16% VRE). **Klebsiella (2619, 4013, 4065, 7587, 8328).** About one fourth to three fourths of *Klebsiella* bacteremias are nosocomial. Sources include the urinary tract, hepatobiliary tract, and airway. Nosocomial bacteremia isolates include *K. pneumoniae* (in 75–80%) and *K. oxytoca* (in 15–25%). **Pseudomonas (2588, 3455).** Most *Pseudomonas* bacteremias are nosocomial. Important sources are the urinary tract and airway. In the United Kingdom, of >3,000 nosocomial bacteremia isolates in 2003, more than three fourths were *P. aeruginosa*. **Staphylococcus.** *S. aureus* accounts for ~25% of nosocomial bacteremias, and CoNS for another 15%. Of all *S. aureus* strains, ~50% are MRSA.

Infrequent isolates. Infrequent isolates (≤1%) in nosocomia bacteremia include *Aeromonas, Alcaligenes, Bacillus, Bacteroides, Burkholderia cepacia, Campylobacter, Clostridium, Corynebacterium, Haemophilus influenzae* b and non-b, *Listeria, Micrococcus, Morganella, Moraxella, Mycobacterium, Neisseria, Propionibacterium, Providencia, Salmonella,* and *Stenotrophomonas maltophilia*.

Agents of community-acquired bacteremia. In contrast, main agents of community-acquired bacteremia include *E. coli* (in 10–50%), *S. aureus* (in 5–20%), *S. pneumoniae* (in 2–25%), and *Salmonella* (in 0.5–85%).

Infrequent agents are (A–Z) *Brucella* (enzootic areas), *Burkholderia pseudomallei* (endemic areas), *C. pneumoniae* (flulike), *C. burnetii* (flulike), *Klebsiella* (diabetics), *Legionella* (elderly), *M. tuberculosis* (low-income countries), *M. pneumoniae* (flulike), and *N. meningitidis*.

Fungi
Candida **(319, 510, 2122, 3452, 4195, 4627, 5863, 5952, 6920).** *Candida* is the most frequent fungal isolate. Some 5–10% of blood cultures grow *Candida*. Species include *C. albicans* (in 50–70%), *C. glabrata* (in 10–15%), *C. parapsilosis* (in ~10%), *C. krusei* (in ~8%), and *C. tropicalis* (in ~6%).

Others (4195, 5861, 7928). Infrequent fungemia isolates include *Aspergillus* and *Cryptococcus*; yeastlike fungi such as *Geotrichum, Rhodotorula,* and *Trichosporon*; hyaline molds such as *Acremonium, Fusarium, Scedosporium,* and *Paecilomyces*, dematiaceous (pigmented) molds (agents of "phaeohyphomycosis") such as *Exophiala* and *Wangiella*, and zygomycetes such as *Absidia, Mucor,* and *Rhizopus*.

Protozoa
Patients have acquired malaria from intravascular devices (34, 5879). At the Nottingham City Hospital, United Kingdom, in 1999, three patients contracted falciparum malaria likely from flushed intravenous lines; on the same ward were three patients who had acquired falciparum malaria abroad. In Saudi Arabia in 1992, sequential use of syringes on heparin locks caused a nosocomial falciparum malaria outbreak with 20 cases.

NOSOCOMIAL BSI AND SEPSIS
Overview (1230, 2122, 4771, 4867, 6248, 6250, 6272, 8227, 8229). About 70–85% of all BSI are nosocomial, the remainder is community acquired. A source is not identified in >50% of patients. However, in adults in ICU, 65–85% of nosocomial BSI are intravascular device associated. By case mix, hospital unit, and surveillance, rates of catheter-associated BSI are 0.3–1.3 (often 0.5) per 100 device-days, or ~0.5–4.5% (often 1–2%) of catheter carriers. In neonates, by birth weight, rates of BSI from umbilical catheters or CVC are 0–1.6 (often 0.2–1) per 100 device-days. In the United States, rates (aggregate of BSI, bacteremia, and sepsis) rose from $83/10^5$ in 1979 to $240/10^5$ in 2000. More BSI are predicted to occur in the elderly in the near future. By case mix and hospital unit, lethality ranges from 10% to 80%. In the United states, lethality decreased from 28% in 1979 to 18% in 2000.

Agents (234, 1230, 2136, 4993, 5533, 6248, 8227, 8229). Gram-positive bacteria (e.g., staphylococcal skin flora) account for 30–60% of BSI and sepsis cases, gram-negative bacteria for 25–30%, and fungi (e.g., *Candida*) for ~10%. In about one fourth of cases, the etiology is polymicrobial. Causative agents change over time in the hospital, with an early preponderance of *S. aureus* and *E. coli*, and a later wave by *Enterococcus* and *Acinetobacter* (Fig. 18.1). Whether and how cytomegalovirus (CMV), Epstein-Barr virus (EBV), HIV, herpes simplex virus (HSV), *Influenzavirus, Leishmania*, and other agents predispose to BSI is not well known.

Bacteria
Frequent causes of BSI or nosocomial sepsis (234, 2136, 5533, 6318, 8227, 8228) (Table 18.1). Frequent causes of BSI or nosocomial sepsis (>1% of isolates) (arranged by approximate share in various settings) are *Staphylococcus* (CoNS, *S. aureus*), *Streptococcus* (*S. pneumoniae*, others), *E. coli, Enterococcus, Enterobacter, Klebsiella, P. aeruginosa, H. influenzae, Acinetobacter, B. cepacia,* and anaerobes. **Staphylococcus (615, 2390, 4993, 7864).** *S. aureus* and CoNS are the most frequent agents of nosocomial BSI and sepsis. Of all *S. aureus*, 60–70% is

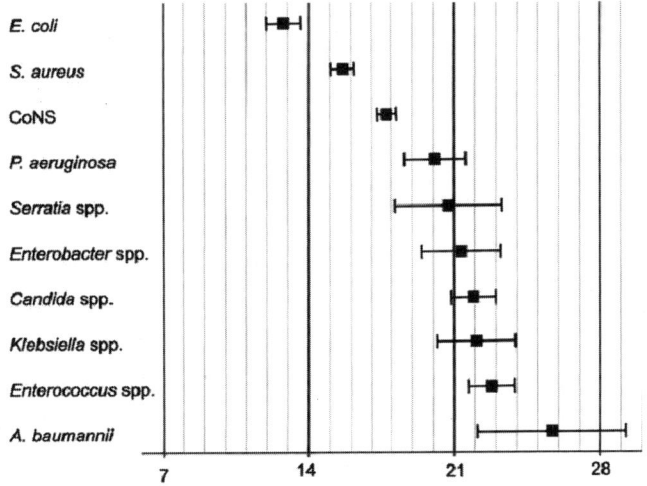

Figure 18.1 Agents from nosocomial bloodstream infections, 49 U.S. hospitals, 1995–2002 ($n = 24{,}179$). Isolates (*y* axis) are given by days from admission (*x* axis). Squares are for means, and lines show standard deviations. From reference 8227. Reproduced with permission by University of Chicago Press.

Table 18.1 Reported relative frequencies and rates of occurrence of nosocomial agentemias (viremia, bacteremia, and fungemia), bloodstream infections, or sepsis, by agent cluster[a]

Cluster	Agent	Agentemia Share (%)	Agentemia Rate of occurrence	Bloodstream infection or sepsis Share (%)	Bloodstream infection or sepsis Rate of occurrence (no. of cases/10^3 admissions)
Air-droplet or skin-blood	*Candida*	5–10	$4/10^3$ discharges $0.7–1.4/10^5$ population	5–10	0.5
	CoNS (*S. epidermidis*)	15		25–75	1.6
	Klebsiella	9–12	$0.8/10^3$ admissions	5–15	2
	S. aureus	25		20 (5–40)	1
	Streptococcus (*S. pneumoniae*, others)	0.3–15		10–15 (3–23)	
Feces-food	*Enterobacter*	4–6	$0.3/10^3$ admissions	5	
	E. coli	6–12	$20–50/10^5$ population	9 (6–27)	0.3
	Enterococcus (with VRE)	3–12	$12/10^5$ population	4–12	0.5
	Proteus	2			
Environmental	*Acinetobacter*	1	$1–3/10^5$ population	3–6	
	Citrobacter	0.8–2			
	Pseudomonas	14–19	$5–6/10^5$ population	4–15	
	Serratia	0.8–1.8	$0.2/10^3$ admissions		

[a]Rates refer to hospital admissions or discharges or to the general population.

MRSA. In U.S. hospitals, the time from admission to BSI is roughly 2–3 weeks. Rates in U.S. hospitals per 1,000 admissions are 1 (*S. aureus*) to 1.6 (CoNS). Rates of CVC-associated *S. epidermidis* BSI/100 device-days are 0.4–0.5 (in ICU) to 1.5 (in burn units). Lethality of catheter-related staphylococcal BSI is ~15%.

For infrequent bacteria (≤1% of isolates) see the section on nosocomial bacteremia above.

Fungi

Frequent causes of BSI (>1% of isolates) (2136, 5533, 8227, 8228) (Table 18.1) are *Candida* and *Malassezia*. In U.S. hospitals, the mean time from admission to *Candida* BSI is roughly 3 weeks. Of catheter-associated BSI, 5–10% are due to *Candida* and ≤2% are due to *Malassezia*. For infrequent fungi (≤1% of isolates), see the section on nosocomial fungemia above.

18.3 SURGICAL SITE AND WOUND INFECTIONS

Surgical sites are body parts intentionally incised under surgical conditions. Wounds are disruptions of skin or mucosa, either acute from injury (e.g., abrasion and burn), or chronic from spontaneous processes (e.g., hypoperfusion, pressure, and inflammation).

Exposure (http://www.census.gov) (Box VI.1). Global statistics are not publicly available. Worldwide, surgical procedures likely exceed 200 million/year. In the United States in 2001, short-stay hospitals reported 24 million surgical procedures, for a rate of $8,500/10^5$. Surgery increasingly is performed in outpatient settings.

Infections (433, 815, 4788, 5309, 7001, 8024, 8197). Wound infections are manifest by pain, inflammation, or drainage.

Surgical site infections (SSI) (Box 18.2) are manifest ~2–60 days from surgery, by pain, inflammation, wound dehiscence, abscess formation, or fever, but chiefly purulent drainage. SSI account for ~15% of nosocomial infections. Given average lengths of stay of 5–8 days, 33–50% of SSI are diagnosed after hospital discharge. By type of surgery, site (clean or contaminated), and surveillance (hospital, ambulatory, and days of follow-up), reported SSI rates range from 0.05 to 50/1,000 procedures. A crude estimate is of 1–2% SSI from hospitalization and a further 1–2% during ambulatory follow-up. For implants, see section 18.6.

Prevention (2124, 3294, 6483, 6600, 7364, 8024). Preventive measures include good preoperative practice (judicious indication, short hospital stay, restrictive use of antibiotics, site preparation), good surgical practice (skill, hygiene, and short time in theater), and good postoperative practice (good hand hygiene, good site care, limited patient transfers, and ambulatory follow-up). The effectiveness of single-use and reusable gowns and drapes is not well established.

> **Box 18.2** Agents of surgical site infections, by agent cluster
>
> Relative frequency and risks are shown in parentheses.
>
> Droplet-air *Klebsiella* (2–4%), *Morganella* (1%)
> Feces-food *Bacteroides* (1%, abdominal surgery), *Citrobacter* (1–2%), clostridia (0–1%), *Enterobacter* (1–4%), *Enterococcus* (5–15%, also VRE), *E. coli* (5–20%), *Proteus* (0–3%)
> Environmental *C. tetani*, environmental mycobacteria, *Pseudomonas* (10–25%), *Serratia* (0–18%)
> Skin-blood Prions (ear-nose-throat and neurosurgery, very rare); HBV, HCV; *Corynebacterium* (4–6%), *Propionibacterium* (0–2%), *S. aureus* (10–50%, many MRSA), CoNS (5–25%), *Streptococcus* (0–3%); *Candida* (9–12%)

WOUND INFECTIONS

Any wound should prompt review of tetanus vaccination and query of rabies exposure. Acute (traumatic) wounds include abrasions, open fractures, gun shot wounds, and burns. For animal bites, see chapter 1; for human bites, see section 13.5.

Acute wound infections (815, 896, 4857). Sources include the environment, hands, droplets, and surrounding skin.

The main aerobic agents of infected wounds are *Staphylococcus* (*S. aureus*, in burns: >20%, CoNS), *Streptococcus* (viridans, fecal, and group C *Streptococcus* [GCS]), and *E. coli*.

Less frequent are *Acinetobacter*, *Aeromonas* (mud), *Bacillus*, *Corynebacterium*, *Enterobacter* (burns: 10%), *Enterococcus* (burns: 10%), *Klebsiella*, *Proteus*, *Providencia*, *Pseudomonas* (burns: ~20%), *Stenotrophomonas*, *Vibrio vulnificus* (marine waters or foods), as well as *Candida*.

Anaerobic agents have been isolated from 20–70% (typically 50%) of infected wounds, mainly *Bacteroides* (abscesses), *Clostridium* (e.g., *C. histolyticum* and *C. perfringens*), and *Peptostreptococcus*, infrequently *Fusobacterium*, *Prevotella*, *Propionibacterium*, and *Veillonella*.

PRIONS AND SURGERY

Creutzfeldt-Jakob disease (CJD). Sporadic (classical) CJD (606, 1525, 2156, 7729, 8030, 8177, 8390). About 300 iatrogenic CJD cases have been reported, mainly because of dura mater implants and human growth hormone. Few cases have been suspected from neurosurgery by stereotactic electrodes used on patients with sporadic CJD. This neurosurgical mode is supported by experiments in mice and monkeys. In contrast, general surgery on patients with sporadic CJD does not seem to constitute a significant nosocomial risk (Table 14.2). In Europe, two case-control studies did not detect risks from surgery, dental work, or other medical interventions, unlike a study in Australia with 241 cases and 784 community controls that found a significant association of surgery with sporadic CJD. **Variant CJD (2539, 3331, 6091).** An emerging, putative hazard is surgery on patients who are incubating or ill with variant CJD. In variant CJD, infective prion likely accumulates in some peripheral organs or tissues during the (later) incubation period, including blood, tonsils, spleen, lymph nodes, enteric plaques, retina, and optic nerve. Of concern, therefore, are interventions with reusable instruments on such tissues or organs, mainly tonsillectomy and appendectomy. To prevent iatrogenic transmission of variant CJD, disposable instruments have been advocated for adenotonsillectomy and appendectomy in the United Kingdom since 2001. For decontamination of instruments, see section 18.2.

VIRUSES AND SURGERY

Viruses rarely mimick surgical conditions, e.g., appendicitis from CMV, or jaundice from hepatitis viruses. Surgery may reactivate latent infections, e.g., by *Herpesviridae*. For infections in or from health workers, see section 12.6. Evidence for nosocomial transmission of viruses seems limited to HBV and HCV.

HBV (4972). In Italy in 1994–1999, significant risks of acute hepatitis B ($n = 3,120$) cases compared with acute hepatitis A ($n = 7,158$) controls were invasive procedures, including abdominal, oral, and gynecological surgery.

HCV (950, 4972). Suspected risks include abdominal, ophthalmological, gynecological, and obstetric surgery, including legally induced abortion and uterine curettage.

BACTERIA AND SURGERY

Risks (2124). Risks are modified by patient condition, type of facility, type and duration of intervention, and site stratified by expected degree of contamination:

- Clean (intact surface, healthy skin), e.g., mastectomy, hernia repair, coronary bypass, knee endoprosthesis
- Contaminated (area colonized), e.g., cholecystectomy, surgical reduction of fracture

- Dirty (wound, spilled bowel content), e.g., gun shot wound, ruptured appendicitis

Rates (1230, 2655, 2678, 3278, 3552, 5113, 5451, 5891, 8024) (Fig. 18.2). Crude SSI rates are 2–4% in North America and West Europe, but 3–20% in low-income countries. For healthy persons, clean sites, and short (≤ 2 h) interventions in high-income countries, expected SSI rates are 2–3% (Table 18.2). In patients with comorbidities, hours-long surgery at contaminated sites doubles, triples, or quadruples rates. SSIs double lethality and increase risks of readmittance fivefold. Ranges (rounded) of SSI rates in North America and West Europe are summarized below for representative interventions. Ranges are for 95% CI, severity scores (low versus high), or percentiles (25th versus to 75th).

- General surgery: head and neck (2–5%), hernia (0.5–4%), struma (0.5%), solid organ transplant (4–14%).
- Visceral surgery: appendectomy (1–4%), cholecystectomy (0.5–3%), small bowel (5–12%), colon (4–11%). Rates in colorectal surgery can exceed 10%, despite bowel preparation and preoperative antibiotic prophylaxis.
- Cardiovascular surgery: coronary bypass graft (1–5%), vascular (6–7%), and vene stripping (0.2%). In Sweden, rates from coronary bypass graft reached 30%, including leg, deep sternal, and mediastinal infections (7278).
- Orthopedic surgery (365, 3278, 7439): arthroscopy (0.01–0.5%), osteosynthesis (1–4%), hip prosthesis, or total hip or knee replacement (1–5%, typically <2%).
- Gynecological surgery: breast (0.5–4%), hysterectomy (vaginal, 1–2; abdominal, 1–5%), Caesarean section (1–8%, typically 2–4%). In France, the rates from Caesarean section were 2–3%, including abdominal, uterine, and pelvic infections (433).
- Urologic surgery: prostate surgery (1–8%), kidney surgery (1–5%).
- Neurosurgery: craniotomy (1–2.5%), ventricular shunt (4–6%).

Bacteria (273, 2720, 5891, 8024)
About 40–55% of SSI are polymicrobial, in particular, necrotic tissue infections. Visceral SSI are mainly caused by bowel flora, including anaerobes such as *Bacteroides fragilis* and *Peptostreptococcus*.

Frequent agents of SSI. Frequent agents of SSI (>5% of isolates, Box 18.2) are (by relative frequency) *S. aureus* (10–50%, MRSA can constitute >50%), *Pseudomonas* (10–25%), CoNS (5–25%), *E. coli* (5–20%), and *Enterococcus* (5–15%, including VRE). ***S. aureus* (3294).** In hospital patients, the density of *S. aureus* in the nose correlates with its prevalence on the skin, and preoperative skin

Figure 18.2 SSI, United Kingdom, 1997–2000. Percentage of operations infected (*y* axis, overall 4% or 2,074/48,522), is given by site (*x* axis). Dots represent participating hospitals. Box plot represent percentiles (right upper corner). From reference 5891. Reproduced with permission by Public Health Laboratory Service.

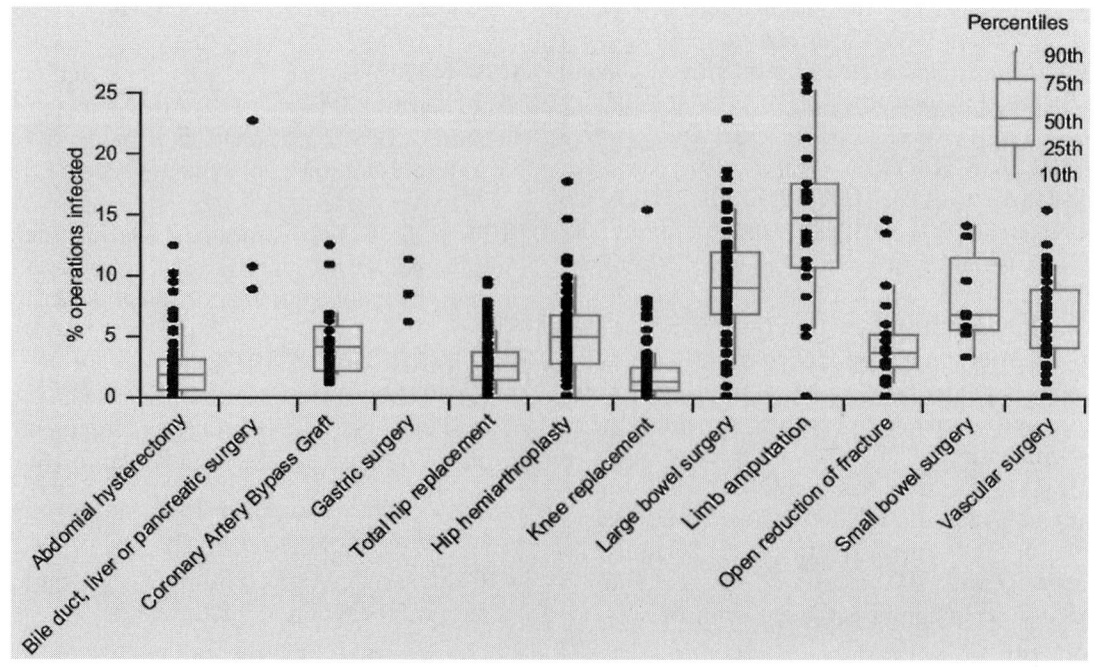

Table 18.2 SSI, United States, 1992–1998[a]

Intervention	Low-risk patients (risk score 0)[b]		Higher-risk patients (risk score ≥1)[b]	
	No. of patients	% with SSI[c]	No. of patients	% with SSI[c]
Cholecystectomy	23,891	0.5	18,924	1–5
Appendectomy	4,449	1	7,078	3–6
Small bowel surgery	823	6	3,069	8–15
Cardiac surgery	1,021	1	17,295	2–3
Vascular surgery	3,579	1	43,110	2–5
Cesarean section	59,921	3	21,561	5–9
Prostatectomy	1,648	1	1,306	3

[a]From reference 2678.
[b]Risk score is determined from the duration of intervention and patient condition.
[c]Numbers are rounded to the nearest decimal point.

carriage correlates with SSI rates, for attack rates of 2–9% in noncarriers and 6–31% in carriers. Occasionally, carrier health workers have caused outbreaks of SSI.

Infrequent agents of SSI. Infrequent agents (≤5%) include (A–Z): *Acinetobacter*, *Bacteroides* (1%), *Citrobacter* (1–2%), *Clostridium* (0–1%), *Corynebacterium* (4–6%), *Enterobacter* (1–4%), environmental mycobacteria, *Klebsiella* (2–4%), *Morganella* (1%), *Nocardia*, *Propionibacterium* (0–2%), *Proteus* (0–3%), *Serratia* (0–18%), and *Streptococcus* (0–3%). **Acinetobacter (4725).** In Baltimore, Md., in 2003, high-pressure lavage with sterile saline for wound debridement caused an outbreak of *A. baumannii* with eight wound infections; likely source was a disposable suction canister insert that to save cost was disposed only when full rather than after each patient. **Clostridium (7475).** Species of clostridia are infrequent causes of SSI, typically manifest as gas gangrene. Sources of *C. tetani* can be "external" wounds of skin and soft tissue, or "internal" wounds, e.g., from bowel surgery. In Bombay, India, in 1954–1962, the incidence of postoperative tetanus was 0.25/1,000 surgical procedures per year (6698). **Mycobacterium.** *M. fortuitum* (962, 1306, 1479, 3067, 6576, 6786) has complicated punch biopsy, breast augmentation surgery, laparoscopy, thoracotomy, and bypass surgery. In 39,455 breast augmentation procedures over 3 1/2 years, rates were 0.6% for all SSI, and 0.01% for SSI by *M. fortuitum* and *M. xenopi* (323). Of 3,244 patients undergoing microdiscectomy for disc hernia, 58 (1.8%) contracted *M. xenopi* spinal infections from instruments contaminated in water from a stagnant hotwater tank. **Nocardia (8046).** The hands of an anesthetist were the source of *N. farcinica* sternal infections in 5 (5%) of 87 patients submitted to coronary bypass graft. **S. pyogenes (GAS) (250, 4039).** GAS is a rare cause of SSI. However, postoperative outbreaks by staff-to-patient spread have been reported.

FUNGI AND SURGERY

Fungal agents of SSI include *C. albicans* (in 6–7%), other *Candida* spp. (in 3–5%), mainly *C. parapsilosis*, rarely *C. krusei*, *C. tropicalis*, also *Torulopsis glabrata*, and *Aspergillus*.

18.4 TRANSFUSIONS

Blood is both a fluid organ or tissue and a bioproduct. Donations (450 ml) are processed to "units," including packed erythrocytes (190 ml), plasma (200 ml), platelets (50 ml), cryoprecipitate (10 ml), and Hyper-Ig.

Exposure (1240, 2784, 2852, 7051). Worldwide, donations exceed 75 million units per year. In the United States, ~13 million blood units are transfused annually to ~4.5 million recipients.

Exposure is reduced in one-time recipients and cumulative in repeat recipients such as hemophiliacs A or B who lack genes for clotting factors VIII or IX. In the United States, ~0.02% of live male births are hemophiliacs, and the prevalence in the male population is ~$13/10^5$.

Safety. Measures to assure safety of supply include donor screening, good manufacturing practice, recipient screening, and posttransfusion surveillance.

- Donors (1962, 2784, 2852, 3611, 6187, 8420) (Table 18.3) are screened by history and tests. Answers that may exclude from donation include lifestyle (sex with high-risk groups, injection drug use, imprisonment, tattooing), international travel, HIV infection, malaria (e.g., for 3 years from recovery), tuberculosis (e.g., for 2 years from cure), syphilis (e.g., for 1 year from treatment), attenuated vaccines (e.g., for 3 months from administration), herpes (e.g., for 4 weeks from recovery), and flu (e.g., to recovery). Donations from test-positive donors (D+) are discarded. By selection, donors (voluntary or paid, first or repeat) are not representative of the population. In the United States in 2001, of first donors 0.08% tested positive for HBsAg, 0.3% for anti-HCV, and 0.01% for anti-HIV, prevalence that was clearly below population prevalence. Test-negative donors (incubating, viremia below detection) escape detection and constitute a residual risk. Reported "window periods" (infective but test-negative donors) by NAT are 7 days for HCV, about 11 days for HIV, and 16–22 days for HBV but up to 51 days for anti-HTLV, 59 days for HBsAg, and 70 days for anti-HCV (Table 18.3). NAT clearly shortens windows and lowers residual risks.

- Manufacturing (2852, 4025, 6187) aims to minimize risks by inactivating residual agents (HBV, HCV, HIV), including by detergents and fractionation steps. For efficient production of Ig, plasma is pooled, with a theoretical risk that a single infective donor could contaminate a pool.
- Recipients are screened for incompatibilities. K. Landsteiner (1868–1943) in 1900–1901 described ABO blood groups. Now, >100 erythrocyte antigens are recognized. Judicial indications assure that benefits from transfusion outweigh risks. Infection risks cumulate; recipients of multiple or repeat transfusions are at greater risk than one-time and single-unit recipients.
- Surveillance. Possible targets for surveillance include test-positive donations, conversions in repeat donations, infections in recipients within 3–6 months posttransfusion, and late or past infections (look-back studies).

Transfusion-associated infections (Box 18.3). Infections in recipients can be nosocomial (by procedure), reactivated (in latently infected, often immune-impaired recipients), or transfusion-transmitted (by infective donation). Discordant D+R− pairs (donor test-positive, recipient test-negative) should prompt recipient surveillance. Ideally, "null" blood for eventual testing is kept from donors and pretransfusion recipients.

For transfusion-transmission, a requirement is viable agents in donor ("agentemia," includes prionemia, viremia, bacteremia, fungemia, parasitemia) and donation. Supportive evidence is survival of an agent in stored product, an incubation period that is compatible with the transfusion date, identical strains in donor, donation, and exposed recipients, no other risks in infected recipient, and clustered cases from a single infective donor.

TRANSFUSION-TRANSMITTED PRIONS
Sporadic (classic) CJD (926, 999, 2852, 8203). There is no evidence for transmission through blood or blood products.

Variant CJD (999, 2852, 4474, 5794, 5916, 8204). Biological, experimental, and clinical evidence shows that variant CJD is transfusion transmissible. A patient with variant CJD who died in 2003 had received blood in the United Kingdom in 1996, from a donor diagnosed with variant CJD in 1999. As a precaution, donors are deferred who have spent a cumulative period of time in the United Kingdom or other European countries that have reported cases of bovine spongiform encephalopathy (BSE). Morover, donated blood is leukodepleted in the United Kingdom and some other countries.

TRANSFUSION-TRANSMITTED VIRUSES
In theory, any undetected viremia could cause transfusion-transmitted infections. However, for this, viremia needs to remain high, remain inapparent, and remain over time. Therefore, the list of confirmed agents is considerably shorter than the theoretical list. Most high-income countries focus donation screening on HBV, HCV, and HIV.

Droplet-Air Cluster
In many respiratory viral infections, viremia appears to be short lived and limited to the time around disease manifestation. Transfusion-transmission is reported for parvovirus B19 (PVB19) and suspected for varicella-zoster virus (VZV) (4134).

PVB19 (4438, 8361). Blood from inapparent donors can contain and transmit PVB19. Initially high viremia ($>10^9$

Table 18.3 Viral infections in United States population, in tissue donors, and in blood donors, 2001[a]

Virus	Window days[b]	Prevalence (%)			No. of conversions/ 10^5 donor years[c]			Residual rate/ 10^5 donations[d]	
		Population	Tissue donors	Blood donors[e]	Population	Tissue donors	Blood donors	Tissue donors	Blood donors
HBV	34–59	0.4	0.2	0.08	28	18	1	1–3	0.05–0.5
HCV	7–82	1.8	1.1	0.3	9	12	0.5–2.5	0.2–2.4	0–0.08
HIV	11–22	0.2	0.09	0.01	14	30	1–3	0.6–1.8	0–0.1
HTLV	51	Low	0.07	0.01–0.02	?	5.6	0.2	0.8	0.03

[a]Adapted from reference 8420.
[b]Number of days after infection that infective donors can test negative by NAT (shortest period), antigen test, or antibody tests (longest period).
[c]Number of conversions in repeat blood donors. Overall tissue donor rates were calculated from their age- and sex-specific rates.
[d]Number of conversions during the window period.
[e]First-time blood donors.

> **Box 18.3** Agents from blood or blood products, by agent cluster
>
> Vehicles and remarks are listed in parentheses.
>
> | | |
> |---|---|
> | Droplet-air | PVB19, possibly VZV; *Klebsiella* (platelets and erythrocytes) |
> | Feces-food | HAV, possibly HEV; *Enterobacter* (platelets and erythrocytes), *Y. enterocolitica* (erythrocytes) |
> | Zoonotic | CTFV, TBEV, WNV, possibly *Hantavirus*; *Babesia*, *Leishmania* (visceral), *Plasmodium* (all species infective to humans and erythrocytes), *T. cruzi* |
> | Environmental | *Pseudomonas* (platelets and erythrocytes), *Serratia* (platelets and erythrocytes) |
> | Skin-blood | variant CJD; GBV-C, HBV, HCV, HIV, herpesviruses (mainly CMV), HTLV; *Staphylococcus* (platelets and erythrocytes); *Candida* |

DNA copies per ml) is followed by low levels ($<10^6$ copies/ml) that persist for >1 month; NAT can amplify viral DNA in blood from immune-competent individuals up to 2½ years.

- Donors (3746). Donations are not routinely screened for PVB19. In the United States, 0.1% (11/9,568) of blood units tested positive for PVB19 by NAT or seroassay for Ig.
- Recipients (2851, 3746, 4025, 8351). PVB19 has been transmitted by blood products, especially pooled factors VIII and IX concentrates. Two weeks after infusion of 5 units of solvent-detergent-treated plasma, a 36-year-old woman with myasthenia gravis developed acute, symptomatic PVB19 infection; high levels of PVB19-DNA in several lots triggered a product recall. Of 11 recipients with NAT-positive blood, only one became infected. This low rate was explained by neutralizing antibodies in donors or recipients. In the United States, the rate of transfusional PVB19 infection is $\sim 10/10^5$ units.

Feces-Food Cluster

HAV (813, 5225). By NAT, viremia lasts ~ 1 to >12 (typically 3) months; it begins from ~ 4 (typically 2) weeks before jaundice or peak transaminitis (d_0) and extends for $\sim ½$ to 2–3 (occasionally >12) months after d_0. Sporadic transfusion-transmission was suspected in hemophiliacs.

HEV (117, 1476). Viremia seems to last ≥ 2 (occasionally >4) weeks. Transfusion-transmission is suspected in endemic areas, for instance in children with sickle-cell anemia.

Zoonotic Cluster

Transfusion-transmission is reported for Colorado tick fever virus (CTFV) (3981), West Nile virus (WNV), and tick-borne encephalitis virus (TBEC), (7898), and suspected for *Hantavirus* (8324).

WNV (1240, 5786). Transfusion-transmitted infections have emerged in the United States. In 2002–2003, 23 patients were confirmed to have acquired WNV from transfused erythrocytes (13 or 57%), platelets (7 or 30%), or fresh-frozen plasma (3 or 13%). Maxima of donation-transfusion intervals were 5 days for platelets, 33 days for erythrocytes, and 44 days for fresh-frozen plasma. In 2003, of ~ 6 million blood units screened by NAT, ≥ 818 ($<0.015\%$) donations amplified WNV. However, six transfusion-transmitted infections had escaped screening because of viremia below detection level.

Skin-Blood Cluster

Overview (2792, 4134, 5883, 6688, 7052) (Table 18.3). Transfusion-transmission has been reported for HBV, HCV, herpesviruses (CMV, EBV, human herpes virus 6 [HHV6], human herpes virus 7 [HHV7], human herpes virus 8 [HHV8], and HSV), and retroviruses (HIV, human T-lymphotropic virus [HTLV]), and innocuous GBV-C. For blood safety, the focus is on HBV, HCV, and HIV.

In 12 Latin American countries in 1997, prevalence per 10^5 donations ($n \sim 1.58$ million) was 70–360 for HIV, 130–850 for HCV, and 150–1,020 for HBV. In contrast in the United Kingdom in 2000, the aggregated prevalence of the viral trio was $10/10^5$ donors (252/2,548,244).

Before recombinant clotting factors became available in the 1990s, hemophiliacs were at high risk of transfusional infections, for reported prevalence of 30% for HBV markers, 60–90% for anti-HCV, and 35–45% for HIV.

CMV (4134, 5698). CMV is transfusion transmissible, likely from reactivation of CMV in blood monocytes that remain latently infected for life.

- Donors (5698, 6837). Reported seroprevalence in donors is 40–100%. In Taiwan in 1989–1990, 90% (2,597/2,824) of voluntary blood donors tested positive for anti-CMV IgG, and 0.2% (7) had anti-CMV IgM.
- Recipients (4134, 5418, 5698, 6398). From 1–65% of donations from reactive (D+) donors cause CMV infection in susceptible (R−) recipients. In immune-competent R−, transfusion-transmitted infection is

generally inapparent or mild, mononucleosis-like. R− at risk of high rates of transmission or severe CMV disease include pregnant women, low-birth-weight (<1.2 kg) infants, transplant recipients (organ and stem cells), and immune-impaired patients. For them, options include donations from D− (impractical if donor seroprevalence is >90%), filtered or leukocyte-depleted products, and preemptive treatment with ganciclovir.

GBV-C. Transfusion-transmission is confirmed but apparently innocuous.

- Donors (4816, 7941). Prevalence by NAT was ~1% in donors in Japan, and in the People's Republic of China, it was 0.7% (1/150) in voluntary donors and 8% (21/265) in professional donors.
- Recipients (6672). Recipients of multiple transfusions are at increased risk. In Germany, marker (RNA, anti-GBV-C) prevalence is 4% (2/51) in hemophiliacs and 33% (17/51) in other multiply-transfused recipients.

HBV (999, 2612, 2784, 2852, 5913). Reported "window" periods are 34–49 days (by NAT) to 45–59 days (by HBsAg and anti-HBc IgM). Reported residual risks (from window period) in high-income countries are ~0.05–0.5/10^5 donations.

- Donors (2783, 5883, 5913, 7240). Reported HBsAg prevalence per 10^5 donors is 20–60 in the United States and 2.5 in the United Kingdom (21.5 in new donors and 0.3 in repeat donors). In contrast in Indonesia, 9% (338/3,839, 95% CI 8–10) of voluntary blood donors tested positive for HBsAg. In France, rates of HBsAg conversion in repeat blood donors per 10^5 person-years decreased from 6 (95% CI 4–8) in 1992–1994 to 1 (0.7–1.6) in 2001–2003.
- Recipients (2851, 6187, 7022). In the United States, the transfusion-transmitted HBV infection rate is 0.7–3.2/10^5 units. In the United Kingdom, the same rate is 0.25–1/10^5 units. In the United Kingdom in 1991–1997, 0.6% (24/4,185) of reported acute hepatitis B cases were transfusional with a decrease from 5 in 1991 to 1 in 1997.

HCV (999, 1297, 2784, 2852, 4979, 5913, 6585). Without sensitive donor screening, HCV is a transfusion hazard. Reported window periods are 66–82 days by anti-HCV, but only 7–12 days by NAT. In high-income countries that use NAT for screening, residual risks are extremely low (≤0.08/10^5 donations). In the United States in 1999–2000, ~0.4/10^5 donations tested positive by NAT only.

- Donors (12, 1318, 2783, 5883, 5913, 6585, 8156, 8420). Patients with chronic (subclinical) hepatitis C can amplify virus by NAT for up to 25 years after exposure. Individuals with a history of transfusion have an up to 10-fold increased risk of being infected. Voluntary blood donors are 6–10 times less frequently seroreactive than the population. In contrast, commercial donors are several times more often reactive than voluntary donors. Reported anti-HCV prevalence per 10^5 donors is 70–200 in the United States, 15 in France (81 in first-time donors, 2 in repeat donors), and 7 in the United Kingdom (55 in first-time donors, 1 in repeat donors). For comparison, reported seroprevalence in donors in low-income countries is 1.5–2.5%. In France, seroconversion rates in repeat donors per 10^5 person-years decreased from 2.5 (95% CI 1–4.5) in 1992–1994 to 0.4 (95% CI 0.2–1.3) in 2001–2003.
- Recipients (6187, 7023). Screening has greatly reduced transfusion-transmitted HCV infections. In the United Kingdom, currently the rate of acute hepatitis C from transfusion erythrocytes is 0.03/10^5 units. From transfusions in the United Kingdom of the 1980s–1990s, 3–7% of HCV infections were considered transfusion associated.

HIV (999, 1297, 2784, 2852, 5913). Reported window periods are 16–22 days for anti-HIV, and 11–12 days for RNA. In high-income countries that use NAT, residual risks are very low (0–0.1/10^5 donations). In the United States in 1999–2000, ~0.05/10^5 donations tested positive by NAT only.

- Donors (2783, 5426, 5883, 5913, 6774, 7017). Reported seroprevalence per 10^5 donors is ≤20 in the United States, 2 in France (5 in first-time donors, 1 in repeat donors), and 0.6 in the United Kingdom (2 in first-time donors, 0.4 in repeat donors). In sub-Saharan Africa, seroprevalence in donors ranged from 1% (10/704) in Gabon, to 6% (155/2,610) in Ethiopia, and 7% (319/4,761) in Tanzania. In Africa in 1995, however, close to one fourth of 2.5 million blood transfusions were not screened for HIV antibody. In France, seroconversion rates in repeat blood donors per 10^5 person-years decreased from 3 (95% CI 2–4) in 1992–1994 to 1 (95% CI 0.5–1.5) in 2001–2003.
- Recipients (2344, 2851, 6187). Rates of transfusion-transmitted HIV infections per 10^5 units are 0.04–0.5 in the United States, and 0.025 in the United Kingdom. In Romania by the end of 1990, >400 children had contracted HIV by transfusion of unscreened blood.

HTLV (2851, 4717, 5320). HTLV is transfusion transmissible, from reactivation of latently infected lymphocytes. Cell-free blood products do not transmit HTLV.

- Donors (9, 5912, 7244, 8420). Donors in or from endemic areas should be screened. Reported seroprevalence per 10^5 donors are 10–25 in the United States, 30 in Italy (an endemic area), and 1 in France (4 in first-time donors, 0.1 in repeat donors).
- Recipients (1973, 2851, 4717). Some 40–60% of recipients of infective blood seroconvert, after a median period of 51 days. In the United States, transfusion-transmitted HTLV infection rates are 0.05–0.4/10^5 units. In Brazil in 1991–1995, 29% (15/52) of patients with tropical spastic paraparesis (that is associated with HTLV1) had a history of transfusion, and transfusion was more important than risks from unsafe sex or injection drug use. Intervals from transfusion to symptoms were ½–30 years, with medians of 6 years (from last transfusion) to 10 years (from first transfusion).

TRANSFUSION-TRANSMITTED BACTERIA

Risks (1242, 2852, 3619, 4131, 5272, 6162, 6187). Blood products can contain bacteria or bacterial endotoxins. Platelets are a growth medium for bacteria when stored at 20–24°C for >3 days. The prevalence of bacterially contaminated platelets is ~0.3–1/1,000 units.

Reactions from contaminated products in recipients are typically immediate and include chills, fever, and septic shock. Lethality is high (60–100%). In high-income countries, rates of transfusional bacteremia or BSI per 10^5 transfused units are 0.02–0.2 for red blood cell products and 1–20 for platelets. The sepsis rate from transfused platelets is 1/10^5 recipients.

Agents (1242, 5272, 6162). For contaminated donations, bacteremia in donors needs to be inapparent and persistent. Nosocomial infection can result from inadequate handling of products or equipment, or inadequate preparation of the site.

- Frequent transfusion-associated bacteria (by relative frequency from erythrocytes E or platelets P) are: *Y. enterocolitica* (E: 50%), *Staphylococcus* (P: CoNS 10%; E and P: *S. aureus* 4–17%), *Serratia* (E and P: 8–15%, *S. marcescens* and *S. liquefaciens*), *Pseudomonas* (E and P: 6–12%), *Klebsiella* (E and P: 4–17%), and *Enterobacter* (E and P: 6–8%).
- Infrequently isolated are (A–Z): *Bacillus* (P), *Brucella* (endemic areas), *Clostridium* (E and P), *Enterococcus* (E), *Ehrlichia* (4933), *E. coli* (P), *Propionibacterium* (E), *Providencia* (E), *Rickettsia* (4933), *Salmonella* (P), *Streptococcus* (P), and *Treponema pallidum pallidum*.

Y. enterocolitica (720, 4288, 7206). Mild, unrecognized diarrhea can cause asymptomatic bacteremia in donors. *Y. enterocolitica* can survive or even grow in units kept at 0–4°C. Infections in recipients can result in fatal septic shock.

T. pallidum pallidum (1005, 5643). Seroprevalence in donors is 0.1–0.3 in high-income countries, but 0.3–13 in low-income countries. However, transfusional syphilis (from inapparent treponemia) is rare in high-income countries.

TRANSFUSION-TRANSMITTED FUNGI

Instances are rare. A case of transfusion-associated *C. parapsilosis* was reported in a woman with neoplasia. Identical strains were isolated from the transfused red blood cell unit but not from the donor. Possible sources included transient donor fungemia or contamination during blood collection (5924).

TRANSFUSION-TRANSMITTED PROTOZOA

Transfusion-transmission requires parasitemic donors, and survival in donations during storage. *Babesia*, *Leishmania*, *Plasmodium*, and *Trypanosoma cruzi* meet these requirements. For *Toxoplasma*, transfusion-transmission is limited to rare instances, when tachyzoites circulate in peripheral blood (3756).

Babesia (2852, 3292, 4933). Over 40 transfusion-transmitted *B. microti* infections are reported in the United States, including from erythrocytes and platelets. *B. microti* can survive in blood components for up to 35 days.

- Donors (3499, 4329, 6715, 8006). Inapparently infected donors are a challenge for blood bank safety. Whether recall of recent tick bites can reliably predict infective donors is uncertain. In Connecticut in 1997–1998, 4% (1,284/30,669) of donors reported tick bites in the preceding 6 months, but *B. microti* antibodies were as prevalent in donors recalling tick bites (0.4%, 3/848) as in donors not recalling bites (0.3%, 3/1,000). In contrast in Germany, *B. divergens* antigenemia was more frequent in persons with a history of tick bites (12%, 26/225) than in control blood donors (2%, 2/120).
- Recipients (1960, 3292, 4933). An inapparently infected donor exposed six recipients, one adult, one child, four neonates; three recipients became parasitemic. The risk of transfusional babesiosis is ~0.6/10^5 units. Unlike tick-borne babesiosis, which is seasonal, transfusional babesiosis is perennial.

Leishmania (2951). Under conditions of blood banking, *Leishmania* can remain infective for ≥15 days, including in whole blood, packed red blood cells, and platelets.

- Donors (4271, 4584, 5654). *L. infantum* and *L. donovani* parasitemias can be inapparent. In Brazil, 9% of 1,194 volunteer blood donors were seroreactive to *L. donovani*. Also in Brazil, *L. donovani* DNA was amplified from blood of 24% (5/21) of asymptomatic but seroreactive donors. In southern France, 76 (13%) of 565 blood donors were reactive in Western blot, and buffy coats from nine reactors grew promastigotes in culture. Screening of donors in or from highly enzootic-endemic areas should be considered.
- Recipients (4584). Cases of transfusional visceral leishmaniasis have been reported outside enzootic-endemic areas in North America and West Europe. In infected areas, multiply transfused patients are at increased risk of infection.

Plasmodium (563, 2523, 3950, 5255, 6961). As blood stages are largely intraerythrocytic, transfusional risks are limited to products with erythrocytes. The infectious dose is low, probably 1–10 asexual parasites per blood unit.

- Donors (563, 3950, 6517). For parasitemia prevalence in endemic areas, see chapter 20. Screening should be tailored to local needs and could include history, antigen or antibody tests, or possibly NAT. In hyperendemic areas, serology likely detects partially immune rather than infective (parasitemic) donors. In North America and West Europe, travelers are excluded from donation for 6 months after leaving malarious areas; immigrants are excluded for 3 years.
- Recipients (999, 5255). In high-income contries, transfusion-transmitted malaria rates are $\leq 0.03/10^5$ units. In the United States in 1963–1999, 93 transfusional malaria cases were reported: 33 (35%) by *P. falciparum*, 25 (27%) each by *P. vivax* and *P. malariae*, and 5 (5%) by *P. ovale*; 3 (3%) cases were mixed, and in 2 (2%) the species was unknown. Lethality was 11% (10/93). Well-documented risks in nonmalarious areas contrast with poorly known risks in endemic areas where chemoprophylaxis of recipients is an alternative or addition to donor screening.

T. cruzi (999, 8099). Infectivity of latently infected, seroreactive individuals could be detected by xenodiagnosis (by allowing laboratory reduvids to feed on subjects), which is impractical. In enzootic countries without national blood bank policy, risks from transmission can reach 10–20%. In high-income countries with significant numbers of Latin American immigrants, *T. cruzi* is an emerging blood transfusion hazard.

- Donors (999, 3035, 3270, 4330, 6688, 8099). Donor seroprevalence in Latin America ranges broadly from $\sim 0.1\%$ to $\geq 5\%$. Prevalence of 1–5% has been reported in Argentina, Colombia, Costa Rica, Honduras, Mexico, Paraguay, and Peru, prevalence of >5% in Bolivia and Guatemala. In Mexico, donor prevalence ranges from 0.2 to 2.8%. In U.S. blood donors, 0.01–0.2% are seroreactive, and 7–14% report birth or stays in enzootic areas. Donor screening may include history, antibodies, and hemoculture and NAT on reactive donors.
- Recipients (6688). Rates of transfusion-transmitted *T. cruzi* infections reported in Latin America range broadly, from zero in five countries to a high of $480/10^5$ units in Costa Rica.

TRANSFUSION-TRANSMITTED HELMINTHS

Microfilariae (335) (early larvae) that circulate in peripheral (diurnal and nocturnal) blood can survive in banked blood. Under experimental conditions, counts of motile *Loa loa* microfilariae in blood decreased by 66% during storage for 18 days, from 1,564/ml to 1,032/ml. Transfusional microfilaremia can cause fever and rash. However, microfilariae cannot develop further in humans (they need to be taken up by a vector; see chapter 4).

18.5 TRANSPLANTS

Transplants (grafts) are living, replacing organs, tissues, or cells. In autologous grafts, donor (D) and recipient (R) are identical. In allogeneic grafts, D and R are different humans. In xenotransplants, D is mammals. Organs are solid, delineated, multifunctional body parts, transplanted as such (e.g., kidney) or as parts (e.g., bone, cornea, skin). Tissues (e.g., fascia) are soft, amorphous, connecting body parts. Cells (e.g., sperms and stem cells) are separate, small living units. For blood, see "Transfusions" above.

Infections. Transplants can become colonized from procurement. Unlike implants (see "Implants" below), transplants can carry agents in parenchyma, blood vessels, or cells from latently infected (D+) donors. Transplant-associated infections can be nosocomial (during insertion), reactivated (by impaired immunity in latently infected [R+] recipients), or transplant transmitted (from D+ to R−). For the latter, criteria are the same as for transfusion-transmission (see section 18.4).

Theoretical risks from xenotransplants are mammalian viruses such as porcine endogenous retrovirus (PERV) (2180, 3254) and encephalomyocarditisvirus (EMCV) (870). For reactivated infections, see section 14.6.

Prevention. Preventive measures include donor evaluation, good procurement and storage practices, recipient evaluation, pretransplant vaccines, posttransplant exposure avoidance, and surveillance.

- Donor screening (6651) for infectivity (D+, D−). Screening could include exposure history (Box IV.1), with a focus on lifestyle (sex with high-risk groups, injection drug use, imprisonment, tattoos), bites by animals, international travel, vaccines, and past infections (prions, HIV, syphilis, tuberculosis, malaria), physical examination, tuberculin skin test, and blood tests for CMV, EBV, HBV, HCV HIV, HTLV, *T. pallidum*, and *T. gondii*. Test-negative "window" periods are the same as with blood donors (Table 18.3). For tissues or cells preserved for months, donation screening before use may be added to detect contaminants from storage. Donation screening can replace donor screening, if the latter is impracticable, e.g., ejaculate screening for targeted STI before in vitro fertilization.
- Recipient screening for susceptibility (R−, R+). It could include review of vaccines and the same program as with donors.
- Vaccines (348, 1167) to consider for pretransplant review and updates include diphtheria, tetanus, pertussis$_{acellular}$ (dTp$_a$), HBV, *Influenzavirus*, measles, mumps, rubella (MMR), polio, and VZV, in stem cell recipients with an emphasis on vaccines for encapsulated agents (Hib, *N. meningitidis*, and *S. pneumoniae*).
- Exposure avoidance (7012) should cover hospital (health workers, environment, and visitors), domicile (household members for *Mycobacterium*, showers for *Legionella*, air-conditioning for *Aspergillus*, and pets for zoonoses), and leisure (sex, drugs, and travel).
- Chemoprophylaxis (1167) or preemptive therapy (active infection and no disease yet) (6771, 6924) should be considered during graft-versus-host reactions and in R− from D+. Target opportunists include CMV, fungi, and *Toxoplasma*.

SOLID ORGAN TRANSPLANTS

Exposure (http://www.census.gov/prod/2004pubs/04statab/health). The first heart transplantation was performed in South Africa in 1967. In the United States in 2003 (1990) the reported numbers of organs transplants were kidney >15,000 (>9,000), liver >5,600 (>2,500), heart >2,000 (>2,000), pancreas >1,300 (60), and lung >1,000 (200). In 2003, 1-year survival (and numbers of people waiting for that organ) were: kidney 98% (58,400), pancreas 95% (>4,000), heart 87%, (>3,500), liver 85% (17,500), and lung 82% (>3,900).

Infections (2421, 4726, 5754, 6453, 7008) (Box 18.4). About 20–70% of organ transplant recipients develop bacterial infections (UTI, respiratory tract infection [RTI], intra-abdominal), and 1–19% develop fungal diseases. Risk modifiers include recipient susceptibility, type of suppressive treatment, type of transplant, and time.

- Time (5754, 6453, 7008). Initially (weeks 0–4 posttransplant), SSI (see section 18.3) and HSV reactivation dominate. During months 1–6, opportunists (e.g., *Legionella*, *Listeria*, *Nocardia*, *Aspergillus*, *Candida*, *Pneumocystis*, and *Toxoplasma*), viruses (e.g., CMV, EBV, HBV, and HCV), and *Mycobacterium* are prominent. After >6 months, most recipients do well or are diagnosed with outpatient infections, e.g., UTI or pneumonia. About 10–15% develop late reactivations, mainly zoster, and 5–10% continue immune-suppressive therapy.
- Organ. An infection profile by organ is beyond the scope of this book. A summary follows below. Chronic infections that lead to transplantation may persist beyond transplantation.

Kidney transplant recipients (599, 4726, 5688, 5754). Typical are UTI (mainly due to *E. coli*) and infections by CMV (reactivated or primary) and polyoma BK

Box 18.4 Organ transplant-associated agents, by agent cluster	
TT, transplant transmitted.	
Droplet-air	AdV, *Influenzavirus*, PIV, PVB19, RSV; *B. cepacia*, *Legionella*, *Klebsiella*, *M. tuberculosis*, *Pseudomonas*; *Aspergillus*, *Cryptococcus*, *Histoplasma* (TT), *Pneumocystis*
Feces-food	EBV, enteric AdV, CMV, HCV (could be TT), *Rotavirus*; *C. difficile*, *Enterobacter*, *Enterococcus*, *E. coli*, *Listeria*, *Proteus*, *Salmonella*; microsporidia; *T. gondii* (can be TT)
Zoonotic	LCMV (TT), rabies virus (TT), WNV (TT); *Ehrlichia*, *Francisella*; *Leishmania* (can be TT), *Plasmodium* (can be TT), *T. cruzi* (can be TT)
Environmental	Environmental mycobacteria; *S. stercoralis* (TT?)
Skin-blood	BKV, CMV (can be TT), EBV (can be TT), HBV, HCV (TT?), HHV6, HHV8 (can be TT), HIV (can be TT), VZV; *Candida*

virus. A rare but serious risk is invasive disease from reactivated *Strongyloides stercoralis.*

Liver transplant recipients (6924). Typical are recurrent hepatitis C, CMV disease (reactivated or primary), bacteremia by resistant enteric bacteria such as VRE and *Pseudomonas, Candida* fungemia (nosocomial), and invasive *Aspergillus* disease.

Heart transplant recipients (2959, 6771, 7487). Typical infectious complications are pneumonia (including by *Legionella, M. tuberculosis,* and environmental mycobacteria), bacterial sepsis, and CMV disease (reactivated or primary).

Lung transplant recipients (856, 1332, 1791, 1839, 2858, 7487). Typical are pneumonia due to *B. cepacia* (in recipients transplanted because of cystic fibrosis) and *Legionella,* invasive *S. pneumoniae* disease (in 6%, for a rate of ~2/100 person-years), invasive *Aspergillus* disease (attack rates up to 10–20%), and *Pneumocystis* pneumonia.

Droplet-Air Cluster

Viruses (2595, 7008, 8012). Lung, heart, and other organ transplant recipients are exposed to the full diversity of respiratory viruses. Respiratory viruses reported in recipients include AdV, *Influenzavirus,* parainfluenzavirus (PIV), PVB19, and respiratory syncytial virus (RSV).

Bacteria. Reactivated or acquired respiratory bacterial agents reported in lung, heart, and other transplant recipients include *B. cepacia* (cystic fibrosis), *Klebsiella, Legionella, M. tuberculosis,* and *Pseudomonas* (cystic fibrosis). Paired organs such as lungs provide an opportunity to compare self- with non-self-transplantational infections. **Legionella (5754, 7487).** At a tertiary care center in the United States, rates of *Legionella* pneumonia per 1,000 recipients were 0.2 for kidney recipients, 0.3 for liver recipients, but 1.9 for heart recipients and 2.1 for lung recipients. Microbiological diagnoses included *L. pneumophila* serogroups 1, 3, 4, 5, and 6 and *L. micdadei.* Posttransplant *Legionella* pneumonia may herald rejection reaction. **M. tuberculosis (5260, 5754).** Disease rates in recipients in high-income countries are 1–6%, that is 20–70 times higher than in the population. The main mechanism is reactivation (R+). Symptoms and sites can be atypical, and reactivated tuberculosis can contribute to allograft malfunction.

Fungi. Reactivated or acquired respiratory fungi reported in lung, heart, and other transplant recipients include *Aspergillus, Cryptococcus, Histoplasma,* and *Pneumocystis.* **Aspergillus (856, 2857, 6924, 7008).** Invasive *Aspergillus* disease is a transplantation hazard, in particular, for lung and liver recipients. Risks include spores in air, colonization (frequent in lung recipients), massive immunosuppression, and renal dysfunction. Disease is typically manifest in the first few months posttransplant. **Cryptococcus (3514).** In 178 reviewed cases, disease was manifest from 2 days to 12 years (median, 1½ years) posttransplant. In half (87) of cases, the CNS was the only site affected. Disease rate was 28/1,000 recipients, and lethality was 42%. Whether infections are acquired or reactivated is not known. **Histoplasma (4423, 7679).** Transplantational infections are infrequent, even in endemic areas. Transplant-transmission has been documented. **Pneumocystis (2858, 3257, 3363, 4726, 6065).** *Pneumocystis* pneumonia (PCP) is a transplantation hazard. PCP can be manifest from 6 weeks to 16 years (typically 5 months) posttransplant. Without chemoprophylaxis, 5–25% of organ recipients can develop PCP. In Cleveland, Ohio, in 1987–1996, 2% (25/1,299) of organ recipients developed PCP, for a rate of 5/1,000 transplant-years (14.5 in year 1, ~2 in following years). Rates per 1,000 transplant-years were highest (22) in lung recipients and lowest (~1) in kidney recipients. Molecular and epidemiological data in kidney recipients and outbreaks suggest that up to >50% of PCP can be acquired nosocomially from source patients (children, HIV-infected).

Feces-Food Cluster

Infectious abdominal complications in liver, intestinal, renal, and other transplant recipients include diarrhea (attack rates, 10–40%), intra-abdominal abscesses, esophagitis, and colitis. Recipients are exposed to the spectrum of enteric agents. Intestinal transplant rejection episodes may coincide with diarrhea episodes.

Viruses (5967, 8416). Reported agents of viral enteritis or extraintestinal disease include CMV, EBV, enteric AdV, and *Rotavirus.*

Bacteria (599, 4726, 8416). Reported agents of bacterial enteritis, UTI, or extraintestinal disease include *C. difficile, Enterobacter, E. faecalis* (diagnosed in 22% or 47/213 of kidney recipients in 1 year), *E. coli* (in 36% or 76/213 of kidney recipients), *Listeria, Proteus,* and *Salmonella.* **Listeria (2194, 2890, 5754, 7008).** The disease is typically manifest 2–6 months posttransplant. About two thirds of cases are manifest as CNS infection. Lethality is ~8%. Food is a vehicle for nosocomial clusters in immunecompromised patients. **Salmonella (5754).** The most frequent manifestation is BSI. The rate of non-Typhi infections in kidney recipients is ~20 times greater than in the population.

Fungi. Reported agents of enteric and extraintestinal disease are *Candida* (esophagitis) and microsporidia. ***En-***

cephalitozoon (2607, 4234, 5120, 6700). *E. cuniculi* can cause diarrhea and invasive disease in organ recipients.

Protozoa (8416). Reported agents of enteric and extraintestinal disease are *Cryptosporidium*, *Giardia*, and *Toxoplasma*. **Toxoplasma (2596, 3075, 3756, 5754, 6220).** *Toxoplasma* infections can be reactivated or transplant transmitted. The risk of reactivation in R+ is 1–2%. In 31 kidney recipients with toxoplasmosis, sources were undetermined in 61% (19), endogenous (reactivation) in 7% (2), and likely an infected transplant in 32% (10). Any organ could serve as a vehicle, but heart is preponderant. Rates of acquisition in D+R− pairs are 1–30% for kidney, 20% for liver, and 50–60% for heart. Among 119 heart recipients, 14 were D+R− pairs; of the 14 susceptible recipients, 7 did not receive chemoprophylaxis, and 4 developed toxoplasmosis 20–32 days posttransplant confirmed by *T. gondii* cysts in myocardium from biopsy or necropsy.

Zoonotic Cluster

Sources include unrecognized infections in human donations and posttransplant exposure. Porcine, simian, and bovine materials are increasingly being considered alternatives to scarce human materials.

Viruses. Lymphocytic choriomeningitis virus (LCMV) (1249). In the United States in 2005, liver, lungs, and two kidneys from a test-negative donor caused disease in four recipients. The likely source of LCMV was a test-positive hamster kept by the deceased donor. **Rabies virus (1239, 3244).** In the United States in 2004, liver, two kidneys, and iliac artery from a donor incubating unrecognized bat-mediated rabies transmitted the virus to four recipients who became ill 21–27 days posttransplant and died of encephalitis. Rabies was confirmed in donor and recipients by histopathology, electron microscopy, serology, or other tests. Similarly in Germany in 2005, rabies was confirmed in two of six recipients (two kidneys, two corneae, one lung, one liver) from a donor with a postportem diagnosis of rabies. **WNV (1200, 3604).** In the United States, two kidneys, one liver, and one heart from an inapparently infected donor transmitted WNV to four recipients who became ill 7–17 days posttransplant.

Bacteria (6520). Impaired immunity predisposes recipients to unusually severe disease of high lethality. Special precautions are advised for them, including for foods, pets, and leisure activities. Agents that have been identified in recipients include *Ehrlichia* and *Francisella*.

Protozoa. *Leishmania* **(3272).** About 30 transplant-associated cases of visceral leishmaniasis (VL) have been reported, mainly in kidney recipients. Disease was manifest 3–156 (median, 12) months posttransplant. Leishmaniasis months (3–36) posttransplant is compatible with reactivation and transplant-transmission, whereas manifestation after >3 years suggests acquisition in enzootic-endemic areas. ***Plasmodium.*** Transplant-associated malaria due to *P. falciparum*, *P. vivax*, and *P. malariae* has been reported in kidney, liver, and heart recipients (368, 2404, 3408, 4308, 5501, 7615). In Turkey, the rate of posttransplant malaria in kidney recipients was 3% (11/420), but 10 of the 11 patients with malaria had received transplants in India. Transplantational malaria outside malarious areas in nontraveled recipients strongly suggests transplant-transmission. ***T. cruzi*** **(1108, 3955, 6237, 8380).** *T. cruzi* can be transplant transmitted. Infections have been reported in kidney recipients living in enzootic areas, as well as in recipients outside enzootic areas, from immigrant donors. Although *T. cruzi* latently infects heart muscle cells and neural cells of the esophagus or colon, the kidney is the vehicle for most transplant-transmitted cases.

Environmental Cluster

Mycobacteria **(5754).** Environmental mycobacteria reported in organ recipients include *M. avium-M. intracellulare*, *M. chelonae*, *M. fortuitum*, and *M. kansasii*. Infections are manifest days to years posttransplant. ***Nocardia*** **(5754, 6028).** *Nocardia* is an uncommon cause of invasive diseases in kidney and heart recipients. *Nocardia* can become manifest any time posttransplant.

Strongyloides **(5688).** Massive and disseminated disease are complications in immune-impaired kidney transplant recipients. Why this complication is not observed in heart, liver, lung, or pancreas transplant recipients is unclear. A possible explanation is larvae dormant in kidney that are transplant transmitted and become reactivated by immune-suppressive treatment.

Skin-Blood Cluster

Viruses. Reactivated viruses include HBV, HCV, HIV, *Herpesviridae* (CMV, HHV8, HSV, and VZV), and polyomaviruses (BK polyomavirus [BKV] and JC polyomavirus [JCV]). Transplant-transmission is confirmed for CMV, EBV, HIV, and HHV8, and suspected for HCV (Box 18.4). **CMV (599, 2288, 4726, 5754, 5967, 6452, 7008, 8416).** Posttransplant CMV disease is diverse, including mononucleosis-like illness, pneumonia, hepatitis, colitis, and chorioretinitis. Reactivated CMV disease is typically manifest within 30–60 days posttransplant, rarely after 5–6 months. By chemoprophylaxis and organ, reported disease rates are ∼10–75%. D (+ or −) and R (+ or −) constellations influence disease expression and rates. By 3–28 (mean, 8) weeks posttransplant, 13% (24/192) of recipients had developed CMV disease: 8% (2/24) of D+R+, 46% (11/24) of D−R+ (both groups likely by reactivation),

33% (8/24) of D−R− (likely by primary infection), and 13% (3/24) of D+R− (possibly transplant transmitted). Among 146 liver recipients, lethality was lowest in D−R− (likely primary disease), intermediate in D−R+ or D+R+ (odds ratios of 2–3, likely reactivations), and highest in D+R− (odds ratio of 4.5, likely by transplant). **EBV (2923, 3609, 4884, 7008).** Posttransplant infections can be reactivated, transplant transmitted, or acquired (primary). EBV was transmitted by liver, causing lymphoproliferative disease in R−. Reactivated disease in R+ is typically manifest 2–6 months posttransplant. In kidney transplant recipients, reactivation in the first week of immune-suppressive treatment appears to be associated with graft rejection. **HBV (5781, 7008).** In ≥80% of R+ liver recipients, HBV is reactivated posttransplant. Reactivated HBV is typically manifest within 30–60 days posttransplant. **HCV (6585, 7008).** HCV can cause recurrent hepatitis C and cirrhosis in R+ liver recipients. Reactivated hepatitis C is typically manifest in 30–60 days posttransplant. Although infections in recipients are mainly reactivated, transmission by transplantation or accompanying transfusion is likely, as a history of transplantation is a significant risk for HCV infection. **HHV6 (7008).** Reactivation of HHV6 has been recognized increasingly, typically within 6 weeks posttransplant. **HHV8 (2648, 3357, 3677, 6184).** HHV8 transplant-transmission has been reported. Of 90 R−, 10 (11%) seroconverted in 6–7 months posttransplant. In the United States, Kaposi's sarcoma is diagnosed in 0.5% of transplant recipients. In Germany, 22 (21%) of 107 transplant recipients had anti-HHV8 IgG, compared with 0.4% (1/236) of blood donors. **HIV (2069).** In Pennsylvania 0.3% (2/583) of donors and 1.7% (18/1,043) of recipients were HIV infected. Of 18 HIV-positive recipients, 7 had pretransplant antibodies, while 11 seroconverted posttransplant. Sources for 11 seroconverters were unknown in eight, high-risk blood donors in 2, and a D+ in 1. **HSV (5754, 7008).** Disease manifestations include mucosal lesions and pneumonia. Reported disease rates are 1–53%. HSV is reactivated and manifest typically within 1 month posttransplant. **BKV (3344, 4164, 5296, 7008).** BKV-associated nephropathy is an emerging disease in kidney recipients. It is diagnosed 2–213 (mean, 42) weeks posttransplant, in 1–7% of kidney recipients. Manifestations include pyuria, viruria, tubulointerstitial nephritis, and graft failure. **JCV (4164).** JCV-associated progressive multifocal leukoencephalopathy has occasionally been reported in transplant recipients. **VZV (2880, 5754, 7008).** Most (90–100%) transplant recipients are latently infected (R+) and at risk of reactivation; a small number is R− and at risk of primary infection. Disease is manifest in 1–15% of recipients, for a rate of 2.7/100 transplant-years. In a large series of 869 organ recipients, zoster attack rates were 9% (75) overall: 6% (15/263) in liver recipients, 7% (32/434) in kidney recipients, 15% (8/53) in lung recipients, and 17% (20/119) in heart recipients. Disease has typically been manifest 6–9 months posttransplant.

Fungi (5754, 5781, 7008). Disease is typically manifest in the postoperative period. In liver recipients, the bowel is a source of *Candida*, and a significant proportion of abdominal infections is due to *Candida*. The rate of invasive *Candida* disease is 10–320/1,000 recipients.

PARTIAL ORGAN, TISSUE, AND CELL TRANSPLANTS

Partial organs and tissue transplants from human donors include cornea, bone and cartilage, epidermis and fascia, heart valves and vascular grafts, and embryos. Cell transplants include hematopoietic stem cells and sperma.

Exposure (1167, 3890) (http://www.census.gov/prod/2004pubs/04statab/health). In the United States in the 2000s, annual records are of 1.2 million bone graft procedures, 200,000 sperma donations, >46,000 cornea grafts, >20,000 stem cell grafts, 5,000 tendon grafts, 3,250 m^2 skin grafts, 3,000 heart valve grafts, and 2,500 embryo transfers.

Infections (Box 18.5). Agents associated with transplantation of partial organs, tissues, and cells include prions,

---

Box 18.5 Agents after or from partial organs, tissues, or cell transplants, by cluster

TT, transplant transmitted.

Droplet-air	AdV, *Influenzavirus*, PIV, *Rhinovirus*, RSV, VZV; *Legionella*, *M. tuberculosis* (can be TT); *Aspergillus*, *Pneumocystis*
Feces-food	*Citrobacter*, *Clostridium*, *Enterobacter*, *Enterococcus* (including VRE), *E. coli*, *Listeria*; *T. gondii* (can be TT)
Zoonotic	Rabies virus (TT); *Plasmodium* (can be TT)
Environmental	Environmental mycobacteria, *Nocardia*, *Pseudomonas*, *Stenotrophomonas*; *Fusarium*, *Mucor*, *Rhizopus*; *Strongyloides*
Skin-blood	Prions (TT), CMV (can be TT), EBV (can be TT), HBV (can be TT), HCV (can be TT), HHV6, HPV (TT?), HSV, HTLV (can be TT), polyomaviruses BK and JC; *Staphylococcus* (CoNS, TT?); *Candida*

viruses, and protozoa. Seroprevalence in 11,391 U.S. tissue donors in 2000–2002 was 0.2% for HBV (by HBsAg), 1.1% for HCV (by anti-HCV), 0.09% for HIV (by anti-HIV) (Table 18.3) (8420).

Bone, Cartilage, and Tendon

The focus is on bacteria (623, 2110, 2325, 4465, 7502, 7788). Bone and its products (powder and spongiosa) may grow pretransplant bacteria, including *Aeromonas*, *Bacillus*, *B. cepacia*, *E. coli*, *Klebsiella*, and *S. epidermidis*. Infection rates in recipients are comparable to rates in prosthetic implants. By size and type of the graft, infection rates in recipients of culture-negative bone allografts ($n = 324$) from a large U.S. hospital bone bank were 4–5%. In Taiwan, 5% (12/262) of grafts grew bacteria during surgery; infection rates were 2% (4/250) in recipients of culture-negative allografts, 75% (9/12) in recipients of contaminated grafts, and 5% overall.

Clostridium **(265).** Although rare, 26 bone and cartilage transplant-associated infections were recorded in the United States, including *C. sordellii*.

Mycobacterium **(2110, 6337).** In the 1940s, *M. tuberculosis* osteomyelitis was reported from frozen rib allografts. For 19 patients infected with *M. fortuitum* after open-heart surgery, the suspected source was bone wax and graft.

Cornea and Dura Mater

Prions. Cornea and dura mater are rare vehicles. **Cornea (845, 2057, 3219, 3379, 3890, 4207).** Cases of CJD by cornea from unrecognized D+ have been reported. For one case in Germany the incubation period was 30 years. Proposed donor exclusion criteria include death from unknown neurological disease or death at psychiatric clinics. On the other hand, the projected prevalence of CJD among ~45,000 U.S. cornea donors is ~1 when assuming that 90% of CJD cases are incubating and inapparent. **Dura mater (928, 2110, 3125, 4208, 5325).** Cases of CJD by lyophilized dura mater from unrecognized D+ have been reported. The lifetime risk for recipients to develop CJD is estimated at 0.03–0.05%. By 2000, 114 transplant-transmitted cases were reported. Reported incubation periods range from 14 months to 22 years (median, 10 years).

Viruses. Cornea is a rare vehicle for CMV, HBV, HSV, and rabies. **CMV (2110).** Following allografts from D+, 8% (2/25) of R− seroconverted, a finding that suggests transmission by cornea. **Rabies virus (1239, 3379, 3443, 3653).** Cornea from unrecognized D+ is a rare vehicle of rabies in recipients.

Bacteria (2110, 3477, 5185). Although ~5–15% of corneae grow bacteria on retrieval, as an avascular structure and after rinsing in disinfectant, the cornea is not an efficient vehicle. At a cornea bank, *B. cepacia* in trypan blue dye was found to have contaminated 28 of 169 corneae; however, no postgraft infections were recorded.

In Vitro Fertilization

Infections (1491, 2665, 3537) predispose for infertility that motivates couples for in vitro fertilization. In women this includes bacterial vaginosis (by *Gardnerella*, *Mycoplasma*, and *Prevotella*), inapparent endometrial infection, and pelvic inflammatory disease. Donor and recipient screens could include CMV, HBV, HCV, HIV, HSV, HPV, *Chlamydia trachomatis*, *Neisseria gonorrhoeae*, *Mycoplasma hominis*, *Treponema pallidum*, *Ureaplasma*, *Candida* (*C. albicans* and *C. glabrata*), and *Trichomonas*. Appropriate treatments can reduce or eliminate infection risks associated with in vitro fertilization and embryo transfer. For STI, see section 14.7.

Ejaculate (1491, 4383, 5715). Ejaculate can contain viruses ("virospermia", e.g., CMV, HBV, HIV, HPV, HSV, possibly HCV), bacteria ("bacteriospermia", e.g., *C. trachomatis*, *Ureaplasma urealyticum*, possibly *T. pallidum*), and parasites (*Trichomonas vaginalis* and *Schistosoma haematobium*). In The Netherlands, PCR amplified *C. trachomatis* in semen from 4% (4/97) of asymptomatic donors 20–45 years of age processed for insemination. Although some of these agents may predispose to male or parental hypofertility, a significant, detrimental effect on in vitro fertilization is considered unlikely, perhaps because semen is cryopreserved before use.

Stem Cells

Stem cells (565, 1167) here are hematopoietic precursor cells, whether from bone marrow, placenta, umbilical cord or peripheral blood, and whether allogeneic (from twins, siblings, registry) or autologous. By impaired phagocytosis and indwelling devices, recipients are at high risk of infection. At Duke University, North Carolina, in 1990–1998, of 485 children having received 510 stem cell allografts, 276 (57%) contracted 585 infections. Recovery and posttransplant infections progress through three broad phases:

- In month 0–1, cellular immune depletion is reversed by successful engraftment and sustained counts of neutrophils ($>500/\mu l$ and platelets ($\geq 20,000/\mu l$). Nosocomial infections are typical, including by *Enterococcus*, *Staphylococcus* (CoNS, *S. aureus*), gram-negative rods, and *Candida*.

- In months 1–3, graft-versus-host disease (GVHD) may ensue. Typical agents are CMV, encapsulated bacteria (*S. pneumoniae*, *H. influenzae*, and *N. meningitidis*), and fungi (*Aspergillus* and *Pneumocystis*).

- In months 4–24, immune competence recovers (more rapidly in autografts than allografts). Typical are CMV,

VZV, EBV, and vaccine-preventable agents (measles virus, *S. pneumoniae*, and *C. tetani*).

A detailed review of infections in recipients is beyond the scope of this book. A summary by agent clusters follows.

Droplet-air cluster. About 5–10% of recipients develop pneumonia, for a rate of ~6/1,000 neutropenia-days (1902). In up to 70% of cases, no agent may be identified. **Viruses (565, 812, 1167, 7924).** Respiratory viruses are a hazard for stem cell recipients, in particular, in the first year posttransplant, and including community-acquired viruses. Agents of lower RTI or pneumonia in stem cell recipients include AdV (may account for 8% of infections in pediatric recipients), CMV, *Influenzavirus*, HSV, PIV, *Rhinovirus*, and RSV.

- PIV (1581). Person-to-person spread is a risk in clinics that are frequently visited by family members of recipients. At a United Kingdom bone marrow transplant unit, PIV3 caused outbreaks in 1995 (for 4 months) and 1996 (for 1 month) with 15 infections in recipients 7–153 days posttransplant.
- RSV (3153, 7366). RSV has caused outbreaks in recipients and on hematology wards. At a U.S. bone marrow center in 1990, RSV infected 19% (31/199) recipients in 13 weeks; 78% (14/18) with pneumonia died.
- VZV (1167, 3113, 3173). Reactivation of VZV is a hazard. Of 1,186 stem cell recipients, 216 (18%) reactivated VZV in 4 days to 11 years posttransplant (86% within 18 months). In a randomized vaccine trial, the zoster rate in recipients of the control arm was 29/100 and year. R− should be advised to avoid exposure.

Bacteria. Bacterial pneumonia in stem cell recipients can be reactivated or acquired.

- *Legionella* (3154, 5630). *Legionella* should always be considered in recipients with pneumonia. Because *L. pneumophila* non-1 serogroups and species other than *L. pneumophila* can infect recipients, detection should not be limited to urine test. Sources can be nosocomial (see section 17.7) or in the community (see section 6.2). In an outbreak at a bone marrow transplantation unit, the attack rate was 17% (4/23).
- *M. tuberculosis* (8358). The population rate of *M. tuberculosis* predicts disease rates in recipients. The overall attack rate is ~0.5% (52/13 881). Risks include allograft, GVHD, and total body irradiation.

Fungi

- *Aspergillus* (131, 565, 1167, 2857, 4749, 7902, 7906). *Aspergillus* causes significant disease in stem cell recipients. Risks include allograft, posttransplant pre-engraftment neutropenia, and GVHD. In Seattle in 1993–1998, 359 recipients suffered 375 episodes of invasive disease, for rates per 100 per year of 1–6 in autograft recipients and 10–12 in allografts. In pediatric recipients, 5% (28/585) of all infections were due to *Aspergillus*. On autopsy, *Aspergillus* was detected in 17% (25/149) of recipients. Not all infections are invasive. About 75–80% of *A. fumigatus* isolates and ~20% of *A. flavus* represent invasion, while remaining fractions are from colonization. Molecular and epidemiological evidence suggests that perhaps up to one third of infections are nosocomials while the rest are community acquired.
- *Pneumocystis* (5017, 5500, 7055). Stem cell recipients are susceptible to PCP. Some 8% of recipients may develop PCP. Time to diagnosis is ~5–16 (typically 10) months. In Seattle, Wash., in 1993–1996, by chemoprophylaxis, PCP rates in allograft recipients were ~0.3–5/100 person-years.

Feces-food cluster. Bacteria (565, 1167, 1321, 1902). Agents of enteric infections or BSI in stem cell recipients include *Citrobacter*, *C. difficile*, *Enterobacter*, *Enterococcus* (including VRE), *E. coli*, and *Listeria*. Antibiotics make stem cell recipients susceptible to *C. difficile*. In pediatric recipients, 4% (22/585) of all infections were due to *C. difficile*. Corticosteroids increase susceptibility of recipients to *L. moncytogenes*, for an attack rate in recipients of 0.4%. **Protozoa.** Manifestations of *T. gondii* (1167, 4971, 6959) are diverse and include pneumonitis with respiratory distress. Disease is typically manifest in the first 1–3 months posttransplant. Disease can result from reactivation (most, in R+), primary infection (in D−R−), or transplant-transmission (rare, in D+R−). The value of D and R screening is uncertain. The reported disease rate in R+ is 2%.

Zoonotic cluster. Impaired immunity facilitates reactivation of latent zoonotic infections (see "Solid Organ Transplants" above). Falciparum malaria has been reported in a stem cell recipient, more likely by transplant-transmission than by reactivation (4318). D and R in or from malarious areas are proposed to receive antimalarials before cell collection and conditioning, whether patent parasitemia is present or not.

Environmental cluster. Bacteria (1902, 3985). Stem cell recipients are susceptible to hospital wet agents such as *Pseudomonas* and *Stenotrophomonas*. Outbreaks are a threat for hematology units. *Nocardia* (7705) is an uncommon cause of invasive disease in recipients. At three centers, 27 cases were diagnosed in 25 years, for a rate of 3/1,000 per year. The median time to diagnosis was 30 weeks.

Fungi (4749, 5498). *Fusarium*, *Mucor*, and *Rhizopus* have been isolated from stem cell recipients. In Brasilian and U.S. hospitals, the cumulative incidence of invasive *Fusarium* disease was ~0.5–1%.

Helminths (1167). Recipients with unexplained eosinophilia should be evaluated for *Strongyloides*.

Skin-blood cluster. About 18–22% of recipients develop BSI, for rates of ~12–19/1,000 neutropenia-days (1902). **Viruses.** Evidence exists for transplant-transmission of CMV and EBV. These viruses can latently infect peripheral leukocytes.

- CMV (565, 1167, 2934, 8382). After engraftment, during months 1–3, CMV is a critical agent that can cause pneumonia, retinitis, hepatitis, or colitis, and predispose for other opportunists. Of 239 allograft recipients, 19% (46) were diagnosed with CMV infections after a median of 50 days. In pediatric recipients, 4% (23/585) of all infections were due to CMV. In Cairo, Egypt, 39% (11/28) of recipients tested positive for CMV by NAT posttransplant, compared with 6% (2/35) of nongrafted candidates from the same center. This difference could be due to reactivation or transplant-transmission. For D+R− pairs and R+ of allografts, chemoprophylaxis or preemptive treatment with ganciclovir should be considered.
- EBV (1748, 3080) can be transmitted by stem cells, and EBV is a cause of posttransplant lymphoproliferative disease.
- HBV (7389, 8382). Over 25 months, six patients contracted acute hepatitis B from stem cells grafts contaminated in a cryopreservation tank through leakage of bags. In Cairo, Egypt, 11% (3/28) of stem cell recipients tested positive for HBV by NAT posttransplant, compared with 3% (1/35) of nongrafted candidates from the same center.
- HCV. In Cairo, Egypt, 21% (6/28) of stem cell recipients tested positive for HCV by NAT posttransplant, compared with 6% (2/35) of nongrafted candidates from the same center (8382).
- HHV6 (8345). Likely from reactivation, HHV6 was reported to cause viremia and rash in 35% of R+ within 1 month posttranplant.
- HPV. With increasing time posttransplant, warts become increasingly prevalent in recipients.
- HSV (1167). Reactivated HSV is a significant cause of morbidity in stem cell recipients. Disease can be localized (oropharyngeal, pneumonia, and keratitis) or disseminated. R+ can shed HSV, becoming a nosocomial source. For allografted R+, acyclovir prophylaxis is recommended; for R−, exposure avoidance.
- BKV and JCV (565, 2221, 3344, 4164). In pediatric recipients, 11% (63/585) of all infections were due to BKV or JCV. Besides AdV and toxins, reactivated BKV is a cause of hemorrhagic cystitis in recipients. Reported rates of BKV cystitis in recipients are 10–14%. BKV cystitis becomes manifest 1–84 (typically 9) days posttransplant. JCV-associated progressive multifocal leukoencephalopathy has occasionally been reported in stem cell recipients.
- VZV (7458). Stem cell recipients are at risk of reactivation and disseminated disease. Chemoprophylaxis with aciclovir seems to effectively suppress reactivation.

Bacteria (1167, 1902, 5431). Stem cell recipients are susceptible to *Staphylococcus* (CoNS, *S. aureus*). CoNS is the leading cause of BSI in recipients. Sources of CoNS are nosocomial. CoNS was found to contaminate stem cell preparations. Streptococci are also reported in recipients. **Fungi (565, 1167, 1902, 7784, 7902).** Candida infects about 5–25% of stem cell recipients. In pediatric recipients, 10% (56/585) of all infections were due to *Candida*. Sources can be endogenous or nosocomial. A risk is posttransplant, pre-engraftment neutropenia that may last 10–18 (tyically 15) days.

Heart Valves and Vascular Grafts
As human-derived and synthetic cardiovascular grafts are commonly treated together, see section 18.6.

Skin Grafts
Infected sites such as vascular ulcers and burns can be the reason for grafting and constitute sources for graft infections.

Viruses (2110, 5927). Skin allografts are a suspected but unconfirmed vehicle for viruses. Donor screening could focus on HIV and HPV. In HIV-infected patients, survival of skin grafts is impaired.

Bacteria (1666, 7645). Skin flora and nosocomial wet bacteria are to be expected on skin allografts. Of 132 recipients of full-thickness or split skin grafts for traumatic, burn, or other skin defects, 31 (24%) lost grafts because of infections by *P. aeruginosa* (in 58%), *S. aureus*, *Enterobacter*, *Enterococcus*, and *Acinetobacter*. Pretransplant treatment with disinfectants or antibiotics can reduce bacterial risks.

18.6 IMPLANTS

Implants are synthetic devices intended for permanent placement in the human body. Hip endoprosthesis was introduced in 1960, the intrauterine device in 1970.

Exposure. In the United States alone, implants per year comprise 2 million osteosynthetic implants, 600,000 joint protheses, 450,000 vascular implants, 300,000 pacemakers-defibrillators, 130,000 pairs of mammary implants, 85,000 mechanical heart valves, and 40,000 cerebrospinal fluid shunts.

Infections (372, 1750) (Box 18.6). Implants, unlike transplants (see section 18.5) can be sterilized for use. Implant-associated infections ("implantitis") are therefore nosocomial or endogenous (at implant sites or from distant foci) rather than implant transmitted. Most (one half to two thirds) implantitis is due to either *S. aureus* or CoNS. For acute surgical site infections, see section 18.3.

CARDIOVASCULAR IMPLANTS

Cardiac implants (372, 1000) include prosthetic heart valves, pacemaker leads, and defibrillator leads. Arterial implants include synthetic vascular grafts, synthetic patches, vascular stents, and intraaortic balloon pumps. Infections can be manifest by fever, endocarditis, aneurysm, embolism, and septic shock.

Prosthetic Heart Valves (1000, 5207)

Worldwide, >370,000 prosthetic heart valves are implanted per year. About half are synthetic, most others are biosynthetic (tissue), made from human, porcine, or bovine valves fixed on a synthetic ring. Synthetic valves are not intrinsically infected but thrombogenic, requiring lifelong anticoagulation. Conversely, natural valves from HBsAg-positive donors have transmitted HBV to recipients.

Prosthetic valve endocarditis (PVE) (1349, 1750, 3371, 3829, 5183). PVE is the main, life-threatening complication of prosthetic heart valves. This is not surprising, as infected valves are a reason for replacement and a potential source for prosthetis infection. PVE accounts for 1–15% of all infective endocarditis. By follow-up period (2–24 months) and surgery (primary, revision), 1–3% of recipients develop PVE, for overall rates of 0.3–0.6/100 patient-years. Lethality is 22% in the hospital and >30% overall. **Agents (1349, 3829, 3988, 5183, 5388, 8070).** In early PVE, nosocomial agents dominate. In late PVE, the agents resemble native-valve endocarditis (3829). By onset (first 2 months versus after >12 months), the main agents are *S. aureus* and CoNS (~65% versus ~45%), viridans (*Streptococcus mitis, S. oralis, S. sanguis,* and *S. gordonii*) and other streptococci (0–3% versus 40%), and *Enterococcus* (7–12%).

Infrequent agents include *Bartonella quintana, Corynebacterium* (3–5%), gram-negative rods (3–11%), "HACEK" agents (~6%, **H**aemophilus aphrophilus, **A**ctinobacillus actinomycetemcomitans, **C**ardiobacterium hominis, **E**ikenella corrodens, and **K**ingella kingae), *Pasteurella multocida,* and fungi (1–12%, *Aspergillus, Candida*).

Pacemakers and Defibrillators (372, 1015, 3829)

Worldwide, >3.4 milion persons carry pacemakers or defibrillators, and 0.5 million are implanted each year. Batteries are placed in a subcutaneous pouch; leads are intracardiac. By device type, implant year, and antibiotic prophylaxis, reported infection rates are 0.1–20% (often 1–8%). About 90% are pouch infections, and 10% are endocarditis.

Lead endocarditis (372, 1015, 1703, 1750, 2098, 5013, 5681). About 0.5% of carriers develop endocarditis, for a rate of 0.55/1,000 recipients per year. Some 10% of implants eventually fail; in about one fourth of failures, removal is necessary because of infection. Lethality is 8–30%. **Agents (372, 2098, 3829).** Main agents of lead endocaritis are *S. aureus* and CoNS (in 70–90%), *Streptococcus* (~15%, *S. anginosus,* others), *Enterococcus* (~10%, *E. faecalis*), and *Corynebacterium*. Essentially, these represent skin flora that can ascend from infected pouches. In 13%, infections are polymicrobial.

Uncommon agents include *Actinobacillus, Brucella, Enterobacter, E. coli, Klebsiella, Haemophilus parainfluenzae, Mycobacterium, Peptostreptococcus, Propionibacterium, Pseudomonas, Serratia; Aspergillus, Candida,* and *Torulopsis.*

Stents and Other Vascular Implants

Stents (372). Stents are small metal mesh tubes inserted into vessels to keep flow open. In the United States, >400,000 stents are implanted each year. Stent infections are rare (<1 of 10,000), but if they occur, they are life-threatening, including aneurysm, embolism, and sepsis.

Box 18.6 Main implant-associated agents, by cluster

Droplet-air	*K. pneumoniae, M. tuberculosis, S. pneumoniae; Aspergillus*
Feces-food	*Enterococcus* (including *E. faecalis,* VRE), *E. coli, Salmonella*
Zoonotic	*Bartonella, Pasteurella*
Environmental	*Actinomyces,* environmental mycobacteria, *P. aeruginosa*
Skin-blood	*Corynebacterium, Propionibacterium, Staphylococcus* (typically in one half to two thirds: CoNS, *S. aureus,* MRSA), *Streptococcus* (GAS, viridans); *Candida*

Vascular implants (422, 1750, 1999). Types of vascular implants include coronary artery stents, peripheral vascular stents, and cadaveric veins or arteries (e.g., aortoiliac) for bypasses. Complications can be manifest from days to 2–5 years postimplant. Manifestations include bleeding, "mycotic" aneurism, and sepsis. Risks vary with site (high for inguina), surgery (high for revision), and underlying morbidity (high for diabetes). Reported 5-year infection rates are 2–6%. Treatment is difficult, often requiring surgery. Two-year survival is <60%. A majority of infections is due to *Staphylococcus*. For hemodialysis, see section 18.7.

OSTEOSYNTHETIC AND ORTHOPEDIC IMPLANTS (1750, 8412)

"Motility" implants include metallic plates, nails, and fixation pins for osteosynthesis, and metals and ceramics for osteosynthetic replacement of joints, e.g., hip. Infection (implantitis) is suspected from instability, pain, and inflammation and confirmed by imaging, revision surgery, and microbiology (culture and NAT from periprosthetic tissue and removed implant).

Infection is maintained in biofilm that forms when floating (planctonic) bacteria settle on fibrin-coated implant surfaces and secret glycocalyx. Bacteria in biofilms are sheltered from antibiotics and immune attack. Treatment options include removal of implant or salvage antimicrobial combination therapy for 3–6 months.

Osteosynthesis (1750, 3278)

By case mix, body part, operative method, and geography, 1–4% of osteosynthetic implants become infected (see section 18.3). Rates are higher for revision than primary surgery, and higher for external pins than internal plates. Over 50% of infections are due to *S. aureus* (>40%) and CoNS (>10%).

Endoprostheses (1750, 2271, 4343, 4405, 7439, 8153)

Worldwide, there are ~1 million hip and >0.25 million knee replacements each year. Infection risks vary by joint, time period, type and duration of intervention, implant material, and comorbidities, in particular, diabetes, overweight, and malignancy. Historical prosthesis infection rates were 5–10%, current 10-year rates in high-income countries are 0.5–5% (typically <2.5%). Yet, >10% of joint prostheses may require revision surgery, mostly for biomechanical failure. **Agents (2077, 2271, 4343, 4405, 8153, 8412).** Agent pattern varies by months postimplant: after <1 month, *Staphylococcus* dominates; after 1–24 months, anaerobics and polymicrobials dominate and onset is often insidious; and after >24 months, "odd" hematogenously seeded agents become more frequent.

Main agents are *Staphylococcus* (in 40–70%, *S. aureus*, MRSA, and CoNS), polymicrobials (in 10–15%), anaerobes (8–10%, mainly *Propionibacterium*), *Streptococcus* (5–15%, GAS), and *Enterococcus*.

Infrequent and unusual agents include *Citrobacter freundii*, *H. influenzae*, mycobacteria (*M. tuberculosis*, environmental, e.g., *M. fortuitum*), *Mycoplasma*, *Salmonella* (mainly hip), and *Streptococcus anginosus*.

NEUROSENSORY IMPLANTS (6518)

Neurosensory implants include shunts for hydrocephalus, and cochlear implants. Neurosurgery carries a risk of site infection (see section 18.3), epidural, subdural, or brain abscess, and meningoencephalitis by a wide agent spectrum that includes *Staphylococcus*, enterobacteria, and *P. aeruginosa*.

Cerebrospinal Fluid (CSF) Shunts (372, 1750, 5132, 7944)

Shunts are subcutaneously inserted tubings that drain CSF from brain ventricles to peritoneum (ventriculoperitoneal shunt) or heart atrium (ventriculoatrial shunt), or from spinal cord lumen to peritoneum (lumboperitoneal shunt). Complications include endocarditis, nephritis, and less frequently meningitis. By shunt type and surgery (primary or revision), reported infection rates are 2–29%; for ventriculoatrial shunts, 2–9%. **Agents (372, 4783, 5199, 7944).** Major agents are *Staphylococcus* (in one half to two thirds, *S. aureus*, CoNS), *Propionibacterium acnes* (should not be readily rejected as a contaminant), and gram-negative rods (in up to 25%), including *E. coli*, *K. pneumoniae*, and *P. aeruginosa*. Treatment often necessitates shunt removal.

Cochlear Implants (2659, 6177)

Cochlear implants are devices for improving hearing. In the United States in 20 years, ~60,000 cochlear implants were placed, ~10,000 children carry an implant, and ~1 million people with impaired hearing are candidates. **Agents (1217, 2659, 6177).** Some implants increase the risk of invasive *S. pneumoniae* disease. *Pseudomonas* is an agent of chronic cochlear implant infection. Vaccines for potential recipients include *S. pneumoniae* and *H. influenzae* b (for children).

INTRAUTERINE DEVICES (3713, 7584)

IUD are flexible, metal or plastic devices that release copper or hormones for fertility control. Worldwide, ~160 million (15%) women of reproductive age wear IUD. Contraindications include sex with multiple partners, a history of ectopic pregnancy or pelvic inflammatory disease, postpartal endometritis, septic abortion, impaired immunity, and genital actinomycosis. Removed IUD have yielded cervicovaginal flora (e.g., *Lactobacillus*, *G. vaginalis*, *C. albicans*), and pathogens such as *Staphylococcus* (CoNS, *S. aureus*), *E. coli*, *Enterococcus*, *Peptostreptococcus*, and *S. agalactiae*. Discussed complications include bacterial vaginosis, increased carriage (*C. trachomatis*, *S. agalactiae*, and *Actinomyces*), and ascending abdominopelvic diseases. However, when complying with contraindications and good insertion practice, IUD-associated infections appear to be very rare.

***Actinomyces* (332, 2399, 5705, 5833).** Women with IUD appear at increased risk of vaginal carriage. In 0–30% of women with IUD, *Actinomyces* has been isolated from cervical smears. In case-control studies, the proportion of colonized women was 1–3% in IUD wearers and 0–0.2% in nonwearers. Abdominopelvic *A. israelii* disease is a rare complication of prolonged IUD use.

***C. trachomatis* (2329).** Of 327 IUD wearers, 19 (6%) tested positive for genital *C. trachomatis* (17 were asymptomatic, 2 had pelvic inflammatory disease [PID]). For prevention of PID, preimplant screening, treatment, and counseling are advised.

PID (2323, 2941, 5212, 6915, 7584). Unsafe sex and overdiagnosis in IUD wearers, and condom use in control groups are likely confounders of observational studies. If an increased risk of PID exists for IUD wearers, it is likely small and limited to insertion. Once in place, wearers who do not engage in high-risk sex acquire infections at a rate of <1.5/1,000 women-years. In Kenya, 636 IUD wearers were monitored for 24 months. PID was diagnosed in 2% (3/156) of HIV-infected women and 0.4% (2/493) of noninfected women; IUD were considered appropriate for women who had access to care. Of 200 Greek women who inserted IUD despite a high (60%) prevalence of lower genital infections, none developed PID after 36 months of observation.

BREAST IMPLANTS (1750, 5933)

In the United States in 2000, at least 2 million women received breast implants. The typical material is silicone. Infections have complicated 2–2.5% of implants. Two thirds of infections develop early (0–6 weeks postsurgery); the remaining occur late (after months to years).

Agents. The main agent of early infections is *S. aureus*. It has caused toxic shock syndrome in recipients. Late infections have been poorly documented. Reported agents include *Bacteroides*, *Enterococcus*, environmental mycobacteria (see section 17.6), *K. pneumoniae*, *Pasteurella*, *P. aeruginosa*, and *Staphylococcus* (*S. aureus*, CoNS).

18.7 DIALYSIS

Dialysis is the process of removing metabolites from blood by semipermeable membranes and hyperosmolarity. The automate is the dialyzer (blood-washing machine). Dialysis is invasive, as it requires vascular (hemodialysis [HD]) or peritoneal (peritoneal dialysis [PD]) access. Indications are acute, for acute renal failure, or chronic, for end-stage renal disease. Only chronic dialysis is reviewed here.

Exposure. Worldwide, >1 million persons are on dialysis, 70–85% on HD, 15–30% on PD.

Infections (593, 3069, 3315, 5166, 7493, 7776) (Box 18.7). In most patients with end-stage renal disease, immunity is impaired and anergy may cause false-negative tuberculin skin test reactions. Impaired immunity and vascular access make dialysis patients susceptible to infections. Frequent infections in dialysis patients are access-site infections and pneumonias. Tuberculosis rates are 10- to 25-fold higher in dialysis patients than in high-income populations. Dialysis-associated infections can be reactivated or acquired nosocomially from workers, patients, or dialysis equipment.

Prevention (172, 3315, 7492, 7776, 8270). Preventive measures include educating patients and staff about access-site care, vaccines for patients and staff (focusing on HBV, influenza, and *S. pneumoniae*), routine testing of patients and staff for HBV and HCV, and surveillance. For HBV- and HCV-infected dialysis patients, cohorting is recommended, including dedicated room or unit sector, dialyzers, and staff. Immune-impaired dialysis patients exposed to infective tuberculosis should be treated for latent *M. tuberculosis* infection, regardless of skin test results. If diagnosed tuberculosis disease, dialysis needs to be performed in isolation, until treatment has achieved clinical improvement and negative sputum cultures. Nasal carriers of *S. aureus* in dialysis centers need special attention.

HEMODIALYSIS (172, 3069, 7493)

In the United States in 2000, >3,600 centers cared for >240,000 HD patients. Of all infections, about one half to three fourths are access-site infections, pneumonia, and UTI. Bacteremias may account for 10%; BSI are less frequent, but the most frequent infectious cause of death. Lethality of HD patients can exceed 20% per year.

Access-Site Infections

Infections (372, 593, 7493). Vascular access for HD includes arteriovenous fistulas, catheters, and synthetic grafts. By access type and center, reported infection rates per 100 patient-months are 0.6–12 (often 3), with a low

> **Box 18.7** Dialysis-associated agents and infections, by cluster
>
> Droplet-air *Klebsiella, M. tuberculosis*
> Feces-food   *Enterobacter, Enterococcus* (including VRE), *E. coli*
> Environmental Wet cluster: e.g., *Acinetobacter, B. cepacia,* environmental mycobacteria, *Pseudomonas, Serratia, Stenotrophomonas*
> Skin-blood   HBV, HCV, GBV-C; *Staphylococcus* (about two thirds, CoNS, *S. aureus*, including MRSA)

for arteriovenous fistulas, and a high for noncuffed catheters. About 70% of HD patients are hospitalized within 2 years for access-site complications that frequently require site change.

Agents (372, 739, 3789, 7493). Main agents of access-site infections and access-related bacteremias are *Staphylococcus* (in ~50–85%, *S. aureus*, CoNS), *Enterococcus* (in 5–10%), gram-negative rods (10–20%, e.g., *Enterobacter* in 2–5%, *E. coli* in 2–3%, *Klebsiella* in 2–4%, and *Pseudomonas* in 2%), and fungi (in 0.5–1%). Resistant agents are a concern, including MRSA, VRE, *Acinetobacter*, and *Stenotrophomonas*. Wet bacteria such as *B. cepacia* and *M. chelonae* have caused outbreaks on HD units.

Viremia
The main hazards are HBV, HCV, and HIV. Other agents reported in HD patients include CMV, HHV8 (2648), and GBV-C (hepatitis G virus).

HBV (172). HBsAg prevalence in HD patients in the United States fell from 7.8% in 1976 to 0.9% in 1999. Carriers of HBsAg are infectious, carriers of HBsAg-HBeAg are highly infectious from blood, with 10^{8-9} virions per ml. At room temperature, HBV survives on surfaces for ≥7 days. Outbreaks in HD units have been reported.

HCV (172, 1863, 2465, 7492, 8270). Infection risks include increasing time on HD, rooms or equipment shared with infected patients, and contaminated dialysis equipment. Worldwide, 1–80% of HD patients are seroreactive: 7–10% in North America, 1–2% in northern Europe, 6% in western Europe, 25% in southern Europe, and 25–35% in eastern Europe, and 40–80% in low-income countries. In Spain, of new, marker-negative HD patients, 7% (8/114) seroconverted in 18–56 months (7/8 converters were also NAT positive). Outbreaks in HD units have been reported.

GBV-C (3468, 4816, 8270). GBV-C is prevalent in dialysis units, but there is no evidence of harm. In Taiwan, 25% (40/160) of HD patients and 8% (3/40) of healthy staff tested positive for antibodies or nucleic acid, and the infection rate was 2.6/100 patients per year.

HIV (172, 2157, 8270). In the United States, 1.4% of HD patients are infected. In high-income countries, HIV transmission in dialysis units seems rare. Outbreaks have been reported in Egypt and Colombia, however. At two centers in Egypt in 1993, syringes shared by HD patients caused 39 infections.

Bacteremia and BSI
Risks (172, 1990, 7365). Reported BSI rates in HD patients are 0.7–3.6 (typically 2) per 100 patient-months.

Agents (1990, 2953, 7365). Causative agents include *Staphylococcus* (in ~60–70%, *S. aureus*, MRSA, and CoNS), *Enterococcus* (in ~10%), *Enterobacter, Klebsiella,* and *Serratia*. **T. pallidum pallidum (6640).** In Saudi Arabia in 1996–2000, 5% (10/187) of HD patients were initially reactive, and 2% (3) seroconverted after 10–14 (mean, 12) months. Latent syphilis in HD patients can be a source of nosocomial spread, and seroscreening is an option.

PERITONEAL DIALYSIS
Overview (603, 7776). Forms of PD include continuous ambulatory PD (CAPD, the most common), continuous machine-cycled PD (CCPD), automated PD (APD), and continuous flow PD (CFPD). Sealing the tunnel at the site where the peritoneal catheter exits the skin is critical. Complications are exit-site infections and peritonitis. Their rates can reach 0.3–1 per person per year. By good site and connection care, one third to one half of patients on CAPD can avoid peritonitis.

Agents (592, 2145, 8058). Agents of both exit-site infections and peritonitis mirror skin and bowel floras and contaminants from dialysis fluid. The main agent is *Staphylococcus* (in 25–95%, CoNS, *S. aureus*). Other reported agents include *Pseudomonas* (in 5–15%), *E. coli* (in 5–10%), environmental mycobacteria (in ~5%, e.g., *M. chelonae* from the dialyzer), *Enterococcus* (in 2–7%), and *K. pneumoniae* (in 2–5%), *Corynebacterium* (nondiphtheriae, in 0–9%), as well as *C. albicans* (in ~5%).

18.8 INTENSIVE CARE

ICU (6318) are hospital units that monitor vital signs continuously, 24 h/day, 7 days/week. By patients, ICU are grouped as neonatal, medical, surgical, combined, or other.

Exposure. Devices frequently utilized in ICU (usage rates per 100 patient-days) include bladder catheters (20–90), CVCs, (40–80), and machines for assisted ventilation (30–50).

Infections (1901, 2195, 2954, 6248-6250, 6318, 7658, 7836, 7837). A review of infections in ICU is beyond the scope of this book. On any given day, 10–45% of patients in ICU have at least one infection. As patients with community-acquired severe infections such as pneumonia or sepsis are likely admitted to ICU, nosocomial (hospital-acquired) infections should be reported separately. In Europe in April 1992, point prevalence in ICU was 45% (4,501/10,038) for all infections and 20% (2,064/10,038) for nosocomial infections. By case mix and ICU type, frequent nosocomial infections in ICU are pneumonia (relative share, 20–45%), UTI (15–30%), and BSI (15–40%).

By case mix and ICU type, infection rates per 100 device-days are 0.35–15 (often 1–2) for ventilator-associated pneumonia, 0.05–8 (often 1) for catheter-associated UTI, and 0.05–10 (often 0.2–1) for catheter-associated BSI. For nosocomial pneumonias, see section 17.5; for nosocomial UTI, see section 17.4; and for BSI, see section 18.2.

Agents (4320, 5336, 7658, 7836). Viruses from pneumonia in ICU are often community acquired, e.g., AdV, *Influenzavirus*, PIV, and RSV. In contrast, ICU-acquired infections are frequently polymicrobial, and predominantly due to nosocomial agents (see Box VI.2 and Table 18.1).

Frequent nosocomial agents in ICU (relative frequency, >5%) include *S. aureus* (30%), *P. aeruginosa* (24–30%), CoNS (20%), *Candida* and other yeasts (17%), *E. coli* (7–13%), *Enterococcus* (7–12%), *Acinetobacter* (10%), *Klebsiella* (4–17%, often 6–8%), and *Enterobacter* (low to 13%).

Antimicrobial resistance. Antimicrobial resistance is prevalent among many nosocomial agents and of particular concern in ICU (see Fig. 17.1). A few examples follow:

- *Acinetobacter* (1571). In Spain in 1997–1998, 8% (153/1836) of consecutive ICU patients grew *A. baumannii* resistant to carbapenem; colonization or infection risks included recent carbapenem use or recent colonization.
- *Enterobacter* (1230). In the United States in 1998–2004, 28% of 5,328 isolates from ICU were ESβL producers and resistant to third generation cephalosporins.
- *Enterococcus* (1230, 1430). In the United States in 1998–2004, 14% of 14,140 isolates from ICU were VRE. In Perth, Australia, in 2001, VRE (*E. faecium*) colonized or infected 68 patients in ICU, and one strain colonized 0.9% (169/19,658) of patients on 23 wards. The outbreak was controlled by screening all hospitalized patients, rapid laboratory detection (in 30–48 h, by culture and PCR), isolation of carriers, and cohorting of contacts.
- *Staphylococcus* (1230). In the United States in 1998–2004, 53% of 22,890 *S. aureus* isolates from ICU were MRSA.

Outbreaks in ICUs. Reports of outbreaks are numerous, in particular, from neonatal ICU. Outbreaks have included viruses such as *Influenzavirus* (6527), *Rhinovirus* (7688), *Rotavirus* (8151), and RSV (1619); bacteria such as *Acinetobacter* (5091), *Citrobacter* (7472), *Enterobacter*, *Enterococcus* (1430), *Klebsiella* (2656), *Pseudomonas* (2905), *Serratia* (7166), and *Stenotrophomonas* (6373); and fungi such as *Malassezia* (1320).

SECTION VII
Agents

19 Taxonomic Overview
20 Genera A to Z

19

Taxonomic Overview

Diversity (3225, 7371). Earth is incredibly beautiful and diverse. Less than 2 million of ~4–100 million species are cataloged. About 1,200 agents can colonize or infect humans: prions, >200 viruses (4% of 5,000), >500 bacteria (8% of 6,000), >60 protists (<0.1% of 0.1–0.2 million), >200 fungi (0.2% of 0.1 million), ~290 helminths (0.7% of >40,000), and arthropods (<0.01% of >1 million). Taxonomy of many proteobacteria, protists, and fungi is in flux, and a "tree of life" is a continuous "construction site." For reference, Table 20.1 provides a simple taxonomic overview. A summary of basic units follows.

Prions (6029). Prions are misfolded, transmissible proteins that withstand ordinary heat treatment. Hosts, histopathology, and proteomics are used to define phenotypes.

Viruses (7748). Viruses are biochemical units characterized by a core from nucleic acid (RNA or DNA) and a shell from protein, without or with an envelope. For replication, viruses need living units (cells). Taxonomy uses hosts, cytopathology, ultrastructure, genomics, phylogeny, and response to antivirals such as nucleoside antagonists (e.g., acyclovir, lamivudine, ribavirin), enzyme inhibitors (e.g., neuraminidases, proteases, reverse transcriptases), and interferon-α. Available vaccines include mumps, measles, rubella (MMR), polio, varicella, hepatitis A, hepatitis B, influenza, Japanese encephalitis, rabies, tick-borne encephalitis, and yellow fever.

Bacteria. Bacteria are basic living units characterized by free RNA and DNA in protoplasm, an outer membrane, and a peptidoglycan cell wall. Taxonomy uses hosts, in vitro growth and metabolism, staining and morphology, genomics, phylogeny, and response to antimycobacterials (e.g., isoniazid) and antibiotics such as β-lactams (e.g., penicillin, aminopenicillin-anti-β-lactamase combinations, and cephalosporins), macrolides (e.g., erythromycin), quinolones, and aminoglycosides (e.g., streptomycin).

Gram-negative proteobacteria have thin walls that do not retain Gram stain. Gram-positive bacteria have thick (firmicute) walls that retain stain. Available vaccines include diphtheria, tetanus, pertussis$_{acellular}$ (DTP$_a$), *Haemophilus influenzae* b, bacillus-Calmette-Guérin (BCG) (for *Mycobacterium tuberculosis*), *Neisseria meningitidis* (A, C, W135, Y), *Streptococcus pneumoniae*, *Salmonella enterica* serovar Typhi, and *Vibrio cholerae*.

Protists (4300). Protists are eukaryotes featuring a nucleus and organelles. Protists include ancestral, aquatic, unicellular organisms, straminopiles (with tripartite, hollow hairs), amebas (motile by pseudopodia), and protozoa (with organelles such as mitochondria, alveoli, flagella, kinetoplasts, and chloroplasts). Taxonomy is in flux, using ultrastructure, genomics, and phylogeny, rather than traditional light microscopy and response to antiprotozoals such as antiamebics (e.g., nitroimidazoles), antileishmanials (e.g., meglumine antimoniate), antimalarials (e.g., artemisinins and quinolines), and antitrypanosomials (e.g., benznidazole and melarsoprol). Vaccines for humans are not yet available.

Fungi (5251, 5859). Fungi are eukaryotes with chitinous cell walls, plasma membranes with ergosterol, and asexual (buds, conidia) or sexual (spores, in asci or basidia) reproduction. Taxonomy uses growth on substrates, reproduction, ultrastructure, genomics, phylogeny, and response to antifungals such as triazoles (e.g., fluconazole), amphotericin B, and terbinafine. Yeast are unicellular and budding. Dimorphic fungi are yeastlike at body temperature, but form filaments (hyphae) in soil or culture. Zygomycetes form nonseptate hyphae. Molds form septate hyphae that are translucent (hyaline) or pigmented (dematiaceous). Pigmented molds can release colorful microcultures (grains) from fistules in tissue. Dermatophytes are molds that utilize keratin. Microsporidia are unicellular, intracellular eukaryotes that by phylogeny and chitinous spores formed in polar tubuli belong to fungi.

Helminths (1816). Helminths are soft-bodied metazoa. In 1758, C. Linné (1707–1778) named six worms: *Ascaris lumbricoides*, *Diphyllobothrium latum*, *Dracunculus medinensis*, *Enterrobius vermicularis*, *Fasciola hepatica*, and *Taenia solium*. Although nematodes seem in a clade with arthropods, and platyhelminths are related to molluscs, helminths are retained as a group here.

Density of eggs in feces can be a surrogate measure of adult worm load. Infections in the community are often distributed unevenly (overdispersed), with few individuals carrying most of the worm load. Exposure "hot spots" can perhaps explain overdispersion, e.g., popular defecation sites. Anthelminthics include benzimidazoles (e.g., albendazole and mebendazole) for intestinal nematodes and tissue cestodes, ivermectine for intestinal and tissue nematodes and for tissue cestodes, and praziquantel for schistosomes.

20

Genera A to Z

Entries typically describe modes of spread or acquisition (by droplet-air, by feces-food, from (in)vertebrates, from the environment, or by skin-blood), risks, clinical impact (reported cases, rates per 10^5 population), outbreaks, and control or preventive measures. For taxonomy, see Table 20.1. For acronyms, see appendix 2.

ABSIDIA (*Zygomycota*: *Mucorales*) (1427, 5861). These fungi inhabit soil and plant debris. Acquisition is from inhalation or trauma. *A. corymbifera* can colonize hospitalized patients and cause invasive disease (zygomycosis) in patients with neutropenia, diabetes, or other immune impairments.

ACANTHAMOEBA (763, 4139, 4777, 4957, 6653, 6927, 7925) (Amoebozoa: Acanthopodida). These amebas dwell in soil, water, and dust, as trophozoites or cysts. Cysts are tenacious, resisting free chlorine of up to 1.6 mg/liter. Several species have been reported in humans, including *A. castellani* and *A. polyphaga*. **SPREAD**: is by water contact or splash (keratitis), or by inhalation (encephalitis). **RISKS**: for keratitis: wearing contact lenses, rinsing contact lenses with water, outdoor exposure (fishing), corneal abrasions. **CLINICAL INFORMATION**: Manifestations are keratitis (in immune-competent hosts), subacute granulomatous amebic encephalitis (mainly in immune-impaired hosts), rarely disseminated disease. The incubation period assumed for encephalitis is weeks to months. Trophozoites or cysts in corneal scrapes, cerebrospinal fluid, or brain biopsy confirm the clinical diagnosis. Encephalitis lethality is high. Treatment options include combinations of antifungals and antibiotics. **IMPACT**: Encephalitis cases are sporadic. In the 1980s, the incidence of amebic keratitis was estimated at $<0.2/10^5$/year. **OUTBREAKS**: A keratitis outbreak followed contamination of tap water from floods.

ACINETOBACTER (583, 604, 1769, 4725, 5915, 7000, 7740) (γ-*Proteobacteria*: *Pseudomonadales*, taxonomy uncertain). These tenacious, gram-negative bacteria are typically multidrug-resistant (MDR). There are >10 named species and >30 genospecies. Phenotypes of *A. baumannii* and *A. calcoaceticus* are virtually indistinguishable. This complex inhabits soil, water, vegetables, and nosohabitats. *Acinetobacter* can colonize human skin, the respiratory tract of patients, and temporarily the hands of health workers. **ACQUISITION**: Mainly nosocomial, from

Table 20.1 Simplified taxonomy of human-infective agents (HIA), selected zoonotic or animal-infective agents (AIA), and environmental agents (EIA)

Main taxa	Subordinate taxa and remarks
Prions	**HIA:** Creutzfeldt-Jakob disease, kuru. **AIA:** Bovine spongiform encephalopathy, scrapie, chronic wasting disease
Viruses	
RNA, unenveloped	
Astroviridae	*Mamastrovirus* (**HIA:** human astrovirus; **AIA:** mammalian astroviruses), also *Avastrovirus*
Caliciviridae	**HIA:** *Norovirus, Sapovirus.* **AIA:** *Lagovirus* (rabbits), *Vesivirus* (swine)
Hepeviridae	**HIA:** *Hepevirus* (HEV)
Picornaviridae	**HIA:** *Enterovirus* (e.g., echovirus or poliovirus), *Hepatovirus* (hepatitis A virus), *Rhinovirus.* **AIA:** *Aphthovirus* (foot-and-mouth disease virus), *Cardiovirus* (encephalomyocarditis virus)
Reoviridae	**HIA:** *Reovirus, Rotavirus.* **AIA:** *Coltivirus* (Colorado tick fever virus), *Orbivirus* (bovine bluetongue virus)
RNA, enveloped	
Orthomyxoviridae	**HIA:** *Influenzavirus*
Retroviridae	*Lentivirus* (**HIA:** human immunodeficiency virus; **AIA:** simian and feline immunodeficiency viruses), *Deltaretrovirus* (**HIA:** human T-lymphotropic virus; **AIA:** simian T-lymphotropic viruses). **AIA:** *Alpharetrovirus* (avian leukosis virus), *Betaretrovirus* (simian retrovirus 1 type D), *Gammaretrovirus* (feline leukemia virus), *Deltaretrovirus* (bovine leukemia virus), *Spumavirus* (foamy viruses)
Mononegavirales	
Bornaviridae	**HIA:** *Bornavirus*
Filoviridae	**HIA:** *Filovirus* (Ebola virus, Marburg virus)
Paramyxoviridae	**HIA:** *Morbillivirus* (measles), *Pneumovirus* (RSV), *Respirovirus* (P1V1, P1V3), *Rubulavirus* (mumps P1V2, P1V4), *Metapneumovirus.* **AIA:** *Avulavirus* (NDV); *Henipavirus* (Hendravirus and Nipahvirus), *Morbillivirus* (canine distemper and rinderpest viruses), *Respirovirus* (Sendaivirus)
Rhabdoviriade	**AIA:** *Lyssavirus* (rabies and bat lyssaviruses), *Vesiculovirus* (vesicular stomatitis virus)
Nidovirales	
Coronaviridae	**HIA:** *Coronavirus* (human CoV, SARS-CoV) **AIA:** *Torovirus*
Vector-vertebrate group	
Arenaviridae	**AIA:** *Arenavirus* (GUAV, JUNV, Lassavirus, LCMV, MACV, Sabia virus)
Bunyaviridae	**AIA:** *Hantavirus, Nairovirus* (CCHFV), *Orthobunyavirus* (Bunyamweravirus, California encephalitis virus group [INKV, JCV, LACV, SSHV, and TAHV], OROV), *Phlebovirus* (Rift Valley fever virus and sandfly fever viruses)
Flaviviridae	**HIA:** *Hepacivirus* (HCV, possibly GBV-C). **AIA:** *Flavivirus* (DENV, JEV, KFDV, MVEV, OHFV, POWV, SLEV, TBEV, WNV, YFV, and Zika virus), *Pestivirus* (classical swine fever virus and bovine viral diarrhea virus)
Togaviridae	**HIA:** *Rubivirus* (rubellavirus). **AIA:** *Alphavirus* (BFV, CHIKV, EEEV, Mayaro, ONNV, RRV, SFV, SINV, VEEV, and WEEV)
DNA, unenveloped	
Adenoviridae	*Mastadenovirus* (**HIA:** human adenovirus)
Circoviridae	**HIA:** SEN virus and TT virus
Papillomaviridae	**HIA:** *Papillomavirus* (HPV)
Parvoviridae	**HIA:** *Erythrovirus* (PVB19). **AIA:** Canine, murine, and simian parvoviruses
Polyomaviridae	*Polyomavirus* (**HIA:** polyomaviruses BK and JC, **AIA:** simian virus 40)
DNA, enveloped	
Hepadnaviridae	**HIA:** *Orthohepadnavirus* (HBV); *Avihepadnavirus*
Herpesviridae	
α	*Simplexvirus* (**HIA:** HSV, **AIA:** SHV), *Varicellovirus* (**HIA:**VZV). **AIA:** MDV, gallid herpesvirus 1.
β	**HIA:** *Cytomegalovirus* (CMV); *Roseolovirus* (HHV6 and HHV7)
γ	**HIA:** *Lymphocryptovirus* (EBV); *Rhadinovirus* (HHV8)
Poxviridae	**HIA:** *Orthopoxvirus* (vaccinia, variola), *Molluscipoxvirus* (Molluscum contagiosum) **AIA:** *Orthopoxvirus* (cowpox, ectromelia, monkeypox), *Parapoxvirus* (orf, pseudocowpox), *Avipoxvirus* (fowlpox); *Leporipoxvirus* (myxoma); *Yatapoxvirus*

(continued)

Table 20.1 (continued)

Main taxa	Subordinate taxa and remarks
Bacteria	
Proteobacteria	
α	
Rickettsiales	**AIA:** *Anaplasma, Ehrlichia, Neorickettsia, Orientia, Rickettsia, Wolbachia*
Rhizobiales	**AIA:** *Bartonella, Brucella*
β	
Burkholderiales	**HIA:** *Bordetella.* **EIA:** *Alcaligenes, Burkholderia, Ralstonia*
Neisseriales	**HIA:** *Eikenella, Kingella, Neisseria*
Nitrosomonadales	**AIA:** *Spirillum*
γ	
Legionellales	**AIA:** *Coxiella.* **EIA:** *Legionella*
Enterobacteriales	**HIA, EIA, or AIA:** *Citrobacter, Enterobacter, Escherichia, Klebsiella, Morganella, Plesiomonas, Proteus, Providencia, Salmonella, Serratia, Shigella, Yersinia*
Pasteurellales	**HIA:** *Haemophilus.* **AIA:** *Pasteurella.* **EIA:** *Actinobacillus*
Pseudomonadales	**HIA:** *Acinetobacter, Moraxella, Pseudomonas*
Other orders	**HIA:** *Aeromonas, Vibrio, Cardiobacterium.* **AIA:** *Francisella.* **EIA:** *Stenotrophomonas*
ε	
Campylobacterales	**HIA:** *Campylobacter, Helicobacter*
Actinobacteria	
Actinomycetales	**HIA:** *Actinomyces, Corynebacterium, Mycobacterium, Propionibacterium.* **EIA:** *Actinomadura, Nocardia, Rhodococcus, Streptomyces, Tropheryma*
Bifidobacteriales	**HIA:** *Bifidobacterium, Gardnerella*
Gram positive (Firmicutes)	
Anaeroplasmatales	**AIA:** *Erysipelothrix*
Bacillales	**HIA:** *Staphylococcus.* **EIA:** *Bacillus, Listeria*
Clostridiales	**HIA:** *Clostridium, Peptostreptococcus*
Lactobacillales	**HIA:** *Enterococcus, Lactobacillus, Streptococcus*
Mycoplasmatales	**HIA:** *Mycoplasma, Ureaplasma*
Other bacteria	
Spirochaetales	**HIA:** *Treponema.* **AIA:** *Borrelia, Leptospira*
Chlamydiales	**HIA:** *Chlamydia*
Bacteroidales	**HIA:** *Bacteroides, Porphyromonas, Prevotella*
Flavobacteriales	**AIA:** *Capnocytophaga*
Fusobacterales	**EIA:** *Fusobacterium*
Fungi	
Microsporidia	**AIA:** *Encephalitozoon, Enterocytozoon, Nosema*
Zygomycota	
Entomophthorales	**EIA:** *Basidiobolus*
Mucorales	**EIA:** *Absidia, Cunninghamella, Mucor, Rhizopus*
Ascomycota	
Pneumocystidales	**HIA:** *Pneumocystis jirovecii,* **AIA:** *Pneumocystis carinii*
Saccharomycetales	**EIA:** *Candida, Geotrichum, Saccharomyces*
Molds Hyaline	
Eurotiales	**EIA:** *Aspergillus, Paecilomyces, Penicillium*
Hypocreales	**EIA:** *Acremonium, Fusarium*
Onygenales	**EIA:** *Blastomyces, Coccidioides, Histoplasma.* **HIA:** *Epidermophyton.* **AIA:** *Microsporum, Trichophyton*
Other orders	**EIA:** *Scedosporium; Sporothrix*
Pigmented	
Chaetothyriales	**EIA:** *Exophiala, Fonsecaea, Phialophora, Wangiella*
Other orders	**EIA:** *Cladophialophora, Cladosporium, Leptosphaeria, Madurella*

(continued)

Table 20.1 Simplified taxonomy of human-infective agents (HIA) and selected zoonotic or animal-infective agents (AIA)[a] (continued)

Main taxa	Subordinate taxa and remarks
Basidiomycota	
Tremellales	**EIA:** *Cryptococcus, Trichosporon*
Sporidiales	**EIA:** *Rhodotorula*
Agaricales, Boletales	Edible mushrooms
Plants	
Sporophyta	Non-vascular: liverworts, hornworts, mosses; Vascular: club mosses, horsetails, ferns
Spermatophyta	Gymnosperms (naked seeds): cycads, ginkgo, ephedras, order Coniferales. Angiosperms: paleoherbs, monocots, basic dicots, caryophyllids, rosids, sympetals
Protists-protozoa	
Straminopila	**HIA:** *Blastocystis*. **EIA:** oomycetes, algae (phaeophytes, xanthophytes), diatoms
Mesomycetozoa	**EIA:** *Rhinosporidium seeberi*, fish protists
Amoebozoa	**HIA:** *Entamoeba*. **EIA:** Acanthopodida (*Acanthamoeba, Balamuthia, Hartmannella*), Heterolobosea (*Naegleria, Vahlkampfia*)
Euglenozoa	**HIA:** Diplomonadida (1-2 flagella: *Giardia*), Trichomonadida (≥3 flagella: *Dientamoeba, Trichomonas*). **AIA:** Kinetoplastida (*Leishmania, Trypanosoma*)
Alveolata	
Ciliata	**AIA:** *Balantidium*
Apicomplexa	**HIA or AIA:** Eucoccidiorida: *Cryptosporidium, Cyclospora, Isospora, Toxoplasma*. **AIA:** Haemosporidia: *Plasmodium*, Piroplasmorida: *Babesia, Theileria*
Dinoflagellata	**EIA:** *Pfiesteria*
Invertebrates	
Mollusca	Snails (Gastropoda), squids-octopuses (Cephalopoda), clams (Bivalvia)
Platyhelmintha	
Trematoda	Digenea: **AIA:** *Clonorchis, Fasciola, Heterophyes, Opisthorchis, Paragonimus*. **HIA:** *Schistosoma*
Cestoda	**AIA:** Pseudophyllidea (shed eggs): *Diphyllobothrium, Spirometra* Cyclophyllidea (shed proglottids): *Dipylidium, Echinococcus, Taenia*. **HIA:** *Hymenolepis*
Nematoda	
Ascaridida	**HIA:** *Ascaris* **AIA:** *Anisakis, Baylisascaris, Toxascaris, Toxocara, Pseudoterranova*
Oxyurida	**HIA:** *Enterobius*
Rhabditida	**HIA:** *Strongyloides*
Strongylida	**HIA:** *Ancylostoma, Necator* **AIA:** *Angiostrongylus, Oesophagostomum, Trichostrongylus*
Spirurida	**HIA:** *Dracunculus*. **AIA:** *Gnathostoma*, Filariidae (*Loa, Mansonella, Onchocerca, Wuchereria*)
Enoplida	**HIA:** *Trichuris* **AIA:** *Capillaria, Trichinella*
Arthropoda	
Hexapoda (insects)	Anoplura (lice), Diptera (flies, mosquitoes); Hemiptera (bugs), Siphonaptera (fleas)
Arachnida (spiders)	Acari (ticks, mites)
Crustacea (crayfish)	Decapoda (crabs, lobsters, shrimp), Pentastomida
Vertebrates	Aves (birds), Pisces (fish), Amphibia, Reptilia, Mammalia: marsupials (e.g., opossum), "Afroplacentals" (e.g., elephant), "Gondwanoplacentals" (e.g., armadillo), "Laurasioplacentals" (e.g., primates, bats)

hands or clothes of health workers, rarely in the community. **RISKS:** assisted ventilation, intravascular catheters, prior antibiotics. **CLINICAL INFORMATION:** An incubation period is not known, but in hospitals, the time to first acquisition is 1–50 (typically 10–25) days, and in war wounds the time from injury to agent recovery was 3–12 (median 6) days. Manifestations include pneumonia, bloodstream, surgical site, and wound (burn, war) infections. By site and strain, lethality is 15–45% or higher. About 10–50% of isolates are insensitive or resistant to carbapenems (e.g., imipenem), and ~5–55% are MDR. Treatment is difficult, an option is imipenem plus aminoglycoside. **IMPACT:** As a nosocomial agent. *Acinetobacter* accounts for 1.5% of nosocomial bloodstream infections. **OUTBREAKS:** Nosocomial outbreaks are a threat, including in the intensive care unit, and from hands or machines.

ACREMONIUM (3921, 4666, 7928) (*Ascomycota*: *Hypocreales*). Of these soil-dwelling molds, *A. falciforme*, *A. kiliense*, and *A. recifei* have been isolated in humans. Manifestations include onychomycosis, eumycetoma, keratitis, and invasive disease (hyalohyphomycosis). In Iran, *Acremonium* is grown from 4% of toenail onychomycosis. *Acremonium* in eumycetoma produces white grains; its relative frequency in this condition can reach 10%.

ACTINOBACILLUS (γ-*Proteobacteria*: *Pasteurellales*) (1713, 5471). *A. actinomycetemcomitans* is part of the oropharyngeal flora. It is a cause of periodontitis, and a rare cause of endocarditis. In households, it can spread person-to-person.

ACTINOMADURA (4513, 4666, 4927, 5362) (*Actinobacteria*: *Actinomycetales*). These branching bacteria inhabit warm soils. Mainly *A. madurae* and *A. pelletieri* are isolated in humans. ACQUISITION: By skin trauma. RISKS: Farm, field, and home work in rural warmer areas of Africa, Latin America, and Asia. CLINICAL INFORMATION: The incubation period is 1–5 (typically 2) years. Manifestation is actinomycetoma. Sites include lower legs or arms (two thirds of cases in India), but also covered body parts. Grains of *A. madurae* are white, yellow, or pink; grains of *A. pelletieri* are red. IMPACT: Cases are sporadic. By geography, actinomycetomas account for <10% to >90% of (bacterial and fungal) mycetomas. Among actinomycetomas, relative frequencies are 10–40% for *A. madurae* and 25–80% for *A. pelletieri*.

ACTINOMYCES (90, 2399, 2557, 5471, 6033) (*Actinobacteria*: *Actinomycetales*). These *branching* bacteria colonize buccal and other mucosa of mammals and humans. Of >30 species, *A. israelii* is most frequently isolated in humans. ACQUISITION: Most infections are endogenous; some result from skin trauma, bites, or a fist-fight. In contrast, the famous "grass in the mouth" is a myth rather than a source. RISKS: Intrauterine devices may predispose to vaginal colonization. Immune-impaired patients seem susceptible. CLINICAL INFORMATION: Manifestations include cevicofacial, thoracic, abdominal, and pelvic abscesses, and actinomycetoma. *A. israelii* in actinomycetoma produces white or yellow grains. IMPACT: Infections are sporadic. In Germany, 13% (1,575/12,253) of cervicofacial specimens grew *Actinomyces*.

ADENOVIRUS (4038, 6350, 6490, 6589, 7924) (unenveloped DNA viruses: *Adenoviridae*). The genus *Mastadenovirus* includes human (AdV), bovine, canine, and porcine adenoviruses. Of AdV, there are >45 serotypes; some can persist in tonsils or in the bowel. AdV circulates worldwide. SPREAD: Infections can be reactivated or acquired, from hands or droplets, likely from aerosols, objects, and tap water. The infectious dose is low (five virions). AdV is typically shed in droplets or stools for 7–14 days, limiting infectivity to ≤2 weeks that straddle late incubation to recovery. RISKS: crowded barracks, daycare centers, poorly chlorinated swimming pools. CLINICAL INFORMATION: Most infections are inapparent. The incubation period is 3–12 days. Manifestations are diverse and include the common cold, pharyngitis, bronchitis (e.g., by types 3, 4, or 7), pneumonia, glandular fever, sporadic and epidemic keratoconjunctivitis (e.g., by types 8 or 19), diarrhea (e.g., by types 31, 40, and 41), and invasive disease in immune-impaired hosts (lethality up to 60%). Confirmation is by culture or nucleic acid amplification test, or by antibody or antigen tests. IMPACT: For military populations, seroconversion rates of 6–10% per week and attack rates of 5–10% per week are reported. OUTBREAKS: Venues for respiratory outbreaks include military barracks and dormitories, and nursing homes. Epidemic keratoconjunctivitis has occurred in communities and eye clinics.

AEROMONAS (2070, 3585, 5898, 7694, 8315) (γ-*Proteobacteria*: *Aeromonadales*). These gram-negative rods inhabit fresh- and seawater, shellfish, fish, vegetables, salads, and other foods. Species frequent in humans, foods, and water are *A. hydrophila*, *A. caviae*, and *A. veronii*. ACQUISITION: is via skin trauma or from foods. RISKS: international travel, untreated drinking water. Food can be contaminated by rinsing with unsafe water, or by crop irrigation. *Aeromonas* can multiply in foods stored at +4°C. CLINICAL INFORMATION: The incubation period is 8–48 hours. Manifestations: wound infection, diarrhea, and invasive disease in immune-impaired hosts. IMPACT: Reported yield from diagnostic stool specimens is ~0.5–2.5%. OUTBREAKS: An outbreak occurred among rugby teams exposed to mud.

ALCALIGENES (673) (β-*Proteobacteria*: *Burkholderiales*). These are gram-negative, motile (flagellated) rods. *A. faecalis* is isolated from water, rarely from humans.

ALPHARETROVIRUS (5782, 7586) (enveloped RNA virus: *Retroviridae*). The genus includes avian leukosis virus (ALV) that is oncogenic in poultry. Spread is horizontally (hen-to-hen) and vertically (hen-to-egg). ALV can contaminate avian cell lines, but there is no evidence of harm to humans.

ALPHAVIRUS (unenveloped RNA viruses: *Togaviridae*). The genus comprises arthropod-borne viruses, including eastern equine encephalitis virus, Venezuelan equine encephalitis virus, and western equine encephalitis virus with a tropism for brain, and Barmah forest virus, Chikungunyan virus, Mayaro virus, O'nyong-nyong virus, Ross River virus, and Sindbis virus, with a tropism for joints.

Barmah forest virus (BFV) (714, 4617, 8342) circulates in Australia, in mosquitoes and marsupials. SPREAD: via mosquito bite. RISKS: visit to or residence in endemic area. CLINICAL INFORMATION: Most infections are inapparent. The incubation period is 7–9 days. Manifestations: flulike illness, (vesiculous) rash, arthralgia, lethary. In almost one half of cases, illness lasts >6 months. IMPACT: In Australia, ~700–900 cases are reported annually, for rates of 3–6/10^5 and year. Rates peak at age 45–54 years. OUTBREAKS: Recent outbreaks occurred in 2002 (Gippsland, Victoria, 50 cases), 1995 (New South Wales, >200 cases), 1992–1993 (Western Australia), and 1991–1992 (Northern Territory, 187 cases).

Chikungunya virus (CHIKV) (1917, 4219, 5973, 7461, 7762) circulates in sub-Saharan Africa, India, and Southeast Asia, in canopy mosquitoes and tree-dwelling primates (Africa), and in urban *Aedes aegypti* and humans (Asia). SPREAD: via mosquito bite, rarely in laboratories. RISKS: visit to or residence in endemic area, rainy season. CLINICAL INFORMATION: At least 40% of infections are inapparent. The incubation period is 1–12 (typically 3–5) days. Manifestations: flulike illness, rash (can mimic dengue), arthritis. Joint stiffness can persist for months or years. Lethality is negligible. IMPACT: In enzootic-endemic areas, 5–50% of adults can be seroreactive. OUTBREAKS: Outbreaks have occurred in West, East, and South Africa, India, and Southeast Asia, sometimes after years of silence. CHIKV reappeared in Indonesia in 2001, after a gap of nearly 20 years; in Java, Lombok, Sulawesi, and Sumatra in 2001–2003, 24 outbreaks caused >5,800 cases. In western Java, attack rates reached 0.3–0.7%. In Barsi Town, Maharashtra state, India, in 1973, an epidemic caused >20,000 suspected cases, for an attack rate of 32%.

Eastern equine encephalomyelitis virus (EEEV) (1679, 1888, 4197) circulates in the Americas, in swamp birds and *Culiseta* mosquitoes (North America), and in small mammals and *Culex* mosquitoes (Latin America). SPREAD: is via mosquito bite (*Aedes, Culex*, and *Coquillitidea*). RISKS: year-round in tropical areas, summer to fall in temperate climates. CLINICAL INFORMATION: Likely ≥90% of infections are inapparent. The incubation period is 5–15 days. Manifestation is by encephalitis. Confirmation is by nucleic acid amplification test, virus isolation, or serology (conversion). Lethality is 30–50% (55–80% in elderly, 25–35% at 20–59 years of age). Some 20–35% of survivors have neurological sequelae. IMPACT: In enzootic areas of Latin America, 0–4% of healthy residents are seroreactive. In the United States in 1955–1990, 191 human cases were reported, for a rate of 0.002–0.004/10^5 and year. OUTBREAKS: Outbreaks in humans can precede, accompany, or follow epizootics. In the United States in 1989, 14 East Coast states reported 9 human and 196 equine cases.

Mayaro virus (MAYV) (1842, 3771, 7517) circulates in tropical Latin America, in canopy mosquitoes and mammals. SPREAD: is mainly via mosquito bites, occasionally in the laboratory (by inhalation). RISKS: domicile in tropical forests. CLINICAL INFORMATION: The incubation period is ~3–6 days. Manifestations: flulike illness, rash, and arthralgia that can last months. IMPACT: Most cases are sporadic. In enzootic areas, up to 6% of residents can be seroreactive. OUTBREAKS: Outbreaks have occurred in the Amazon. In an outbreak in rural Pará, Brazil, in 1977–1978 that was likely carried by canopy mosquitoes (*Haemagogus*), ~20% of 4,000 exposed inhabitants were infected, and marmosets (*Calithrix argentata*) served as amplifying hosts.

O'nyong-nyong virus (ONNV) (3976, 4579, 6596, 7762) circulates in Africa, in *Anopheles* mosquitoes and apparently humans as natural host. SPREAD: is via mosquito bite. CLINICAL INFORMATION: The presumed incubation period is 5–15 days. Manifestations: fever, rash, lymphadenopathy, arthralgia. OUTBREAKS: In East Africa in 1959–1962, epidemic ONNV caused 0.75–2 million cases. After decades of silence, epidemic ONNV reemerged in Uganda in 1996–1997, for attack rates up to 29% in residents near lakes and swamps.

Ross River virus (RRV) (4617, 6477, 8342) circulates in Australia and parts of the Pacific, in mosquitoes (*Aedes* and *Culex*), marsupials, perhaps horses and fruit bats. SPREAD: is via mosquito bite. RISKS: domicile in rural areas and outdoor activity. CLINICAL INFORMATION: Some 25–95% of infections are inapparent. The incubation period is 3–21 (often 9) days. Manifestations: fever, rash, (epidemic) arthralgia. Recovery can take 6 months. IMPACT: Seroprevalence in enzootic areas can reach 30%. In Australia in interepidemic years, ~1,500–3,200 cases are reported per year, for rates of ~7–17/10^5 per year. OUTBREAKS: Many outbreaks are reported. In 1979–1980, an epidemic hit the South Pacific (Fiji, New Caledonia, Rarotonga, and Samoa) with >50,000 cases. Recent outbreaks in Australia occurred in 2002 (117 cases or 25/10^5 in several states) and 1990–1991 (368 cases or 238/10^5 in Northern Territory).

Semliki Forest virus (SFV) (4821) circulates in countries with warm climates, in *Aedes* mosquitoes, and mammals. SFV is widely used in laboratories. The putative incubation period is 5–15 days. Manifestations are flulike.

Sindbisvirus (SINV) (946, 4154, 4187). Lineages of SINV circulate in Africa (Ethiopian), Eurasia (Paleoarctic), and Australia (Australian), in birds, mammals, and mosquitoes. Migratory birds can carry SINV over vast territories. SPREAD: is via *Aedes* mosquito bite. CLINICAL INFORMATION: Most (95%) infections are inapparent. The incubation period is 3–11 (typically 7) days. Manifestations ("Karelia", "Ockelbo" or "Pogosta" disease): flulike illness, rash, and arthritis. In half of the cases, arthralgia persists for >1 year. IMPACT: In enzootic areas, 0.5–8% of residents are seroreactive. In Scandinavia, reported disease rates are $0.1–18/10^5$ per year, in outbreaks up to 80 per 10^5 person-years.

Venezuelan equine encephalitis virus (VEEV) (456, 2247, 5131, 6174, 7985) circulates in the New World, enzootically (avirulent ID-F strains) in *Culex* and small mammals, and epizootically (virulent IAB and IC strains) in equids. *Aedes* or other mosquitoes carry VEEV to humans. SPREAD: is via mosquito bite, rarely via aerosols, a capability that makes VEEV a potential bioweapon. RISKS: rural domicile and forest work. CLINICAL INFORMATION: >99% of infections are inapparent. The incubation period is 1–5 days. Manifestations: flulike illness, encephalitis (in ~4%), and abortion. Lethality is 0.4–1.7%. Sequelae are uncommon. IMPACT: In Latin America, by age and exposure, 0–75% of healthy residents can be seroreactive. OUTBREAKS: Epizootics and edemics in 1955–1959, 1962–1969, and 1971 have caused tens of thousands of cases in equids and humans. Incompletely inactivated equine vaccines are suspected to have contributed to epizootics in the 1960s. After a 19-year gap, epidemic VEEV emerged in Venezuela in 1992–1993. In Venezuela and Colombia in 1995, an epidemic caused 75,000 cases in people of all ages, for attack rates of up to 30% in some municipalities; heavy rains had produced high vector densities. Commercial vaccines are available for equids but not humans.

Western equine encephalomyelitis virus (WEEV) (349, 3385, 6204) circulates in the New World, in birds and mosquitoes: *Culex* in North America, *Aedes* in Latin America. SPREAD: is via mosquito bite. RISKS: rural domicile, farm work, and outdoor activities. CLINICAL INFORMATION: In children, >95% of infections are inapparent; this proportion is even greater in adults. The incubation period is 4–10 days. Manifestations: flulike illness, encephalitis. Lethality is 3%. Sequelae are common in infants. IMPACT: In California residents in 1995, seroprevalence was 1% (9/690) in Imperial valley and 0.5% (5/1,066) in Sacramento valley. OUTBREAKS: North America recorded epidemics in 1941 (>3,400 cases; rate, $167/10^5$), 1975 (300 cases), and 1987 (37 cases in five states). In California, despite epizootic transmission in 1983 and 1993–1994, cases in humans were not reported.

ANAPLASMA (α-*Proteobacteria*: *Rickettsiales*). *Anaplasma* spp. are gram-negative, intracellular, tick-borne ancestral bacteria of mammals having undergone several taxonomic revisions (check *Ehrlichia* or *Rickettsia* as well). *A. bovis* and *A. marginale* circulate in cattle and their ticks (*Boophilus* and *Dermacentor*).

A. phagocytophilum (539, 909, 1872, 2068, 7080, 7182, 7203, 8238) (ex-*Ehrlichia phagocytophila*, *E. equi*) circulates in North America and Europe, in small and larger mammals, and ticks. SPREAD: is via tick bite. RISKS: rural domicile, dog ownership, age 40–60 years, male sex, and spring to fall seasons. *A. phagocytophilum* is a hazard for blood banking, because it survives in blood at 4°C for 18 days. CLINICAL INFORMATION: Many infections are inapparent or mild. The incubation period is 5–21 (typically 11) days. Manifestations (human granulocytic "ehrlichiosis"): flulike illness, also vomiting and diarrhea, rarely multiorgan failure. Reported lethality is 0.3–1%. About 50–85% of patients recall recent tick exposure. Confirmation is by microscopy of blood smear (agents in neutrophils), blood culture, seroconversion (two specimens, 2–3 weeks apart), or nucleic acid amplification test. IMPACT: Most cases have been reported in the United States (449 in 1986–1997, 1,091 in 1997–2001, 789 in 2001–2002), few (>60) in western Europe. Seroprevalence in healthy adults from enzootic areas is 0–20%, often 0.5–3.5%. Reported disease rates range broadly by location and age; in the United States, the national average is $\sim 0.1/10^5$ per year. Reported infection (seroconversion) rates are 0.8–5%.

ANCYLOSTOMA and NECATOR (Nematoda: Strongylida: Ancylostomatidae). These are soil-transmitted nematodes.

A. braziliense, *A. caninum*, and *A. ceylanicum* (2244, 2578, 6018, 7547, 7794) are worms that parasitize dogs and cats (final hosts, shed eggs with feces). *A. caninum* is cosmopolitean, *A. braziliense* and *A. ceylanicum* occur in countries with warm climates. SPREAD: is via contact of unprotected skin with polluted soil. RISKS: walking barefoot, lying on beach sand, and sprinkling fecally polluted lawns. CLINICAL INFORMATION: Humans are dead-end hosts (except few patent *A. ceylanicum* infections). The incubation period (in an outbreak in travelers, from departure to first rash) was 5–35 (mean, 15–16) days. Manifestations: cutaneous larva migrans. Diagnosis is clinical (or from removed larva). *A. caninum* is a cause of eosinophilic enteritis confirmed by colonoscopy or laparotomy.

A. duodenale and *Necatur americanus* (134, 898, 1835, 3441, 6500, 7541, 8103) are hookworms (*A. duodenale* with toothed mouth and *N. americanus* with bladed mouth) that circulate in warmer climates, in soil, and in humans who shed eggs with feces. In moist soil, fresh feces, or on human skin, eggs develop to infective larvae (L3) in 1–2 days. Life span of adults is 1 year (*A. duodenale*) to 3–5 years (*N. americanus*). SPREAD: is via skin contact with fecally polluted soil; *A. duodenale* can also be acquired from breastmilk or foods. RISKS: residence in endemic area, high settlement density, outdoor work, no toilet at domicile, no footwear, human feces for fertilizer, and sandy soils. Shoes are protective. CLINICAL INFORMATION: Adults locate in the duodenum. Daily egg output is 5,000–10,000/female of *N. americanus* to 10,000–30,000/female of *A. duodenale*. The prepatent period is 5–8 weeks, in hypobiotic *A. duodenale* months. Many (more than one third) light infections are inapparent. Hookworm eggs can be detected by microscopy of fresh stool samples. Larvae from cultured stool samples permit identification of species. Fecal egg counts are linearly correlated with intestinal blood loss and nonlinearly with worm burden that is 1 to >100 (often 5–10). By age, species, and iron diet, egg counts >3,000–5,000 per g of feces define heavy infections. By geography, coinfections are possible of *N. americanus* with *A. duodenale, Ascaris, Trichuris,* or *Schistosoma*. The incubation period (to abdominal pain) is 2–6 weeks. Manifestations: itchy skin at portal of entry, fleeting blood eosinophilia, abdominal pain, occult blood loss (vampire worm), and iron deficiency anemia. Daily blood loss is 0.1–0.4 (mean, 0.3) ml per 10 adult *N. americanus*, and 0.5–3 (mean, 1.5) ml per 10 adult *A. duodenale* (fivefold higher). Pregnant women are susceptible to iron deficiency. Based on age, worm species, iron diet, and the definition of anemia used, the proportion of anemia attributable to hookworms is ~3–22%. Treatment options include benzimidazoles and pyrantel pamoate. In West Africa, mebendazole-resistant *N. americanus* has been reported. **IMPACT:** Worldwide, 3.2 billion people are at risk and >500 million are infected, for an overall prevalence of 15% and a range of 3–95%. In Chad, 33% of 1,000 school children were infected and the mean egg count was 180/g. In Kenya, 78% of 1,738 school children were infected including 9% with heavy (>1,250 eggs/g) infection. In People's Republic of China in 1988–1992, trom ~1.5 million tests, 190–200 million people were infected (17%) including 2.7% with heavy infections. **OUTBREAKS:** Outbreaks have affected troops and tunnel workers (in the 1880s). Treatment of all children or women of childbearing age should be considered in areas where ≥70% of school children are infected, or ≥10% have heavy infections. However, as rates of reinfection are high, sanitation and health education should complement mass treatment campaigns.

ANGIOSTRONGYLUS (Nematoda: Strongylida). These worms circulate in rodents (final hosts, e.g., rats), their feces, and terrestrial snails and slugs (intermediate hosts). Shrimp, crabs, frogs, fish, horses, and dogs can act as transport hosts. Of >15 species, *A. cantonensis* and *A. costaricensis* infect humans. **ACQUISITION:** is from foods, likely also from handling snails or slugs. **RISKS:** snails for food, children who play with snails, larvae-containing slime on unwashed vegetables, salads, or fruits, raw vegetable juices, poorly cooked transport hosts (land crabs, freshwater prawns, and frogs).

A. cantonensis (3992, 6017, 6963, 7579-7581, 7949, 8295) originated in East Asia and has expanded into Southeast Asia, the Pacific, Australia, Africa, and the Caribbean (where it overlaps with *A. costaricensis*). **CLINICAL INFORMATION:** The incubation period is 1–45 (typically 14) days. Manifestation (eosinophilic meningitis): headache, fever, meningoencephalitis, rarely iridocyclitis. Eosinophilia in blood and cerebrospinal fluid and serology are supportive. Confirmation is by visualizing larvae in cerebrospinal fluid (in 10% of cases). Lethality in hospitalized children is ~5%. **IMPACT:** Sporadic and epidemic cases. **OUTBREAKS:** Outbreaks have affected travelers, migrants, patrons of a restaurant, fishermen, and the community.

A. costaricensis (4090, 5188) is enzootic in Latin America. **CLINICAL INFORMATION:** The putative incubation period is ≤24 days. Manifestations include acute abdominal pain (can mimic appendicitis), intestinal obstruction, and palpable abdominal mass. Diagnosis can only be confirmed histopathologically. **IMPACT:** Not known. **OUTBREAKS:** An outbreak in Guatemala in 1994–1995 caused 22 cases.

ANISAKIS AND PSEUDOTERRANOVA (336, 1007, 1606, 4877, 5703, 6226, 7294) (Nematoda: Ascaridida). *A. simplex* (herringworm) and *P. decipiens* sl (codworm) circulate in marine mammals (final hosts), their feces (eggs), small crustaceans (first intermediate hosts, e.g., copepods and krill), and marine fish, large crustaceans, or squid (second intermediate hosts). Larvae from fish and humans measure 1–3 cm and are readily visible. **ACQUISITION:** is by eating viable larvae with marine fish or squid. **RISKS:** raw seafood. Freezing ($-20°C$ for ≥7 days) kills larvae. **CLINICAL INFORMATION:** The incubation period is 1 h to 14 days, often few to 12 h. Manifestations: (anisakiasis) include sudden urticaria, angioedema, and anaphylaxis (seafood allergy), also acute abdominal pain (can mimic appendicitis), rarely bowel obstruction. Disease from *P. decipiens* is milder, with tingling throat, gastralgia, and regurgitation of larvae. Eosinophilia is supportive. Specific immunoglobulin E in radioimmunoassay, and visualization of larvae on endoscopy or histology are diagnostic. **IMPACT:** Thousands of cases have been reported in communities habitually eating raw fish, mainly in East Asia (Japan and Korea), less in northern and southern Europe, few in North America (Alaska and Hawaii). Disease rates can reach $4/10^5$ per year. **OUTBREAKS:** Food-borne outbreaks have occurred. The Netherlands have controlled anisakiasis by a legal requirement for freezing raw herring.

APHTHOVIRUS (486, 2722) (unenveloped RNA viruses: *Picornaviridae*). The genus includes foot-and-mouth disease virus (FMDV) that circulates worldwide, in cloven-hoofed, domestic and wild mammals. **SPREAD:** Although highly infective among mammals via contact, droplets, aerosols, and objects, FMDV rarely infects humans, presumably via aerosols, broken skin, or milk. RISKS: Winds can carry the virus long distances. CLINICAL INFORMATION: The presumed incubation period is 2–6 days. IMPACT: At least 40 infections in humans are documented. OUTBREAKS: In the United Kingdom in 2001, an epizootic caused ~2,100 confirmed animal (mainly sheep) cases; 4.2 million animals were killed and disposed of to contain the epizootic.

ARCOBACTER (7757) (ε-*Proteobacteria*). *A. butzleri* is related to *Campylobacter*. In Belgium, diagnostic yield from submitted stool samples is 0.1% (84/67,599).

ARENAVIRUS (776, 5694) (enveloped RNA viruses: *Arenaviridae*). *Arenavirus* includes lymphocytic choriomeningitis virus, and agents of viral hemorrhagic fevers (VHFs) in the Old World (Lassa virus) and New World (guanarito, Junin, Machupo, and Sabia viruses).
 Guanaritovirus (GUAV) (1815, 6544) circulates in central Venezuela, in wild rodents. SPREAD: presumably from contact with rodents or inhalation of rodent aerosols; interhuman spread is uncertain. RISKS: farm work and peridomestic rodent contacts. CLINICAL INFORMATION: The incubation period is 7–14 days. Manifestations (Venezuelan hemorrhagic fever): fever, vomiting, bleeding. Lethality can reach 33%. IMPACT: Not well known. OUTBREAKS: Out-breaks can occur every 4–5 years.
 Junín virus (JUNV) (3158, 4668, 8029) circulates in northcentral Argentina in wild rodents. SPREAD: Presumably from contact with rodents or inhalation of rodent aerosols. RISKS: farm work, rodent contact, and April-June season. CLINICAL INFORMATION: Subclinical infections occur. The incubation period is 7–14 days. Manifestations (Argentinian hemorrhagic fever): flulike illness, bleeding. Leukopenia and thrombopenia are suggestive. Confirmation is by nucleic acid amplification test or other tests. Lethality is >15%, with treatment <1%. IMPACT: In enzootic areas up to 12% of residents can be seroreactive. OUTBREAKS: In the 1950s–1980s, there were annual outbreaks in Argentina, with attack rates decreasing from 7 to 1/1,000 per year.
 Lassa virus (LASV) (339, 3040, 6256, 8131) circulates West Africa (mainly Guinea, Liberia, Nigeria, and Sierra Leone), in rodents, their excretions, and the environment. SPREAD: is via (i) contact with rodents or their excreta (aerosolized rodent urine is not a confirmed mode), (ii) consumption of rodent-polluted foods (or multimammate rats, considered by some a delicacy), (iii) droplets from patients, (iv) blood, body fluids and tissues from patients. Virus can be shed in urine for 3–9 weeks and in semen for 3 months. The risk of secondary spread on long-distance flights and from imported cases seems low. Of 149 exposed persons, none contracted disease, and only one (0.7%) was seroreactive, a physician who had examined the index patient. RISKS: residence in enzootic areas, travel to epidemic areas, patient care, and needle sharing. The first reported cases (1969–1972) included nurses and physicians. CLINICAL INFORMATION: 80% of infections are inapparent or mild. The incubation period is 5–16 days. Manifestations (Lassa fever): fever, vomiting, pharyngitis, conjunctivitis, periorbital edema, bleeding, cerebral edema, and multiorgan failure. Confirmation is by serology (immunoglobulin M), nucleic acid amplification test, or culture. Ribavirin is a treatment option. By age, setting, and denominator, lethality is 1% (community) to 15–30% (hospital). Hearing deficits persist in up to 29% of survivors. IMPACT: Infections can be sporadic, endemic, or epidemic. Estimates are of 0.1–13 million cases per year. In enzootic areas, 4–55% of residents are seroreactive, and infection rates can reach 5–22% per year. OUTBREAKS: Outbreaks occur at intervals in enzootic areas.
 Lymphocytic choriomeningitis virus (LCMV) (467, 1249, 4759, 5010, 6433) circulates in mice and other rodents worldwide. ACQUISITION: is presumably from contact with rodents or their excreta, or inhalation of aerosols; in pregnancy, there is a risk of intrauterine transmission. CLINICAL INFORMATION: The putative incubation period is 1 1/2–10 days; for meningeal symptoms it is up to 21 days. Manifestations: flulike illness, less frequently, aseptic meningitis. IMPACT: In urban areas of the United States, ~5% of residents can be seroreactive. Of randomly selected residents ($n = 504$) of Nova Scotia, Canada, 4% were seroreactive.
 Machupo virus (MACV) (6547, 7828) circulates in rodents in Bolivia. SPREAD: is likely by contact with rodents or their excrements, or inhalation of rodent aerosols; interhuman spread is rare but reported. CLINICAL INFORMATION: The incubation period is 7–14 days. Manifestation (Bolivian hemorrhagic fever): flulike illness, bleeding (petechiae and epistaxis). Diagnostic tests are not commercially available. Lethality is 15–30%. IMPACT: Not known. OUTBREAKS: In 1994, an outbreak caused seven cases in one family, including six deaths, and three further cases.

ASCARIS (Nematoda: Ascaridida). The genus includes closely related *A. suum* (in swine) and *A. lumbricoides* (in humans).
 A. lumbricoides (900, 1835, 2299, 3002, 3084, 3441, 7499, 7541, 7689) circulates in tropical and temperate climates, in humans (final host), their feces (eggs), soil, and foods. Eggs need 10–55 days to embryonate and be infective (L3 larvae). Life span of female adults is 1–1 1/2 years. SPREAD: is via ingestion of embryonated eggs from foods, utensils, or soil, possibly via inhalation of eggs in household dust. Females produce 0.2–0.25 million eggs per day. In Jamaica, human uptake was estimated to

~10–20 eggs per child per year. The theoretical reproduction number (R_0) is four to five cases. **RISKS:** unsafe drinking water, no sanitation, promiscuous defecation, crowding, geophagia, wastewater irrigation, vegetable gardening, and pig ownership. **CLINICAL INFORMATION:** The prepatent period is 2–3 months. Adults locate in the small bowel. Most infections are inapparent or mild. Acute manifestations include fleeting pneumonitis, ileal obstruction (40–90% of all complications). Putative chronic manifestations include anorexia, malabsorption, growth retardation, and asthma. Eggs on microscopy of stool samples, and expulsed worms (spontaneous, on treatment) are diagnostic. Fecal egg counts are indicative of worm burden: counts <5,000/g define mild infections, counts >50,000/g define heavy infections. Disease complication rates are indicative of endemicity. Lethality of bowel obstruction is 0–9%. **IMPACT:** Worldwide, 4.2 billion people are at risk and >1.1 billion are infected (about one third children), for a prevalence of ~25%, and a range of 5–95% by age and geography. In 1,738 school children in Kenya, prevalence was 42% for all infections and 4.5% for heavy (>20,000 eggs/g) infections. In northwestern Iran, where the temperature in winter can fall to −28°C, the prevalence was >50%. In People's Republic of China in 1988–1992, from ~1.5 million tests, 530 million were infected, for prevalences of 47% of all infections of 1.8% of heavy infections. Disease impact is inadequately known. There are 120–350 million cases per year. By age and geography, rates of surgery for bowel obstruction are 0–300/10^5 per year. **OUTBREAKS:** Control measures for soil-transmitted helminths include community (mass) treatments, hand hygiene, boiling of drinking water, and improved sanitation. Ascariasis is controlled in most areas in high-income countries, although local pockets of transmission may persist.

ASPERGILLUS (1882, 3233, 4233, 4430, 4582, 4813, 5834, 7050) (*Ascomycota: Eurotiales*). These hyaline, mycotoxin-producing molds inhabit soil, plant debris, stables, and buildings. Filaments in soil form infective spores (conidia) that are released on disturbance and remain airborne. Of 150–200 species, mainly *A. fumigatus*, *A. flavus*, *A. niger*, and *A. terreus* are isolated in humans. **ACQUISITION:** is via inhalation of conidia in dust, animal dust, or water. Reported concentrations are 0.2–15 conidia per m^3 in outdoor air, and up to 30 CFU/m^3 in rooms. **RISKS:** Inhalation of conidia is a routine event. Immune-impaired patients are susceptible to invasive disease (e.g., stem cell recipients, neutropenia, human immunodeficiency virus infection, malnourishment). **CLINICAL INFORMATION:** Colonization is difficult to distinguish from invasion; 50–90% of isolates from lower respiratory tract reflect colonization rather than infection. The sensitivity of culture is low. Evidence for invasion is the microscopic presence of *Aspergillus* in needle aspirate or biopsy. The putative incubation period is 3 days to 3 weeks. Manifestations include allergy (wheeze), onychomycosis, eumycetoma, necrotizing lung disease, and dissemination. Grains in eumycetoma are white (*A. nidulans*) or green (*A. flavus*). Treatment options include voriconazole and amphotericin B. Lethality of invasive disease can reach 60%. **IMPACT:** In cystic fibrosis patients in Europe, the prevalence of allergic bronchopulmonary aspergillosis is 8% (range: 2% in Sweden, 14% in Belgium). In autopsy series, the prevalence of invasive disease has increased in the past two decades, from ≤0.4% to 4%. In the community, the rate of invasive disease is 1.2/10^5 per year. **OUTBREAKS:** Outbreaks are reported in hospitals.

ASTROVIRUS See Mamastrovirus.

AVIPOXVIRUS (enveloped double-stranded DNA virus: *Poxviridae*). The genus unites canarypoxvirus and fowlpoxvirus.

AVULAVIRUS (enveloped RNA viruses: *Mononegavirales: Paramyxoviridae*). A prominent member is **Newcastle disease virus** (NDV) (1069, 3747) that is related to mumps virus. NDV is enzootic in birds, including poultry. **SPREAD:** is via inhalation of bird dust or aerosols, contact with birds, feathers, or carcasses, and occasionally in the laboratory, via mucosal splash. **CLINICAL INFORMATION:** The incubation period is 1–2 days. Manifestation: conjunctivitis (typically unilateral).

BABESIA (2455, 2796, 3290, 3332, 3410, 3979, 4097) (Alveolata: Apicomplexa: Piroplasmorida). These are intraerythrocytic, pear-shaped protozoa that circulate worldwide, in birds, mammals, and ticks. Sporozoites (from ticks) and merozoites (from blood) are infective. By morphology and host, >100 species are described. Few species are confirmed in humans, mainly murine *B. microti* (holarctic), and bovine *B. bigemina* and *B. divergens*, while *B. canis* and *B. microtis*-like spp. are emerging. **SPREAD:** is via tick bite, rarely via transfusion, or intrauterine. **RISKS:** domicile in tick-infested area, outdoor activities, and tick season. About 30% of patients recall tick bites. Splenectomized persons are susceptible. **CLINICAL INFORMATION:** Some 25–50% of infections are inapparent. The incubation period is 1–6 (often 3) weeks from tick bite, and up to 9 weeks from transfusion. Manifestations: flulike illness (in 80–90%), hemolysis (hematocrit <35%, in ~60%), or fulminant disease. Confirmation is by microscopy of blood smear or nucleic acid amplification test, possibly serology or culture. Parasitemia in normosplenic patients can reach 20% but is typically low (<1%). Parasitemia can persist. Lethality is 6.5% (North America) to 42% (Europe). Treatment options include drug combinations, e.g., clindamycin and quinine, or azithromycin and atovaquone. IMPACT: Seroprevalence is 0–0.6%; in frequently tick-exposed populations, it is 4–9%. In residents of Long Island (N.Y.), the seroconversion rate was 0.1/100 per year. In residents of Block Island (Rhode Island), the disease rate was 0.2/100 per year. There are >300 cases in the United States (1969–2000, mainly *B. microti*), and ~30 in Europe (1957–2000, mainly *B. bigemina* in splenectomized patients). OUTBREAKS: Vaccines are available for cattle but not for humans.

BACILLUS (*Bacteria*: *Bacillales*). These are gram-positive rods that form heat-resistant endospores and inhabit soil and plants. *B. thuringiensis* is used for biocontrol of insects. *B. anthracis*, *B. cereus*, and *B. subtilis* (in immune-impaired patients) are infective to humans.

B. anthracis (411, 1763, 3555, 5847, 6678, 7072, 7822, 8264) circulates in grazing mammals that ingest spores and become ill and die, their carcasses that release spores, and soil, a reservoir in which spores remain viable for years. Spores are inactivated by heat: boiling for 10 min, moist heat (105°C) for 10 minutes, or dry heat (150°C) for 10 minutes. SPREAD: is via (i) injury or contact with infected animals, carcasses, or animal products, (ii) insect bite, (iii) ingestion of contaminated meat, (iv) inhalation of spores outdoors and in laboratories. RISKS: livestock contacts, butchering, cuts on hands, work with animals or animal products. Sources in sporadic cases can be elusive. For inhalational anthrax, the infective dose is ~8,000 spores. CLINICAL INFORMATION: The incubation period is 9 h to 12 days (inoculation), 1–10 days (inhalation), and up to 100 days (animal experiments). Manifestations (anthrax): can be cutaneous (skin edema, eschar, and "pustula maligna"), enteric (dysentery), pulmonary (cough and widened mediastinum), and systemic (sepsis). Lethality ranges from 1.5–3.% in outbreaks to 45% (treated) and 100% (untreated) in inhalational anthrax. IMPACT: Estimates are of 2,000–20,000 human cases per year. Spores are a potential bioweapon. In high-income countries, any human or animal case would be unusual. In 1950–2001, alerts prompted 38 investigations in the United States, and one each in Haiti, Paraguay, and Kazakhstan. In the 1930s, the disease rate in enzootic areas of the former Soviet Union was 40–60/10^5 per year. OUTBREAKS: In Zimbabwe in 1978–1980, an epidemic caused 9,445 cases. In Kazakhstan in 1997–1998, an outbreak caused 73 cases. Vaccines are licensed for veterinary use. Options for postexposure prophylaxis include ciprofloxacin and doxycycline.

B. cereus (2669, 2913, 7384, 7723) inhabits soil, dust, plant debris, and foods. Heat activates germination of spores, and production of toxins. *B. cereus* grows at pH 4.3–9.3 and 4–50°C; psychrophilic strains can grow at 4–8°C, e.g., refrigerated milk. ACQUISITION: is from foods, in hospitals also from contaminated machines. RISKS: Frequently contaminated foods include rice and other cereals, spices, peas, and beans, but also milk, dried milk products, and infant foods. Heat (95°C for 35 min) kills bacteria, but not endospores that germinate (at 25–30°C) when cooked food is slowly cooled, producing toxins. The diarrhea toxin is inactivated at 56°C for 5 min, the emetic toxin survives 126°C for 1.5 hours and remains active when foods, e.g., rice, are reheated. CLINICAL INFORMATION: The incubation period is 1/2–12 hours for emetic toxin, and 6–24 h for diarrhea toxin. Manifestations: acute food poisoning, invasive disease in hospitalized patients. IMPACT: Not well known. OUTBREAKS: *B. cereus* is a cause of food-borne and nosocomial outbreaks.

BACTEROIDES (*Bacteria*: *Bacteroidales*) (1901, 2124, 2818, 4360, 7009). These gram-negative, anaerobic, bile-resistant rods circulate in mammals, sewage, and water, and colonize the buccal cavity, colon, and female genital tract of humans. Of several species, *B. fragilis* and *B. thetaiotaomicron* are isolated in humans. SPREAD: Infections are endogenous, but nosocomial acquisition seems possible. RISKS: aspiration, breakdown of natural barriers, and bowel spill. CLINICAL INFORMATION: An incubation period is not reported. Manifestations: wound infection, acute inflammation (e.g., appendicitis, cholecystitis, and endometritis), tissue abscess (dental, diverticular, subphrenic, lung, and brain), and bacteremia (in two thirds from an abdominal source). Lethality of *B. fragilis* bacteremia is ~20%. *Bacteroides* disease is typically polymicrobial and may require surgery; antimicrobial options include metronidazole, clindamycin, and β-lactam/anti-β-lactamase combinations. IMPACT: *Bacteroides* accounts for 2–3% of bacteremia isolates and up to 7% of nosocomial isolates.

BALAMUTHIA (1854, 6716, 8072) (6927) (Amoebozoa: Acanthopodida). *B. mandrillaris* is an ameba free-living in soil as trophozoites or cysts. *B. mandrillaris* is separated from *Acanthamoeba* by fastidious growth and ultrastructure. SPREAD: via inhalation of dust or skin trauma. Manifestations: encephalitis (mainly children, can be immune impaired or competent). Granuloma at the entry site may precede encephalitis. IMPACT: Some 100 cases.

BALANTIDIUM (1909, 2238, 7778) (Alveolata: Ciliata: Vestibuliferida). *B. coli* circulates in tropical and temperate climates, in pigs, other mammals, and humans who shed cysts and trophozoites with feces. SPREAD: is via pig contact or tap water. RISKS: poor sanitation, poor housing. CLINICAL INFORMATION: Most infections are inapparent. The incubation period is 5–24 (typically 12) days. Manifestations: diarrhea (watery and dysentery), rarely appendicitis or, in immune-impaired hosts, pulmonary. Confirmation is by microscopy of feces. IMPACT: In enzootic rural areas, prevalence is typically ≤1%, occasionally ≥10%.

BARTONELLA (852, 911, 4166, 7385) (α-*Proteobacteria*: *Rhizobiales*). These gram-negative bacteria parasitize mammalian erythrocytes and are transmitted by arthropods. Confirmation is by nucleic acid amplification test from blood or biopsy, or by blood culture with subculture into shell vials. Of healthy community members 0–20% are seroreactive; but by test and geography, there is serological cross-reactivity within the genus or α-proteobacteria. The main species infective to humans are *B. bacilliformis*, *B. henselae*, and *B. quintana*. Species rare or suspected in humans include *B. clarridgeiae* and *B. elisabethae*.

B. bacilliformis (182, 1299, 1566, 2182, 4068, 4837) circulates in the northwestern Andes of South America, in sandflies and unknown wild mammals, perhaps rodents. SPREAD: is via sandfly bite. RISKS: domicile in or visit to endemic areas. CLINICAL INFORMATION: About 10–55% of infections are inapparent. The incubation period is not known; in D. A. Carrión's (1857–1885) self-inoculation to which he succumbed in 1885, it was 21 days. Manifestations: can be acute, as (Oroya) fever and hemolytic anemia, or chronic, as subcutaneous, vascular proliferations (verruga peruviana). Lethality of Oroya fever is 1-50%. IMPACT: Reported seroprevalence in endemic areas is 45–75%. OUTBREAKS: Outbreaks have occurred in Peru and Ecuador.

B. henselae (2283, 3615, 4024, 6263) circulates in cats and cat fleas worldwide; the agent has also been reported in dogs and *Ixodes* ticks. SPREAD: via cat flea, cat scratch, cat bite, infrequently via dog contact. RISKS: cat ownership, work with cats. CLINICAL INFORMATION: Inapparent infections seem common in children. The incubation period is 3–10 days (skin lesion) to 3–50 (typically 14) days (lymphadenopathy). Manifestations: include skin lesions and lymphadenopathy (cat scratch disease), vascular proliferations (in immune-impaired hosts), and endocarditis, perhaps also inflammatory bowel disease. Coagulase-negative *Staphylococcus* manifestations complicate ~2% of cat scratch disease. IMPACT: By age and geography, 6-9% or more of healthy community members may have elevated antibody titers to *B. henselae*. Reported rates of cat scratch disease, by geography and out- or inpatient settings are 0.7–9/10^5 per year.

B. elisabethae (1532, 3348, 4899) has been isolated from rodents and humans. SPREAD: is presumed through cat contacts. CLINICAL INFORMATION: A likely, rare manifestation is endocarditis. IMPACT: High seroprevalence (~30%) have been reported in injection drug users in North America and in orienteer runners in northern Europe.

B. (ex-*Rickettsia*, ex-*Rochalimaea*) quintana (2470, 2471, 3617, 4851, 5563, 6114) circulates focally, in body lice and humans. SPREAD: is via body lice. RISKS: homelessness, crowding, unsanitary housing, lousiness, injection drug use, cat contact. CLINICAL INFORMATION: Inapparent infections occur. The incubation period is 15–38 days (from inoculation experiments, 6–22 days). Manifestations: febrile illness (trench or quintan fever), endocarditis, bacteremia, in human immunodeficiency virus-infected persons also bacillary angiomatosis. Confirmation is by direct immunofluorescence of blood smear (rapid) or by blood culture (can take 45 days). IMPACT: In a rural community of the Peruvian Andes, 12% (24/194) of residents were seroreactive, and 19% (36) were louse infested; lice amplified *B. quintana* by nucleic acid amplification test. In World Wars I and II, epidemics caused ~1 million cases of trench fever. After years of silence, cases resurged in the 1990s, in urban North America and West Europe. In Seattle in 1993, 10 homeless, human immunodeficiency virus-negative, inner-city residents were diagnosed with *B. quintana* bacteremia.

BASIDIOBOLUS (6238) (*Zygomycota*: *Entomophthorales*). This ribbonlike fungus inhabits soil, plant debris, and animal feces. ACQUISITION: is likely from inhalation, trauma, or insect bite. Manifestations (zygomycosis): include subcutaneous nodules and invasive disease.

BAYLISASCARIS (2674, 5011, 6434, 6624) (Nematoda: Ascaridida). *B. procyonis* circulates in raccoons (final hosts), their feces (contain eggs), and rodents, other mammals, and birds (intermediate hosts). Eggs in soil take 2–4 weeks to become infective. SPREAD: is by uptake of eggs via hands dirty from soil or wood, or via geophagia, e.g., by chewing on wood chips. RISKS: dirty hands from garden, play, or work and ownership of infected pet rabbits. Manifestations: encephalitis (neural larva migrans) and ocular lesions (ocular larva migrans). Encephalitis can be fatal.

BETARETROVIRUS (enveloped RNA viruses: *Retroviridae*).

Simian retrovirus type D (SRVD) (4350) is enzootic in Asian macaques (*Macaca*). SRVD was isolated in blood, saliva, and urine from infected animals. Infections in humans have been reported, likely from secretions or contact.

BLASTOCYSTIS (275, 1462, 3669, 4079, 4314, 5454) (Protists: Straminopila). *B. "hominis"* circulates worldwide, in vertebrates and their feces, including birds (e.g., chicken), amphibians, rodents (e.g., rats), cattle, pigs, and primates. SPREAD: is via hands, animal contacts, foods, or tap water. RISKS: drinking unboiled water in low-income countries, travel to endemic areas, living in institutions. Individuals with latent hepatitis B virus and *Helicobacter pylori* infections, and immune-impaired individuals seem susceptible. CLINICAL INFORMATION: Prepatent and incubation periods have not been determined. About 85–100% infections are inapparent. Pathogenicity of *B. hominis* is debated ("a protist in search of diarrhea"); coinfections with confirmed pathogens confound an association with diarrhea. Among 6,422 Japanese, 30 (0.5%) were infected; all infections were inapparent, except for "one who reported flatus and one who reported mild abdominal discomfort" (3428). IMPACT: Reported fecal prevalence is 0.5–30% (often 1–10%) in high-income countries and 10–80% (often 30–50%) in low-income countries. OUTBREAKS: An outbreak is reported in a day-care center.

BLASTOMYCES (487, 1061, 1625, 2054, 4339, 6023) (*Ascomycota*: *Onygenales*). *B. dermatitidis* inhabits soil and woody plants in parts of North America, Africa, and Southwest Asia. Molds produce infective spores (conidia). Dogs can become infected like humans. SPREAD: is by inhalation of spores in dust, inoculation with soil, via dog bites, and intrauterine, possibly via household contact. RISKS: domiciles near foci, outdoor activities, construction and other earth-disturbing work. African Americans seem more susceptible than Caucasians. CLINICAL INFORMATION: Over 50% of infections are inapparent. The incubation period is from 1–5 weeks (inoculation) to 4–15 weeks (inhalation). Years of latency can separate infection from first symptoms. Manifestations: can be cutaneous, pulmonary (cough, fever, night sweat, and pleuritic pain), or systemic (invasive disease). Confirmation is by cytology, histology, or culture. IMPACT: In North America, infection rates per 10^5 per year are 0.2–2 overall and 12–200 in endemic areas. OUTBREAKS: Outbreaks have occurred near freshwater bodies.

BORDETELLA (β-*Proteobacteria*: *Burkholderiales*). These gram-negative, toxin-producing rods colonize the respiratory tract of birds, mammals, and humans. The main human pathogen is *B. pertussis*.

B. bronchiseptica (2104) colonizes or infects dogs (kennel cough), cats, guinea pigs, rabbits (snuffles), pigs (atrophic rhinitis), mice, and rats. Human respiratory tract or invasive infections occur sporadically. At risk are human immunodeficiency virus-infected individuals who own pets.

B. parapertussis (3209, 3236, 4361) has a host range apparently limited to sheep and humans. Manifestations: milder form of pertussis, without lymphocytosis. IMPACT: As a differential diagnosis of cough. In Poland, the infection rate was ~1–7/10^5 per year. OUTBREAKS: Pertussis vaccine may be ineffective against this agent. In a highly vaccinated (four doses in 98%) population in Finland, *B. parapertussis* was detected by culture or PCR from 11% (60/564) of outpatients with paroxysmal cough. In Poland in 1995–2002, 14 of 17 confirmed *B. parapertussis* infections were in individuals with documented vaccination (up to four doses by age 18 months).

B. pertussis (664, 1195, 1250, 2179, 6656, 6907, 6954, 8144, 8222). Humans are the only host for *B. pertussis*. Reservoir is a small proportion (0.5–3%) of nasopharyngeal carriers among infants, adolescents, and elderly. SPREAD: is via droplets from carriers or patients. Infectivity builds up 1–2 weeks before cough onset (d_0) and fades in the 3 weeks after d_0. Effective treatment for 5 days abrogates infectivity. Secondary attack rates in households can reach 30–50%. RISKS: crowding, a case at home or in class, and vaccine noncompliance. CLINICAL INFORMATION: About 50–60% of infections in adults are inapparent. The incubation period is 4–21 (often 7–10) days. Manifestations: (pertussis) include paroxysmal, persistent (>2 weeks) cough (in 100%), cyanosis (in two thirds), inspiratory whoop (in 50%), posttussive vomiting (in 50%), and lymphocytosis. Complications include apnoea, pneumonia (in 5–30%), encephalopathy (seizures in 1–3%), and malnutrition. Some 20% of patients are hospitalized. Lethality is ~0.05–3% (highs at age <2 months and in low-income countries). Diagnosis is confirmed by culture or nucleic acid amplification test from nasopharyngeal swabs or washings. Macrolides are an option for treatment and postexposure prophylaxis. IMPACT: In the prevaccine era of the 1950s, disease rates in high-income countries were 150–1,000/10^5 per year. In the placebo arm of a vaccine trial, the rate of culture-confirmed pertussis in infants 5-11 months of age reached ~2,500/10^5 per year. In the 2000s, disease rates in countries with good vaccine coverage (three or more doses in >80% of preschool children) are ~0.5–10/10^5 per year. In the United States in 1997–2000, 28,187 cases were reported, for mean rates per 10^5 per year of 56 in infants, 4–6 in children and youths, and 0.8 in adults. In poorly vaccinated countries, rates remain at 100–1,000/10^5 per year. Worldwide in the 2000s, there were 20–40 million cases per year. With waning immunity 10–15 years after vaccination or natural infection, youths and adults can become carriers, sources, and victims. Disease rates in youths and adults can exceed 100/10^5 per year. Of cough in adults that lasts >2 weeks, 7–32% (often 25%) is due to *B. pertussis*. OUTBREAKS: Venues for outbreak include schools, institutions, work places, urban, rural, and minority communities in high- and low-income countries, hospitals, and nursing homes. Waves of pertussis can go through communities at intervals of 3–5 years. In outbreaks, attack rates in children in low-income countries can reach 20-70%. Vaccines protect from disease and reduce transmission, although colonization may not be prevented equally well. By endemicity, the first vaccine dose can be given at 6 weeks of age.

BORNAVIRUS (BDV) (1696, 6257) (enveloped RNA viruses: *Mononegavirales*: *Bornaviridae*) BDV is enzootic in central Europe, mainly in horses and sheep. SPREAD: is presumably from salivary, nasal, or conjunctival secretions. CLINICAL INFORMATION: The mammalian incubation period is ≥4 weeks. Manifestations: BDV is neurotropic. Putative associations include mood disorders and schizophrenia. IMPACT: Sporadic in humans.

BORRELIA (1023, 7111) (*Bacteria*: *Spirochaetales*). These helical bacteria exhibit rotating and flexing motility. The genus includes agents of Lyme disease and relapsing fevers (Table 20.2). Treatment options include tetracyclines, β-lactams, and macrolides.

B. burgdorferi sl (909, 3256, 4817, 4933, 5909, 7128), the agent of Lyme disease, circulates in North America and Eurasia, in *Ixodes* ticks, mammals, and birds. *B. burgdorferi* ss in North America and *B. afzelii*, *B. burgdorferi* ss, and *B. garinii* in Eurasia are infective to humans. Occurrence in humans is unconfirmed for *B. andersonii* and *B. bissettii* in North America and for *B. lusitaniae*, *B. japonica*, and *B. valaisiana* in Eurasia. SPREAD: is via tick bite, occasionally by insects, possibly by intrauterine transmission. RISKS: domicile close to foci or in enzootic areas, large property, tick abundance, outdoor activities near foci, and spring to fall season. Infections in humans overlap with vector tick ranges. Because *B. burgdorferi* survives in blood components for several weeks, it is a potential hazard for blood safety. CLINICAL INFORMATION: Of infections 50–98% are inapparent. The incubation period is 1–180 (often 10–21) days. Manifestations (Lyme disease): vary regionally and include erythema migrans (in 60–90%), neuroborreliosis (in 10–80%, often by *B. garinii*), arthritis (in 5–50%, often by *B. burgdorferi* ss), carditis or cardiac arrhythmia (in 0.5–5%), and acrodermatitis (in 0–3%, often by *B. afzelii*). Less than 30% of cases in North America but >60% in Europe recall a tick bite. Erythema in Europe migrates slowly and remains for 2–6 weeks, whereas in North America it migrates fast and fades within days. Confirmation is difficult and based on PCR from biopsy (skin, synovia) and immunoglobulin M and G antibodies in blood or cerebrospinal fluid (two-step testing or conversion in paired sera). Removed ticks are a diagnostic aid. Because questing ticks can harbor several agents, mixed infections should be considered. IMPACT: By test and geography, seroprevalence in North America and Eurasia is ~1–15% (often 3–6%), in people living near foci, 5–45% (often <20%). Seroconversion rates in exposed populations are 1–3% per year. By location, season, diagnostic criteria, and case ascertainment, reported disease rates are 1–1,000/10^5 per year. OUTBREAKS: Except the outbreak of arthritis in Lyme, Connecticut, in 1972, few outbreaks have been reported. Preventive measures include posting and avoidance of foci, protective clothes, repellents, search for ticks when leaving a focus, prompt removal of attached ticks, possibly postexposure prophylaxis with antibiotics, in particular, if removed ticks test positive for *B. burgdorferi* sl. A Lyme disease recombinant vaccine was available in the United States in 1998–2002.

B. recurrentis (956, 5089, 6099, 6114, 7252), the agent of louse-borne relapsing fever (LBRF), circulates in foci, in body lice (*Pediculus humanus corporis*) and humans. SPREAD: On feeding, body lice excret *B. recurrentis* with feces; inoculation is by scratching. Intrauterine transmission can occur. RISKS: domicile in or visit to underserved, remote areas, poor body hygiene among civilian or military populations, crowding (e.g., in prison), homelessness, displacement by war or disaster. CLINICAL INFORMATION: The incubation period is 2–10 (often 4–8) days. Manifestations: fever (in ~100%) that lasts ~5 days and relapses in 6–8 days, flulike illness (in 50–90%), bleeding (petechia, overt in 10–25%), and jaundice. Confirmation is by microscopy (blood smear and buffy coat). A shock-like (Jarisch-Herxheimer) reaction

Table 20.2 *Borrelia*: tick-borne relapsing fever (TBRF), louse-borne relapsing fever (LBRF), and Lyme disease

Parameter	TBRF	LBRF	Lyme disease
Vector	*Ornithodoros* (soft) ticks	*Pediculus* body louse	*Ixodes* (hard) ticks
Geography	Tropical and temperate climate areas	Tropical areas	Northern hemisphere
Agent	Tick specific, e.g., *B. duttonii* (East Africa), *B. hermsii* (North America), *B. hispanica* (Mediterranean), *B. persica* (Asia)	*B. recurrentis*	*B. burgdorferi* sensu lato (sl)
Skin eruption	Usually none	Louse bites	Erythema migrans
No. of fever relapses	0–15 (typically 2–3)	Few	None
Blood smear	Agent seen	Agent seen	Negative
Reservoir	Rodents; for *B. duttoni*, humans	Humans	Small mammals
Risk	Rural cabins (rodent and tick infested)	Crowding, poor hygiene	Outdoor activity

complicates 5–50% of treatments. Treated lethality is 2–6%. IMPACT: Foci exist at the horn of Africa (Ethiopia, Somalia, and Sudan), and in the South American Andes. OUTBREAKS: In World War II, LBRF swept through North Africa, causing 2 million civilian and military cases, for attack rates of 2-30%. "The epidemic was finally brought under control by mass treatment with arsenic and DDT, after 30,000 had died" (956). In Ethiopia in 1991, an outbreak occurred in two camps for prisoners of war with >650 cases. Control is based on prompt treatment of cases and on delousing of people and clothes.

B. duttonii (in East and southern Africa), ***B. crocidurae*** (in West Africa), ***B. hermsii*** (in North America), ***B. venezuelensis*** (in Latin America), ***B. persica*** (in Asia), ***B. hispanica*** (in the Mediterranean) and further putative species are agents of tick-borne relapsing fever (TBRF) (831, 2255, 3962, 4289, 6726) (5772, 7315, 7553) that circulate in *Ornithodorus* (soft) ticks and small mammals. Humans are incidental hosts, except *B. duttoni* for which humans are the principal host. SPREAD: is via tick bite or coxal fluid, rarely intrauterine. RISKS: domicile in or visit to rural enzootic areas, sleeping on mud floor, cleaning out rodent-infested cabins, outdoor activities. CLINICAL INFORMATION: The incubation period is 2–18 (often 7) days. Manifestations (TBRF): fever that lasts 2–7 (3) days and relapses after 4–14 (7) days and meningism. The number of fever relapses is 0–15, typically 2–3. Confirmation is by microscopy (blood smear and buffy coat) or nucleic acid amplification test (NAT). Complications include bleeding, convulsion, and spontaneous abortion. Lethality is 0–8%. IMPACT: In East and West Africa, blood smears from ~1–2% of healthy children can demonstrate borreliae by microscopy (NAT can double this prevalence). In Senegal, spirochetes (*B. crocidurae* by NAT) were detected by microscopy in 0.4% (33 of 7,750) of adults suspected to have malaria. Disease rates apparently reach 5% per year (*B. crocidurae*, West Africa), even 16% (*B. duttoni*, East Africa). In the United States in 1990–2000, 247 cases of TBRF were reported. OUTBREAKS: Venues in the United States were rural cabins: in New Mexico in 2002 (11 cases, attack rate 28%), in Colorado in 1995 (11 cases, attack rate 48%), and in Arizona in 1990 (15 cases among >10,000 visitors overnighting in cabins of Grand Canyon National Park).

BRUCELLA (α-*Proteobacteria*: *Rhizobiales*) (2637, 3162, 4552, 4978, 4983, 7879, 8307). These intracellular, coccoid, gram-negative bacteria circulate worldwide, in marine and terrestrial, wild and domestic mammals and their secretions. Infective to humans are ***B. abortus*** from cattle and wild ungulates (seven biovars, moderately virulent), ***B. canis*** from dogs (not in routine diagnostic program, likely underdiagnosed), ***B. melitenis*** from goat, sheep, camel, and wild ungulates (three biovars, highly virulent, relative frequency in humans 90%), and ***B. suis*** from swine, reindeer, caribou, and rodents (biovars 1, 3, and 5 highly virulent, low or unknown virulence of biovars 2 and 4). *B. neotomae* (in rodents) and *B. ovis* (in sheep) are not infective to humans. Gram-labile brucellae are easily misidentified. SPREAD: is (i) via ingestion of raw milk, nonpasteurized dairy products, or meat, (ii) via inhalation of aerosols generated during abortion or delivery, (iii) via injury from work with animals or carcasses, (iv) via laboratory aerosols, (v) via transfusion or placental cells, (vi) occasionally by mother-to-child transmission (intrauterine and breastmilk) or sexually. RISKS: drinking raw milk, eating fresh, unpasteurized cheese, dairy products from enzootic areas, livestock husbandry, work with animal contacts, laboratory work. CLINICAL INFORMATION: About 50–90% of infections are inapparent. The incubation period ranges from days to 5 months; a typical figure is 3–8 weeks. Manifestations: can be acute, gradual, or chronic and include recurring (undulant) fever (in 60–100%), night sweats, malaise, and weight loss. Complications include arthritis, sacroiliitis, spondylitis (in 6–38%), hepatitis (in 8–14%), endocarditis (in <2%), and neurobrucellosis (in <2%), in early pregnancy also fetal loss (in up to 40%). Confirmation is preferably by culture or nucleic acid amplification test from blood. Blood must be cultured for ≥4 weeks. Treatment options include doxycycline combined with rifampin or aminoglycoside. IMPACT: In enzootic areas, seroprevalence is 1–25% (often 2–8%). Reported disease rates are 2–540 (often 10–30) per 10^5 per year. OUTBREAKS: Venues for outbreaks include slaugtherhouses, farms, and laboratories. A major outbreak vehicle is unpasteurized cheese. Epizootics (abortion storms) have occurred in herds.

BRUGIA (Nematoda: Spirurida). These filariids circulate in Asia in mosquitoes that carry infective (L3) larvae, and final mammalian hosts that harbor adult worms in lymphatics, and microfilariae in peripheral blood. ***B. malayi*** and in Indonesia ***B. timori*** are infective to humans. *B. pahangi*, which is enzootic in cats and dogs, is not confirmed in humans. ***B. malayi*** (4116, 4280, 5027, 8366) occurs in Southeast Asia. Host for a "periodic" strain are humans, hosts for a "subperiodic" (zoonotic) strain are monkeys, felids, and humans. SPREAD: is via *Anopheles* or *Mansonia* bite. CLINICAL INFORMATION: Many infections are inapparent. The presumed prepatent period is 3–6 months, the presumed incubation period is 6–12 months. Manifestations can be acute (fever and lymphadenitis) or chronic (lymphedema, "elephantiasis"). Confirmation is by visualizing microfilariae in night blood, or by nucleic acid amplification test, specific anti-immunoglobulin E, or antigen card test. IMPACT: Some ~13 million persons are infected, including ~3 million with complications. The prevalence of microfilaremia in endemic areas is 0–1.5% (often 0.5%).

BURKHOLDERIA (β-*Proteobacteria*: *Burkholderiales*). *Burkholderia* are soil-dwelling, gram-negative, glucose nonfermenting rods. Of ~40 species, mainly *B. cepacia* and *B. pseudomallei* are isolated in humans.

  B. cepacia (1499, 1966, 4459, 4529, 6831, 6880) inhabits soil, plant roots, and nutrient-poor water. This agent is able to degrade oil and pesticides. **SPREAD**: is likely via inhalation (dust and aerosols), perhaps via droplets. **RISKS**: *B. cepacea* colonizes or infects the airway of 3–50% of cystic fibrosis patients. Patients with malignancies are susceptible. **CLINICAL INFORMATION**: An incubation period is not documented. Manifestations: deteriorating lung function, sepsis. Attributable lethality can exceed 20%. **IMPACT**: *B. cepacia* accounts for 0.1–0.2% of nosocomial infection isolates. The rate of *B. cepacia* recovery from respiratory specimens in intensive care units is 1.4/100 discharges. **OUTBREAKS**: Sources implicated in nosocomial outbreaks included contaminated machines and solutions and colonized patients.

  B. mallei (7083) causes "glanders" in equids. Infections in humans have resulted from contact with infected horses or from laboratory exposure.

  B. pseudomallei (1331, 1682, 1684, 1730, 6087) is an exotoxin-producing agent that circulates in subtropical and tropical areas of Australasia and perhaps Latin America, in soil, plants, freshwater, and mammals. **SPREAD**: is via (i) skin trauma or contact with soil or muddy water (in one fourth of Australian cases), (ii) inhalation of dust, (iii) aspiration by swimming in contaminated water, (iv) nosocomial or laboratory exposure, (v) sex, breastmilk, (vi) animal contact or insect bite. **RISKS**: Outdoor activities, walking barefoot, work in rice fields. Predisposing (in 45–65%) are diabetes, alcoholism, end-stage renal disease, and immune impairment. **CLINICAL INFORMATION**: Most infections are asymptomatic. The incubation period is days to months (even years), after inoculation 1–21 (typically 9) days. Manifestations (melioidosis): include soft-tissue infection, pneumonia (can mimick tuberculosis), and sepsis. Confirmation is by culture. Lethality of invasive disease is 10–40% (often 15%). **IMPACT**: Because of cross-reactivity in the genus, e.g., with *B. mallei* or *B. thailandensis*, serosurveys should be interpreted with caution. In Thailand, high seroprevalence has been reported in rural (18%) *and* urban (4%) populations. Disease rates in endemic areas are ~2–40 (typically 20) per 10^5 and year. **OUTBREAKS**: Outbreaks have been reported in Australia.

CALICIVIRUSES (small-round-structured viruses). See Norovirus.

CALIFORNIA ENCEPHALITIS VIRUS GROUP (INKV, JCV, LACV, SSHV, AND THV). See Orthobunyavirus.

CAMPYLOBACTER (1011, 2263, 2984, 3009, 4162, 5112, 6574) (ε-*Proteobacteria*: *Campylobacterales*). These are twisted, enterotropic rods with darting and spinning motility. Of several species, mainly (in ~90%) *C. jejuni* is found in humans, infrequently *C. coli*, rarely *C. fetus* or *C. lari*. *C. jejuni* circulates in birds and mammals, their feces and fodder, and in humans, sewage, water, and foods. In water, heat (65°C for 3 min) kills the agent, as does free chlorine (0.3 mg/liter at 25°C). **SPREAD**: is via foods, tap water, and animal contact. Poultry is the vehicle for one half or more of sporadic cases. **RISKS**: include consumption of raw milk, untreated tap water, undercooked poultry, barbecued pork or sausage, or salad vegetables; handling of raw poultry, work with animals or animal carcasses, living or working on a farm, dog or cat contacts; travel to countries with warm climates, and summer time. Humans shed *Campylobacter* for 0–12 (typically 2–4) weeks. **CLINICAL INFORMATION**: Some two thirds of infections are inapparent. By infective dose, the incubation period is 1–10 (typically 2–5) days. Manifestations: acute diarrhea, abdominal cramps (in 50–85%), fever (40–75%), overt or microscopically bloody stools. In immune-competent patients, the infection is self-limiting. Complications: dehydration, cholecystitis, sepsis, and Guillain-Barré syndrome. Some 10% of patients are hospitalized. Attributable lethality of food-borne disease is 0.1–1%. **IMPACT**: Over 95% of cases are sporadic. The reported disease rate in high-income countries is ~10–120/10^5 and year; corrected for underreporting, rates are up to 40 times higher. In low-income countries, the disease rate in children is 0.5–2 per child per year, and the average number of lifetime episodes is >5 per person. By age, location, and season, yield in diagnostic stool samples is 1–7% in high-income countries and 5–20% in preschool children with diarrhea in low-income countries. **OUTBREAKS**: Vehicles most frequently implicated in outbreaks are tap water, milk, and poultry. In the United Kingdom in 1995–1999, 50 *Campylobacter* outbreaks were reported (2% of all outbreaks in the period), with cases numbering 2–89 per outbreak.

CANDIDA (*Ascomycota*: *Saccharomycetales*). These opportunistic yeasts are ubiquitous in the environment (soil, bird feces, and plastic surfaces) and colonize birds and other vertebrates. Of >200 species, the most frequent in humans are *C. albicans*, *C. glabrata*, *C. parapsilosis*, and *C. tropicalis*. The four can be part of the human flora, and they can cause invasive disease. By geography, relative frequencies in candidemia are: *C. albicans*, 45–65%; *C. glabrata*, 10–15%; *C. parapsilosis*, 10–20%; and *C. tropicalis*, 3–15%.

  C. albicans (214, 1528, 2134, 2311, 2456, 3452, 3921, 4244, 4700) is part of the flora of skin, bowel, and vagina. **SPREAD**: is endogenous or acquired, likely via contact. **RISKS**: for colonization and disease include recent or current use of antibiotics, vascular devices, hemodialysis, and impaired immunity, e.g., by diabetes, neutropenia, or transplantation. CLINICAL INFORMATION: Colonization predisposes to infection. The putative incubation period is a few (2–5) days. Manifestations: onychomycosis, intertrigo, vulvovaginitis (with pruritus, white and thick ["curdy"] discharge, and inflammation), and balanitis; in immune-impaired or critically ill patients, also fungemia and meningitis. Invasive disease is confirmed by culture from usually sterile sites and biopsy. By case mix and type of hospital unit, attributable lethality of invasive disease is 10–50%, for a mortality of $\sim 1/10^5$. IMPACT: By age, sex, and geography, 3–30% of toenail onychomycosis and 50–85% of fingernail onychomycosis are due to *Candida* (mainly *C. albicans*). By age and pregnancy status, $\sim$2–10% of women of childbearing age are vaginally colonized, and *Candida* vaginitis is diagnosed in 20–25% of women with vaginal symptoms. In metropolitan San Francisco in 1992–1993, the rate of invasive *Candida* disease was $18/10^5$ and year. In Calgary, Canada, invasive disease rates per 10^5 per year were 3 overall, with peaks of 20 at extremes of age ($<$1, $>$75 years). In the United Kingdom in 2003, candidemia rates per 10^5 were 2.5, with highs in infants ($\sim$10) and at age $>$75 years (5.5 in females and $\sim$11 in males) (Fig. 20.1). Impact in hospitals is considerable. *Candida* accounts for 5–10% of bloodstream infections. Candidemia rates are 0.1–4/1,000 admissions or 0.02–0.1/1,000 patient-days (10–20 times higher in intensive care units).

C. parapsilosis (754, 884, 1473) can colonize plastic and hands of healthy persons. RISKS: stays in intensive care unit, colonized hands of health workers, impaired immunity, e.g., by low birth weight, diabetes, injection drug use, or malignancy. CLINICAL INFORMATION: Diseases due to *C. parapsilosis* include onychomycosis (mainly of fingernails), fungemia, endocarditis, and device-associated infections. OUTBREAKS: A nosocomial outbreak has caused 22 bloodstream infections.

CAPILLARIA (Nematoda: Enoplida). These worms circulate in vertebrates. *C. hepatica* and *C. philippensis* can parasitize humans.

C. hepatica (3767, 6633) circulates worldwide, in rodents, e.g., rats (final hosts that hold eggs in liver), and carnivores and scavengers that prey on rodents (transport hosts that shed eggs fecally). Eggs need to embryonate in soil for 2–6 weeks. SPREAD: is via fecally polluted soil (geophagia) or foods. CLINICAL INFORMATION: Manifestations (hepatic capillariasis): hepatomegaly, fever eosinophilia, rarely fatal hepatic necrosis. Confirmation is by visualizing eggs (*Trichuris*-like) in liver biopsy. IMPACT: Rare ($\sim$40 human cases reported).

C. philippensis (388, 1648) circulates in Asia and Egypt, in birds and humans (final hosts) who shed eggs (occasionally larvae) with feces, and freshwater or brackish fish (intermediate hosts). SPREAD: is via ingestion of larvae in fish or by larval autoinfection. CLINICAL INFORMATION: In experimental infection, the prepatent period is 4–6 weeks. Manifestations (intestinal capillariasis): diarrhea, weight loss, eosinophilia. Confirmation is by visualizing eggs (*Trichuris*-like) in stool. IMPACT: Infrequent. In Luzon, Philippines, in 1967–1970, an epidemic caused >1,400 cases; lethality was 6–7%.

CAPNOCYTOPHAGA (755, 6599, 7312) (*Bacteria: Flavobacteriales*). These gram-negative, flexible rods are part of the buccal flora of mammals. *C. canimorsus* colonizes dogs, and cats, *C. gingivalis* colonizes humans. ACQUISITION: infections are endogenous or from bites (in $\sim$55%), scratch (in $\sim$10%), or contact with dogs (saliva and droplets). CLINICAL INFORMATION: The incubation is 1–8 days. Manifestations: periodontitis, wound infection, invasive disease (e.g., sepsis, meningitis, and endocarditis). Immune-impaired hosts (asplenia, alcoholism, and suppressive treatment) are susceptible. Lethality of invasive disease is $\sim$30%. IMPACT: Sporadic.

CARDIOBACTERIUM (γ-*Proteobacteria*: *Cardiobacteriales*). *C. hominis* is part of the oropharyngeal flora and a sporadic cause of endocarditis.

CARDIOVIRUS (870) (unenveloped RNA viruses: *Picornaviridae*). A member is encephalomyocarditisvirus (EMCV) that circulates feco-orally among rats and mice. EMCV can jump to pigs and occasionally humans. In pigs, EMCV can cause myocarditis and chronic infections important for xenotransplants.

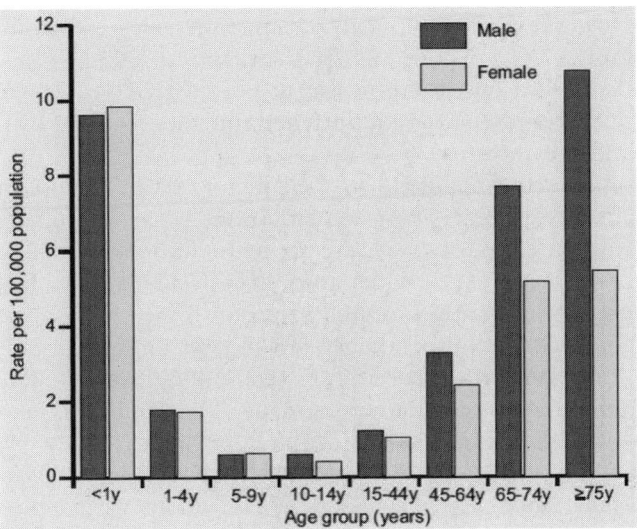

Figure 20.1 Candidemia reports, England, Wales, and Northern Ireland, 2003 ($n = 1,380$). Rates are given per 10^5 population (y axis) by age (x axis, years) and sex. From reference 3452. Reproduced with permission by Public Health Laboratory Service.

CHIKUNGUNYA VIRUS (CHIKV). *See Alphavirus.*

CHLAMYDIA* AND *CHLAMYDOPHILA (Bacteria: *Chlamydiales*). These are intracellular, inclusion-forming bacteria sensitive to macrolides, tetracyclines, and fluoroquinolones. Chlamydias latently infect vertebrates. Cross-protection between *Chlamydia* and *Chlamydophila* is unlikely. Hosts of *Chlamydia* include humans (*C. trachomatis*), pigs (*C. suis*), and mice (*C. muridarum*). For *C. trachomatis* humans are exclusive hosts, with a predilection for eyes (serovars A–C), genitals (D–K), or lymph nodes (L1–3). Hosts of *Chlamydophila* include humans (*C. pneumoniae*), birds and humans (*C. psittaci*), cats and rarely humans (*C. felis*), ruminants and rarely humans (*C. abortus*), guinea pigs (*C. caviae*), and ruminants and marsupials (*C. pecorum*).

C. trachomatis, **ocular (serovars A–C)** (139, 653, 2200, 2509, 4599, 6498, 6647, 6659) *C. trachomatis* serovars A–C circulate in low-income countries, mainly in arid areas and preschool children. **SPREAD**: is via skin or hand contact, droplets, face-seeking flies, or objects, e.g., towels. **RISKS**: include shortage of water, poor facial cleanliness, flies on faces, towel sharing, lack of toilets, lack of garbage collection, abundance of flies, feces around domiciles, crowding, proximity to livestock, and no access to treatment. **CLINICAL INFORMATION**: About 5–30% of laboratory-confirmed infections are inapparent. Disease seems to require reinfections. The incubation period is 5–10 days. Manifestations: trachoma, a follicular conjunctivitis. Stages are active trachoma with ≥5 tarsal follicules (TF) or intense inflammation (TI), tarsal scars (TS), and sequelae of trichiasis (TT) or corneal opacity (CO). Diagnosis is clinical. **IMPACT**: Trachoma is endemic in 48 countries of Africa, South Asia, and the western Pacific. About 150 million people have active trachoma, for a prevalence of 3%. In some communities, the prevalence of active trachoma (TF and TI) in children can exceed 50%. Clinical surveys may overestimate occurrence, as <55% of clinically diagnosed TF and TI is laboratory confirmed. Prevalence >5% (TI in children 0–9 years of age) or >20% (TF) defines levels considered a public health problem. About 4% of blindness worldwide is attributed to trachoma. **OUTBREAKS**: Outbreaks are not a feature of trachoma. Prevention promotes "SAFE": "S"urgery (for TT), "A"ntibiotics (for TF, TI), "F"acial cleanliness (for children), and "E"nvironmental improvements (tap water, toilets that keep off flies).

C. trachomatis, **genital (serovars D–K)** (60, 3720, 4011, 5059, 5400) circulate in humans worldwide. **SPREAD**: is via sex (sexually transmitted infection). **RISKS**: include being adolescent, nonmarried, nulliparous, and having multiple sex partners. **CLINICAL INFORMATION**: Infections are inapparent in 20–90% of men and 40–90% of women. Inapparent infections can persist for months or years. Some 15% of individuals are repeatedly infected, after a median interval of 6 months. The putative incubation period is 1–7 weeks. Manifestations: genital discharge disease (cervicitis in women and urethritis and proctitis in men), neonatal conjunctivitis. Untreated, complications include pelvic inflammatory disease (in ≤40% of infections) and ectopic pregnancy. Of laparoscopically confirmed pelvic inflammatory disease, 15–65% is due to *C. trachomatis*. Confirmation is by nucleic acid amplification test, culture, or other test from urine (office- or self-collected) or smear (cervical, urethral). **IMPACT**: *C. trachomatis* is endemic in all sexually active populations (see sections 14.7, 13.6, and 13.7). By age, setting, and test, infection prevalence reported for high-income countries is 1–15% (often 3–5%) and infection rates are 100–400/10^5 per year. Underreporting is likely. Rates are highest in inner-city populations and adolescents. **OUTBREAKS**: By age, endemicity, and risk mix, universal or targeted screening is recommended. Proposed targets include sexually active females 15–25 years of age and females with a new or more than one sex partner who had not used condoms in the preceding 3 months.

C. trachomatis, **lymphatic (serovars L1–3)** (492, 493, 7710) circulates locally in sexually active adults. **SPREAD**: is via sex (sexually transmitted infection). Sex partners need to be contacted and evaluated. **CLINICAL INFORMATION**: The incubation period is 3 days to 6 (often 4) weeks. Lymphgranuloma venereum (LGV) is manifest by a papule at genitals or rectum that can ulcerate, regional adenopathy (buboes, in ~90%) that can become purulent and fistulous, and proctocolitis (in ~5%). **IMPACT**: LGV is usually rare in North America and West Europe, and most cases are imported. However, pockets of local transmission have persisted in groups that practice high-risk sex, and in 2003 LGV has reemerged in urban western Europe. **OUTBREAKS**: Recent outbreaks are reported among homosexual men and cocaine users.

Chlamydophila abortus (4959) is a rare cause of abortion in pregnant women. **SPREAD**: is via contact with infected cows, sheep or goats, or their abortion products. In The Netherlands, an infected woman had preterm stillbirth. Her only exposure were visits to the goat farm her husband operated and washing his clothes.

C. pneumoniae (3791, 4027, 4960, 6684, 6860, 7559) biovars circulate in humans (TWAR), horses, and koalas. **SPREAD**: is via droplets or hands, likely via aerosols, occasionally in hospitals. **CLINICAL INFORMATION**: About 50–90% of endemic infections are inapparent. Reinfections are frequent. The incubation period is 7–30 days. Manifestations: include pharyngitis, bronchitis, sinusitis, flulike illness, and community-acquired pneumonia. Diagnosis is serologically (immunoglobulin G) or by nucleic acid amplification test (from blood or bronchoalveolar fluid). Lethality of pneumonia in the elderly is ~3%. A discussed late complication of infection is atherosclerosis. IMPACT: Reported seroprevalence is low in preschool children, 20–75% in adolescents, and 50–100% in adults. Infection rates in households per 100 person-years are 6–9 in school children and ~2 in adolescents and adults. Diagnostic yield in outpatients with respiratory symptoms is ~1%. OUTBREAKS: Venues for outbreaks include the community, households, schools, the military, and nursing homes. Reported epidemic rates are 3–14/10^5 per year.

C. psittaci (1166, 1826, 3531, 5801, 6723, 8183) circulates in birds, mammals, and humans. The agent resists drying. Of eight serovars, all seem infective to humans. SPREAD: is via inhalation of bird dust or contact with colonized, incubating, or sick birds. RISKS: From 65% to 85% of patients mention bird leisure or work contacts. CLINICAL INFORMATION: Up to 40% of infections are inapparent. The incubation period is 5–21 days. Manifestations (ornithosis, psittacosis): flulike illness, atypical pneumonia, hepatitis, and endocarditis. Lethality in the preantibiotic era was 15–20%, with treatment it is now <1%, although in a community outbreak in Australia it reached 6%. IMPACT: Reported disease rates per 10^5 per year are 0.02–0.05 in the United States, 0.5–1.5 in Australia, and ~2.5 in Switzerland. In an enzootic area of Italy, the rate of hospitalized ornithosis cases was 13/10^5 per year. OUTBREAKS: Venues for outbreaks include communities, families, farms, abattoirs, aviaries, and a customs office.

CITROBACTER (1991, 3011) (γ-*Proteobacteria*: *Enterobacteriales*). These gram-negative rods are related to *Salmonella* and circulate in mammals, manure, sewage, soil, and water. Of >10 species, mainly *C. diversus*, *C. freundii*, and *C. koseri* are found in humans. *Citrobacter* can colonize the human intestinal, genitourinary, and respiratory tracts. SPREAD: Infections are endogenous or acquired, likely via contact. RISKS: neonates, impaired immunity. CLINICAL INFORMATION: The incubation period is not known. Manifestations: sepsis, meningitis. Lethality of invasive disease is 30–55%. IMPACT: *Citrobacter* accounts for ~2% of nosocomial urinary tract infections and ~1% each for surgical site infection, nosocomial pneumonias, and bloodstream infections. OUTBREAKS: Main outbreak settings are hospitals, in particular neonatal ICU.

CLADOPHIALOPHORA AND CLADOSPORIUM (23, 2245) (*Ascomycota*). These pigmented molds inhabit soil and plants. SPREAD: is likely via trauma or inhalation. Manifestations: chromomycosis (in immune-competent hosts) and invasive disease (in immune-impaired hosts). In Madagascar, of 170 fungi isolated from histopathologically confirmed chromomycosis cases, 38% were *Cladophialophora carrionii*.

CLONORCHIS (OPISTHORCHIS) SINENSIS (1818, 4570, 5472, 8355) (Trematoda: Digenea). *C. sinensis* circulates in East Asia (People's Republic of China, Korea, Taiwan, Vietnam, and eastern Siberia), in fish-eating mammals and humans (final hosts, shed eggs), freshwater snails (first intermediate hosts), and fish, mainly *Cyprinoidea* (second hosts, harbor-infective metacercariae). SPREAD: is via uptake of viable metacercariae from fish; hands and kitchen utensils can cross-contaminate other foods. RISKS: domicile close to rivers, habitual eating of raw fish, in particular, by males (male:female ratio of 2–3 :1). CLINICAL INFORMATION: The prepatent period is ~3–4 weeks. Adults locate in bile ducts. Life span of adults is ~20 years. Infections can remain silent for decades. Manifestations: cholecystitis, cholangitis, gallbladder and duct stones, and jaundice. *C. sinensis* can be oncogenic, and a late complication of heavy infection is cholangiocarcinoma. Confirmation is by visualizing operculate eggs in stool or duodenal fluid. Egg counts >10,000/g feces define heavy infection. A treatment option is praziquantel. IMPACT: Some 7–35 million people are infected (in People's Republic of China 3–15 million). By geography, diet, and control, the infection prevalence in enzootic-endemic areas is 0.1–30%, often 1–5%. In Guangxi, southern People's Republic of China, the overall prevalence was 32% (491/1,552), that of heavy infections was 4% (57). No cases have been reported in Japan since 1991.

CLOSTRIDIUM (*Firmicutes*: *Clostridiales*). These anaerobic, endospore-forming gram-positive rods circulate in soil, plants, grazing mammals, and manure. Of >160 species, *C. botulinum*, *C. difficile*, *C. perfringens*, and *C. tetani* are mainly identified in humans. *C. novyi* (2392) and *C. sordellii* (3947) are contaminants of street opium and heroin, causing myonecrosis (gas gangrene) and sepsis in injection drug users.

C. botulinum (22, 862, 1207, 2510, 2580, 3054, 3794, 7014, 7774) spores are ubiquitous in soil, plants, aquatic sediments, fish bowels, animal carcasses, and farm products. Types A-G produce potent, color- and odorless botulinum toxins A-G. Most cases in humans are due to toxins A, B, or E. Heat inactivates bacteria (60°C for a few minutes), toxin (85°C for 5 min), and spores (120°C for 25 min). Conditions favorable for the production of toxin in foods are: anaerobic, nonacidic (pH >4), nonsalty (NaCl <3–10%), and high water activity (usually controlled by NaCl). SPREAD: is via (i) uptake of preformed toxin from foods (food botulism), (ii) uptake of spores that germinate temporarily colonizes bowel (infant botulism), (iii) inoculation (wound botulism), (iv) reactivated endogenous colonization, (v) inhalation of intentionally released, weaponized toxins or agents. RISKS: toxin from home-preserved foods, spores in street-illicit drugs (injection drug use), spores in honey (infant botulism). CLINICAL INFORMATION: By toxin and dose, incubation periods are 1 h to 12 (often 1) days (food-borne) to 3 weeks (endogenous). Manifestation (neurotoxic): muscle weakness (in ~90%), dysphagia (in ~80%), ophthalmoplegia (in 75–80%, diplopia, ptosis), and descending paralysis. Toxin can be identified in serum, feces, and leftover foods. Bacteria can be detected in feces (in ~50% of food-borne cases). By toxin and dose, lethality is 0-30% (often 5–10%). IMPACT: Disease rates per 10^5 per year are, in general, <0.06 in North America and West Europe, but 2–8.5 in Alaska, up to 1 in the Republic of Georgia, and up to 2 in Poland. More than 1,000 cases of infant botulism have been reported, most in the United States, ~50 in Europe. OUTBREAKS: A single case is a clinical and epidemiological emergency that requires immediate care and reporting. Numerous outbreaks have been documented in North America (766 in the United States in 1899–1977, 160 in 1990–2000), Asia (154 in Georgia in 1980-2002, 986 in People's Republic of China in 1958–1983), and Europe (737 in France in 1956–2000, and 112 in Italy in 1992–1996), few in Africa (5 in 1959–2002). In two thirds of outbreaks, there is only one case, and often there are only two to four cases per outbreak. Recent vehicles for outbreaks included a church supper in Texas, homemade asparagus in France, and commercially tinned fish in tomato sauce in South Africa.

C. difficile (434, 462, 4940, 5477, 6276, 7440) spores are ubiquitous and resilient to disinfectants. *C. difficile* can colonize the human bowel. Strains can produce toxins A (enterotoxin) or B (cytotoxin). SPREAD: Infections are endogenous or acquired in the community (one third) or nosocomially (two thirds), via hands, contact, tubings, or instruments. RISKS: Hospitalization for >2 weeks, frequent, recent, or current use of antimicrobials, possibly diapers. Susceptibility is increased after age 60 years. CLINICAL INFORMATION: Most (60–95%) infections are inapparent. An incubation period has not been reported, but >2 weeks can elapse from first use of antibiotics to the appearance of *C. difficile*-associated diarrhea (CDAD). Manifestations of CDAD can range from self-limited diarrhea to fulminant, bloody (pseudomembranous) colitis. About 20–25% of cases relapse. Confirmation is difficult and based on screening for *C. difficile* common antigen by enzyme-linked immunosorbent assay followed by nucleic acid amplification test for toxins A and B genes and culture. By diagnostic criteria and case mix, lethality of CDAD is 1–60% (often 10%). IMPACT: By antibiotics policy and ward, disease rates in hospitals are 1–5/1,000 admissions. In Perth, Australia, reduced use of third generation cephalosporins paralleled decreasing CDAD rates per 1,000 discharges from 2–3 in 1993–1998 to ~1 in 2000. OUTBREAKS: Outbreaks have occurred in hospitals. In the United Kingdom in 1992–2000, 13% (176/1,369) of infectious diarrhea outbreaks in hospitals were due to CDAD.

C. perfringens (=*welchii*) (3364, 4566, 6362, 6612, 7170) spores are ubiquitous in soil, animals, feces, and foods. Types A–E produce toxins (α–ε, enterotoxic) and gas. *C. perfringens* colonizes the human bowel and the female genital tract. SPREAD: is via foods or skin trauma. Infections can also arise endogenously. RISKS: Food that is precooked and served cold, and contaminated, anaerobic wounds. For food poisoning, >10^6–10^8 bacteria per g food are needed: enterotoxin is only formed in vivo, after ingestion of bacteria. In parallel with enterotoxin, spores are formed. CLINICAL INFORMATION: The incubation period is 2–24 h. Manifestations include food poisoning (diarrhea and abdominal cramps), gas gangrene (muscular pain, myonecrosis, and septic shock), endometritis (mainly from criminal abortion), and necrotizing enteritis (pigbel of Papua New Guinea). Lethality of gas gangrene is 30–60%. Confirmation is by enterotoxin assay from stool and by culture of clinical materials. IMPACT: A major agent of food poisoning (see section III). The reported rate of endometritis from legal abortion is 0.1%. OUTBREAKS: *C. perfringens* is a frequent cause of food-borne outbreaks. In Finland in 1975–1999, 20% (238) of all reported food-borne outbreaks were due to *C. perfringens*. Outbreak settings include restaurants, social events, conferences, camps, schools, prisons, hospitals, and homes.

C. tetani (1158, 1286, 4931, 5747, 5792, 6049, 6472, 6562, 7475) is widespread in soil. Spores are dispersed with dust and animal feces. Killing needs heat (121°C for 10 min in an autoclave), or formalin (3% for 24 h). In anaerobic wounds, spores germinate, producing neurotoxin (tetanospasmin). SPREAD: is via (i) trauma (e.g., puncture, foreign object, and burn). (ii) wound colonization (e.g., decubitus ulcer, frostbite, and gingivitis), (iii) animal bite (e.g., dog, snake, and insect), perhaps human bite, and (iv) dirty procedures (e.g., umbilical cord cut, circumcision, illegal abortion, and piercing). Portals include feet, legs, hands, arms, head, injection sites, and surgical sites. RISKS: include not being vaccinated, walking barefoot, penetrating wound, home birth and delivery, and nonprofessional cutting of the umbilical cord. CLINICAL INFORMATION: The incubation period is 2–60 (typically 5–15) days. Tetanus is diagnosed clinically, from spasms, e.g., "risus sardonicus," "trismus," and "opisthotonus." Hippocrates in 400 BC described a man with a dart wound, locked jaw, and backward bending who died. Complications include arrhythmia, laryngeal spasm, and apnea. By age and vaccination status, lethality is 2–90% (often 10–30%). IMPACT: The global number of tetanus deaths is 0.3 million per year (including 0.25 million neonates). In the 20 countries that report 90% of neonatal tetanus deaths, median mortality is 3/1,000 live births. In high-income countries, reported tetanus rates are <0.1/10^5 per year (<0.02 in the United States and ≥0.05 in much of West Europe). OUTBREAKS: Toxoid-adsorbed vaccine became available in World War II. Neonatal and adult tetanus are vaccine preventable, yet both persist: neonatal tetanus in low-income countries and adult tetanus in injection drug users and the elderly in high-income countries. With neither booster nor natural infection, antitoxin titers decline with time, leaving 40% or more of elderly susceptible (titer <0.01–0.15 IU/ml). Vaccine in pregnancy effectively prevents tetanus in babies.

COCCIDIOIDES (1654, 2416, 4042, 5851, 6413) (*Ascomycota: Onygenales*). These thermally dimorphic fungi thrive in arid, alkaline soils where infective arthroconidia are produced. Recently, morphologically identical *C. posadasii* was separated from prototype *C. immitis*. The former appears to range in the southwestern United States, Mexico, Venezuela, and Argentina, the latter in California only. SPREAD: is via inhalation of aerosolized arthroconidia; animal-to-person and person-to-person spread do not occur. RISKS: Residence in or visit to endemic areas, dust storms and earthquakes, winter season, tillage of soil by farm, excavation, and construction work, e.g., bulldozing or digging telephone posts, military training, all-terrain vehicle driving, and model airplane flying. CLINICAL INFORMATION: Some 60% of infections are inapparent or mild. The incubation period is 1–3 weeks, and occasionally up to 7 weeks. Manifestations: dry cough, flulike, pneumonia, chronic lung disease (can mimic tuberculosis), erythema nodosum, and disseminated disease (smoking, diabetes, and elderly). In ~5% of infections, residues are apparent on chest radiographs. Confirmation is by nucleic acid amplification test, biopsy, culture, or serology. IMPACT: In endemic areas of the United States, disease rates are ~15-85/10^5 per year. OUTBREAKS: Venues for outbreaks include military training camps, archeological digging sites, and construction sites.

COLTIVIRUS (unenveloped RNA viruses: *Reoviridae*). These are tick-borne viruses of rodents. Members include Colorado tick fever virus (CTFV) in North America, and Eyach virus in Europe.

Colorado tick fever virus (CTFV) (3981) circulates in rodents and wood ticks (*Dermacentor andersoni*). Preferred habitat are open stands of ponderosa pine. SPREAD: is via tick bite, occasionally in the laboratory or transfusion. RISKS: CTFV can persist in peripheral blood cells for 3–4 months. CLINICAL INFORMATION: The incubation period is 3–10 (typically 5) days. Manifestations: flulike illness. A rare complication is encephalitis, mainly in children. Confirmation is by nucleic acid amplification test or serology.

CRIMEAN-CONGO HEMORRHAGIC FEVER VIRUS (CCHFV). *See* Nairovirus.

CORONAVIRUS (enveloped RNA viruses: *Nidovirales*) (3402, 8051). Coronavirus is widespread in vertebrates, including chicken (avian infectious bronchitis virus), rats, pigs (porcine epidemic diarrhea virus), cats and dogs (feline and canine coronaviruses). There is much genetic variability. Agents in humans are human coronavirus and severe acute respiratory syndrome coronavirus.

Human coronavirus (HCoV) (269, 2164, 2303, 7676) is a respiratory virus of humans that circulates worldwide. SPREAD: is via droplets, perhaps objects, including in hospitals. RISKS: In temperate climates, transmission peaks in winter. Preschool children, elderly, and patients with comorbidities are susceptible. CLINICAL INFORMATION: Inapparent infections are likely. The putative incubation period is ~3 days. Manifestations: rhinitis, common cold, bronchiolitis, flulike illness, and pneumonia. Diagnosis is by nucleic acid amplification test from nasopharyngeal fluid. IMPACT: High seroprevalence (90%) and infection rates (>1 per person per year) were reported. By seroconversion, HCoV was the only agent identified in 4% of children with acute respiratory illness. OUTBREAKS: A community outbreak has been reported.

Severe acute respiratory syndrome coronavirus (SARS-CoV) (1308, 1375, 2803, 4237, 4466, 4483, 7272, 8276, 8354, 8398) emerged in 2003, with severe acute respiratory syndrome (SARS), likely from a species jump in rural People's Republic of China. A suspected reservoir are bats (or palm civets). SPREAD: is via (i) droplets or hand contacts with patients, (ii) likely hospital and laboratory aerosols, (iii) contacts with animals on markets, (iv) possibly polluted surfaces or objects. Only 10% of spread occurs before onset of symptoms (d_0). Viral load peaks *after* d_0, and from d_0, SARS-CoV is shed in sputum for 2–7 (median, 3) weeks and in stools for 2–18 (median, 4) weeks. Infectivity decreases during reconvalescence and is minimal for the last 10 days after fever has resolved. RISKS: In outbreaks, "super-spreaders" can be highly infective in the first week of illness. In Toronto, the 20-day attack rate in quarantined contacts was 1%. CLINICAL INFORMATION: Silent seroreactivities in healthy adults suggest inapparent infections. The incubation period is 2–14 (typically 4–8) days. Manifestations: fever (in 95–100%), flulike illness (in 50–70%), rapidly worsening dyspnea (in 30–80%), and diarrhea (in 30–70%). Confirmation is by nucleic acid amplification test (nasal, throat, lower respiratory tract, or stool samples), or serology (conversion, fourfold rise). By time and material, diagnostic yield is 30–65%. Of probable SARS cases, 45% tested positive by nucleic acid amplification test from nasopharyngeal fluids and 28% from stools. Lethality is 5–30% (typically 10%). **IMPACT**: In pre-SARS Hong Kong, the seroprevalence was ~2%. **OUTBREAKS**: The SARS pandemic began in Guangdong Province, People's Republic of China, in XI/2002, and by VIII/2003, >8,000 probable cases were reported from 31 countries, mostly (95%) People's Republic of China, Hong Kong, Singapore, and Taiwan. Epidemic spread, and escape from laboratories in Asia raised concerns that SARS-CoV could be weaponized.

CORYNEBACTERIUM (Actinobacteria: Actinomycetales) (2557). These are aerobe, spore-nonforming, gram-positive rods ("diphtheroids," "coryneforms") that inhabit mammalian skin or mucosa. Of ≥20 species, *C. diphtheriae*, *C. jeikeium*, *C. pseudotuberculosis*, and *C. ulcerans* are isolated in humans.

C. diphtheriae (1789, 1943, 4003, 4568, 4931, 5051, 6195, 7865) colonizes human throat, nasopharynx, and skin. There are four biotypes (e.g., gravis), and toxigenic (phage-infected) strains that secrete exotoxin; some strains may harbor the phage without expressing toxin. **SPREAD**: is via saliva (kissing), droplets, and body contact. Infectivity is moderate. Cutaneous diphtheria is also infective. In theory (R_0), a source could generate three to seven new cases. **RISKS**: not being vaccinated (e.g., minorities), contact with a case, crowding, poor living condition, injection drug use, travel to and from epidemic areas, and migration. Alcoholism predisposes to severe course. **CLINICAL INFORMATION**: A frequently quoted incubation period is 2–5 days. Manifestations of toxigenic diphtheria: include membraneous rhinitis or tonsillitis, swollen (bull) neck, and membranous skin ulcer. Complications include croup and myocarditis (in ~10–20% of pharyngeal and ~5% of skin diphtheria). By age and immune status, lethality is 0.5-30% (often 5–10%). Manifestations of nontoxigenic diphtheria: include pharyngitis, endocarditis, and skin lesions. Lethality can reach levels of toxigenic diphtheria. In the United Kingdom in 1995–1996, of 265 nontoxigenic isolates, 93% (247) were from throat, 4% (10) were from skin, 0.4% (1) were from blood, and the rest (7) were from other or unknown sites. **IMPACT**: Vaccines have greatly reduced diphtheria rates in high-income countries. Typical rates approach zero (<$0.05/10^5$ per year). In the United States in 1980–1994, 41 (unlinked) cases of respiratory diphtheria were reported with 4 (10%) deaths in unvaccinated children. **OUTBREAKS**: Outbreaks were frequent in the prevaccine era, but remain a threat for poorly vaccinated groups. In 1990–1998, epidemics surged through the ex-Soviet Union, causing >157,000 cases and 5,000 deaths. Toxoid-adsorbed vaccine became available in World War II. While vaccines protect well from disease they are not designed to prevent carriage. In a school outbreak in Texas in 1967, attack rates were 1% (2/205) in vaccinated students (≥3 doses in 10 years), 11% (10/91) in incompletely vaccinated students, but 30% (3/10) in nonvaccinated students. In contrast, the respective proportions of carriers were 35% (71/205), 20% (18/91), and nil (0/10). Without vaccine or natural booster, antitoxin titers decline with time, leaving 20–50% or more of elderly susceptible (titers, <0.01 IU/ml). Sustained vaccination is needed to maintain herd immunity and interrupt transmission. Case management includes isolation, standard precautions, laboratory prealert and workup, antibiotic and antitoxin therapy, prompt reporting, and contact tracing for postexposure prophylaxis (antibiotics and vaccine updates).

C. jeikeium (7939) is part of human skin flora. **SPREAD**: (droplet air and skin-blood) is apparently via contact. Manifestations: bacteremia, endocarditis, mainly in patients with devices or impaired immunity. **OUTBREAKS**: Nosocomial outbreaks have been reported.

C. pseudotuberculosis (5800, 8335) occurs in cattle, sheep, goats, houseflies, and soil. Manifestations in livestock include abscesses, mastitis, and invasive disease. Sporadic human infections have been documented, mainly lymphadenitis from occupational exposure to sheep.

C. ulcerans (3174, 4887, 7897) occurs in cattle and humans. Like *C. diphtheriae*, *C. ulcerans* can host toxigenic phages. **SPREAD**: is via contact with infected mammals, or ingestion of raw milk. In some patients, the history is blank for these modes. Manifestations: pharyngotonsillitis (can mimick diphtheria), rarely skin lesions. Nontoxigenic *C. ulcerans* can cause chronic pulmonary disease. **IMPACT**: Sporadic. Contacts of toxigenic cases should be traced, treated, and vaccinated like diphtheria cases.

COXIELLA (910, 1096, 2085, 3243, 4633, 6121, 7071, 7484, 7755) (γ-Proteobacteria: Legionellales). *C. burnetii* is an intracellular bacterium that circulates worldwide, in hard ticks, birds, domestic and wild mammals, their secretions (urine, feces, birth products, and milk), soil, and dust. Sporelike life forms are able to survive in tick feces, wool, sand, tap water, and salted meat for months to years. **SPREAD**: is via (i) inhalation of dust, (ii) inhalation of aerosols from animal birth, animal dust, wool dust, (iii) tick bite (rare), (iv) inhalation of laboratory aerosols, (v) ingestion of raw dairy products, (vi) sex (rare). **RISKS**: work with infected animals, animal dust. Infective placenta can yield up to 10^9 agents/g. The infective dose can be as low as one inhaled agent. **CLINICAL INFORMATION**: From 45% to 95% of infections are inapparent or mild. The incubation period is 1–6 (typically 2–3) weeks.

Manifestations (Q fever): can be acute or chronic and include headache (in 95%), flulike illness (in 80%), atypical pneumonia, and hepatitis. Complications include meningoencephalitis (in 1%), myocarditis (in 1%), and chronic endocarditis. Confirmation is by serology or nucleic acid amplification test from blood, urine, or tissue. In France, of 1,383 hospitalized Q fever patients, 77% (1,070) were acute (seroconversion, immunoglobulin (Ig) M) and 23% (313) were chronic (phase I IgG titers). Treatment options include tetracyclines or macrolide plus rifampin combination. IMPACT: In enzootic areas, seroprevalence is 0.5-60% (often 5–10%). By surveillance and area, reported rates of acute Q fever are $0.1–50/10^5$ per year. OUTBREAKS: Outbreaks have affected civilian and military, rural and urban communities. In 18 outbreaks from 1981 to 2000, case loads were 3–415 (mean, 64) per outbreak, with a high in Switzerland in 1983 with 415 cases. Sources include dust, herds, animals (on farms, pets, at school, in clinics and research), stables, abattoirs, animal products, manufacturing plants, and a shelter for the homeless.

COXSACKIEVIRUS. *See* Enterovirus.

CREUTZFELDT-JAKOB DISEASE (CJD). *See* Prions.

CRIMEAN-CONGO HEMORRHAGIC FEVER VIRUS (CCHFV). *See* Nairovirus.

CUNNINGHAMELLA (1511, 1751) (*Zygomycota*: *Mucorales*). These filamentous fungi inhabit soil. *C. bertholletiae* has been isolated in humans. ACQUISITION: is by inhalation. Manifestations (zygomycosis): rhinocerebral, pulmonary, and invasive disease in immune-impaired hosts. Lethality can exceed 80%.

CRYPTOCOCCUS (696, 2036, 3358, 3678, 5079, 7442) (*Basidiomycota*: *Tremellales*). *Cryptococcus* is a genus of encapsulated, yeastlike fungi. Of >30 species, *C. laurentii* and *C. neoformans* have been diagnosed in humans. Of *C. neoformans*, three varieties have been described: *C. neoformans grubii* (a worldwide opportunist), *C. neoformans neoformans* (an opportunist mainly in parts of Europe), and *C. neoformans gattii* (now *C. gattii*, a primary pathogen in warmer climates). *Cryptococcus* is ubiquitous in seed-eating birds, bird guano, soil, and dust. ACQUISITION: is by inhalation of spores, rarely by needle stick or organ transplant. RISKS: bird dust, bird droppings, work with birds. CLINICAL INFORMATION: Perhaps one third of infections are inapparent. The putative incubation period is 6–10 weeks. Manifestations: include skin lesions, pneumonia, meningitis, fungemia, and disseminated disease. Most cases are in hosts with impaired immunity. In Alabama in 1992–1994, the disease rate was 1,950 times higher in human immunodeficiency-infected than uninfected individuals. In France in 1985–1993, 84% (827/990) of cases had AIDS, and 16% (163) had malignancies or other immune deficiencies. Confirmation is by culture, antigen test from cerebrospinal fluid or serum, and biopsy. Lethality is 4–6% in high-income countries, and 40–100% in Africa. IMPACT: In the pre-AIDS era, disease rates were $<0.1/10^5$ per year. In the 1990s, disease rates in endemic areas rose to $1–7/10^5$ per year. Highly active antiretroviral treatment has decreased rates in the 2000s to $0.4-1.3/10^5$ per year. In Europe, cryptococcosis is the opportunistic infection that defines 2–4% of AIDS cases. The lifetime risk of *Cryptococcus* infection in organ transplant recipients is 3–4%. OUTBREAKS: On Vancouver Island, British Columbia, in 1999–2002, an outbreak of *C. neoformans gattii* caused ≥59 cases and 2 deaths.

CRYPTOSPORIDIUM (309, 597, 1369, 2813, 3352, 3505, 3560, 6446, 7608) (Alveolata: Eucoccidiorida). These are oocyst-forming protozoa that parasitize the bowel of mammals. Oocysts from feces are immediately infective (sporulated). There are ~10 species, including *C. canis*, *C. felis*, and *C. muris* from name-telling hosts, *C. parvum* (ex-genotype 2) from bovines and humans, and *C. hominis* (ex-*C. parvum* genotype 1) from humans. Oocysts withstand cold or freezing; in water, inactivation requires heat (64–72°C for 1–2 min) or high levels of free chlorine. SPREAD: is via (i) tap water or (less commonly) foods, (ii) contact with cases, (iii) contact with animals, (iv) swallowing of water from swimming pools or recreational lakes. RISKS: drinking tap water or raw milk, swimming in polluted pools or freshwater, visits to farms and contact with farm animals (cattle and calves), contact with a diarrhea case in the household, changing diapers of a child with diarrhea, international travel, and summer and fall transmission season. Shedding continues for up to 15 days after resolution of diarrhea. The infective $dose_{50}$ for immune-competent persons is ~10 oocysts. CLINICAL INFORMATION: The prepatent period (in animals) is 5½ days (*C. parvum*) to 9 days (*C. hominis*). The incubation period is 2–28 (typically 6–10) days. Manifestations: include self-limited diarrhea, abdominal cramps, nausea, and fever (in 40%) in immune-competent hosts, and persisting or life-threatening diarrhea in immune-impaired hosts. In the United States, >50% of cases are non-HIV-infected persons. Confirmation is by microscopy of stained stools, fecal antigen test, and possibly nucleic acid amplification test. In hospitalized children with chronic diarrhea, attributable lethality can reach ~6%. IMPACT: Infection prevalences are 1–3% in high-income countries, and 3–10% in low-income countries. Yield from stools in low-income countries is 1.5–8.5% (healthy children) to 2.5–25% (children with diarrhea).

In high-income countries, disease rates, by geography, age, season, and reporting are $1-24/10^5$ per year (low in the United States in 1998–2002). In low-income countries, infection is acquired early in life, after age one year. In a periurban community of Peru, the infection rate in children was 2–40/100 child-years and 0–40% of infections were associated with diarrhea. OUTBREAKS: Outbreaks have been reported from drinking water, foods, and swimming pools. In the United States, only 7–14% of cases are outbreak related.

CYCLOSPORA (Alveolata: Eucoccidiorida). *Cyclospora* is a genus with >10 species of oocyst-forming protozoa.

C. cayetanensis (597, 1232, 3285, 3354, 3359, 4506, 7124, 7880) circulates worldwide, in humans, sewage, drinking water, and foods. Oocysts are not infective when shed (encased sporocysts need to evolve to sporozoites). In the environment, sporulation takes days to weeks; it is slowed by 4°C, and arrested by freeze (−20°C for 24 h) or heat (60°C for 1 h). SPREAD: is via tap water or foods. By immune vigor, shedding ceases with resolution of diarrhea, or persists for >1 month. RISKS: unsafe water and foods, international travel, hand contact with soil, high-transmission season. CLINICAL INFORMATION: In low-income countries, 70–90% of infections in children are inapparent. The incubation period is 1–13 (typically 7–8) days. Manifestations: self-limited diarrhea, in immune-impaired hosts chronic or severe diarrhea, fatigue, and fever. Confirmation is by microscopy of stained stool specimens, or nucleic acid amplification test from foods. A treatment option is cotrimoxazole. IMPACT: Enteric infections are prevalent in <0.5% of people in high-income countries, and 0.5–30% (often 1–3%) in low-income countries. In the United States in 1997-2002, surveillance suggested a downward trend to rates of $0.1-0.4/10^5$ per year. In low-income countries, infection rates in children reach 0.1–0.3 per child-year. OUTBREAKS: Reported vehicles include drinking water, raspberries, fresh basil, and mesclun lettuce.

CYTOMEGALOVIRUS (CMV) (1822, 2611, 5109, 6641, 7106, 8272, 8332) (enveloped DNA viruses: β-*Herpesviridae*). CMV circulates worldwide in humans; reservoirs are latently infected neonates, children, and adults. Infections persist for life. SPREAD: Infections are reactivated or acquired via (i) body contact, sex, and mother-to-child (intrauterine, breastmilk), (ii) transfusion and transplant, (iii) objects. RISKS: CMV is shed in saliva, urine, semen, vaginal secretions, and breastmilk. CMV can be present in periodontitis lesions, blood (viremia), tissues, and organs. Infected neonates can shed CMV intermittently for up to 6 years. A major source of CMV in households are children in day care. Neonates and immune-impaired hosts are susceptible. CLINICAL INFORMATION: In children, more than three fourths of infections are inapparent. The incubation period is ~4–10 (often 6) weeks (perinatal), 3–12 weeks (by transfusion), and 1–4 months (by transplant). Manifestations: vary by immune vigor and include malaise, fever (mononucleosis-like), transaminitis, pneumonitis, retinitis, colitis, and congenital disease. Confirmation is by nucleic acid amplification test, antigen test, serology (immunoglobulin M, rise in 2–6 weeks after infection) or culture; diagnostic materials include urine, saliva, and blood. IMPACT: Infections are frequently acquired early in life. Seroprevalence increases with age, to reach 50–90% in adults. Seroconversion rates are 2–26% per year, among U.S. sexually active female adolescents 14/100 person-years. OUTBREAKS: Outside human immunodeficiency virus-infected communities. Outbreaks have been poorly documented.

DELTARETROVIRUS (enveloped RNA viruses: *Retroviridae*). The genus includes human T-lymphotropic virus (HTLV) and simian T-lymphotropic viruses.

HTLV1, 2 (3833, 5912, 7525) HTLV circulates in humans. SPREAD: is mother-to-child and by sex and transfusion. CLINICAL INFORMATION: Many infections are inapparent. However, "silent" seroreactivities reported in the past may represent cross-reactivities, including with *Plasmodium* and helminths. HTLV1 coinfections with human immunodeficiency virus, hepatitis C virus, and *Strongyloides* have been reported. The incubation period is months to years. Manifestations: HTLV1 causes adult T-cell (CD41) leukemia, tropical spastic paraparesis, and perhaps other inflammatory diseases. HTLV2 is a cause of T-cell (CD81) leukemia. IMPACT: The lifetime risk of leukemia in HTLV1-infected persons is 1–5%. By age, sex, ethnicity, and geography, seroprevalence is ~1–17% in endemic areas of Africa, Asia, and Latin America, and 0.1–3% in North America and West Europe.

DENGUE VIRUS (DENV). See Flavivirus.

DICROCOELIUM (Trematoda: Digenea).
D. dendriticum (5116, 5472, 5656) is a biliary fluke that occurs worldwide, in domestic and wild ruminants (final hosts, shed eggs), terrestrial snails (first intermediate hosts, >90 species), and ants (second hosts, *Formica* spp.). SPREAD: is via uptake of metacercariae with ants paralyzed on grass shafts. In contrast, eating eggs with liver from infected final hosts results in innocuous egg passage (pseudoinfection). Confirmation is by visualizing operculate eggs in stools (transiently in pseudoinfection and persistently in true infection). IMPACT: True dicrocoeliasis in humans is rare. In villagers in the Red River delta of Vietnam, the fecal prevalence was 0.1% (1/721).

DIENTAMOEBA (Euglenozoa: Trichomonadida).

D. fragilis (2759, 5476, 8215, 8216) is a "flagellate without flagellum," and it lacks a cyst stage. *D. fragilis* circulates in tropical and temperate climates, in humans who shed trophozoites with feces. **SPREAD:** is via hands and body contact. A proposed vehicle are eggs of *Enterobius*. **RISKS:** life in closed communities or institutions and international travel. **CLINICAL INFORMATION:** Prepatent and incubation periods are not known. From 10% to 85% of infections are inapparent. Manifestations: abdominal pain, diarrhea, eosinophilia (in 5–30%). Confirmation is by visualizing trophozoites in stained stools (preferably >1 specimen, or by culture. **IMPACT:** Diagnostic yield is 1–10% (often 2–4%).

DIPHYLLOBOTHRIUM (1923, 2084, 5564, 6570, 6767, 7408) (Cestoda: Pseudophyllidea). These cestodes include freshwater species (e.g., *D. latum* and *D. dendriticum*) and marine species (e.g., *D. pacificum*). Cycles exist in the Old and New Worlds, in fish-eating mammals and humans (final hosts, shed proglottids but mainly eggs in feces), krill (first intermediate hosts), and fish (second hosts, harbor infective plerocercoid larvae). The life span of adults is 5–15 years. Heat (56°C for 5 min) or freezing (−18°C for 24 h) kills larvae, likely also salting. **SPREAD:** is by ingestion of viable larvae from poorly cooked or raw fish. **CLINICAL INFORMATION:** Many infections are inapparent. The prepatent period is 3 weeks. The reported incubation period is 1 week to 6 months. Manifestations: are poorly defined and may include flatulence, diarrhea, and abdominal discomfort. A frequently quoted but rarely substantiated complication is malabsorption of vitamin B12. Confirmation is by visualizing operculate eggs in stool samples from exposed persons. A treatment option is praziquantel. **IMPACT:** Infections are sporadic in Asia, North and South America (Argentina, Brazil, Chile, and Peru), and Europe. In Europe, ~500 infections are diagnosed per year, mainly in Balticum and Scandinavia. In São Paulo, the diagnostic yield in people who reported raw fish as a diet was 0.5% (13/2,505). **OUTBREAKS:** Family clusters and household outbreaks have been reported. In the Lake Como area, Italy, in 1999, six cases were reported in four months. In the United States in 1980, salmon was the vehicle for an outbreak with >30 infections.

DIPYLIDIUM (Cestoda: Cyclophyllidea).
D. caninum (5130) circulates worldwide, in neglected dogs and cats, and their fleas. **SPREAD:** is by incidentally ingesting infective fleas. Manifestations: diarrhea. **IMPACT:** Rare.

DIROFILARIA (Nematoda: Spirurida). These filarial worms circulate in mosquitoes and mammals. There are >25 species. Of these, *D. immitis* and *D. repens* have been identified in humans who are dead-end hosts. Serosurveys in enzootic areas suggest infection prevalence of 3–21%. In Spain, the rate of pulmonary dirofilariasis is ~4/10^5 per year.
D. immitis (1054, 5197, 6069) circulates in warm climates worldwide, in mosquitoes, dogs, and other canids. Worms in the pulmonary artery release microfilariae into blood of host mammals. **SPREAD:** is by mosquito bite. Manifestations: pulmonary nodules (coins), rarely genital nodules. Diagnosis is by biopsy or wait-and-see strategy (to avoid lung biopsy). **IMPACT:** Sporadic. Reported cases are ~100 in the United States, >20 in Japan, and >10 in Europe.
D. repens (1054, 5702, 6069) circulates in the Old World, in mosquitoes, dogs, cats, and wild carnivores. Worms in the subcutis release microfilariae into blood of host mammals. **SPREAD:** is by mosquito bite. Manifestations: subcutaneous, ocular, or genital nodules, rarely pulmonary nodules. Diagnosis is by biopsy. **IMPACT:** Sporadic. Reported cases are ~800 in Europe, Central Asia, and Sri Lanka. In Europe, autochthonous cases occurred in Italy (two thirds), France (one fourth, mainly Corsica), Greece, and Spain.

DRACUNCULUS (Nematoda: Spirurida). These filaria-like worms parasitize snakes and mammals. Of about a dozen species, only *D. medinensis* (Guinea worm) (1028, 8122) is infective to humans. This species circulates in sub-Saharan Africa, in humans (final host, release larvae into water from broken skin), and tiny freshwater crustaceans (intermediate hosts, e.g., *Metacyclops*). **SPREAD:** is by drinking polluted water from shallow sources. **CLINICAL INFORMATION:** The prepatent and incubation periods are 10–14 months. Manifestations (dracunculiasis): a soft tissue lesion (on the leg in >85%) through which female parts emerge and release larvae, pain, and superinfection. **IMPACT:** Preeradication, there were ~3.5 million cases in 20 countries. An eradication program was launched in 1980 that advocated safe drinking water (cloth filtering or boiling), secured sites (e.g., borehole wells), and monthly temephos applications (against crustaceans). By 2004, disease was eliminated in Asia (India, Pakistan, Uzbekistan, and Yemen) and confined in Africa to 11 countries (nine in West Africa, Ethiopia, and Sudan). Of 16,026 cases reported in 2004, ~45% each were from Ghana (7,275) and Sudan (7,266). **OUTBREAKS:** Community outbreaks have occurred.

EASTERN EQUINE ENCEPHALOMYELITIS VIRUS (EEEV). *See* Alphavirus.

EBOLAVIRUS (EBOV). *See* Filovirus.

ECHINOCOCCUS (Cestoda: Cyclophyllidea: Taeniidae). Larvae from four species can infect humans: monocystic

E. granulosus and polycystic *E. multilocularis*, rarely *E. oligarthrus* and *E. vogeli*.

E. granulosus (2119, 2187, 3902, 4223, 4628, 6140, 7454, 7510). At least eight genotypes ("G") are recognized: G1 ("sheep" strain) on all continents, in dogs and other canids (final hosts), and sheep, cattle, goat, pig, camel, and macropods (intermediate hosts); G5 ("cattle" strain) in dogs and bovids; G7 ("pig" strain) in dogs and pigs; G4 ("horse" strain) in dogs and horses; G6 ("camel" strain) in dogs and camels and bovids; and G8 ("Nordic" or "cervid" strain) in wolf, dog, and reindeer. Final canid hosts harbor adults in intestine and shed eggs with feces. Eggs survive at 7°C for >6 months, at 21°C for >7 weeks, and at 40°C for a few hours. **SPREAD:** is by ingestion of eggs, presumably from (i) fur of final hosts, (ii) polluted soil, (iii) fruits, vegetables, or cross-contaminated foods (hands, utensils, pests, and flies), (iv) tap water. Inhalation of egg-ladden dust is a possible mode. **RISKS:** dog ownership, dog feces in or around premises, dogs that lick kitchen utensils, children who play with dogs, farming, home slaughter, handling offal, feeding offal to dogs, and a history of past infection. **CLINICAL INFORMATION:** Many (up to 40%) infections are inapparent for years. The presumed incubation period is 2–5 years. Manifestations (cystic echinococcosis), by cyst size (≤7.5 cm in ~90%) and site (55–90% in liver, and 10–30% in lung) include abdominal pain, allergy (ruptured cyst from trauma), and space-occupying lesion. Confirmation is by imaging, serology, surgery, and histology; nucleic acid amplification test is being developed. Cysts may regress spontaneously. Treatment options include albendazole or mebendazole. **IMPACT:** There are ~2–3 million infections worldwide. By imaging or serology, infection prevalence in enzootic areas is 0.1–10% (often 1–3%). By surgery or case reports, disease rates are 0.5–10/10^5 per year, focally (South America, East Africa, central People's Republic of China, southern, central, and eastern Europe) 20–80/10^5 per year.

E. multilocularis (460, 1887, 2119, 2869, 3901, 5488, 6142, 7947) circulates in the Northern Hemisphere, in foxes (final sylvatic host), occasionally dogs and cats (final synanthropic host) that shed infective eggs with feces, and rodents (intermediate hosts). Eggs survive at −18°C for months, at −80°C for 4 days. **SPREAD:** is by ingestion of eggs, presumably from (i) fur, (ii) soil, (iii) fecally polluted wild berries, mushrooms, or fallen fruits. **RISKS:** farmhouse domicile, farm and forest work, outdoor activities, vegetables from private gardens, eating unwashed wild berries, chewing grass, ownership of free-roaming dogs or cats, and dog or cat contacts. Proglottids are occasionally demonstrated in the perianal region of dogs, and dogs can roll in fox feces. In Tibet, fenced pastures likely increased infection risks for pastoralists. **CLINICAL INFORMATION:** Some infections are inapparent. From pediatric cases, the incubation period is estimated at 5–15 years. Commensurate with the site (liver in >90%), manifestations (alveolar echinococcosis) include abdominal pain, hepatomegaly, and jaundice. Confirmation is by imaging, serology, surgery, and histopathology. Some infections seem self-limited, but, in general, growth is relentlessly progressive, cancerlike. Untreated lethality is >90%, with medical treatment and surgery, 10-year survival is 80%. **IMPACT:** There are ~0.1–0.3 million infections worldwide. Prevalence in enzootic areas ranges from 0.001–0.5% (western Europe) to 5–15% (boreal Eurasia). Disease rates per 10^5 per year are 0.02–1 (western Europe) to 100–200 (boreal Eurasia). Foxes have brought *E. multilocularis* into some urban areas. Programs have controlled transmission on some islands (Cyprus, Iceland, Alaskan St. Lawrence, and Tasmania).

ECHINOSTOMA (Trematoda: Digenea) (1288, 2884, 8356). These flukes circulate in Asia, in birds, mammals, and humans (final hosts, shed eggs with feces), freshwater snails (first intermediate hosts), and molluscs, crustaceans, and freshwater fish (second hosts). Over a dozen species can infect humans, notably *E. ilocanum* and *E. malayanum*. **SPREAD:** is by uptake of viable metacercariae from second hosts. **CLINICAL INFORMATION:** The prepatent period is ~3 weeks. From infection in a volunteer, the incubation period is 10 days. Adults locate in the small bowel. Manifestations: abdominal cramps, and watery diarrhea. Confirmation is by visualizing operculate eggs in stool (look *Fasciola*-like). **IMPACT:** In enzootic-endemic areas infection prevalence reported is 2–50%.

ECHOVIRUS. *See* Enterovirus.

EHRLICHIA (α-*Proteobacteria*: *Rickettsiales*) (2067). These are intracellular ancestral bacteria of repeatedly changed taxonomy. Check *Coxiella*, *Anaplasma*, *Orientia*, or *Rickettsia* as well.

E. canis (851) is closely related to if not synonymous with *E. chaffeensis*. As its species name suggests, the agent circulates in dogs and dog ticks (*Rhipicephalus sanguineus*) worldwide.

E. chaffeensis (1872, 2068, 7108, 7182, 8297) is closely related to if not synonymous with *Cowdria ruminantium*. *E. chaffeensis* circulates in North America, and perhaps elsewhere, in deer and ticks that carry the agent to humans. **SPREAD:** is via tick bite. **RISKS:** 80–90% of cases recall recent tick exposure. Males account for two thirds of cases. *Ehrlichia* can survive in blood components for 11–14 days. **CLINICAL INFORMATION:** Over 90% of infections are inapparent. The incubation period is 1–21 (often 7–10) days. *E. chaffeensis* invades monocytes. Manifestations (human monocytic ehrlichiosis): flulike illness, also vomiting, diarrhea, cough, and septic shock. Reported lethality is ~3%. Confirmation is by PCR and microscopy of blood smear. IMPACT: Reported seroprevalence is 0.1–0.5%, in pockets >10%. However, serosurveys are likely confounded by cross-reactivities within Rickettsiales. In the United States, there were 742 reported cases counted in 1986–1997 seasons, 487 in 1997–2001, and 358 in 2001–2002. Sporadic infections are reported in Latin America and Europe. Disease rates range broadly by age and area, for a national United States average of ∼0.06 per 10^5 per year in 2001–2002.

E. ewingii (1872, 7182, 8298) circulates in North America, in deer, canids, and ticks. Unlike *E. chaffeensis*, *E. ewingii* invades neutrophils. In the United States, few cases were reported in the 1999–2000 season, and <30 cases in 2001–2002.

EIKENELLA (5770, 7972) (β-*Proteobacteria*: *Neisseriales*). *Eikenella* is a genus of gram-negative rods. *E. corrodens* is part of the human oral, enteric, and genital flora. SPREAD: Infections are endogenous or acquired via human bites. Manifestations: periodontitis, bite-wound infection, abscess, and endocarditis.

ENCEPHALITOZOON. See *Microsporidia*.

ENDOGENOUS VIRUSES. Endogenous viruses are incomplete viruses (proviruses) (150, 3254, 6572). They are integrated into the genome and neither leave nor enter cells for replication. They are considered relicts ("fossil DNA") of ancient germ-cell infections. Taxonomy is unresolved. Examples are Baboon endogenous virus, endogenous feline leukemia viruses, porcine endogenous retrovirus (PERV), and human endogenous retroviruses. Although seemingly innocuous for humans, PERV is scrutinized in xenotransplants.

ENTAMOEBA (1469) (Ameboza, unclear taxonomy). *Entamoeba* has ≥15 species, including pathogenic *E. histolytica* (cysts with four nuclei), opportunistic *E. gingivalis* (no cysts), and commensals with 8-nucleated cysts (*E. coli*) or 4-nucleated cysts (*E. dispar*, *E. hartmanni*, and *E. moshkovskii*). *E. histolytica* cysts and trophozoites are morphologically indistinguishable from *E. dispar* and *E. moshkovskii*, whereas *E. hartmanni* is smaller.

E. gingivalis (4555) colonizes the human buccal mucosa. Diagnosis is by microscopy of mouth wash. *E. gingivalis* is a cause of gingivitis and periodontal disease ("oral amebiasis"), mainly in human immunodeficiency virus-infected persons.

E. histolytica (471, 560, 703, 2662, 2831, 4482, 6279, 7114) circulates mainly in warmer climates in sewage, water, and foods and in humans who harbor trophozoites in colon and shed cysts in feces. Cysts are inactivated by heat (>55°C). SPREAD: is by uptake of viable cysts via tap water, foods, hands in contact with patients, anal sex, rarely nosocomially. RISKS: residence in or travel to endemic areas, untreated tap water, raw or handled foods, crowded housing, sex among men, and presence of *Giardia*. Chlorinated drinking water and washing hands before eating decrease risks. CLINICAL INFORMATION: About 80–90% infections are inapparent. Males might be carriers more often than females. Of carriers, 5–20% develop disease in 2–24 months. The incubation period is days to years, often 3 weeks. Manifestations: of invasive disease include colitis (dysentery) and amebic liver abscess (ALA). In ALA, male:female ratios are 1:1 in infants, but 4–9:1 in adults. Confirmation is by visualizing hematophagous forms in fresh stool or colonic fluid, serology, imaging, fine-needle aspiration, and nucleic acid amplification test (NAT) (cysts in stool). ALA is an emergency; lethality of treated ALA is 1–3%. Treatment options include nitroimidazoles and luminal cysticidals (e.g., diloxanide furoate). IMPACT: By age and geography, fecal prevalences of *E. histolytica/dispar* are 1–50% in low-income countries and 0–4% in high-income countries. By setting and case mix, *E. dispar*-to-*E. histolytica* ratios are 10:1 to 0.5:1, often ∼3:1. By *E. histolytica*-specific methods, the prevalence in low-income countries is 1–15%, and perhaps 1% worldwide. Invasive disease causes ∼50 million cases per year and 0.1 million deaths per year. In Vietnam, the rate of ALA is ∼20/10^5 per year. Seroprevalence that reflects past invasive disease is 7–8%. OUTBREAKS: Outbreaks are reported from drinking water, on farms, in households, urban homosexual communities, rural communities, tourists, a chiropractic clinic, and institutions.

E. moshkovskii (145) is a free-living ameba of worldwide occurrence in wet soils, lake, and river sediments, tidal pools, brackish coastal waters, and sewage. In Bangladesh, by NAT on stools, 21% of 109 preschool children tested positive for *E. moshkovskii* (16% for *E. histolytica* and 36% for *E. dispar*). Modes of spread are unknown.

ENTEROBACTER (γ-*Proteobacteria*: *Enterobacteriales*). These gram-negative rods circulate in the bowel of vertebrates, in sewage, soil, water, and plants. There are >10 species.

E. cloacae (2827, 3283, 3832, 4464, 7320, 7550, 8357) is an opportunist that frequently colonizes the human bowel, including of babies. SPREAD: Infections are endogenous or acquired via hands, body contacts, or contaminated solutions or instruments. RISKS: invasive procedures, indwelling devices, assisted ventilation, crowding of colonized patients, and soiled hands of health workers. CLINICAL INFORMATION: An incubation period is not known. Manifestations: wound infection, urinary tract infection (UTI), bloodstream infection (BSI), and invasive disease, in particular, in neonates. By age and comorbidity, lethality of invasive disease is 7–80% (often 33%). IMPACT: *Enterobacter* accounts for ∼5% of nosocomial UTI, ∼10% of nosopneumonias, 6–7% of surgical site infections, and ~5% of BSI. The rate of *Enterobacter* BSI in neonates is 0.5/1,000 live births. **OUTBREAKS:** Most outbreaks have occurred in neonatal intensive care unit.

E. sakazakii (yellow-pigmented *E. cloacae*) (3807, 4184, 7698) is widespread in the home and food industry environments. It is a cause of sporadic and epidemic illness in neonates.

ENTEROBIUS (Nematoda: Oxyurida).

E. (=Oxyuris) vermicularis (47, 1325, 4492, 7030, 7253) occurs worldwide in humans who shed eggs perianally. Life span of adults is 1½–3½ months. **SPREAD:** is by uptake of eggs via hands, fingernails, or objects taken into the mouth, or via inhalation of egg-ladden dust, perhaps via foods. Modes allow for auto- and household-reinfections. **RISKS:** crowding and poor personal hygiene. **CLINICAL INFORMATION:** The prepatent period is ~1 month. Confirmation is by visualizing eggs on anal Scotch tapes (ideally 1–3 obtained early in the morning). Most (80%) to few (10%) infections are inapparent. A typical burden is 20 worms per person. The incubation period is 2 days to 4 weeks. Manifestations: perianal itch, vulvovaginitis, in females also cystitis. The role of *E. vermicularis* in appendicitis and enuresis is uncertain. Treatment options include benzimidazoles and pyrantel pamoate. **IMPACT:** By age, setting, and test, prevalence in children is 1–60% (often 5–20%). **OUTBREAKS:** Control in schools or institutions is achieved through simultaneous treatment of classes, households, or departments.

ENTEROCOCCUS (616, 1275, 1986, 2604, 2757, 8178) (*Firmicutes*: *Lactobacillales*) These gram-positive cocci occur worldwide, in (in)vertebrates, sewage, soil, water, plants, and foods. Of 12–19 species, *E. faecalis* and *E. faecium* colonize humans, contributing substantially to enteric flora and bowel biomass (up to 10^8 CFU/g). *Enterococcus* is resilient, surviving heat (60°C for 30 min), salinity (6.5% NaCl), and acidic pH, and it is intrinsically resistant to antimicrobials, including β-lactams. Vancomycin-resistant *Enterococcus* (VRE) was reported in 1988 (7669). **SPREAD:** Infections can be endogenous but are more often acquired, via hands, skin contact, animal contact, foods, objects, or from the environment. About 90% of VRE are acquired nosocomially. Hands of health workers can spread VRE. Likely reservoirs for VRE are humans, hospitals (mainly in the United States), and livestock (mainly in Europe). Food is an emerging, worrisome vehicle of VRE. **RISKS:** invasive procedures, stay in intensive care unit, long hospital stay, interfacility transfers, recent use of antimicrobials that facilitate overgrowth. **CLINICAL INFORMATION:** Clinical and exposure data are needed to distinguish colonization, infection, and disease. The incubation period is not known, but a typical time to becoming newly colonized is 5 days. Manifestations: nosocomial infections, e.g., of urinary tract, surgical sites, or bloodstream, also peritonitis and endocarditis. The role of *Enterococcus* in food poisoning is not clear. By syndrome, lethality in the hospital is 10–50% (often 15%). **IMPACT:** Main impact is in hospitals (see section VI). **OUTBREAKS:** With VRE as marker, outbreaks have been detected in hospitals. In Europe, VRE also circulates in the community, likely promoted by avoparcin as a growth promoter in food mammals.

ENTEROCYTOZOON. See *Microsporidia*.

ENTEROVIRUS (EV) (3462) (unenveloped RNA viruses: *Picornaviridae*). *Enterovirus* includes ≥68 cosmopolitan serotypes: 29 of coxsackievirus (A1–22, A24, B1–6), 31 of echovirus (1–7, 9, 11–27, 29–34), 4 of enterovirus (EV 68–71), hepatitis A virus (identical with EV72, see *Hepatovirus*), poliovirus (3), and swine vesicular disease virus (evolved from coxsackievirus B). EVs are resistant to ethanol but sensitive to free chlorine. Infections are confirmed by virus isolation, nucleic acid amplification test, or serology (immunoglobulin M, conversion, increased titer in paired sera).

Coxsackie-, echo-, and enterovirus (605, 1186, 1378, 2943, 3470, 3651, 3958, 4432, 5548, 5832, 6350, 7798) circulate worldwide, in humans, their droplets and feces, and in water. However, surveillance in Finland over 20 years showed different serotypes in clinical materials and sewage samples. Prevailing serotypes vary over time and by geography. Molecular evidence suggests that rapid global spread is possible. In the United States in 2000–2001, among 1,862 typed nonpolio isolates, frequent serotypes were EV18 (22%) and EV13 (21%). In Australia in 1991–2000, of 11,275 isolates, 68% were not typed, while frequent types were echoviruses (22%) and coxsackie B viruses (6%). In the United Kingdom in 1975–1994, of 40,366 typed isolates, frequent serotypes were EV11 (12%), EV22 (8%) and coxsackie B4 virus (7%). **SPREAD:** is via hands, droplets, and fecally polluted water, mainly in the community, but also in hospitals. **RISKS:** EVs are shed in feces for 5–6 weeks. In temperate climates, transmission is seasonal. Handwashing is protective. **CLINICAL INFORMATION:** A majority of infections is inapparent or mild. The incubation period is 2–7 days. Manifestations: are diverse, variable by age and serotype, and can be mucocutaneous (conjunctivitis, herpangina, hand-foot-and-mouth disease), respiratory (bronchiolitis and pleurodynia), systemic (mononucleosis-like illness and viremia with rash), neurological (aseptic meningitis and acute flaccid paralysis), and enteric (diarrhea and perhaps diabetogenic "islanditis"). **IMPACT:** Impact has been inadequately documented. Seroprevalence increases with age. By serotype and epidemic occurrence, 50% of school children and almost 100% of adults can be reactive. In summer, EVs are recovered from 25–50% of infants hospitalized for fever. Reported EV hospitalization rates in infants and children are 0.3–1.40/1,000 per year. OUTBREAKS: Numerous community outbreaks are reported in the Americas, Australasia, and Europe. In Cuba in 2000, echovirus 16 caused 16,943 cases of aseptic meningitis. In New Zealand in 2000, echovirus 33 caused 75 cases of aseptic meningitis or encephalitis, for a rate of $2.6/10^5$. In Taiwan in 1998, EV71 caused 129,106 cases, mainly hand-foot-and-mouth disease and herpangina; in hospitalized children, lethality was 8–31%. In Okinawa in 1994, EV70 caused 7,509 cases of hemorrhagic conjunctivitis. In Gran Canaria, Spain, in 2000 echovirus 13 caused 152 meningitis cases; age of patients ranged from 1 month to 29 years (mean, 5–6 years), and the male:female ratio was 2:1. In Romania in 1999, multiple serotypes caused 4,734 cases of aseptic meningitis.

Poliomyelitis virus (PolioV1-3) (356, 4009, 4030, 5097, 5758, 6013, 6014) circulates in humans, droplets, feces, sewage, and water. SPREAD: is by ingestion, via hands, saliva, droplets from contacts, or polluted tap water. Humans shed virus in respiratory secretions for ≤1 week, and in feces for up to 4–6 weeks (in immune-impaired hosts for months). In theory (R_0), a case could infect five or seven other persons. RISKS: not being vaccinated, having a case in the household, large sibship, and unsafe tap water. Pregnancy and injections in the month before disease onset increase susceptibility. CLINICAL INFORMATION: Of infections 95–99% are inapparent. The incubation period is 2–35 (typically 12) days. Manifestations: fever, aseptic meningitis, flaccid paralysis. By outbreak setting and immunity, lethality is 0.5–11.5%. IMPACT: In the 1980s, polio was endemic in >125 countries, and there were >350,000 cases per year. In 1988, the World Health Assembly resolved to eradicate polio. WHO regions now certified polio-free are the Americas (since 1994), the West Pacific (since 2000), and Europe (since 2002). "Pockets" remain in West, East, and North Africa and Central Asia (Afghanistan, Bangladesh, India, and Pakistan). OUTBREAKS: In 1976–1995, 48 outbreaks caused ~17,000 cases, for a median attack rate of $4/10^5$. In India in 1999, PolioV3 caused 730 confirmed cases. In Albania in 1996, after >10 years of absence, PolioV1 caused 138 cases and 16 (12%) deaths, for an attack rate of $10/10^5$ at age 19–25 years; cases also appeared in Greece and Kosovo, demonstrating potential for rapid spread. Inactivated (IPV) and oral (OPV) vaccines are effective and well tolerated. When in the late 1990s rare OPV-associated paralytic polio began to outweigh risks from wild polio, IPV was recommended to replace OPV primary series in infants. Obstacles to eradication include noncompliance with vaccine programs, and attenuated strains that acquire virulence, first observed in an outbreak in Hispaniola in 2000–2001.

Swine vesicular disease virus (SVDV) (4426) circulates in pigs. Rare human infections occur by contact with swine, from skin abrasions.

EPIDERMOPHYTON (*Ascomycota*: *Onygales*). *E. floccosum* (3557) is a hyaline, keratophilic, anthropophilic mold. Reservoirs are carriers. SPREAD: is poorly known but likely via contact with skin or contaminated surfaces, e.g., saunas. Manifestations: tinea corporis, tinea cruris, occasionally tinea pedis, onychomycosis.

EPSTEIN-BARR VIRUS (EBV OR HUMAN HERPES VIRUS 4). See Lymphocryptovirus.

ERYSIPELOTHRIX (*Firmicutes*: *Anaeroplasmatales*). *E. rhusiopathiae* (897, 7946) is a gram-positive rod that circulates in vertebrates (fish, birds, mammals), their carcasses (at slaughterhouse environments), waste, soil, and fresh and marine waters. SPREAD: is via contact or injury with animals, their products, or waste. RISKS: occupational (e.g., butchers and seafood packers). CLINICAL INFORMATION: The incubation period is 2–7 days. Manifestations: demarcated (erysipeloid) or diffuse skin infection, concomitant or primary sepsis. Lethality of invasive disease is ~40%.

ERYTHROVIRUS (unenveloped DNA viruses: *Parvoviridae*). Prototype is parvovirus B19 (PVB19) (2828, 3369, 5507, 6780, 7494, 8351, 8361). PVB19 circulates in humans worldwide. The virus has an affinity for erythroid precursor cells.

PVB19 resists alcohol and detergents. SPREAD: is via droplets and respiratory secretions, or vertically, rarely via blood products and transplants. PVB19 is shed from incubation to appearance of a rash, for ~1 week in aplastic crisis, and indefinitely in immune-impaired hosts. Infectivity seems moderate, but primary and secondary attack rates of >40% have been reported. RISKS: include children in the household, work with children, and spring and early summer season. CLINICAL INFORMATION: At least 25–50% of infections are inapparent. The incubation period is 4–28 (typically 12–14) days. Manifestations: include rash (in 75–95%, erythema infectiosum, slapped cheek, or fifth disease), fever (in 10%), arthropathy, aplastic crisis (mainly in sickle-cell anemia), chronic aplastic anemia, spontaneous abortion, and fetal hydrops. Viremia lasts 11–53 (typically 18) days. Confirmation is by serology (conversion, immunoglobulin M [IgM], high IgG) or nucleic acid amplification test. IMPACT: In countries that approach measles elimination, erythema infectiosum has emerged as a cause of febrile rash in children. Seroprevalence in high-income countries increases with age, from 2–20% in children to 40–80% in adults and >85% in the elderly. In Dutch blood donors, the infection rate was ~0.6% (95% confidence interval [CI] 0.2–0.7%)

per year. OUTBREAKS: Epidemic waves can go through communities every 4–5 years. Venues for outbreaks include kindergarten, elementary and secondary schools, and hospitals.

ESCHERICHIA (γ-*Proteobacteria*, *Enterobacteriales*). Prototype of these gram-negative rods is *E. coli* (1663, 2486, 2984, 6339).

E. coli occurs worldwide, in birds, mammals, and humans, in feces, sewage, soil, foods, and water. Somatic "O" antigens (>180) define serogroups, flagellar "H" antigens (>60) define serotypes, toxins and biology define uropathic and diarrheogenic biotypes: enteroaggregative *E. coli*, enterohemorrhagic *E. coli*, enteroinvasive *E. coli*, enteropathogenic *E. coli*, and enterotoxigenic *E. coli*. By genetic characteristics, *E. coli* is conspecific with *Shigella*.

E. coli is susceptible to plasmids that transfer antibiotic resistance. Up to one fourth of human isolates are resistant to β-lactam/anti-β-lactmase combinations. *E. coli* is killed by heat (70°C throughout meat for 2 min) or free chlorine. SPREAD: Infections can be endogenous, but most of uropathogenic and diarrheogenic types are acquired, via hand contacts (community and hospital), foods, or tap water. Manifestations: diarrhea, urinary tract and bloodstream infections. IMPACT: *E. coli* is a major cause of diarrhea (infants and travelers). The rate of *E. coli* O157 diarrhea in high-income countries is $\sim$2–3/10^5 per year. OUTBREAKS: Numerous food-borne and other outbreaks have been reported.

Enteroaggregative *E. coli* (EAEC) (50, 3508, 4374, 5576, 5666), e.g., of serogroups O7, O77, O126, O127, adheres to mucosa, in vitro to cells. Epidemiological knowledge is limited. Of healthy persons, 0–30% (typically 10%) are colonized. SPREAD: (feces-food) is likely via water (well, tap). RISKS: domicile in and visits to low-income countries, summer season. CLINICAL INFORMATION: The incubation period in volunteers is 8–18 h. Manifestations: watery, bloody (in up to one third), or persistent diarrhea, and malnutrition. IMPACT: EAEC is recovered from 2–10% of diarrhea cases in high-income countries and from 8–68% (typically 20%) in low-income countries. In periurban Santiago, Chile, the rate of EAEC diarrhea in children 0–47 months of age is 0.1–0.6 per child-year. In Germany, the rate of children in hospital with EAEC is $\sim$8/10^5 per year. OUTBREAKS: Venues included the community, schools, a conference center, a hotel, and a hospital nursery.

Enterohemorrhagic *E. coli* (EHEC) (280, 554, 1513, 2632, 3838, 5998, 7855, 8249), in particular serogroup O157, secretes shiga (vero) toxin. Cattle is a major reservoir. SPREAD: is via hand and skin contacts with animals and patients, and via polluted foods ("burger bug") and tap water, also via recreational waters. RISKS: bovine-derived and contaminated foods and drinks, farm work or visits, contact with cattle, pasture soil, and recreational waters, children in day care. The infectious dose is low (2–700 bacteria in outbreaks). Reconvalescent children shed EHEC in stool for 2 days to 2 months (typically 3 weeks). CLINICAL INFORMATION: Carriage is infrequent (in ≤1%). The incubation period is 1–14 (typically 3–4) days. Manifestations: watery or bloody (in 10–60%, "all blood, no stool") diarrhea, vomiting (in $\sim$50%), and hemolytic-uremic syndrome (HUS, in $\sim$1–10%). In the United States, the EHEC hospitalization rate is 30–40%. By diagnosis, lethality is 0.1–5% (typically 1%). Of HUS cases followed for ≥1 year, $\sim$12% have died or developed end-stage renal disease. IMPACT: In North America and West Europe, EHEC is identified in 0.3–4% of stool specimens. The disease rate rate is 1–10 (often 2)/10^5 and year. OUTBREAKS: In the 1980s–1990s, numerous outbreaks were reported in North America, Japan, Australia, and West Europe. In the United States in 1982–1994, of 69 outbreaks with 2,334 cases (34 per outbreak), 55% (38) were food-borne, 4% (3) were waterborne, 13% (9) were by interhuman contact, and for 28% (19) vehicles or modes of spread were unknown.

Enteroinvasive *E. coli* (EIEC) (2855, 4374, 5349, 5666) can invade the enteric mucosa. The main reservoir is humans. SPREAD: is via foods, tap water, and human contacts. Inapparent infections are unusual. CLINICAL INFORMATION: The incubation period is hours to 6 days. Manifestations: watery or febrile, dysentery-like diarrhea. All ages can be affected. IMPACT: EIEC are infrequent in high-income countries. Recovery from diarrheal stoosl is $\sim$1–3%. In periurban Santiago, Chile, EIEC diarrhea rate in children 0–47 months of age was 0.04–0.06 per child-year. OUTBREAKS: Few outbreaks have been reported.

Enteropathogenic *E. coli* (EPEC) (442, 4374, 5552, 7160, 7536) can adhere to mucosa, destructing microvilli. Reservoirs are cattle and humans (infants and nursing mothers). "Typical" strains (e.g., O55:H6, O86:H34, and O111:H2) carry "adherence factor plasmid" (EAF), while "atypical" strains (e.g., O26:H11, O55:H7) do not. Currently in high-income countries, only 10% of EPEC strains are EAF-positive. SPREAD: is via hands, weaning formula, other foods, or objects, possibly dust or aerosol. RISKS: domicile in and visits to low-income countries. EPEC is shed in stool for up to 2 weeks after reconvalescence. The infective dose in volunteers is high (10^8–10^{10} CFU), but presumably lower in infants. CLINICAL INFORMATION: The incubation period is 2–48 h. Manifestations: watery diarrhea, vomiting, and low-grade fever: Mainly infants and children are affected. Historical lethality was high (25–50%). IMPACT: EPEC is a major cause of diarrhea in infants of low-income countries of whom 2–20% (typically 5–10%) yield the agent. In periurban Santiago, Chile, the EPEC diarrhea rate in children 0–47 months of age is 0.02–0.3 per child-year.

OUTBREAKS: In the past, "typical" strains caused diarrhea outbreaks in infants. In a recent outbreak in Australia, EPEC was isolated from 19 (59%) of 32 infant patients, 14 strains were of a new serotype (O126:H12).

Enterotoxigenic *E. coli* (ETEC) (31, 49, 1722, 1739, 6255, 8092). Humans are the principal reservoir for ETEC. About 8% of healthy adults can be colonized. ETEC secretes heat-stable (ST) and heat-labile (LT) enterotoxins. LT is related to cholera toxin. SPREAD: is via foods and tap water. RISKS: Residence in and travel to low-income countries, warm weather. The infective dose in volunteers is high. ETEC is shed in the stool for <5 days. CLINICAL INFORMATION: In children in low-income countries, 70–80% of infections can be inapparent. The incubation period is 6 h to 3 (typically 1–2) days. Manifestations: watery or dehydrating (in ~5%) diarrhea, fever (in ~20%). Lethality in infants in low-income countries is ~0.2%. IMPACT: ETEC is a major cause of diarrhea in children and travelers. Recovery from diarrhea stools is 10–35%. In preschool children of low-income countries, the number of diarrhea episodes attributed to ETEC is ~210 million per year, for rates of 0.3–1 per child per year, or 0.1–0.6 per child-year. ETEC has been isolated in ~35% of short-term travelers with diarrhea. OUTBREAKS: In 1975–1995, 14 ETEC outbreaks were reported in the United States, and a further seven on cruise ships, causing 5,683 cases (150 per outbreak, excluding one waterborne outbreak with 2,666 cases).

EXOPHIALA (*Ascomycota: Chaetothyriales*). *E. jeanselmei* (90) is a pigmented mold that inhabits soil. It is a cause of black-grain eumycetoma.

FASCIOLA (Trematoda: Digenea). These flukes circulate in grazing mammals and freshwater snails. Mainly *F. hepatica* infects humans, while *F. gigantica* is occasionally reported from humans in tropical and subtropical parts of Africa and Asia, where enzootic areas overlap with *F. hepatica*.

F. *hepatica* (1459, 1689, 1723, 2241, 6501, 8339) was first illustrated by F. Redi (1627–1697) in his *Omne Vivum ex Ovo* (All Life from Life) in 1668, and named by C. Linné in 1758. By 1882, its strange life cycle was elucidated: from sheep and cattle (final hosts, shed eggs in feces) to freshwater snails (first intermediate hosts) and pasture plants (second hosts, with gluey metacercariae). *F. hepatica* is enzootic on all continents. In some foci, humans may contribute to the cycle. The life span of adults is ~5–10 years. SPREAD: is by ingestion of viable metacercariae with foods. RISKS: salad plants from pastures, canals, unfenced home gardens. CLINICAL INFORMATION: The prepatent is ~2–3 months. Adults locate in common bile duct. Inapparent infections exist. Confirmation is by visualizing operculate eggs in stool samples or duodenal fluid; concentration tests need to be repeated to detect irregular and low egg output ($\leq 1/g$ feces), and to exclude pseudoinfection (eggs from liver products). The incubation period is days (invasion) to $1\frac{1}{2}$–3 months (biliary phase). Manifestations: abdominal pain, fever, and eosinophilia (invasion), pain, jaundice, and elevated alkaline phosphatase (biliary phase). Dystopic immatures can cause focal neurological or other signs. A treatment option is triclabendazole. IMPACT: In >60 countries there are ≥ 2.5 million infected people (and >600 million infected livestock). Prevalence is <0.001–3% in high-income countries, and ~2–20% in low-income countries. Around Lake Titicaca at 3,800–4,100 m altitude in Bolivia and Peru, reported prevalence is 15–24%; curiously, waters of the lake itself appear to be free from lymnaeid snails. In the Nile delta of Egypt, reported prevalence is 1–25%. OUTBREAKS: Outbreaks can occur after floods or from common meals.

FASCIOLOPSIS (Trematoda: Digenea).

F. *buski* (1818, 2885) circulates focally in East and Southeast Asia, in mammals (e.g., pigs, bovids, and horses) and humans (final hosts, shed eggs in feces), freshwater snails (first intermediate hosts), and aquatic plants (second hosts, with gluey metacercariae). SPREAD: is via ingestion of viable metacercariae from plants that grow or float in raw surface waters; handling such plants can cross-contaminate other foods. CLINICAL INFORMATION: The prepatent period is 9–13 weeks. Adults locate in the duodenum. Light infections are inapparent. Confirmation: see *F. hepatica* (above). Manifestations: epigastric pain, diarrhea, eosinophilia. IMPACT: Fecal prevalence in endemic areas is 1–70%. In People's Republic of China in the 1990s, there were 1.6–2.2 million infected humans.

FILOVIRUS (enveloped RNA viruses: *Mononegavirales: Filoviridae*). The prototypes are *Ebolavirus* and *Marburgvirus*.

Ebola virus (EBOV) (2462, 4353, 4648, 5074, 8115, 8127) circulates in sub-Saharan Africa, in suspected but unidentified small mammals, occasionally perhaps primates. Biotypes include EBOV-Ivory Coast, EBOV-Reston, EBOV-Sudan, and EBOV-Zaire. SPREAD: is (i) initially via contact or injury with forest mammals, later (ii) via contact with patients and corpses, and (iii) in hospitals, via blood or secretions from patients, including by needle stick and mucosal splash. RISKS: hunting monkeys in the rain forest, unprotected handling of corpses, nosocomial exposure. Patients seem invective for 1–60 days. CLINICAL INFORMATION: Subclinical infections occur (EBOV-Reston, other EBOV). The incubation period is 2–21 (usually 5–14) days. Manifestations: flulike illness, intense weakness, vomiting, diarrhea, rash, and bleeding (can mimick dysentery). Lethality in hospitalized cases is 70–90%. Confirmation is by antibody or antigen test, NAT, or culture, including from blood, saliva, or urine; tests require high-security laboratories. IMPACT: Serosurveys in endemic areas suggest prevalences of 5–10% (reactivities before 1995 are likely confounded by cross-reactivities). To date, >1,800 cases are documented. OUTBREAKS: Outbreaks are widely known. Containment requires isolation in appropriate hospitals and standard precautions. EBOV-Ivory Coast occurred in 1994, when a Swiss research worker contracted disease from necropsy of a dead chimpansee in the Taï forest of Côte d'Ivoire. EBOV-Reston occurred in epizootics among cynomolgus monkeys from the Philippines imported into the United States in 1989 (Virginia), 1990 (Pennsylvania), and 1996 (Texas), and into Italy in 1992. EBOV-Sudan occurred in Sudan in 1976 (284 cases, 151 [53%] deaths) and 1979 (34 cases, 22 [65%] deaths), Uganda in 2000 (425 cases, 224 [53%] deaths), and Sudan in 2004 (17 cases, 7 [41%] deaths). In the 2000 Uganda outbreak, primary attack rate was 0.13%, secondary attack rate in ~5,000 contacts followed for 21 days was 2.5%. The index case in the Sudan 2004 outbreak was a radio technician who had hunted baboon (*Papio anubis*). EBOV-Zaire occurred in Congo (ex-Zaire) in 1976 (318 cases, 280 [88%] deaths), Gabon in 1980 (2 mild infections), Congo in 1995 (Kikwit, 316 cases, 245 [80%] deaths), Gabon in 1996 (91 cases, 66 [73%] deaths), and Gabon and Congo in 2001–2003 (5 outbreaks, 313 cases, 264 [84%] deaths). Index cases in Congo 2001–2003 outbreaks were hunters of primates (gorillas, chimpanzees) and forest antelopes (duikers). At least 10 infection chains ensued, mainly in households, which accounted for most of cases.

Marburg virus (MARV) (491, 612, 2836, 5361, 8125, 8384) circulates in Africa, in as yet unidentified animals. MARV is inactivated by heat and detergents; it survives in blood at ambient temperature for 2 weeks. SPREAD: is via contact with patients, blood, and secretions, mainly in the hospital, rarely in households; spread via contact with animal hosts is suspected. RISKS: contacts with monkeys, mining work in rain forest, patient contacts, nosocomial exposure, laboratory work. CLINICAL INFORMATION: Subclinical infections seem to occur. The incubation period is 2–14 days. Manifestations: fever, bleeding. Lethality is 20–80%. IMPACT: In African rain forest people, seroprevalences are 1–6%. OUTBREAKS: Imported monkeys caused an outbreak in 1967 with 31 cases in Marburg and Frankfurt, Germany, and two cases in Belgrade (ex-Yugoslavia), for a lethality of 23%. Clusters and outbreaks reemerged in South Africa in 1975 (one index case from Zimbabwe, two secondary cases, for a lethality of 33%), Kenya in 1980 (2 cases, lethality 50%), Zimbabwe in 1982 (one case), Kenya in 1987 (one fatal case), Congo (ex-Zaire) in 1998–2000 (149 cases, 123 [82%] deaths), and Angola in 2004–2005 (≥275 cases, 255 [93%] deaths).

FLAVIVIRUS (enveloped RNA viruses: *Flaviviridae*). These are arthropod-borne viruses, mainly DENV, JEV, KFDV, MVEV, OHFV, POWV, SLEV, TBEV, WNV, YFV, and Zikavirus. Given cross-reactivity in the genus, and wide use of YF vaccine, *Flavivirus* serology should be interpreted with caution.

Alkhurma virus (1348) is related to KFDV. It occurs in the Middle East, in mammals and ticks. SPREAD: is likely from vertebrate or tick bite, trauma from handling animal tissue, or drinking of unpasteurized milk. Manifestations: flulike illness, bleeding (VHF). Lethality is 25%. IMPACT: Rare (>20 human cases reported).

Dengue virus (DENV) (2977, 3034, 3208, 5441, 6271, 6932, 7421, 7896, 8100) circulates in tropical and subtropical areas, in mammals and mosquitoes (forest cycles), and humans and *Aedes aegypti* (urban cycle). There are four serotypes that vary in frequency by geography and year. Immunity to the same type is long-lasting, while cross-reactivity or cross-protection to other types is transient. SPREAD: is via mosquito bite, rarely needle stick. RISKS: domicile in or visit to endemic or outbreak areas, mosquito nonproofed housing, discarded cans on premise, pit latrines, and rainy season. CLINICAL INFORMATION: From 50% to 75% of infections are inapparent. The incubation period is 4–10 (often 7) days. Viremia begins 2 days before disease onset and lasts ~1 week. Manifestations: flulike illness, rash (dengue fever, DF), bleeding (hemorrhagic fever, DHF), and shock syndrome (DSS). By denominator, lethality of DHF/DSS is <1% to >20% (often 2–5%). IMPACT: Some 2.5–3 billion people are exposed, there are ~100 million infections per year, and ~50 million cases per year, including 0.25–0.5 million DHF/DSS cases, and >10,000 deaths. By age and season, disease rates are 20–450/10^5 per year. By seroconversions, infection rates can exceed 10% and year. OUTBREAKS: Many epidemics have been reported on mainlands and islands. Preventive measures include elimination of peridomestic mosquito-breeding sites, proofed housing, personal protection, early case detection and reporting, and response teams for indoor spraying. **Latin America.** When *A. aegypti* reinvaded the continent in 1969, epidemics occurred in the Caribbean, e.g., Puerto Rico in 1977 (355,000 cases, several serotypes, no DHF) and Cuba in 1981 (350,000 DENV2 cases, with DHF/DSS), and the mainland, e.g., Colombia in 1971–1972 (450,000 DENV2 infections) and El Salvador in 2000 (16,355 cases, ~10% of residents had evidence of recent infection). **Australasia.** Outbreaks occurred on islands in the Indian Ocean (Comoros, Réunion, and Seychelles) and the Pacific (Micronesia, New Caledonia,

Fiji, and French Polynesia) as well as on mainlands, e.g., Thailand in 1987 (152,840 cases in 67 of 73 provinces, with DHF) and Vietnam in 1998 (119,429 cases in 19 provinces, mainly DENV3 but also DENV1, 2, and 4, with DHF and 342 deaths). North Queesland, Australia, is vulnerable and has experienced repeated outbreaks.

Japanese encephalitis virus (JEV) (108, 358, 3165, 4048, 5895, 7201) circulates in the eastern half of Asia, in birds, pigs, and *Culex* mosquitoes. SPREAD: is via mosquito bite; rarely intrauterine. RISKS: domicile in or visit to enzootic or epidemic areas, domicile close to water or pigs, irrigation rice farming, swine production, summer season. CLINICAL INFORMATION: Most (>99% in children, >95% in adults) infections are inapparent. The incubation period is 4–16 days. Diagnosis is largely serological; IgM is demonstrable 4–7 days after disease onset. Manifestations: fever, encephalitis. Lethality is 10–50%. Of survivors, 40–70% have permanent neurological or mental sequelae. IMPACT: By age and test, seroprevalence in enzootic areas is ~1–4%. Reported cases are 50,000 per year. Reported disease rate in enzootic areas is 10–150/10^5 per year. OUTBREAKS: Many enzootic areas have experienced outbreaks. Examples include Korea in 1949 (5,548 cases, 2,429 [44%] deaths), Uttar Pradesh, India, in 1988 (4,544 cases, 1,413 [31%] deaths), Saipan island in 1990 (10 cases, attack rate 0.025%, postepidemic seroprevalence 4%), Nepal in 1997 (infection rate focally 28%) and 1999 (2,924 cases, 434 (15%) deaths). In Japan, vaccination, vector control, and changes in pig farming reduced cases per year from up to 2,000 in the 1960s to 35 in 1991–1998. Unexpectedly, JE reemerged in southern Japan in August–September 2002 with six cases. Vaccines are available, including formalin-inactived, mouse brain-derived vaccine licensed in the United States. Proposed indications for travelers are stays in rural enzootic areas for >1 month during the transmission season, or of any length during outbreaks. Mosquito avoidance is advised. Impregnated bednets are of proven benefit.

Kunjin virus (KUNV) (1345, 3092) is closely related to WNV. KUNV circulates in Australia and Southeast Asia, in wading birds, other vertebrate hosts, and freshwater mosquitoes (*Culex annulirostris*). Manifestations: flulike illness, mild encephalitis.

Kyasanur Forest disease virus (KFDV) (70) occurs in India, in wild mammals and ticks. SPREAD: is via tick bite. CLINICAL INFORMATION: The incubation period is 2–9 days. Manifestations: fever, meningoencephalitis, bleeding (VHF). Lethality is 3–10%. IMPACT: Epizootics in wild monkeys can precede outbreaks in humans.

Louping ill virus (LIV) (1347) is related to TBEV. LIV is a cause of encephalitis in sheep. Spread is by *Ixodes* ticks. Sporadic infections are documented in shepherds and other occupationally exposed persons.

Murray Valley encephalitis virus (MVEV) (907, 4616, 7065, 8342) circulates in parts of Australia and New Guinea, in birds and *Culex* mosquitoes. SPREAD: is via mosquito bite. CLINICAL INFORMATION: Most (≥98%) infections are inapparent. The incubation period is likley 5–28 days. Manifestations: encephalitis. Lethality is 15%, occasionally up to 30%. Of survivers, 25–50% have neurological sequelae. IMPACT: Sporadic. Reported cases in Australia were 63 in 1975–2000, 5 in 2001, 2 in 2002. OUTBREAKS: Outbreaks occurred in Australia in 1917–1925 (>280 cases), 1950–1951 (in Murray Valley), 1974 (58 cases from all mainland states), and 1993 (nine cases with four deaths in the Kimberleys, following heavy rains and flooding).

Omsk hemorrhagic fever virus (OHFV) (1347) is related to TBEV. OHFV circulates in forest and steppes in southwestern (Omsk) and western Siberia, in rodents and *Dermacentor* ticks. SPREAD: is via tickbite, handling of viremic rodents or their secretions, and in the hospital, via blood or aerosols. RISKS: hunting rodents, gathering mushrooms and berries, fall season (peak in September–October). CLINICAL INFORMATION: The incubation period is 1–10 (typically 3–7) days. Manifestations: fever, general lymphadenopathy, bleeding (VHF). Lethality is 0.5–3%, occasionally 10%.

Powassan virus (POWV) (1178, 2113, 2716) circulates in North America and eastern Russia, in rodents, middle-sized mammals (skunks, weasles), and ticks (*Ixodes* and *Dermacentor*). SPREAD: via tickbite. RISKS: outdoor activities, summer and fall seasons (peak in June–September). Not all patients recall tick bites. Tick attachment for 15 minutes may suffice for transmission. CLINICAL INFORMATION: About one third of infections are inapparent. The incubation period is likely 7–14 days. Manifestations: flulike illness, encephalitis. Lethality is 10-15%. Sequelae can be considerable. IMPACT: In 1958–1998, 27 POWV encephalitis cases were reported in North America.

St. Louis encephalitis virus (SLEV) (1311, 2971, 3737, 6204, 6804) circulates in the Americas, in birds and *Culex* mosquitoes. SPREAD: is via mosquito bite. RISKS: Attack rates are above average in children and the elderly. Transmission is seasonal and focal in the eastern half of the United States, but perennial in the western half and tropical Latin America. Cases peak in late summer (August–September). CLINICAL INFORMATION: Most (>99%) infections are inapparent. The incubation period is 5–15 days. Manifestations: flulike illness, encephalitis. Sequelae seem rare, although 30–50% of patients present neurodeficits on hospital discharge. Lethality is 2–30%. IMPACT: Occurrence is enzootic-epizootic and sporadic-epidemic. In healthy adult residents, reported seroprevalence is 0.8–11% (often 4–5%). Reported epidemic disease rates are 16–37/10^5. OUTBREAKS: The first major outbreak occurred in St. Louis, Mo., in 1933, with 1,097 cases and 221 (20%) deaths. Later outbreaks at unpredictable intervals included the Mississippi and Ohio river basins in 1975 (2,100 cases, 170 [8%] deaths), Florida in 1990 (226 cases), and Louisiana in 2001 (70 cases, 3 [4%] deaths). Urban areas are not exempt from outbreaks, e.g., Corpus Christi, Dallas, and Houston in Texas.

Tick-borne encephalitis virus (TBEV) (3061, 3409, 3788, 4113, 4150, 4171, 4357, 6218, 7262) circulates focally, in ticks and small mammals, in Europe in *Ixodes ricinus*, in Asia in *I. persulcatus*. An envelope protein defines "European," "Far Eastern," and "Siberian" subtypes. Humans are incidental hosts and do not contribute to TBEV recycling. TBEV is inactivated by heat, but resilient in raw milk and butter. SPREAD: is via bite by nymphal or adult ticks, occasionally by raw goat milk (in <1% of cases), viremic blood, or laboratory accident. RISKS: domiciles near foci, outdoor activities for leisure (hiking, bicycling, berry picking, includes urban residents) or work (farm, forest, hunt), summer season. The majority (70–75%) of patients recall recent tick exposure. CLINICAL INFORMATION: From 60% to 95% of infections are inapparent. The incubation period is 2–28 (typically 7–14) days. Manifestations: flulike illness (first phase), meningitis or encephalitis (second phase, in 5–90% of cases). Viremia lasts 1–8 (often 4) days. As virus isolation and NAT are successful only in initial viremia, confirmation is based on serology (IgM, high IgG). Lethality is 0-4% (often 1%) for European subtype, and 5–20% for Asian subtypes. Of survivors of the second phase, a variable proportion (0–46%) has neurological sequelae. IMPACT: Seroprevalence in nonvaccinated, rural populations is 0–30% (often 1–10%). Reported seroconversion rates are 1–2% per year. In >25 countries, there are ~3,000–12,000 cases per year. By season and vaccine status, disease rates per 10^5 per year are 0.3–1 in western Europe and 5–50 (rarely >150) in eastern Europe. In travelers and military units, reported disease rates are 0.1–0.9/1,000 person-months. OUTBREAKS: Outbreaks have been reported. Inactivated vaccines are available and recommended for repeatedly or continuously exposed persons.

Wesselbron virus (364, 1916) is related to YFV. WSLV circulates in sub-Saharan Africa and Thailand, in mosquitoes, rodents, and domestic mammals. WSLV is a cause of febrile illness.

West Nile virus (WNV) (1258, 2798, 2904, 3206, 3471, 8386) circulates in Africa, Eurasia, and the Americas, in mosquitoes (from >10 genera), birds (resident and migratory), and likely mammals (rodents, bats, and horses). WNV can make susceptible birds "drop dead from the sky". SPREAD: is (i) via mosquito bite, (ii) possibly via contact with viremic animals (through broken skin), (iii) rarely intrauterine or via breastmilk, (iv) via blood, transplants, or in the laboratory. RISKS: outdoor and indoor mosquito exposure, high mosquito densities from irrigation, heavy rains, and floods, domicile in areas with high vegetation cover, proximity to dead birds, and summer season. Elderly are susceptible to neuroinvasive disease (Fig. 20.2). CLINICAL INFORMATION: Most (≥85%) infections are inapparent. Viremia lasts 1 week; in immune-impaired individuals it lasts 1 month. The incubation period is 2–14 (often 3–6) days, from transplants 2–21 (often 10) days. Manifestations: include flulike illness, general lymphadenopathy, meningoencephalitis (in <1%), acute flaccid paralysis, and optic neuritis. Confirmation is by serology (IgM or IgG in serum or CSF), NAT, or virus isolation. By denominator, setting, and case mix, lethality is 0.3–16%. In the United States in 2002, lethality was 0.3% (2/704) in febrile cases but 9% (199/2,354) in encephalitis. IMPACT: Seroprevalence in residents in enzootic areas are ~1–30% (reported higher figures are likely confounded by cross-reactivity). Since its appearance in New York in 1999, WNV in four to five seasons has crossed the continent, expanded into Canada, Mexico, and the Caribbean, and has become seasonally endemic. Reported cases in the United States were 21–66/year in 1999–2001, 3,419 (with 180 or 5% deaths) in 2002, and 7,718 (166 or 2%) in 2003, 2,241 (76 or 3%) in 2004, and 2,581 (83 or 3%) in 2005. Population infection rates are ~2.5% per year. OUTBREAKS: Outbreaks brought WNV back to attention, including in Romania in summer 1996 (393 cases hospitalized in Bucharest, 17 [4%] deaths), Tunisia in 1997 (173 cases, 8 [5%] deaths), southern Russia in 1999 (826 suspected and 318 confirmed cases, 40 deaths), New York in 1999 (3,500–13,000 infections, 1,700 febrile cases, 59 neuroinvasive cases, and 7 deaths), and Israel in 2000 (417 cases, 35 [8%] deaths).

Yellow fever virus (YFV) (954, 1188, 1278, 1796, 1841, 2037, 5621, 8112) circulates in tropical Africa and South America, in wild mammals and forest mosquitoes (sylvatic cycles), and humans and *A. aegypti* ("spill-over"

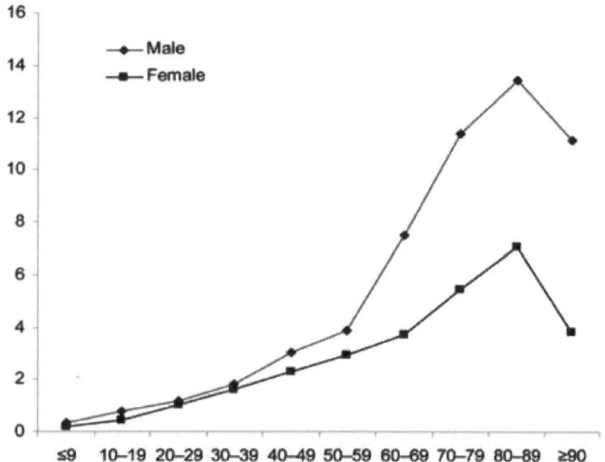

Figure 20.2 Neuroinvasive West Nile virus disease, United States 1999-2004 (n = 7,096). Reported rate per 10^5 population (y axis) by age groups (x axis, years) and gender. From reference 3206.

urban cycle). SPREAD: is via mosquito bite. RISKS: domicile in or visit to enzootic rural area, not being vaccinated, forest and farm work. CLINICAL INFORMATION: From 45% to 85% of infections are inapparent or mild. The incubation period is 3–6 days (in W. Reed's 13 experimental infections in 1900–1901 it was 41 h to 6 days). Manifestations: flulike illness, jaundice, bleeding (VHF), multiorgan failure. Confirmation is by NAT from blood, serology (conversion), histopathology, and virus isolation. Lethality of hospitalized cases is 20–85% (with a high in children). IMPACT: YF is considered a risk in ~44 tropical countries. There are ~200,000 cases per year with 50,000 deaths, mostly (90%) in Africa. Infections are believed to be 10–500 times more frequent than the cases reported. Seroprevalence in enzootic areas is 1–3% (South America) to 20–60% (tropical Africa). The endemic disease rate is 100–200/10^5 per year. OUTBREAKS: Examples of epidemics include Ethiopia in 1960–1962 (100,000 cases, 30,000 deaths), Burkina Faso in 1983 (12,500–17,500 cases, 2,500–3,500 deaths), and Nigeria in 1987 (116,000 cases, 24,000 deaths). Attack rates can reach 1–2%. In Minas Gerais, Brazil, in 2001, YF in a farm worker heralded 31 further confirmed and 81 suspected cases. An outbreak in Sudan in 2003 (162 suspected cases) underscored YFV circulation in East Africa. After >220 passages in culture, 17D YF vaccine was introduced in 1937. This effective vaccine strain is still in use. Indications include residents in and travelers to enzootic and epidemic areas, and laboratory personnel exposed to YFV.

Zika virus (8242) circulates in Africa (e.g., Zika Forest, Uganda) and Asia, in primates and mosquitoes. Humans can become infected. Manifestations: fever, rash.

FONSECAEA (23, 2245, 6551, 6895) (*Ascomycota: Chaetothyriales*). *F. pedrosoi* is a pigmented mold that inhabits soil, rotting wood, and plants, mainly in tropical climates. SPREAD: is via skin trauma. RISKS: farm work, being male (male:female is >9:1). CLINICAL INFORMATION: The presumed incubation period is months. Manifestations: chromomycosis (80% of lesions are on feet or legs), rarely keratitis, sinusitis, or invasive disease. IMPACT: In Madagascar, chromomycosis rate is 0.5/10^5 per year. The relative frequency of *F. pedrosoi* was 62% in 170 culture-confirmed chromomycosis cases.

FOOT-AND-MOUTH DISEASE VIRUS (FMDV). *See* Aphthovirus.

FRANCISELLA (γ-*Proteobacteria: Thiotrichales*).

F. tularensis (909, 2172, 2185, 2347, 3030, 3205, 6202) is a gram-negative coccoid rod that circulates in the Northern Hemisphere, in soil, water, plants, and >250 species of (in)vertebrates, notably arthropods, rodents, and lagomorphs. Of three biovars, A (*tularensis*) is virulent and dominant in North America, B (*palaearctica*) is moderately virulent and dominant in Eurasia, and C (*novicida*) is rare and aquatic. *F. tularensis* is resilient, surviving low temperatures in soil, carcasses, and tap water for up to 3 months. SPREAD: is via (i) animal contact or trauma, (ii) arthropod bite (ticks in America, mosquitoes or deerflies in Europe), (iii) inhalation of dust (Europe), (iv) ingestion of meat or tap water, and (v) in laboratories or veterinary clinics. RISKS: outdoor work, animal contacts, cat ownership, tick bites, being male. Seasonal peaks are different for vector and hunting activities. The infective dose is low (10 bacteria for percutaneous or airborne infections). Inhalation is suspect of intentional release. CLINICAL INFORMATION: From 3% to 30% of infections are inapparent. The incubation period is 1 day to 1 month (typically 2–5 days). Manifestations: (tularemia) vary with portal of entry, can be constitutional (flulike in 80–95%), cutaneous (inoculation ulcer in 10–85%, regional lymphadenitis in 85–95%), and respiratory (pharyngitis in 20–85%, pneumonia in 5–50%, enlarged hili). Complications include erythema nodosum, sepsis, hepatitis, and pericarditis. Confirmation is difficult, consider serology (various tests, positive from 2 weeks after illness onset, can cross-react with *Brucella*, *Proteus*, and *Yersinia*), NAT (from scrapings, sputum, blood), or culture (positive in 10% only and hazardous). By biovar and treatment, lethality is 0.1–30%, with biovar A often 0.5–2%. IMPACT: Seroprevalence in residents in enzootic areas is 0.2–5%. Disease rates in interepidemic periods are 0.02–3.5/10^5 per year, but up to 66/10^5 per year during epidemics. OUTBREAKS: Outbreaks have been associated with ticks, mosquitoes, deerflies, small animals, outdoor activities, polluted foods, and drinking water. Epizootics have been reported in rabbits, hares, and sheep.

FUSARIUM (884, 3682, 5440, 5497) (*Ascomycota: Hypocreales*). These are hyaline molds that produce septate, sickle-shaped macroconidia and inhabit soil, plants, and hospital water. *F. oxysporum* and *F. solani* have been diagnosed in humans. ACQUISITION: is presumed from the environment. CLINICAL INFORMATION: An incubation period is not reported. Manifestations: onychomycosis (fingernails and more often of toenails), eumycetoma (white grains), and keratitis in immune-competent hosts, and violaceous or ecthyma-like skin lesions, fungemia, and invasive disease in immune-impaired hosts (diabetes, malignancy, and transplant). Lethality of invasive disease is 50–75%.

FUSOBACTERIUM (*Bacteroidales*) (1055, 3682). These are gram-negative rods. There are >10 species. *F. necrophorum* and *F. nucleatum* are part of buccal, bowel, and genitourinary flora of animals and humans. SPREAD: Infections seem largely endogenous. Manifestations:

fever that resists antibiotids, and fungemia in immune-compromised hosts (neutropenia and malignancy). *Fusobacterium* has a role in polymicrobial (Plaut-Vincent) tonsillitis. Lethality of invasive disease is 50–65%. Treatment options include amphothericin B and voriconazole.

GARDNERELLA (*Actinobacteria*: *Bifidobacteriales*).
G. vaginalis (214, 4201, 5543) is part of the vaginal flora. Infections are endogenous; sexual spread does not seem to occur. CLINICAL INFORMATION: This agent is associated with bacterial vaginosis that is manifest by increased, thin, malodorous vaginal discharge, absence of *Lactobacillus*, and presence of bacteria with corkscrew motility in wet mounts. Proposed complications of *G. vaginalis*-vaginosis are miscarriage in the second trimester, and pelvic inflammatory disease (PID). IMPACT: Among women in general practice, 10–30% are diagnosed bacterial vaginosis. Of women with vaginal symptoms, 40–50% can yield *G. vaginalis*.

GB VIRUS C (2522, 3468, 4816, 7117) (GBV-C, enveloped RNA viruses: *Flaviviridae*). Named for a patient (G.B.) and after simian GBV-A and GBV-B isolates, and initially misnamed "hepatitis G virus," GBV-C replicates in lymphocytes rather than hepatocytes, and it does not cause hepatitis. SPREAD: is via blood, contact, or sex. CLINICAL INFORMATION: Infections can persist for (up to 16) years, but long-term effects are not known. GBV-C is a "virus in search of disease" or a "commensal virus." IMPACT: Among healthy adults not exposed to blood, GBV-C is amplified by NAT in ~1–4%, and antibodies to GBV-C are detected in 1–16%. Coinfections with HBV, HCV, and HIV are frequent. In HIV-infected individuals, GBV-C seems to be a surrogate of prolonged survival.

GEOTRICHUM (884, 2761) (*Ascomycota*: *Saccharomycetales*). These are opportunistic yeasts. *G. candidum* is important for ripening cheese, and it is an occasional cause of fingernail onychomycosis. In immune-impaired hosts, *G. candidum* and *G. capitatum* can cause invasive disease.

GIARDIA (7452) (*Euglenozoa*: *Diplomonadida*). These are flagellated protozoa visualized in 1681 by A. van Leeuwenhoek (1632–1723). Host-specific species include *G. bovis*, *G. canis*, *G. cati*, and *G. muris*. In contrast, *G. lamblia* sl (=*G. duodenalis*, *G. intestinalis*, "*G. enterica*") is host promiscuous.
G. lamblia sl (1457, 3353, 3423, 3670, 6000, 6279, 7213, 7241) circulates worldwide, in sewage, water, foods, and mammals and humans who harbor trophozoites and shed infective cysts. Cysts survive in water at 4–10°C for months, but are inactivated by heat (70°C for 10 min) or free chlorine. SPREAD: is by ingestion of viable cysts via tap water or fecally polluted foods, hand contacts (e.g., in day care centers and nursing homes), anal sex, possibly pet contacts. Humans can shed cysts or trophozoites for months. RISKS: lack of toilet, patient contact, preschool children in the household, children in day care, handling diapers or dirty linen, drinking tap or surface water, eating raw vegetables, swimming in freshwater, backpacking and camping, sex among men, and travel to endemic areas. Washing hands before eating and breastfeeding decrease risks. CLINICAL INFORMATION: The infective dose is low (~10 cysts). The prepatent perid is 6–21 (typically 14) days. *G. lamblia* locates in the duodenum. From 50% to 100% of infections are inapparent. The incubation period is 1 day to 3 months (typically 1–2 weeks). Manifestations: flatulence, loose, foul-smelling stools, chronic (>2 weeks) diarrhea (in 30%), and malabsorption (fat and vitamins). In endemic areas, the age of first acquisition is ≤6 months. Rates of reinfection posttreatment can reach 100% in 6 months. Preschool children may have experienced several disease episodes. Reinfected adults clear up to three fourths of infections spontaneously. Confirmation is by microscopy of several, concentrated stool or duodenal fluid samples, or by fecal antigen test. Nitroimidazoles are a treatment option. IMPACT: By age and habitat, prevalences are 2–7% in high-income countries, and 3–30% (typically 10%) in low-income countries. By age, case mix, and geography, diagnostic yield is ~2–7% in acute diarrhea, and ~10–20% in chronic diarrhea. In the United States in 1998–2002, reported disease rates were 7–8/10^5 per year (peak of 23.5/10^5 in Vermont in 2002). Northern states tended to report more cases and have higher rates than southern states (Fig. 20.3), a pattern that fits well with *Giardia*'s adaptation to cool climates. In New Zealand, the reported disease rate in 1996–2000 was 41/10^5 per year. OUTBREAKS: Outbreaks have occurred in cities, day care centers, ski resorts, camps, restaurants, and nursing homes, carried by various types of water supplies and foods. In the United States, only 2–12% of reported cases are outbreak related.

GNATHOSTOMA (1287, 1708, 1920, 4085, 4981, 5167, 6379, 6934) (Nematoda: Spirurida). Of ~12 species that parasitize vertebrates, *G. spinigerum* is most frequently diagnosed in humans, followed by *G. doloresi*, *G. hispidum*, *G. malaysiae*, and *G. nipponicum*.
G. spinigerum circulates in warm climates, in cats and dogs (final hosts, harbor adults in the stomach, and shed eggs), copepods (first intermediate hosts), and freshwater fish (second hosts). The cycle is complicated by vertebrate parathenic hosts that, like intermediate hosts, harbor infective larvae (L3) in tissues. Humans are dead-end hosts. SPREAD: is via ingestion of viable L3 from foods (fish), possibly percutaneously, on contact with L3

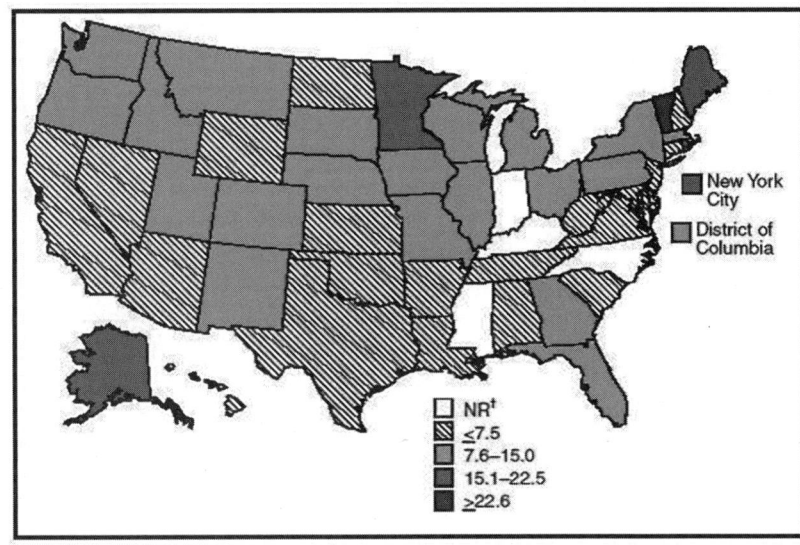

Figure 20.3 Reported giardiasis cases, United States 2002 ($n = 21,3000$). Rates are given per 10^5 population by states. NR, not reporting. From reference 3353.

in foods. RISKS: preference for raw fish, residents and visitors who relish exotic foods in enzootic areas. CLINICAL INFORMATION: The incubation period is hours to 5 months, often 1–10 weeks. Manifestations: can be cutaneous (larva migrans and migratory swellings), visceral (e.g., larvae in eye or brain), or eosinophilia. Confirmation is by biopsy, serology (immunoblot), or surgery. Treatment options include albendazole or ivermectin. IMPACT: In Thailand in the 1990s, ~600 cases per year were laboratory confirmed, and *G. spinigerum* was diagnosed in 6 of ~200,000 surgical materials. In Mexico in 1980–1996, >1,400 cases were recorded from 6 states. OUTBREAKS: Food-borne outbreaks have been reported. At a Korean restaurant in Yangon, Myanmar, in 2001, 38 of 60 emigrants contracted gnathostomiasis from eating raw freshwater fish. In a fishing village in Sinaloa state, Mexico, five adults contracted gnathostomiasis from eating "ceviche" (raw fish).

GUANARITO VIRUS (GUAV). *See* Arenavirus.

HAEMOPHILUS (γ-*Proteobacteria*: *Pasteurellales*). These are gram-negative rods that colonize mucosa of mammals. *H. ducreyi*, *H. influenzae*, and *H. parainfluenzae* are infective to humans.

H. ducreyi (943, 4390, 5007, 7126, 7464) colonizes the human genital tract, at least temporarily (a carrier state is unconfirmed). Most clinical isolates are producing β-lactamase. SPREAD: is via sex (STI). RISKS: sex with prostitutes, visits to endemic or outbreak areas, being uncircumcised. The risk of spread male to female is 60–80%; that female to male is unknown. Assuming infectivity for 5 weeks, and spread to 70% of contacts, models predict that females need to change sex partners ≥18 times per year to maintain *H. ducreyi* in the community. As entry and exit sites for HIV, ulcers in chancroid promote spread of HIV. CLINICAL INFORMATION: Up to 20% of infections are inapparent. The incubation period is 1–25 (typically 7) days (in experimental skin infection 1 day to papule and 3–9 days to pustule). Manifestations (chancroid or ulcus molle): painful, "soft" ulcers (1 in ~30% of males, can be >1), adenopathy (in one fourth to one half). The male:female ratio was 3–25:1 in outbreaks in the United States, but 1.6:1 in an outbreak in Greenland. Confirmation is by NAT or culture from ulcer swab. IMPACT: Endemic in sexually active adults in parts of Africa and Asia, and sporadic in high-income countries (see section 14.7). Worldwide, there are ~7 million cases per year. OUTBREAKS: In the United States in 1981–1987, 4,486 chancroid cases were reported in nine outbreaks (~500 per outbreak); in six outbreaks, prostitutes were involved. In Jackson, Miss., during an epidemic in 1994–1995, the chancroid disease rate was ~$54/10^5$ per year.

H. influenzae (483, 3427, 4035, 4934, 4936, 5820, 6474) colonizes the human respiratory tract, starting at age <4 months. Unencapsulated strains are nontypeable. Polysaccharide in capsulated strains defines serotypes. Of 2,676 community isolates from all continents, 86% (2,305) were nontypeable, 14% (371) were typeable: either b (Hib, 41%), d (26%), or a, c, e or f (33%). Serotyping is useful for epidemiology but results can be inconsistent. In the 2000s, 5–40% of isolates produce β-lactamase and are resistant to ampicillin. SPREAD: is via droplets, starting early in life, rarely nosocomially, e.g., in pulmonary rehabilitation. RISKS: early weaning, preschool age, crowded households, preschool siblings, day care attendance, and parents who are smokers. CLINICAL INFORMATION: The reported incubation period is 4–5 days. Disease by Hib that affects mainly children include epiglottitis, pneumonia, BSI, and meningitis. Disease by other strains include otitis media, sinusitis, bronchitis, purulent conjunctivitis, pneumonia, and BSI. Lethality of invasive Hib disease is 1–14% in high-income countries to 10–25% in low-income countries. **IMPACT:** In the prevaccine era, the global rate of Hib disease in preschool children was 370/10^5 per year; the Hib meningitis rate was 1–95 (often 20–70)/10^5 preschool children per year. In high-income countries, vaccines have reduced Hib disease rates to 0.3-2/10^5 preschool children per year. In the United States in 2000, disease rates per 10^5 preschool children were 0.3 for Hib, 0.8 for non-b or nontypeable strains, and 0.2 for nontyped strains. **OUTBREAKS:** Venues for outbreaks include the community, minorities, day care centers, hospital wards, and nursing homes. Conjugate vaccines are effective against invasive Hib disease and reduce Hib carriage. Vaccines do not prevent disease by non-b or nontypeable strains. Worldwide, a minority (<5%) of children is covered by vaccine. For exposed household members chemoprophylaxis should be considered.

H. parainfluenzae (5681) is part of the upper respiratory tract flora. It is a sporadic cause of endocarditis or other invasive disease.

HAND-AND-MOUTH DISEASE VIRUS. See Enterovirus.

HANTAVIRUS (enveloped RNA viruses: *Bunyaviridae*). A cosmopolitan member is SEOV. Eurasian members hosted by Murinae and Arvicolinae rodent subfamilies are DOBV, HTNV, PUUV, SAAV, and TULV. New World members hosted by *Sigmodontinae* subfamily include ANDV, LNV, and SNV (Table 3.1).

Andes virus (ANDV) (1120, 2583, 2833, 5673) circulates in South America (Argentina, Bolivia, Chile, and Uruguay). Host is *Oligoryzomys longicaudatus*. ANDV is a confirmed cause of HPS (see "SNV"). ANDV is the only *Hantavirus* for which person-to-person spread has been documented.

Bermejo virus (5672) is related to ANDV. It circulates in Bolivia. Putative host is *Oligoryzomys*. It is a cause of HPS (see "SNV").

Dobrava virus (DOBV) (6718, 6877) has emerged in Slovenia. Host are mice (*Apodemus agrarius, A. flavicollis,* and *A. sylvaticus*). DOBV seems widespread in West, East, and South Europe. Manifestations: are of variable severity, but DOBV can cause HFRS (see "HTNV").

Hantaan virus (HTNV) (141, 1390, 4299) circulates in Eurasia, mainly in field mice (*A. agrarius*), but also in *Rattus norvegicus*. In parts of Asia, areas of HTNV and SEOV overlap. **RISKS:** rodent contacts, outdoor work (e.g., by hunters, rangers, biologists, farmers, and troops), rodent-infested housing, and fall season. **CLINICAL INFORMATION:** Infections can be inapparent. The incubation period is 1–6 (typically 2–3) weeks. Manifestations (hemorrhagic fever with renal syndrome, HFRS): fever (in 100%), bleeding (VHF, in 30–70%), oliguria (<500 ml, in about two thirds), acute renal failure. Other hantaviruses that can cause HFRS include DOBV and SEOV. Lethality of HFRS is 10–60%. **IMPACT:** Worldwide, there are perhaps >50,000 cases per/year, mainly in People's Republic of China. In the 1990s, seroprevalence of 1.5–4% was reported from enzootic areas of Russia. In Russia, rates of HFRS per 10^5 per year are ~4 overall, 5 in the European part, 2 in the Asian part. **OUTBREAKS:** Outbreaks have been reported in troops, including in Manchuria in 1932 (12,000 cases in a Japanese army of 1 million), and in Korea in 1951–1954 (>3,200 cases among United Nations troops).

Laguna Negra virus (LNV) (2363, 8190) circulates in Latin America (Bolivia and Gran Chaco of Paraguay). Host is *Calomys laucha*. In Paraguay in 1995–1996, an outbreak caused 27 cases, and 4 (15%) infections among contacts. Human disease appears to be a rather mild febrile illness. In the Chaco, ~35–50% of residents are seroreactive to *Hantavirus*.

Oran virus (5922) is related to ANDV. It circulates in northeastern Argentina. Putative host is *Oligoryzomys*. The reported seroprevalence in residents is 6.5%.

Puumala virus (PUUV) (1481, 3494, 4149, 4664, 5609, 6405) circulates in bank voles (*Clethrionomys*), in Scandinavia, western Europe, and probably the Balkans. In West Europe and the Balkans, PUUV may cocirculate with DOBV and HTNV. **RISKS:** domicile in enzootic area, outdoor work, being male (male:female ratio is 3:1), fall and winter seasons. **CLINICAL INFORMATION:** The incubation period is 10–25 days. Manifestations (epidemic nephropathy): fever (in ≥95%), back pain (in 55–65%), hematuria (macroscopic in 2–7%, microscopic in 60–70%), impaired renal function (in ≥95%). Lethality is <0.05%. **IMPACT:** In Scandinavia, depending on location and season, infection and disease rates are ~5–35/10^5 per year. In West Europe, by geography and surveillance, reported case rates are 0.2–40/10^5 per year (low in Bavaria, high in Ardennes). Seroprevalence in the general population is 0–2%. In World War II, there were 10,000 cases among German troops in Finnish Lapland. Outbreaks may follow conditions that support large rodent populations. Reported venues included military settings (maneuvers and deployments).

Saaremaa virus (SAAV) (4574) emerged in Estonia. Host are mice (*A. agrarius*). SAAV circulates in the Balticum, together with PUUV, and in Denmark. Infections in humans seem to occur.

Seoul virus (SEOV) (100, 1387, 2772, 3311, 3493, 8253) circulates in Eurasia and the Americas, in rats (*Rattus rattus, R. norvegicus*) that shed virus with urine, feces, or saliva. Laboratory rats were occasionally infected. **SPREAD:** is via contact with rodents or inhalation of rodent-generated aerosols, occasionally in laboratories. **RISKS:** as with HTNV. **CLINICAL INFORMATION:**

Infections can be inapparent. The incubation period is 1–6 weeks. Manifestations: see HTNV. Confirmation is by NAT or serology (there may be cross-reactivity within the genus). A possible sequelae of (silent) SEOV infection is hypertensive renal disease. **IMPACT**: See HTNV. In Baltimore in 1986–1988, 0.3% (3/1,180) of an inner city population were seroreactive to SEOV.

Sin Nombre virus (SNV) (281, 498, 2005, 2536, 3346, 8349) emerged in the southwestern United States. It circulates in North America and perhaps Central America. Hosts are deer mice (*Peromyscus maniculatus*). **SPREAD**: is via inhalation of rodent-generated aerosols. **RISKS**: seem mainly peridomestic: cleaning houses from rodent droppings, killing rodents, touching trapped rodents, and the summer season. **CLINICAL INFORMATION**: The incubation period is 9–51 (usually 7–21) days. Manifestation (hantavirus [cardio]pulmonary syndrome, HPS): fever (in ≥95%), respiratory distress (in ≥90%), and hypotension. Lethality is high 25–60%. **IMPACT**: From its appearance in 1993–2003, >350 cases were confirmed in the United States. Reported seroprevalence in exposed groups is 0–13%. **OUTBREAKS**: In May–December 1993, SNV emerged in the four-corners area (Arizona, Colorado, New Mexico, and Utah) of the United States, causing 53 cases and 32 (60%) deaths. In the same area, an outbreak in 1998–1999 caused 42 cases and 16 (38%) deaths. Warm years from El Niño–Southern Oscillation events (ENSO) associated with mass fruiting of pines and large rodent populations likely triggered the outbreaks. In Panama in 1999–2000, an outbreak caused 12 cases and 3 (25%) deaths.

Tula virus (TULV) (6712) emerged in Russia. Host are voles (*Microtus arvalis* and *M. agrestis*). TULV circulates in eastern Europe; in Slovakia, together with DOBV and PUUV. Infection in a human has been reported.

HARTMANNELLA (7925) (Amoebozoa: Euamoebida). These are free-living amebas that inhabit soil, water, and dust, and host bacteria such as *Legionella*. **SPREAD**: is presumed via ingestion, inhalation, or contact. **CLINICAL INFORMATION**: Sporadic keratitis.

HELICOBACTER (ε-*Proteobacteria*: *Campylobacteriales*). These are curved (in culture) or spiral (in biopsy) rods. Hosts for *H. felis* and *H. heilmannii* (ex-*Gastrospirillum hominis*) are domestic mammals such as cats, dogs, and pigs.

H. pylori (722, 924, 4684, 5541, 7092, 7885) occurs worldwide, colonizing human gastric mucosa and oropharynx (dental plaques). Occurrence in the environment is likely. *H. pylori* has accompanied humans for >100,000 years, and it is used as a marker of prehistoric migration. **SPREAD**: is likely via contact in households, inhalation of aerosols from vomiting, uptake of fecally polluted foods or tap water, medical instruments (gastric tubes, endoscopes). Spread by animal contact is doubtful. Saliva is a potential vehicle; *H. pylori* DNA and antibody are demonstrated in saliva. **RISKS**: crowding, a colonized mother, low level of education, unsafe food or water. *H. pylori*-associated hypochlorhydria can predispose to cholera. **CLINICAL INFORMATION**: Most infections are inapparent, although gastritis is diagnosed histologically in 20–25% of infected persons. From experiments and gastric intubation, the incubation period can be as short as 3–7 days. Manifestations: gastritis, gastric and duodenal ulcer, perhaps dyspepsia. Infections can persist for decades, and a long-term complication is gastric adenocarcinoma. Infections can also be cleared, at rates comparable to acquisition, perhaps spontaneously, or when antimicrobials are used for other indications. In new birth cohorts of high-income countries acquisition is declining, and *H. pylori* may ultimately disappear from high-income countries. Diagnostic methods include urea breath test, biopsy, and antigen detection from stool. **IMPACT**: The global infection prevalence is ~50%. In low-income countries, infection is acquired in infancy, and by age 20 years, 70–90% of people are infected. In high-income countries, acquisition is slower, at rates of 0.3–1.4% per year, and at age 50 years, prevalence is typically 25–50%, occasionally 80%. In a representative sample ($n = 2,581$) from the United States in 1988–1991, seroprevalence is 25% (95% CI 22–28%) at age 6–19 years. **OUTBREAKS**: An outbreak of gastritis following gastric intubation has retrospectively been attributed to *H. pylori*.

HENIPAVIRUS (enveloped RNA viruses: *Mononegavirales*: *Paramyxoviridae*). These are measles-related viruses from bats.

Hendra virus (5277, 5755) emerged in Queensland, Australia, in 1994. Host are *Pteropus* fruit bats. **SPREAD**: is from horses to humans; involvement of bats is elusive so far. **CLINICAL INFORMATION**: The incubation period is likely 4–18 days. Manifestations: flulike illness, encephalitis. **OUTBREAKS**: An epizootic in horses in Australia.

Nipah virus (1440, 3463) emerged in Malaysia and Singapore in 1998. The host is *Pteropus* fruit bats. **SPREAD**: is via pig contact and nosocomially, perhaps by contact with patients. **CLINICAL INFORMATION**: Some 10% of infections are subclinical. The incubation period seems short. Manifestations: encephalitis. In Malaysia, Singapore, and Bangladesh. In Malaysia in 1999, an outbreak caused 265 cases of encephalitis with 105 (40%) deaths, mainly among pig farmers.

HEPACIVIRUS (enveloped RNA viruses: *Flaviviridae*). Prototype is hepatitis C virus (HCV) (173, 1063, 1344, 1536, 5993, 6389, 7248, 8011, 8156).

HCV occurs in humans worldwide. There are six major genotypes, and subtypes. Main genotypes are 1 and 2 in West Africa, 4 in Central Africa, and 3 and 6 in Asia. Subtypes in injection drug users (IDU) include 3a and 1a.

HCV is susceptible to glutaraldehyde disinfectant. **SPREAD**: is via reused or shared, or nonsterile injections, ritual instruments, or other materials contaminated with blood, injury from work with infective blood or likely other body fluids, infrequently mother-to-child, by household contact, or sex. A proposed mode is tick bite. **RISKS**: IDU (in >50% of cases in high income countries), having multiple sex partners, sex among men, hemophiliacs receiving blood products of the 1980s. Since tests became available in the 1990s, blood products no longer constitute a significant risk (Fig. 20.4). **CLINICAL INFORMATION**: From 70% to 85% of new infections are inapparent. Confirmation is by third-generation antibody tests or NAT (detection limit ~500 RNA copies per ml). Unfortunately to date, tests cannot discern recent from chronic infection. The incubation period is 6–26 (typically 4–10) weeks. Manifestations: fatigue, arthralgia, jaundice. After follow-up for >20 years, >45% of untreated infections had resolved, 45% had evolved to chronic hepatitis (with persisting viremia), ~0.5–20% to cirrhosis (high estimate from retrospective studies in liver units, low from cohort community studies), and ≤0.05% to hepatocellular carcinoma. In North America, about two thirds of persons are unaware of their HCV infection. Cleared infection does not protect from reinfection. **IMPACT**: Population seroprevalences are 0.5–2% in high-income countries, and 2–5% in low-income countries, for a range of 0% to >20%. Seroprevalence peaks in adults. In France, the seroconversion rate in blood donors is ~2 (95% CI 1–3)/10^5 person-years. By age, geography, and diagnostic criteria, reported rates of acute HC are 1–4/10^5 per year. In North America, 40% of chronic liver disease is attributable to HCV. In IDU, the rate of HCV-associated cirrhosis is ~3/1,000 person-years. **OUTBREAKS**: Nosocomial venues for outbreaks included a pain clinic, emergency room, hemodialysis unit, and oncology ward. Contaminated anti-D immune globulin was an outbreak vehicle.

HEPATITIS A VIRUS (HAV). See Hepatovirus.

HEPATITIS B VIRUS (HBV). See Orthohepadnavirus.

HEPATITIS C VIRUS (HCV). See Hepacivirus.

HEPATITIS D SUBVIRUS (HDV). See Orthohepadnavirus.

HEPATITIS E VIRUS (HCV). See Hepevirus.

"HEPATITIS G" VIRUS. See GB virus C (GBV-C).

HEPATOVIRUS (unenveloped RNA viruses: *Picornaviridae*). Prototype is hepatitis A virus (HAV) (637, 1251, 2393, 3621, 3687, 5210).

HAV circulates worldwide, in humans, feces, fresh and marine waters, and handled foods. HAV is inactivated on surfaces by formalin or bleach (NaOCl), in water by heat (85°C for 1 min) or free chlorine. **SPREAD**: is via contact with incubating or ill persons, or via polluted foods or tap water. **RISKS**: residence in or travel to (hyper)endemic or outbreak areas, patient contacts, food work, and research work. In the United States, reported sources include households (in 14% of cases), sex among men (in 8%), day care (in 8%), IDUs (in 5%), international travel (in 5%), and foods (in 4%); in half of cases, a source was not known. In Europe, travel accounts for 20–40% of sporadic HA cases. The infective dose is 10–100 virus particles. HAV is detected in feces from 2 weeks before disease onset (d_0, jaundice) for several months after d_0, but patients are considered noninfectious 1 week after d_0. **CLINICAL INFORMATION**: From 70% to 90% of infections in children and 30–75% in adults are inapparent. Subclinically infected children are a major reservoir, but there is no chronic carrier state. Anti-HAV IgM confirm recent infection, anti-HAV IgG confirm past infection or vaccination. By infective dose, the incubation period is 2–7 (typically 4) weeks. Manifestations: nausea, fever, jaundice. Lethality is 0.02–0.3% overall, but 1.8-2.5% in patients older than 50 years of age or with chronic liver

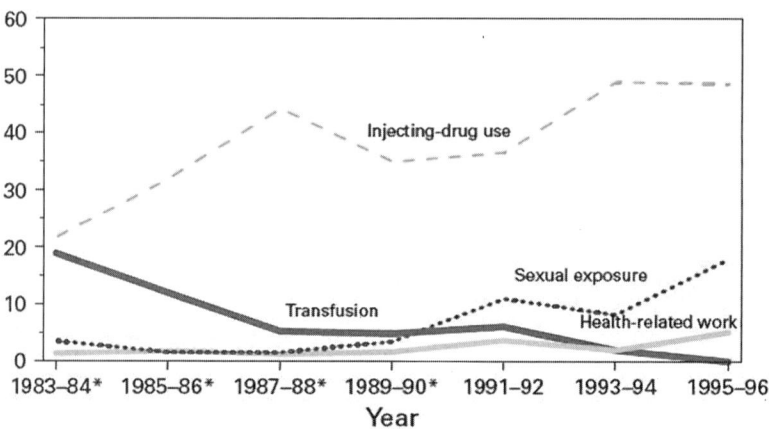

Figure 20.4 Risk groups of acute hepatitis C, United States, 1983-1996. Values are the percentage among all cases (*y* axis) by reporting years (*x* axis) and risks (IDU, sex, transfusion, health work). Asterisks indicate non-A, non-B hepatitis. From reference 173.

disease. IMPACT: Worldwide, 1–10 million new infections occur per year. Three levels of endemicity are described:

(a) HAV is hyperendemic in Africa, where most preschool children become infected, at rates $>30/10^5$ per year. By age 15 years, $\geq$95% of people are seroreactive. As a result, most acute hepatitis in adults is not due to HAV.

(b) HAV is mesoendemic in Latin America and much of Asia where children and youths acquire HAV at rates of $15–30/10^5$ per year. At school age, $\sim$30–50% are seroreactive, and only after age 30 years $\geq$95% of people are reactive. In an area of Nicaragua where >90% of domiciles had indoor tap water, and 40% had flush toilets, the rate of HAV infection in the placebo arm of a vaccine trial was $\sim$15/100 person-years. Outbreaks are a threat in mesoendemic areas, and universal vaccination is recommended.

(c) HAV is hypoendemic in high-income countries. Of children and adolescents, <10–20% are seroreactive, and most nonvaccinated adults remain susceptible. In the United Kingdom, from oral fluid testing and when excluding vaccinees, the population seroprevalence is currently 7–11%. Reported disease rates per 10^5 per year are 1–15 ($\sim$3 in the United States and 2–3 in Germany), although true rates are likely several times higher when corrected for underreporting. Hypoendemic countries should consider targeted vaccination. OUTBREAKS: Venues for outbreaks include populations, homosexual communities, and travel destinations. Attack rates can reach 4–11%. Examples of large epidemics are Greenland in 1970–1974 (4,961 cases, attack rate 11%), Shanghai in 1988 (by raw clams, nearly 300,000 HA cases, attack rate 4%). Effective vaccines are available. In the United States, routine vaccination of children in high-incidence states was paralleled by declining rates of acute HA, from $\sim$10/10^5 per year in 1987–1997 to $\sim$3/10^5 in 2002. Mass vaccination can interrupt outbreaks.

HEPEVIRUS (unenveloped RNA viruses: *Hepeviridae*). Prototype is hepatitis E virus (HEV) (94, 1734, 2201, 4985, 6063). Genotypes are reported in birds, rodents, monkeys, domestic pigs, and humans. HEV is heat stable. Human HEV circulates in feces, sewage, and water, mainly in low-income countries. SPREAD: is via polluted drinking water and by contact, although secondary spread in households is much less frequent in HEV (1–2%) than HAV (15%). RISKS: rural domicile in or visit to endemic area, use of river water for bathing, defecation, and drinking, and contact with pigs. Fecal shedding begins 1 week before illness onset and lasts 2–4 weeks. CLINICAL INFORMATION: Surprisingly, and in contrast to HAV, children largely escape HEV, except in outbreaks. The incubation period is 2–9 weeks (5 weeks in experimental infection). Manifestations: brief viremia, anorexia (in 66–100%), and jaundice (in $\sim$100%). Pregnant women are unusually susceptible, for attack rates twice that of nonpregnant women, fulminant course in 10–20%, abortion, and premature birth. Lethality is 0.2–4% (up to 20% in pregnant women). Tests to discern "Non-A, non-B hepatitis" as HCV or HEV became available in the 1990s. Acute infection is confirmed by NAT or anti-HEV IgM; IgG can persist for years or regress within months. IMPACT: In low-income countries, seroprevalences in healthy adults is, in general, <15–25%, although in rural Southeast Asia and Egypt prevalence >45% has been reported. Large population segments remain susceptible to sporadic or epidemic HEV. In the Kathmandu Valley of Nepal, infections in persons 12–48 years of age monitored for 12 months occurred at a rate of 10/100 person-years, while the disease rate was 4.5/100 person-years. In high-income countries, acute HE is infrequent and mostly travel related, but the disease can be contracted locally. Seroprevalence is typically low (0.5–5%), although in parts of the United States $\sim$20% of blood donors have been reactive. OUTBREAKS: More than 50 outbreaks have been reported, mainly in Africa and Asia, from water, and in adolescents and young adults. Examples include Delhi, India, in 1955–1956 (29,300 jaundice cases, attack rate 2.3%, diagnosed in retrospect), Ahmedabad, India, in 1975–1976 (2,572 cases), Medea, Algeria, in 1980–1981 (788 cases), Somalia in 1988 (11,413 cases), Kanpur, India, in 1991 (79,000 cases, attack rate 3.8%), Islamabad, Pakistan in 1994 (3,827 cases, attack rate 10.4%), and Sudan in 2004 (>6,800 cases).

HERPES SIMPLEX VIRUS (HSV, OR HUMAN HERPES VIRUS). See Simplexvirus.

HETEROPHYES (1289, 8236, 8356) (Trematoda: Digenea). These flukes circulate in Asia and Africa, in carnivores (e.g., cats) and humans (final hosts and shed eggs in feces), freshwater and brackish water snails (first intermediate hosts), and fish (second hosts). Over 20 species have been reported in humans, including *H. heterophyes*, and *H. nocens*. SPREAD: is by uptake of viable metacercariae from undercooked fish. CLINICAL INFORMATION: The prepatent period is 1–2 weeks. Adults locate in the intestine. Most infections are inapparent. Confirmation is by visualizing operculate eggs in stool or duodenal fluid. The reported incubation period is 9 days. Manifestations: abdominal discomfort. IMPACT: In enzootic areas; the reported prevalence in humans is 0.01–11%.

HISTOPLASMA (*Ascomycota*: *Onygenales*). Prototype is *H. capsulatum* (62, 1060, 1233, 1296, 2321, 2990, 4423, 4590, 5193) of which two varieties exist: *H. capsulatum capsulatum* in warm climates, and *H. capsulatum duboisii* in Africa. *H. capsulatum* is a dimorphic fungus: filamentous in soil, yeastlike in human tissue. *H. capsulatum* grows in nitrate- and phosphate-rich soils, often in association with bird and bat excrements. Filaments release spores (micro- and macroconidia). ACQUISITION: is via inhalation of spores from dust, occasionally via transplants. RISKS: domicile in or visit to endemic area, visits to caves, bird- or bat-inhabited buildings or trees, cleaning bird roosts, cutting down trees in which birds have roosted, soil-disturbing activities, e.g., farm work, construction work inside and outside of buildings. CLINICAL INFORMATION: Over 95% of sporadic infections but only 20–50% of epidemic infections are inapparent. The incubation period is 4–18 (often 7-14) days. *H. capsulatum capsulatum* can cause flulike illness, acute or chronic pneumonia (can mimick tuberculosis), and invasive disease (in immune-impaired hosts). For *H. capsulatum duboisii*, skin and bone infections are typical. Confirmation is by culture, biopsy (lung, skin), serology, or antigen test from urine (disseminated disease). IMPACT: In a 1992–1993 population study, the rate of invasive histoplasmosis was $0.7/10^5$ per year. OUTBREAKS: Venues for outbreaks from dust or bat droppings included cities, a school, a hotel, an industrial plant, a prison, a belfry, and caves. In Mason City, Iowa, in 1962, 8,400 residents became infected by dust from bulldozing. For construction and demolition work in endemic areas, protective gear is advised.

HOOKWORM. *See* Ancylostoma.

HUMAN HERPES VIRUS 1, 2 (HERPES SIMPLEX VIRUS, HSV1, 2). *See* Simplexvirus.

HUMAN HERPES VIRUS 3 (VARICELLA-ZOSTER VIRUS, VZV). *See* Varicellovirus.

HUMAN HERPES VIRUS 4 (EPSTEIN-BARR VIRUS, EBV). *See* Lymphocryptovirus.

HUMAN HERPES VIRUS 5 (HHV5). *See* Cytomegalovirus (CMV).

HUMAN HERPES VIRUS 6 (HHV6). *See* Roseolovirus.

HUMAN HERPES VIRUS 7 (HHV7) (enveloped DNA viruses: *Herpesviridae*: β). Persists in human blood cells.

HUMAN HERPES VIRUS 8 (HHV8). *See* Rhadinovirus.

HUMAN IMMUNODEFICIENCY VIRUS (HIV). *See* Lentivirus.

HUMAN PAPILLOMAVIRUS (HPV). *See* Papillomavirus.

HUMAN T-LYMPHOTROPIC VIRUS (HTLV). *See* Deltaretrovirus.

HYMENOLEPIS (Cestoda: Cyclophyllidea). Of these dwarf cestodes, *H. diminuta* and *H. nana* infect humans.
  H. diminuta (4727, 5474) circulates in rodents (final hosts, shed eggs), beetles, flea larvae, and other coprophilic insects (intermediate hosts, carry metacestodes). SPREAD: is via uncooked, beetle-pested foods, or incidental ingestion of fleas. IMPACT: Infections in humans are rare. Fecal prevalence can be 0.5% focally.
  H. nana (2240, 3757, 4626, 6938) circulates worldwide, in rodents and humans (final hosts, shed infective eggs), optionally in coprophilic insects. Life span of adults is weeks or months. SPREAD: is by uptake of eggs, via hands, autoinfection, or fecally polluted foods. RISKS: substandard homes, no sanitation, being a child or an orphan, having an infected sibling, day care. CLINICAL INFORMATION: The prepatent period is 3–4 weeks. Most infections are inapparent. The incubation period is ~2 weeks. Manifestations: vague, perhaps anal itch, abdominal pain. Treatment options include praziquantel and niclosamide. IMPACT: By age and habitat, prevalence in low-income countries is 0.01–20% (typically 0.5–3%). In Peru in 1999, at an elevation of 3,910 m, the prevalence in 338 Quechua schoolchildren was 17%.

INFLUENZAVIRUS (3973) (enveloped RNA viruses: *Orthomyxoviridae*). *Influenzavirus* circulates worldwide, in birds, mammals, and humans. Core proteins define types (A, B, C); envelope hemagglutinins (H1–15) and neuraminidases (N1–9) define A subtypes.
  Avian influenza A virus (1467, 4056, 5813, 7163). Water birds are natural reservoir, and birds support all A subtypes (see section 3.7). SPREAD: is via contact with poultry or other birds that shed virus with excrement or secretions. Avian-to-human spread is confirmed for subtypes A/H5N1, A/H7N2, A/H7N3, A/H7N7, A/H9N2, and A/H10N7. Manifestations: conjunctivitis, flulike illness, pneumonia, or highly lethal disease. OUTBREAKS: Production of vaccines requires new methods, including whole virus, enhanced adjuvants, and reverse genetics.
  Human influenza A virus (876, 2466, 2530, 3152, 3232, 5420, 7402, 7672). To date, only A subtypes H1-3, N1-2 are sustained in humans. SPREAD: is via droplets, aerosols, and hand contacts, probably via objects, rarely via contact with pigs or birds. RISKS: cold weather, indoor life, crowded rooms, public transports. Infectiousness is high. R_0 estimates are of 1.5–2 in seasonal waves and 3–20 in pandemics. Beginning 1 day before illness onset, adults shed virus for ~3–5 days, children shed virus for ~3 weeks, and immune-impaired hosts shed virus for longer periods. The infective dose is low (few virus particles). Droplets are less effective in causing

lower respiratory tract infections (RTIs) than aerosols (<5 (m). **CLINICAL INFORMATION:** By age and setting, 25–65% (typically 50%) of infections are inapparent. The incubation period is 1-4 (typically 2) days. Manifestations: cough, headache, malaise, myalgia, fever (flu-like illness). Diagnosis is supported by rapid (30 min) antigen tests and confirmed by virus isolation, ideally from nasopharyngeal fluids (swab or wash). Comorbidities and viral (RSV, PIV), or bacterial (*N. meningitidis* and *S. pneumoniae*) co- or superinfections can precipitate complications: croup, sinusitis, otitis media, pneumonia, multiorgan failure. Overall lethality is ≤0.01%. Elderly and comorbid persons account for 15% of patients but 70–95% of deaths. **IMPACT:** The attack rate in "regular" seasons is 1–5% in adults, and up to 20% in children. In the 2003–2004 U.S. flu season, 19% (24,649/130,577) of submitted respiratory specimens yielded influenza-viruses (99% A and 1% B); among 7,191 A isolates subtyped, 99.9% were A/H3N2. In the U.S. 2001–2002 flu season, yield had been 16% (15,671/100,671, 87% A, 13% B). By season, influenza viruses account for 5–20% of RTI in children. Hospitalization rates per 10^5 are high (120–1,000) at age <5 years, intermediate (125–250) at age ≥65 years, and low (0–40) at age 5–65 years. **OUTBREAKS:** Disease rates above a threshold define epidemic periods. In the United Kingdom and The Netherlands, the threshold is 50 flulike cases per 10^5 per week over successive weeks. Average epidemics last ≤10 weeks. Serious epidemics can strain health services.

Global spread, high attack rates, and high excess mortality characterize pandemics of which four have occurred: in 1918–1919 (by A/H1N1, "Spanish flu"), 1957–1958 (by A/H2N2, "Asian flu"), 1968–1969 (by A/H3N2, "Hong Kong flu"), and 1977–1978 (by A/H1N1, "Russian flu"). The 1918–1919 pandemic caused >50 million deaths worldwide in 18 months and perhaps arose in a British military camp in France in winter of 1917. Attack rates in pandemics can reach 40–50%. Excess mortality per 10^5 was 218 in 1918–1919, 22 in 1957–1958, and 14 in 1968–1969. Pandemics are unpredictable and believed to arise when a genetically reassorted (antigenic shift) virus hits susceptible populations.

Vaccines became available after World War II. From meta-analyses, vaccines are 80% (95% CI 74–90) effective in children and 77% (95% CI 66–85) in working adults. From randomized trials or cohort studies, effectiveness is 52% (95% CI 29–67) in community elderly and 60% in nursing homes. Vaccine targets include groups at risk of complications (e.g., age 0.5–2 and ≥65 years, cardiopulmonary comorbidity), and likely spreaders (e.g., health workers).

ISOSPORA (Apicomplexa: Eucoccidiorida). Of perhaps 250 species (many nonvalidated) in mammals, only I. belli (1273, 4443) infects humans. This coccidian circulates in warm climates, in humans who shed unsporulated oocysts with feces, and the environment. Unlike *Sarcocystis*, *Isospora* oocysts (contain two sporocysts, each with four sporozoites) need to sporulate to be infective; under optimal conditions, this takes <24 h. **SPREAD:** is likely via foods or tap water, possibly hand contacts or sex. **CLINICAL INFORMATION:** Few (<10%) infections seem to remain inapparent. The incubation period is not known. Manifestations: self-limited diarrhea, urticaria (in 5%), and eosinophilia (in up to 30%), in immune-impaired hosts chronic diarrhea or invasive disease. Confirmation is by visualizing *unsporulated* oocysts in stool or duodenal fluid. A treatment option is co-trimoxazole. **IMPACT:** Reported fecal prevalences are 0–0.4%

JAPANESE ENCEPHALITIS VIRUS (JEV). See Flavivirus.

JUNÍN VIRUS (JUNV). See Arenavirus.

KINGELLA (β-*Proteobacteria*: *Neisseriales*). Of these gram-negative coccobacilli, *K. kingae* (2332, 8306) colonizes the oropharynx of children. **SPREAD:** Infections are endogenous, or acquired via droplets or saliva. Manifestations: bacteremia, septic arthritis, and osteomyelitis. Mainly children (immune-competent) are affected; viral coinfections may cause *K. kingae* to become invasive. **IMPACT:** Of healthy children, 2–14% are colonized. The reported disease rate is $10/10^5$ children per year.

KLEBSIELLA (γ-*Proteobacteria*: *Enterobacteriales*). These capsulated, gram-negative rods are widespread in water, sewage, soil, and plants, but also on mucosa of mammals. In humans, mainly *K. pneumoniae*, *K. oxytoca*, and *K. granulomatis* (ex-*Calymmatobacterium granulomatis*) are isolated.

K. granulomatis (811, 1100, 5532) circulates in humans, mainly in some low-income countries (South Africa, French Guiana, India, and New Guinea) and minority communities. **SPREAD:** is mainly via sex and occasionally via hand and skin contacts or vaginal delivery. **CLINICAL INFORMATION:** The incubation period is 1 day to 1 year (usually 2–8 weeks). Manifestations: ulcerogranulomatous genital and perianal skin lesions (donovanosis), extragenital disease (in ~6%), e.g., otitis, osteomyelitis. Confirmation is by biopsy. Cell culture (since the 1990s) and (noncommercial) NAT are available. A treatment option is azithromycine. **IMPACT:** In Cayenne, French Guiana, in 1970–1980, the disease rate among African American residents was $\sim4/10^5$ per year.

K. pneumoniae (1937, 2656, 4013, 4043, 6048, 7558, 7587) is an opportunist that colonizes human nasopharynx and bowel. Presence on skin, e.g., hands, is transient, but epidemiologically significant. Strains that produce extended-spectrum β-lactamases (ESβL, resistant to cephalosporins) are increasingly isolated in hospitals. SPREAD: Infections can be endogenous or acquired, via hands or contaminated objects; droplets from patients are not a reported vehicle. RISKS: invasive procedures, devices, recent use of β-lactam antibiotics. Impaired immunity (e.g., preterm babies and diabetics) and comorbidity (e.g., chronic obstructive lung disease) predispose to invasive disease. CLINICAL INFORMATION: The incubation period seems short (<48 h). Manifestations: urinary tract infection (UTI), surgical site infection (SSI), pneumonia, bloodstream infection (BSI), meningitis, and *Klebsiella* liver abscess. Pneumonia and BSI are mainly nosocomial but can be community acquired (e.g., in alcoholics). Lethality is 1%, that of invasive disease is 25–50%. IMPACT: For impact in hospitals, see section VI. OUTBREAKS: Numerous nosocomial outbreaks are reported, ~20 in neonatal intensive care units (ICU).

K. oxytoca (609, 1853, 3688, 6207) survives in hot springs, can biodegrade insecticides, and is innately resistant to cephalosporins (due to chromosomal ESβL). Clinically and epidemiologically it behaves like *K. pneumoniae*, with outbreaks from environmental sources and hands as vehicles.

KURU. See prions.

KYASANUR FOREST DISEASE VIRUS (KFDV). See Flavivirus.

LACAZIA (ex-*Loboa*) (*Ascomycota*: *Onygenales*). *L. loboi* (2192, 2405) is a dimorphic fungus that inhabits water and soil in tropical Latin America. SPREAD: is via contact or trauma. RISKS: fresh or marine water work, e.g., fishermen, farmers, gold miners, rubber workers, hunters, dolphin caretakers. Manifestations (lobomycosis): verrucous, vegetative, ulcerated, or keloidlike skin lesions. IMPACT: Over 500 cases reported to date.

LACTOBACILLUS (*Firmicutes*: *Lactobacillales*) (1057). These gram-positive rods colonize the intestinal tract of birds and mammals, and foods from animals and plants. *Lactobacillus* is part of the flora of human buccal and bowel mucosa and of the vagina. In comorbid patients (malignancy and diabetes), *Lactobacillus* can cause bacteremia (>120 cases reported) or endocarditis (>70 cases).

LASSA VIRUS (LASV). See Arenavirus.

LEGIONELLA (γ-*Proteobacteria*: *Legionellales*). These are intracellular, gram-negative bacteria that inhabit natural and artificial waters and muddy soils worldwide. There are >40 species, including *L. pneumophila* (~90% of clinical isolates), *L. bozemanii*, and *L. longbeachae*. *Legionella* can persist in free-living amebas and in biofilms, as "viable but not culturable" agents.

L. pneumophila (2625, 3739, 3751, 5073, 5265) has several serogroups (and >40 subtypes); serogroup 1 accounts for 70–85% of cases. SPREAD: is via inhalation of aerosols, or (micro)aspiration of contaminated water, but not person-to-person. RISKS: hotel and private whirlpools and spas, proximity to cooling towers, poorly used or maintained domestic and hospital water supplies, hot tap water. Comorbidities (lung disease and diabetes), age (>50 years), smoking, alcoholism, impaired immunity (corticoids and transplant recipients), and intubation increase susceceptibility. CLINICAL INFORMATION: Up to 40% of infections are inapparent. The incubation period is 0.5–10 (typically 3–7) days. Manifestations: Pontiac fever (flulike), Legionnaire's disease (pneumonia). In travel-related cases, the female:male ratio is >2:1. Confirming tests are not ideal and include urine antigen test (takes <1 h, 70–90% sensitive, for serogroup 1 only), culture (from lower respiratory tract sample or blood, 10–80% sensitive, takes 3–7 days), and serology (from paired samples, 60–80% sensitive). By setting, case mix, and management, lethality is 1–30%. IMPACT: Most cases are sporadic. Reported disease rates are $0.1–2/10^5$ per year (the United States 10-year average is $\sim 0.5/10^5$ per year). By test and cutoff, reported seroprevalence is 0–20% (often 2%). OUTBREAKS: The first outbreak in Philadelphia in 1976 caused 182 cases and 29 (16%) deaths. Settings for outbreaks included urban aerosol-generating sites, industrial plants, fairs, hotels, office buildings, and hospitals. In Australia in 1991–2000, 22 *L. pneumophila* serogroup 1 outbreaks caused 246 cases (11 per outbreak). In Europe in 2000–2002, 60% (113/189) of reported outbreaks were travel related (315 cases, 3 per outbreak), 20% (38) were community acquired (1,059 cases, 28 per outbreak), 19% (36) were nosocomial (211 cases, 6 per outbreak), and 1% (2) had private home sources (four cases). In Murcia, Spain, in 2001, the "world's largest" legionella outbreak caused 449 confirmed and 636–696 cases.

LEISHMANIA (Euglenozoa: Kinetoplastida) (1758, 1895, 4114, 5275). Over 20 species circulate in Old and New World areas with warm climates, in sandflies (infective promastigotes), mammals, and humans (intracellular amastigotes) (Table 20.3). Treatment options for visceral, disfiguring, disseminated, or relapsing disease are limited and include pentavalent antimonials, miltefosine, pentamidine, and terbinafine. Resistance to antimonials is a problem in India and is emerging in Africa. Preventive measures include sandfly-proofed housing, garbage removal, residual insecticides, animal corrals away from

Table 20.3 Leishmaniases of humans: types, geography, agents, sandfly vectors, risks, and reservoirs

Type[a]	Range	*Leishmania* species	Sandfly vector	Areas of risk	Reservoir
ACL	Asia	*L. tropica*	*Phlebotomus sergenti*	Urban	Humans
ZCL	Africa, Asia	*L. major*	*P. papatasi*	Arid areas	Rodents
	Latin America	*L. braziliensis* sl, *L. mexicana* sl	*Lutzomyia* spp.	Forests, rural	Small mammals
AVL	Sudan, India	*L. donovani*	*P. argentipes*	Urban	Humans
ZVL	Mediterranean	*L. infantum*	*P. perniciosus*	Chapparal	Dogs, carnivores
	Latin America	*L. infantum* (= *L. chagasi*)	*L. longipalpis*	Peridomestic	Dogs, carnivores

[a]L, leishmaniasis; AC, anthroponotic-cutaneous; AV, anthroponotic-visceral; ZC, zoonotic-cutaneous; ZV, zoonotic-visceral.

domiciles, repellents for dogs and humans, impregnated bednets, and prompt case detection and treatment.

Mucocutaneous leishmaniasis (CL) (121, 1820, 1825, 3627, 5582, 6233, 8010, 8303). Agents carried in the Old World by *Phlebotomus* include zoonotic *L. major* and anthroponotic *L. tropica*. Main agents carried in the New World by *Lutzomyia* include zoonotic *L. braziliensis* sl (*L. guyanensis*, *L. panamensis*, and *L. peruviana*) and *L. mexicana* sl (*L. amazonensis* and *L. pifanoi*). Dermotropism is not strict, as *L. tropica* and *L. braziliensis* sl have been reported in visceral infections. **SPREAD**: is via sandfly bite and rarely needle stick. **RISKS**: domicile in and visit to enzootic-endemic areas, substandard housing, solitary homes, tall trees on premises, nocturnal outdoor activities, noncompliance with mosquito protection. Of 310 U.S. soldiers who acquired Old World CL in Iraq, only 17% had ever impregnated uniforms, and only 10% had slept under bednets. **CLINICAL INFORMATION**: Up to 90% of infections are inapparent. The incubation period is 1 day to 6 months (often 4 weeks). Skin manifestations vary by species (virulence), host (immunity), and habitat (humid lowlands and dry highlands). Skin lesions, typically located at exposed parts, can be papulous, nodulous ("dry"), erosive, ulcerous ("wet"), or mucosal ("espundia", ≤20% of cases). Most (≤90%) skin lesions heal spontaneously in 3–18 months. Mucosal lesions can persist for years and spread lymphogenously, hematogenously, or diffusely. Confirmation is by microscopy, NAT, or culture, from scrapings, punch biopsy, or blood buffy coat. Diagnostic yield can be <40%. **IMPACT**: By leishmanin skin testing in enzootic or endemic areas, the prevalence of past or ongoing infection is 2–40%. By clinical examination, the active disease prevalence is 0.05–10%. The reported infection rate is 3–23/100 person-years. In Brazil in 1982–2002, the reported disease rate was 5–23/10^5 per year. Actual disease rates could reach 0.05–2% per year or more. In the 2000s, there were 1–2 million new cases per year (>90% from Algeria; Brazil, Peru; Afghanistan, Iran, Iraq, Saudi Arabia, and Syria). **OUTBREAKS**: Venues for outbreaks included the community, a shanty town, a refugee camp, a coffee plantation, and troops (with attack rates of up to 3%). During an epidemic of zoonotic CL in Sudan in 1986–1987, ~10,000 patients reported to hospitals in 6 months. In Rio Grande do Norte, Brazil, in 1987, 407 zoonotic CL cases occurred in one municipality, for an attack rate of 1.3%. Anthroponotic CL has caused outbreaks in Kabul, Afghanistan, at an altitude of 1,850 m.

Visceral leishmaniasis (VL) (72, 445, 1795, 2646, 7796). Anthroponotic *L. donovani* circulates in *Phlebotomus* and humans in East Africa and the Indian subcontinent. Zoonotic *L. infantum* (=*L. chagasi*) circulates in West Africa, the Mediterranean, Asia, and Latin America, in dogs, humans, and sandflies. Viscerotropism is not strict because *L. donovani* and *L. infantum* can cause mucocutaneous disease. **SPREAD**: is via sandfly bite, rarely by needle stick, organ transplant, blood transfusion, mother-to-child, or perhaps needle-sharing among IDUs. **RISKS**: domicile in or visit to an enzootic-endemic areas, having a case in the household, sleeping downstairs or outdoors in summer, house with mud walls or floors, peridomestic garbage, and dogs or cattle on premises. **CLINICAL INFORMATION**: From 25% to 95% of infections are inapparent or "latent." The incubation period is ≤10 days to ≥2 years (often 2–3 months). Manifestations (kala azar): prolonged fever (in >95%), weight loss ("hot skin and bones"), epistaxis, splenomegaly, and anemia. Signs can be purely mucosal (gingivitis and nasal vegetation). Complications include immune nonresponsiveness (anergy), post-kala azar dermal leishmaniasis (PKDL, in 3–10% of treated cases), and HIV coinfection. Confirmation is by NAT (blood), microscopy (spleen or bone marrow aspirate), or culture (buffy coat). Lethality is 75–95% untreated, but 5–15% with treatment. **IMPACT**: VL occurs in >60 countries. There are ~0.5 million new cases per year (90% in Sudan; Brazil; Bangladesh, India, and Nepal). Reported prevalences of past or current infections in enzootic-endemic areas are 2–25% (by serology) to 5–50% (by nonspecific skin test), while parasitologically confirmed disease prevalences in India were 1.5–13%. By age, location, intensity of transmission, and test, reported infection rates are 1,000–10,000/10^5 per year and disease rates are ~5–650/10^5 per year. **OUTBREAKS**: Massive epidemics occurred in Bihar, India, in 1977 (100,000 cases), Sudan in 1984–1989 (>100,000 deaths) and Bihar in 1991–1992 (250,000 cases). Smaller outbreaks occurred in Emilia-Romagna, Italy, in 1971–1972 (91 infections, 60 cases, and 13 [22%] deaths), in a city in Brazil in 1989–1992, and in a refugee camp in Kenya in 2000.

LENTIVIRUS (3063, 5805) (enveloped RNA viruses: *Retroviridae*). *Lentivirus* includes human (HIV), feline (FIV), and simian (SIV) immunodeficiency viruses. SIV is prevalent in African monkeys. By crossing species via contact, secretions, or possibly monkey foods, SIVs have given rise to HIV.

Human immunodeficiency virus (HIV) (1231, 3105, 3626, 6487, 6763, 7146, 8108). Although of simian origin, reservoirs of HIV1 and HIV2 are limited to humans. Sources of HIV are blood, vaginal secretions, semen, and breastmilk. Of HIV1, a number of subtypes are described. SPREAD: is via sex among men or heterosexual sex, mother-to-child (intrauterine, perinatally, and breastmilk), and via injections (IDU, occupational trauma) or transfusions. Driving forces are in sub-Saharan Africa heterosexual sex (>85% of infections), work (migrant, transport), and mother-to-child transmission (10%); in Asia sex work, IDU, and drug trafficking (in golden triangle); in high-income countries homosexual sex (~38%) and IDU (36%). Viremia is high in initial (primary) and late (AIDS) infection, and low in-between or on treatment. Of HIV infections, 80–100% are spread before HIV is manifest as AIDS. Transmission rates vary with source and range from ≥90% for blood transfusion to virtually nil for insertive oral sex (Table 13.2). RISKS: IDU, sex work, casual sex, unsafe injections, unsafe blood products. In the United States, main risks are male-male sex (overall, 44%; among males, 61%; among females, zero), IDU overall, 16%; males, 15%; females, 19%), and high-risk male-female sex (sex with infected or risk-behaving partner, overall, 34%; males, 17%; females, 78%). CLINICAL INFORMATION: Primary infections can be inapparent or mild, flulike. Infection is confirmed by two-step antibody test, or NAT. In high-income countries, 20–60% of infected individuals are not tested, tested late, or unaware of the result (in the United States, one fourth). Of U.S. adults (age 18–64 years), 10–12% have been tested in the preceding 12 months, and 37–39% have been tested in their lifetime. The incubation period (to AIDS) is 2–6 years in children, 3–9 years in adults in Africa or Asia, and 10–11 years in adults in high-income counries. Manifestations of AIDS include diarrhea, weight loss, fever, reactivated and acquired opportunistic diseases, and HIV-induced malignancies. Lethality is close to 100%, but highly active antiretroviral therapy (HAART) can significantly delay AIDS and prolong survival. In Europe pre-HAART, median survival periods from seroconversion were 8–12 years. IMPACT: To date, ~40 million children and adults are HIV infected worldwide. Infection prevalences in adults are 0.6% in North America, 0.3–0.6% in West and East Europe, and 0.1–30% in low-income countries: 8% in sub-Saharan Africa (<1% in North, 2–6% in West, 5–15% in urban East, 15–30% in urban South Africa), 0.5–4% in Latin America, 0.1–10% in Asia. New infections are ~4–6 million per year (70–100/10^5 per year): 1–2% in high-income countries (including 40,000 each in North America and Europe), two thirds in Africa, and nearly one third in remaining low-income countries. In the United States in 2003, the age-adjusted rate of diagnosed HIV/AIDS was 20/10^5 per year (28 in males, 11 in females). In Europe in 2003, the reported infection rate was 2.5–25/10^5 per year. In a community trial in Uganda in 1994–1996, the HIV1 infection rate reached 1.5/100 person-years. OUTBREAKS: The current pandemic is a mix of outbreaks in regions and groups at risk. Reemergence in high-income countries in the 2000s calls for new preventive strategies, e.g., integrating HIV into routine medical care (including testing).

LEPTOSPHAERIA (90, 4650) (*Ascomycota*: *Pleosporales*) *Leptosphaeria* is a genus of pigmented molds that inhabit soil and plants. *L. senegalensis* and *L. thompkinsii* can cause (black-grain) eumycetoma. Its relative frequency in eumycetoma is 5% (Mali) to 30% (Mauritania).

LEPTOSPIRA (*Bacteria*: *Spirochaetales*) (632, 3064, 3648, 3718, 4279, 5341, 8091). These are flexible, helical bacteria. Prototype is *L. interrogans*.

L. interrogans circulates worldwide, in mammals, urine, warm freshwater, and wet soil. Infected mammals shed *L. interrogans* for life. There are >24 serogroups and >220 serovars. The 16 genospecies do not match with serogroups. Frequent serogroups are Icterohaemorrhagiae, Pomona, Sejroe, Australis, Grippotyphosa, Canicola, Hebdomadis, and Ballum. SPREAD: is via (i) contact of broken skin or mucosa with polluted water or soil, (ii) swallowing of surface water, (iii) contact with infective animals, (iv) tap water, and (v) work-related trauma from bacteremic blood. RISKS: slum, rural, or flooded domicile, open sewers or rats on premise, rodent contact, dog or cat ownership, activities related to water or muddy soil, waste work, no shoeware for field work, and being male. Of 102 cases in Germany in 1997–2000, 30% were leisure related, 30% were occupational, and the remainder were peridomestic. The male:female ratio is 1.2–19 (often 4) to 1. In temperate climates, transmission is seasonal. CLINICAL INFORMATION: In enzootic areas, 60–90% of infections are inapparent. The incubation period is 1–24 (typically 7–14) days. Manifestations: fever (in >90%), flulike illness (in 30–90%), jaundice (in 5–90%), oliguria or acute renal failure (in ≤30%), meningism or aseptic meningitis (in 25%), and bleeding (in ≤5%). Leptospiremia can persist for 6 weeks. By age and severity,

lethality is 0–20% (often 5%). Confirmation is by serology, NAT, or microscopy of blood or urine. IMPACT: About 0.1 million cases are believed to be hospitalized worldwide annually. By intensity of exposure, reported disease rates are 0.1–100 (often 2)/10^5 per year. In the Caribbean, seroconversion rates of 2.9–3.5% per year have been observed. Reported seroprevalences are 0.1–50% (often 1–10%). OUTBREAKS: Outbreaks are reported in urban areas, among troops, at sportive events, from recreational water contacts, and via drinking water. Protective clothing is recommended for work or leisure water exposure.

LISTERIA (*Firmicutes*: *Bacillales*). These are small, gram-positive rods that inhabit soil, water, plants, and foods. In humans, the main species is *L. monocytogenes*.

L. monocytogenes (342, 2548, 2876, 2936, 5483, 5579, 6355, 6884, 7435) is an intracellular opportunist that colonizes the intestinal tracts of mammals worldwide. Of >10 serotypes, the most frequent in humans are 4b, 1/2a, and 1/2b. Curiously, most outbreaks are due to 4b, while most foods yield 1/2a or 1/2b. *L. monocytogenes* survives 10% salt, temperatures of −0.5 to +45°C ("the agent that comes from the cold"), and vacuum packaging, but is killed by pasteurization or microwave cooking. SPREAD: is via foods or mother-to-child, rarely by animal contact or in the hospital. RISKS: unpasteurized milk products, fermented or salted meat products, raw seafood, delicatessen, and raw vegetables. However, most people regularly ingest low numbers of *L. monocytogenes* without harm. The experimental infective dose that affects 50% of the people (ID_{50}) is high, >10^5 bacteria. Neonates, pregnant women, elderly, and immune-impaired hosts are susceptible. Carriers can shed the agent in stools for months. In mothers of infected neonates, high levels are detected in the amniotic fluid, birth canal, urine, and lochia for up to 10 days after delivery. Inapparent infections are frequent. CLINICAL INFORMATION: The incubation period is 5–12 days (neonates), to 3 months (ingestion), often 2–6 weeks. Manifestations: by age and immune competence, are: fever (60–80%), diarrhea (40–80%), sepsis (10–50%), meningoencephalitis (15–80%, meningeal signs often mild or absent initially), and spontaneous abortion. Confirmation is by culture from blood, CSF, meconium, in outbreaks also from foods and the environment. Lethality in immune-impaired hosts is high (20–30%), in the elderly it is occasionally 60–70%. Of survivors of neurolisteriosis, 30% have sequelae. IMPACT: Worldwide cases are estimated to several thousands per year. By age, dietary habits, and surveillance, the sporadic disease rate is 0.05–1.5 (often 0.1–0.5) per 10^5 per year. In France in 10 years, preventive policies for the food industry reduced rates by about two thirds. *L. monocytogenes* can be recovered from the stool samples of 0.5–15% (often 1–4%) of adults.

OUTBREAKS: Many food-borne outbreaks (see section III) and a few nosocomial outbreaks have been reported.

LOA (Nematoda: Spirurida).

L. loa Filariid *L. loa* (81, 5234, 7309, 7530, 7953) circulates in West and Central Africa, in *Chrysops* flies (infective larvae L3) and humans (adults, microfilariae). A monkey reservoir is not known. The life span of adults is 12–17 years. SPREAD: is via fly bite. RISKS: domicile in endemic areas, outdoor work. CLINICAL INFORMATION: Many infections are inapparent. Adult worms migrate through subcutaneous tissues, microfilariae (mf) circulate in blood during daytime. The prepatent period is 1 year. Manifestations: transient, recurring (Calabar) swellings, subconjunctival worm passage, and eosinophilia. Showing photos of subconjunctival *L. loa* is a means to assess community prevalence. Confirmation is by visualizing mf in day blood (thick film, concentration), serology, or NAT. Mf densities range from <35 to 350,000 per ml. By NAT or serology, the ratio of subpatent to patent (microfilaremic) infections is 3:1. Ivermectin and diethylcarbamazine (DEC) are microfilaricidals. In individuals with mf levels >8,000–50,000 per ml, a complication of DEC treatment is encephalitis. IMPACT: Infected people are estimated to 3–13 million. In endemic areas, reported mf prevalences are 0.5–30%.

LYMPHOCRYPTOVIRUS (enveloped DNA viruses: γ *Herpesviridae*). Prototype is Epstein-Barr virus (EBV, or human herpes virus 4, HHV4).

EBV (1303, 1628, 3299, 4631, 4966, 6641) persists in resting B cells and perhaps periodontitis lesions. Humans with infections can shed EBV intermittently for months or years, mainly from saliva, but also from genital secretions. SPREAD: is via kissing, saliva, sex, or transplants (stem cells, solid organs). CLINICAL INFORMATION: Many infections (>90% in children and 30–80% in young adults) are inapparent. The incubation period is 4–7 weeks. Manifestations: tonsillopharyngitis, mononucleosis (fever, cervical adenopathy, and fatigue), hepatitis, uveitis. Confirmation is by microscopy (atypical lymphocytes in blood smear), serology (heterophilic antibodies), NAT, or other test. Oncogenic strains are associated with B-cell lymphoproliferative disease, Burkitt lymphoma, and nasopharyngeal carcinoma. The role of EBV in the pathogenesis of multiple sclerosis is a research topic. IMPACT: In high-income countries, ~65–80% of young adults are seroreactive. In low-income countries, EBV is acquired early in life, and by age 2–4 years, 35–60% of children can be reactive.

LYMPHOCYTIC CHORIOMENINGITIS VIRUS (LCMV). See *Arenavirus*.

LYSSAVIRUS (1235, 1239, 2152, 3250, 4103, 5988, 6470, 7612, 7963, 8104) (enveloped RNA viruses:

Mononegavirales: *Rhabdoviridae*). The genus comprises seven genotypes. Infections in humans are confirmed for classical rabies virus (genotype 1), European bat lyssaviruses (EBLV1 and 2, genotypes 5 and 6), Australian bat lyssavirus (ABLV, genotype 7), and Duvenhagevirus (genotype 4). Maintenance hosts are terrestrial mammals in the Old and New Worlds for rabies virus, bats for rabies virus in America, insectivorous bats for EBLV in Europe and for rare Duvenhage virus in Zimbabwe, and fruit bats for ABLV in Australia. Source animals for rabies in humans can be different from maintenance animals and include incubating or rabid dogs and cats, livestock, wild terrestrial mammals, and bats (vampire bats in South America). Determinaton of virus variants from cryptic rabies patients provides clues to source animal and geographic provenance of the virus. SPREAD: is via bite, scratch, or mucosal splash, rarely via organ transplant or laboratory work, possibly via inhalation of aerosols in bat-inhabited caves. RISKS: domicile in or travel to enzootic rural areas, contact with nonvaccinated (stray) puppies, work with terrestrial mammals in enzootic areas, bat nonproofed housing. Two cases illustrate the range of risks. In Canada in 2000, a school boy died of bat-derived rabies, 25 days after staying in a wildlife sanctuary cottage where his parents had found a bat in the kitchen and his brother had observed a bat in the bathroom. In Sweden in 2000, a teenage girl died of rabies after visiting family in Thailand, where she took care of the family's puppy that one day returned with bite wounds and died two weeks later. CLINICAL INFORMATION: The incubation period is 5 days to 6–10 years (typically 30–60 days); in cornea recipients, the incubation period has been 9–273 days. Manifestations: mainly as encephalitis (unrest, fever, inability to swallow, and hallucination). Confirmation requires combined (NAT, antigen, and serology) and repeat tests on saliva, CSF, skin (nuchal biopsy), and urine. Rabies is almost always fatal. IMPACT: Worldwide, ~50,000 people die of rabies annually. In the United States, mean case reports per year were 24 in 1946–1949, 1–2 in 1962–1965, and 3 in 1970–2000. Cases reported were 1 in 2001 and 3 in 2002. In Europe in 1977–2000, 281 cases were recorded (12 per year); of these, 30 were imported (mainly in West Europe), and 251 were indigenous (mainly in East Europe, including Turkey). Case reports were 12 in 2001 and 7 in 2002. Worldwide, >20,000 mammals are found rabid annually (>7,000 in the United States). OUTBREAKS: Epizootics can occur at irregular intervals. By driving species (fox and dog), terrestric "fronts" can advance at speeds of 40–200 km/year. Prevention for humans includes bat-proofing of housing, avoiding contacts with wild and stray animals, and vaccine. A problem is the recognition of donors of blood and organs who were incubating rabies.

In 1882, L. Pasteur (1822–1895) administered to a 9-year-old boy vaccine for PEP that he had attenuated by continuous passage of wild virus in rabbits for 3 years. Vaccines available today are effective against classical rabies and apparently against bat genotypes. Recommended indications are risks in enzootic areas from work, leisure or domicile, e.g., workers in animal shelters, pet shops, parks, and laboratories, bikers, trekkers, spelunkers, hunters, children in remote areas.

PEP consists of immediate washing of wounds, rabies Ig, and vaccine. Worldwide, about 10 million PEP per year are administered, for a rate of $400/10^5$ per year in enzootic areas. PEP has been administered to family members of cases, health, laboratory, autopsy, and rescue workers, and animal handlers and caretakers.

MACHUPO VIRUS (MACV). See Arenavirus.

MADURELLA (90, 1801, 4666) (*Ascomycota*: *Dothideales*). These are pigmented molds that inhabit soil and thorny plants. *M. grisea* is cosmopolitan, *M. mycetomatis* is limited to arid areas of the Old World. SPREAD: is via microtrauma. RISKS: work on soil or plants with bare skin. CLINICAL INFORMATION: The presumed incubation period is months to years. Manifestations: black-grain eumycetoma. IMPACT: Relative frequencies in eumycetoma are 50–60% (Brazil and India) for *M. grisea*, and 13% (India) to 65–95% (tropical Africa) for *M. mycetomatis*.

MALASSEZIA (321, 2176, 5208, 6733) (*Basidiomycota*: *Tremellales*). These are lipophilic yeasts that colonize dogs, cats, other mammals, and perhaps the environment. Of ≥7 species, *M. furfur*, *M. globosa*, *M. pachydermatis*, and *M. sympodialis* have been isolated in humans. SPREAD: is apparently via contact with colonized humans or mammals (e.g., dogs). Manifestations: tinea (pityriasis) versicolor, seborrhoic dermatitis, rarely invasive disease in immune-impaired or critically ill patients. Confirmation is by microscopy of scotch tapes from skin, elevated specific IgE, and culture (skin, blood). IMPACT: Impact has been poorly documented. At a dermatology clinic in Tripoli, Libya in 1997–1999, tinea versicolor was mycologically confirmed in 15% (322/2,224) of attendees. OUTBREAKS: *M. furfur* and *M. pachydermatis* have caused nosocomial outbreaks.

MAMASTROVIRUS (unenveloped RNA viruses: *Astroviridae*) *Mamastrovirus* includes human, feline, ovine, and porcine astroviruses.

Human astrovirus (ASTV) (1724, 2756, 5569, 6690, 7930) circulates worldwide, in humans, their feces, and water. SPREAD: is likely via foods or tap water. Infectiousness seems high. Humans shed virus for ~1 week; immune-impaired persons shed virus for months. CLINICAL INFORMATION: The incubation period is 1–3 days. Manifestations: diarrhea, mainly in children. IMPACT: Diagnostic yield in stools from children with diarrhea is 2–12%. OUTBREAKS: Venues for outbreaks include child day care centers, schools, military units, transplant units, and homes for the elderly. At 14 schools in Osaka, Japan, in 1991, likely food-borne ASTV caused a point-source outbreak with >4,700 cases.

MANSONELLA (Nematoda: Spirurida; ex-*Acanthocheilonema*, *Dipetalonea*, *Tetrapetalonema*). These are arthrpod-borne filariid worms. There are >70 species of which three infect humans. The pathogenicity of adult worms and microfilariae (mf) is low.

M. ozzardi (466, 6835) circulates in tropical America, in *Culicoides* midges and *Simulium* blackflies, and humans. SPREAD: is via insect bite. RISKS: daytime outdoor activities, e.g., panning gold, rafting. CLINICAL INFORMATION: Most infections are inapparent. Prepatent period and the location of adults are not known. Confirmation is by visualizing mf in blood (thick films) or skin (snips). Mf densities in blood are 50–15,000/ml. Coinfections can occur with other filariae, e.g., *O. volvulus* in South America. IMPACT: By age and location, prevalence is 2.5–80% (often 10–30%).

M. perstans (81, 848, 3880, 7954) circulates in tropical Africa and America, in *Culicoides* midges and humans. SPREAD: is via insect bite. RISKS: daytime outdoor activities. CLINICAL INFORMATION: Most infections are inapparent. Adult worms locate in the peritoneal cavity, mf in peripheral blood. Confirmation is by visualizing mf in blood (thick film, concentration). Mf densities in blood are 1–7,400 (often 100) per ml. Coinfections can occur with other filariae, e.g., *L. loa*, *W. bancrofti*, and *O. volvulus* in Africa, or *M. ozzardi* in South America. IMPACT: Carriers in endemic areas are estimated to >30 million. Reported prevalences are 1–100%, with highs in rain forest people in central Africa and the Amazon.

M. streptocerca (2407) circulates in tropical Africa, in *Culex* mosquitoes, and humans. SPREAD: is via insect bite. CLINICAL INFORMATION: Most infections are inapparent. Adults and mf both dwell in skin. The prepatent period can last 1 year. Attributed manifestations include pruritus and dermatitis. Confirmation is by visualizing mf in skin snips. A typical mf density in skin is 2/mg. Endemic areas overlap with *O. volvulus* and *W. bancrofti*.

MARBURGVIRUS. See Filovirus.

MAREK'S DISEASE VIRUS (MDV) (4247) (enveloped DNA viruses: α-*Herpesviridae*). MDV circulates in chickens worldwide, likely with feather dust. MDV causes epizootics and T-cell lymphomas in chicken. MDV seems able to cross species and infect humans, likely via inhalation.

MEASLES VIRUS. See Morbillivirus.

METAGONIMUS (1288, 4298) (Trematoda: Digenea). These flukes circulate in Asia, in rats, dogs, cats, and humans (final hosts, shed eggs), snails (first intermediate host), and fish (second host, harbor infective metacercariae). Several species have been reported in humans, mainly *M. yokogawai*. SPREAD: is via raw or undercooked freshwater fish. CLINICAL INFORMATION: The prepatent period is 1–2 weeks. Most infections are inapparent. The reported incubation period is 7–10 days. Manifestations: vague, perhaps diarrhea, and cramps. Confirmation is by visualizing operculate eggs in stool or duodenal fluid. IMPACT: The prevalence in endemic areas is 0.2–5%, in minority communities with particular dietary habits >20%. In Korea, infected people are estimated at 120,000.

MASTADENOVIRUS. See Adenovirus.

MAYARO VIRUS (MAYV). See Alphavirus.

MEASLES VIRUS. See Morbillivirus.

METAPNEUMOVIRUS (enveloped RNA viruses: *Mononegavirales*: *Paramyxoviridae*). Prototype is human metapneumovirus (HMPV) (479, 737, 2300, 2524, 4614, 4691, 7715, 8185).

HMPV emerged in 2001 and by 2005 was reported in North America, Australia, and Europe. SPREAD: is likely via respiratory secretions. RISKS: winter season. Children, elderly, and immune-impaired individuals are susceptible. CLINICAL INFORMATION: Inapparent infections seem uncommon; HMPV has been demonstrated in 4% of asymptomatic adults. The incubation period is not known. Manifestations: upper RTI (sore throat, rhinitis, and bronchitis), flulike illness, bronchiolitis, pneumonia. In Canada, 3% of cases were coinfected with *Influenzavirus*, and 1.5% with RSV. Suitable specimens for NAT are nose or throat swabs, and respiratory secretions. IMPACT: By age and test, HMPV accounts for 2–15% (typically 3–5%) of acute RTI in outpatients. In Hong Kong, preschool children were hospitalized for hMPV at a rate of ~440/10^5/year.

METORCHIS (Trematoda: Digenea). *M. conjunctus* (4624, 8356) circulates in North America, in sled dogs, other carnivores, and humans (final hosts, shed eggs), aquatic snails (first intermediate host), and fish (second host, harbor metacercariae). SPREAD: is via raw fish. CLINICAL INFORMATION: Most infections are inapparent. The prepatent period is 4–5 weeks. Adults locate in liver. The incubation period is 1–15 (median, 4–5) days. Manifestations: anorexia, liver dysfunction, fever, eosinophilia. OUTBREAKS: North of Montreal, Canada, in 1993, an outbreak caused 19 cases.

MICROBACTERIUM (163) (*Actinobacteria*: *Actinomycetales*). These coryneform rods are rare causes of nosocomial disease in immune-impaired patients.

MICROSPORIDIA (28, 1924, 3076, 4522, 6700, 7607). These intracellular fungi occur worldwide, in arthropods, fish, and mammals, including livestock, dogs, and cats. Infected animals shed infective spores into the environment. Spores are resilient, resisting freezing ($-24°C$ for 24 h). Of ~1,200 species in >135 genera, mainly *Encephalitozoon* (*E. cuniculi*, *E. hellem*, and *E. intestinalis*) and *Enterocytozoon* (*E. bieneusi*), infrequently *Brachiola*, *Nosema*, *Pleistophora*, and *Trachipleistophora* have been isolated in humans. SPREAD: is presumed via hand contacts and human secretions, or sex, animal contacts or secretions, tap water or foods. Possible modes include by crushed insects, and nosocomially (patient-to-staff). Putative RISKS: sex among men, injection drug use, pet ownership, water contacts (work, pools and hot tubs), wearing contact lenses, travel, organ transplants. CLINICAL INFORMATION: Inapparent infections occur. The incubation period is not known; a laboratory worker developed microsporidial keratitis 3 weeks after mucosal splash from culture supernatant. Manifestations: self-limited diarrhea in immune-competent persons, and protracted diarrhea, sinusitis, keratoconjunctivitis, and invasive, life-threatening disease in immune-impaired patients. Confirmation is by NAT, (electron)microscopy (biopsy, stool), serology, or antigen capture (urine, feces, and aspirate). Albendazole is active against *Encephalitozoon* but inactive against *Enterocytozoon*. IMPACT: By case mix, test, and location, reported prevalence is <0.1% to 15% (by NAT often 5–10%). Microsporidia can account for 5–15% of acute diarrhea and of up to 50% of persistent diarrhea in HIV-infected patients. OUTBREAKS: Microsporidia are considered emerging foodborne agents. A probably waterborne outbreak has been reported.

MICROSPORUM (*Ascomycota*: *Onygales*) (2555, 3049, 4078, 6392). These keratophilic molds are fluorescent under UV (Wood) light and form arthrospores on the outside of hairs (ectothrix). Humans can be infected by anthropophilic (*M. audouinii*), zoophilic (e.g., *M. canis*), or geophilic (e.g., *M. gypseum*) species. SPREAD: is by contact with humans or their personal objects, animals, or soil. CLINICAL INFORMATION: Infections with anthropophilic *M. audouinii* can be inapparent, in particular, in children who are a major reservoir. In contrast, zoophilic species seem to cause inflammatory responses. An incubation period is not known; a baby was diagnosed with *M. canis* scalp infection 35 days after birth. Manifestations: tinea capitis, tinea corporis, infrequently tinea pedis, rarely onychomycosis. Confirmation is by microscopy or culture from brush or scrapings. IMPACT: *M. canis* is prevalent in the Old and New Worlds. *M. audouinii* seems infrequent, occurring focally. In tinea capitis, by age and geography, 25–50% of cases grow *Microsporum*, mainly *M. canis* (90-100% of isolates), infrequently *M. gypseum* (0–10%). In tinea corporis, 5–30% of cases grow *Microsporum*, mainly *M. canis* (67–100%) or *M. gypseum* (0–20%). In tinea pedis, 0.5–10% (often 1–2%) of cases grow *Microsporum*, mainly *M. canis*. OUTBREAKS: Reported settings for outbreaks are the community, a child care center, and hospitals.

MOLLUSCIPOXVIRUS (enveloped DNA viruses: *Poxviridae*). Prototype is **molluscum contagiosum virus** (MCV) (838, 6956).

MCV circulates worldwide, in humans who shed virus from lesions. Sporadic cases are reported in birds, a dog, a horse, and chimpanzees. SPREAD: Infections can be endogenous (self-inoculation) or acquired, via skin contact, sex, contaminated objects or surfaces, rarely by electrolysis (hair removal). RISKS: swimming in pools, other outdoor sports, and casual sex. Children with atopy and patients with impaired immunity are susceptible. CLINICAL INFORMATION: The incubation period is 2 weeks to 2–6 months. Manifestations: papules, nodules, or umbilicated lesions at head, extremities, trunk, genitals, perianal, and mucosal sites. In HIV-infected persons, lesions can be vegetative (giant). Lesions resolve spontaneously within months or years. To prevent spread, genital lesions should be treated; options include cryosurgery, curettage, and podophyllotoxin gel. Relapses are frequent. IMPACT: Reported infection rates are 2/1,000 person-years in high-income countries and ≥20/1,000 and year in low-income countries. OUTBREAKS: Reported outbreak venues include a kibbutz and an outdoor public swimming pool.

MORAXELLA (519, 7775, 7800) (γ-*Proteobacteria*: *Pseudomonadales*). Prototype is *M.* (ex-*Branhamella*, *Neisseria*) *catarrhalis* that colonizes the human respiratory tract. From 80% to 100% of clinical isolates are producers of β-lactamase. SPREAD: Infections are endogenous or acquired, presumably via droplets or respiratory therapy. Manifestations: follicular (epidemic) conjunctivitis, upper RTI (sinusitis, otitis media, laryngitis, and bronchitis), pneumonia. IMPACT: *M. catarrhalis* is considered a frequent pathogen of the respiratory tract, after *S. pneumoniae* and *H. influenzae*. In Australia in a 3-year prospective study, 25% (2,263/9,092) of respiratory specimens grew bacteria, and 1% (118) grew *M. catarrhalis*. Most isolates were from children, 69% (82/118) were community acquired, and 31% (36) were nosocomial. OUTBREAKS: Nosocomial outbreaks have been reported.

MORBILLIVIRUS (enveloped RNA viruses: *Mononegavirales*: *Paramyxoviridae*). Members are measles virus, distemper virus of dogs, and rinderpest virus of cattle.

Measles virus (1252, 1779, 1861, 3516, 4411, 5845, 7714, 8119, 8120) circulates in susceptible humans, mainly nonvaccinated infants. Susceptible individuals are replenished by successive birth cohorts and by migration. **SPREAD:** is via droplets and aerosols, including outpatient waiting rooms and hospitals. **RISKS:** noncompliance with vaccine, domicile in or visit to endemic or outbreak area, poorly ventilated, crowded rooms, winter season. Virus is shed starting 4 days before rash onsets and for 7–11 days. Infectivity is greatest in the few days before rash appears. Primary attack rates in susceptible individuals can exceed 90%, secondary attack rates are 75–85%. Outbreaks can continue over up to 12 propagation generations. **CLINICAL INFORMATION:** Inapparent infections are rare (≤1%) and do not contribute to spread. The incubation period is 6–19 (median 12) days. Manifestations: fever (>38°C), maculopapular rash (for 3–7 days), and cough, conjunctivitis, or coryza. In low-risk areas and interepidemic periods, <10–30% of suspected cases are confirmed measles. In such settings, laboratory confirmation is advised. Tests include serology (IgM, conversion) or NAT from blood or saliva. Hospitalization rates are 5–9% in Europe, and 19% in the United States. Complications include pneumonia (in 5% of cases in high-income countries, ≥10% in low-income countries), otitis media (5–15%), croup, diarrhea, malnutrition, xerophthalmia, encephalitis (0.06–0.3%, in the United States 0.1%), and premature delivery. Lethality is highly variable, 0.04–0.8% in outbreaks in high-income countries (0.04% in New Zealand, 0.2% in the United States, and 0.8% in Ireland), to 0.1–15% in low-income countries (high in infants and malnourished children). **IMPACT:** Current estimates are ~30–40 million cases per year worldwide, and 0.7–0.8 million deaths per year (0.5 million in Africa). Measles is largely controlled in the New World, and most cases in the United States are now linked to imported cases. In West Europe, the overall reported disease rate is $2-3/10^5$ per year, and ~20% of cases are outbreak related. In low-income countries, disease rates can reach $20-50/10^5$ per year. **OUTBREAKS:** Measles epidemics naturally recur in ~2–4 years. Factors facilitating outbreaks are low or declining vaccine coverage (<80–90%), minorities who object vaccination (e.g., orthodox religious groups) or are difficult to reach (e.g., nomads, migrants, and refugees), and vaccine failure (e.g., violated cold chain, vaccinee of age <9 months, and anergy). In rare outbreaks among well (>90%) vaccinated communities, measles lethality is low. Examples of recent outbreaks are in low-income countries Hong Kong in 1988 (80% coverage), Harare, Zimbabwe in 1988 (83%), Burundi in 1999 (likely ~30%; >27,000 cases), and Sri Lanka in 1999–2000 (>90%; >15,000 cases). Examples in high-income countries are New Zealand in 1991 (82%), Luxembourg in 1996 (70–76%), Germany in 1996 and 2003 (<80%), Ireland in 1999–2000 (~80%), southern Italy in 2000 and 2003 (<60%), and southern France (59-84%). Effective and affordable vaccines are available. Coverage in 2003 was 77% worldwide (65% in Africa and >90% in many high-income countries). For sustained interruption of transmission, >95% of the population need to receive two vaccine doses. Coverage >80% extends epidemic intervals to 4–8 years. In outbreaks, vaccines are recommended for adolescents and adults who share rooms, including in boarding schools, correctional and care facilities, and military units.

MORGANELLA (5534, 7601) (γ-*Proteobacteria*: *Enterobacteriales*). Prototype is *M. morganii* that colonizes the human bowel. **SPREAD:** Infections are endogenous or acquired nosocomially. Manifestations: UTI, intra-abdominal infection, SSI, invasive disease. **IMPACT:** Sporadic. **OUTBREAKS:** A nosocomial outbreak is reported.

MUCOR (5861, 6238) (*Zygomycota*: *Mucorales*). These are hyaline, ribbonlike fungi that inhabit soil and release spores into air. **ACQUISITION:** is likely from inhalation, ingestion, or trauma. Manifestations (zygomycosis): skin lesions and invasive disease in patients with neutropenia, diabetes, or other immune impairments, including mycotic embolism.

MUMPS VIRUS (enveloped RNA viruses: *Mononegavirales*: *Paramyxoviridae*: *Rubulavirus*) (1756, 3033, 6243, 7760, 8097). Mumps virus circulates in susceptible humans worldwide. **SPREAD:** is via saliva and droplets, perhaps droplet nuclei. **RISKS:** children, adolescents, and adults who share rooms with cases, including in boarding schools, care and correction facilities, and military units, and noncompliance with vaccination. Virus is shed from saliva. Infectivity begins 2–7 days before parotitis onset and lasts for ~11 days. Secondary attack rates reach 30%. **CLINICAL INFORMATION:** Infections are inapparent in >60% of preschool children and ~30% of susceptible adolescents and adults. The incubation period is 14–24 (typically 21) days. Manifestations: painful swelling of ≥1 salivary gland (parotis, submandibular), headache (viremia), meningeal irritation or meningitis (in 1–30% of cases), encephalitis (0.02–0.3%), deafness (transient in 4%, permanent in ≤1%), epididymoorchitis (children, 3%; adult males, 25%), abortion (in first trimester in 25%), and pancreatitis (4%). In low-risk areas and interepidemic periods, <10% of clinically diagnosed cases are mumps by laboratory tests. EBV, PIV, and AdV can cause mumpslike manifestations. Confirmation is by NAT (from saliva, throat swabs, and CSF), serology (IgM, IgG-conversion), or culture. **IMPACT:** In areas with low vaccine coverage, disease rates are $100-1,000/10^5$ per year, and by age >20 years, seroreactivity approaches 90%. In the United States in 2001–2002, the reported disease rate was $0.1/10^5$ per year. Finland has interrupted transmission since 1996. OUTBREAKS: Epidemics have a natural cycle of 3–5 years. Outbreaks are possible in communities even with high (>80%) vaccine coverage. Possible reasons include violated cold chain, primary vaccine failure, and waned immunity after a single dose. For sustained interruption of transmission, >90% of the population need to receive two vaccine doses.

MYCOBACTERIUM (934) (*Actinobacteria*: *Actinomycetales*). This genus of acid-fast rods includes ~70 species that are characterized by reservoir (mammals and environment), growth speed (rapid if colonies are visible in 1 week, slow, or nonculturable), pigment formation (in light, in the dark, or nonchromogenic), resistance, and genome.

- The *M. tuberculosis* complex includes *M. tuberculosis* (99% of isolates in Europe), *M. africanum* (0.4%), *M. bovis* (0.4%), *M. microti* (rare in humans, recovered from *Microtus agrestis*, cats, llamas, and other mammals), *M. canettii* (rare), and BCG (bacille Calmette-Guérin vaccine, introduced in France in 1921 by A. Calmette and C. Guérin, after attenuation of *M. bovis* by serial passage on bile-imbibed potatoes for 13 years).

- Environmental (atypical) mycobacteria (2298, 3190, 4751) inhabit soil and water in which they survive hot temperature (45°C) and usual concentrations of free chlorine or ozone. Rapid growers are *M. abscessus*, *M. chelonae*, and *M. fortuitum*, slow growers include *M. avium*-*M. intracellulare*, *M. kansasii*, *M. marinum*, and *M. ulcerans*. Modes of spread include contact with water or soil, inhalation of aerosols, inoculation, and ingestion (tap water or raw milk). Comorbidities and impaired immunity predispose to disease. Contamination, pseudoinfection (contaminated clinical materials), and colonization can be difficult to distinguish from infection. A single isolate from an innocuous site suggests contamination or colonization. Repeated isolates from a diseased site confirm infection. Environmental mycobacteria can account for 3–22% of *Mycobacterium* isolates. Reported infection rates in high-income countries are $1-15/10^5$ per year, disease rates $0.1-2/10^5$ per year.

A summary of selected species follows.

M. abscessus (2246, 6782, 7486) is a rapid grower that inhabits soil and water. SPREAD: is by invasive procedures. CLINICAL INFORMATION: The incubation period is 1–20 (median, 5) weeks. Manifestations: SSI, abscesses. IMPACT: *M. abscessus* is recovered from ~5% of children and adolescents with cystic fibrosis, likely from nonnosocomial sources.

M. avium and **M. intracellulare** (*M. avium* complex, MAC) (942, 2926, 3824, 3918, 4144, 7490) are slow growers. *M. avium* is recovered from swampy soils, fresh and hospital water, *M. avium avium* also from birds, *M. avium paratuberculosis* (MAP) also from cattle (including feces and milk), other ruminants, pigs, and humans. SPREAD: is likely via inhalation of aerosols from showers (homes and hospitals), via drinking unpasteurized milk, or via instruments (e.g., endoscopy). Spread via animal contact is uncertain. Manifestations: pulmonary or invasive disease in immune-impaired patients, pulmonary disease and lypmhadenitis in HIV-negative patients. In The Netherlands, *M. avium* was isolated in 50 (56%) of 89 children with cervicofacial lymphadenitis by PCR. MAC has been recovered from feces and from sputum of patients without MAC lung disease. MAP is a proposed cause of inflammatory bowel disease.

M. bovis (619, 1589, 1812, 4480, 5540, 6996) is part of the *M. tuberculosis* complex. It circulates in wildlife and domestic ruminants. SPREAD: Infections are reactivated or acquired from mammalian droplets or aerosols, handling of milk, and ingestion of unpasteurized milk and dairy products. Interhuman spread is neither confirmed nor excluded. RISKS: A likely risk is unpasteurized dairy products taken home from enzootic areas (souvenir cheese). Manifestations: are indistinguishable from *M. tuberculosis* and include pulmonary, cervical, and peritoneal tuberculosis, and lupus vulgaris of the skin. IMPACT: In high-income countries, *M. bovis* in humans is rare because of milk pasteurization and culling of infected herds. Worldwide, ~3% of tuberculosis (2% of pulmonary and 9% of extrapulmonary) is due to *M. bovis*. Its relative share among strains of tuberculosis is ≤1% in the United Kingdom but reached 33% in San Diego, Calif., in 1980–1997, among culture-confirmed pediatric tuberculosis.

M. chelonae (4000, 7940) is a rapid grower that inhabits soil and water. SPREAD: is via invasive procedures, rarely by inhalation. Manifestations: nodulous, draining soft-tissue infections in immune-competent persons, and pulmonary or invasive disease in immune-impaired patients. IMPACT: Voluntary reporting in the United States suggests a disease rate of $0.1-0.3/10^5$ per year.

M. fortuitum (4709, 8221) is a rapid grower that inhabits soil and water. SPREAD: is via invasive procedures, rarely inhalation. Manifestations: skin and soft-tissue infections, and pulmonary disease. OUTBREAKS: At a California pedicure salon, whirlpool footbaths were the source for an outbreak of skin and soft-tissue infections among female customers.

M. genavense (3327) is a slow grower that has been detected in tap water and sick birds. SPREAD: is presumed via ingestion or inhalation. Manifestations: invasive disease in AIDS patients.

M. haemophilum (942, 2287, 6569) is a slow grower. A reservoir for *M. haemophilum* is not known. Manifestations: skin infections, pulmonary and invasive disease, mainly in immune-impaired patients. In The Netherlands, 16 (18%) of 89 children with cervicofacial lymphadenitis were diagnosed with *M. haemophilum* infection by NAT.

M. kansasii (1066, 6363, 6609, 7292) is a slow grower recovered from municipal tap water, infrequently from river or lake water, soil, or dust. Virulence seems to vary by subtypes. **SPREAD:** is via inhalation of aerosols (natural and nosocomial). Manifestations: tuberculosis-like, skin and pulmonary disease, in immune-competent and -impaired hosts. **IMPACT:** Reported disease rates are 0.3–20/10^5 per year; in AIDS patients up to 650–1,100/10^5 per year.

M. leprae (403, 629, 889, 3903, 4962, 7829, 8123) growth is very slow, one division in the mouse footpad taking 2 weeks. Reservoirs are humans, the armadillo, and perhaps soil, vegetation, and water. **SPREAD:** is mainly via nasal secretions or aerosols, rarely via contact, tattoo, or injury. Spread is better explained by "networks" than "chains." **RISKS:** poverty, living in urban slums, no access to care. **CLINICAL INFORMATION:** Latent infections and nasal carriage can be detected by serology, lepromin skin test, or NAT from nasal smear. The incubation period (injury or experimental) is 3 months to 30 years, often 3 (tuberculoid leprosy) to 10 (lepromatous leprosy) years. Manifestations: hypopigmented and hypoesthetic (in 70%) skin patches (1–5 in paucibacillary, >5 or confluent in multibacillary leprosy), acute neuritis or thickened nerves, acute inflammatory reaction, and dry cornea and lagophthalmus. The male:female ratio is 1.5–2:1. Confirmation is by microscopy of smears from nose blow, slit skin (of ear lobes and lesions), or biopsy; up to 70% of patients are smear negative (histology positive). Multidrug therapy (MDT, for 6–24 months) is effective and has a low relapse rate (0.1–1% per year). Options for (observed) MDT include rifampin, clofazimine, ofloxacin, and clarithromycin. Resistance to dapsone, clofazimine, ofloxacin, and rifampin has been reported. **IMPACT:** In endemic areas up to 5% of healthy adults can be infected. In 2004, there were ~0.5 million cases registered for treatment worldwide, for regional prevalences of 1–20/10^5. Variable treatment lengths could confound these estimates, and focally, true prevalence could reach 50–2,000/10^5. In 2004, ~0.5 million new cases were detected (close to 80% in Southeast Asia), for detection rates of 0.4–26.5/10^5. The proportion of new cases with visible disability (ulcer, muscle atrophy, and contracture) can be 2–14%. In an endemic area of Indonesia, the case rate in the nonintervention arm of a prevention trial was 390/10^5 per year. In Texas in 1973–1997, 810 leprosy cases were reported, for a rate of 0.2/10^5 per year. Overall in 2004, leprosy was considered a public health problem in nine countries: Brazil, India, Nepal, and six countries in Central and East Africa. **OUTBREAKS:** Few outbreaks have been documented, mainly among minority and island populations.

M. malmoense (4514) is a slow grower that inhabits water and soil. **SPREAD:** is via ingestion or inhalation. Manifestations: pulmonary (patients with comorbidities, e.g., chronic obstructive pulmonary disease), lymphadenitis, disseminated disease.

M. marinum (333, 3693, 4391, 8277) is a slow grower that inhabits stagnant waters. **SPREAD:** is via skin trauma or water contact. **CLINICAL INFORMATION:** The incubation period is 5 days to 9 months (often 2–3 weeks). Manifestations ("fish tank" or "swimming pool granuloma," "mariner's tb"): ulcerous, solitary nodulous, and spreading nodulous (sporotrichoid, in ~10%) skin lesions, also synovitis and arthritis, rarely disseminated disease in immune-impaired patients.

M. tuberculosis (102, 710, 1237, 2304, 3315, 4891, 7808, 8116) growth is slow, taking 12–18 days to form visible colonies. Strains can be resistant to isoniazin (INH), rifampin (RMP), both (MDR), or other tuberculostatics, either primarily or from previous treatment. **SPREAD:** Infections are reactivated or acquired from human aerosols (droplet nuclei) or droplets (by cough, sneeze, singing, and talking); rarely mother-to-child, nosocomially (e.g., bronchoscopy), or by work injury. In densely populated high-risk areas, cases are mainly community acquired rather than reactivated. **RISKS:** contact with an infective case for hours to months in closed, poorly ventilated spaces, crowding, injection drug use, incarceration, late case detection. Sharing air for >5 days in a room with an open case virtually always results in infection. Risks for MDR include previous tuberculosis, previous treatment, origin from a high-risk country, and noncompliance with treatment. Cases whose sputum is positive by microscopy (open) are most infectious, but smear-negative cases contribute to 15–20% of spread. Open cases expectorate 1–10 million bacteria per ml of sputum. An open case can infect up to 200 or more contacts. In an outbreak at a day care center in Greece, the infection rate reached an astounding 89%. **CLINICAL INFORMATION:** Infection is confirmed by skin conversion to tuberculin. Reactivity takes 2–12 (often 8) weeks to develop. Skin test can be false positive (from BCG, environmental mycobacteria) or false negative (by anergy). About 90% of infections are inapparent. By age and immune competence, the lifetime risk for infection to progress to disease (active tuberculosis) is 10%. The risk is highest in the first year after acquisition, and eight times lower in the next 6 years. The incubation period is 1–12 (median, 2) months. Manifestations: pulmonary (cough >2 weeks, hemoptysis), systemic (fever, weight loss, and night sweats), disseminated (miliary), and organ-specific, e.g., lymphadenitis, meningitis, nephritis, osteomyelitis, and "lupus" of the skin.

Confirmation is by chest X ray, sputum smear, culture, and biopsy. Sputum from active pulmonary disease cases is positive by smear in 50–80% and by culture in ≤85%. In Australia in 2002, frequently culture-positive materials were sputum (in 46% or 325/712), lymph node (in 20% or 142), and bronchoscopic materials (in 14% or 100). In the 1940s–1950s, ~65% of open cases died (in 4 years), 25–33% healed spontaneously, and some became chronic excretors. To date, lethality is 23% worldwide (with HIV coinfections), and 2–8% in high-income countries. Treatment options include INH (introduced in 1952, preferred to treat latent infections), rifampin, pyrazinamide, and ethambutol. Minimum length is 6–9 months. Adequate treatment curbs infectivity in ~2 weeks, but typically three negative sputum smears from three separate days are required to release a patient from isolation. IMPACT: The infection prevalence is ~32% worldwide (35% in Africa, 18% in the Americas, 29–44% in Asia, and 15% in Europe). In 2002, there were 8.8 million new cases, including 3.9 million smear positive. Also in 2002, disease rates per 10^5 were 140 worldwide: 200–1,000 in Africa, 40–60 in Latin America, 25–550 in Asia, and 5–15 in high-income countries. High rates in Africa corresponded with high proportions of HIV coinfections (Fig. 20.5). In the United States in 2003, the reported disease rate was $5/10^5$ (23 in foreign born, 2.7 in United States born). In high-income countries, ~30–55% of active disease cases are foreign born. OUTBREAKS: Venues for recent outbreaks included the community, families, a day care center, a navy ship, homeless shelters, prisons, and hospitals. MDR strains caused outbreaks. In rare instances, smear-negative source cases are implicated in outbreaks. Preventive measures include early case detection and treatment, contact tracing, PEP, and BCG.

M. ulcerans (97, 1851, 5455, 7722, 8107) is a slow grower that is widespread in warm wetlands. SPREAD: is via water or mud contact or skin trauma, perhaps via insect bites. Aerosols from winds or gas bubbles, and floods might disperse the agent in the environment. RISKS: contact with water, mud, or plants, and floods. CLINICAL INFORMATION: A skin test survey suggested inapparent infections. The incubation period is 2–14 (often 6–12) weeks. Manifestations (Buruli ulcer): nodules (in ~5–10% of cases), ulcers (in 20–40%), and osteomyelitis (in 5–10%). About 25–50% of recovered patients have sequelae, including loss of a limb (in 10%) or disfiguring scars. Early recognition is hampered by remote domiciles and reluctance to accept care. IMPACT: Point prevalence can reach 0.1–0.15% focally, the cumulative prevalence (florid and past disease) 1%. A reported disease rate is $22/10^5$ per year. OUTBREAKS: On Phillip Island in temperate Southeast Australia in 1992–1995, an outbreak caused 29 cases, mostly among the elderly; sprinklers for a golf course were the source confirmed by NAT from water samples. In the Sudan in 2002, an out-

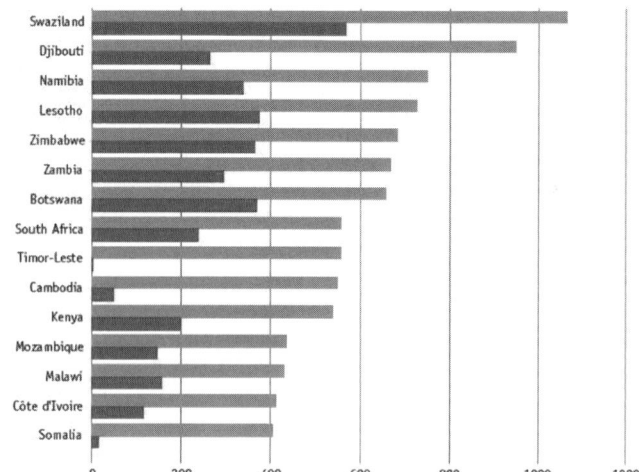

Figure 20.5 Reported tuberculosis cases in 15 countries, 2002: Number of cases (x axis, $/10^5$) are given by country (y axis) and type: all forms and all ages (grey bars) and HIV co-infection at age 15-49 years (red bars). From reference 8116. Reproduced with permission by WHO.

break affected internally displaced persons. BCG vaccination is suggested to have a moderate, short-lived protective effect.

M. xenopi (323, 370, 4706) is a slow grower that inhabits warm tap-water systems, likely in biofilms. SPREAD: is via inhalation or ingestion of tap water in domestic or hospital habitats. Immune-impaired individuals and patients with chronic lung disease are susceptible. Manifestation: lung, bone, and joint disease in HIV-infected and HIV-negative patients. OUTBREAKS: A nosocomial outbreak has been reported.

MYCOPLASMA (2644) (*Firmicutes: Mollicutes: Mycoplasmatales*). These are tiny bacteria that have lost their gram-positive cell wall during evolution. Hosts include plants, insects, birds, and mammals. Of >90 species, *M. genitalium*, *M. hominis*, and *M. pneumoniae* are infective to humans. Mycoplasms are sensitive to tetracyclines, macrolides, and some fluoroquinolones, but, by their lack of a cell wall, not to β-lactams.

M. genitalium (2293, 3580, 4710, 6906) colonizes the human genital tract. SPREAD: is via sex. Manifestations: Colonization and infection can be difficult to separate. *M. genitalis* is an accepted cause of nongonococcal, nonchlamydial urethritis in men, and of cervicitis, endometritis, and pelvic inflammatory disease in women. Detection is by NAT from first void urine, urethral, vaginal, or cervical smear, semen samples, or biopsy. IMPACT: STI (see section 14.7).

M. hominis (221, 5838, 6376) colonizes the human genital tract. SPREAD: is via sex. *M. hominis* seems able to survive inside *Trichomonas vaginalis*. Manifestations: As with *M. genitalium*, colonization can confound the diagnosis of infection. *M. hominis* has been associated with nongonococcal urethritis and balanoposthitis in men, and bacterial vaginosis, premature rupture of membranes, salpingitis, and pelvic inflammatory disease in women. *M. hominis* is a rare cause of invasive disease in immune-impaired patients (e.g., transplant recipients). **IMPACT:** STI (see section 14.7).

M. pneumoniae (787, 1778, 1994, 2235, 3532, 3594, 5022, 6130) colonizes the human oropharynx. **SPREAD:** is via droplets. **RISK:** long contact with a case in a closed room. **CLINICAL INFORMATION:** From 20% to 90% of infections are inapparent. The incubation period is ~2–4 weeks. Manifestations: mimic viral RTI and include cough (in 80–100% of cases), fever (in 60–95%), sore throat (in 25–40%), and radiographic signs of "atypical" pneumonia (in 2–10%). Confirmation is by NAT (from oropharyngeal swabs) or serology. Complications can be cutaneous (in <2%: purpura, Stevens-Johnson syndrome) or neurological (in 0.1–2.5%: encephalitis, Guillain-Barré syndrome). **IMPACT:** Seroprevalence in convenience and population samples is 5–30%. Reported infection rates are 1,000–5,000/10^5 per year, the reported pneumonia rates are 200–600/10^5 per year (high in children). **OUTBREAKS:** Epidemic waves recur every 3–9 years. Venues for outbreaks are communities, colleges, camps, military settings, hospitals, and long-term care facilities. Exposed persons may benefit from macrolide chemoprophylaxis.

MYIASIS. *See section 4.6.*

NAEGLERIA (Amoebozoa: Heterolobosea). These are free-living amebas. Of several species, *N. fowleri* is infective to humans.

N. fowleri (682, 1503, 4777, 4911, 6841) inhabits soil, water, and dust in warm climates, as cysts, ameboid or flagellate life forms. *N. fowleri* tolerates hot-water temperatures (40–45°C), but it is inactivated by free chlorine. **SPREAD:** is by water that gets into the nasopharynx. **RISKS:** submerging in polluted freshwater (swimming, diving, splashing, water skiing, and washing babies), summer months. **CLINICAL INFORMATION:** The incubation period is 1–21 (typically 3–7) days. Manifestations: (primary amebic meningoencephalitis, PAM): fulminant (meningococcal-like) meningitis, with abrupt headache, fever, and stiff neck. Diagnosis is by NAT, microscopy of centrifuged CSF (wet mounts and stained smears), or culture. Over 85% of cases are fatal. Combinations of antifungals (e.g., amphotericin B) and antibiotics (e.g., rifampin) are a treatment option. **IMPACT:** PAM is rare, <200 cases are recorded worldwide. In the United States in 1989–2000, 24 fatal cases were reported through waterborne disease outbreak surveillance, mainly in children; none were reported in 2001 and two in 2002. Recently the first case was reported in Italy in 2003, a 9-year-old boy who swam in a polluted water hole of the Po River. **OUTBREAKS:** Clusters of cases had occurred in Bohemia in the 1960s, from poorly chlorinated indoor swimming pools that had water temperatures of 24°C. Unsuited for swimming are thermally polluted waters, low-level stagnant waters, and sites sign-posted to contain free-living amebas.

NAIROVIRUS (enveloped RNA viruses: *Bunyaviridae*). Prototype is Crimean-Congo hemorrhagic fever virus (CCHFV) (326, 327, 1347, 2222, 5303, 5718, 6976, 8075).

CCHFV circulates in the Old World (Southwest, Central, and East Asia, tropical Africa), in *Hyalomma* ticks, birds (including ostriches), wild mammals (e.g., hares), and livestock (e.g., cattle, sheep, goats, and camels). **SPREAD:** is via (i) work with viremic livestock, (ii) tick bite, or crushing ticks with bare hands, (iii) community contact with incubating patients, (iv) contact with blood or tissue from patients. There are insufficient data to support transmission by animal or patient aerosols. **RISKS:** include tick bites in enzootic areas; animal work (e.g., castration, shearing, butchering, but also ostrich farming, camel breeding, and herding), sleeping outdoors, a case in the family, hospital and laboratory work. In Turkey, 53% of 35 patients had a history of recent tick bite. Viremia persists for 7–8 (occasionally 12) days. **CLINICAL INFORMATION:** By serosurveys, inapparent infections occur. The incubation period is 1–7 days (1–3 days from tick bite and 5–7 days from tissue or blood). Manifestations: fever and pain (in 80% of cases), vomiting or nausea (in 40–80%), and, in a second phase, bleeding (epistaxis, petechiae, in 30–45%). CCHF has been confirmed by NAT (from serum, biopsy), serology (anti-IgM), or culture (biosafety level 4 required). By disease stage and treatment, lethality is 3–70%. Ribavirin therapy seems effective, reducing lethality to <10%. **IMPACT:** Reported seroprevalence in enzootic areas ranges from 0–1% (South Africa and Southwest Asia) to 3–13% (West and Central Africa). **OUTBREAKS:** In South Africa in 1981–1986, 29 locally transmitted cases were recorded in 16 outbreaks. Recent outbreaks occurred in Pakistan in 2000 (six confirmed plus 23 suspected cases), Kosovo in 2001 (18 confirmed and 51 suspected cases), and Mauritania in 2003 (38 cases). Hospital outbreaks (year, secondary cases) were reported in Dubai (1979, 5), Iraq (1979, 2), South Africa (1984, 8), Pakistan (1987, 2; 1994, 3; 2002, 2), Albania (2001, 1), and Mauritania (2003, 15).

NAPLES SANDFLY FEVER VIRUS (SFNV). *See* Phlebovirus.

NECATOR. *See* Ancylostoma.

NEISSERIA (β-*Proteobacteria*: *Neisseriales*). These are gram-negative diplococci. The genus includes commensal *N. lactamica* and *N. catarrhalis* and pathogenic *N. gonorrhoeae* and *N. meningitidis*.

N. gonorrhoeae (gonococcus) (3720, 4011, 4075, 4715, 4951, 5059, 5159, 8043) has humans as the only reservoir. The agent is fragile outside the human body. SPREAD: is via genitogenital, orogenital, and anogenital sex, and mother-to-child. RISKS: for community (see section 14.7), female prostitutes (see section 13.6), homosexual men (see section 13.7). CLINICAL INFORMATION: Many infections (male, 40–60%, female, 5–10%) are inapparent. The incubation period (urethritis) is 2–14 (often 8) days. Manifestations: purulent urethral or vaginal discharge, neonatal conjunctivitis. Untreated, complications include urethral stricture, pelvic inflammatory disease (PID), and infertility. Confirmation is by microscopy and culture from genital swab, or NAT from urine (office- or self-collected). Treatment options include cephalosporins and fluoroquinolones. IMPACT: Disease rates vary by age, sex, geography, reporting, and denominator. The global estimate is $\sim 1,000/10^5$ per year. Rates in high-income countries are 10–10,000 (often 100–1,000)/10^5 per year. Reported rates/10^5 per year are 24 in Canada and 125 in the United States. In a retrospective cohort in Baltimore, Md., the rate of reinfection in STI clinic attendees was 4/100 person-years, and the median time to reinfection was 1 year. By sample and test, infection prevalence in adult females is 0–13% (typically 1%) in high-income countries, and 3–18% in low-income countries. In a representative United States sample of young adults 18–26 years of age, the prevalence by ligase chain reaction on first void urine was 0.4% (95% Cl 0.3–0.6). OUTBREAKS: Outbreaks are rarely reported. Exposed partners (can be more than one per case) are identified through contact tracing; infections can be prevalent in traced partners (>40% in a Swedish study).

N. meningitidis (meningococcus) (647, 4095, 4278, 5885, 5961, 6037, 7709). Humans are the only reservoir. The polysaccharide capsule defines >10 serogroups, mainly A, B, C, W135, and Y (capsule switching can occur). Approximate relative frequencies are in North America: B, 35–50%; C, 30%; Y, 10–35%; and W135, 2–4%, and in West Europe: B, 55–65%; C, 30–40%; Y, 1–3%; and W-135, 1–3%. In New Zealand, B dominates (>85% of cases); in Africa and Asia, A dominates. SPREAD: is via droplets or hand contact. "Close" are contacts in households, child care centers, and from oral secretions (kissing, mouth-to-mouth resuscitation, and intubation). RISKS: a case in the household, crowded sleeping quarters, preschool age, and winter months. Compared with the population, secondary attack rates are increased in households, day care, and school class contacts. The infective period begins 7 days before disease onset (d_0) and ends 24 h after t_0 (treatment onset). Viral coinfections may enhance spread (e.g., by stimulating sneezing and coughing). CLINICAL INFORMATION: A majority of infections is inapparent. The incubation period is 2–10 (often 3–5) days. Manifestations: bacterial meningitis (headache, stiff neck, and altered mental status; can be fulminant with rapid coma), sepsis, metastatic infections. Confirmation is by emergency blood culture, if feasible, microscopy, NAT, and culture from CSF. Lethality is 7–23% (often 10–15%). Sequelae (in $\sim$10–20%): neurological disability, hearing loss, limb loss. IMPACT: Rates of invasive disease per 10^5 per year are 0.5–1.5 in North America, and 0.3–3.6 in West Europe (<1 in Italy and France, 1.5–2.5 in Switzerland, and >3 in the United Kingdom). OUTBREAKS: Although most (>95%) cases in high-income countries are sporadic, outbreaks are a constant threat. The expected number of outbreaks is $\sim$5–15/year in the United States and 2–3/year in Canada. Outbreaks can be of creeping, persisting, or explosive type. By size of the community, attack rates are 10–1,000 (often 100–200)/10^5. Major epidemics (cases, lethality) occurred in Finland in 1973–1974 (1,300 cases, 4.3%), Sao Paulo, Brazil, in 1974 (30,555), Norway in 1975–1978 (404, 13.7%), and Ethiopia in 1989 (41,139, 3.9%). Large epidemics recur in Africa, inside and outside of the meningitis belt. In the United States, three or more primary cases in 3 months (two or more in educational institutions) or community attack rates >10/10^5 are recommended levels to consider use of vaccine. In Africa, a proposed threshold for public health action is an attack rate >15/10^5 and week over 2 consecutive weeks. Polysaccharide (e.g., tetravalent: A, C, Y, and W135) and conjugate vaccines are available, but vaccines for serogroup B are sorely missed. In the United States, conjugate vaccine is recommended for college freshmen living in dormitories, military recruits, travelers to hyperendemic or epidemic areas, exposed microbiologists, susceptible individuals (e.g., asplenia), in some outbreaks, and routinely for adolescents (age 11–12 years or high-school entry). Serogroup A vaccine is universally recommended for infants in sub-Saharan Africa.

Chemoprophylaxis should be given within 24 h to contacts of confirmed or probable cases, either *prolonged* contacts (households, children <6 years of age in same institution, students and recruits in same dormitory) or *massive* contacts (kissing, resuscitation, and intubation).

NEORICKETTSIA (α-*Proteobacteria*: *Rickettsiales*). These are *Ehrlichia*-like intracellular bacteria. *N. risticii* causes Potomac fever in horses in North America and possibly Europe. Horses seem to acquire the agent by ingesting insects or snails parasitized by stages of trematodes that carry *N. risticii*. Of *N. sennetsu* sporadic, flulike human infections are reported in Japan and Malaysia, presumably via ingestion of raw fish.

NEOSPORA (Apicomplexa: Eucoccidiorida). *N. caninum* is a *Toxoplasma*-like protozoan that circulates in dogs (final host, shed cysts), and cattle, goats, sheep, and horses (intermediate hosts). *N. caninum* can cause abortion in livestock. Infections in humans are not documented.

NEWCASTLE DISEASE VIRUS (NDV). See *Avulavirus*.

NOCARDIA (2320, 3782, 6555, 6629) (*Actinobacteria: Actinomycetales*). These are *branching* rod *bacteria* that inhabit water, soil, plant debris, animals, and dust. Many of the >25 species are implicated in infection in humans, including *N. asteroides* sl (*N. asteroides* ss and *N. farcinica*) and *N. brasiliensis*. SPREAD: is via inhalation of dust, plant trauma, or invasive procedure. CLINICAL INFORMATION: The incubation period is 21–45 (often 28) days for SSI, and up to 210 days for transplants. Manifestations: actinomycetoma, pneumonia, invasive disease. Most patients with invasive disease have comorbidities (e.g., pulmonary disease and diabetes) or impaired immunity (e.g., suppressive therapy and AIDS). Provided that contamination can be excluded, gram-stained smear and culture (sputum and tissue) confirm disease. Agents of actinomycetoma (e.g., *N. asteroides* sl, *N. brasiliensis*, *N. caviae*, and *N. transvalensis*) produce white, cream, or yellow grains. IMPACT: By geography, the relative frequency of *N. brasiliensis* sl in actinomycetoma is ~25–90%.

NOROVIRUS (1097, 1213, 2520, 2594, 3132, 3367, 4518) (NoV; unenveloped RNA viruses: *Caliciviridae*). *Norovirus* circulates worldwide, in birds, mammals, humans, and the environment. Of ≥3 genogroups, 2 (GI, GII) are detected in humans. Humans shed NoV with vomit and feces, after recovery from diarrhea for up to 2–3 weeks. NoV resists 0–60°C, including regular laundry, and in food. SPREAD: is via hand contacts (in 85% of United Kingdom outbreaks), inhalation of aerosols (generated by vomiting or explosive diarrhea), foods (in 5% of United Kingdom outbreaks), tap or surface water, or contaminated objects. RISKS: Poor hygiene of body, food, tap water, or recreational water. Infectivity is high, and the infective dose low (<100 viruses). Index infections are often food- or waterborne, secondary spread is often person-to-person. CLINICAL INFORMATION: one fourth to one third of infections are inapparent. The incubation period is 7 h to 5 (typically 1–2) days. Manifestations ("winter vomiting disease"): vomiting (can be explosive), diarrhea (can dehydrate), fever. Confirmation is by NAT (more sensitive than electron microscopy). Illness can last 1–5 days. Lethality is <0.05%. IMPACT: By place and test method, NoV accounts for >60% to >90% of diarrhea outbreaks of nonbacterial etiology. In West Europe, NoV accounts for 8–11% of acute infectious diarrhea in the community. OUTBREAKS: Settings for the many outbreaks have included restaurants, cruise ships, a concert hall, day care centers, schools, youth camps, resorts, a pilgrim tour, hospitals, and homes. In the United Kingdom in 1992–2000, of 1,877 laboratory-confirmed outbreaks (affecting 57,060 persons), main settings were hospitals (40% or 754) and residential-care facilities (39% or 724).

OESOPHAGOSTOMUM (Nematoda: Strongylida). These nematodes occur worldwide, in mammals (e.g., pigs and ruminants) that shed eggs and ingest infective larvae from forage or soil. *O. bifurcum* (7184, 8410) is reported in humans, primarily from West Africa. SPREAD: is via geophagia or soil-polluted foods. CLINICAL INFORMATION: Infections can be inapparent. Manifestations: granulomatous colitis. Eggs in stool are hookworm-like; confirmation, like with *Strongyloides*, requires stool culture. A treatment option is albendazole. IMPACT: Reported focal infection prevalence is 1–15%

OMSK HEMORRHAGIC FEVER VIRUS (OHFV). See *Flavivirus*.

ONCHOCERCA (Nematoda: Spirurida). These arthropod-borne filariid worms infect cattle, deer, and other mammals, e.g., *O. gutturosa*, *O. lienalis*, and *O. ochengi*.
O. volvulus (3861, 3954, 6247, 6368, 7954, 8102) circulates in rural tropical Africa, Arabia, and Latin America, in *Simulium* blackflies that carry infective larvae and in humans who harbor adult worms in subcutaneous nodules and microfilariae (mf) in skin. The life span of adults is 8–15 years, that of mf is ~30 months. SPREAD: is via fly bite (occasional perinatal spread is suspected). RISKS: domicile or work in endemic areas, in particular, along rivers that are *Simulium*-breeding sites. CLINICAL INFORMATION: The prepatent period is ~1 year. The incubation period is ~2 or more months. Manifestations (river blindness): persistent pruritus, papulous, scabies-like dermatitis, depigmented (leopard) skin, lipoma-like nodules (onchocercomas), lymphedema (hanging groin), keratitis, and blindness. Confirmation is by visualizing mf in skin snips (by microscopy of wet mounts) or eye (cornea or anterior chamber, by slit lamp), or by ultrasound (adults in nodules). IMPACT: About 16–18 million people are infected. Areas are hyperendemic, if mf skin prevalence is >60%, nodule prevalence in rapidly assessed male adults is >40%, or if onchocercal blindness

prevalence is >6%. Infection rates can exceed 20% per year. OUTBREAKS: The "onchocerciasis control program" (OCP, 1974–2002) that was based initially on aerial spraying in savannah areas of 11 West African countries, and later adopted mass ivermectin treatments in savannah and forest areas, interrupted transmission in most target areas. Similar programs are ongoing in 19 other countries in Africa and Yemen since 1995 ("African program for onchocerciasis control," APOC) and in six American countries since 1991 ("onchocerciasis elimination program for the Americas," OEPA). OCP, APOC, and OEPA need to continue beyond worm longevity, until adults have died out spontaneously. Transmission has likely been interrupted in foci in Colombia, Ecuador, and Mexico.

O'NYONG-NYONG FEVER VIRUS (ONNV). See Alphavirus.

OPISTHORCHIS (Trematoda: Digenea). These are food-borne biliary flukes that are enzootic in the Old World. *O. felineus* and *O. viverrini* infect humans.

O. felineus (4665, 8347) is enzootic in Russia (including West Siberia), Ukraine, and Kazakhstan, and foci are reported in Belarus, possibly the Baltic states, and Poland. Biology and epidemiology resemble *O. viverrini*. The incubation period is 10 days to 4 weeks. Manifestations: nausea, abdominal pain, fever, arthralgia, and skin rash. IMPACT: About 1.6 million people are infected. Reported infection prevalence is 5–65%.

O. viverrini (3638, 4665, 6034, 7081) circulates in Southeast Asia (Thailand, Laos, and Cambodia), in fish-eating mammals and humans (final hosts, shed eggs with feces), snails (first intermediate hosts), and freshwater fish (second hosts, harbor metacercariae). SPREAD: is via undercooked or raw fish. RISKS: preference for raw fish, water-development projects. CLINICAL INFORMATION: The prepatent period is 2–3 weeks. Adults locate in biliary ducts. Egg counts >10,000/g feces define heavy infections. Most (≥90%) light infections are inapparent. Manifestations: vague, can include flatulence, abdominal pain, and eosinophilia; intrahepatic stones, and recurring cholangitis are not typical. A late complication of heavy infections is cholangiocarcinoma. Confirmation is by visualizing operculate eggs with thickened walls in stool or duodenal fluid. Praziquantel is a treatment option. IMPACT: About 9 million people are infected, including 7 million in Thailand. Reported infection prevalence in enzootic areas is 0–70% (often 10–25%), that of heavy infections is <0.5%.

ORBIVIRUS (nonenveloped RNA viruses: *Reoviridae*). Prototype is bluetongue virus (BTV) (843) that circulates in warm climates, in biting midges and wild ruminants and livestock (sheep, cattle).

ORIENTIA (α-*Proteobacteria: Rickettsiales*). These are intracellular, *Rickettsia*-like rods. Prototype is *O. tsutsugamushi* (3884, 3940, 4137, 4827, 6088, 6535, 6892, 7356). This agent circulates in Australasia, in rodents and mites. SPREAD: is via larval mite (chigger) bite. RISKS: domicile in or travel to enzootic areas, outdoor activities, military training. Transmission is seasonal in temperate climate areas, but perennial in subtropical or tropical areas. CLINICAL INFORMATION: Inapparent infections occur. The incubation period is 5–21 (typically 7–10) days. Manifestations (scrub typhus): flulike illness (in 90–100% of cases), regional or generalized adenopathy (in 20%), skin rash (in 10–95%), and eschar (in 7–95%). Complications are pneumonia and meningoencephalitis. Confirmation is by serology (≥4-fold increase in titer) or NAT. Treatment options include doxycycline and azithromycin; doxycycline resistance has been reported. Lethality in the preantibiotic era was 1–10%, with treatment it is 0.2–0.4%. IMPACT: Reported seroprevalence in enzootic areas is 1–5% (Indonesia and Malaysia) to 20–35% (People's Republic of China, Malaysia, Solomon Islands, and Thailand). In Japan in 2000, 756 cases were reported from 37 of 47 prefectures, for a disease rate of 0.1–7.6 (mean, 0.6)/10^5 per year. Recently, cases have been reported from Sri Lanka.

OROPOUCHE VIRUS (OROV). See Orthobunyavirus.

ORTHOHEPADNAVIRUS (enveloped DNA viruses: *Hepadnaviridae*). The genus includes viruses of woodchucks (*Marmota*), squirrels (*Spermophilus*), and other mammals, but mainly HBV and HBV-associated HDV.

Hepatitis B virus (HBV) (6, 171, 1175, 2612, 3328, 4183, 4251, 4284) occurs worldwide. Blood (serum), saliva, and semen are infectious. There are serotypes (adw, ayw, adr, ayr) and genotypes (A–H) that cluster geographically (A in Africa, North America, and northern Europe; B and C in Asia; D in the Mediterranean and India; and E in sub-Saharan Africa). SPREAD: is via reused or shared, blood-tainted injection materials, ritual procedures (piercing and tattooing), work-related percutaneous or mucosal injury, transfusion of unsafe blood, mother-to-child, close contact, or sex. RISKS: domicile in hyperendemic areas, a case in the household, sex with a carrier, multiple sex partners, sex among men, injection drug use, work exposing to blood, invasive procedures (e.g., hemodialysis). CLINICAL INFORMATION: About 90–95% of infections in neonates and 50–70% of new infections in adults are inapparent. The incubation period is 4–10 weeks. Manifestations: include acute and chronic HB, cirrhosis, and hepatocellular carcinoma (after 35–45 years). Lethality of acute (fulminant) HB can approach 2.5%. The proportion of acute infections that become chronic is 90% in neonates, 30% in preschool children, and 2% in adolescents and adults. About 15–40% of chronic infections progress to cirrhosis. Chronic infections and cirrhosis are correlated with age and endemicity. Markers of HBV infection are antigens (HBsAg and HBeAg), antibodies (anti-HBc and anti-HBs), and viral DNA. The interpretation of single-positive markers is: for HBsAg, acute infection and infectousness (positive ≥6 weeks postexposure); for anti-HBc IgM, new or reactivated infection; for anti-HBc IgG, resolved acute infection; for anti-HBs IgG immunity (natural or from vaccination), titers >10 mIU/ml are considered protective. Suggestive of chronic infection are HBsAg persisting for >6 months plus anti-HBc IgG. Viremia in chronic infection ranges from <100 copies/ml to >10^9 copies/ml. IMPACT: About 2 billion people (one third of the world population) live with markers of past or current HBV infection. About 350–400 million people are carriers: 5–6% worldwide, 8–15% in hyperendemic areas of sub-Saharan Africa, the Amazon, and Southeast and East Asia (in pockets up to >20-30%), 2–7% in mesoendemic areas in Southwest and Southcentral Asia and much of Latin America, and <2% in hypoendemic (high-income) areas. Rates of acute HB/10^5 per year range from >200 (hyperendemic) to 50–100 (mesoendemic) and 1–10 (hypoendemic). In the United States, reported rates of acute HB in 2000–2002 were ~3/10^5 per year. Worldwide, about 320,000 deaths per year are attributed to HBV. OUTBREAKS: Recombinant vaccines protect from acute and chronic infection, and reduce carrier prevalence, perinatal and accidental transmission risks, and rates of hepatocellular carcinoma. Protection lasts at least 15 years. By endemicity and national guidelines, vaccines are recommended for all infants, all adolescents, or groups at risk.

Hepatitis D virus (HDV) (129, 2319) is a defective virus that depends on HBV, causing HBV superinfection or aggravation. Anti-HBs-positive individuals resist HDV. HDV occurs worldwide, endemically in low-income countries, the Mediterranean, and among IDUs, and sporadically in the United States, northern Europe, and among recipients of multiple transfusions. The prevalence of HDV among HBsAg-positive individuals is 1–20% (often 5%).

ORTHOBUNYAVIRUS (enveloped RNA viruses: *Bunyaviridae*). The genus unites >150 viruses that circulate in insects and vertebrates. Representatives infective to humans include Bunyamweravirus (CVV), California encephalitis virus group (INKV, JCV, LACV, SSHV, and TAHV), and Oropouche virus (OROV).

Bunyamwera virus: Cache Valley virus (CVV) (6796) circulates in North America, in mosquitoes, and large, domestic or wild mammals. Infections in humans can be manifest as encephalitis.

California encephalitis virus group (1871, 2230, 3475, 4858, 4907, 5084, 7761):

Inkoo virus (INKV) circulates in the holarctic (Scandinavia, Russia, and Alaska), in herbivores (e.g., caribou and reindeer) and *Aedes* (*Ochlerotatus*) mosquitoes. Manifestations: flulike, occasionally encephalitis. Some 0.5% of residents in enzootic areas can be seroreactive.

Jamestown Canyon virus (JCV) circulates in North America, in herbivores (e.g., cattle and horses) and *Aedes* mosquitoes. Manifestations: flulike, also encephalitis. Some 4–10% of rural residents can be seroreactive.

La Crosse virus (LACV) circulates in North America, in small mammals (chipmunks, squirrels, and rabbits) and *Aedes*. Most (>99%) infections are inapparent. The incubation period is 5–15 days. Manifestations: flulike, encephalitis, mainly children. Virtually all encephalitis cases survive, but ~10% have neurological deficits. In enzootic areas, ~2–10% of residents can be seroreactive, and the disease rate can be 20–30/10^5 per year.

Snowshoe hare virus (SSHV) circulates in the holarctic, in hares and *Aedes* mosquitoes. The putative incubation period is 5–15 days. Manifestations: fever and encephalitis. Some 3.5% of residents in enzootic areas can be seroreactive.

Tahyna virus (TAHV) circulates in Africa, Eurasia, and Australia, in rabbits, hedgehogs, and *Aedes* mosquitoes. Manifestations: fever, also encephalitis.

Oropouche virus (OROV) (391, 5918, 7397, 7414) circulates in tropical Latin America, in midges, sloths, and monkeys (sylvatic cycle), and in peridomestic animals and humans (urban cycle). Some 40% of infections are inapparent. The incubation period is ~3–12 days. Manifestations: dengue-like illness, arthralgia. Seroprevalence in urban and forest residents of the Amazon is ~1–35%. More than 30 outbreaks have been reported. Large epidemics have occurred in Brazil: in Belém in 1991 (11,000 infections) and Belém and Manaus in 1980–1981 (100,000 infections).

ORTHOPOXVIRUS (enveloped DNA viruses: *Poxviridae*). This genus includes cowpox virus (CPXV), ectromelia virus, monkeypox virus (MPXV), vaccinia virus, and variola virus.

Cowpox virus (CPXV) (1570, 5817, 8245) circulates in Eurasia, in rodents (reservoir hosts) and rodent-hunting cats; zoo animals, dogs, and cows can also be infected. SPREAD: is via animal contact or injury, mainly from cats or rodents. CLINICAL INFORMATION: The incubation period is days. Manifestations: painful, nodulous or vesiculous, inflamed skin lesions with raised rim that can be anthrax- or monkeypox-like, and regional adenopathy. Diagnosis is by electron microscopy, NAT, or culture from biopsy. IMPACT: Sporadic.

Monkeypox virus (MPXV) (853, 1221, 1912, 4281) circulates in African rain forest, in rodents and monkeys.

SPREAD: is via animal contact (rodents and monkeys), or via skin contact or droplets from patients. The infective period is 1 week from rash onset. Infectiousness is low. However, up to six infection generations have been reported. The secondary attack rate is ~3%. CLINICAL INFORMATION: The incubation period is 10–14 days. Manifestations: mimic smallpox or varicella, although adenopathy can be prominent. Confirmation is by electron microscopy and NAT from pustules. Reported lethality is 9–17%. IMPACT: In 1970–1995, there were 417 cases in humans. In ex-Zaire in 1996–1997, 511 cases were suspected; after excluding varicella, 304 cases met the case definition. In the same area in 1997, seven current and 81 retrospective cases were identified. OUTBREAKS: Several outbreaks have occurred in the African rain forest. In the United States in 2003, an outbreak caused 87 cases (20 laboratory confirmed) in several states; the source was rodents (likely giant rats, *Cricetomys*) imported as pets from West Africa. Smallpox (vaccinia) vaccine seems to partially protect from MPXV; in Africa, contacts with vaccinia scars had an eightfold lower attack rate than nonvaccinated (scar-free) contacts.

Vaccinia virus (VACV) (497, 5785, 6776, 8237). Vaccination (inoculation with infective cowpox material) has been practiced in People's Republic of China since the tenth century, by B. Jesty (1737–1816) in the United Kingdom in 1774, and 22 years later (1796–1798) by E. Jenner (1749–1823) on two "volunteers" (one he challenged with smallpox material, the other was source for vaccine; he published results in 1798). Derived from cows or horses, VACV has been a source for attenuated, widely used smallpox vaccines. SPREAD: is via contact. RISKS: immune-impaired hosts in households of vaccinees, health and laboratory work. Secondary attack rates can reach 9%. CLINICAL INFORMATION: The incubation period is 5–19 (typically 10–11) days. Lethality in secondary cases can reach 10%. IMPACT: For prevention of bioterrorism and as a biodelivery system.

Variola virus (VPXV) (854, 2100, 3252, 8003, 8360). Variolation (inoculation with infective smallpox material) was performed for centuries. After an intensive campaign and vaccinia mass vaccinations, natural smallpox was eradicated in 1977. Remaining reservoirs for VPXV are biodefense (and bioterror) laboratories. SPREAD: is via respiratory droplets and aerosols. RISKS: How many cases a source case could theoretically generate is debated (for R_0 of ~2–10). Although <20% of spread takes place before disease is manifest, infectivity is high, for secondary attack rates of 25–40%. In Meschede, Germany, in 1970, an electrician returning from Pakistan with incubating smallpox, despite being isolated (for suspected typhoid fever), caused 19 secondary cases (on all three floors of the hospital). During a nosocomial outbreak in Nagoya, Japan, in 1945, a person contracted smallpox just from a coffee break in a laboratory. CLINICAL INFORMATION: The incubation period is 7–17 (typically 10–14) days. Manifestations (smallpox): fever, vesiculous rash (vesicles appear simultaneously, become umbilicated), and bleeding. Illness can last 4 weeks. Lethality is 20–50%. OUTBREAKS: The preeradication era was characterized by numerous smallpox outbreaks on all continents.

PAECILOMYCES (5640, 5861, 7928) (*Ascomycota*: *Eurotiales*).

These are hyaline molds that inhabit soil, plant debris, and worm eggs in soil. Spores in air and can contaminate hospital environments. *P. lilacinus* has been reported in humans. SPREAD: is via skin contact, devices, or inhalation. Manifestations (hyalohyphomycosis): cutaneous (nodulous or necrotic lesions), ocular (keratitis and endophthalmitis), and invasive disease (fungemia) in immune-impaired hosts (neutropenia, transplants, and AIDS). Confirmation is by biopsy and culture. Treatment options include triazoles and voriconazole. IMPACT: Sporadic. OUTBREAKS: *P. lilacinus* in a skin preparation used in a transplantation unit caused an outbreak of invasive disease.

PANTOEA (γ-*Proteobacteria*: *Enterobacteriales*).

These gram-negative bacteria inhabit water, soil, plants, and animals. *P. (= Enterobacter) agglomerans* (= *Erwinia herbicola*) (4093) has caused wound infections and septic arthritis from thorny plants, e.g., cacti, yuccas, or palms.

PAPILLOMAVIRUS (unenveloped DNA viruses: *Papillomaviridae*).

The genus includes papillomaviruses of birds, bovids, canids, and felids.

Human papillomavirus (HPV) (526, 5259, 7194, 7239, 8132, 8166). Humans are the only reservoir. There are >100 genotypes, some (e.g., 6, 11) with a predilection for skin (warts), others for anocervical epithelia. SPREAD: is via skin or surface contact (skin warts), sex, or autoinoculation. Anogenital infections are *not* acquired from surfaces at well-maintained public places. RISKS: walking barefoot at public places; age 15–25 years, multiple sex partners, sex work, and sex among men. Virus is shed from lesions or through desquamation; within cells, HPV resists desiccation, remaining viable for up to 7 days. Skin warts tend to recur, whether from reactivation or reinfection is unclear. Immune-impaired persons are susceptible to anogenital infection, and perhaps cervical and anal dysplasia. CLINICAL INFORMATION: Most cervical and many skin infections are inapparent. The incubation period for genitoanal warts is 4–6 weeks (in women whose husbands returned from Asia) to 24 (often 3) months. Manifestations: skin warts ("common," "flat," and "plantar"), genitoanal warts (condylomata acuminata), cervical dysplasia, and malignancy of cervix, perhaps of anus, skin, head, and neck. Thirteen oncogenic (high risk) types (16, 18, 31, 33, 35, 39, 45, 51, 52, 56, 58, 59, 66) are strongly associated with cervical cancer. Diagnosis is by cytology (pap smear), NAT from scrapings, and serology. IMPACT: For STI in the community, see section 14.7, and for prostitutes, see section 13.6. The lifetime risk of genital HPV infection is ~80%. Of all infections, 5% evolve to genital warts and <1% to invasive cervical cancer. Of all malignancies, 2.5% in high-income countries and 7–8% in low-income countries have been attributed to HPV. OUTBREAKS: Outbreaks do not seem to be reported.

PARACHLAMYDIA (*Bacteria: Chlamydiales*). These are intracellular bacteria that survive in free-living amebas (*Acanthamoeba* and *Hartmanella*) (2277). *Parachlamydia* seems to be an emerging cause of amoeba-related pneumonia.

PARACOCCIDIOIDES (*Ascomycota, Onygenales*).
P. brasiliensis (1036, 3795, 5076, 5831, 6229) is a thermally dimporphic fungus from Latin America, mainly Brazil, that occupies as yet unknown niches. Coffee-growing areas and the nine-banded armadillo are suspected to be involved in its natural cycle. SPREAD: is presumed by inhalation of dust. RISKS: Domicile in endemic areas, outdoor work (farm work and wood cutting). CLINICAL INFORMATION: From skin test surveys, up to 80% of infections are inapparent. The incubation period is not known; the youngest reported case was a 2-year-old child. In immigrants, latent infections can be reactivated after years. Manifestations: acute febrile illness and adenopathy (mainly in children), chronic oropharyngeal lesions, weight loss, and pulmonary, tuberculosis-like disease (mainly in adults). Coinfections with *M. tuberculosis* (in ~5%) and *H. capsulatum* have been reported. The male:female ratio is a striking 10:1 (3:1 in children, 15:1 in adults). Confirmation is by visualizing thick-walled budding yeasts in clinical materials (scrapings, biopsy, aspirate, and broncheal lavage), or by culture or NAT from sputum. Treatment options include systemic antifungals and co-trimoxazole. Lethality in 422 cases treated in Brazil in 1980–1999 was 7.6%. IMPACT: By skin test, the infection prevalence in asymptomatic school children living in an endemic area of Brazil was ~5%. The reported disease rate is $1-3/10^5$/year.

PARAGONIMUS (Trematoda: Digenea) (1037, 1818, 5235, 5544, 7960). These lung flukes circulate in Africa, Asia, and Latin America, in mammals (>50 genera), including dogs and cats (final hosts, shed eggs with sputum or feces), snails (first intermediate hosts), and freshwater crustaceans (second hosts, harbor metacercariae). Of >40 species, >10 have been reported in humans, including *P. mexicanus*, *P. africanus*, and *P. westermanni*. Adults have a life span of up to 20 years. SPREAD: is via ingestion of viable metacercariae in freshwater crabs and crayfish. RISKS: habit of eating raw crabs, cross-contamination via hands and kitchen utensils, traditional oriental medicines. CLINICAL INFORMATION: Adults locate in lung parenchyma. The prepatent period is about 3 months. The incubation period (in outbreaks) is 2–15 days. Manifestations: cough, hemoptysis, tuberculosis-like findings on chest X ray, blood and sputum eosinophilia, and elevated total IgE. Aberrant larvae and aberrant zoonotic species (e.g., *P. skrjabini*) can cause extrapulmonary manifestations, including larva migrans, subcutaneous nodules, and space-occupying lesions of brain and viscera. Confirmation is by visualizing operculate eggs in sputum (concentrates) or stool samples. Treatment options include praziquantel and triclabendazole. IMPACT: In the 1990s, ~21 million people were living with the infection. In enzootic areas, reported infection prevalence by sputum microscopy is 0.2–11%. In Vietnam, the median prevalence of *P. heterotremus* by 14 sputum, stool, or serological surveys was 4%. OUTBREAKS: Outbreaks in Nigeria in 1967–1970 and 1983–1985 were attributed to war and the shortage of food and firewood, forcing people to eat raw crabs. In a mountain area of Henan Province, People's Republic of China, in 1995, four of seven tourists contracted *P. skrjabini* disease from eating raw crabs. Indigenous paragonimiasis reemerged in Japan in the 1980s, after being near to eradication in the 1970s.

PARAINFLUENZAVIRUS (enveloped RNA viruses: *Mononegavirales: Paramyxoviridae*) includes murine (Sendaivirus), bovine, and human viruses (PIV).
PIV (846, 4239, 4731, 5846, 6350, 7402). There are four antigenically and genetically different types from two genera: PIV1 and PIV3 from *Respirovirus*, and PIV2 and PIV4 from *Rubulavirus*. For all four, humans are the only reservoir. Shedding is from respiratory secretions. From large isolates in the United Kingdom and Australia, relative frequencies are PIV3, 65–71%; PIV1, 17–19%; PIV2, 8–10%; and PIV4, 0.1–1%; type was not known for 3–6% of isolates. SPREAD: is via droplets, probably contaminated objects. RISKS: PIV mainly infects young children. Travelers and medical personnel are likely vectors. CLINICAL INFORMATION: The incubation period is 1–8 days. Manifestations: include coryza, laryngitis, croup, bronchitis, fever, bronchiolitis, and pneumonia. Immune-impaired hosts are susceptible. Confirmation is by NAT, virus isolation, or antigen detection, mainly from respiratory specimens. IMPACT: Infections occur in epidemic waves, PIV3 in annual waves with peaks in late spring or early summer, PIV1 and PIV2 in biennial waves with peaks in late fall or early winter. OUTBREAKS: Venues for outbreaks include the community, hospitals (mainly departments for immune-compromised hosts such as stem cell recipients), and institutions. Cohorting and standard precautions are means to reduce spread.

PARAPOXVIRUS (enveloped DNA viruses: *Poxviridae*) (7674). The genus includes orfvirus of sheep and goats, and pseudocowpox virus (PCPV) of cows. SPREAD: is via contact. Farm workers and unskilled butchers are at risk. CLINICAL INFORMATION: The reported incubation period is 5–19 (median, 14) days. Manifestations: papulous, vesiculous, nodulous (milker's nodules), or granulomatous skin lesions.

PARVOVIRUS B19 (PVB19). See Erythrovirus.

PASTEURELLA (γ-*Proteobacteria: Pasteurellales*) (630, 1364, 2232, 3457, 4493, 7889). These are small, gram-negative bacteria that colonize the respiratory and gastrointestinal tracts of mammals and birds worldwide. There are >15 species. *P. multocida* causes "avian cholera." Infective species to humans are *P. haemolytica* (from cattle), *P. pneumotropica* (from rodents), but mainly *P. multocida* (from dogs, cats). SPREAD: is via bite, licking, or contact, likely inhalation of animal aerosols. Because infections are observed in persons without a history of animal exposure, and *P. multocida* can colonize the upper respiratory tract of animal workers, reactivated endogenous infection is an alternative mode. CLINICAL INFORMATION: The incubation period seems short (≤1 day). Manifestations: cutaneous (two thirds of cases, wound infection, cellulitis), pneumonia, BSI, and device-related infections (elderly with underlying disease). Lethality of *Pasteurella* meningitis in infants is about 10%. IMPACT: The incidence of *Pasteurella* bite wound infections in France was ~$50/10^5$ per year.

PENICILLIUM (*Ascomycota*, order *Eurotiales*). These are hyaline molds that inhabit soil and wood. *Penicillium* can metabolize cellulose, contaminate petri dishes, and produce toxins and penicillin G (A. Fleming's famous *P. notatum*). *P. camemberti*, *P. glaucum* (Gorgonzola), and *P. roquefortii* are used for producing name-telling cheeses.

P. marneffei (2955, 7599) is unique by being thermally dimorphic and invasive to humans. *P. marneffei* occurs in Southcentral, Southeast, and East Asia. Wild rodents are a reported reservoir (bamboo rats: *Cannomys*, *Rhizomys*), although soil is a more likely source for humans. SPREAD: is presumed via inhalation. Manifestations ("hyalohyphomycosis," invasive, fungemic disease in HIV-infected persons): fever, weight loss, generalized adenopathy, skin eruptions (brown maculopapules), dyspnea, hepatomegaly, and anemia. Confirmation is by culture (of blood, bone marrow, aspirate, and skin), NAT, or biopsy. Treatment options include amphotericin B, itraconazole, and ketoconazole.

PENTASTOMIDA (2020, 4267, 4597) (Arthropoda: Crustacea). These "tongue worms" are taxonomic "odd balls" as they resemble worms but belong to arthropods. Pentastomids circulate in herbivores (intermediate hosts) and reptiles (final hosts, shed eggs with cough or feces). Of ~70 species in 17 genera mainly *Linguatula serrata* and *Armillifer armillatus* are reported in humans. SPREAD: is by uptake of eggs from foods or by animal contact. CLINICAL INFORMATION: Most infections are inapparent, presenting as tiny calcifications (commas) on radiography. Manifestations: are due to migrating or encysted, space-occupying larvae. IMPACT: Sporadic. By routine radiography in enzootic areas, prevalence of infection in humans is 1–2%.

PEPTOSTREPTOCOCCUS (2124) (*Firmicutes: Clostridiales*). These are anaerobic, gram-positve cocci that are part of the human respiratory flora (*P. magnus* is now *Finegoldia magna*, and *P. micros* is now *Micromonas micros*). SPREAD: Infections are endogenous or related to invasive procedures. Manifestations: periodontitis, subcutaneous abscesses, diabetic foot infections, rarely invasive disease (endocarditis and prosthetic joint infection).

PHIALOPHORA (5734) (*Ascomycota: Chaetothyriales*). These are pigmented molds that inhabit soil and vegetation. SPREAD: is via soil contact, trauma with plants, or perhaps invasive procedures. Manifestations: onychomycosis, chromomycosis, eumycetoma, phaeohyphomycosis (subcutaneous necrotizing nodules), keratitis, endophthalmitis, in immune-impaired hosts also invasive disease.

PHLEBOVIRUS (enveloped RNA viruses: *Bunyaviridae*). These are arthropod-borne viruses of mammals in countries with warm climates. RVFV and sandfly fever virus are infective to humans.

Rift Valley fever virus (RVFV) (120, 1157, 2854, 4632, 8263) circulates in Africa and Asia, in rodents, wildlife, and livestock, and *Aedes* mosquitoes, in particular, floodwater breeders. SPREAD: is via (i) *Culex* bite (bridge viremic livestock and humans), (ii) contact with viremic animals, their blood, body fluids, or tissues, (iii) ingestion of raw milk, (iv) possibly droplets from hospitalized patients. RISKS: living in or visits to epidemic areas, work-related animal contacts, animal dieoffs, abortion storms, and abundance of *Culex*. CLINICAL INFORMATION: Inapparent or mild infections occur. The incubation period is 2–6 days. Manifestations: flulike illness (in >90% of cases), vomiting (in ~50%), jaundice (in ~18%), liver failure (in 1%), bleeding (in 1–7%, VHF), retinitis (in ~5%), and confusion or encephalitis (in 1%). Lethality is <1% overall, but 15–50% in hospitalized and outbreak cases. IMPACT: In enzootic areas, reported seroprevalence is 14–23%. OUTBREAKS: Epizootics have been recognized in Africa since 1931. Interepizootic intervals are 2–4 years in forested areas, and 15–30 years in savanna areas that receive irregular rainfall. Satellite sensing of vegetation is proposed for early warning of epizootics. Epidemics follow floods and epizootics. In Africa in 1930–1990, >30 outbreaks occurred. Major and recent examples include Egypt in 1977–1978 (>18,000 cases, 598 [3%] deaths, attack rates 21.5% in farm areas, and 9% in troops), Egypt in 1993 (600–1,500 infections), East Africa in 1997–1998 (89,000 infections), and the Arabian peninsula in 2000 (884 hospitalized cases and 124 [14%] deaths in Saudia Arabia, 1,087 cases and 121 [11%] deaths in Yemen).

Sandfly fever virus (484, 1934, 3251) circulates in North Africa, South Europe (Cyprus, France, Greece, Italy, Portugal, and Spain), and Southwest and Central Asia, in *Phlebotomus* sandflies that maintain the agent transovarially, and rodents, perhaps bats, and domestic mammals. There are three serotypes: Naples (SFNV), Sicilian (SFSV), and Toscana (TOSV). **SPREAD** is via sandfly bite. **RISKS**: domicile in or visits to enzootic areas, outdoor activities (e.g., farm work, fishing, gardening, and military training), summer season. **CLINICAL INFORMATION**: Many infections are mild or inapparent. The incubation period from volunteer studies is 3–7 days. Manifestations (sandfly, phlebotomus, or pappataci fever): flulike illness, severe headache, acute aseptic meningitis (only TOSV). Confirmation is by serology (IgM or ≥4-fold rise in titer). **IMPACT**: Insecticide campaigns against malaria in South Europe (e.g., Greece and Italy) after World War II drastically reduced vector densities, cases, and seroprevalence. However, there is evidence for the reemergence of TOSV. By age and location, the reported seroprevalence in adults in enzootic areas is 0–55%.

PLASMODIUM (2171, 3201, 4107, 5616, 6665) (Alveolata: Apicomplexa: Haemosporidia). These protozoa circulate in mosquitoes (release infective sporozoites from salivary glands), birds, reptiles, and mammals (harbor liver forms, asexual blood forms, and gametocytes). Of >200 speces, *P. falciparum*, *P. malariae*, *P. ovale*, and *P. vivax* are infective to humans. Rarely, monkey plasmodia have been detected in humans. Of all infections, 0–10% (typically 0.5–5%) by microscopy, and up to 30–60% (typically 10–20%) by PCR are mixed. Antimalarial pressure selects for drug resistance, mainly of *P. falciparum*. **SPREAD**: is via mosquito bite, shared needles, injury from parasitemic blood, transfusion, transplant, mother-to-child, or "induced" (obsolete treatments of neurosyphilis or Lyme disease). **RISKS**: include domicile in or travel to endemic areas, nocturnal outdoor activities (e.g., migrants and troops), sleeping in camps, noncompliance with mosquito protection and chemoprophylaxis, parasitemia in pregnancy, and injection drug use. Mosquitoes can be displaced by winds, aircraft, boat, or baggage. **CLINICAL INFORMATION**: Age, immune status, and parasite species and density modify disease expression. In partially immune residents of malarious areas, parasitemia is often inapparent. Parasitemia in children is used to define levels of endemicity (Table 20.4). In nonimmune persons (travelers and preschool children), most parasitemias are manifest, as flulike illness that stays benign (uncomplicated malaria) or progresses in hours or days to life-threatening (cerebral) malaria (Table 20.5). Partially immune persons, too, can contract clinical malaria, e.g., pregnant women or individuals with coinfections (HIV, pneumonia, and typhoid fever). Confirmation is by microscopy of several blood smears (detection threshold, four parasites per μl in thick smear), rapid tests, or PCR (detects subpatent parasitemias). **IMPACT**: Close to 3 billion people (48% of the world population) are exposed (20-25% in hypoendemic areas, and 60% in meso- or hyperendemic areas). There are ~400–550 million cases per year. By age and geography, disease rates are 1,000–35,000/10^5 per year. **OUTBREAKS**: Malaria outbreaks are a threat in highlands of East Africa and Madagascar, the Amazon, the Caribbean coast of South America, and on the border of North and South Korea. Fight against vectors and case management contain malaria, but areas kept free of malaria are vulnerable to introduced malaria. Individual protection includes mosquito repellents, impregnated clothes, and bednets.

P. falciparum (2046, 2224, 3995, 5678, 6923, 7005, 8403) occurs in tropical Africa, Asia, and Latin America.

Table 20.4 Levels of malaria endemicity and transmission

Parameter	Hyper- or holoendemicity	Mesoendemicity	Hypoendemicity
Transmission	Year round	Seasonal (3–9 months)	Irregular (0–3 months)
Typical habitat	Tropical forest	Dry forest, savanna, steppe	Dry lands, highlands
% of children with parasitemia	>50–>75	10–50% (reservoir in dry period)	<10%
No. of sporozoites /person	>1–3 /day	1 / day-month	<1 /month
Immunity (no. of years needed)	Partially protective (<5)	Variable (5–10)	None
% of patients with fever due to malaria	30	By season, 10–80	<10, if outbreaks >80
Risk of drug resistance	Low	Moderate	High

Table 20.5 Clinical characteristics of four major human-infective *Plasmodium* spp.

Parameter	P. falciparum	P. vivax	P. ovale	P. malariae
Prepatency (days)	5.5–28	8–28	12–21	14–60
Incubation (days) (range)	14–21 (5–365)	14–84 (12–365)	14–365	28–49 (8–210)
Severity	Life-threatening (cerebral, organ failure), anemia	Benign (tertian fever) (Ruptured spleen)[a]	Benign (tertian fever)	Benign (quartan fever) Tropical splenomegaly or nephrotic syndromes[a]
Relapse	No	Yes, from liver	Yes, from liver	Yes, from blood

[a]Rare outcomes.

RISKS: Infected *Anopheles* on average inoculate ~8 viable sporozoites per bite. In western Kenya, the time from birth to first *P. falciparum* parasitemia is 3–4 months. Patent infection predisposes to clinical malaria. Risks for cerebral malaria include treatment delays, ineffective treatment, MDR strains, primary infections, and nonimmunity. Ovalocytosis, sickle cell trait, and other inherited factors are partially protective. CLINICAL INFORMATION: (Table 20.5). Although many (20–80%) parasitemias in partially immune persons can be inapparent, even low levels (<1,000/μl) can cause anemia. Densities in partially immune persons predictive of disease, by age and place are 500–15,000/μl (for 4,000/μl, sensitivity and specificity are 80% each). Sequestration of parasitized erythrocytes results in hypoperfusion, somnolence, respiratory distress, and renal failure (cerebral malaria). Momentous peripheral parasite counts do not predict severity. By age, immunity, delay, and availability of treatment, lethality is 0.1–5% (cerebral malaria up to 40%). Infants in endemic areas are prone to severe anemia (hematocrit <15%, hemoglobin <5 g/dl) rather than cerebral malaria. Infection in pregnancy can result in anemia, premature delivery, low birth weight, and congenital infection. IMPACT: *P. falciparum* relative frequency in parasitemia is 80–100% in Africa, 30–90% in Asia and the Southwest Pacific, and 30% in Latin America. Cases are estimated to 300–660 million per year. By age, season, geography, and prophylaxis, disease rates per 100 per year are 0.5–450 (typically 10–100) in residents in Africa and Asia, 0.1 in Latin America, and 0.5–30 in travelers and troops. OUTBREAKS: In 1908, an epidemic in the Punjab (split in 1947 between Pakistan and India) caused >300,000 deaths, for a mortality of 1,500/10^5. Outbreaks are reported in malaria fringe areas, highlands, newly colonized areas, following heavy rains, around dams, on islands, among troops, in a camp, in cities, a hospital, and among IDU. Attack rates reported in outbreaks are 35% (Tajikistan 1997) and 39% (Kenya, 1997).

P. knowlesi (6918) circulates among wild macaques in Asia. Naturally acquired infections in humans were rare until 2000, when 120 NAT-confirmed manifest cases were detected in residents in Sarawak (Malaysian Borneo).

P. malariae (3854, 4913, 6740, 7839) circulates in Africa, Asia, and Latin America. CLINICAL INFORMATION: Parasite density is often low; subpatent parasitemia can persist for decades (Table 20.5). Manifestations: uncomplicated (quartan) malaria, splenomegaly, rarely nephrotic syndrome. IMPACT: There are tens of millions of cases per year. Its relative frequency in parasitemia is 0–30% (typically 0.5–5%). In Brazil, the *P. malariae* prevalence in 497 residents in the Amazon basin was 1% by microscopy but 12% by nested PCR.

P. ovale (1527, 2336, 3854, 7216) circulates in tropical Africa, Southwest and Southeast Asia, and the Southwest Pacific. CLINICAL INFORMATION: Parasite densities >800/μl seem pyrogenic. Manifestations: uncomplicated (tertian) malaria. IMPACT: There are perhaps 10 million cases per year. In Senegal in 1990–1996, the disease rate was 2–25/100 person-years. Its relative frequency in parasitemia is 0–7% (typically 1%).

P. vivax (170, 2046, 2118, 4984, 5732, 6627, 8403) circulates in tropical and temperate areas of Africa, Asia, and Latin America. West Africa is exempt, as its population lacks the Duffy blood group receptor that *P. vivax* needs for erythrocyte invasion. *P. vivax* reemerged in Henan, People's Republic of China, in the early 1990s, and by 1994–1995, 3% of residents were smear positive, and >10% reported ≥1 clinical episode. Manifestations: uncomplicated (tertian) malaria, rarely ruptured spleen (in ~1%), respiratory distress, and critical illness (Table 20.5). Reported parasite densities are 30 to 52,000/μl (often 1,000–6,000/μl). Without causal treatment (of hypnozoites in liver), *P. vivax* can relapse. IMPACT: Its relative frequency in parasitemia is ≥95% in North Africa, Andean highlands, and Turkey; 30–70% in Latin America, Asia, and the Southwest Pacific; and 0–10% in sub-Saharan Africa. There are ~70–140 million cases per year. By geography, protection, and surveillance, disease rates are 0.5–30 (often 10)/100 per year. OUTBREAKS: Recent outbreaks have been reported in the Peruvian Amazon (with an attack rate of up to 83%), the border (demilitarized) zone between North and South Korea, Singapore (in 1996, two foreign workers as sources for 17 locally acquired cases), and among IDUs.

PLESIOMONAS (γ-*Proteobacteria*: *Enterobacteriales*).
P. shigelloides (6144, 6854, 7591) is widespread in fresh and brackish water, sludge, sewage, fish, seafood,

and mammals. SPREAD: is via polluted foods or tap water. RISKS: international travel, eating undercooked seafood, swimming in untreated waters. CLINICAL INFORMATION: An incubation period has not been documented. Manifestations: possibly acute, self-limited diarrhea, rarely, invasive disease in immune-impaired hosts. Sepsis has a lethality of ~60%. IMPACT: By geography, reported fecal prevalence is 0–6%, with a tendency toward higher yield from diarrheic stool samples and tropical countries. OUTBREAKS: Few food-borne and waterborne outbreaks have been reported.

PNEUMOCYSTIS (*Ascomycota: Pneumocystidales*). *Pneumocystis* is a genus of opportunistic, cyst-forming fungi. *P. carinii* occurs in mammals, *P. jirovecii* in humans.

P. jirovecii (4945, 5205, 6065, 6227, 7441, 7771) colonizes the human respiratory tract, in particular, of infants and immune-impaired hosts. SPREAD: Infections are endogenous or acquired, via droplets (perhaps aerosols) in communities, institutions, and open air; intrauterine transmission is possible. Zoonotic transmission (of *P. carinii*) is considered unlikely. RISKS: recent hospitalization. Malnourished children and immune-impaired hosts are susceptible. CLINICAL INFORMATION: Rising antibody titers in healthy persons suggest inapparent infection. From volunteers, clusters, and neonates, the incubation period is 2–12 weeks. Manifestations (*Pneumocystis* pneumonia, PCP): nonproductive cough, progressive dyspnea, fever. PCP is an AIDS-defining illness that occurs when CD4+ T cell counts are <200/µl. Confirmation is by NAT from oropharyngeal washings, induced sputum, or bronchoalveolar fluid, or by microscopy of stained material. By comorbidities and treatment, lethality is 5–60%. Options for treatment and chemoprophylaxis include co-trimoxazole, and combinations of atovaquone or dapsone with pyrimethamine. IMPACT: Exposure seems ubiquitous, and seroprevalence of 50–100% has been reported in children, including by use of human-derived antigens. In Chile in 1998–2000, *P. jiroveci* was isolated by autopsy and NAT in 52% (45/87) of immune-competent children in the community who died unexpectedly, and in 20% (5/25) of children who died in hospitals. Pre-AIDS, the reported PCP rate in high-income countries was 0.03 (infants 0.3)/10^5 per year. In the 1990s, PCP defined AIDS in two thirds of HIV-infected adults in high-income countries, and in 40–60% of children. Although highly active antiretroviral therapy (HAART) has reduced PCP rates to 0.3–3.5/100 person-years, PCP remains an AIDS-defining opportunistic infection. OUTBREAKS: In the 1940s–1970s, outbreaks were reported in Eurasia and Africa, in prematures, malnourished children, and orphans. In the 1980s, outbreaks in IDU and homosexual men portended AIDS. Since the 1990s, the focus has shifted to nosocomial outbreaks. Restoration of immune competence can largely prevent PCP.

PNEUMOVIRUS (enveloped RNA viruses: *Mononegavirales: Paramyxoviridae*). Prototype is RSV.

Respiratory syncytial virus (RSV) (347, 678, 1950, 3650, 7156, 7402) circulates in humans worldwide. Humans shed RSV with respiratory secretions. SPREAD: is via droplets and hand contact, perhaps aerosols, and via objects (hand-to-nose or hand-to-eye, less hand-to-mouth). RISKS: crowded rooms, smokers in the household, winter season. Shedding begins 1 day after infection and continues for 3–7 days (adults), 2–3 weeks (infants), or several months (immune-compromised hosts). CLINICAL INFORMATION: At least 15% of infections are inapparent. Reinfections are frequent. Confirmation is by antigen test or culture from nasal washings. The incubation period is 2–8 days. Manifestations: flulike illness, bronchiolitis, exacerbation of chronic obstructive lung disease, or pneumonia. Prematures, neonates, immune-impaired hosts, and persons with comorbidities are susceptible. Coinfections with *Influenzavirus* can confound the diagnosis of flulike illness. Lethality is ≤0.1% (3–5% in children with comorbidities). IMPACT: In the United States, 50% of children acquire RSV with the first transmission season, and by age 2 years, most have been infected once. Hospitalization rates in infants, by age, season, and urbanization, are 0.3–25% (typically 1–3%) per year. In Lombok, Indonesia, the rate of severe RSV disease in infants <2 years of age was 1/100 child-years. Year-round in United States adults, 2–6% of hospitalizations for pneumonia are related to RSV. By age and season, RSV is recovered from ~15–90% of patients with lower RTI, and 0–50% (typically 25%) of lower RTI are attributed to RSV. OUTBREAKS: Venues for outbreaks include communities, hospitals, and nursing homes. Epidemic waves recur annually, usually in September–May and last 3–6 months.

POLIOMYELITISVIRUS. See *Enterovirus*.

POLYOMAVIRUS (unenveloped DNA viruses: *Polyomaviridae*). Members are bovine and simian (SV40) viruses, and BK (BKV) and JC (JCV) viruses of humans. SV40, BKV, and JCV can cross-react serologically.

BKV (2221, 3344, 4164) (from patient B.K.) circulates worldwide. Humans shed BKV from respiratory secretions, urine, and feces. SPREAD: is presumably via inhalation (droplets, aerosols), contact, or intrauterine, or via foods and drinking water. CLINICAL INFORMATION: Most infections are inapparent, persistent, and established early in life. Manifestations: are limited to immune-impaired hosts and include hemorrhagic cystitis, nephropathy, pneumonitis, retinitis, encephalitis, and, possibly, autoimmune disease, and malignancy. Past infection is diagnosed serologically, active (replicative) infection is diagnosed by culture, NAT, or electron microscopy from biopsy. IMPACT: Worldwide, 45–95% of adults are seroreactive.

JCV (2189, 4164) (from patient J.C.) circulates worldwide. Humans shed JCV in urine. **SPREAD:** Modes are unknown. **CLINICAL INFORMATION:** Most infections are inapparent, persistent, and established early in life. Manifestations: progressive multifocal leukoencephalopathy, a fatal disease of severely immune-compromised patients. **IMPACT:** Worldwide, 70–80% of adults are seroreactive. The point prevalence of JCV in urine is 5%.

SV40 (2212, 6386, 6798) is enzootic in monkeys. **SPREAD:** is via monkey contact. **RISKS:** animal work. Before recognition in 1963, batches of poliovaccine produced on monkey kidney cell lines were SV40 contained, and some pre-1963 vaccine recipients were exposed. **CLINICAL INFORMATION:** SV40 seems unable to establish persistent or reactivated infection in humans. There is a debated link between SV40 and human malignancies (brain, lymphomas, mesotheliomas, and osteosarcomas). SV40 sequences detected in malignant cells are perhaps explained by contamination of expression vectors that are widely used in laboratories. **IMPACT:** Previously reported seroprevalence of 5% in children and of 2–20% in adults is likely confounded by cross-reactivity with BKV and JCV. Virological evidence does not support SV40 circulation in the community.

POLIOMYELITISVIRUS. See Enterovirus.

PORPHYROMONAS (1466, 5471) (*Bacteria: Bacterioidales*).
These are gram-negative anaerobic rods that are part of the buccal flora of dogs, cats, and humans, including *P. gingivalis* and *P. endodontalis*. Manifestations: gingivitis, periodontitis, infected bite wounds.

POWASSAN VIRUS (POWV). See Flavivirus.

PREVOTELLA (*Bacteria: Bacterioidales*).
These are gram-negative, bile-sensitive anaerobic rods that are part of the buccal flora of mammals, including *P. dentalis*, *P. intermedia*, and *P. nigrescens* in humans. Manifestations: periodontitis, infected bite wounds, subcutaneous abscesses, and device-related infections.

PRIONS (85, 1526, 6016, 6029).
Prions are misfolded proteins that cause transmissible spongiform encephalopathies (TSE). TSE in humans are CJD, Gerstmann-Sträussler-Scheinker disease, kuru, and fatal familial insomnia. TSE in mammals include scrapie (in sheep, goats), BSE (in cattle, goats), CWD (in elk, mule deer), transmissible mink encephalopathy (in captive mink, *Mustela vison*), and feline spongiform encephalopathy (in felines, including cats). Curiously, prions can change phenotype (glycosylation, plaque formation in brain, binding to lymphoid tissues) from passage through hosts. Prions are quite resistant to heat and formaldehyde. For inactivation, vapor heat (134°C) is recommended.

Bovine spongiform encephalopathy (BSE) (1224, 1526, 6995) emerged in the United Kingdom in 1986; by 2003, an epizootic had affected ~200,000 cattle, with collateral bovine cases in Asia (Israel and Japan), North America (Canada and United States) and Europe (20 countries). Suspected source was sheep-derived "meat and bone meal" recycled to cattle in the United Kingdom, a mode that resembles kuru. BSE presumably jumped to humans via foods (e.g., meat balls), causing variant CJD in the United Kingdom. Several prion phenotypes may be involved in the causation of BSE. In 2002, the BSE agent was identified in a goat in France. In goat, BSE could cocirculate with scrapie.

Chronic wasting disease (CWD) (5054, 5055, 8182) is known since the 1970s, from captive and free-ranging mule deer (*Odocoileus hemionus*), white-tailed deer (*O. virginianus*), and Rocky Mountain elk (*Cervus elaphus nelsoni*), in patchy prairie areas of the United States and Canada. Spread is horizontal (herd-to-herd) and vertical (dam-to-offspring, before or after birth). Emerging issues include environmental persistence of causative prions, and species jump (deer-to-cattle).

Creutzfeldt-Jakob disease (CJD) (927, 1526, 2775, 3331, 5325, 5916, 8176) (http://www.cjd.ed.ac.uk). Most (85%) cases of classical CJD are sporadic, 10–15% are familial (inherited), and 0–5% are iatrogenic. Variant CJD has emerged in the United Kingdom in 1996, in the wake of the BSE epizootic. **SPREAD:** Modes for sporadic CJD are unknown. Modes for iatrogenic CJD are injection of growth hormone from cadaveric human brain, transplants of human dura mater or cornea, and stereotactic encephalography. Variant CJD is presumably spread via foods tainted with bovine risk materials (brain, spinal cord). It can be transmitted by transfusion of blood from unrecognized, incubating donors. **CLINICAL INFORMATION:** Incubation periods are 16 months to 30 years (iatrogenic CJD), 4–10 years (begin or peak BSE epizootic to first case of variant CJD), or 5–21 years (variant CJD cases from but outside the United Kingdom). Manifestations: progressive dementia and motor dysfunction (classical CJD), anxiety, insomnia, gait disturbance, and slurred speech (variant CJD). Lethality reaches 100% in 4–14 months, at median ages of 28 years (variant CJD) to 68 years (classical CJD). **IMPACT:** Classical CJD occurs worldwide, at rates of 0.1–1.5 (typically 1)/million and year. An unexplained high rate (2.7–3.9/million and year) was observed in Switzerland in 2001–2002. In the United Kingdom, prion protein was demonstrated in 1 of 8,318 lymphoid tissue (tonsil, appendix) samples, for a prevalence of 120/million (95% CI 0.5–900). **OUTBREAKS:** In the United Kingdom in 1996–2004, an outbreak of variant CJD caused >150 confirmed and probable cases. Further cases, likely exposed in the United Kingdom, were diagnosed in Europe (France, Italy, and Ireland) and North

America (Canada and United States). There is evidence that this epidemic is stabilizing.

Kuru (1526, 2575) is a prion disease of the Fore tribe in Papua New Guinea highlands. Similiarities with scrapie prompted transmission experiments in chimpanzees. **SPREAD**: is via ritual cannibalism. **RISKS**: Preference of Fore women for human brain and viscera, and of men for less infective skeletal muscle could explain female preponderance among kuru patients. **CLINICAL INFORMATION**: The incubation period from infections in infants and point source cannibalistic feasts is 4–40 (typically 10–13) years. Manifestations: ataxia, dysarthria, and shivering tremor. Lethality is 100% in 6–24 months. **IMPACT**: Kuru emerged in eastern Papua New Guinea in the 1900s, was described in 1957, and disappeared in the 1990s.

Scrapie (2909, 3384) is known from sheep since the eighteenth century, from goats since the 1940s. Signs are pruritus and ataxia. Scrapie is fatal. Spread is horizontal (sheep-to-sheep) and vertical (ewe-to-lamb), perhaps from the environment (pasture-to-sheep). It would seem that scrapie does not present risks for humans, neither by contact, nor by products (meat, milk). This situation could change, should BSE jump to sheep.

PROPIONIBACTERIUM (*Actinobacteria: Actinomycetales*). These are gram-positive, anaerobic, coryneform rods that colonize mammals and foods (milk and cheese). *P. acnes* (5629) colonizes human skin (sebaceous follicles) and mucosa (conjunctiva, upper respiratory tract, and bowel). **SPREAD**: Infections are endogenous or perhaps acquired via skin contact. Risks: devices, impaired immunity. Manifestations: acne (frequent in adolescents in high-income countries); skin, eye, and abdominal infections; invasive disease, e.g., endocarditis. A treatment option is benzylpenicillin; resistance is reported to clindamycin (in 15% of 304 isolates from Europe) and erythromycin (in 17%).

PROTEUS (3936, 5534, 6503) (γ-*Proteobacteria: Enterobacteriales*). Proteus inhabits the environment and the human bowel. Mainly isolated in humans are *P. mirabilis*, *P. penneri*, and *P. vulgaris*. **SPREAD**: Infections are endogenous or acquired nosocomially. **RISKS**: recent use of antibiotics and indwelling urinary catheter. Manifestations: UTI, SSI, BSI. **IMPACT**: *P. mirabilis* accounts for ~5% of nosocomial UTI, 3% of SSI, 2% of nosocomial pneumonias, and 1% of BSI. While *P. mirabilis* is usually susceptible to β-lactams, the prevalence of isolates that produce extended-spectrum β-lactamase (ESβL) in North America and West Europe is 7–10%. **OUTBREAKS**: Nosocomial outbreaks have been reported, apparently from cross-contamination (e.g. urine bottles), and including by ESβL-producing strains.

PROVIDENCIA (1406, 5264, 5534) (γ-*Proteobacteria: Enterobacteriales*). *Providencia* colonizes the human bowel. Species in humans include *P. alcalifaciens*, *P. rettgeri*, and *P. stuartii*. **SPREAD**: Infections are endogenous or acquired nosocomially. **CLINICAL INFORMATION**: The incubation period is 1–4 (typically 3) days. Manifestations: UTI, acute diarrhea, BSI. **IMPACT**: *P. stuartii* is prevalent in nursing homes, in patients with indwelling bladder catheters. **OUTBREAKS**: *P. alcalifaciens* has caused food-borne community outbreaks. An nosocomial UTI outbreaks by *P. stuartii* cross-contamination is also reported.

PSEUDOMONAS (γ-*Proteobacteria: Pseudomonadales*). These are motile, glucose nonfermenting gram-negative rods.

P. aeruginosa (192, 690, 2237, 3187, 3876, 4401, 8379) inhabits water, soil, vegetation, and skin and mucosa of animals and humans. *P. aeruginosa* can form biofilms on plastic tubings. **SPREAD**: Infections are endogenous (~80%) or acquired (~20%) via droplets, hand contacts, contaminated instruments, or from water (pool, freshwater). **RISKS**: contaminated swimming pools, recent use of antibiotics, invasive procedures, indwelling devices, long hospital stay, and assisted ventilation. Cystic fibrosis and burn patients and immune-impaired individuals are susceptible. In cystic fibrosis, mucoid phenotypes are difficult to eradicate and predict shortened survival. **CLINICAL INFORMATION**: The incubation period is ½–6 days; in burn patients, the average time to acquisition is 8 days. Manifestations: skin infection, external otitis, infected burn wounds, SSI, nosocomial or community-acquired pneumonia, BSI. Treatment options include third (e.g., ceftazidime) generation or extended-spectrum (e.g., piperacillin) cephalosporins. MDR strains (resistant to ceftazidime, piperacillin, imipenem, and gentamicin or ciprofoxacin) account for 4–8% of isolates. Lethality of invasive disease is 20-60%. **IMPACT**: *P. aeruginosa* accounts for ~15% of nosocomial pneumonias, ~10% of nosocomial UTI, ~8% of SSI, and 3–8% of BSI. At a Swiss university hospital, the disease rate was 0.6–1.5/1,000 admissions. **OUTBREAKS**: Settings for outbreaks are mainly hospitals, less frequently nursing homes and the community.

RABIES VIRUS. See Lyssavirus.

RALSTONIA (1500, 4167) (β-*Proteobacteria: Burkholderiales*). These are gram-negative rods that inhabit moist environments. From contaminated solutions or machinery, species such as *R. pickettii* can colonize or infect humans. Groups at risk include cystic fibrosis patients, device carriers, and patients with malignancies.

REOVIRUS (2755) (unenveloped RNA viruses: *Reoviridae*). *Reovirus* occurs in birds, wild and domestic mammals, and humans, their feces, and sewage. **SPREAD:** is presumably via hand contacts or droplets from humans, or via foods or tap water, apparently not from animals. **CLINICAL INFORMATION:** Infections can be inapparent. The incubation period seems ~1–3 days. Manifestations: can be respiratory (**r**), enteric (**e**), or other (**o**, orphan). **IMPACT:** Sporadic. In Argentina in 1981–2001, only 0.1% (3/2,854) of stool samples from children with acute gastroenteritis tested positive for reovirus by polyacrylamide gel electrophoresis.

RESPIRATORY SYNCYTIAL VIRUS (RSV). *See* Pneumovirus.

RESPIROVIRUS. *See* Parainfluenzavirus.

RHADINOVIRUS (enveloped DNA viruses: *Herpesviridae*). Prototype is HHV8 (human herpes virus 8, Kaposi's sarcoma-associated herpesvirus, or "crazy 8").
 HHV8 (328, 2648, 3478, 3686, 4254, 7376) **SPREAD:** is likely via saliva, sex, shared syringes, transfusion, and organ transplant. **RISKS:** injection drug use, perhaps health work. Persons with impaired immunity are susceptible **CLINICAL INFORMATION:** The incubation period is not known. Manifestations: fever, maculopapular rash (primary infection). HHV8 can be oncogenic: persistent infection is associated with Kaposi's sarcoma, lymphomas, and other rare malignancies. **IMPACT:** By age, test, and endemicity of Kaposi's sarcoma, reported seroprevalences in adults are 0–30%. Of transplant recipients, ~10% seroconverted within 6 months.

RHINOSPORIDIUM (protists: Mesomycetozoea). These agents are related to fish protists ("neither fish nor fungus") and the suspected niche is stagnant freshwaters and wetlands.
 R. seeberi (295, 2513, 2572, 6871, 7882) occurs in warmer parts of Africa, the Americas, Asia, and Europe, in horses, cattle, and humans. *R. seeberi* has not been recovered from the environment, and its reservoir is unknown. **SPREAD:** is likely via water contact. **RISKS:** work- and leisure-related water activities. **CLINICAL INFORMATION:** The incubation period in an outbreak was 4–7 months. Manifestations: polyplike growth on mucosa (nasal, conjunctival, occasionally urethral), lymphatic spread, regional lymphadenitis, rarely hematogenous dissemination. Confirmation is by biopsy, if available by NAT, possibly by dot-Elisa (IgM, salivary IgA). Treatment is surgical, antifungals seem ineffective. **IMPACT:** Mainly sporadic, endemic in parts of India and Sri Lanka. In southern India, the prevalence in school children from an endemic area was 1%. **OUTBREAKS:** In Serbia in 1992–1993, 17 people contracted rhinosporidiosis from swimming in a lake east of Belgrad.

RHINOVIRUS (705, 3651, 4525, 5149, 6350, 7618) (nonenveloped RNA viruses: *Picornaviridae*). There are >100 serotypes. Reservoirs are humans who shed virus from nasal secretions. **SPREAD:** is via hand contacts, droplets, aerosols, perhaps objects. **RISKS:** Transmission is seasonal, with local peaks in fall, winter, or spring. Shedding begins 1 day before illness onset, and fades away, in a majority of cases in 6 days, but among children, 20% shed virus for 21 days, and 1% for 28 days. Infectivity is high, for secondary attack rates of 25–70%. **CLINICAL INFORMATION:** 20–70% of infections are inapparent. The incubation period is 10–16 h. Manifestations: profuse rhinorrhea, stuffed nose, sore throat (common cold), acute otitis media, sinusitis, bronchiolitis, acute or exacerbated asthma, and severe respiratory illness in compromised hosts. The term "cold" is misleading as cold winds and wet feet in volunteer studies failed to produce "cold." **IMPACT:** By age and season, rates of acute viral RTI are 0.5–2/person per year. By age, illness (upper and lower RTI), and season, diagnostic yield from respiratory samples can be 4–9%. Of 329 children followed during the first 2 years of life, 24% were seroreactive by age 6 months, and 91% by age 2 years. **OUTBREAKS:** Settings for infrequently reported outbreaks include the community, hospitals, and a long-term care facilities.

RHIZOPUS (5861, 6238) (*Zygomycota*: *Mucorales*). These zygomycetes inhabit soil, plants, and foods (e.g., wheat, rice, onions, groundnuts, and tomatoes). **ACQUISITION:** is by inhalation, injury, or nosocomially (e.g., from wooden tongue blades, adhesive bands). Manifestation (zygomycosis): skin infection, abscess, sinusitis, and invasive disease in patients with neutropenia, diabetes or other immune impairments.

RHODOCOCCUS (*Actinobacteria*: *Actinomycetales*; ex-*Corynebacterium* or *Nocardia*).
 R. equi (8020) is an opportunist that inhabits soil around farms, freshwater and salt water, reptiles, birds, and marine and terrestrial mammals. **SPREAD:** is likely via inhalation, microtrauma, or contact with colonized herbivores (horses). **CLINICAL INFORMATION:** Invasive disease in immune impaired hosts. **IMPACT:** Sporadic; about 100 cases are reported.

RHODOTORULA (5861) (*Basidiomycota*: *Sporidiales*). These are yeastlike fungi that inhabit soil, air, dairy foods, skin, nails, and mucosa. Manifestations: invasive disease in immune-impaired carriers of devices.

RICKETTSIA (360, 909, 3884, 6381) (α-*Proteobacteria*: *Rickettsiales*). These are arthropod-borne, gram-negative, intracellular bacteria. New diagnostic tools detect new species, for a veritable "species fever." Traditional "typhus group" unites *R. provazekii* and *R. typhi* that are transmitted by lice or fleas. A "spotted fever group" unites >30, mainly tick-borne species, including mite-borne *R. akari* and flea-borne *R. felis* (Table 20.6). For spotted fever rickettsiae, humans are incidental hosts. For transmission, ticks need to be attached for >24 h. Rickettsial infections are confirmed by serology (Western blot, ≥4-fold rise in titer, IgM), NAT (from skin biopsy at tick-bite site, removed ticks), or blood culture. Antibodies can crossreact within the genus. Treatment of choice is docycycline.

R. africae (1106, 3684, 5363, 6116) circulates in Africa and likely the Caribbean, in large mammals and *Amblyomma hebraeum* ticks. **SPREAD:** is via tick bite. Risks: domicile in or visits (for >7 days) to enzootic areas, outdoor activities (e.g., hunting), sleeping on the ground, noncompliance with tick prevention. **CLINICAL INFORMATION:** About one third of infections in travelers are inapparent or mild. The incubation period is 4–12 (typically 5–8) days. Manifestations (African tick fever): fever (in ~100% of cases), flulike illness, inoculation eschar (in 50% 1, in 45% >1, in 5% none), regional adenopathy (in 50–100%), skin rash (in 15–45%), stiff neck. **IMPACT:** Reported seroprevalence in residents in enzootic areas is 0–46% (there is cross-reactivity with *R. conorii*). Of first-time travelers to sub-Saharan Africa, 9–11% can be seroreactive. **OUTBREAKS:** Outbreaks have been observed among travelers and troops.

R. akari (865, 3836, 4124, 6071) circulates in North America and Eurasia, in house mice and *Allodermanyssus sanguineus* mites. **SPREAD:** is via mite bite. Risks: contact with mice, IDU. **CLINICAL INFORMATION:** The incubation period is 7–14 days. Manifestations (rickettsial pox): flulike illness, rash (papulovesicular), inoculation eschar. **IMPACT:** Sporadic. Up to 1980, about 800 cases were reported. In New York, N.Y., in 1980–1989, 13 cases were reported, with an age range of 11 months to 58 years. **OUTBREAKS:** In Manhattan, N. Y., in 1979, five cases occurred in two families who lived in the same low-income, crowded building; occupants had reported seeing mice daily.

R. australis (3479, 6350, 6793) circulates in Australia, in mammals and *Ixodes holocyclus* ticks. **SPREAD:** is via tick bite. Risks: outdoor activities. Manifestations: flulike illness, rash (in ~95% of cases), inoculation eschar (in two thirds), and lymphadenopathy (in 85%). **IMPACT:** Sporadic. In 1991–2000, 72 cases (0–24 [mean 7]/year) were reported in various parts of Australia.

R. conorii sl (86, 242, 1735, 1838, 4138, 6493, 7340, 7663) circulates in dogs, other mammals, and *Rhipicephalus sanguineus* ticks, *R. conorii* ss in the Mediterranean, Africa, Southwest Asia, and India; *R. conorii* sl in Israel and Portugal, *R. pumilo* in Central Asia. North of the Alps, *R. conorii* ss is periodically introduced by dogs (and their ticks) returning from Mediterranean holidays. **SPREAD:** is via tick bite. Risks: warm season, dog ownership, animal contact, and visit to enzootic areas. **CLINICAL INFORMATION:** Many infections are inapparent. The incubation period is 1–16 (typically 6) days. Manifestations (Mediterranean, Astrakhan, and Israeli spotted fevers): fever (in ~100% of cases), rash (in 95%), inoculation eschar (in Mediterranean in 30–90%, in

Table 20.6 Selected arthropod-borne rickettsiae: vector, disease, and range

Vector	*Rickettsia* species	Disease	Range
Lice			
Pediculus	R. prowazekii	Epidemic typhus	Africa, Andes, United States
Fleas			
Ctenocephalides	R. felis	Pseudotyphus	United States
Xenopsylla	R. typhi	Murine typhus	Africa, America, Europe
Mites			
Allodermanyssus	R. akari	Rickettsialpox	United States, Eurasia
Ticks			
Amblyomma	R. africae	African tick bite fever	Africa, Caribbean
Dermacentor	R. rickettsii	American spotted fevers	Americas
	R. sibirica	Siberian tick typhus	Eurasia (Russia, China)
	R. slovaca	Spotted fevers	Europe, Southwest Asia
Haemaphysalis	R. japonica	Japanese tick typhus	Japan
	R. heilongjiangensis	Spotted fever	China
Ixodes	R. australis	Queensland tick typhus	Australia
	R. helvetica	"Tick fever"	Europe, Thailand
Rhipicephalus	R. conorii ss	Mediterranean spotted fever	Mediterranean, Africa, India
	R. conorii sl	Israeli spotted fever	Israel, Portugal

Astrakhan in 25%, in Israel in none), lymphadenopathy (in 30%), vomiting and meningism (in 10%). Lethality is 0.5–2.5%. IMPACT: By area, reported seroprevalence in humans is 0-70% (often 15%). The disease rate in enzootic areas is ~1–50/10^5 per year. OUTBREAKS: Household clusters and outbreaks are reported. In the Crimea, southwestern Russia in 1996–1997, an outbreak of Mediterranean spotted fever caused ≥110 cases. In the Astrakhan area close to the Caspian sea in 1983–1989, and outbreak of Astrakhan spotted fever caused 321 cases.

R. felis (762, 2312, 4746, 5584, 6260) circulates in mammals and fleas (*Ctenocephalides felis*, also *Pulex irritans*), probably worldwide. In California and Texas, opossums are likely hosts. SPREAD: is via cat flea. Manifestations: flulike illness, rash. IMPACT: Human or flea infections are reported in Ethiopia, the United States, Central and South America, and southern and western Europe.

R. heilongjiangensis (4944) has been identified in *Dermacentor sylvarum* ticks from the Russian Far East and People's Republic of China, and in humans with acute febrile illness. In Central Asia, a variety of rickettsiae circulate, including *R. akari*, *R. conorii*, *R. japonica*, *R. mongolotimonae*, *R. heilongjiangensis*, and *R. sibirica*.

R. helvetica (78, 2475, 5437) circulates in northern, western, and southern Europe and Thailand, in mammals, and in *Ixodes ricinus* ticks. SPREAD: is via tick bite. Manifestations: fever, myocarditis. IMPACT: Sporadic, reported since 1998. In eastern France, 35 (9%) of 379 forest workers were seroreactive to *R. helvetica*.

R. japonica (1041, 3640, 5466) circulates in southwestern Japan and perhaps other parts of Asia, in rodents, dogs, and *Haemaphysalis longicornis* ticks. SPREAD: is via tick bite. RISKS: seasonal. CLINICAL INFORMATION: The incubation period is 4–7 days. Manifestations: flulike illness, rash, inoculation eschar (in 90% of cases). IMPACT: Sporadic. In Japan from description in 1984 to 2003, >400 cases were reported. In Korea, 20% (676/3,401) of febrile patients were reactive to *R. japonica* in IFA. On Luzon and Samar Islands, Philippines, 1% (2/157) of febrile patients were reactive to *R. japonica* in IFA. However, cross-reactivity could confound these latter results.

R. prowazekii (4580, 4812, 5126, 5412, 6114, 6119, 6235, 7339, 7610, 8417) circulates focally in body lice (*Pediculus humanus*) and humans, and in flying squirrels in the United States. Current foci exist in East African highlands and in the South American Andes. SPREAD: is via lice feces that are rubbed or scratched into skin or eye. RISKS: cold weather, no change of clothes, crowding in prisons, camps, or hospitals, lack of water and soap, louse infestation, conflict and disaster situations, visits to endemic or epidemic areas. CLINICAL INFORMATION: Infections can be latent (in lymphatic tissues) for years.

The incubation period is ~10–14 days. Manifestations (epidemic or louse-borne typhus, LBT): abrupt fever (in ~100%), petechiae (in ~50%), cough (in 40–60%), stiff neck, drowsiness, or coma (in 17–23%). Lethality is 6–30% (untreated) to <0.5–3% (treated). Reactivation (Brill-Zinsser disease) is characterized by abrupt fever, rash, and antibody to *R. prowazekii* (high IgG, low IgM). IMPACT: In a rural village of the Peruvian Andes in 1998, 20% (39/194) of inhabitants were louse infested, and 19% (36/194) were seroreactive to *R. prowazekii*. In eastern Algeria in 2000, a woman was diagnosed with sero-confirmed LBT. In the 1990s, cases of Brill-Zinsser disease occurred in North America and Europe. In 1999, a man from New Mexico contracted LBT in Texas, confirming local persistence of the agent. In the United States in 1976–2002, 41 infections were documented from exposure to flying squirrels or their nests. OUTBREAKS: Devastating epidemics occurred in World Wars I (millions died in Russian labor and prison camps) and II (China in 1940–1946 reported 124,552 cases and 5,642 [4.5%] deaths). More recently, outbreaks occurred in Uganda in 1973–1976 (>300 cases), Bolivia in 1981 (at an altitude of 3,800 m, 22 cases), Burundi in 1995–1997 (during civil war, >45,500 clinical cases and *R. prowazekii* DNA amplified in lice), and Russia in the winter of 1997–1998 (in a psychiatric hospital with failed heating, night temperatures of −10°C, lice-infested staff and patients, and 29 cases). Prevention is based on body hygiene and control of lice.

R. rickettsii (1809, 3332, 3740, 5184, 6284, 6794, 7545) circulates in the Americas, in birds, small and medium-sized mammals (e.g., dogs), and *Dermacentor variabilis* ticks, in South America also *Amblyomma*. SPREAD: is via tick bite. RISKS: outdoor activities (e.g., military training), detached housing, dog ownership, warm season. CLINICAL INFORMATION: From 30% to 80% of infections are inapparent. The incubation period is 2–14 (typically 7) days. Manifestations (Rocky Mountain and Brazilian spotted fevers): flulike illness, skin rash (in 65–90%, begins at ankles or wrists), lymphadenopathy (in ~25%), stupor (in ~25%), stiff neck (in ~18%); inoculation eschars are rare. Lethality is 20–80% (untreated) to 2–6% (with treatment, can occasionally reach 19%). In the United States, lethality is highest at age >40 years. IMPACT: By enzootic area, seroprevalence in healthy residents is 3% (Long Island, N. Y., 22/671) to 4% (Brazil, 22/525). Among Long Island residents, the seroconversion rate was 924/10^5 per year. By area and surveillance (passive, active), disease rates are 0.2–15/10^5 per year. In the United States, reported cases (per 10^5 per year) were 495 (0.2) in 2000, 695 (0.3) in 2001, and 1,104 (0.4) in 2002. OUTBREAKS: Family clusters seem frequent.

R. sibirica (1367, 4388, 6493) circulates in Eurasia, in small mammals, *Dermacentor nuttallii*, *Haemaphysalis concinna*, and likely further ticks. SPREAD: is via tick bite. Risks: rural domicile in enzootic area, warm season. Manifestations (Siberian tick typhus): flulike illness, inoculation eschar, skin rash. IMPACT: In parts of North Asia, up to 50% of local people can be seroreactive.

R. slovaca (1134, 5653, 6118) circulates in southern, western, and eastern Europe, and Southwest Asia, in mammals and *Dermacentor marginatus* ticks. SPREAD: is via tick bite. Tick attachment is typically at the head (in scalp). RISKS: Tick bites appear to cluster in cooler months. CLINICAL INFORMATION: The incubation period is 4½–7 days. Manifestations: mainly regional lymphadenopathy, also necrotic erythema at portal of entry, rarely fever (in ~10%) or rash ("spotless"). Sequelae include asthenia, and alopecia areata at the portal of entry. IMPACT: Sporadic.

R. typhi (665, 1211, 2728, 3271, 4137, 4176, 4471, 6896) circulates in warm climates, in rodents and their fleas, in the southwestern United States also in free-ranging cats, dogs, and opossums and their fleas. SPREAD: is via flea feces that are rubbed into broken skin or mucosa, possibly by flea bites. RISKS: contacts with rats or other rodents (including through grain sacks and in warehouses), contact with cats or other animals, cargo work in port cities, stays in camps, visits to enzootic areas, warm season. CLINICAL INFORMATION: Inapparent infections are likely. The incubation period is 5½–14 days. Manifestations (murine, endemic, or flea-borne typhus, FBT): fever or flulike illness (in ~100%), rash (in 0–80%, often 50%), vomiting and stiff neck (in up to 50%), and cough (in 0–40%). Lethality is 0–3.8%. IMPACT: Sporadic or endemic. Recent case reports are from Brazil, Israel, Sri Lanka, Thailand, and the United States. By age and location, reported disease rates are 0.4–28/10^5 per year. Seroprevalence in residents of enzootic areas is 0–35%. OUTBREAKS: Although easily overlooked, outbreaks have been reported. In Hawaii in 2002, an outbreak caused 25 laboratory-confirmed and 22 probable cases.

ROSEOLOVIRUS (enveloped DNA viruses: β-*Herpesviridae*). Prototype is human herpes virus 6 (HHV6) of which A and B variants exist.

HHV6 (1014, 2517, 5749, 8345, 8389) latently infects human cells, either in salivary glands (HHV6-B), or peripheral blood monocytes (mainly HHV6-B, also HHV6-A). Humans shed HHV6 with saliva for prolonged periods. SPREAD: is via saliva or respiratory secretions, and mother-to-child. Infectivity is high. RISKS: include having older siblings and being female. CLINICAL INFORMATION: Most intrauterine infections seem inapparent (unlike related CMV), while most (>90%) postnatal infections are manifest. The incubation period is ~10–15 days. Acute primary infections by HHV6-A in infants (exanthema subitum) include running nose (in 65%), fever (in >50%), and roseola (rash on defervescence, in >20%). HHV6-A and HHV6-B can be reactivated in patients with impaired immunity (malignancy, transplant, and AIDS), causing viremia and disseminated disease (e.g., bone marrow suppression, pneumonitis, retinitis, and encephalitis). Confirmation is by NAT (from saliva, blood, or CSF), serology, or culture. IMPACT: HHV6 is acquired in early childhood. Seroprevalence increases with age; from 40% at age 1 year to 77% at age 2 years, to approach 100% in older children. OUTBREAKS: Venues for outbreaks include day care centers, an orphanage, and hospitals.

ROSS RIVER VIRUS (RRV). See Alphavirus.

ROTAVIRUS (RV) (208, 668, 2410, 5726, 6910, 7091, 7835) (unenveloped RNA viruses: *Reoviridae*). Capsid and "wheel" proteins define group (A–G) and serotype (G, P) antigens. Groups A–G circulate in birds and mammals, groups A–C in humans (A, worldwide; B, mainly in epidemics in Asia; and C, regionally). Frequent group A serotypes are P4G2, P8G1, P8G3, and P8G4, while P8G9 is emerging. SPREAD: is via hand contacts, droplets, and possibly aerosols, and via foods, tap water, or objects. Zoonotic spread seems insignificant. RISKS: contact with a case, day care, crowded domicile. In children, fecal shedding begins 3–5 days before diarrhea onset (d_0) and continues for 7–14 days *after* cessation of diarrhea. Infectiousness is high. By tissue culture infectious doses ($TCID_{50}$), infectious particles are highly concentrated in diarrheic stools (10^6 $TCID_{50}$/ml), while the infective dose is low (1–10 $TCID_{50}$/ml). CLINICAL INFORMATION: By age and test, the proportion of inapparent infections is 10–75% (high in the first and second year of life). The incubation period is 1–4 (in volunteers up to 6) days. Manifestations: watery or dehydrating (cholera-like) diarrhea (in one third up to 20 bowel movements/24 h), vomiting, and fever. Confirmation is by antigen detection from stool, or NAT. IMPACT: By test, specimen (watery, soft), and case mix (acute diarrhea or not, children or adults, in- or outpatients), diagnostic yield is 10–70%. Due probably to polymicrobial infections, the fraction of diarrhea that is attributable to RV is only 5–10%. By age 3 years, 60–90% of children worldwide will have been infected. Primary infections are the most frequent cause of *severe* (hospitalized) diarrhea worldwide, while reinfections are milder. The disease rate in preschool children is ~25% per year, for 138 million diarrhea episodes (111 million at home, 23 million visiting clinics, 2 million hospitalized, including ~0.5 million deaths). Rates are lower in high-income countries (5–9% per year) than in low-income countries (100–120% per child), and >80% of deaths are in low-income countries. OUTBREAKS: Though mainly an infection of infants, adults can be affected. Venues for outbreaks include the community, schools, long-term care, and travel groups. Examples of large epidemics are Micronesia in 1964 (nearly 3,500 cases), People's Republic of China in 1982–1983 (group B, several epidemics, >1 million cases), Japan in 1988 (group C, Fukui city schools, 675 cases), and Tirana, Albania, in XII/2000 to I/2001 (waterborne, >900 cases). A first generation vaccine was withdrawn from the marked for perceived or real risk of intussusception.

RUBIVIRUS (enveloped RNA viruses: *Togaviridae*). *Rubivirus* is a "stranger among togavirids" (Table 20.1).
  Rubella virus (417, 1781, 2296, 3033, 4215, 5109, 5942, 8096, 8407) circulates in susceptible humans worldwide. **SPREAD**: is via droplets and mother-to-child. **RISKS**: noncompliance with vaccine programs, contact with a case (friends, school mates, family, and colleagues), crowded working and living conditions. Shedding begins 7–13 days before rash onset (d_0) and continues for 17–19 days; congenitally infected babies shed virus for ≥1 year, including from urine. For worker safety, infectivity is stated to last from 7 days before d_0 to 7 days thereafter. Infectivity is moderate to high (R_0 is 3–8). **CLINICAL INFORMATION**: 10–50% of infections are inapparent. The incubation period is 7–27 (typically 14–21) days. Postnatal rubella is manifest by rash (in ~100%), adenopathy (in 75%), fever (in 50%), and arthralgia. Congenital rubella is manifest by cataract, deafness, neurological, and cardiac defects. Case definitions can predict only ~20% of sporadic cases, and in high-income countries with high vaccine coverage and low disease rates, ≤3–48% of reported cases are laboratory confirmed as rubella. Confirmation by NAT or serology (IgM and IgG) from saliva or serum is therefore essential. **IMPACT**: In high-income countries, rubella has shifted from children to young adults. Among nonvaccinated young women, ≥80% are now susceptible. In low-income countries, children are frequently infected, and most, but not all, pregnant women are immune. The latest reported disease rates in high-income countries per 10^5 per year range from <0.01 (United States) to ~1 (Australia) and ~2 (Germany). In epidemic years, population disease rates can reach 15–200/10^5 per year. **OUTBREAKS**: A pandemic occurred in 1963–1965. Rubella epidemics recur in natural cycles every ~3–5 years. Venues for outbreaks are the community, households, minorities, religious groups, colleges, worksites, production halls, ships, a cinema, troops, prisons, and clinic waiting rooms. Acre state, Brazil, in 2000, experienced 391 confirmed cases, for an attack rate of 150/10^5. Bishkek City and Chui Oblast, Kyrgyzstan, in 2001, reported 326 confirmed cases, for an attack rate of 129/10^5. Effective vaccines are available. In areas with high vaccination coverage, susceptible immigrants can become reservoirs and victims of postnatal and congenital rubella.

RUBULAVIRUS (PARAMYXOVIRIDAE). See *Mumps virus* and *Parainfluenzavirus 2 and 4 (PIV2, PIV4)*.

SACCHAROMYCES (*Ascomycota*: *Saccharomycetales*). These are yeasts well known from baking and fermenting sugar (*S. uvarum* and *S. cerevisiae*). *S. cerevisiae* can also colonize human mucosa and cause fungemia or invasive disease in carriers of devices and individuals with impaired immunity.

ST. LOUIS ENCEPHALITIS VIRUS (SLEV). See *Flavivirus*.

SALMONELLA (γ-*Proteobacteria*: *Enterobacteriales*). These are gram-negative rods. Prototype is *S. enterica* that features >2,450 serotypes.
  Non-Typhi serovars (382, 1052, 2151, 2252, 4828, 7855, 7881) circulate worldwide, in birds, reptiles, wild and domestic mammals, and humans, their feces, sewage, hands, and foods. Of worldwide isolates typed in 1995 ($n = 264,195$), 67% (176,256) were *S. enterica* serovar Enteritidis, and 16% were Typhimurium, and these two serotypes have remained dominant ever since. Phage (definitive) types (DT), and infrequent (<2%) serotypes are useful markers of vehicles and sources. Examples are serovar Agona in oat cereals and dried beef, serovar Berta in soft cheese, serovar Ealing in milk powder, serovar Goldcoast in paté and sausage, serovar Hadar in turkey, serovar Livingstone in fish, serovar Napoli in chocolate, serovar Oranienburg in black pepper, serovar Stourbridge from unpasteurized goat cheese, and serovar Virchow in poultry. Salmonellae survive in water for days, in soil for 2–14 weeks, in ripening cheese for 7–10 months, and in manure and feeds for years. Heat kills salmonellae (in milk pasteurization, in water 65°C for 3 min, in foods, 60°C for 2 min). Resistance to ampicillin and co-trimoxazole is widespread and resistance to quinolones and MDR is emerging. **SPREAD**: is via foods, animal contacts, and exceptionally, under poor hygienic conditions, by hand contact. **RISKS**: travel to high-risk (tropical) countries, summer season. Shedding in stool continues for 4 weeks (in 40–50% of cases), for 8–12 weeks (in 5–15%), or for 9–12 months (in <5%, mainly infants). Shedding can be intermittent. Antimicrobials prolong rather than abrogate shedding. **CLINICAL INFORMATION**: By infective dose, the incubation period is 6 h to 5 days, typically 1–2 days, rarely (without secondary spread) 16–27 days. Manifestations: include diarrhea (in >90%), fever (in 70–80%), cramps, occult blood loss (in ~40% by microscopy), and bactermia and metastatic infections (in ~3–5%, mainly infants). Major non-Typhi, non-Paratyphi invasive serovars are Typhimurium, Enteritidis, Heidelberg, and Choleraesuis. Lethality of food-borne salmonellosis is 0.8–3% (with a high for invasive disease). **IMPACT**: Diagnostic yield in

submitted stools is ~0.5–5%. High-income countries report disease or laboratory isolation rates per 10^5 per year of 10–100 (United States, 15; Spain, 17; Switzerland, 30; Australia, 40). The rate of invasive disease in the United States is ~$1/10^5$ per year. **OUTBREAKS:** Numerous outbreaks are reported by a variety of vehicles, including raw eggs (and products), raw milk (and products), poultry, pork, pastry, raw vegetables, and sprouts. However, most (90%) infections are sporadic.

Serovar Typhi (1661, 4393, 5597, 5742, 6291, 7144, 7537, 7681, 7860, 8343). Humans are the only living reservoir. Serovar Typhi shares capsular Vi antigen with serovars Paratyphi C and Dublin and with *Citrobacter freundii*. Resistance to co-trimoxazole and ampicillin is widespread, and resistance to quinolones and third-generation cephalosporins is emerging. **SPREAD:** is via foods, tap water, or close contact. **RISKS:** include unsafe tap water, lack of toilets, no handwashing, no use of soap, raw sewage discharge in vicinity, foods handled by carriers, foods from stalls, flies on foods, sharing foods from the same plate, a case or carrier in the household, and domicile in or travel to areas with poor sanitation. By gastric acidity (antacids and gastrectomy), the infective dose is 10^6–10^3 bacteria. Serovar Typhi is shed in feces from incubation to recovery; ~10% of patients shed serovar Typhi for ~3 months, and by age and treatment, 1–5% become long-term (>1 year) carriers. The New York cook carrier "typhoid Mary" in the 1900s was source for 53 typhoid cases. **CLINICAL INFORMATION:** By infective dose, the incubation period is 3–60 (typically 7–28) days. Manifestations (typhoid fever): persistent fever (in 90–100%), bacteremia (50–90%), rose spots (0–50%), and reduced sensorium. Complications include jaundice (in up to 30%), intestinal bleeding (in 4–15%) or perforation (in 1–2%), myocarditis (in 5%), and encephalopathy (in 0.5–1.5%). Confirmation is by culture (blood, stool, and duodenal fluid). By treatment, 5–15% of patients relapse, typically 2–3 weeks after defervescence. Lethality is ≤1% (in complicated cases up to 10%). **IMPACT:** Of worldwide *Salmonella* isolates in 1995 ($n = 264{,}195$), ~1% (3,572) were serovar Typhi. There were ~22 million cases of typhoid and paratyphoid fever and 0.2 million deaths worldwide in 2000. Disease rates per 10^5 per year are <10 in high-income countries (United States, 0.1; France, 0.2; Australia, 4; and Italy, 1, in the south up to 7), but 10–1,000 in low-income countries. In high-income countries, 75–95% of cases are imported, and few (<10%) are outbreak related. In controls of 20 vaccine trials, the median rate was $75/10^5$ person-years. In Delhi, India, in 1995–1996, the disease rate was $980/10^5$ person-years (2,730 at age <5 years, 1,170 at 5–18 years, and 110 at 19–40 years). **OUTBREAKS:** In the city of Hamburg in 1885–1888, a waterborne typhoid outbreak caused 15,804 cases with 1,214 (8%) deaths. In the United States in 1960–1999, 54 outbreaks caused 957 cases (18 per outbreak), with attack rates of 0.3–80% (median, 23%). Of outbreaks with vehicle known, 26 were food borne (including nine by fresh salads, four by seafood, and four by meat), and six were water borne. In Tajikistan in 1997, MDR serovar Typhi caused 8,901 cases. In Nepal in 2002, a waterborne outbreak caused 5,963 cases.

Vaccines (inactivated and attenuated) are available, with 50–70% efficacy for 2–5 years.

SAPOVIRUS (SaV) (3132, 6353) (unenveloped RNA viruses: *Caliciviridae*). SaV circulates worldwide, in humans and the environment. SaV is less frequent than but comparable to NoV (see *Norovirus*).

SARCOCYSTIS (2554) (*Alveolata*: *Apicomplexa*: *Eucoccidiorida*). These are oocyst-forming coccidian protozoa that circulate worldwide, in mammals (final hosts, shed oocysts), and birds and mammals (intermediate hosts, harbor cysts in tissue).

S. hominis (ex-*S. bovihominis*, *Isospora hominis*) and **S. suihominis** (1935, 6713). Humans are final hosts who shed oocysts (or free sporozoites) with feces. **SPREAD:** is via ingestion of undercooked beef (*S. hominis*), pork (*S. suihominis*), or venison. **CLINICAL INFORMATION:** The prepatent period (in volunteers) is 10–12 days. The incubation period is hours to 1 week. Manifestations (intestinal sarcocystosis): watery diarrhea and eosinophilic enteritis. Confirmation is by microscopy of stool or duodenal biopsy. Unlike *Isospora*, oocysts of *S. hominis* are sporulated and infective when shed. **IMPACT:** Sporadic. The fecal prevalence is ≤0.5%

Sarcocystis sp. (282, 8250). Humans are intermediate hosts who carry cysts in tissue (muscle). **SPREAD:** is via ingestion of sporulated oocysts from mammals, or foods fecally polluted by dogs, cats, or other mammals. **CLINICAL INFORMATION:** The presumed incubation period is 1–3 weeks. Manifestations (tissue sarcocystosis): fever, myalgia, fleeting rash, and blood eosinophilia. Confirmation is by tissue (muscle) biopsy. **IMPACT:** Sporadic. By geography, reported prevalence in enzootic areas by autopsy is 0–20%. **OUTBREAKS:** In rural Malaysia in 1993, 7 of 15 U.S. military personnel contracted muscular sarcocystosis; reported exposures included extensive contact with soil, drinking untreated water, and consumption of lizard meat, and fresh vegetables.

SARCOPTES. *See section 4.6.*

SARS-COV. *See Coronavirus.*

SCEDOSPORIUM (4666, 7143, 7928) (*Ascomycota*: *Microascales*). These are pigmented molds that inhabit soil. *S. apiospermum* (=*Pseudallescheria boydii*) and *S.*

prolificans have been isolated in humans. The former seems less virulent than the latter, but more widespread, including in cattle and poultry manure, sewage, swamps, and coastal tidelands. *Scedosporium* can colonize the respiratory tract of cystic fibrosis patients and transplant recipients. **SPREAD**: is via injury, inhalation of dust, or invasive care. Manifestations: wound infection, septic arthritis, white-grain eumycetoma, in immune-impaired hosts invasive disease. Lethality of invasive disease is high (~60%).

SCHISTOSOMA (4654, 7225, 7670) (Trematoda: Digenea). These are tissue flukes that circulate in mammals and humans (final hosts, harbor adults in viscera, pass eggs in urine or feces), and aquatic snails (intermediate hosts, release infective cercariae into water). Of ≥15 species, *S. haematobium*, *S. intercalatum*, and *S. mansoni* infect humans, and *S. japonicum*, *S. malayensis*, and *S. mekongi* infect mammals *and* humans. In parts of Africa, where *S. haematobium* and *S. mansoni* coexist, mixed infections occur. Life span of adult worms in humans is 3–8 years, on occasion 30–37 years. **SPREAD**: is via contact with stagnant freshwater. **RISKS**: domicile close to foci, work- or leisure-related water contacts (e.g., rice farming, fishing, swimming, and washing), dam and irrigation projects, discharge of raw sewage into freshwater, raw feces for fertilizer, and adventure travel (rafting and canoeing). Infective water sites are focal, seasonal, and vary with human use. **CLINICAL INFORMATION**: first-line treatment is with praziquantel. Of chronically infected, untreated residents in endemic areas, ~10% will develop disease complications. **CONTROL**: Preventive and control measures include sanitation, provision of tap water, education about defecation, mass or targeted praziquantel treatments, and snail elimination by water management and molluscicides.

S. haematobium (898, 913, 2163, 3178, 4340, 5951, 8103) circulates in >50 countries of Africa and Southwest Asia, in humans who shed eggs in urine, and freshwater *Bulinus* snails. **CLINICAL INFORMATION**: Adults locate in pelvic venules. The prepatent period is 10–12 weeks. From 20% to 50% of light infections are inapparent or latent. The incubation period is 10–12 weeks (first hematuria) to years (complications). Manifestations (urinary schistosomiasis): dysuria, cystitis, micro- or macrohematuria, and anemia. A history of water contact in endemic areas plus hematuria is suggestive. Confirmation is by visualizing eggs (with a terminal spine) in repeated early-morning urine filtrates. Egg counts >50/10 ml define heavy infection. Complications include obstructive uropathy (hydroureter, hydronephrosis, diagnosed by ultrasound), inflammation from dystopic eggs (e.g., transverse myelitis, epididymitis, and cervicitis), and carcinoma of the bladder. **IMPACT**: Over 430 million people live in infected areas, >110 million are infected, ~50–90 million have the disease, and there are ~0.16 million attributable deaths per year. By age and habitat, infection prevalence can be 0–100%. In Egypt in the 1990s, prevalence was 0–2% in the Nile delta but 5–14% in middle and upper governorates. In Chad, of 1,017 children 8–13 years of age, 23% were infected, and 6% had heavy infections. Reinfection rates in clinical studies were high (30–80% in 6–7 months). **OUTBREAKS**: Outbreaks of acute schistosomiasis have been reported in travelers. Targeted treatment (e.g., of school children) is recommended when infection prevalence is ≥50% in school surveys, or macrohematuria prevalence is ≥30%.

S. intercalatum (2636, 6282, 7383) is curiously limited to ~10 countries in central Africa. Final hosts are humans, intermediate hosts are *Bulinus* snails (also host *S. haematobium*). *S. intercalatum* can hybridize with *S. haematobium*. Urban foci exist. The prepatent period is 5–7 weeks. Manifestations (colonorectal schistosomiasis): resemble intestinal schistosomiasis but lesions preferentially locate in the sigmoid or rectum. Unlike *S. mansoni*, eggs in stool are fusiform and lack a lateral spine.

S. japonicum (189, 4344, 4398, 4399, 6044, 6417) circulates in People's Republic of China, Indonesia, and the Philippines, in mammals (e.g., pigs, cattle, and cats) and humans (shed eggs with feces), and freshwater *Oncomelania* snails (release cercariae). **CLINICAL INFORMATION**: The prepatent period is 3–10 weeks. The incubation period is 2–12 (typically 6) weeks (acute infection) to 30 years (complications). Manifestations: can be acute (Katayama fever) by fever and eosinophilia, or chronic (hepatocolonic schistosomiasis) by diarrhea, colitis, anemia, hepatosplenomegaly. Complications include hepatic fibrosis and neural schistosomiasis. Fibrosis and possible progression to liver cancer are suspected to be enhanced by HBV or HCV coinfection. A history of water contact in enzootic-endemic areas should trigger tests. Confirmation is by visualizing rounded eggs with a lateral knob in repeated stool specimens or rectal biopsy. **IMPACT**: In People's Republic of China over 30 years, impressive efforts brought infections down to 0.9 million in five provinces; prevalence in remaining infected areas is 5–8%. In a treatment trial in Hunan Province, People's Republic of China, in 1996–1998, the reinfection rate was 22%. In the Philippines, *S. japonicum* is enzootic-endemic in ≥5 islands (Bohol, Leyte, Mindanao, Mindoro, and Samar), for an overall prevalence of 4–5%. Decade-long control efforts have eliminated *S. japonicum* in Japan.

S. malayensis is related to *S. japonicum*. It is enzootic in the forests of the Malaysian peninsula. Infections in humans are rare and incidental.

S. mansoni (429, 900, 2214, 2714, 3776, 3924, 4809, 7399) circulates in >50 countries of Africa, South America, and Southwest Asia, in humans (shed eggs in feces) and freshwater *Biomphalaria* snails. **CLINICAL INFORMATION:** Adult worms locate in mesenteric veins. The prepatent period is 5–8 weeks. At least 40–50% of infections are inapparent or latent. The incubation period is hours (dermatitis) to 2–10 weeks (fever) or 30 years (complications). Manifestations: can be acute and local (swimmer's itch) by a fleeting, pruriginous skin rash at the portal of entry, acute and systemic (Katayama fever) by fever and blood eosinophilia, or chronic (colonic schistosomiasis) by diarrhea, dysentery, appendicitis, and anemia. Complications include hepatic fibrosis, portal hypertension, myelitis, and coinfections with HBV, HCV, *Salmonella*, and soil-transmitted helminths. A history of water contacts in endemic areas should trigger tests. Confirmation is by visualizing eggs with a lateral spine in repeated stool samples or rectal biopsy. Egg counts >400–500/g define heavy infections. **IMPACT:** Nearly 400 million people live in infected areas, >50 million are infected, 4–9 million have the disease, and there are ~0.13 million attributable deaths per year. Prevalence varies broadly by age, place, and time. In parts of metropolitan Belo Horizonte, Brazil, prevalence is 9–12%. In Egypt in the 1990s, infection prevalence was 18–43% in the Nile delta, but 0.5–4% in the middle and upper governorates. In western Kenya, of 1,738 school children, 22% were infected, and 4.5% had heavy infections. In Uganda in 1998–2000, the prevalence was 20% in 13,798 schoolchildren, and 48% in 9,829 community members. Reinfection rates in clinical studies were high (40–70% after 5–12 months). At altitudes of 1,800–2,200 m in Ethiopia in 1997, the infection rate was 20% per year. Similarly, in irrigated areas of Sudan in 1988–1989, infection rates were 15–58% per year. **OUTBREAKS:** Outbreaks have occurred at a holiday resort in Brazil, following floods, near a dam, and among travelers. Mass treatment and snail control have eliminated *S. mansoni* in most Caribbean islands, notably Puerto Rico and St. Lucia. Obstacles are insensitive tests to detect lightly infected carriers and anthelminthic resistance.

S. mekongi (330, 7176, 7655) circulates in Cambodia and Laos, in mammals and humans, and *Neotricula* snails. Manifestations: hepatosplenomegaly, portal hypertension. In foci along the Mekong River prevalence can reach 15–50%.

Zoonotic schistosomes (83, 1131, 3426, 4368). Avian schistosomes (*Gigantobilharzia*, *Trichobilharzia*) from temperate freshwaters do not complete development in humans, some mammalian schistosomes (e.g., *S. bovis* and *S. mattheei*) from tropical freshwaters only occasionally do. Their larvae cause self-limited cercarial dermatitis characterized by pruritis, rash, and eosinophilia shortly after exposure to infective freshwater.

SERRATIA (322, 1016, 2233, 2427, 2953, 5652, 7226, 7863) (γ-*Proteobacteria*: *Enterobacteriales*). These are gram-negative rods that inhabit water, plants, even plastic (e.g., blood bags), and some members can degrade hydrocarbons in gasoline and lubricating oil. Of >10 species mainly *S. marcescens* is isolated in humans. Strains can produce ESβL. **SPREAD:** Infections are endogenous or acquired, likely via hand or skin contacts, including in hospitals, possibly via inhalation of aerosols. **RISKS:** recent use of antibiotics, invasive procedures, exposure to contaminated solutions or medical equipments, assisted ventilation, and impaired immunity. *S. marcescens* can colonize skin, respiratory tract, and urinary tract of device carriers, e.g., bladder catheters. Hospital patients can carry *S. marcescens* for at least 1–2 months. **CLINICAL INFORMATION:** Outbreaks suggest incubation periods from 1 day to 3–4 weeks. Manifestations: nosocomial UTI, RTI, SSI, eye infection, and invasive disease (e.g., sepsis). Confirmation is by culture. **IMPACT:** *S. marcescens* accounts for ~1% each of nosocomial UTI, SSI, and BSI. From 0% to 60% of hospitalized patients can be colonized. Nosocomial *S. marcescens* bacteremia rates per 100 patient-days are 0.002–0.01, in outbreaks up to 0.8. **OUTBREAKS:** Reported sources or vehicles for outbreaks include sinks, urine containers and urinals, milk bottles, solutions (including disinfectants), instruments (laryngoscopes and eye droppers), devices (electronic and monitoring), and inadequately sterilized theatre linen. An epicenter are neonatal ICUs.

SHIGELLA (33, 723, 2981, 3946, 4072, 6853, 8129) (γ-*Proteobacteria*: *Enterobacteriales*). *Shigella* circulates worldwide, in humans (the only host), their feces, hands, and foods. Four species and a number of serotypes are recognized although *Shigella* is genomically a single species that is conspecific with *Escherichia coli*. Relative frequencies among all isolates in high- (low-)income countries are 70–80% (15%) for *S. sonnei*, 15–25% (55–60%) for *S. flexneri*, 1–6% (1–6%) each for *S. dysenteriae* and *S. boydii*. Of *S. dysenteriae*, type 1 is particularly virulent for severe disease and high epidemic potential. *Shigella* is inactivated by heat ($\geq 65°C$), but survives freezing ($-20°C$) and acidity (e.g., in fruit juices). Resistance to ampicillin and cotrimoxazol is frequent, and resistance to quinolones is emerging. **SPREAD:** is person-to-person (via hands, 80% in the United States) and via fecally polluted foods. The infective dose is low. By species, 10–100 bacteria cause illness in 10–40% of volunteers. Shedding is for ~1 week, occasionally for 11 weeks. The risk of interhuman spred is high: reported secondary attack rates are 20–70%. **RISKS:** poor housing, lack of tap water, no hand hygiene, no soap for washing hands, poor catering practices, attending day care, living in institutions, holiday camps, or military camps. Transmission can be seasonal. **CLINICAL INFORMATION:** From 25% to 55% of infections are inapparent. The incubation period is hours to 8 (typically 2) days. Manifestations: diarrhea (in ~100%), cramps (in 30–85%), fever (in 20–80%), vomiting (in 20–50%), dysentery (in 10–35%), and pus cells or erythrocytes on microscopy of feces (in 60–95%). In the United States, ~10% of cases are hospitalized. Lethality is 0.05–0.7% (in epidemics in low-income countries 1–7%). **IMPACT:** Worldwide, there are ~140–165 million cases per year (91 million in Asia), and 0.6–1.1 million deaths per year (0.4 million in Asia). In high-income countries, reported disease rates per 10^5 per year are 2–10, with a high (8–36) in preschool children, and a low (~1) in the elderly; in the United States in 2000–2002, rates were 7–8. In low-income countries, dysentery rates reach 200–2,700/10^5 per year, or 0.2 per child-year. By age and case mix, diagnostic yield of stool cultures is ~0.2% (high-income countries) to 5–15% (low-income countries). **OUTBREAKS:** Pandemics were described in the 1960s–1980s, affecting Latin America, Africa, and Southeast Asia. Epidemic S. dysenteriae type 1 waves recur at intervals of ~10 years. Venues for outbreaks include communities, minorities, schools, and camps. In a district in Sierra Leone in 1999, an outbreak caused 4,218 dysentery cases, for an attack rate of 7.5%. Preventive and control measures include provision of tap water and sanitation, promotion of hand hygiene, safe water storage, and water disinfection by end users, provision of safe foods, exclusion of ill persons from food work, recall of contaminated products, and prompt isolation and treatment of cases.

SICILIAN SANDFLY FEVER VIRUS (SFSV). See Phlebovirus.

SIMPLEXVIRUS (enveloped DNA viruses: α-Herpesviridae). Simplexvirus includes human (HSV or HHV) and simian (SHV) herpes viruses. **Herpes simplex virus** (HSV) (3944, 6513, 7106, 7907) circulates worldwide. Humans shed virus type 1 (HSV1) or type 2 (HSV2) from mucocutaneous lesions, saliva, or genital secretions. Shedding is for 1–8 weeks after primary infection, and intermittently thereafter. From genital sites, HSV2 is shed for more days than HSV1. HSV becomes latent in root ganglia, HSV1 of the head (e.g., N. trigeminus), HSV2 of the pelvis. Treatment options include nucleoside analogues (acyclovir, famciclovir, and valacyclovir).

HSV1 (205, 5941, 8290). **SPREAD:** is via lip, hand, and skin contacts, and orogenital sex, rarely via contact with objects (mattresses and instruments). **CLINICAL INFORMATION:** About 90% of primary infections are inapparent. The incubation period is 2–12 (typically 4) days; in an outbreak among wrestlers it was 4–11 days. Manifestations: vesiculous lesions at lips (labial herpes), buccal mucosa (cold sore), eye (ocular herpes, a significant cause of blindness), fingers (herpetic whitlow), and genitals (HSV1 accounts for a fraction of genital herpes, focally up to 30–50%). **IMPACT:** In a nationally representative United States survey in 1988–1994, seroprevalence among persons ≥12 years of age was 51% (95% CI 49–53) for HSV1 alone, 5% (95% CI 5–6) for HSV2 only, and 17% (95% CI 15–18) for both. The rate of HSV1 acquisition by sexually active United States female adolescents is ~3/100 person-years. Because preceding HSV1 seems to modify acquisition of HSV2, "a decent interval between kissing and intercourse" has been suggested (5941). **OUTBREAKS:** Outbreaks are reported in wrestlers (herpes gladiatorum).

HSV2 (784, 2435, 2711, 6990, 7538). **SPREAD:** is via genitogenital and anogenital sex; a rare mode is traditional Jewish circumcision (oral suctioning of blood after foreskin cutting). **RISKS:** for the community, see section 14.7; for prostitutes, see section 13.6; for homosexual men, see section 13.7. Most infected persons are unaware of their HSV2 infection. Shedding is from lesions, as well as from intact skin (subclinical shedding). Shedding is shorter in recurrent (mean 7 days) than primary infections (11 days). By PCR, subclinical shedding is detected on 20–25% of all latent days. **CLINICAL INFORMATION:** From 20% to 90% of primary infections are inapparent. The incubation period is 2–12 (typically 4) days. Manifestations: painful vesiculous or ulcerous lesions at genitals or anus, regional adenopathy, and fever. Confirmation is by culture, PCR, antigen capture, or serology. Diagnosis should include typing, as HSV1:HSV2 ratio and age-specific prevalence of genital HSV1 infections is indicative of high-risk sex. Coinfections with other STI are frequent. Genital ulcers enhance HIV transmission. Pain shooting into buttocks or hips can herald reactivation. Complications include neonatal infection and invasive disease (e.g., aseptic meningitis) in immune-impaired patients. **IMPACT:** By age 35 years, seroprevalence is 30–90% in Africa, 10–55% in the Americas, 5–35% in Europe, and 0–30% in Asia. In U.S. adults, the overall HSV2 seroprevalence is ~22%, with a range of ~0.5–45% by sex and ethnicity. HSV2 prevalence is negligible in persons who have never been sexually active. The rate of HSV2 acquisition by sexually active United States female adolescents is ~4/100 person-years. In Italy in 1993–1997, point prevalence of cervical HSV shedding by antigen capture was 8% (357/4,565) in females attending clinics and 4% (4/92) in asymptomatic pregnant women.

SHV (3485, 3681) is a species complex that includes cercopithecine herpesvirus 1 (CeHV1) reported in humans. CeHV1 was first isolated from Dr. "B" in 1934, hence its former name, herpesvirus B. CeHV-1 is enzootic in macaques that shed virus with oral, conjunctival, or genital secretions. **SPREAD:** is via bite, scratch, or mucosal splash. **RISKS:** animal work, children who keep macaques as pets, tourism to temples inhabited by free-roaming macaques. **CLINICAL INFORMATION:** The incubation period is 2 days to 5 weeks. Manifestations: vesicles at inoculation site (inconsistent), flulike illness, and encephalomyelitis. Lethality in the preantiviral era was >70%. IMPACT: About 40–50 cases in humans.

SINDBIS VIRUS (SINV). *See* Alphavirus.

SPIRILLUM (6889) (β-*Proteobacteria, Nitrosomonadales*). *S. minus* is a spiral rod bacterium from rats. SPREAD: is via rat contact or bite. CLINICAL INFORMATION: The incubation period is ~1 week to 2 months. Manifestations (sodoku, spirillary rat-bite fever): skin lesion at portal of entry, regional adenopathy, and fever. *S. minus* is visible in dark-field microscopy of blood or aspirate. IMPACT: Sporadic.

SPIROMETRA (561, 790, 5699) (Cestoda: Pseudophyllidea). These tapeworms circulate in swine, dogs, and cats (final hosts, shed eggs), and snakes, amphibians, and freshwater crustaceans (intermediate hosts, harbor procercoid larvae). SPREAD: is via ingestion of copepod-polluted water or undercooked snakes or frogs, via handling of infective tissues, or by applying frogs as a poultice for open sores. Manifestations (sparganosis): skin nodules, space-occupying mass in skin, eye, or brain. IMPACT: Some 300 cases have been reported, mainly from East Asia, rarely in the Americas and Europe.

SPOROTHRIX (*Ascomycota: Ophiostomatales*). These are thermally dimorphic fungi that inhabit soil, wood, and plants, in particular, hay and sphagnum moss. Molds in soil produce spores (conidia). Prototype is **S. schenckii** (1522, 1810, 3850, 4591, 4647, 5721, 7942). SPREAD: is via microtrauma (e.g., thorn, splinter, or fishhook), scratch or bite by cats or other vertebrates (from contaminated claws or teeth), possibly by inhalation of environmental aerosols. A carpet layer developed bursal sporotrichosis after puncturing his knee with a carpet tack. Abrasions can be minimal and not perceived by patients, in particular, children. RISKS: outdoor activities (e.g., farm or wood work, horticulture), cat ownership. CLINICAL INFORMATION: Infections can be subclinical or self-limited. The incubation period is 1–9 (typically 2–3) weeks. Manifestations: subcutaneous nodules, skin ulcers, regional lymphadenitis, tuberculosis-like lung disease, rarely invasive disease. Confirmation is by microscopy and culture from biopsy or fine-needle aspiration. Treatment options include itraconazole and oral potassium iodide solution. IMPACT: In endemic areas, reported disease rates are $50–100/10^5$ per year. OUTBREAKS: Numerous outbreaks are reported, including in households, mines, and tree nursery workers, and in association with hay, peat moss, and timber. In the Witwatersrand gold mine of South Africa in 1941–1944, an outbreak caused 2,825 cases; the implicated source was the timber used for shoring mine tunnels. In the United States in 1988, an outbreak caused 84 cases among persons handling seedlings packed in sphagnum moss. The duration of exposure was 1–210 (median, 12) hours, and the risk of infection increased with increasing length of exposure.

SPUMAVIRUS (enveloped RNA viruses: *Retroviridae*). The genus includes feline (FeFV) and simian (SiFV) foamy viruses. **Simian foamy virus** (SiFV) (3743, 8243) is enzootic in monkeys in central Africa. SPREAD: is via monkey contacts or secretions, likely via consumption of monkey meat. RISKS: hunt for or handling of monkeys, work with monkeys in research centers or zoos. SiFV can contaminate monkey kidney cell lines. CLINICAL INFORMATION: Sporadic. Disease manifestations in humans are not known.

STAPHYLOCOCCUS (*Firmicutes: Bacillales*). These are gram-positive cocci. Of many species, *S. aureus* (coagulase-positive) and coagulase-negative staphylococci (CoNS) such as *S. epidermidis* are mainly infective to humans.

S. aureus (303, 476, 1047, 2327, 3588, 4243, 6549, 7998) can colonize humans worldwide, mainly in the nose, temporarily also on the hands and skin. *S. aureus* produces golden (aureus) colonies, enzymes (coagulase, β-lactamase), and toxins (exfoliative, enteric, and cytotoxic). *S. aureus* survives 10–49°C but is killed by pasteurization. Enterotoxins (emetic and pyrogenic) are inactivated only at 120°C for 20–40 min. Penicillin resistance has been known since 1942 (the year penicllin G was introduced), methicillin-resistant *S. aureus* (MRSA) since 1961 (1 year after methicillin was introduced). SPREAD: Infections are endogenous or acquired from hand and skin contacts in community and care settings (cross-infection), or via ingestion of enterotoxin-loaded foods. RISKS: for colonization, infection, or invasion include contact with an infective person, a health worker in the household, recent use of antibiotics, recent hospitalization, injection drug use, carrying a device, extremes of age, and underlying illness. Nasal coinfection with *Rhinovirus* enhances shedding of *S. aureus* into air. Desquamation of *S. aureus* from skin may contribute to nasal carriage. CLINICAL INFORMATION: The incubation period is ½–12 (typically 2–5) hours (food poisoning) or 1–14 days (perinatal infection and outbreaks). Manifestations: food poisoning, toxic shock syndrome (TSS, three fourths menstrual), pyodermia (impetigo and cellulitis), abscess, RTI, BSI (in up to 60% with endocarditis), and bone and joint infections. Lethality varies from nil (food poisoning) to 4% (TSS) and 20–38% (invasive disease, 20% in days 0–30, plus 18% in months 2–12; MRSA can double the figures). IMPACT: Staphylococcal food poisoning occurs worldwide. *S. aureus* and MRSA are major agents in hospitals, although MRSA has escaped into the community. The invasive disease rate is $\sim 20–30/10^5$ per year, the rate of TSS is $\sim 1–3/10^5$ per year.

In an outbreak among military trainees, the rate of MRSA skin infections was ~1/100 person-weeks, compared with a baseline cellulitis rate of 0.3/100 person-weeks. **OUTBREAKS:** Epidemic clones can disseminate rapidly. Preventive and control measures include food and hand hygiene, judicious use of antibiotics, screening of hospital transfer and high-risk patients, isolation of MRSA patients, hand hygiene, standard precautions, and contact tracing.

Staphylococcus, **coagulase-negative (CoNS)** (615, 736, 2390, 3571, 3967, 6082, 6157, 7391, 7864). Of coagulase-negative species, *S. epidermidis* and *S. saprophyticus* are mainly isolated in humans. *S. epidermidis* is part of the skin flora. CoNS also colonize mucosa (nose and conjunctiva). *S. epidermidis* is frequently resistant to methicillin. Treatment options for such strains include vancomycin and linezolid. **SPREAD:** Infections are endogenous or acquired from hand and skin contacts, possibly via polluted air. **RISKS:** carrying an intravascular device, being critically ill, a neonate, or an immune-impaired patient. **CLINICAL INFORMATION:** An incubation period is not documented. Manifestations: SSI (*S. epidermidis*), UTI (*S. saprophyticus*), device-related infections, and invasive disease (BSI, sepsis, native valve endocarditis, and meningitis). Confirmation is by culture. Recovery of identical strains from >1 blood culture helps to separate contamination from infection. Reported lethality of BSI is 16%. **IMPACT:** CoNS account for ~4% of nosocomial UTI, ~14% of SSI, and ~30% of nosocomial BSI. Rates of BSI due to CoNS are ~0.05/100 hospital-days, or 0.3/100 inpatients. **OUTBREAKS:** Nosocomial clusters and outbreaks are reported. Compliance with hand hygiene reduces nosocomial spread.

STENOTROPHOMONAS (248, 1859, 2532, 3914, 6773) (γ-*Proteobacteria*: *Xanthomonadales*). *S.* (ex-*Pseudomonas*) *maltophilia* inhabits soil, water, sewage, and foods, and hospital tap water. **SPREAD:** is presumably via hand contacts (cross-infection). A variable fraction of humans shed *S. maltophilia* in the feces. **RISKS:** indwelling devices (e.g., central venous catheters), recent use of antibiotics, recent surgery, admittance to ICU, mechanical ventilation, tracheostomy, prolonged hospital stay. Cystic fibrosis patients are susceptible. **CLINICAL INFORMATION:** About half of hospital isolates reflect colonization. An incubation period is not documented. Manifestations: SSI, pneumonia, BSI, endocarditis. Nearly half of pneumonia due to *S. maltophilia* is polymicrobial. Main associates are *Acinetobacter* and *Pseudomonas aeruginosa*. Treatment options include combinations, e.g., of β-lactams/anti-β-lactamases, and aminoglycosides. Atttributable lethality of invasive disease is ~20–25%. **IMPACT:** *S. maltophilia* accounts for 0.5–1% of nosocomial infection isolates. Infection rates are ≤0.1/100 admissions, or ≤1.8/100 patient-days. **OUTBREAKS:** Many nosocomial clusters and outbreaks are reported, including neonatal and surgical ICU, and transplant units.

STREPTOBACILLUS (*Fusobacteria*: *Fusobacterales*). *S. moniliformis* (1243, 2910, 5570, 7518) is a gram-negative rod that colonizes the nasopharynx and oral cavity of rats, other rodents, cats, and dogs that prey on rodents. **SPREAD:** is via bite, scratch, or contact with rats and other mammals, or via foods or fecally polluted tap water. **RISKS:** substandard housing, persons who handle rodents, farmers, pet owners. **CLINICAL INFORMATION:** The incubation period is 1–30 (typically 2–10) days. Manifestations (rat-bite or Haverhill fever): fever, rash, sepsis, septic arthritis, endocarditis. Confirmation is by culture of blood or synovial fluid. Untreated lethality is up 10%, in endocarditis up to 50%. **IMPACT:** Sporadic. **OUTBREAKS:** In Haverhill, Mass. in 1926, milk polluted by rats was implicated in an outbreak with 86 cases. In the United Kingdom in 1983, a waterborne outbreak caused 304 cases.

STREPTOCOCCUS (2284, 7171) (*Firmicutes*: *Lactobacillales*). These are gram-positive cocci. There are >50 species. Modern taxonomy is based on molecular methods; cell wall carbohydrate serogroups are shared by some species and are not expressed by others (Table 20.7). **CLINICAL INFORMATION:** Confirmation is by culture. *S. pyogenes* (GAS) and *S. agalactiae* (GBS) remain sensitive to β-lactams, while sensitivity of viridans and other streptococci is variable, and a large fraction of *S. pneumoniae* is penicillin resistant.

S. agalactiae (group B, GBS) (692, 2730, 3130, 4594, 5019, 6567, 6702, 6707) colonizes bowel and genitourinary tract of humans and bovids. **SPREAD:** Infections are endogenous or acquired via hand or skin contact, sex, or perinatally, including in hospitals, rarely via animal contacts. Of 767 initially GBS-negative women, 45% (344) became colonized in 12 months. **RISKS:** intravascular devices, having multiple sex partners, African American ethnicity (vaginal acquisition); premature rupture of membranes (perinatal acquisition). Comorbidities (diabetes, decubitus, and neurogenic bladder) and impaired immunity increase susceptibility. **CLINICAL INFORMATION:** An incubation period is not reported. Hospital acquisition time is 4–59 (typically 17) days. Manifestations: invasive disease (sepsis, endocarditis, and spondylodiscitis) in adults with comorbidities, and neonatal sepsis (of early or late [after ≥7 days] onset). Lethality is ~10% (adults), ~25% (neonates), or ~35% (endocarditis). **IMPACT:** By geography and test, prevalence is 5–50% in delivering women, and 10–30% in nonpregnant women of comparable age. Invasive GBS disease rates are 2–7/10^5/year overall, in elderly ~20/10^5 per year, in

Table 20.7 Overview of *Streptococcus* spp. by hemolysis on blood agar (β for complete), Lancefield serogroups (A-W), and major hosts[a]

Lysis	Species	Lancefield serogroup(s)	Major host(s)
β	*S. pyogenes*	A	Humans
	S. agalactiae	B	Humans, bovines
	S. dysgalactiae subsp. *equisimilis*	A, C, G, L	Humans, mammals
	S. equi		
	subsp. *equi*	C	Mammals
	subsp. *zooepidemicus*	C	Mammals, humans
	S. canis	G	Dogs, humans
	S. porcinus	E, P, U, V, or none	Swine, humans
Non-β	*S. pneumoniae*	None	Humans
	S. dysgalactiae subsp. *dysgalactiae*	C	Horses, cattle, sheep, pigs
	S. bovis sl		
	S. equinus	D	Equines, bovines
	S. gallolyticus	D	Humans, koalas
	S. infantarius	D	Humans, bovines
	S. suis	R, S, T	Swine, humans
	Viridans ("oral") streptococci[b]	A, C, G, F, or none	Humans, mammals

[a]From reference 2284.
[b]Includes species in groups anginosus-milleri, mitis, mutans, salivarius, and sanguinus.

neonates 0.5–1/1,000 live births, in hospitals 0.05–0.1/100 admissions. Prevention strategies include screening, treatment of women at risk, and intrapartum antibiotics.

S. canis, S. anginosus, and S. dysgalactiae subsp. *equisimilis* express group G antigen (GGS) (1512, 7304) (Table 20.7). GGS colonize domestic animals. Dog bite has resulted in *C. canis* sepsis. Patients with comorbidities (malignancy and diabetes) are susceptible. Manifestations: cellulitis, sepsis.

S. dysgalactiae subsp. *dysgalactiae* and *equisimilis* and **S. equi** subsp. *equi* and *zooepidemicus* can express group C antigen (**GCS**) (2191, 8256). **S. bovis** complex (*S. equinus*, *S. gallolyticus*, and *S. infantarius*) expresses group D antigen (**GDS**) (6671, 6885, 7560) (Table 20.7). GCS and GDS colonize or infect mammals. *S. dysgalactiae equisimilis*, *S. equi zooepidemicus*, and *S. bovis* sl have been recovered from colonized or infected humans. Erythromycin-resistance is reported in GCS and GDS. **SPREAD**: Infections are endogenous or acquired via foods, droplets, or contacts with animals. **RISKS**: Exposure to animals or their products was implicated in 24% (21/88) of cases of GCS bacteremia. Manifestations: pharyngitis, invasive disease. *S. bovis* sl is increasingly recognized as a cause of BSI, endocarditis, and meningitis. Patients with advanced liver disease are susceptible to *S. bovis* sl. **IMPACT**: In Israel in 1980–2000, *S. bovis* sl accounted for ~1% of all bacteremias.

S. pneumoniae (681, 726, 1656, 5508, 5525, 5526, 6816, 7640) colonizes the human nasopharynx worldwide (see section 14.1). Capsule polysaccharides define some 100 serotypes. Dominant serotypes change over time. Many strains are penicillin resistant. **SPREAD**: is via droplets, other respiratory secretions, or hands, rarely nosocomially. **RISKS**: for colonization: crowding. For invasive disease: age <2 years, day care, minority community, nursing home resident, sickle cell disease, impaired immunity. Risks for invasion by penicillin-resistant strains: hospitalization, recent (past 3 months) use of β-lactams. Clones can spread city-to-city and country-to-country. **CLINICAL INFORMATION**: Of newly acquired strains, 15% result in disease. Outbreaks suggest incubation periods of 1–14 days. Diseases by continuity or aspiration include otitis media, sinusitis, conjunctivitis, and pneumonia. Diseases by dissemination (invasion) include BSI, meningitis, endocarditis, and septic arthritis. By age and case mix, lethality of invasive disease is 1% to >40%. In the United States in 1993–1999, lethality in children was 2%. In Australia in 2001, lethality was 9% overall: 1% (5/512) at age <5 years, 7% (38/529) at age 5–65 years, and 20% (82/405) at age >65 years. **IMPACT**: Worldwide, there are ≥2 million deaths per year due to *S. pneumoniae*. In high-income countries, by age mix, case definition, and vaccine coverage, invasive disease rates per 10^5 per year are 1–100 (typically 10–25) overall, 60–100 in preschool children and the elderly, and 1 in adults. In the United States, the reported invasive disease rate in 2003 was 1.7/10^5. Pneumococcal meningitis occurs at a rate of 1–7/10^5 per year. **OUTBREAKS**: Outbreaks, common in the preantibiotic era, have reemerged, with reported attack rates >1%. A 23-valent polysaccharide vaccine that covers ~85–90% of prevalent serotypes, protects from invasive disease, and can be given from age ≥2 years. A

7-valent conjugate vaccine that covers ~40–65% of prevalent serotypes, protects from invasive disease, reduces colonization by covered serotypes, and can be given from age ≥6 weeks.

S. pyogenes (group A, GAS) (1197, 1658, 3813, 4379, 4544, 5282, 5337, 6341, 7506, 7852) colonizes the pharynx, vagina, and anus of humans worldwide. Humans shed GAS with respiratory and wound secretions. S. pyogenes is equipped with an array of virulence factors. **SPREAD:** is via droplets, hands, and skin contacts. Molecular epidemiology suggests that virulent GAS is acquired rather than endogenous. In close-knit communities or schools, new strains can be exchanged within 2–28 weaks. **RISKS:** Crowded living, rapid gathering of persons. Although not part of residual skin flora, GAS on hands or skin is readily spread by contact. Scarlet fever is highly infective (R_0 of 4–8). Infectivity begins 7 days before disease onset and continues for 24 hours after treatment onset. **CLINICAL INFORMATION:** About 60% of respiratory colonizations remain inapparent, 40% go on to pharyngitis. By syndrome, the incubation period is 12 hours to 6 (typically 1–2) days (food-borne streptococcal pharyngitis), 1–3 days (invasive disease), 2–4 days (scarlet fever), or 2–33 (typically 10) days (impetigo). Manifestations: are diverse and include pharyngitis (mainly high-income countries), impetigo (mainly low-income countries), cellulitis, erysipelas, SSI, scarlet fever, acute rheumatic fever, pneumonia, and invasive disease, e.g., necrotizing fasciitis, puerperal or other sepsis, toxic shock syndrome (TSS), meningitis, and endocarditis. By geography, age, and case mix, lethality of invasive disease is 3–18%: 6% in acute rheumatic fever in low-income countries, 13–58% in necrotizing fasciitis in high-income countries, 30–80% in TSS. **IMPACT:** GAS is present in the throat of 20–45% of healthy persons (see section 14.1). In The Netherlands in 1992–1996, 8% (880/10,985) of GAS isolates were from patients with invasive disease. In high-income countries, by setting and reporting, rates are ~2/100 person-years (streptococcal impetigo), 0.3–66 (typically 2–4)/10^5 and year (invasive GAS disease), and 0.4/10^5 and year (acute rheumatic fever). In India, the rate of GAS pharyngitis in school age children was ~1 per child-year, and the rate of acute rheumatic fever was ~54/10^5 per year. **OUTBREAKS:** S. pyogenes has caused outbreaks of pneumonia, rheumatic fever, invasive disease, of contact-borne impetigo, and of food- and droplet-borne pharyngitis. In a GAS pneumonia outbreak, attack rate was 0.7%. In food-borne pharyngitis outbreaks, primary attack rates reached 10–85%, while secondary attack rates were lower (2–8%, presumably from droplets). Any invasive case on a surgery or obstetrical ward should prompt infection control measures and enhanced surveillance. Antibiotic treatment of patients and carriers can curb outbreaks in schools and hospitals. There is uncertainty whether to provide chemoprophylaxis to households with an invasive GAS disease case.

S. suis (4057, 4738, 5798, 7188, 7825) is a commensal of pigs. **SPREAD:** is via pig contact, microtrauma, or ingestion of uncooked pork products. **RISKS:** Hunters, pig farmers, pig transporters, abattoir and raw pork meat workers. **CLINICAL INFORMATION:** Throats of workers can be colonized with S. suis. The likely incubation period is a few to 24 h. Manifestations: bacteremia, sepsis, septic shock, and other invasive diseases in immune-impaired hosts.

Viridans or "oral" Streptococcus (530, 957, 3712, 4595) are part of buccal, pharyngeal, bowel, and vaginal flora of mammals and humans. They express A, C, G, F, or none of group antigens (Table 20.7). Species groups include "anginosus-milleri" (S. anginosus, S. constellatus, and S. intermedius), "mitis" (e.g., S. mitis and S. oralis), "mutans" (e.g., S. cricetus, S. macacae, and S. rattus of name-giving mammals), "salivarius" (e.g., S. salivarius), and "sanguinis" (e.g., S. sanguinus and S. gordonii). **SPREAD:** largely endogenous. **CLINICAL INFORMATION:** Viridans streptococci prevent colonization with pathogenic bacteria, but by gene shuffling act as a resistance reservoir. Viridans streptococci form biofilms on teeth (dental plaques) and are involved in periodontitis. Source for hematogenous spread is buccal cavity (dental procedures) and bowel. Manifestations: nosocomial BSI, endocarditis, intra-abdominal abscess, perforating appendicitis (anginosus-milleri group). **IMPACT:** In Finland in 1998–2001, 5% (108/2,038) of isolates from nosocomial BSI were viridans streptococci, mainly of mitis group. Of 607 nonduplicate endocarditis isolates from United Kingdom reference laboratories in 1996–2000, 86% (522) were viridans streptococci, mainly S. oralis (24% or 145), S. sanguis (18% or 110), and S. gordonii (9% or 55).

STREPTOMYCES (90, 2076) (Actinobacteria: Actinomycetales). These are branching, aerobic, soil-dwelling rods that produce antimicrobials (e.g., amphothericin, ivermectin, spiramycin, and streptomycin). There are >3,000 species. **SPREAD:** via microtrauma. Manifestations: actinomycetoma, rarely invasive disease in immune-impaired hosts. Grains from S. somaliensis fistules are yellow or brown. **IMPACT:** The relative frequency of S. somaliensis in actinomycetoma case series ranged from 4% (in Senegal) to 10% (in Mali), 38% (in Niger), and 52% (in Mauritania)

STRONGYLOIDES (6925) (Nematoda: Rhabditida). These are small nematodes that are free-living in soil and parasitize vertebrates. There are >50 species, including S. fuelleborni (in primates and humans), S. ratti (in rats),

S. stercoralis (in humans), and *S. westeri* (in horses). Zoonotic larvae occasionally cause skin eruptions and allergic reactions.

S. fuelleborni (316, 2964, 5701) occurs in tropical Africa (in primates and forest peoples) and Papua New Guinea (subsp. *kellyi*; no animal reservoir known). SPREAD: is by skin contact with soil, rarely via breastmilk. CLINICAL INFORMATION: Focal. Manifestations: like *S. stercoralis*. However, eggs rather than larvae are shed with feces.

S. stercoralis (2732, 3969, 5985, 6361, 6390, 6879, 6940, 7231, 7407) circulates in warm and temperate climates, in humans who shed larvae with feces and soil. Under optimal conditions, larvae in soil develop to infective (L3) larvae in a few to 6 days. The life span of adults is perhaps 1 year. SPREAD: is by skin contact with infective soil, hand contact (person-to-person). Transmission by latently infected kidney transplants is a possibility. External (ano-oral) and internal (duodenorectal) autoinfection can perpetuate infections for >50 years. RISKS: contact of bare skin with infective soil, sewage, or garbage, outdoor work or leisure activities, infected household members, substandard housing in endemic areas, lack of toilets or sanitation, camps, and travel to endemic areas. CLINICAL INFORMATION: Adults locate in the duodenum. The prepatent period is 3 weeks. Confirmation is by visualizing larvae in stool samples (fresh and fixed, three specimens), duodenal fluid, or sputum. At least one fourth of infections are inapparent. The incubation period is not known. Manifestations: itchy, migrating skin eruptions (larva currens, in 0–80% of cases), undulant blood eosinophilia (in 15–80%), abdominal pain (in 5–60%), and chronic diarrhea. Complications: massive (hyper) or invasive (disseminated) disease, mainly in immune-impaired (corticosteroids, transplant recipients) or HTLV1-coinfected hosts. Lethality of invasive disease is ~50%. Treatment options are ivermectin or benzimidazoles. Treatment failures should prompt tests for HTLV1. IMPACT: By habitat and test method, prevalences in endemic areas are ~0.4–40% (typically 2–10%), for a world estimate of 0.5–1.5%. In high-income countries, local transmission is reported in Canada (in the 1980s), southeastern United States (up to the 1990s, prevalence 0.4–4%), Queensland (Australia, in the 1990s), West Europe (Italy, Spain to date, Belgium, France up to the 1990s, United Kingdom in the 1980s, up to latitude 53°N).

SUIPOXVIRUS (enveloped DNA viruses: *Poxviridae*). *Suipoxvirus* includes swinepoxvirus (SWPV) in pigs.

TAENIA (3593, 3691) (Cestoda: Cyclophyllidea). *Taenia* circulates worldwide, in herbivores (intermediate hosts) that eat eggs and harbor larvae (cysticerci) in tissues, and carnivores or humans (final hosts) who eat larvae, harbor adults in the bowel, and shed egg-containing proglottids. Three species infect humans: *T. asiatica*, *T. saginata*, and *T. solium*. All three can coexist in Yunnan (People's Republic of China) and Vietnam. Eggs are microscopically indistinguishable, but species can be identified from purged scolices, proglottids, or by antigen test or NAT from stools. Larvae in meat are inactivated by heat (56°C for 1 min) or freeze (-18°C for 30 min). Treatment options for adult worms include niclosamide or praziquantel, followed by purge.

T. asiatica (2309) circulates in East Asia (People's Republic of China, Korea, and Taiwan) and Southeast Asia (Indonesia and Vietnam), in pigs, cattle, goats, and monkeys (intermediate hosts, harbor cysticerci in viscera, mainly liver), and humans (final hosts, shed motile proglottids, ~1 per day). SPREAD: is via undercooked pig viscera. MANIFESTATIONS: vague, anal pruritus, mild abdominal pain.

T. saginata (529) circulates worldwide, in cattle (intermediate hosts, harbor cysticerci in muscle or other organs), and humans (final hosts, shed motile proglottis, ~6–7/day). There are ~100,000 eggs/proglottid. Life span of adults is 20–30 years. SPREAD: is via undercooked beef meat. CLINICAL INFORMATION: Adults locate in the small bowel. The prepatent period is 10–14 weeks. Most infections are asymptomatic, although proglottids can be seen in stools or underwear. Carriers are detected by a history of proglottid passage, perianal adhesive tape test, stool tests for eggs or antigen, or NAT. Manifestations: vague, anal pruritus, mild abdominal pain.

T. solium (1855, 1857, 2440, 2622, 3492, 4636, 5407, 7938, 8192, 8418) circulates in pork-consuming areas, in pigs (intermediate hosts, harbor larvae in muscle and other organs) and humans (final hosts), who shed nonmotile proglottids (~6–7/day) and infective eggs. There are ~80,000 eggs per proglottid. Life span is 20–30 years for adult worms, and weeks to 1–2 years for larvae. SPREAD: Uptake of viable larvae from undercooked pork results in intestinal infection. Uptake of eggs results in cysticercosis; sources of eggs are foods fecally polluted by carriers, dirty hands, ano-oral autoinfection, and duodenogastric regurgitating or vomiting induced by traditional anthelminthics. RISKS: for intestinal infection: pork diet, preference for raw pork, lack of meat inspection (cannibalism was a suspected ancestral risk). Risks for cysticercosis: carrier food workers or household aids, poor hand and kitchen hygiene, fecally contaminated foods (e.g., vegetables), history of passing proglottids or of *Taenia* treatments. CLINICAL INFORMATION: Adults locate in the small bowel. The prepatent period is 9–10 weeks. Most infections are asymptomatic. Screening for carriers is by history (seeing proglottids) and stool testing. Manifestations are vague and mild and include abdominal discomfort. Larvae locate in eye, brain, or other tissues, causing space-occupying lesions (cysticercosis). It takes ~8–10 weeks for larvae to be demonstrable in tissue. The incubation period is 4–5 years. Manifestations vary by site, number and viability of cysts ("active," "degenerating," or calcified). Manifestations of neurocysticercosis include headache and adult-onset epilepsy. Diagnosis is by biopsy, antibody or antigen capture tests from serum or CSF, and imaging. Treatment options for active larvae include albendazole or praziquantel. In a series from Los Angeles in 1988–1990, lethality was 6% (8/138). In 0–15% of cases, intestinal infection and cysticercosis occur simultaneously. IMPACT: There are 5–10 million intestinal infections, 5–50 million tissue infections, and 0.5 million neurocysticercosis deaths per year. In enzootic-endemic areas, by sampling and test, carrier prevalences are ~0.2–2% (typically ≤1%), and (past or active) tissue infection prevalences are ~0.3–30% (typically 10%). In low-income countries, neurocysticercosis accounts for ~10% of neurological admissions, and 10–70% of seizures. In North America and West Europe, cysticercosis is only exceptionally acquired locally and mainly imported by immigrants. In southern California, intestinal infection and cysticercosis are prevalent in ~1–2% of Hispanic migrants, for a neurocysticercosis rate of ~$0.6/10^5$ per year. OUTBREAKS: In the United States in 1990–1991, migrant carrier workers caused an outbreak in Jewish households with six neurocysticercosis cases and 5 inapparent infections. Preventive measures include identification and treatment of carriers, hygiene education, sanitation, meat inspection, and good pig husbandry.

THEILERIA (1633) (Alveolata: Apicomplexa: Piroplasmorida). These are tick-borne, intraerythrocytic, *Babesia*-like protozoa that parasitize wild and domestic mammals. There are >30 species. In cattle, *Theileria* spp. cause "Texas fever," "east coast fever," and "Mediterranean coast fever." Infections in humans have not been reported.

TICK-BORNE ENCEPHALITIS VIRUS (TBEV).
See Flavivirus.

TOSCANA SANDFLY FEVER VIRUS (TOSV).
See Phlebovirus.

TOXOCARA (Nematoda: Ascaridida). These are *Ascaris*-related nematodes. Of >10 species, human infections are confirmed for *T. canis* (from dogs) and *T. cati* (from cats), and suspected for *T. pteropodis* (from bats), and *T. vitulorum* (from buffalo). Related genera are *Toxascaris leonina* and *Baylisascaris procyonis*.

T. canis (193, 1899, 2305, 2843, 3540, 5661, 7219, 7222, 7785) circulates worldwide, in dogs (final hosts, shed eggs, mainly puppies), soil, and a broad range of vertebrates (intermediate or transport hosts, harbor larvae), e.g., pigs, lambs, rodents, chickens, pigeons, and even earthworms. Eggs are hardy, surviving cold in clay soil for up to 2 years. Under favorable conditions, eggs embryonate and become infective in ~9 days. SPREAD: is via uptake of embryonated eggs from dog feces (mainly puppies), soils (playing on the ground, geophagia), or perhaps recreational waters; in adults, foods are a more likely source, including fecally polluted, egg-carrying vegetables, salads, or fish, and larvae in undercooked meats or viscera of transport hosts (e.g., rabbits) or folk medicines (e.g., raw snails). RISKS: dog ownership, puppies in the home, kennel work, farm work, hunting, habitual geophagia, playing in public parks (sandboxes), and unwashed home-grown vegetables. CLINICAL INFORMATION: Many infections are inapparent. The incubation period is not known; a volunteer given ~100 infective eggs had hypereosinophilia after 13 days. Manifestations: hepatomegaly and blood eosinophilia (visceral larva migrans), granuloma of the eye (ocular larva migrans), skin allergy, asthma, rarely space-occupying lesion of the brain. Diagnosis is serological (high IgG to excretory-secretory antigen in ELISA), or by biopsy. Treatment options include benzimidazoles and ivermectin. IMPACT: By age and test, reported seroprevalences are 1–25% in high-income countries, and 2–90% in tropical countries. In the United States, the prevalence of ocular toxocariasis is ~$7–10/10^5$. In a highly endemic area of Brazil, the seroconversion rate was 18% per year.

T. cati (2114, 2415, 6537) circulates worldwide in cats (final hosts, shed eggs). SPREAD: is likely via ingestion of eggs from hand contacts with cats or their feces, or by geophagia. RISKS: cat ownership. CLINICAL INFORMATION: Visceral and ocular larva migrans are clinically indistinguishable from *T. canis*. IMPACT: *T. cati* to *T. canis* ratios in toxocariasis infection and disease are not known but believed to be well <1. NAT might resolve this issue.

TOXOPLASMA (Alveolata: Apicomplexa: Eucoccidiorida). Prototype is *T. gondii*.

T. gondii (383, 649, 2091, 3733, 4063, 5155, 6215, 7923) circulates worldwide, in birds and most mammals (intermediate hosts, harbor tissue cysts), and felids (mainly cats, final hosts, shed oocysts in feces). Oocysts (contain sporozoites), tissue cysts (contain bradyzoites), and tachyzoites (free-living in blood) can all be infective. *T. gondii* can invade almost any mammalian cell type. Tissue cysts are inactivated by heat (70°C for 10 min microwave cooking may take longer), or freeze (−20°C for 3 days). SPREAD: is (i) via foods, by cysts in meats (pork, mutton; source for 30–60% of infections in high-income countries) or by oocysts in fecally polluted vegetables or drinking water, (ii) by hands, from handling raw foods, cats (mainly kitten) or their litter, (iii) from the environment by ingestion or inhalation of oocysts from soil or dust (main mode in low-income countries), (iv) by solid organ, tissue and cell transplants, or in laboratory and research facilities, by injury or handling of infective materials, (v) mother-to-child, in tachyzoitemic pregnant women. RISKS: cat ownership, contact with cats or their litter, houses with dusty concrete floors, work with soil or raw vegetables, gardening, geophagia, unsafe tap water, poorly cooked meats, tasting raw meat products, eating unwashed vegetables or fruits, stays in low-income countries, adventure travel, jungle training. CLINICAL INFORMATION: Most infections are inapparent (in outbreaks ≤25%). Congenital infections can be inapparent at birth and become manifest after years. The infective dose is unknown. The incubation period is 3 days to 3 (typically 1–2) weeks (outbreaks, nosocomial spread), or months to years (congenital). Manifestations vary by age and immune competence. Acute primary infections in immune-competent hosts can cause adenopathy, lassitude, and fever. Intrauterine infections can cause stillbirth, hydrocephalus, intracranial calcifications, and late-onset chorioretinitis. Encephalitis or brain abscess are AIDS defining. Confirmation is by serology (IgM, high IgG), NAT (from whole blood, CSF, and amniotic fluid), histology (lymph node biopsy and placenta), rarely culture. Treatment options include pyrimethamine in combination with sulfonamide and folinic acid, and spiramycin. IMPACT: By age, diet, and living conditions, seroprevalence in adults is 15–40% in North America, 10–65% in Europe, and 5–85% in low-income countries, for a world median of ~33%. In a national United States sample in 1999–2000, seroprevalence was 16% (95% CI 14–18%) overall, 9% (95% CI 6–12) at age 12–19 years, and 20% (95% CI 16–25) at age 40–49 years. Reported seroconversion rates are 0.1–3% per year. OUTBREAKS: Vehicles for outbreaks included drinking water, goat milk, undercooked meat, rare hamburger, rare venison, raw pork liver, soil, and dust in a riding stable. Settings included a municipality, farms, families, and a camp.

TREPONEMA (*Bacteria*: *Spirochaetales*) (2815, 6917). These are screwlike bacteria. *T. pallidum* (three subspecies) and *T. carateum* are pathogenic to humans. Dark-field microscopy of smears from skin or genital lesions is diagnostic but insensitive. Antibodies appear 14–21 days after exposure. Rapid plasma reagin (RPR) and venereal disease research laboratory (VDRL) tests have been widely used for screening. Sensitivity of these nontreponemal tests is 78–86% for primary syphilis, 100% for secondary syphilis, and 95–98% for latent syphilis. In the absence of cross-reacting nonvenereal treponematoses, specificity of these tests is good (98–99%). Confirming tests use *Treponema* antigens and include fluorescent treponemal antibody absorption (FTA-abs), hemagglutination (TPHA), and *T. pallidum* particle agglutination (TPPA) tests. Penicillin remains first-line treatment.

T. carateum (4689, 8247) causes pinta (a nonvenereal treponematosis). *T. carateum* circulates in young adults, in rural, arid Latin America. SPREAD: is via contact. CLINICAL INFORMATION: The reported incubation period is 2–3 weeks. Manifestations: mottled discoloration of the skin. IMPACT: Despite mass treatments in the 1940s–1960s, foci persist.

T. pallidum endemicum (2599, 7675) causes endemic syphilis (bejel, a nonvenereal treponematosis). *T. pallidum endemicum* circulates in children and latently infected adults, in rural, arid Africa and West Asia. SPREAD: is via hand and skin contacts, flies, and shared objects (e.g., cups). RISKS: nomads, pastoralists. Manifestations: erosive lesions of skin and mucosa. IMPACT: Despite mass treatments in the 1940s–1960s, foci persist.

T. pallidum pallidum (1236, 1608, 1965, 2815, 5802, 6640, 7476, 7975) causes syphilis (lues). *T. pallidum pallidum* circulates in sexually active, promiscuous humans worldwide. SPREAD: is via sex, transplacental, or contact with skin lesions or body fluids, rarely via transfusion, dialysis, or needle-stick injury. RISKS: sex among men, prostitution, injection drug use, underprivileged minorities. In France in 2000–2002, of 642 syphilis cases (primary, secondary, early-latent), 84% (538) were homo- or bisexual men, 13% (82) were heterosexual men, and 3% (22) were heterosexual females. Infectivity of primary, secondary, and early-latent syphilis is high, with transmission rates of 20–80% (among sex partners typically 60%). CLINICAL INFORMATION: The incubation period is 10–90 (typically 21) days (primary syphilis), 4–10 weeks (secondary syphilis) and years (tertiary syphilis). Manifestations: is in stages (primary, secondary, latent, tertiary). Signs of primary syphilis are ulcer at portal of entry and adenopathy. Signs of secondary syphilis are variable skin eruptions, including macular rash and condylomata lata. Early-latent (≤1 year from secondary) and late-latent syphilis are silent. Signs of tertiary syphilis (reached by ~35% of untreated cases) include gummata, aortitis, tabes dorsalis, and encephalopathy. For intrauterine and congenital syphilis, see section 14.7. In the United Kingdom in 1994–1997, of 139 women treated for syphilis in pregnancy, 0.7% (1) had primary, 3% (4) had secondary, 19% (26) had early-latent, and 78% (108) had late-latent or undetermined syphilis. In West Australia in 1996–1999, of 196 syphilis cases, 7% (14) had primary, 16% (32) had secondary, and 77% (150) had latent syphilis. Serology is the main tool for screening (RPR, VDRL) and confirming (FTA-abs, TPHA) syphilis. Over 50% of cases are HIV coinfected. IMPACT: There are ~12 million new cases per year worldwide, for a crude rate of $200/10^5$ per year. In high-income countries, preantibiotic rates were $50–200/10^5$ per year. Public health programs reduced rates to currently 0.2–6/10⁵ per year. In the United States in 2000–2002, reported rates were 2.2–2.4/10⁵ per year for primary and secondary syphilis, and 11.5–11.7/10⁵ per year for all stages. In 2002, rates/10⁵ were 3.8 in men and 1.1 in women, for a rate ratio of 3.5 (Fig. 20.6). **OUTBREAKS:** Outbreaks occurred among urban homosexual and heterosexual males and drug users, and in prisons. In eastern Europe, syphilis resurged in the early 1990s. In Russia, notifications rose from lows of 2–4/10⁵ in the 1960s–1980s to 263/10⁵ in 1995. Preventive and control measures include promotion of safe sex, early detection and treatment of cases, contact tracing, and offering screening at sites where sex and drugs are sold.

T. pallidum pertenue (112, 237, 371, 6739, 7426) causes yaws (a nonvenereal treponematosis). *T. pallidum pertenue* circulates in children and latently infected adults, in rural, humid Africa, Latin America, and Asia. **SPREAD:** is via skin and hand contacts, rarely via shared objects. **RISKS:** remote minorities. **CLINICAL INFORMATION:** The incubation period is 9–90 (typically 21) days. Portal of entry can be a scratched insect bite. Manifestations: multiple, papillomatous skin lesions, hyperkeratosis, destructive chondroosteitis. **IMPACT:** Despite mass treatments in the 1940s–1960s, foci persist. Focal prevalences are 0.3–6% (clinically) to 3.5–20% (serologically). **OUTBREAKS:** In South African mines in the 1980s, an outbreak occurred at 1,630 m below sea level. More recently, an outbreak in a village in southern Thailand caused 54 cases, for an attack rate of 23%.

TRICHINELLA (745, 1475, 2082, 5917, 5994, 6447, 6657, 6994, 7952). (Nematoda: Enoplida) circulates in carnivorous, scavenging or cannibalistic, terrestrial and marine mammals that take up tissue larvae from prey. In the predator intestine, larvae rapidly develop into adults; females release larvae that invade tissues. Human-infective are encapsulating *T. britovi, T. nativa, T. nelsoni,* and *T. spiralis,* and nonencapsulating *T. pseudospiralis.* France seems the only country that has documented *T. spiralis, T. britovi,* and *T. pseudospiralis* in humans. **SPREAD:** is via larvae in undercooked meats (pork, horse, and game) or meat products (e.g., sausages). **RISKS:** preference for raw meat or game, home-prepared or individually imported products (souvenirs and gifts). Larvae are killed by heat (71°C throughout for 1 min), or freeze (−15°C, cuts of ≤15 cm for ≥3 weeks, cuts of 16–69 cm for ≥4 weeks). Adequately heated meat changes color from red to gray, and texture from tight to lose. **CLINICAL INFORMATION:** From 25% to 99% of infections are inapparent. Larvae can be demonstrated in muscle ~1 week after infection. Larvae calcify in tissues after ~5–18 months. The incubation period is 1 day (allergy) to 4 (typically 1–2) weeks (invasion). By infective dose, species, and age, manifestations include abrupt diarrhea (in 0–35%), fever (in 40–100%), allergic facial or eyelid edema (in 30-100%), myalgia (in 30–90%), shock, and eosinophilia (in 50–100%). A Danish couple contracted trichinellosis from eating roasted pork in Serbia: she with life-threatening cardiopulmonary complications and 2,000 larvae per g in muscle biopsy, he inapparently, with eosinophilia, and a single larva in muscle biopsy. Elevated muscle enzymes and anti-*Trichinella* Ig E, IgM, and IgG corroborate, and larvae in biopsy (from deltoid muscle) or leftover foods confirm diagnosis. Treatment options in the acute phase include benzimidazoles, antihistamines, and corticosteroids Lethality from large series is 0.2–1%. **IMPACT:** Worldwide, ~11 million people are infected. In Henan, an enzootic province of China, the infection prevalence by random muscle biopsy in non-trichinellosis surgery patients was 2.5% (26/1,048). There are 4,000–6,000 new cases per year worldwide. By geography, disease rates are 0.01–10 (typically 0.1–2)/10⁵ per year. **OUTBREAKS:** Main epidemic vehicle is undercooked pork or pork products. Alternative vehicles include horse meat, game

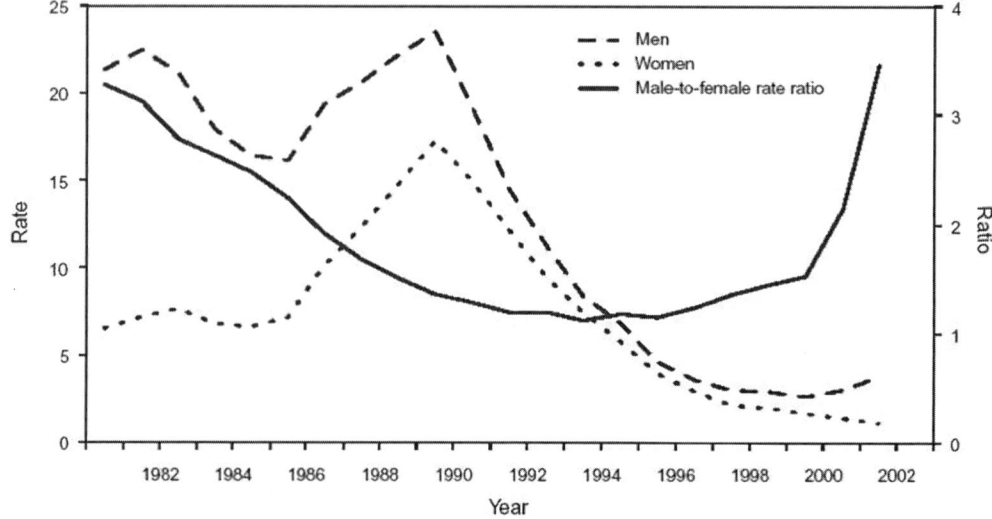

Figure 20.6 Reported primary and secondary syphilis, United States, 1982–2002: rates are given per 10⁵ (left *y* axis), by years (*x* axis) and sex. The male-to-female rate ratio is also given (right *y* axis). From reference 1218.

(e.g., boar and bear), and ethnic and speciality foods. Attack rates in outbreaks have ranged from 2% to 36%. In a few epidemics, case numbers have exceeded 200–500.

T. britovi (2634, 2824, 5994) is enzootic in temperate Eurasia, in wild carnivores (Canidae, Felidae, Ursidae), generally at elevations >500 m. *T. britovi* also infects boars, domestic pigs, horses, and humans.

T. nativa (4625, 5134, 6011, 6994) is enzootic in the Holarctic, including Greenland and Svalbard (Spitzbergen), in wild carnivores (*Ursidae*, *Mustelidae*, *Felidae*, and *Canidae*) and marine mammals (seals and walrus). Limit to the south seems the January −5°C isotherm. Larvae in muscle resist freezing. *T. nativa* infects indigenous peoples in the Arctic, and leisure hunters. A man shot a black bear (*Ursus americanus*) in Canada, field dressed it, and transported meat on ice to Tennessee, where he cooked the meat at an outdoor grill party where he and a woman who ate bear steaks rare contracted *T. nativa* trichinellosis.

T. nelsoni (5994) is enzootic in tropical Africa, in wild carnivores (*Hyaenidae*, *Felidae*). Larvae in muscle resist heat (up to 56°C for 1 h), but are sensitive to cold. *T. nelsoni* occasionally infects Suidae. Human infections are poorly documented.

T. papuae (5663) is enzootic in wild pigs in New Guinea. Human infections are reported in gardening and hunting Melanesian communities in Western province of Papua New Guinea.

T. pseudospiralis (223, 3510, 3744, 6107) seems enzootic worldwide, in small mammals (rodents and marsupials) and raptor and carrion-feeding birds. *T. pseudospiralis* also infects pigs and humans. Infections in humans are reported in New Zealand (one case, perhaps from pork or Tasmanian wallaby meat), Thailand (59 outbreak cases, from wild pig) and France (four outbreak cases, from wild boar).

T. spiralis (733, 2606, 5995, 6447) circulates in temperate and warm climates, in domestic mammals and wildlife, including boars, bears, and rodents. *T. spiralis* has a high affinity for domestic pigs, rats, and mice. In the United States in 1997–2001, of 72 reported cases, 12 (17%) had commercial pork products as source (four imported), and 9 (13%) had home-raised pork as source. In France and Italy, horse meat is a source.

TRICHOMONAS (Euglenozoa:Trichomonadida).

T. vaginalis (214, 3859, 3983, 5856, 6735, 7040, 8043, 8395) colonizes the human urogenital tract. *T. vaginalis* is fragile in the environment and highly sensitive to desiccation or free chlorine. **SPREAD**: is via vaginal sex, rarely perinatally, very rarely (if at all) from wet surfaces. *T. vaginalis* is shed with urine, genital secretions, and semen. **RISKS**: multiple sex partners (see section 14.7), women in prison, and a history of multiple, induced abortions. **CLINICAL INFORMATION**: About 50% of infections are inapparent (up to 90% in males, 25–50% in females). The reported incubation period is 4–28 days. Manifestations: dysuria, discharge, urethritis, and vaginitis. Suspected complications include infertility and low birth weight. In Africa, *T. vaginalis* increases (perhaps doubles) the risk of HIV transmission. Confirmation is by microscopy (wet mounts have a sensitivity of only 40–60%), culture, or NAT from urine (office- or self-collected) or swab. Nitroimidazoles are a treatment option. Partner treatment can decrease reinfection rates. **IMPACT**: By age, sex, setting, and test, infection prevalences in adults are 3–48%. Of females coming to office with vaginal symptoms, 15–20% are diagnosed with trichomoniasis. New cases are estimated to >170 million per year worldwide. Reported infection rates are 1.4–1.6/100 person-years in the United States and 1/100 person-years in China (among 16,797 females followed for 132,946 person-years).

TRICHOPHYTON (148, 2176, 3557, 4078, 4326, 4653, 6392) (*Ascomycota*: *Onygales*). These are keratophilic, nonfluorescent molds that form arthrospores inside hair shafts (endothrix). Species can be anthropophilic (e.g., *T. mentagrophytes* var. *interdigitale*), zoophilic (e.g., *T. mentagrophytes* var. *mentagrophytes*), or geogphilic (e.g., *T. terrestre*) (Table 20.8). **SPREAD**: by species is by contact with humans (hairs, desquamation) or their personal objects, animals, or soil. **CLINICAL INFORMATION**: Inapparent infections are frequent (in >50%) and are reservoir for anthropophilic species. Zoophilic species may be more often manifest than anthropophilic species, although zoophilic and geophilic species can be carried silently on scalp, skin, feet, and nails as well. The incubation period is 5–7 weeks or longer. Manifestations: tinea capitis, tinea corporis, tinea pedis (interdigital or moccasin-type), and onychomycosis (tinea unguium and finger and toe nails). Diagnosis is by microscopy or culture from hair brush or scrapings. **IMPACT**: The prevalence of dermatophytic infections in children and adults is ∼0–10% (typically 2–3%). By age and location, *Trichophyton* is cultured from ∼0.5–70% of cases of tinea capitis, ∼10–70% of tinea corporis, ∼90–95% of tinea pedis, and ∼20–75% of tinea unguium. Relative frequencies vary by geography. In North America and western Europe, *T. tonsurans* seems to replace *Microsporum* as the main agent of tinea capitis. **OUTBREAKS**: *T. tonsurans* has caused outbreaks of tinea corporis in a rehabilitation facility and on a pediatric ward.

TRICHOSPORON (263, 884, 2761, 5861, 5921, 6921, 7234, 7928) (*Basidiomycota*: *Tremellales*). These are yeast-like fungi recovered from soil, water, foods, and air. Several of the >15 species can colonize or infect humans, including *T. asahii*, *T. asteroides*, *T. cutaneum*, and *T. mucoides*. **SPREAD**: is likely via ingestion or inhalation, or from previously colonized sites. **RISKS**: intravascular

Table 20.8 Agents of tinea with crude relative frequencies, by source and type of tinea

Source	Fungus	Crude relative frequencies (%) within each type of tinea			
		Tinea capitis	Tinea corporis	Tinea pedis	Tinea unguium
Humans	T. mentagrophytes		Up to 40	Up to 80	10–40
	T. rubrum	<5	20–35	20–70	0–90 (mainly toenails)
	T. tonsurans	0–90		<5	<5
	T. violaceum	Up to 65	5–70	10–15	0–35
Animals	T. equinum		<5		
	T. verrucosum	Up to 30	Up to 20		
Environment	T. terrestre			<5	

devices, impaired immunity (neutropenia, transplant recipients, corticosteroids). CLINICAL INFORMATION: *Trichosporon* is a cause of contamination, colonization, infection, or invasive disease. An incubation period has not been reported. Manifestations: tinea pedis, fingernail onychomycosis, and folliculitis (by *T. asteroides* and *T. cutaneum*), hairshaft nodules of scalp or pubic hair ("white piedra," by *T. ovoides* and *T. inkin*), summer-type hypersensitivity pneumonitis (by *T. dermatis* and *T. asahii*), nosocomial UTI, and invasive disease in immune-impaired hosts ("trichosporonosis," by *T. asahii* and *T. mucoides*). Treatment options are limited and include amphotericin B, triazoles, and fluconazole. Lethality of invasive disease can reach 80%. OUTBREAKS: A nosocomial *T. mucoides* pseudooutbreak was traced to bronchoscopes contaminated from reprocessing.

TRICHOSTRONGYLUS (517, 768) (Nematoda: Strongylida). *Trichostrongylus* circulates worldwide, in herbivores, rodents, and primates (final hosts, shed eggs), and soil in which eggs develop to infective larvae (L3). Species such as *T. axei* from sheep and horses, and *T. colubriformis* from sheep and goats have also been reported in humans. Life span of adults is ≥7 years. SPREAD: is via ingestion of L3 from dirty hands (soil, manure, and animal contacts) or unwashed vegetables. CLINICAL INFORMATION: The prepatent period is 3–4 weeks. Manifestations: abdominal discomfort, mild diarrhea, and eosinophilia. Confirmation is by visualizing hookwormlike eggs in stools. IMPACT: Sporadic or focal. In Australia, five infections (0.01%) were diagnosed from >46,000 stool tests.

TRICHURIS (Nematoda: Enoplida). This nematode circulates in warm climates worldwide, in mammals (shed eggs), and soil (harbors infective eggs). Eggs need 3–4 weeks (at 25°C) to embryonate and become infective. Heat (>52°C) and freeze (below −9°C) inactivate eggs. Species include *T. muris* (in rodents), *T. suis* (in pigs), *T. vulpis* (in dogs and cats), and *T. trichiura* (in monkeys and humans). Although infections in humans with *T. vulpis* have been documented, the principal species in humans is *T. trichiura*. Life span of adults is several years.

T. trichiura (528, 900, 1835, 2074, 7165, 7499, 8103). SPREAD: is via ingestion of embryonated eggs from foods or dirty hands. In Jamaica, the estimated dose was 6–60 eggs per child per year. RISKS: domicile in or travel to endemic areas, domicile in urban slums or close to refuse dumps, no sanitation, use of raw wastewater or human feces in agriculture, vegetable gardening, and geophagia. CLINICAL INFORMATION: Adults colonize the large bowel. Worm burden is 1–1,000 (often 50) per person. Typically, it is overdispersed, with a few people in a community carrying a high burden and most carrying a low burden. The prepatent period is 4–12 weeks. Confirmation is by visualizing eggs in stools or adults on rectocolonoscopy. Many light infections are inapparant. Egg counts >10,000/g feces define heavy infection. Coinfections with *Ascaris* and hookworm are frequent. Putative manifestations include abdominal pain, diarrhea or dysentery, iron-deficiency anemia, and retarded growth. Treatment options include benzimidazoles (for several days) and ivermectin. IMPACT: Worldwide, 3,200 million people are at risk, and >550 million are infected, for a crude infection prevalence of 17%. By age and geography, infection prevalence in low-income countries is 1–98%, (typically 20–30%). In western Kenya, 21–95% (overall 55%) of 1,738 school children were infected, and 0–15% (overall 4%) had infections with >1,000 eggs/g feces. In People's Republic of China in 1988–1992, based on ~1.5 million tests, ~19% of the population (202–222 million) were infected, and 0.2% had heavy infections. Pockets of transmission persist in parts of Europe. OUTBREAKS: In communities with a prevalence in school children of ≥70% or heavy infections of ≥10%, systematic treatment of preschool children and women of childbearing age is recommended.

TROPHERYMA (2096, 4663, 4667, 6117) (*Actinobacteria*: *Actinomycetales*). *T. whippelii* is a fastidious rod related to soil-dwelling actinomycetes, culturable only since 2000. NAT demonstrated *T. whippelii* in wastewater from sewage treatment plants in Germany. SPREAD: a suspected mode is foods. **CLINICAL INFORMATION:** Studies of saliva and duodenal biopsy from healthy persons suggest that *T. whippelii* is part of the buccal flora and that inapparent infections occur. Manifestations (Whipple's disease): diverse, can include enteric (diarrhea, weight loss), cardiac (endocarditis), neurological, and other symptoms and signs.

TRYPANOSOMA (2993, 5448, 7899) (Euglenozoa: Kinetoplastida). These are arthroprod-borne, flagellated protozoa. Species from mammals include *T. brucei brucei*, *T. brucei rhodesiense*, *T. cruzi*, *T. congolense*, *T. evansi*, *T. lewisi* (rats), *T. rangeli*, and *T. vivax*. Species isolated in humans are in Africa, *T. brucei gambiense* and *T. brucei rhodesiense*; in Latin America, *T. cruzi* and *T. rangeli*; and in India, *T. evansi*.

***T. brucei* sl** (709, 1337, 3520, 5449, 6122, 6467, 7174) circulates in Africa, in tsetse flies (inoculate infective metacyclic forms with blood meals), wildlife (herbivores, carnivores, rodents, and primates) and domestic mammals (carry blood forms). **SPREAD:** is via fly bite, with *T. brucei gambiense* rarely by needle stick or congenitally. **CLINICAL INFORMATION:** The prepatent period is 1–2 weeks. The incubation period is 5 days (chancre) to 10–21 days (adenopathy fever). Screening is clinical and by serology, e.g., "card agglutination test for trypanosomiasis" (CATT). Confirmation is by microscopy of smears from blood, node aspirate, or CSF (detection threshold ≥ 10 parasites/μl), or by NAT. Centrifugation of blood or CSF improves yield. *T. brucei brucei*, *T. brucei gambiense*, and *T. brucei rhodesiense* are microscopically indistinguishable. Differentiation of zoonotic *T. brucei* ss from anthroponotic *T. brucei gambiense* and *T. brucei rhodesiense* requires molecular tests (a human serum resistance [SRA] gene seems specific for *T. brucei rhodesiense*) or "blood incubation infectivity test" (BIIT). Treatment options are limited and include pentamidine or suramin (early stage) and melarsoprol (neuroinvasive stage). **IMPACT:** There are ~260 foci of human African trypanosomiasis (HAT) in 36 countries of sub-Saharan Africa. The prevalence of confirmed infections in these areas is 0.2–6.5% (typically 0.5–3%). New HAT cases are estimated at 40,000–100,000/year. In rural enzootic-endemic areas, seroprevalence can reach 20%.

T. brucei gambiense (3538, 4698) circulates in forest areas in West and Central Africa (from Senegal to Uganda). Humans are the main vertebrate reservoir. **RISKS:** rural domicile in endemic areas, daytime peridomestic activities, in particular, along water courses. Manifestations (West African, protracted form of HAT): inoculation chancre (in $\leq$25% of cases), regional (nuchal) adenopathy (in 85%), rash, pruritus, and fever, after months followed by signs of encephalitis (headache, unsteady gait, and daytime somnolence). By treatment regime and compliance, 1–30% of treatments fail or relapse. Lethality is 100% without treatment and 1–2.5% with treatment. **OUTBREAKS:** In southern Sudan in 1997–1999, *T. brucei gambiense* resurged, with 3,785 new cases detected in Equatoria Province. Early detection and treatment of cases is a key control measure, and its lack is a major reason for outbreaks.

T. brucei rhodesiense (3517, 5161, 5162) circulates in savanna in East Africa (east of Rift Valley, from Ethiopia to Botswana). Game and domestic mammals are the main vertebrate reservoirs, humans are tangental hosts. **RISKS:** "going into the bush," for herding, hunting, or honey collection, tourism ("safari") in tsetse territory. The estimated infective dose is ~350 parasites. Manifestations (East African, acute form of HAT, an emergency): inoculation chancre (in 20–90%), regional adenopathy, fever, and meningoencephalitis. Untreated, lethality is ~100. **OUTBREAKS:** Numerous outbreaks have occurred, often from moving cattle for trade, or from civilian and military crises. In Uganda in 1976–1983, an epidemic caused 19,974 cases, for a disease rate of 90–1,200/10^5 per year. In 1990, an epidemic in Uganda and Kenya caused ~0.5 million cases.

T. cruzi (226, 1785, 1936, 2938, 5140, 5319, 5461, 7520, 8099) is enzootic in the Americas, from the southern United States over central and tropical South America (zymodeme I) to Patagonia in the southern cone (zymodeme II). Vector is triatomine bugs that while feeding excrete infective metacyclic forms with feces on skin. Hosts are parasitemic wild and domestic mammals. **SPREAD:** is via bug feces, transfusion, organ transplant, laboratory accident, mother-to-child, occasionally likely by ingestion of contaminated foods. **RISKS:** rural domicile in enzootic areas, substandard, bug-infested housing, history of exposure to bugs. **CLINICAL INFORMATION:** The Brazilian physician C.R.J. Chagas (1879–1934) described the agent, disease, vector, and hosts (1285). The incubation period is 1–24 days (acute phase) to years (late phase). Signs of acute Chagas disease are edema at the inoculation site (Romaña's sign, in only 35–45% of cases) and fever (in ~85%, lasts 2–3 weeks). The acute phase evolves to latent infection that may remain asymptomatic for life. However, 8–30% of latently infected people develop chronic Chagas disease after years or decades. Signs can be cardiac (arrhythmia, cardiomegaly, mainly zymodeme I) or enteric (megaesophagus, megacolon, mainly zymodeme II). Confirmation is by serology plus NAT, parasitology (xenodiagnosis), or histopathology. Treatment options are limited to benznidazole or nifurtimox, indicated for the acute phase, congenital infection, and perhaps chronic disease. Reported lethality of acute disease is 5%. **IMPACT:** In the 1980s (preeradication), 100 million people were at risk, and 17–18 million were infected in 18 enzootic countries. Control has reduced infections to ~10 million in 2000. Peridomestic transmission seems interrupted in Uruguay, Chile, and much (8 of

12 states) of Brazil. Seroprevalence is low (<1%) in French Guiana, Guyana, and Suriname, intermediate (1–5%) in Guatemala, Mexico, Argentina, Brazil, Chile, and Ecuador, and high (8–50%) in Paraguay, northeastern Argentina, and other enzootic areas. A threat to control is sylvatic *T. infestans* that bridges sylvatic and peridomestic habitats. In rural Guatemala, the infection rate is 0.5–3.8/100 inhabitants per year. **OUTBREAKS**: Peridomestic bugs have caused outbreaks with 8–20 acute cases. Surprisingly, of 205 acute cases recorded in 1968–2000, 111 (54%) were considered food borne. Preventive measures include improved housing, pyrethroid house spraying, exclusion of domestic mammals from premises, and health education.

T. evansi (3568, 8126) circulates in tropical countries, in horses (surra), livestock, dogs and cats, and tabanid flies and other hematophagous insects that transmit *T. evansi* mechanically. Humans are reported to be naturally resistant, but infection in a human was documented in India in 2005.

T. rangeli (2993) circulates in Latin America, in triatomine bugs and vertebrate animals. Geography, vectors, and reservoir hosts (e.g., Edentata, Marsupialia, Rodentia, Carnivora, and Primata) broadly overlap with *T. cruzi*. **SPREAD**: is via bug feces, like for *T. cruzi*. Infections in humans are innocuous; >2,600 are recorded (>1,140 in Venezuela and >1,100 in Guatemala).

TSUKAMURELLA (6732) (*Actinobacteria: Actinomycetales*). These are *Nocardia*-related bacteria that inhabit sediments, wastewater, and occasionally piped water. *Tsukamurella* can cause invasive disease in immune impaired hosts. The most frequently isolated species is *T. paurometabola*.

TTV (556, 6541) (unenveloped DNA viruses: *Circoviridae*). TTV derives its name from "transfusion-transmitted," "Torque Teno," or patient "TT." TTV is prevalent in 2–100% of healthy persons worldwide (10–70% in North America and Europe). **SPREAD**: is via blood transfusion, but additional, unknown modes are likely. TTV can be detected in saliva, feces, breastmilk, vaginal fluid, and semen. **CLINICAL INFORMATION**: TTV is an orphan virus "in search of disease." TTV is not associated with hepatitis, as originally thought. Because of its high prevalence, coincidental associations with prevalent other viruses are predictable, e.g., HBV or HCV.

UREAPLASMA (*Firmicutes: Mycoplasmatales*) (5, 2700, 8344). *U. urealyticum* colonizes the urogenital tract of humans worldwide. There are >10 serovars in two biovars. **SPREAD**: is via sex. **CLINICAL INFORMATION**: Inapparent infections occur. An incubation period is not known, although it appears to be longer than in gonococcal urethritis. Suspected manifestations: urethritis in men, with less copious, less purulent discharge than gonococcal urethritis, preterm labor. Detection is by NAT from urine, swab (urethral, vaginal, and cervical), or amniotic fluid. Lethality in immune-competent patients is minimal.

VAHLKAMPFIA (7925) (Amoebozoa: Heterolobosea). These amebas are free-living in water, river sediment, soil, and around roots in arid soils, where concentration can vary seasonally. *Vahlkampfia* is occasionally recovered from keratitis in contact lens wearers.

VARICELLOVIRUS (enveloped double-stranded DNA viruses of *Herpesviridae*). Prototype is VZV (or HHV3) that circulates in humans worldwide.

Varicella-zoster virus (VZV) (867, 1780, 2880, 4881, 5989, 6222, 6790, 7269, 7604). **SPREAD**: is via droplets, aerosols, possibly contaminated objects. Aerosols are generated in the throat and from skin lesions. **RISKS**: siblings in day care or kindergarten, a case in the household, health work. Infectivity is high (R_0 is 7–11), and secondary attack rates in nonvaccinated communities are 30–100%. Seronegative pregnant women, other adults, and hosts with impaired immunity are susceptible to complications. Reactivation risks include age >50 years and impaired immunity (malignancy, transplants). **CLINICAL INFORMATION**: By infective dose, the incubation period is 10–20 (often 14–17) days. Most primary infections are manifest as varicella (chicken pox), with typically 20–200 vesicles. Complications in 1–15% (often 3.5–5.5%) of cases include bacterial skin infections (e.g., impetigo), otitis media, pneumonia, dissemination, and encephalitis. Varicella lethality is <0.01% in high-income countries (mainly in adults) but 1% in outbreaks in low-income countries, and 4–34% in immune-impaired hosts. Treatment options include specific VZV-Ig and antivirals. After primary infection, VZV becomes latent in dorsal root ganglia. Reactivation results in zoster (shingles), with linear vesicles at ocular, thoracid, inguinal, or other sites, and postherpetic neuralgia. **IMPACT**: In temperate climates, the disease rate in children is high (~9–14% per year), and by age 15 years, ≥90% are seroreactive (latently infected); ≤5–10% of adults remain susceptible. In some tropical areas such as the Caribbean and Southcentral and Southeast Asia, infections are curiously delayed, and 15–25% of young adults remain susceptible. This age shift is important for migrant health workers in West Europe. In California, varicella-related mortality per 10^5 per year decreased from 0.07 in 1988–1994 (prevaccine) to 0.04 in 1995–2000 (with vaccine). **OUTBREAKS**: Outbreak venues included the community, day care centers, and schools. Effective vaccines are available. Indications should follow national guidelines. As a history of varicella reliably predicts immunity, indications could be targeted to susceptible individuals whose history is blank for varicella or who test negative for anti-VZV IgG, e.g., (i) children on entry into child care or primary school, or adolescents on leaving school, (ii) non-pregnant females who plan to become pregnant, (iii) health and social workers, (iv) persons at risk of complications, and their family and household contacts.

VEILLONELLA (tentatively assigned to β-*Proteobacteria*: *Neisseriales*). These are anaerobic, gram-negative cocci that are part of the mouth, bowel, and vaginal flora of mammals and humans. *V. parvula* (633) has been recovered from or causally implicated in sinusitis and invasive disease (bacteremia, endocarditis, septic arthritis, and meningitis).

VENEZUELAN EQUINE ENCEPHALITIS VIRUS (VEEV). See Alphavirus.

VESICULOVIRUS (enveloped RNA viruses: *Mononegavirales*: *Rhabdoviridae*). *Vesiculovirus* includes chandipuravirus and vesicular stomatitis virus.

Chandipura virus (6108) is endemic in rural India and West Africa. SPREAD: is via sandfly bite. Manifestations: fever, vomiting, encephalitis. IMPACT: Sporadic or epidemic. OUTBREAKS: An outbreak in India in 2003 caused 329 cases (six confirmed virologically) and 183 (56%) deaths.

Vesicular stomatitis virus (VSV) (6057, 6195) circulates in the New World, in horses, cattle, and pigs (could be confused with foot-and-mouth-disease, see *Aphthovirus*). During epizootics, humans can become infected. SPREAD: is presumably via contact or droplets. Animal-to-animal spread seems via contact or sandfly bites. CLINICAL INFORMATION: The incubation period is ~2–6 days. Manifestations: vesicular lesions and flulike illness (could be confused with hand-foot-mouth-disease; see *Enterovirus*).

VIBRIO (167, 5209) (γ-*Proteobacteria*: *Vibrionales*). *Vibrio* is an aquatic, motile ("vibrating"), halophilic rod. There are >30 species. By relative frequency, the main isolates from humans include *V. parahaemolyticus* (in 30–35%), *V. cholerae* (non-O1/non-O139 in ~15%, O1 in 0–50%, O139 in 0–30%), *V. vulnificus* (in 5–20%), and *V. alginolyticus* (in 0–7%). In Florida in 1981–1988, rates of *Vibrio* illness per 10^5 per year were 9.5 for raw oyster eaters with liver disease, 0.9 for healthy raw oyster eaters, and 0.2 for non-raw oyster eaters. Patients with hepatic disease, prior gastric surgery, or taking antacids should avoid raw seafood. *Vibrio* is killed by boiling (100°C for 10 s); shells should be opened for frying.

V. alginolyticus (2823, 5586) circulates in marine waters and shellfish, and it is recovered from aquarium seawater. SPREAD: is via water contact, swallowing water, or trauma (e.g., coral reef). CLINICAL INFORMATION: The incubation period is ~24 h. Manifestations: wound infection, cellulitis, otitis externa and media, rarely invasive disease in immune-impaired hosts.

V. cholerae (1030, 1470, 6194, 6506, 7887, 8114) circulates in brackish and estuarine warm waters, marine life, humans who shed the agent with feces, sewage, and tap water. Somatic O antigens define >100 serogroups; a virus encodes for cholera toxin. Toxigenic *V. cholerae* O1 (biotypes "classical," "El Tor") and O139 cause epidemic cholera, nontoxigenic O1 and O139, as well as non-O1 serogroups ("nonagglutinable" or NAG, e.g., *V. cholerae* O141) cause sporadic cholera that is clinically indistinguishable from epidemic cholera. NAGs are recovered not only from humans but also from waterfowl, wildlife, and domestic animals. SPREAD: is via drinking water, foods, or hand contacts, including occasionally nosocomially. RISKS: handled and leftover foods, raw seafood, seafood imported from endemic areas, unsafe tap water, long distance to a water source, substandard housing, camps, gatherings, a case in the household, poor hand hygiene, bathing in contaminated freshwater, cholera season, visits to outbreak areas. The infectious dose is 10^6–10^8 bacteria (volunteers) to 10^3–10^5 (in users of antacids, endemic areas). CLINICAL INFORMATION: Most (90%) infections are inapparent or mild, 8% are moderate, and 2% are severe, requiring emergency treatment. Carriers exist. The incubation period is 4 h to 8½ (often ½–5) days. Manifestations: watery or profuse diarrhea (rice water), dehydration, hypothermia, and shock. Water loss can reach 0.5–1 liter/h. By rapidity of rehydration, lethality is 0.1–15%, in endemic areas ~1.5% overall. Enteric coinfections seem frequent (in up to 20% of cases in endemic areas). *V. cholerae* non-O1 can cause invasive disease. IMPACT: In 2003 (2002, 2001), 45 (52, 58) countries reported 111,575 (142,311, 184,311) cases, including 1.7% (3.2%, 1.5%) deaths. By age and surveillance, disease rates are 30–700 (typically 100–300)/10^5 per year in low-income countries, and 0.2–0.3/10^5 per year in endemic pockets in high-income countries. OUTBREAKS: Pandemics were recorded in 1817–1896 (first to fifth), 1899–1923 (sixth), and since 1960 (seventh). When the seventh pandemic hit South America in 1991, ~750,000 cholera cases ensued. In 1992, *V. cholerae* O139 emerged in Bangladesh and India. Epidemic waves recur at intervals. Examples of epidemics with >1,000 cases are: Peru in 1991 (16,400 cases, 0.4% deaths), Bangladesh in 1991–1992 (107,300, 1.4%), Guinea-Bissau in 1994 (15,878, 2%), Nigeria in 1996 (1,384, 7%), Uganda in 1997–1998 (6,228), India in 1998 (16,500, 1.7%), Dhaka (Bangladesh) in 2002 (30,000), and Yap (Micronesia) in 2000–2001 (3,400, after a 10-year gap). Outbreaks have affected all continents, including Europe, e.g., Italy in 1994 (12 cases) and Ukraine in 1994–1995 (1,370 cases,

2.3% deaths). Reported attack rates in outbreaks are 1–3.5%. Preventive measures include safe tap water and foods, sanitation, educating hand washing (households and food handlers), and surveillance. Effective vaccines are available. Oral vaccines can contribute to curb outbreaks and are an accepted measure in emergency situations.

V. parahaemolyticus (1006, 4216, 4337, 7621) circulates worldwide, in warm, coastal waters, sediments, marine invertebrates (plankton, bivalves, and crustaceans), and fish. In opened bivalves, *V. parahaemolyticus* is killed by heat (boiling for 2–3 min). SPREAD: is via seafood, and skin contact with seawater. RISKS: preference for raw seafood (e.g., oysters), mishandled seafoods, transmission season. Food can be contaminated by hands, marine water used for washing or sprinkling foods, likely also flies. Infectivity seems low, the infective dose is high ($\geq 10^5$ particles), and secondary spread is not reported. CLINICAL INFORMATION: Up to 30% of infections are inapparent. The incubation period is ½ (often 12) hours to 4 days (diarrheal disease), or 1–10 days (otitis). Manifestations: diarrheal disease (in 50–100%, can include vomiting and fever), wound infection (in 0–30%), otitis (in swimmers), and invasive disease (e.g., BSI, in 0–10%). Confirmation is by culture from stools, blood, or wound specimens. Diarrhea is usually self-limited. By invasiveness, reported lethality is 0.04–33%. IMPACT: The prevalence in diagnostic stool samples is <1–3%. In the United States, *V. parahaemolyticus* accounts for 30–35% of clinical *Vibrio* isolates. Where raw seafood is popular (e.g., Japan, Korea, Singapore, and Taiwan), *V. parahaemolyticus* (and *V. vulnificus*) can account for 20–65% of bacterial causes of food poisoning (cases and outbreaks). In Vietnam in 1997–1999, the disease rate was $18/10^5$ person-years. OUTBREAKS: Venues for food-borne outbreaks included the community, a boarding school, a restaurant, a conference, a hotel, an island resort, aircraft, ships, and military personnel. A clone (O3:K6) emerged in Japan or Taiwan in the mid-1990s that has dispersed internationally meanwhile.

V. vulnificus (770, 3464, 4843, 5586) circulates worldwide, in coastal, warm seawaters, sediments, and marine life (plankton, bivalves, and crustaceans). Salinity of >3% seems to hamper growth. SPREAD: is via raw seafood, contact or trauma with marine waters, or handling of or trauma from fish, oysters, or crabs. RISKS: preference for raw or undercooked seafoods, contact with marine waters or sealife for work (fishing, pisciculture, marketing, and catering) or leisure (swimming), warm season (V–X in the United States). CLINICAL INFORMATION: The incubation period is 3–4 (often 12–24) hours to 10–12 days. Manifestations: diarrhea, wound infection (in ~30–70% of cases, from trauma or hematogenous spread), necrotizing fasciitis (up to 50%), and invasive disease (in 25–65%), e.g., sepsis, in both comorbid (liver disease and diabetes) and immune-competent patients. Lethality of invasive disease is high (25–70%), even with adequate treatment. Confirmation is by culture from stool, blood, or wound swabs. IMPACT: In enzootic-endemic areas, *V. vulnificus* accounts for 5–20% of *Vibrio* isolates. Reported disease rates are $0.2–1.2/\ 10^5$ per year.

WANGIELLA (Ascomycota: Chaetothyriales). *W. dermatitidis* (548, 1317) is a pigmented fungus that inhabits soil. SPREAD: is likely via soil contact. Manifestations: skin infection, external otitis, keratitis, invasive disease (fungemia and brain abscess) in compromised hosts, e.g., from indwelling devices and CSF eosinophilia.

WESTERN EQUINE ENCEPHALOMYELITIS VIRUS (WEEV). See Alphavirus.

WEST NILE VIRUS (WNV). See Flavivirus.

WOLBACHIA (1647) (α-Proteobacteria: Rickettsiales). These are intracellular, gram-negative coccobacilli symbiontic in filariids. *Wolbachia* is suspected of being involved in inflammatory responses to filariae.

WUCHERERIA (Nematoda: Spirurida). Prototype is *W. bancrofti*.

W. bancrofti (506, 1940, 5514, 6150, 6911, 8124) circulates in warm climates, in mosquitoes that inject infective larvae (L3), and humans who harbor adults in lymphatic organs and microfilariae (mf) in peripheral blood. Microfilaremia is mainly nocturnal (peak at 2100–0300 h), rarely diurnal ("subperiodic" Pacific strain), and correlated with peak vector acitivity. Life span is 1½–25 months for mf, and 5–10 (rarely up to 40) years for adults. SPREAD: is via mosquito bite. Passage of mf via umbilical cord blood is reported, not, however, passage of adult worms. RISKS: domicile or long (>3 months) stays in endemic areas, domicile close to urban foci, non-mosquito-proofed housing, bednets not available, defective, or not used. CLINICAL INFORMATION: The prepatent period is 9–12 months. Many infections (without or with patent microfilaremia) are inapparent. The incubation period is 3–18 months. Manifestations (lymphatic filariasis) can be acute (epididymitis, lymphangitis, and fever) or chronic (after year-long silent infection or recurrent acute episodes), including hydrocele, lymphedema (elephantiasis), internal fistules that cause chyluria, and infertility. Confirmation is by ultrasound (motile adults), visualizing mf in thick smears or filtrates of night blood, antigen capture, or NAT. IMPACT: About 1.2–2 billion people are considered at risk, >110 million are infected in ~75 countries (~40 in Africa, 7 in Latin

America, 17 in Asia, and >10 in the Pacific), and ∼40 million have chronic disease. By age, geography, and test, infection prevalence is 0.5–55%, and disease point prevalences are ∼1–15%. In 1,829 Tanzanian school children, prevalences were 17% by microfilaremia, and 44% by antigen test. Reported rates are 1–13% per year for new infections and 7–10% per year for acute episodes. Infections can be cleared spontaneously at rates comparable to acquisition rates. OUTBREAKS: Mosquito control measures include indoor residual insecticides, window screens, impregnated bednets, and breeding-site destruction (container collection, polystyrene beads in latrine pits). Control was successful in Trinidad and Tobago, Santa Catarina state (Brazil), People's Republic of China, southern Japan, Taiwan, and Australia. Worldwide elimination was launched in 1998, using annual community treatments with single doses of ivermectin, albendazole, or diethylcarbamazine, singly or in combination.

YATAPOXVIRUS (enveloped DNA viruses: *Poxviridae*). A member is tanapoxvirus (1911, 7175) that appears to circulate in primates in tropical Africa. Modes of acquisition are unknown. Proposed are animal contacts and hematophagous insects. Manifestations: fever, vesiculous, umbilicated skin lesions. IMPACT: Sporadic, or epidemic. A differential diagnosis of smallpox. OUTBREAKS: Outbreaks occurred along the Tana River, Kenya, in 1957 and 1962.

YELLOW FEVER VIRUS (YFV). See Flavivirus.

YERSINIA (162, 720, 2879, 6974) (γ-*Proteobacteria*: *Enterobacteriales*). These are gram-negative, bipolar (safety pin) coccoid rods with ∼10 species. *Y. enterocolitica* (most frequent), *Y. pseudotuberculosis* (infrequent), and *Y. pestis* (rare) are infective to humans. This trio has a preference for lymphatic tissues (mesenteric and regional lymph nodes, tonsils) and broadly shares antigens (with *Escherichia*, *Salmonella*, *Vibrio*, even *Brucella*), making serological diagnosis difficult. Treatment options include aminoglycosides (e.g., streptomycin), tetracyclines, and fluoroquinolones.

Y. enterocolitica (366, 720, 2253, 4311, 6154) circulates in temperate climates, in cold-blooded vertebrates, wild and domestic mammals (e.g., pigs), manure, soil, freshwater, tap water, and foods. The somatic O antigen defines ∼60 serogroups (O:3 and O:9 are most frequent in humans). There are six biovars (virulent 2, 3, 4, 5, and 1B, and environmental apathogenic 1A). *Y. enterocolitica* grows at 0–4°C (refrigerator temperature), a niche that is relevant for cold foods and blood banking. SPREAD: is mainly via foods or tap water, infrequently via contact with infected humans or mammals or by blood transfusion. RISKS: drinking untreated tap water, eating raw milk, vegetables, or undercooked meat products, and work and leisure contacts with animals. There may be a peak in winter. The infectious dose is high (10^6 particles). Convalescent humans shed the agent for 2–3 weeks, on occasion for months. CLINICAL INFORMATION: From 25% to 80% of infections are inapparent. The incubation period is 1–10 (typically 3–7) days. Manifestations: watery (infrequently bloody) diarrhea, pseudoappendicitis, sepsis, and immunoreactive disease (arthritis and erythema nodosum). Confirmation is by culture from stool, blood, aspirate, food leftovers, or companion animals. Biovar and serogroup should be determined. Lethality attributable to food-borne yersiniosis is 0.1–0.8%. IMPACT: Diagnostic yield from stools is typically low (0.5–1%), with extremes of 0.2–8% (includes apathogenic biovar). Most infections are diagnosed in small children, with an occasional minor second peak in adolescents. In high-income countries, disease rates are 0.4–14 (often 1–10)/10^5 and year. OUTBREAKS: Outbreaks are reported from milk and ethnic foods, in households, and on an oil tanker.

Y. pestis (98, 796, 1206, 2564, 3553, 4531, 5633, 6136, 8118) circulates focally in Africa, the Americas, and Asia, in small mammals (rodents and lagomorphs) and their fleas (sylvatic plague), occasionally in peridomestic mammals (e.g., rats, cats, dogs, "urban plague"). Except soil around rodent burrows, *Y. pestis* does not survive free-living. SPREAD: is via (i) fleas that regurgitate *Y. pestis* on feeding attempts, (ii) scratch, bite, or droplets from incubating or ill mammals (e.g., cats), (iii) handling of animal carcasses, (iv) droplets from humans with pneumonic plague, (v) human fleas, (vi) ingestion of meat from infected camels or rodents. RISKS: domicile near or visit to a focus or epizootic area, rodent-infested housing, work with enzootic mammals (hunting, skinning, and veterinary), flea bites, cat or dog ownership, work with infective patients or clinical materials, and warm season. CLINICAL INFORMATION: Seroreactions suggest the occurrence of inapparent infections. The incubation period is ½–8 days (inoculation) to 2–3 days (inhalation). Manifestations: fever and regional adenopathy (bubo, drains portal of entry), pneumonia (primary if from droplets, secondary if from sepsis), and invasive disease (sepsis, meningitis, coagulopathy, or "black death"). In the United States in 1947–1996, of 390 reported cases, 84% were bubonic, 13% were septic, and 2% were pneumonic. In Kazakhstan in 1990–2002, the male to female ratio in 19 cases was 2.8 to 1. Confirmation is by antigen detection (aspirate), culture (blood, aspirate, sputum; takes 48 h for visible growth), possibly serology (paired sera, four-fold increase in titer). Lethality of untreated bubonic plague is 40–60%. By site (bubo, pneumonia, and sepsis) and delay, treated lethality is 0–70% (often 5–7%). IMPACT: In the past 50 years worldwide, case reports on average were 1,700/year. In 2003 (2002, 2001), 9 (13, 12) countries reported 2,118 (1,925, 2,671) cases, with 9% (9%, 7%) deaths. In enzootic areas, reported disease rates per 10^5 per year are 1–4 in interepidemic periods and 77–4,500 during epidemics. **OUTBREAKS**: Pandemics occurred in 541–750 (first, "Justinian," biovar "Antiqua," from East Africa), 1330 to end-1600 (second, "Black Death," biovar "Medievalis," from Central Asia), and 1855 to present (third, biovar "Orientalis"). Examples of outbreaks (cases and details) include Manchuria in 1911 (60,000, pneumonic), Madagascar in 1991 (170, in port shantytown), Zaire in 1992 (191, lethality 41%), Peru in 1992–1994 (1,151, lethality 4.7%), Mozambique in 1994 (226, by *Mastomys* for food), India 1994 (876, >0.6 million fleeing in panic), Madagascar in 1997 (18, lethality 44%), Ecuador in 1998 (12 deaths, at altitude of 3,300 m), and Algeria in 2003 (five, bubonic, near Oran).

Vaccines are not commercially available. Prophylactic measures include avoiding enzootic-epizootic areas, rodent control on premises, keeping pets at close range, repellents, impregnated clothing, protective clothes when handling dead animals and for patient care, public alerts at campgrounds, and preexposure chemoprophylaxis. For PEP from exposure to pneumonic plague (by cats and humans), doxycycline or quinolones are recommended.

Y. pseudotuberculosis (720, 3632, 5509, 6009) circulates in temperate climates, in birds, wild and domestic mammals, manure, water, and fodder. In soil, *Y. pseudotuberculosis* survives for up to 18 months, in meat at 4°C for 4 months. Humans are infrequently affected. **SPREAD**: is via ingestion of fecally polluted foods or tap water, or by animal contact. Interhuman spread is not reported. **RISKS**: school children, adolescents, and young adults are mainly affected. Convalescent humans shed the agent for 2–3 weeks, if untreated occasionally for months. However, carriage seems rare. **CLINICAL INFORMATION**: About two thirds of infections are inapparent. The incubation period is 3–7 days. Manifestations: diarrhea (in 90% of cases), fever (in 90%), pseudoappendicitis (mesenteric adenitis, in 75%), sepsis, and immunoreactive disease (arthritis). Confirmation is by culture from stool or blood. **IMPACT**: Diagnostic yield from submitted stools in high-income countries is <0.5%. The reported disease rate is <$0.1/10^5$ per year. **OUTBREAKS**: Vehicles for outbreaks were milk (homogenized or reconstituted) and iceberg lettuce. Venues included schools, restaurants, and a summer camp.

APPENDIX 1
EXPOSURE CHECKLIST

Remember the goal "To efficiently recognize and manage infectious agents and diseases."

A patient might volunteer details of exposure. Alternatively, a structured interview like the one below might provide insights.

SUSCEPTIBILITY, COLONIZATION, AND HIGH-RISK GROUPS

- Demography:
  - ☐ age
  - ☐ country of birth
  - ☐ domicile, year when moved to this domicile
- Susceptibility:
  - ☐ pregnant
  - ☐ IDU (ever, current)
  - ☐ HIV-infected
  - ☐ carries device
  - ☐ minority
  - ☐ other:
- Past infections:
  - ☐ chickenpox
  - ☐ hepatitis (A, B, C)
  - ☐ STI (e.g., syphilis)
  - ☐ tuberculosis
  - ☐ typhoid
  - ☐ other:
- Vaccines: all doses of:
  - ☐ HBV
  - ☐ influenza
  - ☐ MMR
  - ☐ polio
  - ☐ varicella
  - ☐ BCG
  - ☐ DTP
  - ☐ Hib
  - ☐ pneumococci
  - ☐ other:

NOSOCOMIAL EXPOSURE

- Antimicrobials in past 3 months:
  - ❑ β-lactams
  - ❑ macrolides
  - ❑ quinolones
  - ❑ antimalarials
  - ❑ other:
- Interventions in past 3 months:
  - ❑ injection
  - ❑ blood test
  - ❑ emergency visit
  - ❑ dentistry
  - ❑ surgery
  - ❑ other:

EXPOSURE IN THE LOCAL COMMUNITY

- Foods: any in past 48 h:
  - ❑ raw milk
  - ❑ raw eggs
  - ❑ seafood
  - ❑ "exotic-ethnic,"
  - ❑ other:
- Animals: any touching in past month of:
  - ❑ dog
  - ❑ cat
  - ❑ livestock
  - ❑ rodent
  - ❑ reptile
  - ❑ fish
  - ❑ bird
  - ❑ other:

  Ever:
  - ❑ tick bite
  - ❑ dog, cat, or bat attack
  - ❑ other:
- Environment: any skin contact in past month with:
  - ❑ soil
  - ❑ saltwater
  - ❑ freshwater
  - ❑ plants
  - ❑ sharps
  - ❑ other:
- Current season:
  - ❑ cold
  - ❑ warm
  - ❑ rainy
- Domicile: current:
  - ❑ home with tap water, flush toilet
  - ❑ number in household
  - ❑ prison, nursing home, other:
- People: any contact with ill person in past month:
  - ❑ at home
  - ❑ at work

❏ in day care
　　❏ at school
　　❏ other:
- Lifestyle: ever:
　　❏ in prison
　　❏ IDU
　　❏ diagnosed STI
　　❏ tested for HIV
　　❏ sex with same sex
　　❏ forced to have sex
- Work: currently:
　　❏ unemployed
　　❏ retired
　　❏ in education
　　❏ other:
- Current type of work:
　　❏ construction
　　❏ manufacture, maintenance
　　❏ military, guard
　　❏ farm, abattoir
　　❏ catering
　　❏ health, lab
　　❏ waste
　　❏ transport
　　❏ class, clerk, store
　　❏ other:
- Leisure: activity in past week:
　　❏ visit to fairs
　　❏ dined out
　　❏ outdoors
　　❏ indoor sports
　　❏ night club
　　❏ other:

DISPLACED OR IMPORTED AGENTS AND INFECTIONS

- Regional commuting:
　　❏ by private car
　　❏ by bus, train, tram, ferryboat
　　❏ other:
- Visits in past month to:
　　❏ beach
　　❏ park
　　❏ forest
　　❏ cave
　　❏ hotel (accommodation)
　　❏ other:
- International
　All continents and countries visited:
　All international flights in past year:
- Goods or gifts: in past month:
　　❏ any souvenir or gift from abroad
　　❏ any foods brought home
　　❏ other:

APPENDIX 2
ACRONYMS

GENERAL

BCG	Bacillus Calmette Guérin
BSE	Bovine spongiform encephalopathy
BSI	Bloodstream infection(s)
BSL	Biosafety level
CDC	Centers for Disease Control and Prevention
CFU	Colony-forming unit(s)
CJD	Creutzfeldt-Jakob disease
CI	Confidence interval
CoNS	Coagulase-negative *Staphylococcus*
CSF	Cerebrospinal fluid
d_0	First day of illness
D+, D−	Donor: seroreactive (infected), seronegative
DT	Definitive type (*Salmonella* phage type)
dTp_a	Diphtheria (adult), tetanus, pertussis$_{acellular}$ (adult)
e_0	First day of exposure
EAEC	Enteroaggregative *Escherichia coli*
EHEC	Enterohemorrhagic *Escherichia coli*
EIEC	Enteroinvasive *Escherichia coli*
ELISA	Enzyme-linked immunosorbent assay
EPEC	Enteropathogenic *Escherichia coli*
ESβL	Extended-spectrum β-lactamases
ETEC	Enterotoxigenic *Escherichia coli*
ex	formerly
FTA-abs	Fluorescent *Treponema* antibody test
GAS, GBS	Group A, group B *Streptococcus*
HF	Hemorrhagic fever
HGE	Human granulocytic ehrlichiosis
Hib	*Haemophilus influenzae* serotype b vaccine
HME	Human monocytic ehrlichiosis

ICU	Intensive care unit(s)
ID (ID$_{50}$)	Infective dose (infects 50% of those exposed)
IDU	Injection drug use/r(s)
IFA	Immunofluorescence assay
Ig	Immunoglobulin(s)
LBRF	Louse-borne relapsing fever
L3	Third stage (infective) larva(e)
MDR	Multidrug resistance
MIC	Minimum inhibitory concentration (in vitro)
MMR	measles, mumps, rubella vaccine
MRSA, MSSA	Methicillin-resistant (MRSA) or sensitive (MSSA) *S. aureus*
n =	Number examined
NAT	Nucleic acid amplification test(s)
PEP	Postexposure prophylaxis
R+, R−	Recipient: seroreactive (infected), seronegative
R_0	Theoretical reproduction number
RPR	Rapid plasma reagin (syphilis) test
RT(I)	Respiratory tract (infection)
SARS	Severe acute respiratory syndrome
sl, ss	sensu lato (complex of >1 species), sensu stricto (1 species)
sp., spp.	species (singular), species (plural)
SSI	Surgical site infection(s)
STI	Sexually transmitted infection(s)
TBRF	Tick-borne relapsing fever
t_0	First day of treatment
UT(I)	Urinary tract (infection)
var.	variant
VRE	Vancomycin-resistant *Enterococcus*
WHO	World Health Organization

VIRUSES

AdV	Adenovirus
AIBV	Avian infectious bronchitis virus
ALV	Avian leukosis virus
ANDV	Andes virus
ASTV	Human astrovirus
BaEV	Baboon endogenous virus
BFV	Barmah Forest virus
BKV	Polyoma BK virus
BLV	Bovine leukemia virus
BTV	Bluetongue virus
CCHFV	Crimean-Congo hemorrhagic fever virus
CHIKV	Chikungunya virus
CMV	Cytomegalovirus
CPXV	Cowpox virus
CSFV	Classical swine fever virus

CTFV	Colorado tick fever virus
DOBV	Dobrava virus
DENV	Dengue virus
EBLV	European bat lyssavirus
EBV	Epstein-Barr virus
EEEV	Eastern equine encephalomyelitis virus
FeLV	Feline leukemia virus
FIV	Feline immunodeficiency virus
FMDV	Foot-and-mouth disease virus
GBV-C	GB virus-C (hepatitis G virus)
GUAV	Guanarito virus (Venezuelan HF)
HA(V)	Hepatitis A (virus)
HB(V), HBsAg	Hepatitis B (virus), hepatitis B surface antigen
HC(V)	Hepatitis C (virus)
HE(V)	Hepatitis E (virus)
HF(V)	Hemorrhagic fever/virus
HHV	Human herpes virus
HIV	Human immunodeficiency virus
HPV	Human papillomavirus
HSV	Herpes simplex virus
HTNV	Hantaan virus
HTLV	Human T-lymphotropic virus
INKV	Inkoo virus
JCV	Polyoma JC virus
JEV	Japanese encephalitis virus
JUNV	Junin virus (Argentinian HF)
KFD(V)	Kyasanur Forest disease (virus)
LCV	La Crosse virus
LCMV	Lymphocytic choriomeningitis virus
LIV	Louping ill virus
LNV	Laguna negra virus
MAYV	Mayaro virus
MACV	Machupo virus (Bolivian HF)
MDV	Marek's disease virus
MPXV	Monkeypox virus
MVEV	Murray Valley encephalitis virus
NDV	Newcastle disease virus
NoV	*Norovirus*
OHFV	Omsk hemorrhagic fever virus
ONNV	O'nyong-nyong virus
OROV	Oropouche virus
PCPV	Pseudocowpox virus
PERV	Porcine endogenous retrovirus
PIV	Parainfluenza virus
PUUV	Puumala virus
PVB19	Parvovirus B19

RRV	Ross River virus
RSV	Respiratory syncytial virus
RVFV	Rift Valley fever virus
SAAV	Saarema virus
SARS-CoV	SARS-associated coronavirus
SFNV	Sandfly fever Naples virus
SFSV	Sandfly fever Sicilian virus
SFV	Semliki Forest virus
SHV	Simian herpesvirus
SiFV	Simian foamy virus
SINV	Sindbis virus
SIV	Simian immunodeficiency virus
SLEV	St. Louis encephalitis virus
SNV	Sin Nombre virus
SPV	Simian parvovirus
SSHV	Snowshoe hare virus
SV40	Simian virus 40
SEOV	Seoul virus
TAHV	Tahyna virus
TBEV	Tick-borne encephalitis virus
TOSV	Sandfly fever Toscana virus
VEEV	Venezuelan equine encephalitis virus
VHF	Viral hemorrhagic fever
VSV	Vesicular stomatitis virus
VZV	Varicella-zoster virus
WEEV	Western equine encephalitis virus
WNV	West Nile virus
YFV	Yellow fever virus

GLOSSARY

Agent Infectious disease agents are chemical entities (prions and viruses) or living (cellular) units that are capable of residing on (colonization) or invading into (infection) living cells. Agents are submicroscopic (prions and viruses), microscopic (bacteria, fungi, and protozoa) or macroscopic (helminthes and ectoparasites).

Attack rate The rate at which new cases occur in a defined group of susceptible persons in a short period (typically few multiples of the incubation period). Primary attack rate is calculated from all initially and simultaneously exposed persons. Secondary attack rate is calculated from exposed persons after lapse of one incubation period.

Avian Bird related.

Breteau index The number of water collections that contain mosquito larvae per 100 houses examined. The index is a crude measure of peridomestic mosquito risk. However, as small (e.g., a 10-ml can) and large (e.g., a 100-liter barrel) water collections are treated equally, the index is a poor measure of mosquito abundance.

Canine Dog related.

Carrier An individual who harbors an agent inapparently beyond the incubation and recovery periods, typically for >3–12 months, eventually for life. Shedding carriers pass viable agents with droplets, feces, or urine, or from skin. Shedding can be continuous, intermittent, or limited to periods of reactivation. Nonshedding carriers are infective from blood or transplants. Carriage usually follows infection and underscores persistence; a single, cross-sectional survey cannot differentiate colonization and carriage.

Case In this book, a synonym for patient, that is, a manifestly ill person. Levels of certainty can be attached, e.g., laboratory-confirmed (definitive), meeting a definition (probable), or compatible with a known disease (suspected). The first case in a chain is called source or index case. Epidemiologically unlinked simultaneous cases (within one incubation period) are called coprimary cases.

Clinical Bedside findings (history, symptoms, and signs from physical examination) and rapid diagnostic tools (e.g., dip-stick tests).

Clone A community of agents that descended from defined, ideally single-unit, ancestors. Compared with isolate or strain, a clone exhibits least variability of phenotype and genotype.

Cohorting Placing patients with the same disease in the same room, on the same ward, or under the care of the same team.

Coliforms All (total) aerobic and facultative anaerobic, non-spore-forming, gram-negative rods that ferment lactose and produce gas within 48 h of culture at 35°C. Fecal coliforms are coliforms that grow and produce gas within 24 h at 44.5°C.

Colonization The innocuous presence of agents (commensals, opportunists, and rarely virulent) on surfaces (epithelia and mucosa). Although, in general, there is no need for treatment, colonized individuals can be infective. Unlike carriage, colonization is linked to exposure (e.g., hospitalization and delivery). Unlike infection, colonization is not compatible with tissue damage, invasion, or a systemic immune response. However, colonization may evolve to infection.

Commensal An innocuous, nonvirulent agent that multiplies and stays on surfaces of immune-competent hosts. Commensals are parts of the flora that is acquired beginning with the first day of life.

Communicable Infectious by any mode, including vector, injection, tranfusion, transplant, or experiment.

Confidence interval (CI) Delineates the range into which a population value is likely to fall when a procedure is repeated many times. The 95% CI provides this range for 95 of 100 rounds.

Contagious Infectious from aerosols, droplets, feces, hands, or skin manifestations.

Contamination The presence of an agent on inanimate surfaces (instrument and clothes), vehicles (foods and solutions), or skin remote from its reservoir (misplaced). On the skin, contamination can be difficult to distinguish from colonization. However, contamination of the skin is short lived and the misplaced agent will fail to be recovered from repeat samples.

Continent A large land mass, here Africa, America, Asia, Australia, and Europe. Depending on need, Asia and Australia are summarized as "Australasia," Australia and Europe as "Eurasia." The Americas means North and Latin America. The Indian subcontinent includes Bangladesh, Bhutan, India, Nepal, and Pakistan.

Control A continued public health effort that aims to sustainably reduce disease transmission to an acceptable, predefined level. Unlike elimination or eradication, the agent remains present at a low level and in reservoirs.

Cross-contamination The transfer of an agent from one surface to another, by hands, foods, or instruments, typically in kitchens or hospitals.

Cross-infection The transfer of an agent from one individual to another, by hands, solutions, or instruments, typically in hospitals.

Denominator The population that generates an outcome of interest (e.g., infections, cases, or deaths). By purpose, denominators are the national (general) population, the fraction that is exposed (e.g., that lives in a malarious area) or the fraction that is at risk (e.g., IDU).

Disaster An extreme (out of usual range) event, either natural or man-made. Typically it affects a significant number of persons (say $>1,000$).

Disease A defined condition of ill health. An infectious disease is the result of an imbalanced host-agent interaction that becomes manifest. Acute disease is manifest within hours or days, subacute disease is manifest within weeks, and chronic disease is manifest after months or years, by insiduous tissue damage.

Effect The result of an influence, e.g., an agent, medication, or intervention.

Efficacy (adjective "efficacious") A beneficial effect achieved under ideal (study) conditions.

Effectiveness (effective) A beneficial effect achieved under usual (real-life and -time) conditions, including noncompliance and erroneous applications.

Efficiency ("efficient" or "cost-effective") A beneficial result achieved under usual conditions and with optimal use of available resources (money, personnel, materials, and time).

Elimination The sustained reduction of the disease rate to zero level. The agent may still survive at an inaccessible reservoir (e.g., wildlife).

Endemic The continuous, expected presence of an agent, infection, or disease in a community or area. National surveillance can define "baseline" levels for time periods (time series) and areas, and upper limits (early warning) that characterize epidemics. Endemicity can be stratified into low (hypoendemic), intermediate (mesoendemic), and high (hyperendemic) levels. Meso- or hyperendemicity corresponds to a level that is colloquially referred to as "common" or "frequent" (e.g., prevalence $>5\%$ or rates $>100/10^5$/year).

Endogenous In epidemiology characterizes agents or infections that arise from a preexisting source (e.g., colonized bowel or throat). In virology, endogenous means the innocuous integration of (defective) viral nucleic acid into mammalian nucleic acid, without expression or production of viral particles.

Entomological inoculation rate (EIR) Measures the number of infective arthropod bites that a resident receives in an endemic-enzootic area over a given period. In malariology, the EIR can be expressed as numbers of sporozoites per person per year.

Enzootic The continuous, expected presence of an agent, infection, or disease in an animal population or area. Use of "endemic" for animals is ethymologically incorrect. Unfortunately, there is no accepted term for the steady presence of an agent in the environment (e.g., "entellic").

Epidemic An outbreak of larger scale, with many cases (e.g., >100) or a larger area involved (e.g., district, interstate, or international). Epidemics involving >1 continent are called pandemics.

Epizootic The sudden appearance or unexpected increase of animal cases at a larger scale, say >100.

Eradication The sustained public health effort that has lead to complete removal of an agent from all reservoirs. Once achieved, further measures are no longer necessary.

Evaluation The planned follow-up of procedures and interventions for outcome effects.

Exposure The venues or mechanisms that lead to encounters of agents and hosts at a place and in a time. Exposure links environment (habitat and season), host (susceptibility), and agent (virulence) with time (duration and frequency). Results from exposure include rejection, tolerance, or invasion.

Feline Cat-related.

Genospecies A species that is identified solely from differences of the genome. Genotypes are defined by a smaller proportion (say $>8–14\%$) of nucleotide differences.

Habitat Infectious disease habitats (settings and milieus) are places in which agents, hosts, and environment coexist in equilibrium. Infection biohabitats can be wetlands (e.g., lakes and marshes), forests (evergreen, deciduous and forest savanna), grasslands (bush savanna, tall-grass and short-grass prairie), barren lands (desert, alpine and polar tundra). Infection community habitats (day-use only) include day care centers, schools, shopping malls, municipal centers, and public places. Infection domiciliary habitats (overnight stay) include homes and institutions (e.g., prisons and orphanages). Nosocomial habitats include practices, health centers, and hospitals.

Hazard A factor that can cause harm. Environmental hazards include infective female mosquitoes and fungal spores in air. Unlike risk, hazard is immanent, a threat that has not materialized yet. In practice, hazard and risk are often used interchangeably.

Horizontal Spread of an agent among individuals of the same generation, e.g., sex partners.

Host Life form (plant, animal, and human) that grants access to an agent. A maintenance or **reservoir** host is a host that is relevant for long-term survival and circulation of an agent, for instance, by persistent and inapparent viremia or parasitemia, or intestinal colonization with shedding. Momentary presence of an agent in a host or a high seroprevalence in an animal population suggests but cannot prove reservoir status. Die-offs (e.g., in rats) although spectacular are not usually compatible with reservoir status. Pivotal for reservoir status is age.

Immunity The coordinated defense response of a host to an infectious agent. A measurable immune response (antibody titer or cellular skin reaction) can indicate sensitization (priming), past infection, overreaction, cross-reaction (false response), or protection. Protective immunity results in clearance of current and resistance to future infections. Concomitant (partially protective) immunity results in disease resolution and tolerance of inapparent infection. Whether concomitant immunity protects from future infection is debated. The immune system is competent when its responses are timely, vigorous, and balanced (predictable). The immune system is compromised or impaired when its response is slow, weak, or absent (anergy and deficiency). Causes can be congenital or acquired (infections, malignancies, and treatments). In autoimmune disease, the system overreacts and no longer distinguishes foreign (agents) from self.

Import Places of acquisition and diagnosis are dissociated, either between countries or between political subunits of the same country.

Incidence The number of new infections, cases, or deaths that arise from an exposed and susceptible population in a specified time. In national populations, the fractions that are nonsusceptible (immune) or nonexposed are mostly unknown and ignored. Examples are population incidence (per 10^5 per year), attack rates (per 100 exposed), and mortality (deaths per 10^5 per year). If in a group of people exposure is of variable length, person-times of exposure are calculated, and the resulting rate is called incidence density. Incidence and incidence density provide estimates of probabilities for events to occur ("absolute" risk).

Incubation period The time from exposure to first symptoms (e.g., diarrhea, body temperature >38.0°C) or signs (e.g., rash and stiff neck). Reported periods vary with infective dose, portal of entry, and host immune competence, and definition of presenting manifestation.

Index case The first (primary) case in a series of cases.

Infection A condition in which agents in tissue cause damage (granuloma, inflammation, necrosis) and a host response (activation of immune cells, secretory or systemic Ig). In clinical practice, infection is often the demonstration of an unwanted agent desirable to treat. Infection requires a sufficient dose and a susceptible host. Infections can be inapparent (latent) or manifest (disease). To separate inapparent infection from colonization would require demonstration of a host response (e.g., by biopsy), which is often impracticable. Furthermore, colonization can evolve to infection if host immune competence deteriorates or if an agent acquires virulence. Colonization and inapparent infections are beneficial for agent survival and recycling while fulminant disease and resistant hosts are detrimental to agent recycling.

Infectivity The capacity of an agent to invade and replicate in a host. Measures of infectivity are the **infective dose** (ID, e.g., the dose that infects 50% of persons, the ID_{50}), the entomological inoculation rate (EIR), and the attack rate. The duration of infectiousness (**infective period**) varies with exit site (shedding, e.g., from saliva, sputum, feces, urine, and lochia), and host immunity (reconvalescence, carrier, and immune impairment). Shedding can be intermittent, and the infective period can extend for years.

Infectious Capable of spread.

Invasive Breaking through natural barriers (intact cell lines). In invasive disease, agents are recovered from usually sterile sites (e.g., blood, CSF). Hematogenous spread causes disseminated (systemic) or metastatic (remote site) disease. Invasive procedures are instrumentations through barriers, e.g., injections and vascular devices.

Invertebrates Animals that lack a spinal column, including arthropods, molluscs, and helminths.

Isolate A group of cultured agents that derives from a natural source and a single colony on a plate. Although monospecific, an isolate can represent a mix of phenotypes or genotypes.

Isolation The containment of a suspected or confirmed infective person until risks of spread are minimal. Unlike quarantine, infectiousness is suspected from exposure, history, immune status, or symptoms and signs, and investigated by laboratory tests. Antimicrobial treatment typically shortens isolation time.

Latency Inapparent infections that persist for months, years, or life. Latent agents can remain dormant, with little or no metabolic activity (e.g., *Plasmodium vivax* hypnozoites). Latent viruses are characterized by the presence of viral genome (NAT is positive) in the absence of replication (culture or test for reverse transcriptase are negative). Latency may or may not be associated with cellular damage.

Lethality or case fatality ratio The proportion of deaths out of 100 cases. Critical is the definition of "cases": restriction to hospitalized cases inflates lethality, inclusion of mild and poorly defined community cases deflates it.

Mesophilic agents Grow at temperatures of 15–40°C (usual range of ambient or body temperatures).

Minimum field infection rate (MFIR) The proportion of mosquitoes caught in the field over a period (e.g., 1 year) that is infective. As large numbers are tested in pools, a formula is needed to calculate MFIR as a percentage: MFIR = 100 * (number of positive pools /number of individuals tested).

Mortality The number of deaths per 10^5 population per year.

Murine Mouse related.

Niche A small-scale habitat, a shelter place that offers protection from competition and local survival.

Noninvasive agents Restricted to surfaces and niches populated by "normal" flora, such as skin.

Nosocomial. For definition, see section VI.

Odds A way to express likelihood by the ratio: "it will happen"/"it will not happen." **Chance**, the conventional way, is to express the same ratio as: "it will happen"/("it will happen" *plus* "it will not happen"). For instance, if out of 10 interventions 2 result in death, the chance of death is 2 /(2 + 8) or 0.2 (20%), while the odds of death are 2 /8 or 1 in 4 (0.25).

Opportunist An agent that is innocuous in normal hosts but infective if normal barriers break down (because of damage by foreign body or device) or the immune system is impaired (because of treatments or infections in immune-compromised hosts).

Outbreak The sudden appearance or unexplained increase of cases or infections. An outbreak is usually described as an incident in which two or more people contract the same infection or disease from a common exposure. Outbreaks are smaller than epidemics, limited by number (say to 2–99 cases) and extent (say a district, restaurant, school class). If a link among cases is suspected (e.g., microbiologically) but not confirmed epidemiologically (e.g., in a case-control study), grouped cases are called clusters.

Pandemic An epidemic that affects more than one continent. Similarly, **panzootic** is an epizootic that affects more than one continent.

Paraclinical All diagnostic procedures that are not available at the bed side, including endoscopy, imaging, laboratory tests, ultrasound, and X ray.

Pasteurization A method to destruct unwanted pathogens in foods without depreciating nutritious quality. With milk this means abrupt heat (to >71.8°C for 15 s) and rapid cooling (to <8°C). The term is now expanded to radiation.

Persistence Presence (of an agent, symptom) for months, years, or life. Shedding is not a prerequisite.

Phylogenesis The evolutionary (developmental) history of a taxon.

Porcine Swine related.

Portal of entry Part of the body through which an agent enters a host. Major portals are (un)broken skin, alveoli of the lung, and enteric mucosa. Minor portals include buccal and gastric mucosa and genital epithelia.

Pseudoinfection is an infection that is misdiagnosed ("spurious") because of a false-positive laboratory test, e.g., contaminated staining material. **Pseudooutbreak** is an outbreak that is misdiagnosed because of enhanced surveillance or grouped pseudoinfections.

Prenatal The period from after conception up to birth.

Prepatent period The time from exposure to first detection of an agent in the host (e.g., from blood, feces, or skin). The prepatent period varies with the sensitivity of a laboratory test. The prepatent period can be shorter, equally long, or longer than the incubation period.

Prevalence A measure for the presence of a condition at a moment (point-prevalence, e.g., a day) or in a period (period-prevalence, e.g., a year). Here, "frequent" generally means a prevalence >5%.

Primary A case without previous known contact. **Co-primary** Initial cases from common exposure whose disease onset is separated by less than one incubation period, e.g., in meningococcal disease <24 h.

Psychrophilic agents can grow at temperatures <0°C.

Quarantine A measure that restricts free movement of exposed persons. Exposure is ascertained from the history (e.g., contact with a case) or by predefined criteria. Unlike isolation, the infection status (incubating, infectious) of a person is not known at the time the quarantine is issued. Quarantine can be at home or dedicated sites (transit halls, hotels, and camps). Often it includes self-reporting of symptoms and monitoring of temperature.

Reactivation The transition from latency to manifest infection. Recovery of the causative agent is not a requirement. Suspected triggers include deteriorating immune competence and stress.

Receptivity An increased probability of transmission in an area or community. Unlike vulnerability, all ingredients for transmission are in place (e.g., weather, vector, susceptible individuals), except the agent itself.

Relapse The transition from latency to manifest infection that is accompanied by recovery of the causative agent.

Reproductive number. The basic (R_0) and actual (R) reproductive numbers are measures of infectiousness. R_0 is the theoretical number of new cases the source case could generate in a fully susceptible (nonimmune) population. At $R_0 < 1$, an an agent will disappear. At $R_0 = 1$, there is equilibrium (endemicity). At $R_0 > 1$, new cases will exceed recovered cases. $R_0 > 5$ signals high infectivity, $R_0 > 10$ signals exponential case accrual.

Reservoir An abiotic (environmental) or biotic (invertebrates and vertebrates) holding place for an agent. From there, the agent attempts to disperse and to return later. While source marks origin, and vehicle marks transportation, reservoir characterizes persistence. Ideal reservoir hosts carry (and shed) an agent for life. Views are divided whether "transport" or bridging hosts are part of a reservoir.

Resistance. A host is resistant who denies access (innate resistance) to an agent or clears infection efficiently (acquired resistance). Intact barriers are a very effective mechanisms of innate resistance. In acquired resistance, the immune system must identify and memorize targets (antigens), a process that may need repeated exposure. An agent is resistant if it is able to survive concentrations of an antimicrobial that are usually adequate for inactivation. In vivo antimicrobial resistance may not be correlated with resistance in vitro, as the latter is influenced by bioavailability (absorption and tissue penetration).

Risk The probability for a harm to occur. Unlike hazard, harm has materialized, and the probability of occurrence can be quantified. In a broader sence (that is synonymous with hazard), risk characterizes factors with a potential for harm. "Absolute" risk is harm per (10^2, 10^5) persons exposed over time. "Relative" risk (or risk ratio) is the ratio of an increased risk to a baseline (background) risk.

Saprophytes Agents that thrive on decaying or dead organic materials.

Screening A procedure to sort out individuals with a particular characterstic from all others. Screening can involve a highly (99.9%) sensitive but nonspecific test in a first step that is followed by a highly specific (99.9%) but insensitive test in a second step ("two-step procedure").

Secondary A case who follows contact with a primary case, after a full incubation period, e.g., in meningococcal disease after >24 h.

Simian Monkey related.

Sources are starting points for agents, e.g., soil, hosts, or colonized humans. While reservoir marks persistence, and vehicle marks transportation, source characterizes origin. For *S. enterica* serovar *Enteritidis*, the reservoir are animals, the source can be a poultry flock, and the vehicle can be raw eggs. Viewed from humans, sources can be outside the body (exogenous) or inside (endogenous).

Species An idealized set of individuals with identical relevant characteristics, including their ancestors, genes, ecologic niches, and phenotypes. For higher life forms, the capacity to produce fertile offspring is a characteristic of a species. Modern taxonomy aims to converge phylogeny (ancestry), evolution (life over geological times), biology (reproduction), morphology (ultrastructure), and practical needs (names).

Sporadic Single cases, dotted like the solitary Sporades Islands in the Aegean sea.

Strain A population of cultured agents that is well characterized beyond the species level, by cultural (e.g., drug resistance), animal experimental (e.g., host specificity), molecular (genome), or other evidence. Strains exhibit less phenotypic or genotypic variability than isolates.

Stratification A method of making homogenous (comparable) layers ("strata" in Latin), e.g., of geographic zones, people, or data, for selection or analysis.

Susceptibility The property of an agent or host to be sensitive to influences. Host susceptibility can be biological (genetic makeup and immune system), physiological (low birth weight, pregnancy, and old age), or acquired (nutritional and treatment). Conversely, vaccines reduce or abolish susceptibility to an agent, an infection, or a disease.

Taxon A unit of classification, a tool to arrange biodiversity. In a taxon, predefined characteristics are common to all its members. Taxons include classes, orders, families, genera, and species.

Terrorism A method of causing fear or panic by brutal acts among unpredictable targets. Bioterrorism deploys infectious disease agents for terrorism, including genetically modified (weaponized) agents.

Thermophilic agents These grow at heat (40–70°C). Such temperatures are achieved during composting.

Transmissibility The possibility of parenteral agent transfer. Unlike hosts that shed agents spontaneously, transfer of agents from latently infected hosts requires vectors (mosquito and tick), interventions (instrument, transfusion, and transplant), or experiment. For instance, classical CJD is transmissible but not contagious.

Transmission The passage of an agent from a source (donor) to a host (recipient). Modes describe the ways agents use. Major modes are human-to-human, animal-to-human, environment-to-human, and vehicle-to-human. Transmission by vehicles is particularly difficult to demonstrate epidemiologically.

Transmission potential (TP) The sum of infective agents (e.g., larvae) an exposed individual could receive from an infective vector in a given period, e.g., year (annual TP). TP is calculated from the average proportion of infective vectors multiplied by the average biting (landing) rate on volunteers.

Transovarial Passage of an agent via eggs from one arthropod generation to the next.

Transplantation The replacement of failing body parts by living organs, tissues, or cells, from self (autotransplant), living or dead other humans (allotransplant), or mammals (xenotransplant).

Transstadial Passage of an agent through developmental arthropod stages, e.g., larva-to-pupa.

Tropism Preference of an agent for a particular tissue, e.g., nerve cells (neurotropism).

Type A maintained, preserved, reference organism of known origin (place, time, and lineage), structure (macroscopic and ultrastructure), biology (culture, antigens, and enzyme activity), and genome. Types include biotypes, serotypes, zymotypes, and genotypes. If common characteristics are less certain or stable, -var is used instead of -type (e.g., biovar).

Vector An animate carrier of agents. Vectors can be "mechanical," that is, simply transporting (e.g., *Shigella* by houseflies), or "cyclic" (e.g., *Plasmodium* in *Anopheles*), that is, requiring intrinsic development (infectivity reached only after an "intrinsic incubation period").

Vehicle A vessel of transportation for agents. Vehicles are mainly inanimate (e.g., foods, tap water, and instruments), but the term is also used for hands, blood, and excretions. Daily objects that are vehicles are also called "fomites."

Vertebrates Animals that have a spinal column.

Vertical Passage of an agent over two generations, e.g., intrauterine, from mother to child.

Vulnerability A state of increased probability of transmission in an area or community, provided conditions become favorable (e.g., rise in temperature, influx of a vector or of susceptibles) and an agent is introduced.

Waste Material for disposal, including sewage. In health care, this includes organic and inorganic materials from practices, hospitals, laboratories, and research facilities. By source, waste is variously labeled "biomedical," "infectious," or "clinical." Grouping is important for prevention, reprocessing, and incineration. Proposed groups are linen, instruments, sharps, nonsharp disposables, biomaterials (tissues, excretions, and secretions), toxic and radioactive chemicals.

Xenodiagnosis The use of laboratory-reared, hematophagous arthropods for diagnostic purposes. *Trypanosoma*-free triatomine bugs are used to demonstrate subpatent parasitemia in latent Chagas infections. After feeding and elapse of the intrinsic incubation period, bugs are dissected and examined microscopically.

References

CDC	Centers for Disease Control and Prevention
MMWR	*Morbidity Mortality Weekly Report*
MOH	Ministry of Health
PHLS	Public Health Laboratory Service
RKI	Robert Koch Institut
WER	*Weekly Epidemiologic Record*
WHO	World Health Organisation

1. 1990. Cryptosporidiosis in England and Wales: prevalence and clinical and epidemiological features. Public Health Laboratory Service Study Group. *BMJ* **300:**774-7.
2. 1995. Public health impact of Rwandan refugee crisis: what happened in Goma, Zaire, in July, 1994? Goma Epidemiology Group. *Lancet* **345:**339-44.
3. 1996. Foodborne outbreak of diarrheal illness associated with Cryptosporidium parvum—Minnesota, 1995. *MMWR* **45:**783-4.
4. **AAAS (American Academy for the Advancement of Science).** 1991. Malaria and development in Africa. A cross-sectoral approach. U.S. Agency for International Development. Africa Bureau, Washington, D.C.
5. **Aaltone, R., J. Jalava, E. Laurikainen, U. Karkkainen, and A. Alanen.** 2002. Cervical ureaplasma urealyticum colonization: comparison of PCR and culture for its detection and association with preterm birth. *Scand J Infect Dis* **34:**35-40.
6. **AAP (American Academy of Pediatrics).** 2003. Red Book, 26th ed. American Academy of Pediatrics, Elk Grove Village, IL 60009-0927.
7. **Aaskov, J. G., J. U. Mataika, G. W. Lawrence, V. Rabukawaqa, M. M. Tucker, J. A. Miles, and D. A. Dalglish.** 1981. An epidemic of Ross river virus infection in Fiji, 1979. *Am J Trop Med Hyg* **30:**1053-9.
8. **Abbas, B., and H. Agab.** 2002. A review of camel brucellosis. *Prev Vet Med* **55:**47-56.
9. **Abbaszadegan, M. R., M. Gholamin, A. Tabatabaee, R. Farid, M. Houshmand, and M. Abbaszadegan.** 2003. Prevalence of human T-lymphotropic virus type 1 among blood donors from Mashhad, Iran. *J Clin Microbiol* **41:**2593-5.
10. **Abdel-Haq, N. M., B. I. Asmar, W. M. Abuhammour, and W. J. Brown.** 2000. Yersinia enterocolitica infection in children. *Pediatr Infect Dis J* **19:**954-8.
11. **Abdelnoor, A. M., R. Batshoun, and B. M. Roumani.** 1983. The bacterial flora of fruits and vegetables in Lebanon and the effect of washing on the bacterial content. *Zentralbl Bakteriol Mikrobiol Hyg [B]* **177:**342-9.
12. **Abdourakhmanov, D. T., A. S. Hasaev, F. J. Castro, and J. Guardia.** 1998. Epidemiologic and clinical aspects of hepatitis C virus infection in the Russian Republic of Daghestan. *Eur J Epidemiol* **14:**549-53.
13. **Abdur Rab, M., T. W. Freeman, S. Rahim, N. Durrani, A. Simon-Taha, and M. Rowland.** 2003. High altitude epidemic malaria in Bamian province, central Afghanistan. *East Mediterr Health J* **9:**232-9.
14. **Abe, N., M. Nagoshi, K. Takami, Y. Sawano, and H. Yoshikawa.** 2002. A survey of Blastocystis sp. in livestock, pets, and zoo animals in Japan. *Vet Parasitol* **106:**203-12.
15. **Abe, N., Y. Nishikawa, A. Yasukawa, and K. Haruki.** 1999. Entamoeba histolytica outbreaks in institutions for the mentally retarded. *Jpn J Infect Dis* **52:**135-6.
16. **Abe, N., Z. Wu, and H. Yoshikawa.** 2003. Zoonotic genotypes of Blastocystis hominis detected in cattle and pigs by PCR with diagnostic primers and restriction fragment length polymorphism analysis of the small subunit ribosomal RNA gene. *Parasitol Res* **90:**124-8.
17. **Abe, T., K. Yamaki, T. Hayakawa, H. Fukuda, Y. Ito, H. Kume, T. Komiya, K. Ishihara, and K. Hirai.** 2002. A seroepidemiological study of the risk of Q fever infection in Japanese veterinarians. *Eur J Epidemiol* **17:**1029-32.
18. **Abeck, D., and M. Mempel.** 1998. Staphylococcus aureus colonization in atopic dermatitis and its therapeutic implications. *Br J Dermatol* **139:**13-6.
19. **Abed-Benamara, M., I. Achir, F. Rodhain, and C. Perez-Eid.** 1997. [First Algerian case of human otomyiasis from Chrysomya bezziana]. *Bull Soc Pathol Exot* **90:**172-5.
20. **Aberg, J. A., J. E. Gallant, J. Anderson, J. M. Oleske, H. Libman, J. S. Currier, V. E. Stone, and J. E. Kaplan.** 2004. Primary Care Guidelines for the Management of Persons Infected with Human Immunodeficiency Virus: Recommendations of the HIV Medicine Association of the Infectious Diseases Society of America. *Clin Infect Dis* **39:**609-29.
21. **Abgrall, S., C. Rabaud, and D. Costagliola.** 2001. Incidence and risk factors for toxoplasmic encephalitis in human immunodeficiency virus-infected patients before and during the highly active antiretroviral therapy era. *Clin Infect Dis* **33:**1747-55.

22. Abgueguen, P., V. Delbos, J. M. Chennebault, S. Fanello, O. Brenet, P. Alquier, J. C. Granry, and E. Pichard. 2003. Nine cases of foodborne botulism type B in France and literature review. *Eur J Clin Microbiol Infect Dis.* **22:**749–52.
23. Abliz, P., K. Fukushima, K. Takizawa, and K. Nishimura. 2004. Identification of pathogenic dematiaceous fungi and related taxa based on large subunit ribosomal DNA D1/D2 domain sequence analysis. *FEMS Immunol Med Microbiol* **40:**41-9.
24. Abo-Shehada, M. N., H. Anshassi, G. Mustafa, and Z. Amr. 1999. Prevalence of Surra among camels and horses in Jordan. *Prev Vet Med* **38:**289-93.
25. Abraham, C. D., C. J. Conde-Glez, A. Cruz-Valdez, L. Sanchez-Zamorano, C. Hernandez-Marquez, and E. Lazcano-Ponce. 2003. Sexual and demographic risk factors for herpes simplex virus type 2 according to schooling level among Mexican youths. *Sex Transm Dis* **30:**549-55.
26. Abraham, S. N., and R. V. Lawande. 1982. Incidence of free-living amoebae in the nasal passages of local population in Zaria, Nigeria. *J Trop Med Hyg* **85:**217-22.
27. Abrahamian, F. M., C. V. Pollack, F. LoVecchio, R. Nanda, and R. W. Carlson. 2000. Fatal tetanus in a drug abuser with "protective" antitetanus antibodies. *J Emerg Med* **18:**189-93.
28. Abreu-Acosta, N., J. Lorenzo-Morales, Y. Leal-Guio, N. Coronado-Alvarez, P. Foronda, J. Alcoba-Florez, F. Izquierdo, N. Batista-Diaz, C. D. Aguila, and B. Valladares. 2005. Enterocytozoon bieneusi (microsporidia) in clinical samples from immunocompetent individuals in Tenerife, Canary Islands, Spain. *Trans R Soc Trop Med Hyg* **99:**848-55.
29. Abu-Elteen, K. H. 1999. Incidence and distribution of Candida species isolated from human skin in Jordan. *Mycoses* **42:**311-7.
30. Abu-Elteen, K. H., and R. M. Abu-Alteen. 1998. The prevalence of Candida albicans populations in the mouths of complete denture wearers. *New Microbiol* **21:**41-8.
31. Abu-Elyazeed, R., T. F. Wierzba, A. S. Mourad, L. F. Peruski, B. A. Kay, M. Rao, A. M. Churilla, A. L. Bourgeois, A. K. Mortagy, S. M. Kamal, S. J. Savarino, J. R. Campbell, J. R. Murphy, A. Naficy, and J. D. Clemens. 1999. Epidemiology of enterotoxigenic Escherichia coli diarrhea in a pediatric cohort in a periurban area of lower Egypt. *J Infect Dis* **179:**382-9.
32. Abu-Elyazeed, R. R., J. K. Podgore, N. S. Mansour, and M. E. Kilpatrick. 1993. Field trial of 1% niclosamide as a topical antipenetrant to Schistosoma mansoni cercariae. *Am J Trop Med Hyg* **49:**403-9.
33. Abu-Elyazeed, R. R., T. F. Wierzba, R. W. Frenck, S. D. Putnam, M. R. Rao, S. J. Savarino, K. A. Kamal, L. F. Peruski, Jr., I. A. Abd-El Messih, S. A. El-Alkamy, A. B. Naficy, and J. D. Clemens. 2004. Epidemiology of Shigella-associated diarrhea in rural Egyptian children. *Am J Trop Med Hyg* **71:**367-72.
34. Abulrahi, H. A., E. A. Bohlega, R. E. Fontaine, S. M. al-Seghayer, and A. A. al-Ruwais. 1997. Plasmodium falciparum malaria transmitted in hospital through heparin locks. *Lancet* **349:**23-5.
35. Acar, J. F. 1999. Resistance patterns of Haemophilus influenzae. *J Chemother* **11:**44-50.
36. Aceijas, C., G. V. Stimson, M. Hickman, and T. Rhodes. 2004. Global overview of injecting drug use and HIV infection among injecting drug users. *AIDS* **18:**2295-303.
37. Achukwi, M. D., W. Harnett, and A. Renz. 2000. Onchocerca ochengi transmission dynamics and the correlation of O. ochengi microfilaria density in cattle with the transmission potential. *Vet Res* **31:**611-21.
38. (ACIP), Advisory Committee on Immunization Practices. 1999. Prevention of hepatitis A through active or passive immunization: recommendations of the Advisory Committee on Immunization Practices (ACIP). *MMWR* **48 (RR-12):**1-37.
39. Ackerman, Z., E. Ackerman, and O. Paltiel. 2000. Intrafamilial transmission of hepatitis C virus: a systematic review. *J Viral Hepat* **7:**93-103.
40. Ackermann, R., K. Krüger, M. Roggendorf, B. Rehse-Kupper, M. Mortter, M. Schneider, and I. Vukadinovic. 1986. Die Verbreitung der Frühsommer-Meningoenzephalitis in der Bundesrepublik Deutschland. *Deutsche Medizinische Wochenschrift* **111:**927-33.
41. Ackermann, R., W. Stille, W. Blumenthal, E. B. Helm, K. Keller, and O. Baldus. 1972. [Syrian hamsters as vectors of lymphocytic choriomeningitis]. *Dtsch Med Wochenschr* **97:**1725-31.
42. Ackers, M. L., B. E. Mahon, E. Leahy, B. Goode, T. Damrow, P. S. Hayes, W. F. Bibb, D. H. Rice, T. J. Barrett, L. Hutwagner, P. M. Griffin, and L. Slutsker. 1998. An outbreak of Escherichia coli O157:H7 infections associated with leaf lettuce consumption. *J Infect Dis* **177:**1588-93.
43. Ackers, M. L., N. D. Puhr, R. V. Tauxe, and E. D. Mintz. 2000. Laboratory-based surveillance of Salmonella serotype Typhi infections in the United States: antimicrobial resistance on the rise. *JAMA* **283:**2668-73.
44. Ackers, M. L., S. Schoenfeld, J. Markman, M. G. Smith, M. A. Nicholson, W. DeWitt, D. N. Cameron, P. M. Griffin, and L. Slutsker. 2000. An outbreak of Yersinia enterocolitica O:8 infections associated with pasteurized milk. *J Infect Dis* **181:**1834-7.
45. Ackland, J. R., D. A. Worswick, and B. P. Marmion. 1994. Vaccine prophylaxis of Q fever. A follow-up study of the efficacy of Q-Vax (CSL) 1985-1990. *Med J Aust* **160:**704-8.
46. Acosta, C. J., C. M. Galindo, J. Kimario, K. Senkoro, H. Urassa, C. Casals, M. Corachan, N. Eseko, M. Tanner, H. Mshinda, F. Lwilla, J. Vila, and P. L. Alonso. 2001. Cholera outbreak in southern Tanzania: risk factors and patterns of transmission. *Emerg Infect Dis* **7(3):**583-7.
47. Acosta, M., D. Cazorla, and M. Garvett. 2002. [Enterobiasis among schoolchildren in a rural population from Estado Falcon, Venezuela, and its relation with socioeconomic level]. *Invest Clin* **43:**173-81.
48. Acuno-Soto, R., L. Calderón-Romero, D. Romero-López, and A. Bravo-Lindoro. 2000. Murine typhus in Mexico City. *Trans R Soc Trop Med Hyg* **94:**45.
49. Adachi, J. A., C. D. Ericsson, Z. D. Jiang, M. W. DuPont, S. R. Pallegar, and H. L. DuPont. 2002. Natural history of enteroaggregative and enterotoxigenic Escherichia coli infection among US travelers to Guadalajara, Mexico. *J Infect Dis* **185:**1681-3.
50. Adachi, J. A., Z. D. Jiang, J. J. Mathewson, M. P. Verenkar, S. Thompson, F. Martinez-Sandoval, R. Steffen, C. D. Ericsson, and H. L. DuPont. 2001. Enteroaggregative Escherichia coli as a major etiologic agent in traveler's diarrhea in 3 regions of the world. *Clin Infect Dis* **32:**1706-9.
51. Adachi, J. A., J. J. Mathewson, Z. D. Jiang, C. D. Ericsson, and H. L. DuPont. 2002. Enteric pathogens in Mexican sauces of popular restaurants in Guadalajara, Mexico, and Houston, Texas. *Ann Intern Med* **136:**884-7.
52. Adachi, M., K. Manji, R. Ichimi, H. Nishimori, K. Shindo, N. Matsubayashi, R. L. Mbise, A. Massawe, Q. Liu, F. Kawamoto, Y. Chinzei, and M. Sakurai. 2000. Detection of congenital

malaria by polymerase-chain-reaction methodology in Dar es Salaam, Tanzania. *Parasitol Res* **86**:615-8.

53. **Adad, S. J., R. V. de Lima, Z. T. Sawan, M. L. Silva, M. A. de Souza, J. C. Saldanha, V. A. Falco, A. H. da Cunha, and E. F. Murta.** 2001. Frequency of Trichomonas vaginalis, Candida sp and Gardnerella vaginalis in cervical-vaginal smears in four different decades. *Sao Paulo Med J* **119**:200-5.

54. **Adak, G. K., S. M. Meakins, H. Yip, B. A. Lopman, and S. J. O'Brien.** 2005. Disease risks from foods, England and Wales, 1996-2000. *Emerg Infect Dis* **11**:365-72.

55. **Adak, T., V. P. Sharma, and V. S. Orlov.** 1998. Studies on the Plasmodium vivax relapse pattern in Delhi, India. *Am J Trop Med Hyg* **59**:175-9.

56. **Adamkiewicz, T. V., M. Berkovitch, C. Krishnan, and et al.** 1998. Infection due to Yersinia enterocolitica in a series of patients with b-thalassemia: incidence and predisposing factors. *Clin Infect Dis* **27**:1362-6.

57. **Adams, B. B.** 2002. Dermatologic disorders of the athlete. *Sports Med* **32**:309-21.

58. **Adams, B. B.** 2002. Tinea corporis gladiatorum. *J Am Acad Dermatol* **47**:286-90.

59. **Adams, D.** 2001. Catgut sutures—possible BSE risk. *Aust Vet J* **79**:245-6.

60. **Adams, E. J., A. Charlett, W. J. Edmunds, and G. Hughes.** 2004. Chlamydia trachomatis in the United Kingdom: a systematic review and analysis of prevalence studies. *Sex Transm Infect* **80**:354-62.

61. **Adams, M. S., A. M. J. Croft, D. A. Winfield, and P. R. Richards.** 1997. An outbreak of rubella in British troops in Bosnia. *Epidemiol Infect* **118**:253-7.

62. **Adderson, E. E.** 2004. Histoplasmosis in a pediatric oncology center. *J Pediatr* **144**:100-6.

63. **Addiss, D. G., J. P. Davis, M. LaVenture, P. J. Wand, M. A. Hutchinson, and R. M. McKinney.** 1989. Community-acquired Legionnaires' disease associated with a cooling tower: evidence for longer-distance transport of Legionella pneumophila. *Am J Epidemiol* **130**:557-68.

64. **Addiss, D. G., J. P. Davis, B. D. Meade, D. G. Burstyn, M. Meissner, J. A. Zastrow, J. L. Berg, P. Drinka, and R. Phillips.** 1991. A pertussis outbreak in a Wisconsin nursing home. *J Infect Dis* **164**:704-10.

65. **Addiss, D. G., J. M. Stewart, R. J. Finton, S. P. Wahlquist, R. M. Williams, J. W. Dickerson, H. C. Spencer, and D. D. Juranek.** 1991. Giardia lamblia and Cryptosporidium infections in child day-care centers in Fulton County, Georgia. *Pediatr Infect Dis J* **10**:907-11.

66. **Addiss, D. G., J. C. Yashuk, D. E. Clapp, and P. A. Blake.** 1989. Outbreaks of diarrhoeal illness on passenger cruise ships, 1975-85. *Epidemiol Infect* **103**:63-72.

67. **Adekoya, N., and R. S. Hopkins.** 2005. Racial disparities in nationally notifiable diseases—United States, 2002. *MMWR* **54**:9-11.

68. **Adelson, M. E., R. V. Rao, R. C. Tilton, K. Cabets, E. Eskow, L. Fein, J. L. Occi, and E. Mordechai.** 2004. Prevalence of Borrelia burgdorferi, Bartonella spp., Babesia microti, and Anaplasma phagocytophila in Ixodes scapularis ticks collected in Northern New Jersey. *J Clin Microbiol* **42**:2799-801.

69. **Adesina, O. A., and H. A. Odelola.** 1991. Ecological distribution of Chikungunya haemagglutination inhibition antibodies in human and domestic animals in Nigeria. *Trop Geogr Med* **43**:271-5.

70. **Adhikari Prabha, M. R., M. G. Prabhu, C. V. Raghuveer, M. Bai, and M. A. Mala.** 1993. Clinical study of 100 cases of Kyasanur Forest disease with clinicopathological correlation. *Indian J Med Sci* **47**:124-30.

71. **Adib, S. M., H. Al-Takash, and C. Al-Hajj.** 1999. Tuberculosis in Lebanese jails: prevalence and risk factors. *Eur J Epidemiol* **15**:253-60.

72. **Adini, I., M. Ephros, J. Chen, and C. L. Jaffe.** 2003. Asymptomatic visceral leishmaniasis, northern Israel. *Emerg Infect Dis* **9**:397-8.

73. **Adler, A. I., and J. Altman.** 1993. An outbreak of mud-wrestling-induced pustular dermatitis in college students. Dermatitis palaestrae limosae. *JAMA* **269**:502-4.

74. **Adler, H., S. Vonstein, P. Deplazes, C. Stieger, and R. Frei.** 2002. Prevalence of Leptospira spp. in various species of small mammals caught in an inner-city area in Switzerland. *Epidemiol Infect* **128**:107-9.

75. **Adler, S. P.** 1986. Molecular epidemiology of cytomegalovirus: evidence for viral transmission to parents from children infected at a day care center. *Pediatr Infect Dis* **5**:315-8.

76. **Adler, S. P.** 1988. Molecular epidemiology of cytomegalovirus: viral transmission among children attending a day care center, their parents, and caretakers. *J Pediatr* **112**:366-372.

77. **Adler, S. P., J. W. Finney, A. M. Manganello, and A. M. Best.** 2004. Prevention of child-to-mother transmission of cytomegalovirus among pregnant women. *J Pediatr* **145**:485-91.

78. **Aeschlimann, A., W. Burgdorfer, H. Matile, O. Peter, and R. Wyler.** 1979. Aspects nouveaux du rûle de vecteur joué par Ixodes ricinus L. en Suisse. *Acta Trop* **36**:81-191.

79. **Afrane, Y. A., E. Klinkenberg, P. Drechsel, K. Owusu-Daaku, R. Garms, and T. Kruppa.** 2004. Does irrigated urban agriculture influence the transmission of malaria in the city of Kumasi, Ghana? *Acta Trop* **89**:125-34.

80. **Agarwal, M., and G. Shukla.** 1999. Cholera epidemiology. *Lancet* **353**:2068-9.

81. **Agbolade, M., and D. O. Akinboye.** 2001. Loa loa and Mansonella perstans infections in Ijebu north, western Nigeria: a parasitological study. *Jpn J Infect Dis* **54**:108-10.

82. **Agerton, T., S. Valway, B. Gore, C. Pozsik, B. Plikaytis, C. Woodley, and I. Onorato.** 1997. Transmission of a highly drug-resistant strain (strain W1) of Mycobacterium tuberculosis. Community outbreak and nosocomial transmission via a contaminated bronchoscope. *JAMA* **278**:1073-7.

83. **Agrawal, M. C., S. Gupta, and J. George.** 2000. Cercarial dermatitis in India. *Bull WHO* **78**:278.

84. **Aguilera, J. F., A. Perrocheau, C. Meffre, and S. Hahne.** 2002. Outbreak of serogroup w135 meningococcal disease after the Hajj Pilgrimage, europe, 2000. *Emerg Infect Dis* **8**:761-7.

85. **Aguzzi, A., and M. Heikenwalder.** 2003. Prion diseases: Cannibals and garbage piles. *Nature* **423**:127-9.

86. **Aharonowitz, G., S. Koton, S. Segal, E. Anis, and M. S. Green.** 1999. Epidemiological characteristics of spotted fever in Israel over 26 years. *Clin Infect Dis* **29**:1321-2.

87. **Ahlfors, K., S. A. Ivarsson, and S. Harris.** 1999. Report on a long-term study of maternal and congenital cytomegalovirus infection in Sweden. Review of prospective studies available in the literature. *Scand J Infect Dis* **31**:443-57.

88. Ahlm, C., O. A. Alexeyev, F. Elgh, B. Aava, G. Wadell, A. Tarnvik, P. Juto, and T. Palo. 1997. High prevalence of hantavirus antibodies in bank voles (Clethrionomys glareolus) captured in the vicinity of households afflicted with nephropathia epidemica. *Am J Trop Med Hyg* **56**:674-8.

89. Ahlm, C., K. Wallin, A. Lundkvist, F. Elgh, P. Juto, M. Merza, and A. Tarnvik. 2000. Serologic evidence of Puumala virus infection in wild moose in northern Sweden. *Am J Trop Med Hyg* **62**:106-11.

90. Ahmed, A. O., W. Van Leeuwen, A. Fahal, W. Van De Sande, H. Verbrugh, and A. Van Belkum. 2004. Mycetoma caused by Madurella mycetomatis: a neglected infectious burden. *Lancet Infect Dis* **4**:566-74.

91. Ahmed, H. J., H. H. Mohammed, M. W. Yusuf, S. F. Ahmed, and G. Huldt. 1988. Human toxoplasmosis in Somalia. Prevalence of Toxoplasma antibodies in a village in the lower Scebelli region and in Mogadishu. *Trans R Soc Trop Med Hyg* **82**:330-2.

92. Ahmed, R. E., H. H. Geuenich, and H. E. Muller. 1984. [Pathogen distribution in waste water sprinkler irrigation]. *Zentralbl Bakteriol Mikrobiol Hyg [B]* **179**:151-61.

93. Ahmed, S., and L. Gruer. 2001. "Clostridium novyi and Co: the drug injector outbreaks" - conference summary and recommendations. *Eurosurveillance Weekly* **46**:3-5.

94. Ahn, J. M., S. G. Kang, D. Y. Lee, S. J. Shin, and H. S. Yoo. 2005. Identification of Novel Human Hepatitis E Virus (HEV) Isolates and Determination of the Seroprevalence of HEV in Korea. *J Clin Microbiol* **43**:3042-8.

95. Aho, M., M. Kurki, H. Rautelin, and T. U. Kosunen. 1989. Waterborne outbreak of Campylobacter enteritis after outdoors infantry drill in Utti, Finland. *Epidemiol Infect* **103**:133-41.

96. Aidara-Kane, A., A. Ranaivo, A. Spiegel, M. Catteau, and J. Rocourt. 2000. [Microbiological quality of street-vendor ice cream in Dakar]. *Dakar Med* **45**:20-4.

97. Aiga, H., T. Amano, S. Cairncross, J. A. Domako, O. K. Nanas, and S. Coleman. 2004. Assessing Water-Related Risk Factors for Buruli Ulcer: A Case-Control Study in Ghana. *Am J Trop Med Hyg* **71**:387-392.

98. Aikimbajev, A., T. Meka-Mechenko, G. Temiralieva, J. Bekenov, Z. Sagiyev, K. Kaljan, and A. K. Mukhambetova. 2003. Plague peculiarities in Kazakhstan at the present time. *Przegl Epidemiol* **57**:593-8.

99. Aintablian, N., P. Walpita, and M. H. Sawyer. 1998. Detection of Bordetella pertussis and respiratory synctial virus in air samples from hospital rooms. *Infect Control Hosp Epidemiol* **19**:918-23.

100. Aitichou, M., S. S. Saleh, A. K. McElroy, C. Schmaljohn, and M. S. Ibrahim. 2005. Identification of Dobrava, Hantaan, Seoul, and Puumala viruses by one-step real-time RT-PCR. *J Virol Methods* **124**:21-6.

101. Aitken, C., and D. J. Jeffries. 2001. Nosocomial spread of viral disease. *Clin Microbiol Rev* **14**:528-46.

102. Aivazis, V., G. Pardalos, P. Kirkou-Thanou, K. Starmouli, and E. Roilides. 2004. Tuberculosis outbreak in a day care centre: always a risk. *Acta Paediatr* **93**:140.

103. Ajello, L., and L. Polonelli. 1985. Imported paracoccidioidomycosis: a public health problem in non-endemic areas. *Eur J Epidemiol* **1**:160-5.

104. Aka, N. A. D., A. C. E. Allabi, G. Dreyfuss, D. Kinde-Gazard, L. Tawo, D. Rondelaud, B. Bouteille, G. Avode, S. Y. Anagonou, M. Gninafon, A. Massougbodji, and M. Dumas. 1999. Observations épidémiologiques sur le premier cas de paragonimose humaine et les hôtes intermédiaires potentiels de Paragonimus sp. au Bénin. *Bull Soc Pathol Exot* **92**:191-4.

105. Akahane, H., K. Shibue, A. Shimizu, and S. Toshitani. 1998. Human gnathostomiasis caused by Gnathostoma doloresi, with particular reference to the parasitological investigation of the causative agent. *Ann Trop Med Parasitol* **92**:721-6.

106. Akazawa, M., J. L. Sindelar, and A. D. Paltiel. 2003. Economic costs of influenza-related work absenteeism. *Value Health* **6**:107-15.

107. Akhondi, H., and A. R. Rahimi. 2002. Haemophilus aphrophilus endocarditis after tongue piercing. *Emerg Infect Dis* **8**:850-1.

108. Akiba, T., K. Osaka, S. Tang, S. Tang, M. Nakayama, A. Yamamoto, I. Kurane, N. Okabe, and T. Umenai. 2001. Analysis of Japanese encephalitis epidemic in western Nepal in 1997. *Epidemiol Infect* **126**:81-8.

109. Akihara, S., T. G. Phan, T. A. Nguyen, G. Hansman, S. Okitsu, and H. Ushijima. 2005. Existence of multiple outbreaks of viral gastroenteritis among infants in a day care center in Japan. *Arch Virol* **150**:2061-75.

110. Akin, F., M. Spraker, R. Aly, J. Leyden, W. Raynor, and W. Landin. 2001. Effects of breathable disposable diapers: reduced prevalence of Candida and common diaper dermatitis. *Pediatr Dermatol* **18**:282-90.

111. Akogun, O. B. 1999. Onchocerciasis in Taraba State, Nigeria: clinical-epidemiological study of at-risk males in Bakundi District. *Zentralbl Bakteriol* **289**:371-9.

112. Akogun, O. B. 1999. Yaws and syphilis in the Garkida area of Nigeria. *Zentralbl Bakteriol* **289**:101-7.

113. Akoua-Koffi, C., K. D. Ekra, A. B. Kone, N. S. Dagnan, V. Akran, K. L. Kouadio, Y. G. Loukou, K. Odehouri, J. Tagliante-Saracino, and A. Ehouman. 2002. Détection et gestion de l'épidémie de fièvre jaune en Côte d'Ivoire, 2001. *Med Trop* **62**:305-9.

114. al Bustan, M. A., E. E. Udo, and T. D. Chugh. 1996. Nasal carriage of enterotoxin-producing Staphylococcus aureus among restaurant workers in Kuwait City. *Epidemiol Infect* **116**:319-22.

115. al-Ahmadi, K. S., H. E. el Bushra, and A. S. al-Zahrani. 1998. An outbreak of food poisoning associated with restaurant-made mayonnaise in Abha, Saudi Arabia. *J Diarrhoeal Dis Res* **16**:201-4.

116. Al-Doory, Y., and A. F. DiSalvo. 1992. Blastomycosis. Plenum, New York.

117. al-Fawaz, I., S. al-Rasheed, M. al-Mugeiren, A. al-Salloum, M. al-Sohaibani, and S. Ramia. 1996. Hepatitis E virus infection in patients from Saudi Arabia with sickle cell anaemia and beta-thalassemia major: possible transmission by blood transfusion. *J Viral Hepat* **3**:203-5.

118. al-Ghamdi, M., S. al-Sabty, A. Kannan, and B. Rowe. 1989. An outbreak of food poisoning in a workers' camp in Saudi Arabia caused by Salmonella minnesota. *J Diarrhoeal Dis Res* **7**:18-20.

119. Al-Ghamdi, M. S., F. El-Morsy, Z. H. Al-Musafa, M. Al-Ramadhan, and M. Hanif. 1999. Antibiotic resistance of Escherichia coli isolated from poultry workers, patients and chicken in the eastern province of Saudi Arabia. *Trop Med Int Health* **4**:278-83.

120. Al-Hazmi, M., E. Ayobanji, M. Abdurahman, S. Banzal, J. Ashraf, A. El-Bushra, A. Hazmi, M. Abdullah, H. Abbo, A. Elamin, T. Al-Sammani el, M. Gadour, C. Menon, M. Hamza, I. Rahim, M. Hafez, M. Jambavalikar, H. Arishi, and A. Aqeel. 2003. Epidemic Rift valley fever in Saudi Arabia: a clinical study of severe illness in humans. *Clin Infect Dis* **36:**245-52.

121. Al-Jawabreh, A., L. F. Schnur, A. Nasereddin, J. M. Schwenkenbecher, Z. Abdeen, F. Barghuthy, H. Khanfar, W. Presber, and G. Schonian. 2004. The recent emergence of Leishmania tropica in Jericho (A'riha) and its environs, a classical focus of L. major. *Trop Med Int Health* **9:**812-6.

122. Al-Khatib, I., A. Ju'ba, N. Kamal, N. Hamed, N. Hmeidan, and S. Massad. 2003. Impact of housing conditions on the health of the people at al-Ama'ri refugee camp in the West Bank of Palestine. *Int J Environ Health Res* **13:**315-26.

123. al-Lahham, A. B., M. Abu-Saud, and A. A. Shehabi. 1990. Prevalence of Salmonella, Shigella and intestinal parasites in food handlers in Irbid, Jordan. *J Diarrhoeal Dis Res* **8:**160-2.

124. al-Quarawi, S. N., H. E. el Bushra, R. E. Fontaine, S. A. Bubshait, and N. A. el Tantawy. 1995. Typhoid fever from water desalinized using reverse osmosis. *Epidemiol Infect* **114:**41-50.

125. al-Salihi, F. L., J. P. Curran, and J. Wang. 1974. Neonatal Trichomonas vaginalis: report of three cases and review of the literature. *Pediatrics* **53:**196-200.

126. Al-Shamahy, H. A., C. J. Whitty, and S. G. Wright. 2000. Risk factors for human brucellosis in Yemen: a case control study. *Epidemiol Infect* **125:**309-13.

127. Al-Shammari, S., T. Khoja, F. El-Khwasky, and A. Gad. 2001. Intestinal parasitic diseases in Riyadh, Saudi Arabia: prevalence, sociodemographic and environmental associates. *Trop Med Int Health* **6:**184-9.

128. Al-Tikriti, S. K., F. Al-Ani, F. J. Jurji, H. Tantawi, M. Al-Moslih, N. Al-Janabi, M. I. Mahmud, A. Al-Bana, H. Habib, H. Al-Munthri, S. Al-Janabi, A. L.-J. K, M. Yonan, F. Hassan, and D. I. Simpson. 1981. Congo/Crimean haemorrhagic fever in Iraq. *Bull WHO* **59:**85-90.

129. Al-Traif, I., A. Ali, M. Dafalla, W. Al-Tamimi, and L. Qassem. 2004. Prevalence of hepatitis delta antibody among HBsAG carriers in Saudi Arabia. *Ann Saudi Med* **24:**343-4.

130. Alamanos, Y., V. Maipa, S. Levidiotou, and E. Gessouli. 2000. A community waterborne outbreak of gastro-enteritis attributed to Shigella sonnei. *Epidemiol Infect* **125:**499-503.

131. Alangaden, G. J., M. Wahiduzzaman, and P. H. Chandrasekar. 2002. Aspergillosis: the most common community-acquired pneumonia with gram-negative bacilli as copathogens in stem cell transplant recipients with graft-versus-host disease. *Clin Infect Dis* **35:**659-64.

132. Albanese, G., C. Venturi, and G. Galbiati. 2001. Treatment of larva migrans cutanea (creeping eruption): a comparison between albendazole and traditional therapy. *Int J Dermatol* **40:**67-71.

133. Alberdi, M. P., A. R. Walker, and K. A. Urquhart. 2000. Field evidence that roe deer (Capreolus capreolus) are a natural host for Ehrlichia phagocytophila. *Epidemiol Infect* **124:**315-23.

134. Albonico, M., R. J. Stoltzfus, L. Savioli, J. M. Tielsch, H. M. Chwaya, E. Ercole, and G. Cancrini. 1998. Epidemiological evidence for a differential effect of hookworm species, Ancylostoma duodenale or Necator americanus, on iron status of children. *Int J Epidemiol* **27:**530-7.

135. Albrecht, H., H. J. Stellbrink, J. Petersen, A. Patzak, H. Jager, and H. Greten. 1994. [Disseminated histoplasmosis in AIDS]. *Dtsch Med Wochenschr* **119:**657-62.

136. Alcabes, P., B. O'Sullivan, E. Nadal, and M. Mouzon. 1988. An outbreak of Salmonella gastroenteritis in an urban jail. *Infect Control Hosp Epidemiol* **9:**542-7.

137. Alcais, A., L. Abel, C. David, M. E. Torrez, P. Flandre, and J. P. Dedet. 1997. Risk factors for onset of cutaneous and mucocutaneous leishmaniasis in Bolivia. *Am J Trop Med Hyg* **57:**79-84.

138. Alcoba-Florez, J., E. Perz-Roth, S. Gonzalez-Linares, and S. Mendez-Alvarez. 2005. Outbreak of Shigella sonnei in a rural hotel in La Gomera, Canary Islands, Spain. *Int Microbiol* **8:**133-6.

139. Alemayehu, W., M. Melese, E. Fredlander, A. Worku, and P. Courtright. 2005. Active trachoma in children in central Ethiopia: association with altitude. *Trans R Soc Trop Med Hyg* **99:**840-3.

140. Alexander, J. P., Jr., L. E. Chapman, M. A. Pallansch, W. T. Stephenson, T. J. Torok, and L. J. Anderson. 1993. Coxsackievirus B2 infection and aseptic meningitis: a focal outbreak among members of a high school football team. *J Infect Dis* **167:**1201-5.

141. Alexeyev, O. A., F. Elgh, A. V. Zhestkov, G. Wadell, and P. Juto. 1996. Hantaan and puumala virus antibodies in blood donors in Samara, an HFRS-endemic region in European Russia. *Lancet* **347:**1483.

142. Alford, C. A., S. Stagno, R. F. Pass, and W. J. Britt. 1990. Congenital and perinatal cytomegalovirus infections. *Rev Infect Dis* **12 Suppl 7:**S745-53.

143. Alfurayh, O., A. Sabeel, M. N. Al Ahdal, K. Almeshari, G. Kessie, M. Hamid, and D. M. Dela Cruz. 2000. Hand contamination with hepatitis C virus in staff looking after hepatitis C-positive hemodialysis patients. *Am J Nephrol* **20:**103-6.

144. Alghaithy, A. A., N. E. Bilal, M. Gedebou, and A. H. Weily. 2000. Nasal carriage and antibiotic resistance of Staphylococcus aureus isolates from hospital and non-hospital personnel in Abha, Saudi Arabia. *Trans R Soc Trop Med Hyg* **94:**504-7.

145. Ali, I. K. M., M. B. Hossain, S. Roy, P. F. Ayeh-Kumi, W. A. Petri, Jr., R. Haque, and C. G. Clark. 2003. Entamoeba moshkovskii infections in children in Bangladesh. *Emerg Infect Dis* **9:**580-4.

146. Ali, M., Y. Wagatsuma, M. Emch, and R. F. Breiman. 2003. Use of a geographic information system for defining spatial risk for dengue transmission in Bangladesh: role for Aedes albopictus in an urban outbreak. *Am J Trop Med Hyg* **69:**634-40.

147. Ali, R., A. W. Mounts, U. D. Parashar, M. Sahani, M. Lye, M. M. Isa, K. Balathevan, M. T. Arif, and T. G. Ksiazek. 2001. Nipah virus infection among military personnel involved in pib culling during an outbreak of encephalitis in Malaysia, 1998-1999. *Emerg Infect Dis* **7:**759-761.

148. Ali-Shtayeh, M. S., A.-A. M. Salameh, S. I. Abu-Ghdeib, R. M. Jamous, and H. Khraim. 2002. Prevalence of tinea capitis as well as of asymptomatic carriers in school children in Nablus area (Palestine). *Mycoses* **45:**188-94.

149. Alkaya, G. S., R. M. Hockberg, J. Thompson, A. P. Nazitto, L. A. Pizzurro, F. F. Schady, M. A. McPherson, R. L. Coshnear, A. K. Goodman, S. M. Friedman, S. Schultz, S. J. Millian, and D. J. Sencer. 1985. Rubella outbreak among office workers—New York city. *MMWR* **34:**455-9.

150. Allan, J. S., S. R. Broussard, M. G. Michaels, T. E. Starzl, K. L. Leighton, E. M. Whitehead, A. G. Comuzzie, R. E. Lanford, M. M. Leland, W. M. Switzer, and W. Heneine. 1998. Amplification of simian retroviral sequences from human recipients of baboon liver transplants. *AIDS Res Hum Retroviruses* **14**:821-4.

151. Allan, T., T. Horgan, H. Scaife, E. Koch, S. Nowicki, M. K. Parrish, and E. Salehi. 2001. Outbreak of legionnaires' disease among automotive plant workers - Ohio, 2001. *MMWR* **50**:357-359.

152. Allander, T., A. Gruber, M. Naghavi, A. Beyene, T. Soderstrom, M. Bjorkholm, L. Grillner, and M. A. Persson. 1995. Frequent patient-to-patient transmission of hepatitis C virus in a haematology ward. *Lancet* **345**:603-7.

153. Allen, A. M., G. R. Irwin, J. J. Karwacki, D. C. Warren, and R. S. Levine. 1975. Epidemic hepatitis B: a sustained outbreak in a large military population. *Am J Epidemiol* **102**:545-52.

154. Allen, K. D., and H. T. Green. 1989. An outbreak of Trichuris trichiura in a mental handicap hospital. *J Hosp Infect* **13**:161-6.

155. Allerberger, F., N. Al-Jazrawi, P. Kreidl, M. P. Dierich, G. Feierl, I. Hein, and M. Wagner. 2003. Barbecued Chicken Causing a Multi-State Outbreak of Campylobacter jejuni Enteritis. *Infection* **31**:19-23.

156. Allerberger, F., A. Liesegang, K. Grif, D. Khaschabi, R. Prager, J. Danzl, F. Hock, J. Ottl, M. P. Dierich, C. Berghold, I. Neckstaller, H. Tschape, and I. Fisher. 2003. Occurrence of Salmonella enterica serovar Dublin in Austria. *Wien Med Wochenschr* **153**:148-52.

157. Allos, B. M. 2001. Campylobacter jejuni Infections: update on emerging issues and trends. *Clin Infect Dis* **32**:1201-6.

158. Almallah, Y. Z., C. D. Rennie, J. Stone, and M. J. Lancashire. 2000. Urinary tract infection and patient satisfaction after flexible cystoscopy and urodynamic evaluation. *Urology* **56**:37-9.

159. Almeda, J., J. Casabona, B. Simon, M. Gerard, D. Rey, V. Puro, and T. Thomas. 2004. Proposed recommendations for the management of HIV post-exposure prophylaxis after sexual, injecting drug or other exposures in Europe. *Eur Surveill* **9**:35–40.

160. Almeida, L. M. 2001. the epidemiology of hepatitis A in Rio de Janeiro: environmental and domestic risk factors. *Epidemiol Infect* **127**:327-333.

161. Almog, R., M. Low, D. Cohen, G. Robin, S. Ashkenazi, H. Bercovier, M. Gdalevich, Y. Samuels, I. Ashkenazi, J. Shemer, A. Eldad, and M. S. Green. 1999. Prevalence of anti-hepatitis A antibodies, hepatitis B viral markers, and anti-hepatitis C antibodies among immigrants from the former USSR who arrived in Israel during 1990-1991. *Infection* **27**:212-7.

162. Alonso, J. M. 1999. Interactions écologiques des Yersinia au sein de l'hôte réservoir commun, le rongeur. *Bull Soc Pathol Exot* **92**:414-7.

163. Alonso-Echanove, J., S. S. Shah, A. J. Valenti, S. N. Dirrigl, L. A. Carson, M. J. Arduino, and W. R. Jarvis. 2001. Nosocomial outbreak of Microbacterium species bacteremia among cancer patients. *J Infect Dis* **184**:754-60.

164. Alonso-Sanz, M., F. Chaves, F. Dronda, S. Catalan, and A. Gonzalez-Lopez. 1995. [Intestinal parasitoses in the prison population in the Madrid area (1991-1993)]. *Enferm Infecc Microbiol Clin* **13**:90-5.

165. Alrajhi, A. A., I. Rahim, M. Akood, and M. Hazmi. 1999. Chloroquine-resistant Plasmodium falciparum cerebral malaria in a chloroquine-susceptible area. *J Infect Dis* **180**:1738-41.

166. Altaf, A., S. Luby, A. J. Ahmed, N. Zaidi, A. J. Khan, S. Mirza, J. McCormick, and S. Fisher-Hoch. 1998. Outbreak of Crimean-Congo haemorrhagic fever in Quetta, Pakistan: contact tracing and risk assessment. *Trop Med Int Health* **3**:878-82.

167. Altekruse, S. F., R. D. Bishop, L. M. Baldy, S. G. Thompson, S. A. Wilson, B. J. Ray, and P. M. Griffin. 2000. Vibrio gastroenteritis in the US Gulf of Mexico region: the role of raw oysters. *Epidemiol Infect* **124**:489-95.

168. Altekruse, S. F., N. J. Stern, P. I. Fields, and D. L. Swerdlow. 1999. Campylobacter jejuni - an emerging foodborne pathogen. *Emerg Infect Dis* **5**:28-35.

169. Altekruse, S. F., B. B. Timbo, J. C. Mowbray, N. H. Bean, and M. E. Potter. 1998. Cheese-associated outbreaks of human illness in the United States, 1973 to 1992: sanitary manufacturing practices protect consumers. *J Food Prot* **61**:1405-7.

170. Alten, B., S. S. Caglar, F. M. Simsek, and S. Kaynas. 2003. Effect of insecticide-treated bednets for malaria control in Southeast Anatolia-Turkey. *J Vector Ecol* **28**:97-107.

171. Alter, M. J. 2003. Epidemiology of hepatitis B in Europe and worldwide. *J Hepatol* **39 Suppl 1**:S64-9.

172. Alter, M. J., R. L. Lyerla, J. I. Tokars, E. R. Miller, and M. J. Arduino. 2001. Recommendations for preventing transmission of infections among chronic hemodialysis patients. *MMWR* **50 (RR-5)**:1-46.

173. Alter, M. J., and H. S. Margolis. 1998. Recommendations for prevention and control of hepatitis C virus (HCV) infection and HCV-related chronic disease. *MMWR* **47(RR-19)**:1-40.

174. Alvarado-Esquivel, C., E. Sablon, S. Martinez-Garcia, and S. Estrada-Martinez. 2005. Hepatitis virus and HIV infections in inmates of a state correctional facility in Mexico. *Epidemiol Infect* **133**:679-85.

175. Alvseike, O., T. Leegard, P. Aavitsland, and J. Lassen. 2002. Trend of multiple drug resistant Salmonella Typhimurium in Norway. *Eurosurveillance* **7**:5-7.

176. Alweis, R. L., K. DiRosario, E. Conidi, K. C. Kain, R. Olans, and J. L. Tully. 2004. Serial nosocomial transmission of Plasmodium falciparum malaria from patient to nurse to patient. *Infect Control Hosp Epidemiol* **25**:55-9.

177. Aly, R. 1994. Ecology and epidemiology of dermatophyte infections. *J Am Acad Dermatol* **31**:S21-5.

178. Aly, R. 1999. Ecology, epidemiology and diagnosis of tinea capitis. *Pediatr Infect Dis J* **18**:180-5.

179. Alzeer, A., A. Mashlah, N. Fakim, N. Al-Sugair, M. Al-Hedaithy, S. Al-Majed, and G. Jamjoom. 1998. Tuberculosis is the commonest cause of pneumonia requiring hospitalization during Hajj (pilgrimage to Makkah). *J Infect* **36**:303-6.

180. Amahmid, O., S. Asmama, and K. Bouhoum. 1999. The effect of waste water reuse in irrigation on the contamination level of food crops by Giardia cysts and Ascaris eggs. *Int J Food Microbiol* **49**:19-26.

181. Amankwa, J. A., P. Bloch, J. Meyer-Lassen, A. Olsen, and N. O. Christensen. 1994. Urinary and intestinal schistosomiasis in the Tono Irrigation Scheme, Kassena/Nankana District, upper east region, Ghana. *Trop Med Parasitol* **45**:319-23.

182. Amano, Y., J. Rumbea, J. Knobloch, J. Olson, and M. Kron. 1997. Bartonellosis in Ecuador: serosurvey and current status of cutaneous verrucous disease. *Am J Trop Med Hyg* **57**:174-9.

183. **Amass, S. F., and D. A. Scholz.** 1998. Acute nonfatal erysipelas in sows in a commercial farrow-to-finish operation. *J Am Vet Med Assoc* **212:**708-9.
184. **Amin, O. M.** 2002. Seasonal prevalence of intestinal parasites in the United States during 2000. *Am J Trop Med Hyg* **66:**799-803.
185. **Amir, L. H., H. Harris, and L. Andriske.** 1999. An audit of mastitis in the emergency department. *J Hum Lact* **15:**221-4.
186. **Ammatuna, P., G. Campisi, L. Giovannelli, D. Giambelluca, C. Alaimo, S. Mancuso, and V. Margiotta.** 2001. Presence of Epstein-Barr virus, cytomegalovirus and human papillomavirus in normal oral mucosa of HIV-infected and renal transplant patients. *Oral Dis* **7:**34-40.
187. **Ammon, A., L. R. Petersen, and H. Karch.** 1999. A large outbreak of hemolytic uremic syndrome caused by an unusual sorbitol-fermenting strain of Escherichia coli O157:H. *J Infect Dis* **179:**1274-7.
188. **Amornkul, P. N., H. Takahashi, A. K. Bogard, M. Nakata, R. Harpaz, and P. V. Effler.** 2004. Low risk of measles transmission after exposure on an international airline flight. *J Infect Dis* **189 Suppl 1:**81-5.
189. **Amorosa, V., D. Kremens, M. S. Wolfe, T. Flanigan, K. M. Cahill, K. Judy, S. Kasner, and E. Blumberg.** 2005. Schistosoma mansoni in family 5 years after safari. *Emerg Infect Dis* **11:**339-41.
190. **Amvros'eva, T. V., Z. F. Bogush, O. N. Kazinets, V. D'Iakonova O, N. V. Poklonskaia, G. P. Golovneva, and R. M. Sharko.** 2004. [Outbreak of enteroviral infection in Vitebsk during pollution of water supply by enteroviruses]. *Vopr Virusol* **49:**30-4.
191. **Anaissie, E. J., R. T. Kuchar, J. H. Rex, A. Francesconi, M. Kasai, F. M. Muller, M. Lozano-Chiu, R. C. Summerbell, M. C. Dignani, S. J. Chanock, and T. J. Walsh.** 2001. Fusariosis associated with pathogenic fusarium species colonization of a hospital water system: a new paradigm for the epidemiology of opportunistic mold infections. *Clin Infect Dis* **33:**1871-8.
192. **Anaissie, E. J., S. R. Penzak, and M. C. Dignani.** 2002. The hospital water supply as a source of nosocomial infections: a plea for action. *Arch Intern Med* **162:**1483-92.
193. **Anaruma Filho, F., P. P. Chieffi, C. R. S. Correa, E. D. Camargo, E. P. Real da Silveira, and J. J. B. Aranha.** 2003. Human toxocariasis: incidence among residents in the outskirts of Campinas, state of São Paulo, Brazil. *Rev Inst Med Trop Sao Paulo* **45:**293-4.
194. **Anastassopoulou, C. G., D. Paraskevis, V. Sypsa, M. Psichogiou, A. Katsoulidou, N. Tassopoulos, A. Skoutelis, M. Malliori, and A. Hatzakis.** 1998. Prevalence patterns and genotypes of GB virus C/hepatitis G virus among imprisoned intravenous drug users. *J Med Virol* **56:**246-52.
195. **Ancelle, T., J. Dupouy-Camet, J. Desenclos, E. Maillot, S. Savage-Houze, F. Charlet, J. Drucker, and A. Moren.** 1998. A multifocal outbreak of trichinellosis linked to horse meat imported from North America to France in 1993. *Am J Trop Med Hyg* **59:**615-9.
196. **Anda, P., J. Segura del Pozo, J. M. Diaz Garcia, R. Escudero, F. J. Garcia Pena, M. C. Lopez Velasco, R. E. Sellek, M. R. Jimenez Chillaron, L. P. Sanchez Serrano, and J. F. Martinez Navarro.** 2001. Waterborne outbreak of tularemia associated with crayfish fishing. *Emerg Infect Dis* **7:**575-82.
197. **Andersen, B. M., H. Haugen, M. Rasch, A. Heldal Haugen, and A. Tageson.** 2000. Outbreak of scabies in Norwegian nursing homes and home care patients: control and prevention. *J Hosp Infect* **45:**160-4.
198. **Andersen, F. L., H. Ouhelli, and M. Kachani.** 1997. Compendium on cystic echinococcosis in Africa and in middle eastern countries with special reference to Morocco. Brigham Young University, Provo, Utah.
199. **Andersen, J., L. Berthelsen, B. Bech Jensen, and I. Lind.** 1998. Dynamics of the meningococcal carrier state and characteristics of the carrier strains: a longitudinal study within three cohorts of military recruits. *Epidemiol Infect* **121:**85-94.
200. **Anderson, A. D., V. D. Garrett, J. Sobel, S. S. Monroe, R. L. Fankhauser, K. J. Schwab, J. S. Bresee, P. S. Mead, C. Higgins, J. Campana, and R. I. Glass.** 2001. Multistate Outbreak of Norwalk-like Virus Gastroenteritis Associated with a Common Caterer. *Am J Epidemiol* **154:**1013-1019.
201. **Anderson, A. D., A. G. Heryford, J. P. Sarisky, C. Higgins, S. S. Monroe, R. S. Beard, C. M. Newport, J. L. Cashdollar, G. S. Fout, D. E. Robbins, S. A. Seys, K. J. Musgrave, C. Medus, J. Vinje, J. S. Bresee, H. M. Mainzer, and R. I. Glass.** 2003. A waterborne outbreak of Norwalk-like virus among snowmobilers—Wyoming, 2001. *J Infect Dis* **187:**303-6.
202. **Anderson, A. D., B. Smoak, E. Shuping, C. Ockenhouse, and B. Petruccelli.** 2005. Q fever and the US military. *Emerg Infect Dis* **11:**1320-2.
203. **Anderson, B., N. J. Bodsworth, R. A. Rohrsheim, and B. J. Donovan.** 1994. Hepatitis B virus infection and vaccination status of high risk people in Sydney: 1982 and 1991. *Med J Aust* **161:**368-71.
204. **Anderson, B. J.** 1999. The effectiveness of valacyclovir in preventing reactivation of herpes gladiatorum in wrestlers. *Clin J Sport Med* **9:**86-90.
205. **Anderson, B. J.** 2003. The epidemiology and clinical analysis of several outbreaks of herpes gladiatorum. *Med Sci Sports Exerc* **35:**1809-1814.
206. **Anderson, B. S., and H. P. Minette.** 1986. Leptospirosis in Hawaii: shifting trends in exposure, 1907-1984. *Int J Zoonoses* **13:**76-88.
207. **Anderson, E. C., and L. W. Rowe.** 1998. The prevalence of antibody to the viruses of bovine virus diarrhoea, bovine herpes virus 1, rift valley fever, ephemeral fever and bluetongue and to Leptospira sp in free-ranging wildlife in Zimbabwe. *Epidemiol Infect* **121:**441-9.
208. **Anderson, E. J., and S. G. Weber.** 2004. Rotavirus infection in adults. *Lancet Infect Dis* **4:**91-9.
209. **Anderson, G. D., and D. R. Lee.** 1976. Salmonella in horses: a source of contamination of horsemeat in a packing plant under federal inspection. *Appl Environ Microbiol* **31:**661-3.
210. **Anderson, J. E.** 2003. Condom use and HIV risk among US adults. *Am J Public Health* **93:**912-4.
211. **Anderson, L. C., S. L. Leary, and P. J. Manning.** 1983. Rat-bite fever in animal research laboratory personnel. *Lab Anim Sci* **33:**292–4.
212. **Anderson, L. J., S. M. Gillespie, T. J. Torok, E. S. Hurwitz, C. J. Tsou, and G. W. Gary.** 1990. Risk of infection following exposures to human parvovirus B19. *Behring Inst Mitt* **85:**60-3.
213. **Anderson, M. J., E. Lewis, I. M. Kidd, S. M. Hall, and B. J. Cohen.** 1984. An outbreak of erythema infectiosum associated with human parvovirus infection. *J Hyg (Lond)* **93:**85-93.
214. **Anderson, M. R., K. Klink, and A. Cohrssen.** 2004. Evaluation of vaginal complaints. *JAMA* **291:**1368-79.

215. **Anderson, R. L.** 1989. Iodophor antiseptics: intrinsic microbial contamination with resistant bacteria. *Infect Control Hosp Epidemiol* **10:**443-6.

216. **Andersson, M. A., M. Nikulin, U. Koljalg, M. C. Andersson, F. Rainey, K. Reijula, E. L. Hintikka, and M. Salkinoja-Salonen.** 1997. Bacteria, molds, and toxins in water-damaged building materials. *Appl Environ Microbiol* **63:**387-93.

217. **Andersson von Rosen, I., L. Gotherfors, S. Schmeisser, A. Tarnvik, and C. Svanborg Eden.** 1990. Outbreak of Haemophilus influenzae type b meningitis in a day care center. *Pediatr Infect Dis J* **9:**326-32.

218. **Ando, K., K. Ishikura, T. Nakakugi, Y. Shimono, T. Tamai, M. Sugawa, W. Limviroj, and Y. Chinzei.** 2001. Five cases of Diphyllobothrium nihonkaiense infection with discovery of plerocercoids from an infective source, Oncorhynchus masou ishikawae. *J Parasitol* **87:**96-100.

219. **Andoh, K., K. Yamanaka, and T. Akashi.** 2002. [The significance of tuberculin skin test in the investigation of mass outbreak of tuberculosis in schools]. *Kekkaku* **77:**589-95.

220. **Andrade-Narvaez, F. J., S. B. Canto Lara, N. R. Van Wynsberghe, E. A. Rebollar-Tellez, A. Vargas-Gonzalez, and N. E. Albertos-Alpuche.** 2003. Seasonal transmission of Leishmania (Leishmania) mexicana in the state of Campeche, Yucatan Peninsula, Mexico. *Mem Inst Oswaldo Cruz* **98:**995-8.

221. **Andrade-Rocha, F. T.** 2003. Ureaplasma urealyticum and Mycoplasma hominis in men attending for routine semen analysis. Prevalence, incidence by age and clinical settings, influence on sperm characteristics, relationship with the leukocyte count and clinical value. *Urol Int* **71:**377-81.

222. **Andre-Fontaine, G., X. Peslerbe, and J. P. Ganiere.** 1992. Occupational hazard of unnoticed leptospirosis in water ways maintenance staff. *Eur J Epidemiol* **8:**228-32.

223. **Andrews, J. R., R. Ainsworth, and D. Abernethy.** 1994. Trichinella pseudospiralis in humans: description of a case and its treatment. *Trans R Soc Trop Med Hyg* **88:**200-3.

224. **Andzhaparidze, A. G., V. Karetnyi Iu, L. I. Korzaia, M. S. Balaian, and I. P. Titova.** 1989. [Epizootic hepatitis A among African green monkeys kept in a vivarium]. *Vopr Virusol* **34:**292-6.

225. **Anez, N., H. Carrasco, H. Parada, G. Crisante, A. Rojas, N. Gonzalez, J. L. Ramirez, P. Guevara, C. Rivero, R. Borges, and J. V. Scorza.** 1999. Acute Chagas' disease in western Venezuela: a clinical, seroparasitologic, and epidemiologic study. *Am J Trop Med Hyg* **60:**215-22.

226. **Anez, N., G. Crisante, A. Rojas, H. Carrasco, H. Parada, Y. Yepez, R. Borges, P. Guevara, and J. L. Ramirez.** 2001. Detection and significance of inapparent infection in Chagas disease in western Venezuela. *Am J Trop Med Hyg* **65:**227-32.

227. **Ang, L. H.** 2000. Outbreak of giardiasis in a daycare nursery. *Commun Dis Public Health* **3:**212-3.

228. **Ang, L. H.** 2000. Outbreak of hepatitis A in a special needs school in Kent: 1999. *Commun Dis Public Health* **3:**139-40.

229. **Ang, P., N. Rattana-Apiromyakij, and C. L. Goh.** 2000. Retrospective study of Mycobacterium marinum skin infections. *Int J Dermatol* **39:**343-7.

230. **Angeloni, V. L., R. A. Keller, and D. H. Walker.** 1997. Rickettsialpox-like illness in a traveler. *Mil Med* **162:**636-9.

231. **Angulo, F. J., J. Getz, J. P. Taylor, K. A. Hendricks, C. L. Hatheway, S. S. Barth, H. M. Solomon, A. E. Larson, E. A. Johnson, L. N. Nickey, and A. A. Ries.** 1998. A large outbreak of botulism: the hazardous baked potato. *J Infect Dis* **178:**172-7.

232. **Angulo, F. J., S. Tippen, D. J. Sharp, B. J. Payne, C. Collier, J. E. Hill, T. J. Barrett, R. M. Clark, E. E. Geldreich, H. D. Donnell, Jr., and D. L. Swerdlow.** 1997. A community waterborne outbreak of salmonellosis and the effectiveness of a boil water order. *Am J Public Health* **87:**580-4.

233. **Anish, E. J.** 2004. Viral hepatitis: sports-related risk. *Curr Sports Med Rep* **3:**100-6.

234. **Annane, D., E. Bellissant, and J. M. Cavaillon.** 2005. Septic shock. *Lancet* **365:**63-78.

235. **Anonymous.** 2003. Water, sanitation and drainage: ensuring better provision with limited resources. *Environ Urbanization* **15:**3-10.

236. **Ansart, S., O. Pajot, J. P. Grivois, V. Zeller, E. Klement, L. Perez, P. Bossi, F. Bricaire, and E. Caumes.** 2004. Pneumonia among travelers returning from abroad. *J Travel Med* **11:**87-91.

237. **Anselmi, M., J. M. Moreira, C. Caicedo, R. Guderian, and G. Tognoni.** 2003. Community participation eliminates yaws in Ecuador. *Trop Med Int Health* **8:**634-8.

238. **Antai, S. P.** 1988. Study of the Bacillus flora of Nigerian spices. *Int J Food Microbiol* **6:**259-61.

239. **Anthony, B. F., E. L. Kaplan, L. W. Wannamaker, and S. S. Chapman.** 1976. The dynamics of streptococcal infections in a defined population of children: serotypes associated with skin and respiratory infections. *Am J Epidemiol* **104:**652-66.

240. **Anthony, R. L., M. J. Bangs, N. Hamzah, H. Basri, Purnomo, and B. Subianto.** 1992. Heightened transmission of stable malaria in an isolated population in the highlands of Irian Jaya, Indonesia. *Am J Trop Med Hyg* **47:**346-56.

241. **Antinori, S., L. Galimberti, E. Gianelli, S. Calattini, M. Piazza, P. Morelli, M. Moroni, M. Galli, and M. Corbellino.** 2004. Prospective observational study of fever in hospitalized returning travelers and migrants from tropical areas, 1997-2001. *J Travel Med* **11:**135-42.

242. **Anton, E., B. Font, T. Munoz, I. Sanfeliu, and F. Segura.** 2003. Clinical and laboratory characteristics of 144 patients with mediterranean spotted fever. *Eur J Clin Microbiol Infect Dis* **22:**126-8.

243. **Antona, D.** 2002. Le tétanos en France en 2000 et 2001. *Bull Epidémiol Hebdomadaire* **40:**197-9.

244. **Antonio-Nkondjio, C., P. Awono-Ambene, J. C. Toto, J. Y. Meunier, S. Zebaze-Kemleu, R. Nyambam, C. S. Wondji, T. Tchuinkam, and D. Fontenill.** 2002. High malaria transmission intensity in a village close to Yaounde, the capital city of Cameroon. *J Med Entomol* **39:**350-5.

245. **Anyiwo, C. E., A. O. Coker, and S. O. Daniel.** 1982. Pseudomonas aeruginosa in postoperative wounds from chlorhexidine solutions. *J Hosp Infect* **3:**189-91.

246. **Ao, T., N. Sam, R. Manongi, G. Seage, and S. Kapiga.** 2003. Social and behavioural determinants of consistent condom use among hotel and bar workers in Northern Tanzania. *Int J STD AIDS* **14:**688-96.

247. **Aoki, T., N. Koizumi, and H. Watanabe.** 2001. A case of leptospirosis probably caused by drinking contaminated well-water after an earthquake. *Jpn J Infect Dis* **54:**243-4.

248. **Apisarnthanarak, A., V. J. Fraser, W. M. Dunne, J. R. Little, J. Hoppe-Bauer, J. L. Mayfield, and L. B. Polish.** 2003. Stenotrophomonas maltophilia intestinal colonization in hospitalized oncology patients with diarrhea. *Clin Infect Dis* **37:**1131-5.

249. Appawu, M. A., S. K. Dadzie, A. Baffoe-Wilmot, and M. D. Wilson. 2001. Lymphatic filariasis in Ghana: entomological investigation of transmission dynamics and intensity in communities served by irrigation systems in the Upper East Region of Ghana. *Trop Med Int Health* **6**:511-6.

250. Aragon, T., M. Katz, L. Mintz, D. Vugia, S. Waterman, D. Bradshaw, T. Lacey, M. Sanders, and D. Dwyer. 1999. Nosocomial group A streptococcal infections associated with asymptomatic health-care workers - Maryland and California. *MMWR* **49**:163-166.

251. Aragon, T. J., S. Novotny, W. Enanoria, D. J. Vugia, A. Khalakdina, and M. H. Katz. 2003. Endemic cryptosporidiosis and exposure to municipal tap water in persons with acquired immunodeficiency syndrome (AIDS): a case-control study. *BMC Public Health* **3**:2.

252. Arai, T., N. Ikejima, T. Itoh, S. Sakai, T. Shimada, and R. Sakazaki. 1980. A survey of Plesiomonas shigelloides from aquatic environments, domestic animals, pets and humans. *J Hyg (Lond)* **84**:203-11.

253. Arambulo, P. V., 3rd, B. D. Cabrera, T. S. Osteria, and J. C. Baltazar. 1977. A comparative study of Trichomonas vaginalis prevalence in Filipino women. *Southeast Asian J Trop Med Public Health* **8**:298-302.

254. Aramburu Guarda, J., C. Ramal Asayag, and R. Witzig. 1999. Malaria reemergence in the Peruvian Amazon region. *Emerg Infect Dis* **5**:209-15.

255. Aramini, J. J., C. Stephen, J. P. Dubey, C. Engelstoft, H. Schwantje, and C. S. Ribble. 1999. Potential contamination of drinking water with Toxoplasma gondii oocysts. *Epidemiol Infect* **122**:305-15.

256. Aranaz, A., L. De Juan, N. Montero, C. Sanchez, M. Galka, C. Delso, J. Alvarez, B. Romero, J. Bezos, A. I. Vela, V. Briones, A. Mateos, and L. Dominguez. 2004. Bovine tuberculosis (Mycobacterium bovis) in wildlife in Spain. *J Clin Microbiol* **42**:2602-8.

257. Arankalle, V. A., M. K. Goverdhan, and K. Banerjee. 1994. Antibodies against hepatitis E virus in Old World monkeys. *J Viral Hepat* **1**:125-9.

258. Araújo, A., L. F. Ferreira, N. Guidon, N. Maues Da Serra Freire, K. J. Reinhard, and K. Dittmar. 2000. Ten thousand years of head lice infection. *Parasitol Today* **16**:269.

259. Araujo, F. R., C. P. Araujo, M. R. Werneck, and A. Gorski. 2000. [Cutaneous larva migrans in children in a school of center-western Brazil]. *Rev Saude Publica* **34**:84-5.

260. Arav-Boger, R. 2000. Cat-bite tularemia in a seventeen-year-old girl treated with ciprofloxacin. *Pediatr Infect Dis J* **19**:583-4.

261. Arce Arnaez, A., I. Rodero Garduno, J. Inigo Martinez, M. Burgoa Arenales, and E. Guevara Alemany. 2004. [Hepatitis A outbreak in a day care center and household transmission]. *An Pediatr (Barc)* **60**:222-7.

262. Archer, R. M. B., and E. Moretto. 1994. Ocorrência de Vibrio parahaemolyticus em Mexilhões (Perna perna, Linnaeus, 1758) de banco natural do litoral do município de Palhoça, Santa Catarina, Brazil. *Cadernos de Saúde Pública* **10**:379-86.

263. Archer-Dubon, C., R. Orozco-Topete, J. Leyva-Santiago, R. Arenas, J. Carbajosa, and A. Ysunza. 2003. Superficial mycotic infections of the foot in a native pediatric population: a pathogenic role for Trichosporon cutaneum? *Pediatr Dermatol* **20**:299-302.

264. Archibald, L. K., A. Corl, B. Shah, M. Schulte, M. J. Arduino, S. Aguero, D. J. Fisher, B. W. Stechenberg, S. N. Banerjee, and W. R. Jarvis. 1997. Serratia marcescens outbreak associated with extrinsic contamination of 1% chlorxylenol soap. *Infect Control Hosp Epidemiol* **18**:704-9.

265. Archibald, L. K., D. B. Jernigan, and K. M.A. 2002. Update: allograft-associated bacterial infections - United States, 2002. *MMWR* **51**:207-210.

266. Archibold, O. W. 1995. Ecology of world vegetation. Chapman & Hall, London.

267. Arcieri, R., A. M. Dionisi, A. Caprioli, P. Lopalco, R. Prato, C. Germinario, C. Rizzo, A. M. Larocca, S. Barbuti, D. Greco, and I. Luzzi. 1999. Direct detection of Clostridium perfringens enterotoxin in patients' stools during an outbreak of food poisoning. *FEMS Immunol Med Microbiol* **23**:45-8.

268. Arday, D. R., D. D. Kanjarpane, and P. W. Kelley. 1989. Mumps in the US army 1980-86: should recruits be immunized? *Am J Epidemiol* **79**:471-4.

269. Arden, K. E., M. D. Nissen, T. P. Sloots, and I. M. Mackay. 2005. New human coronavirus, HCoV-NL63, associated with severe lower respiratory tract disease in Australia. *J Med Virol* **75**:455-62.

270. Arfi, C., L. Dehen, E. Benassaia, P. Faure, D. Farge, P. Morel, and L. Dubertret. 1999. [Dermatologic consultation in a precarious situation: a prospective medical and social study at the Hopital Saint-Louis in Paris]. *Ann Dermatol Venereol* **126**:682-6.

271. Arfons, L., A. J. Ray, and C. J. Donskey. 2005. Clostridium difficile infection among health care workers receiving antibiotic therapy. *Clin Infect Dis* **40**:1384-5.

272. Arguin, P. M. 1999. Human rabies prevention - United States, 1999. Recommendations of the Advisory Committee on Immunization Practices (ACIP). *MMWR* **49 (RR-1)**:1-21.

273. Arias, C. A., G. Quintero, B. E. Vanegas, C. L. Rico, and J. F. Patino. 2003. Surveillance of surgical site infections: decade of experience at a Colombian tertiary care center. *World J Surg* **27**:529-33.

274. Arikawa, J., K. Yoshimatsu, and H. Kariwa. 2001. Epidemiology and epizootiology of hantavirus infection in Japan. *Jpn J Infect Dis* **54**:95-102.

275. Arisue, N., T. Hashimoto, H. Yoshikawa, Y. Nakamura, G. Nakamura, F. Nakamura, T. A. Yano, and M. Hasegawa. 2002. Phylogenetic position of Blastocystis hominis and of stramenopiles inferred from multiple molecular sequence data. *J Eukaryot Microbiol* **49**:42-53.

276. Arita, I., Z. Jezek, L. Khodakevich, and K. Ruti. 1985. Human monkeypox: a newly emerged orthopoxvirus zoonosis in the tropical rain forests of Africa. *Am J Trop Med Hyg* **34**:781-9.

277. Armand-Lefevre, L., R. Ruimy, and A. Andremont. 2005. Clonal comparison of Staphylococcus aureus isolates from healthy pig farmers, human controls, and pigs. *Emerg Infect Dis* **11**:711-4.

278. Armengaud, A., N. Kessalis, J. C. Desenclos, E. Maillot, P. Brousse, P. Brouqui, H. Tixier-Dupont, D. Raoult, P. Provensal, and Y. Obadia. 1997. Urban outbreak of Q fever, Briançon, France, march to june 1996. *Eurosurveillance* **2**:12-15.

279. Armstrong, C. W., S. R. Jenkins, L. Kaufman, T. M. Kerkering, B. S. Rouse, and G. B. Miller, Jr. 1987. Common-source outbreak of blastomycosis in hunters and their dogs. *J Infect Dis* **155**:568-70.

280. Armstrong, G. L., J. Hollingsworth, and J. G. Morris, Jr. 1996. Emerging foodborne pathogens: Escherichia coli O157:H7 as a model of entry of a new pathogen into the food supply of the developed world. *Epidemiol Rev* **18**:29-51.

281. Armstrong, L. R., S. R. Zaki, M. J. Goldoft, R. L. Todd, A. S. Khan, R. F. Khabbaz, T. G. Ksiazek, and C. J. Peters. 1995. Hantavirus pulmonary syndrome associated with entering or cleaning rarely used, rodent-infested structures. *J Infect Dis* **172**:1166.

282. Arness, M. K., J. D. Brown, J. P. Dubey, R. C. Neafie, and D. E. Granstrom. 1999. An outbreak of acute eosinophilic myositis attributed to human Sarcocystis parasitism. *Am J Trop Med Hyg* **61**:548-53.

283. Arness, M. K., B. H. Feighner, M. L. Canham, D. N. Taylor, S. S. Monroe, T. J. Cieslak, E. L. Hoedebecke, C. S. Polyak, J. C. Cuthie, R. L. Fankhauser, C. D. Humphrey, T. L. Barker, C. D. Jenkins, and D. R. Skillman. 2000. Norwalk-like viral gastroenteritis outbreak in U.S. Army trainees. *Emerg Infect Dis* **6**:204-7.

284. Arnez, M., T. Luznik-Bufon, T. Avsic-Zupanc, E. Ruzic-Sabljic, M. Petrovec, S. Lotric-Furlan, and F. Strle. 2003. Causes of febrile illnesses after a tick bite in Slovenian children. *Pediatr Infect Dis J* **22**:1078-83.

285. Arnon, S. S., R. Schechter, T. V. Inglesby, D. A. Henderson, J. G. Bartlett, M. S. Ascher, E. Eitzen, A. D. Fine, J. Hauer, M. Layton, S. Lillibridge, M. T. Osterholm, T. O'Toole, G. Parker, T. M. Perl, P. K. Russell, D. L. Swerdlow, and K. Tonat. 2001. Botulinum toxin as a biological weapon: medical and public health management. *JAMA* **285**:1059-70.

286. Arnow, P. M., R. L. Andersen, P. D. Mainous, and E. J. Smith. 1978. Pumonary aspergillosis during hospital renovation. *Am Rev Respir Dis* **118**:49-53.

287. Arnow, P. M., T. Chou, D. Weil, E. N. Shapiro, and C. Kretzschmar. 1982. Nosocomial Legionnaires' disease caused by aerosolized tap water from respiratory devices. *J Infect Dis* **146**:460-7.

288. Arnow, P. M., S. Garcia-Houchins, M. B. Neagle, J. L. Bova, J. J. Dillon, and T. Chou. 1998. An outbreak of bloodstream infections arising from hemodialysis equipment. *J Infect Dis* **178**:783-91.

289. Arnow, P. M., S. G. Houchins, and G. Pugliese. 1991. An outbreak of tinea corporis in hospital personnel caused by a patient with Trichophyton tonsurans infection. *Pediatr Infect Dis J* **10**:355-9.

290. Arnow, P. M., S. G. Houchins, J. M. Richards, and R. Chudy. 1991. Aspergillus fumigatus contamination of lymphokine-activated killer cells infused into cancer patients. *J Clin Microbiol* **29**:1038-41.

291. Arnow, P. M., M. Sadigh, C. Costas, D. Weil, and R. Chudy. 1991. Endemic and epidemic aspergillosis associated with in-hospital replication of Aspergillus organisms. *J Infect Dis* **164**:998-1002.

292. Arnow, P. M., M. Smaron, and V. Ormiste. 1984. Brucellosis in a group of travelers to Spain. *JAMA* **251**:505-7.

293. Aronson, N., M. Ananthakrishnan, W. Bernstein, L. Hochberg, M. Marovich, C. Ockenhouse, I. Yoon, P. Weina, P. Benson, J. Fischer, D. Hack, C. Hawkes, M. Polhemus, G. Wortmann, P. McEvoy, R. Neafie, R. DeFraites, and B. L. Herwaldt. 2004. Update: cutaneous leishmaniasis in U.S. military personnel—southwest/central Asia, 2002-2004. *MMWR* **53**:264-5.

294. Arora, N. K., S. K. Panda, S. K. Nanda, I. H. Ansari, S. Joshi, R. Dixit, and R. Bathla. 1999. Hepatitis E infection in children: study of an outbreak. *J Gastroenterol Hepatol* **14**:572-7.

295. Arseculeratne, S. N. 2005. Rhinosporidiosis: what is the cause? *Curr Opin Infect Dis* **18**:113-8.

296. Arsenault, J., C. Girard, P. Dubreuil, D. Daignault, J. R. Galarneau, J. Boisclair, C. Simard, and D. Belanger. 2003. Prevalence of and carcass condemnation from maedi-visna, paratuberculosis and caseous lymphadenitis in culled sheep from Quebec, Canada. *Prev Vet Med* **59**:67-81.

297. Arshi, S., H. Sadeghi, A. Majidpour, Z. Zarifi, M. Nouraei, H. Sezavar, and R. Ghasemi. 2003. A simple mistake responsible for 153 cases of muscular cold abscesses. *Vaccine* **21**:4120-1.

298. Arthur, R. R., M. S. el-Sharkawy, S. E. Cope, B. A. Botros, S. Oun, J. C. Morrill, R. E. Shope, R. G. Hibbs, M. A. Darwish, and I. Z. Imam. 1993. Recurrence of Rift valley fever in Egypt. *Lancet* **342**:1149-50.

299. Arvanitidou, M., P. Mamassi, and A. Vayona. 2004. Epidemiological evidence for vaccinating wastewater treatment plant workers against hepatitis A and hepatitis B virus. *Eur J Epidemiol* **19**:259-62.

300. Arvidson, M., D. Hellberg, and P. A. Mardh. 1996. Sexual risk behavior and history of sexually transmitted diseases in relation to casual travel sex during different types of journeys. *Acta Obstet Gynecol Scand* **75**:490-4.

301. Arvin, A. M., C. M. Koropchak, and A. E. Wittek. 1983. Immunologic evidence of reinfection with varicella-zoster virus. *J Infect Dis* **148**:200-5.

302. Asano, Y., T. Yoshikawa, M. Ihira, H. Furukawa, K. Suzuki, and S. Suga. 1999. Spread of varicella-zoster virus DNA to family members and environments from siblings with varicella in a household. *Pediatrics* **103**:e61.

303. Asao, T., Y. Kumeda, T. Kawai, T. Shibata, H. Oda, K. Haruki, H. Nakazawa, and S. Kozaki. 2003. An extensive outbreak of staphylococcal food poisoning due to low-fat milk in Japan: estimation of enterotoxin A in the incriminated milk and powdered skim milk. *Epidemiol Infect* **130**:33-40.

304. Asaolu, S. O., I. E. Ofoezie, P. A. Odumuyiwa, O. A. Sowemimo, and T. A. Ogunniyi. 2002. Effect of water supply and sanitation on the prevalence and intensity of Ascaris lumbricoides among pre-school-age children in Ajebandele and Ifewara, Osun State, Nigeria. *Trans R Soc Trop Med Hyg* **96**:600-4.

305. Asari, S., M. Deguchi, K. Tahara, M. Taniike, M. Toyokawa, I. Nishi, M. Watanabe, Y. Iwatani, and K. Makimoto. 2003. Seroprevalence survey of measles, rubella, varicella, and mumps antibodies in health care workers and evaluation of a vaccination program in a tertiary care hospital in Japan. *Am J Infect Control* **31**:157-62.

306. Asato, R., K. Taira, M. Nakamura, J. Kudaka, K. Itokazu, and M. Kawanaka. 2004. Changing epidemiology of angiostrongyliasis cantonensis in Okinawa prefecture, Japan. *Jpn J Infect Dis* **57**:184-6.

307. Ash, R. J., B. Mauck, and M. Morgan. 2002. Antibiotic resistance of gram-negative bacteria in rivers, United States. *Emerg Infect Dis* **8**:713-6.

308. Ashbolt, R., R. Givney, J. E. Gregory, G. Hall, R. Hundy, M. Kirk, I. McKay, L. Meuleners, G. Millard, J. Raupach, P. Roche, N. Prasopa-Plaizier, M. K. Sama, R. Stafford, N. Tomaska, L. Unicomb, and C. L. Williams. 2002. Enhancing foodborne disease surveillance across Australia in 2001: the OzFoodNet working group. *Commun Dis Intell* **26**:375-406.

309. Ashbolt, R. H., D. J. Coleman, A. Misrachi, J. M. Conti, and M. D. Kirk. 2003. An outbreak of cryptosporidiosis associated

with an animal nursery at a regional fair. *Commun Dis Intell* 27:244-8.
310. **Ashdown, L. R.** 1979. Nosocomial infection due to Pseudomonas pseudomallei: two cases and an epidemiologic study. *Rev Infect Dis* 1:891-4.
311. **Ashdown, L. R.** 1992. Melioidosis and safety in the clinical laboratory. *J Hosp Infect* 21:301-6.
312. **Ashford, D. A., J. di Pietra, J. Lingappa, C. Woods, H. Noll, B. Neville, R. Weyant, S. L. Bragg, R. A. Spiegel, J. Tappero, and B. A. Perkins.** 2004. Adverse events in humans associated with accidental exposure to the livestock brucellosis vaccine RB51. *Vaccine* 22:3435-9.
313. **Ashford, D. A., R. A. Hajjeh, M. F. Kelley, L. Kaufman, L. Hutwagner, and M. M. McNeil.** 1999. Outbreak of histoplasmosis among cavers attending the National Speleological Society Annual Convention, Texas, 1994. *Am J Trop Med Hyg* 60:899-903.
314. **Ashford, D. A., R. M. Kaiser, R. A. Spiegel, B. A. Perkins, R. S. Weyant, S. L. Bragg, B. Plikaytis, C. Jarquin, J. O. De Lose Reyes, and J. J. Amador.** 2000. Asymptomatic infection and risk factors for leptospirosis in Nicaragua. *Am J Trop Med Hyg* 63:249-54.
315. **Ashford, R. F. U., and D. C. Shanson.** 1978. El Tor cholera: a cautionary tale. *Lancet* 1 (**March 11**):550.
316. **Ashford, R. W., G. Barnish, and M. E. Viney.** 1992. Strongyloides fuelleborni kellyi: infection and disease in Papua New Guinea. *Parasitol Today* 8:314-8.
317. **Ashford, R. W., G. D. Reid, and T. M. Butynski.** 1990. The intestinal faunas of man and mountain gorillas in a shared habitat. *Ann Trop Med Parasitol* 84:337-40.
318. **Askling, H. H., J. Nilsson, A. Tegnell, R. Janzon, and K. Ekdahl.** 2005. Malaria risk in travelers. *Emerg Infect Dis* 11:436-41.
319. **Asmundsdottir, L. R., H. Erlendsdottir, and M. Gottfredsson.** 2002. Increasing incidence of candidemia: results from a 20-year nationwide study in iceland. *J Clin Microbiol* 40:3489-92.
320. **Aspinall, T. V., D. Marlee, J. E. Hyde, and P. F. Sims.** 2002. Prevalence of Toxoplasma gondii in commercial meat products as monitored by polymerase chain reaction—food for thought? *Int J Parasitol* 32:1193-9.
321. **Aspiroz, C., M. Ara, M. Varea, A. Rezusta, and C. Rubio.** 2002. Isolation of Malassezia globosa and M. sympodialis from patients with pityriasis versicolor in Spain. *Mycopathologia* 154:111-7.
322. **Assadian, O., A. Berger, C. Aspock, S. Mustafa, C. Kohlhauser, and A. M. Hirschl.** 2002. Nosocomial outbreak of Serratia marcescens in a neonatal intensive care unit. *Infect Control Hosp Epidemiol* 23:457-61.
323. **Astagneau, P., N. Desplaces, V. Vincent, V. Chicheportiche, A. Botherel, S. Maugat, K. Lebascle, P. Leonard, J. Desenclos, J. Grosset, J. Ziza, and G. Brucker.** 2001. Mycobacterium xenopi spinal infections after discovertebral surgery: investigation and screening of a large outbreak. *Lancet* 358:747-51.
324. **Asumu, P. N., and J. M. Milleliri.** 2004. Situation de la trypanosomiase en Guinée équatoriale. *Med Trop* 64:121.
325. **Aszkenasy, O. M.** 2000. A community outbreak of hepatitis A in a religious community in Indiana: failure of immune serum globulin to prevent the spread of infection. *Epidemiol Infect* 124:309-13.
326. **Athar, M. N., H. Z. Baqai, M. Ahmad, M. A. Khalid, N. Bashir, A. M. Ahmad, A. H. Balouch, and K. Bashir.** 2003. Short report: Crimean-Congo hemorrhagic fever outbreak in Rawalpindi, Pakistan, February 2002. *Am J Trop Med Hyg* 69:284-7.
327. **Athar, M. N., M. A. Khalid, A. M. Ahmad, N. Bashir, H. Z. Baqai, M. Ahmad, A. H. Balouch, and K. Bashir.** 2005. Crimean-Congo hemorrhagic fever outbreak in Rawalpindi, Pakistan, February 2002: contact tracing and risk assessment. *Am J Trop Med Hyg* 72:471-3.
328. **Atkinson, J., B. R. Edlin, E. A. Engels, A. H. Kral, K. Seal, C. J. Gamache, D. Whitby, and T. R. O'Brien.** 2003. Seroprevalence of Human Herpesvirus 8 among Injection Drug Users in San Francisco. *J Infect Dis* 187:974-81.
329. **Atlas, R. M., J. F. Williams, and M. K. Huntington.** 1995. Legionella contamination of dental-unit waters. *Appl Environ Microbiol* 61:1208-13.
330. **Attwood, S. W., I. Campbell, E. S. Upatham, and D. Rollinson.** 2004. Schistosomes in the Xe Kong river of Cambodia: the detection of Schistosoma mekongi in a natural population of snails and observations on the intermediate host's distribution. *Ann Trop Med Parasitol* 98:221-30.
331. **Attye, A., P. Auger, and J. Joly.** 1990. Incidence of occult athlete's foot in swimmers. *Eur J Epidemiol* 6:244-7.
332. **Aubert, J. M., M. J. Gobeaux-Castadot, and M. C. Boria.** 1980. Actinomyces in the endometrium of IUD users. *Contraception* 21:577-83.
333. **Aubry, A., O. Chosidow, E. Caumes, J. Robert, and E. Cambau.** 2002. Sixty-three cases of Mycobacterium marinum infection: clinical features, treatment, and antibiotic susceptibility of causative isolates. *Arch Intern Med* 162:1746-52.
334. **Aubry-Damon, H., K. Grenet, P. Sall-Ndiaye, D. Che, E. Cordeiro, M. E. Bougnoux, E. Rigaud, Y. Le Strat, V. Lemanissier, L. Armand-Lefevre, M. Delzescaux, J. C. Desenclos, M. Lienard, and A. Andremont.** 2004. Antimicrobial resistance in commensal flora of pig farmers. *Emerg Infect Dis* 10:873-9.
335. **AuBuchon, J. P., and W. H. Dzik.** 1983. Survival of Loa loa in banked blood. *Lancet* 1:647-8.
336. **Audicana, M. T., I. J. Ansotegui, L. F. de Corres, and M. W. Kennedy.** 2002. Anisakis simplex: dangerous - dead and alive? *Trends in Parasitology* 18:20-5.
337. **Auer, C.** 1990. Health status of children living in a squatter area of Manila, Philippines, with particular emphasis on intestinal parasitoses. *Southeast Asian J Trop Med Public Health* 21:289-300.
338. **Auerbach, S. B., B. Schwartz, D. Williams, M. G. Fiorilli, A. A. Adimora, R. F. Breiman, and W. R. Jarvis.** 1992. Outbreak of invasive group A streptococcal infections in a nursing home. Lessons on prevention and control. *Arch Intern Med* 152:1017-22.
339. **Aufiero, P., N. Karabulut, D. Rumowitz, S. Shah, J. Nsubuga, B. Piepszak, R. D. Salter, E. Bresnitz, C. R. Lacy, C. Robertson, and C. Tan.** 2004. Imported Lassa fever - New Jersey, 2004. *MMWR* 53:894-7.
340. **Auger, P., G. Marquis, J. Joly, and A. Attye.** 1993. Epidemiology of tinea pedis in marathon runners: prevalence of occult athlete's foot. *Mycoses* 36:35-41.
341. **Aureli, P., M. Di Cunto, A. Maffei, G. De Chiara, G. Franciosa, L. Accorinti, A. M. Gambardella, and D. Greco.** 2000. An outbreak in Italy of botulism associated with a dessert made with mascarpone cream cheese. *Eur J Epidemiol* 16:913-8.
342. **Aureli, P., G. C. Fiorucci, D. Caroli, G. Marchiaro, O. Novara, L. Leone, and S. Salmaso.** 2000. An outbreak of febrile gas-

troenteritis associated with corn contaminated by Listeria monocytogenes. *N Engl J Med* **342:**1236-41.

343. **Aureli, P., G. Franciosa, and A. L. Fenicia.** 2002. Infant botulism and honey in Europe: a commentary. *Pediatr Infect Dis J* **21:**866-8.

344. **Austin, D. J., M. J. Bonten, R. A. Weinstein, S. Slaughter, and R. M. Anderson.** 1999. Vancomycin-resistant enterococci in intensive-care hospital settings: transmission dynamics, persistence, and the impact of infection control programs. *Proc Natl Acad Sci USA* **96:**6908-13.

345. **Autorino, G. L., A. Battisti, V. Deubel, G. Ferrari, R. Forletta, A. Giovannini, R. Lelli, S. Murri, and M. T. Scicluna.** 2002. West Nile virus Epidemic in Horses, Tuscany Region, Italy. *Emerg Infect Dis* **8:**1372-8.

346. **Avashia, S. B., J. M. Petersen, C. M. Lindley, M. E. Schriefer, K. L. Gage, M. Cetron, T. A. DeMarcus, D. K. Kim, J. Buck, J. A. Montenieri, J. L. Lowell, M. F. Antolin, M. Y. Kosoy, L. G. Carter, M. C. Chu, K. A. Hendricks, D. T. Dennis, and J. L. Kool.** 2004. First reported prairie dog-to-human tularemia transmission, Texas, 2002. *Emerg Infect Dis* **10:**483-6.

347. **Avendano, L. F., M. A. Palomino, and C. Larranaga.** 2003. Surveillance for respiratory syncytial virus in infants hospitalized for acute lower respiratory infection in Chile (1989 to 2000). *J Clin Microbiol* **41:**4879-82.

348. **Avery, R. K., and P. Ljungman.** 2001. Prophylactic measures in the solid-organ recipient before transplantation. *Clin Infect Dis* **33 Suppl 1:**S15-21.

349. **Aviles, G., M. S. Sabattini, and C. J. Mitchell.** 1992. Transmission of western equine encephalomyelitis virus by Argentine Aedes albifasciatus (Diptera: Culicidae). *J Med Entomol* **29:**850-3.

350. **Awofeso, N., M. Fennell, Z. Waliuzzaman, C. O'Connor, D. Pittam, L. Boonwaat, S. de Kantzow, and W. D. Rawlinson.** 2001. Influenza outbreak in a correctional facility. *Aust N Z J Public Health* **25:**443-6.

351. **Ayadi, A., F. Makni, and M. Ben Said.** 1997. Etat actuel de la fasciolose en Tunisie. *Bull Soc Fr Parasitol* **15:**27-32.

352. **Ayaya, S. O., K. K. Kamar, and R. Kakai.** 2001. Aetiology of tinea capitis in school children. *East Afr Med J* **78:**531-535.

353. **Aye, T. T., and P. Siriarayapon.** 2004. Typhoid fever outbreak in Madaya Township, Mandalay Division, Myanmar, September 2000. *J Med Assoc Thai* **87:**395-9.

354. **Aye, T. T., T. Uchida, X. Z. Ma, F. Iida, T. Shikata, H. Zhuang, and K. M. Win.** 1992. Complete nucleotide sequence of a hepatitis E virus isolated from the Xinjiang epidemic (1986-1988) of China. *Nucleic Acids Res* **20:**3512.

355. **Ayliffe, G. A., A. M. Geddes, J. E. Pearson, and T. C. Williams.** 1979. Spread of Salmonella typhi in a maternity hospital. *J Hyg (Lond)* **82:**353-9.

356. **Aylward, R. B., A. Acharya, S. England, M. Agocs, and J. Linkins.** 2003. Global health goals: lessons from the worldwide effort to eradicate poliomyelitis. *Lancet* **362:**909-14.

357. **Ayora-Talavera, G., J. M. Cadavieco-Burgos, and A. B. Canul-Armas.** 2005. Serologic evidence of human and swine influenza in Mayan persons. *Emerg Infect Dis* **11:**158-61.

358. **Ayukawa, R., H. Fujimoto, M. Ayabe, H. Shoji, R. Matsui, Y. Iwata, H. Fukuda, K. Ochi, K. Noda, Y. Ono, K. Sakai, Y. Takehisa, and K. Yasui.** 2004. An unexpected outbreak of Japanese encephalitis in the Chugoku district of Japan, 2002. *Jpn J Infect Dis* **57:**63-6.

359. **Ayyildiz, A., A. E. Aktas, and H. Yazgi.** 2003. Nasopharyngeal carriage rate of Haemophilus influenzae in children aged 7-12 years in Turkey. *Int J Clin Practice* **57:**686-8.

360. **Azad, A. f., and C. B. Beard.** 1998. Rickettsial pathogens and their arthropod vectors. *Emerg Infect Dis* **4:**179-86.

361. **Azad, A. F., S. Radulovic, J. A. Higgins, B. H. Noden, and J. M. Troyer.** 1997. Flea-borne rickettsioses: ecologic considerations. *Emerg Infect Dis* **3:**319-27.

362. **Azevedo, R. A., A. E. Silva, M. L. Ferraz, L. F. Marcopito, and R. G. Baruzzi.** 1996. [Prevalence of serologic markers of hepatitis B and D viruses in children of the Caiabi and Txucarramae tribes from the Indian Reservation of Xingu, central Brazil]. *Rev Soc Bras Med Trop* **29:**431-9.

363. **Azimi, P. H., R. R. Roberto, J. Guralnik, T. Livermore, S. Hoag, S. Hagens, and N. Lugo.** 1986. Transfusion-acquired hepatitis A in a premature infant with secondary nosocomial spread in an intensive care nursery. *Am J Dis Child* **140:**23-7.

364. **Baba, S. S., A. H. Fagbami, and C. K. Ojeh.** 1999. Preliminary studies on the use of solid-phase immunosorbent techniques for the rapid detection of Wesselsbron virus (WSLV) IgM by haemagglutination-inhibition. *Comp Immunol Microbiol Infect Dis* **22:**71-9.

365. **Babcock, H. M., C. Carroll, M. Matava, P. L'Ecuyer, and V. Fraser.** 2003. Surgical site infections after arthroscopy: Outbreak investigation and case control study. *Arthroscopy* **19:**172-81.

366. **Babic-Erceg, A., Z. Klismanic, M. Erceg, D. Tandara, and M. Smoljanovic.** 2003. An outbreak of Yersinia enterocolitica O:3 infections on an oil tanker. *Eur J Epidemiol* **18:**1159-61.

367. **Babiker, H. A., A. M. Abdel-Muhsin, L. C. Ranford-Cartwright, G. Satti, and D. Walliker.** 1998. Characteristics of Plasmodium falciparum parasites that survive the lengthy dry season in eastern Sudan where malaria transmission is markedly seasonal. *Am J Trop Med Hyg* **59:**582-90.

368. **Babinet, J., F. Gay, D. Bustos, M. Dubarry, D. Jaulmes, L. Nguyen, and M. Gentilini.** 1991. Transmission of Plasmodium falciparum by heart transplant. *BMJ* **303:**1515-6.

369. **Bacaner, N., B. Stauffer, D. R. Boulware, P. F. Walker, and J. S. Keystone.** 2004. Travel medicine considerations for North American immigrants visiting friends and relatives. *JAMA* **291:**2856-64.

370. **Bachmeyer, C., L. Blum, S. Stelianides, B. Benchaa, N. Gruat, and O. Danne.** 2002. Mycobacterium xenopi pulmonary infection in an HIV infected patient under highly active antiretroviral treatment. *Sex Transm Infect* **78:**60-1.

371. **Backhouse, J. L., B. J. Hudson, P. A. Hamilton, and S. I. Nesteroff.** 1998. Failure of penicillin treatment of yaws on Karkar Island, Papua New Guinea. *Am J Trop Med Hyg* **59:**388-92.

372. **Baddour, L. M., M. A. Bettmann, A. F. Bolger, A. E. Epstein, P. Ferrieri, M. A. Gerber, M. H. Gewitz, A. K. Jacobs, M. E. Levison, J. W. Newburger, T. J. Pallasch, W. R. Wilson, R. S. Baltimore, D. A. Falace, S. T. Shulman, L. Y. Tani, and K. A. Taubert.** 2003. Nonvalvular cardiovascular device-related infections. *Circulation* **108:**2015-31.

373. **Baddour, L. M., S. M. Gaia, R. Griffin, and R. Hudson.** 1986. A hospital cafeteria-related food-borne outbreak due to Bacillus cereus: unique features. *Infect Control* **7:**462-5.

374. **Baden, L. R., W. Thiemke, A. Skolnik, R. Chambers, J. Strymish, H. S. Gold, R. C. Moellering, Jr., and G. M. Eliopoulos.** 2001. Prolonged colonization with vancomycin-

resistant Enterococcus faecium in long-term care patients and the significance of "clearance". *Clin Infect Dis* **33**:1654-60.

375. **Bader, M., A. H. Pedersen, R. Williams, J. Spearman, and H. Anderson.** 1977. Venereal transmission of shigellosis in Seattle-King county. *Sex Transm Dis* **4**:89-91.

376. **Badiaga, S., P. Brouqui, and D. Raoult.** 2005. Autochthonous epidemic typhus associated with Bartonella quintana bacteremia in a homeless person. *Am J Trop Med Hyg* **72**:638-9.

377. **Badiaga, S., J. Delmont, P. Brouqui, F. Janbon, J. Durant, A. Bosseray, D. Malvy, E. Bonnet, A. Sotto, S. Dydymski, and D. Peyramond.** 1999. [Imported dengue: study of 44 cases observed from 1994 to 1997 in 9 university hospital centers. Infectio-Sud-France group]. *Pathol Biol (Paris)* **47**:539-42.

378. **Badilla, X., V. Pérez-Herra, L. Quirós, A. Morice, E. Jimenez, E. Saenz, F. Salazar, R. Fernandez, L. Orciari, P. Yager, S. Whitfield, and C. E. Rupprecht.** 2003. Human rabies: a reemerging disease in Costa Rica? *Emerg Infect Dis* **9**:721-3.

379. **Badrinath, P., T. Sundkvist, H. Mahgoub, and R. Kent.** 2004. An outbreak of Salmonella enteritidis phage type 34a infection associated with a Chinese restaurant in Suffolk, United Kingdom. *BMC Public Health* **4**:40.

380. **Bae, H. G., C. Drosten, P. Emmerich, R. Colebunders, P. Hantson, S. Pest, M. Parent, H. Schmitz, M. A. Warnat, and M. Niedrig.** 2005. Analysis of two imported cases of yellow fever infection from Ivory Coast and The Gambia to Germany and Belgium. *J Clin Virol* **33**:274-80.

381. **BAG (Bundesamt für Gesundheit).** 1997. Chemisches Monitoring von Strassenheroin und -cocain in der Stadt Bern (1995-1996). *Bull Bundesamt Gesundheit* **20**:8-9.

382. **BAG (Bundesamt für Gesundheit).** 2004. Campylobacter und Salmonella - Stand Ende 2003. *Bulletin Bundesamt für Gesundheit* **40**:737-40.

383. **Bahia-Oliveira, L. M., J. L. Jones, J. Azevedo-Silva, C. C. Alves, F. Orefice, and D. G. Addiss.** 2003. Highly endemic, waterborne toxoplasmosis in north Rio de Janeiro state, Brazil. *Emerg Infect Dis* **9**:55-62.

384. **Bailey, G. D., B. A. Vanselow, M. A. Hornitzky, S. I. Hum, G. J. Eamens, P. A. Gill, K. H. Walker, and J. P. Cronin.** 2003. A study of the foodborne pathogens: Campylobacter, Listeria and Yersinia, in faeces from slaughter-age cattle and sheep in Australia. *Commun Dis Intell* **27**:249-57.

385. **Bailey, J. V., J. Kavanagh, C. Owen, K. A. McLean, and C. J. Skinner.** 2000. Lesbians and cervical screening. *Br J Gen Pract* **50**:481-2.

386. **Baillargeon, J., M. F. Kelley, C. T. Leach, G. Baillargeon, and B. H. Pollock.** 2004. Methicillin-resistant Staphylococcus aureus infection in the Texas prison system. *Clin Infect Dis* **38**:e92-5.

387. **Bailly, J. L., A. Beguet, M. Chambon, C. Henquell, and H. Peigue-Lafeuille.** 2000. Nosocomial transmission of echovirus 30: molecular evidence by phylogenetic analysis of the VP1 encoding sequence. *J Clin Microbiol* **38**:2889-92.

388. **Bair, M. J., K. P. Hwang, T. E. Wang, T. C. Liou, S. C. Lin, C. R. Kao, T. Y. Wang, and K. K. Pang.** 2004. Clinical features of human intestinal capillariasis in Taiwan. *World J Gastroenterol* **10**:2391-3.

389. **Baird, J. K., H. Basri, P. Weina, J. D. MaGuire, M. J. Barcus, H. Picarema, I. R. Elyazar, E. Ayomi, and Sekartuti.** 2003. Adult Javanese migrants to Indonesian Papua at high risk of severe disease caused by malaria. *Epidemiol Infect* **131**:791-7.

390. **Baird, R. W., H. Teichtahl, H. M. Ednie, A. Tasiopoulos, N. Ryanf, and D. Gee.** 1999. A fluffy white traveller: imported Coccidiodes immitis infection in an Australian tourist. *Pathology* **31**:47-50.

391. **Baisley, K. J., D. M. Watts, L. E. Munstermann, and M. L. Wilson.** 1998. Epidemiology of endemic Oropouche virus transmission in upper Amazonian Peru. *Am J Trop Med Hyg* **59**:710-6.

392. **Bakari, M., E. Lyamuya, F. Mugusi, E. Aris, S. Chale, P. Magao, R. Jossiah, M. Janabi, A. Swai, N. Pallangyo, E. Sandstrom, F. Mhalu, G. Biberfeld, and K. Pallangyo.** 2000. The prevalence and incidence of HIV-1 infection and syphilis in a cohort of police officers in Dar es Salaam, Tanzania: a potential population for HIV vaccine trials. *AIDS* **14**:313-20.

393. **Bakari, M., W. Urassa, K. Pallangyo, A. Swai, F. Mhalu, G. Biberfeld, and E. Sandstrom.** 2004. The natural course of disease following HIV-1 infection in dar es salaam, Tanzania: a study among hotel workers relating clinical events to CD4 T-lymphocyte counts. *Scand J Infect Dis* **36**:466-73.

394. **Baker, D. G.** 1998. Natural pathogens of laboratory mice, rats, and rabbits and their effects on research. *Clin Microbiol Rev* **11**:231-66.

395. **Baker, K. H., and J. P. Hegarty.** 2001. Presence of Helicobacter pylori in drinking water is associated with clinical infection. *Scand J Infect Dis* **33**:744-6.

396. **Baker, M., D. Martin, C. Kieft, N. Jones, and D. Lennon.** 1999. The evolving meningococcal disease epidemic in New Zealand. *N Z Public Health Rep* **6**:57-61.

397. **Baker, M., A. McNicholas, N. Garrett, N. Jones, J. Stewart, V. Koberstein, and D. Lennon.** 2000. Household crowding a major risk factor for epidemic meningococcal disease in Auckland children. *Pediatr Infect Dis J* **19**:983-90.

398. **Baker, M., P. Taylor, E. Wilson, and P. Short.** 1998. A case of diphtheria in Auckland - implications for disease control. *N Z Public Health Rep* **5**:73-6.

399. **Baker, W. M., B. M. Simone, J. T. Niemann, and A. Daly.** 1986. Special event medical care: the 1984 Los Angeles Summer Olympics experience. *Ann Emerg Med* **15**:185-90.

400. **Bakhshi, S. S.** 2001. Code of practice for funeral workers: managing infection risk and body bagging. *Commun Dis Public Health* **4**:283-7.

401. **Bakir, M., A. Yagci, N. Ulger, C. Akbenlioglu, A. Ilki, and G. Soyletir.** 2001. Asymtomatic carriage of Neisseria meningitidis and Neisseria lactamica in relation to Streptococcus pneumoniae and Haemophilus influenzae colonization in healthy children: apropos of 1400 children sampled. *Eur J Epidemiol* **17**:1015-8.

402. **Bakker, M. I., M. Hatta, A. Kwenang, P. R. Klatser, and L. Oskam.** 2002. Epidemiology of leprosy on five isolated islands in the Flores Sea, Indonesia. *Trop Med Int Health* **7**:780-7.

403. **Bakker, M. I., M. Hatta, A. Kwenang, B. H. Van Benthem, S. M. Van Beers, P. R. Klatser, and L. Oskam.** 2005. Prevention of leprosy using rifampicin as chemoprophylaxis. *Am J Trop Med Hyg* **72**:443-8.

404. **Balaka, B., A. D. Agbere, P. Bonkoungou, K. Kessie, K. Assimadi, and K. Agbo.** 2000. Paludism congénital-maladie à Plasmodium falciparum chez le nouveau-né à risque infectieux. *Arch Pediatr* **7**:243-8.

405. **Balayeva, N. M., M. E. Eremeeva, F. Ignatovich, N. V. Rudakov, T. A. Reschetnikova, I. E. Samoilenko, V. K. Yastrebov, and D. Raoult.** 1996. Biological and genetic characterization of Rickettsia sibirica strains isolated in the endemic area of the north Asian tick typhus. *Am J Trop Med Hyg* **1996**:685-92.

406. **Balbino, V. Q., C. B. Marcondes, B. Alexander, L. K. Luna, M. M. Lucena, A. C. Mendes, and P. P. Andrade.** 2001. First report of Lutzomyia (Nyssomyia) umbratilis Ward & Frahia, 1977 outside of Amazonian Region, in Recife, State of Pernambuco, Brazil (Diptera: Psychodidae: Phlebotominae). *Mem Inst Oswaldo Cruz* **96:**315-7.

407. **Balcarek, K. B., R. Bagley, G. A. Cloud, and R. F. Pass.** 1990. Cytomegalovirus infection among employees of a children's hospital. No evidence for increased risk associated with patient care. *JAMA* **263:**840-4.

408. **Baldari, M., A. Tamburro, G. Sabatinelli, R. Romi, C. Severini, G. Cuccagna, G. Fiorilli, M. P. Allegri, C. Buriani, and M. Toti.** 1998. Malaria in Maremma, Italy. *Lancet* **351:**1246-7.

409. **Baldo, E. T., V. Y. Belizario, W. U. De Leon, H. H. Kong, and D. I. Chung.** 2004. Infection status of intestinal parasites in children living in residential institutions in Metro Manila, the Philippines. *Korean J Parasitol* **42:**67-70.

410. **Baldo, V., A. Floreani, T. Menegon, G. Angiolelli, and R. Trivello.** 2000. Prevalence of antibodies against hepatitis C virus in the elderly: a seroepidemiological study in a nursing home and in an open population. The Collaborative Group. *Gerontology* **46:**194-8.

411. **Bales, M. E., A. L. Dannenberg, P. S. Brachman, A. F. Kaufmann, P. C. Klatsky, and D. A. Ashford.** 2002. Epidemiologic response to anthrax outbreaks: field investigations, 1950-2001. *Emerg Infect Dis* **8:**1163-74.

412. **Balfour, C. L., and H. H. Balfour, Jr.** 1986. Cytomegalovirus is not an occupational risk for nurses in renal transplant and neonatal units. Results of a prospective surveillance study. *JAMA* **256:**1909-14.

413. **Balkhy, H. H., Z. A. Memish, S. Bafaqeer, and M. A. Almuneef.** 2004. Influenza a common viral infection among Hajj pilgrims: time for routine surveillance and vaccination. *J Travel Med* **11:**82-6.

414. **Ball, R., and M. Van Wey.** 1997. Tuberculosis skin test conversion among health care workers at a military medical center. *Mil Med* **162:**338-43.

415. **Ball, T. M., and A. L. Wright.** 1999. Health care costs of formula-feeding in the first year of life. *Pediatrics* **103:**870-6.

416. **Balogun, M. A., M. E. Ramsay, C. K. Fairley, M. Collins, and J. Heptonstall.** 1999. Acute hepatitis B infection in England and Wales, 1985-96. *Epidemiol Infect* **122:**125-31.

417. **Banatvala, J. E., and D. W. G. Brown.** 2004. Rubella. *Lancet* **363:**1127-37.

418. **Banatvala, N., A. R. Magnano, M. L. Cartter, T. J. Barrett, W. F. Bibb, L. L. Vasile, P. Mshar, M. A. Lambert-Fair, J. H. Green, N. H. Bean, and R. V. Tauxe.** 1996. Meat grinders and molecular epidemiology: two supermarket outbreaks of Escherichia coli O157:H7 infection. *J Infect Dis* **173:**480-3.

419. **Bancroft, W. H., P. W. Kelley, and E. T. Takafuji.** 1990. The military and hepatitis B. *Vaccine* **8 Suppl:**S33-6; discussion S41-3.

420. **Bandaranayake, D. R., C. E. Salmond, and M. I. Tobias.** 1991. Occupational risk of hepatitis B for police and customs personnel. *Am J Epidemiol* **134:**1447-53.

421. **Bandres, J. C., J. J. Mathewson, C. D. Ericsson, and H. L. Dupont.** 1992. Trimethoprim/sulfamethoxazole remains active against enterotoxigenic Escherichia coli and Shigella species in Guadalajara, Mexico. *Am J Med Sci* **303:**289-91.

422. **Bandyk, D. F., M. L. Novotney, B. L. Johnson, M. R. Back, and S. R. Roth.** 2001. Use of rifampin-soaked gelatin-sealed polyester grafts for in situ treatment of primary aortic and vascular prosthetic infections. *J Surg Res* **95:**44-9.

423. **Banerjee, S. N., M. Banerjee, K. Fernando, W. Burgdorfer, and T. G. Schwan.** 1998. Tick-borne relapsing fever in British Columbia, Canada: first isolation of Borrelia hermsii. *J Clin Microbiol* **36:**3505-8.

424. **Baneth, G., G. Dank, E. Keren-Kornblatt, E. Sekeles, I. Adini, C. L. Eisenberger, L. F. Schnur, R. King, and C. L. Jaffe.** 1998. Emergence of visceral leishmaniasis in central Israel. *Am J Trop Med Hyg* **59:**722-5.

425. **Banish, L. D., R. Sims, M. Bush, D. Sack, and R. J. Montali.** 1993. Clearance of Shigella flexneri carriers in a zoologic collection of primates. *J Am Vet Med Assoc* **203:**133-6.

426. **Banks, M., R. Bendall, S. Grierson, G. Heath, J. Mitchell, and H. Dalton.** 2004. Human and porcine hepatitis E virus strains, United Kingdom. *Emerg Infect Dis* **10:**953-5.

427. **Barbaree, J. M., R. F. Breiman, and A. P. Dufour.** 1993. Legionella. Current status and emerging perspectives. American Society for Microbiology, Washington, D.C.

428. **Barber, D. A., P. B. Bahnson, R. Isaacson, C. J. Jones, and R. M. Weigel.** 2002. Distribution of Salmonella in swine production ecosystems. *J Food Prot* **65:**1861-8.

429. **Barbosa, C. S., A. L. Domingues, F. Abath, S. M. Montenegro, U. Guida, J. Carneiro, B. Tabosa, C. N. Moraes, and V. Spinelli.** 2001. [An outbreak of acute schistosomiasis at Porto de Galinhas beach, Pernambuco, Brazil]. *Cad Saude Publica* **17:**725-8.

430. **Barbosa, F. S., and D. P. Pereira Da Costa.** 1981. Incapacitating effects of schistosomiasis mansoni on the productivity of sugar-cane cutters in northeastern Brazil. *Am J Epidemiol* **114:**102-11.

431. **Barbosa-Cesnik, C., K. Schwartz, and B. Foxman.** 2003. Lactation mastitis. *JAMA* **289:**1609-12.

432. **Barbour, A. G., C. R. Nichols, and T. Fukushima.** 1976. An outbreak of giardiasis in a group of campers. *Am J Trop Med Hyg* **25:**384-9.

433. **Barbut, F., B. Carbonne, F. Truchot, C. Spielvogel, D. Jannet, I. Goderel, V. Lejeune, and J. Milliez.** 2004. [Surgical site infections after cesarean section: results of a five-year prospective surveillance]. *J Gynecol Obstet Biol Reprod (Paris)* **33:**487-96.

434. **Barbut, F., M. Delmee, J. S. Brazier, J. C. Petit, I. R. Poxton, M. Rupnik, V. Lalande, C. Schneider, P. Mastrantonio, R. Alonso, E. Kuipjer, and M. Tvede.** 2003. A European survey of diagnostic methods and testing protocols for Clostridium difficile. *Clin Microbiol Infect* **9:**989-96.

435. **Barbut, F., and J. C. Petit.** 2001. Epidemiology of Clostridium difficile-associated infections. *Clin Microbiol Inf* **7:**405-10.

436. **Bard, D., and J. Lambrozo.** 1992. Les méningo-encéphalites et encéphalites à amibes libres. *Méd Mal Infect* **22:**698-705.

437. **Barker, J., and S. F. Bloomfield.** 2000. Survival of Salmonella in bathrooms and toilets in domestic homes following salmonellosis. *J Appl Microbiol* **89:**137-44.

438. **Barker, T. L., A. L. Richards, E. Laksono, J. L. Sanchez, B. H. Feighner, W. Z. McBride, M. V. Rubertone, and K. C. Hyams.** 2001. Serosurvey of Borrelia burgdorferi infection among U.S. military personnel: a low risk of infection. *Am J Trop Med Hyg* **65:**804-9.

439. **Barker, W. H., J. B. Weissman, V. R. Dowell, L. Gutmann, and D. A. Kautter.** 1977. Type B botulism outbreak caused by a commercial food product. West Virginia and Pennsylvania, 1973. *JAMA* **237**:456-9.

440. **Barker-Hudson, P., B. H. Kay, R. E. Jones, I. D. Fanning, and L. D. Smythe.** 1993. Surveillance of mosquitoes and arbovirus infection at the Ross River Dam (Stage 1), Australia. *J Am Mosq Control Assoc* **9**:389-99.

441. **Barlough, J. E., G. H. Reubel, J. E. Madigan, L. K. Vredevoe, P. E. Miller, and Y. Rikihisa.** 1998. Detection of Ehrlichia risticii, the agent of Potomac horse fever, in freshwater stream snails (Pleuroceridae: Juga spp.) from northern California. *Appl Environ Microbiol* **64**:2888-93.

442. **Barlow, R. S., R. G. Hirst, R. E. Norton, C. Ashhurst-Smith, and K. A. Bettelheim.** 1999. A novel serotype of enteropathogenic Escherichia coli (EPEC) as a major pathogen in an outbreak of infantile diarrhoea. *J Med Microbiol* **48**:1123-5.

443. **Barnes, G. H., and A. T. Edwards.** 1992. An investigation into an outbreak of Salmonella enteritidis phage-type 4 infection and the consumption of custard slices and trifles. *Epidemiol Infect* **109**:397-403.

444. **Barnett, E. D.** 2004. Infectious disease screening for refugees resettled in the United States. *Clin Infect Dis* **39**:833-41.

445. **Barnett, P. G., S. P. Singh, C. Bern, A. W. Hightower, and S. Sundar.** 2005. Virgin soil: the spread of visceral leishmaniasis into Uttar Pradesh, India. *Am J Trop Med Hyg* **73**:720-725.

446. **Baro, T., J. M. Torres-Rodriguez, M. H. De Mendoza, Y. Morera, and C. Alia.** 1998. First identification of autochthonous Cryptococcus neoformans var. gattii isolated from goats with predominantly severe pulmonary disease in Spain. *J Clin Microbiol* **36**:458-61.

447. **Baron, R. C., M. H. Hatch, K. Kleeman, and J. N. MacCormack.** 1982. Aseptic meningitis among members of a high school football team. An outbreak associated with echovirus 16 infection. *JAMA* **248**:1724-7.

448. **Baron, R. C., F. D. Murphy, H. B. Greenberg, C. E. Davis, D. J. Bregman, G. W. Gary, J. M. Hughes, and L. B. Schonberger.** 1982. Norwalk gastrointestinal illness: an outbreak associated with swimming in a recreational lake and secondary person-to-person transmission. *Am J Epidemiol* **115**:163-72.

449. **Baron, S., E. Njamkepo, E. Grimprel, P. Begue, J. C. Desenclos, J. Drucker, and N. Guiso.** 1998. Epidemiology of pertussis in French hospitals in 1993 and 1994: thirty years after a routine use of vaccination. *Pediatr Infect Dis J* **17**:412-8.

450. **Barongo, L. R., M. W. Borgdorff, F. F. Mosha, A. Nicoll, H. Grosskurth, K. P. Senkoro, J. N. Newell, J. Changalucha, A. H. Klokke, J. Z. Killewo, et al.** 1992. The epidemiology of HIV-1 infection in urban areas, roadside settlements and rural villages in Mwanza Region, Tanzania. *AIDS* **6**:1521-8.

451. **Barralet, J., R. Stafford, C. Towner, and P. Smith.** 2004. Outbreak of Salmonella Singapore associated with eating sushi. *Commun Dis Intell* **28**:527-8.

452. **Barrasso, R., J. De Brux, O. Croissant, and G. Orth.** 1987. High prevalence of papillomavirus-associated penile intraepithelial neoplasia in sexual partners of women with cervical intraepithelial neoplasia. *N Engl J Med* **317**:916-23.

453. **Barraza, E. M., S. L. Ludwig, J. C. Gaydos, and J. F. Brundage.** 1999. Reemergence of adenovirus type 4 acute respiratory disease in military trainees: report of an outbreak during a lapse in vaccination. *J Infect Dis* **179**:1531-3.

454. **Barre, N., G. Garris, and E. Camus.** 1995. Propagation of the tick Amblyomma variegatum in the Caribbean. *Rev Sci Tech* **14**:841-55.

455. **Barrera Oro, J. G., and K. T. McKee, Jr.** 1991. Toward a vaccine against Argentine hemorrhagic fever. *Bull Pan Am Health Organ* **25**:118-26.

456. **Barrera, R., C. Ferro, J. C. Navarro, J. Freier, J. Liria, R. Salas, M. Ahumada, C. Vasquez, M. Gonzalez, W. Kang, J. Boshell, and S. C. Weaver.** 2002. Contrasting sylvatic foci of Venezuelan equine encephalitis virus in northern South America. *Am J Trop Med Hyg* **67**:324-34.

457. **Barrera, R., M. E. Grillet, Y. Rangel, J. Berti, and A. Ache.** 1999. Temporal and spatial patterns of malaria reinfection in northeastern Venezuela. *Am J Trop Med Hyg* **61**:784-90.

458. **Barreto, A., M. Aragon, and P. R. Epstein.** 1995. Bubonic plague outbreak in Mozambique, 1994. *Lancet* **345**:983-4.

459. **Bartholomew, C., W. C. Saxinger, J. W. Clark, M. Gail, A. Dudgeon, B. Mahabir, B. Hull-Drysdale, F. Cleghorn, R. C. Gallo, and W. A. Blattner.** 1987. Transmission of HTLV-I and HIV among homosexual men in Trinidad. *JAMA* **257**:2604-8.

460. **Bartholomot, G., D. A. Vuitton, S. Harraga, Z. Shi da, P. Giraudoux, G. Barnish, Y. H. Wang, C. N. MacPherson, and P. S. Craig.** 2002. Combined ultrasound and serologic screening for hepatic alveolar echinococcosis in central China. *Am J Trop Med Hyg* **66**:23-9.

461. **Bartie, C., and K. P. Klugman.** 1997. Exposures to Legionella pneumophila and Chlamydia pneumoniae in South African Mine Workers. *Int J Occup Environ Health* **3**:120-127.

462. **Bartlett, J. G.** 2002. Antibiotic-associated diarrhea. *N Engl J Med* **348**:334-9.

463. **Bartlett, J. G., S. F. Dowell, L. A. Mandell, T. M. File Jr, D. M. Musher, and M. J. Fine.** 2000. Practice guidelines for the management of community-acquired pneumonia in adults. Infectious Diseases Society of America. *Clin Infect Dis* **31**:347-82.

464. **Bartlett, M. S., S. H. Vermund, R. Jacobs, P. J. Durant, M. M. Shaw, J. W. Smith, X. Tang, J. J. Lu, B. Li, S. Jin, and C. H. Lee.** 1997. Detection of Pneumocystis carinii DNA in air samples: likely environmental risk to susceptible persons. *J Clin Microbiol* **35**:2511-3.

465. **Bartlett, P. C., L. A. Vonbehren, R. P. Tewari, R. J. Martin, L. Eagleton, M. J. Isaac, and P. S. Kulkarni.** 1982. Bats in the belfry: an outbreak of histoplasmosis. *Am J Public Health* **72**:1369-72.

466. **Bartoloni, A., G. Cancrini, F. Bartalesi, D. Marcolin, M. Roselli, C. C. Arce, and A. J. Hall.** 1999. Mansonella ozzardi infection in Bolivia: prevalence and clinical associations in the Chaco region. *Am J Trop Med Hyg* **61**:830-3.

467. **Barton, L. L., and M. B. Mets.** 2001. Congenital lymphocytic choriomeningitis virus infection: decade of rediscovery. *Clin Infect Dis* **33**:370-4.

468. **Bartram, J., N. Thyssen, A. Gowers, K. Pond, and T. Lack.** 2002. Water and health in Europe. *WHO Reg Publ Eur Ser* **93**:1-222.

469. **Barwick, R. S., D. A. Levy, G. F. Craun, M. J. Beach, and R. L. Calderon.** 2000. Surveillance for waterborne-disease outbreaks—United States, 1997-1998. *MMWR* **49 (SS-4)**:1-21.

470. **Barwick, R. S., H. O. Mohammed, M. E. White, and R. B. Bryant.** 2003. Factors associated with the likelihood of Giardia spp. and Cryptosporidium spp. in soil from dairy farms. *J Dairy Sci* **86**:784-91.

471. **Barwick, R. S., A. Uzicanin, S. Lareau, N. Malakmadze, P. Imnadze, M. Iosava, N. Ninashvili, M. Wilson, A. W. Hightower, S. Johnston, H. Bishop, W. A. Petri, Jr., and D. D. Juranek.** 2002. Outbreak of amebiasis in Tbilisi, republic of Georgia, 1998. *Am J Trop Med Hyg* **67:**623-31.

472. **Basanez, M. G., R. C. Collins, C. H. Porter, M. P. Little, and D. Brandling-Bennett.** 2002. Transmission intensity and the patterns of Onchocerca volvulus infection in human communities. *Am J Trop Med Hyg* **67:**669-79.

473. **Bassa, A. G., A. A. Hoosen, J. Moodley, and A. Bramdev.** 1993. Granuloma inguinale (donovanosis) in women. An analysis of 61 cases from Durban, South Africa. *Sex Transm Dis* **20:**164-7.

474. **Basset, D., C. Girou, I. P. Nozais, F. D'Hermies, C. Hoang, R. Gordon, and A. D'Alessandro.** 1998. Neotropical echinococcosis in Suriname: Echinococcus oligarthrus in the orbit and Echinococcus vogeli in the abdomen. *Am J Trop Med Hyg* **59:**787-90.

475. **Basset, D., J. P. Guyonnet, P. Bastien, M. A. Montis, G. Baggieri, P. Callamand, I. Millot, G. Serres, M. C. Genoux, D. Rieu, J. P. Dedet, and D. M. Jarry.** 1994. Foyer endémique d'anguillulose autochtone dans un camp de gitans de l'Hérault. *Bull Epidémiol Hebdomadaire* **24 (14 June):**109.

476. **Bassetti, S., W. E. Bischoff, M. Walter, B. A. Bassetti-Wyss, L. Mason, B. A. Reboussin, R. B. D'Agostino, Jr., J. M. Gwaltney, Jr., M. A. Pfaller, and R. J. Sherertz.** 2005. Dispersal of Staphylococcus aureus into the air associated with a rhinovirus infection. *Infect Control Hosp Epidemiol* **26:**196-203.

477. **Bassetti, S., M. Hoffmann, H. C. Bucher, U. Fluckiger, and M. Battegay.** 2002. Infections requiring hospitalization of injection drug users who participated in an injection opiate maintenance program. *Clin Infect Dis* **34:**711-3.

478. **Bassinet, L., M. Matrat, E. Njamkepo, S. Aberrane, B. Housset, and N. Guiso.** 2004. Nosocomial pertussis outbreak among adult patients and healthcare workers. *Infect Control Hosp Epidemiol* **25:**995-7.

479. **Bastien, N., D. Ward, P. Van Caeseele, K. Brandt, S. H. Lee, G. McNabb, B. Klisko, E. Chan, and Y. Li.** 2003. Human metapneumovirus infection in the Canadian population. *J Clin Microbiol* **41:**4642-6.

480. **Bastien, P., D. Basset, and J. P. Dédet.** 1995. Hétérophyose et diarrhée chez le voyageur: à propos d'un cas observé chez un enfant au retour d'un séjour en Egypte. *Med Trop* **55:**243-5.

481. **Bastos, F. I., C. Barcellos, C. M. Lowndes, and S. R. Friedman.** 1999. Co-infection with malaria and HIV in injecting drug users in Brazil: a new challenge to public health? *Addiction* **94:**1165-74.

482. **Basu, A., P. Garg, S. Datta, S. Chakraborty, T. Bhattacharya, A. Khan, S. Ramamurthy, S. K. Bhattacharya, S. Yamasaki, Y. Takeda, and G. B. Nair.** 2000. Vibrio cholerae O139 in Calcutta, 1992-1998: incidence, antibiograms, and genotypes. *Emerg Infect Dis* **6:**139-47.

483. **Bath, S., K. Bisgard, T. Murphy, K. Shutt, and N. Rosenstein.** 2002. Progress toward elimination of Haemophilus influenzae type b invasive disease among infants and children - United States, 1998-2000. *MMWR* **51:**234-7.

484. **Batieha, A., E. K. Saliba, R. Graham, E. Mohareb, Y. Hijazi, and P. Wijeyaratne.** 2000. Seroprevalence of West Nile, Rift Valley, and Sandfly arboviruses in Hashimiah, Jordan. *Emerg Infect Dis* **6:**356-62.

485. **Battey, Y. M., R. B. Wallace, B. C. Allan, and B. M. Keeffe.** 1970. Gastro-enteritis in Australia caused by a marine vibrio. *Med J Aust* **feb 28:**430-3.

486. **Bauer, K.** 1997. Foot- and-mouth disease as zoonosis. *Arch Virol Suppl* **13:**95-7.

487. **Baumgardner, D. J., B. P. Buggy, B. J. Mattson, J. S. Burdick, and D. Ludwig.** 1992. Epidemiology of blastomycosis in a region of high endemicity in north central Wisconsin. *Clin Infect Dis* **15:**629-35.

488. **Baumgardner, D. J., and J. S. Burdick.** 1991. An outbreak of human and canine blastomycosis. *Rev Infect Dis* **13:**898-905.

489. **Baumgartner, A., and J. Danuser.** 2003. Vorkommen der Zoonoseerreger Campylobacter, Salmonella und Yersinia enterocolitica in Schweinemastbetrieben und auf rohem Schweinefleisch. *Bull BAG* **23 (2 jun):**398-9.

490. **Baumler, A. J., B. M. Hargis, and R. M. Tsolis.** 2000. Tracing the origins of Salmonella outbreaks. *Science* **287:**50-2.

491. **Bausch, D. G., M. Borchert, T. Grein, C. Roth, R. Swanepoel, M. L. Libande, A. Talarmin, E. Bertherat, J. J. Muyembe-Tamfum, B. Tugume, R. Colebunders, K. M. Konde, P. Pirad, L. L. Olinda, G. R. Rodier, P. Campbell, O. Tomori, T. G. Ksiazek, and P. E. Rollin.** 2003. Risk factors for Marburg hemorrhagic fever, Democratic Republic of the Congo. *Emerg Infect Dis* **9:**1531-7.

492. **Bauwens, J. E., M. F. Lampe, R. J. Suchland, K. Wong, and W. E. Stamm.** 1995. Infection with Chlamydia trachomatis lymphogranuloma venereum serovar L1 in homosexual men with proctitis: molecular analysis of an unusual case cluster. *Clin Infect Dis* **20:**576-81.

493. **Bauwens, J. E., H. Orlander, M. P. Gomez, M. Lampe, S. Morse, W. E. Stamm, R. Cone, R. Ashley, P. Swenson, and K. K. Holmes.** 2002. Epidemic Lymphogranuloma venereum during epidemics of crack cocaine use and HIV infection in the Bahamas. *Sex Transm Dis* **29:**253-9.

494. **Bavaro, M. F., D. J. Kelly, G. A. Dasch, B. R. Hale, and P. Olson.** 2005. History of U.S. military contributions to the study of rickettsial diseases. *Mil Med* **170:**49-60.

495. **Bavastrelli, M., M. Midulla, D. Rossi, M. Salzano, E. Calzolari, C. Midulla, S. Sanguigni, A. Torre, and O. Giardini.** 1998. Sexually active adolescents and young adults: a high-risk group for Chlamydia trachomatis infection. *J Travel Med* **5:**57-60.

496. **Bawden, M. P., D. D. Slaten, and J. D. Malone.** 1995. Falciparum malaria in a displaced Haitian population. *Trans R Soc Trop Med Hyg* **89:**600-3.

497. **Baxby, D.** 1999. Edward Jenner's inquiry; a bicentenary analysis. *Vaccine* **17:**301-7.

498. **Bayard, V., P. T. Kitsutani, E. O. Barria, L. A. Ruedas, D. S. Tinnin, C. Munoz, I. B. de Mosca, G. Guerrero, R. Kant, A. Garcia, L. Caceres, F. G. Gracio, E. Quiroz, Z. de Castillo, B. Armien, M. Libel, J. N. Mills, A. S. Khan, S. T. Nichol, P. E. Rollin, T. G. Ksiazek, and C. J. Peters.** 2004. Outbreak of hantavirus pulmonary syndrome, Los Santos, Panama, 1999-2000. *Emerg Infect Dis* **10:**1635-42.

499. **Bazex, J., H. Jouas, M. Cornac, and Y. Donati.** 1987. Donovanose: à propos de deux observations. *Méd Mal Infect* **17:**128-30.

500. **Bean, N. H., J. S. Goulding, C. Lao, and F. J. Angulo.** 1996. Surveillance for foodborne-disease outbreaks—United States, 1988-1992. *MMWR CDC Surveill Summ* **45:**1-66.

501. Bean, N. H., E. K. Maloney, M. E. Potter, P. Korazemo, B. Ray, J. P. Taylor, S. Seigler, and J. Snowden. 1998. Crayfish: a newly recognized vehicle for vibrio infections. *Epidemiol Infect* **121**:269-73.

502. Beard, C. B., G. Pye, F. J. Steurer, R. Rodriguez, R. Campman, A. T. Peterson, J. Ramsey, R. A. Wirtz, and L. E. Robinson. 2003. Chagas disease in a domestic transmission cycle, southern Texas, USA. *Emerg Infect Dis* **9**:103-5.

503. Beasley, R. P., and L. Y. Hwang. 1983. Postnatal infectivity of hepatitis B surfaceantigen-carrier mothers. *J Infect Dis* **147**:185-90.

504. Beati, L., L. Humair, A. Aeschlimann, and D. Raoult. 1994. Identification of spotted fever group rickettsiae isolated from Dermacentor marginatus and Ixodes ricinus ticks collected in Switzerland. *Am J Trop Med Hyg* **51**:138-48.

505. Beatty, M. E., T. Jack, S. Sivapalasingam, S. S. Yao, I. Paul, B. Bibb, K. D. Greene, K. Kubota, E. D. Mintz, and J. T. Brooks. 2004. An Outbreak of Vibrio cholerae O1 infections on Ebeye Island, Republic of the Marshall Islands, associated with use of an adequately chlorinated water source. *Clin Infect Dis* **38**:1-9.

506. Beau de Rochars, M. V., M. D. Milord, Y. St Jean, A. M. Desormeaux, J. J. Dorvil, J. G. Lafontant, D. G. Addiss, and T. G. Streit. 2004. Geographic distribution of lymphatic filariasis in Haiti. *Am J Trop Med Hyg* **71**:598-601.

507. Beaufoy, A. 1993. Infections in intravenous drug users: a two-year review. *Can J Infect Control* **8**:7-9.

508. Beaver, P. C. 1962. Toxocariasis (VLM) in relationship to tropical eosinophilia. *Bull Soc Pathol Exot* **55**:555-76.

509. Beck-Sague, C., S. W. Dooley, M. D. Hutton, J. Otten, A. Breeden, J. T. Crawford, A. E. Pitchenik, C. Woodley, G. Cauthen, and W. R. Jarvis. 1992. Hospital outbreak of multidrug-resistant Mycobacterium tuberculosis infections. Factors in transmission to staff and HIV-infected patients. *JAMA* **268**:1280-6.

510. Beck-Sague, C., and W. R. Jarvis. 1993. Secular trends in the epidemiology of nosocomial fungal infections in the United States, 1980-1990. National Nosocomial Infections Surveillance System. *J Infect Dis* **167**:1247-51.

511. Beck-Sague, C. M., W. R. Jarvis, J. H. Brook, D. H. Culver, A. Potts, E. Gay, B. W. Shotts, B. Hill, R. L. Anderson, and M. P. Weinstein. 1990. Epidemic bacteremia due to Acinetobacter baumannii in five intensive care units. *Am J Epidemiol* **132**:723-33.

512. Beck-Sague, C. M., W. R. Jarvis, J. A. Fruehling, C. E. Ott, M. T. Higgins, and F. L. Bates. 1991. Universal precautions and mortuary practitioners: influence on practices and risk of occupationally acquired infection. *J Occup Med* **33**:874-8.

513. Beckendorf, R., S. A. Klotz, N. Hinkle, and W. Bartholomew. 2002. Nasal myiasis in an intensive care unit linked to hospital-wide mouse infestation. *Arch Intern Med* **162**:638-40.

514. Becker, H., G. Schaller, W. von Wiese, and G. Terplan. 1994. Bacillus cereus in infant foods and dried milk products. *Int J Food Microbiol* **23**:1-15.

515. Becker, K. M., G. E. Glass, W. Brathwaite, and J. M. Zenilman. 1998. Geographic epidemiology of gonorrhea in Baltimore, Maryland, using a geographic information system. *Am J Epidemiol* **147**:709-716.

516. Becker, S. I., R. D. Smalligan, J. D. Frame, H. Kleanthous, T. J. Tibbitts, T. P. Monath, and K. C. Hyams. 1999. Risk of Helicobacter pylori infection among long-term residents in developing countries. *Am J Trop Med Hyg* **60**:267-70.

517. Becquet, R., J. Poirriez, E. Dei-Cas, E. Dutoit, S. Deblock, M. Abdellatifi, and A. Vernes. 1982. Contribution à l'étude de la trichostrongylose humaine (à propos de 71 observations). *Ann Soc Belg Med Trop* **62**:139-55.

518. Beecham, H. J., 3rd, M. L. Cohen, and W. E. Parkin. 1979. Salmonella typhimurium. Transmission by fiberoptic upper gastrointestinal endoscopy. *JAMA* **241**:1013-5.

519. Beekmann, S. E., K. P. Heilmann, S. S. Richter, J. Garcia-de-Lomas, and G. V. Doern. 2005. Antimicrobial resistance in Streptococcus pneumoniae, Haemophilus influenzae, Moraxella catarrhalis and group A beta-haemolytic streptococci in 2002-2003. Results of the multinational GRASP Surveillance Program. *Int J Antimicrob Agents* **25**:148-56.

520. Begier, E. M., K. Frenette, N. L. Barrett, P. Mshar, S. Petit, D. J. Boxrud, K. Watkins-Colwell, S. Wheeler, E. A. Cebelinski, A. Glennen, D. Nguyen, and J. L. Hadler. 2004. A high-morbidity outbreak of methicillin-resistant Staphylococcus aureus among players on a college football team, facilitated by cosmetic body shaving and turf burns. *Clin Infect Dis* **39**:1446-53.

521. Begue, R. E., R. Meza, G. Castellares, C. Cabezas, B. Vasquez, A. Ballardo, J. Cam, and J. L. Sanchez. 1995. Outbreak of diarrhea due to Vibrio parahaemolyticus among military personnel in Lima, Peru. *Clin Infect Dis* **21**:1513-4.

522. Behets, F., J. Andriamiadana, D. Rasamilalao, N. Ratsimbazafy, D. Randrianasolo, G. Dallabetta, and M. Cohen. 2001. Sexually transmitted infections and associated sociodemographic and behavioural factors in women seeking primary care suggest Madagascar's vulnerability to rapid HIV spread. *Trop Med Int Health* **6**:202-11.

523. Behets, F. M., J. Andriamiadana, D. Randrianasolo, R. Randriamanga, D. Rasamilalao, C. Y. Chen, J. B. Weiss, S. A. Morse, G. Dallabetta, and M. S. Cohen. 1999. Chancroid, primary syphilis, genital herpes, and lymphogranuloma venereum in Antananarivo, Madagascar. *J Infect Dis* **180**:1382-5.

524. Behroozan, D. S., M. M. Christian, and R. L. Moy. 2000. Mycobacterium fortuitum infection following neck liposuction: A case report. *Dermatol Surg* **26**:588-90.

525. Beilenson, P., D. Rose, D. Dunning, W. Brathwaite, K. West, F. Meyers, J. Krick, D. Akers, R. Miazad, A. Bhatia, and D. Dwyer. 1998. Epidemic of congenital syphilis - Baltimore, 1996-1997. *MMWR* **47**:904-7.

526. Bekkers, R. L., L. F. Massuger, J. Bulten, and W. J. Melchers. 2004. Epidemiological and clinical aspects of human papillomavirus detection in the prevention of cervical cancer. *Rev Med Virol* **14**:95-105.

527. Belabbes, E.-H., A. Bouguermouh, A. Benatallah, and G. Illoul. 1985. Epidemic non-A, non-B viral hepatitis in Algeria: strong evidence for its spreading by water. *J Med Virol* **16**:257-63.

528. Belizario, V. Y., M. E. Amarillo, W. U. de Leon, A. E. de los Reyes, M. G. Bugayong, and B. J. Macatangay. 2003. A comparison of the efficacy of single doses of albendazole, ivermectin, and diethylcarbamazine alone or in combinations against Ascaris and Trichuris spp. *Bull WHO* **81**:35-42.

529. Beljaev, A. E. 2000. Taenia saginata. *N Engl J Med* **342**:1139; author reply 1139-40.

530. Belko, J., D. A. Goldmann, A. Macone, and A. K. M. Zaidi. 2002. Clinically significant infections with organisms of the Streptococcus milleri group. *Pediatr Infect Dis J* **21**:715-26.

531. **Bell, B. P.,** M. Goldoft, P. M. Griffin, M. A. Davis, D. C. Gordon, P. I. Tarr, C. A. Bartleson, J. H. Lewis, T. J. Barrett, J. G. Wells, et al. 1994. A multistate outbreak of Escherichia coli O157:H7-associated bloody diarrhea and hemolytic uremic syndrome from hamburgers. The Washington experience. *JAMA* **272:**1349-53.

532. **Bell, D. M.** 2004. Public health interventions and SARS spread, 2003. *Emerg Infect Dis* **10:**1900-6.

533. **Bell, J. C.,** L. R. Jorm, M. Williamson, N. H. Shaw, D. L. Kazandjian, R. Chiew, and A. G. Capon. 1996. Legionellosis linked with a hotel car park—how many were infected? *Epidemiol Infect* **116:**185-92.

534. **Bell, L. M.,** S. J. Naides, P. Stoffman, R. L. Hodinka, and S. A. Plotkin. 1989. Human parvovirus B19 infection among hospital staff members after contact with infected patients. *N Engl J Med* **321:**485-91.

535. **Beller, M.,** A. Ellis, S. H. Lee, M. A. Drebot, S. A. Jenkerson, E. Funk, M. D. Sobsey, O. D. Simmons, 3rd, S. S. Monroe, T. Ando, J. Noel, M. Petric, J. P. Middaugh, and J. S. Spika. 1997. Outbreak of viral gastroenteritis due to a contaminated well. *JAMA* **278:**563-568.

536. **Beller, M.,** and B. D. Gessner. 1994. An outbreak of tinea corporis gladiatorum on a high school wrestling team. *J Am Acad Dermatol* **31:**197-201.

537. **Bellin, E. Y.,** D. D. Fletcher, and S. M. Safyer. 1993. Association of tuberculosis infection with increased time in or admission to the New York City jail system. *JAMA* **269:**2228-31.

538. **Belliot, G.,** H. Laveran, and S. S. Monroe. 1997. Outbreak of gastroenteritis in military recruits associated with serotype 3 astrovirus infection. *J Med Virol* **51:**101-6.

539. **Belongia, E. A.,** C. M. Gale, K. D. Reed, P. D. Mitchell, M. Vandermause, M. F. Finkel, J. J. Kazmierczak, and J. P. Davis. 2001. Population-based incidence of human granulocytic ehrlichiosis in northwestern Wisconsin, 1997-1999. *J Infect Dis* **184:**1470-4.

540. **Belongia, E. A.,** J. L. Goodman, E. J. Holland, C. W. Andres, S. R. Homann, R. L. Mahanti, M. W. Mizener, A. Erice, and M. T. Osterholm. 1991. An outbreak of herpes gladiatorum at a high-school wrestling camp. *N Engl J Med* **325:**906-10.

541. **Belongia, E. A.,** K. L. MacDonald, G. L. Parham, K. E. White, J. A. Korlath, M. N. Lobato, S. M. Strand, K. A. Casale, and M. T. Osterholm. 1991. An outbreak of Escherichia coli O157:H7 colitis associated with consumption of precooked meat patties. *J Infect Dis* **164:**338-43.

542. **Belongia, E. A.,** M. T. Osterholm, J. T. Soler, D. A. Ammend, J. E. Braun, and K. L. MacDonald. 1993. Transmission of Escherichia coli O157:H7 infection in Minnesota child day-care facilities. *JAMA* **269:**883-8.

543. **Beltrami, E. M.,** F. Alvarado-Ramy, S. E. Critchley, A. L. Panlilio, D. M. Cardo, W. A. Bower, M. J. Alter, J. E. Kaplan, B. Lushniak, D. K. Henderson, K. A. Struble, and A. Macher. 2001. Updated U.S. public health service guidelines for the management of occupational exposures to HBV, HCV, and HIV and recommendations for postexposure prophylaxis. *MMWR* **50 (RR-11):**1-52.

544. **Beltrami, E. M.,** A. Kozak, I. T. Williams, A. M. Saekhou, M. L. Kalish, O. V. Nainan, S. L. Stramer, M. C. Fucci, D. Frederickson, and D. M. Cardo. 2003. Transmission of HIV and hepatitis C virus from a nursing home patient to a health care worker. *Am J Infect Control* **31:**168-75.

545. **Beltrami, J. F.,** T. A. Farley, J. T. Hamrick, D. A. Cohen, and D. H. Martin. 1998. Evaluation of the Gen-Probe PACE 2 assay for the detection of asymptomatic Chlamydia trachomatis and Neisseria gonorrhoeae infections in male arrestees. *Sex Transm Dis* **25:**501-4.

546. **Belza, M. J.** 2004. Prevalence of HIV, HTLV-I and HTLV-II among female sex workers in Spain, 2000-2001. *Eur J Epidemiol* **19:**279-82.

547. **Ben Salah, A. B.,** R. Ben Ismail, F. Amri, S. Chlif, F. Ben Rzig, H. Kharrat, H. Hadhri, M. Hassouna, and K. Dellagi. 2000. Investigation of the spread of human visceral leishmaniasis in central Tunisia. *Trans R Soc Trop Med Hyg* **94:**382-6.

548. **Benaoudia, F.,** M. Assouline, Y. Pouliquen, A. Bouvet, and E. Gueho. 1999. Exophiala (Wangiella) dermatitidis keratitis after keratoplasty. *Med Mycol* **37:**53-6.

549. **Bender, B. S.,** R. Bennett, B. E. Laughon, W. B. Greenough, 3rd, C. Gaydos, S. D. Sears, M. S. Forman, and J. G. Bartlett. 1986. Is Clostridium difficile endemic in chronic-care facilities? *Lancet* **2:**11-3.

550. **Bender, J. B.** 2005. Compendium of measures to prevent disease associated with animals in public settings, 2005. *MMWR* **54 (RR-4):**1-12.

551. **Bender, J. B.,** C. W. Hedberg, J. M. Besser, D. J. Boxrud, K. L. MacDonald, and M. T. Osterholm. 1997. Surveillance for Escherichia coli O157:H7 infections in Minnesota by molecular subtyping. *N Engl J Med* **337:**388-94.

552. **Bender, J. B.,** and S. A. Shulman. 2004. Reports of zoonotic disease outbreaks associated with animal exhibits and availability of recommendations for preventing zoonotic disease transmission from animals to people in such settings. *J Am Vet Med Assoc* **224:**1105-9.

553. **Bender, J. B.,** S. A. Shulman, G. A. Averbeck, G. C. Pantlin, and B. E. Stromberg. 2005. Epidemiologic features of Campylobacter infection among cats in the upper midwestern United States. *J Am Vet Med Assoc* **226:**544-7.

554. **Bender, J. B.,** K. E. Smith, A. A. McNees, T. R. Rabatsky-Ehr, S. D. Segler, M. A. Hawkins, N. L. Spina, W. E. Keene, M. H. Kennedy, T. J. Van Gilder, and C. W. Hedberg. 2004. Factors Affecting Surveillance Data on Escherichia coli O157 Infections Collected from FoodNet Sites, 1996-1999. *Clin Infect Dis* **38 Suppl 3:**S157-64.

555. **Bender, J. B.,** and D. T. Tsukayama. 2004. Horses and the risk of zoonotic infections. *Vet Clin North Am Equine Pract* **20:**643-53.

556. **Bendinelli, M.,** M. Pistello, F. Maggi, C. Fornai, G. Freer, and M. L. Vatteroni. 2001. Molecular properties, biology, and clinical implications of TT virus, a recently identified widespread infectious agent of humans. *Clin Microbiol Rev* **14:**98-113.

557. **Benenson, M. W.,** E. T. Takafuji, W. H. Bancroft, S. M. Lemon, M. C. Callahan, and D. A. Leach. 1980. A military community outbreak of hepatitis type A related to transmission in a child care facility. *Am J Epidemiol* **112:**471-81.

558. **Benenson, M. W.,** E. T. Takafuji, S. M. Lemon, R. L. Greenup, and A. J. Sulzer. 1982. Oocyst-transmitted toxoplasmosis associated with ingestion of contaminated water. *N Engl J Med* **307:**666-9.

559. **Benet, A.,** A. Mai, F. Bockarie, M. Lagog, P. Zimmerman, M. P. Alpers, J. C. Reeder, and M. J. Bockarie. 2004. Polymerase chain reaction diagnosis and the changing pattern of vector ecology and malaria transmission dynamics in Papua New Guinea. *Am J Trop Med Hyg* **71:**277-84.

560. Benetton, M. L., A. V. Goncalves, M. E. Meneghini, E. F. Silva, and M. Carneiro. 2005. Risk factors for infection by the Entamoeba histolytica/E. dispar complex: An epidemiological study conducted in outpatient clinics in the city of Manaus, Amazon Region, Brazil. *Trans R Soc Trop Med Hyg* **99**:532-40.

561. Bengtson, S. D., and F. Rogers. 2001. Prevalence of sparganosis by county of origin in Florida feral swine. *Vet Parasitol* **97**:239-42.

562. Benin, A. L., R. F. Benson, K. E. Arnold, A. E. Fiore, P. G. Cook, L. K. Williams, B. Fields, and R. E. Besser. 2002. An outbreak of travel-associated legionnaires disease and Pontiac fever: the need for enhanced surveillance of travel-associated legionellosis in the United States. *J Infect Dis* **185**:237-243.

563. Benito, A., and J. M. Rubio. 2001. Usefulness of seminested polymerase chain reaction for screening blood donors at risk for malaria in Spain. *Emerg Infect Dis* **7**:1068.

564. Benjamin, B., and S. H. Annobil. 1992. Childhood brucellosis in southwestern Saudi Arabia: a 5-year experience. *J Trop Pediatr* **38**:167-72.

565. Benjamin, D. K., W. C. Miller, S. Bayliff, L. Martel, K. A. Alexander, and P. L. Martin. 2002. Infections diagnosed in the first year after pediatric stem cell transplantation. *Pediatr Infect Dis J* **21**:227-34.

566. Benjelloun, S., B. Bahbouhi, N. Bouchrit, L. Cherkaoui, N. Hda, J. Mahjour, and A. Benslimane. 1997. Seroepidemiological study of an acute hepatitis E outbreak in Morocco. *Res Virol* **148**:279-87.

567. Benkel, D. H., E. M. McClure, D. Woolard, J. V. Rullan, G. B. Miller, Jr., S. R. Jenkins, J. H. Hershey, R. F. Benson, J. M. Pruckler, E. W. Brown, M. S. Kolczak, R. L. Hackler, B. S. Rouse, and R. F. Breiman. 2000. Outbreak of Legionnaires' disease associated with a display whirlpool spa. *Int J Epidemiol* **29**:1092-8.

568. Benki, S., S. B. Mostad, B. A. Richardson, K. Mandaliya, J. K. Kreiss, and J. Overbaugh. 2004. Cyclic shedding of HIV-1 RNA in cervical secretions during the menstrual cycle. *J Infect Dis* **189**:2192-201.

569. Bennett, C. M., C. Dalton, M. Beers-Deeble, A. Milazzo, E. Kraa, D. Davos, M. Puech, A. Tan, and M. W. Heuzenroeder. 2003. Fresh garlic: a possible vehicle for Salmonella Virchow. *Epidemiol Infect* **131**:1041-8.

570. Bennett, J., M. Schooley, H. Traverso, S. B. Agha, and J. R. Boring, 3rd. 1996. Bundling, a newly identified risk factor for neonatal tetanus: implications for global control. *Int J Epidemiol* **25**:879-84.

571. Bennett, N. M., J. Buffington, and F. M. LaForce. 1992. Pneumococcal bacteremia in Monroe County, New York. *Am J Public Health* **82**:1513-6.

572. Bennett, S. N., D. E. Peterson, D. R. Johnson, W. N. Hall, B. Robinson-Dunn, and S. Dietrich. 1994. Bronchoscopy-associated Mycobacterium xenopi pseudoinfections. *Am J Respir Crit Care Med* **150**:245-50.

573. Benson, C. A., J. E. Kaplan, H. Masur, A. Pau, and K. K. Holmes. 2004. Treating opportunistic infections among HIV-exposed and infected children: recommendations from CDC, the National Institutes of Health, and the Infectious Diseases Society of America. *MMWR* **53 (RR-15)**:1-112.

574. Bentley, R., M. Daly, and T. Harris. 1980. Toxocara infection among veterinarians. *Vet Rec* **106**:277-8.

575. Benzerroug, E. H., P. G. Janssens, and P. Ambroise-Thomas. 1991. [Seroepidemiological study of malaria in the Algerian Sahara]. *Bull WHO* **69**:713-23.

576. Beran, J., L. Asokliene, I. Lucenko, I. Jansone, I. Velicko, and E. Pujate. 2004. Tickborne encephalitis in Europe: Czech Republic, Lithuania and Latvia. *Eurosurveillance Weekly* **8**:7-12.

577. Berard, H., and M. Laille. 1990. [40 cases of dengue (serotype 3) occurring in a military camp during an epidemic in New Caledonia (1989). The value of vector control]. *Med Trop (Mars)* **50**:423-8.

578. Bercault, N., and T. Boulain. 2001. Mortality rate attributable to ventilator-associated nosocomial pneumonia in an adult intensive care unit: a prospective case-control study. *Crit Care Med* **29**:2303-9.

579. Berdal, B. P., O. Scheel, A. R. Ogaard, T. Hoel, T. J. Gutteberg, and G. Anestad. 1992. Spread of subclinical Chlamydia pneumoniae infection in a closed community. *Scand J Infect Dis* **24**:431-6.

580. Berger, A., H. W. Doerr, I. Scharrer, and B. Weber. 1997. Follow-up of four HIV-infected individuals after administration of hepatitis C virus and GBV-C/hepatitis G virus contaminated intravenous immunoglobulin: evidence for HCV but not for GBV-C/HGV transmission. *J Med Virol* **53**:25-30.

581. Berger, J. R., and N. J. David. 1993. Creutzfeldt-Jakob disease in a physician: a review of the disorder in health care workers. *Neurology* **43**:205-6.

582. Berghold, C., C. Kornschober, and S. Weber. 2003. A regional outbreak of S. Enteritidis phage type 5, traced back to the flocks of an egg producer, Austria. *Eur Surveill* **8**:195-8.

583. Bergogne-Berezin, E., and K. J. Towner. 1996. Acinetobacter spp. as nosocomial pathogens: microbiological, clinical, and epidemiological features. *Clin Microbiol Rev* **9**:148-65.

584. Bergquist, N. R. 2002. Schistosomiasis: from risk assessment to control. *Trends Parasitol* **18**:309-14.

585. Bergson, C. L., and N. C. Fernandes. 2001. Tinea capitis: study of asymptomatic carriers and sick adolescents, adults and elderly who live with children with the disease. *Rev Inst Med Trop Sao Paulo* **43**:87-91.

586. Bergstein, J. M., E. J. t. Baker, C. Aprahamian, M. Schein, and D. H. Wittmann. 1995. Soft tissue abscesses associated with parenteral drug abuse: presentation, microbiology, and treatment. *Am Surg* **61**:1105-8.

587. Bergstrom, S., and B. Hederstedt. 1992. Materno-fetal transmission of syphilis in Mozambican parturients. *Genitourin Med* **68**:141.

588. Berkelman, R. L. 2003. Human illness associated with use of veterinary vaccines. *Clin Infect Dis* **37**:407-14.

589. Berlau, J., H. Aucken, H. Malnick, and T. Pitt. 1999. Distribution of Acinetobacter species on skin of healthy humans. *Eur J Clin Microbiol Infect Dis* **18**:179-83.

590. Berlau, J., H. M. Aucken, E. Houang, and T. L. Pitt. 1999. Isolation of Acinetobacter spp. including A. baumannii from vegetables: implications for hospital-acquired infections. *J Hosp Infect* **42**:201-4.

591. Berlinberg, C. D., S. R. Weingarten, L. B. Bolton, and S. H. Waterman. 1989. Occupational exposure to influenza—introduction of an index case to a hospital. *Infect Control Hosp Epidemiol* **10**:70-3.

592. Berman, S. J. 2001. Infections in patients with end-stage renal disease. An overview. *Infect Dis Clin North Am* **15**:709-20, vii.

593. Berman, S. J., E. W. Johnson, C. Nakatsu, M. Alkan, R. Chen, and J. LeDuc. 2004. Burden of infection in patients with end-stage renal disease requiring long-term dialysis. *Clin Infect Dis* **39:**1747-53.

594. Bern, C., B. Hernandez, M. B. Lopez, M. J. Arrowood, M. A. de Mejia, A. M. de Merida, A. W. Hightower, L. Venczel, B. L. Herwaldt, and R. E. Klein. 1999. Epidemiologic studies of Cyclospora cayetanensis in Guatemala. *Emerg Infect Dis* **5:**766-74.

595. Bern, C., B. Hernandez, M. B. Lopez, M. J. Arrowood, A. M. De Merida, and R. E. Klein. 2000. The contrasting epidemiology of Cyclospora and Cryptosporidium among outpatients in Guatemala. *Am J Trop Med Hyg* **63:**231-5.

596. Bern, C., A. B. Joshi, S. N. Jha, M. L. Das, A. Hightower, G. D. Thakur, and M. B. Bista. 2000. Factors associated with visceral leishmaniasis in Nepal: bed-net use is strongly protective. *Am J Trop Med Hyg* **63:**184-8.

597. Bern, C., Y. Ortega, W. Checkley, J. M. Roberts, A. G. Lescano, L. Cabrera, M. Verastegui, R. E. Black, C. Sterling, and R. H. Gilman. 2002. Epidemiologic differences between cyclosporiasis and cryptosporidiosis in Peruvian children. *Emerg Infect Dis* **8:**581-5.

598. Bern, C., M. A. Pallansch, H. E. Gary, Jr., J. P. Alexander, T. J. Torok, R. I. Glass, and L. J. Anderson. 1992. Acute hemorrhagic conjunctivitis due to enterovirus 70 in American Samoa: serum-neutralizing antibodies and sex-specific protection. *Am J Epidemiol* **136:**1502-6.

599. Bernabeu-Wittel, M., M. Naranjo, J. M. Cisneros, E. Canas, M. A. Gentil, G. Algarra, P. Pereira, F. J. Gonzalez-Roncero, A. de Alarcon, and J. Pachon. 2002. Infections in renal transplant recipients receiving mycophenolate versus azathioprine-based immunosuppression. *Eur J Clin Microbiol Infect Dis* **21:**173-80.

600. Bernabeu-Wittel, M., J. Pachon, A. Alarcon, L. F. Lopez-Cortes, P. Viciana, M. E. Jimenez-Mejias, J. L. Villanueva, R. Torronteras, and F. J. Caballero-Granado. 1999. Murine typhus as a common cause of fever of intermediate duration: a 17-year study in the south of Spain. *Arch Intern Med* **159:**872-6.

601. Bernard, K. W., P. L. Graitcer, T. van der Vlugt, J. S. Moran, and K. M. Pulley. 1989. Epidemiological surveillance in Peace Corps Volunteers: a model for monitoring health in temporary residents of developing countries. *Int J Epidemiol* **18:**220-6.

602. Bernard, R. P. 1965. The Zermatt typhoid outbreak in 1963. *J Hyg (Lond)* **63:**537-63.

603. Bernardini, J., J. L. Holley, J. R. Johnston, J. A. Perlmutter, and B. Piraino. 1991. An analysis of ten-year trends in infections in adults on continuous ambulatory peritoneal dialysis (CAPD). *Clin Nephrol* **36:**29-34.

604. Bernards, A. T., H. I. Harinck, L. Dijkshoorn, T. J. van der Reijden, and P. J. van den Broek. 2004. Persistent Acinetobacter baumannii? Look inside your medical equipment. *Infect Control Hosp Epidemiol* **25:**1002-4.

605. Bernit, E., X. De Lamballerie, C. Zandotti, P. Berger, V. Veit, N. Schleinitz, P. De Micco, J. R. Harle, and R. N. Charrel. 2004. Prospective investigation of a large outbreak of meningitis due to echovirus 30 during summer 2000 in marseilles, france. *Medicine (Baltimore)* **83:**245-53.

606. Bernoulli, C., J. Siegfried, G. Baumgartner, F. Regli, T. Rabinowicz, D. C. Gajdusek, and C. J. Gibbs, Jr. 1977. Danger of accidental person-to-person transmission of Creutzfeldt-Jakob disease by surgery. *Lancet* **1:**478-9.

607. Bert, F., E. Maubec, B. Bruneau, P. Berry, and N. Lambert-Zechovsky. 1998. Multi-resistant Pseudomonas aeruginosa outbreak associated with contaminated tap water in a neurosurgery intensive care unit. *J Hosp Infect* **39:**53-62.

608. Berthelot, P., F. Grattard, C. Amerger, M. C. Frery, F. Lucht, B. Pozzetto, and P. Fargier. 1999. Investigation of a nosocomial outbreak due to Serratia marcescens in a maternity hospital. *Infect Control Hosp Epidemiol* **20:**233-6.

609. Berthelot, P., F. Grattard, H. Patural, A. Ros, H. Jelassi-Saoudin, B. Pozzetto, G. Teyssier, and F. Lucht. 2001. Nosocomial colonization of premature babies with Klebsiella oxytoca: probable role of enteral feeding procedure in transmission and control of the outbreak with the use of gloves. *Infect Control Hosp Epidemiol* **22:**148-51.

610. Berthelot, P., F. Grattard, A. Ros, F. Lucht, and B. Pozzetto. 1998. Nosocomial legionellosis outbreak over a three-year period: investigation and control. *Clin Microbiol Inf* **4:**385-91.

611. Bertherat, E., A. Renaut, R. Nabias, G. Dubreuil, and M. C. Georges-Courbot. 1999. Leptospirosis and Ebola virus infection in five gold-panning villages in northeastern Gabon. *Am J Trop Med Hyg* **60:**610-5.

612. Bertherat, E., A. Talarmin, and H. Zeller. 1999. [Democratic Republic of the Congo: between civil war and the Marburg virus. International Committee of Technical and Scientific Coordination of the Durba Epidemic]. *Med Trop* **59:**201-4.

613. Berthier, M., J. L. Fauchère, J. Perrin, B. Grignon, and D. Oriot. 1996. Fulminant meningitis due to Bacillus anthracis in 11-year-old girl during ramadan. *Lancet* **347:**828.

614. Berthoud, F., and S. Berthoud. 1975. [18 cases of anguilluliasis diagnosed at Geneva]. *Schweiz Med Wochenschr* **105:**1110-5.

615. Bertrand, X., S. Lallemand, M. Thouverez, K. Boisson, and D. Talon. 2002. [Bacteremia caused by coagulase-negative staphylococci: incidence, frequency of teicoplanin resistance and molecular epidemiology]. *Pathol Biol (Paris)* **50:**552-9.

616. Bertrand, X., M. Thouverez, P. Bailly, C. Cornette, and D. Talon. 2000. Clinical and molecular epidemiology of hospital Enterococcus faecium isolates in eastern France. Members of Reseau Franc-Comtois de Lutte contr les Infections Nosocomiales. *J Hosp Infect* **45:**125-34.

617. Besansky, N. J., C. A. Hill, and C. Costantini. 2004. No accounting for taste: host preference in malaria vectors. *Trends Parasitol* **20:**249-51.

618. Besser, R. E., S. M. Lett, J. T. Weber, M. P. Doyle, T. J. Barrett, J. G. Wells, and P. M. Griffin. 1993. An outbreak of diarrhea and hemolytic uremic syndrome from Escherichia coli O157:H7 in fresh-pressed apple cider. *JAMA* **269:**2217-20.

619. Besser, R. E., B. Pakiz, J. M. Schulte, S. Alvarado, E. R. Zell, T. A. Kenyon, and I. M. Onorato. 2001. Risk factors for positive mantoux tuberculin skin tests in children in San Diego, California: evidence for boosting and possible foodborne transmission. *Pediatrics* **108:**305-10.

620. Besser, T. E., M. Goldoft, L. C. Pritchett, R. Khakhria, D. D. Hancock, D. H. Rice, J. M. Gay, W. Johnson, and C. C. Gay. 2000. Multiresistant Salmonella Typhimurium DT104 infections of humans and domestic animals in the Pacific Northwest of the United States. *Epidemiol Infect* **124:**193-200.

621. Betancourt, W. Q., and J. B. Rose. 2004. Drinking water treatment processes for removal of Cryptosporidium and Giardia. *Vet Parasitol* **126:**219-34.

622. **Bethony, J., J. T. Williams, H. Kloos, J. Blangero, L. Alves-Fraga, G. Buck, A. Michalek, S. Williams-Blangero, P. T. Loverde, R. Correa-Oliveira, and A. Gazzinelli.** 2001. Exposure to Schistosoma mansoni infections in a rural area in Brazil. II: household risk factors. *Trop Med Int Health* **6:** 136-45.

623. **Bettin, D., C. Harms, J. Polster, and T. Niemeyer.** 1998. High incidence of pathogenic microorganisms in bone allografts explanted in the morgue. *Acta Orthop Scand* **69:**311-4.

624. **Betz, T. G., B. L. Davis, P. V. Fournier, J. A. Rawlings, L. B. Elliot, and D. A. Baggett.** 1982. Occupational dermatitis associated with straw itch mites (Pyemotes ventricosus). *JAMA* **247:**2821-3.

625. **Beumer, R. R., M. C. te Giffel, E. Spoorenberg, and F. M. Rombouts.** 1996. Listeria species in domestic environments. *Epidemiol Infect* **117:**437-42.

626. **Beuret, C.** 2003. A simple method for isolation of enteric viruses (noroviruses and enteroviruses) in water. *J Virol Methods* **107:**1-8.

627. **Beuret, C., A. Baumgartner, and J. Schluep.** 2003. Virus-contaminated oysters: a three-month monitoring of oysters imported to Switzerland. *Appl Environ Microbiol* **69:**2292-7.

628. **Beuret, C., D. Kohler, and T. Luthi.** 2000. Norwalk-like virus sequences detected by reverse transcription- polymerase chain reaction in mineral waters imported into or bottled in Switzerland. *J Food Prot* **63:**1576-82.

629. **Beyene, D., A. Aseffa, M. Harboe, D. Kidane, M. Macdonald, P. R. Klatser, G. A. Bjune, and W. C. Smith.** 2003. Nasal carriage of Mycobacterium leprae DNA in healthy individuals in Lega Robi village, Ethiopia. *Epidemiol Infect* **131:**841-8.

630. **Beytout, J., H. Laurichesse, F. Gachignat, C. Chanal, and M. Rey.** 1993. Risque infectieux des blessures d'origine animale. Intérêt de la prévention des pasteurelloses. *Méd Mal Infect* **23 (spécial):**526-9.

631. **Bhalla, A., N. J. Pultz, D. M. Gries, A. J. Ray, E. C. Eckstein, D. C. Aron, and C. J. Donskey.** 2004. Acquisition of nosocomial pathogens on hands after contact with environmental surfaces near hospitalized patients. *Infect Control Hosp Epidemiol* **25:**164-7.

632. **Bharti, A. R., J. E. Nally, J. N. Ricaldi, M. A. Matthias, M. M. Diaz, M. A. Lovett, P. N. Levett, R. H. Gilman, M. R. Willig, E. Gotuzzo, and J. M. Vinetz.** 2003. Leptospirosis: a zoonotic disease of global importance. *Lancet Infect Dis* **3:**757-71.

633. **Bhatti, M. A., and M. O. Frank.** 2000. Veillonella parvula meningitis: case report and review of Veillonella infections. *Clin Infect Dis* **31:**839-40.

634. **Bhopal, R. S.** 1993. Geographical variation of Legionnaires' disease: a critique and guide to future research. *Int J Epidemiol* **22:**1127-36.

635. **Bhopal, R. S., R. J. Fallon, E. C. Buist, R. J. Black, and J. D. Urquhart.** 1991. Proximity of the home to a cooling tower and risk of non-outbreak Legionnaires' disease. *BMJ* **302:**378-83.

636. **Bi, P., S. Tong, K. Donald, K. Parton, and J. Ni.** 2002. Climatic, reservoir and occupational variables and the transmission of haemorrhagic fever with renal syndrome in China. *Int J Epidemiol* **31:**189-93.

637. **Bialek, S. R., D. A. Thoroughman, D. Hu, E. P. Simard, J. Chattin, J. E. Cheek, and B. P. Bell.** 2004. Hepatitis A incidence and hepatitis A vaccination among American Indians and Alaska Natives, 1990-2001. *Am J Public Health* **94:**996-1001.

638. **Bianli, X., C. Zaolin, H. Qingxia, and L. Hui.** 2001. Epidemiological survey of Trichinella infection in some areas of Henan province. *Parasite* **8:**S71-3.

639. **Bielaszewska, M., J. Janda, K. Blahova, H. Minarikova, E. Jikova, M. A. Karmali, J. Laubova, J. Sikulova, M. A. Preston, R. Khakhria, H. Karch, H. Klazarova, and O. Nyc.** 1997. Human Escherichia coli O157:H7 infection associated with the consumption of unpasteurized goat's milk. *Epidemiol Infect* **119:**299-305.

640. **Bienzle, U., C. H. Coester, J. Knobloch, and I. Guggenmoos-Holzmann.** 1984. Protozoal enteric infections in homosexual men. *Klin Wochenschr* **62:**323-7.

641. **Bienzle, U., F. Ebert, and M. Dietrich.** 1978. Cutaneous leishmaniasis in Eastern Saudi Arabia. Epidemiological and clinical features in a nonimmune population living in an endemic area. *Tropenmed Parasitol* **29:**188-93.

642. **Biggar, R. J., J. P. Woodall, P. D. Walter, and G. E. Haughie.** 1975. Lymphocytic choriomeningitis outbreak associated with pet hamsters. Fifty-seven cases from New York State. *JAMA* **232:**494-500.

643. **Bigham, J. M., M. T. Hutcheon, D. M. Patrick, and A. J. Pollard.** 2001. Death from invasive meningococcal disease following close contact with a case of primary meningococcal conjunctivitis - Langley, British Columbia, 1999. *Can Commun Dis Rep* **27:**13-18.

644. **Bile, K., A. Isse, O. Mohamud, P. Allebeck, L. Nilsson, H. Norder, I. K. Mushahwar, and L. O. Magnius.** 1994. Contrasting roles of rivers and wells as sources of drinking water on attack and fatality rates in a hepatitis E epidemic in Somalia. *Am J Trop Med Hyg* **51:**466-74.

645. **Bile, K., O. Mohamud, C. Aden, A. Isse, H. Norder, L. Nilsson, and L. O. Magnius.** 1992. The risk for hepatitis A, B, and C at two institutions for children in Somalia with different socioeconomic conditions. *Am J Trop Med Hyg* **47:**357-64.

646. **Billette de Villemeur, T.** 1997. Le point sur la maladie de Creutzfeldt-Jakob iatrogène après traitement par hormone de croissance extractive en France: aspects cliniques, épidémiologiques et neuropathologiques. *Bull Epidém Hebdomadaire* **28:**130-131.

647. **Bilukha, O. O., and N. Rosenstein.** 2005. Prevention and control of meningococcal disease. Recommendations of the Advisory Committee on Immunization Practices (ACIP). *MMWR* **54 (RR-7):**1-21.

648. **Bin, H., Z. Grossman, S. Pokamunski, M. Malkinson, L. Weiss, P. Duvdevani, C. Banet, Y. Weisman, E. Annis, E. Gandaku, V. Yahalom, M. Hindyieh, L. Shulman, and E. Mendelson.** 2001. West Nile fever in Israel 1999-2000: from geese to humans. *Ann N Y Acad Sci* **951:**127-42.

649. **Binquet, C., M. Wallon, C. Quantin, L. Kodjikian, J. Garweg, J. Fleury, F. Peyron, and M. Abrahamowicz.** 2003. Prognostic factors for the long-term development of ocular lesions in 327 children with congenital toxoplasmosis. *Epidemiol Infect* **131:**1157-68.

650. **Binswanger, I. A., A. H. Kral, R. N. Bluthenthal, D. J. Rybold, and B. R. Edlin.** 2000. High prevalence of abscesses and cellulitis among community-recruited injection drug users in San Francisco. *Clin Infect Dis* **30:**579-81.

651. **Bircher, A. J., B. Gysi, H. R. Zenklusen, and R. Aerni.** 2000. [Eosinophilic esophagitis associated with recurrent urticaria: is the worm Anisakis simplex involved?]. *Schweiz Med Wochenschr* **130:**1814-9.

652. Bird, J., R. Browning, R. P. Hobson, F. M. MacKenzie, J. Brand, and I. M. Gould. 1998. Multiply-resistant Klebsiella pneumoniae: failure of spread in community-based elderly care facilities. *J Hosp Infect* **40**:243-7.

653. Bird, M., C. R. Dawson, J. S. Schachter, Y. Miao, A. Shama, A. Osman, A. Bassem, and T. M. Lietman. 2003. Does the diagnosis of trachoma adequately identify ocular chlamydial infection in trachoma-endemic areas? *J Infect Dis* **187**:1669-73.

654. Birkhead, G., and a. W. Group. 1998. Prevention of invasive group A streptococcal disease among household contacts of case-patients. Is prophylaxis warranted? *JAMA* **279**:1206-1210.

655. Birkhead, G., E. N. Janoff, R. L. Vogt, and P. D. Smith. 1989. Elevated levels of immunoglobulin A to Giardia lamblia during a waterborne outbreak of gastroenteritis. *J Clin Microbiol* **27**:1707-10.

656. Birkhead, G., R. L. Vogt, E. M. Heun, J. T. Snyder, and B. A. McClane. 1988. Characterization of an outbreak of Clostridium perfringens food poisoning by quantitative fecal culture and fecal enterotoxin measurement. *J Clin Microbiol* **26**:471-4.

657. Birkhead, G. S., D. L. Morse, W. C. Levine, J. K. Fudala, S. F. Kondracki, H. G. Chang, M. Shayegani, L. Novick, and P. A. Blake. 1993. Typhoid fever at a resort hotel in New York: a large outbreak with an unusual vehicle. *J Infect Dis* **167**:1228-32.

658. Birmingham, K. 2000. Were some CJD victims infected by vaccines? *Nature* **408**:3-4.

659. Birmingham, M. E., L. A. Lee, N. Ndayimirije, S. Nkurikiye, B. S. Hersh, J. G. Wells, and M. S. Deming. 1997. Epidemic cholera in Burundi: patterns of transmission in the Great Rift Valley Lake region. *Lancet* **349**:981-5.

660. Bisbini, P., E. Leoni, and A. Nanetti. 2000. An outbreak of Salmonella Hadar associated with roast rabbit in a restaurant. *Eur J Epidemiol* **16**:613-8.

661. Bischoff, W. E., S. Bassetti, B. A. Bassetti-Wyss, M. L. Wallis, B. K. Tucker, B. A. Reboussin, R. B. D'Agostino, Jr., M. A. Pfaller, J. M. Gwaltney, Jr., and R. J. Sherertz. 2004. Airborne dispersal as a novel transmission route of coagulase-negative staphylococci: interaction between coagulase-negative staphylococci and rhinovirus infection. *Infect Control Hosp Epidemiol* **25**:504-11.

662. Bise, G., and R. Coninx. 1997. Epidemic typhus in a prison in Burundi. *Trans R Soc Trop Med Hyg* **91**:133-4.

663. Biselli, R., A. Fattorossi, P. M. Matricardi, R. Nisini, T. Stroffolini, and R. D'Amelio. 1993. Dramatic reduction of meningococcal meningitis among military recruits in Italy after introduction of specific vaccination. *Vaccine* **11**:578-81.

664. Bisgard, K. M., F. B. Pascual, K. R. Ehresmann, C. A. Miller, C. Cianfrini, C. E. Jennings, C. A. Rebmann, J. Gabel, S. L. Schauer, and S. M. Lett. 2004. Infant pertussis: who was the source? *Pediatr Infect Dis J* **23**:985-9.

665. Bishara, J., D. Hershkovitz, P. Yagupsky, T. Lazarovitch, I. Boldur, T. Kra-Oz, and S. Pitlik. 2004. Murine typhus among Arabs and Jews in Israel 1991-2001. *Eur J Epidemiol* **19**:1123-6.

666. Bisharat, N., V. Agmon, R. Finkelstein, R. Raz, G. Ben-Dror, L. Lerner, S. Soboh, R. Colodner, D. N. Cameron, D. L. Wykstra, D. L. Swerdlow, and J. J. Farmer, 3rd. 1999. Clinical, epidemiological, and microbiological features of Vibrio vulnificus biogroup 3 causing outbreaks of wound infection and bacteraemia in Israel. Israel Vibrio Study Group. *Lancet* **354**:1421-4.

667. Bisharat, N., J. Strahilewitz, M. Ephros, and R. Raz. 1998. Outbreak of acute schistosomiasis among Israeli rafters on the Omo river in Ethiopia. *Am J Trop Med Hyg* **59**:504.

668. Bishop, R., and G. Barnes. 1996. Rotavirus infection - the need for a vaccine. *Commun Dis Intell* **20**:296-8.

669. Bishop, R. F., D. J. S. Cameron, A. A. Veenstra, and G. L. Barnes. 1979. Diarrhea and rotavirus infection associated with differing regimens for postnatal care of newborn babies. *J Clin Microbiol* **9**:525-9.

670. Bisno, A. L., M. A. Gerber, J. M. Gwaltney, Jr., E. L. Kaplan, and R. H. Schwartz. 2002. Practice guidelines for the diagnosis and management of group A streptococcal pharyngitis. *Clin Infect Dis* **35**:113-25.

671. Bisoffi, Z., A. Matteelli, D. Aquilini, G. Guaraldi, G. Magnani, G. Orlando, G. Gaiera, T. Jelinek, and R. H. Behrens. 2003. Malaria clusters among illegal Chinese immigrants to Europe through Africa. *Emerg Infect Dis* **9**:1177-8.

672. Bittencourt, A. L., E. Mota, R. Ribeiro Filho, L. G. Fernandes, P. R. de Almeida, I. Sherlock, J. Maguire, J. Piesman, and C. W. Todd. 1985. Incidence of congenital Chagas' disease in Bahia, Brazil. *J Trop Pediatr* **31**:242-8.

673. Bizet, J., and C. Bizet. 1997. Strains of Alcaligenes faecalis from clinical material. *J Infect* **35**:167-9.

674. Bjerregaard, P., R. Steinglass, D. M. Mutie, G. Kimani, M. Mjomba, and V. Orinda. 1993. Neonatal tetanus mortality in coastal Kenya: a community survey. *Int J Epidemiol* **22**:163-9.

675. Bjoersdorff, A., S. Bergstrom, R. F. Massung, P. D. Haemig, and B. Olsen. 2001. Ehrlichia-infected ticks on migrating birds. *Emerg Infect Dis* **7**:877-9.

676. Bjorland, J., R. T. Bryan, W. Strauss, G. V. Hillyer, and J. B. McAuley. 1995. An outbreak of acute fascioliasis among Aymara Indians in the Bolivian altiplano. *Clin Infect Dis* **21**:1228-33.

677. Bjorvatn, B., and S. G. Gundersen. 1980. Rabies exposure among Norwegian missionaries working abroad. *Scand J Infect Dis* **12**:257-64.

678. Black, C. P. 2003. Systematic review of the biology and medical management of respiratory syncytial virus infection. *Respir Care* **48**:209-31; discussion 231-3.

679. Black, R. E., L. Cisneros, M. M. Levine, A. Banfi, H. Lobos, and H. Rodriguez. 1985. Case-control study to identify risk factors for paediatric endemic typhoid fever in Santiago, Chile. *Bull WHO* **63**:899-904.

680. Black, R. E., R. J. Jackson, T. Tsai, M. Medvesky, M. Shayegani, J. C. Feeley, K. I. MacLeod, and A. M. Wakelee. 1978. Epidemic Yersinia enterocolitica infection due to contaminated chocolate milk. *N Engl J Med* **298**:76-9.

681. Black, S., H. Shinefield, R. Baxter, R. Austrian, L. Bracken, J. Hansen, E. Lewis, and B. Fireman. 2004. Postlicensure surveillance for pneumococcal invasive disease after use of heptavalent pneumococcal conjugate vaccine in northern California Kaiser Permanente. *Pediatr Infect Dis J* **23**:485-9.

682. Blackburn, B. G., G. F. Craun, J. S. Yoder, V. Hill, R. L. Calderon, N. Chen, S. H. Lee, D. A. Levy, and M. J. Beach. 2004. Surveillance for waterborne-disease outbreaks associated with drinking water—United States, 2001-2002. *MMWR SS* **53**:23-45.

683. Blackmore, C. A., K. Limpakarnjanarat, J. G. Rigau-Perez, W. L. Albritton, and J. R. Greenwood. 1985. An outbreak of

chancroid in Orange County, California: descriptive epidemiology and disease-control measures. *J Infect Dis* **151**:840-4.

684. **Blackmore, C. G. M., L. M. Stark, W. C. Jeter, R. L. Oliveri, R. G. Brooks, L. A. Conti, and S. T. Wiersma.** 2003. Surveillance results from the first west nile virus transmission season in Florida, 2001. *Am J Trop Med Hyg* **69**:141-50.

685. **Blackmore, D. K., and L. Schollum.** 1982. The occupational hazards of leptospirosis in the meat industry. *N Z Med J* **95**:494-7.

686. **Blackmore, D. K., and L. M. Schollum.** 1982. Risks of contracting leptospirosis on the dairy farm. *N Z Med J* **95**:649-52.

687. **Blackwell, V., and F. Vega-Lopez.** 2001. Cutaneous larva migrans: clinical features and management of 44 cases presenting in the returning traveller. *Br J Dermatol* **145**:434-7.

688. **Blake, P. A., M. L. Rosenberg, J. Florencia, J. B. Costa, L. do Prado Quintino, and E. J. Gangarosa.** 1977. Cholera in Portugal, 1974. II. Transmission by bottled mineral water. *Am J Epidemiol* **105**:344-8.

689. **Blanc, D. S., T. Parret, B. Janin, P. Raselli, and P. Francioli.** 1997. Nosocomial infections and pseudoinfections from contaminated bronchoscopes: two-year follow up using molecular markers. *Infect Control Hosp Epidemiol* **18**:134-6.

690. **Blanc, D. S., C. Petignat, B. Janin, J. Bille, and P. Francioli.** 1998. Frequency and molecular diversity of Pseudomonas aeruginosa upon admission and during hospitalization: a prospective epidemiologic study. *Clin Microbiol Infect* **4**:242-247.

691. **Blanc, D. S., D. Pittet, C. Ruef, A. F. Widmer, K. Muhlemann, C. Petignat, S. Harbarth, R. Auckenthaler, J. Bille, R. Frei, R. Zbinden, P. Moreillon, P. Sudre, and P. Francioli.** 2002. Molecular epidemiology of predominant clones and sporadic strains of methicillin resistant Staphylococcus aureus in Switzerland and comparison with European epidemic clones. *Clin Microbiol Infect* **8**:419-26.

692. **Blancas, D., M. Santin, M. Olmo, F. Alcaide, J. Carratala, and F. Gudiol.** 2004. Group B streptococcal disease in nonpregnant adults: incidence, clinical characteristics, and outcome. *Eur J Clin Microbiol Infect Dis* **23**:168-73.

693. **Blanche, S.** 2000. [Accidental HIV exposure of children through injury with discarded syringes]. *Arch Pediatr* **7**:83-6.

694. **Blanco Ramos, J. R., J. A. Oteo Revuelta, V. Martinez de Artola, E. Ramalle Gomara, A. Garcia Pineda, and V. Ibarra Cucalon.** 1998. [Seroepidemiology of Bartonella henselae infection in a risk group]. *Rev Clin Esp* **198**:805-9.

695. **Blancou, J.** 1997. Organisation internationale de la lutte contre les anthropozoonoses. *Med Trop* **57** (**suppl**):37S-43S.

696. **Blaschke-Hellmessen, R.** 2000. [Cryptococcus species—etiological agents of zoonoses or sapronosis?]. *Mycoses* **43 Suppl 1**:48-60.

697. **Blaser, M. J.** 1999. Where does Helicobacter pylori come from and why is it going away? *JAMA* **282**:2260-2.

698. **Blasi, F., A. Boschini, R. Cosentini, D. Legnani, C. Smacchia, C. Ghira, and L. Allegra.** 1994. Outbreak of Chlamydia pneumoniae infection in former injection-drug users. *Chest* **105**:812-5.

699. **Blasi, F., P. Tarsia, C. Arosio, L. Fagetti, and L. Allegra.** 1998. Epidemiology of Chlamydia pneumoniae. *Clin Microbiol Infect* **4 Suppl 4**:S1-S6.

700. **Blatt, S. P., M. D. Parkinson, E. Pace, P. Hoffman, D. Dolan, P. Lauderdale, R. A. Zajac, and G. P. Melcher.** 1993. Nosocomial Legionnaires' disease: aspiration as a primary mode of disease acquisition. *Am J Med* **95**:16-22.

701. **Blaxhult, A., O. Kirk, C. Pedersen, M. Dietrich, S. E. Barton, et al.** 2000. Regional differences in presentation of AIDS in Europe. *Epidemiol Infect* **125**:142-51.

702. **Blessmann, J., I. K. Ali, P. A. Nu, B. T. Dinh, T. Q. Viet, A. L. Van, C. G. Clark, and E. Tannich.** 2003. Longitudinal study of intestinal Entamoeba histolytica infections in asymptomatic adult carriers. *J Clin Microbiol* **41**:4745-50.

703. **Blessmann, J., P. Van Linh, P. A. Nu, H. D. Thi, B. Muller-Myhsok, H. Buss, and E. Tannich.** 2002. Epidemiology of amebiasis in a region of high incidence of amebic liver abscess in central Vietnam. *Am J Trop Med Hyg* **66**:578-83.

704. **Bloch, A. B., S. L. Stramer, J. D. Smith, H. S. Margolis, H. A. Fields, T. W. McKinley, C. P. Gerba, J. E. Maynard, and R. K. Sikes.** 1990. Recovery of hepatitis A virus from a water supply responsible for a common source outbreak of hepatitis A. *Am J Public Health* **80**:428-30.

705. **Blomqvist, S., M. Roivainen, T. Puhakka, M. Kleemola, and T. Hovi.** 2002. Virological and serological analysis of rhinovirus infections during the first two years of life in a cohort of children. *J Med Virol* **66**:263-8.

706. **Bloom, S., A. Rguig, A. Berraho, L. Zniber, N. Bouazzaoui, Z. Zaghloul, S. Reef, A. Zidouh, M. Papania, and J. Seward.** 2005. Congenital rubella syndrome burden in Morocco: a rapid retrospective assessment. *Lancet* **365**:135-41.

707. **Blotta, M. H., R. L. Mamoni, S. J. Oliveira, S. A. Nouer, P. M. Papaiordanou, A. Goveia, and Z. P. Camargo.** 1999. Endemic regions of paracoccidioidomycosis in Brazil: a clinical and epidemiologic study of 584 cases in the southeast region. *Am J Trop Med Hyg* **61**:390-4.

708. **Blow, J. A., M. J. Turell, A. L. Silverman, and E. D. Walker.** 2001. Stercorarial shedding and transtadial transmission of hepatitis B virus by common bed bugs (Hemiptera: Cimicidae). *J Med Entomol* **38**:694-700.

709. **Blum, J., and C. Burri.** 2002. Treatment of late stage sleeping sickness caused by T. b. gambiense: a new approach to the use of an old drug. *Swiss Med Wkly* **132**:51-6.

710. **Blumberg, H. M., M. K. Leonard, Jr., and R. M. Jasmer.** 2005. Update on the treatment of tuberculosis and latent tuberculosis infection. *JAMA* **293**:2776-84.

711. **Blumberg, H. M., M. Sotir, M. Erwin, R. Bachman, and J. A. Shulman.** 1998. Risk of house staff tuberculin skin test conversion in an area with a high incidence of tuberculosis. *Clin Infect Dis* **27**:826-33.

712. **Blumenthal, D. S., D. Taplin, and M. G. Schultz.** 1976. A community outbreak of scabies. *Am J Epidemiol* **104**:667-72.

713. **Blumenthal, U. J., E. Cifuentes, S. Bennett, M. Quigley, and G. Ruiz-Palacios.** 2001. The risk of enteric infections associated with wastewater reuse: the effect of season and degree of storage of wastewater. *Trans R Soc Trop Med Hyg* **95**:131-7.

714. **Blumer, C., P. Roche, J. Spencer, M. Lin, A. Milton, C. Bunn, H. Gidding, J. Kaldor, M. Kirk, R. Hall, T. Della-Porta, R. Leader, and P. Wright.** 2003. Australia's notifiable diseases status, 2001. *Commun Dis Intell* **27**:1-78.

715. **Boase, J., S. Lipsky, P. Simani, S. Smith, and C. Skilton.** 1999. Outbreak of Salmonella serotype Muenchen infections associated with unpasteurized orange juice - United States and Canada, June 1999. *MMWR* **48**:582-585.

716. Boccia, D., A. E. Tozzi, B. Cotter, C. Rizzo, T. Russo, G. Buttinelli, A. Caprioli, M. L. Marziano, and F. M. Ruggeri. 2002. Waterborne outbreak of norwalk-like virus gastroenteritis at a tourist resort, Italy. *Emerg Infect Dis* **8**:563-8.

717. Bock, N. N., J. P. Mallory, N. Mobley, B. DeVoe, and B. B. Taylor. 1998. Outbreak of tuberculosis associated with a floating card game in the rural south: lessons for tuberculosis contact investigations. *Clin Infect Dis* **27**:1221-6.

718. Bock, N. N., M. J. Sotir, P. L. Parrott, and H. M. Blumberg. 1999. Nosocomial tuberculosis exposure in an outpatient setting: evaluation of patients exposed to healthcare providers with tuberculosis. *Infect Control Hosp Epidemiol* **20**:421-5.

719. Bockarie, M. J., L. Tavul, W. Kastens, E. Michael, and J. W. Kazura. 2002. Impact of untreated bednets on prevalence of Wuchereria bancrofti transmitted by Anopheles farauti in Papua New Guinea. *Med Vet Entomol* **16**:116-9.

720. Bockemuhl, J., and P. Roggentin. 2004. [Intestinal yersiniosis. Clinical importance, epidemiology, diagnosis, and prevention]. *Bundesgesundheitsblatt Gesundheitsforschung Gesundheitsschutz* **47**:685-91.

721. Bockemühl, J., and A. Triemer. 1974. Ecology and epidemiology of Vibrio parahaemolyticus on the coast of Togo. *Bull WHO* **51**:353-60.

722. Bode, G., P. Marchildon, J. Peacock, H. Brenner, and D. Rothenbacher. 2002. Diagnosis of Helicobacter pylori infection in children: comparison of a salivary immunoglobulin G antibody test with the [(13)C]urea breath test. *Clin Diagn Lab Immunol* **9**:493-5.

723. Boehme, C., T. Iglesias, A. Loyola, L. Soto, G. Rodriguez, P. Reydet, and V. Illesca. 2002. [Comparison of Shigella susceptibility to commonly used antimicrobials in the Temuco Regional Hospital, Chile 1990 - 2001]. *Rev Med Chil* **130**:1021-6.

724. Boelaert, M., B. Criel, J. Leeuwenburg, W. Van Damme, D. Le Ray, and P. Van der Stuyft. 2000. Visceral leishmaniasis control: a public health perspective. *Trans R Soc Trop Med Hyg* **94**:465-71.

725. Boelee, E., and H. Laamrani. 2004. Environmental control of schistosomiasis through community participation in a Moroccan oasis. *Trop Med Int Health* **9**:997-1004.

726. Bogaert, D., R. De Groot, and P. W. Hermans. 2004. Streptococcus pneumoniae colonisation: the key to pneumococcal disease. *Lancet Infect Dis* **4**:144-54.

727. Bogaert, D., M. N. Engelen, A. J. Timmers-Reker, K. P. Elzenaar, P. G. Peerbooms, R. A. Coutinho, R. de Groot, and P. W. Hermans. 2001. Pneumococcal carriage in children in the netherlands: a molecular epidemiological study. *J Clin Microbiol* **39**:3316-20.

728. Bogaert, D., A. van Belkum, M. Sluijter, A. Luijendijk, R. de Groot, H. C. Rumke, H. A. Verbrugh, and P. W. Hermans. 2004. Colonisation by Streptococcus pneumoniae and Staphylococcus aureus in healthy children. *Lancet* **363**:1871-2.

729. Bogaerts, J., B. Vuylsteke, W. Martinez Tello, V. Mukantabana, J. Akingeneye, M. Laga, and P. Piot. 1995. Simple algorithms for the management of genital ulcers: evaluation in a primary health care center in Kigali, Rwanda. *Bull WHO* **73**:761-7.

730. Bogdan, C., G. Schonian, A. L. Banuls, M. Hide, F. Pratlong, E. Lorenz, M. Rollinghoff, and R. Mertens. 2001. Visceral leishmaniasis in a German child who had never entered a known endemic area: case report and review of the literature. *Clin Infect Dis* **32**:302-6.

731. Bohlen, L. M., K. Muhlemann, O. Dubuis, C. Aebi, and M. G. Tauber. 2000. Outbreak among drug users caused by a clonal strain of group A streptococcus. *Emerg Infect Dis* **6**:175-9.

732. Bohmer, C. J., E. C. Klinkenberg-Knol, E. J. Kuipers, M. C. Niezen-de Boer, H. Schreuder, F. Schuckink-Kool, and S. G. Meuwissen. 1997. The prevalence of Helicobacter pylori infection among inhabitants and healthy employees of institutes for the intellectually disabled. *Am J Gastroenterol* **92**:1000-4.

733. Boireau, P., I. Vallee, T. Roman, C. Perret, L. Mingyuan, H. R. Gamble, and A. Gajadhar. 2000. Trichinella in horses: a low frequency infection with high human risk. *Vet Parasitol* **93**:309-20.

734. Boiro, L., O. K. Konstaninov, and A. D. Numerov. 1987. Isolement du virus de la fièvre de la vallée du Rift à partir de chéiroptères en république de Gunée. *Bull Soc Pathol Exot* **80**:62-7.

735. Boisier, P., L. Rahalison, M. Rasolomaharo, M. Ratsitorahina, M. Mahafaly, M. Razafimahefa, J. M. Duplantier, and S. Chanteau. 2002. Epidemiologic features of four successive annual outbreaks of bubonic plague in Mahajanga, Madagascar. *Emerg Infect Dis* **8**:311-6.

736. Boisson, K., M. Thouverez, D. Talon, and X. Bertrand. 2002. Characterisation of coagulase-negative staphylococci isolated from blood infections: incidence, susceptibility to glycopeptides, and molecular epidemiology. *Eur J Clin Microbiol Infect Dis* **21**:660-5.

737. Boivin, G., G. De Serres, S. Côté, R. Gilca, Y. Abed, L. Rochette, M. G. Bergeron, and P. Dery. 2003. Human metapneumovirus infections in hospitalized children. *Emerg Infect Dis* **9**:634-40.

738. Bokhout, M. 1987. Rubella outbreak among unimmunized male high school students in Wabush/Labrador city - Newfoundland. *Can Dis Wkly Rep* **13**:199-202.

739. Bolan, G., A. L. Reingold, L. A. Carson, V. A. Silcox, C. L. Woodley, P. S. Hayes, A. W. Hightower, L. McFarland, J. W. Brown, 3rd, N. J. Petersen, et al. 1985. Infections with Mycobacterium chelonei in patients receiving dialysis and using processed hemodialyzers. *J Infect Dis* **152**:1013-9.

740. Boland, M., G. Sayers, T. Coleman, C. Bergin, N. Sheehan, E. Creamer, M. O'Connell, L. Jones, and W. Zochowski. 2004. A cluster of leptospirosis cases in canoeists following a competition on the River Liffey. *Epidemiol Infect* **132**:195-200.

741. Bolduc, D., L. F. Srour, L. Sweet, A. Neatby, E. Galanis, S. Isaacs, and G. Lim. 2004. Severe outbreak of Escherichia coli O157:H7 in health care institutions in Charlottetown, Prince Edward Island, fall 2002. *Can Commun Dis Rep* **30**:81-8.

742. Bollag, U. 1980. Practical evaluation of a pilot immunization campaign against typhoid fever in a Cambodian refugee camp. *Int J Epidemiol* **9**:121-2.

743. Bolland, J. M., and D. Moehle McCallum. 2002. Touched by homelessness: an examination of hospitality for the down and out. *Am J Public Health* **92**:116-8.

744. Bollini, P., J. D. Laporte, and T. W. Harding. 2002. HIV prevention in prisons. Do international guidelines matter? *Eur J Public Health* **12**:83-9.

745. Bolpe, J., and R. Boffi. 2001. Human trichinellosis in Argentina. Review of the casuistry registered from 1990 to 1999. *Parasite* **8**:S78-80.

746. Bolton, F. J., S. B. Surman, K. Martin, D. R. A. Wareing, and T. J. Humphrey. 1999. Presence of campylobacter and salmonella in sand from bathing beaches. *Epidemiol Infect* **122**:7-13.

747. **Bolyard, E. A., O. C. Tablan, W. W. Williams, M. L. Pearson, C. N. Shapiro, and S. D. Deitchmann.** 1998. Guideline for infection control in healthcare personnel, 1998. Hospital Infection Control Practices Advisory Committee. *Infect Control Hosp Epidemiol* **19**:407-63.

748. **Bonametti, A. M., N. Passos Jdo, E. M. da Silva, and A. L. Bortoliero.** 1996. [Outbreak of acute toxoplasmosis transmitted thru the ingestion of ovine raw meat]. *Rev Soc Bras Med Trop* **30**:21-5.

749. **Bonanni, P.** 1998. Report on working group 1: Albania, Andorra, Canada, France, Italy, Moldavia, Portugal, Poland, Romania and Spain. *Vaccine* **16 Suppl 9**:S58-S60.

750. **Bonanni, P., and G. Bonaccorsi.** 2001. Vaccination against hepatitis B in health care workers. *Vaccine* **19**:2389-94.

751. **Bonanni, P., R. Colombai, G. Franchi, A. Lo Nostro, N. Comodo, and E. Tiscione.** 1998. Experience of hepatitis A vaccination during an outbreak in a nursery school of Tuscany, Italy. *Epidemiol Infect* **121**:377-80.

752. **Bonanni, P., A. Franzin, C. Staderini, M. Pitta, G. Garofalo, R. Cecconi, M. G. Santini, P. Lai, and B. Innocenti.** 2005. Vaccination against hepatitis A during outbreaks starting in schools: what can we learn from experiences in central Italy? *Vaccine* **23**:2176-80.

753. **Bonardi, S., F. Brindani, G. Pizzin, L. Lucidi, M. D'Incau, E. Liebana, and S. Morabito.** 2003. Detection of Salmonella spp., Yersinia enterocolitica and verocytotoxin-producing Escherichia coli O157 in pigs at slaughter in Italy. *Int J Food Microbiol* **85**:101-10.

754. **Bonassoli, L. A., M. Bertoli, and T. I. Svidzinski.** 2005. High frequency of Candida parapsilosis on the hands of healthy hosts. *J Hosp Infect* **59**:159-62.

755. **Bonatti, H., D. W. Rossboth, D. Nachbaur, M. Fille, C. Aspock, I. Hend, K. Hourmont, L. White, H. Malnick, and F. J. Allerberger.** 2003. A series of infections due to Capnocytophaga spp in immunosuppressed and immunocompetent patients. *Clin Microbiol Infect* **9**:380-7.

756. **Boneva, R. S., T. M. Folks, and L. E. Chapman.** 2001. Infectious disease issues in xenotransplantation. *Clin Microbiol Rev* **14**:1-14.

757. **Bonhomme, M. G., W. Rojanapithayakorn, P. J. Feldblum, and M. J. Rosenberg.** 1994. Incidence of sexually transmitted diseases among massage parlour employees in Bangkok, Thailand. *Int J STD AIDS* **5**:214-7.

758. **Bonifacio, N., M. Saito, R. H. Gilman, F. Leung, N. C. Chavez, J. C. Huarcaya, and C. V. Quispe.** 2002. High risk for tuberculosis in hospital physicians, Peru. *Emerg Infect Dis* **8**:747-8.

759. **Bonnet, D., G. Nguyen, J. J. De Pina, G. Martet, J. Miltgen, A. Cuguilliere, D. Verrot, T. Lonjon, M. Civatte, and M. Morillon.** 2002. [American pulmonary histoplasmosis. Prospective study with 232 soldiers after a 2-year assignment in Guiana]. *Med Trop (Mars)* **62**:33-8.

760. **Bonten, M. J., M. K. Hayden, C. Nathan, J. van Voorhis, M. Matushek, S. Slaughter, T. Rice, and R. A. Weinstein.** 1996. Epidemiology of colonisation of patients and environment with vancomycin-resistant enterococci. *Lancet* **348**:1615-9.

761. **Boost, M. V., M. M. O'Donoghue, and J. S. Dooley.** 2001. Prevalence of carriage of antimicrobial resistant strains of Streptococcus pneumoniae in primary school children in Hong Kong. *Epidemiol Infect* **127**:49-55.

762. **Boostrom, A., M. S. Beier, J. A. Macaluso, K. R. Macaluso, D. Sprenger, J. Hayes, S. Radulovic, and A. F. Azad.** 2002. Geographic Association of Rickettsia felis-Infected Opossums with Human Murine Typhus, Texas. *Emerg Infect Dis* **8**:549-54.

763. **Booton, G. C., D. J. Kelly, Y. W. Chu, D. V. Seal, E. Houang, D. S. Lam, T. J. Byers, and P. A. Fuerst.** 2002. 18S ribosomal DNA typing and tracking of Acanthamoeba species isolates from corneal scrape specimens, contact lenses, lens cases, and home water supplies of Acanthamoeba keratitis patients in Hong Kong. *J Clin Microbiol* **40**:1621-5.

764. **Booy, R.** 1995. Outbreak of group C meningococcal disease in Australian Aboriginal children. *Lancet* **346**:572-3.

765. **Borau, J., R. T. Czap, K. A. Strellrecht, and R. A. Venezia.** 2000. Long-term control of Legionella species in potable water after a nosocomial legionellosis outbreak in an intensive care unit. *Infect Control Hosp Epidemiol* **21**:602-3.

766. **Borchardt, M. A., M. E. Stemper, and J. H. Standridge.** 2003. Aeromonas isolates from human diarrheic stool and groundwater compared by pulsed-field gel electrophoresis. *Emerg Infect Dis* **9**.

767. **Boreham, P. F., and R. E. Phillips.** 1986. Giardiasis in Mount Isa, north-west Queensland. *Med J Aust* **144**:524-8.

768. **Boreham, R. F., M. J. McCowan, A. E. Ryan, A. M. Allworth, and J. M. Robson.** 1995. Human trichostrongyliasis in Queensland. *Pathology* **27**:182-5.

769. **Borella, P., M. T. Montagna, V. Romano-Spica, S. Stampi, G. Stancanelli, M. Triassi, R. Neglia, I. Marchesi, G. Fantuzzi, D. Tato, C. Napoli, G. Quaranta, P. Laurenti, E. Leoni, G. De Luca, C. Ossi, M. Moro, and G. Ribera D'Alcala.** 2004. Legionella infection risk from domestic hot water. *Emerg Infect Dis* **10**:457-64.

770. **Borenstein, M., and F. Kerdel.** 2003. Infections with Vibrio vulnificus. *Dermatol Clin* **21**:245-8.

771. **Borg, M. A., and A. Portelli.** 1999. Hospital laundry workers—an at-risk group for hepatitis A? *Occup Med (Lond)* **49**: 448-50.

772. **Borgen, K., M. Sorum, H. Kruse, and Y. Wasteson.** 2000. Persistence of vancomycin-resistant enterococci (VRE) on Norwegian broiler farms. *FEMS Microbiol Lett* **191**:255-8.

773. **Borges, R., and J. Mendes.** 2002. Epidemiological aspects of head lice in children attending day care centres, urban and rural schools in Uberlandia, central Brazil. *Mem Inst Oswaldo Cruz* **97**:189-92.

774. **Borghans, J. G., and J. L. Stanford.** 1973. Mycobacterium chelonei in abscesses after injection of diphtheria- pertussis-tetanus-polio vaccine. *Am Rev Respir Dis* **107**:1-8.

775. **Borgnolo, G., B. Hailu, A. Ciancarelli, M. Almaviva, and T. Woldemariam.** 1993. Louse-borne relapsing fever. A clinical and an epidemiological study of 389 patients in Asella Hospital, Ethiopia. *Trop Geogr Med* **45**:66-9.

776. **Borio, L., T. Inglesby, C. J. Peters, A. L. Schmaljohn, J. M. Hughes, P. B. Jahrling, T. Ksiazek, K. M. Johnson, A. Meyerhoff, T. O'Toole, M. S. Ascher, J. Bartlett, J. G. Breman, E. M. Eitzen, Jr., M. Hamburg, J. Hauer, D. A. Henderson, R. T. Johnson, G. Kwik, M. Layton, S. Lillibridge, G. J. Nabel, M. T. Osterholm, T. M. Perl, P. Russell, and K. Tonat.** 2002. Hemorrhagic fever viruses as biological weapons: medical and public health management. *JAMA* **287**:2391-405.

777. **Bormane, A., I. Lucenko, A. Duks, V. Mavtchoutko, R. Ranka, K. Salmina, and V. Baumanis.** 2004. Vectors of tick-borne diseases and epidemiological situation in Latvia in 1993-2002. *Int J Med Microbiol* **293 Suppl 37**:36-47.

778. **Bornstein, N., D. Marmet, M. Surgot, M. Nowicki, A. Arslan, J. Esteve, and J. Fleurette.** 1989. Exposure to Legionellaceae at

a hot spring spa: a prospective clinical and serological study. *Epidemiol Infect* **102**:31-6.

779. **Borroto, R. J., and R. Martinez-Piedra.** 2000. Geographical patterns of cholera in Mexico, 1991-1996. *Int J Epidemiol* **29**:764-72.

780. **Borup, L. H., J. S. Peters, and C. R. Sartori.** 2003. Onchocerciasis (river blindness). *Cutis* **72**:297-302.

781. **Bosak, P. J., L. M. Reed, and W. J. Crans.** 2001. Habitat preference of host-seeking Coquillettidia perturbans (Walker) in relation to birds and eastern equine encephalomyelitis virus in New Jersey. *J Vector Ecol* **26**:103-9.

782. **Bosch, A., G. Sanchez, F. Le Guyader, H. Vanaclocha, L. Haugarreau, and R. M. Pinto.** 2001. Human enteric viruses in Coquina clams associated with a large hepatitis A outbreak. *Water Sci Technol* **43**:61-5.

783. **Bosch, X.** 1998. Hepatitis C outbreak astounds Spain. *Lancet* **351**:1415.

784. **Boselli, F., G. Chiossi, M. Bortolamasi, and A. Gallinelli.** 2005. Prevalence and determinants of genital shedding of herpes simplex virus among women attending Italian colposcopy clinics. *Eur J Obstet Gynecol Reprod Biol* **118**:86-90.

785. **Boshuizen, H. C., S. E. Neppelenbroek, H. van Vliet, J. F. Schellekens, J. W. den Boer, M. F. Peeters, and M. A. Conyn-van Spaendonck.** 2001. Subclinical Legionella infection in workers near the source of a large outbreak of Legionnaires disease. *J Infect Dis* **184**:515-8.

786. **Bosi, C., A. Davin-Regli, R. Charrel, B. Rocca, D. Monnet, and C. Bollet.** 1996. Serratia marcescens nosocomial outbreak due to contamination of hexetidine solution. *J Hosp Infect* **33**:217-24.

787. **Bosnak, M., B. Dikici, V. Bosnak, O. Dogru, I. Ozkan, A. Ceylan, and K. Haspolat.** 2002. Prevalence of Mycoplasma pneumoniae in children in Diyarbakir, the south-east of Turkey. *Pediatr Int* **44**:510-2.

788. **Bossi, P., A. Tegnell, A. Baka, A. Werner, F. van Loock, J. Hendriks, H. Maidhof, and G. Gouvras.** 2004. Bichat guidelines for the clinical management of botulism and bioterrorism-related botulism. *Eur Surveill* **9**.

789. **Botros, B. A., D. M. Watts, A. K. Soliman, A. W. Salib, M. I. Moussa, H. Mursal, C. Douglas, and M. Farah.** 1989. Serological evidence of dengue fever among refugees, Hargeysa, Somalia. *J Med Virol* **29**:79-81.

790. **Botterel, F., and P. Bouree.** 2003. Ocular Sparganosis : A Case Report. *J Travel Med* **10**:245-246.

791. **Bottiger, M., and E. Herrstrom.** 1992. Isolation of polioviruses from sewage and their characteristics: experience over two decades in Sweden. *Scand J Infect Dis* **24**:151-5.

792. **Botto, H., and Jury de la Conférence de Consensus sur les Infections Urinaires Nosocomiales de l'Adulte.** 2003. Infections urinaires nosocomiales de l'adulte: conférence de consensus 2002, texte court. *Méd Mal Infect* **33**:370-5.

793. **Bottone, E. J.** 1999. Yersinia enterocolitica: overview and epidemiologic correlates. *Microbes Infect* **1**:323-33.

794. **Bou, R., A. Dominguez, D. Fontanals, I. Sanfeliu, I. Pons, J. Renau, V. Pineda, E. Lobera, C. Latorre, M. Majo, and L. Salleras.** 2000. Prevalence of Haemophilus influenzae pharyngeal carriers in the school population of Catalonia. Working Group on invasive disease caused by Haemophilus influenzae. *Eur J Epidemiol* **16**:521-6.

795. **Bouhoum, K., and J. Schwartzbrod.** 1998. Epidemiological study of intestinal helminthiasis in a Marrakech raw sewage spreading zone. *Zentralbl Hyg Umweltmed* **200**:553-61.

796. **Boulanger, L. L., P. Ettestad, J. Fogarty, D. T. Dennis, D. Romig, and G. J. Mertz.** 2004. Gentamicin and tetracyclines for the treatment of human plague: review of 75 cases in New Mexico, 1985-1999. *Clin Infect Dis* **38**:663-9.

797. **Boulware, D. R.** 2004. Influence of hygiene on gastrointestinal illness among wilderness backpackers. *J Travel Med* **11**:27-33.

798. **Bouma, M. J., S. D. Parvez, R. Nesbit, and A. M. Winkler.** 1996. Malaria control using permethrin applied to tents of nomadic Afghan refugees in northern Pakistan. *Bull WHO* **74**:413-21.

799. **Bouma, M. J., and H. J. van der Kaay.** 1994. Epidemic malaria in India and the El Niño southern oscillation. *Lancet* **344**:1638-9.

800. **Bouree, P., P. Espinoza, O. Coco Cianci, and P. Loue.** 1988. [Prevalence of parasitic diseases and HBV and HIV viruses among black Africans in prison. (Study of 116 subjects)]. *Bull Soc Pathol Exot Filiales* **81**:173-82.

801. **Bourgault, A. M., A. Yechouron, C. Gaudreau, H. Gilbert, and F. Lamothe.** 1998. Should all stool specimens be routinely tested for Clostridium difficile? *Clin Microbiol Infect* **5**:219-23.

802. **Bourgeade, A., Y. Nosny, M. Olivier-Paufique, and B. Faugère.** 1989. A propos de 32 cas d'oedèmes localisés récidivants au retour des tropiques. *Bull Soc Pathol Exot* **82**:21-8.

803. **Bourke, A. T., Y. N. Cossins, B. R. Gray, T. J. Lunney, N. A. Rostron, R. V. Holmes, E. R. Griggs, D. J. Larsen, and V. R. Kelk.** 1986. Investigation of cholera acquired from the riverine environment in Queensland. *Med J Aust* **144**:229-34.

804. **Bouros, D., J. Demoiliopoulos, P. Panagou, N. Yiatromanolakis, M. Moschos, A. Paraskevopoulos, D. Demoiliopoulos, and N. M. Siafakas.** 1995. Incidence of tuberculosis in Greek armed forces from 1965-1993. *Respiration* **62**:336-40.

805. **Boussaa, S., S. Guernaoui, B. Pesson, and A. Boumezzough.** 2005. Seasonal fluctuations of phlebotomine sand fly populations (Diptera: Psychodidae) in the urban area of Marrakech, Morocco. *Acta Trop* **95**:86-91.

806. **Boussery, G., M. Boelaert, J. V. Peteghem, P. Ejikon, and K. Henckaerts.** 2001. Visceral leishmaniasis (kala-azar) outbreak in Somali refugees and Kenyan shepherds, Kenya. *Emerg Infect Dis* **7(3)**:603-4.

807. **Bouvet, E., J. Choin, M. Bourdais, and G. Rykner.** 1995. Lutte contre la pédiculose dans les écoles à Paris. *Bull Épidémiol Hebdomadaire* **14**:61-2.

808. **Bouza, E., R. San Juan, P. Munoz, A. Voss, and J. Kluytmans.** 2001. A European perspective on nosocomial urinary tract infections I. Report on the microbiology workload, etiology and antimicrobial susceptibility (ESGNI-003 study). *Clin Microbiol Inf* **7**:523-31.

809. **Bouza, E., R. San Juan, A. Voss, and J. Kluytmans.** 2001. A European perspective onnosocomial urinary tract infections II. Report on incidence, clinical characteristics and outcome (ESGNI-004 study). *Clin Microbiol Infect* **7**:532-42.

810. **Bovallius, A., B. Bucht, R. Roffey, and P. Anas.** 1978. Long-range air transmission of bacteria. *Appl Environ Microbiol* **35**:1231-2.

811. **Bowden, F. J., S. N. Tabrizi, S. M. Garland, and C. K. Fairley.** 2002. Infectious diseases. 6: Sexually transmitted infections: new diagnostic approaches and treatments. *Med J Aust* **176**:551-7.

812. **Bowden, R. A.** 1997. Respiratory virus infections after marrow transplant: the Fred Hutchinson Cancer Research Center experience. *Am J Med* **102**:27-30; discussion 42-3.

813. **Bower, W. A., O. V. Nainan, X. Han, and H. S. Margolis.** 2000. Duration of viremia in hepatitis A virus infection. *J Infect Dis* **182:**12-7.

814. **Bowie, W. R., A. S. King, D. H. Werker, J. L. Isaac-Renton, A. Bell, S. B. Eng, and S. A. Marion.** 1997. Outbreak of toxoplasmosis associated with municipal drinking water. The BC Toxoplasma Investigation Team. *Lancet* **350:**173-7.

815. **Bowler, P. G., B. I. Duerden, and D. G. Armstrong.** 2001. Wound microbiology and associated approaches to wound management. *Clin Microbiol Rev* **14:**244-69.

816. **Bown, K. J., M. Begon, M. Bennett, Z. Woldehiwet, and N. H. Ogden.** 2003. Seasonal Dynamics of Anaplasma phagocytophila in a Rodent-Tick (Ixodes trianguliceps) System, United Kingdom. *Emerg Infect Dis* **9:**63-70.

817. **Boyce, J. M., and D. Pittet.** 2002. Guidelines for hand hygiene in health-care settings. Recommendations of the healthcare infection control practices advisory committee and the HICPAC/SHEA/APIC/IDSA hand gygiene task force. *MMWR* **51 (RR-16):**1-45.

818. **Boyce, T. G., D. Koo, D. L. Swerdlow, T. M. Gomez, B. Serrano, L. N. Nickey, F. W. Hickman-Brenner, G. B. Malcolm, and P. M. Griffin.** 1996. Recurrent outbreaks of Salmonella Enteritidis infections in a Texas restaurant: phage type 4 arrives in the United States. *Epidemiol Infect* **117:**29-34.

819. **Boyce, T. G., E. D. Mintz, K. D. Greene, J. G. Wells, J. C. Hockin, D. Morgan, and R. V. Tauxe.** 1995. Vibrio cholerae O139 Bengal infections among tourists to Southeast Asia: an intercontinental foodborne outbreak. *J Infect Dis* **172:**1401-4.

820. **Boyer, K. M., R. S. Munford, G. O. Maupin, C. P. Pattison, M. D. Fox, A. M. Barnes, W. L. Jones, and J. E. Maynard.** 1977. Tick-borne relapsing fever: an interstate outbreak originating at Grand Canyon national park. *Am J Epidemiol* **105:**469-79.

821. **Brachman, P. S., H. Gold, S. A. Plotkin, F. R. Fekety, and M. Werrin.** 1962. Field evaluation of a human anthrax vaccine. *Am J Public Health* **52:**632-645.

822. **Brack, M.** 1987. Agents transmissible from simians to man. Springer-Verlag, Berlin.

823. **Bradaric, N., V. Punda-Polic, I. Milas, I. Ivic, D. Grgic, N. Radosevic, and I. Petric.** 1996. Two outbreaks of typhoid fever related to the war in Bosnia and Herzegovina. *Eur J Epidemiol* **12:**409-12.

824. **Braddy, C. M., and J. E. Blair.** 2005. Colonization of personal digital assistants used in a health care setting. *Am J Infect Control* **33:**230-2.

825. **Bradford, D. L.** 1983. Syphilis case-finding in an Australian men's sauna club. *Med J Aust* **2:**561-4.

826. **Bradley, D. J., and D. C. Warhurst.** 1997. Guidelines for the prevention of malaria in travellers from the United Kingdom. *CDR Rev* **7:**R137-R152.

827. **Bradley, K., M. Grubbs, M. Lytle, M. Crutcher, K. Smith, and P. Keim.** 2001. Tularemia - Oklahoma, 2000. *MMWR* **50:**704-706.

828. **Brady, M. T., J. Evans, and J. Cuartas.** 1990. Survival and disinfection of parainfluenza viruses on environmental surfaces. *Am J Infect Control* **18:**18-23.

829. **Braga, L. L., Y. Mendonca, C. A. Paiva, A. Sales, A. L. Cavalcante, and B. J. Mann.** 1998. Seropositivity for and intestinal colonization with Entamoeba histolytica and Entamoeba dispar in individuals in northeastern Brazil. *J Clin Microbiol* **36:**3044-5.

830. **Bragonier, R., P. Nasveld, and A. Auliffe.** 2002. Plasmodium malariae in East Timor. *Southeast Asian J Trop Med Public Health* **33:**689-90.

831. **Brahim, H., J. D. Perrier-Gros-Claude, D. Postic, G. Baranton, and R. Jambou.** 2005. Identifying relapsing fever borrelia, Senegal. *Emerg Infect Dis* **11:**474-5.

832. **Braithwaite, R. L., T. Stephens, C. Sterk, and K. Braithwaite.** 1999. Risks associated with tattooing and body piercing. *J Public Health Policy* **20:**459-70.

833. **Brajac, I., K. Loncarek, L. Stojnic-Sosa, and F. Gruber.** 2005. Delayed onset of warts over tattoo mark provoked by sunburn. *J Eur Acad Dermatol Venereol* **19:**247-8.

834. **Brajac, I., L. Stojnic-Sosa, L. Prpic, K. Loncarek, and F. Gruber.** 2004. The epidemiology of Microsporum canis infections in Rijeka area, Croatia. *Mycoses* **47:**222-6.

835. **Brandão-Filho, S. P., M. E. Brito, F. G. Carvalho, E. A. Ishikawa, E. Cupolillo, L. Floeter-Winter, and J. J. Shaw.** 2003. Wild and synanthropic hosts of Leishmania (Viannia) braziliensis in the endemic cutaneous leishmaniasis locality of Amaraji, Pernambuco state, Brazil. *Trans R Soc Trop Med Hyg* **97:**291-6.

836. **Brandel, J. P., M. Preece, P. Brown, E. Croes, J. L. Laplanche, Y. Agid, R. Will, and A. Alperovitch.** 2003. Distribution of codon 129 genotype in human growth hormone-treated CJD patients in France and the U.K. *Lancet* **362:**128-30.

837. **Brassard, P., J. Bruneau, K. Schwartzman, M. Senecal, and D. Menzies.** 2004. Yield of tuberculin screening among injection drug users. *Int J Tuberc Lung Dis* **8:**988-93.

838. **Braue, A., G. Ross, G. Varigos, and H. Kelly.** 2005. Epidemiology and impact of childhood molluscum contagiosum: a case series and critical review of the literature. *Pediatr Dermatol* **22:**287-94.

839. **Brault, A. C., A. M. Powers, C. L. Chavez, R. N. Lopez, M. F. Cachon, L. F. Gutierrez, W. Kang, R. B. Tesh, R. E. Shope, and S. C. Weaver.** 1999. Genetic and antigenic diversity among eastern equine encephalitis viruses from North, Central, and South America. *Am J Trop Med Hyg* **61:**579-86.

840. **Braun, T. I., T. Fekete, and A. Lynch.** 1988. Strongyloidiasis in an institution for mentally retarded adults. *Arch Intern Med* **148:**634-6.

841. **Bravo, J. R., M. G. Guzmán, and G. P. Kouri.** 1987. Why dengue haemorrhagic fever in Cuba? I. Individual risk factors for dengue haemorrhagic fever/dengue shock syndrome (DHF/DSS). *Trans R Soc Trop Med Hyg* **81:**816-820.

842. **Brazier, J. S., M. Gal, V. Hall, and T. Morris.** 2004. Outbreak of Clostridium histolyticum infections in injecting drug users in England and Scotland. *Eur Surveill* **9:**15–6.

843. **Breard, E., C. Hamblin, S. Hammoumi, C. Sailleau, G. Dauphin, and S. Zientara.** 2004. The epidemiology and diagnosis of bluetongue with particular reference to Corsica. *Res Vet Sci* **77:**1-8.

844. **Breathnach, A. S., A. de Ruiter, G. M. Holdsworth, N. T. Bateman, D. G. O'Sullivan, P. J. Rees, D. Snashall, H. J. Milburn, B. S. Peters, J. Watson, F. A. Drobniewski, and G. L. French.** 1998. An outbreak of multi-drug-resistant tuberculosis in a London teaching hospital. *J Hosp Infect* **39:**111-7.

845. **Bredehorn, T., F. Wilhelm, C. Wiederhold, and G. I. Duncker.** 2001. [Incidence of potential transmitters of Creutzfeldt-Jakob disease. A study of a collective of potential cornea donors]. *Ophthalmologe* **98:**269-72.

846. **Breese Hall, C.** 2001. Respiratory syncytial virus and parainfluenza virus. *N Engl J Med* **344:**1917-28.

847. **Breese, P. L., F. N. Judson, K. A. Penley, and J. M. Douglas, Jr.** 1995. Anal human papillomavirus infection among homosex-

ual and bisexual men: prevalence of type-specific infection and association with human immunodeficiency virus. *Sex Transm Dis* **22:**7-14.

848. **Bregani, E. R., A. Rovellini, and P. Tarsia.** 2003. Effects of thiabendazole in Mansonella perstans filariasis. *Parasitologia* **45:**151-3.

849. **Breiman, R. F., B. S. Fields, G. N. Sanden, L. Volmer, A. Meier, and J. S. Spika.** 1990. Association of shower use with Legionnaires' disease. Possible role of amoebae. *JAMA* **263:**2924-6.

850. **Breiman, R. F., J. S. Spika, V. J. Navarro, P. M. Darden, and C. P. Darby.** 1990. Pneumococcal bacteremia in Charleston County, South Carolina. A decade later. *Arch Intern Med* **150:**1401-5.

851. **Breitschwerdt, E. B., B. C. Hegarty, and S. I. Hancock.** 1998. Sequential evaluation of dogs naturally infected with Ehrlichia canis, Ehrlichia chaffeensis, Ehrlichia equi, Ehrlichia ewingii, or Bartonella vinsonii. *J Clin Microbiol* **36:**2645-51.

852. **Breitschwerdt, E. B., and D. L. Kordick.** 2000. Bartonella infection in animals: carriership, reservoir potential, pathogenicity, and zoonotic potential for human infection. *Clin Microbiol Rev* **13:**428-38.

853. **Breman, J. G., and D. A. Henderson.** 1998. Poxvirus dilemmas—monkeypox, smallpox, and biologic terrorism. *N Engl J Med* **339:**556-9.

854. **Breman, J. G., and D. A. Henderson.** 2002. Diagnosis and management of smallpox. *N Engl J Med* **346:**1300-1308.

855. **Bremer, V., K. Leitmeyer, E. Jensen, U. Metzel, H. Meczulat, E. Weise, D. Werber, H. Tschaepe, L. Kreienbrock, S. Glaser, and A. Ammon.** 2004. Outbreak of Salmonella Goldcoast infections linked to consumption of fermented sausage, Germany 2001. *Epidemiol Infect* **132:**881-7.

856. **Brenier-Pinchart, M. P., B. Lebeau, G. Devouassoux, P. Mondon, C. Pison, P. Ambroise-Thomas, and R. Grillot.** 1998. Aspergillus and lung transplant recipients: a mycologic and molecular epidemiologic study. *J Heart Lung Transplant* **17:**972-9.

857. **Brennan, M., P. Strebel, H. George, W. K. Yih, R. Tachdjian, S. M. Lett, P. Cassiday, G. Sanden, and M. Wharton.** 2000. Evidence for transmission of pertussis in schools, Massachusetts, 1996: epidemiologic data supported by pulsed-field gel electrophoresis studies. *J Infect Dis* **181:**210-5.

858. **Brenner, M. A., and M. B. Patel.** 2003. Cutaneous larva migrans: the creeping eruption. *Cutis* **72:**111-5.

859. **Brès, P. L. J.** 1986. A century of progress in combating yellow fever. *Bull WHO* **64:**775-86.

860. **Bresee, J. S., E. E. Mast, P. J. Coleman, M. J. Baron, and L. B. Schonberger.** 1996. Hepatitis C virus infection associated with administration of intravenous immune globulin. A cohort study. *JAMA* **276:**1563-7.

861. **Bresnitz, E., C. Grant, S. Ostrawski, C. Morris, J. Calabria, B. Reetz, and S. Clugston.** 2001. Outbreak of pneumococcal pneumonia among unvaccinated residents of a nursing home - New Jersey, April 2001. *MMWR* **50:**707-710.

862. **Brett, M. M., G. Hallas, and O. Mpamugo.** 2004. Wound botulism in the UK and Ireland. *J Med Microbiol* **53:**555-61.

863. **Brett, M. M., J. Hood, J. S. Brazier, B. I. Duerden, and S. J. Hahne.** 2005. Soft tissue infections caused by spore-forming bacteria in injecting drug users in the United Kingdom. *Epidemiol Infect* **133:**575-82.

864. **Brett, M. M., J. McLauchlin, A. Harris, S. O'Brien, N. Black, R. J. Forsyth, D. Roberts, and F. J. Bolton.** 2005. A case of infant botulism with a possible link to infant formula milk powder: evidence for the presence of more than one strain of Clostridium botulinum in clinical specimens and food. *J Med Microbiol* **54:**769-76.

865. **Brettman, L. R., S. Lewin, R. S. Holzman, W. D. Goldman, J. S. Marr, P. Kechijian, and R. Schinella.** 1981. Rickettsialpox: report of an outbreak and a contemporary review. *Medicine (Baltimore)* **60:**363-72.

866. **Breuer, B., S. M. Friedman, E. S. Millner, M. A. Kane, R. H. Snyder, and J. E. Maynard.** 1985. Transmission of hepatitis B virus to classroom contacts of mentally retarded carriers. *JAMA* **254:**3190-5.

867. **Breuer, J.** 2005. Varicella vaccination for healthcare workers. *BMJ* **330:**433-4.

868. **Breuer, T., D. H. Benkel, R. L. Shapiro, W. N. Hall, M. M. Winnett, M. J. Linn, J. Neimann, T. J. Barrett, S. Dietrich, F. P. Downes, D. M. Toney, J. L. Pearson, H. Rolka, L. Slutsker, and P. M. Griffin.** 2001. A multistate outbreak of Escherichia coli O157:H7 infections linked to alfalfa sprouts grown from contaminated seeds. *Emerg Infect Dis* **7:**977-982.

869. **Breugelmans, J. G., P. Zucs, K. Porten, S. Broll, M. Niedrig, A. Ammon, and G. Krause.** 2004. SARS transmission and commercial aircraft. *Emerg Infect Dis* **10:**1502-3.

870. **Brewer, L. A., H. C. Lwamba, M. P. Murtaugh, A. C. Palmenberg, C. Brown, and M. K. Njenga.** 2001. Porcine encephalomyocarditis virus persists in pig myocardium and infects human myocardial cells. *J Virol* **75:**11621-9.

871. **Brewer, T. F., D. Vlahov, E. Taylor, D. Hall, A. Munoz, and B. F. Polk.** 1988. Transmission of HIV-1 within a statewide prison system. *AIDS* **2:**363-7.

872. **Brewster, D.** 1999. Environmental management for vector control. Is it worth a dam if it worsens malaria? *BMJ* **319:**651-2.

873. **Brewster, D. H., M. I. Brown, D. Robertson, G. L. Houghton, J. Bimson, and J. C. Sharp.** 1994. An outbreak of Escherichia coli O157 associated with a children's paddling pool. *Epidemiol Infect* **112:**441-7.

874. **Briand, S., H. Khalifa, C. L. Peter, O. J. Khatib, F. K. Bolay, B. A. Woodruff, and M. A. Anderson.** 2003. Cholera epidemic after increased civil conflict - Monrovia, Liberia, June-September 2003. *MMWR* **52:**1093-5.

875. **Bridges, C. B., J. M. Katz, W. H. Seto, P. K. Chan, D. Tsang, W. Ho, K. H. Mak, W. Lim, J. S. Tam, M. Clarke, S. G. Williams, A. W. Mounts, J. S. Bresee, L. A. Conn, T. Rowe, J. Hu-Primmer, R. A. Abernathy, X. Lu, N. J. Cox, and K. Fukuda.** 2000. Risk of influenza A (H5N1) infection among health care workers exposed to patients with influenza A (H5N1), Hong Kong. *J Infect Dis* **181:**344-8.

876. **Bridges, C. B., M. J. Kuehnert, and C. B. Hall.** 2003. Transmission of influenza: implications for control in health care settings. *Clin Infect Dis* **37:**1094-101.

877. **Bridges, C. B., W. Lim, J. Hu-Primmer, L. Sims, K. Fukuda, K. H. Mak, T. Rowe, W. W. Thompson, L. Conn, X. Lu, N. J. Cox, and J. M. Katz.** 2002. Risk of influenza A (H5N1) infection among poultry workers, Hong Kong, 19971–998. *J Infect Dis* **185:**1005-10.

878. **Bridges, C. B., W. W. Thompson, M. I. Meltzer, G. R. Reeve, W. J. Talamonti, N. J. Cox, H. A. Lilac, H. Hall, A. Klimov, and**

K. Fukuda. 2000. Effectiveness and cost-benefit of influenza vaccination of healthy working adults. A randomized controlled trial. *JAMA* **284**:1655-63.
879. Bridges, E. M. 1997. World soils, 3rd edition ed. Cambridge University Press, Cambridge, United Kingdom.
880. Briedis, D. J., and H. G. Robson. 1978. Epidemiologic and clinical features of sporadic Salmonella enteric fever. *Can Med Assoc J* **119**:1183-7.
881. Briggs, P. M., B. G. Delta, S. R. Keener, J. L. Freeman, J. L. Hunter, and J. W. Ezzell. 1988. Human cutaneous anthrax - North Carolina, 1987. *MMWR* **37**:413-414.
882. Bright, C. 1998. Life out of bounds. W.W. Norton & Co. Ltd., London.
883. Briley, R. T., J. H. Teel, and J. P. Fowler. 2001. Nontypical Bacillus cereus outbreak in a child care center. *J Environ Health* **63**:9-11, 21.
884. Brilhante, R. S., R. A. Cordeiro, D. J. Medrano, M. F. Rocha, A. J. Monteiro, C. S. Cavalcante, T. E. Meireles, and J. J. Sidrim. 2005. Onychomycosis in Ceara (Northeast Brazil): epidemiological and laboratory aspects. *Mem Inst Oswaldo Cruz* **100**:131-5.
885. Brinkmann, U. K., R. Korte, and B. Schmidt-Ehry. 1988. The distribution and spread of schistosomiasis in relation to water resources development in Mali. *Trop Med Parasitol* **39**:182-5.
886. Brisabois, A., V. Lafarge, A. Brouillaud, M. L. de Buyser, C. Collette, B. Garin-Bastuji, and M. F. Thorel. 1997. [Pathogenic organisms in milk and milk products: the situation in France and in Europe]. *Rev Sci Tech* **16**:452-71.
887. Briss, P. A., L. J. Fehrs, R. A. Parker, P. F. Wright, E. C. Sannella, R. H. Hutcheson, and W. Schaffner. 1994. Sustained transmission of mumps in a highly vaccinated population: assessment of primary vaccine failure and waning vaccine-induced immunity. *J Infect Dis* **169**:77-82.
888. Brisseau, J. M., J. P. Cebron, T. Petit, M. Marjolet, P. Cuilliere, J. Godin, and J. Y. Grolleau. 1988. Chagas' myocarditis imported into France. *Lancet* **1**:1046.
889. Britton, W. J., and D. N. Lockwood. 2004. Leprosy. *Lancet* **363**:1209-19.
890. Brocks, K. M., U. B. Johansen, H. O. Jorgensen, L. R. Ravnborg, and E. L. Svejgaard. 1999. Tinea pedis and onychomycosis in Danish soldiers before and after service in ex-Yugoslavia. *Mycoses* **42**:475-8.
891. Brodine, S. K., M. A. Shafer, R. A. Shaffer, C. B. Boyer, S. D. Putnam, F. S. Wignall, R. J. Thomas, B. Bales, and J. Schachter. 1998. Asymptomatic sexually transmitted disease prevalence in four military populations: application of DNA amplification assays for Chlamydia and gonorrhea screening. *J Infect Dis* **178**:1202-4.
892. Brodsky, R. E., H. C. Spencer jr., and M. G. Schultz. 1974. Giardiasis in American travelers to the Soviet Union. *J Infect Dis* **130**:319-23.
893. Broholm, K. A., L. Sjodin, I. Backlund, B. Johansson, H. Norder, and L. Magnius. 2001. [Hepatitis B outbreak in a day care center affected several families. It could have been prevented by vaccination of all children]. *Lakartidningen* **98**:2337-8, 2341-2.
894. Bronowicki, J. P., V. Venard, C. Botte, N. Monhoven, I. Gastin, L. Chone, H. Hudziak, B. Rihn, C. Delanoe, A. LeFaou, M. A. Bigard, P. Gaucher, and B. Rhin. 1997. Patient-to-patient transmission of hepatitis C virus during colonoscopy. *N Engl J Med* **337**:237-40.
895. Brook, I. 2002. Microbiology of polymicrobial abscesses and implications for therapy. *J Antimicrob Chemother* **50**:805-10.
896. Brook, I., and E. H. Frazier. 1990. Aerobic and anaerobic bacteriology of wounds and cutaneous abscesses. *Arch Surg* **125**:1445-51.
897. Brooke, C. J., and T. V. Riley. 1999. Erysipelothrix rhusiopathiae: bacteriology, epidemiology and clinical manifestations of an occupational pathogen. *J Med Microbiol* **48**:789-99.
898. Brooker, S., M. Beasley, M. Ndinaromtan, E. M. Madjiouroum, M. Baboguel, E. Djenguinabe, S. I. Hay, and D. A. Bundy. 2002. Use of remote sensing and a geographical information system in a national helminth control programme in Chad. *Bull WHO* **80**:783-9.
899. Brooker, S., S. Clarke, J. K. Njagi, S. Polack, B. Mugo, B. Estambale, E. Muchiri, P. Magnussen, and J. Cox. 2004. Spatial clustering of malaria and associated risk factors during an epidemic in a highland area of western Kenya. *Trop Med Int Health* **9**:757-66.
900. Brooker, S., E. A. Miguel, S. Moulin, A. I. Luoba, D. A. Bundy, and M. Kremer. 2000. Epidemiology of single and multiple species of helminth infections among school children in Busia District, Kenya. *East Afr Med J* **77**:157-61.
901. Brooker, S., N. Mohammed, K. Adil, S. Agha, R. Reithinger, M. Rowland, I. Ali, and J. Kolaczinski. 2004. Leishmaniasis in refugee and local pakistani populations. *Emerg Infect Dis* **10**:1681-4.
902. Brookes, S. M., J. N. Aegerter, G. C. Smith, D. M. Healy, T. A. Jolliffe, S. M. Swift, I. J. Mackie, J. S. Pritchard, P. A. Racey, N. P. Moore, and A. R. Fooks. 2005. European bat lyssavirus in Scottish bats. *Emerg Infect Dis* **11**:572-8.
903. Brooks, J. T., D. Bergmire-Sweat, M. Kennedy, K. Hendricks, M. Garcia, L. Marengo, J. Wells, M. Ying, W. Bibb, P. M. Griffin, R. M. Hoekstra, and C. R. Friedman. 2004. Outbreak of Shiga toxin-producing Escherichia coli O111:H8 infections among attendees of a high school cheerleading camp. *Clin Infect Dis* **38**:190-8.
904. Brooks, J. T., S. Y. Rowe, P. Shillam, D. M. Heltzel, S. B. Hunter, L. Slutsker, R. M. Hoekstra, and S. P. Luby. 2001. Salmonella Typhimurium Infections Transmitted by Chlorine-pretreated Clover Sprout Seeds. *Am J Epidemiol* **154**:1020-1028.
905. Brooks, S. E., R. O. Veal, M. Kramer, L. Dore, N. Schupf, and M. Adachi. 1992. Reduction in the incidence of Clostridium difficile-associated diarrhea in an acute care hospital and a skilled nursing facility following replacement of electronic thermometers with single-use disposables. *Infect Control Hosp Epidemiol* **13**:98-103.
906. Broom, A. K., M. D. A. Lindsay, A. J. Plant, A. E. Wright, R. J. Condon, and J. S. Mackenzie. 2002. Epizootic activity of Murray valley encephalitis virus in an Aboriginal community in the southeast Kimberley region of Western Australia: results of cross-sectional and longitudinal serologic studies. *Am J Trop Med Hyg* **67**:319-23.
907. Broom, A. K., M. D. A. Lindsay, A. E. Wright, D. W. Smith, and J. S. Mackenzie. 2003. Epizootic activity of Murray valley encephalitis and Kunjin viruses in an aboriginal community in the southeast Kimberley region of western Australia: results of mosquito fauna and virus isolation studies. *Am J Trop Med Hyg* **69**:277-83.

908. **Broome, C. V., M. LaVenture, H. S. Kaye, A. T. Davis, H. White, B. D. Plikaytis, and D. W. Fraser.** 1980. An explosive outbreak of Mycoplasma pneumoniae infection in a summer camp. *Pediatrics* **66:**884-8.

909. **Brouqui, P., F. Bacellar, G. Baranton, R. J. Birtles, A. Bjoersdorff, J. R. Blanco, G. Caruso, M. Cinco, P. E. Fournier, E. Francavilla, M. Jensenius, J. Kazar, H. Laferl, A. Lakos, S. Lotric Furlan, M. Maurin, J. A. Oteo, P. Parola, C. Perez-Eid, O. Peter, D. Postic, D. Raoult, A. Tellez, Y. Tselentis, and B. Wilske.** 2004. Guidelines for the diagnosis of tick-borne bacterial diseases in Europe. *Clin Microbiol Infect* **10:**1108-32.

910. **Brouqui, P., S. Badiaga, and D. Raoult.** 2004. Q fever outbreak in homeless shelter. *Emerg Infect Dis* **10:**1297-9.

911. **Brouqui, P., P. Houpikian, H. T. Dupont, P. Toubiana, Y. Obadia, V. Lafay, and D. Raoult.** 1996. Survey of the seroprevalence of Bartonella quintana in homeless people. *Clin Infect Dis* **23:**756-9.

912. **Brouqui, P., A. Stein, H. T. Dupont, P. Gallian, S. Badiaga, J. M. Rolain, J. L. Mege, B. La Scola, P. Berbis, and D. Raoult.** 2005. Ectoparasitism and vector-borne diseases in 930 homeless people from Marseilles. *Medicine (Baltimore)* **84:**61-8.

913. **Brouwer, K. C., P. D. Ndhlovu, Y. Wagatsuma, A. Munatsi, and C. J. Shiff.** 2003. Epidemiological assessment of Schistosoma haematobium-induced kidney and bladder pathology in rural Zimbabwe. *Acta Trop* **85:**339-47.

914. **Brown, A., S. Bolisetty, P. Whelan, D. Smith, and G. Wheaton.** 2002. Reappearance of human cases due to Murray valley encephalitis virus and Kunjin virus in Central Australia after an absence of 26 years. *Commun Dis Intell* **26:**39-44.

915. **Brown, C. M., J. W. Cann, G. Simons, R. L. Fankhauser, W. Thomas, U. D. Parashar, and M. J. Lewis.** 2001. Outbreak of Norwalk virus in a Caribbean island resort: application of molecular diagnostics to ascertain the vehicle of infection. *Epidemiol Infect* **126:**425-32.

916. **Brown, C. M., P. J. Nuorti, R. F. Breiman, A. L. Hathcock, B. S. Fields, H. B. Lipman, G. C. Llewellyn, J. Hofmann, and M. Cetron.** 1999. A community outbreak of Legionnaires' disease linked to hospital cooling towers: an epidemiological method to calculate dose of exposure. *Int J Epidemiol* **28:**353-9.

917. **Brown, D., J. Gray, P. MacDonald, A. Green, D. Morgan, G. Christopher, R. Glass, and R. Turcios.** 2002. Outbreak of acute gastroenteritis associated with Norwalk-like viruses among British military personnel - Afghanistan, May 2002. *MMWR* **51:**477-9.

918. **Brown, D. J., H. Mather, L. M. Browning, and J. E. Coia.** 2003. Investigation of human infections with Salmonella enterica serovar Java in Scotland and possible association with imported poultry. *Eurosurveillance* **8:**35-40.

919. **Brown, F. M., E. W. Moharebb, F. Yousif, Y. Sultan, and N. I. Girgis.** 1996. Angiostrongylus eosinophilic meningitis in Egypt. *Lancet* **348:**964-5.

920. **Brown, G. W., A. Shirai, M. Jegathesan, D. S. Burke, J. C. Twartz, J. P. Saunders, and D. L. Huxsoll.** 1984. Febrile illness in Malaysia—an analysis of 1,629 hospitalized patients. *Am J Trop Med Hyg* **33:**311-5.

921. **Brown, J., K. Hort, R. Bouwman, A. Capon, N. Bansal, I. Goldthorpe, K. Chant, and S. Vemulpad.** 2001. Investigation and control of a cluster of cases of Legionnaires disease in western Sydney. *Commun Dis Intell* **25:**63-6.

922. **Brown, K. E., Z. Liu, G. Gallinella, S. Wong, I. P. Mills, and G. O'Sullivan M.** 2004. Simian parvovirus infection: a potential zoonosis. *J Infect Dis* **190:**1900-7.

923. **Brown, L. M.** 2000. Helicobacter pylori: epidemiology and routes of transmission. *Epidemiol Rev* **22:**283-97.

924. **Brown, L. M., T. L. Thomas, J. L. Ma, Y. S. Chang, W. C. You, W. D. Liu, L. Zhang, D. Pee, and M. H. Gail.** 2002. Helicobacter pylori infection in rural China: demographic, lifestyle and environmental factors. *Int J Epidemiol* **31:**638-45.

925. **Brown, L. S., Jr., D. P. Drotman, A. Chu, C. L. Brown, Jr., and D. Knowlan.** 1995. Bleeding injuries in professional football: estimating the risk for HIV transmission. *Ann Intern Med* **122:**273-4.

926. **Brown, P.** 2000. BSE and transmission through blood. *Lancet* **356:**955-6.

927. **Brown, P.** 2001. Afterthoughts about bovine spongiforme encephalopathy and variant Creutzfeldt-Jakob disease. *Emerg Infect Dis* **7:**598-600.

928. **Brown, P., M. Preece, J. P. Brandel, T. Sato, L. McShane, I. Zerr, A. Fletcher, R. G. Will, M. Pocchiari, N. R. Cashman, J. H. d'Aignaux, L. Cervenakova, J. Fradkin, L. B. Schonberger, and S. J. Collins.** 2000. Iatrogenic Creutzfeldt-Jakob disease at the millennium. *Neurology* **55:**1075-81.

929. **Brown, R. L.** 1991. Successful treatment of primary amebic meningoencephalitis. *Arch Intern Med* **151:**1201-2.

930. **Brown, V., M. Abdir Issak, M. Rossi, P. Barboza, and A. Paugam.** 1998. Epidemic of malaria in north-eastern Kenya. *Lancet* **352:**1356-7.

931. **Brown, V., G. Jacquier, C. Bachy, D. Bitar, and D. Legros.** 2002. [Management of cholera epidemics in a refugee camp]. *Bull Soc Pathol Exot* **95:**351-4.

932. **Brown, V., B. Larouze, G. Desve, J. J. Rousset, M. Thibon, A. Fourrier, and V. Schwoebel.** 1988. Clinical presentation of louse-borne relapsing fever among Ethiopian refugees in northern Somalia. *Ann Trop Med Parasitol* **82:**499-502.

933. **Brown, Z. A., J. Benedetti, R. Ashley, S. Burchett, S. Selke, S. Berry, L. A. Vontver, and L. Corey.** 1991. Neonatal herpes simplex virus infection in relation to asymptomatic maternal infection at the time of labor. *N Engl J Med* **324:**1247-52.

934. **Brown-Elliott, B. A., D. E. Griffith, and R. J. Wallace, Jr.** 2002. Newly described or emerging human species of nontuberculous mycobacteria. *Infect Dis Clin North Am* **16:**187-220.

935. **Bruce, B. B., M. A. Blass, H. M. Blumberg, J. L. Lennox, C. del Rio, and C. R. Horsburgh, Jr.** 2000. Risk of Cryptosporidium parvum transmission between hospital roommates. *Clin Infect Dis* **31:**947-50.

936. **Bruce, M. G., N. E. Rosenstein, J. M. Capparella, K. A. Shutt, B. A. Perkins, and M. Collins.** 2001. Risk factors for meningococcal disease in college students. *JAMA* **286:**688-93.

937. **Brudney, K., and J. Dobkin.** 1991. Resurgent tuberculosis in New York City. Human immunodeficiency virus, homelessness, and the decline of tuberculosis control programs. *Am Rev Respir Dis* **144:**745-9.

938. **Brugha, R., J. Heptonstall, P. Farrington, S. Andren, K. Perry, and J. Parry.** 1998. Risk of hepatitis A infection in sewage workers. *Occup Environ Med* **55:**567-9.

939. **Brugha, R., I. B. Vipond, M. R. Evans, Q. D. Sandifer, R. J. Roberts, R. L. Salmon, E. O. Caul, and A. K. Mukerjee.** 1999. A community outbreak of food-borne small round-structured virus gastroenteritis caused by a contaminated water supply. *Epidemiol Infect* **122:**145-154.

940. **Brugha, R. F., A. J. Howard, G. R. Thomas, R. Parry, L. R. Ward, and S. R. Palmer.** 1995. Chaos under canvas: a Salmonella enteritidis PT 6B outbreak. *Epidemiol Infect* **115:**513-7.

941. Bruguera, M., J. C. Saiz, S. Franco, M. Gimenez-Barcons, J. M. Sanchez-Tapias, S. Fabregas, R. Vega, N. Camps, A. Dominguez, and L. Salleras. 2002. Outbreak of nosocomial hepatitis C virus infection resolved by genetic analysis of HCV RNA. *J Clin Microbiol* **40**:4363-6.

942. Bruijnesteijn van Coppenraet, L. E., E. J. Kuijper, J. A. Lindeboom, J. M. Prins, and E. C. Claas. 2005. Mycobacterium haemophilum and lymphadenitis in children. *Emerg Infect Dis* **11**:62-8.

943. Bruisten, S. M., I. Cairo, H. Fennema, A. Pijl, M. Buimer, P. G. Peerbooms, E. Van Dyck, A. Meijer, J. M. Ossewaarde, and G. J. van Doornum. 2001. Diagnosing genital ulcer disease in a clinic for sexually transmitted diseases in Amsterdam, The Netherlands. *J Clin Microbiol* **39**:601-5.

944. Brummer, E., E. Castaneda, and A. Restrepo. 1993. Paracoccidioidomycosis: an update. *Clin Microbiol Rev* **6**:89-117.

945. Brummer-Korvenkontio, M., H. Henttonen, and A. Vaheri. 1982. Hemorrhagic fever with renal syndrome in Finland: ecology and virology of nephropathia epidemica. *Scand J Infect Dis* 36 (**Suppl**):88-91.

946. Brummer-Korvenkontio, M., O. Vapalahti, P. Kuusisto, P. Saikku, T. Manni, P. Koskela, T. Nygren, H. Brummer-Korvenkontio, and A. Vaheri. 2002. Epidemiology of Sindbis virus infections in Finland 1981-96: possible factors explaining a peculiar disease pattern. *Epidemiol Infect* **129**:335-45.

947. Brundage, J. F., J. D. Gunzenhauser, J. N. Longfield, M. V. Rubertone, S. L. Ludwig, F. A. Rubin, and E. L. Kaplan. 1996. Epidemiology and control of acute respiratory diseases with emphasis on group A beta-hemolytic streptococcus: a decade of U.S. Army experience. *Pediatrics* **97**:964-70.

948. Bruneau, A., H. Rodrigue, J. Ismael, R. Dion, and R. Allard. 2004. Outbreak of E. coli O157:H7 associated with bathing at a public beach in the Montreal-Centre region. *Can Commun Dis Rep* **30**:133-6.

949. Bruning-Fann, C. S., S. M. Schmitt, S. D. Fitzgerald, J. S. Fierke, P. D. Friedrich, J. B. Kaneene, K. A. Clarke, K. L. Butler, J. B. Payeur, D. L. Whipple, T. M. Cooley, J. M. Miller, and D. P. Muzo. 2001. Bovine tuberculosis in free-ranging carnivores from Michigan. *J Wildl Dis* **37**:58-64.

950. Brusaferro, S., F. Barbone, P. Andrian, G. Brianti, L. Ciccone, A. Furlan, D. Gnesutta, S. Stel, E. Zamparo, P. Toniutto, P. Ferroni, and V. Gasparini. 1999. A study on the role of the family and other risk factors in HCV transmission. *Eur J Epidemiol* **15**:125-32.

951. Brusin, S. 2000. The communicable disease surveillance system in the Kosovar refugee camps in the former Yugoslav Republic of Macedonia April-August 1999. *J Epidemiol Community Health* **54**:52-7.

952. Bryan, J. A., J. D. Lehmann, I. F. Setiady, and M. H. Hatch. 1974. An outbreak of hepatitis-A associated with recreational lake water. *Am J Epidemiol* **99**:145-54.

953. Bryan, J. P., M. Iqbal, S. Tsarev, I. A. Malik, J. F. Duncan, A. Ahmed, A. Khan, A. R. Rafiqui, R. H. Purcell, and L. J. Legters. 2002. Epidemic of hepatitis E in a military unit in Abbottabad, Pakistan. *Am J Trop Med Hyg* **67**:662-8.

954. Bryant, J. K., H. C. Wang, C. Cabezas, G. Ramirez, D. Watts, K. Russell, and A. D. Barrett. 2003. Enzootic transmission of yellow fever virus in Peru. *Emerg Infect Dis* **9**:926-33.

955. Bryce, J., C. Boschi-Pinto, K. Shibuya, and R. E. Black. 2005. WHO estimates of the causes of death in children. *Lancet* **365**:1147-52.

956. Bryceson, A. D. M., E. H. O. Parry, P. L. Perine, D. A. Warrell, D. Vukotich, and C. S. Leithead. 1970. Louse-borne relapsing fever. A clinical and laboratory study of 62 cases in Ethiopia and a reconsideration of the literature. *Q J Med* **39**:129-70.

957. Bryskier, A. 2002. Viridans group streptococci: a reservoir of resistant bacteria in oral cavities. *Clin Microbiol Infect* **8**:65-9.

958. Buavirat, A., K. Page-Shafer, G. J. van Griensven, J. S. Mandel, J. Evans, J. Chuaratanaphong, S. Chiamwongpat, R. Sacks, and A. Moss. 2003. Risk of prevalent HIV infection associated with incarceration among injecting drug users in Bangkok, Thailand: case-control study. *BMJ* **326**:308.

959. Buchwald, D. S., and M. J. Blaser. 1984. A review of human salmonellosis: II. Duration of excretion following infection with nontyphi Salmonella. *Rev Infect Dis* **6**:345-56.

960. Buck, C., A. Llopis, E. Nájera, and M. Terris. 1988. The challenge of epidemiology. Issues and selected readings. Pan American Health Organization, Washington, D.C.

961. Buckley, B. 1980. Q fever epidemic in Victorian general practice. *Med J Aust* **1**:593-5.

962. Buckley, R., M. W. Cobb, S. Ghurani, N. F. Brock, and R. R. Harford. 1997. Mycobacterium fortuitum infection occurring after a punch biopsy procedure. *Pediatr Dermatol* **14**:290-2.

963. Buczek, A., D. Markowska-Gosik, D. Widomska, and I. M. Kawa. 2004. Pediculosis capitis among schoolchildren in urban and rural areas of eastern Poland. *Eur J Epidemiol* **19**:491-5.

964. Buehler, J. W., J. T. Holloway, R. A. Goodman, and R. K. Sikes. 1983. Gnat sore eyes: seasonal, acute conjunctivitis in a southern state. *South Med J* **76**:587-9.

965. Buehler, J. W., J. N. Kuritsky, G. W. Gorman, A. W. Hightower, C. V. Broome, and R. K. Sikes. 1985. Prevalence of antibodies to Legionella pneumophila among workers exposed to a contaminated cooling tower. *Arch Environ Health* **40**:207-10.

966. Buhariwalla, F., B. Cann, and T. J. Marrie. 1996. A dog-related outbreak of Q fever. *Clin Infect Dis* **23**:753-755.

967. Buijs, J., G. Borsboom, J. J. van Gemund, A. Hazebroek, P. A. M. van Dongen, F. van Knapen, and H. J. Neijens. 1994. Toxocara seroprevalence in 5-year-old elementary schoolchildren: relation with allergic asthma. *Am J Epidemiol* **140**:839-47.

968. Buishi, I., T. Walters, Z. Guildea, P. Craig, and S. Palmer. 2005. Reemergence of canine Echinococcus granulosus infection, Wales. *Emerg Infect Dis* **11**:568-71.

969. Buisson, Y., P. Coursaget, R. Bercion, D. Anne, T. Debord, and R. Roue. 1994. Hepatitis E virus infection in soldiers sent to endemic regions. *Lancet* **344**:1165-6.

970. Bula, C. J., J. Bille, and M. P. Glauser. 1995. An epidemic of food-borne listeriosis in western Switzerland: description of 57 cases involving adults. *Clin Infect Dis* **20**:66-72.

971. Bulkow, L. R., R. J. Singleton, R. A. Karron, and L. H. Harrison. 2002. Risk factors for severe respiratory syncytial virus infection among Alaska native children. *Pediatrics* **109**:210-6.

972. Bull, A., S. K. Crerar, and M. Y. Beers. 2002. Australia's imported food program - a valuable source of information on micro-organisms in foods. *Commun Dis Intell* **26**:28-32.

973. Bullock, P. M., T. R. Ames, R. A. Robinson, B. Greig, M. A. Mellencamp, and J. S. Dumler. 2000. Ehrlichia equi infection of horses from Minnesota and Wisconsin: detection of seroconversion and acute disease investigation. *J Vet Intern Med* **14**:252-7.

974. **Bulterys, M.** 2001. Preventing vertical HIV transmission in the year 2000: progress and prospects—a review. *Placenta* **22 Suppl A:**S5-S12.

975. **Bulterys, M., M. G. Fowler, K. K. Van Rompay, and A. P. Kourtis.** 2004. Prevention of mother-to-child transmission of HIV-1 through breast-feeding: past, present, and future. *J Infect Dis* **189:**2149-53.

976. **Buma, A. H., P. Beutels, P. van Damme, G. Tormans, E. van Doorslaer, and A. Leentvaar-Kuijpers.** 1998. An economic evaluation of hepatitis A vaccination in Dutch military personnel. *Mil Med* **163:**564-7.

977. **Bundesen, H. N., F. O. Tonney, and I. D. Rawlings.** 1934. The outbreak of amebiasis in Chicago during 1933. Sequence of events. *JAMA* **102:**367-72.

978. **Bunikis, J., J. Tsao, C. J. Luke, M. G. Luna, D. Fish, and A. G. Barbour.** 2004. Borrelia burgdorferi Infection in a Natural Population of Peromyscus Leucopus Mice: A Longitudinal Study in an Area Where Lyme Borreliosis Is Highly Endemic. *J Infect Dis* **189:**1515-23.

979. **Bunn, J. E., W. G. MacKay, J. E. Thomas, D. C. Reid, and L. T. Weaver.** 2002. Detection of Helicobacter pylori DNA in drinking water biofilms: implications for transmission in early life. *Lett Appl Microbiol* **34:**450-4.

980. **Bunnag, T., K. Klongkamnuankarn, S. Thirachandra, P. Impand, and S. Sornmani.** 1982. Seroepidemiology of amoebiasis in the villagers in Phichit Province and urban slum dwellers in Bangkok, Thailand. *Southeast Asian J Trop Med Public Health* **13:**541-6.

981. **Bunnell, J. E., C. L. Hice, D. M. Watts, V. Montrueil, R. B. Tesh, and J. M. Vinetz.** 2000. Detection of pathogenic Leptospira spp. infections among mammals captured in the Peruvian Amazon basin region. *Am J Trop Med Hyg* **63:**255-8.

982. **Burdon, J. T., P. J. Stanley, G. Lloyd, and N. C. Jones.** 1994. A case of Japanese encephalitis. *J Infect* **28:**175-9.

983. **Bureau-Chalot, F., E. Piednoir, C. Pierrat, B. Santerne, and O. Bajolet.** 2003. [Nosocomial Burkholderia cepacia outbreak in an intensive pediatric care unit]. *Arch Pediatr* **10:**882-6.

984. **Burek, V., L. Misic-Mayerus, and T. Maretic.** 1992. Antibodies to Borrelia burgdorferi in various population groups in Croatia. *Scand J Infect Dis* **24:**683-4.

985. **Burger, J.** 1999. American Indians, hunting and fishing rates, risk, and the Idaho National Engineering and Environmental Laboratory. *Environ Res* **80:**317-29.

986. **Burgess, I. F.** 2004. Human lice and their control. *Annu Rev Entomol* **49:**457-81.

987. **Burke, D. M., D. C. Shackley, and P. H. O'Reilly.** 2002. The community-based morbidity of flexible cystoscopy. *Br J Urol* **89:**347-9.

988. **Burke, J. P.** 2003. Infection control - a problem for patient safety. *N Engl J Med* **348:**651-6.

989. **Burket, C. T., C. N. Vann, R. R. Pinger, C. L. Chatot, and F. E. Steiner.** 1998. Minimum infection rate of Amblyomma americanum (Acari: Ixodidae) by Ehrlichia chaffeensis (Rickettsiales: Ehrlichieae) in southern Indiana. *J Med Entomol* **35:**653-9.

990. **Burkhart, C. N.** 2003. Fomite transmission with head lice: a continuing controversy. *Lancet* **361:**99-100.

991. **Burkot, T., and K. Ichimori.** 2002. The PacELF programme: will mass drug administration be enough? *Trends Parasitol* **18:**109-15.

992. **Burkot, T. R., B. S. Schneider, N. J. Pieniazek, C. M. Happ, J. S. Rutherford, S. B. Slemenda, E. Hoffmeister, G. O. Maupin, and N. S. Zeidner.** 2000. Babesia microti and Borrelia bissettii transmission by Ixodes spinipalpis ticks among prairie voles, Microtus ochrogaster, in Colorado. *Parasitology* **121:**595-9.

993. **Burney, M. I., A. Ghafoor, M. Saleen, P. A. Webb, and J. Casals.** 1980. Nosocomial outbreak of viral hemorrhagic fever caused by Crimean Hemorrhagic fever-Congo virus in Pakistan, January 1976. *Am J Trop Med Hyg* **29:**941-7.

994. **Burns, D. A.** 1987. An outbreak of scabies in a residential home. *Br J Dermatol* **117:**359-61.

995. **Burns, D. N., R. J. Wallace, Jr., M. E. Schultz, Y. S. Zhang, S. Q. Zubairi, Y. J. Pang, C. L. Gibert, B. A. Brown, E. S. Noel, and F. M. Gordin.** 1991. Nosocomial outbreak of respiratory tract colonization with Mycobacterium fortuitum: demonstration of the usefulness of pulsed-field gel electrophoresis in an epidemiologic investigation. *Am Rev Respir Dis* **144:** 1153-9.

996. **Burridge, M. J.** 2001. Ticks (Acari: Ixodidae) spread by the international trade in reptiles and their potential roles in dissemination of diseases. *Bull Entomol Res* **91:**3-23.

997. **Burridge, M. J., and C. W. Schwabe.** 1977. Hydatid disease in New Zealand: an epidemiological study of transmission among Maoris. *Am J Trop Med Hyg* **26:**258-65.

998. **Busani, L., C. Graziani, A. Battisti, A. Franco, A. Ricci, D. Vio, E. Digiannatale, F. Paterlini, M. D'Incau, S. Owczarek, A. Caprioli, and I. Luzzi.** 2004. Antibiotic resistance in Salmonella enterica serotypes Typhimurium, Enteritidis and Infantis from human infections, foodstuffs and farm animals in Italy. *Epidemiol Infect* **132:**245-51.

999. **Busch, M. P., S. H. Kleinman, and G. J. Neomo.** 2003. Current and emerging infectious risks of blood transfusions. *JAMA* **289:**959-62.

1000. **Butany, J., M. J. Collins, D. E. Demellawy, V. Nair, N. Israel, S. W. Leong, and M. A. Borger.** 2005. Morphological and clinical findings in 247 surgically excised native aortic valves. *Can J Cardiol* **21:**747-55.

1001. **Butel, J. S.** 2000. Simian virus 40, poliovirus vaccines, and human cancer: research progress versus media and public interests. *Bull WHO* **78:**195-8.

1002. **Butel, J. S., and J. A. Lednicky.** 1999. Cell and molecular biology of simian virus 40: implications for human infections and disease. *J Natl Cancer Inst* **91:**119-34.

1003. **Butera, S. T., J. Brown, M. E. Callahan, S. M. Owen, A. L. Matthews, D. D. Weigner, L. E. Chapman, and P. A. Sandstrom.** 2000. Survey of veterinary conference attendees for evidence of zoonotic infection by feline retroviruses. *J Am Vet Med Assoc* **217:**1475-9.

1004. **Butler, T.** 1989. The black death past and present. 1. Plague in the 1980s. *Trans R Soc Trop Med Hyg* **83:**458-60.

1005. **Butsashvili, M., T. Tsertsvadze, L. A. McNutt, G. Kamkamidze, R. Gvetadze, and N. Badridze.** 2001. Prevalence of hepatitis B, hepatitis C, syphilis and HIV in Georgian blood donors. *Eur J Epidemiol* **17:**693-5.

1006. **Butt, A. A., K. E. Aldridge, and C. V. Sanders.** 2004. Infections related to the ingestion of seafood Part I: Viral and bacterial infections. *Lancet Infect Dis* **4:**201-12.

1007. **Butt, A. A., K. E. Aldridge, and C. V. Sanders.** 2004. Infections related to the ingestion of seafood. Part II: parasitic infections and food safety. *Lancet Infect Dis* **4:**294-300.

1008. **Buttery, J. P., S. J. Alabaster, R. G. Heine, S. M. Scott, R. A. Crutchfield, A. Bigham, S. N. Tabrizi, and S. M. Garland.**

1998. Multiresistant Pseudomonas aeruginosa outbreak in a pediatric oncology ward related to bath toys. *Pediatr Infect Dis J* **17:**509-13.

1009. **Buttner, D. W., G. von Laer, E. Mannweiler, and M. Buttner.** 1982. Clinical, parasitological and serological studies on onchocerciasis in the Yemen Arab Republic. *Tropenmed Parasitol* **33:**201-12.

1010. **Butz, A. M., P. Fosarelli, J. Dick, T. Cusack, and R. Yolken.** 1993. Prevalence of rotavirus on high-risk fomites in day-care facilities. *Pediatrics* **92:**202-5.

1011. **Butzler, J. P.** 2004. Campylobacter, from obscurity to celebrity. *Clin Microbiol Infect* **10:**868-76.

1012. **Bwayo, J., F. Plummer, M. Omari, A. Mutere, S. Moses, J. Ndinya-Achola, P. Velentgas, and J. Kreiss.** 1994. Human immunodeficiency virus infection in long-distance truck drivers in east Africa. *Arch Intern Med* **154:**1391-6.

1013. **Byington, C. L., K. K. Rittichier, K. E. Bassett, H. Castillo, T. S. Glasgow, J. Daly, and A. T. Pavia.** 2003. Serious bacterial infections in febrile infants younger than 90 days of age: the importance of ampicillin-resistant pathogens. *Pediatrics* **111:**964-8.

1014. **Byington, C. L., D. M. Zerr, E. W. Taggart, L. Nguy, D. R. Hillyard, K. C. Carroll, and L. Corey.** 2002. Human herpesvirus 6 infection in febrile infants ninety days of age and younger. *Pediatr Infect Dis J* **21:**996-9.

1015. **Byrd, C. L., B. L. Wilkoff, C. J. Love, T. D. Sellers, K. T. Turk, R. Reeves, R. Young, B. Crevey, S. P. Kutalek, R. Freedman, R. Friedman, J. Trantham, M. Watts, J. Schutzman, J. Oren, J. Wilson, F. Gold, N. E. Fearnot, and H. J. Van Zandt.** 1999. Intravascular extraction of problematic or infected permanent pacemaker leads: 1994-1996. U.S. Extraction Database, MED Institute. *Pacing Clin Electrophysiol* **22:**1348-57.

1016. **Byrne, A. H., C. M. Herra, H. Aucken, and C. T. Keane.** 2001. Rate of carriage of Serratia marcescens in patients with and without evidence of infection. *Scand J Infect Dis* **33:**822-6.

1017. **Byrne, K., and R. A. Nichols.** 1999. Culex pipiens in London Underground tunnels: differentiation between surface and subterranean populations. *Heredity* **82:**7-15.

1018. **Byrne, N. J., and R. H. Behrens.** 2004. Airline crews' risk for malaria on layovers in urban sub-Saharan Africa: risk assessment and appropriate prevention policy. *J Travel Med* **11:**359-63.

1019. **Byth, S.** 1980. Palm island mystery disease. *Med J Aust* **2:**40-2.

1020. **Cabanes, F. J., M. L. Abarca, and M. R. Bragulat.** 1997. Dermatophytes isolated from domestic animals in Barcelona, Spain. *Mycopathologia* **137:**107-13.

1021. **Cabrera, M. A., A. A. Paula, L. A. Camacho, M. C. Marzochi, S. C. Xavier, A. V. da Silva, and A. M. Jansen.** 2003. Canine visceral leishmaniasis in Barra de Guaratiba, Rio de Janeiro, Brazil: assessment of risk factors. *Rev Inst Med Trop Sao Paulo* **45:**79-83.

1022. **Cacciapuoti, B., L. Ciceroni, C. Maffei, F. Di Stanislao, P. Strusi, L. Calegari, R. Lupidi, G. Scalise, G. Cagnoni, and G. Renga.** 1987. A waterborne outbreak of leptospirosis. *Am J Epidemiol* **126:**535-45.

1023. **Cadavid, D., and A. G. Barbour.** 1998. Neuroborreliosis during relapsing fever: review of the clinical manifestations, pathology, and treatment of infections in humans and experimental animals. *Clin Infect Dis* **26:**151-64.

1024. **Cadilhac, P., and F. Roudot-Thoraval.** 1994. Evaluation du risque de contamination, par le virus de l'hépatite A, du personnel travaillant en égouts. Enquête transversale. *Bull Epidémiol Hebdomadaire* **31:**139-141.

1025. **Caiaffa, W. T., D. Vlahov, N. M. Graham, J. Astemborski, L. Solomon, K. E. Nelson, and A. Munoz.** 1994. Drug smoking, Pneumocystis carinii pneumonia, and immunosuppression increase risk of bacterial pneumonia in human immunodeficiency virus-seropositive injection drug users. *Am J Respir Crit Care Med* **150:**1493-8.

1026. **Caicedo, L. D., M. I. Alvarez, M. Delgado, and A. Cardenas.** 1999. Cryptococcus neoformans in bird excreta in the city zoo of Cali, Colombia. *Mycopathologia* **147:**121-4.

1027. **Cairncross, S., and R. G. Feachem.** 1983. Environmental health engineering in the tropics. John Wiley & Sons, New York.

1028. **Cairncross, S., R. Muller, and N. Zagaria.** 2002. Dracunculiasis (Guinea worm disease) and the eradication initiative. *Clin Microbiol Rev* **15:**223-46.

1029. **Cairns, L., D. Blythe, A. Kao, D. Pappagianis, L. Kaufman, J. Kobayashi, and R. Hajjeh.** 2000. Outbreak of coccidioidomycosis in Washington state residents returning from Mexico. *Clin Infect Dis* **30:**61-4.

1030. **Calain, P., J. P. Chaine, E. Johnson, M. L. Hawley, M. J. O'Leary, H. Oshitani, and C. L. Chaignat.** 2004. Can oral cholera vaccination play a role in controlling a cholera outbreak? *Vaccine* **22:**2444-51.

1031. **Caldas de Castro, M., Y. Yamagata, D. Mtasiwa, M. Tanner, J. Utzinger, J. Keiser, and B. H. Singer.** 2004. Integrated urban malaria control: a case study in dar es salaam, Tanzania. *Am J Trop Med Hyg* **71:**103-17.

1032. **Calder, L., L. Hampton, D. Prentice, M. Reeve, A. Vaughan, R. Vaughan, A. Harrison, L. Voss, A. J. Morris, H. Singh, and V. Koberstein.** 2000. A school and community outbreak of tuberculosis in Auckland. *N Z Med J* **113:**71-4.

1033. **Calder, L., G. Simmons, C. Thornley, P. Taylor, K. Pritchard, G. Greening, and J. Bishop.** 2003. An outbreak of hepatitis A associated with consumption of raw blueberries. *Epidemiol Infect* **131:**745-51.

1034. **Calder, R. A., P. Duclos, M. H. Wilder, V. L. Pryor, and W. J. Scheel.** 1991. Mycobacterium tuberculosis transmission in a health clinic. *Bull Int Union Tuberc Lung Dis* **66:**103-6.

1035. **Calisher, C. H.** 1994. Medically important arboviruses of the United States and Canada. *Clin Microbiol Rev* **7:**89-116.

1036. **Calle, D., D. S. Rosero, L. C. Orozco, D. Camargo, E. Castaneda, and A. Restrepo.** 2001. Paracoccidioidomycosis in Colombia: an ecological study. *Epidemiol Infect* **126:**309-15.

1037. **Calvopina, M., R. H. Guderian, W. Paredes, and P. J. Cooper.** 2003. Comparison of two single-day regimens of triclabendazole for the treatment of human pulmonary paragonimiasis. *Trans R Soc Trop Med Hyg* **97:**451-4.

1038. **Cam, P. D., N. Sorel, L. C. Dan, E. Larher, S. Tassin, J. P. Barbier, and M. Miégeville.** 2001. Contribution à l'épidémiologie de Cyclospora cayetanensis à partir d'une étude sur 12 mois réalisée sur l'eau de distribution à Hanoï (Viêt-Nam). *Méd Mal Infect* **31:**591-6.

1039. **Camargo, L. M., M. U. Ferreira, H. Krieger, E. P. De Camargo, and L. P. Da Silva.** 1994. Unstable hypoendemic malaria in Rondonia (western Amazon region, Brazil): epidemic outbreaks and work-associated incidence in an agro-industrial rural settlement. *Am J Trop Med Hyg* **51:**16-25.

1040. **Camargo, L. M., E. Noronha, J. M. Salcedo, A. P. Dutra, H. Krieger, L. H. Pereira da Silva, and E. P. Camargo.** 1999. The epidemiology of malaria in Rondonia (Western Amazon region, Brazil): study of a riverine population. *Acta Trop* **72:**1-11.

1041. **Camer, G. A., M. Alejandria, M. Amor, H. Satoh, Y. Muramatsu, H. Ueno, and C. Morita.** 2003. Detection of Antibodies against Spotted Fever Group Rickettsia (SFGR), Typhus Group Rickettsia (TGR), and Coxiella burnetii in Human Febrile Patients in the Philippines. *Jpn J Infect Dis* **56:**26-8.

1042. **Camicas, J. L., J. P. Cornet, J. P. Gonzalez, M. L. Wilson, F. Adam, and H. G. Zeller.** 1994. [Crimean-Congo hemorrhagic fever in Senegal. Latest data on the ecology of the CCHF virus]. *Bull Soc Pathol Exot* **87:**11-6.

1043. **Caminero, J. A., M. J. Pena, M. I. Campos-Herrero, J. C. Rodriguez, I. Garcia, P. Cabrera, C. Lafoz, S. Samper, H. Takiff, O. Afonso, J. M. Pavon, M. J. Torres, D. van Soolingen, D. A. Enarson, and C. Martin.** 2001. Epidemiological evidence of the spread of a Mycobacterium tuberculosis strain of the Beijing genotype on Gran Canaria island. *Am J Respir Crit Care Med* **164:**1165-70.

1044. **Campagnolo, E. R., M. C. Warwick, H. L. Marx, Jr., R. P. Cowart, H. D. Donnell, Jr., M. D. Bajani, S. L. Bragg, J. E. Esteban, D. P. Alt, J. W. Tappero, C. A. Bolin, and D. A. Ashford.** 2000. Analysis of the 1998 outbreak of leptospirosis in Missouri in humans exposed to infected swine. *J Am Vet Med Assoc* **216:**676-82.

1045. **Campbell, G., R. Lanciotti, B. Bernard, and H. Lu.** 2002. Laboratory-acquired West Nile virus infections - United States, 2002. *MMWR* **51:**1133-5.

1046. **Campbell, G. L., W. C. Reeves, J. L. Hardy, and B. F. Eldridge.** 1992. Seroepidemiology of California and Bunyamwera serogroup bunyavirus infections in humans in California. *Am J Epidemiol* **136:**308-19.

1047. **Campbell, K. M., A. F. Vaughn, K. L. Russell, B. Smith, D. L. Jimenez, C. P. Barrozo, J. R. Minarcik, N. F. Crum, and M. A. Ryan.** 2004. Risk factors for community-associated methicillin-resistant Staphylococcus aureus infections in an outbreak of disease among military trainees in San Diego, California, in 2002. *J Clin Microbiol* **42:**4050-3.

1048. **Campbell, L. A., C. C. Kuo, and J. T. Grayston.** 1998. Chlamydia pneumoniae and cardiovascular disease. *Emerg Infect Dis* **4:**571-9.

1049. **Campese, C., and B. Decludt.** 2002. Notified cases of legionnaires' disease in France in 2001. *Eurosurveillance* **7:**121-6.

1050. **Campo, N., R. Brizzolara, N. Sinelli, F. Puppo, A. Campelli, F. Indiveri, and A. Picciotto.** 2000. Hepatitis G virus infection in intravenous drug users with or without human immunodeficiency virus infection. *Hepatogastroenterology* **47:**1385-8.

1051. **Campos-Bueno, A., G. Lopez-Abente, and A. M. Andres-Cercadillo.** 2000. Risk factors for Echinococcus granulosus infection: a case-control study. *Am J Trop Med Hyg* **62:**329-34.

1052. **Camps, N., A. Dominguez, M. Company, M. Perez, J. Pardos, T. Llobet, M. A. Usera, and L. Salleras.** 2005. A foodborne outbreak of Salmonella infection due to overproduction of egg-containing foods for a festival. *Epidemiol Infect* **133:**817-22.

1053. **Camps, N., N. Follia, S. Berrón, L. De la Fuente, and J. A. Vázquez.** 1998. An outbreak of invasive meningococcal disease probably associated with an indoor swimming pool. *Clin Microbiol Infect* **4:**349-350.

1054. **Cancrini, G., R. Romi, S. Gabrielli, L. Toma, D. I. P. M, and P. Scaramozzino.** 2003. First finding of Dirofilaria repens in natural population of Aedes albopictus. *Med Vet Entomol* **17:**448-51.

1055. **Candoni, A., C. Fili, R. Trevisan, F. Silvestri, and R. Fanin.** 2003. Fusobacterium nucleatum: a rare cause of bacteremia in neutropenic patients with leukemia and lymphoma. *Clin Microbiol Infect* **9:**1112-5.

1056. **Cannon, C. G., and C. C. Linnemann, Jr.** 1992. Yersinia enterocolitica infections in hospitalized patients: the problem of hospital-acquired infections. *Infect Control Hosp Epidemiol* **13:**139-43.

1057. **Cannon, J. P., T. A. Lee, J. T. Bolanos, and L. H. Danziger.** 2005. Pathogenic relevance of Lactobacillus: a retrospective review of over 200 cases. *Eur J Clin Microbiol Infect Dis* **24:**31-40.

1058. **Cannon, M. J., S. C. Dollard, D. K. Smith, R. S. Klein, P. Schuman, J. D. Rich, D. Vlahov, and P. E. Pellett.** 2001. Blood-borne and sexual transmission of human herpesvirus 8 in women with or at risk for human immunodeficiency virus infection. *N Engl J Med* **344:**637-43.

1059. **Cannon, R. O., J. R. Poliner, R. B. Hirschhorn, D. C. Rodeheaver, and P. R. Silverman.** 1991. A multistate outbreak of Norwalk virus gastroenteritis associated with consumption of commercial ice. *J Infect Dis* **164:**860-863.

1060. **Cano, M. V., and R. A. Hajjeh.** 2001. The epidemiology of histoplasmosis: a review. *Semin Respir Infect* **16:**109-18.

1061. **Cano, M. V., G. F. Ponce-de-Leon, S. Tippen, M. D. Lindsley, M. Warwick, and R. A. Hajjeh.** 2003. Blastomycosis in Missouri: epidemiology and risk factors for endemic disease. *Epidemiol Infect* **131:**907-14.

1062. **Canova, C. R., W. Brunner, and W. H. Reinhart.** 1993. Brucellose: Fallbericht und Zusammenstellung von 10 Fällen (1973-1992) am Kantonsspital Chur. *Schweiz Med Wochenschr* **123:**2370-7.

1063. **Cantaloube, J. F., P. Gallian, H. Attoui, P. Biagini, P. De Micco, and X. de Lamballerie.** 2005. Genotype distribution and molecular epidemiology of hepatitis C virus in blood donors from southeast france. *J Clin Microbiol* **43:**3624-9.

1064. **Cantella, R., A. Colichon, L. Lopez, C. Wu, A. Goldfarb, E. Cuadra, C. Latorre, R. Kanashiro, M. Delgado, and Z. Piscoya.** 1974. Toxoplasmosis in Peru. Geographic prevalence of Toxoplasma gondii antibodies in Peru studied by indirect fluorescent antibody technique. *Trop Geogr Med* **26:**204-9.

1065. **Canto-Lara, S. B., N. R. Van Wynsberghe, A. Vargas-Gonzalez, F. F. Ojeda-Farfan, and F. J. Andrade-Narvaez.** 1999. Use of monoclonal antibodies for the identification of Leishmania spp. isolated from humans and wild rodents in the State of Campeche, Mexico. *Mem Inst Oswaldo Cruz* **94:**305-9.

1066. **Canueto-Quintero, J., F. J. Caballero-Granado, M. Herrero-Romero, A. Dominguez-Castellano, P. Martin-Rico, E. V. Verdu, D. S. Santamaria, R. C. Cerquera, and M. Torres-Tortosa.** 2003. Epidemiological, clinical, and prognostic differences between the diseases caused by Mycobacterium kansasii and Mycobacterium tuberculosis in patients infected with human immunodeficiency virus: a multicenter study. *Clin Infect Dis* **37:**584-90.

1067. **Cao, W. C., Q. M. Zhao, P. H. Zhang, Y. Yang, X. M. Wu, B. H. Wen, X. T. Zhang, and J. D. Habbema.** 2003. Prevalence of Anaplasma phagocytophila and Borrelia burgdorferi in Ixodes persulcatus ticks from northeastern China. *Am J Trop Med Hyg* **68:**547-50.

1068. **Caporaso, N., A. Ascione, and T. Stroffolini.** 1998. Spread of hepatitis C virus infection within families. Investigators of an Italian Multicenter Group. *J Viral Hepat* **5:**67-72.

1069. **Capua, I., and D. J. Alexander.** 2004. Human health implications of avian influenza viruses and paramyxoviruses. *Eur J Clin Microbiol Infect Dis* **23:**1-6.

1070. **Caputo, R., K. De Boulle, J. Del Rosso, and R. Nowicki.** 2001. Prevalence of superficial fungal infections among sports-active individuals: results from the Achilles survey, a review of the literature. *J Eur Acad Dermatol Venerol* **15:**312-6.

1071. **Caraballo, A. J.** 1996. Outbreak of vampire bat biting in a Venezuelan village. *Rev Saude Publica* **30:**483-4.

1072. **Carapetis, J. R., C. Connors, D. Yarmirr, V. Krause, and B. J. Currie.** 1997. Success of a scabies control program in an Australian aboriginal community. *Pediatr Infect Dis J* **16:**494-9.

1073. **Carbonara, S., S. Babudieri, B. Longo, G. Starnini, R. Monarca, B. Brunetti, M. Andreoni, G. Pastore, V. De Marco, and G. Rezza.** 2005. Correlates of Mycobacterium tuberculosis infection in a prison population. *Eur Respir J* **25:**1070-6.

1074. **Carcamo, C., T. Hooton, M. H. Wener, N. S. Weiss, R. Gilman, J. Arevalo, J. Carrasco, C. Seas, M. Caballero, and K. K. Holmes.** 2005. Etiologies and manifestations of persistent diarrhea in adults with HIV-1 infection: a case-control study in Lima, Peru. *J Infect Dis* **191:**11-9.

1075. **Cardo, D. M., D. H. Culver, C. A. Ciesielski, P. U. Srivastava, R. Marcus, D. Abiteboul, J. Heptonstall, G. Ippolito, F. Lot, P. S. McKibben, and D. M. Bell.** 1997. A case-control study of HIV seroconversion in health care workers after percutaneous exposure. Centers for Disease Control and Prevention Needlestick Surveillance Group. *N Engl J Med* **337:**1485-90.

1076. **Cardona-Castro, N., G. Ortega-Rodriguez, and P. Agudelo-Florez.** 1998. Evaluation of three Mycobacterium leprae monoclonal antibodies in mucus and lymph samples from Ziehl-Neelsen stain negative leprosy patients and their household contacts in an Indian community. *Mem Inst Oswaldo Cruz* **93:**487-90.

1077. **Cardoso, L., H. D. Schallig, F. Neto, N. Kroon, and M. Rodrigues.** 2004. Serological survey of Leishmania infection in dogs from the municipality of Peso da Regua (Alto Douro, Portugal) using the direct agglutination test (DAT) and fast agglutination screening test (FAST). *Acta Trop* **91:**95-100.

1078. **Carey, J., M. Motyl, and D. C. Perlman.** 2001. Catheter-related bacteremia due to Streptomyces in a patient receiving holistic infusions. *Emerg Infect Dis* **7:**1043-1045.

1079. **Carleton, R. E., and M. K. Tolbert.** 2004. Prevalence of Dirofilaria immitis and gastrointestinal helminths in cats euthanized at animal control agencies in northwest Georgia. *Vet Parasitol* **119:**319-26.

1080. **Carlier, J. P., C. Henry, V. Lorin, and M. R. Popoff.** 2001. Le botulisme en France à la fin du deuxième millénaire (1998-2000). *Bull Epidémiol Hebdomadaire* **9:**1-8.

1081. **Carlin, F., V. Broussolle, S. Perelle, S. Litman, and P. Fach.** 2004. Prevalence of Clostridium botulinum in food raw materials used in REPFEDs manufactured in France. *Int J Food Microbiol* **91:**141-5.

1082. **Carlton, J. T., and J. B. Geller.** 1993. Ecological roulette: the global transport of nonindigenous marine organisms. *Science* **261:**78-82.

1083. **Carman, W. F., A. G. Elder, L. A. Wallace, K. McAulay, A. Walker, G. D. Murray, and D. J. Stott.** 2000. Effects of influenza vaccination of health-care workers on mortality of elderly people in long-term care: a randomised controlled trial. *Lancet* **355:**93-7.

1084. **Carme, B., C. Aznar, B. de Thoisy, R. Bouynes, M. Demar, A. Motard, and P. Néron.** 2001. Le réservoir de parasite animal de T. gondii en Guyane. Etude sérologique chez les mammifères sauvages non carnivores. *Méd Mal Infect* **31 suppl 2:**312s-3s.

1085. **Carme, B., M. Duda, A. Datry, and M. Gentilini.** 1981. La filariose de Médine (dracunculose) au décours de vacances en Afrique de l'ouest. Conséquences épidémiologiques. *Nouv Presse Med* **10:**2711-3.

1086. **Carmona, C., R. Perdomo, A. Carbo, C. Alvarez, J. Monti, R. Grauert, D. Stern, G. Perera, S. Lloyd, R. Bazini, M. A. Gemmell, and L. Yarzabal.** 1998. Risk factors associated with human cystic echinococcosis in Florida, Uruguay: results of a mass screening study using ultrasound and serology. *Am J Trop Med Hyg* **58:**599-605.

1087. **Carneiro, F. F., E. Cifuentes, M. M. Tellez-Rojo, and I. Romieu.** 2002. The risk of Ascaris lumbricoides infection in children as an environmental health indicator to guide preventive activities in Caparao and Alto Caparao, Brazil. *Bull WHO* **80:**40-6.

1088. **Carnevale, P., P. Guillet, V. Robert, D. Fontenille, J. Doannio, M. Coosemans, and J. Mouchet.** 1999. Diversity of malaria in rice growing areas of the Afrotropical region. *Parasitologia* **41:**273-6.

1089. **Carney, E., S. B. O'Brien, J. J. Sheridan, D. A. McDowell, I. S. Blair, and G. Duffy.** 2006. Prevalence and level of Escherichia coli O157 on beef trimmings, carcasses and boned head meat at a beef slaughter plant. *Food Microbiol* **23:**52-9.

1090. **Carosi, G., A. Maccabruni, F. Castelli, and P. Viale.** 1986. Accidental and transfusion malaria in Italy. *Trans R Soc Trop Med Hyg* **80:**667-8.

1091. **Carpio, A.** 2002. Neurocysticercosis: an update. *Lancet Infect Dis* **2:**751-62.

1092. **Carrada Bravo, T.** 1981. [Typhoid fever and anti-typhoid vaccination. In memory of S. Morones-Alba and A. Celis-Salazar]. *Salud Publica Mex* **23:**103-58.

1093. **Carrasco, J., A. Morrison, and C. Ponce.** 1998. Behaviour of Lutzomyia longipalpis in an area of southern Honduras endemic for visceral/atypical cutaneous leishmaniasis. *Ann Trop Med Parasitol* **92:**869-76.

1094. **Carrasquilla, G., M. Banguero, P. Sanchez, F. Carvajal, R. H. Barker, Jr., G. W. Gervais, E. Algarin, and A. E. Serrano.** 2000. Epidemiologic tools for malaria surveillance in an urban setting of low endemicity along the Colombian Pacific coast. *Am J Trop Med Hyg* **62:**132-7.

1095. **Carrat, F., C. Sahler, S. Rogez, M. Leruez-Ville, F. Freymuth, C. Le Gales, M. Bungener, B. Housset, M. Nicolas, and C. Rouzioux.** 2002. Influenza burden of illness. *Arch Intern Med* **162:**1842-8.

1096. **Carrieri, M. P., H. Tissot-Dupont, D. Rey, P. Brousse, H. Renard, Y. Obadia, and D. Raoult.** 2002. Investigation of a slaughterhouse-related outbreak of Q fever in the French Alps. *Eur J Clin Microbiol Infect Dis* **21:**17-21.

1097. **Carrique-Mas, J., Y. Andersson, B. Petersen, K. O. Hedlund, N. Sjogren, and J. Giesecke.** 2003. A norwalk-like virus waterborne community outbreak in a Swedish village during peak holiday season. *Epidemiol Infect* **131:**737-44.

1098. Carstensen, L., M. Vaarst, and A. Roepstorff. 2002. Helminth infections in Danish organic swine herds. *Vet Parasitol* **106**:253-64.

1099. Carter, A. O., A. A. Borczyk, J. A. Carlson, B. Harvey, J. C. Hockin, M. A. Karmali, C. Krishnan, D. A. Korn, and H. Lior. 1987. A severe outbreak of Escherichia coli O157:H7—associated hemorrhagic colitis in a nursing home. *N Engl J Med* **317**:1496-500.

1100. Carter, J. S., F. J. Bowden, I. Bastian, G. M. Myers, K. S. Sriprakash, and D. J. Kemp. 1999. Phylogenetic evidence for reclassification of Calymmatobacterium granulomatis as Klebsiella granulomatis comb. nov. *Int J Syst Bacteriol* **49 Pt 4**:1695-700.

1101. Carter, R., K. N. Mendis, and D. Roberts. 2000. Spatial targeting of interventions against malaria. *Bull WHO* **78**:1401-11.

1102. Carter, S., K. Horn, G. Hart, M. Dunbar, A. Scoular, and S. MacIntyre. 1997. The sexual behaviour of international travellers at two Glasgow GUM clinics. Glasgow genitourinary medicine. *Int J STD AIDS* **8**:336-8.

1103. Cartmill, T. D., H. Panigrahi, M. A. Worsley, D. C. McCann, C. N. Nice, and E. Keith. 1994. Management and control of a large outbreak of diarrhoea due to Clostridium difficile. *J Hosp Infect* **27**:1-15.

1104. Cartwright, K. A., J. M. Stuart, and P. M. Robinson. 1991. Meningococcal carriage in close contacts of cases. *Epidemiol Infect* **106**:133-41.

1105. Cartwright, R. Y. 2003. Food and waterborne infections associated with package holidays. *J Appl Microbiol* **94 Suppl**:12S-24S.

1106. Caruso, G., C. Zasio, F. Guzzo, C. Granata, V. Mondardini, E. Guerra, E. Macri, and P. Benedetti. 2002. Outbreak of African tick-bite fever in six Italian tourists returning from South Africa. *Eur J Clin Microbiol Infect Dis* **21**:133-6.

1107. Carvalheiro, C. G., M. M. Mussi-Pinhata, A. Y. Yamamoto, C. B. De Souza, and L. M. Maciel. 2005. Incidence of congenital toxoplasmosis estimated by neonatal screening: relevance of diagnostic confirmation in asymptomatic newborn infants. *Epidemiol Infect* **133**:485-91.

1108. Carvalho, M. F., M. F. de Franco, and V. A. Soares. 1997. Amastigotes forms of Trypanosoma cruzi detected in a renal allograft. *Rev Inst Med Trop Sao Paulo* **39**:223-6.

1109. Casadevall, A., and J. R. Perfect. 1998. Cryptococcus neoformans. American Society for Microbiology Press, Washington, D.C.

1110. Casal, M., and M. M. Casal. 2001. Multicenter study of incidence of Mycobacterium marinum in humans in Spain. *Int J Tuberc Lung Dis* **5**:197-9.

1111. Cascio, A., C. Colomba, S. Antinori, M. Orobello, D. Paterson, and L. Titone. 2002. Pediatric visceral leishmaniasis in Western Sicily, Italy: a retrospective analysis of 111 cases. *Eur J Clin Microbiol Infect Dis* **21**:277-82.

1112. Cashman, N. R. 2001. Transmissible spongiform encephalopathies: vaccine issues. *Dev Biol* **106**:445-61.

1113. Casin, I., D. Vexiau-Robert, P. De La Salmoniere, A. Eche, B. Grandry, and M. Janier. 2002. High prevalence of Mycoplasma genitalium in the lower genitourinary tract of women attending a sexually transmitted disease clinic in Paris, France. *Sex Transm Dis* **29**:353-9.

1114. Castanera, M. B., M. A. Lauricella, R. Chuit, and R. E. Gurtler. 1998. Evaluation of dogs as sentinels of the transmission of Trypanosoma cruzi in a rural area of northwestern Argentina. *Ann Trop Med Parasitol* **92**:671-83.

1115. Castell Monsalve, J., J. V. Rullan, E. F. Peiro Callizo, and A. Nieto-Sandoval Alcolea. 1996. [Epidemic outbreak of 81 cases of brucellosis following the consumption of fresh cheese without pasteurization]. *Rev Esp Salud Publica* **70**:303-11.

1116. Castellani Pastoris, M., R. Lo Monaco, P. Goldoni, B. Mentore, G. Balestra, L. Ciceroni, and P. Visca. 1999. Legionnaires' disease on a cruise ship linked to the water supply system: clinical and public health implications. *Clin Infect Dis* **28**:33-8.

1117. Castelli, F., S. Caligaris, A. Matteelli, A. Chiodera, G. Carosi, and G. Fausti. 1993. 'Baggage malaria' in Italy: cryptic malaria explained? *Trans R Soc Trop Med Hyg* **87**:394.

1118. Castelli, F., A. Matteelli, S. Caligaris, M. Gulletta, I. el-Hamad, C. Scolari, G. Chatel, and G. Carosi. 1999. Malaria in migrants. *Parassitologia* **41**:261-5.

1119. Castillo, C., L. Sanhueza, M. Tager, S. Munoz, G. Ossa, and P. Vial. 2002. [Seroprevalence of antibodies against hantavirus in 10 communities of the IX Region of Chile where hantavirus infection were diagnosed]. *Rev Med Chil* **130**:251-8.

1120. Castillo, C., E. Villagra, L. Sanhueza, M. Ferres, J. Mardones, and G. J. Mertz. 2004. Prevalence of antibodies to hantavirus among family and health care worker contacts of persons with hantavirus cardiopulmonary syndrome: lack of evidence for nosocomial transmission of Andes virus to health care workers in Chile. *Am J Trop Med Hyg* **70**:302-4.

1121. Castillo, D., C. Paredes, C. Zanartu, J. Castillo, R. Mercado, V. Munoz, and H. Schenone. 2000. [Environmental contamination with Toxocara sp. eggs in public squares and parks from Santiago, Chile, 1999]. *Bol Chil Parasitol* **55**:86-91.

1122. Castle, P. E., M. Schiffman, M. C. Bratti, A. Hildesheim, R. Herrero, M. L. Hutchinson, A. C. Rodriguez, S. Wacholder, M. E. Sherman, H. Kendall, R. P. Viscidi, J. Jeronimo, J. E. Schussler, and R. D. Burk. 2004. A population-based study of vaginal human papillomavirus infection in hysterectomized women. *J Infect Dis* **190**:458-67.

1123. Castor, M. L., E. A. Wagstrom, R. N. Danila, K. E. Smith, T. S. Naimi, J. M. Besser, K. A. Peacock, B. A. Juni, J. M. Hunt, J. M. Bartkus, S. R. Kirkhorn, and R. Lynfield. 2005. An outbreak of Pontiac fever with respiratory distress among workers performing high-pressure cleaning at a sugar-beet processing plant. *J Infect Dis* **191**:1530-7.

1124. Castro, M. B., W. L. Nicholson, V. L. Kramer, and J. E. Childs. 2001. Persistent infection in Neotoma fuscipes (Muridae: Sigmodontinae) with Ehrlichia phagocytophila sensu lato. *Am J Trop Med Hyg* **65**:261-7.

1125. Casulli, A., M. T. Manfredi, G. La Rosa, A. R. Di Cerbo, A. Dinkel, T. Romig, P. Deplazes, C. Genchi, and E. Pozio. 2005. Echinococcus multilocularis in red foxes (Vulpes vulpes) of the Italian Alpine region: is there a focus of autochthonous transmission? *Int J Parasitol* **35**:1079-83.

1126. **CATMAT (Committee to Advise on Tropical Medicine and Travel).** 1998. Statement on Japanese encephalitis vaccine. *Can Comm Dis Rep* **24 (ACS-3)**:1-8.

1127. Cattand, P. 2001. L'épidémiologie de la trypanosomiase humaine Africaine: une histoire multifactorielle complexe. *Med Trop* **61**:313-22.

1128. Cattani, P., M. Capuano, F. Cerimele, I. L. La Parola, R. Santangelo, C. Masini, D. Cerimele, and G. Fadda. 1999. Human herpesvirus 8 seroprevalence and evaluation of nonsexual transmission routes by detection of DNA in clinical specimens from human immunodeficiency virus-negative patients from central and southern Italy, with and without Kaposi's sarcoma. *J Clin Microbiol* **37:**1150-1153.

1129. **Caumes, E., J. Carriere, G. Guermonprez, F. Bricaire, M. Danis, and M. Gentilini.** 1995. Dermatoses associated with travel to tropical countries: a prospective study of the diagnosis and management of 269 patients presenting to a tropical disease unit. *Clin Infect Dis* **20:**542-8.

1130. **Caumes, E., N. Ehya, J. Nguyen, and F. Bricaire.** 2001. Typhoid and paratyphoid Fever: a 10-year retrospective study of 41 cases in a parisian hospital. *J Travel Med* **8:**293-7.

1131. **Caumes, E., S. Felder-Moinet, C. Couzigou, C. Darras-Joly, P. Latour, and N. Leger.** 2003. Failure of an ointment based on IR3535 (ethyl butylacetylaminopropionate) to prevent an outbreak of cercarial dermatitis during swimming races across Lake Annecy, France. *Ann Trop Med Parasitol* **97:**157-63.

1132. **Causer, L. M., R. D. Newman, A. M. Barber, J. M. Roberts, G. Stennies, P. B. Bloland, M. E. Parise, and R. W. Steketee.** 2002. Malaria surveillance - United States, 2000. *MMWR* **51 (SS-5):**1-21.

1133. **Cavalieri d'Oro, L., E. Merlo, E. Ariano, M. G. Silvestri, A. Ceraminiello, E. Negri, and C. La Vecchia.** 1999. Vibrio cholerae outbreak in Italy. *Emerg Infect Dis* **5:**300-1.

1134. **Cazorla, C., M. Enea, F. Lucht, and D. Raoult.** 2003. First Isolation of Rickettsia slovaca from a Patient, France. *Emerg Infect Dis* **9:**135.

1135. **CDC.** 1978. Nosocomial outbreak of Rhizopus infections associated with Elastoplast* wound dressings - Minnesota. *MMWR* **27:**33-4.

1136. **CDC.** 1981. Anthrax contamination of Haitian goatskin products. *MMWR* **30:**338.

1137. **CDC.** 1981. Diphyllobothriasis associated with salmon - United States. *MMWR* **30:**331-8.

1138. **CDC.** 1983. Group C streptococcal infections associated with eating homemade cheese - New Mexico. *MMWR* **32:**510-516.

1139. **CDC.** 1983. Interstate importation of measles following transmission in an airport - California, Washington, 1982. *MMWR* **32:**210, 215-6.

1140. **CDC.** 1991. Multistate outbreak of Salmonella poona infections - United States and Canada, 1991. *MMWR* **40:**549-552.

1141. **CDC.** 1992. Outbreak of type E botulism associated with an uneviscerated, salt- cured fish product—New Jersey, 1992. *MMWR* **41:**521-2.

1142. **CDC.** 1992. Population-based mortality assessment - Baidoa and Afgoi, Somalia, 1992. *MMWR* **41:**913-7.

1143. **CDC.** 1993. Outbreaks of Mycoplasma pneumoniae respiratory infection - Ohio, Texas, and New York, 1993. *MMWR* **42:**931-9.

1144. **CDC.** 1993. Tuberculosis in imported nonhuman primates - United States, June 1990-May 1993. *MMWR* **42:**572-576.

1145. **CDC.** 1994. Bacillus cereus food poisoning associated with fried rice at wto child day care centers - Virginia, 1993. *MMWR* **43:**177-178.

1146. **CDC.** 1994. Clostridium perfringens gastroenteritis associated with corned beef served at St. Patrick's day meals - Ohio and Virginia, 1993. *MMWR* **43:**137, 143-4.

1147. **CDC.** 1994. Outbreak of Shigella flexneri 2a infections on a cruise ship. *MMWR* **43:**657.

1148. **CDC.** 1995. Escherichia coli O157:H7 outbreak at a summer camp - Virginia, 1994. *MMWR* **44:**419-21.

1149. **CDC.** 1996. Measles outbreak among school-aged children - Juneau, Alaska, 1996. *MMWR* **45:**777-80.

1150. **CDC.** 1996. Vibrio vulnificus infections associated with eating raw oysters - Los Angeles, 1996. *MMWR* **45:**621-4.

1151. **CDC.** 1997. Nonhuman primate spumavirus infections among persons with occupational exposure - United States, 1996. *MMWR* **46:**129-31.

1152. **CDC.** 1997. Outbreak of staphylococcal food poisoning associated with precooked ham -Florida, 1997. *MMWR* **46:**1189-91.

1153. **CDC.** 1998. Foodborne outbreak of cryptosporidiosis - Spokane, Washington, 1997. *MMWR* **47:**565-567.

1154. **CDC.** 1998. Outbreak of influenza A infection - Alaska and the Yukon Territory, June-July 1998. *MMWR* **48:**638.

1155. **CDC.** 1998. Outbreak of Vibrio parahaemolyticus infections associated with eating raw oysters - Pacific Northwest, 1997. *MMWR* **47:**457-62.

1156. **CDC.** 1998. Plesiomonas shigelloides and Salmonella serotype Hartford infections associated with a contaminated water supply - Livingston county, New York, 1996. *MMWR* **47:**395-397.

1157. **CDC.** 1998. Rift valley fever - East Africa, 1997-1998. *MMWR* **47:**261-4.

1158. **CDC.** 1998. Tetanus among injecting-drug users - California, 1997. *MMWR* **47:**149-51.

1159. **CDC.** 1999. Biosafety in microbiological and biomedical laboratories, 4th ed ed. US Government Printing Office, Washington, D.C.

1160. **CDC.** 1999. Blastomycosis acquired occupationally during prairie dog relocation - Colorado, 1998. *MMWR* **48:**98-100.

1161. **CDC.** 1999. Outbreak of Escherichia coli O157:H7 and Campylobacter among attendees of the Washington county fair - New York, 1999. *MMWR* **48:**803-5.

1162. **CDC.** 1999. Outbreak of Vibrio parahaemolyticus infection associated with eatingraw oysters and clams harvested from Long Island sound - Connecticut, New Jersey, and New York, 1998. *MMWR* **48:**48-51.

1163. **CDC.** 1999. Outbreaks of Shigella sonnei infection associated with eating fresh parsley - United States and Canada, July-August 1998. *MMWR* **48:**285-9.

1164. **CDC.** 1999. Update: multistate outbreak of listeriosis - United States, 1998-1999. *MMWR* **47:**1117-8.

1165. **CDC.** 1999. Update: recommendations to prevent hepatitis B virus transmission - United States. *MMWR* **48:**33-34.

1166. **CDC.** 2000. Compendium of measures to control Chlamydia psittaci infection among humans (psittacosis) and pet birds (avian chlamydiosis), 2000. *MMWR* **49 (RR-8):**1-18.

1167. **CDC.** 2000. Guidelines for preventing opportunistic infections among hematopoietic stem cell transplant recipients: recommendations of CDC, the Infectious Disease Society of America, and the American Society of Blood and Marrow Transplantation. *MMWR* **49 (RR-10):**1-94.

1168. **CDC.** 2000. Human ingestion of Bacillus anthracis-contaminated meat - Minnesota, August 2000. *MMWR* **49:**813-6.

1169. CDC. 2000. Human rabies - California, Georgia, Minnesota, New York, and Wisconsin, 2000. *MMWR* **49:**1111-5.

1170. CDC. 2000. Legionnaires' disease associated with potting soil - California, Oregon, and Washington, May-June 2000. *MMWR* **49:**777-8.

1171. CDC. 2000. Outbreak of Escherichia coli O157:H7 infection associated with eating fresh cheese curds - Wisconsin, June 1998. *MMWR* **49:**911-3.

1172. CDC. 2000. Outbreaks of Salmonella serotype Enteritidis infection associated with eating raw or undercooked shell eggs - United States, 19996-1998. *MMWR* **49:**73-79.

1173. CDC. 2000. Targeted tuberculin testing and treatment of latent tuberculosis infection. *MMWR* **49 (RR-6):**1-51.

1174. CDC. 2001. Botulism outbreak associated with eating fermented food - Alaska, 2001. *MMWR* **550:**680-682.

1175. CDC. 2001. Hepatitis B outbreak in a state correctional facility, 2000. *MMWR* **50:**529-532.

1176. CDC. 2001. HIV/AIDS surveillance report 2001, vol. 13(2). Department of Health and Human Services, CDC, Atlanta, Georgia.

1177. CDC. 2001. Methicillin-resistant Staphylococcus aureus skin or soft tissue infections in a state prison—Mississippi, 2000. *MMWR* **50:**919-22.

1178. CDC. 2001. Outbreak of Powassan encephalitis - Maine and Vermont, 1999-2001. *MMWR* **50:**761-4.

1179. CDC. 2001. Outbreaks of Escherichia coli O157:H7 infections among children associated with farm visits - Pennsylvania and Washington, 2000. *MMWR* **50:**293-297.

1180. CDC. 2001. Prevalence of risk behaviors for HIV infection among adults - United States, 1997. *MMWR* **50:**262-5.

1181. CDC. 2001. Shigellosis outbreak associated with an unchlorinated fill-and-drain wading pool - Iowa, 2001. *MMWR* **50:**797-800.

1182. CDC. 2001. Underdiagnosis of dengue - Laredo, Texas, 1999. *MMWR* **50:**57-9.

1183. CDC. 2001. Update: investigation of bioterrorism-related anthrax and interim guidelines for exposure management and antimicrobial therapiy, October 2001. *MMWR* **50:**909-919.

1184. CDC. 2001. Update: outbreak of acute febrile respiratory illness among college students - Acapulco, Mexico, March 2001. *MMWR* **50:**359-360.

1185. CDC. 2002. Enterobacter sakazakii infections associated with the use of powdered infant formula - Tennessee, 2001. *MMWR* **51:**298-300.

1186. CDC. 2002. Enterovirus surveillance - United States, 2000-2001. *MMWR* **51:**1047-9.

1187. CDC. 2002. Exophiala infection from contaminated injectable steroids prepared by a compounding pharmacy - United States, July-November 2002. *MMWR* **51:**1109-12.

1188. CDC. 2002. Fatal yellow fever in a traveler returning from Amazonas, Brazil, 2002. *MMWR* **51:**324-5.

1189. CDC. 2002. Measles outbreak among internationally adopted children arriving in the United States, February-March 2001. *MMWR* **51:**1115-6.

1190. CDC. 2002. Multistate outbreak of Escherichia coli O157:H7 infections associated with eating ground beef - United States, June-July 2002. *MMWR* **51:**637-9.

1191. CDC. 2002. Multistate outbreak of Salmonella serotype Poona infections associated with eating cantaloupe from Mexico - United states and Canada, 2000-2002. *MMWR* **51:**1044-7.

1192. CDC. 2002. Outbreak of Campylobacter jejuni infections associated with drinking unpasteurized milk procured through a cow-leasing program - Wisconsin, 2001. *MMWR* **51:**548-9.

1193. CDC. 2002. Outbreak of listeriosis - northeastern United States, 2002. *MMWR* **51:**950-1.

1194. CDC. 2002. Outbreaks of Salmonella serotype Enteritidis infection associated with eating shell eggs - United States, 1999-2001. *MMWR* **51:**1149-52.

1195. CDC. 2002. Pertussis - United States, 1997-2000. *MMWR* **51:**73-6.

1196. CDC. 2002. Pertussis in an infant adopted from Russia—May 2002. *MMWR* **51:**394-5.

1197. CDC. 2002. Prevention of invasive group A streptococcal disease among household contacts of case patients and among postpartum and postsurgical patients: recommendations from the Centers for Disease Control and Prevention. *Clin Infect Dis* **35:**950-9.

1198. CDC. 2002. Provisional surveillance summary of the West Nile Virus epidemic - United States, January-November 2002. *MMWR* **51**.

1199. CDC. 2002. Rabies in a beaver - Florida, 2001. *MMWR* **51:**481-2.

1200. CDC. 2002. Update: investigations of West Nile virus infections in recipients of organ transplantation and blood transfusion. *MMWR* **51:**833-6.

1201. CDC. 2002. West Nile Virus activity—United States, 2001. *MMWR* **51:**497-501.

1202. CDC. 2003. Absence of transmission of the d9 measles virus - region of the Americas, November 2003-March 2003. *MMWR* **52:**228-9.

1203. CDC. 2003. Cutaneous leishmaniasis in U.S. military personnel - southwest/central Asia, 2002-2003. *MMWR* **52:**1009-12.

1204. CDC. 2003. Hepatitis A outbreak associated with green onions at a restaurant - Monaca, Pennsylvania, 2003. *MMWR* **52:**1155-7.

1205. CDC. 2003. HIV testing - United Staes, 2001. *MMWR* **52:**540-5.

1206. CDC. 2003. Imported plague—New York City, 2002. *MMWR* **52:**725-8.

1207. CDC. 2003. Infant botulism - New York city, 2001-2002. *MMWR* **52:**21-4.

1208. CDC. 2003. Local transmission of Plasmodium vivax malaria - Palm beach county, Florida, 2003. *MMWR* **52:**908-11.

1209. CDC. 2003. Multistate outbreak of monkeypox - Illinois, Indiana, and Wisconsi, 2003. *MMWR* **52:**537-40.

1210. CDC. 2003. Multistate outbreak of Salmonella serotype Typhimurium infections associated with drinking unpasteurized milk - Illinois, Indiana, Ohio, and Tennessee, 2002-2003. *MMWR* **52:**613-5.

1211. CDC. 2003. Murine typhus - Hawaii, 2002. *MMWR* **52:**1224-6.

1212. CDC. 2003. Nonfatal dog bite-related injuries treated in hospital emergency departments - United States, 2001. *MMWR* **52:**605-10.

1213. **CDC.** 2003. Norovirus activity - United States, 2002. *MMWR* **52:**41-5.

1214. **CDC.** 2003. Outbreak of botulism type E associated with eating a beached whale - Western Alaska, July 2002. *MMWR* **52:**24-5.

1215. **CDC.** 2003. Outbreak of severe rotavirus gastroenteritis among children - JAMAica, 2003. *MMWR* **52:**1103-5.

1216. **CDC.** 2003. Pertussis outbreak among adults at an oil refinery - Illinois, August-October 2002. *MMWR* **52:**1-4.

1217. **CDC.** 2003. Pneumococcal vaccination for cochlear implant candidates and recipients: updated recommendations of the advisory committee on immunization practices. *MMWR* **52:**739-40.

1218. **CDC.** 2003. Primary and secondary syphilis - United States, 2002. *MMWR* **52:**1117-20.

1219. **CDC.** 2003. Reptile-associated salmonellosis - selected states, 1998-2002. *MMWR* **52:**1206-9.

1220. **CDC.** 2003. Transmission of hepatitis B and C virus in outpatient settings - New York, Oklahoma, and Nebraska, 2000-2002. *MMWR* **52:**901-6.

1221. **CDC.** 2003. Update: multistate outbreak of monkeypox - Illinois, Indiana, Kansas, Missouri, Ohio, and Wisconsin, 2003. *MMWR* **52:**561-4.

1222. **CDC.** 2003. Update: severe acute respiratory syndrome—worldwide and United States, 2003. *MMWR* **52:**664-5.

1223. **CDC.** 2003. Wound botulism among black tar heroin users—Washington, 2003. *MMWR* **52:**885-6.

1224. **CDC.** 2004. Bovine spongiform encephalopathy in a dairy cow - Washington state, 2003. *MMWR* **52:**1280-5.

1225. **CDC.** 2004. Chlamydia screening among sexually active young female enrollees of health plans—United States, 1999-2001. *MMWR* **53:**983-5.

1226. **CDC.** 2004. Day care-related outbreaks of rhamnose-negative Shigella sonnei—six states, June 2001-March 2003. *MMWR* **53:**60-3.

1227. **CDC.** 2004. Diagnosis and management of foodborne illnesses. *MMWR* **53 (RR-4):**1-33.

1228. **CDC.** 2004. Inadvertent intradermal adiminstration of tetanus toxoid-containing vaccines instead of tuberculosis skin tests. *MMWR* **53:**662-4.

1229. **CDC.** 2004. Measles outbreak in a boarding school - Pennsylvania, 2003. *MMWR* **53:**306-9.

1230. **CDC.** 2004. National Nosocomial Infections Surveillance (NNIS) System Report, data summary from January 1992 through June 2004, issued October 2004. *Am J Infect Control* **32:**470-85.

1231. **CDC.** 2004. Number of persons tested for HIV—United States, 2002. *MMWR* **53:**1110-3.

1232. **CDC.** 2004. Outbreak of cyclosporiasis associated with snow peas - Pennsylvania, 2004. *MMWR* **53:**876-8.

1233. **CDC.** 2004. Outbreak of histoplasmosis among industrial plant workers—Nebraska, 2004. *MMWR* **53:**1020-2.

1234. **CDC.** 2004. An outbreak of norovirus gastroenteritis at a swimming club - Vermont, 2004. *MMWR* **53:**793-5.

1235. **CDC.** 2004. Recovery of a patient from clinical rabies—Wisconsin, 2004. *MMWR* **53:**1171-3.

1236. **CDC.** 2004. Transmission of primary and secondary syphilis by oral sex—Chicago, Illinois, 1998-2002. *MMWR* **53:**966-8.

1237. **CDC.** 2004. Trends in Tuberculosis - United States 1998-2003. *MMWR* **53:**209-14.

1238. **CDC.** 2004. Tuberculosis outbreak in a cummunity hospital - District of Columbia, 2002. *MMWR* **53:**214-6.

1239. **CDC.** 2004. Update: investigation of rabies infections in organ donor and transplant recipients - Alabama, Arkansas, Oklahoma, and Texas, 2004. *MMWR* **53:**615-6.

1240. **CDC.** 2004. Update: West Nile virus screening of blood donations and transfusion-associated transmission - United States, 2003. *MMWR* **53:**281-4.

1241. **CDC.** 2005. Escherichia coli O157:H7 Infections Associated with Ground Beef from a U.S. Military Installation —- Okinawa, Japan, February 2004. *MMWR* **54:**40-42.

1242. **CDC.** 2005. Fatal bacterial infections associated with platelet transfusions—United States, 2004. *MMWR* **54:**168-70.

1243. **CDC.** 2005. Fatal rat-bite fever—Florida and Washington, 2003. *MMWR* **53:**1198-202.

1244. **CDC.** 2005. HIV prevalence, unrecognized infection, and HIV testing among men who have sex with men—five U.S. cities, June 2004-April 2005. *MMWR* **52:**597-601.

1245. **CDC.** 2005. HIV transmission in the adult film industry—Los Angeles, California, 2004. *MMWR* **54:**923-6.

1246. **CDC.** 2005. Inadvertent laboratory exposure to Bacillus anthracis—California, 2004. *MMWR* **54:**301-4.

1247. **CDC.** 2005. Infectious disease and dermatologic conditions in evacuees and rescue workers after hurricane Katrina - multiple states, August-September, 2005. *MMWR* **58:**961-4.

1248. **CDC.** 2005. Legionnaires disease associated with potable water in a hotel—Ocean City, Maryland, October 2003-February 2004. *MMWR* **54:**165-8.

1249. **CDC.** 2005. Lymphocytic choriomeningitis virus infection in organ transplant recipients - Massachusetts, Rhode Island, 2005. *MMWR* **54:**537-9.

1250. **CDC.** 2005. Outbreaks of pertussis associated with hospitals—Kentucky, Pennsylvania, and Oregon, 2003. *MMWR* **54:**67-71.

1251. **CDC.** 2005. Positive test results for acute hepatitis A virus infection among persons with no recent history of acute hepatitis—United States, 2002-2004. *MMWR* **54:**453-6.

1252. **CDC.** 2005. Progress in reducing measles mortality—worldwide, 1999-2003. *MMWR* **54:**200-3.

1253. **CDC.** 2005. Rapid health response, assessment, and surveillance after a tsunami—Thailand, 2004-2005. *MMWR* **54:**61-4.

1254. **CDC.** 2005. Shigella flexneri serotype 3 infections among men who have sex with men—Chicago, Illinois, 2003-2004. *MMWR* **54:**820-2.

1255. **CDC.** 2005. Transmission of hepatitis B virus among persons undergoing blood glucose monitoring in long-term-care facilities—Mississippi, North Carolina, and Los Angeles County, California, 2003-2004. *MMWR* **54:**220-3.

1256. **CDC.** 2005. Tularemia associated with a hamster bite—Colorado, 2004. *MMWR* **53:**1202-3.

1257. **CDC.** 2005. Tularemia transmitted by insect bites—Wyoming, 2001-2003. *MMWR* **54:**170-3.

1258. **CDC.** 2005. Update: West Nile virus activity—United States, 2005. *MMWR* **54:**1105-6.

1259. **CDC** 1987. Western equine encephalitis—United States and Canada, 1987. *MMWR* **36:**655-9.

1260. CDC. 1995. Update: management of patients with suspected viral hemorrhagic fever— United States. *MMWR* **44**:475-9.

1261. CDC. 1998. Multistate outbreak of Salmonella serotype Agona infections linked to toasted oats cereal - United States, April-May, 1998. *MMWR* **47**:462-463.

1262. CDC. 1998. Rubella among crew members of commercial cruise ships—Florida, 1997. *MMWR* **46**:1247-50.

1263. CDC. 1999. Outbreak of poliomyelitis - Angola, 1999. *MMWR* **48**:327-9.

1264. CDC. 2000. Monitoring hospital-acquired infections to promote patient safety - United States 1990-1999. *MMWR* **49**:149-153.

1265. CDC. 2000. Preventing pneumococcal disease among infants and young children. *MMWR* **49 RR-9**:1-35.

1266. CDC. 2001. Public health and injection drug use. *MMWR* **50**:377.

1267. CDC. 2004. Investigation of rabies infections in organ donor and transplant recipients - Alabama, Arkansas, Oklahoma, and Texas, 2004. *MMWR* **53**:586-9.

1268. CDC. 2004. Update: measles among children adopted from China. *MMWR* **53**:459.

1269. Cecere, M. C., R. E. Gurtler, D. M. Canale, R. Chuit, and J. E. Cohen. 2002. Effects of partial housing improvement and insecticide spraying on the reinfestation dynamics of Triatoma infestans in rural northwestern Argentina. *Acta Trop* **84**:101-16.

1270. Cecil, J. A., M. R. Howell, J. J. Tawes, J. C. Gaydos, K. T. McKee Jr, T. C. Quinn, and C. A. Gaydos. 2001. Features of Chlamydia trachomatis and Neisseria gonorrhoeae Infection in Male Army Recruits. *J Infect Dis* **184**:1216-9.

1271. Celiksoz, A., M. Acioz, S. Degerli, A. Alim, and C. Aygan. 2005. Egg positive rate of Enterobius vermicularis and Taenia spp. by cellophane tape method in primary school children in Sivas, Turkey. *Korean J Parasitol* **43**:61-4.

1272. Cerny, Z. 2001. Changes of the epidemiology and the clinical picture of tularemia in Southern Moravia (the Czech Republic) during the period 1936-1999. *Eur J Epidemiol* **17**:637-42.

1273. Certad, G., A. Arenas-Pinto, L. Pocaterra, G. Ferrara, J. Castro, A. Bello, and L. Nunez. 2003. Isosporiasis in Venezuelan adults infected with human immunodeficiency virus: clinical characterization. *Am J Trop Med Hyg* **69**:217-22.

1274. Cetinkaya, B., M. Karahan, E. Atil, R. Kalin, T. De Baere, and M. Vaneechoutte. 2002. Identification of Corynebacterium pseudotuberculosis isolates from sheep and goats by PCR. *Vet Microbiol* **88**:75-83.

1275. Cetinkaya, Y., P. Falk, and G. Mayhall. 2000. Vancomycin-resistant enterococci. *Clin Microbiol Rev* **686-707**.

1276. Cetre, J. C., D. Baratin, F. Tissot Guerraz, M. C. Nicolle, E. Reverdy, P. Parvaz, J. Motin, and M. Sepetjan. 1988. [Nosocomial septicemia and pseudobacteremia caused by Serratia marcescens]. *Presse Med* **17**:1255-8.

1277. Cetron, M. S., L. Chitsulo, J. J. Sullivan, J. Pilcher, M. Wilson, J. Noh, V. C. Tsang, A. W. Hightower, and D. G. Addiss. 1996. Schistosomiasis in lake Malawi. *Lancet* **348**:1274-8.

1278. Cetron, M. S., A. A. Marfin, K. G. Julian, D. J. Gubler, D. J. Sharp, R. S. Barwick, L. H. Weld, R. Chen, R. D. Clover, J. Deseda-Tous, V. Marchessault, P. A. Offit, and T. P. Monath. 2002. Yellow fever vaccine. Recommendations of the advisory committee on immunization practices (ACIP), 2002. *MMWR* **51 (RR-17)**:1-11.

1279. Chabasse, D., G. Bertrand, J. P. Leroux, N. Gauthey, and P. Hocquet. 1985. Bilharziose à Schistosoma mansoni évolutive découverte 37 ans après l'infestation. *Bull Soc Pathol Exot* **78**:643-7.

1280. Chadee, D. D. 1998. Tungiasis among five communities in south-western Trinidad, West Indies. *Ann Trop Med Parasitol* **92**:107-13.

1281. Chadee, D. D., J. C. Beier, and R. Doon. 1999. Re-emergence of Plasmodium malariae in Trinidad, West Indies. *Ann Trop Med Parasitol* **93**:467-75.

1282. Chadee, D. D., and U. Kitron. 1999. Spatial and temporal patterns of imported malaria cases and local transmission in Trinidad. *Am J Trop Med Hyg* **61**:513-7.

1283. Chadee, D. D., and R. Martinez. 2000. Landing periodicity of Aedes aegypti with implications for dengue transmission in Trinidad, West Indies. *J Vector Ecol* **25**:158-63.

1284. Chadee, d. D., and S. C. Rawlins. 1997. Dermatobia hominis myiasis in humans in Trinidad. *Trans R Soc Trop Med Hyg* **91**:57.

1285. Chagas, C. 1909. Nova tripanosomiase humana. Estudos sobre e morfologia e o ciclo evolutivo do Schizotrypanum cruzi n.gen.n.sp. agente etiologico de nova entidade morbida do homem. *Mem Inst Oswaldo Cruz* **1**:159-218.

1286. Chai, F., D. R. Prevots, X. Wang, M. Birmingham, and R. Zhang. 2004. Neonatal tetanus incidence in China, 1996-2001, and risk factors for neonatal tetanus, Guangxi Province, China. *Int J Epidemiol* **33**:551-7.

1287. Chai, J. Y., E. T. Han, E. H. Shin, J. H. Park, J. P. Chu, M. Hirota, F. Nakamura-Uchiyama, and Y. Nawa. 2003. An outbreak of gnathostomiasis among Korean emigrants in Myanmar. *Am J Trop Med Hyg* **69**:67-73.

1288. Chai, J. Y., and S. H. Lee. 2002. Food-borne intestinal trematode infections in the Republic of Korea. *Parasitol Int* **51**:129-54.

1289. Chai, J. Y., J. H. Park, E. T. Han, E. H. Shin, J. L. Kim, S. M. Guk, K. S. Hong, S. H. Lee, and H. J. Rim. 2004. Prevalence of Heterophyes nocens and Pygydiopsis summa infections among residents of the western and southern coastal islands of the Republic of Korea. *Am J Trop Med Hyg* **71**:617-22.

1290. Chakrabarty, A. N., and S. G. Dastidar. 2001. Is soil an alternative source of leprosy infection? *Acta Leprol* **12**:79-84.

1291. Chakraborty, R., M. Iturriza-Gomara, R. Musoke, T. Palakudy, A. D'Agostino, and J. Gray. 2004. An epidemic of enterovirus 71 infection among HIV-1-infected orphans in Nairobi. *AIDS* **18**:1968-70.

1292. Challacombe, S. J., and L. L. Fernandes. 1995. Detecting Legionella pneumophila in water systems: a comparison of various dental units. *J Am Dent Assoc* **126**:603-8.

1293. Chalmers, R. M., S. M. Parry, R. L. Salmon, R. M. Smith, G. A. Willshaw, and T. Cheasty. 1999. The surveillance of vero cytotoxin-producing Escherichia coli O157 in Wales, 1990 to 1998. *Emerg Infect Dis* **5**:566-9.

1294. Chalmers, R. M., R. L. Salmon, G. A. Willshaw, T. Cheasty, N. Looker, I. Davies, and C. Wray. 1997. Vero-cytotoxin-producing Escherichia coli O157 in a farmer handling horses. *Lancet* **349**:1816.

1295. Chaloner, J. H., and L. P. Ormerod. 2002. Assessment of the impact of BCG vaccination on tuberculosis incidence in South Asian adult immigrants. *Commun Dis Public Health* **5**:338-40.

1296. Chamany, S., S. A. Mirza, J. W. Fleming, J. F. Howell, W. S. Lenhart, V. D. Mortimer, M. A. Phelan, M. D. Lindsley, N. J. Iqbal, L. J. Wheat, M. E. Brandt, D. W. Warnock, and R. A. Hajjeh. 2004. A large histoplasmosis outbreak among high school students in Indiana, 2001. *Pediatr Infect Dis J* **23**:909-14.

1297. Chamberland, M. E., H. J. Alter, M. P. Busch, G. Nemo, and M. Ricketts. 2001. Emerging infectious disease issues in blood safety. *Emerg Infect Dis* **7**(3:552-3.

1298. Chamberland, M. E., L. J. Conley, T. J. Bush, C. A. Ciesielski, T. A. Hammett, and H. W. Jaffe. 1991. Health care workers with AIDS. National surveillance update. *JAMA* **266**:3459-62.

1299. Chamberlin, J., L. Laughlin, S. Gordon, S. Romero, N. Solorzano, and R. L. Regnery. 2000. Serodiagnosis of Bartonella bacilliformis infection by indirect fluorescence antibody assay: test development and application to a population in an area of bartonellosis endemicity. *J Clin Microbiol* **38**:4269-71.

1300. Chamot, E., P. Chatelanat, L. Humair, A. Aeschlimann, and J. Bowessidjaou. 1987. Cinq cas de fièvre boutonneuse méditerranéenne en Suisse. *Ann Parasitol Hum Comp* **62**:371-9.

1301. Champion, J. K., A. Taylor, S. Hutchinson, S. Cameron, J. McMenamin, A. Mitchell, and D. Goldberg. 2004. Incidence of Hepatitis C Virus Infection and Associated Risk Factors among Scottish Prison Inmates: A Cohort Study. *Am J Epidemiol* **159**:514-9.

1302. Champsaur, H., E. Questiaux, J. Prevot, M. Henry-Amar, D. Goldszmidt, M. Bourjouane, and C. Bach. 1984. Rotavirus carriage, asymptomatic infection, and disease in the first two years of life. I. Virus shedding. *J Infect Dis* **149**:667-74.

1303. Chan, C. W., A. K. Chiang, K. H. Chan, and A. S. Lau. 2003. Epstein-Barr virus-associated infectious mononucleosis in Chinese children. *Pediatr Infect Dis J* **22**:974-8.

1304. Chan, E. S., J. Aramini, B. Ciebin, D. Middleton, R. Ahmed, M. Howes, I. Brophy, I. Mentis, F. Jamieson, F. Rodgers, M. Nazarowec-White, S. C. Pichette, J. Farrar, M. Gutierrez, W. J. Weis, L. Lior, A. Ellis, and S. Isaacs. 2002. Natural or raw almonds and an outbreak of a rare phage type of Salmonella enteritidis infection. *Can Commun Dis Rep* **28**:97-9.

1305. Chan, J., C. Baxter, and W. M. Wenman. 1989. Brucellosis in an inuit child, probably related to caribou meat consumption. *Scand J Infect Dis* **21**:337-8.

1306. Chan, K. H., K. S. Mann, and W. H. Seto. 1991. Infection of a shunt by Mycobacterium fortuitum: case report. *Neurosurgery* **29**:472-4.

1307. Chan, K. P., K. T. Goh, C. Y. Chong, E. S. Teo, G. Lau, and A. E. Ling. 2003. Epidemic hand, foot and mouth disease caused by human enterovirus 71, Singapore. *Emerg Infect Dis* **9**:78-85.

1308. Chan, P. K. S., W. K. To, K. C. Ng, R. K. Y. Lam, T. K. Ng, R. C. W. Chan, a. Wu, W. C. Yu, N. Lee, D. S. Hui, S. T. Lai, E. K. L. Hon, J. J. Y. Sung, and J. S. Tam. 2004. Laboratory diagnosis of SARS. *Emerg Infect Dis* **10**:825-31.

1309. Chan, P. W., L. C. Lum, Y. F. Ngeow, and M. Y. Yasim. 2001. Mycoplasma Pneumoniae infection in Malaysian children admitted with community acquired pneumonia. *Southeast Asian J Trop Med Public Health* **32**:397-401.

1310. Chandler, B., M. Beller, S. Jenkerson, J. Middaugh, C. Roberts, E. Reisdorf, M. Rausch, R. E. Savage, and J. Davis. 2000. Outbreaks of Norwalk-like viral gastroenteritis - Alaska and Wisconsin, 1999. *MMWR* **49**:207-211.

1311. Chandler, L. J., R. Parsons, and Y. Randle. 2001. Multiple genotypes of St. Louis encephalitis virus (Flaviviridae: Flavivirus) circulate in Harris county, Texas. *Am J Trop Med Hyg* **64**:12-9.

1312. Chandra Shekhar, K., and R. Pathmanathan. 1987. Schistosomiasis in Malaysia. *Rev Infect Dis* **9**:1026-37.

1313. Chandrasekaran, S., M. Mallika, and V. V. Pankajalakshmi. 1995. Studies on the incidence of leptospirosis and possible transmission of Leptospira during leptospiraemia. *Indian J Pathol Microbiol* **38**:133-7.

1314. Chandre, F., F. Darriet, M. Darder, A. Cuany, J. M. Doannio, N. Pasteur, and P. Guillet. 1998. Pyrethroid resistance in Culex quinquefasciatus from west Africa. *Med Vet Entomol* **12**:359-66.

1315. Chang, C. C., B. B. Chomel, R. W. Kasten, R. M. Heller, H. Ueno, K. Yamamoto, V. C. Bleich, B. M. Pierce, B. J. Gonzales, P. K. Swift, W. M. Boyce, S. S. Jang, H. J. Boulouis, Y. Piemont, G. M. Rossolini, M. L. Riccio, G. Cornaglia, L. Pagani, C. Lagatolla, L. Selan, and R. Fontana. 2000. Bartonella spp. isolated from wild and domestic ruminants in North America. *Emerg Infect Dis* **6**:306-11.

1316. Chang, C. C., B. B. Chomel, R. W. Kasten, V. Romano, and N. Tietze. 2001. Molecular evidence of Bartonella spp. in questing adult Ixodes pacificus ticks in California. *J Clin Microbiol* **39**:1221-6.

1317. Chang, C. L., D. S. Kim, D. J. Park, H. J. Kim, C. H. Lee, and J. H. Shin. 2000. Acute cerebral phaeohyphomycosis due to Wangiella dermatitidis accompanied by cerebrospinal fluid eosinophilia. *J Clin Microbiol* **38**:1965-6.

1318. Chang, H. C., M. W. Yu, C. F. Lu, Y. H. Chiu, and C. J. Chen. 2001. Risk factors associated with hepatitis C virus infection in Taiwanese government employees. *Epidemiol Infect* **126**:291-9.

1319. Chang, H. G., M. Eidson, C. Noonan-Toly, C. V. Trimarchi, R. Rudd, B. J. Wallace, P. F. Smith, and D. L. Morse. 2002. Public health impact of reemergence of rabies, New York. *Emerg Infect Dis* **8**:909-13.

1320. Chang, H. J., H. L. Miller, N. Watkins, M. J. Arduino, D. A. Ashford, G. Midgley, S. M. Aguero, R. Pinto-Powell, C. F. von Reyn, W. Edwards, M. M. McNeil, and W. R. Jarvis. 1998. An epidemic of Malassezia pachydermatis in an intensive care nursery associated with colonization of health care workers' pet dogs. *N Engl J Med* **338**:706-11.

1321. Chang, J., R. Powles, J. Mehta, N. Paton, J. Treleaven, and B. Jameson. 1995. Listeriosis in bone marrow transplant recipients: incidence, clinical features, and treatment. *Clin Infect Dis* **21**:1289-90.

1322. Chang, L. Y., C. C. King, K. H. Hsu, H. C. Ning, K. C. Tsao, C. C. Li, Y. C. Huang, S. R. Shih, S. T. Chiou, P. Y. Chen, H. J. Chang, and T. Y. Lin. 2002. Risk factors of enterovirus 71 infection and associated hand, foot, and mouth disease/herpangina in children during an epidemic in Taiwan. *Pediatrics* **109**:e88.

1323. Chang, L. Y., K. C. Tsao, S. H. Hsia, S. R. Shih, C. G. Huang, W. K. Chan, K. H. Hsu, T. Y. Fang, Y. C. Huang, and T. Y. Lin. 2004. Transmission and clinical features of enterovirus 71 infections in household contacts in Taiwan. *JAMA* **291**:222-7.

1324. Chang, Y.-F., J. E. McMahon, D. L. Hennon, R. E. LaPorte, and J. H. Coben. 1997. Dog bite incidence in the city of Pittsburgh: a capture-recapture approach. *Am J Public Health* **87**.

1325. Changsap, B., C. Nithikathkul, P. Boontan, S. Wannapinyosheep, N. Vongvanich, and C. Poister. 2002. Enterobiasis in primary schools in Bang Khun Thian District,

Bangkok, Thailand. *Southeast Asian J Trop Med Public Health* **33 Suppl 3**:72-5.

1326. **Chaniotis, B., G. Gozalo Garcia, and Y. Tselentis.** 1994. Leishmaniasis in greater Athens, Greece. Entomological studies. *Ann Trop Med Parasitol* **88**:659-63.

1327. **Chantal, J., M. H. Bessiere, B. Le Guenno, J. F. Magnaval, and P. Dorchies.** 1996. [Serologic screening of certain zoonoses in the abattoir personnel in Djibouti]. *Bull Soc Pathol Exot* **89**:353-7.

1328. **Chanteau, S., L. Ratsifasoamanana, B. Rasoamanana, L. Rahalison, J. Randriambelosoa, J. Roux, and D. Rabeson.** 1998. Plague, a reemerging disease in Madagascar. *Emerg Infect Dis* **4**:101-4.

1329. **Chao, H. J., D. K. Milton, J. Schwartz, and H. A. Burge.** 2002. Dustborne fungi in large office buildings. *Mycopathologia* **154**:93-106.

1330. **Chaoprasong, C., N. Chanthadisai, U. Buasap, S. Tirawatnapong, and A. Wattanathum.** 2002. Mycoplasma pneumoniae community-acquired pneumonia at three hospitals in Bangkok. *J Med Assoc Thai* **85**:643-7.

1331. **Chaowagul, W., Y. Suputtamongkol, D. A. B. Dance, A. Rajchanuvong, J. Pattara-arechachai, and N. J. White.** 1993. Relapse in melioidosis: incidence and risk factors. *J Infect Dis* **168**:1181-5.

1332. **Chaparro, C., J. Maurer, C. Gutierrez, M. Krajden, C. Chan, T. Winton, S. Keshavjee, M. Scavuzzo, E. Tullis, M. Hutcheon, and S. Kesten.** 2001. Infection with Burkholderia cepacia in cystic fibrosis: outcome following lung transplantation. *Am J Respir Crit Care Med* **163**:43-8.

1333. **Chapman, L. E., M. L. Wilson, D. B. Hall, B. LeGuenno, E. A. Dykstra, K. Ba, and S. P. Fisher-Hoch.** 1991. Risk factors for Crimean-Congo hemorrhagic fever in rural northern Senegal. *J Infect Dis* **164**:686-92.

1334. **Chapman, P. A., c. A. Siddons, A. T. Cerdan Malo, and M. A. Harkin.** 1997. A 1-year study of Escherichia coli O157 in cattle, sheep, pigs and poultry. *Epidemiol Infect* **119**:245-50.

1335. **Chapman, P. A., C. A. Siddons, A. T. Cerdan Malo, and M. A. Harkin.** 2000. A one year study of Escherichia coli O157 in raw beef and lamb products. *Epidemiol Infect* **124**:207-13.

1336. **Chapman, P. J. C., P. R. Wilkinson, and R. N. Davidson.** 1988. Acute schistosomiasis (Katayama fever) among British air crew. *BMJ* **297**:1101.

1337. **Chappuis, F., E. Stivanello, K. Adams, S. Kidane, A. Pittet, and P. A. Bovier.** 2004. Card agglutination test for trypanosomiasis (CATT) end-dilution titer and cerebrospinal fluid cell count as predictors of human African Trypanosomiasis (Trypanosoma brucei gambiense) among serologically suspected individuals in southern Sudan. *Am J Trop Med Hyg* **71**:313-7.

1338. **Chareonsook, O., H. M. Foy, A. Teeratkul, and N. Silarug.** 1999. Changing epidemiology of dengue hemorrhagic fever in Thailand. *Epidemiol Infect* **122**:161-6.

1339. **Chareonviriyaphap, T., M. J. Bangs, and S. Ratanatham.** 2000. Status of malaria in Thailand. *Southeast Asian J Trop Med Public Health* **31**:225-37.

1340. **Chareonviriyaphap, T., A. Prabaripai, M. J. Bangs, and B. Aum-Aung.** 2003. Seasonal abundance and blood feeding activity of Anopheles minimus Theobald (Diptera: Culicidae) in Thailand. *J Med Entomol* **40**:876-81.

1341. **Chariyalertsak, S., P. Vanittanakom, K. E. Nelson, T. Sirisanthana, and N. Vanittanakom.** 1996. Rhizomys sumatrensis and Cannomys badius, new natural animal hosts of Penicillium marneffei. *J Med Vet Mycol* **34**:105-10.

1342. **Charlebois, E. D., D. R. Bangsberg, N. J. Moss, M. R. Moore, A. R. Moss, H. F. Chambers, and F. Perdreau-Remington.** 2002. Population-based community prevalence of methicillin-resistant Staphylococcus aureus in the urban poor of San Francisco. *Clin Infect Dis* **34**:425-33.

1343. **Charles, P. E., H. Zeller, B. Bonnotte, A. L. Decasimacker, J. B. Bour, P. Chavanet, and B. Lorcerie.** 2003. Imported West Nile virus infection in Europe. *Emerg Infect Dis* **9**:750.

1344. **Charles, P. G., P. W. Angus, J. J. Sasadeusz, and M. L. Grayson.** 2003. Management of healthcare workers after occupational exposure to hepatitis C virus. *Med J Aust* **179**:153-7.

1345. **Charles, P. G., J. Leydon, K. A. O'Grady, and B. R. Speed.** 2001. A case of Kunjin virus encephalitis in a traveller returning from the Northern Territory. *Commun Dis Intell* **25**:155-7.

1346. **Charlwood, J. D., J. Pinto, P. R. Ferrara, C. A. Sousa, C. Ferreira, V. Gil, and V. E. Do Rosario.** 2003. Raised houses reduce mosquito bites. *Malar J* **2**:45.

1347. **Charrel, R. N., H. Attoui, A. M. Butenko, J. C. Clegg, V. Deubel, T. V. Frolova, E. A. Gould, T. S. Gritsun, F. X. Heinz, M. Labuda, V. A. Lashkevich, V. Loktev, A. Lundkvist, D. V. Lvov, C. W. Mandl, M. Niedrig, A. Papa, V. S. Petrov, A. Plyusnin, S. Randolph, J. Suss, V. I. Zlobin, and X. de Lamballerie.** 2004. Tick-borne virus diseases of human interest in Europe. *Clin Microbiol Infect* **10**:1040-55.

1348. **Charrel, R. N., and X. De Lamballerie.** 2003. Le virus Alkhurma (famille Flaviviridae, genre Flavivirus): un pathogène émergent responsable de fièvres hémorrhagiques au Moyen-Orient. *Med Trop* **63**:296-9.

1349. **Chastre, J., and J. L. Trouillet.** 1995. Early infective endocarditis on prosthetic valves. *Eur Heart J* **16 Suppl B**:32-8.

1350. **Chatel, G., M. Gulletta, A. Matteelli, A. Marangoni, L. Signorini, O. Oladeji, and S. Caligaris.** 1999. Short report: Diagnosis of tick-borne relapsing fever by the quantitative buffy coat fluorescence method. *Am J Trop Med Hyg* **60**:738-9.

1351. **Chatel, G., M. Gulletta, C. Scolari, E. Bombana, I. El-Hamad, A. Matteelli, and G. Carosi.** 1999. Short report: neurocysticercosis in an Italian traveler to Latin America. *Am J Trop Med Hyg* **60**:255-6.

1352. **Chattopadhyay, U. K., S. Dutta, A. Deb, and D. Pal.** 2001. Verotoxin-producing Escherichia coli—an environment-induced emerging zoonosis in and around Calcutta. *Int J Environ Health Res* **11**:107-12.

1353. **Chaturvedi, U. C., A. Mathur, A. Chandra, S. K. Das, H. O. Tandon, and U. K. Singh.** 1980. Transplacental infection with Japanese encephalitis virus. *J Infect Dis* **141**:712-5.

1354. **Chaturvedi, V., R. Ramani, S. Gromadzki, B. Rodeghier, H. G. Chang, and D. L. Morse.** 2000. Coccidioidomycosis in New York State. *Emerg Infect Dis* **6**:25-9.

1355. **Chau, T. T., N. T. Mai, N. H. Phu, C. Luxemburger, L. V. Chuong, P. P. Loc, T. T. Trang, H. Vinh, B. M. Cuong, D. J. Waller, D. X. Sinh, N. P. Day, T. T. Hien, and N. J. White.** 2002. Malaria in injection drug abusers in Vietnam. *Clin Infect Dis* **34**:1317-22.

1356. **Chaudhuri, A. K., G. Cassie, and M. Silver.** 1975. Outbreak of food-borne type-A hepatitis in Greater Glasgow. *Lancet* **2**:223-5.

1357. Chauve, C. M. 1997. Importance in France of the infestation by Dirofilaria (Nochtiella) repens in dogs. *Parassitologia* **39:**393-5.

1358. Chavasse, D. C., R. P. Shier, O. A. Murphy, S. R. Huttly, S. N. Cousens, and T. Akhtar. 1999. Impact of fly control on childhood diarrhoea in Pakistan: community-randomised trial. *Lancet* **353:**22-5.

1359. Chaves, F., F. Dronda, M. D. Cave, M. Alonso-Sanz, A. Gonzalez-Lopez, K. D. Eisenach, A. Ortega, L. Lopez-Cubero, I. Fernandez-Martin, S. Catalan, and J. H. Bates. 1997. A longitudinal study of transmission of tuberculosis in a large prison population. *Am J Respir Crit Care Med* **155:**719-25.

1360. Cheek, J. E., R. Baron, H. Atlas, D. L. Wilson, and R. D. Crider, Jr. 1995. Mumps outbreak in a highly vaccinated school population. Evidence for large-scale vaccination failure. *Arch Pediatr Adolesc Med* **149:**774-8.

1361. Cheek, J. E., P. Young, L. Branch, K. M. Dupnik, S. T. Kelly, J. M. Sharp, D. M. Toney, J. S. Breese, R. S. Beard, and S. Bulens. 2002. Norwalk-like virus-associated gastroenteritis in a large, high-density encampment - Virginia, July 2001. *MMWR* **51:**661-3.

1362. Cheesbrough, J. S., J. Green, C. I. Gallimore, P. A. Wright, and D. W. Brown. 2000. Widespread environmental contamination with Norwalk-like viruses (NLV) detected in a prolonged hotel outbreak of gastroenteritis. *Epidemiol Infect* **125:**93-8.

1363. Chen, G. G. 1985. [Epidemiologic survey of malaria at Wei-xi County in Yunnan Province]. *Zhonghua Liu Xing Bing Xue Za Zhi* **6:**208-10.

1364. Chen, H. I., K. Hulten, and J. E. Clarridge, 3rd. 2002. Taxonomic subgroups of Pasteurella multocida correlate with clinical presentation. *J Clin Microbiol* **40:**3438-41.

1365. Chen, K. T., C. J. Chen, and J. P. Chiu. 2001. A school waterborne outbreak involving both Shigella sonnei and Entamoeba histolytica. *J Environ Health* **64:**9-13, 26.

1366. Chen, L. H., and M. E. Wilson. 2005. Nosocomial dengue by mucocutaneous transmission. *Emerg Infect Dis* **11:**775.

1367. Chen, M., M. Y. Fan, D. Z. Bi, J. Z. Zhang, and Y. P. Huang. 1998. Detection of Rickettsia sibirica in ticks and small mammals collected in three different regions of China. *Acta Virol* **42:**61-4.

1368. Chen, M., Y. Lu, X. Hua, and K. E. Mott. 1994. Progress in assessment of morbidity due to Clonorchis sinensis infection: a review of recent literature. *Trop Dis Bull* **91:**R7-R65.

1369. Chen, X.-M., J. S. Keithly, C. V. Paya, and N. F. LaRusso. 2002. Cryptosporidiosis. *N Engl J Med* **346:**1723-31.

1370. Chen, Y. S., W. R. Lin, Y. C. Liu, C. L. Chang, V. L. Gan, W. K. Huang, T. S. Huang, S. R. Wann, H. H. Lin, S. S. Lee, C. K. Huang, C. Chin, Y. S. Lin, and M. Y. Yen. 2002. Residential water supply as a likely cause of community-acquired Legionnaires' disease in an immunocompromised host. *Eur J Clin Microbiol Infect Dis* **21:**706-9.

1371. Cheng, A. C., J. N. Hanna, R. Norton, S. L. Hills, J. Davis, V. L. Krause, G. Dowse, T. J. Inglis, and B. J. Currie. 2003. Melioidosis in northern Australia, 2001-02. *Commun Dis Intell* **27:**272-7.

1372. Cheng, H. S., and Y. H. Shieh. 2000. Investigation on subclinical aspects related to intestinal parasitic infections among Thai laborers in Taipei. *J Travel Med* **7:**319-24.

1373. Cheng, H. S., and L. C. Wang. 1999. Amoebiasis among institutionalized psychiatric patients in Taiwan. *Epidemiol Infect* **122:**317-22.

1374. Cheng Immergluck, L., S. Kanungo, A. Schwartz, A. McIntyre, P. C. Schreckenberger, and P. S. Diaz. 2004. Prevalence of Streptococcus pneumoniae and Staphylococcus aureus nasopharyngeal colonization in healthy children in the United States. *Epidemiol Infect* **132:**159-66.

1375. Cheng, P. K., D. A. Wong, L. K. Tong, S. M. Ip, A. C. Lo, C. S. Lau, E. Y. Yeung, and W. W. Lim. 2004. Viral shedding patterns of coronavirus in patients with probable severe acute respiratory syndrome. *Lancet* **363:**1699-700.

1376. Cherian, T., M. C. Steinhoff, L. H. Harrison, D. Rohn, L. K. McDougal, and J. Dick. 1994. A cluster of invasive pneumococcal disease in young children in child care. *JAMA* **271:**695-7.

1377. Chernin, E. 1989. Richard Pearson Strong and the iatrogenic plague disaster in Bilbid prison, Manila, 1906. *Rev Infect Dis* **11:**996-1004.

1378. Cheshier, R., E. Tu, and C. Glaser. 2003. Outbreaks of aseptic meningitis associated with echoviruses 9 and 30 and preliminary surveillance reports on enterovirus activity - United States, 2003. *MMWR* **52:**761-4.

1379. Cheung, Y. F., C. F. Chan, C. W. Lee, and Y. L. Lau. 1994. An outbreak of Pneumocystis carinii pneumonia in children with malignancy. *J Paediatr Child Health* **30:**173-5.

1380. Chhotray, G. P., B. B. Pal, H. K. Khuntia, N. R. Chowdhury, S. Chakraborty, S. Yamasaki, T. Ramamurthy, Y. Takeda, S. K. Bhattacharya, and G. B. Nair. 2002. Incidence and molecular analysis of Vibrio cholerae associated with cholera outbreak subsequent to the super cyclone in Orissa, India. *Epidemiol Infect* **128:**131-8.

1381. Chiari Cde, A., and D. P. Neves. 1984. [Human toxoplasmosis acquired by ingestion of goat's milk]. *Mem Inst Oswaldo Cruz* **79:**337-40.

1382. Chibo, D., M. A. Riddell, M. G. Catton, and C. J. Birch. 2005. Applicability of oral fluid collected onto filter paper for detection and genetic characterization of measles virus strains. *J Clin Microbiol* **43:**3145-9.

1383. Chichino, G., A. M. Bernuzzi, A. Bruno, C. Cevini, C. Atzori, A. Malfitano, and M. Scaglia. 1992. Intestinal capillariasis (Capillaria philippensis) acquired in Indonesia: a case report. *Am J Trop Med Hyg* **47:**10-2.

1384. Chien, N. T., G. Dundoo, M. H. Horani, P. Osmack, J. H. Morley, and A. M. Di Bisceglie. 1999. Seroprevalence of viral hepatitis in an older nursing home population. *J Am Geriatr Soc* **47:**1110-3.

1385. Chikhi-Brachet, R., F. Bon, L. Toubiana, P. Pothier, J. C. Nicolas, A. Flahault, and E. Kohli. 2002. Virus diversity in a winter epidemic of acute diarrhea in France. *J Clin Microbiol* **40:**4266-72.

1386. Childs, J. E., G. E. Glass, G. W. Korch, T. G. Ksiazek, and J. W. Leduc. 1992. Lymphocytic choriomeningitis virus infection and house mouse (Mus musculus) distribution in urban Baltimore. *Am J Trop Med Hyg* **47:**27-34.

1387. Childs, J. E., G. E. Glass, T. G. Ksiazek, C. A. Rossi, J. G. Oro, and J. W. Leduc. 1991. Human-rodent contact and infection with lymphocytic choriomeningitis and Seoul viruses in an inner-city population. *Am J Trop Med Hyg* **44:**117-21.

1388. Childs, J. E., J. W. Krebs, T. G. Ksiazek, G. O. Maupin, K. L. Gage, P. E. Rollin, P. S. Zeitz, J. Sarisky, R. E. Enscore, J. C. Butler, et al. 1995. A household-based, case-control study of environmental factors associated with hantavirus pulmonary syndrome in the southwestern United States. *Am J Trop Med Hyg* **52:**393-7.

1389. **Chimbari, M. J., E. Chirebvu, and B. Ndlela.** 2004. Malaria and schistosomiasis risks associated with surface and sprinkler irrigation systems in Zimbabwe. *Acta Trop* **89:**205-13.

1390. **Chin, C., T. S. Chiueh, W. C. Yang, T. H. Yang, C. M. Shih, H. T. Lin, K. C. Lin, J. C. Lien, T. F. Tsai, S. L. Ruo, S. T. Nichol, T. G. Ksiazek, P. E. Rollin, C. J. Peters, T. N. Wu, and C. Y. Shen.** 2000. Hantavirus infection in Taiwan: the experience of a geographically unique area. *J Med Virol* **60:**237-47.

1391. **Chin-Hong, P. V., E. Vittinghoff, R. D. Cranston, S. Buchbinder, D. Cohen, G. Colfax, M. Da Costa, T. Darragh, E. Hess, F. Judson, B. Koblin, M. Madison, and J. M. Palefsky.** 2004. Age-Specific prevalence of anal human papillomavirus infection in HIV-negative sexually active men who have sex with men: the EXPLORE study. *J Infect Dis* **190:**2070-6.

1392. **Chinai, R.** 2002. Mumbai slum dwellers' sewage project goes nationwide. *Bull WHO* **80:**684-5.

1393. **Chinchilla, M., E. Castro, M. Alfaro, and E. Portilla.** 1979. [Free living amebae that can cause meningoencephalitis. Ist findings in Costa Rica]. *Rev Latinoam Microbiol* **21:**135-42.

1394. **Ching, H. L.** 1984. Fish tapeworm infections (diphyllobothriasis) in Canada, particularly British Columbia. *Can Med Assoc J* **130:**1125-7.

1395. **Chiou, C. S., W. B. Hsu, H. L. Wei, and J. H. Chen.** 2001. Molecular epidemiology of a Shigella flexneri outbreak in a mountainous township in Taiwan, Republic of China. *J Clin Microbiol* **39:**1048-56.

1396. **Chippaux, J. P., B. Bouchité, M. Boussinesq, S. Ranque, T. Baldet, and M. Demanou.** 1998. Impact of repeated large scale ivermectin treatments on the transmission of Loa loa. *Trans R Soc Trop Med Hyg* **92:**454-8.

1397. **Chirico, J., H. Eriksson, O. Fossum, and D. Jansson.** 2003. The poultry red mite, Dermanyssus gallinae, a potential vector of Erysipelothrix rhusiopathiae causing erysipelas in hens. *Med Vet Entomol* **17:**232-4.

1398. **Chironna, M., C. Germinario, D. De Medici, A. Fiore, S. Di Pasquale, M. Quarto, and S. Barbuti.** 2002. Detection of hepatitis A virus in mussels from different sources marketed in Puglia region (South Italy). *Int J Food Microbiol* **75:**11-8.

1399. **Chironna, M., C. Germinario, P. L. Lopalco, F. Carrozzini, S. Barbuti, and M. Quarto.** 2003. Immunity to diphtheria among refugees in southern Italy. *Vaccine* **21:**3157-61.

1400. **Chironna, M., C. Germinario, P. L. Lopalco, F. Carrozzini, S. Barbuti, and M. Quarto.** 2003. Prevalence rates of viral hepatitis infections in refugee Kurds from Iraq and Turkey. *Infection* **31:**70-4.

1401. **Chironna, M., C. Germinario, P. L. Lopalco, M. Quarto, and S. Barbuti.** 2000. HBV, HCV and HDV infections in Albanian refugees in Southern Italy (Apulia region). *Epidemiol Infect* **125:**163-7.

1402. **Chironna, M., P. Lopalco, R. Prato, C. Germinario, S. Barbuti, and M. Quarto.** 2004. Outbreak of infection with hepatitis A virus (HAV) associated with a foodhandler and confirmed by sequence analysis reveals a new HAV genotype IB variant. *J Clin Microbiol* **42:**2825-8.

1403. **Chirurgi, V. A., S. E. Oster, A. A. Goldberg, and R. E. McCabe.** 1992. Nosocomial acquisition of beta-lactamase—negative, ampicillin- resistant enterococcus. *Arch Intern Med* **152:**1457-61.

1404. **Chisolm, S., R. L. Cohen, J. Cortesi, Z. Fabrizi, E. Leskovac, P. A. Thomas, S. Schultz, J. A. McDonald, J. D. Farris, P. F. King, J. Brough, D. K. Heydinger, B. D'Amond, M. Fenstersheib, C. Fazekas, M. J. Wilson, L. G. Dales, and J. Chin.** 1985. Rubella outbreaks in prisons - New York city, West Virginia, California. *MMWR* **34:**615-8.

1405. **Chiu, C. H., T. L. Wu, L. H. Su, C. Chu, J. H. Chia, A. J. Kuo, M. S. Chien, and T. Y. Lin.** 2002. The emergence in Taiwan of fluoroquinolone resistance in Salmonella enterica serotype choleraesuis. *N Engl J Med* **346:**413-9.

1406. **Chlibek, R., J. Jirous, and J. Beran.** 2002. Diarrhea outbreak among Czech army field hospital personnel caused by Providencia alcalifaciens. *J Travel Med* **9:**151-2.

1407. **Chmielewska-Badora, J.** 1998. Seroepidemiologic study on Lyme borreliosis in the Lublin region. *Ann Agric Environ Med* **5:**183-6.

1408. **Cho, S. Y., Y. Kong, and S. Y. Kang.** 1997. Epidemiology of paragonimiasis in Korea. *Southeast Asian J Trop Med Public Health* **28 (suppl 1):**32-6.

1409. **Chobot, S., J. Malis, H. Sebakova, M. Pelikan, O. Zatloukal, P. Palicka, and D. Kocurova.** 1997. Endemic incidence of infections caused by Mycobacterium kansasii in the Karvina district in 1968-1995 (analysis of epidemiological data—review). *Cent Eur J Public Health* **5:**164-73.

1410. **Choi, D. W.** 1984. Clonorchis sinensis: life cycle, intermediate hosts, transmission to man and geographical distribution in Korea. *Arzneim-Forsch / Drug Res* **34:**1145-51.

1411. **Choi, K. H., H. Liu, Y. Guo, L. Han, J. S. Mandel, and G. W. Rutherford.** 2003. Emerging HIV-1 epidemic in China in men who have sex with men. *Lancet* **361:**2125-6.

1412. **Choi, W. Y., H. W. Nam, N. H. Kwak, W. Huh, Y. R. Kim, M. W. Kang, S. Y. Cho, and J. P. Dubey.** 1997. Foodborne outbreaks of human toxoplasmosis. *J Infect Dis* **175:**1280-2.

1413. **Chokephaibulkit, K., M. Uiprasertkul, P. Puthavathana, P. Chearskul, P. Auewarakul, S. F. Dowell, and N. Vanprapar.** 2005. A child with avian influenza A (H5N1) infection. *Pediatr Infect Dis J* **24:**162-6.

1414. **Chomel, B. B., R. C. Abbott, R. W. Kasten, K. A. Floyd-Hawkins, P. H. Kass, C. A. Glaser, N. C. Pedersen, and J. E. Koehler.** 1995. Bartonella henselae prevalence in domestic cats in California: risk factors and association between bacteremia and antibody titers. *J Clin Microbiol* **33:**2445-50.

1415. **Chomel, B. B., E. E. DeBess, D. M. Mangiamele, K. F. Reilly, T. B. Farver, R. K. Sun, and L. R. Barrett.** 1994. Changing trends in the epidemiology of human brucellosis in California from 1973 to 1992: a shift toward foodborne transmission. *J Infect Dis* **170:**1216-23.

1416. **Chongsuvivatwong, V., S. Pas-Ong, W. Ngoathammatasna, D. McNeil, K. Vithsupakorn, V. Bridhikitti, P. Jongsuksuntigul, and C. Jeradit.** 1994. Evaluation of hookworm control program in southern Thailand. *Southeast Asian J Trop Med Public Health* **25:**745-51.

1417. **Chosidow, O.** 2000. Scabies and pediculosis. *Lancet* **355**.

1418. **Chou, J. H., P. H. Hwang, and M. D. Malison.** 1988. An outbreak of type A foodborne botulism in Taiwan due to commercially preserved peanuts. *Int J Epidemiol* **17:**899-902.

1419. **Choudat, D., C. Le Goff, B. Delemotte, G. Paul, V. Mady, J. Fages, and F. Conso.** 1987. Occupational exposure to animals and antibodies against Pasteurella multocida. *Br J Ind Med* **44:**829-33.

1420. **Chow, T. K., J. R. Lambert, M. L. Wahlqvist, and B. H. Hsu-Hage.** 1995. Helicobacter pylori in Melbourne Chinese immigrants: evidence for oral- oral transmission via chopsticks. *J Gastroenterol Hepatol* **10**:562-9.

1421. **Choy, J. L., M. Mayo, A. Janmaat, and B. J. Currie.** 2000. Animal melioidosis in Australia. *Acta Trop* **74**:153-8.

1422. **Chretien, J. H., J. G. Esswein, M. A. McGarvey, and A. deStwolinski.** 1976. Rubella: pattern of outbreak in a university. *South Med J* **69**:1042-4.

1423. **Christensen, P. B., H. B. Krarup, H. G. Niesters, H. Norder, O. B. Schaffalitzky de Muckadell, B. Jeune, and J. Georgsen.** 2001. Outbreak of Hepatitis B among injecting drug users in Denmark. *J Clin Virol* **22**:133-41.

1424. **Christensen, S. E., R. C. Wolfmeyer, S. M. Suver, C. D. Hill, and S. F. F. Britton.** 2001. Influenza B virus outbreak on a cruise ship - northern Europe, 2000. *MMWR* **50**:137-40.

1425. **Christenson, B., M. Bottiger, A. Svensson, and S. Jeansson.** 1992. A 15-year surveillance study of antibodies to herpes simplex virus types 1 and 2 in a cohort of young girls. *J Infect* **25**:147-54.

1426. **Christenson, B., S. P. Sylvan, and B. Noreen.** 1997. Carriage of multiresistant Streptococcus pneumoniae among children attending day-care centres in the Stockholm area. *Scand J Infect Dis* **29**:555-8.

1427. **Christiaens, G., M. P. Hayette, D. Jacquemin, P. Melin, J. Mutsers, and P. De Mol.** 2005. An outbreak of Absidia corymbifera infection associated with bandage contamination in a burns unit. *J Hosp Infect* **61**:88.

1428. **Christian, P., S. K. Khatry, and K. P. West, Jr.** 2004. Antenatal anthelmintic treatment, birthweight, and infant survival in rural Nepal. *Lancet* **364**:981-3.

1429. **Christiann, F., P. Rayet, O. Patey, D. B. Ngueodjibaye, J. F. Theron-le Gargasson, and C. Lafaix.** 1997. Lyme borreliosis in central France: a sero-epidemiologic examination involving hunters. *Eur J Epidemiol* **13**:855.

1430. **Christiansen, K. J., P. A. Tibbett, W. Beresford, J. W. Pearman, R. C. Lee, G. W. Coombs, I. D. Kay, F. G. O'Brien, S. Palladino, C. R. Douglas, P. D. Montgomery, T. Orrell, A. M. Peterson, F. P. Kosaras, J. P. Flexman, C. H. Heath, and C. A. McCullough.** 2004. Eradication of a large outbreak of a single strain of vanB vancomycin-resistant Enterococcus faecium at a major Australian teaching hospital. *Infect Control Hosp Epidemiol* **25**:384-90.

1431. **Christie, B.** 2000. Gangrene bug "killed" 35 heroin users. *BMJ* **320**:1690.

1432. **Christie, C. D., K. M. Garrison, L. Kiely, R. K. Gupta, J. Heubi, and C. D. Marchant.** 2001. A trial of acellular pertussis vaccine in hospital workers during the Cincinnati pertussis epidemic of 1993. *Clin Infect Dis* **33**:997-1003.

1433. **Christie, C. D., A. M. Glover, M. J. Willke, M. L. Marx, S. F. Reising, and N. M. Hutchinson.** 1995. Containment of pertussis in the regional pediatric hospital during the Greater Cincinnati epidemic of 1993. *Infect Control Hosp Epidemiol* **16**:556-63.

1434. **Christie, C. D. C., M. L. Marx, J. A. Daniels, and M. P. Adcock.** 1997. Pertussis containment in schools and day care centers during the Cincinnati epidemic of 1993. *Am J Public Health* **87**:460-2.

1435. **Christmann, D., and T. Staub-Schmidt.** 1996. Encéphalite à tiques d'Europe centrale et de l'est. *Presse Med* **25**:420-3.

1436. **Christopher, F. L., M. J. Hepburn, and R. A. Frolichstein.** 2002. Pertussis in a military and military beneficiary population: case series and review of the literature. *Mil Med* **167**:215-8.

1437. **Christopher, G. W., M. B. Agan, T. J. Cieslak, and P. E. Olson.** 2005. History of U.S. military contributions to the study of bacterial zoonoses. *Mil Med* **170**:39-48.

1438. **Christopher, G. W., and E. M. Eitzen, Jr.** 1999. Air evacuation under high-level biosafety containment: the aeromedical isolation team. *Emerg Infect Dis* **5**:241-6.

1439. **Christova, I., J. Van De Pol, S. Yazar, E. Velo, and L. Schouls.** 2003. Identification of Borrelia burgdorferi sensu lato, Anaplasma and Ehrlichia species, and spotted fever group Rickettsiae in ticks from Southeastern Europe. *Eur J Clin Microbiol Infect Dis* **22**:535-42.

1440. **Chua, K. B., W. J. Bellini, P. A. Rota, B. H. Harcourt, A. Tamin, S. K. Lam, T. G. Ksiazek, P. E. Rollin, S. R. Zaki, W. Shieh, C. S. Goldsmith, D. J. Gubler, J. T. Roehrig, B. Eaton, A. R. Gould, J. Olson, H. Field, P. Daniels, A. E. Ling, C. J. Peters, L. J. Anderson, and B. W. Mahy.** 2000. Nipah virus: a recently emergent deadly paramyxovirus. *Science* **288**:1432-5.

1441. **Chua, S. H., and W. K. Cheong.** 1995. Genital ulcer disease in patients attending a public sexually transmitted disease clinic in Singapore: an epidemiologic study. *Ann Acad Med Singapore* **24**:510-4.

1442. **Chung, L. Y., B. H. Fang, J. H. Chang, S. M. Chye, and C. M. Yen.** 2004. The infectivity and antigenicity of Toxocara canis eggs can be retained after long-term preservation. *Ann Trop Med Parasitol* **98**:251-60.

1443. **Chung, W. C., K. C. Chang, and S. H. Horng.** 1978. Epidemiology of Enterobius vermicularis infection among orphans in orphanages in Taipei City. *Zhonghua Min Guo Wei Sheng Wu Xue Za Zhi* **11**:30-6.

1444. **Chung, Y. K., and F. Y. Pang.** 2002. Dengue virus infection rate in field populations of female Aedes aegypti and Aedes albopictus in Singapore. *Trop Med Int Health* **7**:322-30.

1445. **Chunge, R. N.** 1986. A study of head lice among primary schoolchildren in Kenya. *Trans R Soc Trop Med Hyg* **80**:42-6.

1446. **Church, R. E., and J. Knowelden.** 1978. Scabies in Sheffield: a family infestation. *Br Med J* **1**:761-3.

1447. **Churchill, D. R., C. Morris, A. Fakoya, S. G. Wright, and R. N. Davidson.** 1996. Clinical and laboratory features of patients with loiasis (Loa loa filariasis) in the U.K. *J Infect* **33**:103-9.

1448. **Ciccozzi, M., M. E. Tosti, G. Gallo, P. Ragni, C. Zotti, P. Lopalco, G. Ara, M. Sangalli, E. Balocchini, A. S. Szklo, and A. Mele.** 2002. Risk of hepatitis A infection following travel. *J Viral Hepat* **9**:460-5.

1449. **Ciceroni, L., A. Pinto, C. Rossi, C. Khoury, L. Rivosecchi, E. Stella, and B. Cacciapuoti.** 1988. Rickettsiae of the spotted fever group associated with the host-parasite system Oryctolagus cuniculi/Rhipicephalus pusillus. *Zentralbl Bakteriol Mikrobiol Hyg [A]* **269**:211-7.

1450. **Ciceroni, L., E. Stepan, A. Pinto, P. Pizzocaro, G. Dettori, L. Franzin, R. Lupidi, S. Mansueto, A. Manera, A. Ioli, L. Marcuccio, R. Grillo, S. Ciarrocchi, and M. Cinco.** 2000. Epidemiological trend of human leptospirosis in Italy between 1994 and 1996. *Eur J Epidemiol* **16**:79-86.

1451. **Ciesielski, C., D. Marianos, C. Y. Ou, R. Dumbaugh, J. Witte, R. Berkelman, B. Gooch, G. Myers, C. C. Luo, G. Schochetman, et al.** 1992. Transmission of human immunodeficiency virus in a dental practice. *Ann Intern Med* **116**:798-805.

1452. **Ciesielski, S., D. Esposito, J. Protiva, and M. Piehl.** 1994. The incidence of tuberculosis among North Carolina migrant farmworkers, 1991. *Am J Public Health* **84:**1836-8.

1453. **Ciesielski, S. D., J. R. Seed, J. C. Ortiz, and J. Metts.** 1992. Intestinal parasites among North Carolina migrant farmworkers. *Am J Public Health* **82:**1258-62.

1454. **Cieslak, P. R., T. J. Barrett, P. M. Griffin, K. F. Gensheimer, G. Beckett, J. Buffington, and M. G. Smith.** 1993. Escherichia coli O157:H7 infection from a manured garden. *Lancet* **342:**367.

1455. **Cieslak, P. R., S. J. Noble, D. J. Maxson, L. C. Empey, O. Ravenholt, G. Legarza, J. Tuttle, M. P. Doyle, T. J. Barrett, J. G. Wells, A. M. McNamara, and P. M. Griffin.** 1997. Hamburger-associated Escherichia coli O157:H7 infection in Las Vegas: a hidden epidemic. *Am J Public Health* **87:**176-80.

1456. **Cifuentes, E., M. Gomez, U. Blumenthal, M. M. Tellez-Rojo, I. Romieu, G. Ruiz-Palacios, and S. Ruiz-Velazco.** 2000. Risk factors for Giardia intestinalis infection in agricultural villages practicing wastewater irrigation in Mexico. *Am J Trop Med Hyg* **62:**388-92.

1457. **Cifuentes, E., L. Suarez, M. Espinosa, L. Juarez-Figueroa, and A. Martinez-Palomo.** 2004. Risk of Giardia Intestinalis infection in children from an artificially recharged groundwater area in Mexico City. *Am J Trop Med Hyg* **71:**65-70.

1458. **Cilla, G., E. Pérez-Trallero, C. Gutiérrez, C. Part, and M. Gomáriz.** 1996. Seroprevalence of Toxocara infection in a middle-class and disadvantaged children in northern Spain (Gipuzkoa, Basque country). *Eur J Epidemiol* **12:**541-3.

1459. **Cilla, G., E. Serrano-Bengoechea, A. Cosme, L. Abadia, and E. Perez-Trallero.** 2002. Decrease in human fascioliasis in Gipuzkoa (Spain). *Eur J Epidemiol* **17:**819-21.

1460. **Cinco, M., F. Barbone, M. Grazia Ciufolini, M. Mascioli, M. Anguero Rosenfeld, P. Stefanel, and R. Luzzati.** 2004. Seroprevalence of tick-borne infections in forestry rangers from northeastern Italy. *Clin Microbiol Infect* **10:**1056-61.

1461. **Cinpinski, D., B. Bibler, R. Kebabjian, R. Georgesen, P. Kishel, D. Finkenbinder, N. Bloomenrader, C. Otto, M. J. Beach, J. Roberts, L. Mirel, K. Day, and K. Bauer.** 2003. Surveillance data from swimming pool inspections - selected states and counties, United States, May-September 2002. *MMWR* **52:**513-6.

1462. **Cirioni, O., A. Giacometti, D. Drenaggi, F. Ancarani, and G. Scalise.** 1999. Prevalence and clinical relevance of Blastocystis hominis in diverse patient cohorts. *Eur J Epidemiol* **15:**389-93.

1463. **Cisak, E., J. Sroka, J. Zwolinski, and J. Uminski.** 1998. Seroepidemiologic study on tick-borne encephalitis among forestry workers and farmers from the Lublin region (eastern Poland). *Ann Agric Environ Med* **5:**177-81.

1464. **Cislakova, L., H. Prokopcakova, M. Stef'kovic, and M. Halanova.** 1997. [Encephalitozoon cuniculi—clinical and epidemiologic significance. Results of a preliminary serologic study in humans]. *Epidemiol Mikrobiol Imunol* **46:**30-3.

1465. **Cisneros-Castolo, M., L. Hernández-Ruiz, I. E. Ibarra-Robles, I. H. Fernández-Gárate, and J. Escobedo-De la Peña.** 2001. Prevalence of hepatitis B virus infection and related risk factors in a rural community of Mexico. *Am J Trop Med Hyg* **65:**759-63.

1466. **Citron, D. M., S. Hunt Gerardo, M. C. Claros, F. Abrahamian, D. Talan, and E. J. Goldstein.** 1996. Frequency of isolation of Porphyromonas species from infected dog and cat bite wounds in humans and their characterization by biochemical tests and arbitrarily primed-polymerase chain reaction fingerprinting. *Clin Infect Dis* **23 Suppl 1:**S78-82.

1467. **Claas, E. C., Y. Kawaoka, J. C. de Jong, N. Masurel, and R. G. Webster.** 1994. Infection of children with avian-human reassortant influenza virus from pigs in Europe. *Virology* **204:**453-7.

1468. **Claesson, B. E., N. G. Svensson, L. Gotthardsson, and B. Garden.** 1992. A foodborne outbreak of group A streptococcal disease at a birthday party. *Scand J Infect Dis* **24:**577-86.

1469. **Clark, C. G., and L. S. Diamond.** 1997. Intraspecific variation and phylogenetic relationships in the genus Entamoeba as revealed by ribotyping. *J Eukaryot Microbiol* **44:**142-54.

1470. **Clark, C. G., A. N. Kravetz, V. V. Alekseenko, D. Krendelev Yu, and W. M. Johnson.** 1998. Microbiological and epidemiological investigation of cholera epidemic in Ukraine during 1994 and 1995. *Epidemiol Infect* **121:**1-13.

1471. **Clark, K. L., P. W. Kelley, R. A. Mahmoud, M. B. Goldenbaum, G. S. Meyer, L. J. Fetters, and M. R. Howell.** 1999. Cost-effective syphilis screening in military recruit applicants. *Mil Med* **164:**580-4.

1472. **Clark, M., P. Riben, and E. Nowgesic.** 2002. The association of housing density, isolation and tuberculosis in Canadian first nations communities. *Int J Epidemiol* **31:**940-5.

1473. **Clark, T. A., S. A. Slavinski, J. Morgan, T. Lott, B. A. Arthington-Skaggs, M. E. Brandt, R. M. Webb, M. Currier, R. H. Flowers, S. K. Fridkin, and R. A. Hajjeh.** 2004. Epidemiologic and molecular characterization of an outbreak of Candida parapsilosis bloodstream infections in a community hospital. *J Clin Microbiol* **42:**4468-72.

1474. **Clasen, T. F., J. Brown, S. Collin, O. Suntura, and S. Cairncross.** 2004. Reducing Diarrhea through the Use of Household-Based Ceramic Water Filters: A Randomized, Controlled Trial in Rural Bolivia. *Am J Trop Med Hyg* **70:**651-657.

1475. **Clausen, M. R., C. N. Meyer, T. Krantz, C. Moser, G. Gomme, L. Kayser, J. Albrectsen, C. M. Kapel, and I. C. Bygbjerg.** 1996. Trichinella infection and clinical disease. *Q J Med* **89:**631-6.

1476. **Clayson, E. T., K. S. Myint, R. Snitbhan, D. W. Vaughn, B. L. Innis, L. Chan, P. Cheung, and M. P. Shrestha.** 1995. Viremia, fecal shedding, and IgM and IgG responses in patients with hepatitis E. *J Infect Dis* **172:**927-33.

1477. **Clayson, E. T., M. P. Shrestha, D. W. Vaughn, R. Snitbhan, K. B. Shrestha, C. F. Longer, and B. L. Innis.** 1997. Rates of hepatitis E virus infection and disease among adolescents and adults in Kathmandu, Nepal. *J Infect Dis* **176:**763-6.

1478. **Clayson, E. T., D. W. Vaughn, B. L. Innis, M. P. Shrestha, R. Pandey, and D. B. Malla.** 1998. Association of hepatitis E virus with an outbreak of hepatitis at a military training camp in Nepal. *J Med Virol* **54:**178-82.

1479. **Clegg, H. W., P. Bertagnoll, A. W. Hightower, and W. B. Baine.** 1983. Mammaplasty-associated mycobacterial infection: a survey of plastic surgeons. *Plast Reconstr Surg* **72:**165-9.

1480. **Clement, J., G. Neild, S. L. Hinrichsen, J. A. Crescente, and M. Van Ranst.** 1999. Urban leptospirosis versus urban hantavirus infection in Brazil. *Lancet* **354:**2003-4.

1481. **Clement, J., P. Underwood, D. Ward, J. Pilaski, and J. LeDuc.** 1996. Hantavirus outbreak during military manoeuvres in Germany. *Lancet* **347:**336.

1482. **Clements, C. J., and F. T. Cutts.** 1995. The epidemiology of measles: thirty years of vaccination, p. 13-33. *In* V. ter Meulen and M. A. Billeter (ed.), Measles virus. Springer Verlag, Berlin.

1483. **Clemett, R. S., R. A. Allardyce, H. J. E. Williamson, A. C. Stewart, and R. R. Hidajat.** 1987. Ocular toxocara canis infections: diagnosis by enzyme immunoassay. *Aust N Z J Ophthalmol* **15:**145-50.

1484. **Cliff, J. L., P. Zinkin, and A. Martelli.** 1986. A hospital outbreak of cholera in Maputo, Mozambique. *Trans R Soc Trop Med Hyg* **80:**473-6.

1485. **Coates, D.** 1976. Hygiene of crockery and cutlery from tuberculosis patients [letters]. *Lancet* **2:**633.

1486. **Cobben, N. A., M. Drent, M. Jonkers, E. F. Wouters, M. Vaneechoutte, and E. E. Stobberingh.** 1996. Outbreak of severe Pseudomonas aeruginosa respiratory infections due to contaminated nebulizers. *J Hosp Infect* **33:**63-70.

1487. **Cobelens, F. G., J. Groen, A. D. Osterhaus, A. Leentvaar-Kuipers, P. M. Wertheim-van Dillen, and P. A. Kager.** 2002. Incidence and risk factors of probable dengue virus infection among Dutch travellers to Asia. *Trop Med Int Health* **7:**331-8.

1488. **Cobelens, F. G., S. Kooij, A. Warris-Versteegen, and L. G. Visser.** 2000. Typhoid fever in group travelers: opportunity for studying vaccine efficacy. *J Travel Med* **7:**19-24.

1489. **Cobelens, F. G., H. van Deutekom, I. W. Draayer-Jansen, A. C. Schepp-Beelen, P. J. van Gerven, R. P. van Kessel, and M. E. Mensen.** 2000. Risk of infection with Mycobacterium tuberculosis in travellers to areas of high tuberculosis endemicity. *Lancet* **356:**461-5.

1490. **Cobelens, F. G. J., H. J. van Schothorst, P. M. E. Wertheim-Van Dillen, R. J. Ligtlhelm, I. S. Paul-Steenstra, and P. P. van Thiel.** 2004. Epidemiology of hepatitis B infection among expatriates in Nigeria. *Clin Infect Dis* **38:**370-6.

1491. **Coccia, M. E., F. Cammilli, L. Ginocchioni, and F. Rizzello.** 2004. Role of infection in in vitro fertilization treatment. *Ann N Y Acad Sci* **1034:**219-35.

1492. **Cocco, P. L., A. Caperna, and F. Vinci.** 2003. Occupational risk factors for the sporadic form of Creutzfeldt-Jakob disease. *Med Lav* **94:**353-63.

1493. **Cockerill, F. R., 3rd, K. L. MacDonald, R. L. Thompson, F. Roberson, P. C. Kohner, J. Besser-Wiek, J. M. Manahan, J. M. Musser, P. M. Schlievert, J. Talbot, B. Frankfort, J. M. Steckelberg, W. R. Wilson, and M. T. Osterholm.** 1997. An outbreak of invasive group A streptococcal disease associated with high carriage rates of the invasive clone among school-aged children. *JAMA* **277:**38-43.

1494. **Cody, S. H., S. L. Abbott, A. A. Marfin, B. Schulz, P. Wagner, K. Robbins, J. C. Mohle-Boetani, and D. J. Vugia.** 1999. Two outbreaks of multidrug-resistant Salmonella serotype typhimurium DT104 infections linked to raw-milk cheese in Northern California. *JAMA* **281:**1805-10.

1495. **Cody, S. H., M. K. Glynn, J. A. Farrar, K. L. Cairns, P. M. Griffin, J. Kobayashi, M. Fyfe, R. Hoffman, A. S. King, J. H. Lewis, B. Swaminathan, R. G. Bryant, and D. J. Vugia.** 1999. An outbreak of Escherichia coli O157:H7 infection from unpasteurized commercial apple juice. *Ann Intern Med* **130:**202-9.

1496. **Cody, S. H., O. V. Nainan, R. S. Garfein, H. Meyers, B. P. Bell, C. N. Shapiro, E. L. Meeks, H. Pitt, E. Mouzin, M. J. Alter, H. S. Margolis, and D. J. Vugia.** 2002. Hepatitis C virus transmission from an anesthesiologist to a patient. *Arch Intern Med* **162:**345-50.

1497. **Coelho, L. M., C. Y. Dini, M. H. Milman, and S. M. Oliveira.** 2001. Toxocara spp. eggs in public squares of Sorocaba, Sao Paulo State, Brazil. *Rev Inst Med Trop Sao Paulo* **43:**189-91.

1498. **Coello, R., J. Jiménez, M. García, P. Arroyo, D. Minguez, C. Fernandez, F. Cruzet, and C. Gaspar.** 1994. Prospective study of infection, colonization and carriage of methicillin-resistant Staphylococcus aureus in an outbreak affecting 990 patients. *Eur J Clin Microbiol Infect Dis* **13:**74-81.

1499. **Coenye, T., V. P., J. R. W. Govan, and J. J. Lipuma.** 2001. Minireview. Taxonomy and identification of the Burkholderia cepacia complex. *J Clin Microbiol* **39:**3427-36.

1500. **Coenye, T., T. Spilker, R. Reik, P. Vandamme, and J. J. Lipuma.** 2005. Use of PCR analyses to define the distribution of Ralstonia species recovered from patients with cystic fibrosis. *J Clin Microbiol* **43:**3463-6.

1501. **Coester, C. H., U. Bienzle, H. G. Hoffmann, E. Koehn, and I. Guggenmoos-Holzmann.** 1984. Syphilis, hepatitis A and hepatitis B seromarkers in homosexual men. *Klin Wochenschr* **62:**810-3.

1502. **Coetzee, N., D. Yach, R. Blignaut, and S. A. Fisher.** 1990. Measles vaccination coverage and its determinants in a rapidly growing peri-urban area. *S Afr Med J* **78:**733-7.

1503. **Cogo, P. E.** 2004. Fatal Naegleria fowleri meningoencephalitis, Italy. *Emerg Infect Dis* **10:**1835-7.

1504. **Cohen, B. J., L. Jin, D. W. G. Brown, and M. Kitson.** 1999. Infection with wild-type mumps virus in army recruits temporally associated with MMR vaccine. *Epidemiol Infect* **123:**251-5.

1505. **Cohen, D., M. Ferne, T. Rouach, and S. Bergner-Rabinowitz.** 1987. Food-borne outbreak of group G streptococcal sore throat in an Israeli military base. *Epidemiol Infect* **99:**249-55.

1506. **Cohen, D., M. Green, C. Block, R. Slepon, R. Ambar, S. S. Wasserman, and M. M. Levine.** 1991. Reduction of transmission of shigellosis by control of houseflies (Musca domestica). *Lancet* **337:**993-7.

1507. **Cohen, D., T. Sela, R. Slepon, M. Yavzori, R. Ambar, N. Orr, G. Robin, O. Shpielberg, A. Eldad, and M. Green.** 2001. Prospective cohort studies of shigellosis during military field training. *Eur J Clin Microbiol Infect Dis* **20:**123-6.

1508. **Cohen, H. A., J. Amir, A. Matalon, R. Mayan, S. Beni, and A. Barzilai.** 1997. Stethoscopes and otoscopes—a potential vector of infection? *Fam Pract* **14:**446-9.

1509. **Cohen, J.** 2003. The next frontier for HIV/AIDS. *Science* **301:**1650-62.

1510. **Cohen, J. I., D. S. Davenport, J. A. Stewart, S. Deitchman, J. K. Hilliard, and L. E. Chapman.** 2002. Recommendations for prevention of and therapy for exposure to B virus (Cercopithecine herpesvirus 1). *Clin Infect Dis* **35:**1191-203.

1511. **Cohen-Abbo, A., P. M. Bozeman, and C. C. Patrick.** 1993. Cunninghamella infections: review and report of two cases of Cunninghamella pneumonia in immunocompromised children. *Clin Infect Dis* **17:**173-7.

1512. **Cohen-Poradosu, R., J. Jaffe, D. Lavi, S. Grisariu-Greenzaid, R. Nir-Paz, L. Valinsky, M. Dan-Goor, C. Block, B. Beall, and A. E. Moses.** 2004. Group G streptococcal bacteremia in Jerusalem. *Emerg Infect Dis* **10:**1455-60.

1513. **Coia, J. E.** 1998. Clinical, microbiological and epidemiological aspects of Escherichia coli O157 infection. *FEMS Immunol Med Microbiol* **20:**1-9.

1514. **Coia, J. E., J. C. Sharp, D. M. Campbell, J. Curnow, and C. N. Ramsay.** 1998. Environmental risk factors for sporadic Escherichia coli O157 infection in Scotland: results of a descriptive epidemiology study. *J Infect* **36:**317-21.

1515. **Coimbra, C. E. A., M. M. Borges, and N. M. Flowers.** 1992. Sero-epidemiological survey for Chags' disease among the Xavánte Indians of central Brazil. *Ann Trop Med Parasitol* **86:**567-8.

1516. **Coker, A. O., R. D. Isokpehi, B. N. Thomas, K. O. Amisu, and C. L. Obi.** 2002. Human campylobacteriosis in developing countries. *Emerg Infect Dis* **8:**237-44.

1517. **Coker, R.** 2004. Compulsory screening of immigrants for tuberculosis and HIV. *BMJ* **328:**298-300.

1518. **Coker, R., and K. L. van Weezenbeek.** 2001. Mandatory screening and treatment of immigrants for latent tuberculosis in the USA: just restraint? *Lancet Infect Dis* **1:**270-6.

1519. **Colebunders, R., P. De Serrano, A. Van Gompel, H. Wynants, K. Blot, E. Van den Enden, and J. Van den Ende.** 1993. Imported relapsing fever in European tourists. *Scand J Infect Dis* **25:**533-6.

1520. **Colebunders, R., J. L. Mariage, J. C. Coche, B. Pirenne, S. Kempinaire, P. Hantson, A. Van Gompel, M. Niedrig, M. Van Esbroeck, R. Bailey, C. Drosten, and H. Schmitz.** 2002. A Belgian traveler who acquired yellow fever in the Gambia. *Clin Infect Dis* **35:**e113-6.

1521. **Coleman, R. E., T. Monkanna, K. J. Linthicum, D. A. Strickman, S. P. Frances, P. Tanskul, T. M. Kollars, Jr., I. Inlao, P. Watcharapichat, N. Khlaimanee, D. Phulsuksombati, N. Sangjun, and K. Lerdthusnee.** 2003. Occurrence of Orientia tsutsugamushi in small mammals from Thailand. *Am J Trop Med Hyg* **69:**519-24.

1522. **Coles, F. B., A. Schuchat, J. R. Hibbs, S. F. Kondracki, I. F. Salkin, D. M. Dixon, H. G. Chang, R. A. Duncan, N. J. Hurd, and D. L. Morse.** 1992. A multistate outbreak of sporotrichosis associated with sphagnum moss. *Am J Epidemiol* **136:**475-87.

1523. **Collins, C. H., and D. A. Kennedy.** 1999 (4th ed). Laboratory-acquired infections: history, incidence, causes and preventions. Butterworth Heinemann, Oxford.

1524. **Collins, J. E.** 1997. Impact of changing consumer lifestyles on the emergence/reemergence of foodborne pathogens. *Emerg Infect Dis* **3:**471-9.

1525. **Collins, S., M. G. Law, A. Fletcher, A. Boyd, J. Kaldor, and C. L. Masters.** 1999. Surgical treatment and risk of sporadic Creutzfeldt-Jakob disease: a case-control study. *Lancet* **353:**693-7.

1526. **Collins, S. J., V. A. Lawson, and C. L. Masters.** 2004. Transmissible spongiform encephalopathies. *Lancet* **363:**51-61.

1527. **Collins, W. E., and G. M. Jeffery.** 2002. A restrospective examination of sporozoite-induced and throphozoite-induced infections with Plasmodium ovale: development of parasitologic and clinical immunity during primary infection. *Am J Trop Med Hyg* **66:**492-502.

1528. **Colombo, A. L., J. Perfect, M. DiNubile, K. Bartizal, M. Motyl, P. Hicks, R. Lupinacci, C. Sable, and N. Kartsonis.** 2003. Global distribution and outcomes for Candida species causing invasive candidiasis: results from an international randomized double-blind study of caspofungin versus amphotericin B for the treatment of invasive candidiasis. *Eur J Clin Microbiol Infect Dis* **22:**470-4.

1529. **Colon, L. E.** 1991. Keratoconjunctivitis due to adenovirus type 8: report on a large outbreak. *Ann Ophthalmol* **23:**63-5.

1530. **Coluzzi, M.** 2000. [Malaria eradication in Calabria, residual anopheles and transmission risk]. *Parassitologia* **42:**211-7.

1531. **Comer, J. A., T. Diaz, D. Vlahov, E. Monterroso, and J. E. Childs.** 2001. Evidence of rodent-associated Bartonella and Rickettsia infections among intravenous drug users from central and east Harlem, New York city. *Am J Trop Med Hyg* **65:**855-60.

1532. **Comer, J. A., C. Flynn, R. L. Regnery, D. Vlahov, and J. E. Childs.** 1996. Antibodies to Bartonella species in inner-city intravenous drug users in Baltimore, Md. *Arch Intern Med* **156:**2491-5.

1533. **Comer, J. A., C. D. Paddock, and J. E. Childs.** 2001. Urban zoonoses caused by Bartonella, Coxiella, Ehrlichia, and Rickettsia species. *Vector Borne Zoonotic Dis* **1:**91-118.

1534. **Comer, J. A., T. Tzianabos, C. Flynn, D. Vlahov, and J. E. Childs.** 1999. Serologic evidence of rickettsialpox (Rickettsia akari) infection among intravenous drug users in inner-city Baltimore, Maryland. *Am J Trop Med Hyg* **60:**894-8.

1535. **commission, I.** 1978. Ebola haemorrhagic fever in Zaire, 1976. Report of an International Commission. *Bull WHO* **56:**271-93.

1536. **Comstock, R. D., S. Mallonee, J. L. Fox, R. L. Moolenaar, T. M. Vogt, J. E. Perz, B. P. Bell, and J. M. Crutcher.** 2004. A large nosocomial outbreak of hepatitis C and hepatitis B among patients receiving pain remediation treatments. *Infect Control Hosp Epidemiol* **25:**576-83.

1537. **Conaty, S., P. Bird, G. Bell, E. Kraa, G. Grohmann, and J. M. McAnulty.** 2000. Hepatitis A in New South Wales, Australia from consumption of oysters: the first reported outbreak. *Epidemiol Infect* **121:**121-30.

1538. **Conias, S., and P. Wilson.** 1998. Epidemic cutaneous sporotrichosis: report of 16 cases in Queensland due to mouldy hay. *Australas J Dermatol* **39:**34-7.

1539. **Coninx, R., B. Eshaya-Chauvin, and H. Reyes.** 1995. Tuberculosis in prisons. *Lancet* **346:**1238-9.

1540. **Coninx, R., D. Maher, H. Reyes, and M. Grzemska.** 2000. Tuberculosis in prisons in countries with high prevalence. *BMJ* **320:**440-2.

1541. **Conlon, L., K. Pranica, L. Donart, M. Proctor, E. Simone, L. Lucht, T. Boers, and J. P. Davis.** 2001. Norwalk-like virus outbreaks at two summer camps - Wisconsin, June 2001. *MMWR* **50:**642-643.

1542. **Conn, J. E., R. C. Wilkerson, M. N. Segura, R. T. de Souza, C. D. Schlichting, R. A. Wirtz, and M. M. Povoa.** 2002. Emergence of a new neotropical malaria vector facilitated by human migration and changes in land use. *Am J Trop Med Hyg* **66:**18-22.

1543. **Connelly, B. L., L. R. Stanberry, and D. I. Bernstein.** 1993. Detection of varicella-zoster virus DNA in nasopharyngeal secretions of immune household contacts of varicella. *J Infect Dis* **168:**1253-5.

1544. **Connolly, M. A., M. Gayer, M. J. Ryan, P. Salama, P. Spiegel, and D. L. Heymann.** 2004. Communicable diseases in complex emergencies: impact and challenges. *Lancet* **364:**1974-83.

1545. **Connor, M. P., and A. D. Green.** 1995. Runway malaria in a British serviceman. *J R Soc Med* **88:**415P-416P.

1546. **Conrad, D. A., and H. B. Jenson.** 2002. Management of acute bacterial rhinosinusitis. *Curr Opin Pediatr* **14:**86-90.

1547. **Constable, P. J., and J. M. Harrington.** 1982. Risks of zoonoses in a veterinary service. *BMJ* **284:**246-8.

1548. **Constantine, D. G.** 2003. Geographic translocation of bats: known and potential problems. *Emerg Infect Dis* **9:**17-21.

1549. **Conte, D., M. Fraquelli, D. Prati, A. Colucci, and E. Minola.** 2000. Prevalence and clinical course of chronic hepatitis C virus (HCV) infection and rate of HCV vertical transmission in a cohort of 15,250 pregnant women. *Hepatology* **31:**751-5.

1550. **Conti Diaz, I. A.** 1989. Epidemiology of sporotrichosis in Latin America. *Mycopathologia* **108:**113-6.

1551. **Conway, D. J., A. Hall, K. S. Anwar, M. L. Rahman, and D. A. Bundy.** 1995. Household aggregation of Strongyloides stercoralis infection in Bangladesh. *Trans R Soc Trop Med Hyg* **89:**258-61.

1552. **Conwill, D. E., S. B. Werner, S. K. Dritz, M. Bissett, E. Coffey, G. Nygaard, L. Bradford, F. R. Morrison, and M. W. Knight.** 1982. Legionellosis. The 1980 San Francisco outbreak. *Am Rev Respir Dis* **126:**666-9.

1553. **Conzelmann-Auer, C., U. Ackermann-Liebrich, C. Herzog, and A. Bächlin.** 1992. Hepatitis-A-Ausbruch in einem Kindergarten. *Schweiz Med Wochenschr* **122:**1559-66.

1554. **Cook, A. J., R. E. Gilbert, W. Buffolano, J. Zufferey, E. Petersen, P. A. Jenum, W. Foulon, A. E. Semprini, and D. T. Dunn.** 2000. Sources of toxoplasma infection in pregnant women: European multicentre case-control study. European Research Network on Congenital Toxoplasmosis. *BMJ* **321:**142-7.

1555. **Cook, G. C.** 1994. Fatal yellow fever contracted at the hospital for tropical diseases, London, UK, in 1930. *Trans R Soc Trop Med Hyg* **88:**712-3.

1556. **Cook, G. C., and A. D. Bryceson.** 1988. Longstanding infection with Schistosoma mansoni. *Lancet* **1:**127.

1557. **Cook, K. A., T. E. Dobbs, W. G. Hlady, J. G. Wells, T. J. Barrett, N. D. Puhr, G. A. Lancette, D. W. Bodager, B. L. Toth, C. A. Genese, A. K. Highsmith, K. E. Pilot, L. Finelli, and D. L. Swerdlow.** 1998. Outbreak of Salmonella serotype Hartford infections associated with unpasteurized orange juice. *JAMA* **280:**1504-9.

1558. **Cook, R. L., R. A. Royce, J. C. Thomas, and B. H. Hanusa.** 1999. What's driving an epidemic? The spread of syphilis along an interstate highway in rural North Carolina. *Am J Public Health* **89:**369-73.

1559. **Cooke, R. P., T. Riordan, D. M. Jones, and M. J. Painter.** 1989. Secondary cases of meningococcal infection among close family and household contacts in England and Wales, 1984-7. *BMJ* **298:**555-8.

1560. **Cookson, B., A. P. Johnson, B. Azadian, J. Paul, G. Hutchinson, M. Kaufmann, N. Woodford, M. Malde, B. Walsh, A. Yousif, et al.** 1995. International inter- and intrahospital patient spread of a multiple antibiotic-resistant strain of Klebsiella pneumoniae. *J Infect Dis* **171:**511-3.

1561. **Cookson, S. T., J. L. Corrales, J. O. Lotero, M. Regueira, N. Binsztein, M. W. Reeves, G. Ajello, and W. R. Jarvis.** 1998. Disco fever: epidemic meningococcal disease in northeastern Argentina associated with disco patronage. *J Infect Dis* **178:**266-9.

1562. **Coolahan, L. M., and M. H. Levy.** 1993. The prevalence of tuberculosis infection in New South Wales police recruits, 1987-1990. *Med J Aust* **159:**369-72.

1563. **Cooles, P., and H. Paul.** 1989. Rat bites and diabetic foot in the West Indies. *BMJ* **298:**868.

1564. **Cooney, M. K., J. P. Fox, and C. E. Hall.** 1975. The Seattle Virus Watch. VI. Observations of infections with and illness due to parainfluenza, mumps and respiratory syncytial viruses and Mycoplasma pneumoniae. *Am J Epidemiol* **101:**532-51.

1565. **Cooper, B. S., S. P. Stone, C. C. Kibbler, B. D. Cookson, J. A. Roberts, G. F. Medley, G. Duckworth, R. Lai, and S. Ebrahim.** 2004. Isolation measures in the hospital management of methicillin resistant Staphylococcus aureus (MRSA): systematic review of the literature. *BMJ* **329:**533.

1566. **Cooper, P., R. Guderian, P. Orellana, C. Sandoval, H. Olalla, M. Valdez, M. Calvopina, A. Guevara, and G. Griffin.** 1997. An outbreak of bartonellosis in Zamora Chinchipe province in Ecuador. *Trans R Soc Trop Med Hyg* **91:**544-6.

1567. **Cooper, R. I., and T. Neuhauser.** 1998. Images in clinical medicine. Borreliosis. *N Engl J Med* **338:**231.

1568. **Coosemans, M. H.** 1985. [Comparison of malarial endemicity in a rice-growing area and a cotton-growing area of the Rusizi Plain, Burundi]. *Ann Soc Belg Med Trop* **65 Suppl 2:**187-200.

1569. **Coppo, A., M. Colombo, C. Pazzani, R. Bruni, K. A. Mohamud, K. H. Omar, S. Mastrandrea, A. M. Salvia, G. Rotigliano, and F. Maimone.** 1995. Vibrio cholerae in the horn of Africa: epidemiology, plasmids, tetracycline resistance gene amplification, and comparison between O1 and non-O1 strains. *Am J Trop Med Hyg* **53:**351-9.

1570. **Coras, B., S. Essbauer, M. Pfeffer, H. Meyer, J. Schroder, W. Stolz, M. Landthaler, and T. Vogt.** 2005. Cowpox and a cat. *Lancet* **365:**446.

1571. **Corbella, X., A. Montero, M. Pujol, M. A. Dominguez, J. Ayats, M. J. Argerich, F. Garrigosa, J. Ariza, and F. Gudiol.** 2000. Emergence and rapid spread of carbapenem resistance during a large and sustained hospital outbreak of multiresistant Acinetobacter baumannii. *J Clin Microbiol* **38:**4086-95.

1572. **Corbett, E. L., G. J. Churchyard, S. Charalambos, B. Samb, V. Moloi, T. C. Clayton, A. D. Grant, J. Murray, R. J. Hayes, and K. M. De Cock.** 2002. Morbidity and mortality in South African gold miners: impact of untreated disease due to human immunodeficiency virus. *Clin Infect Dis* **34:**1251-8.

1573. **Corbett, E. L., G. J. Churchyard, M. Hay, P. Herselman, T. Clayton, B. Williams, R. Hayes, D. Mulder, and K. M. De Cock.** 1999. The impact of HIV infection on Mycobacterium kansasii disease in South African gold miners. *Am J Respir Crit Care Med* **160:**10-4.

1574. **Corcoles Jimenez, M. P., T. Ruiz Gomez, and D. Garcia Olmo.** 1996. [Phlebitis following venipuncture. Study of a surgical field]. *Rev Enferm* **19:**13-6.

1575. **Corey, L., and H. H. Handsfield.** 2000. Genital herpes and public health: addressing a global problem. *JAMA* **283:**791-4.

1576. **Corey, L., and K. K. Holmes.** 1980. Sexual transmission of hepatitis A in homosexual men: incidence and mechanism. *N Engl J Med* **302:**435-8.

1577. **Cornwall, J., G. Cameron, and R. B. Ellis-Pegler.** 1993. The effects of World Health Organization chemotherapy on imported leprosy in Auckland, New Zealand, 1983-90. *Lepr Rev* **64:**236-49.

1578. **Corredor, A., R. S. Nicholls, S. Duque, P. Munoz de Hoyos, C. A. Alvarez, R. H. Guderian, H. H. Lopez, and G. I. Palma.** 1998. Current status of onchocerciasis in Colombia. *Am J Trop Med Hyg* **58:**594-8.

1579. Correia, A. M., G. Gonçalves, J. Reis, J. M. Cruz, and J. A. Castro e Freitas. 2001. An outbreak of legionnaires' disease in a municipality in northern Portugal. *Eurosurveillance* **6**:121-4.

1580. Corriere, C., C. Zarro, P. E. Connelly, B. J. Tortella, and R. F. Lavery. 2000. A national survey of air medical infectious disease control practices. *Air Med J* **19**:8-12.

1581. Cortez, K. J., D. D. Erdman, T. C. Peret, V. J. Gill, R. Childs, A. J. Barrett, and J. E. Bennett. 2001. Outbreak of human parainfluenza virus 3 infections in a hematopoietic stem cell transplant population. *J Infect Dis* **184**:1093-7.

1582. Corwin, A., K. Jarot, I. Lubis, K. Nasution, S. Suparmawo, A. Sumardiati, S. Widodo, S. Nazir, G. Orndorff, and Y. Choi. 1995. Two years' investigation of epidemic hepatitis E virus transmission in West Kalimantan (Borneo), Indonesia. *Trans R Soc Trop Med Hyg* **89**:262-5.

1583. Corwin, A., A. Ryan, W. Bloys, R. Thomas, B. Deniega, and D. Watts. 1990. A waterborne outbreak of leptospirosis among United States military personnel in Okinawa, Japan. *Int J Epidemiol* **19**:743-8.

1584. Corwin, A. L., H. B. Khiem, E. T. Clayson, K. S. Pham, T. T. Vo, T. Y. Vu, T. T. Cao, D. Vaughn, J. Merven, T. L. Richie, M. P. Putri, J. He, R. Graham, F. S. Wignall, and K. C. Hyams. 1996. A waterborne outbreak of hepatitis E virus transmission in southwestern Vietnam. *Am J Trop Med Hyg* **54**:559-62.

1585. Corwin, A. L., R. P. Larasati, M. J. Bangs, S. Wuryadi, S. Arjoso, N. Sukri, E. Listyaningsih, S. Hartati, R. Namursa, Z. Anwar, S. Chandra, B. Loho, H. Ahmad, J. R. Campbell, and K. R. Porter. 2001. Epidemic dengue transmission in southern Sumatra, Indonesia. *Trans R Soc Trop Med Hyg* **95**:257-265.

1586. Corwin, A. L., R. Soderquist, M. Edwards, A. White, J. Beecham, P. Mills, R. P. Larasati, D. Subekti, T. Ansari, J. Burans, and B. Oyofo. 1999. Shipboard impact of a probable Norwalk virus outbreak from coastal Japan. *Am J Trop Med Hyg* **61**:898-903.

1587. Corwin, A. L., W. Soeprapto, P. S. Widodo, E. Rahardjo, D. J. Kelly, G. A. Dasch, J. G. Olson, A. Sie, R. P. Larasati, and A. L. Richards. 1997. Short report: surveillance of rickettsial infections in Indonesian military personnel during peace keeping operations in Cambodia. *Am J Trop Med Hyg* **57**:569-70.

1588. Corwin, A. L., N. T. Tien, K. Bounlu, J. Winarno, M. P. Putri, K. Laras, R. P. Larasati, N. Sukri, T. Endy, H. A. Sulaiman, and K. C. Hyams. 1999. The unique riverine ecology of hepatitis E virus transmission in South- East Asia. *Trans R Soc Trop Med Hyg* **93**:255-60.

1589. Cosivi, O., J. M. Grange, C. J. Daborn, M. C. Raviglione, T. Fujikura, D. Cousins, R. A. Robinson, H. F. Huchzermeyer, I. de Kantor, and F. X. Meslin. 1998. Zoonotic tuberculosis due to Mycobacterium bovis in developing countries. *Emerg Infect Dis* **4**:59-70.

1590. Cosivi, O., F. X. Meslin, C. J. Daborn, and J. M. Grange. 1995. Epidemiology of Mycobacterium bovis infection in animals and humans, with particular reference to Africa. *Rev Sci Tech* **14**:733-46.

1591. Cosme, A., E. Ojeda, G. Cilla, J. Torrado, L. Alzate, X. Beristain, V. Orive, and J. Arenas. 2001. Fasciolasis hepatobiliar. Estudio de una serie de 37 pacientes. *Gastroenterol Hepatol* **24**:375-80.

1592. Costa, S. F., M. Newbaer, C. R. Santos, M. Basso, I. Soares, and A. S. Levin. 2001. Nosocomial pneumonia: importance of recognition of aetiological agents to define an appropriate initial empirical therapy. *Int J Antimicrob Agents* **17**:147-50.

1593. Cotch, M. F., S. L. Hillier, R. S. Gibbs, and D. A. Eschenbach. 1998. Epidemiology and outcomes associated with moderate to heavy Candida colonization during pregnancy. Vaginal Infections and Prematurity Study Group. *Am J Obstet Gynecol* **178**:374-80.

1594. Coton, T., B. Chaudier, P. Rey, S. Molinier, B. Wade, V. Sang, X. Lemaitre, and C. Gras. 1999. [Indigenous strongyloidiasis: apropos of a case]. *Med Trop (Mars)* **59**:100.

1595. Cotor, F., O. Zavate, M. Finichiu, G. Avram, and A. Ivan. 1983. Enterovirus contamination of swimming pool water; correlation with bacteriological indicators. *Virologie* **34**:251-6.

1596. Cotte, L., M. Rabodonirina, F. Chapuis, F. Bailly, F. Bissuel, C. Raynal, P. Gelas, F. Persat, M. A. Piens, and C. Trepo. 1999. Waterborne outbreak of intestinal microsporidiosis in persons with and without human immunodeficiency virus infection. *J Infect Dis* **180**:2003-8.

1597. Cotter, S. M., S. Sansom, T. Long, E. Koch, S. Kellerman, F. Smith, F. Averhoff, and B. P. Bell. 2003. Outbreak of Hepatitis A among Men Who Have Sex with Men: Implications for Hepatitis A Vaccination Strategies. *J Infect Dis* **187**:1235-40.

1598. Couldwell, D. L., G. J. Dore, J. L. Harkness, D. J. Marriott, D. A. Cooper, R. Edwards, Y. Li, and J. M. Kaldor. 1996. Nosocomial outbreak of tuberculosis in an outpatient HIV treatment room. *Aids* **10**:521-5.

1599. Coura, J. R., A. C. Junqueira, O. Fernandes, S. A. Valente, and M. A. Miles. 2002. Emerging Chagas disease in Amazonian Brazil. *Trends Parasitol* **18**:171-6.

1600. Coursaget, P., Y. Buisson, N. Enogat, R. Bercion, J. M. Baudet, P. Delmaire, D. Prigent, and J. Desrame. 1998. Outbreak of enterically-transmitted hepatitis due to hepatitis A and hepatitis E viruses. *J Hepatol* **28**:745-50.

1601. Courtin, F., S. Dupont, D. G. Zeze, V. Jamonneau, B. Sane, B. Coulibaly, G. Cuny, and P. Solano. 2005. [Human African trypanosomiasis: urban transmission in the focus of Bonon (Cote d'Ivoire)]. *Trop Med Int Health* **10**:340-6.

1602. Coutinho, R. A., P. Albrecht-van Lent, N. Lelie, H. Nagelkerke, H. Kuipers, and T. Rijsdijk. 1983. Prevalence and incidence of hepatitis A among male homosexuals. *Br Med J (Clin Res Ed)* **287**:1743-5.

1603. Coutinho, Z. F., D. Silva Dd, M. Lazera, V. Petri, R. M. Oliveira, P. C. Sabroza, and B. Wanke. 2002. Paracoccidioidomycosis mortality in Brazil (1980-1995). *Cad Saude Publica* **18**:1441-54.

1604. Couto, A. A., V. S. Calvosa, R. Lacerda, F. Castro, E. Santa Rosa, and J. M. Nascimento. 2001. [Control of malaria transmission in a gold-mining area in Amapa State, Brazil, with participation by private enterprise]. *Cad Saude Publica* **17**:897-907.

1605. Coutsoudis, A., K. Pillay, L. Kuhn, E. Spooner, W. Y. Tsai, and H. M. Coovadia. 2001. Method of feeding and transmission of HIV-1 from mothers to children by 15 months of age: prospective cohort study from Durban, South Africa. *AIDS* **15**:379-87.

1606. Couture, C., L. Measures, J. Gagnon, and C. Desbiens. 2003. Human intestinal anisakiosis due to consumption of raw salmon. *Am J Surgical Pathol* **27**:1167-72.

1607. Couturier, E., Y. Brossard, C. Larsen, M. Larsen, C. Du Mazaubrun, J. Paris-Llado, R. Gillot, R. Henrion, G. Breart, and J. B. Brunet. 1992. HIV infection at outcome of pregnancy in the Paris area, France. *Lancet* **340:**707-9.

1608. **Couturier, E., A. Michel, A. L. Basse-Guérineau, and C. Semaille.** 2004. Surveillance de la syphilis en France métropolitaine, 2000-2002. *Bull Epidémiol Hebdomadaire* **3 (13 Jan):**9-12.

1609. **Covacci, A., J. L. Telford, G. Del Giudice, J. Parsonnet, and R. Rappuoli.** 1999. Helicobacter pylori virulence and genetic geography. *Science* **284:**1328-33.

1610. **Covert, T. C., M. R. Rodgers, A. L. Reyes, and G. N. Stelma, Jr.** 1999. Occurrence of nontuberculous mycobacteria in environmental samples. *Appl Environ Microbiol* **65:**2492-6.

1611. **Cowden, J. M.** 1997. Scottish outbreak of Escherichia coli O157 November-December 1996. *Eurosurveillance* **2:**1-2.

1612. **Cowden, J. M., M. O'Mahony, C. L. Bartlett, B. Rana, B. Smyth, D. Lynch, H. Tillett, L. Ward, D. Roberts, R. J. Gilbert, et al.** 1989. A national outbreak of Salmonella typhimurium DT 124 caused by contaminated salami sticks. *Epidemiol Infect* **103:**219-25.

1613. **Cowell, N. A., M. T. Hansen, A. J. Langley, T. M. Graham, and J. R. Bates.** 2002. Outbreak of staphylococcal enterotoxin food poisoning. *Commun Dis Intell* **26:**574-5.

1614. **Cowen, A. E.** 2001. The clinical risks of infection associated with endoscopy. *Can J Gastroenterol* **15:**321-31.

1615. **Cowgill, K. D., C. E. Lucas, R. F. Benson, S. Chamany, E. W. Brown, B. S. Fields, and D. R. Feikin.** 2005. Recurrence of legionnaires disease at a hotel in the United States Virgin Islands over a 20-year period. *Clin Infect Dis* **40:**1205-7.

1616. **Cowie, B. C., J. Adamopoulos, K. Carter, and H. Kelly.** 2005. Hepatitis E infections, Victoria, Australia. *Emerg Infect Dis* **11:**482-4.

1617. **Cox, F. E. G.** 1996. The Wellcome trust illustrated history of tropical diseases. The Wellcome Trust, London.

1618. **Cox, R. A., C. Mallaghan, C. Conquest, and J. King.** 1995. Epidemic methicillin-resistant Staphylococcus aureus: controlling the spread outside hospital. *J Hosp Infect* **29:**107-19.

1619. **Cox, R. A., P. Rao, and C. Brandon-Cox.** 2001. The use of palivizumab monoclonal antibody to control an outbreak of respiratory syncytial virus infection in a special care baby unit. *J Hosp Infect* **48:**186-92.

1620. **Craig, P. S., M. T. Rogan, and J. C. Allan.** 1996. Detection, screening and community epidemiology of taeniid cestode zoonoses: cystic echinococcosis, alveolar echinococcosis and neurocysticercosis. *Adv Parasitol* **38:**169-250.

1621. **Craig, S. C., G. Broughton, 2nd, J. Bean, and K. T. McKee, Jr.** 1999. Rubella outbreak, Fort Bragg, North Carolina, 1995: a clash of two preventive strategies. *Mil Med* **164:**616-8.

1622. **Craig, S. C., P. R. Pittman, T. E. Lewis, C. A. Rossi, E. A. Henchal, R. A. Kuschner, C. Martinez, K. F. Kohlhase, J. C. Cuthie, G. E. Welch, and J. L. Sanchez.** 1999. An accelerated schedule for tick-borne encephalitis vaccine: the American Military experience in Bosnia. *Am J Trop Med Hyg* **61:**874-8.

1623. **Cramer, E. H., D. Forney, A. L. Dannenberg, M. A. Widdowson, J. S. Bresee, S. Monroe, R. S. Beard, H. White, S. Bulens, E. Mintz, C. Stover, E. Isakbaeva, J. Mullins, J. Wright, V. Hsu, W. Chege, and J. Varma.** 2002. Outbreaks of gastroenteritis associated with noroviruses on cruise ships - United States, 2002. *MMWR* **51:**1112-5.

1624. **Crampin, M., G. Willshaw, R. Hancock, T. Djuretic, C. Elstob, A. Rouse, T. Cheasty, and J. Stuart.** 1999. Outbreak of Escherichia coli O157 infection associated with a music festival. *Eur J Clin Microbiol Infect Dis* **18:**286-8.

1625. **Crampton, T. L., R. B. Light, G. M. Berg, M. P. Meyers, G. C. Schroeder, E. S. Hershfield, and J. M. Embil.** 2002. Epidemiology and clinical spectrum of blastomycosis diagnosed at Manitoba hospitals. *Clin Infect Dis* **34:**1310-6.

1626. **Crans, W. J., D. F. Caccamise, and J. R. McNelly.** 1994. Eastern equine encephalomyelitis virus in relation to the avian community of a coastal cedar swamp. *J Med Entomol* **31:**711-28.

1627. **Craven, P. C., D. C. Mackel, W. B. Baine, W. H. Barker, and E. J. Gangarosa.** 1975. International outbreak of Salmonella Eastbourne infection traced to contaminated chocolate. *Lancet* **1:**788-92.

1628. **Crawford, D. H., A. J. Swerdlow, C. Higgins, K. McAulay, N. Harrison, H. Williams, K. Britton, and K. F. Macsween.** 2002. Sexual history and epstein-barr virus infection. *J Infect Dis* **186:**731-6.

1629. **Cree, L., R. House, and J. M. Cowden.** 2003. Has licensing improved hygiene in butchers' shops? *Commun Dis Publ Health* **6:**275-6.

1630. **Creighton, S., M. Tenant-Flowers, C. B. Taylor, R. Miller, and N. Low.** 2003. Co-infection with gonorrhoea and chlamydia: how much is there and what does it mean? *Int J STD AIDS* **14:**109-13.

1631. **Crespo, P. S.** 2004. Surveillance of cryptosporidiosis in Spain from 1995 to 2003. *Eurosurveill Weekly* **8:**5-7.

1632. **Cretnik, T. Z., P. Vovko, M. Retelj, B. Jutersek, T. Harlander, J. Kolman, and M. Gubina.** 2005. Prevalence and nosocomial spread of methicillin-resistant Staphylococcus aureus in a long-term-care facility in Slovenia. *Infect Control Hosp Epidemiol* **26:**184-90.

1633. **Criado-Fornelio, A., A. Martinez-Marcos, A. Buling-Sarana, and J. C. Barba-Carretero.** 2003. Molecular studies on Babesia, Theileria and Hepatozoon in southern Europe. Part I. Epizootiological aspects. *Vet Parasitol* **113:**189-201.

1634. **Crippa, M., O. Rais, and L. Gern.** 2002. Investigations on the mode and dynamics of transmission and infectivity of Borrelia burgdorferi sensu stricto and Borrelia afzelii in Ixodes ricinus ticks. *Vector Borne Zoonotic Dis* **2:**3-9.

1635. **Cristiano, K., G. Pisani, M. Wirz, and G. Gentili.** 1999. Hepatitis G virus in intramuscular and intravenous immunoglobulin products manufactured in Europe. *Transfusion* **39:**428.

1636. **Critchley, E. M. R., P. J. Hayes, and P. E. Isaacs.** 1989. Outbreak of botulism in north west England and Wales, June, 1989. *Lancet* **ii:**849-53.

1637. **Crnich, C. J., and D. G. Maki.** 2002. The promise of novel technology for the prevention of intravascular device-related bloodstream infection. I. Pathogenesis and short-term devices. *Clin Infect Dis* **34:**1232-42.

1638. **Croese, J.** 1995. Seasonal influence on human enteric infection by Ancylostoma caninum. *Am J Trop Med Hyg* **53:**158-61.

1639. **Crofts, N., G. Cooper, T. Stewart, P. Kiely, P. Coghlan, P. Hearne, and J. Hocking.** 1997. Exposure to hepatitis A virus among blood donors, injecting drug users and prison entrants in Victoria. *J Viral Hepat* **4:**333-8.

1640. **Crofts, N., J. L. Hopper, D. S. Bowden, A. M. Breschkin, R. Milner, and S. A. Locarnini.** 1993. Hepatitis C virus infection among a cohort of Victorian injecting drug users. *Med J Aust* **159:**237-41.

1641. Crofts, N., T. Stewart, P. Hearne, X. Y. Ping, A. M. Breshkin, and S. A. Locarnini. 1995. Spread of bloodborne viruses among Australian prison entrants. *BMJ* **310:**285-8.

1642. Crompton, D. W. 2000. The public health importance of hookworm disease. *Parasitology* **121 Suppl:**S39-50.

1643. Crook, L. D., and B. Tempest. 1992. Plague. A clinical review of 27 cases. *Arch Intern Med* **152:**1253-6.

1644. Crook, P. 2001. Catgut company BSE-safe since 1988. *Aust Vet J* **79:**246.

1645. Crosby, R., R. J. DiClemente, and A. Mettey. 2003. Correlates of recent unprotected anal sex among men having sex with men attending a large sex resort in the South. *Sex Transm Dis* **30:**909-13.

1646. Cross, E. R., and K. C. Hyams. 1990. Tuberculin skin testing in US Navy and Marine Corps personnel and recruits, 1980-86. *Am J Public Health* **80:**435-8.

1647. Cross, H. F., M. Haarbrink, G. Egerton, M. Yazdanbakhsh, and M. J. Taylor. 2001. Severe reactions to filarial chemotherapy and release of Wolbachia endosymbionts into blood. *Lancet* **358:**1873-5.

1648. Cross, J. H. 1990. Intestinal capillariasis. *Parasitol Today* **6:**26-8.

1649. Crowcroft, N., D. Brown, R. Gopal, and D. Morgan. 2002. Current management of patients with viral haemorrhagic fevers in the United Kingdom. *Eurosurveillance* **7:**44-8.

1650. Crowcroft, N. S., A. Infuso, D. Ilef, B. Le Guenno, J. C. Desenclos, F. Van Loock, and J. Clement. 1999. Risk factors for human hantavirus infection: Franco-Belgian collaborative case-control study during 1995-6 epidemic. *BMJ* **318:**1737-8.

1651. Crowcroft, N. S., A. Vyse, D. W. Brown, and D. P. Strachan. 1998. Epidemiology of Epstein-Barr virus infection in pre-adolescent children: application of a new salivary method in Edinburgh, Scotland. *J Epidemiol Community Health* **52:** 101-4.

1652. Crowcroft, N. S., B. Walsh, K. L. Davison, and U. Gungabissoon. 2001. Guidelines for the control of hepatitis A virus infection. *Commun Dis Public Health* **4:**213-27.

1653. Cruickshank, J. G., N. F. Lightfoot, K. H. Sugars, G. Colman, M. D. Simmons, J. Tolliday, and E. H. Oakley. 1982. A large outbreak of streptococcal pyoderma in a military training establishment. *J Hyg (Lond)* **89:**9-21.

1654. Crum, N., C. Lamb, G. Utz, D. Amundson, and M. Wallace. 2002. Coccidioidomycosis outbreak among United States navy seals training in a Coccidioides immitis-endemic area - Coalinga, California. *J Infect Dis* **186:**865-8.

1655. Crum, N. F., N. E. Aronson, E. R. Lederman, J. M. Rusnak, and J. H. Cross. 2005. History of U.S. military contributions to the study of parasitic diseases. *Mil Med* **170:**17-29.

1656. Crum, N. F., C. P. Barrozo, F. A. Chapman, M. A. Ryan, and K. L. Russell. 2004. An outbreak of conjunctivitis due to a novel unencapsulated Streptococcus pneumoniae among military trainees. *Clin Infect Dis* **39:**1148-54.

1657. Crum, N. F., H. M. Chun, M. A. Favata, and B. R. Hale. 2003. Gastrointestinal Schistosomiasis japonicum infections in immigrants from the Island of Leyte, Philippines. *J Travel Med* **10:**131-2.

1658. Crum, N. F., B. R. Hale, D. A. Bradshaw, J. D. Malone, H. M. Chun, W. M. Gill, D. Norton, C. T. Lewis, A. A. Truett, C. Beadle, J. L. Town, M. R. Wallace, D. J. Morris, E. K. Yasumoto, K. L. Russell, E. L. Kaplan, C. Van Beneden, and R. Gorwitz. 2003. Outbreak of group A streptococcal pneumonia among marine corps recruits - California, November 1-December 20, 2002. *MMWR* **52:**106-9.

1659. Crum, N. F., M. Potter, and D. Pappagianis. 2004. Seroincidence of Coccidioidomycosis during Military Desert Training Exercises. *J Clin Microbiol* **42:**4552-5.

1660. Crump, J. A., P. M. Griffin, and F. J. Angulo. 2002. Bacterial contamination of animal feed and its relationship to human foodborne illness. *Clin Infect Dis* **35:**859-65.

1661. Crump, J. A., S. P. Luby, and E. D. Mintz. 2004. The global burden of typhoid fever. *Bull WHO* **82:**346-53.

1662. Crump, J. A., D. R. Murdoch, and M. G. Baker. 2001. Emerging infectious diseases in an island ecosystem: the New Zealand perspective. *Emerg Infect Dis* **7:**767-772.

1663. Crump, J. A., A. C. Sulka, A. J. Langer, C. Schaben, A. S. Crielly, R. Gage, M. Baysinger, M. Moll, G. Withers, D. M. Toney, S. B. Hunter, R. M. Hoekstra, S. K. Wong, P. M. Griffin, and T. J. Van Gilder. 2002. An outbreak of Escherichia coli O157:H7 infections among visitors to a dairy farm. *N Engl J Med* **347:**555-60.

1664. Csángó, P. A., E. Blakstad, G. C. Kirtz, J. E. Pedersen, and B. Czettel. 2004. Tick-borne encephalitis in southern Norway. *Emerg Infect Dis* **10:**533-4.

1665. Csango, P. A., S. Haraldstad, J. E. Pedersen, G. Jagars, and I. Foreland. 1997. Respiratory tract infection due to Chlamydia pneumoniae in military personnel. *Scand J Infect Dis Suppl* **104:**26-9.

1666. Csonge, L., S. Pellet, A. Szenes, and J. Istvan. 1995. Antibiotics in the preservation of allograft and xenograft skin. *Burns* **21:**102-5.

1667. Csonka, G., and J. Pace. 1985. Endemic nonvenereal treponematosis (bejel) in Saudi Arabia. *Rev Infect Dis* **7 Suppl 2:**S260-5.

1668. Cuadros, J., M. J. Calvente, A. Benito, J. Arevalo, M. A. Calero, J. Segura, and J. M. Rubio. 2002. Plasmodium ovale Malaria Acquired in Central Spain. *Emerg Infect Dis* **8:**1506-8.

1669. Cubitt, W. D., D. K. Mitchell, M. J. Carter, M. M. Willcocks, and H. Holzel. 1999. Application of electronmicroscopy, enzyme immunoassay, and RT-PCR to monitor an outbreak of astrovirus type 1 in a paediatric bone marrow transplant unit. *J Med Virol* **57:**313-21.

1670. Cuetara, M. S., A. del Palacio, M. Pereiro, E. Amor, C. Alvarez, and A. R. Noriega. 1997. Prevalence of undetected tinea capitis in a school survey in Spain. *Mycoses* **40:**131-7.

1671. Cuetara, M. S., A. Del Palacio, M. Pereiro, and A. R. Noriega. 1998. Prevalence of undetected tinea capitis in a prospective school survey in Madrid: emergence of new causative fungi. *Br J Dermatol* **138:**658-60.

1672. Cui, J., and Z. Q. Wang. 2001. Outbreaks of human trichinellosis caused by consumption of dog meat in China. *Parasite* **8 (suppl):**S74-S77.

1673. Cui, J., Z. Q. Wang, F. Wu, and X. X. Jin. 1997. Epidemiological and clinical studies on an outbreak of trichinosis in central China. *Ann Trop Med Parasitol* **91:**481-8.

1674. Cui, J., Z. Q. Wang, F. Wu, and X. X. Jin. 1998. An outbreak of paragonimiosis in Zhengzhou city, China. *Acta Trop* **70:**211-6.

1675. Culpepper, R., R. Nolan, S. S. Chapman, and A. Kenney. 2001. Methicillin-resistant Staphylococcus aureus skin or soft tissue infections in a state prison - Mississippi, 2000. *MMWR* **50:**919-922.

1676. **Cummings, K., E. Barrett, J. C. Mohle-Boetani, J. T. Brooks, J. Farrar, T. Hunt, A. Fiore, K. Komatsu, S. B. Werner, and L. Slutsker.** 2001. A multistate outbreak of Samonella enterica serotype Baildon associated with domestic raw tomatoes. *Emerg Infect Dis* **7:**1046-1048.

1677. **Cunha, S., M. Freire, C. Eulalio, J. Critosvao, E. Netto, W. D. Johnson, Jr., S. G. Reed, and R. Badaro.** 1995. Visceral leishmaniasis in a new ecological niche near a major metropolitan area of Brazil. *Trans R Soc Trop Med Hyg* **89:**155-8.

1678. **Cunningham, A. L., G. S. Grohman, J. Harkness, C. Law, D. Marriott, B. Tindall, and D. A. Cooper.** 1988. Gastrointestinal viral infections in homosexual men who were symptomatic and seropositive for human immunodeficiency virus. *J Infect Dis* **158:**386-91.

1679. **Cupp, E. W., K. Klingler, H. K. Hassan, L. M. Viguers, and T. R. Unnasch.** 2003. Transmission of eastern equine encephalomyelitis virus in central Alabama. *Am J Trop Med Hyg* **68:**495-500.

1680. **Curran, K. L., J. B. Kidd, J. Vassallo, and V. L. Van Meter.** 2000. Borrelia burgdorferi and the causative agent of human granulocytic ehrlichiosis in deer ticks, Delaware. *Emerg Infect Dis* **6:**408-11.

1681. **Currie, B., L. O'Connor, and B. Dwyer.** 1993. A new focus of scrub typhus in tropical Australia. *Am J Trop Med Hyg* **49:**425-9.

1682. **Currie, B. J., D. A. Fisher, D. M. Howard, J. N. Burrow, D. Lo, S. Selva-Nayagam, N. M. Anstey, S. E. Huffam, P. L. Snelling, P. J. Marks, D. P. Stephens, G. D. Lum, S. P. Jacups, and V. L. Krause.** 2000. Endemic melioidosis in tropical northern Australia: a 10-year prospective study and review of the literature. *Clin Infect Dis* **31:**981-6.

1683. **Currie, B. J., D. A. Fisher, D. M. Howard, J. N. Burrow, S. Selvanayagam, P. L. Snelling, N. M. Anstey, and M. J. Mayo.** 2000. The epidemiology of melioidosis in Australia and Papua New Guinea. *Acta Trop* **74:**121-7.

1684. **Currie, B. J., T. J. Inglis, and A. M. Vannier.** 2004. Laboratory exposure to Burkholderia pseudomallei - Los Angeles, California, 2003. *MMWR* **53:**988-90.

1685. **Currie, B. J., and S. P. Jacups.** 2003. Intensity of rainfall and severity of melioidosis, Australia. *Emerg Infect Dis* **9:**1538-42.

1686. **Currie, B. J., M. Mayo, N. M. Anstey, P. Donohoe, A. Haase, and D. J. Kemp.** 2001. A cluster of melioidosis cases from an endemic region is clonal and is linked to the water supply using molecular typing of Burkholderia pseudomallei isolates. *Am J Trop Med Hyg* **65:**177-9.

1687. **Currier, R. W., C. A. Herron, S. L. Hendricks, and W. J. Zimmermann.** 1983. A trichinosis outbreak in Iowa. *JAMA* **249:**3196-9.

1688. **Currier, R. W., W. A. Johnson, W. A. Rowley, and C. W. Laudenbach.** 1995. Internal ophthalmomyiasis and treatment by laser photocoagulation: a case report. *Am J Trop Med Hyg* **52:**311-3.

1689. **Curtale, F., Y. A. Hassanein, and L. Savioli.** 2005. Control of human fascioliasis by selective chemotherapy: Design, cost and effect of the first public health, school-based intervention implemented in endemic areas of the Nile Delta, Egypt. *Trans R Soc Trop Med Hyg* **99:**599-609.

1690. **Curtis, A. B., R. Ridzon, R. Vogel, S. McDonough, J. Hargreaves, J. Ferry, S. Valway, and I. M. Onorato.** 1999. Extensive transmission of Mycobacterium tuberculosis from a child. *N Engl J Med* **341:**1491-5.

1691. **Curtis, C. F.** 2002. Restoration of malaria control in the Madagascar highlands by DDT spraying. *Am J Trop Med Hyg* **66:**1.

1692. **Curtis, C. F., and A. E. Mnzava.** 2000. Comparison of house spraying and insecticide-treated nets for malaria control. *Bull WHO* **78:**1389-400.

1693. **Cutts, F. T., S. E. Robertson, J.-L. Diaz-Ortega, and R. Samuel.** 1997. Control of rubella and congenital rubella syndrome (CRS) in developing countries, part 1: burden of disease from CRS. *Bull WHO* **75:**55-68.

1694. **Cyran, W.** 1999. [Abscess formation after intra-gluteal injection. Series: legal cases from praxis no 5: defective injections]. *Fortschr Med* **117:**48-9.

1695. **Czechowicz, R. T., T. P. Millard, H. R. Smith, R. E. Ashton, S. B. Lucas, and R. J. Hay.** 1999. Reactivation of cutaneous leishmaniasis after surgery. *Br J Dermatol* **141:**1113-6.

1696. **Czygan, M., W. Hallensleben, M. Hofer, S. Pollak, C. Sauder, T. Bilzer, I. Blumcke, P. Riederer, B. Bogerts, P. Falkai, M. J. Schwarz, E. Masliah, P. Staeheli, F. T. Hufert, and K. Lieb.** 1999. Borna disease virus in human brains with a rare form of hippocampal degeneration but not in brains of patients with common neuropsychiatric disorders. *J Infect Dis* **180:**1695-9.

1697. **D'Alessio, D., T. E. Minor, C. I. Allen, A. A. Tsiatis, and D. B. Nelson.** 1981. A study of the proportions of swimmers among well controls and children with enterovirus-like illness shedding or not shedding an enterovirus. *Am J Epidemiol* **113:**533-41.

1698. **D'Alessio, D. J., R. H. Heeren, S. L. Hendricks, P. Ogilvie, and M. L. Furcolow.** 1965. A starling roost as the source of urban epidemic histoplasmosis in an area of low incidence. *Am Rev Respir Dis* **92:**725-731.

1699. **D'Amelio, R., C. Molica, R. Biselli, and T. Stroffolini.** 2001. Surveillance of infectious diseases in the Italian military as pre-requisite for tailored vaccination programme. *Vaccine* **19:**2006-11.

1700. **D'Andrea, P. S., L. S. Maroja, R. Gentile, R. Cerqueira, A. Maldonado Junior, and L. Rey.** 2000. The parasitism of Schistosoma mansoni (Digenea-Trematoda) in a naturally infected population of water rats, Nectomys squamipes (Rodentia-Sigmodontinae) in Brazil. *Parasitology* **120** (Pt 6):573-82.

1701. **D'Aoust, J. Y., D. W. Warburton, and A. M. Sewell.** 1985. Salmonella typhimurium phage-type 10 from cheddar cheese implicated in a major Canadian foodborne outbreak. *J Food Prot* **48:**1062-1066.

1702. **D'Avanzo, N. J., V. M. Morris, T. R. Carter, J. M. Maillard, P. M. Scanlon, G. M. Stennies, M. Wilson, P. D. M. MacDonald, and R. D. Newman.** 2002. Congenital malaria as a result of Plasmodium malariae - North Carolina, 2000. *MMWR* **51:**164-5.

1703. **Da Costa, A., G. Kirkorian, K. Isaaz, and P. Touboul.** 2000. [Secondary infections after pacemaker implantation]. *Rev Med Intern* **21:**256-65.

1704. **da Rocha, E. M., G. Fontes, A. C. Brito, T. R. Silva, Z. Medeiros, and C. M. Antunes.** 2000. [Bancroftian filariasis in urban areas of Alagoas State, Northeast Brazil: study in the general population]. *Rev Soc Bras Med Trop* **33:**545-51.

1705. **da Silva, A. A., R. N. Cutrim, M. T. e. A. M. T. de Britto e Alves, L. C. Coimbra, S. R. Tonial, and D. P. Borges.** 1997. Water-contact patterns and risk factors for Schistosoma mansoni infection in a rural village of northeast Brazil. *Rev Inst Med Trop Sao Paulo* **39:**91-6.

1706. **Dabernat, H., M. A. Plisson-Saune, C. Delmas, M. Seguy, G. Faucon, R. Pelissier, H. Carsenti, C. Pradier, M. Roussel-Delvallez, J. Leroy, M. J. Dupont, F. De Bels, and P. Dellamonica.** 2003. Haemophilus influenzae carriage in children attending French day care centers: a molecular epidemiological study. *J Clin Microbiol* **41:**1664-72.

1707. **Dadzie, K. Y., G. De Sole, and J. Remme.** 1992. Ocular onchocerciasis and the intensity of infection in the community. IV. The degraded forest of Sierra Leone. *Trop Med Parasitol* **43:**75-9.

1708. **Daengsvang, S.** 1981. Gnathostomiasis in Southeast Asia. *Southeast Asian J Trop Med Public Health* **12:**319-32.

1709. **Daffos, F., F. Forestier, M. Capella-Pavlovsky, P. Thulliez, C. Aufrant, D. Valenti, and W. L. Cox.** 1988. Prenatal management of 746 pregnancies at risk for congenital toxoplasmosis. *N Engl J Med* **318:**271-5.

1710. **Dagan, R., N. Givon-Lavi, O. Zamir, M. Sikuler-Cohen, L. Guy, J. Janco, P. Yagupsky, and D. Fraser.** 2002. Reduction of nasopharyngeal carriage of Streptococcus pneumoniae after administration of a 9-valent pneumococcal conjugate vaccine to toddlers attending day care centers. *J Infect Dis* **185:**927-36.

1711. **Dagan, R., M. Sikuler-Cohen, O. Zamir, J. Janco, N. Givon-Lavi, and D. Fraser.** 2001. Effect of a conjugate pneumococcal vaccine on the occurrence of respiratory infections and antibiotic use in day-care center attendees. *Pediatr Infect Dis J* **20:**951-8.

1712. **Dahle, U. R., P. Sandven, E. Heldal, T. Mannsaaker, and D. A. Caugant.** 2003. Deciphering an outbreak of drug-resistant Mycobacterium tuberculosis. *J Clin Microbiol* **41:**67-72.

1713. **Dahlen, G., F. Widar, R. Teanpaisan, P. N. Papapanou, V. Baelum, and O. Fejerskov.** 2002. Actinobacillus actinomycetemcomitans in a rural adult population in southern Thailand. *Oral Microbiol Immunol* **17:**137-42.

1714. **Dahlstrand, S., O. Ringertz, and B. Zetterberg.** 1971. Airborne tularemia in Sweden. *Scand J Infect Dis* **3:**7-16.

1715. **Dailloux, M., M. Albert, C. Laurain, S. Andolfatto, A. Lozniewski, P. Hartemann, and L. Mathieu.** 2003. Mycobacterium xenopi and drinking water biofilms. *Appl Environ Microbiol* **69:**6946-8.

1716. **Dallal, R. M., B. G. Harbrecht, A. J. Boujoukas, C. A. Sirio, L. M. Farkas, K. K. Lee, and R. L. Simmons.** 2002. Fulminant Clostridium difficile: an underappreciated and increasing cause of death and complications. *Ann Surg* **235:**363-72.

1717. **Dalle, F., L. Dumont, N. Franco, D. Mesmacque, D. Caillot, P. Bonnin, C. Moiroux, O. Vagner, B. Cuisenier, S. Lizard, and A. Bonnin.** 2003. Genotyping of Candida albicans oral strains from healthy individuals by polymorphic microsatellite locus analysis. *J Clin Microbiol* **41:**2203-5.

1718. **Dallman, P. R.** 1998. Plant life in the world's Mediterranean climates. California, Chile, South Africa, Australia, and the Mediterranean Basin. California Native Plant Society, Berkeley, Los Angeles.

1719. **Dalsgaard, A., N. Frimodt-Moller, B. Bruun, L. Hoi, and J. L. Larsen.** 1996. Clinical manifestations and molecular epidemiology of Vibrio vulnificus infections in Denmark. *Eur J Clin Microbiol Infect Dis* **15:**227-32.

1720. **Dalton, C. B., C. C. Austin, J. Sobel, P. S. Hayes, W. F. Bibb, L. M. Graves, B. Swaminathan, M. E. Proctor, and P. M. Griffin.** 1997. An outbreak of gastroenteritis and fever due to Listeria monocytogenes in milk. *N Engl J Med* **336:**100-5.

1721. **Dalton, C. B., J. Gregory, M. D. Kirk, R. J. Stafford, R. Givney, E. Kraa, and D. Gould.** 2004. Foodborne disease outbreaks in Australia, 1995 to 2000. *Commun Dis Intell* **28:**211-24.

1722. **Dalton, C. B., E. D. Mintz, J. G. Wells, C. A. Bopp, and R. V. Tauxe.** 1999. Outbreaks of enterotoxigenic Escherichia coli infection in American adults: a clinical and epidemiologic profile. *Epidemiol Infect* **123:**9-16.

1723. **Dalton, J. P. e.** 1999. Fasciolosis. CABI Publishing, Wallingford, Oxon, U.K.

1724. **Dalton, R. M., E. R. Roman, A. A. Negredo, I. D. Wilhelmi, R. I. Glass, and A. Sanchez-Fauquier.** 2002. Astrovirus acute gastroenteritis among children in Madrid, Spain. *Pediatr infect Dis J* **21:**1038-44.

1725. **Daly, J. M., J. R. Newton, and J. A. Mumford.** 2004. Current perspectives on control of equine influenza. *Vet Res* **35:** 411-23.

1726. **Damascelli, B., G. Patelli, L. F. Frigerio, R. Lanocita, F. Garbagnati, A. Marchiano, C. Spreafico, G. Di Tolla, L. Monfardini, and G. Porcelli.** 1997. Placement of long-term central venous catheters in outpatients: study of 134 patients over 24,596 catheter days. *AJR Am J Roentgenol* **168:**1235-9.

1727. **Damborg, P., K. E. Olsen, E. Moller Nielsen, and L. Guardabassi.** 2004. Occurrence of Campylobacter jejuni in pets living with human patients infected with C. jejuni. *J Clin Microbiol* **42:**1363-4.

1728. **Damian, M. S., W. Dorndorf, H. Burkardt, I. Singer, B. Leinweber, and W. Schachenmayr.** 1994. [Polyneuritis and myositis in Trypanosoma gambiense infection]. *Dtsch Med Wochenschr* **119:**1690-3.

1729. **Dan, R., and S. M. Chang.** 1990. A prospective study of primary Epstein-Barr virus infections among university students in Hong Kong. *Am J Trop Med Hyg* **42:**380-385.

1730. **Dance, D. A.** 2000. Ecology of Burkholderia pseudomallei and the interactions between environmental Burkholderia spp. and human-animal hosts. *Acta Trop* **74:**159-68.

1731. **Dance, D. A. B., M. D. Smith, H. M. Aucken, and T. L. Pitt.** 1999. Imported melioidosis in England and Wales. *Lancet* **353:**208.

1732. **Dancer, S. J., D. McNair, P. Finn, and A. B. Kolsto.** 2002. Bacillus cereus cellulitis from contaminated heroin. *J Med Microbiol* **51:**278-81.

1733. **Dancer, S. J., and W. C. Noble.** 1991. Nasal, axillary, and perineal carriage of Staphylococcus aureus among women: identification of strains producing epidermolytic toxin. *J Clin Pathol* **44:**681-4.

1734. **Daniel, H. D., A. Warier, P. Abraham, and G. Sridharan.** 2004. Age-wise exposure rates to hepatitis E virus in a southern Indian patient population without liver disease. *Am J Trop Med Hyg* **71:**675-8.

1735. **Daniel, S. A., K. Manika, M. Arvanmdou, and A. Antoniadis.** 2002. Prevalence of Rickettsia conorii and Rickettsia typhi infections in the population of northern Greece. *Am J Trop Med Hyg* **66:**76-9.

1736. **Daniels, M. J., M. R. Hutchings, and A. Greig.** 2003. The risk of disease transmission to livestock posed by contamination of farm stored feed by wildlife excreta. *Epidemiol Infect* **130:**561-8.

1737. **Daniels, N. A., D. A. Bergmire-Sweat, K. J. Schwab, K. A. Hendricks, S. Reddy, S. M. Rowe, R. L. Fankhauser, S. S. Monroe, R. L. Atmar, R. I. Glass, and P. Mead.** 2000. A foodborne outbreak of gastroenteritis associated with Norwalk-like viruses: first molecular traceback to deli sandwiches contaminated during preparation. *J Infect Dis* **181:**1467-70.

1738. **Daniels, N. A., L. C. MacKinnon, S. M. Rowe, N. H. Bean, P. M. Griffin, and P. S. Mead.** 2002. Foodborne disease outbreaks in United States schools. *Pediatr Infect Dis J* **2002:**623-8.

1739. **Daniels, N. A., J. Neimann, A. Karpati, U. D. Parashar, K. D. Greene, J. G. Wells, A. Srivastava, R. V. Tauxe, E. D. Mintz, and R. Quick.** 2000. Traveler's diarrhea at sea: three outbreaks of waterborne enterotoxigenic Escherichia coli on cruise ships. *J Infect Dis* **181:**1491-5.

1740. **Daniels, N. A., B. Ray, A. Easton, N. Marano, E. Kahn, A. L. McShan, 2nd, L. Del Rosario, T. Baldwin, M. A. Kingsley, N. D. Puhr, J. G. Wells, and F. J. Angulo.** 2000. Emergence of a new Vibrio parahaemolyticus serotype in raw oysters: a prevention quandry. *JAMA* **284:**1541-5.

1741. **Danis, K., M. Fitzgerald, J. Connell, M. Conlon, and P. G. Murphy.** 2004. Lessons from a pre-season influenza outbreak in a day school. *Commun Dis Public Health* **7:**179-83.

1742. **Dankner, W. M., S. A. Spector, J. Fierer, and C. E. Davis.** 1987. Malassezia fungemia in neonates and adults: complication of hyperalimentation. *Rev Infect Dis* **9:**743-53.

1743. **Danovaro-Holliday, M. C., C. W. LeBaron, C. Allensworth, R. Raymond, T. G. Borden, A. B. Murray, J. P. Icenogle, and S. E. Reef.** 2000. A large rubella outbreak with spread from the workplace to the community. *JAMA* **284:**2733-9.

1744. **Dar, F. K., R. Bayoumi, T. al Karmi, A. Shalabi, F. Beidas, and M. M. Hussein.** 1993. Status of imported malaria in a control zone of the United Arab Emirates bordering an area of unstable malaria. *Trans R Soc Trop Med Hyg* **87:**617-9.

1745. **Dar, L., S. Broor, S. Sengupta, I. Xess, and P. Seth.** 1999. The first major outbreak of dengue hemorrhagic fever in Delhi, India. *Emerg Infect Dis* **5:**589-590.

1746. **Darchenkova, N. N., T. I. Dergacheva, and Zherikhina, II.** 1992. [The spread of Phlebotomus papatasi Scop., 1786 through the territory of Central Asia and southern Kazakhstan]. *Med Parazitol (Mosk)* **4:**30-3.

1747. **Darelid, J., L. Bengtsson, B. Gastrin, H. Hallander, S. Lofgren, B. E. Malmvall, A. M. Olinder-Nielsen, and A. C. Thelin.** 1994. An outbreak of Legionnaires' disease in a Swedish hospital. *Scand J Infect Dis* **26:**417-25.

1748. **Darenkov, I. A., M. A. Marcarelli, G. P. Basadonna, A. L. Friedman, K. M. Lorber, J. G. Howe, J. Crouch, M. J. Bia, A. S. Kliger, and M. I. Lorber.** 1997. Reduced incidence of Epstein-Barr virus-associated posttransplant lymphoproliferative disorder using preemptive antiviral therapy. *Transplantation* **64:**848-52.

1749. **Darmstadt, G. L., and J. S. Francis.** 2000. Tungiasis in a young child adopted from South America. *Pediatr Infect Dis J* **19:**485-7.

1750. **Darouiche, R. O.** 2004. Treatment of infections associated with surgical implants. *N Engl J Med* **350:**1422-9.

1751. **Darrisaw, L., G. Hanson, D. H. Vesole, and S. C. Kehl.** 2000. Cunninghamella infection post bone marrow transplant: case report and review of the literature. *Bone Marrow Transplant* **25:**1213-6.

1752. **Das Gupta, R., and J. F. Guest.** 2002. A model to estimate the cost benefit of an occupational vaccination programme for influenza with Influvac in the U.K. *Pharmacoeconomics* **20:**475-84.

1753. **Datta, P., M. Laga, F. A. Plummer, J. O. Ndinya-Achola, P. Piot, G. Maitha, A. R. Ronald, and R. C. Brunham.** 1988. Infection and disease after perinatal exposure to Chlamydia trachomatis in Nairobi, Kenya. *J Infect Dis* **158:**524-8.

1754. **Daubin, C., S. Vincent, A. Vabret, D. du Cheyron, J. J. Parienti, M. Ramakers, F. Freymuth, and P. Charbonneau.** 2005. Nosocomial viral ventilator-associated pneumonia in the intensive care unit: a prospective cohort study. *Intensive Care Med* **31:**1116-22.

1755. **Davenport, D. S., D. R. Johnson, G. P. Holmes, D. A. Jewett, S. C. Ross, and J. K. Hilliard.** 1994. Diagnosis and management of human B virus (Herpesvirus simiae) infections in Michigan. *Clin Infect Dis* **19:**33-41.

1756. **Davidkin, I., S. Jokinen, A. Paananen, P. Leinikki, and H. Peltola.** 2005. Etiology of mumps-like illnesses in children and adolescents vaccinated for measles, mumps, and rubella. *J Infect Dis* **191:**719-23.

1757. **Davies, A. L., D. O'Flanagan, R. L. Salmon, and T. J. Coleman.** 1996. Risk factors for Neisseria meningitidis carriage in a school during a community outbreak of meningococcal infection. *Epidemiol Infect* **117:**259-66.

1758. **Davies, C. R., P. Kaye, S. L. Croft, and S. Sundar.** 2003. Leishmaniasis: new approaches to disease control. *BMJ* **326:**377-82.

1759. **Davies, C. R., E. A. Llanos-Cuentas, P. Campos, J. Monge, P. Villaseca, and C. Dye.** 1997. Cutaneous leishmaniasis in the Peruvian Andes: risk factors identified from a village cohort study. *Am J Trop Med Hyg* **56:**85-95.

1760. **Davies, F. G., K. J. Linthicum, and A. D. James.** 1985. Rainfall and epizootic Rift valley fever. *Bull WHO* **63:**941-3.

1761. **Davies, H. D., C. Adair, A. McGeer, D. Ma, S. Robertson, M. Mucenski, L. Kowalsky, G. Tyrell, and C. J. Baker.** 2001. Antibodies to capsular polysaccharides of group B Streptococcus in pregnant Canadian women: relationship to colonization status and infection in the neonate. *J Infect Dis* **184:**285-91.

1762. **Davies, H. D., A. McGeer, B. Schwartz, K. Green, D. Cann, A. E. Simor, and D. E. Low.** 1996. Invasive group A streptococcal infections in Ontario, Canada. Ontario Group A Streptococcal Study Group. *N Engl J Med* **335:**547-54.

1763. **Davies, J. C.** 1982. A major epidemic of anthrax in Zimbabwe. *Cent Afr J Med* **28:**291-8.

1764. **Davies, J. W., W. R. Simon, E. J. Bowmer, A. Mallory, and K. G. Cox.** 1972. Typhoid at sea: epidemic aboard an ocean liner. *Can Med Assoc J* **106:**877-83.

1765. **Davies, M., C. Bruce, K. Bewley, M. Outlaw, V. Mioulet, G. Lloyd, and C. Clegg.** 2003. Poliovirus type 1 in working stocks of typed human rhinoviruses. *Lancet* **361:**1187-8.

1766. **Davis, D. S., and P. H. Elzer.** 2002. Brucella vaccines in wildlife. *Vet Microbiol* **90:**533-44.

1767. **Davis, H., J. P. Taylor, J. N. Perdue, G. N. Stelma, Jr., J. M. Humphreys, Jr., R. Rowntree, 3rd, and K. D. Greene.** 1988. A shigellosis outbreak traced to commercially distributed shredded lettuce. *Am J Epidemiol* **128**:1312-21.

1768. Davis, H., J. M. Vincent, and J. Lynch. 2002. Tick-borne relapsing fever caused by Borrelia turicatae. *Pediatr Infect Dis J* **21**:703-5.

1769. Davis, K. A., K. A. Moran, C. K. McAllister, and P. J. Gray. 2005. Multidrug-resistant Acinetobacter extremity infections in soldiers. *Emerg Infect Dis* **11**:1218-24.

1770. Davis, K. A., J. J. Stewart, H. K. Crouch, C. E. Florez, and D. R. Hospenthal. 2004. Methicillin-resistant Staphylococcus aureus (MRSA) nares colonization at hospital admission and its effect on subsequent MRSA infection. *Clin Infect Dis* **39**:776-82.

1771. Davis, R. M., W. A. Orenstein, J. A. Frank, Jr., J. J. Sacks, L. G. Dales, S. R. Preblud, K. J. Bart, N. M. Williams, and A. R. Hinman. 1986. Transmission of measles in medical settings. 1980 through 1984. *JAMA* **255**:1295-8.

1772. Davis, R. M., E. D. Whitman, W. A. Orenstein, S. R. Preblud, L. E. Markowitz, and A. R. Hinman. 1987. A persistent outbreak of measles despite appropriate prevention and control measures. *Am J Epidemiol* **126**:438-49.

1773. Davis, S., M. Begon, L. De Bruyn, V. S. Ageyev, N. L. Klassovskiy, S. B. Pole, N. Viljugrein, N. C. Stenseth, and H. Leirs. 2004. Predictive thresholds for plague in Kazakhstan. *Science* **304**:736-8.

1774. Davison, K. L., N. Andrews, J. M. White, M. E. Ramsay, N. S. Crowcroft, A. A. Rushdy, E. B. Kaczmarski, P. N. Monk, and J. M. Stuart. 2004. Clusters of meningococcal disease in school and preschool settings in England and Wales: what is the risk? *Arch Dis Child* **89**:256-60.

1775. Davos, D. E., C. F. Cargill, M. R. Kyrkou, J. A. Jamieson, and G. E. Rich. 1981. Outbreak of brucellosis at a South-Australian abattoir. 2. Epidemiological investigations. *Med J Aust* **2**:657-60.

1776. Dawar, M., L. Moody, J. D. Martin, C. Fung, J. Isaac-Renton, and D. M. Patrick. 2002. Two outbreaks of botulism associated with fermented salmon roe - British Columbia, August 2001. *Can Commun Dis Rep* **28**:45-9.

1777. Dawson, A., R. Griffin, A. Fleetwood, and N. J. Barrett. 1995. Farm visits and zoonoses. *Commun Dis Rep CDR Rev* **5**:R81-6.

1778. Daxboeck, F., R. Krause, and C. Wenisch. 2003. Laboratory diagnosis of Mycoplasma pneumoniae infection. *Clin Microbiol Infect* **9**:263-73.

1779. Dayan, G., M. Papania, S. Redd, P. Rota, J. Rota, S. Liffick, L. Lowe, and W. Bellini. 2004. Epidemiology of measles, United States, 2001-2003. *MMWR* **53**:713-6.

1780. Dayan, G. H., M. S. Panero, R. Debbag, A. Urquiza, M. Molina, S. Prieto, M. Del Carmen Perego, G. Scagliotti, D. Galimberti, G. Carroli, C. Wolff, D. S. Schmid, V. Loparev, D. Guris, and J. Seward. 2004. Varicella seroprevalence and molecular epidemiology of varicella-zoster virus in Argentina, 2002. *J Clin Microbiol* **42**:5698-704.

1781. Dayan, G. H., L. Zimmerman, L. Shteinke, K. Kasymbekova, A. Uzicanin, P. Strebel, and S. Reef. 2003. Investigation of a rubella outbreak in Kyrgyzstan in 2001: implications for an integrated approach to measles elimination and prevention of congenital rubella syndrome. *J Infect Dis* **187 Suppl 1**:S235-40.

1782. de Albuquerque, M. C., F. M. da Silva, C. C. Soares, M. Volotao Ede, and N. Santos. 2003. Adenoviruses isolated from civilian and military personnel in the city of Rio de Janeiro, Brazil. *Rev Inst Med Trop Sao Paulo* **45**:233-6.

1783. de Almeida, L. M., M. Amaku, R. Soares Azevedo, S. Cairncross, and E. Massad. 2002. The intensity of transmission of hepatitis A and heterogeneities in socio-environmental risk factors in Rio de Janeiro, Brazil. *Trans R Soc Trop Med Hyg* **96**:605-10.

1784. de Andrade, A. L., C. M. Martelli, R. M. Oliveira, J. R. Arias, F. Zicker, and L. Pang. 1995. High prevalence of asymptomatic malaria in gold mining areas in Brazil. *Clin Infect Dis* **20**:475.

1785. de Andrade, A. L., F. Zicker, R. M. de Oliveira, S. Almeida Silva, A. Luquetti, L. R. Travassos, I. C. Almeida, S. S. de Andrade, J. G. de Andrade, and C. M. Martelli. 1996. Randomised trial of efficacy of benznidazole in treatment of early Trypanosoma cruzi infection. *Lancet* **348**:1407-13.

1786. De Andrade, A. L., F. Zicker, R. M. De Oliveira, I. G. Da Silva, S. A. Silva, S. S. De Andrade, and C. M. Martelli. 1995. Evaluation of risk factors for house infestation by Triatoma infestans in Brazil. *Am J Trop Med Hyg* **53**:443-7.

1787. de Arruda, M. E., C. Aragaki, F. Gagliardi, and R. W. Haile. 1996. A seroprevalence and descriptive epidemiological study of malaria among Indian tribes of the Amazon basin of Brazil. *Ann Trop Med Parasitol* **90**:135-43.

1788. De Benedictis, J., E. Chow-Shaffer, A. Costero, G. G. Clark, J. D. Edman, and T. W. Scott. 2003. Identification of the people from whom engorged Aedes aegypti took blood meals in Florida, Puerto Rico, using polymerase chain reaction-based DNA profiling. *Am J Trop Med Hyg* **68**:437-46.

1789. de Benoist, A. C., J. M. White, A. Efstratiou, C. Kelly, G. Mann, B. Nazareth, C. J. Irish, D. Kumar, and N. S. Crowcroft. 2004. Imported cutaneous diphtheria, United Kingdom. *Emerg Infect Dis* **10**:511-3.

1790. de Boer, R. 2002. Allergens, Der p 1, Der f 1, Fel d 1 and Can f 1, in newly bought mattresses for infants. *Clin Exp Allergy* **32**:1602-5.

1791. de Bruyn, G., T. P. Whelan, M. S. Mulligan, G. Raghu, and A. P. Limaye. 2004. Invasive pneumococcal infections in adult lung transplant recipients. *Am J Transplant* **4**:1366-71.

1792. de Castro, L., P. Rodrigues Ddos, R. Flauzino, M. Moura, and J. P. Leite. 1994. An outbreak of diarrhoea associated with rotavirus serotype 1 in a day care nursery in Rio de Janeiro, Brazil. *Mem Inst Oswaldo Cruz* **89**:5-9.

1793. de Chabalier, F., M. H. Djingarey, A. Hassane, and J. P. Chippaux. 2000. Meningitis seasonal pattern in Africa and detection of epidemics: a retrospective study in Niger, 1990-98. *Trans R Soc Trop Med Hyg* **94**:664-8.

1794. de Clercq, D., J. Vercruysse, M. Sene, I. Seck, C. S. Sall, A. Ly, and V. R. Southgate. 2000. The effects of irrigated agriculture on the transmission of urinary schistosomiasis in the Middle and Upper Valleys of the Senegal River basin. *Ann Trop Med Parasitol* **94**:581-90.

1795. De Doncker, S., V. Hutse, S. Abdellati, S. Rijal, B. M. Singh Karki, S. Decuypere, D. Jacquet, D. Le Ray, M. Boelaert, S. Koirala, and J. C. Dujardin. 2005. A new PCR-ELISA for diagnosis of visceral leishmaniasis in blood of HIV-negative subjects. *Trans R Soc Trop Med Hyg* **99**:25-31.

1796. de Filippis, A. M. B., R. M. R. Nogueira, H. G. Schatzmayr, D. S. Tavares, A. V. Jabor, S. C. Diniz, J. C. Oliveira, E. Moreira, M. P. Miagostovich, E. V. Costa, and R. Galler. 2002. Outbreak of jaundice and hemorrhagic fever in the Southeast of Brazil in 2001: detection and molecular characterization of yellow fever. *J Med Virol* **68**:620-7.

1797. **de Freitas, R. B., D. Wong, F. Boswell, M. F. de Miranda, A. C. Linhares, J. Shirley, and U. Desselberger.** 1990. Prevalence of human parvovirus (B19) and rubella virus infections in urban and remote rural areas in northern Brazil. *J Med Virol* **32**:203-8.

1798. **de Goede, E., M. Martens, S. Van Rooy, and I. VanMoerkerke.** 1995. A case of systemic strongyloidiasis in an ex-coal miner with idiopathic colitis. *Eur J Gastroenterol Hepatol* **7**:807-9.

1799. **de Graaf, R., G. van Zessen, H. Houweling, R. J. Ligthelm, and R. van den Akker.** 1997. Sexual risk of HIV infection among expatriates posted in AIDS endemic areas. *AIDS* **11**:1173-81.

1800. **de Graaf, R., I. Vanwesenbeeck, G. van Zessen, C. J. Straver, and J. H. Visser.** 1994. Male prostitutes and safe sex: different settings, different risks. *AIDS Care* **6**:277-88.

1801. **de Hoog, G. S., D. Adelmann, A. O. Ahmed, and A. van Belkum.** 2004. Phylogeny and typification of Madurella mycetomatis, with a comparison of other agents of eumycetoma. *Mycoses* **47**:121-30.

1802. **de Hoog, G. S., A. Buiting, C. S. Tan, A. B. Stroebel, C. Ketterings, E. J. de Boer, B. Naafs, R. Brimicombe, M. K. Nohlmans-Paulssen, G. T. Fabius, et al.** 1993. Diagnostic problems with imported cases of mycetoma in The Netherlands. *Mycoses* **36**:81-7.

1803. **de Juanes, J. R., A. Gil, A. Gonzalez, M. P. Arrazola, M. San-Martin, and J. Esteban.** 2004. Seroprevalence of pertussis antibody among health care personnel in Spain. *Eur J Epidemiol* **19**:69-72.

1804. **de Kantor, I. N., and V. Ritacco.** 1994. Bovine tuberculosis in Latin America and the Caribbean: current status, control and eradication programs. *Vet Microbiol* **40**:5-14.

1805. **de Klerk, P. F.** 2002. Carcass disposal: lessons from The Netherlands after the foot and mouth disease outbreak of 2001. *Rev Sci Tech* **21**:789-96.

1806. **de la Torre Molina, R., J. Perez Aparicio, M. Hernandez Bienes, R. Jurado Perez, A. Martinez Ruso, and E. Morales Franco.** 2000. [Anisakiasis in fresh fish sold in the north of Cordoba]. *Rev Esp Salud Publica* **74**:517-26.

1807. **de Lalla, F., J. W. Ezzell, G. Pellizzer, E. Parenti, A. Vaglia, F. Marranconi, and A. Tramarin.** 1992. Familial outbreak of agricultural anthrax in an area of northern Italy. *Eur J Clin Microbiol Infect Dis* **11**:839-42.

1808. **de Lalla, F., G. Rizzardini, G. A. Cairoli, E. Rinaldi, D. Santoro, and A. Ostinelli.** 1988. Outbreak of amoebiasis in tourists returning from Thailand. *Lancet* **2**:847.

1809. **De Lemos, E. R. S., F. B. F. Alvarenga, M. L. Cintra, M. C. Ramos, C. D. Paddock, T. L. Ferebee, S. R. Zaki, F. C. Ferreira, R. C. Ravagnani, R. D. Machado, M. A. Guimaraes, and J. R. Coura.** 2001. Spotted fever in Brazil: a seroepidemiological study and description of clinical cases in an endemic area in the state of São Paulo. *Am J Trop Med Hyg* **65**:329-34.

1810. **de Lima Barros, M. B., A. de Oliveira Schubach, M. C. Galhardo, T. M. Schubach, R. S. dos Reis, M. J. Conceicao, and A. C. do Valle.** 2003. Sporotrichosis with widespread cutaneous lesions: report of 24 cases related to transmission by domestic cats in Rio de Janeiro, Brazil. *Int J Dermatol* **42**:677-81.

1811. **de Lima Barros, M. B., T. M. Pacheco Schubach, M. C. Gutierrez Galhardo, A. de Oliviera Schubach, P. C. Monteiro, R. S. Reis, R. M. Zancope-Oliveira, M. dos Santos Lazera, T. Cuzzi-Maya, T. C. Blanco, K. B. Marzochi, B. Wanke, and A. C. do Valle.** 2001. Sporotrichosis: an emergent zoonosis in Rio de Janeiro. *Mem Inst Oswaldo Cruz* **96**:777-9.

1812. **de Lisle, G. W., R. G. Bengis, S. M. Schmitt, and D. J. O'Brien.** 2002. Tuberculosis in free-ranging wildlife: detection, diagnosis and management. *Rev Sci Tech* **21**:317-34.

1813. **De Los Angeles Pando, M., S. Maulen, M. Weissenbacher, R. Marone, R. Duranti, L. M. Peralta, H. Salomon, K. Russell, M. Negrete, S. S. Estani, S. Montano, J. L. Sanchez, and M. M. Avila.** 2003. High human immunodeficiency virus type 1 seroprevalence in men who have sex with men in Buenos Aires, Argentina: risk factors for infection. *Int J Epidemiol* **32**:735-40.

1814. **de los Rios Martin, R., N. Garcia Marin, J. Sanz Moreno, and E. Ballester Orcal.** 2001. [Mumps in a urban area of the Community of Madrid. Vaccination status, diagnosis and intervention measures]. *Aten Primaria* **28**:10-6.

1815. **de Manzione, N., R. A. Salas, H. Paredes, O. Godoy, L. Rojas, F. Araoz, C. F. Fulhorst, T. G. Ksiazek, J. N. Mills, B. A. Ellis, C. J. Peters, and R. B. Tesh.** 1998. Venezuelan hemorrhagic fever: clinical and epidemiological studies of 165 cases. *Clin Infect Dis* **26**:308-13.

1816. **de Meeûs, T., and F. Renaud.** 2002. Parasites within the new phylogeny of eukaryotes. *Trends Parasitol* **18**:247-51.

1817. **de Noray, G., C. Capuano, and M. Abel.** 2003. [Campaign to eradicate yaws on Santo Island, Vanuatu in 2001]. *Med Trop (Mars)* **63**:159-62.

1818. **De, N. V., K. D. Murrell, D. Cong le, P. D. Cam, V. Chau le, N. D. Toan, and A. Dalsgaard.** 2003. The food-borne trematode zoonoses of Vietnam. *Southeast Asian J Trop Med Public Health* **34 Suppl 1**:12-34.

1819. **de Oliveira, A. G., A. L. Falcao, and R. P. Brazil.** 2000. [First record of finding Lutzomyia longipalpis (Lutz & Neiva, 1912) in the urban area of Brazil]. *Rev Saude Publica* **34**:654-5.

1820. **de Oliveira Guerra, J. A., S. Talhari, M. G. Paes, M. Garrido, and J. M. Talhari.** 2003. [Clinical and diagnostic aspects of American tegumentary leishmaniasis in soldiers simultaneously exposed to the infection in the Amazon Region]. *Rev Soc Bras Med Trop* **36**:587-90.

1821. **De Oliveira-Garcia, D., M. Dall'Agnol, M. Rosales, A. C. Azzuz, M. B. Martinez, and J. A. Giron.** 2002. Characterization of Flagella Produced by Clinical Strains of Stenotrophomonas maltophilia. *Emerg Infect Dis* **8**:918-23.

1822. **de Ory, F., R. Ramírez, L. García Comas, P. Leon, M. J. Sagues, and J. C. Sanz.** 2004. Is there a change in cytomegalovirus seroepidemiology in Spain? *Eur J Epidemiol* **19**:85-9.

1823. **De, P., A. E. Singh, T. Wong, and W. Yacoub.** 2003. Outbreak of Neisseria gonorrhoeae in Northern Alberta, Canada. *Sex Transm Dis* **30**:497-501.

1824. **De, P., A. E. Singh, T. Wong, W. Yacoub, and A. M. Jolly.** 2004. Sexual network analysis of a gonorrhoea outbreak. *Sex Transm Infect* **80**:280-5.

1825. **de Pita-Pereira, D., C. R. Alves, M. B. Souza, R. P. Brazil, A. L. Bertho, F. Barbosa Ade, and C. C. Britto.** 2005. Identification of naturally infected Lutzomyia intermedia and Lutzomyia migonei with Leishmania (Viannia) braziliensis in Rio de

Janeiro (Brazil) revealed by a PCR multiplex non-isotopic hybridisation assay. *Trans R Soc Trop Med Hyg* **99**:905-13.

1826. De Schrijver, K. 1995. A psittacosis outbreak in Belgian customs officers. *Eurosurveillance* **0**(Sep):3.

1827. de Schrijver, K., K. Dirven, K. Van Bouwel, L. Mortelmans, P. Van Rossom, T. De Beukelaar, C. Vael, M. Fajo, O. Ronveaux, M. F. Peeters, A. Van der Zee, A. Bergmans, M. Ieven, and H. Goossens. 2003. An outbreak of Legionnaire's disease among visitors to a fair in Belgium in 1999. *Public Health* **117**:117-24.

1828. De Schrijver, K., I. Maes, P. Van Damme, J. Tersago, E. Moes, and M. Van Ranst. 2005. An outbreak of nosocomial hepatitis B virus infection in a nursing home for the elderly in Antwerp (Belgium). *Acta Clin Belg* **60**:63-9.

1829. De Schryver, A., and A. Meheus. 1989. International travel and sexually transmitted diseases. *World Health Stat Q* **42**:90-9.

1830. De Serres, G., T. L. Cromeans, B. Levesque, N. Brassard, C. Barthe, M. Dionne, H. Prud'homme, D. Paradis, C. N. Shapiro, O. V. Nainan, and H. S. Margolis. 1999. Molecular confirmation of hepatitis A virus from well water: epidemiology and public health implications. *J Infect Dis* **179**:37-43.

1831. De Serres, G., B. Levesque, R. Higgins, M. Major, D. Laliberte, N. Boulianne, and B. Duval. 1995. Need for vaccination of sewer workers against leptospirosis and hepatitis A. *Occup Environ Med* **52**:505-7.

1832. De Serres, G., R. Shadmani, B. Duval, N. Boulianne, P. Dery, M. Douville Fradet, L. Rochette, and S. A. Halperin. 2000. Morbidity of pertussis in adolescents and adults. *J Infect Dis* **182**:174-9.

1833. de Silva, A. M., W. P. Dittus, P. H. Amerasinghe, and F. P. Amerasinghe. 1999. Serologic evidence for an epizootic dengue virus infecting toque macaques (Macaca sinica) at Polonnaruwa, Sri Lanka. *Am J Trop Med Hyg* **60**:300-6.

1834. De Silva, L. M., D. L. Mulcahy, and K. R. Kamath. 1984. A family outbreak of toxoplasmosis: a serendipitous finding. *J Infect* **8**:163-7.

1835. de Silva, N. R., S. Brooker, P. J. Hotez, A. Montresor, D. Engels, and L. Savioli. 2003. Soil-transmitted helminth infections: updating the global picture. *Trends Parasitol* **19**:547-51.

1836. de Silva, S., P. Saykao, H. Kelly, C. R. MacIntyre, N. Ryan, J. Leydon, and B. A. Biggs. 2002. Chronic Strongyloides stercoralis infection in Laotian immigrants and refugees 7-20 years after resettlement in Australia. *Epidemiol Infect* **128**:439-44.

1837. de Sousa, O. V., R. H. Vieira, F. G. de Menezes, C. M. dos Reis, and E. Hofer. 2004. Detection of Vibrio parahaemolyticus and Vibrio cholerae in oyster, Crassostrea rhizophorae, collected from a natural nursery in the Coco river estuary, Fortaleza, Ceara, Brazil. *Rev Inst Med Trop Sao Paulo* **46**:59-62.

1838. de Sousa, R., S. D. Nobrega, F. Bacellar, and J. Torgal. 2003. Mediterranean spotted fever in Portugal: risk factors for fatal outcome in 105 hospitalized patients. *Ann N Y Acad Sci* **990**:285-94.

1839. De Soyza, A., A. McDowell, L. Archer, J. H. Dark, S. J. Elborn, E. Mahenthiralingam, K. Gould, and P. A. Corris. 2001. Burkholderia cepacia complex genomovars and pulmonary transplantation outcomes in patients with cystic fibrosis. *Lancet* **358**:1780-1.

1840. de Swart, R. L., P. M. Wertheim-van Dillen, R. S. van Binnendijk, C. P. Muller, J. Frenkel, and A. D. Osterhaus. 2000. Measles in a Dutch hospital introduced by an immuno-compromised infant from Indonesia infected with a new virus genotype. *Lancet* **355**:201-2.

1841. de Thoisy, B., P. Dussart, and M. Kazanji. 2004. Wild terrestrial rainforest mammals as potential reservoirs for flaviviruses (yellow fever, dengue 2 and St Louis encephalitis viruses) in French Guiana. *Trans R Soc Trop Med Hyg* **98**:409-12.

1842. de Thoisy, B., J. Gardon, R. A. Salas, J. Morvan, and M. Kazanji. 2003. Mayaro virus in wild mammals, French Guiana. *Emerg Infect Dis* **9**:1327-9.

1843. De Valk, H., E. Delarocque-Astagneau, G. Colomb, S. Ple, E. Godard, V. Vaillant, S. Haeghebaert, P. H. Bouvet, F. Grimont, P. Grimont, and J. C. Desenclos. 2000. A community-wide outbreak of Salmonella enterica serotype Typhimurium infection associated with eating a raw milk soft cheese in France. *Epidemiol Infect* **124**:1-7.

1844. De Valk, H., V. Vaillant, C. Jacquet, J. Rocourt, F. Le Querrec, F. Stainer, N. Quelquejeu, O. Pierre, V. Pierre, J. C. Desenclos, and V. Goulet. 2001. Two consecutive nationwide outbreaks of listeriosis in France, October 1999-February 2000. *Am J Epidemiol* **154**:944-950.

1845. de Vincenzi, I. 1994. A longitudinal study of human immunodeficiency virus transmission by heterosexual partners. European Study Group on Heterosexual Transmission of HIV. *N Engl J Med* **331**:341-6.

1846. De Wals, P., L. Hertoghe, I. Borlee-Grimee, S. De Maeyer-Cleempoel, G. Reginster-Haneuse, A. Dachy, A. Bouckaert, and M. F. Lechat. 1981. Meningococcal disease in Belgium. Secondary attack rate among household, day-care nursery and pre-elementary school contacts. *J Infect* **3**:53-61.

1847. de Wazieres, B., H. Gil, D. A. Vuitton, and J. L. Dupond. 1998. Nosocomial transmission of dengue from a needlestick injury. *Lancet* **351**:498.

1848. de Wit, M. A., M. P. Koopmans, L. M. Kortbeek, W. J. Wannet, J. Vinje, F. van Leusden, A. I. Bartelds, and Y. T. van Duynhoven. 2001. Sensor, a population-based cohort study on gastroenteritis in the Netherlands: incidence and etiology. *Am J Epidemiol* **154**:666-74.

1849. de Wit, M. A., M. P. Koopmans, and Y. T. van Duynhoven. 2003. Risk factors for norovirus, Sapporo-like virus, and group A rotavirus gastroenteritis. *Emerg Infect Dis* **9**:1563-70.

1850. Deane, L. M. 1992. Simian malaria in Brazil. *Mem Inst Oswaldo Cruz* **87**:1-20.

1851. Debacker, M., J. Aguiar, C. Steunou, C. Zinsou, W. M. Meyers, A. Guedenon, J. T. Scott, M. Dramaix, and F. Portaels. 2004. Mycobacterium ulcerans disease (Buruli ulcer) in rural hospital, Southern Benin, 1997-2001. *Emerg Infect Dis* **10**:1391-8.

1852. Debast, S. B., W. J. Melchers, A. Voss, J. A. Hoogkamp-Korstanje, and J. F. Meis. 1995. Epidemiological survey of an outbreak of multiresistant Serratia marcescens by PCR-fingerprinting. *Infection* **23**:267-71.

1853. Decre, D., B. Burghoffer, V. Gautier, J. C. Petit, and G. Arlet. 2004. Outbreak of multi-resistant Klebsiella oxytoca involving strains with extended-spectrum β-lactamases and strains with extended-spectrum activity of the chromosomal β-lactamase. *J Antimicrob Chemother* **54**:881-888.

1854. Deetz, T. R., M. H. Sawyer, G. Billman, F. L. Schuster, and G. S. Visvesvara. 2003. Successful treatment of balamuthia amoebic encephalitis: presentation of 2 cases. *Clin Infect Dis* **37**:1304-12.

1855. DeGiorgio, C., S. Pietsch-Escueta, V. Tsang, G. Corral-Leyva, L. Ng, M. T. Medina, S. Astudillo, N. Padilla, P. Leyva, L. Martinez, J. Noh, M. Levine, R. del Villasenor, and F. Sorvillo. 2005. Sero-prevalence of Taenia solium cysticercosis and Taenia solium taeniasis in California, USA. *Acta Neurol Scand* **111**:84-8.

1856. Degremont, A., and N. Lorenz. 1990. [Imported diseases in Switzerland: development and perspectives]. *Ther Umsch* **47**:772-9.

1857. Del Brutto, O. H., J. Sotelo, and G. C. Román. 1998. Neurocysticercosis. A clinical handbook. Swets & Zeitlinger Publishers, Lisse, Abingdon, Exton, Tokyo.

1858. Del Giudice, P., P. Dellamonica, J. Durant, V. Rahelinrina, M. P. Grobusch, K. Janitschke, A. Dahan-Guedj, and Y. Le Fichoux. 2001. A case of gnathostomiasis in a European traveller returning from Mexico. *Br J Dermatol* **145**:487-9.

1859. del Toro, M. D., J. Rodriguez-Bano, M. Herrero, A. Rivero, M. A. Garcia-Ordonez, J. Corzo, and R. Perez-Cano. 2002. Clinical epidemiology of Stenotrophomonas maltophilia colonization and infection: a multicenter study. *Medicine (Baltimore)* **81**:228-39.

1860. Delafosse, A., and A. A. Doutoum. 2004. Prevalence of Trypanosoma evansi infection and associated risk factors in camels in eastern Chad. *Vet Parasitol* **119**:155-64.

1861. Delaporte, E., C. A. Wyler-Lazarevic, J. L. Richard, and P. Sudre. 2004. [Contribution of unvaccinated siblings to a measles outbreak in Switzerland]. *Rev Epidemiol Sante Publique* **52**:493-501.

1862. Delarocque-Astagneau, E. 2001. Epidemic of hepatitis A among homosexual men in Paris, 2000. *Eurosurveillance* **46**:6-8.

1863. Delarocque-Astagneau, E., N. Baffoy, V. Thiers, N. Simon, H. de Valk, S. Laperche, A. M. Courouce, P. Astagneau, C. Buisson, and J. C. Desenclos. 2002. Outbreak of hepatitis C virus infection in a hemodialysis unit: potential transmission by the hemodialysis machine? *Infect Control Hosp Epidemiol* **23**:328-34.

1864. Delarocque-Astagneau, E., J. C. Desenclos, P. Bouvet, and P. A. Grimont. 1998. Risk factors for the occurrence of sporadic Salmonella enterica serotype enteritidis infections in children in France: a national case- control study. *Epidemiol Infect* **121**:561-7.

1865. Delgado, O., P. Guevara, S. Silva, E. Belfort, and J. L. Ramirez. 1996. Follow-up of a human accidental infection by Leishmania (Viannia) braziliensis using conventional immunologic techniques and polymerase chain reaction. *Am J Trop Med Hyg* **55**:267-72.

1866. Delhaes, L., B. Bourel, L. Scala, B. Muanza, E. Dutoit, F. Wattel, D. Gosset, D. Camus, and E. Dei-Cas. 2001. Case report: recovery of Calliphora vicinia first-instar larvae from a human traumatic wound associated with a progressive necrotizing bacterial infection. *Am J Trop Med Hyg* **64**:159-61.

1867. Delmont, J., P. Brouqui, P. Poullin, and A. Bourgeaade. 1994. Harbour-acquired Plasmodium falciparum malaria. *Lancet* **344**:330-1.

1868. Delpech, V., J. McAnulty, and K. Morgan. 1998. A salmonellosis outbreak linked to internally contaminated pork meat. *Aust N Z J Public Health* **22**:243-6.

1869. DeMatteo, D., C. Major, B. Block, R. Coates, M. Fearon, E. Goldberg, S. M. King, M. Millson, M. O'Shaughnessy, and S. E. Read. 1999. Toronto street youth and HIV/AIDS: prevalence, demographics, and risks. *J Adolesc Health* **25**:358-66.

1870. Dembert, M. L., W. B. Lawrence, W. G. Weinberg, D. D. Granger, R. D. Sanderson, P. D. Garst, J. J. Eighmy, and T. E. Wells. 1985. Epidemiology of human rabies post-exposure prophylaxis at the US naval facility, Subic bay, Philippines. *Am J Epidemiol* **75**:1440-1.

1871. Demikhov, V. G., and V. G. Chaitsev. 1995. [Neurologic characteristics of diseases caused by Inkoo and Tahyna viruses]. *Vopr Virusol* **40**:21-5.

1872. Demma, L. J., R. C. Holman, J. H. McQuiston, J. W. Krebs, and D. L. Swerdlow. 2005. Epidemiology of human ehrlichiosis and anaplasmosis in the United States, 2001-2002. *Am J Trop Med Hyg* **73**:400-9.

1873. Demma, L. J., M. S. Traeger, W. L. Nicholson, C. D. Paddock, D. M. Blau, M. E. Eremeeva, G. A. Dasch, M. L. Levin, J. Singleton, Jr., S. R. Zaki, J. E. Cheek, D. L. Swerdlow, and J. H. McQuiston. 2005. Rocky Mountain spotted fever from an unexpected tick vector in Arizona. *N Engl J Med* **353**:587-94.

1874. Demmler, G. J., M. D. Yow, S. A. Spector, S. G. Reis, M. T. Brady, D. C. Anderson, and L. H. Taber. 1987. Nosocomial cytomegalovirus infections within two hospitals caring for infants and children. *J Infect Dis* **156**:9-16.

1875. Den Boer, J. W., A. Van Belkum, F. Vlaspolder, and F. J. M. Van Breukelen. 1998. Legionnaire's disease and saunas. *Lancet* **351**:114.

1876. Den Boer, J. W., E. P. Yzerman, J. Schellekens, K. D. Lettinga, H. C. Boshuizen, J. E. Van Steenbergen, A. Bosman, S. Van Den Hof, H. A. Van Vliet, M. F. Peeters, R. J. Van Ketel, P. Speelman, J. L. Kool, and M. A. Conyn-Van Spaendonck. 2002. A large outbreak of legionnaires' disease at a flower show, The Netherlands, 1999. *Emerg Infect Dis* **8**:37-43.

1877. Deneen, V. C., P. A. Belle-Isle, C. M. Taylor, L. L. Gabriel, J. B. Bender, J. H. Wicklund, C. W. Hedberg, and M. T. Osterholm. 1998. Outbreak of cryptosporidiosis associated with a water sprinkler fountain - Minnesota, 1997. *MMWR* **47**:856-860.

1878. Deneen, V. C., J. M. Hunt, C. R. Paule, R. I. James, R. G. Johnson, M. J. Raymond, and C. W. Hedberg. 2000. The impact of foodborne calicivirus disease: the Minnesota experience. *J Infect Dis* **181 Suppl 2**:S281-3.

1879. Denic, S., J. Abramson, R. Anandakrishnan, M. Krishnamurthy, and H. Dosik. 1988. The first report of familial adult T-cell leukemia lymphoma in the United States. *Am J Hematol* **27**:281-3.

1880. Denis, M., J. Refregier-Petton, M. J. Laisney, G. Ermel, and G. Salvat. 2001. Campylobacter contamination in French chicken production from farm to consumers. Use of a PCR assay for detection and identification of Campylobacter jejuni and Camp. coli. *J Appl Microbiol* **91**:255-67.

1881. Dennehy, P. H., S. M. Nelson, S. Spangenberger, J. S. Noel, S. S. Monroe, and R. I. Glass. 2001. A prospective case-control study of the role of astrovirus in acute diarrhea among hospitalized young children. *J Infect Dis* **184**:10-5.

1882. Denning, D. W. 2001. Chronic forms of pulmonary aspergillosis. *Clin Microbiol Infect* **7**:25-31.

1883. Dennis, D. T., T. V. Inglesby, D. A. Henderson, J. G. Bartlett, M. S. Ascher, E. Eitzen, A. D. Fine, A. M. Friedlander, J. Hauer, M. Layton, S. R. Lillibridge, J. E. McDade, M. T.

Osterholm, T. O'Toole, G. Parker, T. M. Perl, P. K. Russell, and K. Tonat. 2001. Tularemia as a biological weapon: medical and public health management. *JAMA* **285:**2763-73.

1884. Dennis, D. T., R. P. Smith, J. J. Welch, C. G. Chute, B. Anderson, J. L. Herndon, and C. F. von Reyn. 1993. Endemic giardiasis in New Hampshire: a case-control study of environmental risks. *J Infect Dis* **167:**1391-5.

1885. Dentinger, C. M., W. A. Bower, O. V. Nainan, S. M. Cotter, G. Myers, L. M. Dubusky, S. Fowler, E. D. Salehi, and B. P. Bell. 2001. An outbreak of hepatitis A associated with green onions. *J Infect Dis* **183:**1273-6.

1886. Denton, M., and K. G. Kerr. 1998. Microbiological and clinical aspects of infection associated with Stenotrophomonas maltophilia. *Clin Microbiol Rev* **11:**57-80.

1887. Deplazes, P., D. Hegglin, S. Gloor, and T. Romig. 2004. Wilderness in the city: the urbanization of Echinococcus multilocularis. *Trends Parasitol* **20:**77-84.

1888. Deresiewicz, R. L., S. J. Thaler, L. Hsu, and A. A. Zamani. 1997. Clinical and neuroradiographic manifestations of eastern equine encephalitis. *N Engl J Med* **336:**1867-74.

1889. Derlet, R. W., and J. R. Carlson. 2002. An analysis of human pathogens found in horse/mule manure along the John Muir Trail in Kings Canyon and Sequoia and Yosemite National Parks. *Wilderness Environ Med* **13:**113-8.

1890. Des Jarlais, D. C., T. Diaz, T. Perlis, D. Vlahov, C. Maslow, M. Latka, R. Rockwell, V. Edwards, S. R. Friedman, E. Monterroso, I. Williams, and R. S. Garfein. 2003. Variability in the Incidence of Human Immunodeficiency Virus, Hepatitis B Virus, and Hepatitis C Virus Infection among Young Injecting Drug Users in New York City. *Am J Epidemiol* **157:**467-71.

1891. Desenclos, J. C., M. Bourdiol-Razès, B. Rolin, P. Garandeau, P. Chaud, G. Daurat, J. Ducos, F. Jaffredo, V. Thiers, and C. Brechot. 1998. Transmission nosocomiale du VHC documentée lors de l'investigation d'une épidémie hospitalière. *Bull Epidémiol Hebdomadaire* **7:**25-7.

1892. Desenclos, J. C., P. Bouvet, E. Benz-Lemoine, F. Grimont, H. Desqueyroux, I. Rebiere, and P. A. Grimont. 1996. Large outbreak of Salmonella enterica serotype paratyphi B infection caused by a goats' milk cheese, France, 1993: a case finding and epidemiological study. *BMJ* **312:**91-4.

1893. Desenclos, J. C., K. C. Klontz, M. H. Wilder, O. V. Nainan, H. S. Margolis, and R. A. Gunn. 1991. A multistate outbreak of hepatitis A caused by the consumption of raw oysters. *Am J Public Health* **81:**1268-72.

1894. Desenclos, J. C., and L. MacLafferty. 1993. Community wide outbreak of hepatitis A linked to children in day care centres and with increased transmission in young adult men in Florida 1988-9. *J Epidemiol Community Health* **47:**269-73.

1895. Desjeux, P. 2001. The increase in risk factors for leishmaniasis worldwide. *Trans R Soc Trop Med Hyg* **95:**239-243.

1896. Desjeux, P., and J. Alvar. 2002-3. Leishmania/HIV co-infections: epidemiology in Europe. *Ann Trop Med Parasitol* **97 suppl 1:**S3-15.

1897. Desmyter, J., J. W. LeDuc, K. M. Johnson, F. Brasseur, C. Deckers, and C. van Ypersele de Strihou. 1983. Laboratory rat associated outbreak of haemorrhagic fever with renal syndrome due to Hantaan-like virus in Belgium. *Lancet* **2:**1445-8.

1898. Desplaces, N., M. Marinescu, and B. Festy. 1986. Les Yersinia dans les selles et les aliments. *Méd Mal Infect* **4:**193-200.

1899. Despommier, D. 2003. Toxocariasis: clinical aspects, epidemiology, medical ecology, and molecular aspects. *Clin Microbiol Rev* **16:**265-72.

1900. Desvois, L., A. Gregory, T. Ancelle, and J. Dupouy-Camet. 2001. Enquête sur l'incidence de la bothriocéphalose en Haute-Savoie (1993-2000). *Bull Epidémiol Hebdomadaire* **45:**1-4.

1901. Dettenkofer, M., W. Ebner, T. Els, R. Babikir, C. Lucking, K. Pelz, H. Ruden, and F. Daschner. 2001. Surveillance of nosocomial infections in a neurology intensive care unit. *J Neurol* **248:**959-64.

1902. Dettenkofer, M., S. Wenzler-Rottele, R. Babikir, H. Bertz, W. Ebner, E. Meyer, H. Ruden, P. Gastmeier, and F. D. Daschner. 2005. Surveillance of nosocomial sepsis and pneumonia in patients with a bone marrow or peripheral blood stem cell transplant: a multicenter project. *Clin Infect Dis* **40:**926-31.

1903. Deutz, A., K. Fuchs, N. Nowotny, H. Auer, W. Schuller, D. Stunzner, H. Aspock, U. Kerbl, and J. Kofer. 2003. [Seroepidemiological studies of zoonotic infections in hunters—comparative analysis with veterinarians, farmers, and abattoir workers]. *Wien Klin Wochenschr* **115 Suppl 3:**61-7.

1904. Deutz, A., K. Fuchs, W. Schuller, N. Nowotny, H. Auer, H. Aspock, D. Stunzner, U. Kerbl, C. Klement, and J. Kofer. 2003. [Seroepidemiological studies of zoonotic infections in hunters in southeastern Austria—prevalences, risk factors, and preventive methods]. *Berl Munch Tierarztl Wochenschr* **116:**306-11.

1905. Deutz, A., J. Spergser, P. Wagner, R. Rosengarten, and J. Kofer. 2005. [Mycobacterium avium subsp. paratuberculosis in wild animal species and cattle in Styria/Austria]. *Berl Munch Tierarztl Wochenschr* **118:**314-20.

1906. Develoux, M., A. Chegou, A. Prual, and M. Olivar. 1994. Malaria in the oasis of Bilma, Republic of Niger. *Trans R Soc Trop Med Hyg* **88:**644.

1907. Develoux, M., V. Robert, A. Djibo, and L. Monjour. 1992. [Seroepidemiological study of visceral leishmaniasis in school children in the Iferouane oasis (Niger)]. *Bull Soc Pathol Exot* **85:**302-3.

1908. Devera, R., C. Perez, and Y. Ramos. 1998. [Enterobiasis in students from Ciudad Bolivar, Venezuela]. *Bol Chil Parasitol* **53:**14-8.

1909. Devera, R., I. Requena, V. Velasquez, H. Castillo, R. Guevara, M. De Sousa, C. Marin, and M. Silva. 1999. [Balantidiasis in a rural community from Bolivar State, Venezuela]. *Bol Chil Parasitol* **54:**7-12.

1910. Dhanda, V., F. M. Rodrigues, and S. N. Ghosh. 1970. Isolation of Chandipura virus from sandflies in Aurangabad. *Indian J Med Res* **58:**179-80.

1911. Dhar, A. D., A. E. Werchniak, Y. Li, J. B. Brennick, C. S. Goldsmith, R. Kline, I. Damon, and S. N. Klaus. 2004. Tanapox infection in a college student. *N Engl J Med* **350:**361-6.

1912. Di Giulio, D. B., and P. B. Eckburg. 2004. Human monkeypox: an emerging zoonosis. *Lancet Infect Dis* **4:**15-25.

1913. Di Pentima, M. C., L. Y. Hwang, C. M. Skeeter, and M. S. Edwards. 1999. Prevalence of antibody to Trypanosoma cruzi in pregnant Hispanic women in Houston. *Clin Infect Dis* **28:**1281-5.

1914. Di Silverio, A., V. Brazzelli, G. Brandozzi, G. Barbarini, A. Maccabruni, and S. Sacchi. 1991. Prevalence of dermatophytes and yeasts (Candida spp., Malassezia furfur) in HIV patients. A study of former drug addicts. *Mycopathologia* **114**:103-7.

1915. Diallo, D. A., S. N. Cousens, N. Cuzin-Ouattara, I. Nebie, E. Ilboudo-Sanogo, and F. Esposito. 2004. Child mortality in a West African population protected with insecticide-treated curtains for a period of up to 6 years. *Bull WHO* **83**:85-91.

1916. Diallo, M., P. Nabeth, K. Ba, A. A. Sall, Y. Ba, M. Mondo, L. Girault, M. O. Abdalahi, and C. Mathiot. 2005. Mosquito vectors of the 1998-1999 outbreak of Rift Valley Fever and other arboviruses (Bagaza, Sanar, Wesselsbron and West Nile) in Mauritania and Senegal. *Med Vet Entomol* **19**:119-26.

1917. Diallo, M., J. Thonnon, M. Traore-Lamizana, and D. Fontenille. 1999. Vectors of Chikungunya virus in Senegal: current data and transmission cycles. *Am J Trop Med Hyg* **60**:281-6.

1918. Diamond, C., C. Speck, M. L. Huang, L. Corey, R. W. Coombs, and J. N. Krieger. 2000. Comparison of assays to detect cytomegalovirus shedding in the semen of HIV-infected men. *J Virol Methods* **90**:185-91.

1919. Dias, J. C. 1993. [The clinical, social and occupational aspects of Chagas disease in an endemic area under the control of the state of Minas Gerais, Brazil]. *Rev Soc Bras Med Trop* **26**:93-9.

1920. Diaz Camacho, S. P., K. Willms, C. de la Cruz Otero Mdel, M. L. Zazueta Ramos, S. Bayliss Gaxiola, R. Castro Velazquez, I. Osuna Ramirez, A. Bojorquez Contreras, E. H. Torres Montoya, and S. Sanchez Gonzales. 2003. Acute outbreak of gnathostomiasis in a fishing community in Sinaloa, Mexico. *Parasitol Int* **52**:133-40.

1921. Diaz, R., R. I. Gomez, N. Garcia, J. A. Valdivia, and D. van Soolingen. 2001. Molecular epidemiological study on transmission of tuberculosis in a hospital for mentally handicapped patients in Havana, Cuba. *J Hosp Infect* **49**:30-6.

1922. DiCarlo, R. P., B. S. Armentor, and D. H. Martin. 1995. Chancroid epidemiology in New Orleans men. *J Infect Dis* **172**:446-52.

1923. Dick, T. A., P. A. Nelson, and A. Choudhury. 2001. Diphyllobothriasis: update on human cases, foci, patterns and sources of human infections and future considerations. *Southeast Asian J Trop Med Public Health* **32 Suppl 2**:59-76.

1924. Didier, E. S., M. E. Stovall, L. C. Green, P. J. Brindley, K. Sestak, and P. J. Didier. 2004. Epidemiology of microsporidiosis: sources and modes of transmission. *Vet Parasitol* **126**:145-66.

1925. Diel, R., S. Rusch-Gerdes, and S. Niemann. 2004. Molecular epidemiology of tuberculosis among immigrants in Hamburg, Germany. *J Clin Microbiol* **42**:2952-60.

1926. Dienstag, J. L., F. M. Davenport, R. W. McCollum, A. V. Hennessy, G. Klatskin, and R. H. Purcell. 1976. Nonhuman primate-associated viral hepatitis type A. Serologic evidence of hepatitis A virus infection. *JAMA* **236**:462-4.

1927. Dierick, K., E. Van Coillie, I. Swiecicka, G. Meyfroidt, H. Devlieger, A. Meulemans, G. Hoedemaekers, L. Fourie, M. Heyndrickx, and J. Mahillon. 2005. Fatal Family Outbreak of Bacillus cereus-Associated Food Poisoning. *J Clin Microbiol* **43**:4277-9.

1928. Dierksen, K. P., M. Inglis, and J. R. Tagg. 2000. High pharyngeal carriage rates of Streptococcus pyogenes in Dunedin school children with a low incidence of rheumatic fever. *N Z Med J* **113**:496-9.

1929. DiGiacomo, R. F., and M. E. Thouless. 1986. Epidemiology of naturally occurring rotavirus infection in rabbits. *Lab Anim Sci* **36**:153-6.

1930. Digoutte, J. P., H. Plassart, J. J. Salaun, G. Heme, L. Ferrara, and M. Germain. 1981. A propos de trois cas de fièvre jaune contractée au Sénégal. *Bull WHO* **59**:759-66.

1931. Dille, J. H. 1999. A worksite influenza immunization program. Impact on lost work days, health care utilization, and health care spending. *Am Assoc Occupational Health Nurses J* **47**:301-9.

1932. Dinesh, D. S., A. Ranjan, A. Palit, K. Kishore, and S. K. Kar. 2001. Seasonal and nocturnal landing/biting behaviour of Phlebotomus argentipes (Diptera: Psychodidae). *Ann Trop Med Parasitol* **95**:197-202.

1933. Dinkel, A., E. M. Njoroge, A. Zimmermann, M. Walz, E. Zeyhle, I. E. Elmahdi, U. Mackenstedt, and T. Romig. 2004. A PCR system for detection of species and genotypes of the Echinococcus granulosus-complex, with reference to the epidemiological situation in eastern Africa. *Int J Parasitol* **34**:645-53.

1934. Dionisio, D., F. Esperti, A. Vivarelli, and M. Valassina. 2003. Epidemiological, clinical and laboratory aspects of sandfly fever. *Curr Opin Infect Dis* **16**:383-8.

1935. Dionisio, D., M. Santucci, C. E. Comin, S. Di Lollo, A. Orsi, M. Gabbrielli, D. Milo, P. G. Rogasi, M. Meli, and S. Vigano. 1992. [Isosporiasis and sarcocystosis. The current findings]. *Recent Prog Med* **83**:719-25.

1936. Diosque, P., A. M. Padilla, R. O. Cimino, R. M. Cardozo, O. S. Negrette, J. D. Marco, R. Zacca, C. Meza, A. Juarez, H. Rojo, R. Rey, R. M. Corrales, J. R. Nasser, and M. A. Basombrio. 2004. Chagas disease in rural areas of Chaco Province, Argentina: epidemiologic survey in humans, reservoirs, and vectors. *Am J Trop Med Hyg* **71**:590-3.

1937. Dipersio, J. R., L. M. Deshpande, D. J. Biedenbach, M. A. Toleman, T. R. Walsh, and R. N. Jones. 2005. Evolution and dissemination of extended-spectrum beta-lactamase-producing Klebsiella pneumoniae: Epidemiology and molecular report from the SENTRY Antimicrobial Surveillance Program (1997-2003). *Diagn Microbiol Infect Dis* **51**:1-7.

1938. Dippold, L., R. Lee, C. Selman, S. Monroe, and C. Henry. 2003. A gastroenteritis outbreak due to norovirus associated with a Colorado hotel. *J Environ Health* **66**:13-7, 26; quiz 27-8.

1939. Dire, D. J., D. E. Hogan, and M. W. Riggs. 1994. A prospective evaluation of risk factors for infections from dog-bite wounds. *Acad Emerg Med* **1**:258-66.

1940. Dissanayake, S. 2001. In Wuchereria bancrofti filariasis, asymptomatic microfilaraemia does not progress to amicrofilaraemic lymphatic disease. *Int J Epidemiol* **30**:394-9.

1941. Dissanayake, S. 2004. Relative lack of clinical disease among household contacts of tuberculosis patients compared to leprosy households. *Trans R Soc Trop Med Hyg* **98**:156-64.

1942. Ditmars, D. M., Jr., and P. Maguina. 1998. Neck skin sporotrichosis after electrolysis. *Plast Reconstr Surg* **101**:504-6.

1943. Dittmann, S., M. Wharton, C. Vitek, M. Ciotti, A. Galazka, S. Guichard, I. Hardy, U. Kartoglu, S. Koyama, J. Kreysler, B. Martin, D. Mercer, T. Ronne, C. Roure, R. Steinglass, P. Strebel, R. Sutter, and M. Trostle. 2000. Successful control of epidemic diphtheria in the states of the Former Union of Soviet Socialist Republics: lessons learned. *J Infect Dis* **181 Suppl 1**:S10-22.

1944. Divizia, M., C. Gnesivo, R. Amore Bonapasta, G. Morace, G. Pisani, and A. Pana. 1993. Hepatitis A virus identification in an outbreak by enzymatic amplification. *Eur J Epidemiol* **9**:203-8.

1945. **Dixon, D. M., I. F. Salkin, R. A. Duncan, N. J. Hurd, J. H. Haines, M. E. Kemna, and F. B. Coles.** 1991. Isolation and characterization of Sporothrix schenckii from clinical and environmental sources associated with the largest U.S. epidemic of sporotrichosis. *J Clin Microbiol* **29:**1106-13.

1946. **Dixon, K. E., C. H. Llewellyn, A. P. A. Travassos da Rosa, and J. F. Travassos da Rosa.** 1981. A multidisciplinary program of infectious disease surveillance along the transamazon highway in Brazil: epidemiology of arbovirus infections. *Bull Pan Am Health Organ* **15:**11-25.

1947. **Dixon, K. E., R. N. Nang, D. H. Kim, Y. J. Hwang, J. W. Park, J. W. Huh, and Y. K. Cho.** 1996. A hospital-based, case-control study of risk factors for hemorrhagic fever with renal syndrome in soldiers of the armed forces of the Republic of Korea. *Am J Trop Med Hyg* **54:**284-8.

1948. **Dixon, L., S. Pearson, and D. J. Clutterbuck.** 2002. Chlamydia trachomatis infection and non-gonococcal urethritis in homosexual and heterosexual men in Edinburgh. *Int J STD AIDS* **13:**425-6.

1949. **Dixon, T. C., M. Meselson, J. Guillemin, and P. C. Hanna.** 1999. Anthrax. *N Engl J Med* **341:**815-26.

1950. **Djelantik, I. G. G., B. D. Gessner, S. Soewignjo, M. Steinhoff, A. Sutanto, A. Widjaya, M. Linehan, V. Moniaga, and Ingerani.** 2003. Incidence and clinical features of hospitalization because of respiratory syncytial virus lower respiratory illness among children less than two years of age in a rural Asian setting. *Pediatr Infect Dis J* **22:**150-6.

1951. **Djibo, A., and A. Cenac.** 2000. [Congenital malaria. Parasitological and serological studies in Niamey (Niger)]. *Sante* **10:**183-7.

1952. **Djupesland, P. G., G. Bjune, E. A. Hoiby, J. K. Gronnesby, and R. Mundal.** 1997. Serogroup B meningococcal disease in the Norwegian armed forces. *Eur J Public Health* **7:**261-266.

1953. **Djuretic, T., P. G. Wall, and G. Nichols.** 1997. General outbreaks of infectious intestinal disease associated with milk and dairy products in England and Wales: 1992 to 1996. *Commun Dis Rep CDR Rev* **7:**R41-5.

1954. **Djuretic, T., P. G. Wall, M. J. Ryan, H. S. Evans, G. K. Adak, and J. M. Cowden.** 1996. General outbreaks of infectious intestinal disease in England and Wales 1992 to 1994. *Commun Dis Rep CDR Rev* **6:**R57-63.

1955. **Do, A. N., B. J. Ray, S. N. Banerjee, A. F. Illian, B. J. Barnett, M. H. Pham, K. A. Hendricks, and W. R. Jarvis.** 1999. Bloodstream infection associated with needleless device use and the importance of infection-control practices in the home health care setting. *J Infect Dis* **179:**442-8.

1956. **do Canto, C. L., C. F. Granato, E. Garcez, L. S. Villas Boas, M. C. Fink, M. P. Estevam, and C. S. Pannuti.** 2000. Cytomegalovirus infection in children with Down syndrome in a day-care center in Brazil. *Rev Inst Med Trop Sao Paulo* **42:**179-83.

1957. **Do Carmo, L. S., C. Cummings, V. R. Linardi, R. S. Dias, J. M. De Souza, M. J. De Sena, D. A. Dos Santos, J. W. Shupp, R. K. Pereira, and M. Jett.** 2004. A case study of a massive staphylococcal food poisoning incident. *Foodborne Pathog Dis* **1:**241-6.

1958. **do Nascimento, S. M., R. H. dos Fernandes Vieira, G. N. Theophilo, D. Dos Prazeres Rodrigues, and G. H. Vieira.** 2001. Vibrio vulnificus as a health hazard for shrimp consumers. *Rev Inst Med Trop Sao Paulo* **43:**263-6.

1959. **Dobos, K. M., F. d. Quinn, D. A. Ashford, C. R. Horsburgh, and C. H. King.** 1999. Emergence of a unique group of necrotizing mycobacterial diseases. *Emerg Infect Dis* **5:**367-78.

1960. **Dobroszycki, J., B. L. Herwaldt, F. Boctor, J. R. Miller, J. Linden, M. L. Eberhard, J. J. Yoon, N. M. Ali, H. B. Tanowitz, F. Graham, L. M. Weiss, and M. Wittner.** 1999. A cluster of transfusion-associated babesiosis cases traced to a single asymptomatic donor. *JAMA* **281:**927-30.

1961. **Dodd, L. G.** 1991. Balantidium coli infestation as a cause of acute appendicitis. *J Infect Dis* **163:**1392.

1962. **Dodd, R. Y., E. P. t. Notari, and S. L. Stramer.** 2002. Current prevalence and incidence of infectious disease markers and estimated window-period risk in the American Red Cross blood donor population. *Transfusion* **42:**975-9.

1963. **Dodhia, H., J. Kearney, and F. Warburton.** 1998. A birthday party, home-made ice cream, and an outbreak of Salmonella enteritidis phage type 6 infection. *Commun Dis Public Health* **1:**31-4.

1964. **Doherty, J. F., N. Price, A. H. Moody, S. G. Wright, and M. J. Glynn.** 1995. Fascioliasis due to imported khat. *Lancet* **345:**462.

1965. **Doherty, L., K. A. Fenton, J. Jones, T. C. Paine, S. P. Higgins, D. Williams, and A. Palfreeman.** 2002. Syphilis: old problem, new strategy. *BMJ* **325:**153-6.

1966. **Doit, C., C. Loukil, A. M. Simon, A. Ferroni, J. E. Fontan, S. Bonacorsi, P. Bidet, V. Jarlier, Y. Aujard, F. Beaufils, and E. Bingen.** 2004. Outbreak of Burkholderia cepacia bacteremia in a pediatric hospital due to contamination of lipid emulsion stoppers. *J Clin Microbiol* **42:**2227-30.

1967. **Doleans, A., H. Aurell, M. Reyrolle, G. Lina, J. Freney, F. Vandenesch, J. Etienne, and S. Jarraud.** 2004. Clinical and environmental distributions of Legionella strains in France are different. *J Clin Microbiol* **42:**458-60.

1968. **Doll, J. M., P. S. Zeitz, P. Ettestad, A. L. Bucholtz, T. Davis, and K. Gage.** 1994. Cat-transmitted fatal pneumonic plague in a person who traveled from Colorato to Arizona. *Am J Trop Med Hyg* **51:**109-14.

1969. **Doller, P. C., K. Dietrich, N. Filipp, S. Brockmann, C. Dreweck, R. Vonthein, C. Wagner-Wiening, and A. Wiedenmann.** 2002. Cyclosporiasis outbreak in Germany associated with the consumption of salad. *Emerg Infect Dis* **8:**992-4.

1970. **Dolo, G., O. J. Briet, A. Dao, S. F. Traore, M. Bouare, N. Sogoba, O. Niare, M. Bagayogo, D. Sangare, T. Teuscher, and Y. T. Toure.** 2004. Malaria transmission in relation to rice cultivation in the irrigated Sahel of Mali. *Acta Trop* **89:**147-59.

1971. **Domergue Than Trong, E., V. Descamps, E. Larger, M. Grossin, S. Belaich, and B. Crickx.** 2001. [Mycobacterium kansasii skin infection at insulin injection sites]. *Ann Dermatol Venereol* **128:**250-2.

1972. **Domingues, D., L. T. Tavira, A. Duarte, A. Sanca, E. Prieto, and F. Exposto.** 2002. Ureaplasma urealyticum biovar determination in women attending a family planning clinic in Guine-Bissau, using polymerase chain reaction of the multiple-banded antigen gene. *J Clin Lab Anal* **16:**71-5.

1973. **Domingues, R. B., M. R. Muniz, M. L. G. Jorge, M. S. Mayo, A. Saez-Alquezar, D. F. Chamone, M. Scaff, and P. E. Marchiori.** 1997. Human T cell lymphotropic virus type-1-associated myelopathy/tropical spastic paraparesis in Sao Paulo, Brazil: association with blood transfusion. *Am J Trop Med Hyg* **57:**56-9.

1974. Domínguez, A., N. Cardeñosa, C. Izquierdo, F. Sánchez, N. Margall, J. A. Vazquez, and L. Salleras. 2001. Prevalence of Neisseria meningitidis carriers in school population of Catalonia, Spain. *Epidemiol Infect* **127:**425-33.

1975. Donahue, J. G., P. W. Choo, J. E. Manson, and R. Platt. 1995. The incidence of herpes zoster. *Arch Intern Med* **155:**1605-9.

1976. Donaldson, A. I. 1997. Risks of spreading foot and mouth disease through milk and dairy products. *Rev Sci Tech* **16:**117-24.

1977. Dondorp, A. M., P. N. Newton, M. Mayxay, W. Van Damme, F. M. Smithuis, S. Yeung, A. Petit, A. J. Lynam, A. Johnson, T. T. Hien, R. McGready, J. J. Farrar, S. Looareesuwan, N. P. Day, M. D. Green, and N. J. White. 2004. Fake antimalarials in Southeast Asia are a major impediment to malaria control: multinational cross-sectional survey on the prevalence of fake antimalarials. *Trop Med Int Health* **9:**1241-6.

1978. Donnelly, C. A., A. C. Ghani, G. M. Leung, A. J. Hedley, C. Fraser, S. Riley, L. J. Abu-Raddad, L. M. Ho, T. Q. Thach, P. Chau, K. P. Chan, T. H. Lam, L. Y. Tse, T. Tsang, S. H. Liu, J. H. Kong, E. M. Lau, N. M. Ferguson, and R. M. Anderson. 2003. Epidemiological determinants of spread of causal agent of severe acute respiratory syndrome in Hong Kong. *Lancet* **361:**1761-66.

1979. Donnio, P. Y., C. Le Goff, J. L. Avril, P. Pouedras, and S. Gras-Rouzet. 1994. Pasteurella multocida: oropharyngeal carriage and antibody response in breeders. *Vet Res* **25:**8-15.

1980. Donohoe, M. 2003. Causes and health consequences of environmental degradation and social injustice. *Soc Sci Med* **56:**573-87.

1981. Donovan, B. 2002. Rising prevalence of genital Chlamydia trachomatis infection in heterosexual patients at the Sydney sexual health center, 1994-2000. *Commun Dis Intell* **26:**51-4.

1982. Donovan, B. 2004. Sexually transmissible infections other than HIV. *Lancet* **363:**545-56.

1983. Donovan, B., N. J. Bodsworth, R. Rohrsheim, A. McNulty, and J. W. Tapsall. 2001. Characteristics of homosexually-active men with gonorrhoea during an epidemic in Sydney, Australia. *Int J STD AIDS* **12:**437-43.

1984. Donovan, S. M., N. Mickiewicz, R. D. Meyer, and C. B. Panosian. 1995. Imported echinococcosis in southern California. *Am J Trop Med Hyg* **53:**668-71.

1985. Donowitz, L. G., F. J. Marsik, K. A. Fisher, and R. P. Wenzel. 1981. Contaminated breast milk: A source of Klebsiella bacteremia in a newborn intensive care unit. *Rev Infect Dis* **3:**716-20.

1986. Donskey, C. J., T. K. Chowdhry, M. T. Hecker, C. K. Hoyen, J. A. Hanrahan, A. M. Hujer, R. A. Hutton-Thomas, C. C. Whalen, R. A. Bonomo, and L. B. Rice. 2000. Effect of antibiotic therapy on the density of vancomycin-resistant enterococci in the stool of colonized patients. *N Engl J Med* **343:**1925-32.

1987. Dooley, D. P. 2005. History of U.S. military contributions to the study of viral hepatitis. *Mil Med* **170:**71-6.

1988. Dooley, D. P., P. S. Bostic, and M. L. Beckius. 1997. Spook house sporotrichosis. A point-source outbreak of sporotrichosis associated with hay bale props in a Halloween haunted-house. *Arch Intern Med* **157:**1885-7.

1989. Dooley, S. W., M. E. Villarino, M. Lawrence, L. Salinas, S. Amil, J. V. Rullan, W. R. Jarvis, A. B. Bloch, and G. M. Cauthen. 1992. Nosocomial transmission of tuberculosis in a hospital unit for HIV- infected patients. *JAMA* **267:**2632-4.

1990. Dopirak, M., C. Hill, M. Oleksiw, D. Dumigan, J. Arvai, E. English, E. Carusillo, S. Malo-Schlegel, J. Richo, K. Traficanti, B. Welch, and B. Cooper. 2002. Surveillance of hemodialysis-associated primary bloodstream infections: the experience of ten hospital-based centers. *Infect Control Hosp Epidemiol* **23:**721-4.

1991. Doran, T. I. 1999. The role of Citrobacter in clinical disease of children: review. *Clin Infect Dis* **28:**384-94.

1992. Dore, G. J., Y. Li, A. McDonald, and J. M. Kaldor. 2001. Spectrum of AIDS-defining illnesses in Australia, 1992 to 1998: influence of country/region of birth. *J Acquir Immune Defic Syndr* **26:**283-90.

1993. Dore, K., J. Buxton, B. Henry, F. Pollari, D. Middleton, M. Fyfe, R. Ahmed, P. Michel, A. King, C. Tinga, and J. B. Wilson. 2004. Risk factors for Salmonella typhimurium DT104 and non-DT104 infection: a Canadian multi-provincial case-control study. *Epidemiol Infect* **132:**485-93.

1994. Dorigo-Zetsma, J. W., B. Wilbrink, H. van der Nat, A. I. Bartelds, M. L. Heijnen, and J. Dankert. 2001. Results of molecular detection of Mycoplasma pneumoniae among patients with acute respiratory infection and in their household contacts reveals children as human reservoirs. *J Infect Dis* **183:**675-8.

1995. Dorko, E., S. Viragova, E. Pilipcinec, and L. Tkacikova. 2003. Candida—agent of the diaper dermatitis? *Folia Microbiol (Praha)* **48:**385-8.

1996. Dorny, P., N. Speybroeck, S. Verstraete, M. Baeke, A. De Becker, D. Berkvens, and J. Vercruysse. 2002. Serological survey of Toxoplasma gondii, feline immunodeficiency virus and feline leukaemia virus in urban stray cats in Belgium. *Vet Rec* **151:**626-9.

1997. Dorny, P., F. Vercammen, J. Brandt, W. Vansteenkiste, D. Berkvens, and S. Geerts. 2000. Sero-epidemiological study of Taenia saginata cysticercosis in Belgian cattle. *Vet Parasitol* **88:**43-9.

1998. Dorsch, M. M., A. S. Cameron, and B. S. Robinson. 1983. The epidemiology and control of primary amoebic meningoencephalitis with particular reference to South Australia. *Trans R Soc Trop Med Hyg* **77:**372-7.

1999. Dosluoglu, H. H., G. R. Curl, R. J. Doerr, F. Painton, and S. Shenoy. 2001. Stent-related iliac artery and iliac vein infections: two unreported presentations and review of the literature. *J Endovasc Ther* **8:**202-9.

2000. Douba, M., A. Mowakeh, and A. Wali. 1997. Current status of cutaneous leishmaniasis in Aleppo, Syrian Arab republic. *Bull WHO* **75:**253-9.

2001. Doubt, J., and E. M. Wallace. 1984. Scabies outbreak in a nursing home - Ontario. *Can Dis Weekly Rep* **10:**5-6.

2002. Douglas, M. W., G. Lum, J. Roy, D. A. Fisher, N. M. Anstey, and B. J. Currie. 2004. Epidemiology of community-acquired and nosocomial bloodstream infections in tropical Australia: a 12-month prospective study. *Trop Med Int Health* **9:**795-804.

2003. Douglas, M. W., K. Mulholland, V. Denyer, and T. Gottlieb. 2001. Multi-drug resistant Pseudomonas aeruginosa outbreak in a burns unit - an infection control study. *Burns* **27:**131-5.

2004. Douglas, M. W., J. L. Walters, and B. J. Currie. 2002. Occupational infection with herpes simplex virus type 1 after a needlestick injury. *Med J Aust* **176:**240.

2005. **Douglass, R. J., A. J. Kuenzi, C. Y. Williams, S. J. Douglass, and J. N. Mills.** 2003. Removing deer mice from buildings and the risk for human exposure to sin nombre virus. *Emerg Infect Dis* **9**:390-2.

2006. **Dounias, G., E. Kypraiou, G. Rachiotis, E. Tsovili, and S. Kostopoulos.** 2005. Prevalence of hepatitis B virus markers in municipal solid waste workers in Keratsini (Greece). *Occup Med (Lond)* **55**:60-3.

2007. **Douvin, C., D. Simon, H. Zinelabidine, V. Wirquin, L. Perlemuter, and D. Dhumeaux.** 1990. An outbreak of hepatitis B in an endocrinology unit traced to a capillary-blood-sampling device. *N Engl J Med* **322**:57-8.

2008. **Dowd, S. E., D. John, J. Eliopolus, C. P. Gerba, J. Naranjo, R. Klein, B. Lopez, M. de Mejia, C. E. Mendoza, and I. L. Pepper.** 2003. Confirmed detection of Cyclospora cayetanesis, Encephalitozoon intestinalis and Cryptosporidium parvum in water used for drinking. *J Water Health* **1**:117-23.

2009. **Dowell, S. F., C. Groves, K. B. Kirkland, H. G. Cicirello, T. Ando, Q. Jin, J. R. Gentsch, S. S. Monroe, C. D. Humphrey, C. Slemp, et al.** 1995. A multistate outbreak of oyster-associated gastroenteritis: implications for interstate tracing of contaminated shellfish. *J Infect Dis* **171**:1497-503.

2010. **Dowell, S. F., R. Mukunu, T. G. Ksiazek, A. S. Khan, P. E. Rollin, and C. J. Peters.** 1999. Transmission of Ebola hemorrhagic fever: a study of risk factors in family members, Kikwit, Democratic Republic of the Congo, 1995. Commission de Lutte contre les Epidemies a Kikwit. *J Infect Dis* **179 Suppl 1**:S87-91.

2011. **Dowell, S. F., T. J. Torok, J. A. Thorp, J. Hedrick, D. D. Erdman, S. R. Zaki, C. J. Hinkle, W. L. Bayer, and L. J. Anderson.** 1995. Parvovirus B19 infection in hospital workers: community or hospital acquisition? *J Infect Dis* **172**:1076-9.

2012. **Dowell, S. F., C. G. Whitney, C. E. Wright, C. E. Rose, Jr., and A. Schuchat.** 2003. Seasonal patterns of invasive pneumococcal disease. *Emerg Infect Dis* **9**:573-9.

2013. **Downdall, N.** 2000. "Is there a doctor on the aircraft?" Top 10 in-flight medical emergencies. *BMJ* **321**:1336—7.

2014. **Downs, A. M., I. Harvey, and C. T. Kennedy.** 1999. The epidemiology of head lice and scabies in the UK. *Epidemiol Infect* **122**:471-7.

2015. **Dowse, G.** 2000. Case report: murine typhus acquired in Bali. *Commun Dis Intell* **24**:394.

2016. **Dowsett, S. A., L. Archila, V. A. Segreto, C. R. Gonzalez, A. Silva, K. A. Vastola, R. D. Bartizek, and M. J. Kowolik.** 1999. Helicobacter pylori infection in indigenous families of Central America: serostatus and oral and fingernail carriage. *J Clin Microbiol* **37**:2456-60.

2017. **Doyle, A., D. Barataud, A. Gallay, J. M. Thiolet, S. Le Guyaguer, E. Kohli, and V. Vaillant.** 2004. Norovirus foodborne outbreaks associated with the consumption of oysters from the Etang de Thau, France, December 2002. *Eur Surveill* **9**:24–26.

2018. **Doyle, M. P., and J. L. Schoeni.** 1987. Isolation of Escherichia coli O157:H7 from retail fresh meats and poultry. *Appl Environ Microbiol* **53**:2394-6.

2019. **Doyle, T. J., and R. T. Bryan.** 2000. Infectious disease morbidity in the US region bordering Mexico, 1990-1998. *J Infect Dis* **182**:1503-10.

2020. **Drabick, J. J.** 1987. Pentastomiasis. *Rev Infect Dis* **9**:1087-94.

2021. **Draganescu, N., M. Duca, E. Girjabu, I. Popescu-Pretor, S. Raducanu, L. Deleanu, and E. Totescu.** 1977. Epidemic outbreak caused by West Nile virus in the crew of a Romanian cargo ship passing the Suez Canal and the Red Sea on route to Yokohama. *Virologie* **28**:259-62.

2022. **Dragon, D. C., D. E. Bader, J. Mitchell, and N. Woollen.** 2005. Natural dissemination of Bacillus anthracis spores in northern Canada. *Appl Environ Microbiol* **71**:1610-5.

2023. **Drakeley, C., D. Schellenberg, J. Kihonda, C. A. Sousa, A. P. Arez, D. Lopes, J. Lines, H. Mshinda, C. Lengeler, J. A. Schellenberg, M. Tanner, and P. Alonso.** 2003. An estimation of the entomological inoculation rate for Ifakara: a semi-urban area in a region of intense malaria transmission in Tanzania. *Trop Med Int Health* **8**:767-774.

2024. **Drew, W. L.** 1993. Cytomegalovirus as a sexually transmitted disease, p. 92-100. *In* Y. Becker and E. S. Huang (ed.), Molecular aspects of human cytomegalovirus disease. Springer-Verlag, Berlin.

2025. **Dreyer, G., A. Santos, J. Noroes, A. Rocha, and D. Addiss.** 1996. Amicrofilaraemic carriers of adult Wuchereria bancrofti. *Trans R Soc Trop Med Hyg* **90**:288-9.

2026. **Drinka, P., J. T. Faulks, C. Gauerke, B. Goodman, M. Stemper, and K. Reed.** 2001. Adverse events associated with methicillin-resistant Staphylococcus aureus in a nursing home. *Arch Intern Med* **161**:2371-7.

2027. **Drinka, P. J., S. Gravenstein, M. Schilling, P. Krause, B. A. Miller, and P. Shult.** 1998. Duration of antiviral prophylaxis during nursing home outbreaks of influenza A: a comparison of 2 protocols. *Arch Intern Med* **158**:2155-9.

2028. **Drinka, P. J., P. Krause, L. Nest, B. M. Goodman, and S. Gravenstein.** 2003. Risk of acquiring influenza A in a nursing home from a culture-positive roommate. *Infect Control Hosp Epidemiol* **24**:872-4.

2029. **Driver, C. R., J. S. Jones, L. Cavitt, B. J. Weathers, S. E. Valway, and I. M. Onorato.** 1995. Tuberculosis in a day-care center, Kentucky, 1993. *Pediatr Infect Dis J* **14**:612-6.

2030. **Driver, C. R., S. E. Valway, W. M. Morgan, I. M. Onorato, and K. G. Castro.** 1994. Transmission of Mycobacterium tuberculosis associated with air travel. *JAMA* **272**:1031-5.

2031. **Drobeniuc, J., M. O. Favorov, C. N. Shapiro, B. P. Bell, E. E. Mast, A. Dadu, D. Culver, P. Iarovoi, B. H. Robertson, and H. S. Margolis.** 2001. Hepatitis E virus antibody prevalence among persons who work with swine. *J Infect Dis* **184**:1594-7.

2032. **Drobniewski, F.** 1995. Tuberculosis in prisons - forgotten plague. *Lancet* **346**:948-9.

2033. **Drobniewski, F., Y. Balabanova, V. Nikolayevsky, M. Ruddy, S. Kuznetzov, S. Zakharova, A. Melentyev, and I. Fedorin.** 2005. Drug-resistant tuberculosis, clinical virulence, and the dominance of the Beijing strain family in Russia. *JAMA* **293**:2726-31.

2034. **Drobniewski, F., E. Tayler, N. Ignatenko, J. Paul, M. Connolly, P. Nye, T. Lyagoshina, and C. Besse.** 1996. Tuberculosis in Siberia: 1. An epidemiological and microbiological assessment. *Tuber Lung Dis* **77**:199-206.

2035. **Drolet, M. J., R. Boisvert, S. Dery, and D. Laliberte.** 1999. [Epidemiological study of a tuberculosis case in a large manufacturing enterprise in Quebec]. *Can J Public Health* **90**:156-9.

2036. **Dromer, F., S. Mathoulin, B. Dupont, and A. Laporte.** 1996. Epidemiology of cryptococcosis in France: a 9-year survey (1985-1993). French Cryptococcosis Study Group. *Clin Infect Dis* **23**:82-90.

2037. Drosten, C., B. M. Kummerer, H. Schmitz, and S. Gunther. 2003. Molecular diagnostics of viral hemorrhagic fevers. *Antiviral Res* **57**:61-87.

2038. Drouet, E., A. Boibieux, S. Michelson, R. Ecochard, F. Biron, D. Peyramond, R. Colimon, and G. Denoyel. 1993. Polymerase chain reaction detection of cytomegalovirus DNA in peripheral blood leukocytes as a predictor of cytomegalovirus disease in HIV-infected patients. *AIDS* **7**:665-8.

2039. Drucker, E., P. G. Alcabes, and P. A. Marx. 2001. The injection century: massive unsterile injections and the mergence of human pathogens. *Lancet* **358**:1989-1992.

2040. Druilhe, P., J. F. Trape, J. P. Leroy, C. Godard, and M. Gentilini. 1980. [Two accidental human infections by Plasmodium cynomolgi bastianellii. A clinical and serological study]. *Ann Soc Belg Med Trop* **60**:349-54.

2041. Drusin, L. M., B. G. Ross, K. H. Rhodes, A. N. Krauss, and R. A. Scott. 2000. Nosocomial ringworm in a neonatal intensive care unit: a nurse and her cat. *Infect Control Hosp Epidemiol* **21**:605-7.

2042. du Moulin, G. C., K. D. Stottmeier, P. A. Pelletier, A. Y. Tsang, and J. Hedley-Whyte. 1988. Concentration of Mycobacterium avium by hospital hot water systems. *JAMA* **260**:1599-601.

2043. Dua, V. K., N. Nanda, N. C. Gupta, P. K. Kar, S. K. Subbarao, and V. P. Sharma. 2000. Investigation of malaria prevalence at National Thermal Power Corporation, Shaktinagar, Sonbhadra District (Uttar Pradesh), India. *Southeast Asian J Trop Med Public Health* **31**:818-24.

2044. Duany, R., M. A. Cruz, S. Atherley, J. A. Suarez, V. Sneller, L. Vaamonde, K. Mavunda, E. Sfakianaki, E. Jennings, R. Sanderson, D. J. Katz, R. Hopkins, P. Fiorella, and W. G. Hlady. 1998. Outbreaks of group B meningococcal disease - Florida, 1995 and 1997. *MMWR* **47**:833-837.

2045. Duarte, E. C., and C. J. Fontes. 2002. [Association between reported annual gold mining extraction and incidence of malaria in Mato Grosso-Brazil, 1985-1996]. *Rev Soc Bras Med Trop* **35**:665-8.

2046. Duarte, E. C., T. W. Gyorkos, L. Pang, and M. Abrahamowicz. 2004. Epidemiology of malaria in a hypoendemic Brazilian Amazon migrant population: a cohort study. *Am J Trop Med Hyg* **70**:229-37.

2047. Dubey, J. P. 1994. Toxoplasmosis. *J Am Vet Med Assoc* **205**:1593-8.

2048. Dubey, J. P. 2000. Sources of Toxoplasma gondii infection in pregnancy. *BMJ* **321**:127-8.

2049. Dubey, J. P., H. R. Gamble, D. Hill, C. Sreekumar, S. Romand, and P. Thuilliez. 2002. High prevalence of viable Toxoplasma gondii infection in market weight pigs from a farm in Massachusetts. *J Parasitol* **88**:1234-8.

2050. Dubey, J. P., E. A. Rollor, K. Smith, O. C. Kwok, and P. Thulliez. 1997. Low seroprevalence of Toxoplasma gondii in feral pigs from a remote island lacking cats. *J Parasitol* **83**:839-41.

2051. Dubey, J. P., W. J. Saville, J. F. Stanek, and S. M. Reed. 2002. Prevalence of Toxoplasma gondii antibodies in domestic cats from rural Ohio. *J Parasitol* **88**:802-3.

2052. Dubey, J. P., P. Thulliez, S. Romand, O. C. Kwok, S. K. Shen, and H. R. Gamble. 1999. Serologic prevalence of Toxoplasma gondii in horses slaughtered for food in North America. *Vet Parasitol* **86**:235-8.

2053. Dubinsky, P., K. Havasiova-Reiterova, B. Petko, I. Hovorka, and O. Tomasovicova. 1995. Role of small mammals in the epidemiology of toxocariasis. *Parasitology* **110 (Pt 2)**:187-93.

2054. Ducrest, V., C. Chuard, and C. Regamey. 2000. [Blastomycosis 30 years after living in Africa]. *Rev Med Suisse Romande* **120**:51-3.

2055. Duenas-Barajas, E., J. E. Bernal, D. R. Vaught, V. R. Nerurkar, P. Sarmiento, R. Yanagihara, and D. C. Gajdusek. 1993. Human retroviruses in Amerindians of Colombia: high prevalence of human T cell lymphotropic virus type II infection among the Tunebo Indians. *Am J Trop Med Hyg* **49**:657-63.

2056. Duffy, E. A., L. M. Lucia, J. M. Kells, A. Castillo, S. D. Pillai, and G. R. Acuff. 2005. Concentrations of Escherichia coli and genetic diversity and antibiotic resistance profiling of Salmonella isolated from irrigation water, packing shed equipment, and fresh produce in Texas. *J Food Prot* **68**:70-9.

2057. Duffy, P., J. Wolf, G. Collins, A. G. DeVoe, B. Streeten, and D. Cowen. 1974. Letter: Possible person-to-person transmission of Creutzfeldt-Jakob disease. *N Engl J Med* **290**:692-3.

2058. Duffy, P. E., H. Le Guillouzic, R. F. Gass, and B. L. Innis. 1990. Murine typhus identified as a major cause of febrile illness in a camp for displaced Khmers in Thailand. *Am J Trop Med Hyg* **43**:520-6.

2059. Dufour, A., M. Alary, C. Poulin, F. Allard, L. Noel, G. Trottier, D. Lepine, and C. Hankins. 1996. Prevalence and risk behaviours for HIV infection among inmates of a provincial prison in Quebec City. *AIDS* **10**:1009-15.

2060. Dugan, V. G., S. E. Little, D. E. Stallknecht, and A. D. Beall. 2000. Natural infection of domestic goats with Ehrlichia chaffeensis. *J Clin Microbiol* **38**:448-9.

2061. Duggan, A. J., and M. P. Hutchinson. 1966. Sleeping sickness in Europeans: a review of 109 cases. *J Trop Med Hyg* **69**:124-31.

2062. Duh, D., M. Petrovec, A. Bidovec, and T. Avsic-Zupanc. 2005. Cervics as Babesiae hosts, Slovenia. *Emerg Infect Dis* **11**:1121-3.

2063. Duh, D., M. Petrovec, T. Trilar, and T. Avsic-Zupanc. 2003. The molecular evidence of Babesia microti infection in small mammals collected in Slovenia. *Parasitology* **126**:113-7.

2064. Dukers, N. H., S. M. Bruisten, J. A. van den Hoek, J. B. de Wit, G. J. van Doornum, and R. A. Coutinho. 2000. Strong decline in herpes simplex virus antibodies over time among young homosexual men is associated with changing sexual behavior. *Am J Epidemiol* **152**:666-73.

2065. Dukers, N. H., N. Renwick, M. Prins, R. B. Geskus, T. F. Schulz, G. J. Weverling, R. A. Coutinho, and J. Goudsmit. 2000. Risk factors for human herpesvirus 8 seropositivity and seroconversion in a cohort of homosexual men. *Am J Epidemiol* **151**:213-24.

2066. Dumett, R. 1993. Disease and mortality among gold miners of Ghana: colonial government and mining company attitudes and policies, 1900-1938. *Soc Sci Med* **37**:213-32.

2067. Dumler, J. S., A. F. Barbet, C. P. Bekker, G. A. Dasch, G. H. Palmer, S. C. Ray, Y. Rikihisa, and F. R. Rurangirwa. 2001. Reorganization of genera in the families Rickettsiaceae and Anaplasmataceae in the order Rickettsiales: unification of some species of Ehrlichia with Anaplasma, Cowdria with Ehrlichia and Ehrlichia with Neorickettsia, descriptions of six new species combinations and designation of Ehrlichia equi and 'HGE agent' as subjective synonyms of Ehrlichia phagocytophila. *Int J Syst Evol Microbiol* **51**:2145-65.

2068. **Dumler, J. S., and D. H. Walker.** 2001. Tick-borne ehrlichioses. *Lancet Infect Dis* **April:**21-8.

2069. **Dummer, J. S., S. Erb, M. K. Breinig, M. Ho, C. R. Rinaldo, Jr., P. Gupta, M. V. Ragni, A. Tzakis, L. Makowka, D. Van Thiel, et al.** 1989. Infection with human immunodeficiency virus in the Pittsburgh transplant population. A study of 583 donors and 1043 recipients, 1981-1986. *Transplantation* **47:**134-40.

2070. **Dumontet, S., K. Krovacek, S. B. Svenson, V. Pasquale, S. B. Baloda, and G. Figliuolo.** 2000. Prevalence and diversity of Aeromonas and Vibrio spp. in coastal waters of southern Italy. *Comp Immunol Microbiol Inf Dis* **23:**53-72.

2071. **Dunais, B., C. Pradier, H. Carsenti, M. Sabah, G. Mancini, E. Fontas, and P. Dellamonica.** 2003. Influence of child care on nasopharyngeal carriage of Streptococcus pneumoniae and Haemophilus influenzae. *Pediatr Infect Dis J* **22:**589-92.

2072. **Dunlap, B. G., and M. L. Thies.** 2002. Giardia in beaver (Castor canadensis) and nutria (Myocastor coypus) from east Texas. *J Parasitol* **88:**1254-8.

2073. **Dunn, B. E., H. Cohen, and M. J. Blaser.** 1997. Helicobacter pylori. *Clin Microbiol Rev* **10:**720-41.

2074. **Dunn, J. J., S. T. Columbus, W. E. Aldeen, M. Davis, and K. C. Carroll.** 2002. Trichuris vulpis recovered from a patient with chronic diarrhea and five dogs. *J Clin Microbiol* **40:**2703-4.

2075. **Dunn, R. A., W. N. Hall, J. V. Altamirano, S. E. Dietrich, B. Robinson-Dunn, and D. R. Johnson.** 1995. Outbreak of Shigella flexneri linked to salad prepared at a central commissary in Michigan. *Public Health Rep* **110:**580-6.

2076. **Dunne, E. F., W. J. Burman, and M. L. Wilson.** 1998. Streptomyces pneumonia in a patient with human immunodeficiency virus infection: case report and review of the literature on invasive Streptomyces infections. *Clin Infect Dis* **27:**93-6.

2077. **Dupon, M., A. Lortat-Jacob, N. Desplaces, J. Gaudias, V. Dacquet, H. Carsenti, and P. Dellamonica.** 2001. Secondary prosthetic joint infection: diagnostic criteria, treatment. *Méd Mal Infect* **31:**123-130.

2078. **Dupon, M., A. M. Rogues, M. Malou, C. d'Ivernois, and J. Y. Lacut.** 1992. Scrub typhus: an imported rickettsial disease. *Infection* **20:**153-4.

2079. **DuPont, H. L., E. J. Gangarosa, L. B. Reller, W. E. Woodward, R. W. Armstrong, J. Hammond, K. Glaser, and G. K. Morris.** 1970. Shigellosis in custodial institutions. *Am J Epidemiol* **92:**172-9.

2080. **DuPont, H. L., M. M. Levine, R. B. Hornick, and S. B. Formal.** 1989. Inoculum size in shigellosis and implications for expected mode of transmission. *J Infect Dis* **159:**1126-8.

2081. **DuPont, H. L., and R. Steffen.** 2001. Textbook of travel medicine and health, vol. 2nd ed. BC Decker Inc., London.

2082. **Dupouy-Camet, J.** 2000. Trichinellosis: a worldwide zoonosis. *Vet Parasitol* **93:**191-200.

2083. **Dupouy-Camet, J., T. Ancelle, I. Vicens, M. E. Bougnoux, F. Mougin, and C. Tourte-Schaefer.** 1990. Transmission de la giardiase dans une crèche: analyse des facteurs de risque et controle. *Méd Mal Infect* **20:**197-202.

2084. **Dupouy-Camet, J., and R. Peduzzi.** 2004. Current situation of human diphyllobothriasis in Europe. *Eurosurveillance* **9:**31-5.

2085. **Dupuis, G., J. Petite, O. Peter, and M. Vouilloz.** 1987. An important outbreak of human Q fever in a Swiss Alpine valley. *Int J Epidemiol* **16:**282-7.

2086. **Durand, A. M.** 2004. Scrub typhus in the republic of Palau, Micronesia. *Emerg Infect Dis* **10:**1838-40.

2087. **Durand, B., V. Chevalier, R. Pouillot, J. Labie, I. Marendat, B. Murgue, H. Zeller, and S. Zientara.** 2002. West nile virus outbreak in horses, southern france, 2000: results of a serosurvey. *Emerg Infect Dis* **8:**777-82.

2088. **Durand, J. P., M. Bouloy, L. Richecoeur, C. N. Peyrefitte, and H. Tolou.** 2003. Rift valley fever virus infection among French troops in Chad. *Emerg Infect Dis* **9:**751-2.

2089. **Durand, J. P., L. Richecoeur, C. Peyrefitte, J. P. Boutin, B. Davoust, H. Zeller, M. Bouloy, and H. Tolou.** 2002. La fièvre de la vallée du rift: infections sporadiques de militaires français hors des zones d'épidémies actuellement connues. *Med Trop* **62:**291-4.

2090. **Durante Mangoni, E., C. Severini, M. Menegon, R. Romi, G. Ruggiero, and G. Majori.** 2003. Case report: An unusual late relapse of Plasmodium vivax malaria. *Am J Trop Med Hyg* **68:**159-60.

2091. **Durlach, R. A., F. Kaufer, L. Carral, and J. Hirt.** 2003. Toxoplasmic lymphadenitis—clinical and serologic profile. *Clin Microbiol Infect* **9:**625-31.

2092. **Durrheim, D. N.** 1995. Taxi rank malaria. *BMJ* **311:**1507.

2093. **Durrheim, D. N., L. E. Braack, S. Waner, and S. Gammon.** 1998. Risk of malaria in visitors to the Kruger National Park, South Africa. *J Travel Med* **5:**173-7.

2094. **Durso, L. M., K. Reynolds, N. Bauer, Jr., and J. E. Keen.** 2005. Shiga-toxigenic Escherichia coli O157:H7 infections among livestock exhibitors and visitors at a Texas County Fair. *Vector Borne Zoonotic Dis* **5:**193-201.

2095. **Dusfour, I., R. E. Harbach, and S. Manguin.** 2004. Bionomics and systematics of the oriental Anopheles sundaicus complex in relation to malaria transmission and vector control. *Am J Trop Med Hyg* **71:**518-24.

2096. **Dutly, F., and M. Altwegg.** 2001. Whipple's disease and "Tropheryma whippelii". *Clin Microbiol Rev* **14:**561-83.

2097. **Dutz, W., E. Jennings-Khodadad, C. Post, E. Kohout, I. Nazarian, and H. Esmaili.** 1974. Marasmus and Pneumocystis carinii pneumonia in institutionalised infants. Observations during an endemic. *Z Kinderheilkd* **117:**241-58.

2098. **Duval, X., C. Selton-Suty, F. Alla, M. Salvador-Mazenq, Y. Bernard, M. Weber, F. Lacassin, P. Nazeyrolas, C. Chidiac, B. Hoen, and C. Leport.** 2004. Endocarditis in Patients with a Permanent Pacemaker: A 1-Year Epidemiological Survey on Infective Endocarditis due to Valvular and/or Pacemaker Infection. *Clin Infect Dis* **39:**68-74.

2099. **Dwight, P. J., M. Naus, P. Sarsfield, and B. Limerick.** 2000. An outbreak of human blastomycosis: the epidemiology of blastomycosis in the Kenora catchment region of Ontario, Canada. *Can Commun Dis Rep* **26:**82-91.

2100. **Dworetzky, M.** 2002. Smallpox, October 1945. *N Engl J Med* **346:**1329.

2101. **Dworkin, M. S., H. R. Gamble, D. S. Zarlenga, and P. O. Tennican.** 1996. Outbreak of trichinellosis associated with eating cougar jerky. *J Infect Dis* **174:**663-6.

2102. **Dworkin, M. S., C. E. Jennings, J. Roth-Thomas, J. E. Lang, C. Stukenberg, and J. R. Lumpkin.** 2002. An Outbreak of Varicella among children attending preschool and elementary school in Illinois. *Clin Infect Dis* **35:**102-4.

2103. **Dworkin, M. S., P. C. Shoemaker, C. L. Fritz, M. E. Dowell, and D. E. Anderson, Jr.** 2002. The epidemiology of tick-borne relapsing fever in the United States. *Am J Trop Med Hyg* **66:**753-8.

2104. **Dworkin, M. S., P. S. Sullivan, S. E. Buskin, R. D. Harrington, J. Olliffe, R. D. MacArthur, and C. E. Lopez.** 1999. Bordetella bronchiseptica infection in human immunodeficiency virus-infected patients. *Clin Infect Dis* **28:**1095-9.

2105. **Dworkin, M. S., J. W. Ward, D. L. Hanson, J. L. Jones, and J. E. Kaplan.** 2001. Pneumococcal disease among human immunodeficiency virus-infected persons: incidence, risk factors, and impact of vaccination. *Clin Infect Dis* **32:**794-800.

2106. **Dwyer, D. M., E. G. Klein, G. R. Istre, M. G. Robinson, D. A. Neumann, and G. A. McCoy.** 1987. Salmonella newport infections transmitted by fiberoptic colonoscopy. *Gastrointest Endosc* **33:**84-7.

2107. **Dykewicz, C. A., V. M. Dato, S. P. Fisher-Hoch, M. V. Howarth, G. I. Perez-Oronoz, S. M. Ostroff, H. Gary, Jr., L. B. Schonberger, and J. B. McCormick.** 1992. Lymphocytic choriomeningitis outbreak associated with nude mice in a research institute. *JAMA* **267:**1349-53.

2108. **Eamsila, C., S. P. Frances, and D. Strickman.** 1994. Evaluation of permethrin-treated military uniforms for personal protection against malaria in northeastern Thailand. *J Am Mosq Control Assoc* **10:**515-21.

2109. **Earhart, K. C., C. Beadle, L. K. Miller, M. W. Pruss, G. C. Gray, E. K. Ledbetter, and M. R. Wallace.** 2001. Outbreak of influenza in highly vaccinated crew of U.S. navy ship. *Emerg Infect Dis* **7:**463-465.

2110. **Eastlund, T.** 1995. Infectious disease transmission through cell, tissue, and organ transplantation: reducing the risk through donor selection. *Cell Transplantation* **4:**455-77.

2111. **Ebeja, A. K., P. Lutumba, D. Molisho, G. Kegels, C. Miaka Mia Bilenge, and M. Boelaert.** 2003. La maladie de sommeil dans la region Ville de Kinshasa: une analyse retrospective des donnees de surveillance sur la periode 1996-2000. *Trop Med Int Health* **8:**949-955.

2112. **Ebel, G. D., A. P. Dupuis, 2nd, D. Nicholas, D. Young, J. Maffei, and L. D. Kramer.** 2002. Detection by Enzyme-Linked Immunosorbent Assay of Antibodies to West Nile virus in Birds. *Emerg Infect Dis* **8:**979-82.

2113. **Ebel, G. D., and L. D. Kramer.** 2004. Short report: duration of tick attachment required for transmission of powassan virus by deer ticks. *Am J Trop Med Hyg* **71:**268-71.

2114. **Eberhard, M. L., and E. Alfano.** 1998. Adult Toxocara cati infections in U.S. children: report of four cases. *Am J Trop Med Hyg* **59:**404-6.

2115. **Eberhart-Phillips, J., R. E. Besser, M. P. Tormey, D. Koo, D. Feikin, M. R. Araneta, J. Wells, L. Kilman, G. W. Rutherford, P. M. Griffin, R. Baron, and L. Mascola.** 1996. An outbreak of cholera from food served on an international aircraft. *Epidemiol Infect* **116:**9-13.

2116. **Eberhart-Phillips, J., N. Walker, N. Garrett, D. Bell, D. Sinclair, W. Rainger, and M. Bates.** 1997. Campylobacteriosis in New Zealand: results of a case-control study. *J Epidemiol Community Health* **51:**686-91.

2117. **Ebisawa, I., M. Takayanagi, and M. Kigawa.** 1988. Some factors affecting isolation of Clostridium tetani from human and animal stools. *Jpn J Exp Med* **58:**233-41.

2118. **Echeverri, M., A. Tobon, G. Alvarez, J. Carmona, and S. Blair.** 2003. Clinical and laboratory findings of Plasmodium vivax malaria in Colombia, 2001. *Rev Inst Med Trop Sao Paulo* **45:**29-34.

2119. **Eckert, J., and P. Deplazes.** 2004. Biological, epidemiological, and clinical aspects of echinococcosis, a zoonosis of increasing concern. *Clin Microbiol Rev* **17:**107-35.

2120. **Edelhofer, R., E. M. Heppe-Winger, A. Hassl, and H. Aspöck.** 1989. Toxoplasma-Infektionen bei jagdbaren Wildtieren in Ostösterreich. *Mitt Österr Ges Tropenmed Parasitol* **11:**119-23.

2121. **Edeling, W. M., J. J. Verweij, C. I. Ponsioen, and L. G. Visser.** 2004. [Outbreak of amoebiasis in a Dutch family; tropics unexpectedly nearby]. *Ned Tijdschr Geneeskd* **148:**1830-4.

2122. **Edgeworth, J. D., D. F. Treacher, and S. J. Eykyn.** 1999. A 25-year study of nosocomial bacteremia in adult intensive care unit. *Crit Care Med* **27:**1421-8.

2123. **Edlin, B. R., J. I. Tokars, M. H. Grieco, J. T. Crawford, J. Williams, E. M. Sordillo, K. R. Ong, J. O. Kilburn, S. W. Dooley, K. G. Castro, et al.** 1992. An outbreak of multidrug-resistant tuberculosis among hospitalized patients with the acquired immunodeficiency syndrome. *N Engl J Med* **326:**1514-21.

2124. **Edmiston, C. E., C. J. Krepel, G. R. Seabrook, and W. G. Jochimsen.** 2002. Anaerobic infections in the surgical patient: microbial etiology and therapy. *Clin Infect Dis* **35 (suppl 1):**S112-8.

2125. **Edmunds, W. J., M. Brisson, and J. D. Rose.** 2001. The epidemiology of herpes zoster and potential cost-effectiveness of vaccination in England and Wales. *Vaccine* **19:**3076-90.

2126. **Edungbola, L. D.** 1982. Cutaneous myiasis due to tumbu-flu, Cordylobia anthropophaga in Ilorin, Kwara state, Nigeria. *Acta Trop* **39:**355-62.

2127. **Edungbola, L. D., and S. Watts.** 1984. An outbreak of dracunculiasis in a peri-urban community of Ilorin, Kwara State, Nigeria. *Acta Trop* **41:**155-63.

2128. **Edwards, A. T., M. Roulson, and M. J. Ironside.** 1988. A milk-borne outbreak of serious infection due to Streptococcus zooepidemicus (Lancefield Group C). *Epidemiol Infect* **101:**43-51.

2129. **Effler, P., M. Isaacson, L. Arntzen, R. Heenan, P. Canter, T. Barrett, L. Lee, C. Mambo, W. Levine, A. Zaidi, and P. M. Griffin.** 2001. Factors contributing to the emergence of Escherichia coli O157 in Africa. *Emerg Infect Dis* **7:**812-9.

2130. **Effler, P. V., L. Pang, P. Kitsutani, V. Vorndam, M. Nakata, T. Ayers, J. Elm, T. Tom, P. Reiter, J. G. Rigau-Perez, J. M. Hayes, K. Mills, M. Napier, G. G. Clark, and D. J. Gubler.** 2005. Dengue fever, Hawaii, 2001-2002. *Emerg Infect Dis* **11:**742-9.

2131. **Efstratiou, A., K. H. Engler, I. K. Mazurova, T. Glushkevich, J. Vuopio-Varkila, and T. Popovic.** 2000. Current approaches to the laboratory diagnosis of diphtheria. *J Infect Dis* **181 Suppl 1:**S138-45.

2132. **Efuntoye, M. O., and S. O. Fashanu.** 2001. Fungi isolated from skins and pens of healthy animals in Nigeria. *Mycopathologia* **153:**21-3.

2133. **Egger, M., N. Low, G. D. Smith, B. Lindblom, and B. Herrmann.** 1998. Screening for chlamydial infections and the risk of ectopic pregnancy in a county in Sweden: ecological analysis. *BMJ* **316:**1776-80.

2134. **Eggimann, P., J. Garbino, and D. Pittet.** 2003. Epidemiology of Candida species infections in critically ill non-immunosuppressed patients. *Lancet Infect Dis* **3:**685-702.

2135. **Eggimann, P., S. Hugonnet, H. Sax, S. Touveneau, J. C. Chevrolet, and D. Pittet.** 2002. Ventilator-associated pneumonia: risks and rates. *Swiss Med Wkly* **132 (suppl 130):**S19.

2136. **Eggimann, P., and D. Pittet.** 2002. Overview of catheter-related infections with special emphasis on prevention based on educational programs. *Clin Microbiol Infect* **8:**295-309.

2137. **Egoz, N., S. Shihab, L. Leitner, and M. Lucian.** 1988. An outbreak of typhoid fever due to contamination of the municipal water supply in northern Israel. *Isr J Med Sci* **24:**640-3.

2138. **Egoz, N., M. Shmilovitz, B. Kretzer, M. Lucian, V. Porat, and R. Raz.** 1991. An outbreak of Shigella sonnei infection due to contamination of a municipal water supply in northern Israel. *J Infect* **22:**87-93.

2139. **Ehresmann, K. R., C. W. Hedberg, M. B. Grimm, C. A. Norton, K. L. MacDonald, and M. T. Osterholm.** 1995. An outbreak of measles at an international sporting event with airborne transmission in a domed stadium. *J Infect Dis* **171:**679-83.

2140. **Eichmann, A.** 1993. [Sexually transmissible diseases following travel in tropical countries]. *Schweiz Med Wochenschr* **123:**1250-5.

2141. **Eichner, M., and K. Dietz.** 1996. Eradication of poliomyelitis: when can one be sure that polio virus transmission has been terminated? *Am J Epidemiol* **143:**816-22.

2142. **Eijkhout, H. W., J. W. M. Van der Meer, C. G. M. Kallenberg, R. S. Weening, J. T. van Dissel, et al.** 2001. The effect of two different dosages of intravenous immunoglobulin on the incidence of recurrent infections in patients with primary hypogammaglobulinemia. A randomized, double-blind, multicenter crossover trial. *Ann Intern Med* **135:**165-74.

2143. **Eisele, M., J. Heukelbach, E. Van Marck, H. Mehlhorn, O. Meckes, S. Franck, and H. Feldmeier.** 2003. Investigations on the biology, epidemiology, pathology and control of Tunga penetrans in Brazil: I. Natural history of tungiasis in man. *Parasitol Res* **90:**87-99.

2144. **Eisen, L., R. J. Eisen, C. C. Chang, J. Mun, and R. S. Lane.** 2004. Acarologic risk of exposure to Borrelia burgdorferi spirochaetes: long-term evaluations in north-western California, with implications for Lyme borreliosis risk-assessment models. *Med Vet Entomol* **18:**38-49.

2145. **Eisenberg, E. S., M. Ambalu, G. Szylagi, V. Aning, and R. Soeiro.** 1987. Colonization of skin and development of peritonitis due to coagulase-negative staphylococci in patients undergoing peritoneal dialysis. *J Infect Dis* **156:**478-82.

2146. **Eisenberg, M. S., K. Gaarslev, W. Brown, M. Horwitz, and D. Hill.** 1975. Staphylococcal food poisoning aboard a commercial aircraft. *Lancet* **2:**595-9.

2147. **Eisenhut, M., T. F. Schwarz, and B. Hegenscheid.** 1999. Seroprevalence of dengue, chikungunya and Sindbis virus infections in German aid workers. *Infection* **27:**82-5.

2148. **Eitrem, R., S. Vene, and B. Niklasson.** 1990. Incidence of sand fly fever among Swedish United Nations soldiers on Cyprus during 1985. *Am J Trop Med Hyg* **43:**207-11.

2149. **Ejlertsen, T., B. Gahrn-Hansen, P. Sogaard, O. Heltberg, and W. Frederiksen.** 1996. Pasteurella aerogenes isolated from ulcers or wounds in humans with occupational exposure to pigs: a report of 7 Danish cases. *Scand J Infect Dis* **28:**567-70.

2150. **Ekdahl, K., and Y. Andersson.** 2004. Regional risks and seasonality in travel-associated campylobacteriosis. *BMC Infect Dis* **4:**54.

2151. **Ekdahl, K., B. de Jong, R. Wollin, and Y. Andersson.** 2005. Travel-associated non-typhoidal salmonellosis: geographical and seasonal differences and serotype distribution. *Clin Microbiol Infect* **11:**138-44.

2152. **Ekdahl, K., and M. Grandien.** 2000. A case of rabies diagnosed in Sweden. *Eurosurveillance Weekly* **28:**1.

2153. **Ekman, M. R., J. T. Grayston, R. Visakorpi, M. Kleemola, C. C. Kuo, and P. Saikku.** 1993. An epidemic of infections due to Chlamydia pneumoniae in military conscripts. *Clin Infect Dis* **17:**420-5.

2154. **El Bashir, H., E. Haworth, M. Zambon, S. Shafi, J. Zuckerman, and R. Booy.** 2004. Influenza among U.K. pilgrims to Hajj, 2003. *Emerg Infect Dis* **10:**1882-3.

2155. **el Fari, M., Y. Graser, W. Presber, and H. J. Tietz.** 2000. An epidemic of tinea corporis caused by Trichophyton tonsurans among children (wrestlers) in Germany. *Mycoses* **43:**191-6.

2156. **el Hachimi, K. H., M. P. Chaunu, L. Cervenakova, P. Brown, and J. F. Foncin.** 1997. Putative neurosurgical transmission of Creutzfeldt-Jakob disease with analysis of donor and recipient: agent strains. *C R Acad Sci III* **320:**319-28.

2157. **El Sayed, N. M., P. J. Gomatos, C. Beck-Sague, U. Dietrich, H. von Briesen, S. Osmanov, J. Esparza, R. R. Arthur, M. H. Wahdan, and W. R. Jarvis.** 2000. Epidemic transmission of human immunodeficiency virus in renal dialysis centers in Egypt. *J Infect Dis* **181:**91-7.

2158. **El Tayeb, A. B., T. Y. Morishita, and E. J. Angrick.** 2004. Evaluation of Pasteurella multocida isolated from rabbits by capsular typing, somatic serotyping, and restriction endonuclease analysis. *J Vet Diagn Invest* **16:**121-5.

2159. **el-Azazy, O. M., and E. M. Scrimgeour.** 1997. Crimean-Congo haemorrhagic fever virus infection in the western province of Saudi Arabia. *Trans R Soc Trop Med Hyg* **91:**275-8.

2160. **El-Bouri, K. W., A. M. Lewis, C. A. Okeahialam, D. Wright, A. Tanna, and D. H. Joynson.** 1998. A community outbreak of invasive and non-invasive group A beta-haemolytic streptococcal disease in a town in South Wales. *Epidemiol Infect* **121:**515-21.

2161. **El-Hamad, I., C. Casalini, A. Matteelli, S. Casari, M. Bugiani, M. Caputo, E. Bombana, C. Scolari, R. Moioli, C. Scarcella, and G. Carosi.** 2001. Screening for tuberculosis and latent tuberculosis infection among undocumented immigrants at an unspecialised health service unit. *Int J Tuberc Lung Dis* **5:**712-6.

2162. **El-Hassan, A. M., and E. E. Zijlstra.** 2001. Leishmaniasis in Sudan. 1. Cutaneous leishmaniasis. *Trans R Soc Trop Med Hyg* **94 suppl 1:**S1-S17.

2163. **El-Khoby, T., N. Galal, A. Fenwick, R. Barakat, A. El-Hawey, Z. Nooman, M. Habib, F. Abdel-Wahab, N. S. Gabr, H. M. Hammam, M. H. Hussein, N. N. Mikhail, B. L. Cline, and G. T. Strickland.** 2000. The epidemiology of schistosomiasis in Egypt: summary findings in nine governorates. *Am J Epidemiol* **62 suppl to 2:**88-99.

2164. **El-Sahly, H. M., R. L. Atmar, W. P. Glezen, and S. B. Greenberg.** 2000. Spectrum of clinical illness in hospitalized patients with "common cold" virus infections. *Clin Infect Dis* **31:**96-100.

2165. **el-Sherbini, M., S. al-Agili, H. el-Jali, M. Aboshkiwa, and M. Koha.** 1999. Isolation of Yersinia enterocolitica from cases of acute appendicitis and ice-cream. *East Mediterr Health J* **5:**130-5.

2166. **Elamin, E. A., S. Elias, A. Daugschies, and M. Rommel.** 1992. Prevalence of Toxoplasma gondii antibodies in pastoral camels (Camelus dromedarius) in the Butana plains, mid-Eastern Sudan. *Vet Parasitol* **43:**171-5.

2167. **Elbers, A. R., U. Vecht, A. D. Osterhaus, J. Groen, H. J. Wisselink, R. J. Diepersloot, and M. J. Tielen.** 1999. Low prevalence of antibodies against the zoonotic agents Brucella abortus, Leptospira spp., Streptococcus suis serotype II, hantavirus, and lymphocytic choriomeningitis virus among veterinarians and pig farmers in the southern part of The Netherlands. *Vet Q* **21:**50-4.

2168. **Elder, A. G., B. O'Donnell, E. A. McCruden, I. S. Symington, and W. F. Carman.** 1996. Incidence and recall of influenza in a cohort of Glasgow healthcare workers during the 1993-4 epidemic: results of serum testing and questionnaire. *BMJ* **313:**1241-2.

2169. **Eldridge, B. F., C. Glaser, R. E. Pedrin, and R. E. Chiles.** 2001. The first reported case of California encephalitis in more than 50 years. *Emerg Infect Dis* **7:**451-2.

2170. **Elewski, B. E.** 2000. Tinea capitis: a current perspective. *J Am Acad Dermatol* **42:**1-20; quiz 21-4.

2171. **Eliades, M. J., S. Shah, P. Nguyen-Dinh, R. D. Newman, A. M. Barber, J. M. Roberts, S. Mali, M. E. Parise, and R. Steketee.** 2005. Malaria surveillance—United States, 2003. *MMWR* **54 (SS-2):**25-40.

2172. **Eliasson, H., J. Lindback, J. P. Nuorti, M. Arneborn, J. Giesecke, and A. Tegnell.** 2002. The 2000 tularemia outbreak: a case-control study of risk factors in disease-endemic and emergent areas, Sweden. *Emerg Infect Dis* **8:**956-60.

2173. **Elifson, K. W., J. Boles, W. W. Darrow, and C. E. Sterk.** 1999. HIV seroprevalence and risk factors among clients of female and male prostitutes. *J Acquir Immune Defic Syndr Hum Retrovirol* **20:**195-200.

2174. **Eliseev, L. N., M. V. Strelkova, and Zherikhina, II.** 1991. [The characteristics of the epidemic activation of a natural focus of zoonotic cutaneous leishmaniasis in places with a sympatric dissemination of Leishmania major, L. turanica and L. gerbilli]. *Med Parazitol (Mosk)* issue 3:24-9.

2175. **Elizaga, M. L., R. A. Weinstein, and M. K. Hayden.** 2002. Patients in long-term care facilities: a reservoir for vancomycin-resistant enterococci. *Clin Infect Dis* **34:**441-6.

2176. **Ellabib, M. S., Z. Khalifa, and K. Kavanagh.** 2002. Dermatophytes and other fungi associated with skin mycoses in Tripoli, Libya. *Mycoses* **45:**101-4.

2177. **Ellerbeck, E. F., D. Vlahov, J. P. Libonati, M. E. Salive, and T. F. Brewer.** 1989. Gonorrhea prevalence in the Maryland state prisons. *Sex Transm Dis* **16:**165-7.

2178. **Elliott, D. J., S. C. Eppes, and J. D. Klein.** 2001. Teratogen update: Lyme disease. *Teratology* **64:**276-81.

2179. **Elliott, E., P. McIntyre, G. Ridley, A. Morris, J. Massie, J. McEniery, and G. Knight.** 2004. National study of infants hospitalized with pertussis in the acellular vaccine era. *Pediatr Infect Dis J* **23:**246-52.

2180. **Elliott, R. B., L. Escobar, O. Garkavenko, M. C. Croxson, B. A. Schroeder, M. McGregor, G. Ferguson, N. Beckman, and S. Ferguson.** 2000. No evidence of infection with porcine endogenous retrovirus in recipients of encapsulated porcine islet xenografts. *Cell Transplant* **9:**895-901.

2181. **Ellis, A., M. Preston, A. Borczyk, B. Miller, P. Stone, B. Hatton, A. Chagla, and J. Hockin.** 1998. A community outbreak of Salmonella berta associated with a soft cheese product. *Epidemiol Infect* **120:**29-35.

2182. **Ellis, B. A., L. D. Rotz, J. A. Leake, F. Samalvides, J. Bernable, G. Ventura, C. Padilla, P. Villaseca, L. Beati, R. Regnery, J. E. Childs, J. G. Olson, and C. P. Carrillo.** 1999. An outbreak of acute bartonellosis (Oroya fever) in the Urubamba region of Peru, 1998. *Am J Trop Med Hyg* **61:**344-9.

2183. **Ellis, D. H., and T. J. Pfeiffer.** 1990. Ecology, life cycle, and infectious propagule of Cryptococcus neoformans. *Lancet* **336:**923-5.

2184. **Ellis, D. H., and T. J. Pfeiffer.** 1990. Natural habitat of Cryptococcus neoformans var. gattii. *J Clin Microbiol* **28:**1642-4.

2185. **Ellis, J., P. C. Oyston, M. Green, and R. W. Titball.** 2002. Tularemia. *Clin Microbiol Rev* **15:**631-46.

2186. **Ellis, S. E., C. S. Coffey, E. F. Mitchel, Jr., R. S. Dittus, and M. R. Griffin.** 2003. Influenza- and respiratory syncytial virus-associated morbidity and mortality in the nursing home population. *J Am Geriatr Soc* **51:**761-7.

2187. **Elmahdi, I. E., Q. M. Ali, M. M. Magzoub, A. M. Ibrahim, M. B. Saad, and T. Romig.** 2004. Cystic echinococcosis of livestock and humans in central Sudan. *Ann Trop Med Parasitol* **98:**473-9.

2188. **Elnaiem, D. A., H. K. Hassan, and R. D. Ward.** 1999. Associations of Phlebotomus orientalis and other sandflies with vegetation types in the eastern Sudan focus of kala-azar. *Med Vet Entomol* **13:**198-203.

2189. **Elphick, G. F., W. Querbes, J. A. Jordan, G. V. Gee, S. Eash, K. Manley, A. Dugan, M. Stanifer, A. Bhatnagar, W. K. Kroeze, B. L. Roth, and W. J. Atwood.** 2004. The human polyomavirus, JCV, uses serotonin receptors to infect cells. *Science* **306:**1380-3.

2190. **Elsayed, E. A., N. Mousa, A. Dabbagh, H. El-Bushra, F. Mahoney, S. Haithami, H. El-Sakka, G. Sabitenelli, S. Agbo, R. Nandy, and L. Cairns.** 2004. Emergency measles control activities - Darfur, Sudan, 2004. *MMWR* **53:**897-9.

2191. **Elsayed, S., O. Hammerberg, V. Massey, and Z. Hussain.** 2003. Streptococcus equi subspecies equi (Lancefield group C) meningitis in a child. *Clin Microbiol Infect* **9:**869-72.

2192. **Elsayed, S., S. M. Kuhn, D. Barber, D. L. Church, S. Adams, and R. Kasper.** 2004. Human case of lobomycosis. *Emerg Infect Dis* **10:**715-8.

2193. **Elshibly, S., I. Kallings, D. Hellberg, and P. A. Mardh.** 1996. Sexual risk behaviour in women carriers of Mycoplasma hominis. *Br J Obstet Gynaecol* **103:**1124-8.

2194. **Elsner, H. A., W. Tenschert, L. Fischer, and P. M. Kaulfers.** 1997. Nosocomial infections by Listeria monocytogenes: analysis of a cluster of septicemias in immunocompromised patients. *Infection* **25:**135-9.

2195. **Elward, A. M., D. K. Warren, and V. J. Fraser.** 2002. Ventilator-associated pneumonia in pediatric intensive care unit patients: risk factors and outcomes. *Pediatrics* **109:**758-64.

2196. **Elzi, L., M. Decker, M. Battegay, J. Rutishauser, and J. Blum.** 2004. Chest pain after travel to the tropics. *Lancet* **363:**1198.

2197. **Embil, J., P. Warren, M. Yakrus, R. Stark, S. Corne, D. Forrest, and E. Hershfield.** 1997. Pulmonary illness associated with exposure to Mycobacterium-avium complex in hot tub water. Hypersensitivity pneumonitis or infection? *Chest* **111:**813-6.

2198. **Emeribe, A. O.** 1988. Gambiense trypanosomiasis acquired from needle scratch. *Lancet* **1:**470-1.

2199. **Emerson, P. M., S. Cairncross, R. L. Bailey, and D. C. W. Mabey.** 2000. Review of the evidence base for the 'F' and 'E' components of the SAFE strategy for trachoma control. *Trop Med Int Health* **5:**515-27.

2200. Emerson, P. M., S. W. Lindsay, N. Alexander, M. Bah, S. M. Dibba, H. B. Faal, K. O. Lowe, K. P. McAdam, A. A. Ratcliffe, G. E. Walraven, and R. L. Bailey. 2004. Role of flies and provision of latrines in trachoma control: cluster-randomised controlled trial. *Lancet* **363**.

2201. Emerson, S. U., and R. H. Purcell. 2004. Running like water—the omnipresence of hepatitis E. *N Engl J Med* **351**:2367-8.

2202. Emmerson, A. M. 2001. Emerging waterborne infections in health-care settings. *Emerg Infect Dis* **7**:272-6.

2203. Empana, J. P., M. D. Perrin, B. Pilon, and D. Ilef. 2000. Epidémie de shigellose à Shigella sonnei dans un institut médico éducatif spécialisé (département de l'Aisne, novembre 1998 - mars 1999). *Bull Epidémiol Hebdomadaire* **10**:43-4.

2204. Encarnacion, C. F., M. F. Giordano, and H. W. Murray. 1994. Onchocerciasis in New York City. The Moa-Manhattan connection. *Arch Intern Med* **154**:1749-51.

2205. Enders, G., E. Miller, J. Cradock-Watson, I. Bolley, and M. Ridehalgh. 1994. Consequences of varicella and herpes zoster in pregnancy: prospective study of 1739 cases. *Lancet* **343**:1548-51.

2206. Eng, T. R., D. B. Fishbein, H. E. Talamante, D. B. Hall, G. F. Chavez, J. G. Dobbins, F. J. Muro, J. L. Bustos, M. de los Angeles Ricardy, and A. Munguia. 1993. Urban epizootic of rabies in Mexico: epidemiology and impact of animal bite injuries. *Bull WHO* **71**:615-24.

2207. Engberg, J., F. M. Aarestrup, D. E. Taylor, P. Gerner-Smidt, and I. Nachamkin. 2001. Quinolone and macrolide resistance in Campylobacter jejuni and C. coli: resistance mechanisms and trends in human isolates. *Emerg Infect Dis* **7**:24-34.

2208. Engberg, J., P. Gerner-Smidt, F. Scheutz, E. Moller Nielsen, S. L. On, and K. Molbak. 1998. Water-borne Campylobacter jejuni infection in a Danish town - a 6-week continuous source outbreak. *Clin Microbiol Inf* **4**:648-56.

2209. Engel, G. A., L. Jones-Engel, M. A. Schillaci, K. G. Suaryana, A. Putra, A. Fuentes, and R. Henkel. 2002. Human exposure to herpesvirus B-seropositive macaques, Bali, Indonesia. *Emerg Infect Dis* **8**:789-95.

2210. Engelkens, H. J., A. P. Oranje, and E. Stolz. 1989. Early yaws, imported in The Netherlands. *Genitourin Med* **65**:316-8.

2211. Engels, D., C. Urbani, A. Belotto, F. Meslin, and L. Savioli. 2003. The control of human (neuro)cysticercosis: which way forward? *Acta Trop* **87**:177-82.

2212. Engels, E. A., J. Chen, R. P. Viscidi, K. V. Shah, R. W. Daniel, N. Chatterjee, and M. A. Klebanoff. 2004. Poliovirus vaccination during pregnancy, maternal seroconversion to Simian virus 40, and risk of childhood cancer. *Am J Epidemiol* **160**:306-16.

2213. Engels, E. A., W. M. Switzer, W. Heneine, and R. P. Viscidi. 2004. Serologic evidence for exposure to simian virus 40 in North American zoo workers. *J Infect Dis* **190**:2065-9.

2214. Enk, M. J., A. Amorim, and V. T. Schall. 2003. Acute schistosomiasis outbreak in the metropolitan area of Belo Horizonte, Minas Gerais: alert about the risk of unnoticed transmission increased by growing rural tourism. *Mem Inst Oswaldo Cruz* **98**:745-50.

2215. Enocksson, E., B. Wretlind, G. Sterner, and B. Anzen. 1990. Listeriosis during pregnancy and in neonates. *Scand J Infect Dis Suppl* **71**:89-94.

2216. Enserink, M. 2000. Has leishmaniasis become endemic in the US? *Science* **290**:1881—2.

2217. Enserink, M., and J. Kaiser. 2004. Biodefense research. Accidental anthrax shipment spurs debate over safety. *Science* **304**:1726-7.

2218. Ensink, J. H., W. van der Hoek, M. Mukhtar, Z. Tahir, and F. P. Amerasinghe. 2005. High risk of hookworm infection among wastewater farmers in Pakistan. *Trans R Soc Trop Med Hyg* **99**:809-818.

2219. Eono, P., C. Polaert, and J. P. Louis. 1999. [Malaria in expatriates in Abidjan]. *Med Trop (Mars)* **59**:358-64.

2220. Epstein, P. R., T. E. Ford, and R. R. Colwell. 1993. Marine ecosystems. *Lancet* **342**:1216-9.

2221. Erard, V., B. Storer, L. Corey, J. Nollkamper, M. L. Huang, A. Limaye, and M. Boeckh. 2004. BK virus infection in hematopoietic stem cell transplant recipients: frequency, risk factors, and association with postengraftment hemorrhagic cystitis. *Clin Infect Dis* **39**:1861-5.

2222. Ergönül, Ö., A. Celikbas, B. Dokuzoguz, S. Eren, N. Baykam, and H. Esener. 2004. Characteristics of patients with Crimean-Congo hemorrhagic fever in a recent outbreak in Turkey and impact of oral ribavirin therapy. *Clin Infect Dis* **39**:284-7.

2223. Erhart, A., N. D. Thang, T. H. Bien, N. M. Tung, N. Q. Hung, L. X. Hung, T. Q. Tuy, N. Speybroeck, L. D. Cong, M. Coosemans, and U. D'Alessandro. 2004. Malaria epidemiology in a rural area of the Mekong Delta: a prospective community-based study. *Trop Med Int Health* **9**:1081-90.

2224. Erhart, A., N. D. Thang, N. Q. Hung, V. Toi le, X. Hung le, T. Q. Tuy, D. Cong le, N. Speybroeck, M. Coosemans, and U. D'Alessandro. 2004. Forest malaria in Vietnam: a challenge for control. *Am J Trop Med Hyg* **70**:110-8.

2225. Ericsson, H., A. Eklow, M. L. Danielsson-Tham, S. Loncarevic, L. O. Mentzing, I. Persson, H. Unnerstad, and W. Tham. 1997. An outbreak of listeriosis suspected to have been caused by rainbow trout. *J Clin Microbiol* **35**:2904-7.

2226. Erkens, K., M. Lademann, K. Tintelnot, M. Lafrenz, U. Knaben, and E. C. Reisinger. 2002. Histoplasmose-Gruppenerkrankung bei Fledermausforschern nach Kubaaufenthalt. *Dtsch Med Wochenschr* **127**:21-5.

2227. Ernould, J. C., A. Kaman, R. Labbo, D. Couret, and J. P. Chippaux. 2000. Recent urban growth and urinary schistosomiasis in Niamey, Niger. *Trop Med Int Health* **5**:431-7.

2228. Ernst, E., and A. White. 1997. Life-threatening adverse reactions after acupuncture? A systematic review. *Pain* **71**:123-6.

2229. Ernst, N. S., J. A. Hernandez, R. J. MacKay, M. P. Brown, J. M. Gaskin, A. D. Nguyen, S. Giguere, P. T. Colahan, M. R. Troedsson, G. R. Haines, I. R. Addison, and B. J. Miller. 2004. Risk factors associated with fecal Salmonella shedding among hospitalized horses with signs of gastrointestinal tract disease. *J Am Vet Med Assoc* **225**:275-81.

2230. Erwin, P. C., T. F. Jones, R. R. Gerhardt, S. K. Halford, A. B. Smith, L. E. Patterson, K. L. Gottfried, K. L. Burkhalter, R. S. Nasci, and W. Schaffner. 2002. La Crosse encephalitis in Eastern Tennessee: clinical, environmental, and entomological characteristics from a blinded cohort study. *Am J Epidemiol* **155**:1060-5.

2231. Esaki, H., A. Morioka, K. Ishihara, A. Kojima, S. Shiroki, Y. Tamura, and T. Takahashi. 2004. Antimicrobial susceptibility of Salmonella isolated from cattle, swine and poultry (2001-2002): report from the Japanese Veterinary Antimicrobial Resistance Monitoring Program. *J Antimicrob Chemother* **53**:266-70.

2232. Escande, F., and C. Lion. 1993. Epidémiologie (1985-1992) des infections à Pasteurella et bactéries apparentées. *Méd Mal Infect* **23**:520-525.

2233. Esel, D., M. Doganay, N. Bozdemir, O. Yildiz, T. Tezcaner, B. Sumerkan, B. Aygen, and A. Selcuklu. 2002. Polymicrobial ventriculitis and evaluation of an outbreak in a surgical intensive care unit due to inadequate sterilization. *J Hosp Infect* **50**:170-4.

2234. Espana, A., M. J. Serna, M. Rubio, P. Redondo, and E. Quintanilla. 1993. Secondary urticaria due to toxocariasis: possibly caused by ingesting raw cattle meat? *J Investig Allergol Clin Immunol* **3**:51-2.

2235. Esposito, S., R. Cavagna, S. Bosis, R. Droghetti, N. Faelli, and N. Principi. 2002. Emerging role of Mycoplasma pneumoniae in children with acute pharyngitis. *Eur J Clin Microbiol Infect Dis* **21**:607-10.

2236. Essey, M. A., and M. A. Koller. 1994. Status of bovine tuberculosis in North America. *Vet Microbiol* **40**:15-22.

2237. Estahbanati, H. K., P. P. Kashani, and F. Ghanaatpisheh. 2002. Frequency of Pseudomonas aeruginosa serotypes in burn wound infections and their resistance to antibiotics. *Burns* **28**:340-8.

2238. Esteban, J. G., C. Aguirre, R. Angles, L. R. Ash, and S. Mas-Coma. 1998. Balantidiasis in Aymara children from the northern Bolivian Altiplano. *Am J Trop Med Hyg* **59**:922-7.

2239. Esteban, J. G., C. Aguirre, A. Flores, W. Strauss, R. Angles, and S. Mas-Coma. 1998. High Cryptosporidium prevalences in healthy Aymara children from the northern Bolivian Altiplano. *Am J Trop Med Hyg* **58**:50-5.

2240. Esteban, J. G., C. González, M. D. Bargues, R. Angles, C. Sanchez, C. Naquira, and S. Mas-Coma. 2002. High fascioliasis infection in children linked to a man-made irrigation zone in Peru. *Trop Med Int Health* **7**:339-48.

2241. Esteban, J. G., C. Gonzalez, F. Curtale, C. Munoz-Antoli, M. A. Valero, M. D. Bargues, M. el-Sayed, A. A. el-Wakeel, Y. Abdel-Wahab, A. Montresor, D. Engels, L. Savioli, and S. Mas-Coma. 2003. Hyperendemic fascioliasis associated with schistosomiasis in villages in the Nile Delta of Egypt. *Am J Trop Med Hyg* **69**:429-37.

2242. Esteban, J. I., J. Gomez, M. Martell, B. Cabot, J. Quer, J. Camps, A. Gonzalez, T. Otero, A. Moya, and R. Esteban. 1996. Transmission of hepatitis C virus by a cardiac surgeon. *N Engl J Med* **334**:555-60.

2243. Estebanez, P., N. K. Russell, M. D. Aguilar, I. Cifuentes, M. V. Zunzunegui, and K. McPherson. 2001. Determinants of HIV prevalence amongst female IDU in Madrid. *Eur J Epidemiol* **17**:573-80.

2244. Esterre, P., and F. Agis. 1985. [Beach sand nematodes in Guadeloupe: associated public health problems]. *Bull Soc Pathol Exot Filiales* **78**:71-8.

2245. Esterre, P., A. Andriantsimahavandy, E. R. Ramarcel, and J. L. Pecarrere. 1996. Forty years of chromoblastomycosis in Madagascar: a review. *Am J Trop Med Hyg* **55**:45-7.

2246. Estivariz, C. 2004. Nontuberculous mycobacterial infections after cosmetic surgery - Santo Domingo, Dominican Republic, 2003-2004. *MMWR* **53**:509.

2247. Estrada-Franco, J. G., R. Navarro-Lopez, J. E. Freier, D. Cordova, T. Clements, A. Moncayo, W. Kang, C. Gomez-Hernandez, G. Rodriguez-Dominguez, G. V. Ludwig, and S. C. Weaver. 2004. Venezuelan equine encephalitis virus, southern Mexico. *Emerg Infect Dis* **10**:2113-21.

2248. Estrada-Garcia, T., J. F. Cerna, M. R. Thompson, and C. Lopez-Saucedo. 2002. Faecal contamination and enterotoxigenic Escherichia coli in street-vended chili sauces in Mexico and its public health relevance. *Epidemiol Infect* **129**:223-6.

2249. Estrada-Garcia, T., C. Lopez-Saucedo, C. Arevalo, L. Flores-Romo, O. Luna, and I. Perez-Martinez. 2005. Street-vended seafood: a risk for foodborne diseases in Mexico. *Lancet Infect Dis* **5**:69-70.

2250. Estrada-Garcia, T., C. Lopez-Saucedo, B. Zamarripa-Ayala, M. R. Thompson, L. Gutierrez-Cogco, A. Mancera-Martinez, and A. Escobar-Gutierrez. 2004. Prevalence of Escherichia coli and Salmonella spp. in street-vended food of open markets (tianguis) and general hygienic and trading practices in Mexico City. *Epidemiol Infect* **132**:1181-4.

2251. Estrada-Pena, A., A. A. Guglielmone, and A. J. Mangold. 2004. The distribution and ecological 'preferences' of the tick Amblyomma cajennense (Acari: Ixodidae), an ectoparasite of humans and other mammals in the Americas. *Ann Trop Med Parasitol* **98**:283-92.

2252. Ethelberg, S., M. Lisby, M. Torpdahl, G. Sorensen, J. Neimann, P. Rasmussen, S. Bang, U. Stamer, H. B. Hansson, K. Nygard, D. L. Baggesen, E. M. Nielsen, K. Molbak, and M. Helms. 2004. Prolonged restaurant-associated outbreak of multidrug-resistant Salmonella Typhimurium among patients from several European countries. *Clin Microbiol Infect* **10**:904-10.

2253. Ethelberg, S., K. E. Olsen, P. Gerner-Smidt, and K. Molbak. 2004. Household outbreaks among culture-confirmed cases of bacterial gastrointestinal disease. *Am J Epidemiol* **159**:406-12.

2254. Etkind, P., S. M. Lett, P. D. Macdonald, E. Silva, and J. Peppe. 1992. Pertussis outbreaks in groups claiming religious exemptions to vaccinations. *Am J Dis Child* **146**:173-6.

2255. Ettestad, P. J., R. E. Voorhees, C. M. Sewell, J. Iralu, J. Cheek, K. J. Secord, D. Mosier, R. E. Enscore, M. E. Schriefer, S. Marshall, R. J. Groves, and C. B. Smelser. 2003. Tickborne relapsing fever outbreak after a family gathering - New Mexico, August 2002. *MMWR* **52**:809-12.

2256. Euler, G. L., K. G. Wooten, A. L. Baughman, and W. W. Williams. 2003. Hepatitis B surface antigen prevalence among pregnant women in urban areas: implications for testing, reporting, and preventing perinatal transmission. *Pediatrics* **111**:1192-7.

2257. Evans, A. C., D. J. Martin, and B. D. Ginsburg. 1991. Katayama fever in scuba divers. A report of 3 cases. *S Afr Med J* **79**:271-4.

2258. Evans, B. G., and D. Abiteboul. 1999. Bilan des infections professionnelles par le VIH dans le monde: les données de la littérature jusqu'en décembre 1997. *Eurosurveillance* **4**:29–32.

2259. Evans, H. S., P. Madden, C. Douglas, G. K. Adak, S. J. O'Brien, T. Djuretic, P. G. Wall, and R. Stanwell-Smith. 1998. General outbreaks of infectious intestinal disease in England and Wales: 1995 and 1996. *Commun Dis Public Health* **1**:165-71.

2260. Evans, M. E., K. L. Hall, and S. E. Berry. 1997. Influenza control in acute care hospitals. *Am J Infect Control* **25**:357-62.

2261. Evans, M. R., W. Lane, J. A. Frost, and G. Nylen. 1998. A campylobacter outbreak associated with stir-fried food. *Epidemiol Infect* **121**:275-9.

2262. Evans, M. R., R. Meldrum, W. Lane, D. Gardner, C. D. Ribeiro, C. I. Gallimore, and D. Westmoreland. 2002. An outbreak of viral gastroenteritis following environmental contamination at a concert hall. *Epidemiol Infect* **129**:355-60.

2263. Evans, M. R., C. D. Ribeiro, and R. L. Salmon. 2003. Hazards of healthy living: bottled water and salad vegetables as risk factors for campylobacter infections. *Emerg Infect Dis* **9**:1219-25.

2264. Evans, M. R., R. J. Roberts, C. D. Ribeiro, D. Gardner, and D. Kembrey. 1996. A milk-borne campylobacter outbreak following an educational farm visit. *Epidemiol Infect* **117**:457-62.

2265. Evans, M. R., R. L. Salmon, L. Nehaul, S. Mably, L. Wafford, M. Z. Nolan-Farrell, D. Gardner, and C. D. Ribeiro. 1999. An outbreak of Salmonella typhimurium DT170 associated with kebab meat and yogurt relish. *Epidemiol Infect* **122**:377-83.

2266. Evans, M. R., D. Shickle, and M. Z. Morgan. 2001. Travel illness in British package holiday tourists: prospective cohort study. *J Infect* **43**:140-7.

2267. Evans, M. R., J. P. Tromans, E. L. Dexter, C. D. Ribeiro, and D. Gardner. 1996. Consecutive salmonella outbreaks traced to the same bakery. *Epidemiol Infect* **116**:161-7.

2268. Evans, M. R., E. J. Wilkinson, R. Jones, K. Mathias, and P. Lenartowicz. 2003. Presumed Pseudomonas folliculitis outbreak in children following an outdoor games event. *Commun Dis Public Health* **6**:18-21.

2269. Eveillard, M., C. Ernst, S. Cuviller, F. X. Lescure, M. Malpaux, I. Defouilloy, M. Gresanleux, M. Duboisset, J. Lienard, and F. Eb. 2002. Prevalence of methicillin-resistant Staphylococcus aureus carriage at the time of admission in two acute geriatric wards. *J Hosp Infect* **50**:122-6.

2270. Eveillard, M., Y. Martin, N. Hidri, Y. Boussougant, and M. L. Joly-Guillou. 2004. Carriage of methicillin-resistant Staphylococcus aureus among hospital employees: prevalence, duration, and transmission to households. *Infect Control Hosp Epidemiol* **25**:114-20.

2271. Eveillard, M., P. Mertl, B. Canarelli, and M. De Lestang. 2002. Risque infectieux après implantations de prothèse de genou. Etude des infections profondes pour une série continue de 210 prothèses totales de genou en première intention. *Bull Epidémiol Hebdomadaire* **26 mars**:53-5.

2272. Evengard, B. 1990. Diagnostic and clinical aspects of schistosomiasis in 182 patients treated at a Swedish ward for tropical diseases during a 10-year period. *Scand J Infect Dis* **22**:585-94.

2273. Evengard, B., K. Petersson, M. L. Engman, S. Wiklund, S. A. Ivarsson, K. Tear-Fahnehjelm, M. Forsgren, R. Gilbert, and G. Malm. 2001. Low incidence of toxoplasma infection during pregnancy and in newborns in Sweden. *Epidemiol Infect* **127**:121-7.

2274. Evenson, M. L., M. W. Hinds, R. S. Bernstein, and M. S. Bergdoll. 1988. Estimation of human dose of staphylococcal enterotoxin A from a large outbreak of staphylococcal food poisoning involving chocolate milk. *Int J Food Microbiol* **7**:311-6.

2275. Everard, C. O., C. N. Edwards, J. D. Everard, and D. G. Carrington. 1995. A twelve-year study of leptospirosis on Barbados. *Eur J Epidemiol* **11**:311-20.

2276. Everard, C. O., and J. D. Everard. 1992. Mongoose rabies in the Caribbean. *Ann N Y Acad Sci* **653**:356-66.

2277. Everett, K. D. E. 2000. Chlamydia and Chlamydiales: more than meets the eye. *Vet Microbiol* **75**:109-26.

2278. Ewald, D. P., G. V. Hall, and C. C. Franks. 2003. An evaluation of a SAFE-style trachoma control program in Central Australia. *Med J Aust* **178**:65-8.

2279. Ewer, K., J. Deeks, L. Alvarez, G. Bryant, S. Waller, P. Andersen, P. Monk, and A. Lalvani. 2003. Comparison of T-cell-based assay with tuberculin skin test for diagnosis of Mycobacterium tuberculosis infection in a school tuberculosis outbreak. *Lancet* **361**:1168-73.

2280. Extremera Montero, F., R. Moyano Acost, B. Gomez Pozo, P. Bermudez Ruiz, J. Lopez Mendez, S. Aguilar Rivas, and J. Ingelmo Martin. 2001. [Exposure to Mycobacterium tuberculosis during a bus travel]. *Med Clin (Barc)* **116**:182-5.

2281. Ezell, H., B. Tramontin, R. Hudson, L. Tengelsen, C. Hahn, K. Smith, J. Bender, D. Boxrud, J. Adams, R. K. Frank, K. Culbertson, T. Besser, D. Rice, R. Gautom, R. Pallipamu, M. Golddoft, J. Grendon, J. Kobayashi, F. Angulo, T. Barrett, S. Rossiter, S. Sivapalasingam, and J. Wright. 2001. Outbreaks of multidrug-resistant Salmonella Typhimurium associated with veterinary facilities - Idaho, Minnesota, and Washington, 1999. *MMWR* **50**:701-704.

2282. Faa, A. G., W. J. McBride, G. Garstone, R. E. Thompson, and P. Holt. 2003. Scrub typhus in the Torres Strait islands of north Queensland, Australia. *Emerg Infect Dis* **9**:480-2.

2283. Fabbi, M., L. De Giuli, M. Tranquillo, R. Bragoni, M. Casiraghi, and C. Genchi. 2004. Prevalence of Bartonella henselae in Italian stray cats: evaluation of serology to assess the risk of transmission of Bartonella to humans. *J Clin Microbiol* **42**:264-8.

2284. Facklam, R. 2002. What happened to the streptococci: overview of taxonomic and nomenclature changes. *Clin Microbiol Rev* **15**:613-30.

2285. Fahrer, H., M. J. Sauvain, E. Zhioua, C. Van Hoecke, and L. E. Gern. 1998. Longterm survey (7 years) in a population at risk for Lyme borreliosis: what happens to the seropositive individuals? *Eur J Epidemiol* **14**:117-23.

2286. Faine, S. 1982. Guidelines for the control of leptospirosis. *WHO offset publication* **67**:1-171.

2287. Fairhurst, R. M., B. M. Kubak, D. A. Pegues, J. D. Moriguchi, K. F. Han, J. C. Haley, and J. A. Kobashigawa. 2002. Mycobacterium haemophilum infections in heart transplant recipients: case report and review of the literature. *Am J Transplant* **2**:476-9.

2288. Falagas, M. E., D. R. Snydman, J. Griffith, R. Ruthazer, and B. G. Werner. 1997. Effect of cytomegalovirus infection status on first-year mortality rates among orthotopic liver transplant recipients. *Ann Intern Med* **126**:275-9.

2289. Falcao, J. P., D. P. Falcao, and T. A. Gomes. 2004. Ice as a vehicle for diarrheagenic Escherichia coli. *Int J Food Microbiol* **91**:99-103.

2290. Falck, G. 1996. Group A streptococcal skin infections after indoor association football tournament. *Lancet* **347**:840-1.

2291. Falco, R. C., D. F. McKenna, T. J. Daniels, R. B. Nadelman, J. Nowakowski, D. Fish, and G. P. Wormser. 1999. Temporal relation between Ixodes Ixodes scapularis abundance and risk for Lyme disease associated with erythema migrans. *Am J Epidemiol* **149**:771-6.

2292. Falcone, V., J. Leupold, J. Clotten, E. Urbanyi, O. Herchenroder, W. Spatz, B. Volk, N. Bohm, A. Toniolo, D. Neumann-Haefelin, and M. Schweizer. 1999. Sites of simian foamy virus persistence in naturally infected African green monkeys: latent provirus is ubiquitous, whereas viral replication is restricted to the oral mucosa. *Virology* **257**:7-14.

2293. Falk, L., H. Fredlund, and J. S. Jensen. 2005. Signs and symptoms of urethritis and cervicitis among women with or without Mycoplasma genitalium or Chlamydia trachomatis infection. *Sex Transm Infect* **81**:73-8.

2294. Falk, P. S., J. Winnike, C. Woodmansee, M. Desai, and C. G. Mayhall. 2000. Outbreak of vancomycin-resistant enterococci in a burn unit. *Infect Control Hosp Epidemiol* **21:**575-82.

2295. Falk, W. A., K. Buchan, M. Dow, J. Z. Garson, E. Hill, M. Nosal, M. Tarrant, R. C. Westbury, and F. M. White. 1989. The epidemiology of mumps in southern Alberta, 1980-1982. *Am J Epidemiol* **130:**736-49.

2296. Falkensammer, B., G. Walder, D. Busch, A. Giessauf, M. Dierich, and R. Wurzner. 2004. Epidemiology of rubella infections in Austria: important lessons to be learned. *Eur J Clin Microbiol Infect Dis* **23:**502-5.

2297. Falkinham, J. O., 3rd. 2002. Nontuberculous mycobacteria in the environment. *Clin Chest Med* **23:**529-51.

2298. Falkinham, J. O., 3rd. 2003. Mycobacterial aerosols and respiratory disease. *Emerg Infect Dis* **9:**763-7.

2299. Fallah, M., A. Mirarab, F. JAMAlian, and A. Ghaderi. 2002. Evaluation of two years of mass chemotherapy against ascariasis in Hamadan, Islamic Republic of Iran. *Bull WHO* **80:**399-402.

2300. Falsey, A. R., D. Erdman, L. J. Anderson, and E. E. Walsh. 2003. Human metapneumovirus infections in young and elderly adults. *J Infect Dis* **187:**785-90.

2301. Falsey, A. R., R. M. McCann, W. J. Hall, M. A. Tanner, M. M. Criddle, M. A. Formica, C. S. Irvine, J. E. Kolassa, W. H. Barker, and J. J. Treanor. 1995. Acute respiratory tract infection in daycare centers for older persons. *J Am Geriatr Soc* **43:**30-6.

2302. Falsey, A. R., and E. E. Walsh. 2000. Respiratory syncytial virus infection in adults. *Clin Microbiol Rev* **13:**371-84.

2303. Falsey, A. R., E. E. Walsh, and F. G. Hayden. 2002. Rhinovirus and coronavirus infection-associated hospitalizations among older adults. *J Infect Dis* **185:**1338-41.

2304. Falzon, D., and A. Infuso. 2004. World Tb day 2004 and current Tb perspectives in Europe: an update from EuroTb. *Eurosurveillance Weekly* **8:**1-3.

2305. Fan, C. K., H. S. Lan, C. C. Hung, W. C. Chung, C. W. Liao, W. Y. Du, and K. E. Su. 2004. Seroepidemiology of Toxocara canis infection among mountain aboriginal adults in Taiwan. *Am J Trop Med Hyg* **71:**216-21.

2306. Fan, C. K., C. W. Liao, M. S. Wu, N. Y. Hu, and K. E. Su. 2004. Prevalence of Pediculus capitis infestation among school children of Chinese refugees residing in mountanous areas of northern Thailand. *Kaohsiung J Med Sci* **20:**183-7.

2307. Fan, C. K., K. E. Su, Y. H. Lin, C. W. Liao, W. Y. Du, and H. Y. Chiou. 2001. Seroepidemiologic survey of Dirofilaria immitis infection among domestic dogs in Taipei City and mountain aboriginal districts in Taiwan (1998-1999). *Vet Parasitol* **102:**113-20.

2308. Fan, M. Y., D. H. Walker, S. R. Yu, and Q. H. Liu. 1987. Epidemiology and ecology of rickettsial diseases in the People's Republic of China. *Rev Infect Dis* **9:**823-40.

2309. Fan, P. C., and W. C. Chung. 1998. Taenia saginata asiatica: epidemiology, infection, immunological and molecular studies. *J Microbiol Immunol Infect* **31:**84-9.

2310. Fandeur, T., B. Volney, C. Peneau, and B. de Thoisy. 2000. Monkeys of the rainforest in French Guiana are natural reservoirs for P. brasilianum/P. malariae malaria. *Parasitology* **120 (Pt 1):**11-21.

2311. Fanello, S., J. P. Bouchara, N. Jousset, V. Delbos, and A. M. LeFlohic. 2001. Nosocomial Candida albicans acquisition in a geriatric unit: epidemiology and evidence for person-to-person transmission. *J Hosp Infect* **47:**46-52.

2312. Fang, R., and D. Raoult. 2003. Antigenic classification of Rickettsia felis by using monoclonal and polyclonal antibodies. *Clin Diagn Lab Immunol* **10:**221-8.

2313. Fankhauser, R. L., S. S. Monroe, J. S. Noel, C. D. Humphrey, J. S. Bresee, U. D. Parashar, T. Ando, and R. I. Glass. 2002. Epidemiologic and molecular trends of "Norwalk-like viruses" associated with outbreaks of gastroenteritis in the United States. *J Infect Dis* **186:**1-7.

2314. Fankhauser, R. L., J. S. Noel, S. S. Monroe, T. Ando, and R. I. Glass. 1998. Molecular epidemiology of "Norwalk-like viruses" in outbreaks of gastroenteritis in the United States. *J Infect Dis* **178:**1571-8.

2315. Fanning, A., and S. Edwards. 1991. Mycobacterium bovis infection in human beings in contact with elk (Cervus elaphus) in Alberta, Canada. *Lancet* **338:**1253-5.

2316. Fantry, G. T., Q. X. Zheng, and S. P. James. 1995. Conventional cleaning and disinfection techniques eliminate the risk of endoscopic transmission of Helicobacter pylori. *Am J Gastroenterol* **90:**227-32.

2317. Faoagali, J. L., and D. Darcy. 1995. Chickenpox outbreak among the staff of a large, urban adult hospital: costs of monitoring and control. *Am J Infect Control* **23:**247-50.

2318. Farah, Z., and A. Fischer. 2004. Milk and meat from the camel: handbook on products and processing. Eidgenössische Technische Hochschule and Hochschulverlag, Zürich, Switzerland.

2319. Farci, P. 2003. Delta hepatitis: an update. *J Hepatol* **39 Suppl 1:**S212-9.

2320. Farina, C., P. Boiron, I. Ferrari, F. Provost, and A. Goglio. 2001. Report of human nocardiosis in Italy between 1993 and 1997. *Eur J Epidemiol* **17:**1019-22.

2321. Farina, C., F. Gnecchi, G. Michetti, A. Parma, C. Cavanna, and P. Nasta. 2000. Imported and autochthonous histoplasmosis in Bergamo province, Northern Italy. *Scand J Infect Dis* **32:**271-4.

2322. Farizo, K. M., P. M. Strebel, R. T. Chen, A. Kimbler, T. J. Cleary, and S. L. Cochi. 1993. Fatal respiratory disease due to Corynebacterium diphtheriae: case report and review of guidelines for management, investigation, and control. *Clin Infect Dis* **16:**59-68.

2323. Farley, T. M., M. J. Rosenberg, P. J. Rowe, J. H. Chen, and O. Meirik. 1992. Intrauterine devices and pelvic inflammatory disease: an international perspective. *Lancet* **339:**785-8.

2324. Farr, W., M. J. Gonzalez, H. Garbauskas, C. E. Zinderman, and J. E. LaMar, 2nd. 2004. Suspected meningococcal meningitis on an aircraft carrier. *Mil Med* **169:**684-6.

2325. Farrington, M., I. Matthews, J. Foreman, K. M. Richardson, and E. Caffrey. 1998. Microbiological monitoring of bone grafts: two years' experience at a tissue bank. *J Hosp Infect* **38:**261-71.

2326. Farshid, M., F. Mitchell, R. Biswas, O. K. Ndimbie, and M. Ding. 1997. Prevalence of hepatitis G virus in hepatitis C virus (HCV)-infected patients and in HCV-contaminated intravenous immunoglobulin products. *J Viral Hepat* **4:**415-9.

2327. Fatkenheuer, G., M. Preuss, B. Salzberger, N. Schmeisser, O. A. Cornely, H. Wisplinghoff, and H. Seifert. 2004. Long Term Outcome and Quality of Care of Patients with Staphylococcus aureus Bacteremia. *Eur J Clin Microbiol Infect Dis* **23:**157-62.

2328. Fattal, B., Y. Wax, M. Davies, and H. I. Shuval. 1986. Health risks associated with wastewater irrigation: an epidemiological study. *Am J Public Health* **76:**977-9.

2329. **Faundes, A., E. Telles, M. L. Cristofoletti, D. Faundes, S. Castro, and E. Hardy.** 1998. The risk of inadvertent intrauterine device insertion in women carriers of endocervical Chlamydia trachomatis. *Contraception* **58**:105-9.

2330. **Faustini, A., P. G. Rossi, and C. A. Perucci.** 2003. Outbreaks of food borne diseases in the Lazio region, Italy: the results of epidemiological field investigations. *Eur J Epidemiol* **18**:699-702.

2331. **Faustini, A., M. Sangalli, M. Fantasia, R. Manganello, E. Mattaccini, R. Trippanera, D. Spera, U. La Rosa, M. T. Topi, F. Forastiere, and C. A. Perucci.** 1998. An outbreak of Salmonella hadar associated with food consumption at a building site canteen. *Eur J Epidemiol* **14**:99-106.

2332. **Faville, R., S. Koop, F. Ogunmodede, R. Lynfield, R. Danila, B. Juni, D. Boxrud, A. Glennen, E. Shade, K. Penterman, and K. Kiang.** 2004. Osteomyelitis/septic arthritis caused by Kingella kingae among day care attendees - Minnesota, 2003. *MMWR* **53**:241-3.

2333. **Favoretto, S. R., C. de Mattos, N. B. Morais, F. A. Alves Araujo, and C. A. de Mattos.** 2001. Rabies in marmosets (Callithrix jacchus), Ceará, Brazil. *Emerg Infect Dis* **7**:1062-5.

2334. **Favorov, M. O., M. Y. Kosoy, S. A. Tsarev, J. E. Childs, and H. S. Margolis.** 2000. Prevalence of antibody to hepatitis E virus among rodents in the United States. *J Infect Dis* **181**:449-55.

2335. **Faye, D., P. J. L. Pereira de Almeida, B. Goossens, S. Osaer, M. Ndao, D. Berkvens, N. Speybroeck, F. Nieberding, and S. Geerts.** 2001. Prevalence and incidence of trypanosomosis in horses and donkeys in the Gambia. *Vet Parasitol* **101**:101-14.

2336. **Faye, F. B., A. Spiegel, A. Tall, C. Sokhna, D. Fontenille, C. Rogier, and J. F. Trape.** 2002. Diagnostic criteria and risk factors for Plasmodium ovale malaria. *J Infect Dis* **186**:690-5.

2337. **Faye, O., D. Fontenille, O. Gaye, N. Sy, J. F. Molez, L. Konate, G. Hebrard, J. P. Herve, J. Trouillet, and S. Diallo.** 1995. [Malaria and rice growing in the Senegal River delta (Senegal)]. *Ann Soc Belg Med Trop* **75**:179-89.

2338. **Fayer, R., J. P. Dubey, and D. S. Lindsay.** 2004. Zoonotic protozoa: from land to sea. *Trends Parasitol* **20**:531-6.

2339. **Fayer, R., E. J. Lewis, J. M. Trout, T. K. Graczyk, M. C. Jenkins, J. Higgins, L. Xiao, and A. A. Lal.** 1999. Cryptosporidium parvum in oysters from commercial harvesting sites in the Chesapeake Bay. *Emerg Infect Dis* **5**:706-10.

2340. **Feachem, R. G.** 1982. Environmental aspects of cholera epidemiology. III Transmission and control. *Trop Dis Bull* **79**:1-47.

2341. **Feder, H. M., P. R. Mitchell, and M. Z. Seeley.** 2003. A warble in Connecticut. *Lancet* **361**:1952.

2342. **Feikin, D. R., J. F. Moroney, D. F. Talkington, W. L. Thacker, J. E. Code, L. A. Schwartz, D. D. Erdman, J. C. Butler, and M. S. Cetron.** 1999. An outbreak of acute respiratory disease caused by Mycoplasma pneumoniae and adenovirus at a federal service training academy: new implications from an old scenario. *Clin Infect Dis* **29**:1545-50.

2343. **Fein, H., S. Naseem, D. P. Witte, V. F. Garcia, A. Lucky, and M. A. Staat.** 2001. Tungiasis in North America: a report of 2 cases in internationally adopted children. *J Pediatr* **139**:744-6.

2344. **Fejes, L.** 1993. [Incidence of Molluscum contagiosum in children with AIDS at the Cervanoda Orphanage, District of Constanta, Romania]. *Bull Soc Pathol Exot* **86**:327-8.

2345. **Fekadu, M.** 1982. Rabies in Ethiopia. *Am J Epidemiol* **115**:266-73.

2346. **Fekety, R., and A. B. Shah.** 1993. Diagnosis and treatment of Clostridium difficile colitis. *JAMA* **269**.

2347. **Feldman, K. A.** 2003. Tularemia. *J Am Vet Med Assoc* **222**:725-30.

2348. **Feldman, K. A., R. E. Enscore, S. L. Lathrop, B. T. Matyas, M. McGuill, M. E. Schriefer, D. Stiles-Enos, D. T. Dennis, L. R. Petersen, and E. B. Hayes.** 2001. An outbreak of primary pneumonic tularemia on Martha's Vineyard. *N Engl J Med* **345**:1601-6.

2349. **Feldman, K. A., D. Stiles-Enos, K. Julian, B. T. Matyas, S. R. Telford, 3rd, M. C. Chu, L. R. Petersen, and E. B. Hayes.** 2003. Tularemia on Martha's Vineyard: Seroprevalence and Occupational Risk. *Emerg Infect Dis* **9**:350-4.

2350. **Feldman, R. E., W. B. Baine, J. L. Nitzkin, M. S. Saslaw, and R. A. Pollard, Jr.** 1974. Epidemiology of Salmonella typhi infection in a migrant labor camp in Dade County, Florida. *J Infect Dis* **130**:335-42.

2351. **Feliciangeli, M. D.** 2004. Natural breeding places of phlebotomine sandflies. *Med Vet Entomol* **18**:71-80.

2352. **Feliciangeli, M. D., and J. Rabinovich.** 1998. Abundance of Lutzomyia ovallesi but not Lu. gomezi (Diptera: Psychodidae) correlated with cutaneous leishmaniasis incidence in north-central Venezuela. *Med Vet Entomol* **12**:121-31.

2353. **Fell, G., O. Hamouda, R. Lindner, S. Rehmet, A. Liesegang, R. Prager, B. Gericke, and L. Petersen.** 2000. An outbreak of Salmonella blockley infections following smoked eel consumption in Germany. *Epidemiol Infect* **125**:9-12.

2354. **Fenstersheib, M. D., M. Miller, C. Diggins, S. Liska, L. Detwiler, S. B. Werner, D. Lindquist, W. L. Thacker, and R. F. Benson.** 1990. Outbreak of Pontiac fever due to Legionella anisa. *Lancet* **336**:35-7.

2355. **Fenton, K., C. Korovessis, A. M. Johnson, A. McCadden, S. McManus, K. Wellings, C. H. Mercer, C. Carder, A. J. Copas, K. Nanchahal, W. Macdowall, G. Ridgway, J. Field, and B. Erens.** 2001. Sexual behaviour in Britain: reported sexually transmitted infections and prevalent genital Chlamydia trachomatis infection. *Lancet* **358**:1851-4.

2356. **Fenton, K. A., C. H. Mercer, S. McManus, B. Erens, K. Wellings, W. Macdowall, C. L. Byron, A. J. Copas, K. Nanchahal, J. Field, and A. M. Johnson.** 2005. Ethnic variations in sexual behaviour in Great Britain and risk of sexually transmitted infections: a probability survey. *Lancet* **365**:1246-55.

2357. **Ferguson, D. D., J. Scheftel, A. Cronquist, K. Smith, A. Woo-Ming, E. Anderson, J. Knutsen, A. K. De, and K. Gershman.** 2005. Temporally distinct Escherichia coli 0157 outbreaks associated with alfalfa sprouts linked to a common seed source—Colorado and Minnesota, 2003. *Epidemiol Infect* **133**:439-47.

2358. **Ferguson, D. V., and G. A. Heidt.** 1981. Survey for rabies, leptospirosis, toxoplasmosis and tularemia in striped skunks (Mephitis mephitis) from three public use areas in northwestern Arkansas. *J Wildl Dis* **17**:515-9.

2359. **Ferguson, G. W., J. M. Shultz, and A. L. Bisno.** 1991. Epidemiology of acute rheumatic fever in a multiethnic, multiracial urban community: the Miami-Dade County experience. *J Infect Dis* **164**:720-5.

2360. **Fernández, J. A., P. López, D. Orozco, and J. Merino.** 2002. Clinical study of an outbreak of legionnaire's disease in Alcoy, southeastern Spain. *Eur J Clin Microbiol Infect Dis* **21**:729-35.

2361. **Fernandez-Martin, J. I., F. Dronda, F. Chaves, M. Alonso-Sanz, S. Catalan, and A. Gonzalez-Lopez.** 1996. [Campylobacter jejuni infections in a prison population coinfected with the human immunodeficiency virus]. *Rev Clin Esp* **196:**16-20.

2362. Fernandez-Soto, P., A. Encinas-Grandes, and R. Perez-Sanchez. 2003. Rickettsia aeschlimannii in Spain: molecular evidence in Hyalomma marginatum and five other tick species that feed on humans. *Emerg Infect Dis* **9:**889-90.

2363. Ferrer, J. F., D. Galligan, E. Esteban, V. Rey, A. Murua, S. Gutierrez, L. Gonzalez, M. Thakuri, L. Feldman, B. Poiesz, and C. E. Jonsson. 2003. Hantavirus infection in people inhabiting a highly endemic region of the Gran Chaco territory, Paraguay: association with Trypanosoma cruzi infection, epidemiological features and haematological characteristics. *Ann Trop Med Parasitol* **97:**269-80.

2364. Ferrera, A., W. J. G. Melchers, J. P. Velema, and M. Figueroa. 1997. Association of infections with human immunodeficiency virus and human papillomavirus in Honduras. *Am J Trop Med Hyg* **57:**138-41.

2365. Ferro, C., J. Boshell, A. C. Moncayo, M. Gonzalez, M. L. Ahumada, W. Kang, and S. C. Weaver. 2003. Natural Enzootic Vectors of Venezuelan equine encephalitis virus, Magdalena Valley, Colombia. *Emerg Infect Dis* **9:**49-54.

2366. Ferro, C., R. Pardo, M. Torres, and A. C. Morrison. 1997. Larval microhabitats of Lutzomyia longipalpis (Diptera: Psychodidae) in an endemic focus of visceral leishmaniasis in Colombia. *J Med Entomol* **34:**719-28.

2367. Ferroni, A., L. Nguyen, B. Pron, G. Quesne, M. C. Brusset, and P. Berche. 1998. Outbreak of nosocomial urinary tract infections due to Pseudomonas aeruginosa in a paediatric surgical unit associated with tap-water contamination. *J Hosp Infect* **39:**301-7.

2368. Ferson, M., P. Paraskevopoulos, S. Hatzi, P. Yankos, M. Fennell, and A. Condylios. 2000. Presumptive summer influenza A: an outbreak on a trans-Tasman cruise. *Commun Dis Intell* **24:**45-7.

2369. Ferson, M. J. 1994. Outbreak of primary herpes stomatitis in a child-care center. *Commun Dis Intell* **18:**141.

2370. Ferson, M. J. 1997. Infection control in child care settings. *Commun Dis Intell* **21:**333-7.

2371. Ferson, M. J., K. Morgan, P. W. Robertson, A. W. Hampson, I. Carter, and W. D. Rawlinson. 2004. Concurrent summer influenza and pertussis outbreaks in a nursing home in Sydney, Australia. *Infect Control Hosp Epidemiol* **25:**962-6.

2372. Ferson, M. J., S. Stringfellow, K. McPhie, C. J. McIver, and A. Simos. 1997. Longitudinal study of rotavirus infection in child-care centres. *J Paediatr Child Health* **33:**157-60.

2373. Fevre, E. M., P. G. Coleman, M. Odiit, J. W. Magona, S. C. Welburn, and M. E. Woolhouse. 2001. The origins of a new Trypanosoma brucei rhodesiense sleeping sickness outbreak in eastern Uganda. *Lancet* **358:**625-8.

2374. Fevre, E. M., R. W. Kaboyo, V. Persson, M. Edelsten, P. G. Coleman, and S. Cleaveland. 2005. The epidemiology of animal bite injuries in Uganda and projections of the burden of rabies. *Trop Med Int Health* **10:**790-8.

2375. Fewtrell, L., and J. Bartram. 2001. Water quality. Guidelines, standards and health: assessment of risk and risk management for water-related infectious disease. IWA Publishing, London.

2376. Fiallo, P., E. Nunzi, G. Bisighini, and G. Vaccari. 1993. Leprosy in an Italian tourist visiting the tropics. *Trans R Soc Trop Med Hyg* **87:**675.

2377. Fichet-Calvet, E., I. Jomaa, R. Ben Ismail, and R. W. Ashford. 2003. Leishmania major infection in the fat sand rat Psammomys obesus in Tunisia: interaction of host and parasite populations. *Ann Trop Med Parasitol* **97:**593-603.

2378. Fielding, J. E. 2005. An outbreak of measles in Adelaide. *Commun Dis Intell* **29:**80-2.

2379. Fields, B. S., T. Haupt, J. P. Davis, M. J. Arduino, P. H. Miller, and J. C. Butler. 2001. Pontiac fever due to Legionella micdadei from a whirlpool spa: possible role of bacterial endotoxin. *J Infect Dis* **184:**1289-92.

2380. Figueiredo, J. F., D. A. Silva, D. D. Cabral, and J. R. Mineo. 2001. Seroprevalence of Toxoplasma gondii infection in goats by the indirect haemagglutination, immunofluorescence and immunoenzymatic tests in the region of Uberlandia, Brazil. *Mem Inst Oswaldo Cruz* **96:**687-92.

2381. Figueroa, J. E., and P. Densen. 1991. Infectious diseases associated with complement deficiencies. *Clin Microbiol Rev* **4:**359-95.

2382. File, T. M. 2003. Community-acquired pneumonia. *Lancet* **362:**1991-2001.

2383. File, T. M., Jr., J. S. Tan, and J. F. Plouffe. 1998. The role of atypical pathogens: Mycoplasma pneumoniae, Chlamydia pneumoniae, and Legionella pneumophila in respiratory infection. *Infect Dis Clin N Am* **12:**569-92.

2384. Filice, C., G. Di Perri, M. Strosselli, E. Brunetti, S. Dughetti, D. H. Van Thiel, and C. Scotti-Foglieni. 1992. Outcome of hepatic amebic abscesses managed with three different therapeutic strategies. *Dig Dis Sci* **37:**240-7.

2385. Findlay, G. H. 1985. Sporotrichosis research in the Transvaal—how it began 60 years ago. *S Afr Med J* **68:**117-8.

2386. Fine, M. J., M. A. Smith, C. A. Carson, S. S. Mutha, S. S. Sankey, L. A. Weissfeld, and W. N. Kapoor. 1996. Prognosis and outcomes of patients with community-acquired pneumonia. A meta-analysis. *JAMA* **275:**134-41.

2387. Finelli, L., D. Swerdlow, K. Mertz, H. Ragazzoni, and K. Spitalny. 1992. Outbreak of cholera associated with crab brought from an area with epidemic disease. *J Infect Dis* **166:**1433-5.

2388. Finger, R., L. J. Anderson, R. C. Dicker, B. Harrison, R. Doan, A. Downing, and L. Corey. 1987. Epidemic infections caused by respiratory syncytial virus in institutionalized young adults. *J Infect Dis* **155:**1335-9.

2389. Fingerle, V., J. L. Goodman, R. C. Johnson, T. J. Kurtti, U. G. Munderloh, and B. Wilske. 1997. Human granulocytic ehrlichiosis in southern Germany: increased seroprevalence in high-risk groups. *J Clin Microbiol* **35:**3244-7.

2390. Finkelstein, R., R. Fusman, I. Oren, I. Kassis, and N. Hashman. 2002. Clinical and epidemiologic significance of coagulase-negative staphylococci bacteremia in a tertiary care university Israeli hospital. *Am J Infect Control* **30:**21-5.

2391. Finn, R., C. Groves, M. Coe, M. Pass, and L. H. Harrison. 2001. Cluster of serogroup C meningococcal disease associated with attendance at a party. *South Med J* **94:**1192-4.

2392. Finn, S. P., E. Leen, L. English, and D. S. O'Briain. 2003. Autopsy findings in an outbreak of severe systemic illness in heroin users following injection site inflammation: an effect of Clostridium novyi exotoxin? *Arch Pathol Lab Med* **127:**1465-70.

2393. Fiore, A. E. 2004. Hepatitis A transmitted by food. *Clin Infect Dis* **38:**705-15.

2394. **Fiore, A. E., J. C. Butler, T. G. Emori, and R. P. Gaynes.** 1999. A survey of methods used to detect nosocomial legionellosis among participants in the National Nosocomial Infections Surveillance System. *Infect Control Hosp Epidemiol* **20:**412-6.

2395. **Fiore, A. E., J. P. Nuorti, O. S. Levine, A. Marx, A. C. Weltman, S. Yeager, R. F. Benson, J. Pruckler, P. H. Edelstein, P. Greer, S. R. Zaki, B. S. Fields, and J. C. Butler.** 1998. Epidemic Legionnaires' disease two decades later: old sources, new diagnostic methods. *Clin Infect Dis* **26:**426-33.

2396. **Fiore, J. R., B. Suligoi, L. Monno, G. Angarano, and G. Pastore.** 2002. HIV-1 shedding in genital tract of infected women. *Lancet* **359:**1525-6.

2397. **Fiori, P. L., S. Mastrandrea, P. Rappelli, and P. Cappuccinelli.** 2000. Brucella abortus infection acquired in microbiology laboratories. *J Clin Microbiol* **38:**2005-6.

2398. **Fiorillo, L., M. Zucker, D. Sawyer, and A. N. Lin.** 2001. The pseudomonas hot-foot syndrome. *N Engl J Med* **345:**335-8.

2399. **Fiorino, A.** 1996. Intrauterine contraceptive device-associated actinomycotic abscess and Actinomyces detection on cervical smear. *Obstet Gynecol* **87:**142-9.

2400. **Firmo, J. O. A., M. F. Lima e Costa, L. E. Guerra, and R. S. Rocha.** 1996. Urban schistosomiasis: morbidity, sociodemographic characteristics and water contact patterns predictive of infection. *Int J Epidemiol* **25:**1292-1300.

2401. **Fischer, B. P., A. Muller, R. Strauss, H. T. Schneider, and E. G. Hahn.** 1998. [Tsutsugamushi fever. Rare rickettsiosis after a stay in the Philippines]. *Dtsch Med Wochenschr* **123:**562-6.

2402. **Fischer, D., A. Veldman, V. Schafer, and M. Diefenbach.** 2004. Bacterial colonization of patients undergoing international air transport: a prospective epidemiologic study. *J Travel Med* **11:**44-8.

2403. **Fischer, J. R., D. E. Stallknecht, P. Luttrell, A. A. Dhondt, and K. A. Converse.** 1997. Mycoplasmal conjunctivitis in wild songbirds: the spread of a new contagious disease in a mobile host population. *Emerg Infect Dis* **3:**69-72.

2404. **Fischer, L., M. Sterneck, M. Claus, A. Costard-Jackle, B. Fleischer, H. Herbst, X. Rogiers, and C. E. Broelsch.** 1999. Transmission of malaria tertiana by multi-organ donation. *Clin Transplant* **13:**491-5.

2405. **Fischer, M., A. Chrusciak Talhari, D. Reinel, and S. Talhari.** 2002. [Sucessful treatment with clofazimine and itraconazole in a 46 year old patient after 32 years duration of disease]. *Hautarzt* **53:**677-81.

2406. **Fischer, P., T. Supali, and R. M. Maizels.** 2004. Lymphatic filariasis and Brugia timori: prospects for elimination. *Trends Parasitol* **20:**351-5.

2407. **Fischer, P., E. Tukesiga, and D. W. Buttner.** 1999. Long-term suppression of Mansonella streptocerca microfilariae after treatment with ivermectin. *J Infect Dis* **180:**1403-5.

2408. **Fischer, P. R.** 1997. Congenital malaria: an African survey. *Clin Pediatr (Phila)* **36:**411-3.

2409. **Fischer, P. R., C. Brunetti, V. Welch, and J. C. Christenson.** 1996. Nosocomial mumps: report of an outbreak and its control. *Am J Infect Control* **24:**13-8.

2410. **Fischer, T. K., P. Valentiner-Branth, H. Steinsland, M. Perch, G. Santos, P. Aaby, K. Molbak, and H. Sommerfelt.** 2002. Protective immunity after natural rotavirus infection: a community cohort study of newborn children in Guinea-Bissau, West Africa. *J Infect Dis* **186:**593-7.

2411. **Fishbein, D. B., and D. Raoult.** 1992. A cluster of Coxiella burnetii infections associated with exposure to vaccinated goats and their unpasteurized dairy products. *Am J Trop Med Hyg* **47:**33-40.

2412. **Fisher, A. A.** 1988. Swimming pool granulomas due to Mycobacterium marinum: an occupational hazard of lifeguards. *Cutis* **41:**397-8.

2413. **Fisher, I. S. T.** 1997. Salmonella enteritidis and S. typhimurium in western Europe for 1993-1995: a surveillance report from Salm-Net. *Eurosurveillance* **2:**4-6.

2414. **Fisher, L., M. Williams, L. Feltmann, D. Donnell, T. Hicks, T. Macias, L. Watson, and C. Jennings.** 1994. Outbreak of measles among Christian science students - Missouri and Illinois, 1994. *MMWR* **43:**463-5.

2415. **Fisher, M.** 2003. Toxocara cati: an underestimated zoonotic agent. *Trends Parasitol* **19:**167-70.

2416. **Fisher, M. C., G. L. Koenig, T. J. White, G. San-Blas, R. Negroni, I. G. Alvarez, B. Wanke, and J. W. Taylor.** 2001. Biogeographic range expansion into South America by Coccidioides immitis mirrors New World patterns of human migration. *Proc Natl Acad Sci USA* **98:**4558-62.

2417. **Fisher, M. C., S. S. Long, K. L. McGowan, E. Kaselis, and D. G. Smith.** 1989. Outbreak of pertussis in a residential facility for handicapped people. *J Pediatr* **114:**934-9.

2418. **Fisher-Hoch, S. P., J. A. Khan, S. Rehman, S. Mirza, M. Khurshid, and J. B. McCormick.** 1995. Crimean Congo-haemorrhagic fever treated with oral ribavirin. *Lancet* **346:**472-5.

2419. **Fisher-Hoch, S. P., J. B. McCormick, R. Swanepoel, A. Van Middlekoop, S. Harvey, and H. G. Kustner.** 1992. Risk of human infections with Crimean-Congo hemorrhagic fever virus in a South African rural community. *Am J Trop Med Hyg* **47:**337-45.

2420. **Fisher-Hoch, S. P., O. Tomori, A. Nasidi, G. I. Perez-Oronoz, Y. Fakile, L. Hutwagner, and J. B. McCormick.** 1995. Review of cases of nosocomial Lassa fever in Nigeria: the high price of poor medical practice. *BMJ* **311:**857-9.

2421. **Fishman, J. A., and R. H. Rubin.** 1998. Infection in organ-transplant recipients. *N Engl J Med* **338:**1741-51.

2422. **Fisker, N., J. Georgsen, T. Stolborg, M. R. Khalil, and P. B. Christensen.** 2002. Low hepatitis B prevalence among preschool children in Denmark: saliva anti-HBc screening in day care centres. *J Med Virol* **68:**500-4.

2423. **Fitzgerald, D. W., F. Behets, A. Caliendo, D. Roberfroid, C. Lucet, J. W. Fitzgerald, and L. Kuykens.** 2000. Economic hardship and sexually transmitted diseases in Haiti's rural Artibonite Valley. *Am J Trop Med Hyg* **62:**496-501.

2424. **Fitzpatrick, P. E., R. L. Salmon, P. R. Hunter, R. J. Roberts, and S. R. Palmer.** 2000. Risk factors for carriage of Neisseria meningitidis during an outbreak in Wales. *Emerg Infect Dis* **6:**65-9.

2425. **Flamaing, J., I. Engelmann, E. Joosten, M. Van Ranst, J. Verhaegen, and W. E. Peetermans.** 2003. Viral lower respiratory tract infection in the elderly: a prospective in-hospital study. *Eur J Clin Microbiol Infect Dis* **22:**720-5.

2426. **Flanigan, T. P., T. G. Schwan, C. Armstrong, L. P. Van Voris, and R. A. Salata.** 1991. Relapsing fever in the US Virgin islands: a previously unrecognized focus of infection. *J Infect Dis* **163:**1391-2.

2427. **Fleisch, F., U. Zimmermann-Baer, R. Zbinden, G. Bischoff, R. Arlettaz, K. Waldvogel, D. Nadal, and C. Ruef.** 2002. Three consecutive outbreaks of Serratia marcescens in a neonatal intensive care unit. *Clin Infect Dis* **34**:767-73.

2428. **Fleischer, B.** 1998. Cholera in Hamburg. *Newsl Int Soc Chemother* **2**:3-4.

2429. **Fleisher, G. R.** 1999. The management of bite wounds. *N Engl J Med* **340**:138-40.

2430. **Fleisher, G. R., P. S. Pasquariello, W. S. Warren, W. S. Zavod, A. B. Korval, H. D. Turner, and E. T. Lennette.** 1981. Intrafamilial transmission of Epstein-Barr virus infections. *J Pediatr* **98**:16-9.

2431. **Fleissner, M. L., J. E. Herrmann, J. W. Booth, N. R. Blacklow, and N. A. Nowak.** 1998. Role of norwalk virus in two foodborne outbreaks of gastroenteritis: definitive virus association. *Am J Epidemiol* **129**:165-172.

2432. **Fleming, C. A., D. Caron, J. E. Gunn, and M. A. Barry.** 1998. A foodborne outbreak of Cyclospora cayetanensis at a wedding: clinical features and risk factors for illness. *Arch Intern Med* **158**:1121-5.

2433. **Fleming, C. A., D. Caron, J. E. Gunn, M. S. Horine, B. T. Matyas, and M. A. Barry.** 2000. An outbreak of Shigella sonnei associated with a recreational spray fountain. *Am J Public Health* **90**:1641-2.

2434. **Fleming, D. M., M. A. Barley, and R. S. Chapman.** 2004. Surveillance of the bioterrorist threat: a primary care response. *Commun Dis Public Health* **7**:68-72.

2435. **Fleming, D. T., G. M. McQuillan, R. E. Johnson, A. J. Nahmias, S. O. Aral, F. K. Lee, and M. E. St Louis.** 1997. Herpes simplex virus type 2 in the United States, 1976 to 1994. *N Engl J Med* **337**:1105-11.

2436. **Fleming, D. W., S. L. Cochi, K. L. MacDonald, J. Brondum, P. S. Hayes, B. D. Plikaytis, M. B. Holmes, A. Audurier, C. V. Broome, and A. L. Reingold.** 1985. Pasteurized milk as a vehicle of infection in an outbreak of listeriosis. *N Engl J Med* **312**:404-7.

2437. **Fletcher, C. L., M. R. Ardern-Jones, and R. J. Hay.** 2002. Widespread bullous eruption due to multiple bed bug bites. *Clin Exp Dermatol* **27**:74-5.

2438. **Fletcher, M., M. E. Levy, and D. D. Griffin.** 2000. Foodborne outbreak of group A rotavirus gastroenteritis among college students - Distric of Columbia, March-April 2000. *MMWR* **49**:1131-3.

2439. **Fliegel, P. E., and W. M. Weinstein.** 1982. Rubella outbreak in a prenatal clinic: management and prevention. *Am J Infect Control* **10**:29-33.

2440. **Flisser, A., E. Sarti, M. Lightowlers, and P. Schantz.** 2003. Neurocysticercosis: regional status, epidemiology, impact and control measures in the Americas. *Acta Trop* **87**:43-51.

2441. **Flood, J., L. Mintz, M. Jay, F. Taylor, and W. L. Drew.** 1995. Hantavirus infection following wilderness camping in Washington State and northeastern California. *West J Med* **163**:162-4.

2442. **Flood, J. M., S. K. Sarafian, G. A. Bolan, C. Lammel, J. Engelman, R. M. Greenblatt, G. F. Brooks, A. Back, and S. A. Morse.** 1993. Multistrain outbreak of chancroid in San Francisco, 1989-1991. *J Infect Dis* **167**:1106-11.

2443. **Flores Hernandez, S., H. Reyes Morales, R. Perez Cuevas, and H. Guiscafre Gallardo.** 1999. The day care center as a risk factor for acute respiratory infections. *Arch Med Res* **30**:216-23.

2444. **Flunker, G., A. Peters, S. Wiersbitzky, S. Modrow, and W. Seidel.** 1998. Persistent parvovirus B19 infections in immunocompromised children. *Med Microbiol Immunol (Berl)* **186**:189-94.

2445. **Flynn, N. M., P. D. Hoeprich, M. M. Kawachi, K. K. Lee, and R. M. Lawrence.** 1979. An unusual outbreak of windborne coccidioidomycosis. *N Engl J Med* **301**:358-361.

2446. **Follmann, E. H., D. G. Ritter, and M. Beller.** 1994. Survey of fox trappers in northern Alaska for rabies antibody. *Epidemiol Infect* **113**:137-41.

2447. **Folz, B. J., B. M. Lippert, C. Kuelkens, and J. A. Werner.** 2000. Hazards of piercing and facial body art: a report of three patients and literature review. *Ann Plast Surg* **45**:374-81.

2448. **Fone, D. L., and R. M. Barker.** 1994. Associations between human and farm animal infections with Salmonella typhimurium DT104 in Herefordshire. *Commun Dis Rep CDR Rev* **4**:R136-40.

2449. **Fonseca, W., B. R. Kirkwood, C. G. Victora, S. R. Fuchs, J. A. Flores, and C. Misago.** 1996. Risk factors for childhood pneumonia among the urban poor in Fortaleza, Brazil: a case—control study. *Bull WHO* **74**:199-208.

2450. **Fontaine, R. E., S. Arnon, W. T. Martin, T. M. Vernon, Jr., E. J. Gangarosa, J. J. Farmer, 3rd, A. B. Moran, J. H. Silliker, and D. L. Decker.** 1978. Raw hamburger: an interstate common source of human salmonellosis. *Am J Epidemiol* **107**:36-45.

2451. **Fontaine, R. E., M. L. Cohen, W. T. Martin, and T. M. Vernon.** 1980. Epidemic salmonellosis from cheddar cheese: surveillance and prevention. *Am J Epidemiol* **111**:247-53.

2452. **Fontaine, R. E., A. E. Najjar, and J. S. Prince.** 1961. The 1958 epidemic in Ethiopia. *Am J Trop Med Hyg* **10**:795-803.

2453. **Fontenille, D., and J. C. Toto.** 2001. Aedes (Stegomyia) albopictus (Skuse), a potential new dengue vector in southern Cameroon. *Emerg Infect Dis* **7**:1066-1067.

2454. **Fooks, A. R., L. M. McElhinney, D. J. Pounder, C. J. Finnegan, K. Mansfield, N. Johnson, S. M. Brookes, G. Parsons, K. White, P. G. McIntyre, and D. Nathwani.** 2003. Case report: isolation of a European bat lyssavirus type 2a from a fatal human case of rabies encephalitis. *J Med Virol* **71**:281-9.

2455. **Foppa, I. M., P. J. Krause, A. Spielman, H. Goethert, L. Gern, B. Brand, and S. R. Telford, 3rd.** 2002. Entomologic and Serologic Evidence of Zoonotic Transmission of Babesia microti, Eastern Switzerland. *Emerg Infect Dis* **8**:722-6.

2456. **Forbes, D., L. Ee, P. Camer-Pesci, and P. B. Ward.** 2001. Faecal candida and diarrhoea. *Arch Dis Child* **84**:328-31.

2457. **Forbes, L. B.** 2000. The occurrence and ecology of Trichinella in marine mammals. *Vet Parasitol* **93**:321-34.

2458. **Ford, N., C. N., and H. Jeanmart.** 2003. Homelessness and hardship in Moscow. *Lancet* **361**:875.

2459. **Ford, P. M., C. White, H. Kaufmann, J. MacTavish, M. Pearson, S. Ford, P. Sankar-Mistry, and P. Connop.** 1995. Voluntary anonymous linked study of the prevalence of HIV infection and hepatitis C among inmates in a Canadian federal penitentiary for women. *CMAJ* **153**:1605-9.

2460. **Forleo-Neto, E., C. F. de Oliveira, E. M. Maluf, C. Bataglin, J. M. Araujo, L. F. Kunz, Jr., A. K. Pustai, V. S. Vieira, R. C. Zanella, M. C. Brandileone, L. M. Mimica, and I. M. Mimica.** 1999. Decreased point prevalence of Haemophilus influenzae type b (Hib) oropharyngeal colonization by mass immunization of Brazilian children less than 5 years old with hib polyribosylribitol phosphate polysaccharide-tetanus toxoid conjugate vaccine in combination with diphtheria-tetanus toxoids-pertussis vaccine. *J Infect Dis* **180**:1153-8.

2461. **Formenty, P., C. Boesch, M. Wyers, C. Steiner, F. Donati, F. Dind, F. Walker, and B. Le Guenno.** 1999. Ebola virus outbreak among wild chimpanzees living in a rain forest of Cote d'Ivoire. *J Infect Dis* **179 Suppl 1**:S120-6.

2462. **Formenty, P., C. Hatz, B. Le Guenno, A. Stoll, P. Rogenmoser, and A. Widmer.** 1999. Human infection due to Ebola virus, subtype Cote d'Ivoire: clinical and biologic presentation. *J Infect Dis* **179 Suppl 1**:S48-53.

2463. **Formica, S., and C. Botto.** 1990. Filariasis focus due to Mansonella ozzardi and Mansonella perstans in the Amazon Federal Territory of Venezuela. *J Trop Med Hyg* **93**:160-5.

2464. **Formiga-Cruz, M., G. Tofino-Quesada, S. Bofill-Mas, D. N. Lees, K. Henshilwood, A. K. Allard, A. C. Conden-Hansson, B. E. Hernroth, A. Vantarakis, A. Tsibouxi, M. Papapetropoulou, M. D. Furones, and R. Girones.** 2002. Distribution of human virus contamination in shellfish from different growing areas in Greece, Spain, Sweden, and the United Kingdom. *Appl Environ Microbiol* **68**:5990-8.

2465. **Forns, X., P. Fernandez-Llama, M. Pons, J. Costa, S. Ampurdanes, F. X. Lopez-Labrador, E. Olmedo, J. Lopez-Pedret, A. Darnell, L. Revert, J. M. Sanchez-Tapias, and J. Rodes.** 1997. Incidence and risk factors of hepatitis C virus infection in a haemodialysis unit. *Nephrol Dial Transplant* **12**:736-40.

2466. **Forster, J.** 2003. Influenza in children: the German perspective. *Pediatr Infect Dis J* **22**:S215-7.

2467. **Forthal, D. N., S. P. Bauer, and J. B. McCormick.** 1987. Antibody to hemorrhagic fever with renal syndrome viruses (Hantaviruses) in the United States. *Am J Epidemiol* **126**:1210-3.

2468. **Foster, G., T. Patterson, F. Howie, V. Simpson, N. Davison, A. Efstratiou, and S. Lai.** 2002. Corynebacterium ulcerans in free-ranging otters. *Vet Rec* **150**:524.

2469. **Foster, S. O., E. L. Palmer, G. W. Gary, Jr., M. L. Martin, K. L. Herrmann, P. Beasley, and J. Sampson.** 1980. Gastroenteritis due to rotavirus in an isolated Pacific island group: an epidemic of 3,439 cases. *J Infect Dis* **141**:32-9.

2470. **Foucault, C., K. Barrau, P. Brouqui, and D. Raoult.** 2002. Bartonella quintana Bacteremia among Homeless People. *Clin Infect Dis* **35**:684-9.

2471. **Foucault, C., J. M. Rolain, D. Raoult, and P. Brouqui.** 2004. Detection of Bartonella quintana by direct immunofluorescence examination of blood smears of a patient with acute trench fever. *J Clin Microbiol* **42**:4904-6.

2472. **Fouchier, R. A., P. M. Schneeberger, F. W. Rozendaal, J. M. Broekman, S. A. Kemink, V. Munster, T. Kuiken, G. F. Rimmelzwaan, M. Schutten, G. J. Van Doornum, G. Koch, A. Bosman, M. Koopmans, and A. D. Osterhaus.** 2004. Avian influenza A virus (H7N7) associated with human conjunctivitis and a fatal case of acute respiratory distress syndrome. *Proc Natl Acad Sci USA* **101**:1356-61.

2473. **Fountain, D., M. Ralston, N. Higgins, J. B. Gorlin, L. Uhl, C. Wheeler, J. H. Antin, W. H. Churchill, and R. J. Benjamin.** 1997. Liquid nitrogen freezers: a potential source of microbial contamination of hematopoietic stem cell components. *Transfusion* **37**:585-91.

2474. **Fournet, F., S. Traore, and J. P. Hervouet.** 1999. Effects of urbanization on transmission of human African trypanosomiasis in a suburban relict forest area of Daloa, Cote d'Ivoire. *Trans R Soc Trop Med Hyg* **93**:130-2.

2475. **Fournier, P. E., C. Allombert, Y. Supputamongkol, G. Caruso, P. Brouqui, and D. Raoult.** 2004. Aneruptive fever associated with antibodies to Rickettsia helvetica in Europe and Thailand. *J Clin Microbiol* **42**:816-8.

2476. **Fournier, P. E., F. Grunnenberger, B. Jaulhac, G. Gastinger, and D. Raoult.** 2000. Evidence of Rickettsia helvetica infection in humans, eastern France. *Emerg Infect Dis* **6**:389-92.

2477. **Fournier, P. E., J. B. Ndihokubwayo, J. Guidran, P. J. Kelly, and D. Raoult.** 2002. Human pathogens in body and head lice. *Emerg Infect Dis* **8**:1515-8.

2478. **Fournier, P. E., V. Roux, E. Caumes, M. Donzel, and D. Raoult.** 1998. Outbreak of Rickettsia africae infections in participants of an adventure race in South Africa. *Clin Infect Dis* **27**:316-23.

2479. **Fournier, S., S. Dubrou, O. Liguory, F. Gaussin, M. Santillana-Hayat, C. Sarfati, J. M. Molina, and F. Derouin.** 2002. Detection of Microsporidia, cryptosporidia and Giardia in swimming pools: a one-year prospective study. *FEMS Immunol Med Microbiol* **33**:209-13.

2480. **Fournier, S., O. Liguory, M. Santillana-Hayat, E. Guillot, C. Sarfati, N. Dumoutier, J. Molina, and F. Derouin.** 2000. Detection of microsporidia in surface water: a one-year follow-up study. *FEMS Immunol Med Microbiol* **29**:95-100.

2481. **Fowler, K. B., S. Stagno, and R. F. Pass.** 1993. Maternal age and congenital cytomegalovirus infection: screening of two diverse newborn populations, 1980-1990. *J Infect Dis* **168**:552-6.

2482. **Fowler, K. B., S. Stagno, R. F. Pass, W. J. Britt, T. J. Boll, and C. A. Alford.** 1992. The outcome of congenital cytomegalovirus infection in relation to maternal antibody status. *N Engl J Med* **326**:663-667.

2483. **Fox, E., J. Bouloumie, J. G. Olson, D. Tible, M. Lluberas, S. O. Shakib, J. P. Parra, and G. Rodier.** 1991. [Plasmodium falciparum travels by train from Ethiopia to Djibouti]. *Med Trop (Mars)* **51**:185-9.

2484. **Fox, J. P., M. K. Cooney, and C. E. Hall.** 1975. The Seattle virus watch. V. Epidemiologic observations of rhinovirus infections, 1965-1969, in families with young children. *Am J Epidemiol* **101**:122-43.

2485. **Fox, K. K., C. Del Rio, K. K. Holmes, E. W. Hook, 3rd, F. N. Judson, J. S. Knapp, G. W. Procop, S. A. Wang, W. L. Whittington, and W. C. Levine.** 2001. Gonorrhoea in the HIV era: a reversal in trends among men who have sex with men. *Am J Public Health* **91**:954-64.

2486. **Foxman, B., S. D. Manning, P. Tallman, R. Bauer, L. Zhang, J. S. Koopman, B. Gillespie, J. D. Sobel, and C. F. Marrs.** 2002. Uropathogenic Escherichia coli are more likely than commensal E coli to be shared between heterosexual sex partners. *Am J Epidemiol* **156**:1133-40.

2487. **Foy, H. M., J. T. Grayston, G. E. Kenny, E. R. Alexander, and R. McMahan.** 1966. Epidemiology of Mycoplasma pneumoniae infection in families. *JAMA* **197**:859-66.

2488. **Fradkin, J. E., L. B. Schonberger, J. L. Mills, W. J. Gunn, J. M. Piper, D. K. Wysowski, R. Thomson, S. Durako, and P. Brown.** 1991. Creutzfeldt-Jakob disease in pituitary growth hormone recipients in the United States. *JAMA* **265**:880-4.

2489. **Frances, S. P., R. D. Cooper, K. L. Rowcliffe, N. Chen, and Q. Cheng.** 2004. Occurrence of Ross River virus and Barmah Forest virus in mosquitoes at Shoalwater Bay military training area, Queensland, Australia. *J Med Entomol* **41**:115-20.

2490. **Frances, S. P., C. Eamsila, and D. Strickman.** 1997. Antibodies to Orientia tsutsugamushi in soldiers in northeastern Thailand. *Southeast Asian J Trop Med Public Health* **28:**666-8.

2491. **Franciosa, G., M. Pourshaban, M. Gianfranceschi, A. Gattuso, L. Fenicia, A. M. Ferrini, V. Mannoni, G. De Luca, and P. Aureli.** 1999. Clostridium botulinum spores and toxin in mascarpone cheese and other milk products. *J Food Prot* **62:**867-71.

2492. **Francis, S., J. Rowland, K. Rattenbury, D. Powell, W. N. Rogers, L. Ward, and S. R. Palmer.** 1989. An outbreak of paratyphoid fever in the UK associated with a fish-and-chip shop. *Epidemiol Infect* **103:**445-8.

2493. **Franco, E., C. Giambi, R. Ialacci, R. C. Coppola, and A. R. Zanetti.** 2003. Risk groups for hepatitis A virus infection. *Vaccine* **21:**2224-33.

2494. **Franco, R. M., and R. Cantusio Neto.** 2002. Occurrence of cryptosporidial oocysts and giardia cysts in bottled mineral water commercialized in the city of Campinas, State of Sao Paulo, Brazil. *Mem Inst Oswaldo Cruz* **97:**205-7.

2495. **Franco, R. M., R. Rocha-Eberhardt, and R. Cantusio Neto.** 2001. Occurrence of Cryptosporidium oocysts and Giardia cysts in raw water from the Atibaia River, Campinas, Brazil. *Rev Inst Med Trop Sao Paulo* **43:**109-11.

2496. **Frangoulis, E., B. Athanasopoulou, and A. Katsambas.** 2004. Etiology of tinea capitis in Athens, Greece — a 6-year (1996-2001) retrospective study. *Mycoses* **47:**208-12.

2497. **Frank, C., M. Hadziandoniou, F. Pratlong, A. Garifallou, and J. A. Rioux.** 1993. Leishmania tropica and Leishmania infantum responsible for cutaneous leishmaniasis in Greece: sixteen autochthonous cases. *Trans R Soc Trop Med Hyg* **87:**184-5.

2498. **Frank, C., I. Schöneberg, G. Krause, H. Claus, A. Ammon, and K. Stark.** 2004. Increase in imported dengue, Germany, 2001-2002. *Emerg Infect Dis* **10:**903-6.

2499. **Frank, C., J. Walter, M. Muehlen, A. Jansen, U. van Treeck, A. M. Hauri, I. Zoellner, E. Schreier, O. Hamouda, and K. Stark.** 2005. Large outbreak of hepatitis A in tourists staying at a hotel in Hurghada, Egypt, 2004 - orange juice implicated. *Eurosurveillance* **10:**135-7.

2500. **Frank, P. T., and K. M. Johnson.** 1970. An outbreak of Venezuelan encephalitis in man in the Panama canal zone. *Am J Trop Med Hyg* **19:**860-5.

2501. **Frank, R. K.** 2001. An outbreak of toxoplasmosis in farmed mink (Mustela vison S.). *J Vet Diagn Invest* **13:**245-9.

2502. **Frank, U., L. Herz, and F. D. Daschner.** 1988. Infection risk of cardiac catheterization and arterial angiography with single and multiple use disposable catheters. *Clin Cardiol* **11:**785-7.

2503. **Franklin, R. P., H. Kinde, M. T. Jay, L. D. Kramer, E. G. Green, R. E. Chiles, E. Ostlund, S. Husted, J. Smith, and M. D. Parker.** 2002. Eastern equine encephalitis virus infection in a horse from California. *Emerg Infect Dis* **8:**283-8.

2504. **Frankowski, B. L., and L. B. Weiner.** 2002. American Academy of Pediatrics. Clinical report. Head lice. *Pediatrics* **110:**638-43.

2505. **Franz, D. R., P. B. Jahrling, A. M. Friedlander, D. J. McClain, D. L. Hoover, W. R. Bryne, J. A. Pavlin, G. W. Christopher, and E. M. Eitzen, Jr.** 1997. Clinical recognition and management of patients exposed to biological warfare agents. *JAMA* **278:**399-411.

2506. **Fraser, D., R. Dagan, L. Naggan, V. Greene, J. El-On, Y. Abu-Rbiah, and R. J. Deckelbaum.** 1997. Natural history of Giardia lamblia and Cryptosporidium infections in a cohort of Israeli Bedouin infants: a study of a population in transition. *Am J Trop Med Hyg* **57:**544-9.

2507. **Fraser, D. W., T. R. Tsai, W. Orenstein, W. E. Parkin, H. J. Beecham, R. G. Sharrar, J. Harris, G. F. Mallison, S. M. Martin, J. E. McDade, C. C. Shepard, and P. S. Brachman.** 1977. Legionnaires' disease: description of an epidemic of pneumonia. *N Engl J Med* **297:**1189-97.

2508. **Fraser, G. G., and K. R. Cooke.** 1991. Endemic giardiasis and municipal water supply. *Am J Public Health* **81:**760-2.

2509. **Fraser-Hurt, N., R. L. Bailey, S. Cousens, D. Mabey, H. Faal, and D. C. Mabey.** 2001. Efficacy of oral azithromycin versus topical tetracycline in mass treatment of endemic trachoma. *Bull WHO* **79:**632-40.

2510. **Frean, J., L. Arntzen, J. Van Den Heever, and O. Perovic.** 2004. Fatal type A botulism in South Africa, 2002. *Trans R Soc Trop Med Hyg* **98:**290-5.

2511. **Frederiksen, B., and S. Samuelsson.** 1992. Feto-maternal listeriosis in Denmark 1981-1988. *J Infect* **24:**277-87.

2512. **Fredlund, H., E. Bäck, L. Sjöberg, and T. E.** 1987. Watermelon as a vehicle of transmission of shigellosis. *Scand J Infect Dis* **19:**219-21.

2513. **Fredricks, D. N., J. A. Jolley, P. W. Lepp, J. C. Kosek, and D. A. Relman.** 2000. Rhinosporidium seeberi: a human pathogen from a novel group of aquatic protistan parasites. *Emerg Infect Dis* **6:**273-82.

2514. **Frees, N., J. Polkowski, R. Farmer, R. Akin, M. J. Bankowski, M. Neuman, V. Negron, N. Feintuch, R. Cremo, J. Wroten, J. Witte, and A. Landay.** 1992. HIV infection, syphilis, and tuberculosis screening among migrant farm workers—Florida, 1992. *MMWR* **41:**723-5.

2515. **Freier, J. E.** 1993. Eastern equine encephalomyelitis. *Lancet* **342:**1281—2.

2516. **Freifeld, A. G., J. Hilliard, J. Southers, M. Murray, B. Savarese, J. M. Schmitt, and S. E. Straus.** 1995. A controlled seroprevalence survey of primate handlers for evidence of asymptomatic herpes B virus infection. *J Infect Dis* **171:**1031-4.

2517. **Freitas, R. B., T. A. Monteiro, and A. C. Linhares.** 2000. Outbreaks of human-herpes virus 6 (HHV-6) infection in day-care centers in Belem, Para, Brazil. *Rev Inst Med Trop Sao Paulo* **42:**305-11.

2518. **Frenkel, J. K.** 1985. Toxoplasmosis. *Pediatr Clin North Am* **32:**917-32.

2519. **Frenkel, J. K., K. M. Hassanein, R. S. Hassanein, E. Brown, P. Thulliez, and R. Quintero-Nunez.** 1995. Transmission of Toxoplasma gondii in Panama City, Panama: a five-year prospective cohort study of children, cats, rodents, birds, and soil. *Am J Trop Med Hyg* **53:**458-68.

2520. **Fretz, R., H. Schmid, U. Kayser, P. Svoboda, M. Tanner, and A. Baumgartner.** 2003. Rapid propagation of norovirus gastrointestinal illness through multiple nursing homes following a pilgrimage. *Eur J Clin Microbiol Infect Dis* **22:**625-7.

2521. **Freudenstein, U., and P. Monk.** 2000. Limitations of national guidelines in the management of an outbreak of tuberculosis. *Commun Dis Public Health* **3:**184-7.

2522. **Frey, S. E., S. M. Homan, M. Sokol-Anderson, M. T. Cayco, P. Cortorreal, C. E. Musial, and A. M. Di Bisceglie.** 2002.

Evidence for probable sexual transmission of the hepatitis G virus. *Clin Infect Dis* **34**:1033-8.

2523. **Frey-Wettstein, M., A. Maier, K. Markwalder, and U. Munch.** 2001. A case of transfusion transmitted malaria in Switzerland. *Swiss Med Wkly* **131**:320.

2524. **Freymouth, F., A. Vabret, L. Legrand, N. Eterradossi, F. Lafay-Delaire, J. Brouard, and B. Guillois.** 2003. Presence of the new human metapneumovirus in French children with bronchiolitis. *Pediatr Infect Dis J* **22**:92-4.

2525. **Friede, A., J. R. Harris, J. M. Kobayashi, F. E. Shaw, Jr., P. C. Shoemaker-Nawas, and M. A. Kane.** 1988. Transmission of hepatitis B virus from adopted Asian children to their American families. *Am J Public Health* **78**:26-9.

2526. **Frieden, I. J.** 1999. Tinea capitis: asymptomatic carriage of infection. *Pediatr Infect Dis J* **18**:186-90.

2527. **Friedman, C. R., R. M. Hoekstra, M. Samuel, R. Marcus, J. Bender, B. Shiferaw, S. Reddy, S. D. Ahuja, D. L. Helfrick, F. Hardnett, M. Carter, B. Anderson, and R. V. Tauxe.** 2004. Risk factors for sporadic Campylobacter infection in the United States: A case-control study in FoodNet sites. *Clin Infect Dis* **38 Suppl 3**:S285-96.

2528. **Friedman, H. B., A. J. Saah, M. E. Sherman, A. E. Busseniers, W. C. Blackwelder, R. A. Kaslow, A. M. Ghaffari, R. W. Daniel, and K. V. Shah.** 1998. Human papillomavirus, anal squamous intraepithelial lesions, and human immunodeficiency virus in a cohort of gay men. *J Infect Dis* **178**:45-52.

2529. **Friedman, L. S., T. F. O'Brien, L. J. Morse, L. W. Chang, W. E. Wacker, D. M. Ryan, and J. L. Dienstag.** 1985. Revisiting the Holy Cross football team hepatitis outbreak (1969) by serological analysis. *JAMA* **254**:774-6.

2530. **Friedman, M. J., and M. W. Attia.** 2004. Clinical predictors of influenza in children. *Arch Pediatr Adolesc Med* **158**:391-4.

2531. **Friedman, M. S., T. Roels, J. E. Koehler, L. Feldman, W. F. Bibb, and P. Blake.** 1999. Escherichia coli O157:H7 outbreak associated with an improperly chlorinated swimming pool. *Clin Infect Dis* **29**:298-303.

2532. **Friedman, N., T. Korman, C. Fairley, J. Franklin, and D. Spelman.** 2002. Bacteraemia due to Stenotrophomonas maltophilia: An Analysis of 45 Episodes. *J Infect* **45**:47.

2533. **Friedman, S. M., S. Schultz, A. Goodman, S. Millian, and L. Z. Cooper.** 1983. Rubella outbreak among office workers - New York city. *MMWR* **32**:349-52.

2534. **Friedman, S. R., D. C. Ompad, C. Maslow, R. Young, P. Case, S. M. Hudson, T. Diaz, E. Morse, S. Bailey, D. C. Des Jarlais, T. Perlis, A. Hollibaugh, and R. S. Garfein.** 2003. HIV prevalence, risk behaviors, and high-risk sexual and injection networks among young women injectors who have sex with women. *Am J Public Health* **93**:902-6.

2535. **Friis, L., L. Engstrand, and C. Edling.** 1996. Prevalence of Helicobacter pylori infection among sewage workers. *Scand J Work Environ Health* **22**:364-8.

2536. **Fritz, C. L., C. F. Fulhorst, B. Enge, K. L. Winthrop, C. A. Glaser, and D. J. Vugia.** 2002. Exposure to rodents and rodent-borne viruses among persons with elevated occupational risk. *J Occup Environ Med* **44**:962-7.

2537. **Fritz, C. L., and J. C. Young.** 2001. (letter). *Am J Trop Med Hyg* **65**:403.

2538. **Frolich, K., J. Wisser, H. Schmuser, U. Fehlberg, H. Neubauer, R. Grunow, K. Nikolaou, J. Priemer, S. Thiede, W. J. Streich, and S. Speck.** 2003. Epizootiologic and ecologic investigations of European brown hares (Lepus europaeus) in selected populations from Schleswig-Holstein, Germany. *J Wildl Dis* **39**:751-61.

2539. **Frosh, A., R. Joyce, and A. Johnson.** 2001. Iatrogenic vCJD from surgical instruments. *BMJ* **322**:1558-9.

2540. **Frost, F. J., T. Muller, G. F. Craun, R. L. Calderon, and P. A. Roefer.** 2001. Paired city cryptosporidium serosurvey in the southwest USA. *Epidemiol Infect* **126**:301-7.

2541. **Frost, J. A., I. A. Gillespie, and S. J. O'Brien.** 2002. Public health implications of campylobacter outbreaks in England and Wales, 1995-9: epidemiological and microbiological investigations. *Epidemiol Infect* **128**:111-8.

2542. **Frost, J. A., M. B. McEvoy, C. A. Bentley, and Y. Andersson.** 1995. An outbreak of Shigella sonnei infection associated with consumption of iceberg lettuce. *Emerg Infect Dis* **1**:26-9.

2543. **Fry, A. M., P. Lurie, M. Gidley, S. Schmink, J. Lingappa, M. Fischer, and N. E. Rosenstein.** 2001. Haemophilus influenzae Type b Disease Among Amish Children in Pennsylvania: Reasons for Persistent Disease. *Pediatrics* **108**:E60.

2544. **Fry, A. M., M. Rutman, T. Allan, H. Scaife, E. Salehi, R. Benson, B. Fields, S. Nowicki, M. K. Parrish, J. Carpenter, E. Brown, C. Lucas, T. Horgan, E. Koch, and R. E. Besser.** 2003. Legionnaires' disease outbreak in an automobile engine manufacturing plant. *J Infect Dis* **187**:1015-8.

2545. **Fryauff, D. J., R. Krippner, P. Prodjodipuro, C. Ewald, S. Kawengian, K. Pegelow, T. Yun, C. von Heydwolff-Wehnert, B. Oyofo, and R. Gross.** 1999. Cyclospora cayetanensis among expatriate and indigenous populations of West Java, Indonesia. *Emerg Infect Dis* **5**:585-8.

2546. **Fryauff, D. J., G. B. Modi, N. S. Mansour, R. D. Kreutzer, S. Soliman, and F. G. Youssef.** 1993. Epidemiology of cutaneous leishmaniasis at a focus monitored by the multinational force and observers in the northeastern Sinai Desert of Egypt. *Am J Trop Med Hyg* **49**:598-607.

2547. **Fryauff, D. J., S. Tuti, A. Mardi, S. Masbar, R. Patipelohi, B. Leksana, K. C. Kain, M. J. Bangs, T. L. Richie, and J. K. Baird.** 1998. Chloroquine-resistant Plasmodium vivax in transmigration settlements of West Kalimantan, Indonesia. *Am J Trop Med Hyg* **59**:513-8.

2548. **Frye, D. M., R. Zweig, J. Sturgeon, M. Tormey, M. LeCavalier, I. Lee, L. Lawani, and L. Mascola.** 2002. An outbreak of febrile gastroenteritis associated with delicatessen meat contaminated with Listeria monocytogenes. *Clin Infect Dis* **35**:943-9.

2549. **Fuchizaki, U., H. Ohta, and T. Sugimoto.** 2003. Diphyllobothriasis. *Lancet Infect Dis* **3**:32.

2550. **Fuentes, L.** 1986. Ecological study of Rocky Mountain spotted fever in Costa Rica. *Am J Trop Med Hyg* **35**:192-6.

2551. **Fujino, T., and Y. Nagata.** 2000. HTLV-I transmission from mother to child. *J Reprod Immunol* **47**:197-206.

2552. **Fujita, K., H. A. Lilly, A. Kidson, and G. A. Ayliffe.** 1981. Gentamicin-resistant Pseudomonas aeruginosa infection from mattresses in a burns unit. *Br Med J (Clin Res Ed)* **283**:219-20.

2553. **Fukushima, H., R. Nakamura, S. Iitsuka, Y. Ito, and K. Saito.** 1985. Presence of zoonotic pathogens (Yersinia spp., Campylobacter jejuni, Salmonella spp., and Leptospira spp.) simultaneously in dogs and cats. *Zentralbl Bakteriol Mikrobiol Hyg [B]* **181**:430-40.

2554. **Fukuyo, M., G. Battsetseg, and B. Byambaa.** 2002. Prevalence of Sarcocystis infection in meat-producing animals in Mongolia. *Southeast Asian J Trop Med Public Health* **33**:490-5.

2555. **Fuller, L. C., F. J. Child, G. Midgley, and E. M. Higgins.** 2003. Diagnosis and management of scalp ringworm. *BMJ* **326:**539-41.

2556. **Funke, G., M. Altwegg, L. Frommelt, and A. von Graevenitz.** 1999. Emergence of related nontoxigenic Corynebacterium diphtheriae biotype mitis strains in Western Europe. *Emerg Infect Dis* **5:**477-80.

2557. **Funke, G., A. von Graevenitz, J. E. Clarridge, 3rd, and K. A. Bernard.** 1997. Clinical microbiology of coryneform bacteria. *Clin Microbiol Rev* **10:**125-59.

2558. **Furness, B. W., M. J. Beach, and J. M. Roberts.** 2000. Giardiasis surveillance - United States, 1992-1997. *MMWR* **49 (SS-7):**1-13.

2559. **Furtado, C., G. K. Adak, J. M. Stuart, P. G. Wall, H. S. Evans, and D. P. Casemore.** 1998. Outbreaks of waterborne infectious intestinal disease in England and Wales, 1992-5. *Epidemiol Infect* **121:**109-19.

2560. **Furuta, T., M. Akiyama, Y. Kato, and O. Nishio.** 2003. [A food poisoning outbreak caused by purple Washington clam contaminated with norovirus (Norwalk-like virus) and hepatitis A virus]. *Kansenshogaku Zasshi* **77:**89-94.

2561. **Furuta, Y., F. Ohtani, H. Aizawa, S. Fukuda, H. Kawabata, and T. Bergstrom.** 2005. Varicella-zoster virus reactivation is an important cause of acute peripheral facial paralysis in children. *Pediatr Infect Dis J* **24:**97-101.

2562. **Fyfe, M., S. T. Yeung, P. Daly, K. Schallie, M. T. Kelly, and S. Buchanan.** 1997. Outbreak of Vibrio parahaemolyticus related to raw oysters in British Columbia. *Can Commun Dis Rep* **23:**145-8.

2563. **Gabaj, M. M., A. M. Gubsi, and M. A. Q. Awan.** 1989. First human infestations in Africa with larvae of American screwworm, Cochliomyia hominivorax Coq. *Ann Trop Med Parasitol* **83:**553-4.

2564. **Gabastou, J. M., J. Proaño, A. Vimos, G. Jaramillo, E. Hayes, K. Gage, M. Chu, J. Guarner, S. Zaki, J. Bowers, C. Guillemard, H. Tamayo, and A. Ruiz.** 2000. An outbreak of plague including cases with probable pneumonic infection, Ecuador, 1998. *Trans R Soc Trop Med Hyg* **94:**387-91.

2565. **Gabbay, Y. B., B. Jiang, C. S. Oliveira, J. D. Mascarenhas, J. P. Leite, R. I. Glass, and A. C. Linhares.** 1999. An outbreak of group C rotavirus gastroenteritis among children attending a day-care centre in Belem, Brazil. *J Diarrhoeal Dis Res* **17:**69-74.

2566. **Gad, A. M., F. M. Feinsod, I. H. Allam, M. Eisa, A. N. Hassan, B. A. Soliman, S. el Said, and A. J. Saah.** 1986. A possible route for the introduction of Rift Valley fever virus into Egypt during 1977. *J Trop Med Hyg* **89:**233-6.

2567. **Gaeta, G. B., and G. Giusti.** 1990. Epidemiology of chronic viral hepatitis in the Mediterranean area: present status and trends. *Infection* **18:**21-5.

2568. **Gaffey, M. J., R. M. Tucker, M. J. Fisch, and D. E. Normansell.** 1989. The seroprevalence of cytomegalovirus among Virginia State prisoners. *Public Health* **103:**303-6.

2569. **Gage, K. L., D. T. Dennis, and T. F. Tsai.** 1996. Prevention of plague. Recommendations of the Advisory Committee on Immunization Practices (ACIP). *MMWR* **45 (suppl RR-14):**1-15.

2570. **Gage, K. L., and M. Y. Kosoy.** 2005. Natural history of plague: perspectives from more than a century of research. *Annu Rev Entomol* **50:**505-28.

2571. **Gaillot, O., C. Maruejouls, E. Abachin, F. Lecuru, G. Arlet, M. Simonet, and P. Berche.** 1998. Nosocomial outbreak of Klebsiella pneumoniae producing SHV-5 extended- spectrum beta-lactamase, originating from a contaminated ultrasonography coupling gel. *J Clin Microbiol* **36:**1357-60.

2572. **Gaines, J. J., J. R. Clay, F. W. Chandler, M. E. Powell, P. A. Sheffield, and A. P. Keller, 3rd.** 1996. Rhinosporidiosis: three domestic cases. *South Med J* **89:**65-7.

2573. **Gajadhar, A. A., J. J. Aramini, G. Tiffin, and J. R. Bisaillon.** 1998. Prevalence of Toxoplasma gondii in Canadian market-age pigs. *J Parasitol* **84:**759-63.

2574. **Gajdusek, D. C.** 1978. Introduction of Taenia solium into West New Guinea with a note on an epidemic of burns from cysticercus epilepsy in the Ekari people of the Wissel lake area. *Papua New Guinea Med J* **21:**329-42.

2575. **Gajdusek, D. C., C. J. Gibbs, and M. Alpers.** 1966. Experimental transmission of a Kuru-like syndrome to chimpanzees. *Nature* **209:**794-6.

2576. **Gajdusek, D. C., and V. Zigas.** 1957. Degenerative disease of the central nervous system in New Guinea. The endemic occurrence of "kuru" in the native population. *N Engl J Med* **257:**974-8.

2577. **Gal, D., M. Mayo, H. Smith-Vaughan, P. Dasari, M. McKinnon, S. P. Jacups, A. I. Urquhart, M. Hassell, and B. J. Currie.** 2004. Contamination of hand wash detergent linked to occupationally acquired melioidosis. *Am J Trop Med Hyg* **71:**360-2.

2578. **Galanti, B., F. M. Fusco, and S. Nardiello.** 2002. Outbreak of cutaneous larva migrans in Naples, southern Italy. *Trans R Soc Trop Med Hyg* **96:**491-2.

2579. **Galazka, A.** 2000. The changing epidemiology of diphtheria in the vaccine era. *J Infect Dis* **181 suppl 1:**S2-9.

2580. **Galazka, A., and A. Przybylska.** 1999. Surveillance of foodborne botulism in Poland: 1960-1998. *Eurosurveillance* **4:**69-72.

2581. **Galbraith, N. S., P. Forbes, and C. Clifford.** 1982. Communicable disease associated with milk and dairy products in England and Wales 1951-80. *Br Med J (Clin Res Ed)* **284:**1761-5.

2582. **Galena, H. J.** 1992. Complications occurring from diagnostic venipuncture. *J Fam Pract* **34:**582-4.

2583. **Galeno, H., J. Mora, E. Villagra, J. Fernandez, J. Hernandez, G. J. Mertz, and E. Ramirez.** 2002. First Human Isolate of Hantavirus (Andes virus) in the Americas. *Emerg Infect Dis* **8:**657-61.

2584. **Galil, K., B. W. Lee, T. Strine, C. Carraher, A. L. Baughman, M. Eaton, J. Montero, and J. Seward.** 2002. Outbreak of varicella at a day-care center despite vaccination. *N Engl J Med* **347:**1909-15.

2585. **Galil, K., L. A. Miller, M. A. Yakrus, R. J. Wallace, Jr., D. G. Mosley, B. England, G. Huitt, M. M. McNeil, and B. A. Perkins.** 1999. Abscesses due to mycobacterium abscessus linked to injection of unapproved alternative medication. *Emerg Infect Dis* **5:**681-7.

2586. **Galimand, M., and A. Dodin.** 1982. Le point sur la mélioidose dans le monde. *Bull Soc Pathol Exot* **75:**375-83.

2587. **Gallagher, E., J. Ryan, L. J. Kelly, Y. Leforban, and M. Wooldridge.** 2002. Estimating the risk of importation of foot-and-mouth disease into Europe. *Vet Rec* **150:**769-72.

2588. **Gallagher, P. G., and C. Watanakunakorn.** 1989. Pseudomonas bacteremia in a community teaching hospital, 1980-1984. *Rev Infect Dis* **11:**846-52.

2589. Gallardo, F., J. Gascón, and J. Ruiz. 1998. Campylobacter jejuni as a cause of traveler's diarrhea: clinical features and antimicrobial susceptibility. *J Travel Med* **5**:23-6.

2590. Gallay, A., F. Van Loock, S. Demarest, J. Van der Heyden, B. Jans, and H. Van Oyen. 2002. Belgian coca-cola-related outbreak: intoxication, mass sociogenic illness, or both? *Am J Epidemiol* **155**:140-7.

2591. Gallego, M., F. Pratlong, R. Fisa, C. Riera, J. A. Rioux, J. P. Dedet, and M. Portus. 2001. The life-cycle of Leishmania infantum MON-77 in the Priorat (Catalonia, Spain) involves humans, dogs and sandflies; also literature review of distribution and hosts of L. infantum zymodemes in the Old World. *Trans R Soc Trop Med Hyg* **95**:269-71.

2592. Galliard, H. 1957. Outbreak of filariasis (Wuchereria malayi) among French and North African servicemen in North Vietnam. *Bull WHO* **16**:601-8.

2593. Gallimore, C. I., M. A. Barreiros, D. W. Brown, J. P. Nascimento, and J. P. Leite. 2004. Noroviruses associated with acute gastroenteritis in a children's day care facility in Rio de Janeiro, Brazil. *Braz J Med Biol Res* **37**:321-6.

2594. Gallimore, C. I., D. Cubitt, N. du Plessis, and J. J. Gray. 2004. Asymptomatic and symptomatic excretion of noroviruses during a hospital outbreak of gastroenteritis. *J Clin Microbiol* **42**:2271-4.

2595. Gallinella, G., E. Manaresi, S. Venturoli, G. L. Grazi, M. Musiani, and M. Zerbini. 1999. Occurrence and clinical role of active parvovirus B19 infection in transplant recipients. *Eur J Clin Microbiol Infect Dis* **18**:811-3.

2596. Gallino, A., M. Maggiorini, W. Kiowski, X. Martin, W. Wunderli, J. Schneider, M. Turina, and F. Follath. 1996. Toxoplasmosis in heart transplant recipients. *Eur J Clin Microbiol Infect Dis* **15**:389-93.

2597. Gallo, G., R. Berzero, N. Cattai, S. Recchia, and G. Orefici. 1992. An outbreak of group A food-borne streptococcal pharyngitis. *Eur J Epidemiol* **8**:292-7.

2598. Galmés Truyols, A., and J. F. Martínez Navarro. 1997. Travel associated legionellosis among European tourists in Spain. *Eurosurveillance* **7**:43-7.

2599. Galoo, E., and P. Schmoor. 1998. [Identification of a focus of bejel in Mauritania]. *Med Trop* **58**:311-2.

2600. Galperine, T., D. Neau, G. Lina, C. Richez, A. L. Cazeau, H. Dutronc, M. Dupon, and J. M. Ragnaud. 2003. [Menstrual staphylococcal toxic shock is still a reality]. *Presse Med* **32**:1121-2.

2601. Galperine, T., D. Neau, M. P. Moiton, Y. Rotivel, and J. M. Ragnaud. 2004. [The risk of rabies in France and the illegal importation of animals from rabid endemic countries]. *Presse Med* **33**:791-2.

2602. Gamage-Mendis, A. C., R. Carter, C. Mendis, A. P. De Zoysa, P. R. Herath, and K. N. Mendis. 1991. Clustering of malaria infections within an endemic population: risk of malaria associated with the type of housing construction. *Am J Trop Med Hyg* **45**:77-85.

2603. Gambarotto, K., M. C. Ploy, F. Dupron, M. Giangiobbe, and F. Denis. 2001. Occurrence of vancomycin-resistant enterococci in pork and poultry products from a cattle-rearing area of France. *J Clin Microbiol* **39**:2354-5.

2604. Gambarotto, K., M. C. Ploy, P. Turlure, C. Grelaud, C. Martin, D. Bordessoule, and F. Denis. 2000. Prevalence of vancomycin-resistant enterococci in fecal samples from hospitalized patients and nonhospitalized controls in a cattle-rearing area of France. *J Clin Microbiol* **38**:620-4.

2605. Gambel, J. M., J. J. Drabick, J. Seriwatana, and B. L. Innis. 1998. Seroprevalence of hepatitis E virus among United Nations mission in Haiti (UNMIH) peacekeepers, 1995. *Am J Trop Med Hyg* **58**:731-6.

2606. Gamble, H. R. 1997. Parasites associated with pork and pork products. *Rev Sci Tech* **16**:496-506.

2607. Gamboa-Dominguez, A., J. De Anda, J. Donis, F. Ruiz-Maza, G. S. Visvesvara, and H. Diliz. 2003. Disseminated encephalitozoon cuniculi infection in a Mexican kidney transplant recipient. *Transplantation* **75**:1898-900.

2608. Gambotti, L., D. Batisse, N. Colin-de-Verdiere, E. Delaroque-Astagneau, J. C. Desenclos, S. Dominguez, C. Dupont, X. Duval, A. Gervais, J. Ghosn, C. Larsen, S. Pol, J. Serpaggi, A. Simon, M. A. Valantin, and A. Velter. 2005. Acute hepatitis C infection in HIV positive men who have sex with men in Paris, France, 2001-2004. *Eurosurveillance* **10**:115-7.

2609. Gammie, A., R. Morris, and A. P. Wyn-Jones. 2002. Antibodies in crevicular fluid: an epidemiological tool for investigation of waterborne disease. *Epidemiol Infect* **128**:245-9.

2610. Gamp, R. 1987. Salmonellose, bedingt durch Frühlingsrollen. *Bulletin Bundesamt für Gesundheit* **17**:141-144.

2611. Gandhi, M. K., and R. Khanna. 2004. Human cytomegalovirus: clinical aspects, immune regulation, and emerging treatments. *Lancet Infect Dis* **4**:725-38.

2612. Ganem, D., and A. M. Prince. 2004. Hepatitis B virus infection - natural history and clinical consequences. *N Engl J Med* **350**:1118-29.

2613. Gangneux, J. P., J. C. Beaucournu, and C. Guiguen. 2002. Be aware of imported but also autochthonous myiasis. *J Travel Med* **9**:278.

2614. Gans, H., R. DeHovitz, B. Forghani, J. Beeler, Y. Maldonado, and A. M. Arvin. 2003. Measles and mumps vaccination as a model to investigate the developing immune system: passive and active immunity during the first year of life. *Vaccine* **21**:3398-405.

2615. Gantz, N., H. Harmon, J. Handy, K. Gershman, J. Butwin, L. Mascola, A. Weltman, R. Groner, A. Cronquist, M. Kainer, and N. Lee. 2003. Methicillin-resistant Staphylococcus aureus infections among competitive sports participants - Colorado, Indiana, Pensylvania, and Los Angeles county, 2000-2003. *MMWR* **33**:793-5.

2616. Garcés, J. M., J. Rubiés-Prat, E. Menoyd, and R. Serrano. 1990. Outbreak of schistosomiasis in a tourist group returning from Mali. *Eur J Clin Microbiol Infect Dis* **1**:58.

2617. Garcia, A., F. Exposto, E. Prieto, M. Lopes, A. Duarte, and R. Correia da Silva. 2004. Association of Trichomonas vaginalis with sociodemographic factors and other STDs among female inmates in Lisbon. *Int J STD AIDS* **15**:615-8.

2618. Garcia, A., and J. G. Fox. 2003. The rabbit as a new reservoir host of enterohemorrhagic Escherichia coli. *Emerg Infect Dis* **9**:1592-7.

2619. Garcia de la Torre, M., J. Romero-Vivas, J. Martinez-Beltran, A. Guerrero, M. Meseguer, and E. Bouza. 1985. Klebsiella bacteremia: an analysis of 100 episodes. *Rev Infect Dis* **7**:143-50.

2620. Garcia, H. H., R. Araoz, R. Gilman, R. H. Gilman, J. Valdez, A. E. Gonzalez, C. Gavidia, M. L. Bravo, and V. C. Tsang.

1998. Increased prevalence of cysticercosis and taeniasis among professional fried pork vendors and the general population of a village in the Peruvian highlands. *Am J Trop Med Hyg* **59**:902-05.

2621. Garcia, H. H., R. H. Gilman, A. E. Gonzalez, M. Verastegui, S. Rodriguez, C. Gavidia, V. C. Tsang, N. Falcon, A. G. Lescano, L. H. Moulton, T. Bernal, and M. Tovar. 2003. Hyperendemic human and porcine Taenia solium infection in Peru. *Am J Trop Med Hyg* **68**:268-75.

2622. Garcia, H. H., A. E. Gonzalez, C. A. W. Evans, and R. H. Gilman. 2003. Taenia solium cysticercosis. *Lancet* **361**:547-56.

2623. Garcia, P. J., S. Chavez, B. Feringa, M. Chiappe, W. Li, K. U. Jansen, C. Carcamo, and K. K. Holmes. 2004. Reproductive tract infections in rural women from the highlands, jungle and coastal regions of Peru. *Bull WHO* **82**:483-92.

2624. Garcia, S., F. Iracheta, F. Galvan, and N. Heredia. 2001. Microbiological survey of retail herbs and spices from Mexican markets. *J Food Prot* **64**:99-103.

2625. Garcia-Fulgueiras, A., C. Navarro, D. Fenoll, J. Garcia, P. Gonzales-Diego, T. Jimenez-Bunuelas, M. Rodriguez, R. Lopez, F. Pacheco, J. Ruiz, M. Segovia, B. Balandron, and C. Pelaz. 2003. Legionnaires' disease outbreak in Murcia, Spain. *Emerg Infect Dis* **9**:915-21.

2626. Garcia-Fulgueiras, A., S. Sanchez, J. J. Guillen, B. Marsilla, A. Aladuena, and C. Navarro. 2001. A large outbreak of Shigella sonnei gastroenteritis associated with consumption of fresh pasteurised milk cheese. *Eur J Epidemiol* **17**:533-8.

2627. Garcia-Migura, L., E. Pleydell, S. Barnes, R. H. Davies, and E. Liebana. 2005. Characterization of Vancomycin-Resistant Enterococcus faecium Isolates from Broiler Poultry and Pig Farms in England and Wales. *J Clin Microbiol* **43**:3283-9.

2628. Garcia-Noval, J., J. C. Allan, C. Fletes, E. Moreno, F. DeMata, R. Torres-Alvarez, H. Soto de Alfaro, P. Yurrita, H. Higueros-Morales, F. Mencos, and P. S. Craig. 1996. Epidemiology of Taenia solium taeniasis and cysticercosis in two rural Guatemalan communities. *Am J Trop Med Hyg* **55**:282-9.

2629. Garcia-Perez, A. L., J. Barandika, B. Oporto, I. Povedano, and R. A. Juste. 2003. Anaplasma phagocytophila as an abortifacient agent in sheep farms from northern Spain. *Ann N Y Acad Sci* **990**:429-32.

2630. Gardner, G., A. L. Frank, and L. H. Taber. 1984. Effects of social and family factors on viral respiratory infection and illness in the first year of life. *J Epidemiol Community Health* **38**:42-8.

2631. Garenne, M., and P. Aaby. 1990. Pattern of exposure and measles mortality in Senegal. *J Infect Dis* **161**:1088-94.

2632. Garg, A. X., R. S. Suri, N. Barrowman, F. Rehman, D. Matsell, M. P. Rosas-Arellano, M. Salvadori, R. B. Haynes, and W. F. Clark. 2003. Long-term renal prognosis of diarrhea-associated hemolytic uremic syndrome. A systematic review, meat-analysis, and meta-regression. *JAMA* **290**:1360-70.

2633. Garg, P. K., S. Perry, M. Dorn, L. Hardcastle, and J. Parsonnet. 2005. Risk of intestinal helminth and protozoan infection in a refugee population. *Am J Trop Med Hyg* **73**:386-91.

2634. Gari-Toussaint, M., N. Tieulié, J. L. Baldin, P. Marty, J. Dupouy-Camet, P. Delaunay, J. G. Fuzibet, Y. Le Fichoux, and E. Pozio. 2004. Trichinellose à Trichinella britovi dans les Alpes-Maritimes après consommation de viande de sanglier congelée, automne 2003. *Bull Epidémiol Hebdomadaire* **21 (18 mai)**:87-8.

2635. Garin, B., A. Aidara, A. Spiegel, P. Arrive, A. Bastaraud, J. L. Cartel, R. B. Aissa, P. Duval, M. Gay, C. Gherardi, M. Gouali, T. G. Karou, S. L. Kruy, J. L. Soares, F. Mouffok, N. Ravaonindrina, N. Rasolofonirina, M. T. Pham, M. Wouafo, M. Catteau, C. Mathiot, P. Mauclere, and J. Rocourt. 2002. Multicenter study of street foods in 13 towns on four continents by the food and environmental hygiene study group of the international network of Pasteur and associated institutes. *J Food Prot* **65**:146-52.

2636. Garin, D., J. C. Chapalain, J. Thierry, J. D. Perrier Gros Claude, F. Peyron, and D. Courtois. 1990. Le point sur Schistosoma intercalatum. *Med Trop* **50**:433-40.

2637. Garin-Bastuji, B., and F. Delcueillerie. 2001. Les brucelloses humaine et animale en France en l'an 2000. Situation épidémiologique - programmes de contrôle et d'éradication. *Méd Mal Infect* **31 suppl 2**:202-16.

2638. Garland, J. S., K. Henrickson, and D. G. Maki. 2002. The 2002 Hospital Infection Control Practices Advisory Committee Centers for Disease Control and Prevention guideline for prevention of intravascular device-related infection. *Pediatrics* **110**:1009-13.

2639. Garland, S. M., S. Mackay, S. Tabrizi, and S. Jacobs. 1996. Pseudomonas aeruginosa outbreak associated with a contaminated blood-gas analyser in a neonatal intensive care unit. *J Hosp Infect* **33**:145-51.

2640. Garnacho-Montero, J., C. Ortiz-Leyba, F. J. Jiménez-Jiménez, A. E. Barrero-Almodovar, J. L. Garcia-Garmendia, I. M. Bernabeu-Wittel, S. L. Gallego-Lara, and J. Madrazo-Osuna. 2003. Treatment of multidrug-resistant Acinetobacter baumannii ventilator-associated pneumonia (VAP) with intravenous colistin: a comparison with imipenem-susceptible VAP. *Clin Infect Dis* **36**:1111-8.

2641. Garner, J. S. 1997. Guidelines for isolation precautions in hospitals, Atlanta, Georgia.

2642. Garnett, B. T., R. J. Delahay, and T. J. Roper. 2002. Use of cattle farm resources by badgers (Meles meles) and risk of bovine tuberculosis (Mycobacterium bovis) transmission to cattle. *Proc R Soc Lond B Biol Sci* **269**:1487-91.

2643. Garnham, P. C. C. 1945. Malaria epidemics at exceptionally high altitudes in Kenya. *BMJ* **2(14 jul)**:45–47.

2644. Garnier, M., X. Foissac, P. Gaurivaud, F. Laigret, J. Renaudin, C. Saillard, and J. M. Bove. 2001. Mycoplasmas, plants, insect vectors: a matrimonial triangle. *C R Acad Sci* **324**:923-8.

2645. Garrett, D. O., L. C. McDonald, A. Wanderley, C. Wanderley, P. Miller, J. Carr, M. Arduino, L. Sehulster, R. Anderson, and W. R. Jarvis. 2002. An outbreak of neonatal deaths in Brazil associated with contaminated intravenous fluids. *J Infect Dis* **186**:81-6.

2646. Garrote, J. I., M. P. Gutierrez, R. L. Izquierdo, M. A. Duenas, P. Zarzosa, C. Canavate, M. E. Bali, A. Almaraz, M. A. Bratos, C. Berbel, A. Rodriguez-Torres, and A. O. Domingo. 2004. Seroepidemiologic study of Leishmania infantum infection in Castilla-Leon, Spain. *Am J Trop Med Hyg* **71**:403-406.

2647. Garten, R. J., S. Lai, J. Zhang, W. Liu, J. Chen, D. Vlahov, and X. F. Yu. 2004. Rapid transmission of hepatitis C virus among young injecting heroin users in Southern China. *Int J Epidemiol* **33**:182-8.

2648. Gartner, B. C., A. Kloss, H. Kaul, U. Sester, K. Roemer, H. Pees, H. Kohler, and N. Mueller-Lantzsch. 2003. Risk of occupational human herpesvirus 8 infection for health care workers. *J Clin Microbiol* **41**:2156-7.

2649. Gascon, J., M. Alvarez, M. Eugenia Valls, J. Maria Bordas, M. Teresa Jimenez De Anta, and M. Corachan. 2001. [Cyclosporiasis: a clinical and epidemiological study in travellers with imported Cyclospora cayetanensis infection]. *Med Clin (Barc)* **116:**461-4.

2650. Gascon, J., M. Corachan, J. A. Bombi, M. E. Valls, and J. M. Bordes. 1995. Cyclospora in patients with traveller's diarrhea. *Scand J Infect Dis* **27:**511-4.

2651. Gascon, J., T. Marcos, J. Vidal, A. Garcia-Forcada, and M. Corachan. 1995. Cytomegalovirus and Epstein-Barr Virus Infection as a Cause of Chronic Fatigue Syndrome in Travelers to Tropical Countries. *J Travel Med* **2:**41-44.

2652. Gasem, M. H., W. M. Dolmans, M. M. Keuter, and R. R. Djokomoeljanto. 2001. Poor food hygiene and housing as risk factors for typhoid fever in Semarang, Indonesia. *Trop Med Int Health* **6:**484-90.

2653. Gassem, M. A. 1999. Study of the micro-organisms associated with the fermented bread (khamir) produced from sorghum in Gizan region, Saudi Arabia. *J Appl Microbiol* **86:**221-5.

2654. Gasser, R. A., Jr., A. J. Magill, C. N. Oster, and E. C. Tramont. 1991. The threat of infectious disease in Americans returning from Operation Desert Storm. *N Engl J Med* **324:**859-64.

2655. Gastmeier, P., C. Brandt, D. Sohr, R. Babikir, D. Mlageni, F. Daschner, and H. Ruden. 2004. [Surgical site infections in hospitals and outpatient settings. Results of the German nosocomial infection surveillance system (KISS)]. *Bundes-gesundheitsblatt Gesundheitsforschung Gesundheitsschutz* **47:** 339-44.

2656. Gastmeier, P., K. Groneberg, K. Weist, and H. Ruden. 2003. A cluster of nosocomial Klebsiella pneumoniae bloodstream infections in a neonatal intensive care department: Identification of transmission and intervention. *Am J Infect Control* **31:**424-30.

2657. Gastmeier, P., S. Stamm-Balderjahn, S. Hansen, F. Nitzschke-Tiemann, I. Zuschneid, K. Groneberg, and H. Ruden. 2005. How outbreaks can contribute to prevention of nosocomial infection: analysis of 1,022 outbreaks. *Infect Control Hosp Epidemiol* **26:**357-61.

2658. Gastrin, B., A. Kampe, K. G. Nystrom, B. Oden-Johanson, G. Wessel, and B. Zetterberg. 1972. [Salmonella durham epidemic caused by contaminated cocoa]. *Lakartidningen* **69:**5335-8.

2659. Gates, G. A., and R. T. Miyamoto. 2003. Cochlear implants. *N Engl J Med* **349:**421-3.

2660. Gatti, S., C. Cevini, A. Bruno, S. Novati, and M. Scaglia. 1995. Transmission of Entamoeba histolytica within a family complex. *Trans R Soc Trop Med Hyg* **89:**403-5.

2661. Gatti, S., J. C. Petithory, F. Ardoin, C. Pannetier, and M. Scaglia. 2001. Asymptomatic amoebic infection: Entamoeba histolytica or Entamoeba dispar? That is the question. *Bull Soc Pathol Exot* **94:**304-7.

2662. Gatti, S., G. Swierczynski, F. Robinson, M. Anselmi, J. Corrales, J. Moreira, G. Montalvo, A. Bruno, R. Maserati, Z. Bisoffi, and M. Scaglia. 2002. Amebic infections due to the Entamoeba histolytica-Entamoeba dispar complex: a study of the incidence in a remote rural area of Ecuador. *Am J Trop Med Hyg* **67:**123-7.

2663. Gatus, B. J., and M. R. Rose. 1983. Japanese B encephalitis: epidemiological, clinical and pathological aspects. *J Infect* **6:**213–218.

2664. Gaud, M., and M. T. Morgan. 1947-8. Epidemiological study of relapsing fever in North Africa (1943-1945). *Bull WHO* **1:**69-92.

2665. Gaudoin, M., P. Rekha, A. Morris, J. Lynch, and U. Acharya. 1999. Bacterial vaginosis and past chlamydial infection are strongly and independently associated with tubal infertility but do not affect in vitro fertilization success rates. *Fertil Steril* **72:**730-2.

2666. Gaudreau, C., and S. Michaud. 2003. Cluster of erythromycin- and ciprofloxacin-resistant Campylobacter jejuni subsp. jejuni from 1999 to 2001 in men who have sex with men, Québec, Canada. *Clin Infect Dis* **37:**131-6.

2667. Gauert, B. 1998. [Comparative study of the incidence and dissemination of intestinal parasites in child day care centers of the district capital Schwerin]. *Gesundheitswesen* **60:**301-6.

2668. Gaulin, C., M. Frigon, D. Poirier, and C. Fournier. 1999. Transmission of calicivirus by a foodhandler in the presymptomatic phase of illness. *Epidemiol Infect* **123:**475-478.

2669. Gaulin, C., Y. B. Viger, and L. Fillion. 2002. An outbreak of Bacillus cereus implicating a part-time banquet caterer. *Can J Public Health* **93:**353-5.

2670. Gaulin, C., C. Vincent, L. Alain, and J. Ismail. 2002. Outbreak of Salmonella paratyphi B linked to aquariums in the province of Quebec, 2000. *Can Commun Dis Rep* **28:**89-93, 96.

2671. Gaulin, C. D., D. Ramsay, P. Cardinal, and M. A. D'Halevyn. 1999. [Epidemic of gastroenteritis of viral origin associated with eating imported raspberries]. *Can J Public Health* **90:**37-40.

2672. Gauss, C. B., S. Almeria, A. Ortuno, F. Garcia, and J. P. Dubey. 2003. Seroprevalence of Toxoplasma gondii antibodies in domestic cats from Barcelona, Spain. *J Parasitol* **89:**1067-8.

2673. Gauzere, B. A., X. Roblin, P. Blanc, G. Xavierson, and F. Paganin. 1998. [Importation of Plasmodium falciparum malaria, in Reunion Island, from 1993 to 1996: epidemiology and clinical aspects of severe forms]. *Bull Soc Pathol Exot* **91:**95-8.

2674. Gavin, P. J., K. R. Kazacos, T. Q. Tan, W. B. Brinkman, S. E. Byrd, A. T. Davis, M. B. Mets, and S. T. Shulman. 2002. Neural larva migrans caused by the raccoon roundworm Baylisascaris procyonis. *Pediatr Infect Dis J* **21:**971-5.

2675. Gawande, A. V., N. D. Vasudeo, S. P. Zodpey, and D. W. Khandait. 2000. Sexually transmitted infections in long distance truck drivers. *J Commun Dis* **32:**212-5.

2676. Gay, N. J., L. M. Hesketh, K. P. Osborne, C. P. Farrington, P. Morgan-Capner, and E. Miller. 1999. The prevalence of hepatitis B infection in adults in England and Wales. *Epidemiol Infect* **122:**133-8.

2677. Gaydos, C. A., M. R. Howell, B. Pare, K. L. Clark, D. A. Ellis, R. M. Hendrix, J. C. Gaydos, K. T. McKee, Jr., and T. C. Quinn. 1998. Chlamydia trachomatis infections in female military recruits. *N Engl J Med* **339:**739-44.

2678. Gaynes, R. P., D. H. Culver, T. C. Horan, J. R. Edwards, C. Richards, and J. S. Tolson. 2001. Surgical site infection (SSI) rates in the United States, 1992-1998: the National Nosocomial Infections Surveillance System basic SSI risk index. *Clin Infect Dis* **33 Suppl 2:**S69-77.

2679. Gbakima, A. A., M. A. Appawu, S. Dadzie, C. Karikari, S. O. Sackey, A. Baffoe-Wilmot, J. Gyapong, and A. L. Scott. 2005. Lymphatic filariasis in Ghana: establishing the potential for an urban cycle of transmission. *Trop Med Int Health* **10:**387-92.

2680. Gbakima, A. A., B. C. Terry, F. Kanja, S. Kortequee, I. Dukuley, and F. Sahr. 2002. High prevalence of bedbugs Cimex hemipterus and Cimex lectularis in camps for internally displaced persons in Freetown, Sierra Leone: a pilot humanitarian investigation. *West Afr J Med* 21:268-71.

2681. Gdalevich, M., M. Ephros, D. Mimouni, I. Grotto, O. Shpilberg, A. Eldad, and I. Ashkenazi. 2000. Measles epidemic in Israel-successful containment in the military. *Prev Med* 31:649-51.

2682. Gdalevich, M., D. Mimouni, I. Ashkenazi, and J. Shemer. 2000. Rabies in Israel: decades of prevention and a human case. *Public Health* 114:484-7.

2683. Gear, J. S., G. A. Cassel, A. J. Gear, B. Trappler, L. Clausen, A. M. Meyers, M. C. Kew, T. H. Bothwell, R. Sher, G. B. Miller, J. Schneider, H. J. Koornhof, E. D. Gomperts, M. Isaacson, and J. H. Gear. 1975. Outbreak of Marburg virus disease in Johannesburg. *Br Med J* 4:489-93.

2684. Gebo, K. A., A. Srinivasan, T. M. Perl, T. Ross, A. Groth, and W. G. Merz. 2002. Pseudo-outbreak of Mycobacterium fortuitum on a human immunodeficiency virus ward: transient respiratory tract colonization from a contaminated ice machine. *Clin Infect Dis* 35:32-8.

2685. Geddes, D. M. 2001. Of isolates and isolation: Pseudomonas aeruginosa in adults with cystic fibrosis. *Lancet* 358:522-3.

2686. Gehlbach, S. H., J. D. Hamilton, and N. F. Conant. 1973. Coccidioidomycosis. An occupational disease in cotton mill workers. *Arch Intern Med* 131:254-5.

2687. Geiss, H. K., W. Kiehl, and W. Thilo. 1997. A case report of laboratory-acquired diphtheria. *Eurosurveillance* 2:67-8.

2688. Gelfand, H. M., D. R. LeBlanc, J. P. Fox, and D. P. Conwell. 1957. Studies on the development of natural immunity to poliomyelitis in Louisiana. II. Description and analysis of episodes of infection observed in study group households. *Am J Hyg* 65:367-85.

2689. Geltman, P. L., J. Cochran, and C. Hedgecock. 2003. Intestinal parasites among African refugees resettled in Massachusetts and the impact of an overseas pre-departure treatment program. *Am J Trop Med Hyg* 69:657-62.

2690. Gelzer, J., T. Abelin, H. U. Bertschinger, R. Bruppacher, A. E. Metzler, and J. Nicolet. 1983. Wie verbreitet ist Q-Fieber in der Schweiz? *Schweiz Med Wochenschr* 113:892-895.

2691. Geng, E., B. Kreiswirth, C. Driver, J. Li, J. Burzynski, P. DellaLatta, A. LaPaz, and N. W. Schluger. 2002. Changes in the transmission of tuberculosis in New York City from 1990 to 1999. *N Engl J Med* 346:1453-8.

2692. Genobile, D., J. Gaston, G. F. Tallis, J. E. Gregory, J. M. Griffith, M. Valcanis, D. Lightfoot, and J. A. Marshall. 2004. An outbreak of shigellosis in a child care centre. *Commun Dis Intell* 28:225-9.

2693. Genta, R. M. 1989. Global prevalence of strongyloidiasis: critical review with epidemiologic insights into the prevention of disseminated disease. *Rev Infect Dis* 11:755-67.

2694. Gentilini, E., G. Denamiel, A. Betancor, M. Rebuelto, M. Rodriguez Fermepin, and R. A. De Torrest. 2002. Antimicrobial susceptibility of coagulase-negative staphylococci isolated from bovine mastitis in Argentina. *J Dairy Sci* 85:1913-7.

2695. Geoghagen, M., R. Pierre, T. Evans-Gilbert, B. Rodriguez, and C. D. Christie. 2004. Tuberculosis, chickenpox and scabies outbreaks in an orphanage for children with HIV/AIDS in JAMAica. *West Indian Med J* 53:346-51.

2696. George, J. C., and C. Chasted. 2002. Maladies vectorielles à tiques et modifications de l'écosystème en Lorraine. *Bull Soc Pathol Exot* 95:95-9.

2697. George, S., D. Mathai, V. Balraj, M. K. Lalitha, and T. J. John. 1994. An outbreak of anthrax meningoencephalitis. *Trans R Soc Trop Med Hyg* 88:206-7.

2698. Georges, A. J., S. Baize, E. M. Leroy, and M. C. Georges-Courbot. 1998. [Ebola virus: what the practitioner needs to know]. *Med Trop (Mars)* 58:177-86.

2699. Gerbase, A. C., J. T. Rowley, D. H. Heymann, S. F. Berkley, and P. Piot. 1998. Global prevalence and incidence estimates of selected curable STDs. *Sex Transm Infect* 74 Suppl 1:S12-6.

2700. Gerber, S., Y. Vial, P. Hohlfeld, and S. S. Witkin. 2003. Detection of Ureaplasma urealyticum in second-trimester amniotic fluid by polymerase chain reaction correlates with subsequent preterm labor and delivery. *J Infect Dis* 187:518-21.

2701. Gerberding, J. L. 1995. Management of occupational exposures to blood-borne viruses. *N Engl J Med* 332:444-51.

2702. Gerday, E., and C. Grose. 2004. Demographic differences in congenital cytomegalovirus infection in the United States. *J Pediatr* 145:435-6.

2703. Gerding, D. N., S. Johnson, L. R. Peterson, M. E. Mulligan, and J. Silva, Jr. 1995. Clostridium difficile-associated diarrhea and colitis. *Infect Control Hosp Epidemiol* 16:459-77.

2704. Gergen, P. J., G. M. McQuillan, M. Kiely, T. M. Ezzati-Rice, R. W. Sutter, and G. Virella. 1995. A population-based serologic survey of immunity to tetanus in the United States. *N Engl J Med* 332:761-6.

2705. Gerhardt, R. R., K. L. Gottfried, C. S. Apperson, B. S. Davis, P. C. Erwin, A. B. Smith, N. A. Panella, E. E. Powell, and R. S. Nasci. 2001. First isolation of La Crosse virus from naturally infected Aedes albopictus. *Emerg Infect Dis* 7:807-11.

2706. Germanetto, P., Y. Muzellec, and F. Machinot. 1992. Epidémie d'angine à streptocoque d'origine alimentaire dans une collectivité militaire. *Bull Epidémiol Hebdomadaire* 50:237.

2707. Germann, R., M. Schachtele, G. Nessler, U. Seitz, and E. Kniehl. 2003. Cerebral gnathostomiasis as a cause of an extended intracranial bleeding. *Klin Padiatr* 215:223-5.

2708. Gern, L., A. Estrada-Pena, F. Frandsen, J. S. Gray, T. G. Jaenson, F. Jongejan, O. Kahl, E. Korenberg, R. Mehl, and P. A. Nuttall. 1998. European reservoir hosts of Borrelia burgdorferi sensu lato. *Zentralbl Bakteriol* 287:196-204.

2709. Gern, L., and P. F. Humair. 2000. American robins as reservoir hosts for Lyme disease spirochetes. *Emerg Infect Dis* 6:657-8.

2710. Gershon, R. R., K. A. Qureshi, M. A. Barrera, M. J. Erwin, and F. Goldsmith. 2005. Health and safety hazards associated with subways: a review. *J Urban Health* 82:10-20.

2711. Gesundheit, B., G. Grisaru-Soen, D. Greenberg, O. Levtzion-Korach, D. Malkin, M. Petric, G. Koren, M. D. Tendler, B. Ben-Zeev, A. Vardi, R. Dagan, and D. Engelhard. 2004. Neonatal genital herpes simplex virus type 1 infection after Jewish ritual circumcision: modern medicine and religious tradition. *Pediatrics* 114:e259-63.

2712. Getis, A., A. C. Morrison, K. Gray, and T. W. Scott. 2003. Characteristics of the spatial pattern of the dengue vector, Aedes aegypti, in Iquitos, Peru. *Am J Trop Med Hyg* 69:494-505.

2713. Ghebreyesus, T. A., M. Haile, K. H. Witten, A. Getachew, A. M. Yohannes, M. Yohannes, H. D. Teklehaimanot, S. W.

Lindsay, and P. Byass. 1999. Incidence of malaria among children living near dams in northern Ethiopia: community based incidence survey. *BMJ* **319**:663-6.

2714. Ghebreyesus, T. A., K. H. Witten, A. Getachew, M. Haile, M. Yohannes, S. W. Lindsay, and P. Byass. 2002. Schistosome transmission, water-resource development and altitude in northern Ethiopia. *Ann Trop Med Parasitol* **96**:489-95.

2715. Ghendon, Y. 1992. Influenza - its impact and control. *World Health Stat Q* **45**:306-11.

2716. Gholam, B. I., S. Puksa, and J. P. Provias. 1999. Powassan encephalitis: a case report with neuropathology and literature review. *CMAJ* **161**:1419-22.

2717. Ghorpade, A. 2002. Inoculation (tattoo) leprosy: a report of 31 cases. *J Eur Acad Dermatol Venereol* **16**:494-9.

2718. Ghosh, A., A. Chakrabarti, V. K. Sharma, K. Singh, and A. Singh. 1999. Sporotrichosis in Himachal Pradesh (North India). *Trans R Soc Trop Med Hyg* **93**:41-5.

2719. Ghosh, K., C. E. Frew, and D. Carrington. 1992. A family outbreak of Chlamydia pneumoniae infection. *J Infect* **25 Suppl 1**:99-103.

2720. Giacometti, A., O. Cirioni, A. M. Schimizzi, M. S. Del Prete, F. Barchiesi, M. M. D'Errico, E. Petrelli, and G. Scalise. 2000. Epidemiology and microbiology of surgical wound infections. *J Clin Microbiol* **38**:918-22.

2721. Gibb, D. M., R. L. Goodall, D. T. Dunn, M. Healy, P. Neave, M. Cafferkey, and K. L. Butler. 2000. Mother-to-child transmission of hepatitis C virus: evidence for preventable peripartum transmission. *Lancet* **356**:904-7.

2722. Gibbens, J. C., C. E. Sharpe, J. W. Wilesmith, L. M. Mansley, E. Michalopoulou, J. B. Ryan, and M. Hudson. 2001. Descriptive epidemiology of the 2001 foot-and-mouth disease epidemic in Great Britain: the first five months. *Vet Rec* **149**:729-43.

2723. Gibbons, R. V., R. C. Holman, S. R. Mosberg, and C. E. Rupprecht. 2002. Knowledge of bat rabies and human exposure among United States cavers. *Emerg Infect Dis* **8**:532-4.

2724. Gibbs, C. J., Jr., A. Joy, R. Heffner, M. Franko, M. Miyazaki, D. M. Asher, J. E. Parisi, P. W. Brown, and D. C. Gajdusek. 1985. Clinical and pathological features and laboratory confirmation of Creutzfeldt-Jakob disease in a recipient of pituitary-derived human growth hormone. *N Engl J Med* **313**:734-8.

2725. Giboda, M., O. Ditrich, T. Scholz, T. Viengsay, and S. Bouaphanh. 1991. Human Opisthorchis and Haplorchis infections in Laos. *Trans R Soc Trop Med Hyg* **85**:538-40.

2726. Gibson, J. J., C. A. Hornung, G. R. Alexander, F. K. Lee, W. A. Potts, and A. J. Nahmias. 1990. A cross-sectional study of herpes simplex virus types 1 and 2 in college students: occurrence and determinants of infection. *J Infect Dis* **162**:306-12.

2727. Giebink, G. S. 2001. The prevention of pneumococcal disease in children. *N Engl J Med* **345**:1177-83.

2728. Gikas, A., S. Doukakis, J. Pediaditis, S. Kastanakis, A. Psaroulaki, and Y. Tselentis. 2002. Murine typhus in Greece: epidemiological, clinical, and therapeutic data from 83 cases. *Trans R Soc Trop Med Hyg* **96**:250-3.

2729. Gilbert, G. L. 2000. Parvovirus B19 infection and its significance in pregnancy. *Commun Dis Intell* **24**:69-71.

2730. Gilbert, R. 2004. Prenatal screening for group B streptococcal infection: gaps in the evidence. *Int J Epidemiol* **33**:2-8.

2731. Gilbert, R. J., and D. Roberts. 1986. Food hygiene aspects and laboratory methods. *Public Health Laboratory Service Microbiology Digest* **3**:9-11.

2732. Gill, G. V., N. J. Beeching, S. Khoo, J. W. Bailey, S. Partridge, J. W. Blundell, and A. R. Luksza. 2004. A British Second World War veteran with disseminated strongyloidiasis. *Trans R Soc Trop Med Hyg* **98**:382-6.

2733. Gill, G. V., and D. R. Bell. 1979. Strongyloides stercoralis infection in former Far East prisoners of war. *Br Med J* **2**:572-4.

2734. Gill, J., R. Aston, A. J. Vyse, J. M. White, and A. Greenwood. 2002. Susceptibility of young offenders to measles and rubella: an antibody prevalence study using oral fluid samples. *Commun Dis Public Health* **5**:314-7.

2735. Gill, J., L. M. Stark, and G. G. Clark. 2000. Dengue surveillance in Florida, 1997-98. *Emerg Infect Dis* **6**:30-35.

2736. Gill, J. S., M. Bucens, M. Hatton, M. Carey, and G. F. Quadros. 1990. Markers of hepatitis B virus infection in schoolchildren in the Kimberley, Western Australia. *Med J Australia* **153**:34-7.

2737. Gill, O. N., J. D. Coghlan, and I. M. Calder. 1985. The risk of leptospirosis in United Kingdom fish farm workers. Results from a 1981 serological survey. *J Hyg (Lond)* **94**:81-6.

2738. Gillespie, I. A., G. K. Adak, S. J. O'Brien, and F. J. Bolton. 2003. Milkborne general outbreaks of infectious intestinal disease, England and Wales, 1992-2000. *Epidemiol Infect* **130**:461-8.

2739. Gillespie, I. A., G. K. Adak, S. J. O'Brien, M. M. Brett, and F. J. Bolton. 2001. General outbreaks of infectious intestinal disease associated with fish and shellfish, England and Wales, 1992-1999. *Commun Dis Public Health* **4**:117-23.

2740. Gillespie, I. A., C. L. Little, and R. T. Mitchell. 2001. Microbiological examination of ready-to-eat quiche from retail establishments in the United Kingdom. *Commun Dis Public Health* **4**:53-9.

2741. Gillespie, I. A., S. J. O'Brien, and G. K. Adak. 2001. General outbreaks of infectious intestinal diseases linked with private residences in England and Wales, 1992-9: questionnaire study. *BMJ* **323**:1097-8.

2742. Gillespie, I. A., S. J. O'Brien, J. A. Frost, G. K. Adak, P. Horby, A. V. Swan, M. J. Painter, and K. R. Neal. 2002. A Case-Case Comparison of Campylobacter coli and Campylobacter jejuni Infection: A Tool for Generating Hypotheses. *Emerg Infect Dis* **8**:937-42.

2743. Gillespie, S. M., M. L. Cartter, S. Asch, J. B. Rokos, G. W. Gary, C. J. Tsou, D. B. Hall, L. J. Anderson, and E. S. Hurwitz. 1990. Occupational risk of human parvovirus B19 infection for school and day-care personnel during an outbreak of erythema infectiosum. *JAMA* **263**:2061-5.

2744. Gillis, D., I. Grotto, D. Mimouni, M. Huerta, M. Gdalevich, and O. Shpilberg. 2002. Adult infection with hepatitis A despite declining endemicity; in favor of adult vaccination. *Vaccine* **20**:2243-48.

2745. Gilman, R. H., G. S. Marquis, and E. Miranda. 1991. Prevalence and symptoms of Enterobius vermicularis infections in a Peruvian shanty town. *Trans R Soc Trop Med Hyg* **85**:761-4.

2746. Gilman, R. H., G. S. Marquis, E. Miranda, M. Vestegui, and H. Martinez. 1988. Rapid reinfection by Giardia lamblia after treatment in a hyperendemic Third World community. *Lancet* **1**:343-5.

2747. **Gilman, R. H., G. Mondal, M. Maksud, K. Alam, E. Rutherford, J. B. Gilman, and M. U. Khan.** 1982. Endemic focus of Fasciolopsis buski infection in Bangladesh. *Am J Trop Med Hyg* **31:**796-802.

2748. **Gilmore, A., G. Jones, M. Barker, N. Soltanpoor, and J. M. Stuart.** 1999. Meningococcal disease at the University of Southampton: outbreak investigation. *Epidemiol Infect* **123:**185-92.

2749. **Gilmore, A., J. Stuart, and N. Andrews.** 2000. Risk of secondary meningococcal disease in health-care workers. *Lancet* **356:**1654-1655.

2750. **Gilot, B., M. L. Laforge, J. Pichot, and D. Raoult.** 1990. Relationships between the Rhipicephalus sanguineus complex ecology and Mediterranean spotted fever epidemiology in France. *Eur J Epidemiol* **6:**357-62.

2751. **Gingrich, J. B., A. Nisalak, J. R. Latendresse, J. Sattabongkot, C. H. Hoke, J. Pomsdhit, C. Chantalakana, C. Satayaphanta, K. Uechiewcharnkit, and B. L. Innis.** 1992. Japanese encephalitis virus in Bangkok: factors influencing vector infections in three suburban communities. *J Med Entomol* **29:**436-44.

2752. **Ginsburg, C. M., G. Henle, and W. Henle.** 1976. An outbreak of infectious mononucleosis among the personnel of an outpatient clinic. *Am J Epidemiol* **104:**571-5.

2753. **Ginsburg, C. M., G. H. McCracken, Jr., S. Rae, and J. C. Parke, Jr.** 1977. Haemophilus influenzae type b disease. Incidence in a day-care center. *JAMA* **238:**604-7.

2754. **Giojalas, L. C., S. S. Catala, S. N. Asin, and D. E. Gorla.** 1990. Seasonal changes in infectivity of domestic populations of Triatoma infestans. *Trans R Soc Trop Med Hyg* **84:**439-42.

2755. **Giordano, M. O., L. C. Martinez, M. B. Isa, L. J. Ferreyra, F. Canna, J. V. Pavan, M. Paez, R. Notario, and S. V. Nates.** 2002. Twenty year study of the occurrence of reovirus infection in hospitalized children with acute gastroenteritis in Argentina. *Pediatr Infect Dis J* **21:**880-2.

2756. **Giordano, M. O., L. C. Martinez, M. B. Isa, M. Paez Rearte, and S. V. Nates.** 2004. Childhood astrovirus-associated diarrhea in the ambulatory setting in a Public Hospital in Cordoba city, Argentina. *Rev Inst Med Trop Sao Paulo* **46:**93-6.

2757. **Giraffa, G.** 2002. Enterococci from foods. *FEMS Microbiol Rev* **26:**163-71.

2758. **Giraudoux, P., F. Raoul, K. Bardonnet, P. Vuillaume, F. Tourneux, F. Cliquet, P. Delattre, and D. A. Vuitton.** 2001. Alveolar echinococcosis: characteristics of a possible emergence and new perspectives in epidemiosurveillance. *Méd Mal Infect* **31 suppl 2:**247-56.

2759. **Girginkardesler, N., S. Coskun, I. Cuneyt Balcioglu, P. Ertan, and U. Z. Ok.** 2003. Dientamoeba fragilis, a neglected cause of diarrhea, successfully treated with secnidazole. *Clin Microbiol Infect* **9:**110-3.

2760. **Girlich, D., A. Karim, L. Poirel, M. H. Cavin, C. Verny, and P. Nordmann.** 2000. Molecular epidemiology of an outbreak due to IRT-2 beta-lactamase- producing strains of Klebsiella pneumoniae in a geriatric department. *J Antimicrob Chemother* **45:**467-73.

2761. **Girmenia, C., L. Pagano, B. Martino, D. D'Antonio, R. Fanci, G. Specchia, L. Melillo, M. Buelli, G. Pizzarelli, M. Venditti, and P. Martino.** 2005. Invasive infections caused by Trichosporon species and Geotrichum capitatum in patients with hematological malignancies: a retrospective multicenter study from Italy and review of the literature. *J Clin Microbiol* **43:**1818-28.

2762. **Girod, J. C., R. C. Reichman, W. C. Winn, Jr., D. N. Klaucke, R. L. Vogt, and R. Dolin.** 1982. Pneumonic and nonpneumonic forms of legionellosis. The result of a common-source exposure to Legionella pneumophila. *Arch Intern Med* **142:**545-7.

2763. **Girod, R., M. Salvan, F. Simard, L. Andrianaivolambo, D. Fontenille, and S. Laventure.** 1999. [Evaluation of the vectorial capacity of Anopheles arabiensis (Diptera:Culicidae) on the island of Reunion: an approach to the health risk of malaria importation in an area of eradication]. *Bull Soc Pathol Exot* **92:**203-9.

2764. **Gitsch, G., C. Kainz, A. Reinthaller, W. Kopp, G. Tatra, and G. Breitenecker.** 1991. Cervical neoplasia and human papilloma virus infection in prostitutes. *Genitourin Med* **67:**478-80.

2765. **Giuliani, M., G. Palamara, A. Latini, A. Maini, and A. Di Carlo.** 2005. Evidence of an outbreak of syphilis among men who have sex with men in rome. *Arch Dermatol* **141:**100-1.

2766. **Giuliani, M., and B. Suligoi.** 1998. Sentinel surveillance of sexually transmitted diseases in Italy. *Eurosurveillance* **3:**55-58.

2767. **Givon-Lavi, N., R. Dagan, D. Fraser, P. Yagupsky, and N. Porat.** 1999. Marked differences in pneumococcal carriage and resistance patterns between day care centers located within a small area. *Clin Infect Dis* **29:**1274-80.

2768. **Givon-Lavi, N., D. Fraser, N. Porat, and R. Dagan.** 2002. Spread of Streptococcus pneumoniae and antibiotic-resistant S. pneumoniae from day-care center attendees to their younger siblings. *J Infect Dis* **186:**1608-14.

2769. **Gladstone, J. L., and S. J. Millian.** 1981. Rubella exposure in an obstetric clinic. *Obstet Gynecol* **57:**182-6.

2770. **Glaser, J. B., and A. Garden.** 1985. Inoculation of cryptococcosis without transmission of the acquired immunodeficiency syndrome. *N Engl J Med* **313:**266.

2771. **Glaser, L. C., M. V. Wegner, J. P. Davis, M. L. Bunning, A. A. Marfin, G. L. Campbell, B. Bernard, S. W. Lenhart, and M. J. Sotir.** 2003. West Nile virus infection among turkey breeder farm workers - Wisconsin, 2002. *MMWR* **52:**1017-9.

2772. **Glass, G. E., A. J. Watson, J. W. LeDuc, G. D. Kelen, T. C. Quinn, and J. E. Childs.** 1993. Infection with a ratborne hantavirus in US residents is consistently associated with hypertensive renal disease. *J Infect Dis* **167:**614-20.

2773. **Glass, R. I., M. Claeson, P. A. Blake, R. J. Waldman, and N. F. Pierce.** 1991. Cholera in Africa: lessions on transmission and control for Latin America. *Lancet* **338:**791-5.

2774. **Glass, R. I., J. Noel, T. Ando, R. Fankhauser, G. Belliot, A. Mounts, U. D. Parashar, J. S. Bresee, and S. S. Monroe.** 2000. The epidemiology of enteric caliciviruses from humans: a reassessment using new diagnostics. *J Infect Dis* **181 suppl 2:**S254-S261.

2775. **Glatzel, M., C. Rogivue, A. C. Ghani, J. R. Streffer, L. Amsler, and A. Aguzzi.** 2002. Incidence of Creutzfeldt-Jakob disease in Switzerland. *Lancet* **360:**139-41.

2776. **Gleason, W. A., Jr., V. J. Roden, and F. De Castro.** 1975. Letter: Pneumocystis pneumonia in Vietnamese infants. *J Pediatr* **87:**1001-2.

2777. **Gleiser, R. M., G. Schelotto, and D. E. Gorla.** 2002. Spatial pattern of abundance of the mosquito, Ochlerotatus albifasciatus, in relation to habitat characteristics. *Med Vet Entomol* **16**:364-71.

2778. **Glickman, L. T., and P. Schantz.** 1981. Epidemiology and pathogenesis of zoonotic toxocariasis. *Epidemiol Rev* **3**:230-50.

2779. **Gloster, J., H. J. Champion, J. H. Sorensen, T. Mikkelsen, D. B. Ryall, P. Astrup, S. Alexandersen, and A. I. Donaldson.** 2003. Airborne transmission of foot-and-mouth disease virus from Burnside Farm, Heddon-on-the-Wall, Northumberland, during the 2001 epidemic in the United Kingdom. *Vet Rec* **152**:525-33.

2780. **Glover, D. D., and B. Larsen.** 1998. Longitudinal investigation of candida vaginitis in pregnancy: role of superimposed antibiotic use. *Obstet Gynecol* **91**:115-8.

2781. **Glover, D. J., J. DeMain, J. R. Herbold, P. J. Schneider, and M. Bunning.** 2004. Comparative measles incidence among exposed military and nonmilitary persons in Anchorage, Alaska. *Mil Med* **169**:515-7.

2782. **Glynn, J. R., and S. R. Palmer.** 1992. Incubation period, severity of disease, and infecting dose: evidence from a Salmonella outbreak. *Am J Epidemiol* **136**:1369-77.

2783. **Glynn, S. A., M. P. Busch, G. B. Schreiber, E. L. Murphy, D. J. Wright, Y. Tu, and S. H. Kleinman.** 2003. Effect of a national disaster on blood supply and safety. The September 11 experience. *JAMA* **289**:2246-53.

2784. **Glynn, S. A., S. H. Kleinman, D. J. Wright, and M. P. Busch.** 2002. International application of the incidence rate/window period model. *Transfusion* **42**:966-72.

2785. **Go, E. S., C. Urban, J. Burns, B. Kreiswirth, W. Eisner, N. Mariano, K. Mosinka-Snipas, and J. J. Rahal.** 1994. Clinical and molecular epidemiology of acinetobacter infections sensitive only to polymyxin B and sulbactam. *Lancet* **344**:1329-32.

2786. **Gobat, P. F., and T. Jemmi.** 1993. Distribution of mesophilic Aeromonas species in raw and ready-to-eat fish and meat products in Switzerland. *Int J Food Microbiol* **20**:117-20.

2787. **Goddard, J.** 1989. Ticks and tickborne diseases affecting military personnel. United States Air Force (USAF), School of Aerospace Medicine (AFSC), Texas: Brooks Air Force Base.

2788. **Godfrey-Faussett, P., C. Dow, M. E. Black, and A. D. Bryceson.** 1991. Ivermectin in the treatment of onchocerciasis in Britain. *Trop Med Parasitol* **42**:82-4.

2789. **Godfrey-Faussett, P., P. Sonnenberg, S. C. Shearer, M. C. Bruce, C. Mee, L. Morris, and J. Murray.** 2000. Tuberculosis control and molecular epidemiology in a South African gold-mining community. *Lancet* **356**:1066-71.

2790. **Godfroid, J., and A. Käsbohrer.** 2002. Brucellosis in the European Union and Norway at the turn of the twenty-first century. *Vet Microbiol* **90**:135-45.

2791. **Godoy, P., A. Artigues, M. A. Usera, J. L. Gonzalez, N. Pablo, and M. Agusti.** 2000. [Food poisoning outbreak due to the consumption of spaghetti a la carbonara caused by Salmonella enteritidis]. *Enferm Infecc Microbiol Clin* **18**:257-61.

2792. **Goedert, J. J., M. E. Eyster, M. M. Lederman, T. Mandalaki, P. De Moerloose, G. C. White, 2nd, A. L. Angiolillo, N. L. Luban, K. E. Sherman, M. Manco-Johnson, L. Preiss, C. Leissinger, C. M. Kessler, A. R. Cohen, D. DiMichele, M. W. Hilgartner, L. M. Aledort, B. L. Kroner, P. S. Rosenberg, and A. Hatzakis.** 2002. End-stage liver disease in persons with hemophilia and transfusion-associated infections. *Blood* **100**:1584-9.

2793. **Goering, R. V., N. J. Ehrenkranz, C. C. Sanders, and W. E. Sanders, Jr.** 1992. Long term epidemiological analysis of Citrobacter diversus in a neonatal intensive care unit. *Pediatr Infect Dis J* **11**:99-104.

2794. **Goethert, H. K., and S. R. Telford, 3rd.** 2003. Enzootic transmission of Anaplasma bovis in Nantucket cottontail rabbits. *J Clin Microbiol* **41**:3744-7.

2795. **Goethert, H. K., and S. R. Telford, 3rd.** 2003. Enzootic transmission of Babesia divergens among cottontail rabbits on Nantucket Island, Massachusetts. *Am J Trop Med Hyg* **69**:455-60.

2796. **Goethert, H. K., and S. R. Telford, 3rd.** 2003. What is Babesia microti? *Parasitology* **127**:301-9.

2797. **Goettsch, W., E. Geubbels, W. Wannet, M. G. R. Hendrix, J. H. T. Wagenvoort, and A. J. de Neeling.** 2000. MRSA in nursing homes in the Netherlands 1989 to 1998: a developing reservoir? *Eurosurveillance* **5**:28-31.

2798. **Goetz, A. M., and B. A. Goldrick.** 2004. West Nile virus: a primer for infection control professionals. *Am J Infect Control* **32**:101-5.

2799. **Goetz, M. B., H. O'Brien, J. M. Musser, and J. I. Ward.** 1994. Nosocomial transmission of disease caused by nontypeable strains of Haemophilus influenzae. *Am J Med* **96**:342-7.

2800. **Gogoi, S. C., V. Dev, and S. Phookan.** 1996. Morbidity and mortality due to malaria in Tarajulie Tea Estate, Assam, India. *Southeast Asian J Trop Med Public Health* **27**:526-9.

2801. **Gogtay, N. J., S. Desai, V. S. Kadam, K. D. Kamtekar, S. S. Dalvi, and N. A. Kshirsagar.** 2000. Relapse pattern of Plasmodium vivax in Mumbai: a study of 283 cases of vivax malaria. *J Assoc Physicians India* **48**:1085-6.

2802. **Goh, C. L., A. Kamarudin, S. H. Chan, and V. S. Rajan.** 1985. Hepatitis B virus markers in prostitutes in Singapore. *Genitourin Med* **61**:127-9.

2803. **Goh, D. L. M., B. W. Lee, K. S. Chia, B. H. Heng, M. Chen, S. Ma, and C. C. Tan.** 2004. Secondary household transmission of SARS, Singapore. *Emerg Infect Dis* **10**:232-4.

2804. **Goh, K. J., C. T. Tan, N. K. Chew, P. S. Tan, A. Kamarulzaman, S. A. Sarji, K. T. Wong, B. J. Abdullah, K. B. Chua, and S. K. Lam.** 2000. Clinical features of Nipah virus encephalitis among pig farmers in Malaysia. *N Engl J Med* **342**:1229-1235.

2805. **Goh, K. T.** 1981. An outbreak of paratyphoid A in Singapore: clinical and epidemiological studies. *Southeast Asian J Trop Med Public Health* **12**:55-62.

2806. **Goh, K. T.** 2001. Dengue surveillance in Singapore, 2000. *Epidemiol News Bull* **27**:9-13.

2807. **Goh, K. T., Y. W. Chan, L. Y. M. Wong, K. H. Kong, C. J. Oon, and R. Guan.** 1988. The prevalence of hepatitis B virus markers in dental personnel in Singapore. *Trans R Soc Trop Med Hyg* **82**:908-10.

2808. **Goh, K. T., and S. Lam.** 1981. Vibrio infections in Singapore. *Ann Acad Med Singapore* **10**:2-10.

2809. **Goh, K. T., S. Lam, S. Kumarapathy, and J. L. Tan.** 1984. A common source foodborne outbreak of cholera in Singapore. *Int J Epidemiol* **13**:210-5.

2810. **Goh, K. T., S. Lam, and M. K. Ling.** 1987. Epidemiological characteristics of an institutional outbreak of cholera. *Trans R Soc Trop Med Hyg* **81**:230-2.

2811. **Goh, K. T., S. K. Ng, and S. Kumarapathy.** 1985. Disease-bearing insects brought in by international aircraft into Singapore. *Southeast Asian J Trop Med Public Health* **16**:49-53.

2812. Goh, K. T., S. H. Teo, S. Lam, and M. K. Ling. 1990. Person-to-person transmission of cholera in a psychiatric hospital. *J Infect* **20:**193-200.

2813. Goh, S. 2004. Sporadic cryptosporidiosis, North Cumbria, England, 1996-2000. *Emerg Infect Dis* **10:**1007-15.

2814. Goldberg, D. J., J. G. Wrench, P. W. Collier, J. A. Emslie, R. J. Fallon, G. I. Forbes, T. M. McKay, A. C. Macpherson, T. A. Markwick, and D. Reid. 1989. Lochgoilhead fever: outbreak of non-pneumonic legionellosis due to Legionella micdadei. *Lancet* **1:**316-8.

2815. Golden, M. R., C. M. Marra, and K. K. Holmes. 2003. Update on syphilis: resurgence of an old problem. *JAMA* **290:**1510-4.

2816. Goldfarb, L. G., L. Cervenakova, and D. C. Gajdusek. 2004. Genetic studies in relation to kuru: an overview. *Curr Mol Med* **4:**375-84.

2817. Goldman, W. D., and J. S. Marr. 1980. Are air-conditioning maintenance personnel at increased risk of Legionellosis? *Appl Environ Microbiol* **40:**114-6.

2818. Goldstein, E. J. 1996. Anaerobic bacteremia. *Clin Infect Dis* **23 Suppl 1:**S97-101.

2819. Goldstein, E. J., E. P. Pryor, 3rd, and D. M. Citron. 1995. Simian bites and bacterial infection. *Clin Infect Dis* **20:**1551-2.

2820. Goldstein, S. T., M. J. Alter, I. T. Williams, L. A. Moyer, F. N. Judson, K. Mottram, M. Fleenor, P. L. Ryder, and H. S. Margolis. 2002. Incidence and risk factors for acute hepatitis B in the United States, 1982-1998: implications for vaccination programs. *J Infect Dis* **185:**713-9.

2821. Gomes, T. C., M. F. Almeida, L. A. Miura, J. Granja, D. V. Santos, R. M. Oliveira, A. Lopes, B. P. Sequeira, A. A. Rolemberg, A. L. Moraes, and C. S. Santos. 2002. [Intestinal helminthiasis in street population of Rio de Janeiro city]. *Rev Soc Bras Med Trop* **35:**531-2.

2822. Gomez, E., A. Moore, J. Sanchez, J. Kool, P. L. Castellanos, J. M. Feris, M. Kolczak, and O. S. Levine. 1998. The epidemiology of Haemophilus influenzae type b carriage among infants and young children in Santo Domingo, Dominican Republic. *Pediatr Infect Dis J* **17:**782-6.

2823. Gomez, J. M., R. Fajardo, J. F. Patino, and C. A. Arias. 2003. Necrotizing fasciitis due to Vibrio alginolyticus in an immunocompetent patient. *J Clin Microbiol* **41:**3427-9.

2824. Gomez-Garcia, V., J. Hernandez-Quero, and M. Rodriguez-Osorio. 2003. Short report: Human infection with Trichinella britovi in Granada, Spain. *Am J Trop Med Hyg* **68:**463-4.

2825. Gomez-Leon, J., L. Villamil, M. L. Lemos, B. Novoa, and A. Figueras. 2005. Isolation of Vibrio alginolyticus and Vibrio splendidus from aquacultured carpet shell clam (Ruditapes decussatus) larvae associated with mass mortalities. *Appl Environ Microbiol* **71:**98-104.

2826. Gomez-Saladin, E., C. W. Doud, and M. Maroli. 2005. Short report: surveillance of Leishmania sp. among sand flies in Sicily (Italy) using a fluorogenic real-time polymerase chain reaction. *Am J Trop Med Hyg* **72:**138-41.

2827. Goncalves, C. R., T. M. Vaz, D. Leite, B. Pisani, M. Simoes, M. A. Prandi, M. M. Rocha, P. C. Cesar, P. Trabasso, A. von Nowakonski, and K. Irino. 2000. Molecular epidemiology of a nosocomial outbreak due to Enterobacter cloacae and Enterobacter agglomerans in Campinas, Sao Paulo, Brazil. *Rev Inst Med Trop Sao Paulo* **42:**1-7.

2828. Gonçalves, G., A. M. Correia, P. Palminha, H. Rebelo-Andrade, and A. Alves. 2005. Outbreaks caused by parvovirus B19 in three Portuguese schools. *Eurosurveillance* **10:**121-4.

2829. Gonçalves, G., L. Queirós, M. do Carmo Ferreira, M. Pires de Miranda, and H. Rebelo-Andrade. 2004. Oral polio vaccine accidental injection in the north of Portugal. *Eurosurveillance Weekly* **8:**15-6.

2830. Gonçalves, M. A. S., R. J. Sá-Neto, and T. K. Brazil. 2002. Outbreak of aggressions and transmission of rabies in human beings by vampire bats in northeastern Brazil. *Rev Soc Bras Med Trop* **35:**461-4.

2831. Gonin, P., and L. Trudel. 2003. Detection and differentiation of Entamoeba histolytica and Entamoeba dispar isolates in clinical samples by PCR and enzyme-linked immunosorbent assay. *J Clin Microbiol* **41:**237-41.

2832. Gonzalez, A., H. Sagua, L. Cortes, J. Lobo, I. Neira, and J. Araya. 1999. [Human diphyllobothriasis by Diphyllobothrium pacificum. A new case in Antofagasta, Chile]. *Rev Med Chil* **127:**75-7.

2833. Gonzalez Della Valle, M., A. Edelstein, S. Miguel, V. Martinez, J. Cortez, M. L. Cacace, G. Jurgelenas, S. S. Estani, and P. Padula. 2002. Andes virus associated with hantavirus pulmonary syndrome in northern Argentina and determination of the precise site of infection. *Am J Trop Med Hyg* **66:**713-20.

2834. Gonzalez Garcia, J. J., F. Arnalich, J. M. Pena, J. J. Garcia-Alegria, F. Garcia Fernandez, C. Jimenez Herraez, and J. J. Vazquez. 1986. An outbreak of Plasmodium vivax malaria among heroin users in Spain. *Trans R Soc Trop Med Hyg* **80:**549-52.

2835. Gonzalez Hevia, M. A., and M. C. Mendoza. 1995. Differentiation of strains from a food-borne outbreak of Salmonella enterica by phenotypic and genetic typing methods. *Eur J Epidemiol* **11:**479-82.

2836. Gonzalez, J. P., E. Nakoune, W. Slenczka, P. Vidal, and J. M. Morvan. 2000. Ebola and Marburg virus antibody prevalence in selected populations of the Central African Republic. *Microbes Infect* **2:**39-44.

2837. Gonzalez, M. M., E. Gould, G. Dickinson, A. J. Martinez, G. Visvesvara, T. J. Cleary, and G. T. Hensley. 1986. Acquired immunodeficiency syndrome associated with Acanthamoeba infection and other opportunistic organisms. *Arch Pathol Lab Med* **110:**749-51.

2838. Gonzalez Quijada, S., M. Rubio Diaz, J. L. Yanez Ortega, I. Carraminana Martinez, E. Ojeda Fernandez, and J. Lozano Garcia. 2002. [Tularemia: study of 27 patients]. *Med Clin (Barc)* **119:**455-7.

2839. Gonzalez, R., L. De Sousa, R. Devera, A. Jorquera, and E. Ledezma. 1999. Seasonal and nocturnal domiciliary human landing/biting behaviour of Lutzomyia (Lutzomyia) evansi and Lutzomyia (Psychodopygus) panamensis (Diptera; Psychodidae) in a periurban area of a city on the Caribbean coast of eastern Venezuela (Barcelona; Anzoategui State). *Trans R Soc Trop Med Hyg* **93:**361-4.

2840. Gonzalez-Cortes, A., E. J. Gangarosa, C. Parrilla, W. T. Martin, A. M. Espinosa-Ayala, L. Ruiz, D. Bessudo, and H. Hernandez-Arreortua. 1982. Bottled beverages and typhoid fever: the Mexican epidemic of 1972-73. *Am J Public Health* **72:**844-5.

2841. González-Rey, C., S. B. Svenson, L. Bravo, J. Rosinsky, I. Ciznar, and K. Krovacek. 2000. Specific detection of Plesiomonas shigelloides isolated from aquatic environments, animals and human diarrhoeal cases by PCR based on 23S rRNA gene. *FEMS Immunol Med Microbiol* **29**:107-13.

2842. **Goob, T. C., S. M. Yamada, R. E. Newman, and T. M. Cashman.** 1999. Bloodborne exposures at a United States Army Medical Center. *Appl Occup Environ Hyg* **14**:20-5.

2843. **Good, B., C. V. Holland, M. R. H. Taylor, J. Larragy, P. Moriarty, and M. O'Regan.** 2004. Ocular toxocariasis in schoolchildren. *Clin Infect Dis* **39**:173-8.

2844. **Goode, B., K. Caruso, J. Murphy, A. Weber, and J. Burgett.** 1998. Neonatal tetanus - Montana, 1998. *MMWR* **47**:928–930.

2845. **Goodenow, C., J. Netherland, and L. Szalacha.** 2002. AIDS-related risk among adolescent males who have sex with males, females, or both: evidence from a statewide survey. *Am J Public Health* **92**:203-10.

2846. **Goodfellow, A. M., W. E. Hoy, K. S. Sriprakash, M. J. Daly, M. P. Reeve, and J. D. Mathews.** 1999. Proteinuria is associated with persistence of antibody to streptococcal M protein in Aboriginal Australians. *Epidemiol Infect* **122**:67-75.

2847. **Gooding, R. H., and E. S. Krafsur.** 2005. Tsetse genetics: contributions to biology, systematics, and control of tsetse flies. *Annu Rev Entomol* **50**:101-23.

2848. **Goodman, K. A., S. A. Ballagh, and A. Carpio.** 1999. Case-control study of seropositivity for cysticercosis in Cuenca, Ecuador. *Am J Trop Med Hyg* **60**:70-4.

2849. **Goodman, K. J., P. Correa, H. J. Tengana Aux, H. Ramirez, J. P. DeLany, O. Guerrero Pepinosa, M. Lopez Quinones, and T. Collazos Parra.** 1996. Helicobacter pylori infection in the Colombian Andes: a population- based study of transmission pathways. *Am J Epidemiol* **144**:290-9.

2850. **Goodman, R. A., and S. L. Solomon.** 1991. Transmission of infectious diseases in outpatient health care settings. *JAMA* **265**:2377-81.

2851. **Goodnough, L. T., M. E. Brecher, M. H. Kanter, and J. P. AuBuchon.** 1999. Transfusion medicine. First of two parts—blood transfusion. *N Engl J Med* **340**:438-47.

2852. **Goodnough, L. T., A. Shander, and M. E. Brecher.** 2003. Transfusion medicine: looking to the future. *Lancet* **361**:161-9.

2853. **Gopalakrishna, G., P. Choo, Y. S. Leo, B. K. Tay, Y. T. Lim, A. S. Khan, and C. C. Tan.** 2004. SARS transmission and hospital containment. *Emerg Infect Dis* **10**:395-400.

2854. **Gora, D., T. Yaya, T. Jocelyn, F. Didier, D. Maoulouth, S. Amadou, T. D. Ruel, and J. P. Gonzalez.** 2000. The potential role of rodents in the enzootic cycle of Rift Valley fever virus in Senegal. *Microbes Infect* **2**:343-6.

2855. **Gordillo, M. E., G. R. Reeve, J. Pappas, J. J. Mathewson, H. L. DuPont, and B. E. Murray.** 1992. Molecular characterization of strains of enteroinvasive Escherichia coli O143, including isolates from a large outbreak in Houston, Texas. *J Clin Microbiol* **30**:889-93.

2856. **Gordon, J. C., S. w. Gordon, E. Peterson, and R. N. Philip.** 1984. Epidemiology of Rocky Mountain spotted fever in Ohio, 1981: serologic evaluation of canines and rickettsial isolation from ticks associated with human case exposure sites. *Am J Trop Med Hyg* **33**:1026-31.

2857. **Gordon, S. M., and R. K. Avery.** 2001. Aspergillosis in lung transplantation: incidence, risk factors, and prophylactic strategies. *Transpl Infect Dis* **3**:161-7.

2858. **Gordon, S. M., S. P. LaRosa, S. Kalmadi, A. C. Arroliga, R. K. Avery, L. Truesdell-LaRosa, and D. L. Longworth.** 1999. Should prophylaxis for Pneumocystis carinii pneumonia in solid organ transplant recipients ever be discontinued? *Clin Infect Dis* **28**:240-6.

2859. **Gorenflot, A., K. Moubri, E. Precigout, B. Carcy, and T. P. Schetters.** 1998. Human babesiosis. *Ann Trop Med Parasitol* **92**:489-501.

2860. **Gorgolas, M. D., F. Santos-O'Connor, A. L. Unzu, M. L. Fernandez-Guerrero, U. A. De Madrid, T. Garate, R. M. Troyas, and M. P. Grobusch.** 2003. Cutaneous and Medullar Gnathostomiasis in Travelers to Mexico and Thailand. *J Travel Med* **10**:358-361.

2861. **Goritsas, C., I. Plerou, S. Agaliotis, R. Spinthaki, K. Mimidis, D. Velissaris, N. Lazarou, and C. Labropoulou-Karatza.** 2000. HCV infection in the general population of a Greek island: prevalence and risk factors. *Hepatogastroenterology* **47**:782-5.

2862. **Gorman, D. G., D. F. Benson, D. G. Vogel, and H. V. Vinters.** 1992. Creutzfeldt-Jakob disease in a pathologist. *Neurology* **42**:463.

2863. **Gorman, L. J., L. Sanai, A. W. Notman, I. S. Grant, and R. G. Masterton.** 1993. Cross infection in an intensive care unit by Klebsiella pneumoniae from ventilator condensate. *J Hosp Infect* **23**:27-34.

2864. **Gornik, V., K. Behringer, B. Kölb, and M. Exner.** 2000. Erster Giardiasisausbruch im Zusammenhang mit kontaminiertem Drinkwasser in Deutschland. *Bundesgesundheitsblatt Gesundheitsforschung Gesundheitsschutz* **44**:351-7.

2865. **Gorny, R. L., and J. Dutkiewicz.** 2002. Bacterial and fungal aerosols in indoor environment in Central and Eastern European countries. *Ann Agric Environ Med* **9**:17-23.

2866. **Gosbell, I. B., A. D. Ross, and I. B. Turner.** 1999. Chlamydia psittaci infection and reinfection in a veterinarian. *Aust Vet J* **77**:511-3.

2867. **Gotsch, K., J. L. Annest, P. Holmgreen, and J. Gilchrist.** 2002. Nonfatal sports- and recreation-related injuries treated in emergency departments - United States, July 2000-June 2001. *MMWR* **51**:736-40.

2868. **Gottlieb, M. S.** 2001. AIDS - past and future. *N Engl J Med* **344**:1788-91.

2869. **Gottstein, B., F. Saucy, P. Deplazes, J. Reichen, G. Demierre, A. Busato, C. Zuercher, and P. Pugin.** 2001. Is high prevalence of Echinococcus multilocularis in wild and domestic animals associated with disease incidence in humans? *Emerg Infect Dis* **7**:408-12.

2870. **Gotz, H., J. B. de, J. Lindback, P. A. Parment, K. O. Hedlund, M. Torven, and K. Ekdahl.** 2002. Epidemiological investigation of a food-borne gastroenteritis outbreak caused by Norwalk-like virus in 30 day-care centres. *Scand J Infect Dis* **34**:115-21.

2871. **Götz, H. M., R. Nieuwenhuis, T. Ossewaarde, B. Thio, W. van der Meijden, J. Dees, and O. de Zwart.** 2004. Preliminary report of an outbreak of lymphogranuloma venereum in homosexual men in the Netherlands, with implications for other countries in western Europe. *Eurosurveillance Weekly* **8**:1-2.

2872. **Gotz, H. M., A. Tegnell, B. De Jong, K. A. Broholm, M. Kuusi, I. Kallings, and K. Ekdahl.** 2001. A whirlpool associated outbreak of Pontiac fever at a hotel in Northern Sweden. *Epidemiol Infect* **126**:241-7.

2873. Goubau, P. F. J., and C. Munyangeyo. 1983. Fièvre récurrente à tiques et grossesse. *Ann Soc Belg Med Trop* **63**:347-55.

2874. Goujard, J., M. Entat, F. Maillard, E. Mugnier, R. Rappaport, and J. C. Job. 1988. Human pituitary growth hormone (hGH) and Creutzfeldt-Jakob disease: results of an epidemiological survey in France, 1986. *Int J Epidemiol* **17**:423-7.

2875. Goulding, M. R., M. E. Rogers, and S. M. Smitz. 2003. Trends in aging - United States and worldwide. *MMWR* **52**:101-6.

2876. Goulet, V., H. de Valk, O. Pierre, F. Stainer, J. Rocourt, V. Vaillant, C. Jacquet, and J. C. Desenclos. 2001. Effect of prevention measures on incidence of human listeriosis, France, 1987-1997. *Emerg Infect Dis* **7**:983-9.

2877. Goulet, V., J. Rocourt, I. Rebiere, C. Jacquet, C. Moyse, P. Dehaumont, G. Salvat, and P. Veit. 1998. Listeriosis outbreak associated with the consumption of rillettes in France in 1993. *J Infect Dis* **177**:155-60.

2878. Goulston, K. J., O. F. Dent, P. H. Chapuis, G. Chapman, C. I. Smith, A. D. Tait, and C. C. Tennant. 1985. Gastrointestinal morbidity among World War II prisoners of war: 40 years on. *Med J Aust* **143**:6-10.

2879. Gourdon, F., J. Beytout, A. Reynaud, J. P. Romaszko, D. Perre, P. Theodore, H. Soubelet, and J. Sirot. 1999. Human and animal epidemic of Yersinia enterocolitica O:9, 1989-1997, Auvergne, France. *Emerg Infect Dis* **5**:719-21.

2880. Gourishankar, S., J. C. McDermid, G. S. Jhangri, and J. K. Preiksaitis. 2004. Herpes zoster infection following solid organ transplantation: incidence, risk factors and outcomes in the current immunosuppressive era. *Am J Transplant* **4**:108-15.

2881. Gove, S., A. Ali-Salad, M. A. Farah, D. Delaney, M. J. Roble, and J. Walter. 1987. Enterically transmitted non-A, non-B hepatitis - East Africa. *MMWR* **36**:241-4.

2882. Grabau, J. C., S. E. Hughes, E. M. Rodriguez, J. N. Sommer, and E. T. Troy. 2004. Investigation of sudden death from Mycobacterium tuberculosis in a foreign-born worker at a resort hotel. *Heart Lung* **33**:333-7.

2883. Graczyk, T. K., R. Fayer, R. d. Knight, B. Mhangami-Ruwende, J. M. Trout, A. J. Da Silva, and N. J. Pieniazek. 2000. Mechanical transport and transmission of Cryptosporidium parvum oocysts by wild filth flies. *Am J Trop Med Hyg* **63**:178-183.

2884. Graczyk, T. K., and B. Fried. 1998. Echinostomiasis: a common but forgotten food-borne disease. *Am J Trop Med Hyg* **58**:501-4.

2885. Graczyk, T. K., R. H. Gilman, and B. Fried. 2001. Fasciolopsiasis: is it a controllable food-borne disease? *Parasitol Res* **87**:80-3.

2886. Graczyk, T. K., and C. J. Shiff. 2000. Recovery of avian schistosome cercariae from water using penetration stimulant matrix with an unsaturated fatty acid. *Am J Trop Med Hyg* **63**:174-7.

2887. Graczyk, T. K., R. C. Thompson, R. Fayer, P. Adams, U. M. Morgan, and E. J. Lewis. 1999. Giardia duodenalis cysts of genotype A recovered from clams in the Chesapeake Bay subestuary, Rhode River. *Am J Trop Med Hyg* **61**:526-9.

2888. Gragnic, G., J. Julvez, A. Abari, and Y. Alexandre. 1998. HIV-1 and HIV-2 seropositivity among female sex workers in the Tenere Desert, Niger. *Trans R Soc Trop Med Hyg* **92**:29.

2889. Graham, D. R., E. Wu, A. K. Highsmith, and M. L. Ginsburg. 1981. An outbreak of pseudobacteremia caused by Enterobacter cloacae from a phlebotomist's vial of thrombin. *Ann Intern Med* **95**:585-8.

2890. Graham, J. C., S. Lanser, G. Bignardi, S. Pedler, and V. Hollyoak. 2002. Hospital-acquired listeriosis. *J Hosp Infect* **51**:136-9.

2891. Graham, K., N. Mohammad, H. Rehman, M. Farhan, M. Kamal, and M. Rowland. 2002. Comparison of three pyrethroid treatments of top-sheets for malaria control in emergencies: entomological and user acceptance studies in an Afghan refugee camp in Pakistan. *Med Vet Entomol* **16**:199-206.

2892. Graham, K., N. Mohammad, H. Rehman, A. Nazari, M. Ahmad, M. Kamal, O. Skovmand, P. Guillet, R. Allan, M. Zaim, A. Yates, J. Lines, and M. Rowland. 2002. Insecticide-treated plastic tarpaulins for control of malaria vectors in refugee camps. *Med Vet Entomol* **16**:404-8.

2893. Gramiccia, M., and L. Gradoni. 2005. The current status of zoonotic leishmaniases and approaches to disease control. *Int J Parasitol* **35**:1169-80.

2894. Grande, P., A. Cronquist, S. Fernyak, S. H. Huang, I. Bihl, E. Osvald-Doppelhauer, C. Woodfill, D. Vugia, G. Agyekum, J. Kravitz, H. Gillette, G. Armstrong, P. George, L. Finelli, P. Patel, and N. Jain. 2003. Multistate outbreak of hepatitis A among young adult concert attendees - United States, 2003. *MMWR* **52**:844-5.

2895. Grandesso, F., F. Sanderson, J. Kruijt, T. Koene, and V. Brown. 2005. Mortality and malnutrition among populations living in South Darfur, Sudan: results of 3 surveys, September 2004. *JAMA* **293**:1490-4.

2896. Grange, F., B. Levin, E. Pellenq, J. M. Haegy, and J. C. Guillaume. 2001. [Dermatological consultation behind bars: an analysis on a three-year period in a French prison]. *Ann Dermatol Venereol* **128**:513-6.

2897. Grange, J. T., G. W. Baumann, and R. Vaezazizi. 2003. On-site physicians reduce ambulance transports at mass gatherings. *Prehosp Emerg Care* **7**:322-6.

2898. Grani, R., A. Wandeler, F. Steck, and R. Rosli. 1978. [Rabies in a veterinarian]. *Schweiz Med Wochenschr* **108**:593-7.

2899. Granoff, D. M., T. McKinney, E. G. Boies, N. P. Steele, J. Oldfather, J. P. Pandey, and B. K. Suarez. 1986. Haemophilus influenzae type b disease in an Amish population: studies of the effects of genetic factors, immunization, and rifampin prophylaxis on the course of an outbreak. *Pediatrics* **77**:289-95.

2900. Granovsky, M. O., H. L. Minkoff, B. H. Tess, D. Waters, A. Hatzakis, D. E. Devoid, S. H. Landesman, A. Rubinstein, A. M. Di Bisceglie, and J. J. Goedert. 1998. Hepatitis C virus in the mothers and infants cohort study. *Pediatrics* **102**:355-9.

2901. Gransden, W. R., M. Webster, G. L. French, and I. Phillips. 1986. An outbreak of Serratia marcescens transmitted by contaminated breast pumps in a special care baby unit. *J Hosp Infect* **7**:149-54.

2902. Grant, I. R., E. I. Hitchings, A. McCartney, F. Ferguson, and M. T. Rowe. 2002. Effect of commercial-scale high-temperature, short-time pasteurization on the viability of Mycobacterium paratuberculosis in naturally infected cows' milk. *Appl Environ Microbiol* **68**:602-7.

2903. Granum, P. E., K. O'Sullivan, J. M. Tomas, and O. Ormen. 1998. Possible virulence factors of Aeromonas spp. from food and water. *FEMS Immunol Med Microbiol* **21**:131-7.

2904. **Granwehr, B. P., K. M. Lillibridge, S. Higgs, P. W. Mason, J. F. Aronson, G. A. Campbell, and A. D. Barrett.** 2004. West Nile virus: where are we now? *Lancet Infect Dis* **4:**547-56.

2905. **Gras-Le Guen, C., D. Lepelletier, T. Debillon, V. Gournay, E. Espaze, and J. C. Roze.** 2003. Contamination of a milk bank pasteuriser causing a Pseudomonas aeruginosa outbreak in a neonatal intensive care unit. *Arch Dis Child Fetal Neonatal Ed* **88:**F434-5.

2906. **Grave, W., and A. W. Sturm.** 1983. Brucellosis associated with a beauty parlour. *Lancet* **1:**1326-7.

2907. **Gravel, D., M. L. Sample, K. Ramotar, B. Toye, C. Oxley, and G. Garber.** 2002. Outbreak of burkholderia cepacia in the adult intensive care unit traced to contaminated indigo-carmine dye. *Infect Control Hosp Epidemiol* **23:**103-6.

2908. **Gravel-Tropper, D., M. L. Sample, C. Oxley, B. Toye, D. E. Woods, and G. E. Garber.** 1996. Three-year outbreak of pseudobacteremia with Burkholderia cepacia traced to a contaminated blood gas analyzer. *Infect Control Hosp Epidemiol* **17:**737-40.

2909. **Gravenor, M. B., P. Papasozomenos, A. R. McLean, and G. Neophytou.** 2004. A scrapie epidemic in Cyprus. *Epidemiol Infect* **132:**751-60.

2910. **Graves, M. H., and J. M. Janda.** 2001. Rat-bite fever (Streptobacillus moniliformis): a potential emerging disease. *Int J Infect Dis* **5:**151-5.

2911. **Gray, G. C., J. D. Callahan, A. W. Hawksworth, C. A. Fisher, and J. C. Gaydos.** 1999. Respiratory diseases among U.S. military personnel: countering emerging threats. *Emerg Infect Dis* **5:**379-85.

2912. **Gray, G. C., P. R. Goswami, M. D. Malasig, A. W. Hawksworth, D. H. Trump, M. A. Ryan, and D. P. Schnurr.** 2000. Adult adenovirus infections: loss of orphaned vaccines precipitates military respiratory disease epidemics. For the Adenovirus Surveillance Group. *Clin Infect Dis* **31:**663-70.

2913. **Gray, J., R. H. George, G. M. Durbin, A. K. Ewer, M. D. Hocking, and M. E. Morgan.** 1999. An outbreak of Bacillus cereus respiratory tract infections on a neonatal unit due to contaminated ventilator circuits. *J Hosp Infect* **41:**19-22.

2914. **Gray, J. J., T. G. Wreghitt, W. D. Cubitt, and P. R. Elliot.** 1987. An outbreak of gastroenteritis in a home for the elderly associated with astrovirus type 1 and human calicivirus. *J Med Virol* **23:**377-81.

2915. **Gray, R. H., M. J. Wawer, R. Brookmeyer, N. K. Sewankambo, D. Serwadda, F. Wabwire-Mangen, T. Lutalo, X. Li, T. vanCott, and T. C. Quinn.** 2001. Probability of HIV-1 transmission per coital act in monogamous, heterosexual, HIV-1-discordant couples in Rakai, Uganda. *Lancet* **357:**1149-53.

2916. **Grayston, J. T., L. A. Campbell, C. C. Kuo, C. H. Mordhorst, P. Saikku, D. H. Thom, and S. P. Wang.** 1990. A new respiratory tract pathogen: Chlamydia pneumoniae strain TWAR. *J Infect Dis* **161:**618-25.

2917. **Greaves, W. L., W. A. Orenstein, H. C. Stetler, S. R. Preblud, A. R. Hinman, and K. J. Bart.** 1982. Prevention of rubella transmission in medical facilities. *JAMA* **248:**861-4.

2918. **Greaves, W. L., L. M. Rodrigues, B. Anderson, J. Biddle, and W. L. Wittington.** 1986. Outbreak of penicillinase-producing Neisseria gonorrhoeae with an African connection. *South Med J* **79:**420-3.

2919. **Grebaut, P., J. M. Bodo, A. Assona, V. Foumane Ngane, F. Njiokou, G. Ollivier, G. Soula, and C. Laveissiere.** 2001. [Risk factors for human African trypanosomiasis in the Bipindi region of Cameroon]. *Med Trop (Mars)* **61:**377-83.

2920. **Greco, D., G. Allegrini, T. Tizzi, E. Ninu, A. Lamanna, and S. Luzi.** 1987. A waterborne tularemia outbreak. *Eur J Epidemiol* **3:**35-8.

2921. **Green, A. D., C. Mason, and P. M. Spragg.** 2001. Outbreak of cutaneous larva migrans among British military personnel in Belize. *J Travel Med* **8:**267-9.

2922. **Green, K. Y., G. Belliot, J. L. Taylor, J. Valdesuso, J. F. Lew, A. Z. Kapikian, and F. Y. Lin.** 2002. A predominant role for Norwalk-like viruses as agents of epidemic gastroenteritis in Maryland nursing homes for the elderly. *J Infect Dis* **185:**133-146.

2923. **Green, M., M. Kaufmann, J. Wilson, and J. Reyes.** 1997. Comparison of intravenous ganciclovir followed by oral acyclovir with intravenous ganciclovir alone for prevention of cytomegalovirus and Epstein-Barr virus disease after liver transplantation in children. *Clin Infect Dis* **25:**1344-9.

2924. **Green, M. S., E. Anis, D. Gandacu, and I. Grotto.** 2003. The fall and rise of gonorrhoea incidence in Israel: an international phenomenon? *Sex Transm Infect* **79:**116-8.

2925. **Greenberg, J. H.** 1969. Public health problems relating to the Vietnam returnee. *JAMA* **207:**697-702.

2926. **Greenstein, R. J.** 2003. Is Crohn's disease caused by a mycobacterium? Comparisons with leprosy, tuberculosis, and Johne's disease. *Lancet Infect Dis* **3:**507-14.

2927. **Greenwood, M., G. Winnard, and B. Bagot.** 1998. An outbreak of Salmonella enteritidis phage type 19 infection associated with cockles. *Commun Dis Public Health* **1:**35-7.

2928. **Gregersen, P., K. Grunnet, S. A. Uldum, B. H. Andersen, and H. Madsen.** 1999. Pontiac fever at a sewage treatment plant in the food industry. *Scand J Work Environ Health* **25:**291-5.

2929. **Gregg, N. M.** 1941. Congenital cataract following German measles in the mother. *Trans Ophthal Soc Aust* **3:**35-46.

2930. **Greig, J., K. Lalor, C. Ferreira, and E. McCormick.** 2001. An outbreak of Salmonella typhimurium phage type 99 linked to a hotel buffet in Victoria. *Commun Dis Intell* **25:**277-8.

2931. **Grein, T., F. Checchi, J. M. Escriba, A. Tamrat, U. Karunakara, C. Stokes, V. Brown, and D. Legros.** 2003. Mortality among displaced former UNITA members and their families in Angola: a retrospective cluster survey. *BMJ* **327:**650.

2932. **Grein, T., and D. O. O'Flanagan.** 2001. Day-care and meningococcal disease in young children. *Epidemiol Infect* **127:**435-41.

2933. **Greub, G., A. Maziero, G. Kaufmann, C. Colombo, F. Zysset, C. Ruef, and P. Francioli.** 2002. HIV-, HBV- und HCV-Expositionen im medizinischen Bereich in der Schweiz von 1997 bis 2000. *Bull Bundesamt Gesundheit* **40:**692-6.

2934. **Greuter, S., A. Widmer, A. Gratwohl, and P. Reusser.** 1999. Die Zytomegalovirus (CMV)-Infektion und -Erkrankung nach allogener Knochenmarktransplantation (KMT): die Basler Erfahrung bei Patienten mit hämatologischer Neoplasie. *Schweiz Med Wochenschr* **129 suppl 105/II:**9 S.

2935. **Griego, R. D., T. Rosen, I. F. Orengo, and J. E. Wolf.** 1995. Dog, cat, and human bites: a review. *J Am Acad Dermatol* **33:**1019-29.

2936. **Grif, K., G. Patscheider, M. P. Dierich, and F. Allerberger.** 2003. Incidence of fecal carriage of Listeria monocytogenes in three healthy volunteers: a one-year prospective stool survey. *Eur J Clin Microbiol Infect Dis* **22.**

2937. Griffin, D. D., M. Fletcher, M. E. Levy, M. Ching-Lee, R. Nogami, L. Edwards, H. Peters, L. Montague, J. R. Gentsch, and R. I. Glass. 2002. Outbreaks of adult gastroenteritis traced to a single genotype of rotavirus. *J Infect Dis* **185**:1502-5.

2938. Grijalva, M. J., L. Escalante, R. A. Paredes, J. A. Costales, A. Padilla, E. C. Rowland, H. M. Aguilar, and J. Racines. 2003. Seroprevalence and risk factors for Trypanosoma cruzi infection in the Amazon region of Ecuador. *Am J Trop Med Hyg* **69**:380-5.

2939. Grillet, M. E., N. J. Villamizar, J. Cortez, H. L. Frontado, M. Escalona, S. Vivas-Martinez, and M. G. Basanez. 2005. Diurnal biting periodicity of parous Simulium (Diptera: Simuliidae) vectors in the onchocerciasis Amazonian focus. *Acta Trop* **94**:139-58.

2940. Grilli, E. A., M. J. Anderson, and T. W. Hoskins. 1989. Concurrent outbreaks of influenza and parvovirus B19 in a boys' boarding school. *Epidemiol Infect* **103**:359-69.

2941. Grimes, D. A. 2000. Intrauterine device and upper-genital tract infection. *Lancet* **356**:1013-9.

2942. Grimoud, A. M., N. Marty, H. Bocquet, S. Andrieu, J. P. Lodter, and G. Chabanon. 2003. Colonization of the oral cavity by Candida species: risk factors in long-term geriatric care. *J Oral Sci* **45**:51-5.

2943. Grimwood, K., Q. S. Huang, L. G. Sadleir, W. A. Nix, D. R. Kilpatrick, M. S. Oberste, and M. A. Pallansch. 2003. Acute flaccid paralysis from echovirus type 33 infection. *J Clin Microbiol* **41**:2230-2.

2944. Grist, N. R., and J. A. N. Emslie. 1994. Association of clinical pathologists' surveys of infection in British clinical laboratories, 1970-1989. *J Clin Pathol* **47**:391-4.

2945. Grizhebovskii, G. M., G. G. Onishchenko, V. I. Taran, S. I. Ivanov, M. Evchenko Iu, S. S. Galimshin, E. V. Sychugov, E. I. Eremenko, U. N. Bakaev, V. M. Mezentsev, A. F. Briukhanov, and S. L. Protsenko. 2001. [Outbreak of typhoid fever in the Chechen Republic in 2000: epidemiological characterization]. *Zh Mikrobiol Epidemiol Immunobiol* issue 6 (suppl):45-7.

2946. Grob, P. J., B. Bischof, and F. Naeff. 1981. Cluster of hepatitis B transmitted by a physician. *Lancet* **2**:1218-20.

2947. Grobusch, M. P., K. Gobels, D. Teichmann, F. Bergmann, and N. Suttorp. 2001. Early-stage elephantiasis in bancroftian filariasis. *Eur J Clin Microbiol Infect Dis* **20**:835-6.

2948. Grobusch, M. P., N. Mühlberger, T. Jelinek, Z. Bisoffi, M. Corachan, G. Harms, A. Matteelli, G. Fry, C. Hatz, I. Gjorup, M. L. Schmid, J. Knobloch, S. Puente, U. Bronner, A. Kapaun, J. Clerinx, L. N. Nielsen, K. Fleischer, J. Beran, S. da Cunha, M. Schulze, B. Myrvang, and U. Hellgren. 2003. Imported schistosomiasis in Europe: sentinel surveillance data from TropNetEurope. *J Travel Med* **10**:164-9.

2949. Groen, J., P. Koraka, Y. A. Nur, T. Avsic-Zupanc, W. H. Goessens, A. Ott, and A. D. Osterhaus. 2002. Serologic evidence of ehrlichiosis among humans and wild animals in the Netherlands. *Eur J Clin Microbiol Infect Dis* **21**:46-9.

2950. Groen, J., Y. A. Nur, W. Dolmans, R. J. Ligthelm, and A. D. Osterhaus. 1999. Scrub and murine typhus among Dutch travellers. *Infection* **27**:291-2.

2951. Grogl, M., J. L. Daugirda, D. L. Hoover, A. J. Magill, and J. D. Berman. 1993. Survivability and infectivity of viscerotropic Leishmania tropica from Operation Desert Storm participants in human blood products maintained under blood bank conditions. *Am J Trop Med Hyg* **49**:308-15.

2952. Grohmann, G. S., H. B. Greenberg, B. M. Welch, and A. M. Murphy. 1980. Oyster-associated gastroenteritis in Australia: the detection of Norwalk virus and its antibody by immune electron microscopy and radioimmunoassay. *J Med Virol* **6**:11-9.

2953. Grohskopf, L. A., V. R. Roth, D. R. Feikin, M. J. Arduino, L. A. Carson, J. I. Tokars, S. C. Holt, B. J. Jensen, R. E. Hoffman, and W. R. Jarvis. 2001. Serratia liquefaciens bloodstream infections from contamination of epoetin alfa at a hemodialysis center. *N Engl J Med* **344**:1491-7.

2954. Grohskopf, L. A., R. L. Sinkowitz-Cochran, D. O. Garrett, A. H. Sohn, G. L. Levine, J. D. Siegel, B. H. Stover, and W. R. Jarvis. 2002. A national point-prevalence survey of pediatric intensive care unit- acquired infections in the United States. *J Pediatr* **140**:432-8.

2955. Groll, A. H., and T. J. Walsh. 2001. Uncommon opportunistic fungi: new nosocomial threats. *Clin Microbiol Inf* **7 suppl 2**:8-24.

2956. Groseclose, S. L., W. S. Brathwaite, P. A. Hall, F. J. Connor, P. Sharp, W. J. Anderson, R. F. Fagan, J. J. Aponte, G. F. Jones, D. A. Nitschke, M. H. Chang, T. Doyle, R. Dhara, R. A. Jajosky, and J. D. Hatmaker. 2004. Summary of notifiable diseases—United States, 2002. *MMWR* **51**:1-84.

2957. Gross, L. 1996. How Charles Nicolle of the Pasteur Institute discovered that epidemic typhus is transmitted by lice: reminiscences from my years at the Pasteur Institute in Paris. *Proc Natl Acad Sci USA* **93**:10539-40.

2958. Gross, T. P., L. B. Kamara, C. L. Hatheway, P. Powers, J. P. Libonati, S. M. Harmon, and E. Israel. 1989. Clostridium perfringens food poisoning: use of serotyping in an outbreak setting. *J Clin Microbiol* **27**:660-3.

2959. Grossi, P., R. De Maria, A. Caroli, M. S. Zaina, and L. Minoli. 1992. Infections in heart transplant recipients: the experience of the Italian heart transplantation program. Italian Study Group on Infections in Heart Transplantation. *J Heart Lung Transplant* **11**:847-66.

2960. Grotto, I., C. Block, Y. Lerman, M. Wiener, and S. Ashkenazi. 1995. Meningococcal disease in the Israel Defense Force: epidemiologic trends and new challenges. *Isr J Med Sci* **31**:54-8.

2961. Group, O. W. 2003. Foodborne disease in Australia: incidence, notifications and outbreaks. Annual report of the OzFoodNet network, 2002. *Commun Dis Intell* **27**:209-39.

2962. Group, O. W. 2005. Reported foodborne illness and gastroenteritis in Australia: Annual report of the OzFoodNet network, 2004. *Commun Dis Intell* **29**:165-92.

2963. Grove, D. I. 1980. Strongyloidiasis in Allied ex-prisoners of war in south-east Asia. *Br Med J* **280**:598-601.

2964. Grove, D. I. 1996. Human strongyloidiasis. *Adv Parasitol* **38**:251-309.

2965. Grundmann, H., A. Kropec, D. Hartung, R. Berner, and F. Daschner. 1993. Pseudomonas aeruginosa in a neonatal intensive care unit: reservoirs and ecology of the nosocomial pathogen. *J Infect Dis* **168**:943-7.

2966. Grundmann, H., A. Tami, S. Hori, M. Halwani, and R. Slack. 2002. Nottingham Staphylococcus aureus population study: prevalence of MRSA among elderly people in the community. *BMJ* **324**:1365-6.

2967. Gruner, C., P. M. Bittighofer, and K. D. Koch-Wrenger. 1999. [Health risk to workers in recycling plants and on waste disposal sites]. *Schriftenr Ver Wasser Boden Lufthyg* **104**:597-609.

2968. **Gruner, E., E. Bernasconi, R. L. Galeazzi, D. Buhl, R. Heinzle, and D. Nadal.** 1994. Brucellosis: an occupational hazard for medical laboratory personnel. Report of five cases. *Infection* **22:**33-6.

2969. **Gruner, E., M. Opravil, M. Altwegg, and A. von Graevenitz.** 1994. Nontoxigenic Corynebacterium diphtheriae isolated from intravenous drug users. *Clin Infect Dis* **18:**94-6.

2970. **Grunwald, M. H., A. Shai, B. Mosovich, and I. Avinoach.** 2000. Tungiasis. *Australas J Dermatol* **41:**46-7.

2971. **Gruwell, J. A., C. L. Fogarty, S. G. Bennett, G. L. Challet, K. S. Vanderpool, M. Jozan, and J. P. Webb, Jr.** 2000. Role of peridomestic birds in the transmission of St. Louis encephalitis virus in southern California. *J Wildl Dis* **36:**13-34.

2972. **Gsell, O.** 1968. Tularämie in der Schweiz. *Schweiz Med Wochenschr* **98:**380-3.

2973. **Gu, W., G. F. Killeen, C. M. Mbogo, J. L. Regens, J. I. Githure, and J. C. Beier.** 2003. An individual-based model of Plasmodium falciparum malaria transmission on the coast of Kenya. *Trans R Soc Trop Med Hyg* **97:**43-50.

2974. **Guan, L. R.** 1991. Current status of kala-azar and vector control in China. *Bull WHO* **69:**595-601.

2975. **Guan, Y., B. J. Zheng, Y. Q. He, X. L. Liu, Z. X. Zhuang, C. L. Cheung, S. W. Luo, P. H. Li, L. J. Zhang, Y. J. Guan, K. M. Butt, K. L. Wong, K. W. Chan, W. Lim, K. F. Shortridge, K. Y. Yuen, J. S. Peiris, and L. L. Poon.** 2003. Isolation and characterization of viruses related to the SARS coronavirus from animals in southern China. *Science* **302:**276-8.

2976. **Gubler, D. J.** 2003. Aedes albopictus in Africa. *Lancet Infect Dis* **3:**751-2.

2977. **Gubler, D. J., and G. e. Kuno.** 1997. Dengue and dengue hemorrhagic fever. CAB International, Wallingford, U.K.

2978. **Gubler, J., C. Huber-Schneider, E. Gruner, and M. Altwegg.** 1998. An outbreak of nontoxigenic Corynebacterium diphtheriae infection: single bacterial clone causing invasive infection among Swiss drug users. *Clin Infect Dis* **27:**1295-8.

2979. **Gudnadottir, G., I. Hilmarsdottir, and B. Sigurgeirsson.** 1999. Onychomycosis in Icelandic swimmers. *Acta Derm Venereol* **79:**376-7.

2980. **Guerena-Burgueno, F., A. S. Benenson, J. Sepulveda-Amor, M. S. Ascher, D. J. Vugia, and D. Gallo.** 1992. Prevalence of human T cell lymphotropic virus types 1 and 2 (HTLV-1/2) in selected Tijuana subpopulations. *Am J Trop Med Hyg* **47:**127-32.

2981. **Guerin, P. J., C. Brasher, E. Baron, D. Mic, F. Grimont, M. Ryan, P. Aavitsland, and D. Legros.** 2003. Shigella dysenteriae serotype 1 in west Africa: intervention strategy for an outbreak in Sierra Leone. *Lancet* **362:**705-6.

2982. **Guerin, P. J., B. De Jong, E. Heir, V. Hasseltvedt, G. Kapperud, K. Styrmo, B. Gondrosen, J. Lassen, Y. Andersson, and P. Aavitsland.** 2004. Outbreak of Salmonella Livingstone infection in Norway and Sweden due to contaminated processed fish products. *Epidemiol Infect* **132:**889-95.

2983. **Guerra, M. A., E. D. Walker, and U. Kitron.** 2001. Canine surveillance system for Lyme borreliosis in Wisconsin and northern Illinois: geographic distribution and risk factor analysis. *Am J Trop Med Hyg* **65:**546-52.

2984. **Guerrant, R. L., T. Van Gilder, T. S. Steiner, N. M. Thielman, L. Slutsker, R. V. Tauxe, T. Hennessy, P. M. Griffin, H. DuPont, R. B. Sack, P. Tarr, M. Neill, I. Nachamkin, L. B. Reller, M. T. Osterholm, M. L. Bennish, and L. K. Pickering.** 2001. Practice guidelines for the management of infectious diarrhea. *Clin Infect Dis* **32:**331-51.

2985. **Guerrero, A., P. Torres, M. T. Duran, B. Ruiz-Diez, M. Rosales, and J. L. Rodriguez-Tudela.** 2001. Airborne outbreak of nosocomial Scedosporium prolificans infection. *Lancet* **357:**1267-1268.

2986. **Guessous-Idrissi, N., S. Chiheb, A. Hamdani, M. Riyad, M. Bichichi, S. Hamdani, and A. Krimech.** 1997. Cutaneous leishmaniasis: an emerging epidemic focus of Leishmania tropica in north Morocco. *Trans R Soc Trop Med Hyg* **91:**660-3.

2987. **Guest, C., K. C. Spitalny, H. P. Madore, K. Pray, R. Dolin, J. E. Herrmann, and N. R. Blacklow.** 1987. Foodborne Snow Mountain agent gastroenteritis in a school cafeteria. *Pediatrics* **79:**559-63.

2988. **Guevara, P., J. L. Ramirez, E. Rojas, J. V. Scorza, N. Gonzalez, and N. Anez.** 1993. Leishmania braziliensis in blood 30 years after cure. *Lancet* **341:**1341.

2989. **Guex, A. C.** 1999. [Disseminated histoplasmosis within the scope of immune deficiency with suspected HIV infection. HIV infection CDC stage C3. Disseminated histoplasmosis]. *Schweiz Rundsch Med Prax* **88:**917-9.

2990. **Gugnani, H. C., and F. Muotoe-Okafor.** 1997. African histoplasmosis: a review. *Rev Iberoam Micol* **14:**155-9.

2991. **Gugnani, H. C., and C. A. Oyeka.** 1989. Foot infections due to Hendersonula toruloidea and Scytalidium hyalinum in coal miners. *J Med Vet Mycol* **27:**167-79.

2992. **Guha-Sapir, D.** 1991. Rapid assessment of health needs in mass emergencies: review of current concepts and methods. *World Health Stat Q* **44:**171-81.

2993. **Guhl, F., and G. A. Vallejo.** 2003. Trypanosoma (Herpetosoma) rangeli Tejera, 1920: an updated review. *Mem Inst Oswaldo Cruz* **98:**435-42.

2994. **Guibal, F., P. de La Salmoniere, M. Rybojad, S. Hadjrabia, L. Dehen, and G. Arlet.** 2001. High seroprevalence to Bartonella quintana in homeless patients with cutaneous parasitic infestations in downtown Paris. *J Am Acad Dermatol* **44:**219-23.

2995. **Guibourdenche, M., J. P. Darchis, A. Boisivon, E. Collatz, and J. Y. Riou.** 1994. Enzyme electrophoresis, sero- and subtyping, and outer membrane protein characterization of two Neisseria meningitidis strains involved in laboratory-acquired infections. *J Clin Microbiol* **32:**701-4.

2996. **Guignard, S., H. Arienti, L. Freyre, H. Lujan, and H. Rubinstein.** 2000. Prevalence of enteroparasites in a residence for children in the Cordoba Province, Argentina. *Eur J Epidemiol* **16:**287-93.

2997. **Guillet, P., M. C. Germain, T. Giacomini, F. Chandre, M. Akogbeto, O. Faye, A. Kone, L. Manga, and J. Mouchet.** 1998. Origin and prevention of airport malaria in France. *Trop Med Int Health* **3:**700-5.

2998. **Guillet, P., and M. Nathan.** 1999. Aedes albopictus, une menace pour la France? *Méd Trop* **59 suppl 2:**S49–S52.

2999. **Guimaraes, S., and M. I. Sogayar.** 1995. Occurrence of Giardia lamblia in children of municipal day-care centers from Botucatu, Sao Paulo State, Brazil. *Rev Inst Med Trop Sao Paulo* **37:**501-6.

3000. **Guimbao, J., A. Vergara, and J. I. García-Montero.** 2002. Outbreak of pneumococcal disease in a nursing home in Spain. *Eurosurveillance Weekly* **9**(28 Feb)**:**2.

3001. **Gulisano, G., and L. Mariani.** 1996. Amoebic Liver Abscess in a Sicilian Traveler Returning from Bali. *J Travel Med* **3:**174-176.

3002. **Gunawardena, G. S., N. D. Karunaweera, and M. M. Ismail.** 2004. Socio-economic and behavioural factors affecting the prevalence of Ascaris infection in a low-country tea plantation in Sri Lanka. *Ann Trop Med Parasitol* **98:**615-21.

3003. **Gundi, V. A., O. Bourry, B. Davous, D. Raoult, and B. La Scola.** 2004. Bartonella clarridgeiae and B. henselae in dogs, Gabon. *Emerg Infect Dis* **10:**2261-2.

3004. **Gunn, R. A., H. T. Janowski, S. Lieb, E. C. Prather, and H. B. Greenberg.** 1982. Norwalk virus gastroenteritis following raw oyster consumption. *Am J Epidemiol* **115:**348-51.

3005. **Gunn, R. A., and G. Markakis.** 1978. Salmonellosis associated with homemade ice cream. An outbreak report and summary of outbreaks in the United States in 1966 to 1976. *JAMA* **240:**1885-6.

3006. **Gunn, R. A., W. A. Terranova, H. B. Greenberg, R. A. Yashuk, G. W. Gary, J. G. Wells, P. R. Taylor, and R. A. Feldman.** 1980. Norwalk virus gastroenteritis aboard a cruise ship: an outbreak on five consecutive cruises. *Am J Epidemiol* **112:**820-827.

3007. **Gunnlaugsson, G., J. Einarsdottir, F. J. Angulo, S. A. Mentambanar, A. Passa, and R. V. Tauxe.** 1998. Funerals during the 1994 cholera epidemic in Guinea-Bissau, West Africa: the need for disinfection of bodies of persons dying of cholera. *Epidemiol Infect* **120:**7-15.

3008. **Gunther, S., P. Emmerich, T. Laue, O. Kuhle, M. Asper, A. Jung, T. Grewing, J. ter Meulen, and H. Schmitz.** 2000. Imported lassa fever in Germany: molecular characterization of a new lassa virus strain. *Emerg Infect Dis* **6:**466-76.

3009. **Gupta, A.** 2004. Antimicrobial Resistance among Campylobacter Strains, United States, 1997-2001. *Emerg Infect Dis* **10:**1102-9.

3010. **Gupta, A., C. S. Polyak, R. D. Bishop, J. Sobel, and E. D. Mintz.** 2004. Laboratory-confirmed shigellosis in the United States, 1989-2002: epidemiologic trends and patterns. *Clin Infect Dis* **38:**1372-7.

3011. **Gupta, N., A. Yadav, U. Choudhary, and D. R. Arora.** 2003. Citrobacter bacteremia in a tertiary care hospital. *Scand J Infect Dis* **35:**765-8.

3012. **Güraksin, A., and G. Güllülü.** 1997. Prevalence of trachoma in eastern Turkey. *Int J Epidemiol* **26:**436-42.

3013. **Gurfield, A. N., H. J. Boulouis, B. B. Chomel, R. W. Kasten, R. Heller, C. Bouillin, C. Gandoin, D. Thibault, C. C. Chang, F. Barrat, and Y. Piemont.** 2001. Epidemiology of Bartonella infection in domestic cats in France. *Vet Microbiol* **80:**185-98.

3014. **Gurgel-Concalves, R., E. D. Ramalho, M. A. Duarte, A. R. T. Palma, F. Abad-Franch, J. C. Carranza, and C. A. Cuba Cuba.** 2004. Enzootic transmission of Trypanosoma cruzi and T. rangeli in the federal district of Brazil. *Rev Inst Med Trop Sao Paulo* **46:**323-30.

3015. **Gurtler, R. E., M. C. Cecere, D. P. Vazquez, R. Chuit, and J. E. Cohen.** 1996. Host-feeding patterns of domiciliary Triatoma infestans (Hemiptera: Reduviidae) in Northwest Argentina: seasonal and instar variation. *J Med Entomol* **33:**15-26.

3016. **Gurtler, R. E., E. L. Segura, and J. E. Cohen.** 2003. Congenital Transmission of Trypanosoma cruzi Infection in Argentina. *Emerg Infect Dis* **9:**29-32.

3017. **Gurung, R., S. K. Rai, M. Kurokawa, M. K. Shrestha, J. Thakur, C. K. Rai, S. Ruit, and K. Ono.** 2003. Acute hemorrhagic conjunctivitis epidemic—2003 in Nepal. *Nepal Med Coll J* **5:**59-60.

3018. **Gurycova, D., E. Kocianova, V. Vyrostekova, and J. Rehacek.** 1995. Prevalence of ticks infected with Francisella tularensis in natural foci of tularemia in western Slovakia. *Eur J Epidemiol* **11:**469-74.

3019. **Gustafson, P., V. F. Gomes, C. S. Vieira, H. Jensen, R. Seng, R. Norberg, B. Samb, A. Naucler, and P. Aaby.** 2001. Tuberculosis mortality during a civil war in Guinea-Bissau. *JAMA* **286:**599-603.

3020. **Gustafson, P., V. F. Gomes, C. S. Vieira, P. Rabna, R. Seng, P. Johansson, A. Sandstrom, R. Norberg, I. Lisse, B. Samb, P. Aaby, and A. Naucler.** 2004. Tuberculosis in Bissau: incidence and risk factors in an urban community in sub-Saharan Africa. *Int J Epidemiol* **33:**163-72.

3021. **Gustafson, R., M. Forsgren, A. Gardulf, M. Granstrom, and B. Svenungsson.** 1993. Antibody prevalence and clinical manifestations of Lyme borreliosis and tick-borne encephalitis in Swedish orienteers. *Scand J Infect Dis* **25:**605-11.

3022. **Gustafson, T. L., A. L. Booth, R. S. Fricker, E. Cureton, E. W. Fowinkle, R. H. Hutcheson, Jr., and W. Schaffner.** 1987. Disease surveillance and emergency services at the 1982 World's Fair. *Am J Public Health* **77:**861-3.

3023. **Gustafson, T. L., L. Kaufman, R. Weeks, L. Ajello, R. H. Hutcheson, Jr., S. L. Wiener, D. W. Lambe, Jr., T. A. Sayvetz, and W. Schaffner.** 1981. Outbreak of acute pulmonary histoplasmosis in members of a wagon train. *Am J Med* **71:**759-65.

3024. **Gutersohn, T., R. Steffen, P. Van Damme, F. Holdener, and P. Beutels.** 1996. Hepatitis A infection in aircrews: risk of infection and cost-benefit analysis of hepatitis A vaccination. *Aviat Space Environ Med* **67:**153-6.

3025. **Guthmann, J. P., A. J. Hall, S. Jaffar, A. Palacios, J. Lines, and A. Llanos-Cuentas.** 2001. Environmental risk factors for clinical malaria: a case-control study in the Grau region of Peru. *Trans R Soc Trop Med Hyg* **95:**577-83.

3026. **Guthmann, J. P., A. Llanos-Cuentas, A. Palacios, and A. J. Hall.** 2002. Environmental factors as determinants of malaria risk. A descriptive study on the northern coast of Peru. *Trop Med Int Health* **7:**518-25.

3027. **Gutierrez, K. M., M. S. Falkovitz Halpern, Y. Maldonado, and A. M. Arvin.** 1999. The epidemiology of neonatal herpes simplex virus infections in California from 1985 to 1995. *J Infect Dis* **180:**199-202.

3028. **Gutierrez, M., P. Tajada, A. Alvarez, R. De Julian, M. Baquero, V. Soriano, and A. Holguin.** 2004. Prevalence of HIV-1 non-B subtypes, syphilis, HTLV, and hepatitis B and C viruses among immigrant sex workers in Madrid, Spain. *J Med Virol* **74:**521-7.

3029. **Gutierrez, M. C., V. Vincent, D. Aubert, J. Bizet, O. Gaillot, L. Lebrun, C. Le Pendeven, M. P. Le Pennec, D. Mathieu, C. Offredo, B. Pangon, and C. Pierre-Audigier.** 1998. Molecular fingerprinting of Mycobacterium tuberculosis and risk factors for tuberculosis transmission in Paris, France, and surrounding area. *J Clin Microbiol* **36:**486-92.

3030. **Gutiérrez, M. P., M. A. Bratos, J. I. Garrote, A. Duenas, A. Almaraz, R. Alamo, H. Rodriguez Marcos, M. J. Rodriguez Recio, M. F. Munoz, A. Orduna, and A. Rodriguez-Torres.** 2003. Serologic evidence of human infection by Francisella tularensis in the population of Castilla y León (Spain) prior to 1997. *FEMS Immunol Med Microbiol* **35:**165-9.

3031. Gutman, L. T., E. A. Ottesen, T. J. Quan, P. S. Noce, and S. L. Katz. 1973. An inter-familial outbreak of Yersinia enterocolitica enteritis. *N Engl J Med* **288:**1372-7.

3032. Guwatudde, D., M. Nakakeeto, E. C. Jones-Lopez, A. Maganda, A. Chiunda, R. D. Mugerwa, J. J. Ellner, G. Bukenya, and C. C. Whalen. 2003. Tuberculosis in household contacts of infectious cases in Kampala, Uganda. *Am J Epidemiol* **158:**887-98.

3033. Guy, R. J., R. M. Andrews, H. A. Kelly, J. A. Leydon, M. A. Riddell, S. B. Lambert, and M. G. Catton. 2004. Mumps and rubella: a year of enhanced surveillance and laboratory testing. *Epidemiol Infect* **132:**391-8.

3034. Guzmán, M. G., and G. Kourí. 2002. Dengue: an update. *Lancet Infect Dis* **2:**33-42.

3035. Guzman-Bracho, C. 2001. Epidemiology of Chagas disease in Mexico: an update. *Trends Parasitol* **17:**372-6.

3036. Gwaltney, J. M., Jr., M. A. Sande, R. Austrian, and J. O. Hendley. 1975. Spread of Streptococcus pneumoniae in families. II. Relation of transfer of S. pneumoniae to incidence of colds and serum antibody. *J Infect Dis* **132:**62-8.

3037. Gylfe, A., S. Bergström, J. Lundström, and B. Olsen. 2000. Reactivation of Borrelia infection in birds. *Nature* **403:**724-5.

3038. Haake, D. A., M. Dundoo, R. Cader, B. M. Kubak, R. A. Hartskeerl, J. J. Sejvar, and D. A. Ashford. 2002. Leptospirosis, water sports, and chemoprophylaxis. *Clin Infect Dis* **34:**e40-3.

3039. Haas, J. S., M. L. Dean, Y. Y. Hung, and D. J. Rennie. 2003. Differences in mortality among patients with community-acquired pneumonia in California by ethnicity and hospital characteristics. *Am J Med* **114:**660-4.

3040. Haas, W. H., T. Breuer, G. Pfaff, H. Schmitz, P. Kohler, M. Asper, P. Emmerich, C. Drosten, U. Golnitz, K. Fleischer, and S. Gunther. 2003. Imported lassa Fever in Germany: surveillance and management of contact persons. *Clin Infect Dis* **36:**1254-8.

3041. Habbari, K., A. Tifnouti, G. Bitton, and A. Mandil. 2000. Geohelminthic infections associated with raw wastewater reuse for agricultural purposes in Beni-Mellal, Morocco. *Parasitol Int* **48:**249-54.

3042. Habib, A. G. 2003. Tetanus complicating snakebite in northern Nigeria: clinical presentation and public health implications. *Acta Trop* **85:**87-91.

3043. Hackett, C. J. 1984. On the epidemiology of yaws in African miners (1942). *Trans R Soc Trop Med Hyg* **78:**536-8.

3044. Haddad, M. B., T. W. Wilson, K. Ijaz, S. M. Marks, and M. Moore. 2005. Tuberculosis and homelessness in the United States, 1994-2003. *JAMA* **293:**2762-6.

3045. Hadjichristodoulou, C., G. Achileas, P. Yianis, and T. Yianis. 1998. Outbreak of giardiasis among English tourists in Crete. *Lancet* **351:**65-6.

3046. Hadju, V., K. Abadi, L. S. Stephenson, N. N. Noor, H. O. Mohammed, and D. D. Bowman. 1995. Intestinal helminthiasis, nutritional status, and their relationship; a cross-sectional study in urban slum school children in Indonesia. *Southeast Asian J Trop Med Public Health* **26:**719-29.

3047. Hadler, S. C., M. Alcala de Monzon, D. Rivero, M. Perez, A. Bracho, and H. A. Fields. 1992. Epidemiology and long-term consequences of hepatitis delta virus infection in the Yucpa Indians of Venezuela. *Am J Epidemiol* **136:**1507-16.

3048. Hadler, S. C., H. M. Webster, J. J. Erben, J. E. Swanson, and J. E. Maynard. 1980. Hepatitis A in day-care centers. A community-wide assessment. *N Engl J Med* **302:**1222-7.

3049. Haedersdal, M., J. Stenderup, B. Moller, T. Agner, and E. L. Svejgaard. 2003. An outbreak of tinea capitis in a child care centre. *Dan Med Bull* **50:**83-4.

3050. Haeghebaert, S., L. Duché, C. Gilles, B. Masini, M. Dubreuil, J. C. Minet, P. Bouvet, F. Grimont, E. Delarocque Astagneau, and V. Vaillant. 2001. Minced beef and human salmonellosis: review of the investigation of three outbreaks in France. *Eurosurveillance* **6:**21-26.

3051. Haeghebaert, S., F. Le Querrec, P. Bouvet, A. Gallay, and V. Vaillant. 2002. Les toxi-infections alimentaires collectives en France en 2001. *Bull Épidémiol Hebdomadaire* **50:**249-53.

3052. Haeghebaert, S., F. Le Querrec, A. Gallay, P. Bouvet, M. Gomez, and V. Vaillant. 2002. Les toxi-infections alimentaires collectives en France, en 1999 et 2000. *Bull Épidémiol Hebdomadaire* **23:**105-9.

3053. Haeghebaert, S., F. Le Querrec, V. Vaillant, E. Delarocque Astagneau, and P. Bouvet. 1998. Les toxi-infections alimentaires collectives en France en 1997. *Bull Épidémiol Hebdomadaire* **41:**177-181.

3054. Haeghebaert, S., M. R. Popoff, J. P. Carlier, G. Pavillon, and E. Delarocque-Astagneau. 2002. Caractéristiques épidémiologiques du botulisme humain en France, 1991-2000. *Bull Épidémiol Hebdomadaire* **14:**57-9.

3055. Haeghebaert, S., P. Sulern, L. Deroudille, E. Vanneroy-Adenot, O. Bagnis, P. Bouvet, F. Grimont, A. Brisabois, F. Le Querrec, C. Hervy, E. Espie, H. de Valk, and V. Vaillant. 2003. Two outbreaks of Salmonella Enteritidis phage type 8 linked to the consumption of Cantal cheese made with raw milk, France, 2001. *Eurosurveillance* **8:**151-6.

3056. Haelterman, E., M. Boelaert, C. Suetens, L. Blok, M. Henkens, and M. J. Toole. 1996. Impact of a mass vaccination campaign against a meningitis epidemic in a refugee camp. *Trop Med Int Health* **1:**385-92.

3057. Haerer, G., J. Nicolet, L. Bacciarini, B. Gottstein, and M. Giacometti. 2001. Todesursachen, Zoonosen und Reproduktion bei Feldhasen in der Schweiz. *Schweiz Arch Tierheilkd* **143:**193-201.

3058. Haesebrouck, F., F. Pasmans, K. Chiers, D. Maes, R. Ducatelle, and A. Decostere. 2004. Efficacy of vaccines against bacterial diseases in swine: what can we expect? *Vet Microbiol* **100:**255-68.

3059. Haffejee, I. E. 1995. The epidemiology of rotavirus infections: a global perspective. *J Pediatr Gastroenterol Nutr* **20:**275-86.

3060. Hagelskjaer, L., I. Sorensen, and E. Randers. 1998. Streptobacillus moniliformis infection: 2 cases and a literature review. *Scand J Infect Dis* **30:**309-11.

3061. Haglund, M., and G. Gunther. 2003. Tick-borne encephalitis—pathogenesis, clinical course and long-term follow-up. *Vaccine* **21 Suppl 1:**S11-8.

3062. Hagmann, R., J. D. Charlwood, V. Gil, C. Ferreira, V. do Rosario, and T. A. Smith. 2003. Malaria and its possible control on the island of Principe. *Malar J* **2:**15.

3063. Hahn, B. H., G. M. Shaw, K. M. De Cock, and P. M. Sharp. 2000. AIDS as a zoonosis: scientific and public health implications. *Science* **287:**607-14.

3064. Hahn, C., L. Mascola, R. Cader, D. Haake, D. Vugia, C. Easman, B. A. Connor, J. Purdue, K. Hendricks, J. Pape, L. McFarland, M. Eyeson-Annan, P. Buck, H. Artsob, M. Evans, R. Salomon, B. Smyth, T. Coleman, and V. Cardenas. 2001. Update: outbreak of acute febrile illness among athletes participating in eco-challenge-Sabah 2000 - Borneo, Malaysia, 2000. *MMWR* **50:**21-4.

3065. Hahné, M., J. Gray, J. F. Aguilera, N. S. Crowcroft, T. Nichols, E. B. Kaczmarski, and M. E. Ramsay. 2002. W135 meningococcal disease in England and Wales associated with Hajj 2000 and 2001. *Lancet* **359:**582-3.

3066. Hahné, S., J. Macey, G. Tipples, P. Varughese, A. King, R. van Binnendijk, H. Ruijs, J. van Steenbergen, A. Timen, A. M. van Loon, and H. de Melker. 2005. Rubella outbreak in an unvaccinated religious community in the Netherlands spreads to Canada. *Eurosurveillance* **10:**125-7.

3067. Haiavy, J., and H. Tobin. 2002. Mycobacterium fortuitum infection in prosthetic breast implants. *Plast Reconstr Surg* **109:**2124-8.

3068. Haim, M., M. Efrat, M. Wilson, P. M. Schantz, D. Cohen, and J. Shemer. 1997. An outbreak of Trichinella spiralis infection in southern Lebanon. *Epidemiol Infect* **119:**357-62.

3069. Hajjar, J., R. Girard, J. M. Marc, L. Ducruet, M. Beruard, B. Fadel, M. Foret, D. Lerda, C. Roche, M. Vallet, L. Ayzac, and J. Fabry. 2004. [Surveillance of infections in chronic hemodialysis patients]. *Nephrologie* **25:**133-40.

3070. Hajjeh, R., S. McDonnell, S. Reef, C. Licitra, M. Hankins, B. Toth, A. Padhye, L. Kaufman, L. Pasarell, C. Cooper, L. Hutwagner, R. Hopkins, and M. McNeil. 1997. Outbreak of sporotrichosis among tree nursery workers. *J Infect Dis* **176:**499-504.

3071. Hajjeh, R. A., A. Reingold, A. Weil, K. Shutt, A. Schuchat, and B. A. Perkins. 1999. Toxic shock syndrome in the United States: surveillance update, 1979-1996. *Emerg Infect Dis* **5:**807-10.

3072. Hakanen, A., H. Jousimies-Somer, A. Siitonen, P. Huovinen, and P. Kotilainen. 2003. Fluoroquinolone resistance in Campylobacter jejuni isolates in travelers returning to Finland: association of ciprofloxacin resistance to travel destination. *Emerg Infect Dis* **9:**267-70.

3073. Hakanen, A., P. Kotilainen, P. Huovinen, H. Helenius, and A. Siitonen. 2001. Reduced fluoroquinolone susceptibility in Salmonella enterica serotypes in travelers returning from southeast Asia. *Emerg Infect Dis* **7:**996-1003.

3074. Hakansson, C., K. Thoren, G. Norkrans, and G. Johannisson. 1984. Intestinal parasitic infection and other sexually transmitted diseases in asymptomatic homosexual men. *Scand J Infect Dis* **16:**199-202.

3075. Hakim, M., D. Esmore, J. Wallwork, T. A. English, and T. Wreghitt. 1986. Toxoplasmosis in cardiac transplantation. *BMJ* **292:**1108.

3076. Halanova, M., L. Cislakova, A. Valencakova, P. Balent, J. Adam, and M. Travnicek. 2003. Serological screening of occurrence of antibodies to Encephalitozoon cuniculi in humans and animals in Eastern Slovakia. *Ann Agric Environ Med* **10:**117-20.

3077. Hald, T., A. Wingstrand, M. Swanenburg, A. von Altrock, and B. M. Thorberg. 2003. The occurrence and epidemiology of Salmonella in European pig slaughterhouses. *Epidemiol Infect* **131:**1187-203.

3078. Halder, A., M. Mundle, U. K. Bhadra, and B. Saha. 2001. Role of paucibacillary leprosy in the transmission of disease. *Indian J Lepr* **73:**11-5.

3079. Hale, D. C., L. Blumberg, and J. Frean. 2003. Case report: gnathostomiasis in two travelers to Zambia. *Am J Trop Med Hyg* **68:**707-9.

3080. Hale, G., and H. Waldmann. 1998. Risks of developing Epstein-Barr virus-related lymphoproliferative disorders after T-cell-depleted marrow transplants. CAMPATH Users. *Blood* **91:**3079-83.

3081. Haley, C. E., R. C. McDonald, L. Rossi, W. D. Jones, Jr., R. W. Haley, and J. P. Luby. 1989. Tuberculosis epidemic among hospital personnel. *Infect Control Hosp Epidemiol* **10:**204-10.

3082. Haley, R. W., and R. P. Fischer. 2001. Commercial tattooing as a potentially important source of hepatitis C infection. Clinical epidemiology of 626 consecutive patients unaware of their hepatitis C serologic status. *Medicine (Baltimore)* **80:**134-51.

3083. Hall, A., D. J. Conway, K. S. Anwar, and M. L. Rahman. 1994. Strongyloides stercoralis in an urban slum community in Bangladesh: factors independently associated with infection. *Trans R Soc Trop Med Hyg* **88:**527-30.

3084. Hall, A., and C. Holland. 2000. Geographical variation in Ascaris lumbricoides fecundity and its implications for helminth control. *Parasitol Today* **16:**540-4.

3085. Hall, C. B. 2000. Nosocomial respiratory syncytial virus infections: the "Cold War" has not ended. *Clin Infect Dis* **31:**590-6.

3086. Hall, C. B., M. T. Caserta, K. C. Schnabel, C. Boettrich, M. P. McDermott, G. K. Lofthus, J. A. Carnahan, and S. Dewhurst. 2004. Congenital infections with human herpesvirus 6 (HHV6) and human herpesvirus 7 (HHV7). *J Pediatr* **145:**472-7.

3087. Hall, C. B., and R. G. Douglas, Jr. 1981. Modes of transmission of respiratory syncytial virus. *J Pediatr* **99:**100-3.

3088. Hall, C. B., R. G. Douglas, Jr., and J. M. Geiman. 1980. Possible transmission by fomites of respiratory syncytial virus. *J Infect Dis* **141:**98-102.

3089. Hall, C. B., J. M. Geiman, R. Biggar, D. I. Kotok, P. M. Hogan, and G. R. Douglas, Jr. 1976. Respiratory syncytial virus infections within families. *N Engl J Med* **294:**414-9.

3090. Hall, C. J., S. J. Richmond, E. O. Caul, N. H. Pearce, and I. A. Silver. 1982. Laboratory outbreak of Q fever acquired from sheep. *Lancet* **May 1:**1004-1006.

3091. Hall, J. A., J. S. Goulding, N. H. Bean, R. V. Tauxe, and C. W. Hedberg. 2001. Epidemiologic profiling: evaluating foodborne outbreaks for which no pathogen was isolated by routine laboratory testing: United States, 1982-9. *Epidemiol Infect* **127:**381-7.

3092. Hall, R. A., J. H. Scherret, and J. S. Mackenzie. 2001. Kunjin virus: an Australian variant of West Nile? *Ann N Y Acad Sci* **951:**153-60.

3093. Hall, S., K. Galil, B. Watson, and J. Seward. 2000. The use of school-based vaccination clinics to control varicella outbreaks in two schools. *Pediatrics* **105:**e17.

3094. Hall, S. M., A. Pandit, A. Golwilkar, and T. S. Williams. 1999. How do Jains get toxoplasma infection? *Lancet* **354:**486-7.

3095. Hallee, T. J., A. S. Evans, J. C. Niederman, C. M. Brooks, and H. Voegtly. 1974. Infectious mononucleosis at the United

States Military Academy. A prospective study of a single class over four years. *Yale J Biol Med* **47:**182-95.

3096. **Halliday, M. L., L. Y. Kang, T. K. Zhou, M. D. Hu, Q. C. Pan, T. Y. Fu, Y. S. Huang, and S. L. Hu.** 1991. An epidemic of hepatitis A attributable to the ingestion of raw clams in Shanghai, China. *J Infect Dis* **164:**852-9.

3097. **Halm, E. A., and A. S. Teirstein.** 2002. Management of community-acquired pneumonia. *N Engl J Med* **347:**2039-45.

3098. **Halperin, S. A., R. Bortolussi, J. M. Langley, B. J. Eastwood, and G. De Serres.** 1999. A randomized, placebo-controlled trial of erythromycin estolate chemoprophylaxis for household contacts of children with culture- positive bordetella pertussis infection. *Pediatrics* **104:**e42.

3099. **Halpin, K., P. L. Young, H. E. Field, and J. S. Mackenzie.** 2000. Isolation of Hendra virus from pteropid bats: a natural reservoir of Hendra virus. *J Gen Virol* **81:**1927-32.

3100. **Halpin, T. F., and J. A. Molinari.** 2001. Diagnosis and management of Clostridium perfringens sepsis and uterine gas gangrene. *Obstet Gynecol Surv* **57:**53-7.

3101. **Halvorsrud, J., and I. Orstavik.** 1980. An epidemic of rotavirus-associated gastroenteritis in a nursing home for the elderly. *Scand J Infect Dis* **12:**161-4.

3102. **Hamama, A., A. el Marrakchi, and F. el Othmani.** 1992. Occurrence of Yersinia enterocolitica in milk and dairy products in Morocco. *Int J Food Microbiol* **16:**69-77.

3103. **Hamburger, H., and S. Glismann.** 2002. Measles outbreak in North Jutland, Denmark. *Eurosurveillance Weekly* **6:**3-4.

3104. **Hamer, D. H., and B. A. Connor.** 2004. Travel health knowledge, attitudes and practices among United States travelers. *J Travel Med* **11:**23-6.

3105. **Hamers, F. F., and A. M. Downs.** 2004. The changing face of the HIV epidemic in western Europe: what are the implications for public health policies? *Lancet* **364:**83-94.

3106. **Hamill, R. J., E. D. Houston, P. R. Georghiou, C. E. Wright, M. A. Koza, R. M. Cadle, P. A. Goepfert, D. A. Lewis, G. J. Zenon, and J. E. Clarridge.** 1995. An outbreak of Burkholderia (formerly Pseudomonas) cepacia respiratory tract colonization and infection associated with nebulized albuterol therapy. *Ann Intern Med* **122:**762-6.

3107. **Hammami, H., and A. Ayadi.** 2000. Etude de l'infestation naturelle de Lymnaea truncatula Müller par Fasciola hepatica dans les oasis de Tozeur (sud-ouest Tunisien). *Med Trop* **60:**159-62.

3108. **Hammermeister, I., G. Janus, F. Schamarowski, M. Rudolf, E. Jacobs, and M. Kist.** 1992. Elevated risk of Helicobacter pylori infection in submarine crews. *Eur J Clin Microbiol Infect Dis* **11:**9-14.

3109. **Hammerschlag, M. R.** 2001. Mycoplasma pneumoniae infections. *Curr Opin Infect Dis* **14:**181-6.

3110. **Hammond, G. W., M. Slutchuk, J. Scatliff, E. Sherman, J. C. Wilt, and A. R. Ronald.** 1980. Epidemiologic, clinical, laboratory, and therapeutic features of an urban outbreak of chancroid in North America. *Rev Infect Dis* **2:**867-79.

3111. **Hammouda, N. A., W. M. el-Gebali, and M. K. Razek.** 1992. Intestinal parasitic infection among sewage workers in Alexandria, Egypt. *J Egypt Soc Parasitol* **22:**299-303.

3112. **Hamprecht, K., J. Maschmann, M. Vochem, K. Dietz, C. P. Speer, and G. Jahn.** 2001. Epidemiology of transmission of cytomegalovirus from mother to preterm infant by breastfeeding. *Lancet* **357:**513-8.

3113. **Han, C. S., W. Miller, R. Haake, and D. Weisdorf.** 1994. Varicella zoster infection after bone marrow transplantation: incidence, risk factors and complications. *Bone Marrow Transplant* **13:**277-83.

3114. **Han, L. L., F. Popovici, J. P. Alexander, Jr., V. Laurentia, L. A. Tengelsen, C. Cernescu, H. E. Gary, Jr., N. Ion-Nedelcu, G. L. Campbell, and T. F. Tsai.** 1999. Risk factors for West Nile virus infection and meningoencephalitis, Romania, 1996. *J Infect Dis* **179:**230-3.

3115. **Hanberger, H., J. A. Garcia-Rodriguez, M. Gobernado, H. Goossens, L. E. Nilsson, and M. J. Struelens.** 1999. Antibiotic susceptibility among aerobic gram-negative bacilli in intensive care units in 5 European countries. French and Portuguese ICU Study Groups. *JAMA* **281:**67-71.

3116. **Hancox, M.** 2002. Bovine tuberculosis: milk and meat safety. *Lancet* **359:**706-7.

3117. **Handzel, T., D. M. S. Karanja, D. G. Addiss, A. W. Hightower, D. H. Rosen, D. G. Colley, J. Andove, L. Slutsker, and W. E. Secor.** 2003. Geographic distribution of schistosomiasis and soil-transmitted helminths in western Kenya: implications for anthelminthic mass treatment. *Am J Trop Med Hyg* **69:**318-23.

3118. **Hanenberg, R. S., W. Rojanapithayakorn, P. Kunasol, and D. C. Sokal.** 1994. Impact of Thailand's HIV-control programme as indicated by the decline of sexually transmitted diseases. *Lancet* **344:**243-5.

3119. **Hanly, M. G., B. Amaker, and I. Quereshi.** 1998. Visceral leishmaniasis in North West Saudi Arabia: a new endemic focus of L. donovani or further evidence of a changing pathogenic role for L. tropica? *Cent Afr J Med* **44:**202-5.

3120. **Hanna, J.** 1993. Hepatitis A outbreak in a rural town, Atherton tablelands, Queensland, 1992. *Commun Dis Intell* **17:**70-2.

3121. **Hanna, J., and D. Brookes.** 1993. Absenteeism from a child day-care centre during a rotavirus outbreak. *Commun Dis Intell* **17:**350-1.

3122. **Hanna, J. N., I. K. Carney, G. A. Smith, A. E. Tannenberg, J. E. Deverill, J. A. Botha, I. L. Serafin, B. J. Harrower, P. F. Fitzpatrick, and J. W. Searle.** 2000. Australian bat lyssavirus infection: a second human case, with a long incubation period. *Med J Aust* **172:**597-9.

3123. **Hanna, J. N., J. L. Humphreys, S. L. Hills, A. R. Richards, and D. L. Brookes.** 2001. Recognising and responding to outbreaks of hepatitis A associated with child day-care centres. *Aust N Z J Public Health* **25:**525-8.

3124. **Hanna, J. N., S. A. Ritchie, D. P. Eisen, R. D. Cooper, D. L. Brookes, and B. L. Montgomery.** 2004. An outbreak of Plasmodium vivax malaria in Far North Queensland, 2002. *Med J Aust* **180:**24-8.

3125. **Hannah, E. L., E. D. Belay, P. Gambetti, G. Krause, P. Parchi, S. Capellari, R. E. Hoffman, and L. B. Schonberger.** 2001. Creutzfeldt-Jakob disease after receipt of a previously unimplicated brand of dura mater graft. *Neurology* **56:**1080-3.

3126. **Hannah, J., and T. Riordan.** 1988. Case to case spread of cryptosporidiosis; evidence from a day nursery outbreak. *Public Health* **102:**539-44.

3127. **Hannan, M. M., H. Peres, F. Maltez, A. C. Hayward, J. Machado, A. Morgado, R. Proenca, M. R. Nelson, J. Bico, D. B. Young, and B. S. Gazzard.** 2001. Investigation and control of a large outbreak of multi-drug resistant tuberculosis at a central Lisbon hospital. *J Hosp Infect* **47:**91-7.

3128. Hanotier, J., and P. L. Gigase. 1981. Note on a new focus of schistosomiasis (S. mansoni) in Rwanda. *Ann Soc Belg Med Trop* **61:**93-8.

3129. Hanrahan, J. P., D. L. Morse, V. B. Scharf, J. G. Debbie, G. P. Schmid, R. M. McKinney, and M. Shayegani. 1987. A community hospital outbreak of legionellosis. Transmission by potable hot water. *Am J Epidemiol* **125:**639-49.

3130. Hansen, S. M., N. Uldbjerg, M. Kilian, and U. B. Sorensen. 2004. Dynamics of Streptococcus agalactiae colonization in women during and after pregnancy and in their infants. *J Clin Microbiol* **42:**83-9.

3131. Hanslik, T., P. Y. Boelle, and A. Flahault. 2001. Setting up a specific surveillance system of community health during mass gatherings. *J Epidemiol Community Health* **55:**683-4.

3132. Hansman, G. S., L. T. Doan, T. A. Kguyen, S. Okitsu, K. Katayama, S. Ogawa, K. Natori, N. Takeda, Y. Kato, O. Nishio, M. Noda, and H. Ushijima. 2004. Detection of norovirus and sapovirus infection among children with gastroenteritis in Ho Chi Minh City, Vietnam. *Arch Virol* **149:**1673-88.

3133. Happe, S., A. Fischer, C. Heese, D. Reichelt, U. Gruneberg, M. Freund, S. Kloska, S. Evers, and I. W. Husstedt. 2002. [HIV-associated cerebral toxoplasmosis — review and retrospective analysis of 36 patients]. *Nervenarzt* **73:**1174-8.

3134. Haque, R., P. Duggal, I. M. Ali, M. B. Hossain, D. Mondal, R. B. Sack, B. M. Farr, T. H. Beaty, and W. A. Petri, Jr. 2002. Innate and acquired resistance to amebiasis in bangladeshi children. *J Infect Dis* **186:**547-52.

3135. Haque, R., D. Mondal, B. D. Kirkpatrick, S. Akther, B. M. Farr, R. B. Sack, and W. A. Petri, Jr. 2003. Epidemiologic and clinical characteristics of acute diarrhea with emphasis on Entamoeba histolytica infections in preschool children in an urban slum of Dhaka, Bangladesh. *Am J Trop Med Hyg* **69:**398-405.

3136. Harbarth, S., P. Sudre, S. Dharan, M. Cadenas, and D. Pittet. 1999. Outbreak of Enterobacter cloacae related to understaffing, overcrowding, and poor hygiene practices. *Infect Control Hosp Epidemiol* **20:**598-603.

3137. Harcourt-Brown, F. M., and H. K. Holloway. 2003. Encephalitozoon cuniculi in pet rabbits. *Vet Rec* **152:**427-31.

3138. Hardick, J., Y. H. Hsieh, S. Tulloch, J. Kus, J. Tawes, and C. A. Gaydos. 2003. Surveillance of Chlamydia trachomatis and Neisseria gonorrhoeae infections in women in detention in Baltimore, Maryland. *Sex Transm Dis* **30:**64-70.

3139. Hardie, R. M., P. G. Wall, P. Gott, M. Bardhan, and L. R. Bartlett. 1999. Infectious diarrhea in tourists staying in a resort hotel. *Emerg Infect Dis* **5:**168-71.

3140. Hardy, M. A., and H. H. Schmidek. 1968. Epidemiology of tuberculosis aboard a ship. *JAMA* **203:**175-9.

3141. Harger, J. H., S. P. Adler, W. C. Koch, and G. F. Harger. 1998. Prospective evaluation of 618 pregnant women exposed to parvovirus B19: risks and symptoms. *Obstet Gynecol* **91:**413-20.

3142. Harger, J. H., J. M. Ernest, G. R. Thurnau, A. Moawad, E. Thom, M. B. Landon, R. Paul, M. Miodovnik, M. Dombrowski, B. Sibai, P. Van Dorsten, and D. McNellis. 2002. Frequency of congenital varicella syndrome in a prospective cohort of 347 pregnant women. *Obstet Gynecol* **100:**260-5.

3143. Harkness, G. A., D. W. Bentley, M. Mottley, and J. Lee. 1992. Streptococcus pyogenes outbreak in a long-term care facility. *Am J Infect Control* **20:**142-8.

3144. Harley, D., G. Garstone, B. Montgomery, and S. Ritchie. 2001. Locally-acquired Plasmodium falciparum malaria on Darnley Island in the Torres Strait. *Commun Dis Intell* **25:**151-3.

3145. Harley, D., B. Harrower, M. Lyon, and A. Dick. 2001. A primary school outbreak of pharyngoconjunctival fever caused by adenovirus type 3. *Commun Dis Intell* **25:**9-12.

3146. Harley, D., S. Ritchie, D. Phillips, and A. F. van den Hurk. 2000. Mosquito isolates of Ross river virus from Cairns, Queensland, Australia. *Am J Trop Med Hyg* **62:**561-5.

3147. Harms, G., F. Dörner, U. Bienzle, and K. Stark. 2002. Infektionen und Erkrankungen nach Fernreisen. *Dtsch Med Wochenschr* **127:**1748-53.

3148. Harms, G., G. Schonian, and H. Feldmeier. 2003. Leishmaniasis in Germany. *Emerg Infect Dis* **9:**872-5.

3149. Harnett, S. J., K. D. Allen, and R. R. Macmillan. 2001. Critical care unit outbreak of Serratia liquefaciens from contaminated pressure monitoring equipment. *J Hosp Infect* **47:**301-7.

3150. Harpaz, R., B. J. McMahon, H. S. Margolis, C. N. Shapiro, D. Havron, G. Carpenter, L. R. Bulkow, and R. B. Wainwright. 2000. Elimination of new chronic hepatitis B virus infections: results of the Alaska immunization program. *J Infect Dis* **181:**413-8.

3151. Harpaz, R., L. Von Seidlein, F. M. Averhoff, M. P. Tormey, S. D. Sinha, K. Kotsopoulou, S. B. Lambert, B. H. Robertson, J. D. Cherry, and C. N. Shapiro. 1996. Transmission of hepatitis B virus to multiple patients from a surgeon without evidence of inadequate infection control. *N Engl J Med* **334:**549-54.

3152. Harper, S. A., K. Fukuda, T. M. Uyeki, N. J. Cox, and C. B. Bridges. 2005. Prevention and control of influenza. Recommendations of the Advisory Committee on Immunization Practices (ACIP). *MMWR* **54 (RR-8):**1-44.

3153. Harrington, R. D., T. M. Hooton, R. C. Hackman, G. A. Storch, B. Osborne, C. A. Gleaves, A. Benson, and J. D. Meyers. 1992. An outbreak of respiratory syncytial virus in a bone marrow transplant center. *J Infect Dis* **165:**987-93.

3154. Harrington, R. D., A. E. Woolfrey, R. Bowden, M. G. McDowell, and R. C. Hackman. 1996. Legionellosis in a bone marrow transplant center. *Bone Marrow Transplant* **18:**361-8.

3155. Harris, A. R. C., R. J. Russel, and A. D. Charters. 1984. A review of schistosomiasis in immigrants in Western Australia, demonstrating the unusual longevity of Schistosoma mansoni. *Trans R Soc Trop Med Hyg* **78:**385-8.

3156. Harrison, L. H., C. W. Armstrong, S. R. Jenkins, M. W. Harmon, G. W. Ajello, G. B. Miller, Jr., and C. V. Broome. 1991. A cluster of meningococcal disease on a school bus following epidemic influenza. *Arch Intern Med* **151:**1005-9.

3157. Harrison, L. H., D. M. Dwyer, C. T. Maples, and L. Billmann. 1999. Risk of meningococcal infection in college students. *JAMA* **281:**1906-10.

3158. Harrison, L. H., N. A. Halsey, K. T. McKee, Jr., C. J. Peters, J. G. Barrera Oro, A. M. Briggiler, M. R. Feuillade, and J. I. Maiztegui. 1999. Clinical case definitions for Argentine hemorrhagic fever. *Clin Infect Dis* **28:**1091-4.

3159. Harrison, S., and S. Kinra. 2004. Outbreak of Escherichia coli O157 associated with a busy bathing beach. *Commun Dis Public Health* **7:**47-50.

3160. Hart, G. 1992. Factors associated with pediculosis pubis and scabies. *Genitourin Med* **68:**294-5.

3161. Hart, J., U. Spirman, and J. Shattach. 1984. An outbreak of amoebic infection in a kibbutz population. *Trans R Soc Trop Med Hyg* **78:**346-8.

3162. Hasanjani Roushan, M. R., M. Mohrez, S. M. Smailnejad Gangi, M. J. Soleimani Amiri, and M. Hajiahmadi. 2004. Epidemiological features and clinical manifestations in 469 adult patients with brucellosis in Babol, Northern Iran. *Epidemiol Infect* **132:**1109-14.

3163. Hashido, M., F. K. Lee, A. J. Nahmias, H. Tsugami, S. Isomura, Y. Nagata, S. Sonoda, and T. Kawana. 1998. An epidemiologic study of herpes simplex virus type 1 and 2 infection in Japan based on type-specific serological assays. *Epidemiol Infect* **120:**179-86.

3164. Hashimoto, A., S. Kunikane, and T. Hirata. 2002. Prevalence of Cryptosporidium oocysts and giardia cysts in the drinking water supply in Japan. *Water Res* **36:**519-26.

3165. Hashisaki, P., V. Hsu, C. DeBolt, J. Duchin, L. Kidoguchi, M. Leslie, J. Hofmann, A. Marfin, and G. Campbell. 2005. Japanese encephalitis in a U.S. traveler returning from Thailand, 2004. *MMWR* **54:**123-5.

3166. Haslett, T. M., H. D. Isenberg, E. Hilton, V. Tucci, B. G. Kay, and E. M. Vellozzi. 1988. Microbiology of indwelling central intravascular catheters. *J Clin Microbiol* **26:**696-701.

3167. Hassan, A. A., O. Akineden, and E. Usleber. 2005. Identification of Streptococcus canis isolated from milk of dairy cows with subclinical mastitis. *J Clin Microbiol* **43:**1234-8.

3168. Hassanein, K. M., O. M. el-Azazy, and H. M. Yousef. 1997. Detection of Crimean-Congo haemorrhagic fever virus antibodies in humans and imported livestock in Saudi Arabia. *Trans R Soc Trop Med Hyg* **91:**536-7.

3169. Hasselhorn, H. M. 2001. [Prevention of diphtheria in Germany: yesterday, today, tomorrow - an overview]. *Gesundheitswesen* **63:**735-40.

3170. Hassler, D., T. F. Schwarz, and R. Braun. 2002. Dengue-Fieber statt Karnevalsvergnügen in Rio. *Deutsche Medizinische Wochenschrift* **127:**723.

3171. Hastings, L., J. Stuart, N. Andrews, and N. Begg. 1997. A retrospective survey of clusters of meningococcal disease in England and Wales, 1993 to 1995: estimated risks of further cases in household and educational settings. *Commun Dis Rep CDR Rev* **7:**R195-200.

3172. Haswell-Elkins, M. R., P. Sithithaworn, and D. Elkins. 1992. Opisthorchis viverrini and cholangiocarcinoma in northeast Thailand. *Parasitol Today* **8:**86-9.

3173. Hata, A., H. Asanuma, M. Rinki, M. Sharp, R. M. Wong, K. Blume, and A. M. Arvin. 2002. Use of an inactivated varicella vaccine in recipients of hematopoietic-cell transplants. *N Engl J Med* **347:**26-34.

3174. Hatanaka, A., A. Tsunoda, M. Okamoto, K. Ooe, A. Nakamura, M. Miyakoshi, T. Komiya, and M. Takahashi. 2003. Corynebacterium ulcerans Diphtheria in Japan. *Emerg Infect Dis* **9:**752-3.

3175. Hatch, C., J. Sneddon, and G. Jalloh. 2004. A descriptive study of urban rabies during the civil war in Sierra Leone: 1995-2001. *Trop Anim Health Prod* **36:**321-34.

3176. Hatchette, T. F., R. C. Hudson, W. F. Schlech, N. A. Campbell, J. E. Hatchette, S. Ratnam, D. Raoult, C. Donovan, and T. J. Marrie. 2001. Goat-associated Q fever: a new disease in Newfoundland. *Emerg Infect Dis* **7:**413-419.

3177. Hatta, M., S. M. van Beers, B. Madjid, A. Djumadi, M. Y. de Wit, and P. R. Klatser. 1995. Distribution and persistence of Mycobacterium leprae nasal carriage among a population in which leprosy is endemic in Indonesia. *Trans R Soc Trop Med Hyg* **89:**381-5.

3178. Hatz, C. F. 2001. The use of ultrasound in schistosomiasis. *Adv Parasitol* **48:**225-84.

3179. Hatz, C. F., J. M. Bidaux, K. Eichenberger, U. Mikulics, and T. Junghanss. 1995. Circumstances and management of 72 animal bites among long-term residents in the tropics. *Vaccine* **13:**811-5.

3180. Haukenes, G., K. Brinchmann-Hansen, and O. Macovei. 1992. Prevalence of hepatitis B and C and HIV antibodies in children in a Romanian orphanage. *APMIS* **100:**757-61.

3181. Haupt, W. 1999. Rabies - risk of exposure and current trends in prevention of human cases. *Vaccine* **17:**1742-9.

3182. Hauri, A. M., G. L. Armstrong, and Y. J. Hutin. 2004. The global burden of disease attributable to contaminated injections given in health care settings. *Int J STD AIDS* **15:**7-16.

3183. Hauri, A. M., I. Ehrhard, U. Frank, J. Ammer, G. Fell, O. Hamouda, and L. Petersen. 2000. Serogroup C meningococcal disease outbreak associated with discotheque attendance during carnival. *Epidemiol Infect* **124:**69-73.

3184. Hauri, A. M., M. Saehrendt, B. Spangenberg, and P. Roggentin. 2004. A foodborne outbreak of Salmonella enterica subsp. enterica serovar Madelia at a silver anniversary reception. *Eur J Clin Microbiol Infect Dis* **23:**841-3.

3185. Hauri, A. M., M. Schimmelpfennig, M. Walter-Domes, A. Letz, S. Diedrich, J. Lopez-Pila, and E. Schreier. 2005. An outbreak of viral meningitis associated with a public swimming pond. *Epidemiol Infect* **133:**291-8.

3186. Hauschild, A. H., and L. Gauvreau. 1985. Food-borne botulism in Canada, 1971-84. *Can Med Assoc J* **133:**1141-6.

3187. Hauser, A. R., and P. Sriram. 2005. Severe Pseudomonas aeruginosa infections. Tackling the conundrum of drug resistance. *Postgrad Med* **117:**41-8.

3188. Hauser, U., H. Krahl, H. Peters, V. Fingerle, and B. Wilske. 1998. Impact of strain heterogeneity on Lyme disease serology in Europe: comparison of enzyme-linked immunosorbent assays using different species of Borrelia burgdorferi sensu lato. *J Clin Microbiol* **36:**427-36.

3189. Havens, P. L., and C. o. p. AIDS. 2003. Postexposure prophylaxis in children and adolescents for nonoccupational exposure to human immunodeficiency virus. *Pediatrics* **111:**1475-89.

3190. Haverkort, F. 2003. National atypical mycobacteria survey, 2000. *Commun Dis Intell* **27:**180-9.

3191. Hawker, J. I., J. G. Ayres, I. Blair, M. R. Evans, D. L. Smith, E. G. Smith, P. S. Burge, M. J. Carpenter, E. O. Caul, B. Coupland, U. Desselberger, I. D. Farrell, P. J. Saunders, and M. J. Wood. 1998. A large outbreak of Q fever in the West Midlands: windborne spread into a metropolitan area? *Commun Dis Public Health* **1:**180-7.

3192. Hawkes, R. A., C. R. Boughton, and N. D. Naim. 1985. A major outbreak of epidemic polyarthritis in New South Wales during the summer of 1983/1984. *Med J Aust* **143:**330-3.

3193. Hawkes, S., G. J. Hart, A. M. Johnson, C. Shergold, E. Ross, K. M. Herbert, P. Mortimer, J. V. Parry, and D. Mabey. 1994. Risk behaviour and HIV prevalence in international travellers. *AIDS* **8:**247-52.

3194. Hawkes, S., L. Morison, J. Chakraborty, K. Gausia, F. Ahmed, S. S. Islam, N. Alam, D. Brown, and D. Mabey. 2002. Reproductive tract infections: prevalence and risk factors in rural Bangladesh. *Bull WHO* **80:**180-8.

3195. Hawkes, S., B. West, S. Wilson, H. Whittle, and D. Mabey. 1995. Asymptomatic carriage of Haemophilus ducreyi confirmed by the polymerase chain reaction. *Genitourin Med* **71:**224-7.

3196. Hawkins, R. E., J. D. Malone, L. A. Cloninger, P. J. Rozmajzl, D. Lewis, J. Butler, E. Cross, S. Gray, and K. C. Hyams. 1992. Risk of viral hepatitis among military personnel assigned to US Navy ships. *J Infect Dis* **165:**716-9.

3197. Hawley, H. B., D. P. Morin, M. E. Geraghty, J. Tomkow, and C. A. Phillips. 1973. Coxsackievirus B epidemic at a Boy's Summer Camp. Isolation of virus from swimming water. *JAMA* **226:**33-6.

3198. Hay, R. J., C. K. Campbell, R. Wingfield, and Y. M. Clayton. 1983. A comparative study of dermatophytosis in coal miners and dermatological outpatients. *Br J Ind Med* **40:**353-5.

3199. Hay, R. J., Y. M. Clayton, N. De Silva, G. Midgley, and E. Rossor. 1996. Tinea capitis in south-east London—a new pattern of infection with public health implications. *Br J Dermatol* **135:**955-8.

3200. Hay, R. J., and D. W. Mackenzie. 1983. Mycetoma (madura foot) in the United Kingdom—a survey of forty-four cases. *Clin Exp Dermatol* **8:**553-62.

3201. Hay, S. I., C. A. Guerra, A. J. Tatem, A. M. Noor, and R. W. Snow. 2004. The global distribution and population at risk of malaria: past, present, and future. *Lancet Infect Dis* **4:**327-36.

3202. Hayden, F. G. 2002. Introduction: emerging importance of the rhinovirus. *Am J Med* **112 (6A):**1S-3S.

3203. Hayden, F. G., L. V. Gubareva, A. S. Monto, T. C. Klein, M. J. Elliot, J. M. Hammond, S. J. Sharp, and M. J. Ossi. 2000. Inhaled zanamivir for the prevention of influenza in families. Zanamivir Family Study Group. *N Engl J Med* **343:**1282-9.

3204. Hayes, C. G., I. A. Phillips, J. D. Callahan, W. F. Griebenow, K. C. Hyams, S. J. Wu, and D. M. Watts. 1996. The epidemiology of dengue virus infection among urban, jungle, and rural populations in the Amazon region of Peru. *Am J Trop Med Hyg* **55:**459-63.

3205. Hayes, E., S. Marshall, D. Dennis, and K. Feldman. 2002. Tularemia - United States, 1990-2000. *MMWR* **51:**182-4.

3206. Hayes, E. B., N. Komar, R. S. Nasci, S. P. Montgomery, D. R. O'Leary, and G. L. Campbell. 2005. Epidemiology and transmission dynamics of West Nile virus disease. *Emerg Infect Dis* **11:**1167-73.

3207. Hayes, E. B., and J. Piesman. 2003. How can we prevent Lyme disease. *N Engl J Med* **348:**2424-30.

3208. Hayes, J. M., E. Garcia-Rivera, R. Flores-Reyna, G. Suarez-Rangel, T. Rodriguez-Mata, R. Coto-Portillo, R. Baltrons-Orellana, E. Mendoza-Rodriguez, B. F. De Garay, J. Jubis-Estrada, R. Hernandez-Argueta, B. J. Biggerstaff, and J. G. Rigau-Perez. 2003. Risk factors for infection during a severe dengue outbreak in El Salvador in 2000. *Am J Trop Med Hyg* **69:**629-33.

3209. He, Q., M. K. Viljanen, H. Arvilommi, B. Aittanen, and J. Mertsola. 1998. Whooping cough caused by Bordetella pertussis and Bordetella parapertussis in an immunized population. *JAMA* **280:**635-7.

3210. He, Q., M. K. Viljanen, S. Nikkari, R. Lyytikainen, and J. Mertsola. 1994. Outcomes of Bordetella pertussis infection in different age groups of an immunized population. *J Infect Dis* **170:**873-7.

3211. Headington, C. E., C. H. Barbara, B. E. Lambson, D. T. Hart, and D. C. Barker. 2002. Diagnosis of leishmaniasis in Maltese dogs with the aid of the polymerase chain reaction. *Trans R Soc Trop Med Hyg* **96 Suppl 1:**S195-7.

3212. Headrick, M. L., S. Korangy, N. H. Bean, F. J. Angulo, S. F. Altekruse, M. E. Potter, and K. C. Klontz. 1998. The epidemiology of raw milk-associated foodborne disease outbreaks reported in the United States, 1973 through 1992. *Am J Public Health* **88:**1219-21.

3213. Healing, T. D. 1991. Salmonella in rodents: a risk to man? *CDR (Lond Engl Rev)* **1:**R114-6.

3214. Healing, T. D., P. N. Hoffman, and S. E. Young. 1995. The infection hazards of human cadavers. *Commun Dis Rep CDR Rev* **5:**R61-8.

3215. Healy, G. 1989. The impact of cultural and environmental changes on the epidemiology and control of human babesiosis. *Trans R Soc Trop Med Hyg* **83 Suppl:**35-8.

3216. Heap, B. J., and M. L. McCulloch. 1991. Giardiasis and occupational risk in sewage workers. *Lancet* **338:**1152.

3217. Heath, P. T., G. Balfour, A. M. Weisner, A. Efstratiou, T. L. Lamagni, H. Tighe, L. A. O'Connell, M. Cafferkey, N. Q. Verlander, A. Nicoll, and A. C. McCartney. 2004. Group B streptococcal disease in UK and Irish infants younger than 90 days. *Lancet* **363:**292-4.

3218. Heath, P. T., N. K. Nik Yusoff, and C. J. Baker. 2003. Neonatal meningitis. *Arch Dis Child Fetal Neonatal Ed* **88:**F173-8.

3219. Heckmann, J. G., C. J. Lang, F. Petruch, A. Druschky, C. Erb, P. Brown, and B. Neundorfer. 1997. Transmission of Creutzfeldt-Jakob disease via a corneal transplant. *J Neurol Neurosurg Psychiatry* **63:**388-90.

3220. Hedberg, C. W., F. J. Angulo, K. E. White, C. W. Langkop, W. L. Schell, M. G. Stobierski, A. Schuchat, J. M. Besser, S. Dietrich, L. Helsel, P. M. Griffin, J. W. McFarland, and M. T. Osterholm. 1999. Outbreaks of salmonellosis associated with eating uncooked tomatoes: implications for public health. The Investigation Team. *Epidemiol Infect* **122:**385-93.

3221. Hedberg, C. W., J. A. Korlath, J. Y. D'Aoust, K. E. White, W. L. Schell, M. R. Miller, D. N. Cameron, K. L. MacDonald, and M. T. Osterholm. 1992. A multistate outbreak of Salmonella javiana and Salmonella oranienburg infections due to consumption of contaminated cheese. *JAMA* **268:**3203-7.

3222. Hedberg, C. W., W. C. Levine, K. E. White, R. H. Carlson, D. K. Winsor, D. N. Cameron, K. L. MacDonald, and M. T. Osterholm. 1992. An international foodborne outbreak of shigellosis associated with a commercial airline. *JAMA* **268:**3208-12.

3223. Hedberg, C. W., K. E. White, J. A. Johnson, L. M. Edmonson, J. T. Soler, J. A. Korlath, L. S. Theurer, K. L. MacDonald, and M. T. Osterholm. 1991. An outbreak of Salmonella enteritidis infection at a fast-food restaurant: implications for foodhandler-associated transmission. *J Infect Dis* **164:**1135-40.

3224. Hedberg, K., K. E. White, J. C. Forfang, J. A. Korlath, K. A. Friendshuh, C. W. Hedberg, K. L. MacDonald, and M. T. Osterholm. 1989. An outbreak of psittacosis in Minnesota turkey industry workers: implications for modes of transmission and control. *Am J Epidemiol* **130:**569-77.

3225. **Hedges, S. B.** 2002. The origin and evolution of model organisms. *Nat Rev Genet* **3**:838-49.

3226. **Hedlund, K. O., E. Rubilar-Abreu, and L. Svensson.** 2000. Epidemiology of calicivirus infections in Sweden, 1994-1998. *J Infect Dis* **181 suppl 2**:S275-S280.

3227. **Hedrick, R. P.** 1996. Movement of pathogens with the international trade of live fish: problems and solutions. *Rev Sci Tech* **15**:523-31.

3228. **Heffelfinger, J. D., H. S. Weinstock, B. S.M., and E. B. Swint.** 2002. Primary and secondary syphilis - United States, 2000-2001. *MMWR* **51**:971-3.

3229. **Hegazy, A. A., N. M. Darwish, I. A. Abdel-Hamid, and S. M. Hammad.** 1999. Epidemiology and control of scabies in an Egyptian village. *Int J Dermatol* **38**:291-5.

3230. **Heijbel, H., K. Slaine, B. Seigel, P. Wall, S. J. McNabb, W. Gibbons, and G. R. Istre.** 1987. Outbreak of diarrhea in a day care center with spread to household members: the role of Cryptosporidium. *Pediatr Infect Dis J* **6**:532-5.

3231. **Heikel, J., S. Sekkat, F. Bouqdir, H. Rich, B. Takourt, F. Radouani, N. Hda, S. Ibrahimy, and A. Benslimane.** 1999. The prevalence of sexually transmitted pathogens in patients presenting to a Casablanca STD clinic. *Eur J Epidemiol* **15**:711-5.

3232. **Heikkinen, T., T. Ziegler, V. Peltola, P. Lehtinen, P. Toikka, M. Lintu, T. Jartti, T. Juven, J. Kataja, J. Pulkkinen, L. Kainulainen, T. Puhakka, and T. Routi.** 2003. Incidence of influenza in Finnish children. *Pediatr Infect Dis J* **22**:S204-6.

3233. **Heinemann, S., F. Symoens, B. Gordts, H. Jannes, and N. Nolard.** 2004. Environmental investigations and molecular typing of Aspergillus flavus during an outbreak of postoperative infections. *J Hosp Infect* **57**:149-55.

3234. **Heininger, U., C. Braun-Fahrländer, D. Desgrandchamps, J. Glaus, L. Grize, P. Wutzler, and U. B. Schaad.** 2001. Seroprevalence of varicella-zoster virus immunoglobulin G antibodies in Swiss adolescents and risk factor analysis for seronegativity. *Pediatr Infect Dis J* **20**:775-778.

3235. **Heininger, U., J. D. Cherry, K. Stehr, S. Schmitt-Grohe, M. Uberall, S. Laussucq, T. Eckhardt, M. Meyer, and J. Gornbein.** 1998. Comparative Efficacy of the Lederle/Takeda acellular pertussis component DTP (DTaP) vaccine and Lederle whole-cell component DTP vaccine in German children after household exposure. Pertussis Vaccine Study Group. *Pediatrics* **102**:546-53.

3236. **Heininger, U., K. Stehr, S. Schmitt-Grohe, C. Lorenz, R. Rost, P. D. Christenson, M. Uberall, and J. D. Cherry.** 1994. Clinical characteristics of illness caused by Bordetella parapertussis compared with illness caused by Bordetella pertussis. *Pediatr Infect Dis J* **13**:306-9.

3237. **Heinitz, M. L., R. D. Ruble, D. E. Wagner, and S. R. Tatini.** 2000. Incidence of Salmonella in fish and seafood. *J Food Prot* **63**:579-92.

3238. **Heiskanen-Kosma, T., M. Korppi, A. Laurila, C. Jokinen, M. Kleemola, and P. Saikku.** 1999. Chlamydia pneumoniae is an important cause of community-acquired pneumonia in school-aged children: serological results of a prospective, population-based study. *Scand J Infect Dis* **31**:255-9.

3239. **Helfand, R. F., A. S. Khan, M. A. Pallansch, J. P. Alexander, H. B. Meyers, R. A. DeSantis, L. B. Schonberger, and L. J. Anderson.** 1994. Echovirus 30 infection and aseptic meningitis in parents of children attending a child care center. *J Infect Dis* **169**:1133-7.

3240. **Helfand, R. F., D. K. Kim, H. E. Gary, Jr., G. L. Edwards, G. P. Bisson, M. J. Papania, J. L. Heath, D. L. Schaff, W. J. Bellini, S. C. Redd, and L. J. Anderson.** 1998. Nonclassic measles infections in an immune population exposed to measles during a college bus trip. *J Med Virol* **56**:337-41.

3241. **Hellard, M., J. Hocking, J. Willis, G. Dore, and C. Fairley.** 2003. Risk factors leading to Cryptosporidium infection in men who have sex with men. *Sex Transm Infect* **79**:412-4.

3242. **Hellard, M. E., J. S. Hocking, and N. Crofts.** 2004. The prevalence and the risk behaviours associated with the transmission of hepatitis C virus in Australian correctional facilities. *Epidemiol Infect* **132**:409-15.

3243. **Hellenbrand, W., T. Breuer, and L. Petersen.** 2001. Changing epidemiology of Q fever in Germany, 1947-1999. *Emerg Infect Dis* **7**:789-796.

3244. **Hellenbrand, W., C. Meyer, G. Rasch, I. Steffens, and A. Ammon.** 2005. Cases of rabies in Germany following organ transplantation. *Eurosurveillance* **10**:52-3.

3245. **Heller, M. C., J. McClure, N. Pusterla, J. B. Pusterla, and S. Stahel.** 2004. Two cases of Neorickettsia (Ehrlichia) risticii infection in horses from Nova Scotia. *Can Vet J* **45**:421-3.

3246. **Heller, R., M. Kubina, P. Mariet, P. Riegel, G. Delacour, C. Dehio, F. Lamarque, R. Kasten, H. J. Boulouis, H. Monteil, B. Chomel, and Y. Piemont.** 1999. Bartonella alsatica sp. nov., a new Bartonella species isolated from the blood of wild rabbits. *Int J Syst Bacteriol* **49 Pt 1**:283-8.

3247. **Hellyar, A. G.** 1985. The introduction of brucellosis into the Solomon islands. *Trans R Soc Trop Med Hyg* **79**:567-8.

3248. **Helmick, C. G., P. A. Webb, C. L. Scribner, J. W. Krebs, and J. B. McCormick.** 1986. No evidence for increased risk of Lassa fever infection in hospital staff. *Lancet* **2**:1202-5.

3249. **Helvaci, S., S. Gedikoglu, H. Akalin, and H. B. Oral.** 2000. Tularemia in Bursa, Turkey: 205 cases in ten years. *Eur J Epidemiol* **16**:271-6.

3250. **Hemachudha, T., J. Laothamatas, and C. E. Rupprecht.** 2002. Human rabies: a disease of complex neuropathogenetic mechanisms and diagnostic challenges. *Lancet Neurol* **1**:101-9.

3251. **Hemmersbach-Miller, M., P. Parola, R. N. Charrel, J. Paul Durand, and P. Brouqui.** 2004. Sandfly fever due to Toscana virus: an emerging infection in southern France. *Eur J Intern Med* **15**:316-317.

3252. **Henderson, D. A.** 1976. The eradication of smallpox. *Scientific American* **235**:25-33.

3253. **Heneine, W., W. M. Switzer, P. Sandstrom, J. Brown, S. Vedapuri, C. A. Schable, A. S. Khan, N. W. Lerche, M. Schweizer, D. Neumann-Haefelin, L. E. Chapman, and T. M. Folks.** 1998. Identification of a human population infected with simian foamy viruses. *Nat Med* **4**:403-7.

3254. **Heneine, W., A. Tibell, W. M. Switzer, P. Sandstrom, G. V. Rosales, A. Mathews, O. Korsgren, L. E. Chapman, T. M. Folks, and C. G. Groth.** 1998. No evidence of infection with porcine endogenous retrovirus in recipients of porcine islet-cell xenografts. *Lancet* **352**:695-9.

3255. **Heng, B. H., K. T. Goh, D. L. Ng, and A. E. Ling.** 1997. Surveillance of legionellosis and Legionella bacteria in the built environment in Singapore. *Ann Acad Med Singapore* **26**:557-65.

3256. **Hengge, U. R., A. Tannapfel, S. K. Tyring, R. Erbel, G. Arendt, and T. Ruzicka.** 2003. Lyme borreliosis. *Lancet Infect Dis* **3**:489-500.

3257. Hennequin, C., B. Page, P. Roux, C. Legendre, and H. Kreis. 1995. Outbreak of Pneumocystis carinii pneumonia in a renal transplant unit. *Eur J Clin Microbiol Infect Dis* **14:**122-6.

3258. Hennessy, T. W., L. Har Cheng, H. Kassenborg, S. D. Ahuja, J. Mohle-Boetani, R. Marcus, B. Shiferaw, and F. J. Angulo. 2004. Egg Consumption is the Principal Risk Factor for Sporadic Salmonella Serotype Heidelberg Infections: A Case-Control Study in FoodNet Sites. *Clin Infect Dis* **38 Suppl 3:**S237-43.

3259. Hennessy, T. W., C. W. Hedberg, L. Slutsker, K. E. White, J. M. Besser-Wiek, M. E. Moen, J. Feldman, W. W. Coleman, L. M. Edmonson, K. L. MacDonald, and M. T. Osterholm. 1996. A national outbreak of Salmonella enteritidis infections from ice cream. The Investigation Team. *N Engl J Med* **334:**1281-6.

3260. Henning, K. J., E. Bell, J. Braun, and N. D. Barker. 1995. A community-wide outbreak of hepatitis A: risk factors for infection among homosexual and bisexual men. *Am J Med* **99:**132-6.

3261. Henning, P. H., E. B. Tham, A. A. Martin, T. H. Beare, and K. F. Jureidini. 1998. Haemolytic-uraemic syndrome outbreak caused by Escherichia coli O111:H-: clinical outcomes. *Med J Aust* **168:**552-5.

3262. Henriksen, B. M., S. B. Albrektsen, L. B. Simper, and E. Gutschik. 1994. Soft tissue infections from drug abuse. A clinical and microbiological review of 145 cases. *Acta Orthop Scand* **65:**625-8.

3263. Henry, B., C. Plante-Jenkins, and K. Ostrowska. 2001. An outbreak of Serratia marcescens associated with the anesthetic agent propofol. *Am J Infect Control* **29:**312-5.

3264. Henry, M. C., C. Rogier, I. Nzeyimana, S. B. Assi, J. Dossou-Yovo, M. Audibert, J. Mathonnat, A. Keundjian, E. Akodo, T. Teuscher, and P. Carnevale. 2003. Inland valley rice production systems and malaria infection and disease in the savannah of Cote d'Ivoire. *Trop Med Int Health* **8:**449-58.

3265. Henttonen, H., E. Fuglei, C. N. Gower, V. Haukisalmi, R. A. Ims, J. Niemimaa, and N. G. Yoccoz. 2001. Echinococcus multilocularis on Svalbard: introduction of an intermediate host has enabled the local life-cycle. *Parasitology* **123:**547-52.

3266. Hepburn, N. C., and T. J. Brooks. 1991. An outbreak of chickenpox in a military field hospital—the implications for biological warfare. *J R Soc Med* **84:**721-2.

3267. Hepburn, N. C., M. J. Tidman, and J. A. Hunter. 1993. Cutaneous leishmaniasis in British troops from Belize. *Br J Dermatol* **128:**63-8.

3268. Herber, O., and A. Kroeger. 2003. Pyrethroid-impregnated curtains for Chagas' disease control in Venezuela. *Acta Trop* **88:**33-8.

3269. Hernandez, J., J. Bonnedahl, J. Waldenström, H. Palmgren, and B. Olsen. 2003. Salmonella in birds migrating through Sweden. *Emerg Infect Dis* **9:**753-4.

3270. Hernandez-Becerril, N., A. M. Mejia, M. A. Ballinas-Verdugo, V. Garza-Murillo, E. Manilla-Toquero, R. Lopez, S. Trevethan, M. Cardenas, P. A. Reyes, K. Hirayama, and V. M. Monteon. 2005. Blood transfusion and iatrogenic risks in Mexico City. Anti-Trypanosoma cruzi seroprevalence in 43,048 blood donors, evaluation of parasitemia, and electrocardiogram findings in seropositive. *Mem Inst Oswaldo Cruz* **100:**111-6.

3271. Hernández-Cabrera, M., A. Angel-Moreno, E. Santana, M. Bolanos, A. Frances, M. S. Martin-Sanchez, and J. L. Perez-Arellano. 2004. Murine typhus with renal involvement in Canary islands, Spain. *Emerg Infect Dis* **10:**740-3.

3272. Hernandez-Perez, J., M. Yebra-Bango, E. Jimenez-Martinez, C. Sanz-Moreno, V. Cuervas-Mons, L. Alonso Pulpon, A. Ramos-Martinez, and J. Fernandez-Fernandez. 1999. Visceral leishmaniasis (kala-azar) in solid organ transplantation: report of five cases and review. *Clin Infect Dis* **29:**918-21.

3273. Herra, C. M., S. J. Knowles, M. E. Kaufmann, E. Mulvihill, B. McGrath, and C. T. Keane. 1998. An outbreak of an unusual strain of Serratia marcescens in two Dublin hospitals. *J Hosp Infect* **39:**135-41.

3274. Herrera-Basto, E., D. R. Prevots, M. L. Zarate, J. L. Silva, and J. Sepulveda-Amor. 1992. First reported outbreak of classical dengue fever at 1,700 meters above sea level in Guerrero State, Mexico, June 1988. *Am J Trop Med Hyg* **46:**649-53.

3275. Herrero, M. V., W. E. Yarnell, and E. T. Schmidtmann. 2004. Landscape associations of the sand fly, Lutzomyia (Heleocyrtomyia) apache (Diptera: Psychodidae), in the southwestern United States: a geographic information system analysis. *J Vector Ecol* **29:**205-11.

3276. Herrero-Herrero, J. I., R. Ruiz-Beltrán, A. M. Martin-Sánchez, and E. J. Garcia. 1989. Mediterranean spotted fever in Salamanca, Spain. Epidemiological study in patients and serosurvey in animals and healthy human population. *Acta Trop* **46:**335-50.

3277. Herruzo-Cabrera, R., J. Garcia-Caballero, J. M. Martin-Moreno, M. A. Graciani-Perez-Regadera, and J. Perez-Rodriguez. 2001. Clinical assay of N-duopropenide alcohol solution on hand application in newborn and pediatric intensive care units: control of an outbreak of multiresistant Klebsiella pneumoniae in a newborn intensive care unit with this measure. *Am J Infect Control* **29:**162-7.

3278. Herruzo-Cabrera, R., R. Lopez-Gimenez, J. Diez-Sebastian, M. J. Lopez-Acinero, and J. R. Banegas-Banegas. 2004. Surgical site infection of 7301 traumatologic inpatients (divided in two sub-cohorts, study and validation): modifiable determinants and potential benefit. *Eur J Epidemiol* **19:**163-9.

3279. Hersh, B. S., P. E. Fine, W. K. Kent, S. L. Cochi, L. H. Kahn, E. R. Zell, P. L. Hays, and C. L. Wood. 1991. Mumps outbreak in a highly vaccinated population. *J Pediatr* **119:**187-93.

3280. Hersh, B. S., L. E. Markowitz, R. E. Hoffman, D. R. Hoff, M. J. Doran, J. C. Fleishman, S. R. Preblud, and W. A. Orenstein. 1991. A measles outbreak at a college with a prematriculation immunization requirement. *Am J Public Health* **81:**360-4.

3281. Hersh, B. S., F. Popovici, R. C. Apetrei, L. Zolotusca, N. Beldescu, A. Calomfirescu, Z. Jezek, M. J. Oxtoby, A. Gromyko, and D. L. Heymann. 1991. Acquired immunodeficiency syndrome in Romania. *Lancet* **338:**645-9.

3282. Hershberger, E., S. F. Oprea, S. M. Donabedian, M. Perri, P. Bozigar, P. Bartlett, and M. J. Zervos. 2005. Epidemiology of antimicrobial resistance in enterococci of animal origin. *J Antimicrob Chemother* **55:**127-30.

3283. Hervas, J. A., F. Ballesteros, A. Alomar, J. Gil, V. J. Benedi, and S. Alberti. 2001. Increase of Enterobacter in neonatal sepsis: a twenty-two-year study. *Pediatr Infect Dis J* **20:**134-40.

3284. Herve, V., E. Kassa Kelembho, P. Normand, A. Georges, C. Mathiot, and P. Martin. 1992. [Resurgence of yaws in Central African Republic. Role of the Pygmy population as a reservoir of the virus]. *Bull Soc Pathol Exot* **85:**342-6.

3285. Herwaldt, B. L. 2000. Cyclospora cayetanensis: a review, focusing on the outbreaks of cyclosporiasis in the 1990s. *Clin Infect Dis* **31:**1040-57.

3286. **Herwaldt, B. L.** 2001. Laboratory-acquired parasitic infections from accidental exposures. *Clin Microbiol Rev* **14:**659-88.

3287. **Herwaldt, B. L., and M. L. Ackers.** 1997. An outbreak in 1996 of cyclosporiasis associated with imported raspberries. The Cyclospora Working Group. *N Engl J Med* **336:**1548-56.

3288. **Herwaldt, B. L., and M. J. Beach.** 1999. The return of Cyclospora in 1997: another outbreak of cyclosporiasis in North America associated with imported raspberries. Cyclospora Working Group. *Ann Intern Med* **130:**210-20.

3289. **Herwaldt, B. L., K. R. de Arroyave, S. P. Wahlquist, L. J. du Pee, T. R. Eng, and D. D. Juranek.** 1994. Infections with intestinal parasites in Peace Corps volunteers in Guatemala. *J Clin Microbiol* **32:**1376-8.

3290. **Herwaldt, B. L., G. de Bruyn, N. J. Pieniazek, M. Homer, K. H. Lofy, S. B. Slemenda, T. R. Fritsche, D. H. Persing, and A. P. Limaye.** 2004. Babesia divergens-like infection, Washington state. *Emerg Infect Dis* **10:**622-9.

3291. **Herwaldt, B. L., M. J. Grijalva, A. L. Newsome, C. R. McGhee, M. R. Powell, D. G. Nemec, F. J. Steurer, and M. L. Eberhard.** 2000. Use of polymerase chain reaction to diagnose the fifth reported US case of autochthonous transmission of Trypanosoma cruzi, in Tennessee, 1998. *J Infect Dis* **181:**395-9.

3292. **Herwaldt, B. L., D. F. Neitzel, J. B. Gorlin, K. A. Jensen, E. H. Perry, W. R. Peglow, S. B. Slemenda, K. Y. Won, E. K. Nace, N. J. Pieniazek, and M. Wilson.** 2002. Transmission of Babesia microti in Minnesota through four blood donations from the same donor over a 6-month period. *Transfusion* **42:**1154-8.

3293. **Herwaldt, B. L., S. L. Stokes, and D. D. Juranek.** 1993. American cutaneous leishmaniasis in U.S. travelers. *Ann Intern Med* **118:**779-84.

3294. **Herwaldt, L. A.** 2003. Staphylococcus aureus nasal carriage and surgical-site infections. *Surgery* **134:**S2-9.

3295. **Herwaldt, L. A., G. W. Gorman, T. McGrath, S. Toma, B. Brake, A. W. Hightower, J. Jones, A. L. Reingold, P. A. Boxer, P. W. Tang, et al.** 1984. A new Legionella species, Legionella feeleii species nova, causes Pontiac fever in an automobile plant. *Ann Intern Med* **100:**333-8.

3296. **Herwaldt, L. A., S. D. Smith, and C. D. Carter.** 1998. Infection control in the outpatient setting. *Infect Control Hosp Epidemiol* **19:**41-74.

3297. **Heryford, A. G., and S. A. Seys.** 2004. Outbreak of occupational campylobacteriosis associated with a pheasant farm. *J Agric Saf Health* **10:**127-32.

3298. **Heseltine, P. N., M. Ripper, and P. Wohlford.** 1985. Nosocomial rubella—consequences of an outbreak and efficacy of a mandatory immunization program. *Infect Control* **6:**371-4.

3299. **Hess, R. D.** 2004. Routine Epstein-Barr virus diagnostics from the laboratory perspective: still challenging after 35 years. *J Clin Microbiol* **42:**3381-7.

3300. **Heudorf, U.** 1998. [Discussion of prerequisites for food production by the public health office—section 18 of the Federal Epidemiology Regulation and Section 43 of the Infection Control Regulation (draft)]. *Gesundheitswesen* **60:**166-9.

3301. **Heudorf, U., W. Hentschel, M. Hoffmann, C. Luck, and R. Schubert.** 2001. [Legionellas in domestic warm water—effects on the health of residents]. *Gesundheitswesen* **63:**326-34.

3302. **Heukelbach, J., F. A. de Oliveira, L. R. Kerr-Pontes, and H. Feldmeier.** 2001. Risk factors associated with an outbreak of dengue fever in a favela in Fortaleza, north-east Brazil. *Trop Med Int Health* **6:**635-42.

3303. **Heukelbach, J., and H. Feldmeier.** 2004. Ectoparasites—the underestimated realm. *Lancet* **363:**889-91.

3304. **Heukelbach, J., E. Van Haeff, B. Rump, T. Wilcke, R. C. Moura, and H. Feldmeier.** 2003. Parasitic skin diseases: health care-seeking in a slum in north-east Brazil. *Trop Med Int Health* **8:**368-73.

3305. **Heun, E. M., R. L. Vogt, P. J. Hudson, S. Parren, and G. W. Gary.** 1987. Risk factors for secondary transmission in households after a common-source outbreak of Norwalk gastroenteritis. *Am J Epidemiol* **126:**1181-1186.

3306. **Heuvelink, A. E., B. Bleumink, F. L. van den Biggelaar, M. C. Te Giffel, R. R. Beumer, and E. de Boer.** 1998. Occurrence and survival of verocytotoxin-producing Escherichia coli O157 in raw cow's milk in The Netherlands. *J Food Prot* **61:**1597-601.

3307. **Heuvelink, A. E., F. L. van den Biggelaar, J. Zwartkruis-Nahuis, R. G. Herbes, R. Huyben, N. Nagelkerke, W. J. Melchers, L. A. Monnens, and E. de Boer.** 1998. Occurrence of verocytotoxin-producing Escherichia coli O157 on Dutch dairy farms. *J Clin Microbiol* **36:**3480-7.

3308. **Heuvelink, A. E., C. van Heerwaarden, J. T. Zwartkruis-Nahuis, R. van Oosterom, K. Edink, Y. T. van Duynhoven, and E. de Boer.** 2002. Escherichia coli O157 infection associated with a petting zoo. *Epidemiol Infect* **129:**295-302.

3309. **Hewitt, J. H., N. Begg, J. Hewish, S. Rawaf, M. Stringer, and B. Theodore-Gandi.** 1986. Large outbreaks of Clostridium perfringens food poisoning associated with the consumption of boiled salmon. *J Hyg (Lond)* **97:**71-80.

3310. **Hewitt, S., H. Reyburn, R. Ashford, and M. Rowland.** 1998. Anthroponotic cutaneous leishmaniasis in Kabul, Afghanistan: vertical distribution of cases in apartment blocks. *Trans R Soc Trop Med Hyg* **92:**273-4.

3311. **Heyman, P., A. Plyusnina, P. Berny, C. Cochez, M. Artois, M. Zizi, J. P. Pirnay, and A. Plyusnin.** 2004. Seoul hantavirus in Europe: first demonstration of the virus genome in wild Rattus norvegicus captured in France. *Eur J Clin Microbiol Infect Dis* **23:**711-7.

3312. **Heyndrickx, M., D. Vandekerchove, L. Herman, I. Rollier, K. Grijspeerdt, and L. De Zutter.** 2002. Routes for salmonella contamination of poultry meat: epidemiological study from hatchery to slaughterhouse. *Epidemiol Infect* **129:**253-65.

3313. **Hibbs, J. R., and R. A. Gunn.** 1991. Public health intervention in a cocaine-related syphilis outbreak. *Am J Public Health* **81:**1259-62.

3314. **Hickman, M. E., M. A. Rench, P. Ferrieri, and C. J. Baker.** 1999. Changing epidemiology of group B streptococcal colonization. *Pediatrics* **104:**203-9.

3315. **Hickstein, L., C. McPherson, D. Kwalick, V. DeFriez, R. L. Todd, K. Ijaz, C. González, M. Haddad, P. Tribble, M. Arduino, S. Wei, and J. Miller.** 2004. Tuberculosis transmission in a renal dialysis center - Nevada, 2003. *MMWR* **53:**873-5.

3316. **Hide, G.** 1999. History of sleeping sickness in East Africa. *Clin Microbiol Rev* **12:**112-25.

3317. **Hierholzer, J. C., A. Pumarola, A. Rodriguez-Torres, and M. Beltran.** 1974. Occurrence of respiratory illness due to an atypical strain of adenovirus type 11 during a large outbreak in Spanish military recruits. *Am J Epidemiol* **99:**434-42.

3318. **Hilali, A. H., H. Madsen, A. A. Daffalla, M. Wassila, and N. O. Christensen.** 1995. Infection and transmission pattern of Schistosoma mansoni in the Managil irrigation scheme, Sudan. *Ann Trop Med Parasitol* **89:**279-86.

3319. **Hilbink, F., M. Penrose, E. Kovacova, and J. Kazar.** 1993. Q fever is absent from New Zealand. *Int J Epidemiol* **22:**945-9.

3320. **Hilborn, E. D., J. H. Mermin, P. A. Mshar, J. L. Hadler, A. Voetsch, C. Wojtkunski, M. Swartz, R. Mshar, M. A. Lambert-Fair, J. A. Farrar, M. K. Glynn, and L. Slutsker.** 1999. A multistate outbreak of Escherichia coli O157:H7 infections associated with consumption of mesclun lettuce. *Arch Intern Med* **159:**1758-64.

3321. **Hilborn, E. D., P. A. Mshar, T. R. Fiorentino, Z. F. Dembek, T. J. Barrett, R. T. Howard, and M. L. Cartter.** 2000. An outbreak of Escherichia coli O157:H7 infections and haemolytic uraemic syndrome associated with consumption of unpasteurized apple cider. *Epidemiol Infect* **124:**31-6.

3322. **Hildebrand, P., B. M. Meyer-Wyss, S. Mossi, and C. Beglinger.** 2000. Risk among gastroenterologists of acquiring Helicobacter pylori infection: case-control study. *BMJ* **321:**149.

3323. **Hill, A. F., R. J. Butterworth, S. Joiner, G. Jackson, M. N. Rossor, D. J. Thomas, A. Frosh, N. Tolley, J. E. Bell, M. Spencer, A. King, S. Al-Sarraj, J. W. Ironside, P. L. Lantos, and J. Collinge.** 1999. Investigation of variant Creutzfeldt-Jakob disease and other human prion diseases with tonsil biopsy samples. *Lancet* **353:**183-9.

3324. **Hill, A. V.** 2001. The genomics and genetics of human infectious disease susceptibility. *Annu Rev Genomics Hum Genet* **2:**373-400.

3325. **Hill, D. R.** 1989. HIV infection following motor vehicle trauma in central Africa. *JAMA* **261:**3282-3.

3326. **Hill, D. R.** 2000. Health problems in a large cohort of Americans traveling to developing countries. *J Travel Med* **7:**259-66.

3327. **Hillebrand-Haverkort, M. E., A. H. Kolk, L. F. Kox, J. J. Ten Velden, and J. H. Ten Veen.** 1999. Generalized mycobacterium genavense infection in HIV-infected patients: detection of the mycobacterium in hospital tap water. *Scand J Infect Dis* **31:**63-8.

3328. **Hilleman, M. R.** 2001. Overview of the pathogenesis, prophylaxis and therapeusis of viral hepatitis B, with focus on reduction to practical applications. *Vaccine* **19:**1837-48.

3329. **Hillis, W. D.** 1961. An outbreak of infectious hepatitis among chimpanzee handlers at a United States air force base. *Am J Hyg* **73:**316-28.

3330. **Hills, S., J. Piispanen, P. Foley, G. Smith, J. Humphreys, J. Simpson, and G. McDonald.** 2000. Public health implications of dengue in personnel returning from East Timor. *Commun Dis Intell* **24:**365-8.

3331. **Hilton, D. A., A. C. Ghani, L. Conyers, P. Edwards, L. McCardle, D. Ritchie, M. Penney, D. Hegazy, and J. W. Ironside.** 2004. Prevalence of lymphoreticular prion protein accumulation in UK tissue samples. *J Pathol* **203:**733-9.

3332. **Hilton, E., J. DeVoti, J. L. Benach, M. L. Halluska, D. J. White, H. Paxton, and J. S. Dumler.** 1999. Seroprevalence and seroconversion for tick-borne diseases in a high-risk population in the northeast United States. *Am J Med* **106:**404-9.

3333. **Hiltunen-Back, E., O. Haikala, H. Kautiainen, J. Paavonen, and T. Reunala.** 2001. A nationwide sentinel clinic survey of chlamydia trachomatis infection in Finland. *Sex Transm Dis* **28:**252-8.

3334. **Hiltunen-Back, E., T. Rostila, H. Kautiainen, J. Paavonen, and T. Reunala.** 1998. Rapid decrease of endemic gonorrhea in Finland. *Sex Transm Dis* **25:**181-6.

3335. **Himy, R., C. Lemble, B. Fernique, O. Villard, H. Couppie, and M. Kremer.** 1993. [Coprological evaluation of refugees in Strasbourg between January 1986 and December 1990]. *Bull Soc Pathol Exot* **86:**151-3.

3336. **Hindsbo, O., C. V. Nielsen, J. Andreassen, A. L. Willingham, M. Bendixen, M. A. Nielsen, and N. O. Nielsen.** 2000. Age-dependent occurrence of the intestinal ciliate Balantidium coli in pigs at a Danish research farm. *Acta Vet Scand* **41:**79-83.

3337. **Hinman, A. R., D. W. Fraser, R. G. Douglas, G. S. Bowen, A. L. Kraus, W. G. Winkler, and W. W. Rhodes.** 1975. Outbreak of lymphocytic choriomeningitis virus infections in medical center personnel. *Am J Epidemiol* **101:**103-10.

3338. **Hinnebusch, B. J., K. L. Gage, and T. G. Schwan.** 1998. Estimation of vector infectivity rates for plague by means of a standard curve-based competitive polymerase chain reaction method to quantify Yersinia pestis in fleas. *Am J Trop Med Hyg* **58:**562-9.

3339. **Hinton, D. G., A. Shipley, J. W. Galvin, J. T. Harkin, and R. A. Brunton.** 1993. Chlamydiosis in workers at a duck farm and processing plant. *Aust Vet J* **70:**174-6.

3340. **Hira, S. K., B. M. Nkowane, J. Kamanga, D. Wadhawan, D. Kavindele, R. Macuacua, G. Mpoko, M. Malek, D. F. Cruess, and P. L. Perine.** 1990. Epidemiology of human immunodeficiency virus in families in Lusaka, Zambia. *J Acquir Immune Defic Syndr* **3:**83-6.

3341. **Hirabayashi, Y., S. Oka, H. Goto, K. Shimada, T. Kurata, S. P. Fisher-Hoch, and J. B. McCormick.** 1988. An imported case of Lassa fever with late appearance of polyserositis. *J Infect Dis* **158:**872-5.

3342. **Hirakata, Y., K. Arisawa, O. Nishio, and O. Nakagomi.** 2005. Multiprefectural spread of gastroenteritis outbreaks attributable to a single genogroup II norovirus strain from a tourist restaurant in Nagasaki, Japan. *J Clin Microbiol* **43:**1093-8.

3343. **Hirota, W. K., M. B. Duncan, and A. Tsuchida.** 2002. The utility of prescreening for hepatitis A in military recruits prior to vaccination. *Mil Med* **167:**907-10.

3344. **Hirsch, H. H., and J. Steiger.** 2003. Polyomavirus BK. *Lancet Infect Dis* **3:**611-23.

3345. **Hirschhorn, L. R., Y. Trnka, A. Onderdonk, M. L. Lee, and R. Platt.** 1994. Epidemiology of community-acquired Clostridium difficile-associated diarrhea. *J Infect Dis* **169:**127-33.

3346. **Hjelle, B., and G. E. Glass.** 2000. Outbreak of hantavirus infection in the Four Corners region of the United States in the wake of the 1997-1998 El Nino-southern oscillation. *J Infect Dis* **181:**1569-73.

3347. **Hjelle, B., R. F. Khabbaz, G. A. Conway, C. North, D. Green, and J. E. Kaplan.** 1994. Prevalence of human T cell lymphotropic virus type II in American Indian populations of the southwestern United States. *Am J Trop Med Hyg* **51:**11-5.

3348. **Hjelm, E., S. McGill, and G. Blomqvist.** 2002. Prevalence of antibodies to Bartonella henselae, B. elizabethae and B. quintana in Swedish domestic cats. *Scand J Infect Dis* **34:**192-6.

3349. **Hjelm, E., L. Wesslen, H. Gnarpe, J. Gnarpe, C. Nystrom-Rosander, C. Rolf, and G. Friman.** 2001. Antibodies to Chlamydia pneumoniae in young Swedish orienteers. *Scand J Infect Dis* **33:**589-92.

3350. Hlady, W. G., J. V. Bennett, A. R. Samadi, J. Begum, A. Hafez, A. I. Tarafdar, and J. R. Boring. 1992. Neonatal tetanus in rural Bangladesh: risk factors and toxoid efficacy. *Am J Public Health* **82:**1365-9.

3351. Hlady, W. G., and K. C. Klontz. 1996. The epidemiology of Vibrio infections in Florida, 1981-1993. *J Infect Dis* **173:** 1176-83.

3352. Hlavsa, M. C., J. C. Watson, and M. J. Beach. 2005. Cryptosporidiosis surveillance—United States 1999-2002. *MMWR* **54 (SS-1):**1-8.

3353. Hlavsa, M. C., J. C. Watson, and M. J. Beach. 2005. Giardiasis surveillance—United States, 1998-2002. *MMWR Surveill Summ* **54:**9-16.

3354. Ho, A. Y., A. S. Lopez, M. G. Eberhart, R. Levenson, B. S. Finkel, A. J. Da Silva, J. M. Roberts, P. A. Orlandi, C. C. Johnson, and B. L. Herwaldt. 2002. Outbreak of cyclosporiasis associated with imported raspberries, Philadelphia, Pennsylvania, 2000. *Emerg Infect Dis* **8:**783-8.

3355. Ho, G. Y. F., A. M. Y. Nomura, K. Nelson, H. Lee, B. F. Polk, and W. A. Blattner. 1991. Declining seroprevalence and transmission of HTLV-I in Japanese families who immigrated to Hawaii. *Am J Epidemiol* **134:**981-7.

3356. Ho, L., S. K. Tay, S. Y. Chan, and H. U. Bernard. 1993. Sequence variants of human papillomavirus type 16 from couples suggest sexual transmission with low infectivity and polyclonality in genital neoplasia. *J Infect Dis* **168:**803-9.

3357. Ho, M. 1998. Human herpesvirus 8 - let the transplantation physician beware. *N Engl J Med* **339:**1391-1392.

3358. Hoang, L. M., J. A. Maguire, P. Doyle, M. Fyfe, and D. L. Roscoe. 2004. Cryptococcus neoformans infections at Vancouver Hospital and Health Sciences Centre (1997-2002): epidemiology, microbiology and histopathology. *J Med Microbiol* **53:**935-40.

3359. Hoang, L. M. N., M. Fyfe, C. N. Ong, J. Harb, S. Champagne, B. Dixon, and J. Isaac-Renton. 2005. Outbreak of cyclosporiasis in British Columbia associated with imported Thai basil. *Epidemiol Infect* **133:**23-7.

3360. Hobson, R. P., F. M. MacKenzie, and I. M. Gould. 1996. An outbreak of multiply-resistant Klebsiella pneumoniae in the Grampian region of Scotland. *J Hosp Infect* **33:**249-62.

3361. Hochberg, N., and E. T. Ryan. 2004. Medical problems in the returning expatriate. *Clin Occup Environ Med* **4:**205-19.

3362. Hochedez, P., P. Vinsentini, S. Ansart, and E. Caumes. 2004. Changes in the pattern of health disorders diagnosed among two cohorts of French travelers to Nepal, 17 years apart. *J Travel Med* **11:**341-6.

3363. Höcker, B., C. Wendt, A. Nahimana, B. Tönshoff, and P. M. Hauser. 2005. Molecular evidence of Pneumocystis transmission in pediatric transplant unit. *Emerg Infect Dis* **11:** 330-2.

3364. Hocking, A. D. 1997. Foodborne microorganisms of public health significance, 5th ed. Australian Institute of Food Science and Technology Inc., North Sydney.

3365. Hocking, A. D., and M. Faedo. 1992. Fungi causing thread mould spoilage of vacuum packaged Cheddar cheese during maturation. *Int J Food Microbiol* **16:**123-30.

3366. Hodgson, A., T. Smith, S. Gagneux, M. Adjuik, G. Pluschke, N. K. Mensah, F. Binka, and B. Genton. 2001. Risk factors for meningococcal meningitis in northern Ghana. *Trans R Soc Trop Med Hyg* **95:**477-480.

3367. Hoebe, C. J., H. Vennema, A. M. Husman, and Y. T. van Duynhoven. 2004. Norovirus outbreak among primary schoolchildren who had played in a recreational water fountain. *J Infect Dis* **189:**699-705.

3368. Hoebe, C. J., J. H. Wagenvoort, and J. F. Schellekens. 2000. [An outbreak of scarlet fever, impetigo and pharyngitis caused by the same Streptococcus pyogenes type T4M4 in a primary school]. *Ned Tijdschr Geneeskd* **144:**2148-52.

3369. Hoebe, C. J. P. A., E. C. J. Claas, J. E. van Steenbergen, and A. C. M. Kroes. 2002. Confirmation of an outbreak of parvovirus B19 in a primary school using IgM ELISA and PCR on thumb prick blood samples. *J Clin Virol* **25:**303-7.

3370. Hoelzle, L. E., G. Steinhausen, and M. M. Wittenbrink. 2000. PCR-based detection of chlamydial infection in swine and subsequent PCR-coupled genotyping of chlamydial omp1 gene amplicons by DNA-hybridization, RFLP-analysis, and nucelotide sequence analysis. *Epidemiol Infect* **125**.

3371. Hoen, B., F. Alla, C. Selton-Suty, I. Beguinot, A. Bouvet, S. Briancon, J. P. Casalta, N. Danchin, F. Delahaye, J. Etienne, V. Le Moing, C. Leport, J. L. Mainardi, R. Ruimy, and F. Vandenesch. 2002. Changing profile of infective endocarditis: results of a 1-year survey in France. *JAMA* **288:**75-81.

3372. Hoeven-Fritscher, S., and W. Kopp. 1994. [Hepatitis B in persons at high risk for sexually transmitted diseases. Screening and vaccination campaign—acceptance and results]. *Gesundheitswesen* **56:**663-6.

3373. Hoey, J. 1998. Rubella outbreaks on cruise ships. *CMAJ* **158:**516-7.

3374. Hofer, S., S. Gloor, U. Muller, A. Mathis, D. Hegglin, and P. Deplazes. 2000. High prevalence of Echinococcus multilocularis in urban red foxes (Vulpes vulpes) and voles (Arvicola terrestris) in the city of Zurich, Switzerland. *Parasitology* **120 (Pt 2):**135-42.

3375. Hoffbrand, B. I. 1975. Amoebic liver abscess presenting thirty-two years after acute amoebic dysentery. *Proc R Soc Med* **68:**593-4.

3376. Hofflin, J. M., R. H. Sadler, F. G. Araujo, W. E. Page, and J. S. Remington. 1987. Laboratory-acquired Chagas disease. *Trans R Soc Trop Med Hyg* **81:**437-40.

3377. Hoffman, R. E., N. Henderson, K. O'Keefe, and R. C. Wood. 1994. Occupational exposure to human immunodeficiency virus (HIV)-infected blood in Denver, Colorado, police officers. *Am J Epidemiol* **139:**910-7.

3378. Hofmann, H., and C. Kunz. 1984. Arbovirusinfektionen bei Tropenheimkehrern. *Medizin in Entwicklungsländern* **16:**251.

3379. Hogan, R. N., and H. D. Cavanagh. 1995. Transplantation of corneal tissue from donors with diseases of the central nervous system. *Cornea* **14:**547-53.

3380. Hoge, C. W., M. R. Reichler, E. A. Dominguez, J. C. Bremer, T. D. Mastro, K. A. Hendricks, D. M. Musher, J. A. Elliott, R. R. Facklam, and R. F. Breiman. 1994. An epidemic of pneumococcal disease in an overcrowded, inadequately ventilated jail. *N Engl J Med* **331:**643-8.

3381. Hoge, C. W., D. R. Shlim, R. Rajah, J. Triplett, M. Shear, J. G. Rabold, and P. Echeverria. 1993. Epidemiology of diarrhoeal illness associated with coccidian-like organism among travellers and foreign residents in Nepal. *Lancet* **341:**1175-9.

3382. Hogerzeil, H. V., W. J. Terpstra, A. De Geus, and H. Korver. 1986. Leptospirosis in rural Ghana. *Trop Geogr Med* **38:**162-6.

3383. Hohmann, H., S. Panzer, C. Phimpachan, C. Southivong, and F. P. Schelp. 2001. Relationship of intestinal parasites to the environment and to behavioral factors in children in the Bolikhamxay Province of Lao PDR. *Southeast Asian J Trop Med Public Health* **32**:4-13.

3384. Hoinville, L. J. 1996. A review of the epidemiology of scrapie in sheep. *Rev Sci Tech* **15**:827-52.

3385. Hoke, C. H., Jr. 2005. History of U.S. military contributions to the study of viral encephalitis. *Mil Med* **170**:92-105.

3386. Holaday, B., G. Waugh, V. E. Moukaddem, J. West, and S. Harshman. 1995. Fecal contamination in child day care centers: cloth vs paper diapers. *Am J Public Health* **85**:30-3.

3387. Holk, K., S. V. Nielsen, and T. Ronne. 2000. Human leptospirosis in Denmark 1970-1996: an epidemiological and clinical study. *Scand J Infect Dis* **32**:533-8.

3388. Holland, C., and A. K. Carruth. 2001. Exposure risks and tetanus immunization in women of family owned farms. Implications for occupational and environmental health nursing. *AAOHN J* **49**:130-6.

3389. Holland, C., O. C. P., M. R. H. Taylor, G. Hughes, R. W. A. Girdwood, and H. Smith. 1991. Families, parks, gardens and toxocariasis. *Scand J Infect Dis* **23**:225-31.

3390. Holland, C. V., S. O. Asaolu, D. W. Crompton, R. C. Stoddart, R. Macdonald, and S. E. Torimiro. 1989. The epidemiology of Ascaris lumbricoides and other soil-transmitted helminths in primary school children from Ile-Ife, Nigeria. *Parasitology* **99 Pt 2**:275-85.

3391. Holland, C. V., P. O'Lorcain, M. R. Taylor, and A. Kelly. 1995. Sero-epidemiology of toxocariasis in school children. *Parasitology* **110**:535-45.

3392. Holland, G. N. 1999. Reconsidering the pathogenesis of ocular toxoplasmosis. *Am J Ophthalmol* **128**:502-5.

3393. Hollifield, J. L., G. L. Cooper, and B. R. Charlton. 2000. An outbreak of erysipelas in 2-day-old poults. *Avian Dis* **44**:721-4.

3394. Hollyoak, V. A., and R. Freeman. 1995. Pseudomonas aeruginosa and whirlpool baths. *Lancet* **346**:644.

3395. Holman, M. S., D. A. Caporale, J. Goldberg, E. Lacombe, C. Lubelczyk, P. W. Rand, and R. P. Smith. 2004. Anaplasma phagocytophilum, Babesia microti, and Borrelia burgdorferi in Ixodes scapularis, southern coastal Maine. *Emerg Infect Dis* **10**:744-6.

3396. Holman, R. C., A. T. Curns, S. F. Kaufman, J. E. Cheek, R. W. Pinner, and L. B. Schonberger. 2001. Trends in infectious disease hospitalizations among American Indians and Alaska Natives. *Am J Public Health* **91**:425-31.

3397. Holmberg, M., J. N. Mills, S. McGill, G. Benjamin, and B. A. Ellis. 2003. Bartonella infection in sylvatic small mammals of central Sweden. *Epidemiol Infect* **130**:149-57.

3398. Holmes, G. P., J. K. Hilliard, K. C. Klontz, A. H. Rupert, C. M. Schindler, E. Parrish, D. G. Griffin, G. S. Ward, N. D. Bernstein, T. W. Bean, et al. 1990. B virus (Herpesvirus simiae) infection in humans: epidemiologic investigation of a cluster. *Ann Intern Med* **112**:833-9.

3399. Holmes, G. P., J. B. McCormick, S. C. Trock, R. A. Chase, S. M. Lewis, C. A. Mason, P. A. Hall, L. S. Brammer, G. I. Perez-Oronoz, M. K. McDonnell, et al. 1990. Lassa fever in the United States. Investigation of a case and new guidelines for management. *N Engl J Med* **323**:1120-3.

3400. Holmes, J. R., T. Plunkett, P. Pate, W. L. Roper, and W. J. Alexander. 1981. Emetic food poisoning caused by Bacillus cereus. *Arch Intern Med* **141**:766-7.

3401. Holmes, K. K., R. Levine, and M. Weaver. 2004. Effectiveness of condoms in preventing sexually transmitted infections. *Bull WHO* **82**:454-61.

3402. Holmes, K. V. 2003. SARS-associated coronavirus. *N Engl J Med* **348**:1948-51.

3403. Holmgren, E. B., and M. Forsgren. 1990. Epidemiology of tick-borne encephalitis in Sweden 1956-1989: a study of 1 116 cases. *Scand J Infect Dis* **22**:287-95.

3404. Holmstrom, L., B. Nyman, M. Rosengren, S. Wallander, and T. Ripa. 1990. Outbreaks of infections with erythromycin-resistant group A streptococci in child day care centres. *Scand J Infect Dis* **22**:179-85.

3405. Holness, D. L., J. G. DeKoven, and J. R. Nethercott. 1992. Scabies in chronic health care institutions. *Arch Dermatol* **128**:1257-60.

3406. Holsen, D. S., S. Harthug, and H. Myrmel. 1993. Prevalence of antibodies to hepatitis C virus and association with intravenous drug abuse and tattooing in a national prison in Norway. *Eur J Clin Microbiol Infect Dis* **12**:673-6.

3407. Holtby, I., G. M. Tebbutt, J. Green, J. Hedgeley, G. Weeks, and V. Ashton. 2001. Outbreak of Norwalk-like virus infection associated with salad provided in a restaurant. *Commun Dis Public Health* **4**:305-10.

3408. Holzer, B. R., Z. Glück, D. Zambelli, and M. Fey. 1985. Transmission of malaria by renal transplantation. *Transplantation* **39**:315-6.

3409. Holzmann, H. 2003. Diagnosis of tick-borne encephalitis. *Vaccine* **21 Suppl 1**:S36-40.

3410. Homer, M. J., I. Aguilar-Delfin, S. R. Telford, 3rd, P. J. Krause, and D. H. Persing. 2000. Babesiosis. *Clin Microbiol Rev* **13**:451-69.

3411. Honish, L., and K. Bergstrom. 2001. Hepatitis A infected food handler at an Edmonton, Alberta retail food facility: public health protection strategies. *Can Commun Dis Rep* **27**:177-180.

3412. Honish, L., and Q. Nguyen. 2001. Outbreak of Salmonella enteritidis phage type 913 gastroenteritis associated with mung bean sprouts—Edmonton, 2001. *Can Commun Dis Rep* **27**:151-6.

3413. Honish, L., G. Predy, N. Hislop, L. Chui, K. Kowalewska-Grochowska, L. Trottier, C. Kreplin, and I. Zazulak. 2005. An outbreak of E. coli O157:H7 hemorrhagic colitis associated with unpasteurized gouda cheese. *Can J Public Health* **96**:182-4.

3414. Hoogstraal, H. 1979. The epidemiology of tick-borne Crimean-Congo hemorrhagic fever in Asia, Europe, and Africa. *J Med Entomol* **15**:307-417.

3415. Hook, D., B. Jalaludin, and G. Fitzsimmons. 1996. Clostridium perfringens food-borne outbreak: an epidemiological investigation. *Aust N Z J Public Health* **20**:119-22.

3416. Hope Simpson, R. E. 1952. Infectiousness of communicable diseases in the household (measles, chickenpox, and mumps). *Lancet* **2**:549-54.

3417. Hopkins, A. S., J. Whitetail-Eagle, A. L. Corneli, B. Person, P. J. Ettestad, M. DiMenna, J. Norstog, J. Creswell, A. S. Khan, J. G. Olson, K. F. Cavallaro, R. T. Bryan, J. E. Cheek, B. Begay, G. A. Hoddenbach, T. G. Ksiazek, and J. N. Mills. 2002. Experimental evaluation of rodent exclusion methods to reduce hantavirus transmission to residents in a Native American community in New Mexico. *Vector Borne Zoonotic Dis* **2**:61-8.

3418. Hopkins, D. R., J. M. Lane, E. C. Cummings, and J. D. Millar. 1971. Two funeral-associated smallpox outbreaks in Sierra Leone. *Am J Epidemiol* **94**:341-7.

3419. Hopkins, D. R., E. Ruiz-Tiben, T. K. Ruebush, J. Diallo, A. Agle, and P. C. Withers, Jr. 2000. Dracunculiasis eradication: delayed, not denied. *Am J Trop Med Hyg* **62**:163-8.

3420. Hopkins, R. S., G. B. Gaspard, F. P. Williams, Jr., R. J. Karlin, G. Cukor, and N. R. Blacklow. 1984. A community waterborne gastroenteritis outbreak: evidence for rotavirus as the agent. *Am J Public Health* **74**:263-5.

3421. Hopkins, R. S., and D. D. Juranek. 1991. Acute giardiasis: an improved clinical case definition for epidemiological studies. *Am J Epidemiol* **133**:402-7.

3422. Hopperus Buma, A. P., P. P. van Thiel, H. O. Lobel, C. Ohrt, E. J. van Ameijden, R. L. Veltink, D. C. Tendeloo, T. van Gool, M. D. Green, G. D. Todd, D. E. Kyle, and P. A. Kager. 1996. Long-term malaria chemoprophylaxis with mefloquine in Dutch marines in Cambodia. *J Infect Dis* **173**:1506-9.

3423. Hoque, E., V. Hope, R. Scragg, M. Baker, and R. Shrestha. 2004. A descriptive epidemiology of giardiasis in New Zealand and gaps in surveillance data. *N Z Med J* **117**:U1149.

3424. Hoque, M. E., V. T. Hope, R. Scragg, T. Kjellstrom, and R. Lay-Yee. 2001. Nappy handling and risk of giardiasis. *Lancet* **357**:1017-8.

3425. Horak, I. G., J. L. Camicas, and J. E. Keirans. 2002. The Argasidae, Ixodidae and Nuttalliellidae (Acari: Ixodida): a world list of valid tick names. *Exp Appl Acarol* **28**:27-54.

3426. Horak, P., and L. Kolarova. 2001. Bird schistosomes: do they die in mammalian skin? *Trends Parasitol* **17**:66-9.

3427. Horby, P., R. Gilmour, H. C. Wang, and P. McIntyre. 2003. Progress towards eliminating Hib in Australia: an evaluation of Haemophilus influenzae type b prevention in Australia, 1 July 1993 to 30 June 2000. *Commun Dis Intell* **27**:324-41.

3428. Horiki, N., M. Maruyama, Y. Fujita, T. Yonekura, S. Minato, and Y. Kaneda. 1997. Epidemiologic survey of Blastocystis hominis infection in Japan. *Am J Trop Med Hyg* **56**:370-4.

3429. Horman, A., R. Rimhanen-Finne, L. Maunula, C. H. von Bonsdorff, N. Torvela, A. Heikinheimo, and M. L. Hanninen. 2004. Campylobacter spp., Giardia spp., Cryptosporidium spp., noroviruses, and indicator organisms in surface water in southwestern Finland, 2000-2001. *Appl Environ Microbiol* **70**:87-95.

3430. Hornick, R. B. 1985. Selective primary health care: strategies for control of disease in the developing world. XX. Typhoid fever. *Rev Infect Dis* **7**:536-46.

3431. Hornstrup, M. K., and B. Gahrn-Hansen. 1993. Extraintestinal infections caused by Vibrio parahaemolyticus and Vibrio alginolyticus in a Danish county, 1987-1992. *Scand J Infect Dis* **25**:735-40.

3432. Horowitz, H. W., E. Kilchevsky, S. Haber, M. Aguero-Rosenfeld, R. Kranwinkel, E. K. James, S. J. Wong, F. Chu, D. Liveris, and I. Schwartz. 1998. Perinatal transmission of the agent of human granulocytic ehrlichiosis. *N Engl J Med* **339**:375-8.

3433. Horre, R., G. Schumacher, K. Alpers, H. M. Seitz, S. Adler, K. Lemmer, G. S. De Hoog, K. P. Schaal, and K. Tintelno. 2002. A case of imported paracoccidioidomycosis in a German legionnaire. *Med Mycol* **40**:213-6.

3434. Horwitz, M. A., J. S. Marr, M. H. Merson, V. R. Dowell, and J. M. Ellis. 1975. A continuing common-source outbreak of botulism in a family. *Lancet* **ii**:861-3.

3435. Hosoglu, S., M. K. Celen, S. Akalin, M. F. Geyik, Y. Soyoral, and I. H. Kara. 2003. Transmission of hepatitis C by blood splash into conjunctiva in a nurse. *Am J Infect Control* **31**:502-4.

3436. Hospenthal, D. R., K. J. Kwon-Chung, and J. E. Bennett. 1998. Concentrations of airborne Aspergillus compared to the incidence of invasive aspergillosis: lack of correlation. *Med Mycol* **36**:165-8.

3437. Hossain, M. A., K. Z. Hasan, and M. J. Albert. 1994. Shigella carriers among non-diarrhoeal children in an endemic area of shigellosis in Bangladesh. *Trop Geogr Med* **46**:40-2.

3438. Hostetter, M. K., S. Iverson, W. Thomas, D. McKenzie, K. Dole, and D. E. Johnson. 1991. Medical evaluation of internationally adopted children. *N Engl J Med* **325**:479-85.

3439. Hota, B. 2004. Contamination, disinfection, and cross-colonization: are hospital surfaces reservoirs for nosocomial infection? *Clin Infect Dis* **39**:1182-9.

3440. Hotez, P. J., B. Zhan, J. M. Bethony, A. Loukas, A. Williamson, G. N. Goud, J. M. Hawdon, A. Dobardzic, R. Dobardzic, K. Ghosh, M. E. Bottazzi, S. Mendez, B. Zook, Y. Wang, S. Liu, I. Essiet-Gibson, S. Chung-Debose, S. Xiao, D. Knox, M. Meagher, M. Inan, R. Correa-Oliveira, P. Vilk, H. R. Shepherd, W. Brandt, and P. K. Russell. 2003. Progress in the development of a recombinant vaccine for human hookworm disease: the Human Hookworm Vaccine Initiative. *Int J Parasitol* **33**:1245-58.

3441. Hotez, P. J., F. Zheng, X. Long-qi, C. Ming-gang, X. Shu-hua, L. Shu-xian, D. Blair, D. P. McManus, and G. M. Davis. 1997. Emerging and reemerging helminthiases and the public health of China. *Emerg Infect Dis* **3**:303-10.

3442. Houang, E., D. Lam, D. Fan, and D. Seal. 2001. Microbial keratitis in Hong Kong: relationship to climate, environment and contact-lens disinfection. *Trans R Soc Trop Med Hyg* **95**:361-7.

3443. Houff, S. A., R. C. Burton, R. W. Wilson, T. E. Henson, W. T. London, G. M. Baer, L. J. Anderson, W. G. Winkler, D. L. Madden, and J. L. Sever. 1979. Human-to-human transmission of rabies virus by corneal transplant. *N Engl J Med* **300**:603-4.

3444. Houk, V. N. 1980. Spread of tuberculosis via recirculated air in a naval vessel: the Byrd study. *Ann N Y Acad Sci* **353**:10-24.

3445. Hove, T., and J. P. Dubey. 1999. Prevalence of Toxoplasma gondii antibodies in sera of domestic pigs and some wild game species from Zimbabwe. *J Parasitol* **85**:372-3.

3446. Howard, K., and T. J. Inglis. 2003. The effect of free chlorine on Burkholderia pseudomallei in potable water. *Water Res* **37**:4425-32.

3447. Howe, A. D., S. Forster, S. Morton, R. Marshall, K. S. Osborn, P. Wright, and P. R. Hunter. 2002. Cryptosporidium oocysts in a water supply associated with a cryptosporidiosis outbreak. *Emerg Infect Dis* **8**:619-24.

3448. Howe, C., A. Sampath, and M. Spotnitz. 1971. The pseudomallei group: a review. *J Infect Dis* **124**:598-606.

3449. Howie, H., A. Mukerjee, J. Cowden, J. Leith, and T. Reid. 2003. Investigation of an outbreak of Escherichia coli O157 infection caused by environmental exposure at a scout camp. *Epidemiol Infect* **131**:1063-9.

3450. Hoyos, C., J. Romero, J. Solari, and D. Garcia. 1990. [Botulism: the first epidemic outbreak in Peru]. *Rev Gastroenterol Peru* **10**:75-9.

3451. HPA (Health Protection Agency). 2004. Acinetobacter spp bacteremia, England, Wales, and Northern Ireland: 2003. *CDR Weekly* **14:**1-5.

3452. HPA. 2004. Candidaemia reports, England, Wales, and Northern Ireland: 2003. *CDR Weekly* **14:**1-3.

3453. HPA. 2004. Enterococcus spp bacteraemia: England, Wales, and Northern Ireland: 2003. *CDR Weekly* **14:**1-4.

3454. HPA. 2004. Escherichia coli bacteremias, England, Wales, and Northern Ireland: 2003. *CDR Weekly* **14:**1-4.

3455. HPA. 2004. Pseudomonas spp and Stenotrophomonas maltophilia bacteremia: England, Wales, and Northern Ireland: 2003. *CDR Weekly* **14:**1-7.

3456. HPA. 2004. Unusual infections associated with foreign travel - parts 1 to 4, and malaria. *CDR Weekly* **14.**

3457. HPA. 2004. Zoonoses report. United Kingdom 2002, p. 1-64, London.

3458. Hradil, E., K. Hersle, P. Nordin, and J. Faergemann. 1995. An epidemic of tinea corporis caused by Trichophyton tonsurans among wrestlers in Sweden. *Acta Derm Venereol* **75:**305-6.

3459. Hristea, A., S. Hristescu, C. Ciufecu, and A. Vasile. 2001. Seroprevalence of Borrelia burgdorferi in Romania. *Eur J Epidemiol* **17:**891-6.

3460. Hsieh, H. I., J. D. Wang, P. C. Chen, and T. J. Cheng. 2003. Synergistic effect of hepatitis virus infection and occupational exposures to vinyl chloride monomer and ethylene dichloride on serum aminotransferase activity. *Occup Environ Med* **60:**774-8.

3461. Hsieh, Y. H., L. D. Bobo, T. C. Quinn, and S. K. West. 2000. Risk factors for trachoma: 6-year follow-up of children aged 1 and 2 years. *Am J Epidemiol* **152:**204-11.

3462. Hsiung, G. D., and J. R. Wang. 2000. Enterovirus infections with special reference to enterovirus 71. *J Microbiol Immunol Infect* **33:**1-8.

3463. Hsu, V. P., M. J. Hossain, U. D. Parashar, M. M. Ali, T. G. Ksiazek, I. Kuzmin, M. Niezgoda, C. Rupprecht, J. Bresee, and R. F. Breiman. 2004. Nipah virus encephalitis reemergence, Bangladesh. *Emerg Infect Dis* **10:**2082-7.

3464. Hsueh, P. R., C. Y. Lin, H. J. Tang, H. C. Lee, J. W. Liu, Y. C. Liu, and Y. C. Chuang. 2004. Vibrio vulnificus in Taiwan. *Emerg Infect Dis* **10:**1363-8.

3465. Hsueh, P. R., L. J. Teng, P. I. Lee, P. C. Yang, L. M. Huang, S. C. Chang, C. Y. Lee, and K. T. Luh. 1997. Outbreak of scarlet fever at a hospital day care centre: analysis of strain relatedness with phenotypic and genotypic characteristics. *J Hosp Infect* **36:**191-200.

3466. Hsueh, P. R., L. J. Teng, P. C. Yang, H. L. Pan, S. W. Ho, and K. T. Luh. 1999. Nosocomial pseudoepidemic caused by Bacillus cereus traced to contaminated ethyl alcohol from a liquor factory. *J Clin Microbiol* **37:**2280-4.

3467. Hu, Z. 1991. [Observation on prevention of hepatitis B virus transmission between newly-married couples by HBsAg vaccine]. *Zhonghua Liu Xing Bing Xue Za Zhi* **12:**222-5.

3468. Huang, J. J., W. C. Lee, M. K. Ruaan, M. C. Wang, T. T. Chang, and K. C. Young. 2001. Incidence, transmission, and clinical significance of hepatitis G virus infection in hemodialysis patients. *Eur J Clin Microbiol Infect Dis* **20:**374-9.

3469. Huang, P., J. T. Weber, D. M. Sosin, P. M. Griffin, E. G. Long, J. J. Murphy, F. Kocka, C. Peters, and C. Kallick. 1995. The first reported outbreak of diarrheal illness associated with Cyclospora in the United States. *Ann Intern Med* **123:**409-14.

3470. Huang, Q. S., J. M. Carr, W. A. Nix, M. S. Oberste, D. R. Kilpatrick, M. A. Pallansch, M. C. Croxson, J. A. Lindeman, M. G. Baker, and K. Grimwood. 2003. An echovirus type 33 winter outbreak in New Zealand. *Clin Infect Dis* **37:**650-7.

3471. Hubalek, Z., and J. Halouzka. 1999. West Nile fever—a reemerging mosquito-borne viral disease in Europe. *Emerg Infect Dis* **5:**643-50.

3472. Hubalek, Z., W. Sixl, and J. Halouzka. 1998. Francisella tularensis in Dermacentor reticulatus ticks from the Czech Republic and Austria. *Wien Klin Wochenschr* **110:**909-10.

3473. Hubalek, Z., W. Sixl, M. Mikulaskova, B. Sixl-Voigt, W. Thiel, J. Halouzka, Z. Juricova, B. Rosicky, L. Matlova, and M. Honza. 1995. Salmonellae in gulls and other free-living birds in the Czech Republic. *Cent Eur J Public Health* **3:**21-4.

3474. Hubalek, Z., F. Treml, J. Halouzka, Z. Juricova, M. Hunady, and V. Janik. 1996. Frequent isolation of Francisella tularensis from Dermacentor reticulatus ticks in an enzootic focus of tularaemia. *Med Vet Entomol* **10:**241-6.

3475. Hubalek, Z., P. Zeman, J. Halouzka, Z. Juricova, E. Stovickova, H. Balkova, S. Sikutova, and I. Rudolf. 2005. Mosquitoborne viruses, Czech Republic, 2002. *Emerg Infect Dis* **11:**116-8.

3476. Hubert, B., J. Bacou, and H. Belveze. 1989. Epidemiology of human anisakiasis: incidence and sources in France. *Am J Trop Med Hyg* **40:**301-3.

3477. Hudde, T., T. Reinhard, M. Moller, C. Schelle, H. Spelsberg, A. Cepin, and R. Sundmacher. 1997. [Corneoscleral transplant excision in the cadaver. Experiences of the North Rhine Westphalia Lions Cornea Bank 1995 and 1996]. *Ophthalmologe* **94:**780-4.

3478. Hudnall, S. D. 2004. Crazy 8: unraveling human herpesvirus 8 seroprevalence. *Clin Infect Dis* **39:**1059-61.

3479. Hudson, B. J., R. McPetrie, J. Kitchener-Smith, and J. Eccles. 1994. Vesicular rash associated with infection due to Rickettsia australis. *Clin Infect Dis* **18:**118-9.

3480. Hudson, J. A., S. J. Mott, K. M. Delacy, and A. L. Edridge. 1992. Incidence and coincidence of Listeria spp., motile aeromonads and Yersinia enterocolitica on ready-to-eat fleshfoods. *Int J Food Microbiol* **16:**99-108.

3481. Hudspeth, M. K., T. C. Smith, C. P. Barrozo, A. W. Hawksworth, M. A. Ryan, and G. C. Gray. 2001. National Department of Defense Surveillance for Invasive Streptococcus pneumoniae: antibiotic resistance, serotype distribution, and arbitrarily primed polymerase chain reaction analyses. *J Infect Dis* **184:**591-6.

3482. Huerga, H., and R. Lopez-Velez. 2002. Infectious diseases in sub-Saharan African immigrant children in Madrid, Spain. *Pediatr Infect Dis J* **21:**830-4.

3483. Huerta, M., I. Grotto, M. Gdalevich, D. Mimouni, B. Gavrieli, M. Yavzori, D. Cohen, and O. Shpilberg. 2000. A waterborne outbreak of gastroenteritis in the Golan Heights due to enterotoxigenic Escherichia coli. *Infection* **28:**267-71.

3484. Hueston, L., A. Yund, S. Cope, M. Monteville, M. Marchetti, J. Haniotis, J. Clancy, S. Doggett, R. Russell, D. Dwyer, and G. Parker. 1997. Ross river virus in a joint military exercise. *Commun Dis Intell* **21:**193.

3485. Huff, J. L., and P. A. Barry. 2003. B-virus (Cercopithecine herpesvirus 1) infection in humans and macaques: potential for zoonotic disease. *Emerg Infect Dis* **9:**246-50.

3486. Hughes, G., T. Paine, and D. Thomas. 2001. Surveillance of sexually transmitted infections in England and Wales. *Eurosurveillance* **6:**71-81.

3487. **Hughes, J. M., J. M. Boyce, A. R. M. A. Aleem, J. G. Wells, A. S. Rahman, and G. T. Curlin.** 1978. Vibrio parahaemolyticus enterocolitis in Bangladesh: report of an outbreak. *Am J Trop Med Hyg* **27:**106-12.

3488. **Hugot, J. P., K. J. Reinhard, S. L. Gardner, and S. Morand.** 1999. Human enterobiasis in evolution: origin, specificity and transmission. *Parasite* **6:**201-8.

3489. **Huhn, G. D., B. Adam, R. Ruden, L. Hilliard, P. Kirkpatrick, J. Todd, W. Crafts, D. Passaro, and M. S. Dworkin.** 2005. Outbreak of Travel-Related Pontiac Fever among Hotel Guests Illustrating the Need for Better Diagnostic Tests. *J Travel Med* **12:**173-9.

3490. **Hui, A. Y., L. C. Hung, P. C. Tse, W. K. Leung, P. K. Chan, and H. L. Chan.** 2005. Transmission of hepatitis B by human bite—confirmation by detection of virus in saliva and full genome sequencing. *J Clin Virol* **33:**254-6.

3491. **Huilan, S., L. G. Zhen, M. M. Mathan, M. M. Mathew, J. Olarte, R. Espejo, U. Khin Maung, M. A. Ghafoor, M. A. Khan, Z. Sami, et al.** 1991. Etiology of acute diarrhoea among children in developing countries: a multicentre study in five countries. *Bull WHO* **69:**549-55.

3492. **Huisa, B. N., L. A. Menacho, S. Rodriguez, J. A. Bustos, R. H. Gilman, V. C. Tsang, A. E. Gonzalez, and H. H. Garcia.** 2005. Taeniasis and Cysticercosis in Housemaids Working in Affluent Neighborhoods in Lima, Peru. *Am J Trop Med Hyg* **73:**496-500.

3493. **Hujakka, H., V. Koistinen, I. Kuronen, P. Eerikainen, M. Parviainen, A. Lundkvist, A. Vaheri, O. Vapalahti, and A. Narvanen.** 2003. Diagnostic rapid tests for acute hantavirus infections: specific tests for Hantaan, Dobrava and Puumala viruses versus a hantavirus combination test. *J Virol Methods* **108:**117-22.

3494. **Hukic, M., A. Kurt, S. Torstensson, A. Lundkvist, D. Wiger, and B. Niklasson.** 1996. Haemorrhagic fever with renal syndrome in north-east Bosnia. *Lancet* **347:**56-7.

3495. **Huminer, D., K. Symon, I. Groskopf, D. Pietrushka, I. Kremer, P. M. Schantz, and S. D. Pitlik.** 1992. Seroepidemiologic study of toxocariasis and strongyloidiasis in institutionalized mentally retarded adults. *Am J Trop Med Hyg* **46:**278-81.

3496. **Humphries, D. L., L. S. Stephenson, E. J. Pearce, P. H. The, H. T. Dan, and L. T. Khanh.** 1997. The use of human faeces for fertilizer is associated with increased intensity of hookworm infection in Vietnamese women. *Trans R Soc Trop Med Hyg* **91:**518-20.

3497. **Hundy, R. L., and S. Cameron.** 2002. An outbreak of infections with a new Salmonella phage type linked to a symptomatic food handler. *Commun Dis Intell* **26:**562-7.

3498. **Hundy, R. L., and S. Cameron.** 2004. Risk factors for sporadic human infection with shiga toxin-producing Escherichia coli in South Australia. *Commun Dis Intell* **28:**74-9.

3499. **Hunfeld, K. P., A. Lambert, H. Kampen, S. Albert, C. Epe, V. Brade, and A. M. Tenter.** 2002. Seroprevalence of Babesia infections in humans exposed to ticks in midwestern Germany. *J Clin Microbiol* **40:**2431-6.

3500. **Hunfeld, K. P., C. Schmidt, B. Krackhardt, H. G. Posselt, J. Bargon, Y. Yahaf, V. Schafer, V. Brade, and T. A. Wichelhaus.** 2000. Risk of Pseudomonas aeruginosa cross-colonisation in patients with cystic fibrosis within a holiday camp—a molecular-epidemiological study. *Wien Klin Wochenschr* **112:**329-33.

3501. **Hung, T., G. M. Chen, C. G. Wang, H. L. Yao, Z. Y. Fang, T. X. Chao, Z. Y. Chou, W. Ye, X. J. Chang, and S. S. Den.** 1984. Waterborne outbreak of rotavirus diarrhoea in adults in China caused by a novel rotavirus. *Lancet* **1:**1139-42.

3502. **Hunter, L., C. G. Smith, and J. N. MacCormack.** 1994. Brucellosis outbreak at a pork processing plant - North Carolina, 1992. *MMWR* **43:**113-6.

3503. **Hunter, P. R., J. M. Colford, M. W. LeChevallier, S. Binder, and P. S. Berger.** 2001. Waterborne diseases. *Emerg Infect Dis* **7(3):**544.

3504. **Hunter, P. R., G. A. Harrison, and C. A. Fraser.** 1990. Cross-infection and diversity of Candida albicans strain carriage in patients and nursing staff on an intensive care unit. *J Med Vet Mycol* **28:**317-25.

3505. **Hunter, P. R., S. Hughes, S. Woodhouse, Q. Syed, N. Q. Verlander, R. M. Chalmers, K. Morgan, G. Nichols, N. Beeching, and K. Osborn.** 2004. Sporadic cryptosporidiosis case-control study with genotyping. *Emerg Infect Dis* **10:**1241-9.

3506. **Hupertz, V. F., and R. Wyllie.** 2003. Perinatal hepatitis C infection. *Pediatr Infect Dis J* **22:**369-72.

3507. **Huppertz, H. I.** 1986. An epidemic of bacillary dysentery in western Rwanda 1981-1982. *Cent Afr J Med* **32:**79-82.

3508. **Huppertz, H. I., S. Rutkowski, S. Aleksic, and H. Karch.** 1997. Acute and chronic diarrhoea and abdominal colic associated with enteroaggregative Escherichia coli in young children living in western Europe. *Lancet* **349:**1660-2.

3509. **Huq, A., and R. R. Colwell.** 1995. Vibrios in the marine and estuarine environments. *J Mar Biotechnol* **3:**60-3.

3510. **Hurnikova, Z., V. Snabel, E. Pozio, K. Reiterova, G. Hrckova, D. Halasova, and P. Dubinsky.** 2005. First record of Trichinella pseudospiralis in the Slovak Republic found in domestic focus. *Vet Parasitol* **128:**91-8.

3511. **Hurtig, A. K., A. Nicoll, C. Carne, T. Lissauer, N. Connor, J. P. Webster, and L. Ratcliffe.** 1998. Syphilis in pregnant women and their children in the United Kingdom: results from national clinician reporting surveys 1994-7. *BMJ* **317:**1617-9.

3512. **Hurwitz, E. S., M. Haber, A. Chang, T. Shope, S. Teo, M. Ginsberg, N. Waecker, and N. J. Cox.** 2000. Effectiveness of influenza vaccination of day care children in reducing influenza-related morbidity among household contacts. *JAMA* **284:**1677-82.

3513. **Hurwitz, E. S., M. Haber, A. Chang, T. Shope, S. T. Teo, J. S. Giesick, M. M. Ginsberg, and N. J. Cox.** 2000. Studies of the 1996-1997 inactivated influenza vaccine among children attending day care: immunologic response, protection against infection, and clinical effectiveness. *J Infect Dis* **182:**1218-21.

3514. **Husain, S., M. M. Wagener, and N. Singh.** 2001. Cryptococcus neoformans infection in organ transplant recipients: variables influencing clinical characteristics and outcome. *Emerg Infect Dis* **7:**375-81.

3515. **Hussain, A. I., V. Shanmugam, W. M. Switzer, S. X. Tsang, A. Fadly, D. Thea, R. Helfand, W. J. Bellini, T. M. Folks, and W. Heneine.** 2001. Lack of evidence of endogenous avian leukosis virus and endogenous avian retrovirus transmission to measles, mumps, and rubella vaccine recipients. *Emerg Infect Dis* **7:**66-72.

3516. **Hutchins, S. S., M. J. Papania, R. Amler, E. F. Maes, M. Grabowsky, K. Bromberg, V. Glasglow, T. Speed, W. J. Bellini, and W. A. Orenstein.** 2004. Evaluation of the measles clinical case definition. *J Infect Dis* **189 Suppl 1:**153-9.

3517. **Hutchinson, O. C., E. M. Fevre, M. Carrington, and S. C. Welburn.** 2003. Lessons learned from the emergence of a new Trypanosoma brucei rhodesiense sleeping sickness focus in Uganda. *Lancet Infect Dis* **3:**42-5.

3518. **Hutchinson, S. J., D. J. Goldberg, S. M. Gore, S. Cameron, J. McGregor, J. McMenamin, and J. McGavigan.** 1998. Hepatitis B outbreak at Glenochil prison during January to June 1993. *Epidemiol Infect* **121:**185-91.

3519. **Hutin, Y. J., A. M. Hauri, and G. L. Armstrong.** 2003. Use of injections in healthcare settings worldwide, 2000: literature review and regional estimates. *BMJ* **327:**1075.

3520. **Hutin, Y. J., D. Legros, V. Owini, V. Brown, E. Lee, D. Mbulamberi, and C. Paquet.** 2004. Trypanosoma Brucei Gambiense Trypanosomiasis in Terego County, Northern Uganda, 1996: A Lot Quality Assurance Sampling Survey. *Am J Trop Med Hyg* **70:**390-394.

3521. **Hutin, Y. J., M. N. Sombardier, O. Liguory, C. Sarfati, F. Derouin, J. Modai, and J. M. Molina.** 1998. Risk factors for intestinal microsporidiosis in patients with human immunodeficiency virus infection: a case-control study. *J Infect Dis* **178:**904-7.

3522. **Hutin, Y. J. F., V. Pool, E. H. Cramer, O. V. Nainan, J. Weth, I. T. Williams, S. T. Goldstein, K. F. Gensheimer, B. P. Bell, C. N. Shapiro, M. J. Alter, and H. S. Margolis.** 1999. A multistate, foodborne outbreak of hepatitis A. *N Engl J Med* **340:**595-602.

3523. **Hutto, C., R. Ricks, M. Garvie, and R. F. Pass.** 1985. Epidemiology of cytomegalovirus infections in young children: day care vs. home care. *Pediatr Infect Dis* **4:**149-152.

3524. **Hutton, M. D., W. W. Stead, G. M. Cauthen, A. B. Bloch, and W. M. Ewing.** 1990. Nosocomial transmission of tuberculosis associated with a draining abscess. *J Infect Dis* **161:**286-95.

3525. **Hwang, K. P., and E. R. Chen.** 1991. Clinical studies on angiostrongyliasis cantonensis among children in Taiwan. *Southeast Asian J Trop Med Public Health* **22** (**suppl**)**:**194-9.

3526. **Hwang, S. W., T. J. Svoboda, I. J. De Jong, K. J. Kabasele, and E. Gogosis.** 2005. Bed bug infestations in an urban environment. *Emerg Infect Dis* **11:**533-8.

3527. **Hyams, K. C., A. L. Bourgeois, B. R. Merrell, P. Rozmajzl, J. Escamilla, S. A. Thornton, G. M. Wasserman, A. Burke, P. Echeverria, K. Y. Green, et al.** 1991. Diarrheal disease during Operation Desert Shield. *N Engl J Med* **325:**1423-8.

3528. **Hyams, K. C., J. Riddle, M. Rubertone, D. Trump, M. J. Alter, D. F. Cruess, X. Han, O. V. Nainam, L. B. Seeff, J. F. Mazzuchi, and S. Bailey.** 2001. Prevalence and incidence of hepatitis C virus infection in the US military: a seroepidemiologic survey of 21,000 troops. *Am J Epidemiol* **153:**764-70.

3529. **Hyams, K. C., J. Riddle, D. H. Trump, and J. T. Graham.** 2001. Endemic infectious diseases and biological warfare during the gulf war: a decade of analysis and final concerns. *Am J Trop Med Hyg* **65:**664-670.

3530. **Hyams, K. C., D. N. Taylor, G. C. Gray, J. B. Knowles, R. Hawkins, and J. D. Malone.** 1995. The risk of Helicobacter pylori infection among U.S. military personnel deployed outside the United States. *Am J Trop Med Hyg* **52:**109-12.

3531. **Hyde, S. R., and K. Benirschke.** 1997. Gestational psittacosis: case report and literature review. *Mod Pathol* **10:**602-7.

3532. **Hyde, T. B., M. Gilbert, S. B. Schwartz, E. R. Zell, J. P. Watt, W. L. Thacker, D. F. Talkington, and R. E. Besser.** 2001. Azithromycin prophylaxis during a hospital outbreak of Mycoplasma pneumoniae pneumonia. *J Infect Dis* **183:**907-12.

3533. **Hyde, T. B., T. M. Hilger, A. Reingold, M. M. Farley, K. L. O'Brien, and A. Schuchat.** 2002. Trends in incidence and antimicrobial resistance of early-onset sepsis: population-based surveillance in San Francisco and Atlanta. *Pediatrics* **110:**690-5.

3534. **Hyer, R. N., M. R. Howell, M. A. K. Ryan, and J. C. Gaydos.** 2000. Cost-effectiveness analysis of reacquiring and using adenovirus types 4 and 7 vaccines in naval recruits. *Am J Trop Med Hyg* **62:**613-618.

3535. **Hyman, I.** 2004. Setting the stage: reviewing current knowledge on the health of Canadian immigrants: what is the evidence and where are the gaps? *Can J Public Health* **95:**I4-8.

3536. **Hyytiä, E., s. Hielm, and H. Korkeala.** 1998. Prevalence of Clostridium botulinum type E in Finnish fish and fishery products. *Epidemiol Infect* **120:**245-50.

3537. **Ibara, A. S., P. Marcorelles, M. T. Le Martelot, N. Touffet, E. Moalic, G. Hery-Arnaud, J. D. Giroux, and A. M. Le Flohic.** 2004. Two cases of systemic Candida glabrata infection following in vitro fertilization and embryo transfer. *Eur J Clin Microbiol Infect Dis* **23:**53-6.

3538. **Iborra, C., M. Danis, F. Bricaire, and E. Caumes.** 1999. A traveler returning from Central Africa with fever and a skin lesion. *Clin Infect Dis* **28:**679-80.

3539. **Ibrahim, I. N., T. Okabayashi, Ristiyanto, E. W. Lestari, T. Yanase, Y. Muramatsu, H. Ueno, and C. Morita.** 1999. Serosurvey of wild rodents for rickettsioses (spotted fever, murine typhus and Q fever) in Java island, Indonesia. *Eur J Epidemiol* **15:**89-93.

3540. **Iddawela, D. R., P. V. Kumarasiri, and M. S. de Wijesundera.** 2003. A seroepidemiological study of toxocariasis and risk factors for infection in children in Sri Lanka. *Southeast Asian J Trop Med Public Health* **34:**7-15.

3541. **Idesawa, M., N. Sugano, K. Ikeda, M. Oshikawa, M. Takane, K. Seki, and K. Ito.** 2004. Detection of Epstein-Barr virus in saliva by real-time PCR. *Oral Microbiol Immunol* **19:**230-2.

3542. **Iijima, Y., J. O. Oundo, K. Taga, S. M. Saidi, and T. Honda.** 1995. Simultaneous outbreak due to Vibrio cholerae and Shigella dysenteriae in Kenya. *Lancet* **345:**69-70.

3543. **Iivanainen, E., P. J. Martikainen, P. Vaananen, and M. L. Katila.** 1999. Environmental factors affecting the occurrence of mycobacteria in brook sediments. *J Appl Microbiol* **86:**673-81.

3544. **Iivanainen, E., J. Northrup, R. D. Arbeit, M. Ristola, M. L. Katila, and C. F. von Reyn.** 1999. Isolation of mycobacteria from indoor swimming pools in Finland. *APMIS* **107:**193-200.

3545. **Ijaz, K., J. A. Dillaha, Z. Yang, M. D. Cave, and J. H. Bates.** 2002. Unrecognized tuberculosis in a nursing home causing death with spread of tuberculosis to the community. *J Am Geriatr Soc* **50:**1213-8.

3546. **Ijaz, S., E. Arnold, M. Banks, R. P. Bendall, M. E. Cramp, R. Cunningham, H. R. Dalton, T. J. Harrison, S. F. Hill, L. Macfarlane, R. E. Meigh, S. Shafi, M. J. Sheppard, J. Smithson, M. P. Wilson, and C. G. Teo.** 2005. Non-travel-associated hepatitis e in England and wales: demographic, clinical, and molecular epidemiological characteristics. *J Infect Dis* **192:**1166-72.

3547. **Ijumba, J. N., F. C. Shenton, S. E. Clarke, F. W. Mosha, and S. W. Lindsay.** 2002. Irrigated crop production is associated with less malaria than traditional agricultural practices in Tanzania. *Trans R Soc Trop Med Hyg* **96:**476-80.

3548. **Ikeda, R. M., S. F. Kondracki, P. D. Drabkin, G. S. Birkhead, and D. L. Morse.** 1993. Pleurodynia among football players at a high school. An outbreak associated with coxsackievirus B1. *JAMA* **270**:2205-6.

3549. **Ilef, D., A. Infuso, N. Crowcroft, and B. Le Guenno.** 1999. Facteurs de risque de l'infection à hantavirus: une enquête cas-témoins dans les Ardennes belges et françaises. *Bull Epidémiol Hebdomadaire* **8**:30-31.

3550. **Imbert, P., C. Rapp, M. Jagou, A. Saillol, and T. Debord.** 2004. Q fever in travelers: 10 cases. *J Travel Med* **11**:383-5.

3551. **Imrey, P. B., L. A. Jackson, P. H. Ludwinski, A. C. England, 3rd, G. A. Fella, B. C. Fox, L. B. Isdale, M. W. Reeves, and J. D. Wenger.** 1996. Outbreak of serogroup C meningococcal disease associated with campus bar patronage. *Am J Epidemiol* **143**:624-30.

3552. **INCISO.** 2001. Surveillance de l'incidence des infections du site opératoire: analyse et tendances dans le réseau Inciso entre 1998 et 2000. *Bull Epidémiol Hebdomadaire* **25**(19 Jun):1–3.

3553. **Inglesby, T. V., D. T. Dennis, D. A. Henderson, J. G. Bartlett, M. S. Ascher, E. Eitzen, A. D. Fine, A. M. Friedlander, J. Hauer, J. F. Koerner, M. Layton, J. McDade, M. T. Osterholm, T. O'Toole, G. Parker, T. M. Perl, P. K. Russell, M. Schoch-Spana, and K. Tonat.** 2000. Plague as a biological weapon: medical and public health management. Working Group on Civilian Biodefense. *JAMA* **283**:2281-90.

3554. **Inglesby, T. V., D. A. Henderson, J. G. Bartlett, M. S. Ascher, E. Eitzen, A. M. Friedlander, J. Hauer, J. McDade, M. T. Osterholm, T. O'Toole, G. Parker, T. M. Perl, P. K. Russell, and K. Tonat.** 1999. Anthrax as a biological weapon: medical and public health management. Working Group on Civilian Biodefense. *JAMA* **281**:1735-45.

3555. **Inglesby, T. V., T. O'Toole, D. A. Henderson, J. G. Bartlett, M. S. Ascher, E. Eitzen, A. M. Friedlander, J. Gerberding, J. Hauer, J. Hughes, J. McDade, M. T. Osterholm, G. Parker, T. M. Perl, P. K. Russell, and K. Tonat.** 2002. Anthrax as a biological weapon, 2002. Updated recommendations for management. *JAMA* **287**:2236-52.

3556. **Inglis, T. J. J., S. C. Garrow, M. Henderson, A. Clair, J. Sampson, L. O'Reilly, and B. Cameron.** 2000. Burkholderia pseudomallei traced to water treatment plant in Australia. *Emerg Infect Dis* **6**:56-9.

3557. **Ingordo, V., L. Naldi, S. Fracchiolla, and B. Colecchia.** 2004. Prevalence and risk factors for superficial fungal infections among Italian Navy Cadets. *Dermatology* **209**:190-6.

3558. **Inokuma, H., Y. Yoshizaki, Y. Shimada, Y. Sakata, M. Okuda, and T. Onishi.** 2003. Epidemiological survey of Babesia species in Japan performed with specimens from ticks collected from dogs and detection of new Babesia DNA closely related to Babesia odocoilei and Babesia divergens DNA. *J Clin Microbiol* **41**:3494-8.

3559. **Inouye, S., K. Yamashita, S. Yamadera, M. Yoshikawa, N. Kato, and N. Okabe.** 2000. Surveillance of viral gastroenteritis in Japan: pediatric cases and outbreak incidents. *J Infect Dis* **181 suppl 2**:S270-S274.

3560. **Insulander, M., M. Lebbad, T. A. Stenstrom, and B. Svenungsson.** 2005. An outbreak of cryptosporidiosis associated with exposure to swimming pool water. *Scand J Infect Dis* **37**:354-60.

3561. **Ip, F. K., and S. P. Chow.** 1992. Mycobacterium fortuitum infections of the hand. Report of five cases. *J Hand Surg [Br]* **17**:675-7.

3562. **Ippolito, G., V. Puro, and G. De Carli.** 1993. The risk of occupational human immunodeficiency virus infection in health care workers. Italian Multicenter Study. The Italian Study Group on Occupational Risk of HIV infection. *Arch Intern Med* **153**:1451-8.

3563. **Ippolito, G., V. Puro, N. Petrosillo, G. De Carli, G. Micheloni, and E. Magliano.** 1998. Simultaneous infection with HIV and hepatitis C virus following occupational conjunctival blood exposure. *JAMA* **280**:28.

3564. **Iqbal, M., A. Ahmed, A. Qamar, K. Dixon, J. F. Duncan, N. U. Islam, A. Rauf, J. P. Bryan, I. A. Malik, and L. J. Legters.** 1989. An outbreak of enterically transmitted non-A, non-B hepatitis in Pakistan. *Am J Trop Med Hyg* **40**:438-43.

3565. **Iritani, N., Y. Seto, K. Haruki, M. Kimura, M. Ayata, and H. Ogura.** 2000. Major change in the predominant type of "Norwalk-like viruses" in outbreaks of acute nonbacterial gastroenteritis in Osaka City, Japan, between April 1996 and March 1999. *J Clin Microbiol* **38**:2649-54.

3566. **Ironside, J. W., D. A. Hilton, A. Ghani, N. J. Johnston, L. Conyers, L. M. McCardle, and D. Best.** 2000. Retrospective study of prion-protein accumulation in tonsil and appendix tissues. *Lancet* **355**:1693-4.

3567. **Irwin, D. J., J. G. Crawshaw, R. A. Readman, L. Teare, and E. B. Kaczmarski.** 2000. Carriage of Neisseria meningitidis in residents and staff at a residential home for elderly people following a case of invasive disease. *Commun Dis Public Health* **3**:172-4.

3568. **Irwin, P. J., and R. Jefferies.** 2004. Arthropod-transmitted diseases of companion animals in Southeast Asia. *Trends Parasitol* **20**:27-34.

3569. **Irwin, R. S., R. R. Demers, M. R. Pratter, F. L. Garrity, G. Miner, A. Pritchard, and S. Whitaker.** 1980. An outbreak of acinetobacter infection associated with the use of a ventilator spirometer. *Respir Care* **25**:232-7.

3570. **Isaac-Renton, J. L., L. F. Lewis, C. S. Ong, and M. F. Nulsen.** 1994. A second community outbreak of waterborne giardiasis in Canada and serological investigation of patients. *Trans R Soc Trop Med Hyg* **88**:395-9.

3571. **Isaacs, D.** 2003. A ten year, multicentre study of coagulase negative staphylococcal infections in Australasian neonatal units. *Arch Dis Child Fetal Neonatal Ed* **88**:F89-93.

3572. **Isaacson, M.** 1989. Airport malaria: a review. *Bull WHO* **67**:737-43.

3573. **Isaacson, M., J. Frean, J. He, J. Seriwatana, and B. L. Innis.** 2000. An outbreak of hepatitis E in Northern Namibia, 1983. *Am J Trop Med Hyg* **62**:619-25.

3574. **Isaacson, M., and J. A. Frean.** 2001. African malaria vectors in European aircraft. *Lancet* **357**:235.

3575. **Isakbaeva, E. T., N. Khetsuriani, R. S. Beard, A. Peck, D. Erdman, S. S. Monroe, S. Tong, T. G. Ksiazek, S. Lowther, I. Pandya-Smith, L. J. Anderson, J. Lingappa, and M. A. Widdowson.** 2004. SARS-associated coronavirus transmission, United States. *Emerg Infect Dis* **10**:225-31.

3576. **Isakbaeva, E. T., M. A. Widdowson, R. S. Beard, S. N. Bulens, J. Mullins, S. S. Monroe, J. Bresee, P. Sassano, E. H. Cramer, and R. I. Glass.** 2005. Norovirus transmission on cruise ship. *Emerg Infect Dis* **11**:154-8.

3577. **Isenbarger, D. W., L. Bodhidatta, C. W. Hoge, W. Nirdnoy, C. Pitarangsi, U. Umpawasiri, and P. Echeverria.** 1998. Prospective study of the incidence of diarrheal disease and Helicobacter pylori infection among children in an orphanage in Thailand. *Am J Trop Med Hyg* **59**:796-800.

3578. **Ishi, K., F. Suzuku, A. Saito, S. Yoshimoto, and T. Kubota.** 2001. Prevalence of human immunodeficiency virus, hepatitis B and hepatitis C virus antibodies and hepatitis B antigen among commercial sex workers in Japan. *Infect Dis Obstet Gynecol* **9:**215-9.

3579. **Ishida, K., T. Kubota, S. Matsuda, H. Sugaya, M. Manabe, and K. Yoshimura.** 2003. A human case of gnathostomiasis nipponica confirmed indirectly by finding infective larvae in leftover largemouth bass meat. *J Parasitol* **89:**407-9.

3580. **Ishihara, S., M. Yasuda, S. Ito, S. Maeda, and T. Deguchi.** 2004. Mycoplasma genitalium urethritis in men. *Int J Antimicrob Agents* **24 Suppl 1:**S23-7.

3581. **Ishikawa, K., K. Matsui, T. Madarame, S. Sato, K. Oikawa, and T. Uchida.** 1995. Hepatitis E probably contracted via a Chinese herbal medicine, demonstrated by nucleotide sequencing. *J Gastroenterol* **30:**534-8.

3582. **Ishiwata, K., S. P. Diaz Camacho, Amrozi, Y. Horii, N. Nawa, and Y. Nawa.** 1998. Gnathostomiasis in wild boars from Japan. *J Wildl Dis* **34:**155-7.

3583. **Ishizuka, T., and A. Ishizuka.** 1986. A case of diphyllobothriasis due to eating masou-sushi. *Med J Aust* **145:**114.

3584. **Islam, M., M. P. Doyle, S. C. Phatak, P. Millner, and X. Jiang.** 2004. Persistence of enterohemorrhagic Escherichia coli O157:H7 in soil and on leaf lettuce and parsley grown in fields treated with contaminated manure composts or irrigation water. *J Food Prot* **67:**1365-70.

3585. **Isonhood, J. H., and M. Drake.** 2002. Aeromonas species in foods. *J Food Prot* **65:**575-82.

3586. **Israele, V., P. Shirley, and J. W. Sixbey.** 1991. Excretion of the Epstein-Barr virus from the genital tract of men. *J Infect Dis* **163:**1341-3.

3587. **Israil, A., N. Nacescu, C. L. Cedru, C. Ciufecu, and M. Damian.** 1998. Changes in Vibrio cholerae O1 strains isolated in Romania during 1977-95. *Epidemiol Infect* **121:**253-8.

3588. **Issa, N. C., and R. L. Thompson.** 2001. Staphylococcal toxic shock syndrome. Suspicion and prevention are keys to control. *Postgrad Med* **110:**55-6, 59-62.

3589. **Istre, G. R., J. S. Conner, C. V. Broome, A. Hightower, and R. S. Hopkins.** 1985. Risk factors for primary invasive Haemophilus influenzae disease: increased risk from day care attendance and school-aged household members. *J Pediatr* **106:**190-5.

3590. **Istre, G. R., T. S. Dunlop, G. B. Gaspard, and R. S. Hopkins.** 1984. Waterborne giardiasis at a mountain resort: evidence for acquired immunity. *Am J Public Health* **74:**602-4.

3591. **Istre, G. R., and R. S. Hopkins.** 1985. An outbreak of foodborne hepatitis A showing a relationship between dose and incubation period. *Am J Public Health* **75:**280-1.

3592. **Istre, G. R., K. Kreiss, R. S. Hopkins, G. R. Healy, M. Benziger, T. M. Canfield, P. Dickinson, T. R. Englert, R. C. Compton, H. M. Mathews, and R. A. Simmons.** 1982. An outbreak of amebiasis spread by colonic irrigation at a chiropractic clinic. *N Engl J Med* **307:**339-42.

3593. **Ito, A., M. Nakao, and T. Wandra.** 2003. Human taeniasis and cysticercosis in Asia. *Lancet* **362:**1918-20.

3594. **Ito, I., T. Ishida, M. Osawa, M. Arita, T. Hashimoto, T. Hongo, and M. Mishima.** 2001. Culturally verified Mycoplasma pneumoniae pneumonia in Japan: a long-term observation from 1979-99. *Epidemiol Infect* **127:**365-7.

3595. **Itoh, Y., I. Nagano, M. Kunishima, and T. Ezaki.** 1997. Laboratory investigation of enteroaggregative Escherichia coli O untypeable:H10 associated with a massive outbreak of gastrointestinal illness. *J Clin Microbiol* **35:**2546-50.

3596. **Ivanoff, B., and S. E. Robertson.** 1997. Pertussis: a worldwide problem. *Dev Biol Stand* **89:**3-13.

3597. **Ivanova, E. S., N. S. Gvetadze, S. Kigan, and A. N. Nikiforov.** 1996. [Detection of pulmonary tuberculosis in migrants]. *Probl Tuberk* **6:**28-9.

3598. **Ivanova, O. E., T. P. Eremeeva, G. Y. Lipskaya, E. A. Cherkasova, E. V. Gavrilin, and S. G. Drozdov.** 2001. Outbreak of paralytic poliomyelitis in the Chechen Republic in 1995. *Dev Biol* **105:**231-7.

3599. **Ivens, U. I., N. Ebbehoj, O. M. Poulsen, and T. Skov.** 1997. Season, equipment, and job function related to gastrointestinal problems in waste collectors. *Occup Environ Med* **54:**861-7.

3600. **Iversen, A. M., M. Gill, C. L. R. Bartlett, W. D. Cubitt, and D. A. McSwiggan.** 1987. Two outbreaks of foodborne gastroenteritis caused by a small round structured virus: evidence of prolonged infectivity in a food handler. *Lancet* **2:**556-558.

3601. **Iversen, B. G., and T. Jacobsen.** 2002. Outbreak of Pseudomonas infections in Norwegian hospitals traced to contaminated swabs for mouth hygiene. *Eurosurveillance Weekly* **15:**1.

3602. **Iversson, L. B., R. A. Silva, A. P. da Rosa, and V. L. Barros.** 1993. Circulation of eastern equine encephalitis, western equine encephalitis, Ilheus, Maguari and Tacaiuma viruses in equines of the Brazilian Pantanal, South America. *Rev Inst Med Trop Sao Paulo* **35:**355-9.

3603. **Iwamoto, M., G. Hlady, M. Jeter, C. Burnett, C. Drenzek, S. Lance, J. Benson, D. Page, and P. Blake.** 2005. Shigellosis among swimmers in a freshwater lake. *South Med J* **98:**774-8.

3604. **Iwamoto, M., D. B. Jernigan, A. Guasch, M. J. Trepka, C. G. Blackmore, W. C. Hellinger, S. M. Pham, S. Zaki, R. S. Lanciotti, S. E. Lance-Parker, C. A. DiazGranados, A. G. Winquist, C. A. Perlino, S. Wiersma, K. L. Hillyer, J. L. Goodman, A. A. Marfin, M. E. Chamberland, and L. R. Petersen.** 2003. Transmission of West Nile virus from an organ donor to four transplant recipients. *N Engl J Med* **348:**2196-203.

3605. **Iwarson, S.** 1998. Why the Scandinavian countries have not implemented universal vaccination against hepatitis B. *Vaccine* **16 (suppl):**S56-S57.

3606. **Iwasaki, H., T. Yano, S. Kaneko, M. Egi, N. Takada, and T. Ueda.** 2001. [Epidemiological analysis on many cases of tsutsugamushi disease found in Hiroshima Prefecture, Japan]. *Kansenshogaku Zasshi* **75:**365-70.

3607. **Izumiyama, S., I. Furukawa, T. Kuroki, S. Yamai, H. Sugiyama, K. Yagita, and T. Endo.** 2001. Prevalence of Cryptosporidium parvum infections in weaned piglets and fattening porkers in Kanagawa Prefecture, Japan. *Jpn J Infect Dis* **54:**23-6.

3608. **Izurieta, H. S., P. M. Strebel, and P. A. Blake.** 1997. Postlicensure effectiveness of varicella vaccine during an outbreak in a child care center. *JAMA* **278:**1495-9.

3609. **Jabs, W. J., S. Maurmann, H. J. Wagner, M. Muller-Steinhardt, J. Steinhoff, and L. Fricke.** 2004. Time course and frequency of Epstein-Barr virus reactivation after kidney transplantation: linkage to renal allograft rejection. *J Infect Dis* **190:**1600-4.

3610. **Jackson, B. M., T. Payton, G. Horst, T. J. Halpin, and B. K. Mortensen.** 1993. An epidemiologic investigation of a rubella outbreak among the Amish of northeastern Ohio. *Public Health Rep* **108:**436-9.

3611. **Jackson, B. R., M. P. Busch, S. L. Stramer, and J. P. AuBuchon.** 2003. The cost-effectiveness of NAT for HIV, HCV, and HBV in whole-blood donations. *Transfusion* **43:**721-9.

3612. **Jackson, L. A., E. R. Alexander, C. A. DeBolt, P. D. Swenson, J. Boase, M. G. McDowell, M. W. Reeves, and J. D. Wenger.** 1996. Evaluation of the use of mass chemoprophylaxis during a school outbreak of enzyme type 5 serogroup B meningococcal disease. *Pediatr Infect Dis J* **15:**992-8.

3613. **Jackson, L. A., A. F. Kaufmann, W. G. Adams, M. B. Phelps, C. Andreasen, C. W. Langkop, B. J. Francis, and J. D. Wenger.** 1993. Outbreak of leptospirosis associated with swimming. *Pediatr Infect Dis J* **12:**48-54.

3614. **Jackson, L. A., W. E. Keene, J. M. McAnulty, E. R. Alexander, M. Diermayer, M. A. Davis, K. Hedberg, J. Boase, T. J. Barrett, M. Samadpour, and D. W. Fleming.** 2000. Where's the beef? The role of cross-contamination in 4 chain restaurant-associated outbreaks of Escherichia coli O157:H7 in the Pacific Northwest. *Arch Intern Med* **160:**2380-5.

3615. **Jackson, L. A., B. A. Perkins, and J. D. Wenger.** 1993. Cat scratch disease in the United States: an analysis of three national databases. *Am J Public Health* **83:**1707-11.

3616. **Jackson, L. A., A. Schuchat, M. W. Reeves, and J. D. Wenger.** 1995. Serogroup C meningococcal outbreaks in the United States. An emerging threat. *JAMA* **273:**383-9.

3617. **Jackson, L. A., D. H. Spach, D. A. Kippen, N. K. Sugg, R. L. Regnery, M. H. Sayers, and W. E. Stamm.** 1996. Seroprevalence to Bartonella quintana among patients at a community clinic in downtown Seattle. *J Infect Dis* **173:**1023-6.

3618. **Jacobs, M. G., M. G. Brook, W. R. Weir, and B. A. Bannister.** 1991. Dengue haemorrhagic fever: a risk of returning home. *BMJ* **302:**828-9.

3619. **Jacobs, M. R., E. Palavecino, and R. Yomtovian.** 2001. Don't bug me: the problem of bacterial contamination of blood components—challenges and solutions. *Transfusion* **41:**1331-4.

3620. **Jacobs, R. J., P. Rosenthal, and A. S. Meyerhoff.** 2004. Cost effectiveness of hepatitis A/B versus hepatitis B vaccination for US prison inmates. *Vaccine* **22:**1241-8.

3621. **Jacobsen, K. H., and J. S. Koopman.** 2004. Declining hepatitis A seroprevalence: a global review and analysis. *Epidemiol Infect* **132:**1005-22.

3622. **Jacobson, R. L., C. L. Eisenberger, M. Svobodova, G. Baneth, J. Sztern, J. Carvalho, A. Nasereddin, M. E. Fari, U. Shalom, P. Volf, J. Votypka, J. P. Dedet, F. Pratlong, G. Schonian, L. F. Schnur, C. L. Jaffe, and A. Warburg.** 2003. Outbreak of cutaneous leishmaniasis in northern Israel. *J Infect Dis* **188:**1065-73.

3623. **Jacquet, C., B. Catimel, R. Brosch, C. Buchrieser, P. Dehaumont, V. Goulet, A. Lepoutre, P. Veit, and J. Rocourt.** 1995. Investigations related to the epidemic strain involved in the French listeriosis outbreak in 1992. *Appl Environ Microbiol* **61:**2242-6.

3624. **Jacquier, P., P. Hohlfeld, H. Vorkauf, and P. Zuber.** 1995. [Epidemiology of toxoplasmosis in Switzerland: national study of seroprevalence monitored in pregnant women 1990-1991]. *Schweiz Med Wochenschr Suppl* **65:**29S-38S.

3625. **Jafari, M., J. Forsberg, R. O. Gilcher, J. W. Smith, J. M. Crutcher, M. McDermott, B. R. Brown, and J. N. George.** 2002. Salmonella sepsis caused by a platelet transfusion from a donor with a pet snake. *N Engl J Med* **347:**1075-8.

3626. **Jaffar, S., A. D. Grant, J. Whithworth, P. G. Smith, and H. Whittle.** 2004. The natural history of HIV-1 and HIV-2 infections in adults in Africa: a literature review. *Bull WHO* **82:**462-69.

3627. **Jaffe, C. L., G. Baneth, Z. A. Abdeen, Y. Schlein, and A. Warburg.** 2004. Leishmaniasis in Israel and the Palestinian Authority. *Trends Parasitol* **20:**328-32.

3628. **Jahani, M. R., S. A. Motevalian, and M. Mahmoodi.** 2003. Hepatitis B carriers in large vehicle drivers of Iran. *Vaccine* **21:**1948-51.

3629. **Jahrling, P. B., T. W. Geisbert, D. W. Dalgard, E. D. Johnson, T. G. Ksiazek, W. C. Hall, and C. J. Peters.** 1990. Preliminary report: isolation of Ebola virus from monkeys imported to USA. *Lancet* **335:**502-5.

3630. **Jain, S., R. G. Reddy, S. N. Osmani, D. N. Lockwood, and S. Suneetha.** 2002. Childhood leprosy in an urban clinic, Hyderabad, India: clinical presentation and the role of household contacts. *Lepr Rev* **73:**248-53.

3631. **Jain, S. K., D. Persaud, T. M. Perl, M. A. Pass, K. M. Murphy, J. M. Pisciotta, P. F. Scholl, J. F. Casella, and D. J. Sullivan.** 2005. Nosocomial malaria and saline flush. *Emerg Infect Dis* **11:**1097-9.

3632. **Jalava, K., S. Hallanvuo, U. M. Nakari, P. Ruutu, E. Kela, T. Heinasmaki, A. Siitonen, and J. P. Nuorti.** 2004. Multiple outbreaks of Yersinia pseudotuberculosis infections in Finland. *J Clin Microbiol* **42:**2789-91.

3633. **Jalava, K., S. L. W. On, C. S. Harrington, L. P. Andersen, M. L. Hänninen, and P. Vandamme.** 2001. A cultured strain of "Helicobacter heilmannii", a human gastric pathogen, identified as H. bizzozeronii: evidence for zoonotic potential of Helicobacter. *Emerg Infect Dis* **7:**1036-1038.

3634. **Jambou, R., L. Ranaivo, L. Raharimalala, J. Randrianaivo, F. Rakotomanana, D. Modiano, V. Pietra, P. Boisier, L. Rabarijaona, T. Rabe, N. Raveloson, and F. De Giorgi.** 2001. Malaria in the highlands of Madagascar after five years of indoor house spraying of DDT. *Trans R Soc Trop Med Hyg* **95:**14-8.

3635. **Jamgaonkar, A. V., P. N. Yergolkar, G. Geevarghese, G. D. Joshi, M. V. Joshi, and A. C. Mishra.** 2003. Serological evidence for Japanese encephalitis virus and West Nile virus infections in water frequenting and terrestrial wild birds in Kolar District, Karnataka State, India. A retrospective study. *Acta Virol* **47:**185-8.

3636. **Jamieson, J. A., G. E. Rich, M. R. Kyrkou, C. F. Cargill, and D. E. Davos.** 1981. Outbreak of brucellosis at a South-Australian abattoir. 1. Clinical and serological findings. *Med J Aust* **2:**593-6.

3637. **Jamil, B., R. S. Hasan, A. R. Sarwari, J. Burton, R. Hewson, and C. Clegg.** 2005. Crimean-Congo hemorrhagic fever: experience at a tertiary care hospital in Karachi, Pakistan. *Trans R Soc Trop Med Hyg* **99:**577-84.

3638. **Jamornthanyawat, N.** 2002. The diagnosis of human opisthorchiasis. *Southeast Asian J Trop Med Public Health* **33 suppl 3:**86-91.

3639. **Janda, J. M., and S. L. Abbott.** 1998. Evolving concepts regarding the genus Aeromonas: an expanding panorama of species, disease presentations, and unanswered questions. *Clin Infect Dis* **27:**332-44.

3640. **Jang, W. J., J. H. Kim, Y. J. Choi, K. D. Jung, Y. G. Kim, S. H. Lee, M. S. Choi, I. S. Kim, D. H. Walker, and K. H. Park.** 2004. First serologic evidence of human spotted fever group rickettsiosis in Korea. *J Clin Microbiol* **42:**2310-3.

3641. Janini, R., E. Saliba, S. Khoury, O. Oumeish, S. Adwan, and S. Kamhawi. 1995. Incrimination of Phlebotomus papatasi as vector of Leishmania major in the southern Jordan Valley. *Med Vet Entomol* **9**:420-2.

3642. Janisch, T., W. Preiser, A. Berger, U. Mikulicz, B. Thoma, H. Hampl, and H. W. Doerr. 1997. Emerging viral pathogens in long-term expatriates (I): Hepatitis E virus. *Trop Med Int Health* **2**:885-91.

3643. Janisch, T., W. Preiser, A. Berger, M. Niedrig, U. Mikulicz, B. Thoma, and H. W. Doerr. 1997. Emerging viral pathogens in long-term expatriates (II): Dengue virus. *Trop Med Int Health* **2**:934-40.

3644. Janoff, E. N., P. S. Mead, J. R. Mead, P. Echeverria, L. Bodhidatta, M. Bhaibulaya, C. R. Sterling, and D. N. Taylor. 1990. Endemic Cryptosporidium and Giardia lamblia infections in a Thai orphanage. *Am J Trop Med Hyg* **43**:248-56.

3645. Jansa, J. M., J. A. Cayla, D. Ferrer, J. Gracia, C. Pelaz, M. Salvador, A. Benavides, T. Pellicer, P. Rodriguez, J. M. Garces, A. Segura, J. Guix, and A. Plasencia. 2002. An outbreak of Legionnaires' disease in an inner city district: importance of the first 24 hours in the investigation. *Int J Tuberc Lung Dis* **6**:831-8.

3646. Jansen, A., A. Beyer, C. Brandt, M. Hohne, E. Schreier, J. Schulzke, M. Zeitz, and T. Schneider. 2004. [Outbreak of norovirus in berlin - epidemiological and clinical features and prevention]. *Z Gastroenterol* **42**:311-6.

3647. Jansen, A., C. Frank, R. Prager, H. Oppermann, and K. Stark. 2005. [Nation-wide Outbreak of Salmonella Give in Germany, 2004.]. *Z Gastroenterol* **43**:707-13.

3648. Jansen, A., I. Schöneberg, C. Frank, K. Alpers, T. Schneider, and K. Stark. 2005. Leptospirosis in Germany, 1962-2003. *Emerg Infect Dis* **11**:1048-54.

3649. Jara, M., H. W. Hsu, R. B. Eaton, and A. Demaria, Jr. 2001. Epidemiology of congenital toxoplasmosis identified by population-based newborn screening in Massachusetts. *Pediatr Infect Dis J* **20**:1132-5.

3650. Jartti, T. 2004. Respiratory picornaviruses and respiratory syncytial virus as causative agents of acute expiratory wheezing in children. *Emerg Infect Dis* **10**:1095-101.

3651. Jartti, T., P. Lehtinen, T. Vuorinen, M. Koskenvuo, and O. Ruuskanen. 2004. Persistence of rhinovirus and enterovirus RNA after acute respiratory illness in children. *J Med Virol* **72**:695-9.

3652. Jasir, A., A. Noorani, A. Mirsalehian, and C. Schalen. 2000. Isolation rates of Streptococcus pyogenes in patients with acute pharyngotonsillitis and among healthy school children in Iran. *Epidemiol Infect* **124**:47-51.

3653. Javadi, M. A., A. Fayaz, S. A. Mirdehghan, and B. Ainollahi. 1996. Transmission of rabies by corneal graft. *Cornea* **15**:431-3.

3654. Javaloyas, M., D. Garcia-Somoza, and F. Gudiol. 2002. Epidemiology and prognosis of bacteremia: a 10-y study in a community hospital. *Scand J Infect Dis* **34**:436-41.

3655. Jay, M. T., V. Garrett, J. C. Mohle-Boetani, M. Barros, J. A. Farrar, R. Rios, S. Abbott, R. Sowadsky, K. Komatsu, R. Mandrell, J. Sobel, and S. B. Werner. 2004. A Multistate Outbreak of Escherichia coli O157:H7 Infection Linked to Consumption of Beef Tacos at a Fast-Food Restaurant Chain. *Clin Infect Dis* **39**:1-7.

3656. Jeandel, P., R. Josse, and J. P. Durand. 2004. Arthrites virales exotiques: place des alphaviroses. *Med Trop* **64**:81-8.

3657. Jeannel, D., P. Tuppin, G. Brucker, M. Danis, and M. Gentilini. 1991. Imported and autochthonous kala-azar in France. *BMJ* **303**:336-8.

3658. Jefferies, R., U. M. Ryan, C. J. Muhlnickel, and P. J. Irwin. 2003. Two species of canine Babesia in Australia: detection and characterization by PCR. *J Parasitol* **89**:409-12.

3659. Jeggli, S., D. Steiner, H. Joller, A. Tschopp, R. Steffen, and P. Hotz. 2004. Hepatitis E, Helicobacter pylori, and gastrointestinal symptoms in workers exposed to waste water. *Occup Environ Med* **61**:622-7.

3660. Jelfs, J., B. Jalaludin, R. Munro, M. Patel, M. Kerr, D. Daley, S. Neville, and A. Capon. 1998. A cluster of meningococcal disease in western Sydney, Australia initially associated with a nightclub. *Epidemiol Infect* **120**:263-70.

3661. Jelinek, T., Z. Bisoffi, L. Bonazzi, P. Van Thiel, U. Bronner, A. De Frey, S. G. Gundersen, P. McWhinney, and D. Ripamonti. 2002. Cluster of african trypanosomiasis in travelers to Tanzanian national parks. *Emerg Infect Dis* **8**:634-5.

3662. Jelinek, T., G. Dobler, and H. D. Nothdurft. 1998. Evidence of dengue virus infection in a German couple returning from Hawaii. *J Travel Med* **5**:44-5.

3663. Jelinek, T., and T. Löscher. 2001. Clinical features and epidemiology of tick typhus in travelers. *J Travel Med* **8**:57-9.

3664. Jelinek, T., M. Lotze, S. Eichenlaub, T. Loscher, and H. D. Nothdurft. 1997. Prevalence of infection with Cryptosporidium parvum and Cyclospora cayetanensis among international travellers. *Gut* **41**:801-4.

3665. Jelinek, T., N. Mühlberger, G. Harms, M. Corachan, M. P. Grobusch, J. Knobloch, U. Bronner, A. Laferl, A. Kapaun, Z. Bisoffi, J. Clerinx, S. Puente, G. Fry, M. Schulze, U. Hellgren, I. Gjorup, P. Chalupa, C. Hatz, A. Matteelli, M. Schmid, L. N. Nielsen, S. da Cunha, J. Atouguia, B. Myrvang, and K. Fleischer. 2002. Epidemiology and clinical features of imported dengue fever in Europe: sentinel surveillance data from TropNetEurop. *Clin Infect Dis* **35**:1047-52.

3666. Jelinek, T., H. D. Nothdurft, and T. Löscher. 1996. Schistosomiasis in travelers and expatriates. *J Travel Med* **3**:160-4.

3667. Jelinek, T., H. D. Nothdurft, N. Rieder, and T. Loscher. 1995. Cutaneous myiasis: review of 13 cases in travelers returning from tropical countries. *Int J Dermatol* **34**:624-6.

3668. Jelinek, T., H. D. Nothdurft, F. von Sonnenburg, and T. Loscher. 1996. Risk Factors for Typhoid Fever in Travelers. *J Travel Med* **3**:200-203.

3669. Jelinek, T., G. Peyerl, T. Loscher, F. von Sonnenburg, and H. D. Nothdurft. 1997. The role of Blastocystis hominis as a possible intestinal pathogen in travellers. *J Infect* **35**:63-6.

3670. Jelinek, T., and L. T. 2000. Epidemiology of giardiasis in German travelers. *J Travel Med* **7**:70-3.

3671. Jelinek, T., M. Ziegler, and T. Loscher. 1994. [Gnathostomiasis after a stay in Thailand]. *Dtsch Med Wochenschr* **119**: 1618-22.

3672. Jellison, W. L. 1974. Tularemia in North America 1930-1974. University of Montana, Missoula, Montana 59801.

3673. Jemmi, T., S. I. Pak, and M. D. Salman. 2002. Prevalence and risk factors for contamination with Listeria monocytogenes of imported and exported meat and fish products in Switzerland, 1992-2000. *Prev Vet Med* **54**:25-36.

3674. Jenista, J. A., and D. Chapman. 1987. Medical problems of foreign-born adopted children. *Am J Dis Child* **141**:298-302.

3675. **Jenkin, G. A., S. A. Ritchie, J. N. Hanna, and G. V. Brown.** 1997. Airport malaria in Cairns. *Med J Aust* **166**:307-8.

3676. **Jenkins, D. R., A. M. Lewis, and C. J. L. Strachan.** 1990. Imported melioidosis in a British native. *J Infect* **21**:221-2.

3677. **Jenkins, F. J., L. J. Hoffman, and A. Liegey-Dougall.** 2002. Reactivation of and primary infection with human herpesvirus 8 among solid-organ transplant recipients. *J Infect Dis* **185**:1238-43.

3678. **Jenney, A., K. Pandithage, D. A. Fisher, and B. J. Currie.** 2004. Cryptococcus infection in tropical Australia. *J Clin Microbiol* **42**:3865-8.

3679. **Jennings, L. C., T. P. Anderson, A. M. Werno, K. A. Beynon, and D. R. Murdoch.** 2004. Viral etiology of acute respiratory tract infections in children presenting to hospital: role of polymerase chain reaction and demonstration of multiple infections. *Pediatr Infect Dis J* **23**:1003-7.

3680. **Jennings, L. C., and E. C. Dick.** 1987. Transmission and control of rhinovirus colds. *Eur J Epidemiol* **3**:327-35.

3681. **Jensen, K., F. Alvarado-Ramy, J. Gonzalez-Martinez, E. Kraiselburd, and J. Rullan.** 2004. B-virus and free-ranging macaques, Puerto Rico. *Emerg Infect Dis* **10**:494-6.

3682. **Jensen, T. G., B. Gahrn-Hansen, M. Arendrup, and B. Bruun.** 2004. Fusarium fungaemia in immunocompromised patients. *Clin Microbiol Infect* **10**:499-501.

3683. **Jensenius, M., P. E. Fournier, P. Kelly, B. Myrvang, and D. Raoult.** 2003. African tick bite fever. *Lancet Infect Dis* **3**:557-64.

3684. **Jensenius, M., P. E. Fournier, S. Vene, T. Hoel, G. Hasle, A. Z. Henriksen, K. B. Hellum, D. Raoult, and B. Myrvang.** 2003. African tick bite fever in travelers to rural sub-equatorial Africa. *Clin Infect Dis* **36**:1411-7.

3685. **Jensenius, M., T. Hoel, D. Raoult, P. E. Fournier, H. Kjelshus, A. L. Bruu, and B. Myrvang.** 2002. Seroepidemiology of Rickettsia africae infection in Norwegian travellers to rural Africa. *Scand J Infect Dis* **34**:93-6.

3686. **Jenson, H. B.** 2003. Human herpesvirus 8 infection. *Curr Opin Pediatr* **15**:85-91.

3687. **Jenson, H. B.** 2004. The changing picture of hepatitis A in the United States. *Curr Opin Pediatr* **16**:89-93.

3688. **Jeong, S. H., W. M. Kim, C. L. Chang, J. M. Kim, K. Lee, Y. Chong, H. Y. Hwang, Y. W. Baek, H. K. Chung, I. G. Woo, and J. Y. Ku.** 2001. Neonatal intensive care unit outbreak caused by a strain of Klebsiella oxytoca resistant to aztreonam due to overproduction of chromosomal beta-lactamase. *J Hosp Infect* **48**:281-8.

3689. **Jephcott, A. E., N. T. Begg, and I. A. Baker.** 1986. Outbreak of giardiasis associated with mains water in the United Kingdom. *Lancet* **1**:730-2.

3690. **Jereb, J. A.** 2002. Progressing toward tuberculosis elimination. Low-incidence areas of the United States. *MMWR* **51 (RR-05)**:1-16.

3691. **Jeri, C., R. H. Gilman, A. G. Lescano, H. Mayta, M. E. Ramirez, A. E. Gonzalez, R. Nazerali, and H. H. Garcia.** 2004. Species identification after treatment for human taeniasis. *Lancet* **363**:949-50.

3692. **Jernigan, D. B., J. Hofmann, M. S. Cetron, C. A. Genese, J. P. Nuorti, B. S. Fields, R. F. Benson, R. J. Carter, P. H. Edelstein, I. C. Guerrero, S. M. Paul, H. B. Lipman, and R. Breiman.** 1996. Outbreak of Legionnaires' disease among cruise ship passengers exposed to a contaminated whirlpool spa. *Lancet* **347**:494-9.

3693. **Jernigan, J. A., and B. M. Farr.** 2000. Incubation period and sources of exposure for cutaneous Mycobacterium marinum infection: case report and review of the literature. *Clin Infect Dis* **31**:439-43.

3694. **Jernigan, J. A., B. S. Lowry, F. G. Hayden, S. A. Kyger, B. P. Conway, D. H. Groschel, and B. M. Farr.** 1993. Adenovirus type 8 epidemic keratoconjunctivitis in an eye clinic: risk factors and control. *J Infect Dis* **167**:1307-13.

3695. **Jernigan, J. A., Y. Siegman-Igra, R. C. Guerrant, and B. M. Farr.** 1998. A randomized crossover study of disposable thermometers for prevention of Clostridium difficile and other nosocomial infections. *Infect Control Hosp Epidemiol* **19**:494-9.

3696. **Jeronimo, S. M., R. M. Oliveira, S. Mackay, R. M. Costa, J. Sweet, E. T. Nascimento, K. G. Luz, M. Z. Fernandes, J. Jernigan, and R. D. Pearson.** 1994. An urban outbreak of visceral leishmaniasis in Natal, Brazil. *Trans R Soc Trop Med Hyg* **88**:386-8.

3697. **Jessamine, P. G., and R. C. Brunham.** 1990. Rapid control of a chancroid outbreak: implications for Canada. *CMAJ* **142**:1081-5.

3698. **Jesudason, M. V., V. Balaji, U. Mukundan, and C. J. Thomson.** 2000. Ecological study of Vibrio cholerae in Vellore. *Epidemiol Infect* **124**:201-6.

3699. **Jiang, B., H. M. McClure, R. L. Fankhauser, S. S. Monroe, and R. I. Glass.** 2004. Prevalence of rotavirus and norovirus antibodies in non-human primates. *J Med Primatol* **33**:30-3.

3700. **Jiang, J., K. J. Marienau, L. A. May, H. J. Beecham, 3rd, R. Wilkinson, W. M. Ching, and A. L. Richards.** 2003. Laboratory diagnosis of two scrub typhus outbreaks at camp Fuji, Japan in 2000 and 2001 by enzyme-linked immunosorbent assay, rapid flow assay, and western blot assay using outer membrane 56-kd recombinant proteins. *Am J Trop Med Hyg* **69**:60-6.

3701. **Jiang, Z. D., B. Lowe, M. P. Verenkar, D. Ashley, R. Steffen, N. Tornieporth, F. von Sonnenburg, P. Waiyaki, and H. L. DuPont.** 2002. Prevalence of enteric pathogens among international travelers with diarrhea acquired in Kenya (Mombasa), India (Goa), or JAMAica (Montego Bay). *J Infect Dis* **185**:497-502.

3702. **Jimenez, J. F., B. Valladares, J. M. Fernandez-Palacios, F. De Armas, and A. Del Castillo.** 1997. A serologic study of human toxocariasis in the Canary islands (Spain): environmental influences. *Am J Trop Med Hyg* **56**:113-5.

3703. **Jimenez, R. A., M. E. Uran, C. de Bedout, M. Arango, A. M. Tobon, L. E. Cano, and A. Restrepo.** 2002. [Outbreak of acute histoplasmosis in a family group: identification of the infection source]. *Biomedica* **22**:155-9.

3704. **Jimenez, S. M., M. C. Tiburzi, M. S. Salsi, M. E. Pirovani, and M. A. Moguilevsky.** 2003. The role of visible faecal material as a vehicle for generic Escherichia coli, coliform, and other enterobacteria contaminating poultry carcasses during slaughtering. *J Appl Microbiol* **95**:451-6.

3705. **Jimenez-Lucho, V. E., F. Fallon, C. Caputo, and K. Ramsey.** 1995. Role of prolonged surveillance in the eradication of nosocomial scabies in an extended care Veterans Affairs medical center. *Am J Infect Control* **23**:44-9.

3706. **Joce, R. E., J. Bruce, D. Kiely, N. D. Noah, W. B. Dempster, R. Stalker, P. Gumsley, P. A. Chapman, P. Norman, J. Watkins, et al.** 1991. An outbreak of cryptosporidiosis associated with a swimming pool. *Epidemiol Infect* **107**:497-508.

3707. **Johara, M. Y.,** H. Field, A. M. Rashdi, C. Morrissy, B. van der Heide, P. Rota, A. bin Adzhar, J. White, P. Daniels, A. Jamaluddin, and T. Ksiazek. 2001. Nipah virus infection in bats (order Chiroptera) in peninsular Malaysia. *Emerg Infect Dis* **7:**439-441.

3708. **John, D. T.,** and M. J. Howard. 1995. Seasonal distribution of pathogenic free-living amebae in Oklahoma waters. *Parasitol Res* **81:**193-201.

3709. **John, G. C.,** R. W. Nduati, D. A. Mbori-Ngacha, B. A. Richardson, D. Panteleeff, A. Mwatha, J. Overbaugh, J. Bwayo, J. O. Ndinya-Achola, and J. K. Kreiss. 2001. Correlates of mother-to-child human immunodeficiency virus type 1 (HIV-1) transmission: association with maternal plasma HIV-1 RNA load, genital HIV-1 DNA shedding, and breast infections. *J Infect Dis* **183:**206-212.

3710. **Johnsen, C.,** E. Bellin, E. Nadal, and V. Simone. 1991. An outbreak of scabies in a New York City jail. *Am J Infect Control* **19:**162-3.

3711. **Johnson, A. M.,** C. H. Mercer, B. Erens, A. J. Copes, S. McManus, K. Wellings, K. A. Fenton, C. Korovessis, W. Macdowall, K. Nanchahal, S. Purdon, and J. Field. 2001. Sexual behaviour in Britain: partnerships, practices, and HIV risk behaviours. *Lancet* **358:**1835-1842.

3712. **Johnson, A. P.,** M. Warner, K. Broughton, D. James, A. Efsratiou, R. C. George, and D. M. Livermore. 2001. Antibiotic susceptibility of streptococci and related genera causing endocarditis: analysis of UK reference laboratory referrals, January 1996 to March 2000. *BMJ* **322:**395-6.

3713. **Johnson, B. A.** 2005. Insertion and removal of intrauterine devices. *Am Fam Physician* **71:**95-102.

3714. **Johnson, D. E.,** L. C. Miller, S. Iverson, W. Thomas, B. Franchino, K. Dole, M. T. Kiernan, M. K. Georgieff, and M. K. Hostetter. 1992. The health of children adopted from Romania. *JAMA* **268:**3446-51.

3715. **Johnson, I. L.,** J. J. Dwyer, I. D. Rusen, R. Shahin, and B. Yaffe. 2001. Survey of infection control procedures at manicure and pedicure establishments in North York. *Can J Public Health* **92:**134-7.

3716. **Johnson, K. R.,** C. R. Braden, K. L. Cairns, K. W. Field, A. C. Colombel, Z. Yang, C. L. Woodley, G. P. Morlock, A. M. Weber, A. Y. Boudreau, T. A. Bell, I. M. Onorato, S. E. Valway, and P. A. Stehr-Green. 2000. Transmission of Mycobacterium tuberculosis from medical waste. *JAMA* **284:**1683-8.

3717. **Johnson, L. W.** 1995. Communal showers and the risk of plantar warts. *J Fam Pract* **40:**136-8.

3718. **Johnson, M. A.,** H. Smith, P. Joeph, R. H. Gilman, C. T. Bautista, K. J. Campos, M. Cespedes, P. Klatsky, C. Vidal, H. Terry, M. M. Calderon, C. Coral, L. Cabrera, P. S. Parmar, and J. M. Vinetz. 2004. Environmental exposure and leptospirosis, Peru. *Emerg Infect Dis* **10:**1016-22.

3719. **Johnson, N.,** D. W. Lipscomb, R. Stott, G. Gopal Rao, K. Mansfield, J. Smith, L. McElhinney, and A. R. Fooks. 2002. Investigation of a human case of rabies in the United Kingdom. *J Clin Virol* **25:**351-6.

3720. **Johnson, R. E.,** R. E. Newhall, J. R. Papp, J. S. Knapp, C. M. Black, T. L. Gift, R. Steece, L. E. Markowitz, O. J. Devine, C. M. Walsh, S. Wang, D. C. Gunter, K. L. Irwin, S. DeLisle, and S. M. Berman. 2002. Screening tests to detect Chlamydia trachomatis and Neisseria gonorrhoeae infections - 2002. *MMWR* **51 (RR-15):**1-40.

3721. **Johnson, R. N.,** P. G. Lawyer, P. M. Ngumbi, Y. B. Mebrahtu, J. P. Mwanyumba, N. C. Mosonik, S. J. Makasa, J. I. Githure, and C. R. Roberts. 1999. Phlebotomine sand fly (Diptera: Psychodidae) seasonal distribution and infection rates in a defined focus of Leishmania tropica. *Am J Trop Med Hyg* **60:**854-8.

3722. **Johnson, S.,** M. H. Samore, K. A. Farrow, G. E. Killgore, F. C. Tenover, D. Lyras, J. I. Rood, P. DeGirolami, A. L. Baltch, M. E. Rafferty, S. M. Pear, and D. N. Gerding. 1999. Epidemics of diarrhea caused by a clindamycin-resistant strain of Clostridium difficile in four hospitals. *N Engl J Med* **341:**1645-51.

3723. **Johnson, W. M.** 1981. Occupational factors in coccidioidomycosis. *J Occup Med* **23:**367-74.

3724. **Johnston, F.,** V. Krause, N. Miller, and L. Barclay. 1997. An outbreak of influenza B among workers on an oil rig. *Commun Dis Intell* **21:**106.

3725. **Jokipii, A. M.,** M. Hemila, and L. Jokipii. 1985. Prospective study of acquisition of Cryptosporidium, Giardia lamblia, and gastrointestinal illness. *Lancet* **2:**487-9.

3726. **Jokipii, A. M. M.,** and L. Jokipii. 1977. Prepatency of giardiasis. *Lancet* **1 (21 May):**1095-7.

3727. **Jones, B. L.,** L. J. Gorman, J. Simpson, E. T. Curran, S. McNamee, C. Lucas, J. Michie, D. J. Platt, and B. Thakker. 2000. An outbreak of Serratia marcescens in two neonatal intensive care units. *J Hosp Infect* **46:**314-9.

3728. **Jones, F. R.,** J. L. Sanchez, R. Meza, T. M. Batsel, R. Burga, E. Canal, K. Block, J. Perez, C. T. Bautista, J. Escobedo, and S. E. Walz. 2004. Short Report: High Incidence of Shigellosis among Peruvian Soldiers Deployed in the Amazon River Basin. *Am J Trop Med Hyg* **70:**663-665.

3729. **Jones, G.,** R. W. Steketee, R. E. Black, Z. A. Bhutta, and S. S. Morris. 2003. How many child deaths can we prevent this year? *Lancet* **362:**65-71.

3730. **Jones, G. R.,** M. Christodoulides, J. L. Brooks, A. R. Miller, K. A. Cartwright, and J. E. Heckels. 1998. Dynamics of carriage of Neisseria meningitidis in a group of military recruits: subtype stability and specificity of the immune response following colonization. *J Infect Dis* **178:**451-9.

3731. **Jones, I. G.,** and M. Roworth. 1996. An outbreak of Escherichia coli O157 and campylobacteriosis associated with contamination of a drinking water supply. *Public Health* **110:**277-82.

3732. **Jones, J. L.,** D. L. Hanson, M. S. Dworkin, J. E. Kaplan, and J. W. Ward. 1998. Trends in AIDS-related opportunistic infections among men who have sex with men and among injecting drug users, 1991-1996. *J Infect Dis* **178:**114-20.

3733. **Jones, J. L.,** D. Kruszon-Moran, and M. Wilson. 2003. Toxoplasma gondii infection in the United States, 1999-2000. *Emerg Infect Dis* **9:**1371-4.

3734. **Jones, J. L.,** D. Kruszon-Moran, M. Wilson, G. McQuillan, T. Navin, and J. B. McAuley. 2001. Toxoplasma gondii infection in the United States: seroprevalence and risk factors. *Am J Epidemiol* **154:**357-65.

3735. **Jones, J. L.,** A. Lopez, M. Wilson, J. Schulkin, and R. Gibbs. 2001. Congenital toxoplasmosis: a review. *Obstet Gynecol Surv* **56:**296-305.

3736. **Jones, J. S.,** D. Hoerle, and R. Rickse. 1995. Stethoscopes: a potential vector of infection? *Ann Emerg Med* **26:**296-9.

3737. **Jones, S. C.,** J. Morris, G. Hill, M. Alderman, and R. C. Ratard. 2002. St. Louis encephalitis outbreak in Louisiana in 2001. *J La State Med Soc* **154:**303-6.

3738. **Jones, S. R., and R. C. Cushman.** 2004. A field guide to the North American prairie. Houghton Mifflin company, Boston.

3739. **Jones, T. F., R. F. Benson, E. W. Brown, J. R. Rowland, S. C. Crosier, and W. Schaffner.** 2003. Epidemiologic investigation of a restaurant-associated outbreak of pontiac Fever. *Clin Infect Dis* **37**:1292-7.

3740. **Jones, T. F., A. S. Craig, C. D. Paddock, D. B. McKechnie, J. E. Childs, S. R. Zaki, and W. Schaffner.** 1999. Family cluster of Rocky Mountain spotted fever. *Clin Infect Dis* **28**:853-9.

3741. **Jones, T. F., C. L. Woodley, F. F. Fountain, and W. Schaffner.** 2003. Increased incidence of the outbreak strain of Mycobacterium tuberculosis in the surrounding community after an outbreak in a jail. *South Med J* **96**:155-7.

3742. **Jones, T. W., and A. M. Davila.** 2001. Trypanosoma vivax— out of Africa. *Trends Parasitol* **17**:99-101.

3743. **Jones-Engel, L., G. A. Engel, M. A. Schillaci, A. Rompis, A. Putra, K. G. Suaryana, A. Fuentes, B. Beer, S. Hicks, R. White, B. Wilson, and J. S. Allan.** 2005. Primate-to-human retroviral transmission in Asia. *Emerg Infect Dis* **11**:1028-35.

3744. **Jongwutiwes, S., N. Chantachum, P. Kraivichian, P. Siriyasatien, C. Putaporntip, A. Tamburrini, G. La Rosa, C. Sreesunpasirikul, P. Yingyourd, and E. Pozio.** 1998. First outbreak of human trichinellosis caused by Trichinella pseudospiralis. *Clin Infect Dis* **26**:111-5.

3745. **Jongwutiwes, S., C. Putaporntip, T. Iwasaki, T. Sata, and H. Kanbara.** 2004. Naturally acquired Plasmodium knowlesi malaria in human, Thailand. *Emerg Infect Dis* **10**:2211-3.

3746. **Jordan, J., B. Tiangco, J. Kiss, and W. Koch.** 1998. Human parvovirus B19: prevalence of viral DNA in volunteer blood donors and clinical outcomes of transfusion recipients. *Vox Sang* **75**:97-102.

3747. **Jorgensen, P. H., K. J. Handberg, P. Ahrens, H. C. Hansen, R. J. Manvell, and D. J. Alexander.** 1999. An outbreak of Newcastle disease in free-living pheasants (Phasianus colchicus). *Zentralbl Veterinarmed B* **46**:381-7.

3748. **Jorm, L. R., and A. G. Capon.** 1994. Communicable disease outbreaks in long day care centres in western Sydney: occurrence and risk factors. *J Paediatr Child Health* **30**:151-4.

3749. **Jorm, L. R., N. F. Lightfoot, and K. L. Morgan.** 1990. An epidemiological study of an outbreak of Q fever in a secondary school. *Epidemiol Infect* **104**:467-77.

3750. **Jorm, L. R., S. V. Thackway, T. R. Churches, and M. W. Hills.** 2003. Watching the Games: public health surveillance for the Sydney 2000 Olympic Games. *J Epidemiol Community Health* **57**:102-8.

3751. **Joseph, C. A.** 2004. Legionnaires' disease in Europe 2000-2002. *Epidemiol Infect* **132**:417-24.

3752. **Joseph, C. A., E. M. Mitchell, J. M. Cowden, J. C. Bruce, E. J. Threlfall, C. E. Hine, R. Wallis, and M. L. Hall.** 1991. A national outbreak of salmonellosis from yeast flavoured products. *CDR (Lond Engl Rev)* **1**:R16-9.

3753. **Jothikumar, N., R. Paulmurugan, P. Padmanabhan, R. B. Sundari, S. Kamatchiammal, and K. S. Rao.** 2000. Duplex RT-PCR for simultaneous detection of hepatitis A and hepatitis E virus isolated from drinking water samples. *J Environ Monit* **2**:587-90.

3754. **Jouan, A., F. Adam, I. Coulibaly, O. Riou, B. Philippe, E. Ledru, C. Lejan, N. O. Merzoug, T. Ksiazek, and B. Leguenno.** 1990. Épidémie de fièvre de la vallée du Rift en république islamique de Mauritanie. Données géographiques et écologiques. *Bull Soc Pathol Exot* **83**:611-20.

3755. **Joy, R. J. T.** 1999. Malaria in American troops in the south and southwest Pacific in world war II. *Medical History* **43**:192-207.

3756. **Joynson, D. H., and T. G. Wreghitt.** 2001. Toxoplasmosis. A comprehensive clinical guide. Cambridge University Press, Cambridge, U.K.

3757. **Juan, J. O., N. Lopez Chegne, G. Gargala, and L. Favennec.** 2002. Comparative clinical studies of nitazoxanide, albendazole and praziquantel in the treatment of ascariasis, trichuriasis and hymenolepiasis in children from Peru. *Trans R Soc Trop Med Hyg* **96**:193-6.

3758. **Judd, A., M. Hickman, S. Jones, T. McDonald, J. V. Parry, G. V. Stimson, and A. J. Hall.** 2005. Incidence of hepatitis C virus and HIV among new injecting drug users in London: prospective cohort study. *BMJ* **330**:24-5.

3759. **Judd, W., S., C. S. Campbell, E. A. Kellogg, and P. F. Stevens.** 1999. Plant systematics. A phylogenetic approach. Sinauer Associates, Inc. Publishers, Sunderland, Massachusetts.

3760. **Juel-Jensen, B. E.** 1983. Outbreak of chickenpox from a patient with immunosuppressed herpes zoster in hospital. *Br Med J (Clin Res Ed)* **286**:60.

3761. **Julvez, J., and S. Blanchy.** 1988. [Malaria in the islands of the Comoro archipelago. Historical and geophysical aspects. Epidemiologic considerations]. *Bull Soc Pathol Exot Filiales* **81**:847-53.

3762. **Julvez, J., J. Mouchet, A. Michault, A. Fouta, and M. Hamidine.** 1997. [Eco-epidemiology of malaria in Niamey and in the river valley, the Republic of Niger, 1992-1995]. *Bull Soc Pathol Exot* **90**:94-100.

3763. **Jumaa, P., and B. Chattopadhyay.** 1994. Outbreak of gentamicin, ciprofloxacin-resistant Pseudomonas aeruginosa in an intensive care unit, traced to contaminated quivers. *J Hosp Infect* **28**:209-18.

3764. **Jumaian, N., S. A. Kamhawi, M. Halalsheh, and S. K. Abdel-Hafez.** 1998. Short report: outbreak of cutaneous leishmaniasis in a nonimmune population of soldiers in Wadi Araba, Jordan. *Am J Trop Med Hyg* **58**:160-2.

3765. **Juminer, B., G. Borel, H. Mauleon, M. C. Durette-Desset, C. P. Raccurt, M. Roudier, M. Nicolas, and J. M. Perez.** 1993. [Natural murine infestation by Angiostrongylus costaricensis Morera and Cespedes, 1971 in Guadeloupe]. *Bull Soc Pathol Exot* **86**:502-5.

3766. **Juncker-Voss, M., H. Prosl, H. Lussy, U. Enzenberg, H. Auer, H. Lassnig, M. Muller, and N. Nowotny.** 2004. [Screening for antibodies against zoonotic agents among employees of the Zoological Garden of Vienna, Schonbrunn, Austria]. *Berl Munch Tierarztl Wochenschr* **117**:404-9.

3767. **Juncker-Voss, M., H. Prosl, H. Lussy, U. Enzenberg, H. Auer, and N. Nowotny.** 2000. Serological detection of Capillaria hepatica by indirect immunofluorescence assay. *J Clin Microbiol* **38**:431-3.

3768. **Junghanss, T., and N. Weiss.** 1990. [Onchocerciasis in travelers to the tropics]. *Dtsch Med Wochenschr* **115**:1392-6.

3769. **Junod, C.** 1987. [Retrospective study of 1,934 cases of strongyloidiasis diagnosed in Paris (1970-1986). I. Geographic origin. Epidemiology]. *Bull Soc Pathol Exot Filiales* **80**:357-69.

3770. **Junod, C.** 1988. La coccidiose à Isospora belli chez les sujets immuno-compétents (Etude de 40 cas observés à Paris). *Bull Soc Pathol Exot* **81**:317-25.

3771. **Junt, T., J. M. Heraud, J. Lelarge, B. Labeau, and A. Talarmin.** 1999. Determination of natural versus laboratory human infection with Mayaro virus by molecular analysis. *Epidemiol Infect* **123**:511-3.

3772. **Junttila, J., and M. Brander.** 1989. Listeria monocytogenes septicemia associated with consumption of salted mushrooms. *Scand J Infect Dis* **21**:339-42.

3773. **Junttila, J., M. Peltomaa, H. Soini, M. MarJAMAki, and M. K. Viljanen.** 1999. Prevalence of Borrelia burgdorferi in Ixodes ricinus ticks in urban recreational areas of Helsinki. *J Clin Microbiol* **37**:1361-5.

3774. **Jupp, P. G.** 2001. The ecology of West Nile virus in South Africa and the occurrence of outbreaks in humans. *Ann N Y Acad Sci* **951**:143-52.

3775. **Juricova, Z., Z. Hubalek, J. Halouzka, K. Hudec, and J. Pellantova.** 1989. Results of arbovirological examination of birds of the family Hirundinidae in Czechoslovakia. *Folia Parasitol (Praha)* **36**:379-83.

3776. **Kabatereine, N. B., S. Brooker, E. M. Tukahebwa, F. Kazibwe, and A. W. Onapa.** 2004. Epidemiology and geography of Schistosoma mansoni in Uganda: implications for planning control. *Trop Med Int Health* **9**:372-80.

3777. **Kabrane-Lazizi, Y., J. B. Fine, J. Elm, G. E. Glass, H. Higa, A. Diwan, C. J. Gibbs, Jr., X. J. Meng, S. U. Emerson, and R. H. Purcell.** 1999. Evidence for widespread infection of wild rats with hepatitis E virus in the United States. *Am J Trop Med Hyg* **61**:331-5.

3778. **Kabuki, D. Y., A. Y. Kuaye, M. Wiedmann, and K. J. Boor.** 2004. Molecular Subtyping and Tracking of Listeria monocytogenes in Latin-Style Fresh-Cheese Processing Plants. *J Dairy Sci* **87**:2803-12.

3779. **Kaewkes, S.** 2003. Taxonomy and biology of liver flukes. *Acta Trop* **88**:177-86.

3780. **Kagan, L. J., A. E. Aiello, and E. Larson.** 2002. The role of the home environment in the transmission of infectious diseases. *J Community Health* **27**:247-67.

3781. **Kagen, C. N., J. C. Vance, and M. Simpson.** 1984. Gnathostomiasis. Infestation in an Asian immigrant. *Arch Dermatol* **120**:508-10.

3782. **Kageyama, A., K. Yazawa, J. Ishikawa, K. Hotta, K. Nishimura, and Y. Mikami.** 2004. Nocardial infections in Japan from 1992 to 2001, including the first report of infection by Nocardia transvalensis. *Eur J Epidemiol* **19**:383-9.

3783. **Kahn, R. H., D. T. Scholl, S. M. Shane, A. L. Lemoine, and T. A. Farley.** 2002. Screening for syphilis in arrestees: usefulness for community-wide syphilis surveillance and control. *Sex Transm Dis* **29**:150-6.

3784. **Kaic, B., B. Borcic, M. Ljubicic, I. Brkic, and I. Mihaljevic.** 2001. Hepatitis A control in a refugee camp by active immunization. *Vaccine* **19**:3615-9.

3785. **Kain, K. C., and J. S. Keystone.** 1998. Malaria in travellers. Epidemiology, disease and prevention. *Inf Dis Clin N Am* **12**:267-84.

3786. **Kainer, M. A., H. Keshavarz, B. J. Jensen, M. J. Arduino, M. E. Brandt, A. A. Padhye, W. R. Jarvis, and L. K. Archibald.** 2005. Saline-filled breast implant contamination with Curvularia species among women who underwent cosmetic breast augmentation. *J Infect Dis* **192**:170-7.

3787. **Kaiser, A. M., C. Schultsz, G. J. Kruithof, Y. Debets-Ossenkopp, and C. Vandenbroucke-Grauls.** 2004. Carriage of resistant microorganisms in repatriates from foreign hospitals to The Netherlands. *Clin Microbiol Infect* **10**:972-9.

3788. **Kaiser, R.** 2002. Tick-borne encephalitis (TBE) in Germany and clinical course of the disease. *Int J Med Microbiol* **291 Suppl 33**:58-61.

3789. **Kaitwatcharachai, C., K. Silpapojakul, S. Jitsurong, and S. Kalnauwakul.** 2000. An outbreak of Burkholderia cepacia bacteremia in hemodialysis patients: an epidemiologic and molecular study. *Am J Kidney Dis* **36**:199-204.

3790. **Kalashnikova, V. A., E. K. Dzhikidze, Z. K. Stasilevich, and M. G. Chikobava.** 2002. Detection of Campylobacter jejuni in healthy monkeys and monkeys with enteric infections by PCR. *Bull Exp Biol Med* **134**:299-300.

3791. **Kalayoglu, M. V., P. Libby, and G. I. Byrne.** 2002. Chlamydia pneumoniae as an Emerging Risk Factor in Cardiovascular Disease. *JAMA* **288**:2724-31.

3792. **Kaleta, E. F., and E. M. Taday.** 2003. Avian host range of Chlamydophila spp. based on isolation, antigen detection and serology. *Avian Pathol* **32**:435-61.

3793. **Kalima, P., F. X. Emmanuel, and T. Riordan.** 1999. Epidemiology of Streptococcus pneumoniae infections at the Edinburgh City Hospital: 1980-95. *Epidemiol Infect* **122**:251-7.

3794. **Kalluri, P., C. Crowe, M. Reller, L. Gaul, J. Hayslett, S. Barth, S. Eliasberg, J. Ferreira, K. Holt, S. Bengston, K. Hendricks, and J. Sobel.** 2003. An outbreak of foodborne botulism associated with food sold at a salvage store in Texas. *Clin Infect Dis* **37**:1490-5.

3795. **Kalmar, E. M., F. E. Alencar, F. P. Alves, L. W. Pang, G. M. Del Negro, Z. P. Camargo, and M. A. Shikanai-Yasuda.** 2004. Paracoccidioidomycosis: An Epidemiologic Survey in a Pediatric Population from the Brazilian Amazon Using Skin Tests. *Am J Trop Med Hyg* **71**:82-86.

3796. **Kam, K. M., T. H. Leung, Y. Y. Ho, N. K. Ho, and T. A. Saw.** 1995. Outbreak of Vibrio cholerae O1 in Hong Kong related to contaminated fish tank water. *Public Health* **109**:389-95.

3797. **Kamal, I. H., P. Fischer, M. Adly, A. S. El Sayed, Z. S. Morsy, and R. M. Ramzy.** 2001. Evaluation of a PCR-ELISA to detect Wuchereria bancrofti in Culex pipiens from an Egyptian village with a low prevalence of filariasis. *Ann Trop Med Parasitol* **95**:833-41.

3798. **Kamali, A., J. A. Seeley, A. J. Nunn, J. F. Kengeya-Kayondo, A. Ruberantwari, and D. W. Mulder.** 1996. The orphan problem: experience of a sub-Saharan Africa rural population in the AIDS epidemic. *AIDS Care* **8**:509-15.

3799. **Kamat, V.** 2000. Resurgence of malaria in Bombay (Mumbai) in the 1990s: a historical perspective. *Parasitologia* **42**:135-48.

3800. **Kamihama, T., T. Kimura, J. I. Hosokawa, M. Ueji, T. Takase, and K. Tagami.** 1997. Tinea pedis outbreak in swimming pools in Japan. *Public Health* **111**:249-53.

3801. **Kamili, M. A., G. Ali, M. Y. Shah, S. Rashid, S. Khan, and G. Q. Allaqaband.** 1993. Multiple drug resistant typhoid fever outbreak in Kashmir Valley. *Indian J Med Sci* **47**:147-51.

3802. **Kaminsky, R.** 1987. Tsetse ecology in a Liberian rain-forest focus of Gambian sleeping sickness. *Med Vet Entomol* **1**:257-64.

3803. **Kampelmacher, E. H., and L. M. van Noorle Jansen.** 1972. [Further studies on the isolation of L. monocytogenes in clinically healthy individuals]. *Zentralbl Bakteriol [Orig A]* **221**:70-7.

3804. **Kamugisha, C., K. L. Cairns, and C. Akim.** 2003. An outbreak of measles in Tanzanian refugee camps. *J Infect Dis* **187:**S58-62.

3805. **Kan, S. P., H. L. Guyatt, and D. A. Bundy.** 1989. Geohelminth infection of children from rural plantations and urban slums in Malaysia. *Trans R Soc Trop Med Hyg* **83:**817-20.

3806. **Kanamoto, Y., and M. Seno.** 1989. [Respiratory tract infections due to Mycoplasma pneumoniae in elementary school children; a case report]. *Kansenshogaku Zasshi* **63:**1291-5.

3807. **Kandhai, M. C., M. W. Reij, L. G. Gorris, O. Guillaume-Gentil, and M. van Schothorst.** 2004. Occurrence of Enterobacter sakazakii in food production environments and households. *Lancet* **363:**39-40.

3808. **Kane, A., J. Lloyd, M. Zaffran, L. Simonsen, and M. Kane.** 1999. Transmission of hepatitis B, hepatitis C and human immunodeficiency viruses through unsafe injections in the developing world: model-based regional estimates. *Bull WHO* **77:**801-7.

3809. **Kang, G., M. Mathan, B. S. Ramakrishna, E. Mathai, and V. Sarada.** 1994. Human intestinal capillariasis: first report from India. *Trans R Soc Trop Med Hyg* **88:**204.

3810. **Kantakamalakul, W., S. Siritantikorn, P. Thongcharoen, C. Singchai, and P. Puthavathana.** 2003. Prevalence of rabies virus and Hantaan virus infections in commensal rodents and shrews trapped in Bangkok. *J Med Assoc Thai* **86:**1008-14.

3811. **Kao, J. H., C. J. Liu, P. J. Chen, W. Chen, S. C. Hsiang, M. Y. Lai, and D. S. Chen.** 1997. Interspousal transmission of GB virus-C/hepatitis G virus: a comparison with hepatitis C virus. *J Med Virol* **53:**348-53.

3812. **Kapel, C. M., and P. Nansen.** 1996. Gastrointestinal helminths of Arctic foxes (Alopex lagopus) from different bioclimatological regions in Greenland. *J Parasitol* **82:**17-24.

3813. **Kaplan, E. L., J. T. Wotton, and D. R. Johnson.** 2001. Dynamic epidemiology of group A streptococcal serotypes associated with pharyngitis. *Lancet* **358:**1334-7.

3814. **Kaplan, K. M., D. C. Marder, S. L. Cochi, and S. R. Preblud.** 1988. Mumps in the workplace. Further evidence of the changing epidemiology of a childhood vaccine-preventable disease. *JAMA* **260:**1434-8.

3815. **Kapperud, G., S. Gustavsen, I. Hellesnes, A. H. Hansen, J. Lassen, J. Hirn, M. Jahkola, M. A. Montenegro, and R. Helmuth.** 1990. Outbreak of Salmonella typhimurium infection traced to contaminated chocolate and caused by a strain lacking the 60-megadalton virulence plasmid. *J Clin Microbiol* **28:**2597-601.

3816. **Kapperud, G., P. A. Jenum, B. Stray-Pedersen, K. K. Melby, A. Eskild, and J. Eng.** 1996. Risk factors for Toxoplasma gondii infection in pregnancy. Results of a prospective case-control study in Norway. *Am J Epidemiol* **144:**405-12.

3817. **Kapperud, G., J. Lassen, S. M. Ostroff, and S. Aasen.** 1992. Clinical features of sporadic Campylobacter infections in Norway. *Scand J Infect Dis* **24:**741-9.

3818. **Kapperud, G., L. M. Rorvik, V. Hasseltvedt, E. A. Hoiby, B. G. Iversen, K. Staveland, G. Johnsen, J. Leitao, H. Herikstad, Y. Andersson, et al.** 1995. Outbreak of Shigella sonnei infection traced to imported iceberg lettuce. *J Clin Microbiol* **33:**609-14.

3819. **Kapperud, G., E. Skjerve, N. H. Bean, S. M. Ostroff, and J. Lassen.** 1992. Risk factors for sporadic Campylobacter infections: results of a case-control study in southeastern Norway. *J Clin Microbiol* **30:**3117-21.

3820. **Kapperud, G., H. Stenwig, and J. Lassen.** 1998. Epidemiology of Salmonella typhimurium O:4-12 infection in Norway. Evidence of transmission from an avian wildlife reservoir. *Am J Epidemiol* **147:**774-82.

3821. **Kappus, K. D., R. G. Lundgren, Jr., D. D. Juranek, J. M. Roberts, and H. C. Spencer.** 1994. Intestinal parasitism in the United States: update on a continuing problem. *Am J Trop Med Hyg* **50:**705-13.

3822. **Kappus, K. D., J. S. Marks, R. C. Holman, J. K. Bryant, C. Baker, G. W. Gary, and H. B. Greenberg.** 1982. An outbreak of Norwalk gastroenteritis associated with swimming in a pool and secondary person-to-person transmission. *Am J Epidemiol* **116:**834-9.

3823. **Karabiber, N., and F. Aktas.** 1991. Foodborne giardiasis. *Lancet* **337:**376-7.

3824. **Karakousis, P. C., R. D. Moore, and R. E. Chaisson.** 2004. Mycobacterium avium complex in patients with HIV infection in the era of highly active antiretroviral therapy. *Lancet Infect Dis* **4:**557-65.

3825. **Karande, S., H. Kulkarni, M. Kulkarni, A. De, and A. Varaiya.** 2002. Leptospirosis in children in Mumbai slums. *Indian J Pediatr* **69:**855-8.

3826. **Karanja, D. M. S., A. W. Hightower, D. G. Colley, P. N. Mwinzi, K. Galil, J. Andove, and W. E. Secor.** 2002. Resistance to reinfection with Schistosoma mansoni in occupationally exposed adults and effect of HIV-1 co-infection on susceptibility to schistosomiasis: a longitudinal study. *Lancet* **360:**592-6.

3827. **Karch, H., H. Russmann, H. Schmidt, A. Schwarzkopf, and J. Heesemann.** 1995. Long-term shedding and clonal turnover of enterohemorrhagic Escherichia coli O157 in diarrheal diseases. *J Clin Microbiol* **33:**1602-5.

3828. **Karch, S., M. F. Dellile, P. Guillet, and J. Mouchet.** 2001. African malaria vectors in European aircraft. *Lancet* **357:**235.

3829. **Karchmer, A. W., and D. L. Longworth.** 2002. Infections of intracardiac devices. *Infect Dis Clin North Am* **16:**477-505, xii.

3830. **Karita, M., S. Teramukai, and S. Matsumoto.** 2003. Risk of Helicobacter pylori transmission from drinking well water is higher than that from infected intrafamilial members in Japan. *Dig Dis Sci* **48:**1062-7.

3831. **Kark, J. D., and M. Lebiush.** 1981. Smoking and epidemic influenza-like illness in female military recruits: a brief survey. *Am J Public Health* **71:**530-2.

3832. **Kartali, G., E. Tzelepi, S. Pournaras, C. Kontopoulou, F. Kontos, D. Sofianou, A. N. Maniatis, and A. Tsakris.** 2002. Outbreak of infections caused by Enterobacter cloacae producing the integron-associated beta-lactamase IBC-1 in a neonatal intensive care unit of a Greek hospital. *Antimicrob Agents Chemother* **46:**1577-80.

3833. **Kashiwagi, K., N. Furusyo, H. Nakashima, N. Kubo, N. Kinukawa, S. Kashiwagi, and J. Hayashi.** 2004. A decrease in mother-to-child transmission of human T lymphotropic virus type I (HTLV-I) in Okinawa, Japan. *Am J Trop Med Hyg* **70:**158-63.

3834. **Kashiwagi, S., J. Hayashi, H. Ikematsu, S. Nishigori, K. Ishihara, and M. Kaji.** 1982. An outbreak of hepatitis B in members of a high school sumo wrestling club. *JAMA* **248:**213-4.

3835. **Kashiwagi, Y., S. Nemoto, Hisashi Kawashima, K. Takekuma, T. Matsuno, A. Hoshika, and J. Nozaki-Renard.** 2001. Cytomegalovirus DNA among children attending two day-care centers in Tokyo. *Pediatr Int* **43:**493-5.

3836. Kass, E. M., W. K. Szaniawski, H. Levy, J. Leach, K. Srinivasan, and C. Rives. 1994. Rickettsialpox in a New York City hospital, 1980 to 1989. *N Engl J Med* **331:**1612-7.

3837. Kassa, H. 2001. An outbreak of Norwalk-like viral gastroenteritis in a frequently penalized food service operation: a case for mandatory training of food handlers in safety and hygiene. *J Environ Health* **64:**9-12, 33; quiz 37-8.

3838. Kassenborg, H. D., C. W. Hedberg, M. Hoekstra, M. C. Evans, A. E. Chin, R. Marcus, D. J. Vugia, K. Smith, S. Desai Ahuja, L. Slutsker, and P. M. Griffin. 2004. Farm Visits and Undercooked Hamburgers as Major Risk Factors for Sporadic Escherichia coli O157:H7 Infection: Data from a Case-Control Study in 5 FoodNet Sites. *Clin Infect Dis* **38 Suppl 3:**S271-8.

3839. Kassenborg, H. D., K. E. Smith, D. J. Vugia, T. Rabatsky-Ehr, M. R. Bates, M. A. Carter, N. B. Dumas, M. P. Cassidy, N. Marano, R. V. Tauxe, and F. J. Angulo. 2004. Fluoroquinolone-resistant campylobacter infections: eating poultry outside of the home and foreign travel are risk factors. *Clin Infect Dis* **38 Suppl 3:**S279-84.

3840. Kasuga, F., M. Hirota, M. Wada, T. Yunokawa, H. Toyofuku, M. Shibatsuji, H. Michino, T. Kuwasaki, S. Yamamoto, and S. Kumagai. 2004. Archiving of food samples from restaurants and caterers—quantitative profiling of outbreaks of foodborne salmonellosis in Japan. *J Food Prot* **67:**2024-32.

3841. Katavolos, P., P. M. Armstrong, J. E. Dawson, and S. R. Telford III. 1998. Duration of tick attachment required for transmission of granulocytic ehrlichiosis. *J Infect Dis* **177:**1422-5.

3842. Kato, H., H. Kita, T. Karasawa, T. Maegawa, Y. Koino, H. Takakuwa, T. Saikai, K. Kobayashi, T. Yamagishi, and S. Nakamura. 2001. Colonisation and transmission of Clostridium difficile in healthy individuals examined by PCR ribotyping and pulsed-field gel electrophoresis. *J Med Microbiol* **50:**720-7.

3843. Kato, H., H. Uezato, K. Katakura, M. Calvopina, J. D. Marco, P. A. Barroso, E. A. Gomez, T. Mimori, M. Korenaga, H. Iwata, S. Nonaka, and Y. Hashiguchi. 2005. Detection and identification of Leishmania species within naturally infected sand flies in the andean areas of Ecuador by a polymerase chain reaction. *Am J Trop Med Hyg* **72:**87-93.

3844. Katz, A. R., V. E. Ansdell, P. V. Effler, C. R. Middleton, and D. M. Sasaki. 2002. Leptospirosis in Hawaii, 1974-1998: epidemiologic analysis of 353 laboratory-confirmed cases. *Am J Trop Med Hyg* **66:**61-70.

3845. Katz, A. R., D. M. Sasaki, A. H. Mumm, J. Escamilla, C. R. Middleton, and S. E. Romero. 1997. Leptospirosis on Oahu: an outbreak among military personnel associated with recreational exposure. *Mil Med* **162:**101-4.

3846. Katz, D. J., M. A. Cruz, M. J. Trepka, J. A. Suarez, P. D. Fiorella, and R. M. Hammond. 2002. An outbreak of typhoid fever in Florida associated with an imported frozen fruit. *J Infect Dis* **186:**234-9.

3847. Katz, G., L. Rannon, E. Nili, and Y. L. Danon. 1989. West Nile fever—occurrence in a new endemic site in the Negev. *Isr J Med Sci* **25:**39-41.

3848. Katz, J. M., W. Lim, C. B. Bridges, T. Rowe, J. Hu-Primmer, X. Lu, R. A. Abernathy, M. Clarke, L. Conn, H. Kwong, M. Lee, G. Au, Y. Y. Ho, K. H. Mak, N. J. Cox, and K. Fukuda. 1999. Antibody response in individuals infected with avian influenza A (H5N1) viruses and detection of anti-H5 antibody among household and social contacts. *J Infect Dis* **180:**1763-70.

3849. Katzenell, U., J. Shemer, and Y. Bar-Dayan. 2001. Streptococcal contamination of food: an unusual cause of epidemic pharyngitis. *Epidemiol Infect* **127:**179-84.

3850. Kauffman, C. A. 1999. Sporotrichosis. *Clin Infect Dis* **29:**231-7.

3851. Kaufmann, A. F., M. D. Fox, J. M. Boyce, D. C. Anderson, M. E. Potter, W. J. Martone, and C. M. Patton. 1980. Airborne spread of brucellosis. *Ann N Y Acad Sci* **353:**105-14.

3852. Kaul, R., J. Kimani, N. J. Nagelkerke, K. Fonck, E. N. Ngugi, F. Keli, K. S. MacDonald, I. W. Maclean, J. J. Bwayo, M. Temmerman, A. R. Ronald, and S. Moses. 2004. Monthly antibiotic chemoprophylaxis and incidence of sexually transmitted infections and HIV-1 infection in Kenyan sex workers: a randomized controlled trial. *JAMA* **291:**2555-62.

3853. Kauppinen, J., T. Nousiainen, E. Jantunen, R. Mattila, and M. L. Katila. 1999. Hospital water supply as a source of disseminated Mycobacterium fortuitum infection in a leukemia patient. *Infect Control Hosp Epidemiol* **20:**343-5.

3854. Kawamoto, F., Q. Liu, M. U. Ferreira, and I. S. Tantular. 1999. How prevalent are Plasmodium ovale and P. malariae in East Asia? *Parasitol Today* **15:**422-6.

3855. Kay, B., and S. N. Vu. 2005. New strategy against Aedes aegypti in Vietnam. *Lancet* **365:**613-7.

3856. Kay, B. H., and R. A. Farrow. 2000. Mosquito (Diptera: Culicidae) dispersal: implications for the epidemiology of Japanese and Murray Valley encephalitis viruses in Australia. *J Med Entomol* **37:**797-801.

3857. Kay, B. H., W. A. Ives, P. I. Whelan, P. Barker-Hudson, I. D. Fanning, and E. N. Marks. 1990. Is Aedes albopictus in Australia? *Med J Aust* **153:**31-4.

3858. Kay, D., J. M. Fleisher, R. L. Salmon, F. Jones, M. D. Wyer, A. F. Godfree, Z. Zelenauch-Jacquotte, and R. Shore. 1994. Predicting likelihood of gastroenteritis from sea bathing: results from randomised exposure. *Lancet* **344:**905-9.

3859. Kaydos-Daniels, S. C., W. C. Miller, I. Hoffman, M. A. Price, F. Martinson, D. Chilongozi, D. Namakwha, S. Gama, S. Phakati, M. S. Cohen, and M. M. Hobbs. 2004. The use of specimens from various genitourinary sites in men, to detect Trichomonas vaginalis infection. *J Infect Dis* **189:**1926-31.

3860. Kaye, E. M., and E. C. Dooling. 1981. Neonatal herpes simplex meningoencephalitis associated with fetal monitor scalp electrodes. *Neurology* **31:**1045-7.

3861. Kayembe, D. L., D. L. Kasonga, P. K. Kayembe, J. C. Mwanza, and M. Boussinesq. 2003. Profile of eye lesions and vision loss: a cross-sectional study in Lusambo, a forest-savanna area hyperendemic for onchocerciasis in the Democratic Republic of Congo. *Trop Med Int Health* **8:**83-9.

3862. Kayentao, K., M. Kodio, R. D. Newman, H. Maiga, D. Doumtabe, A. Ongoiba, D. Coulibaly, A. S. Keita, B. Maiga, M. Mungai, M. E. Parise, and O. Doumbo. 2005. Comparison of Intermittent Preventive Treatment with Chemoprophylaxis for the Prevention of Malaria during Pregnancy in Mali. *J Infect Dis* **191:**109-16.

3863. Kazadi, W., J. D. Sexton, M. Bigonsa, B. W'Okanga, and M. Way. 2004. Malaria in primary school children and infants in kinshasa, democratic republic of the congo: surveys from the 1980s and 2000. *Am J Trop Med Hyg* **71:**97-102.

3864. Kazakova, S. V., J. C. Hageman, M. Matava, A. Srinivasan, L. Phelan, B. Garfinkel, T. Boo, S. McAllister, J. Anderson, B. Jensen, D. Dodson, D. Lonsway, L. K. McDougal, M. Arduino, V. J. Fraser, G. Killgore, F. C. Tenover, S. Cody, and D. B. Jernigan. 2005. A clone of methicillin-resistant Staphylococcus aureus among professional football players. *N Engl J Med* **352**:468-75.

3865. Kazura, J. W., and M. J. Bockarie. 2003. Lymphatic filariasis in Papua New Guinea: interdisciplinary research on a national health problem. *Trends Parasitol* **19**:260-3.

3866. Kazwala, R. R., C. J. Daborn, L. J. Kusiluka, S. F. Jiwa, J. M. Sharp, and D. M. Kambarage. 1998. Isolation of Mycobacterium species from raw milk of pastoral cattle of the Southern Highlands of Tanzania. *Trop Anim Health Prod* **30**:233-9.

3867. Keady, S., J. Farrar, and J. C. Mohle-Boetani. 2004. Outbreak of Salmonella serotype Enteritidis infections associated with raw almonds - United States and Canada, 2003-2004. *MMWR* **53**:484-7.

3868. Kean, B. H., A. C. Kimball, and W. N. Christenson. 1969. An epidemic of acute toxoplasmosis. *JAMA* **208**:1002-4.

3869. Kean, B. H., D. C. William, and S. K. Luminais. 1979. Epidemic of amoebiasis and giardiasis in a biased population. *Br J Vener Dis* **55**:375-8.

3870. Keane, F. E., B. J. Thomas, C. B. Gilroy, A. Renton, and D. Taylor-Robinson. 2000. The association of Mycoplasma hominis, Ureaplasma urealyticum and Mycoplasma genitalium with bacterial vaginosis: observations on heterosexual women and their male partners. *Int J STD AIDS* **11**:356-60.

3871. Keane, V. P., T. F. O'Rourke, P. Bollini, S. Pampallona, and H. Siem. 1995. Prevalence of tuberculosis in Vietnamese migrants: the experience of the Orderly Departure Program. *Southeast Asian J Trop Med Public Health* **26**:642-7.

3872. Kebabjian, R., B. Bibler, R. Georgesen, P. Kishel, D. Cinpinski, D. Finkenbinder, N. Bloomenrader, C. Otto, M. J. Beach, J. Roberts, L. Mirel, K. Day, K. Bauer, and J. Yoder. 2004. Surveillance data from public spa inspections - United States, May-September 2002. *MMWR* **53**:553-5.

3873. Kee, F., G. McElroy, D. Stewart, P. Coyle, and J. Watson. 1994. A community outbreak of echovirus infection associated with an outdoor swimming pool. *J Public Health Med* **16**:145-8.

3874. Keeffe, E. B. 2004. Occupational risk for hepatitis A: a literature-based analysis. *J Clin Gastroenterol* **38**:440-8.

3875. Keene, W., K. Hedberg, P. Cieslak, S. Schafer, and A. Dechet. 2004. Salmonella serotype Typhimurium outbreak associated with commercially processed egg salad—Oregon, 2003. *MMWR* **53**:1132-4.

3876. Keene, W. E., A. C. Markum, and M. Samadpour. 2004. Outbreak of Pseudomonas aeruginosa infections caused by commercial piercing of upper ear cartilage. *JAMA* **291**:981-5.

3877. Keene, W. E., J. M. McAnulty, F. C. Hoesly, L. P. Williams, Jr., K. Hedberg, G. L. Oxman, T. J. Barrett, M. A. Pfaller, and D. W. Fleming. 1994. A swimming-associated outbreak of hemorrhagic colitis caused by Escherichia coli O157:H7 and Shigella sonnei. *N Engl J Med* **331**:579-84.

3878. Keene, W. E., E. Sazie, J. Kok, D. H. Rice, D. D. Hancock, V. K. Balan, T. Zhao, and M. P. Doyle. 1997. An outbreak of Escherichia coli O157:H7 infections traced to jerky made from deer meat. *JAMA* **277**:1229-31.

3879. Keiser, J., J. Utzinger, M. Caldas de Castro, T. A. Smith, M. Tanner, and B. H. Singer. 2004. Urbanization in sub-saharan Africa and implication for malaria control. *Am J Trop Med Hyg* **71**:118-27.

3880. Keiser, P. B., Y. I. Coulibaly, F. Keita, D. Traore, A. Diallo, D. A. Diallo, R. T. Semnani, O. K. Doumbo, S. F. Traore, A. D. Klion, and T. B. Nutman. 2003. Clinical characteristics of post-treatment reactions to ivermectin/albendazole for Wuchereria bancrofti in a region co-endemic for Mansonella perstans. *Am J Trop Med Hyg* **69**:331-5.

3881. Keita-Perse, O., C. Pradier, S. Tempesta, N. Oran, F. Girard-Pipau, M. R. Popoff, E. Vautor, M. J. Vezolles, and P. Dellamonica. 1999. Outbreak of diarrhea related to Clostridium perfringens in a correctional facility: an epidemiologic investigation. *Clin Microbiol Inf* **5**:714-6.

3882. Keizer, S. T., M. M. Langendam, H. van Deutekom, R. A. Coutinho, and E. J. van Ameijden. 2000. How does tuberculosis relate to HIV positive and HIV negative drug users? *J Epidemiol Community Health* **54**:64-8.

3883. Kelley, P. W., E. T. Takafuji, H. Wiener, W. Milhous, R. Miller, N. J. Thompson, P. Schantz, and R. N. Miller. 1989. An outbreak of hookworm infection associated with military operations in Grenada. *Mil Med* **154**:55-9.

3884. Kelly, D. J., A. L. Richards, J. Temenak, D. Strickman, and G. A. Dasch. 2002. The past and present threat of rickettsial diseases to military medicine and international public health. *Clin Infect Dis* **34**:S145-69.

3885. Kelly, P. J., N. Meads, A. Theobald, P. E. Fournier, and D. Raoult. 2004. Rickettsia felis, Bartonella henselae, and B. clarridgeiae, New Zealand. *Emerg Infect Dis* **10**:967–8.

3886. Kelly-Hope, L. A., D. M. Purdie, and B. H. Kay. 2002. Risk of mosquito-borne epidemic polyarthritis disease among international visitors to Queensland, Australia. *J Travel Med* **9**:211-3.

3887. Kelly-Hope, L. A., A. M. Yapabandara, M. B. Wickramasinghe, M. D. Perera, S. H. Karunaratne, W. P. Fernando, R. R. Abeyasinghe, R. R. Siyambalagoda, P. R. Herath, G. N. Galappaththy, and J. Hemingway. 2005. Spatiotemporal distribution of insecticide resistance in Anopheles culicifacies and Anopheles subpictus in Sri Lanka. *Trans R Soc Trop Med Hyg* **99**:751-61.

3888. Kenawy, M. A., J. C. Beier, and S. el Said. 1986. First record of malaria and associated Anopheles in El Gara Oasis, Egypt. *J Am Mosq Control Assoc* **2**:101-3.

3889. Kennedy, F. M., J. Astbury, J. R. Needham, and T. Cheasty. 1993. Shigellosis due to occupational contact with non-human primates. *Epidemiol Infect* **110**:247-51.

3890. Kennedy, R. H., R. N. Hogan, P. Brown, E. Holland, R. T. Johnson, W. Stark, and J. Sugar. 2001. Eye banking and screening for Creutzfeldt-Jakob disease. *Arch Ophthalmol* **119**:721-6.

3891. Kenny, J. V., and R. J. MacCabe. 1993. Sero-epidemiology of hydatid disease in the non-intervention area of north-east Turkana. *Ann Trop Med Parasitol* **87**:451-7.

3892. Kenny-Walsh, E. 1999. Clinical outcomes after hepatitis C infection from contaminated anti-D immune globulin. Irish Hepatology Research Group. *N Engl J Med* **340**:1228-33.

3893. Kent, C. K., J. K. Chaw, W. Wong, S. Liska, S. Gibson, G. Hubbard, and J. D. Klausner. 2005. Prevalence of rectal, urethral, and pharyngeal chlamydia and gonorrhea detected in 2 clinical settings among men who have sex with men: San Francisco, California, 2003. *Clin Infect Dis* **41**:67-74.

3894. Kent, D. C. 1967. Tuberculosis as a military epidemic disease and its control by the Navy Tuberculosis Control Program. *Dis Chest* **52:**588-94.

3895. Kent, G. P., J. Brondum, R. A. Keenlyside, L. M. LaFazia, and H. D. Scott. 1988. A large outbreak of acupuncture-associated hepatitis B. *Am J Epidemiol* **127:**591-8.

3896. Kent, G. P., J. R. Greenspan, J. L. Herndon, L. M. Mofenson, J. A. Harris, T. R. Eng, and H. A. Waskin. 1988. Epidemic giardiasis caused by a contaminated public water supply. *Am J Public Health* **78:**139-43.

3897. Kenyon, T. A., J. E. Copeland, T. Moeti, R. Oyewo, and N. Binkin. 2000. Transmission of Mycobacterium tuberculosis among employees in a US government office, Gaborone, Botswana. *Int J Tuberc Lung Dis* **4:**962-7.

3898. Kenyon, T. A., S. E. Valway, W. W. Ihle, I. M. Onorato, and K. G. Castro. 1996. Transmission of multidrug-resistant Mycobacterium tuberculosis during a long airplane flight. *N Engl J Med* **334:**933-8.

3899. Kermode, M., N. Crofts, P. Miller, B. Speed, and J. Streeton. 1998. Health indicators and risks among people experiencing homelessness in Melbourne, 1995-1996. *Aust N Z J Public Health* **22:**464-70.

3900. Kermode, M., N. Crofts, B. Speed, P. Miller, and J. Streeton. 1999. Tuberculosis infection and homelessness in Melbourne, Australia, 1995- 1996. *Int J Tuberc Lung Dis* **3:**901-7.

3901. Kern, P., K. Bardonnet, E. Renner, H. Auer, Z. Pawlowski, R. W. Ammann, and D. A. Vuitton. 2003. European echinococcosis registry: human alveolar echinococcosis, Europe, 1982-2000. *Emerg Infect Dis* **9:**343-9.

3902. Kern, P., S. Reuter, K. Buttenschoen, and W. Kratzer. 2001. Diagnostik der zystischen Echinokokkose. *Dtsch Med Wochenschr* **126:**20-3.

3903. Kerr-Pontes, L. R., A. C. Montenegro, M. L. Barreto, G. L. Werneck, and H. Feldmeier. 2004. Inequality and leprosy in Northeast Brazil: an ecological study. *Int J Epidemiol* **33:**262-9.

3904. Kessel, A. S., I. A. Gillespie, S. J. O'Brien, G. K. Adak, T. J. Humphrey, and L. R. Ward. 2001. General outbreaks of infectious intestinal disease linked with poultry, England and Wales, 1992-1999. *Commun Dis Public Health* **4:**171-7.

3905. Keswick, B. H., N. R. Blacklow, G. C. Cukor, H. L. DuPont, and J. L. Vollet. 1982. Norwalk virus and rotavirus in travellers' diarrhoea in Mexico. *Lancet* **1:**109-110.

3906. Ketel, W. B., and A. J. Ognibene. 1971. Japanese B encephalitis in Vietnam. *Am J Med Sci* **261:**271-9.

3907. Keus, K., S. Houston, Y. Melaku, and S. Burling. 2003. Treatment of a cohort of tuberculosis patients using the Manyatta regimen in a conflict zone in south Sudan. *Trans R Soc Trop Med Hyg* **97:**614-8.

3908. Kew, O., V. Morris-Glasgow, M. Landaverde, C. Burns, J. Shaw, Z. Garib, J. Andre, E. Blackman, C. J. Freeman, J. Jorba, R. Sutter, G. Tambini, L. Venczel, C. Pedreira, F. Laender, H. Shimizu, T. Yoneyama, T. Miyamura, H. van Der Avoort, M. S. Oberste, D. Kilpatrick, S. Cochi, M. Pallansch, and C. de Quadros. 2002. Outbreak of poliomyelitis in Hispaniola associated with circulating type 1 vaccine-derived poliovirus. *Science* **296:**356-9.

3909. Keystone, J. S., P. E. Kozarsky, D. O. Freedman, H. Nothdurft, and B. A. Connors. 2004. Travel medicine. Mosby, Elsevier Science.

3910. Khallaayoune, K., and H. Laamrani. 1992. Seasonal patterns in the transmission of Schistosoma haematobium in Attaouia, Morocco. *J Helminthol* **66:**89-95.

3911. Khan, A. S., G. O. Maupin, P. E. Rollin, A. M. Noor, H. H. Shurie, A. G. Shalabi, S. Wasef, Y. M. Haddad, R. Sadek, K. Ijaz, C. J. Peters, and T. G. Ksiazek. 1997. An outbreak of Crimean-Congo hemorrhagic fever in the United Arab Emirates, 1994-1995. *Am J Trop Med Hyg* **57:**519-25.

3912. Khan, A. S., C. L. Moe, R. I. Glass, S. S. Monroe, M. K. Estes, L. E. Chapman, X. Jiang, C. Humphrey, E. Pon, J. K. Iskander, et al. 1994. Norwalk virus-associated gastroenteritis traced to ice consumption aboard a cruise ship in Hawaii: comparison and application of molecular method-based assays. *J Clin Microbiol* **32:**318-22.

3913. Khan, A. S., F. K. Tshioko, D. L. Heymann, B. Le Guenno, P. Nabeth, B. Kerstiens, Y. Fleerackers, P. H. Kilmarx, G. R. Rodier, O. Nkuku, P. E. Rollin, A. Sanchez, S. R. Zaki, R. Swanepoel, O. Tomori, S. T. Nichol, C. J. Peters, J. J. Muyembe-Tamfum, and T. G. Ksiazek. 1999. The reemergence of Ebola hemorrhagic fever, Democratic Republic of the Congo, 1995. Commission de Lutte contre les Epidemies a Kikwit. *J Infect Dis* **179 Suppl 1:**S76-86.

3914. Khan, I. A., and N. J. Mehta. 2002. Stenotrophomonas maltophilia endocarditis: a systematic review. *Angiology* **53:**49-55.

3915. Khan, K., P. Muennig, M. Behta, and J. G. Zivin. 2002. Global drug-resistance patterns and the management of latent tuberculosis infection in immigrants to the United States. *N Engl J Med* **347:**1850-9.

3916. Khan, M. Y., M. W. Mah, and Z. A. Memish. 2001. Brucellosis in pregnant women. *Clin Infect Dis* **32:**1172-7.

3917. Khanna, N., D. Goldenberger, P. Graber, M. Battegay, and A. F. Widmer. 2003. Gastroenteritis outbreak with norovirus in a Swiss university hospital with a newly identified virus strain. *J Hosp Infect* **55:**131-6.

3918. Khare, S., T. A. Ficht, R. L. Santos, J. Romano, A. R. Ficht, S. Zhang, I. R. Grant, M. Libal, D. Hunter, and L. G. Adams. 2004. Rapid and sensitive detection of Mycobacterium avium subsp. paratuberculosis in bovine milk and feces by a combination of immunomagnetic bead separation-conventional PCR and real-time PCR. *J Clin Microbiol* **42:**1075-81.

3919. Khatib, R., M. C. Thirumoorthi, B. Kelly, and K. J. Grady. 1995. Severe psittacosis during pregnancy and suppression of antibody response with early therapy. *Scand J Infect Dis* **27:**519-21.

3920. Khetsuriani, N., K. Bisgard, D. R. Prevots, M. Brennan, M. Wharton, S. Pandya, A. Poppe, K. Flora, G. Dameron, and P. Quinlisk. 2001. Pertussis outbreak in an elementary school with high vaccination coverage. *Pediatr Infect Dis J* **20:**1108-12.

3921. Khosravi, A. R., and P. Mansouri. 2001. Onychomycosis in Tehran, Iran: prevailing fungi and treatment with itraconazole. *Mycopathologia* **150:**9-13.

3922. Khurana, P. S., and D. Litaker. 2000. The dilemma of nosocomial pneumonia: what primary care physicians should know. *Cleve Clin J Med* **67:**25-9, 33-4, 37-8 passim.

3923. Khuroo, M. S., S. Kamili, M. Y. Dar, R. Moecklii, and S. Jameel. 1993. Hepatitis E and long-term antibody status. *Lancet* **341:**1355.

3924. Ki-Zerbo, G. A., M. C. Receveur, D. J. Malvy, F. Djossou, M. Tamboura, and M. Le Bras. 2001. Acute bilharziasis outbreak in a family visiting Mali. *J Travel Med* **8:**319-21.

3925. **Kidenya, V., and M. J. Ferson.** 2000. Typhoid and paratyphoid fever in south-eastern Sydney, 1992-1997. *Commun Dis Intell* **24**:233-6.

3926. **Kiefer, G., M. Battegay, N. Gyr, and C. Hatz.** 2002. [Mansonella perstans filariasis after stay in Cameroon. A 19-year-old patient born in Cameroon, in Switzerland for the last 10 years]. *Schweiz Rundsch Med Prax* **91**:61-6.

3927. **Kiel, F. W., and M. Y. Khan.** 1993. Brucellosis among hospital employees in Saudi Arabia. *Infect Control Hosp Epidemiol* **14**:268-72.

3928. **Kiiamov, F. A., L. S. Orlova, A. Topchin Iu, and G. A. Shalabaev.** 1990. [Cases of cutaneous leishmaniasis infection resulting from the importation of sandflies via transportation means]. *Med Parazitol (Mosk):*40-1.

3929. **Kilgore, P. E., E. D. Belay, D. M. Hamlin, J. S. Noel, C. D. Humphrey, H. E. Gary, Jr., T. Ando, S. S. Monroe, P. E. Kludt, D. S. Rosenthal, J. Freeman, and R. I. Glass.** 1996. A university outbreak of gastroenteritis due to a small round-structured virus: application of mlecular diagnostics to identify the etiologic agent and patterns of transmission. *J Infect Dis* **173**:787-793.

3930. **Kilian, A. H., P. Langi, A. Talisuna, and G. Kabagambe.** 1999. Rainfall pattern, El Nino and malaria in Uganda. *Trans R Soc Trop Med Hyg* **93**:22-3.

3931. **Killalea, D., L. R. Ward, D. Roberts, J. de Louvois, F. Sufi, J. M. Stuart, P. G. Wall, M. Susman, M. Schwieger, P. J. Sanderson, I. S. Fisher, P. S. Mead, O. N. Gill, C. L. Bartlett, and B. Rowe.** 1996. International epidemiological and microbiological study of outbreak of Salmonella agona infection from a ready to eat savoury snack—I: England and Wales and the United States. *BMJ* **313**:1105-7.

3932. **Killick-Kendrick, R., and J. A. Rioux.** 2002. Mark-release-recapture of sand flies fed on leishmanial dogs: the natural life-cycle of Leishmania infantum in Phlebotomus ariasi. *Parassitologia* **44**:67-71.

3933. **Kim, D. C.** 1984. Paragonimus westermani: life cycle, intermediate hosts, transmission to man and geographical distribution in Korea. *Arzneim-Forsch / Drug Res* **34**:1180-3.

3934. **Kim, D. Y., T. B. Stewart, R. W. Bauer, and M. Mitchell.** 2002. Parastrongylus (=Angiostrongylus) cantonensis now endemic in Louisiana wildlife. *J Parasitol* **88**:1024-6.

3935. **Kim, J. S., H. Y. Lee, and Y. K. Ahn.** 1991. [Prevalence of Enterobius vermicularis infection and preventive effects of mass treatment among children in rural and urban areas, and children in orphanages]. *Kisaengchunghak Chapchi* **29**:235-43.

3936. **Kim, J. Y., Y. J. Park, S. I. Kim, M. W. Kang, S. O. Lee, and K. Y. Lee.** 2004. Nosocomial outbreak by Proteus mirabilis producing extended-spectrum beta-lactamase VEB-1 in a Korean university hospital. *J Antimicrob Chemother* **54**:1144-7.

3937. **Kim, L. S., J. Stansell, J. P. Cello, and J. Koch.** 1998. Discrepancy between sex- and water-associated risk behaviors for cryptosporidiosis among HIV-infected patients in San Francisco. *J Acquir Immune Defic Syndr Hum Retrovirol* **19**:44-9.

3938. **Kim, P. E., D. M. Musher, W. P. Glezen, M. C. Rodriguez-Barradas, W. K. Nahm, and C. E. Wright.** 1996. Association of invasive pneumococcal disease with season, atmospheric conditions, air pollution, and the isolation of respiratory viruses. *Clin Infect Dis* **22**:100-6.

3939. **Kim, S. G., E. H. Kim, C. J. Lafferty, and E. Dubovi.** 2005. Coxiella burnetii in bulk tank milk samples, United States. *Emerg Infect Dis* **11**:619-21.

3940. **Kim, Y. S., H. J. Yun, S. K. Shim, S. H. Koo, S. Y. Kim, and S. Kim.** 2004. A comparative trial of a single dose of azithromycin versus doxycycline for the treatment of mild scrub typhus. *Clin Infect Dis* **39**:1329-35.

3941. **Kim-Farley, R., S. Bart, H. Stetler, W. Orenstein, K. Bart, K. Sullivan, T. Halpin, and B. Sirotkin.** 1985. Clinical mumps vaccine efficacy. *Am J Epidemiol* **121**:593-7.

3942. **Kim-Farley, R. J., G. Rutherford, P. Lichfield, S. T. Hsu, W. A. Orenstein, L. B. Schonberger, K. J. Bart, K. J. Lui, and C. C. Lin.** 1984. Outbreak of paralytic poliomyelitis, Taiwan. *Lancet* **2**:1322-4.

3943. **Kimberlin, D. W.** 2004. Neonatal herpes simplex infection. *Clin Microbiol Rev* **17**:1-13.

3944. **Kimberlin, D. W., and D. J. Rouse.** 2004. Clinical practice. Genital herpes. *N Engl J Med* **350**:1970-7.

3945. **Kimmig, P., K. Naser, and W. Frank.** 1991. [Seroepidemiologic studies of human toxocariasis]. *Zentralbl Hyg Umweltmed* **191**:406-22.

3946. **Kimura, A. C.** 2004. Multistate shigellosis outbreak and commercially prepared food, United States. *Emerg Infect Dis* **10**:1147-9.

3947. **Kimura, A. C., J. I. Higa, R. M. Levin, G. Simpson, Y. Vargas, and D. J. Vugia.** 2004. Outbreak of necrotizing fasciitis due to Clostridium sordellii among black-tar heroin users. *Clin Infect Dis* **38**:e87-91.

3948. **Kimura, A. C., V. Reddy, R. Marcus, P. R. Cieslak, J. C. Mohle-Boetani, H. D. Kassenborg, S. D. Segler, F. P. Hardnett, T. Barrett, and D. L. Swerdlow.** 2004. Chicken Consumption Is a Newly Identified Risk Factor for Sporadic Salmonella enterica Serotype Enteritidis Infections in the United States: A Case-Control Study in FoodNet Sites. *Clin Infect Dis* **38 Suppl 3**:S244-52.

3949. **Kimura, H., H. Minakami, K. Sakae, M. Ohbuchi, M. Kuwashima, and K. Otsuki.** 1997. Outbreak of echovirus type 33 infection in Japanese school children. *Pediatr Infect Dis J* **16**:83-4.

3950. **Kinde, G., J. Oke, I. Gnahoui, and A. Massougbodji.** 2000. [The risk of malaria transmission by blood transfusion at Cotonou, Benin]. *Sante* **10**:389-92.

3951. **King, C. C., C. J. Chen, S. L. You, Y. C. Chuang, H. H. Huang, and W. C. Tsai.** 1989. Community-wide epidemiological investigation of a typhoid outbreak in a rural township in Taiwan, Republic of China. *Int J Epidemiol* **18**:254-60.

3952. **King, D.** 2001. Ice machines—an audit of their use in clinical practice. *Commun Dis Public Health* **4**:49-52.

3953. **Kinoti, G. K., and J. M. Mumo.** 1988. Spurious human infection with Schistosoma bovis. *Trans R Soc Trop Med Hyg* **82**:589-90.

3954. **Kirch, A. K., H. P. Duerr, B. Boatin, W. S. Alley, W. H. Hoffmann, H. Schulz-Key, and P. T. Soboslay.** 2003. Impact of parental onchocerciasis and intensity of transmission on development and persistence of Onchocerca volvulus infection in offspring: an 18 year follow-up study. *Parasitology* **127**:327-35.

3955. **Kirchhoff, L. V.** 1993. American trypanosomiasis (Chagas' disease) - a tropical disease now in the United States. *N Engl J Med* **329**:639-44.

3956. **Kirchhoff, L. V., A. A. Gam, and F. C. Gilliam.** 1987. American trypanosomiasis (Chagas' disease) in Central American immigrants. *Am J Med* **82**:915-20.

3957. **Kirk, M. D., C. L. Little, M. Lem, M. Fyfe, D. Genobile, A. Tan, J. Threlfall, A. Paccagnella, D. Lightfoot, H. Lyi, L. McIntyre, L. Ward, D. J. Brown, S. Surnam, and I. S. Fisher.** 2004. An outbreak due to peanuts in their shell caused by Salmonella enterica serotypes Stanley and Newport - sharing molecular information to solve international outbreaks. *Epidemiol Infect* **132**:571-7.

3958. **Kirschke, D. L., T. F. Jones, S. C. Buckingham, A. S. Craig, and W. Schaffner.** 2002. Outbreak of aseptic meningitis associated with echovirus 13. *Pediatr Infect Dis J* **21**:1034-8.

3959. **Kirschke, D. L., T. F. Jones, A. S. Craig, P. S. Chu, G. G. Mayernick, J. A. Patel, and W. Schaffner.** 2003. Pseudomonas aeruginosa and Serratia marcescens contamination associated with a manufacturing defect in bronchoscopes. *N Engl J Med* **348**:214-20.

3960. **Kirschke, D. L., T. F. Jones, C. W. Stratton, J. A. Barnett, and W. Schaffner.** 2003. Outbreak of joint and soft-tissue infections associated with injections from a multiple-dose medication vial. *Clin Infect Dis* **36**:1369-73.

3961. **Kirschner, R. A., Jr., B. C. Parker, and J. O. Falkinham, 3rd.** 1992. Epidemiology of infection by nontuberculous mycobacteria. Mycobacterium avium, Mycobacterium intracellulare, and Mycobacterium scrofulaceum in acid, brown-water swamps of the southeastern United States and their association with environmental variables. *Am Rev Respir Dis* **145**:271-5.

3962. **Kisinza, W. N., P. J. McCall, H. Mitani, A. Talbert, and M. Fukunaga.** 2003. A newly identified tick-borne Borrelia species and relapsing fever in Tanzania. *Lancet* **362**:1283-4.

3963. **Kiss, P., D. De Bacquer, L. Sergooris, M. De Meester, and M. VanHoorne.** 2002. Cytomegalovirus infection: an occupational hazard to kindergarten teachers working with children aged 2.5-6 years. *Int J Occup Environ Health* **8**:79-86.

3964. **Kist, M., H. Langmaack, and M. Just.** 1980. [Spread of Yersinia enterocolitica infection within a hospital]. *Dtsch Med Wochenschr* **105**:185-9.

3965. **Kiszewski, A., A. Mellinger, A. Spielman, P. Malaney, S. E. Sachs, and J. Sachs.** 2004. A global index representing the stability of malaria transmission. *Am J Trop Med Hyg* **70**:486-98.

3966. **Kitahama, S., J. Suzuki, and Y. Kawakami.** 1996. [A case of Tsutsugamushi disease infected by mountain climbing in the Republic of Korea]. *Kansenshogaku Zasshi* **70**:516-9.

3967. **Kitao, T.** 2003. Survey of methicillin-resistant coagulase-negative staphylococci isolated from the fingers of nursing students. *J Infect Chemother* **9**:30-4.

3968. **Kitayaporn, D., C. Uneklabh, B. G. Weniger, P. Lohsomboon, J. Kaewkungwal, W. M. Morgan, and T. Uneklabh.** 1994. HIV-1 incidence determined retrospectively among drug users in Bangkok, Thailand. *Aids* **8**:1443-50.

3969. **Kitchen, L. W., K. K. Tu, and F. T. Kerns.** 2000. Strongyloides-infected patients at Charleston area medical center, West Virginia, 1997-1998. *Clin Infect Dis* **31**:E5-6.

3970. **Kitchen, M. S., C. D. Reiber, and G. B. Eastin.** 1977. An urban epidemic of North American blastomycosis. *Am Rev Respir Dis* **115**:1063-6.

3971. **Kitchener, S., P. A. Leggat, L. Brennan, and B. McCall.** 2002. Importation of dengue by soldiers returning from East Timor to North Queensland, Australia. *J Travel Med* **9**:180-3.

3972. **Kitchener, S., P. Nasveld, B. Russell, and N. Elmes.** 2003. An outbreak of malaria in a forward battalion on active service in East Timor. *Mil Med* **168**:457-9.

3973. **Kitler, M. E., P. Gavinio, and D. Lavanchy.** 2002. Influenza and the work of the World Health Organization. *Vaccine* **20** (suppl):S5-S14.

3974. **Kitvatanachai, S., K. Janyapoon, P. Rhongbutsri, and L. C. Thap.** 2003. A survey on malaria in mobile Cambodians in Aranyaprathet, Sa Kaeo Province, Thailand. *Southeast Asian J Trop Med Public Health* **34**:48-53.

3975. **Kiviranta, H., A. Tuomainen, M. Reiman, S. Laitinen, A. Nevalainen, and J. Liesivuori.** 1999. Exposure to airborne microorganisms and volatile organic compounds in different types of waste handling. *Ann Agric Environ Med* **6**:39-44.

3976. **Kiwanuka, N., E. J. Sanders, E. B. Rwaguma, J. Kawamata, F. P. Ssengooba, R. Najjemba, W. A. Were, M. Lamunu, G. Bagambisa, T. R. Burkot, L. Dunster, J. J. Lutwama, D. A. Martin, C. B. Cropp, N. Karabatsos, R. S. Lanciotti, T. F. Tsai, and G. L. Campbell.** 1999. O'nyong-nyong fever in south-central Uganda, 1996-1997: clinical features and validation of a clinical case definition for surveillance purposes. *Clin Infect Dis* **29**:1243-50.

3977. **Kiyosawa, K., E. Tanaka, T. Sodeyama, K. Yoshizawa, K. Yabu, K. Furuta, H. Imai, Y. Nakano, S. Usuda, K. Uemura, et al.** 1994. Transmission of hepatitis C in an isolated area in Japan: community- acquired infection. The South Kiso Hepatitis Study Group. *Gastroenterology* **106**:1596-602.

3978. **Kjaer, S. K., E. M. de Villiers, B. J. Haugaard, R. B. Christensen, C. Teisen, K. A. Moller, P. Poll, H. Jensen, B. F. Vestergaard, and E. Lynge.** 1988. Human papillomavirus, herpes simplex virus and cervical cancer incidence in Greenland and Denmark. A population-based cross-sectional study. *Int J Cancer* **41**:518-24.

3979. **Kjemtrup, A. M., and P. A. Conrad.** 2000. Human babesiosis: an emerging tick-borne disease. *Int J Parasitol* **30**:1323-37.

3980. **Klapsing, P., J. D. MacLean, S. Glaze, K. L. McClean, M. A. Drebot, R. S. Lanciotti, and G. L. Campbell.** 2005. Ross River virus disease reemergence, Fiji, 2003-2004. *Emerg Infect Dis* **11**:613-5.

3981. **Klasco, R.** 2002. Colorado tick fever. *Med Clin North Am* **86**:435-40.

3982. **Klausner, J. D., T. Aragon, W. T. A. Enanoria, J. K. Mann, V. M. Zapitz, D. Portnoy, S. A. Shallow, K. Israel-Ballard, M. s. Kim, J. O'Connell, and D. J. Vugia.** 2001. Shigella sonnei outbreak among men who have sex with men - San Francisco, California, 2000-2001. *MMWR* **50**:922-6.

3983. **Klausner, J. D., J. T. Baer, K. M. Contento, and G. Bolan.** 1999. Investigation of a suspected outbreak of vaginal trichomoniasis among female inmates. *Sex Transm Dis* **26**:335-8.

3984. **Klausner, J. D., D. Passaro, J. Rosenberg, W. L. Thacker, D. F. Talkington, S. B. Werner, and D. J. Vugia.** 1998. Enhanced control of an outbreak of Mycoplasma pneumoniae pneumonia with azithromycin prophylaxis. *J Infect Dis* **177**:161-6.

3985. **Klausner, J. D., C. Zukerman, A. P. Limaye, and L. Corey.** 1999. Outbreak of Stenotrophomonas maltophilia bacteremia among patients undergoing bone marrow transplantation: association with faulty replacement of handwashing soap. *Infect Control Hosp Epidemiol* **20**:756-8.

3986. **Kleemola, M., P. Saikku, R. Visakorpi, S. P. Wang, and J. T. Grayston.** 1988. Epidemics of pneumonia caused by TWAR, a new Chlamydia organism, in military trainees in Finland. *J Infect Dis* **157**:230-6.

3987. **Klein, B. S., J. M. Vergeront, R. J. Weeks, U. N. Kumar, G. Mathai, B. Varkey, L. Kaufman, R. W. Bradsher, J. F. Stoebig,** and J. P. Davis. 1986. Isolation of Blastomyces dermatitidis in soil associated with a large outbreak of blastomycosis in Wisconsin. *N Engl J Med* **314:**529-34.

3988. Klein, J. L., S. K. Nair, T. G. Harrison, I. Hunt, N. K. Fry, and J. S. Friedland. 2002. Prosthetic valve endocarditis caused by Bartonella quintana. *Emerg Infect Dis* **8:**202-3.

3989. Klein Klouwenberg, P. M., S. Oyakhirome, N. G. Schwarz, B. Glaser, S. Issifou, G. Kiessling, A. Klopfer, P. G. Kremsner, M. Langin, B. Lassmann, M. Necek, M. Potschke, A. Ritz, and M. P. Grobusch. 2005. Malaria and asymptomatic parasitaemia in Gabonese infants under the age of 3 months. *Acta Trop* **95:**81-5.

3990. Klein, R. S., S. W. Warman, G. G. Knackmuhs, S. C. Edberg, and N. H. Steigbigel. 1987. Lack of association of Streptococcus bovis with noncolonic gastrointestinal carcinoma. *Am J Gastroenterol* **82:**540-3.

3991. Klement, E., L. Uliel, I. Engel, T. Hasin, M. Yavzori, N. Orr, N. Davidovitz, N. Lahat, I. Srugo, E. Zangvil, and D. Cohen. 2003. An outbreak of pertussis among young Israeli soldiers. *Epidemiol Infect* **131:**1049-54.

3992. Kliks, M. M., K. Kroenke, and J. M. Hardman. 1982. Eosinophilic radiculomyeloencephalitis: an angiostrongyliasis outbreak in American Samoa related to ingestion of Achatina fulica snails. *Am J Trop Med Hyg* **31:**1114-22.

3993. Kliks, M. M., and N. E. Palumbo. 1992. Eosinophilic meningitis beyond the Pacific basin: the global dispersal of a peridomestic zoonosis caused by Angiostrongylus cantonensis, the nematode lungworm of rats. *Soc Sci Med* **34:**199-212.

3994. Kline, S. E., L. L. Hedemark, and S. F. Davies. 1995. Outbreak of tuberculosis among regular patrons of a neighborhood bar. *N Engl J Med* **333:**222-7.

3995. Klinkenberg, E., F. Konradsen, N. Herrel, M. Mukhtar, W. van der Hoek, and F. P. Amerasinghe. 2004. Malaria vectors in the changing environment of the southern Punjab, Pakistan. *Trans R Soc Trop Med Hyg* **98:**442-9.

3996. Klinkenberg, E., W. van der Hoek, and F. P. Amerasinghe. 2004. A malaria risk analysis in an irrigated area in Sri Lanka. *Acta Trop* **89:**215-25.

3997. Klion, A. D., E. A. Ottesen, and T. B. Nutman. 1994. Effectiveness of diethylcarbamazine in treating loiasis acquired by expatriate visitors to endemic regions: long-term follow-up. *J Infect Dis* **169:**604-10.

3998. Klock, L. E., P. F. Olsen, and T. Fukushima. 1973. Tularemia epidemic associated with the deerfly. *JAMA* **226:**149-52.

3999. Klontz, K. C., N. A. Hynes, R. A. Gunn, M. H. Wilder, M. W. Harmon, and A. P. Kendal. 1989. An outbreak of influenza A/Taiwan/1/86 (H1N1) infections at a naval base and its association with airplane travel. *Am J Epidemiol* **129:**341-8.

4000. Knackmuhs, G., M. Gerwel, C. Patterson, M. Navitski, R. Lawder, A. Monaco, M. Dillon, E. Bresnitz, C. Tan, R. Cooksey, and C. A. Robertson. 2004. Mycobacterium chelonae infections associated with face lifts - New Jersey, 2002-2003. *MMWR* **53:**192-4.

4001. Knap, J., and S. Ryba. 2002. [Active immunization against tick-born encephalitis (TBE) among border guards (1993-2002)]. *Przegl Epidemiol* **56 Suppl 1:**110-6.

4002. Knebel, U., N. Sloot, M. Eikenberg, H. Borsdorf, U. Hoffler, and J. F. Riemann. 2001. Plesiomonas-shigelloides-induzierte Gastroenteritiden - seltene Fälle in der westlichen Welt. *Med Klin (Munich)* **96:**109-13.

4003. Kneen, R., M. D. Nguyen, T. Solomon, N. G. Pham, C. M. Parry, T. T. Nguyen, T. L. Ha, A. Taylor, T. T. Vo, N. P. Day, and N. J. White. 2004. Clinical features and predictors of diphtheritic cardiomyopathy in Vietnamese children. *Clin Infect Dis* **39:**1591-8.

4004. Knezevich, M. 1998. Geophagy as a therapeutic mediator of endoparasitism in a free-ranging group of rhesus macaques (Macaca mulatta). *Am J Primatol* **44:**71-82.

4005. Knightingale, K. W., and E. N. Ayim. 1980. Outbreak of botulism in Kenya after ingestion of white ants. *Br Med J* **281:**1682-3.

4006. Knirsch, C. A., K. Jakob, D. Schoonmaker, J. A. Kiehlbauch, S. J. Wong, P. Della-Latta, S. Whittier, M. Layton, and B. Scully. 2000. An outbreak of Legionella micdadei pneumonia in transplant patients: evaluation, molecular epidemiology, and control. *Am J Med* **108:**290-5.

4007. Knobloch, J., R. Bialek, and J. Hagemann. 1983. [Intestinal protozoal infestation in persons with occupational sewage contact]. *Dtsch Med Wochenschr* **108:**57-60.

4008. Knobloch, J., M. Funke, and U. Bienzle. 1980. Autochthonous amoebic liver abscess in Germany. *Tropenmed Parasitol* **31:**414-6.

4009. Knolle, H. 1995. Übertragung der Poliomyelitis durch Trinkwasser und das Problem der Ausrottung. *Gesundheitswesen* **57:**351-4.

4010. Knowles, S., C. Herra, E. Devitt, A. O'Brien, E. Mulvihill, S. R. McCann, P. Browne, M. J. Kennedy, and C. T. Keane. 2000. An outbreak of multiply resistant Serratia marcescens: the importance of persistent carriage. *Bone Marrow Transplant* **25:**873-7.

4011. Knox, J., S. N. Tabrizi, P. Miller, K. Petoumenos, M. Law, S. Chen, and S. M. Garland. 2002. Evaluation of self-collected samples in contrast to practitioner- collected samples for detection of Chlamydia trachomatis, Neisseria gonorrhoeae, and Trichomonas vaginalis by polymerase chain reaction among women living in remote areas. *Sex Transm Dis* **29:**647-54.

4012. Ko, A. I., M. Galvao Reis, C. M. Ribeiro Dourado, W. D. Johnson, Jr., and L. W. Riley. 1999. Urban epidemic of severe leptospirosis in Brazil. Salvador Leptospirosis Study Group. *Lancet* **354:**820-5.

4013. Ko, W. C., D. L. Paterson, A. J. Sagnimeni, D. S. Hansen, A. Von Gottberg, S. Mohapatra, J. M. Casellas, H. Goossens, L. Mulazimoglu, G. Trenholme, K. P. Klugman, J. G. McCormack, and V. L. Yu. 2002. Community-acquired Klebsiella pneumoniae bacteremia: global differences in clinical patterns. *Emerg Infect Dis* **8:**160-6.

4014. Ko, Y. C., M. J. Chen, and S. M. Yeh. 1992. The predisposing and protective factors against dengue virus transmission by mosquito vector. *Am J Epidemiol* **136:**214-20.

4015. Ko, Y. C., M. S. Ho, T. A. Chiang, S. J. Chang, and P. Y. Chang. 1992. Tattooing as a risk of hepatitis C virus infection. *J Med Virol* **38:**288-91.

4016. Kobayashi, S., T. Morishita, T. Yamashita, K. Sakae, O. Nishio, T. Miyake, Y. Ishihara, and S. Isomura. 1991. A large outbreak of gastroenteritis associated with a small round structured virus among schoolchildren and teachers in Japan. *Epidemiol Infect* **107:**81-6.

4017. Kobler, E., P. Schmuziger, and G. Hartmann. 1979. [Hepatitis following acupuncture]. *Schweiz Med Wochenschr* **109:**1828-9.

4018. **Koch, J., A. Schrauder, K. Alpers, D. Werber, C. Frank, R. Prager, W. Rabsch, S. Broll, F. Feil, P. Roggentin, J. Bockemühl, H. Tschäpe, A. Ammon, and K. Stark.** 2005. Salmonella Agona outbreak from contaminated aniseed, Germany. *Emerg Infect Dis* **11**:1124–1127.

4019. **Koch, T. K., B. O. Berg, S. J. De Armond, and R. F. Gravina.** 1985. Creutzfeldt-Jakob disease in a young adult with idiopathic hypopituitarism. Possible relation to the administration of cadaveric human growth hormone. *N Engl J Med* **313**:731-3.

4020. **Koch, W. C., and S. P. Adler.** 1989. Human parvovirus B19 infections in women of childbearing age and within families. *Pediatr Infect Dis J* **8**:83-7.

4021. **Koch, W. C., J. H. Harger, B. Barnstein, and S. P. Adler.** 1998. Serologic and virologic evidence for frequent intrauterine transmission of human parvovirus B19 with a primary maternal infection during pregnancy. *Pediatr Infect Dis J* **17**:489-94.

4022. **Kocianova, E., O. Kozuch, P. Bakoss, J. Rehacek, and E. Kovacova.** 1993. The prevalence of small terrestrial mammals infected with tick-borne encephalitis virus and leptospirae in the foothills of the southern Bavarian forest, Germany. *Appl Parasitol* **34**:283-90.

4023. **Kock, M., R. Schlacher, F. P. Pichler-Semmelrock, F. F. Reinthaler, U. Eibel, E. Marth, and H. Friedl.** 1998. Airborne microorganisms in the metropolitan area of Graz, Austria. *Cent Eur J Public Health* **6**:25-8.

4024. **Koehler, J. E., C. A. Glaser, and J. W. Tappero.** 1994. Rochalimaea henselae infection. A new zoonosis with the domestic cat as reservoir. *JAMA* **271**:531-5.

4025. **Koenigbauer, U. F., T. Eastlund, and J. W. Day.** 2000. Clinical illness due to parvovirus B19 infection after infusion of solvent/detergent-treated pooled plasma. *Transfusion* **40**:1203-6.

4026. **Koff, R. S., M. M. Slavin, J. D. Connelly, and D. R. Rosen.** 1977. Contagiousness of acute hepatitis B. Secondary attack rates in household contacts. *Gastroenterology* **72**:297-300.

4027. **Koh, W. P., M. B. Taylor, K. Hughes, S. K. Chew, C. W. Fong, M. C. Phoon, K. L. Kang, and V. T. Chow.** 2002. Seroprevalence of IgG antibodies against Chlamydia pneumoniae in Chinese, Malays and Asian Indians in Singapore. *Int J Epidemiol* **31**:1001-1007.

4028. **Koh, Y. M., G. H. Barnes, E. Kaczmarski, and J. M. Stuart.** 1998. Outbreak of meningococcal disease linked to a sports club. *Lancet* **352**:706-7.

4029. **Kohl, K. S., K. Rietberg, S. Wilson, and T. A. Farley.** 2002. Relationship between home food-handling practices and sporadic salmonellosis in adults in Louisiana, United States. *Epidemiol Infect* **129**:267-76.

4030. **Kohler, K. A., W. G. Hlady, K. Banerjee, and R. W. Sutter.** 2003. Outbreak of poliomyelitis due to type 3 poliovirus, northern India, 1999-2000: injections a major contributing factor. *Int J Epidemiol* **32**:272-277.

4031. **Kohn, M. A., T. A. Farley, T. Ando, M. Curtis, S. A. Wilson, Q. Jin, S. S. Monroe, R. C. Baron, L. M. McFarland, and R. I. Glass.** 1995. An outbreak of Norwalk virus gastroenteritis associated with eating raw oysters. Implications for maintaining safe oyster beds. *JAMA* **273**:466-71.

4032. **Kohn, W. G., A. S. Collins, J. L. Cleveland, J. A. Harte, K. J. Eklund, and D. M. Malvitz.** 2003. Guidelines for infection control in dental health-care settings - 2003. *MMWR* **52 (RR-17)**:1-76.

4033. **Koide, M., A. Saito, M. Okazaki, B. Umeda, and R. F. Benson.** 1999. Isolation of Legionella longbeachae serogroup 1 from potting soils in Japan. *Clin Infect Dis* **29**:943-4.

4034. **Koizumi, Y., N. Isoda, Y. Sato, T. Iwaki, K. Ono, K. Ido, K. Sugano, M. Takahashi, T. Nishizawa, and H. Okamoto.** 2004. Infection of a Japanese patient by genotype 4 hepatitis e virus while traveling in Vietnam. *J Clin Microbiol* **42**:3883-5.

4035. **Kojouharova, M., N. Gatcheva, L. Setchanova, S. E. Robertson, and J. D. Wenger.** 2002. Epidemiology of meningitis due to Haemophilus influenzae type b in children in Bulgaria: a prospective, population-based surveillance study. *Bull WHO* **80**:690-5.

4036. **Kolaczinski, J., S. Brooker, H. Reyburn, and M. Rowland.** 2004. Epidemiology of anthroponotic cutaneous leishmaniasis in Afghan refugee camps in northwest Pakistan. *Trans R Soc Trop Med Hyg* **98**:373-8.

4037. **Kolavic, S. A., A. Kimura, S. L. Simons, L. Slutsker, S. Barth, and C. E. Haley.** 1997. An outbreak of Shigella dysenteriae type 2 among laboratory workers due to intentional food contamination. *JAMA* **278**:396-8.

4038. **Kolavic-Gray, S. A., L. N. Binn, J. L. Sanchez, S. B. Cersovsky, C. S. Polyak, F. Mitchell-Raymundo, L. V. Asher, D. W. Vaughn, B. H. Feighner, and B. L. Innis.** 2002. Large Epidemic of Adenovirus Type 4 Infection among Military Trainees: Epidemiological, Clinical, and Laboratory Studies. *Clin Infect Dis* **35**:808-18.

4039. **Kolmos, H. J., R. N. Svendsen, and S. V. Nielsen.** 1997. The surgical team as a source of postoperative wound infections caused by Streptococcus pyogenes. *J Hosp Infect* **35**:207-14.

4040. **Komar, N., D. J. Dohm, M. J. Turell, and A. Spielman.** 1999. Eastern equine encephalitis virus in birds: relative competence of European starlings (Sturnus vulgaris). *Am J Trop Med Hyg* **60**:387-91.

4041. **Komar, N., S. Langevin, S. Hinten, N. Nemeth, E. Edwards, D. Hettler, B. Davis, R. Bowen, and M. Bunning.** 2003. Experimental infection of north american birds with the new york 1999 strain of west nile virus. *Emerg Infect Dis* **9**:311-22.

4042. **Komatsu, K., V. Vaz, C. McRill, T. Colman, A. Comrie, K. Sigel, T. Clark, M. Phelan, and R. Hajjeh.** 2003. Increase in coccidioidomycosis - Arizona, 1998-2001. *MMWR* **52**:109-12.

4043. **Komatsu, M., N. Ikeda, M. Aihara, Y. Nakamachi, S. Kinoshita, K. Yamasaki, and K. Shimakawa.** 2001. Hospital outbreak of MEN-1-derived extended spectrum b-lactamase-producing Klebsiella pneumoniae. *J Infect Chemother* **7**:94-101.

4044. **Komijn, R. E., P. E. W. de Haas, M. M. E. Schneider, T. Eger, J. H. Nieuwenhuijs, R. J. van den Hoek, D. Bakker, F. G. van Zijd Erveld, and D. van Soolingen.** 1999. Prevalence of Mycobacterium aviumin slaughter pigs in the Netherlands and comparison of IS1245 restriction fragment length polymorphism patterns of porcine and human isolates. *J Clin Microbiol* **37**:1254-9.

4045. **Komiya, T., K. Sadamasu, M. I. Kang, S. Tsuboshima, H. Fukushi, and K. Hirai.** 2003. Seroprevalence of Coxiella burnetii infections among cats in different living environments. *J Vet Med Sci* **65**:1047-8.

4046. **Kondrat'ev, V. G., L. A. Bykova, T. N. Poltoratskaia, and S. V. Istratkina.** 1998. [The epidemic situation of tick-borne encephalitis and Lyme disease in the city of Tomsk]. *Med Parazitol (Mosk)*:52-3.

4047. **Kong, P.-M., J. Tapy, P. Calixto, W. J. Burman, R. R. Reves, Z. Yang, and M. D. Cave.** 2002. Skin-test screening and tuberculosis transmission among the homeless. *Emerg Infect Dis* **8:**1280-4.

4048. **Konishi, E., and T. Suzuki.** 2002. Ratios of subclinical to clinical Japanese encephalitis (JE) virus infections in vaccinated populations: evaluation of an inactivated JE vaccine by comparing the ratios with those in unvaccinated populations. *Vaccine* **21:**98-107.

4049. **Koo, D., A. Aragon, V. Moscoso, M. Gudiel, L. Bietti, N. Carrillo, J. Chojoj, B. Gordillo, F. Cano, D. N. Cameron, J. G. Wells, N. H. Bean, and R. V. Tauxe.** 1996. Epidemic cholera in Guatemala, 1993: transmission of a newly introduced epidemic strain by street vendors. *Epidemiol Infect* **116:**121-6.

4050. **Koo, D., K. Maloney, and R. Tauxe.** 1996. Epidemiology of diarrheal disease outbreaks on cruise ships, 1986 through 1993. *JAMA* **275:**545-7.

4051. **Kool, J. L., D. Bergmire-Sweat, J. C. Butler, E. W. Brown, D. J. Peabody, D. S. Massi, J. C. Carpenter, J. M. Pruckler, R. F. Benson, and B. S. Fields.** 1999. Hospital characteristics associated with colonization of water systems by Legionella and risk of nosocomial legionnaires' disease: a cohort study of 15 hospitals. *Infect Control Hosp Epidemiol* **20:**798-805.

4052. **Kool, J. L., M. C. Warwick, J. M. Pruckler, E. W. Brown, and J. C. Butler.** 1998. Outbreak of legionnaires' disease at a bar after basement flooding. *Lancet* **351:**1030.

4053. **Koopman, J. S., and J. Campbell.** 1975. The role of cutaneous diphtheria infections in a diphtheria epidemic. *J Infect Dis* **131:**239-44.

4054. **Koopman, J. S., A. S. Monto, and I. M. Longini, Jr.** 1989. The Tecumseh Study. XVI: Family and community sources of rotavirus infection. *Am J Epidemiol* **130:**760-8.

4055. **Koopmans, M., and D. Brown.** 1999. Seasonality and diversity of Group A rotaviruses in Europe. *Acta Paediatr Suppl* **88:**14-9.

4056. **Koopmans, M., B. Wilbrink, M. Conyn, G. Natrop, H. van der Nat, H. Vennema, A. Meijer, J. van Steenbergen, R. Fouchier, A. Osterhaus, and A. Bosman.** 2004. Transmission of H7N7 avian influenza A virus to human beings during a large outbreak in commercial poultry farms in the Netherlands. *Lancet* **363:**587-93.

4057. **Kopic, J., M. T. Paradzik, and N. Pandak.** 2002. Streptococcus suis infection as a cause of severe illness: 2 cases from Croatia. *Scand J Infect Dis* **34:**683-4.

4058. **Koppe, J. G., D. H. Loewer-Sieger, and H. de Roever-Bonnet.** 1986. Results of 20-year follow-up of congenital toxoplasmosis. *Lancet* **1:**254-6.

4059. **Koram, K. A., S. Owusu-Agyei, D. J. Fryauff, F. Anto, F. Atuguba, A. Hodgson, S. L. Hoffman, and F. K. Nkrumah.** 2003. Seasonal profiles of malaria infection, anaemia, and bednet use among age groups and communities in northern Ghana. *Trop Med Int Health* **8:**793-802.

4060. **Kordick, D. L., K. H. Wilson, D. J. Sexton, T. L. Hadfield, H. A. Berkhoff, and E. B. Breitschwerdt.** 1995. Prolonged Bartonella bacteremia in cats associated with cat-scratch disease patients. *J Clin Microbiol* **33:**3245-51.

4061. **Korenberg, E. I.** 1994. Comparative ecology and epidemiology of Lyme disease and tick-borne encephalitis in the former Soviet Union. *Parasitol Today* **10:**157-60.

4062. **Korenberg, E. I., L. Y. Gorban, Y. V. Kovalevskii, V. I. Frizen, and A. S. Karavanov.** 2001. Risk for human tick-borne encephalitis, borrelioses, and double infection in the pre-Ural region of Russia. *Emerg Infect Dis* **7:**459-62.

4063. **Kortbeek, L. M., H. E. De Melker, I. K. Veldhuijzen, and M. A. Conyn-Van Spaendonck.** 2004. Population-based Toxoplasma seroprevalence study in The Netherlands. *Epidemiol Infect* **132:**839-45.

4064. **Korthuis, P. T., T. R. Jones, M. Lesmana, S. M. Clark, M. Okoseray, G. Ingkokusumo, and F. S. Wignall.** 1998. An outbreak of El Tor cholera associated with a tribal funeral in Irian Jaya, Indonesia. *Southeast Asian J Trop Med Public Health* **29:**550-4.

4065. **Korvick, J. A., C. S. Bryan, B. Farber, T. R. Beam, Jr., L. Schenfeld, R. R. Muder, D. Weinbaum, R. Lumish, D. N. Gerding, and M. M. Wagener.** 1992. Prospective observational study of Klebsiella bacteremia in 230 patients: outcome for antibiotic combinations versus monotherapy. *Antimicrob Agents Chemother* **36:**2639-44.

4066. **Kosatsky, T.** 1984. Household outbreak of Q-fever pneumonia related to a parturient cat. *Lancet* **ii:**1447-9.

4067. **Kosek, M., C. Bern, and R. L. Guerrant.** 2003. The global burden of diarrhoeal disease, as estimated from studies published between 1992 and 2000. *Bull WHO* **81:**197-204.

4068. **Kosek, M., R. Lavarello, R. H. Gilman, J. Delgado, C. Maguina, M. Verastegui, A. G. Lescano, V. Mallqui, J. C. Kosek, S. Recavarren, and L. Cabrera.** 2000. Natural history of infection with Bartonella bacilliformis in a nonendemic population. *J Infect Dis* **182:**865-72.

4069. **Koskiniemi, M., M. Lappalainen, P. Koskela, K. Hedman, P. Ammala, V. Hiilesmaa, and K. Teramo.** 1992. The program for antenatal screening of toxoplasmosis in Finland: a prospective cohort study. *Scand J Infect Dis Suppl* **84:**70-4.

4070. **Kosoy, M. Y., R. L. Regnery, T. Tzianabos, E. L. Marston, D. C. Jones, D. Green, G. O. Maupin, J. G. Olson, and J. E. Childs.** 1997. Distribution, diversity, and host specificity of Bartonella in rodents from the Southeastern United States. *Am J Trop Med Hyg* **57:**578-88.

4071. **Kothari, T., M. P. Reyes, and N. Brooks.** 1977. Pseudomonas cepacia septic arthritis due to intra-articular injections of methylprednisolone. *Can Med Assoc J* **116:**1230, 1232, 1235.

4072. **Kotloff, K. L., J. P. Winickoff, B. Ivanoff, J. D. Clemens, D. L. Swerdlow, P. J. Sansonetti, G. K. Adak, and M. M. Levine.** 1999. Global burden of Shigella infections: implications for vaccine development and implementation of control strategies. *Bull WHO* **77:**651-66.

4073. **Kotwal, R. S., R. B. Wenzel, R. A. Sterling, W. D. Porter, N. N. Jordan, and B. P. Petruccelli.** 2005. An outbreak of malaria in US Army Rangers returning from Afghanistan. *JAMA* **293:**212-6.

4074. **Koulla-Shiro, S., C. Kuaban, and L. Bélec.** 1997. Microbial etiology of acute community-acquired pneumonia in adult hospitalized patients in Yaounde-Cameroon. *Clin Microbiol Infect* **3:**180-186.

4075. **Koumans, E. H., C. M. Black, L. E. Markowitz, E. Unger, A. Pierce, M. K. Sawyer, and J. R. Papp.** 2003. Comparison of Methods for Detection of Chlamydia trachomatis and Neisseria gonorrhoeae Using Commercially Available Nucleic Acid Amplification Tests and a Liquid Pap Smear Medium. *J Clin Microbiol* **41:**1507-11.

4076. Koumans, E. H., D. J. Katz, J. M. Malecki, S. Kumar, S. P. Wahlquist, M. J. Arrowood, A. W. Hightower, and B. L. Herwaldt. 1998. An outbreak of cyclosporiasis in Florida in 1995: a harbinger of multistate outbreaks in 1996 and 1997. Am J Trop Med Hyg **59**:235-42.

4077. Kourtis, A. P., M. Bulterys, S. R. Nesheim, and F. K. Lee. 2001. Understanding the timing of HIV transmission from mother to infant. JAMA **285**:709-12.

4078. Koussidou-Eremondi, T., D. Devliotou-Panagiotidou, O. Mourellou-Tsatsou, and A. Minas. 2005. Epidemiology of dermatomycoses in children living in Northern Greece 1996-2000. Mycoses **48**:11-6.

4079. Koutsavlis, A. T., L. Valiquette, R. Allard, and J. Soto. 2001. Blastocystis hominis: a new pathogen in day-care centres? Can Commun Dis Rep **27**:76-84.

4080. Kovacova, E., J. Kazar, and A. Simkova. 1998. Clinical and serological analysis of a Q fever outbreak in western Slovakia with four-year follow-up. Eur J Clin Microbiol Infect Dis **17**:867-9.

4081. Kovacs, A., S. S. Wasserman, D. Burns, D. J. Wright, J. Cohn, A. Landay, K. Weber, M. Cohen, A. Levine, H. Minkoff, P. Miotti, J. Palefsky, M. Young, and P. Reichelderfer. 2001. Determinants of HIV-1 shedding in the genital tract of women. Lancet **358**:1593-601.

4082. Kovacs, J. A., V. J. Gill, S. Meshnick, and H. Masur. 2001. New insights into transmission, diagnosis, and drug treatment of Pneumocystis carinii pneumonia. JAMA **286**:2450-60.

4083. Kowo, M. P., P. Goubau, E. C. N. Ndam, O. Njoya, S. Sasaki, V. Seghers, and H. Kesteloot. 1995. Prevalence of hepatitis C virus and other blood-borne viruses in Pygmies and neighbouring Bantus in southern Cameroon. Trans R Soc Trop Med Hyg **89**:484-6.

4084. Kozek, W. J., G. Palma, W. Valencia, C. Montalvo, and J. Spain. 1984. Filariasis in Colombia: prevalence of Mansonella ozzardi in the Departamento de Meta, Intendencia del Casanare, and Comisaria del Vichada. Am J Trop Med Hyg **33**:70-2.

4085. Kraivichian, K., S. Nuchprayoon, P. Sitichalernchai, W. Chaicumpa, and S. Yentakam. 2004. Treatment of cutaneous gnathostomiasis with ivermectin. Am J Trop Med Hyg **71**:623-8.

4086. Krajick, K. 2001. Cave biologists unearth buried treasures. Science **293**:2378-81.

4087. Kral, A. H., J. Lorvick, L. Gee, P. Bacchetti, B. Rawal, M. Busch, and B. R. Edlin. 2003. Trends in Human Immunodeficiency Virus Seroincidence among Street- Recruited Injection Drug Users in San Francisco, 1987-1998. Am J Epidemiol **157**:915-22.

4088. Kralj, N., F. Hofmann, M. Michaelis, and H. Berthold. 1998. Zur gegenwärtigen Hepatitis-B-Epidemiologie in Deutschland. Gesundheitswesen **60**:450-5.

4089. Kramer, L. D., and K. A. Bernard. 2001. West Nile virus infection in birds and mammals. Ann N Y Acad Sci **951**:84-93.

4090. Kramer, M. H., G. J. Greer, J. F. Quinonez, N. R. Padilla, B. Hernandez, B. A. Arana, R. Lorenzana, P. Morera, A. W. Hightower, M. L. Eberhard, and B. L. Herwaldt. 1998. First reported outbreak of abdominal angiostrongyliasis. Clin Infect Dis **26**:365-72.

4091. Kramer, M. H., B. L. Herwaldt, G. F. Craun, R. L. Calderon, and D. D. Juranek. 1996. Surveillance for waterborne-disease outbreaks—United States, 1993-1994. MMWR CDC Surveill Summ **45**:1-33.

4092. Kramer, M. H., F. E. Sorhage, S. T. Goldstein, E. Dalley, S. P. Wahlquist, and B. L. Herwaldt. 1998. First reported outbreak in the United States of cryptosporidiosis associated with a recreational lake. Clin Infect Dis **26**:27-33.

4093. Kratz, A., D. Greenberg, Y. Barki, and M. Lifshitz. 2003. Pantoea agglomerans as a cause of septic arthritis after palm tree thorn injury; case report and literature review. Arch Dis Child **88**:542-4.

4094. Kraus, H., and F. Tiefenbrunner. 1975. [Randomised investigations of some Tyrolean swimming pools for the presence of Trichomonas vaginalis and pathogenic fungi (author's transl)]. Zentralbl Bakteriol [Orig B] **160**:286-91.

4095. Krause, G., C. Blackmore, S. Wiersma, C. Lesneski, L. Gauch, and R. S. Hopkins. 2002. Mass Vaccination Campaign Following Community Outbreak of Meningococcal Disease. Emerg Infect Dis **8**:1398-1403.

4096. Krause, G., R. Terzagian, and R. Hammond. 2001. Outbreak of Salmonella serotype Anatum infection associated with unpasteurized orange juice. South Med J **94**:1168-72.

4097. Krause, P. J. 2003. Babesiosis diagnosis and treatment. Vector Borne Zoonotic Dis **3**:45-51.

4098. Krause, P. J., K. McKay, C. A. Thompson, V. K. Sikand, R. Lentz, T. Lepore, L. Closter, D. Christianson, S. R. Telford, D. Persing, J. D. Radolf, and A. Spielman. 2002. Disease-specific diagnosis of coinfecting tickborne zoonoses: babesiosis, human granulocytic ehrlichiosis, and Lyme disease. Clin Infect Dis **34**:1184-91.

4099. Krause, P. J., A. Spielman, S. R. Telford, 3rd, V. K. Sikand, K. McKay, D. Christianson, R. J. Pollack, P. Brassard, J. Magera, R. Ryan, and D. H. Persing. 1998. Persistent parasitemia after acute babesiosis. N Engl J Med **339**:160-5.

4100. Krause, R., Z. Bago, S. Revilla-Fernandez, A. Loitsch, F. Allerberger, P. Kaufmann, K. H. Smolle, G. Brunner, and G. J. Krejs. 2005. Travel-associated rabies in Austrian man. Emerg Infect Dis **11**:719-21.

4101. Krause, R., and E. C. Reisinger. 2005. Candida and antibiotic-associated diarrhoea. Clin Microbiol Infect **11**:1-2.

4102. Krause, V. 2000. Cases of leptospirosis in hunters in the Top End - don't go barefoot. Commun Dis Intell **24**:384.

4103. Krebs, J. W., E. J. Mandel, D. L. Swerdlow, and C. E. Rupprecht. 2004. Rabies surveillance in the United States during 2003. J Am Vet Med Assoc **225**:1837-49.

4104. Krech, T., P. Naumann, C. Wittelsberger, H. H. Reinicke, B. Retzgen, B. Jungnitz, and R. Watermann. 1987. [Diphtheria, an imported disease]. Dtsch Med Wochenschr **112**:541-4.

4105. Krech, U., P. Kohli, and S. Pagon. 1978. [Legionnaire's disease in Switzerland]. Schweiz Med Wochenschr **108**:1653-6.

4106. Kreiss, J. K., N. B. Kiviat, F. A. Plummer, P. L. Roberts, P. Waiyaki, E. Ngugi, and K. K. Holmes. 1992. Human immunodeficiency virus, human papillomavirus, and cervical intraepithelial neoplasia in Nairobi prostitutes. Sex Transm Dis **19**:54-9.

4107. Kremsner, P. G., and S. Krishna. 2002. Antimalarial cocktails-tropical flavours of the month. Lancet **360**:1998-9.

4108. Kriechbaum, A. J., and M. G. Baker. 1996. The epidemiology of imported malaria in New Zealand 1980-92. N Z Med J **109**:405-7.

4109. **Krieger, H., and P. Kimmig.** 1995. [Survival ability of Trichomonas vaginalis in mineral baths]. *Gesundheitswesen* **57:**812-9.

4110. **Krieger, J. N., M. Verdon, N. Siegel, and K. K. Holmes.** 1993. Natural history of urogenital trichomoniasis in men. *J Urol* **149:**1455-8.

4111. **Krisin, H. Basri, D. J. Fryauff, M. J. Barcus, M. J. Bangs, E. Ayomi, H. Marwoto, I. R. Elyazar, T. L. Richie, and J. K. Baird.** 2003. Malaria in a cohort of Javanese migrants to Indonesian Papua. *Ann Trop Med Parasitol* **97:**543-56.

4112. **Kristiansen, K.** 2002. TBE in Denmark—in particular on Bornholm. *Int J Med Microbiol* **291 Suppl 33:**62-3.

4113. **Kriz, B., C. Benes, V. Danielova, and M. Daniel.** 2004. Socioeconomic conditions and other anthropogenic factors influencing tick-borne encephalitis incidence in the Czech Republic. *Int J Med Microbiol* **293 Suppl 37:**63-8.

4114. **Kroeger, A., E. V. Avila, and L. Morison.** 2002. Insecticide impregnated curtains to control domestic transmission of cutaneous leishmaniasis in Venezuela: cluster randomised trial. *BMJ* **325:**810-3.

4115. **Krogstad, D. J., H. C. Spencer, Jr., G. R. Healy, N. N. Gleason, D. J. Sexton, and C. A. Herron.** 1978. Amebiasis: epidemiologic studies in the United States, 1971-1974. *Ann Intern Med* **88:**89-97.

4116. **Kron, M., E. Walker, L. Hernandez, E. Torres, and B. Libranda-Ramirez.** 2000. Lymphatic filariasis in the Philippines. *Parasitol Today* **16:**329-33.

4117. **Krone, M. R., A. Wald, S. R. Tabet, M. Paradise, L. Corey, and C. L. Celum.** 2000. Herpes simplex virus type 2 shedding in human immunodeficiency virus-negative men who have sex with men: frequency, patterns, and risk factors. *Clin Infect Dis* **30:**261-7.

4118. **Krovacek, K., S. Dumontet, E. Eriksson, and S. B. Baloda.** 1995. Isolation, and virulence profiles, of Aeromonas hydrophila implicated in an outbreak of food poisoning in Sweden. *Microbiol Immunol* **39:**655-61.

4119. **Krovacek, K., L. M. Eriksson, C. González-Rey, J. Rosinsky, and I. Ciznar.** 2000. Isolation, biochemical and serological characterisation of Plesiomonas shigelloides from freshwater in Northern Europe. *Comp Immunol Microbiol Inf Dis* **23:**45-51.

4120. **Kruger, A., V. Nurmi, J. Yocha, W. Kipp, T. Rubaale, and R. Garms.** 1999. The Simulium damnosum complex in western Uganda and its role as a vector of Onchocerca volvulus. *Trop Med Int Health* **4:**819-26.

4121. **Kruger, A., A. Rech, X. Z. Su, and E. Tannich.** 2001. Two cases of autochthonous Plasmodium falciparum malaria in Germany with evidence for local transmission by indigenous Anopheles plumbeus. *Trop Med Int Health* **6:**983-5.

4122. **Krumbiegel, P., I. Lehmann, A. Alfreider, G. J. Fritz, D. Boeckler, U. Rolle-Kampczyk, M. Richter, S. Jorks, L. Muller, M. W. Richter, and O. Herbarth.** 2004. Helicobacter pylori determination in non-municipal drinking water and epidemiological findings. *Isotopes Environ Health Stud* **40:**75-80.

4123. **Krumm, C. E., M. M. Conner, and M. W. Miller.** 2005. Relative vulnerability of chronic wasting disease infected mule deer to vehicle collisions. *J Wildl Dis* **41:**503-11.

4124. **Krusell, A., J. A. Comer, and D. J. Sexton.** 2002. Rickettsialpox in north Carolina: a case report. *Emerg Infect Dis* **8:**727-8.

4125. **Kruszewska, D., K. Lembowicz, and S. Tylewska-Wierzbanowska.** 1996. Possible sexual transmission of Q fever among humans. *Clin Infect Dis* **22:**1087-8.

4126. **Kruy, S. L., J. L. Soares, S. Ping, and F. F. Sainte-Marie.** 2001. [Microbiological quality of " ice, ice cream, sorbet" sold on the streets of Phnom Penh; April 1996-April 1997]. *Bull Soc Pathol Exot* **94:**411-4.

4127. **Ksiazek, T. G., J. G. Olson, G. S. Irving, C. S. Settle, R. White, and R. Petrusso.** 1980. An influenza outbreak due to A/USSR/77-like (H1N1) virus aboard a US navy ship. *Am J Epidemiol* **112:**487-94.

4128. **Kuberski, T., T. Flood, and T. Tera.** 1979. Cholera in the Gilbert Island. I. Epidemiological features. *Am J Trop Med Hyg* **28:**677-84.

4129. **Kubli, D., R. Steffen, and M. Schär.** 1987. Importation of poliomyelitis to industrialised nations between 1975 and 1984: evaluation and conclusions for vaccination recommendations. *BMJ* **295:**169-71.

4130. **Kucera, K.** 1967. [Pneumocystosis as an anthropozoonosis]. *Ann Parasitol Hum Comp* **42:**465-81.

4131. **Kuehnert, M. J., V. R. Roth, N. R. Haley, K. R. Gregory, K. V. Elder, G. B. Schreiber, M. J. Arduino, S. C. Holt, L. A. Carson, S. N. Banerjee, and W. R. Jarvis.** 2001. Transfusion-transmitted bacterial infection in the United States, 1998 through 2000. *Transfusion* **41:**1493-9.

4132. **Kuenzi, A. J., R. J. Douglass, D. White, Jr., C. W. Bond, and J. N. Mills.** 2001. Antibody to sin nombre virus in rodents associated with peridomestic habitats in west central Montana. *Am J Trop Med Hyg* **64:**137-46.

4133. **Kuhlencord, A., and W. Bommer.** 1986. Epidemiologie und Pathogenität freibleibender Amöben aus Hallenbädern in Südniedersachsen. *Mitt Österr Ges Tropenmed Parasitol* **8:**1267-74.

4134. **Kuhn, J. E.** 2000. Transfusion-Associated Infections with Cytomegalovirus and Other Human Herpesviruses. *Infusionsther Transfusionsmed* **27:**138-143.

4135. **Kuiper, H., A. P. van Dam, A. W. Moll van Charante, N. P. Nauta, and J. Dankert.** 1993. One year follow-up study to assess the prevalence and incidence of Lyme borreliosis among Dutch forestry workers. *Eur J Clin Microbiol Infect Dis* **12:**413-8.

4136. **Kukkula, M., L. Maunula, E. Silvennoinen, and C. H. Von Bonsdorff.** 1999. Outbreak of viral gastroenteritis due to drinking water contaminated by Norwalk-like viruses. *J Infect Dis* **180:**1771–6.

4137. **Kularatne, S. A., J. S. Edirisingha, I. B. Gawarammana, H. Urakami, M. Chenchittikul, and I. Kaiho.** 2003. Emerging rickettsial infections in Sri Lanka: the pattern in the hilly Central Province. *Trop Med Int Health* **8:**803-11.

4138. **Kuloglu, F., J. M. Rolain, P. E. Fournier, F. Akata, M. Tugrul, and D. Raoult.** 2004. First isolation of Rickettsia conorii from humans in the Trakya (European) region of Turkey. *Eur J Clin Microbiol Infect Dis* **23:**609-14.

4139. **Kumar, R., and D. Lloyd.** 2002. Recent advances in the treatment of Acanthamoeba keratitis. *Clin Infect Dis* **35:**434-41.

4140. **Kumar, V., K. Kishore, A. Palit, S. Keshari, M. C. Sharma, V. N. Das, S. Shivakumar, M. S. Roy, N. K. Sinha, M. Prasad, and S. K. Kar.** 2001. Vectorial efficacy of Phlebotomus argentipes in Kala-azar endemic foci of Bihar (India) under natural and artificial conditions. *J Commun Dis* **33:**102-9.

4141. **Kumlin, U., B. Olsen, M. Granlund, L. G. Elmqvist, and A. Tarnvik.** 1998. Cryptococcosis and starling nests. *Lancet* **351:**1181.

4142. **Kun, J. F. J., P. G. Kremsner, and H. Kretschmer.** 1997. Malaria acquired 13 times in two years in Germany. *N Engl J Med* **337:**1636.

4143. **Kunanusont, C., K. Limpakarnjanarat, and H. M. Foy.** 1990. Outbreak of anthrax in Thailand. *Ann Trop Med Parasitol* **84:**507-12.

4144. **Kunimoto, D. Y., M. S. Peppler, J. Talbot, P. Phillips, and S. D. Shafran.** 2003. Analysis of Mycobacterium avium Complex Isolates from Blood Samples of AIDS Patients by Pulsed-Field Gel Electrophoresis. *J Clin Microbiol* **41:**498-9.

4145. **Kunimoto, D. Y., F. A. Plummer, W. Namaara, L. J. D'Costa, J. O. Ndinya-Achola, and A. R. Ronald.** 1988. Urethral infection with Haemophilus ducreyi in men. *Sex Transm Dis* **15:**37-9.

4146. **Kunins, H. V., A. A. Howard, R. S. Klein, J. H. Arnsten, A. H. Litwin, E. E. Schoenbaum, and M. N. Gourevitch.** 2004. Validity of a self-reported history of a positive tuberculin skin test. A prospective study of drug users. *J Gen Intern Med* **19:**1039-44.

4147. **Kuno, G.** 1995. Review of the factors modulating dengue transmission. *Epidemiol Rev* **17:**321-35.

4148. **Kuntchev, A., M. Kojuharova, S. Gjurova, N. Korsum, and L. Fiore.** 2001. Imported wild poliovirus causing poliomyelitis - Bulgaria, 2001. *MMWR* **50:**1033-5.

4149. **Kunz, A., M. A. Susset, B. Sczepanski, and B. Braun.** 2002. Die Nephropathia epidemica. Wichtige Differenzialdiagnose des akuten Nierenversagens im Endemiegebiet Reutlingen. *Dtsch Med Wochenschr* **127:**1685-9.

4150. **Kunz, C.** 2003. TBE vaccination and the Austrian experience. *Vaccine* **21 Suppl 1:**S50-5.

4151. **Kure, C. F., I. Skaar, and J. Brendehaug.** 2004. Mould contamination in production of semi-hard cheese. *Int J Food Microbiol* **93:**41-9.

4152. **Kuriakose, M., C. K. Eapen, and R. Paul.** 1997. Leptospirosis in Kolenchery, Kerala, India: epidemiology, prevalent local serogroups and serovars and a new serovar. *Eur J Epidemiol* **13:**691-7.

4153. **Kuritsky, J. N., M. T. Osterholm, H. B. Greenberg, J. A. Korlath, J. R. Godes, C. W. Hedberg, J. C. Forfang, A. Z. Kapikian, J. C. McCullough, and K. E. White.** 1984. Norwalk gastroenteritis: a community outbreak associated with bakery product consumption. *Ann Intern Med* **100:**519-21.

4154. **Kurkela, S., T. Manni, A. Vaheri, and O. Vapalahti.** 2004. Causative agent of Pogosta disease isolated from blood and skin lesions. *Emerg Infect Dis* **10:**889-94.

4155. **Kuroki, T., S. Sata, S. Yamai, K. Yagita, Y. Katsube, and T. Endo.** 1998. [Occurrence of free-living amoebae and Legionella in whirlpool bathes]. *Kansenshogaku Zasshi* **72:**1056-63.

4156. **Kuroki, T., K. Yagita, E. Yabuuchi, K. Agata, T. Ishima, Y. Katsube, and T. Endo.** 1998. [Isolation of Legionella and free-living amoebae at hot spring spas in Kanagawa, Japan]. *Kansenshogaku Zasshi* **72:**1050-5.

4157. **Kurtzke, J. F., and K. Hyllested.** 1979. Multiple sclerosis in the Faroe Islands: I. Clinical and epidemiological features. *Ann Neurol* **5:**6-21.

4158. **Kuschner, R. A., A. F. Trofa, R. J. Thomas, C. W. Hoge, C. Pitarangsi, S. Amato, R. P. Olafson, P. Echeverria, J. C. Sadoff, and D. N. Taylor.** 1995. Use of azithromycin for the treatment of Campylobacter enteritis in travelers to Thailand, an area where ciprofloxacin resistance is prevalent. *Clin Infect Dis* **21:**536-41.

4159. **Kusuhara, K., S. Sonoda, K. Takahashi, K. Tokugawa, J. Fukushige, and K. Ueda.** 1987. Mother-to-child transmission of human T-cell leukemia virus type I (HTLV-I): a fifteen-year follow-up study in Okinawa, Japan. *Int J Cancer* **40:**755-7.

4160. **Kutkiene, L., and A. Sruoga.** 2004. Sarcocystis spp. in birds of the order Anseriformes. *Parasitol Res* **92:**171-2.

4161. **Kuusi, M., P. Aavitsland, B. Gondrosen, and G. Kapperud.** 2003. Incidence of gastroenteritis in Norway—a population-based survey. *Epidemiol Infect* **131:**591-7.

4162. **Kuusi, M., J. P. Nuorti, M. L. Hanninen, M. Koskela, V. Jussila, E. Kela, I. Miettinen, and P. Ruutu.** 2005. A large outbreak of campylobacteriosis associated with a municipal water supply in Finland. *Epidemiol Infect* **133:**593-601.

4163. **Kuusi, M., J. P. Nuorti, L. Maunula, N. N. Minh, M. Ratia, J. Karlsson, and C. H. von Bonsdorff.** 2002. A prolonged outbreak of Norwalk-like calicivirus (NLV) gastroenteritis in a rehabilitation centre due to environmental contamination. *Epidemiol Infect* **129:**133-8.

4164. **Kwak, E. J., R. A. Vilchez, P. Randhawa, R. Shapiro, J. S. Butel, and S. Kusne.** 2002. Pathogenesis and management of polyomavirus infection in transplant recipients. *Clin Infect Dis* **35:**1081-7.

4165. **La Scola, B., P. E. Fournier, P. Brouqui, and D. Raoult.** 2001. Detection and culture of Bartonella quintana, Serratia marcescens, and Acinetobacter spp. from decontaminated human body lice. *J Clin Microbiol* **39:**1707-9.

4166. **La Scola, B., and D. Raoult.** 1999. Culture of Bartonella quintana and Bartonella henselae from human samples: a 5-year experience (1993 to 1998). *J Clin Microbiol* **37:**1899-1905.

4167. **Labarca, J. A., W. E. Trick, C. L. Peterson, L. A. Carson, S. C. Holt, M. J. Arduino, M. Meylan, L. Mascola, and W. R. Jarvis.** 1999. A multistate nosocomial outbreak of Ralstonia pickettii colonization associated with an intrinsically contaminated respiratory care solution. *Clin Infect Dis* **29:**1281-6.

4168. **Labbe, A. C., E. Frost, S. Deslandes, A. P. Mendonca, A. C. Alves, and J. Pepin.** 2002. Mycoplasma genitalium is not associated with adverse outcomes of pregnancy in Guinea-Bissau. *Sex Transm Infect* **78:**289-91.

4169. **Labbo, R., A. Fouta, I. Jeanne, I. Ousmane, and J. B. Duchemin.** 2004. Anopheles funestus in Sahel: new evidence from Niger. *Lancet* **363:**660.

4170. **Labombardi, V. J., M. O'Brien A, and J. W. Kislak.** 2002. Pseudo-outbreak of Mycobacterium fortuitum due to contaminated ice machines. *Am J Infect Control* **30:**184-6.

4171. **Labuda, M., E. Eleckova, M. Lickova, and A. Sabo.** 2002. Tick-borne encephalitis virus foci in Slovakia. *Int J Med Microbiol* **291 Suppl 33:**43-7.

4172. **Labuda, M., D. Stunzner, O. Kozuch, W. Sixl, E. Kocianova, R. Schaffler, and V. Vyrostekova.** 1993. Tick-borne encephalitis virus activity in Styria, Austria. *Acta Virol* **37:**187-90.

4173. **Lacerda, R., N. Gravato, W. McFarland, G. Rutherford, K. Iskrant, R. Stall, and N. Hearst.** 1997. Truck drivers in Brazil:

prevalence of HIV and other sexually transmitted diseases, risk behavior and potential for spread of infection. *AIDS* **11 Suppl 1:**S15-9.

4174. **Lacey, S. L., and S. V. Want.** 1995. An outbreak of Enterobacter cloacae associated with contamination of a blood gas machine. *J Infect* **30:**223-6.

4175. **Ladhani, S., C. L. Joannou, D. P. Lochrie, R. W. Evans, and S. M. Poston.** 1999. Clinical, microbial, and biochemical aspects of the exfoliative toxins causing staphylococcal scalded-skin syndrome. *Clin Microbiol Rev* **12:**224-42.

4176. **Laferl, H., P. E. Fournier, G. Seiberl, H. Pichler, and D. Raoult.** 2002. Murine typhus poorly responsive to ciprofloxacin: a case report. *J Travel Med* **9:**103-4.

4177. **Laffer, R. R., R. Frei, and A. F. Widmer.** 2000. [Epidemiology of septicemias in a university hospital over 5 yeaars]. *Schweiz Med Wochenschr* **130:**1471-8.

4178. **Laffon-Leal, S. M., V. M. Vidal-Martinez, and G. Arjona-Torres.** 2000. 'Cebiche'—a potential source of human anisakiasis in Mexico? *J Helminthol* **74:**151-4.

4179. **Laga, M., A. Meheus, and P. Piot.** 1989. Epidemiology and control of gonococcal ophthalmia neonatorum. *Bull WHO* **67:**471-478.

4180. **Lagarde, E., M. Joussemet, J. J. Lataillade, and G. Fabre.** 1995. Risk factors for hepatitis A infection in France: drinking tap water may be of importance. *Eur J Epidemiol* **11:**145-8.

4181. **Lagarde, E., M. Schim Van Der Loeff, C. Enel, B. Holmgren, R. Dray-Spira, G. Pison, J. Piau, V. Delaunay, S. M'Boup, I. Ndoye, M. Coeuret-Pellicer, H. Whittle, and P. Aaby.** 2003. Mobility and the spread of human immunodeficiency virus into rural areas of West Africa. *Int J Epidemiol* **32:**744-752.

4182. **Lahmar, S., H. Debbek, L. H. Zhang, D. P. McManus, A. Souissi, S. Chelly, and P. R. Torgerson.** 2004. Transmission dynamics of the Echinococcus granulosus sheep-dog strain (G1 genotype) in camels in Tunisia. *Vet Parasitol* **121:**151-6.

4183. **Lai, C. L., V. Ratziu, M. F. Yuen, and T. Poynard.** 2003. Viral hepatitis B. *Lancet* **362:**2089-94.

4184. **Lai, K. K.** 2001. Enterobacter sakazakii infections among neonates, infants, children, and adults. Case reports and a review of the literature. *Medicine (Baltimore)* **80:**113-22.

4185. **Lai, K. K., S. A. Fontecchio, A. L. Kelley, Z. S. Melvin, and S. Baker.** 1997. The epidemiology of fecal carriage of vancomycin-resistant enterococci. *Infect Control Hosp Epidemiol* **18:**762-5.

4186. **Lai, S., and A. Efstratiou.** 2002. Report on the sith international meeting of the European laboratory working group on diphtheria, Brussels, Belgium. *Eurosurveillance* **7:**8-12.

4187. **Laine, M., R. Luukkainen, J. Jalava, J. Ilonen, P. Kuusisto, and A. Toivanen.** 2000. Prolonged arthritis associated with sindbis-related (Pogosta) virus infection. *Rheumatology (Oxford)* **39:**1272-4.

4188. **Laird, A. R., V. Ibarra, G. Ruiz-Palacios, M. L. Guerrero, R. I. Glass, and J. R. Gentsch.** 2003. Unexpected detection of animal VP7 genes among common rotavirus strains isolated from children in Mexico. *J Clin Microbiol* **41:**4400-3.

4189. **Laitano, A. C., J. P. Genro, R. Fontoura, S. S. Branco, R. L. Maurer, C. Graeff-Teixeira, J. M. Milanez, L. A. Chiaradia, and J. W. Thome.** 2001. Report on the occurrence of Angiostrongylus costaricensis in southern Brazil, in a new intermediate host from the genus Sarasinula (Veronicellidae, Gastropoda). *Rev Soc Bras Med Trop* **34:**95-7.

4190. **Lakin, D., J. Wurgler, C. Brickley, C. Levy, L. K. Sands, S. J. Englender, and J. Bartzatt.** 1991. Outbreak of relapsing fever - Grand Canyon national park, Arizona, 1990. *MMWR* **40:**296-7, 303.

4191. **Lalitha, M. K., J. Kenneth, A. K. Jana, M. V. Jesudason, K. A. Kuruvilla, K. Jacobson, I. Kuhn, and G. Kronvall.** 1999. Identification of an IV-dextrose solution as the source of an outbreak of Klebsiella pneumoniae sepsis in a newborn nursery. *J Hosp Infect* **43:**70-3.

4192. **Lallemant, M., G. Jourdain, S. Le Coeur, J. Y. Mary, N. Ngo-Giang-Huong, S. Koetsawang, S. Kanshana, K. McIntosh, and V. Thaineua.** 2004. Single-dose perinatal nevirapine plus standard zidovudine to prevent mother-to-child transmission of HIV-1 in Thailand. *N Engl J Med* **351:**217-28.

4193. **Lalvani, A., A. A. Pathan, H. Durkan, K. A. Wilkinson, A. Whelan, J. J. Deeks, W. H. Reece, M. Latif, G. Pasvol, and A. V. Hill.** 2001. Enhanced contact tracing and spatial tracking of Mycobacterium tuberculosis infection by enumeration of antigen-specific T cells. *Lancet* **357:**2017-2021.

4194. **Lam, S. K., K. B. Chua, P. S. Hooi, M. A. Rahimah, S. Kumari, M. Tharmaratnam, S. K. Chuah, D. W. Smith, and I. A. Sampson.** 2001. Chikungunya infection—an emerging disease in Malaysia. *Southeast Asian J Trop Med Public Health* **32:**447-51.

4195. **Lamagni, T. L., B. G. Evans, M. Shigematsu, and E. M. Johnson.** 2001. Emerging trends in the epidemiology of invasive mycoses in England and Wales (1990-9). *Epidemiol Infect* **126:**397-414.

4196. **Lamar, J. E., and M. A. Malakooti.** 2003. Tuberculosis outbreak investigation of a U.S. navy amphibious ship crew and the marine expeditionary unit aboard, 1998. *Mil Med* **168:** 523-7.

4197. **Lambert, A. J., D. A. Martin, and R. S. Lanciotti.** 2003. Detection of North American eastern and western equine encephalitis viruses by nucleic acid amplification assays. *J Clin Microbiol* **41:**379-85.

4198. **Lambert, M., T. Patton, T. Chudzio, J. Machin, and P. Sankar-Mistry.** 1991. An outbreak of rotaviral gastroenteritis in a nursing home for senior citizens. *Can J Public Health* **82:**351-3.

4199. **Lambert, M. L., E. Hasker, A. Van Deun, D. Roberfroid, M. Boelaert, and P. Van der Stuyft.** 2003. Recurrence in tuberculosis: relapse or reinfection? *Lancet Infect Dis* **3:**282-7.

4200. **Lambert, S. B., M. L. Morgan, M. A. Riddell, R. M. Andrews, H. A. Kelly, J. A. Leydon, M. C. Catton, P. A. Lynch, D. K. Gercovich, R. A. Lester, J. A. Carnie, and G. J. Rouch.** 2000. Measles outbreak in young adults in Victoria, 1999. *Med J Aust* **173:**467-71.

4201. **Lamont, R. F., D. J. Morgan, S. D. Wilden, and D. Taylor-Robinson.** 2000. Prevalence of bacterial vaginosis in women attending one of three general practices for routine cervical cytology. *Int J STD AIDS* **11:**495-8.

4202. **Lanata, C. F., C. Tafur, L. Benavente, E. Gotuzzo, and C. Carrillo.** 1990. Detection of Salmonella typhi carriers in food handlers by Vi serology in Lima, Peru. *Bull Pan Am Health Organ* **24:**177-82.

4203. **Landau, Z., and L. Green.** 1999. Chronic brucellosis in workers in a meat-packing plant. *Scand J Infect Dis* **31:**511-2.

4204. **Landen, M. G., M. Beller, E. Funk, H. R. Rolka, and J. Middaugh.** 1998. Measles outbreak in Juneau, Alaska, 1996: implications for future outbreaks. *Pediatrics* **102:**1472.

4205. **Landwehr, D., S. M. Keita, J. M. Ponnighaus, and C. Tounkara.** 1998. Epidemiologic aspects of scabies in Mali, Malawi, and Cambodia. *Int J Dermatol* **37:**588-90.

4206. **Lane, R. S.** 1996. Risk of human exposure to vector ticks (Acari: Ixodidae) in a heavily used recreational area in northern California. *Am J Trop Med Hyg* **55:**165-73.

4207. **Lang, C. J., J. G. Heckmann, and B. Neundorfer.** 1998. Creutzfeldt-Jakob disease via dural and corneal transplants. *J Neurol Sci* **160:**128-39.

4208. **Lang, C. J. G., J. G. Heckmann, V. Querner, B. Neundorfer, J. Kornhuber, M. Buchfelder, and H. A. Kretzschmar.** 2002. Disease latency in Creutzfeldt-Jakob disease via dural grafting: a case report. *Eur J Epidemiol* **17:**1013-4.

4209. **Lange, J. L., K. E. Campbell, and J. F. Brundage.** 2003. Respiratory illnesses in relation to military assignments in the Mojave Desert: retrospective surveillance over a 10-year period. *Mil Med* **168:**1039-43.

4210. **Lange, W. R., and E. Warnock-Eckhart.** 1987. Selected infectious disease risks in international adoptees. *Pediatr Infect Dis J* **6:**447-50.

4211. **Langenberg, W., E. A. Rauws, J. H. Oudbier, and G. N. Tytgat.** 1990. Patient-to-patient transmission of Campylobacter pylori infection by fiberoptic gastroduodenoscopy and biopsy. *J Infect Dis* **161:**507-11.

4212. **Langley, J. M., J. C. LeBlanc, M. Hanakowski, and O. Goloubeva.** 2002. The role of Clostridium difficile and viruses as causes of nosocomial diarrhea in children. *Infect Control Hosp Epidemiol* **23:**660-4.

4213. **Langley, J. M., T. J. Marrie, A. Covert, D. M. Waag, and J. C. Williams.** 1988. Poker players' pneumonia. An urban outbreak of Q fever following exposure to a parturient cat. *N Engl J Med* **319:**354-6.

4214. **Lanzieri, T. M., M. S. Parise, M. M. Siqueira, B. M. Fortaleza, T. C. Segatto, and D. R. Prevots.** 2004. Incidence, clinical features and estimated costs of congenital rubella syndrome after a large rubella outbreak in Recife, Brazil, 1999-2000. *Pediatr Infect Dis J* **23:**1116-22.

4215. **Lanzieri, T. M., T. C. Segatto, M. M. Siqueira, E. C. Santos, L. Jin, and D. R. Prevots.** 2003. Burden of congenital rubella syndrome after a community-wide rubella outbreak, Rio Branco, Acre, Brazil, 2000 to 2001. *Pediatr Infect Dis J* **22:**323-329.

4216. **Laohaprertthisan, V., A. Chowdhury, U. Kongmuang, S. Kalnauwakul, M. Ishibashi, C. Matsumoto, and M. Nishibuchi.** 2003. Prevalence and serodiversity of the pandemic clone among the clinical strains of Vibrio parahaemolyticus isolated in southern Thailand. *Epidemiol Infect* **130:**395-406.

4217. **LaPook, J., A. M. Magun, K. G. Nickerson, and J. I. Meltzer.** 2000. Sheep, watercress, and the internet. *Lancet* **356:**218.

4218. **LaPorte, T., D. Heisey-Grove, P. Kludt, B. T. Matyas, A. Demaria, Jr., R. Dicker, A. De, A. Fiore, O. Nainan, and D. S. Friedman.** 2003. Foodborne transmission of hepatitis A - Massachusetts, 2001. *MMWR* **52:**565-7.

4219. **Laras, K., N. C. Sukri, R. P. Larasati, M. J. Bangs, R. Kosim, Djauzi, T. Wandra, J. Master, H. Kosasih, S. Hartati, C. Beckett, E. R. Sedyaningsih, H. J. Beecham III, and A. L. Corwin.** 2005. Tracking the re-emergence of epidemic chikungunya virus in Indonesia. *Trans R Soc Trop Med Hyg* **99**.

4220. **Lardeux, F., F. Riviere, Y. Sechan, and S. Loncke.** 2002. Control of the Aedes vectors of the dengue viruses and Wuchereria bancrofti: the French Polynesian experience. *Ann Trop Med Parasitol* **96 Suppl 2:**S105-16.

4221. **Lardner, A. J., S. M. Lett, E. Harvey, M. Currier, B. Bracken, F. E. Thompson, F. T. Satalowich, R. H. Hutcheson, G. Birkhead, and K. Hand.** 1992. Human psittacosis linked to a bird distributor in Mississippi - Massachusetts and Tennessee, 1992. *MMWR* **41:**794-7.

4222. **Larghi, A., M. Zubin, A. Crosignani, M. L. Ribero, C. Pipia, P. M. Battezzati, G. Binelli, F. Donato, A. R. Zanetti, M. Podda, and A. Tagger.** 2002. Outcome of an outbreak of acute hepatitis C among healthy volunteers participating in pharmacokinetics studies. *Hepatology* **36:**993-1000.

4223. **Larrieu, E., M. Del Carpio, J. C. Salvitti, C. Mercapide, J. Sustersic, H. Panomarenko, M. Costa, R. Bigatti, J. Labanchi, E. Herrero, G. Cantoni, A. Perez, and M. Odriozola.** 2004. Ultrasonographic diagnosis and medical treatment of human cystic echinococcosis in asymptomatic school age carriers: 5 years of follow-up. *Acta Trop* **91:**5-13.

4224. **Larrieu, E., V. Molina, S. Albarracin, S. Mancini, R. Bigatti, L. Ledesma, C. Chiosso, S. Krivokapich, E. Herrero, and E. Guarnera.** 2004. Porcine and rodent infection with Trichinella, in the Sierra Grande area of Rio Negro province, Argentina. *Ann Trop Med Parasitol* **98:**725-31.

4225. **Larrieu, E. J., M. T. Costa, M. del Carpio, S. Moguillansky, G. Bianchi, and Z. E. Yadon.** 2002. A case-control study of the risk factors for cystic echinococcosis among the children of Rio Negro province, Argentina. *Ann Trop Med Parasitol* **96:**43-52.

4226. **Larrosa, A., M. Cortes-Blanco, S. Martinez, C. Clerencia, L. J. Urdaniz, J. Urban, and J. Garcia.** 2003. Nosocomial outbreak of scabies in a hospital in Spain. *Eur Surveill* **8:**199-203.

4227. **Larsen, S. A., Jr., and D. R. Homer.** 1978. Relation of breast versus bottle feeding to hospitalization for gastroenteritis in a middle-class U.S. population. *J Pediatr* **92:**417-8.

4228. **Larson, E., L. Bobo, R. Bennett, S. Murphy, S. T. Seng, J. T. Choo, and J. Sisler.** 1992. Lack of care giver hand contamination with endemic bacterial pathogens in a nursing home. *Am J Infect Control* **20:**11-5.

4229. **Larsson, P., B. Brinkhoff, and L. Larsson.** 1987. Corynebacterium diphtheriae in the environment of carriers and patients. *J Hosp Infect* **10:**282-6.

4230. **LaRussa, P., S. Steinberg, F. Meurice, and A. Gershon.** 1997. Transmission of vaccine strain varicella-zoster virus from a healthy adult with vaccine-associated rash to susceptible household contacts. *J Infect Dis* **176:**1072-5.

4231. **Lass-Florl, C., P. Rath, D. Niederwieser, G. Kofler, R. Wurzner, A. Krezy, and M. P. Dierich.** 2000. Aspergillus terreus infections in haematological malignancies: molecular epidemiology suggests association with in-hospital plants. *J Hosp Infect* **46:**31-5.

4232. **Lastavica, C. C., M. L. Wilson, V. P. Berardi, A. Spielman, and R. D. Deblinger.** 1989. Rapid emergence of a focal epidemic of Lyme disease in coastal Massachusetts. *N Engl J Med* **320:**133-7.

4233. **Latge, J. P.** 1999. Aspergillus fumigatus and aspergillosis. *Clin Microbiol Rev* **12:**310-50.

4234. **Latib, M. A., M. D. Pascoe, M. S. Duffield, and D. Kahn.** 2001. Microsporidiosis in the graft of a renal transplant recipient. *Transpl Int* **14:**274-7.

4235. **Latif, B. M., J. K. Al-Delemi, B. S. Mohammed, S. M. Al-Bayati, and A. M. Al-Amiry.** 1999. Prevalence of Sarcocystis spp. in meat-producing animals in Iraq. *Vet Parasitol* **84**:85-90.

4236. **Lau, J. T., M. Lau, J. H. Kim, H. Y. Tsui, T. Tsang, and T. W. Wong.** 2004. Probable secondary infections in households of SARS patients in Hong Kong. *Emerg Infect Dis* **10**:235-43.

4237. **Lau, J. T., X. Yang, P. C. Leung, L. Chan, E. Wong, C. Fong, and H. Y. Tsui.** 2004. SARS in three categories of hospital workers, Hong Kong. *Emerg Infect Dis* **10**:1399-404.

4238. **Lau, J. T. F., K. S. Fung, T. W. Wong, J. H. Kim, E. Wong, S. Chung, D. Ho, L. Y. Chan, S. F. Lui, and A. Cheng.** 2004. SARS transmission among hospital workers in Hong Kong. *Emerg Infect Dis* **10**:280-6.

4239. **Lau, S. K., W. K. To, P. W. Tse, A. K. Chan, P. C. Woo, H. W. Tsoi, A. F. Leung, K. S. Li, P. K. Chan, W. W. Lim, R. W. Yung, K. H. Chan, and K. Y. Yuen.** 2005. Human parainfluenza virus 4 outbreak and the role of diagnostic tests. *J Clin Microbiol* **43**:4515-21.

4240. **Laubenthal, H.** 1997. [BSE and heparin and gelatin preparations]. *Anaesthesist* **46**:253-4.

4241. **Laughon, B. E., D. A. Druckman, A. Vernon, T. C. Quinn, B. F. Polk, J. F. Modlin, R. H. Yolken, and J. G. Bartlett.** 1988. Prevalence of enteric pathogens in homosexual men with and without acquired immunodeficiency syndrome. *Gastroenterology* **94**:984-93.

4242. **Laukkanen, R., T. Niskanen, M. Fredriksson-Ahomaa, and H. Korkeala.** 2003. Yersinia pseudotuberculosis in pigs and pig houses in Finland. *Adv Exp Med Biol* **529**:371-3.

4243. **Laupland, K. B., D. L. Church, M. Mucenski, L. R. Sutherland, and H. D. Davies.** 2003. Population-based study of the epidemiology of and the risk factors for invasive Staphylococcus aureus infections. *J Infect Dis* **187**:1452-9.

4244. **Laupland, K. B., D. B. Gregson, D. L. Church, T. Ross, and S. Elsayed.** 2005. Invasive Candida species infections: a 5 year population-based assessment. *J Antimicrob Chemother* **56**:532-7.

4245. **Laurence, B. R.** 1986. Old World blowflies in the New World. *Parasitol Today* **2**:77-9.

4246. **Laurence, B. R.** 1989. The global dispersal of Bancroftian filariasis. *Parasitol Today* **5**:260-4.

4247. **Laurent, S., E. Esnault, G. Dambrine, A. Goudeau, D. Choudat, and D. Rasschaert.** 2001. Detection of avian oncogenic Marek's disease herpesvirus DNA in human sera. *J Gen Virol* **82**:233-40.

4248. **Lauria-Pires, L., M. S. Braga, A. C. Vexenat, N. Nitz, A. Simoes-Barbosa, D. L. Tinoco, and A. R. Teixeira.** 2000. Progressive chronic Chagas heart disease ten years after treatment with anti-Trypanosoma cruzi nitroderivatives. *Am J Trop Med Hyg* **63**:111-8.

4249. **Laurichesse, H., D. Dedman, J. M. Watson, and M. C. Zambon.** 1999. Epidemiological features of parainfluenza virus infections: laboratory surveillance in England and Wales, 1975-1997. *Eur J Epidemiol* **15**:475-484.

4250. **Laussucq, S., A. L. Baltch, R. P. Smith, R. W. Smithwick, B. J. Davis, E. K. Desjardin, V. A. Silcox, A. B. Spellacy, R. T. Zeimis, H. M. Gruft, et al.** 1988. Nosocomial Mycobacterium fortuitum colonization from a contaminated ice machine. *Am Rev Respir Dis* **138**:891-4.

4251. **Lavanchy, D.** 2004. Hepatitis B virus epidemiology, disease burden, treatment, and current and emerging prevention and control measures. *J Viral Hepat* **11**:97-107.

4252. **Laventure, S., J. Mouchet, S. Blanchy, L. Marrama, P. Rabarison, L. Andrianaivolambo, E. Rajaonarivelo, I. Rakotoarivony, and J. Roux.** 1996. [Rice: source of life and death on the plateaux of Madagascar]. *Sante* **6**:79-86.

4253. **Laverdant, C., A. Thabaut, J. Hardelin, P. Cristau, C. Molinie, J. L. Durosoir, H. Essioux, J. P. Daly, P. Larroque, and G. Cathalan.** 1980. Les bilharzioses Africaines de première invasion. *Med Trop* **40**:251-8.

4254. **Lavreys, L., B. Chohan, R. Ashley, B. A. Richardson, L. Corey, K. Mandaliya, J. O. Ndinya-Achola, and J. K. Kreiss.** 2003. Human herpesvirus 8: seroprevalence and correlates in prostitutes in Mombasa, Kenya. *J Infect Dis* **187**:359-63.

4255. **Law, C.** 1990. Sexually transmitted diseases and enteric infections in the male homosexual population. *Semin Dermatol* **9**:178-84.

4256. **Lawn, J. E., S. Cousens, and J. Zupan.** 2005. 4 million neonatal deaths: when? Where? Why? *Lancet* **365**:891-900.

4257. **Lawrence, D. N.** 2004. Outbreaks of Gastrointestinal Diseases on Cruise Ships: Lessons from Three Decades of Progress. *Curr Infect Dis Rep* **6**:115-123.

4258. **Lawrence, D. N., P. A. Blake, J. C. Yashuk, J. G. Wells, W. B. Creech, and J. H. Hughes.** 1979. Vibrio parahaemolyticus gastroenteritis outbreaks aboard two cruise ships. *Am J Epidemiol* **109**:71-80.

4259. **Lawrence, G., J. Leafasia, J. Sheridan, S. Hills, J. Wate, C. Wate, J. Montgomery, N. Pandeya, and D. Purdie.** 2005. Control of scabies, skin sores and haematuria in children in the Solomon islands: another role for ivermectin. *Bull WHO* **83**:34-42.

4260. **Lawrence, G. W., D. Lehmann, G. Anian, C. A. Coakley, G. Saleu, M. J. Barker, and M. W. Davis.** 1990. Impact of active immunisation against enteritis necroticans in Papua New Guinea. *Lancet* **336**:1165-7.

4261. **Lawson, H. W., M. M. Braun, R. I. M. Glass, S. E. Stine, S. S. Monroe, H. K. Atrash, L. E. Lee, and S. J. Englender.** 1991. Waterborne outbreak of Norwalk virus gastroenteritis at a southwest US resort: role of geological formations in contamination of well water. *Lancet* **337**:1200-4.

4262. **Layde, P. M., A. L. Engelberg, H. I. Dobbs, A. C. Curtis, R. B. Craven, P. L. Graitcer, G. V. Sedmak, J. D. Erickson, and G. R. Noble.** 1980. Outbreak of influenza A/USSR/77 at Marquette University. *J Infect Dis* **142**:347-52.

4263. **Layton, M., M. Cartter, E. Bresnitz, S. Wiersma, and L. Mascola.** 2001. Exposure to patients with meningococcal disease on aircrafts - United States, 1999-2001. *MMWR* **50**:485-489.

4264. **Layton, M., M. E. Parise, C. C. Campbell, R. Advani, J. D. Sexton, E. M. Bosler, and J. R. Zucker.** 1995. Mosquito-transmitted malaria in New York City, 1993. *Lancet* **346**:729-31.

4265. **Layton, M. C., M. F. Cantwell, G. J. Dorsinville, S. E. Valway, I. M. Onorato, and T. R. Frieden.** 1995. Tuberculosis screening among homeless persons with AIDS living in single-room-occupancy hotels. *Am J Public Health* **85**:1556-9.

4266. **Lazera, M. S., M. A. Salmito Cavalcanti, A. T. Londero, L. Trilles, M. M. Nishikawa, and B. Wanke.** 2000. Possible primary ecological niche of Cryptococcus neoformans. *Med Mycol* **38**:379-83.

4267. **Lazo, R. F., E. Hidalgo, J. E. Lazo, A. Bermeo, M. Llaguno, J. Murillo, and V. P. Teixeira.** 1999. Ocular linguatuliasis in Ecuador: case report and morphometric study of the larva of Linguatula serrata. *Am J Trop Med Hyg* **60**:405-9.

4268. Le Blancq, S. M., A. Belehu, and W. Peters. 1986. Leishmania in the Old World: 3. The distribution of L. aethiopica zymodemes. *Trans R Soc Trop Med Hyg* **80:**360-6.

4269. Le Blancq, S. M., L. F. Schnur, and W. Peters. 1986. Leishmania in the Old World: 1. The geographical and hostal distribution of L. major zymodemes. *Trans R Soc Trop Med Hyg* **80:**99-112.

4270. Le Coustumier, A. I., A. N. Le Coustumier, M. Artois, A. Audurier, J. Barrat, G. Couetdic, G. Desnoyel, G. Garrigue, B. Jaulhac, P. Laudat, C. Lion, Y. Michel-Briand, H. Monteil, H. De Montclos, C. Tram, M. Weber, and J. L. Widerkehr. 1994. Epidémiologie de la tularémie en France. Modes de transmission inhabituels. Recrudescence en 1993 de la tularémie humaine. *Bulletin Epidémiologique Hebdomadaire* **42 (24 oct):**195-7.

4271. Le Fichoux, Y., J. F. Quaranta, J. P. Aufeuvre, A. Lelievre, P. Marty, I. Suffia, D. Rousseau, and J. Kubar. 1999. Occurrence of Leishmania infantum parasitemia in asymptomatic blood donors living in an area of endemicity in southern France. *J Clin Microbiol* **37:**1953-7.

4272. Le Guenno, B. 1997. [Viral hemorrhagic fevers: what is the risk for travelers?]. *Med Trop (Mars)* **57:**511-3.

4273. Le Guyader, F., F. H. Neill, M. K. Estes, S. S. Monroe, T. Ando, and R. L. Atmar. 1996. Detection and analysis of a small round-structured virus strain in oysters implicated in an outbreak of acute gastroenteritis. *Appl Environ Microbiol* **62:**4268-72.

4274. Le Guyader, F. S., C. Mittelholzer, L. Haugarreau, K. O. Hedlund, R. Alsterlund, M. Pommepuy, and L. Svensson. 2004. Detection of noroviruses in raspberries associated with a gastroenteritis outbreak. *Int J Food Microbiol* **97:**179-86.

4275. Le, T. H., V. D. Nguyen, B. U. Phan, D. Blair, and D. P. McManus. 2004. Case report: unusual presentation of Fasciolopsis buski in a Viet Namese child. *Trans R Soc Trop Med Hyg* **98:**193-4.

4276. Leach, C. T., F. C. Koo, S. G. Hilsenbeck, and H. B. Jenson. 1999. The epidemiology of viral hepatitis in children in south Texas: increased prevalence of hepatitis A along the Texas-Mexico border. *J Infect Dis* **180:**509-13.

4277. Leach, C. T., F. C. Koo, T. L. Kuhls, S. G. Hilsenbeck, and H. B. Jenson. 2000. Prevalence of Cryptosporidium parvum infection in children along the Texas-Mexico border and associated risk factors. *Am J Trop Med Hyg* **62:**656-61.

4278. Leake, J. A. D., M. L. Kone, A. A. Yada, L. F. Barry, G. Traore, A. Ware, T. Coulibaly, A. Berthe, H. Mambu Ma Disu, N. E. Rosenstein, B. D. Plikaytis, K. Esteves, J. Kawamata, J. D. Wenger, D. L. Heymann, and B. A. Perkins. 2002. Early detection and response to meningococcal diseases epidemics in sub-Saharan Africa: appraisal of the WHO strategy. *Bull WHO* **80:**342-9.

4279. Leal-Castellanos, C. B., R. Garcia-Suarez, E. Gonzalez-Figueroa, J. L. Fuentes-Allen, and J. Escobedo-de la Penal. 2003. Risk factors and the prevalence of leptospirosis infection in a rural community of Chiapas, Mexico. *Epidemiol Infect* **131:**1149-56.

4280. Leang, R., D. Socheat, B. Bin, T. Bunkea, and P. Odermatt. 2004. Assessment of disease and infection of lymphatic filariasis in Northeastern Cambodia. *Trop Med Int Health* **9:**1115-20.

4281. Learned, L. A., M. G. Reynolds, D. W. Wassa, Y. Li, V. A. Olson, K. Karem, L. L. Stempora, Z. H. Braden, R. Kline, A. Likos, F. Libama, H. Moudzeo, J. D. Bolanda, P. Tarangonia, P. Boumandoki, P. Formenty, J. M. Harvey, and I. K. Damon. 2005. Extended Interhuman Transmission of Monkeypox in a Hospital Community in the Republic of the Congo, 2003. *Am J Trop Med Hyg* **73:**428-434.

4282. Lebech, M., O. Andersen, N. C. Christensen, J. Hertel, H. E. Nielsen, B. Peitersen, C. Rechnitzer, S. O. Larsen, B. Norgaard-Pedersen, and E. Petersen. 1999. Feasibility of neonatal screening for toxoplasma infection in the absence of prenatal treatment. Danish Congenital Toxoplasmosis Study Group. *Lancet* **353:**1834-7.

4283. Lebessi, E., H. Dellagrammaticas, P. T. Tassios, L. S. Tzouvelekis, S. Ioannidou, M. Foustoukou, and N. J. Legakis. 2002. Extended-spectrum beta-lactamase-producing Klebsiella pneumoniae in a neonatal intensive care unit in the high-prevalence area of Athens, Greece. *J Clin Microbiol* **40:**799-804.

4284. Leblebicioglu, H., and C. Eroglu. 2004. Acute hepatitis B virus infection in Turkey: epidemiology and genotype distribution. *Clin Microbiol Infect* **10:**537-41.

4285. Leclair, J. M., J. Freeman, B. F. Sullivan, C. M. Crowley, and D. A. Goldmann. 1987. Prevention of nosocomial respiratory syncytial virus infections through compliance with glove and gown isolation precautions. *N Engl J Med* **317:**329-34.

4286. Leclerc, H., L. Schwartzbrod, and E. Dei-Cas. 2002. Microbial agents associated with waterborne diseases. *Crit Rev Microbiol* **28:**371-409.

4287. Leclerc, M. C., M. Menegon, A. Cligny, J. L. Noyer, S. Mammadov, N. Aliyev, E. Gasimov, G. Majori, and C. Severini. 2004. Genetic diversity of Plasmodium vivax isolates from Azerbaijan. *Malar J* **3:**40.

4288. Leclercq, A., L. Martin, M. L. Vergnes, N. Ounnoughene, J. F. Laran, P. Giraud, and E. Carniel. 2005. Fatal Yersinia enterocolitica biotype 4 serovar O:3 sepsis after red blood cell transfusion. *Transfusion* **45:**814-8.

4289. Lecompte, Y., and J. F. Trape. 2003. [West African tick-borne relapsing fever]. *Ann Biol Clin (Paris)* **61:**541-8.

4290. Lecour, H., H. Ramos, B. Almeida, and R. Barbosa. 1988. Food-borne botulism. A review of 13 outbreaks. *Arch Intern Med* **148:**578-80.

4291. Leder, K., J. Black, D. O'Brien, Z. Greenwood, K. C. Kain, E. Schwartz, G. Brown, and J. Torresi. 2004. Malaria in travelers: a review of the GeoSentinel surveillance network. *Clin Infect Dis* **39:**1104-12.

4292. Lederberg, J., R. E. Shope, and S. C. Oaks. 1992. Emerging infections. Microbial threats to health in the United States. National Academy Press, Washington, D.C.

4293. Lederer, P., and R. Muller. 1999. [Ornithosis—studies in correlation with an outbreak]. *Gesundheitswesen* **61:**614-9.

4294. LeDoux, M. S. 2000. Tularemia presenting with ataxia. *Clin Infect Dis* **30:**211-2.

4295. LeDuc, J. W., G. A. Smith, J. E. Childs, F. P. Pinheiro, J. I. Maiztegui, B. Niklasson, A. Antoniades, D. M. Robinson, M. Khin, and K. F. Shortridge. 1986. Global survey of antibody to Hantaan-related viruses among peridomestic rodents. *Bull WHO* **64:**139-44.

4296. Lee, A. L., J. Taylor, G. P. Carter, B. Quinn, J. J. Farmer, 3rd, and R. V. Tauxe. 1991. Yersinia enterocolitica O:3: an emerging cause of pediatric gastroenteritis in the United States. *J Infect Dis* **163:**660-3.

4297. **Lee, B. R., S. L. Feaver, C. A. Miller, C. W. Hedberg, and K. R. Ehresmann.** 2004. An elementary school outbreak of varicella attributed to vaccine failure: policy implications. *J Infect Dis* **190**:477-83.

4298. **Lee, G. S., I. S. Cho, Y. H. Lee, H. J. Noh, D. W. Shin, S. G. Lee, and T. Y. Lee.** 2002. Epidemiological study of clonorchiasis and metagonimiasis along the Geum-gang (River) in Okcheon-gun (County), Korea. *Korean J Parasitol* **40**:9-16.

4299. **Lee, H. W., and G. van der Groen.** 1989. Hemorrhagic fever with renal syndrome. *Prog Med Virol* **36**:62-102.

4300. **Lee, J. J., G. F. Leedale, and P. Bradbury.** 2000. An illustrated guide to the protozoa (2nd edition), vol. 1 & 2. Society of Protozoologists, Lawrence, Kansas 66044, USA, PO Box 368.

4301. **Lee, J. S., and K. H. Joo.** 1978. Examination of parasitic contaminants on vegetables in the markets of Seoul. *Korean Cent J. Med* **35**:55-60.

4302. **Lee, J. S., W. J. Lee, S. H. Cho, and H. I. Ree.** 2002. Outbreak of vivax malaria in areas adjacent to the demilitarized zone, South Korea, 1998. *Am J Trop Med Hyg* **66**:13-7.

4303. **Lee, K. K., P. C. Liu, and C. Y. Huang.** 2003. Vibrio parahaemolyticus infectious for both humans and edible mollusk abalone. *Microbes Infect* **5**:481-5.

4304. **Lee, L. A., S. M. Ostroff, H. B. McGee, D. R. Johnson, F. P. Downes, D. N. Cameron, N. H. Bean, and P. M. Griffin.** 1991. An outbreak of shigellosis at an outdoor music festival. *Am J Epidemiol* **133**:608-15.

4305. **Lee, L. H., C. M. LeVea, and P. S. Graman.** 1998. Congenital tuberculosis in a neonatal intensive care unit: case report, epidemiological investigation, and management of exposures. *Clin Infect Dis* **27**:474-7.

4306. **Lee, M. B., and D. Middleton.** 2003. Enteric illness in Ontario, Canada, from 1997-2001. *J Food Prot* **66**:953-61.

4307. **Lee, M. L., C. J. Chen, I. J. Su, K. T. Chen, C. C. Yeh, C. c. Ing, H. L. Chang, Y. C. Wu, M. S. Ho, D. D. Jiang, W. F. Lin, H. C. Lang, T. Y. Lin, M. H. Lai, J. T. Wang, and C. H. Chen.** 2003. Use of quarantine to prevent transmission of severe acute respiratory syndrome - Taiwan, 2003. *MMWR* **52**:680-3.

4308. **Lee, P. C., P. Y. Lee, H. Y. Lei, F. F. Chen, J. Y. Tseng, and Y. T. Ching.** 1994. Malaria infection in kidney transplant recipients. *Transplant Proc* **26**:2099-100.

4309. **Lee, S. H., and S. J. Kim.** 2002. Detection of infectious enteroviruses and adenoviruses in tap water in urban areas in Korea. *Water Res* **36**:248-56.

4310. **Lee, S. H., D. A. Levy, G. F. Craun, M. J. Beach, and R. L. Calderon.** 2002. Surveillance of waterborne-disease outbreaks - United States, 1999-2000. *MMWR* **51** (SS-8):1-48.

4311. **Lee, T. S., S. W. Lee, W. S. Seok, M. Y. Yoo, J. W. Yoon, B. K. Park, K. D. Moon, and D. H. Oh.** 2004. Prevalence, antibiotic susceptibility, and virulence factors of Yersinia enterocolitica and related species from ready-to-eat vegetables available in Korea. *J Food Prot* **67**:1123-7.

4312. **Lee, W. W., M. Singh, and C. L. Tan.** 1996. A recent case of congenital malaria in Singapore. *Singapore Med J* **37**:541-3.

4313. **Leeder, S. R., R. Corkhill, L. M. Irwig, W. W. Holland, and J. R. Colley.** 1976. Influence of family factors on the incidence of lower respiratory illness during the first year of life. *Br J Prev Soc Med* **30**:203-12.

4314. **Leelayoova, S., R. Rangsin, P. Taamasri, T. Naaglor, U. Thathaisong, and M. Mungthin.** 2004. Evidence of Waterborne Transmission of Blastocystis Hominis. *Am J Trop Med Hyg* **70**:658-662.

4315. **Leenders, A. C., A. van Belkum, M. Behrendt, A. Luijendijk, and H. A. Verbrugh.** 1999. Density and molecular epidemiology of Aspergillus in air and relationship to outbreaks of Aspergillus infection. *J Clin Microbiol* **37**:1752-7.

4316. **Leentvaar-Kuijpers, A., J. L. Kool, P. J. Veugelers, R. A. Coutinho, and G. J. van Griensven.** 1995. An outbreak of hepatitis A among homosexual men in Amsterdam, 1991-1993. *Int J Epidemiol* **24**:218-22.

4317. **Lees, D. N., K. Henshilwood, J. Green, C. I. Gallimore, and D. W. Brown.** 1995. Detection of small round structured viruses in shellfish by reverse transcription-PCR. *Appl Environ Microbiol* **61**:4418-24.

4318. **Lefrere, F., C. Besson, A. Datry, P. Chaibi, V. Leblond, J. L. Binet, and L. Sutton.** 1996. Transmission of Plasmodium falciparum by allogeneic bone marrow transplantation. *Bone Marrow Transplant* **18**:473-4.

4319. **Legg, J. P., J. A. Warner, S. L. Johnston, and J. O. Warner.** 2005. Frequency of detection of picornaviruses and seven other respiratory pathogens in infants. *Pediatr Infect Dis J* **24**:611-6.

4320. **Legoff, J., E. Guerot, A. Ndjoyi-Mbiguino, M. Matta, A. Si-Mohamed, L. Gutmann, J. Y. Fagon, and L. Belec.** 2005. High prevalence of respiratory viral infections in patients hospitalized in an intensive care unit for acute respiratory infections as detected by nucleic acid-based assays. *J Clin Microbiol* **43**:455-7.

4321. **Legros, D., M. McCormick, C. Mugero, M. Skinnider, D. D. Bek'Obita, and S. I. Okware.** 2000. Epidemiology of cholera outbreak in Kampala, Uganda. *East Afr Med J* **77**:347-9.

4322. **LeGuerrier, P., P. A. Pilon, D. Deshaies, and R. Allard.** 1996. Pre-exposure rabies prophylaxis for the international traveller: a decision analysis. *Vaccine* **14**:167-76.

4323. **Lehane, L., and G. T. Rawlin.** 2000. Topically acquired bacterial zoonoses from fish: a review. *Med J Aust* **173**:256-9.

4324. **Lehmacher, A., J. Bockemuhl, and S. Aleksic.** 1995. Nationwide outbreak of human salmonellosis in Germany due to contaminated paprika and paprika-powdered potato chips. *Epidemiol Infect* **115**:501-11.

4325. **Lehmann, D., M. T. Tennant, D. T. Silva, D. McAullay, F. Lannigan, H. Coates, and F. J. Stanley.** 2003. Benefits of swimming pools in two remote Aboriginal communities in Western Australia: intervention study. *BMJ* **327**:415-9.

4326. **Leibovici, V., R. Evron, M. Dunchin, N. Strauss-Leviatan, M. Westerman, and A. Ingber.** 2002. Population-based epidemiologic study of tinea pedis in Israeli children. *Pediatr Infect Dis J* **21**:851-3.

4327. **Leibovitz, A., M. Dan, J. Zinger, Y. Carmeli, B. Habot, and R. Segal.** 2003. Pseudomonas aeruginosa and the oropharyngeal ecosystem of tube-fed patients. *Emerg Infect Dis* **9**:956-9.

4328. **Leibovitz, E., M. R. Jacobs, and R. Dagan.** 2004. Haemophilus influenzae: a significant pathogen in acute otitis media. *Pediatr Infect Dis J* **23**:1142-52.

4329. **Leiby, D. A., J. E. Gill, S. T. Johnson, J. Trouern-Trend, R. G. Cable, V. Berardi, M. L. Eberhard, N. J. Pieniazek, and B. L. Herwaldt.** 2002. The natural history of Babesia microti infection in Connecticut blood donors. *Am J Trop Med Hyg* **67** (suppl):122.

4330. **Leiby, D. A., R. M. Herron, Jr., E. J. Read, B. A. Lenes, and R. J. Stumpf.** 2002. Trypanosoma cruzi in Los Angeles and Miami blood donors: impact of evolving donor demographics on seroprevalence and implications for transfusion transmission. *Transfusion* **42**:549-55.

4331. **Leigh, T. R., M. J. Millett, B. Jameson, and J. V. Collins.** 1993. Serum titres of Pneumocystis carinii antibody in health care workers caring for patients with AIDS. *Thorax* **48**:619-21.

4332. **Leighton, C., D. Piper, J. Gunderman-King, V. Rea, K. Gensheimer, J. Randolph, R. Danforth, L. Webber, E. Pritchard, G. Beckett, V. Shinde, R. Facklam, C. Withney, N. Hayes, and B. Flannery.** 2003. Pneumococcal conjunctivitis at an elementary school - Maine, September 20-December 6, 2002. *MMWR* **52**:64-6.

4333. **Leighton, F. A., H. A. Artsob, M. C. Chu, and J. G. Olson.** 2001. A serological survey of rural dogs and cats on the southwestern Canadian prairie for zoonotic pathogens. *Can J Public Health* **92**:67-71.

4334. **Leighton, P. M., and H. M. MacSween.** 1990. Strongyloides stercoralis. The cause of an urticarial-like eruption of 65 years' duration. *Arch Intern Med* **150**:1747-8.

4335. **Leino, T., K. Auranen, J. Jokinen, M. Leinonen, P. Tervonen, and A. K. Takala.** 2001. Pneumococcal carriage in children during their first two years: important role of family exposure. *Pediatr Infect Dis J* **20**:1022-7.

4336. **Lemaitre, N., W. Sougakoff, C. Truffot-Pernot, E. Cambau, J. P. Derenne, F. Bricaire, J. Grosset, and V. Jarlier.** 1998. Use of DNA fingerprinting for primary surveillance of nosocomial tuberculosis in a large urban hospital: detection of outbreaks in homeless people and migrant workers. *Int J Tuberc Lung Dis* **2**:390-6.

4337. **Lemoine, T., P. Germanetto, and P. Giraud.** 1999. Toxi-infection alimentaire collective à Vibrio parahaemolyticus. *Bull Epidémiol Hebdomadaire* **10**:37-8.

4338. **Lemon, S. M., and D. L. Thomas.** 1997. Vaccines to prevent viral hepatitis. *N Engl J Med* **336**:196-204.

4339. **Lemos, L. B., M. Guo, and M. Baliga.** 2000. Blastomycosis: organ involvement and etiologic diagnosis. A review of 123 patients from Mississippi. *Ann Diagn Pathol* **4**:391-406.

4340. **Lengeler, C., J. Utzinger, and M. Tanner.** 2002. Questionnaires, for rapid screening of schistosomiasis in sub-Saharan Africa. *Bull WHO* **80**:235-42.

4341. **Lengerich, E. J., D. G. Addiss, J. J. Marx, B. L. Ungar, and D. D. Juranek.** 1993. Increased exposure to cryptosporidia among dairy farmers in Wisconsin. *J Infect Dis* **167**:1252-5.

4342. **Lenglet, A.** 2005. E-alert 9 August: over 2000 cases so far in Salmonella Hadar outbreak in Spain associated with consumption of pre-cooked chicken, July-August, 2005. *Eurosurveillance Weekly* **10**:1-2.

4343. **Lentino, J. R.** 2003. Prosthetic joint infections: bane of orthopedists, challenge for infectious disease specialists. *Clin Infect Dis* **36**:1157-61.

4344. **Leonardo, L. R., L. P. Acosta, R. M. Olveda, and G. D. Aligui.** 2002. Difficulties and strategies in the control of schistosomiasis in the Philippines. *Acta Trop* **82**:295-9.

4345. **Leoni, E., G. De Luca, P. P. Legnani, R. Sacchetti, S. Stampi, and F. Zanetti.** 2005. Legionella waterline colonization: detection of Legionella species in domestic, hotel and hospital hot water systems. *J Appl Microbiol* **98**:373-9.

4346. **Leoni, E., P. Legnani, M. T. Mucci, and R. Pirani.** 1999. Prevalence of mycobacteria in a swimming pool environment. *J Appl Microbiol* **87**:683-8.

4347. **Leoni, E., P. P. Legnani, M. A. Bucci Sabattini, and F. Righi.** 2001. Prevalence of Legionella spp. in swimming pool environment. *Water Res* **35**:3749-53.

4348. **Lepine, L. A., D. B. Jernigan, J. C. Butler, J. M. Pruckler, R. F. Benson, G. Kim, J. L. Hadler, M. L. Cartter, and B. S. Fields.** 1998. A recurrent outbreak of nosocomial legionnaires' disease detected by urinary antigen testing: evidence for long-term colonization of a hospital plumbing system. *Infect Control Hosp Epidemiol* **19**:905-10.

4349. **Leppard, B., and A. E. Naburi.** 2000. The use of ivermectin in controlling an outbreak of scabies in a prison. *Br J Dermatol* **143**:520-3.

4350. **Lerche, N. W., W. M. Switzer, J. L. Yee, V. Shanmugam, A. N. Rosenthal, L. E. Chapman, T. M. Folks, and W. Heneine.** 2001. Evidence of infection with simian type D retrovirus in persons occupationally exposed to nonhuman primates. *J Virol* **75**:1783-9.

4351. **Lerman, Y., G. Chodick, S. Tepper, G. Livni, and S. Ashkenazi.** 2004. Seroepidemiology of varicella-zoster virus antibodies among health-care workers and day-care-centre workers. *Epidemiol Infect* **132**:1135-8.

4352. **Leroy, E. M., P. Rouquet, P. Formenty, S. Souquiere, A. Kilbourne, J. M. Froment, M. Bermejo, S. Smit, W. Karesh, R. Swanepoel, S. R. Zaki, and P. E. Rollin.** 2004. Multiple Ebola virus transmission events and rapid decline of Central African wildlife. *Science* **303**:387-90.

4353. **Leroy, E. M., P. Telfer, B. Kumulungui, P. Yaba, P. Rouquet, P. Roques, J. P. Gonzalez, T. G. Ksiazek, P. E. Rollin, and E. Nerrienet.** 2004. A serological survey of ebola virus infection in central african nonhuman primates. *J Infect Dis* **190**:1895-9.

4354. **Lertpiriyasuwat, C., J. Kanlayanpotporn, J. Deeying, R. Kijphati, and S. Thepsoontorn.** 2002. Measles outbreak in an orphanage, Bangkok, Thailand, September-October 2000. *J Med Assoc Thai* **85**:653-7.

4355. **Leser, P. G., M. E. Camargo, and R. Baruzzi.** 1977. Toxoplasmosis serologic tests in Brazilian indians (Kren-akorore) of recent contact with civilized man. *Rev Inst Med Trop Sao Paulo* **19**:232-6.

4356. **Leslie, L., C. Arnette, A. Sikder, J. Adams, C. Holbrook, J. Bond, B. King, K. Roberts, M. S. Patrick, C. Palmer, R. Finger, J. W. Tomford, and T. Rushton.** 1995. Histoplasmosis - Kentucky, 1995. *MMWR* **44**:701-703.

4357. **Lesnicar, G., M. Poljak, K. Seme, and J. Lesnicar.** 2003. Pediatric tick-borne encephalitis in 371 cases from an endemic region in Slovenia, 1959 to 2000. *Pediatr Infect Dis J* **22**:612-7.

4358. **Lester, R., S. Beaton, J. Carnie, D. Barbis, and G. Rouch.** 1997. A case of human anthrax in Victoria. *Commun Dis Intell* **21**:47-8.

4359. **Lester, S. C., M. del Pilar Pla, F. Wang, I. Perez Schael, H. Jiang, and T. F. O'Brien.** 1990. The carriage of Escherichia coli resistant to antimicrobial agents by healthy children in Boston, in Caracas, Venezuela, and in Qin Pu, China. *N Engl J Med* **323**:285-9.

4360. **Leszczynski, P., A. van Belkum, H. Pituch, H. Verbrugh, and F. Meisel-Mikolajczyk.** 1997. Vaginal carriage of enterotoxigenic Bacteroides fragilis in pregnant women. *J Clin Microbiol* **35**:2899-903.

4361. **Letowska, I., and W. Hryniewicz.** 2004. Epidemiology and characterization of Bordetella parapertussis strains isolated between 1995 and 2002 in and around Warsaw, Poland. *Eur J Clin Microbiol Infect Dis* **23**:499-501.

4362. **Lettinga, K. D., A. Verbon, G. J. Weverling, J. F. Schellekens, J. W. Den Boer, E. P. Yzerman, J. Prins, W. G. Boersma, R. J. Van Ketel, J. M. Prins, and P. Speelman.** 2002. Legionnaires' disease at a dutch flower show: prognostic factors and impact of therapy. *Emerg Infect Dis* **8:**1448-54.

4363. **Leuenberger, R., and T. Bodmer.** 2000. [Clinical presentation and therapy of Mycobacterium marinum infection as seen in 12 cases]. *Dtsch Med Wochenschr* **125:**7-10.

4364. **Leung, C. C., C. K. Chan, C. M. Tam, W. W. Yew, K. M. Kam, K. F. Au, L. B. Tai, S. M. Leung, and J. Ng.** 2005. Chest radiograph screening for tuberculosis in a Hong Kong prison. *Int J Tuberc Lung Dis* **9:**627-32.

4365. **Leutscher, P. D. C., and S. W. Bagley.** 2003. Health-related challenges in United States peace corps volunteers serving for two years in Madagascar. *J Travel Med* **10:**263-7.

4366. **Lever, F., and C. A. Joseph.** 2003. Travel associated legionnaires' disease in Europe in 2000 and 2001. *Eurosurveillance* **8:**65-72.

4367. **Levesque, B., G. De Serres, R. Higgins, M. A. D'Halewyn, H. Artsob, J. Grondin, M. Major, M. Garvie, and B. Duval.** 1995. Seroepidemiologic study of three zoonoses (leptospirosis, Q fever, and tularemia) among trappers in Quebec, Canada. *Clin Diagn Lab Immunol* **2:**496-8.

4368. **Levesque, B., P. Giovenazzo, P. Guerrier, D. Laverdiere, and H. Prud'Homme.** 2002. Investigation of an outbreak of cercarial dermatitis. *Epidemiol Infect* **129:**379-86.

4369. **Levett, P. N.** 2001. Leptospirosis. *Clin Microbiol Rev* **14:**296-326.

4370. **Levin, A. S., H. H. Caiaffa Filho, S. I. Sinto, E. Sabbaga, A. A. Barone, and C. M. Mendes.** 1991. An outbreak of nosocomial Legionnaires' disease in a renal transplant unit in Sao Paulo, Brazil. Legionellosis Study Team. *J Hosp Infect* **18:**243-8.

4371. **Levin, M. L., W. C. Maddrey, J. R. Wands, and A. L. Mendeloff.** 1974. Hepatitis B transmission by dentists. *JAMA* **228:**1139-40.

4372. **Levine, M. M., R. E. Black, and C. Lanata.** 1982. Precise estimation of the numbers of chronic carriers of Salmonella typhi in Santiago, Chile, an endemic area. *J Infect Dis* **146:**724-6.

4373. **Levine, M. M., H. L. DuPont, M. Khodabandelou, and R. B. Hornick.** 1973. Long-term Shigella-carrier state. *N Engl J Med* **288:**1169-71.

4374. **Levine, M. M., C. Ferreccio, V. Prado, M. Cayazzo, P. Abrego, J. Martinez, L. Maggi, M. M. Baldini, W. Martin, and D. Maneval.** 1993. Epidemiologic studies of Escherichia coli diarrheal infections in a low socioeconomic level peri-urban community in Santiago, Chile. *Am J Epidemiol* **138:**849-69.

4375. **Levine, R. S., A. T. Peterson, and M. Q. Benedict.** 2004. Geographic and ecologic distributions of the Anopheles gambiae complex predicted using a genetic algorithm. *Am J Trop Med Hyg* **70:**105-9.

4376. **Levine, W. C., R. W. Bennett, Y. Choi, K. J. Henning, J. R. Rager, K. A. Hendricks, D. P. Hopkins, R. A. Gunn, and P. M. Griffin.** 1996. Staphylococcal food poisoning caused by imported canned mushrooms. *J Infect Dis* **173:**1263-7.

4377. **Levine, W. C., J. F. Smart, D. L. Archer, N. H. Bean, and R. V. Tauxe.** 1991. Foodborne disease outbreaks in nursing homes, 1975 through 1987. *JAMA* **266:**2105-9.

4378. **Levis, S., J. Garcia, N. Pini, G. Calderon, J. Ramirez, D. Bravo, S. St Jeor, C. Ripoll, M. Bego, E. Lozano, R. Barquez, T. G. Ksiazek, and D. Enria.** 2004. Hantavirus pulmonary syndrome in northwestern Argentina: circulation of Laguna Negra virus associated with Calomys callosus. *Am J Trop Med Hyg* **71:**658-63.

4379. **Levy, M., C. G. Johnson, and E. Kraa.** 2003. Tonsillopharyngitis caused by foodborne group A streptococcus: a prison-based outbreak. *Clin Infect Dis* **36:**175-82.

4380. **Levy, M. H., S. Quilty, L. C. Young, W. Hunt, R. Matthews, and P. W. Robertson.** 2003. Pox in the docks: varicella outbreak in an Australian prison system. *Public Health* **117:**446-51.

4381. **Levy, M. M., M. P. Fink, J. C. Marshall, E. Abraham, D. Angus, D. Cook, J. Cohen, S. M. Opal, J. L. Vincent, and G. Ramsay.** 2003. 2001 SCCM/ESICM/ACCP/ATS/SIS International Sepsis Definitions Conference. *Intensive Care Med* **29:**530-8.

4382. **Levy, P. Y., N. Teysseire, J. Etienne, and D. Raoult.** 2003. A nosocomial outbreak of Legionella pneumophila caused by contaminated transesophageal echocardiography probes. *Infect Control Hosp Epidemiol* **24:**619-22.

4383. **Levy, R., F. Grattard, I. Maubon, A. Ros, and B. Pozzetto.** 2004. Bacterial risk and sperm cryopreservation. *Andrologia* **36:**282-5.

4384. **Levy, R., A. Weissman, G. Blomberg, and Z. J. Hagay.** 1997. Infection by parvovirus B 19 during pregnancy: a review. *Obstet Gynecol Surv* **52:**254-9.

4385. **Lew, J. F., C. L. Moe, S. S. Monroe, J. R. Allen, B. M. Harrison, B. D. Forrester, S. E. Stine, P. A. Woods, J. C. Hierholzer, J. E. Herrmann, et al.** 1991. Astrovirus and adenovirus associated with diarrhea in children in day care settings. *J Infect Dis* **164:**673-8.

4386. **Lew, J. F., D. L. Swerdlow, M. E. Dance, P. M. Griffin, C. A. Bopp, M. J. Gillenwater, T. Mercatante, and R. I. Glass.** 1991. An outbreak of shigellosis aboard a cruise ship caused by a multiple- antibiotic-resistant strain of Shigella flexneri. *Am J Epidemiol* **134:**413-20.

4387. **Lewandowski, C., A. Ognjan, E. Rivers, H. Huitsing, D. Pohlod, H. Lee, and L. D. Saravolatz.** 1992. Health care worker exposure to HIV-1 and HTLV I-II in critically ill, resuscitated emergency department patients. *Ann Emerg Med* **21:**1353-9.

4388. **Lewin, M. R., D. H. Bouyer, D. H. Walker, and D. M. Musher.** 2003. Rickettsia sibirica infection in members of scientific expeditions to northern Asia. *Lancet* **362:**1201-2.

4389. **Lewin, M. R., and M. F. Weinert.** 1999. An eighty-four-year-old man with fever and painless jaundice: a case report and brief review of Clonorchis sinensis infection. *J Travel Med* **6:**207-9.

4390. **Lewis, D. A.** 2003. Chancroid: clinical manifestations, diagnosis, and management. *Sex Transm Infect* **79:**68-71.

4391. **Lewis, F. M., B. J. Marsh, and C. F. von Reyn.** 2003. Fish tank exposure and cutaneous infections due to Mycobacterium marinum: tuberculin skin testing, treatment, and prevention. *Clin Infect Dis* **37:**390-7.

4392. **Lewis, J. W., and R. M. e. Maizels.** 1993. Toxocara and toxocariasis. Clinical., epidemiological and molecular perspectives. Institute of Biology and British Society of Parasitology, London.

4393. **Lewis, M. D., O. Serichantalergs, C. Pitarangsi, N. Chuanak, C. J. Mason, L. R. Regmi, P. Pandey, R. Laskar, C. D.**

Shrestha, and S. Malla. 2005. Typhoid fever: a massive, single-point source, multidrug-resistant outbreak in Nepal. *Clin Infect Dis* **40:**554-61.

4394. Lewis, M. D., A. A. Yousuf, K. Lerdthusnee, A. Razee, K. Chandranoi, and J. W. Jones. 2003. Scrub typhus reemergence in the Maldives. *Emerg Infect Dis* **9:**1638-41.

4395. Lewis, S. M., and B. G. Lewis. 1997. Nosocomial transmission of Trichophyton tonsurans tinea corporis in a rehabilitation hospital. *Infect Control Hosp Epidemiol* **18:**322-5.

4396. Li, J. S., E. D. O'Brien, and C. Guest. 2002. A review of national legionellosis surveillance in Australia, 1991 to 2000. *Commun Dis Intell* **26:**461-8.

4397. Li, Y. L., S. L. Ruo, Z. Tong, Q. R. Ma, Z. L. Liu, K. L. Ye, Z. Y. Zhu, J. B. McCormick, S. P. Fisher-Hoch, and Z. Y. Xu. 1995. A serotypic study of hemorrhagic fever with renal syndrome in rural China. *Am J Trop Med Hyg* **52:**247-51.

4398. Li, Y. S., Y. K. He, Q. R. Zeng, and D. P. McManus. 2003. Epidemiological and morbidity assessment of Schistosoma japonicum infection in a migrant fisherman community, the Dongting lake region, China. *Trans R Soc Trop Med Hyg* **97:**177-81.

4399. Li, Y. S., A. C. Sleigh, A. G. P. Ross, Y. Li, G. M. Williams, M. Tanner, and D. P. McManus. 2000. Two-year impact of praziquantel treatment for Schistosoma japonicum infection in China: re-infection, subclinical disease and fibrosis marker measurements. *Trans R Soc Trop Med Hyg* **94:**191-7.

4400. Li, Y. S., A. C. Sleigh, G. M. Williams, A. G. Ross, S. J. Forsyth, M. Tanner, and D. P. McManus. 2000. Measuring exposure to Schistosoma japonicum in China. III. Activity diaries, snail and human infection, transmission ecology and options for control. *Acta Trop* **75:**279-89.

4401. Li, Z., M. R. Kosorok, P. M. Farrell, A. Laxova, S. E. West, C. G. Green, J. Collins, M. J. Rock, and M. L. Splaingard. 2005. Longitudinal development of mucoid Pseudomonas aeruginosa infection and lung disease progression in children with cystic fibrosis. *JAMA* **293:**581-8.

4402. Li, Z. Y. 1980. Plasmodium knowlesi infection in man (one case report). *Nat Med J. China* **60:**661.

4403. Libman, M. D., J. D. MacLean, and T. W. Gyorkos. 1993. Screening for schistosomiasis, filariasis, and strongyloidiasis among expatriates returning from the tropics. *Clin Infect Dis* **17:**353-9.

4404. Liddell, A. M., S. L. Stockham, M. A. Scott, J. W. Sumner, C. D. Paddock, M. Gaudreault-Keener, M. Q. Arens, and G. A. Storch. 2003. Predominance of Ehrlichia ewingii in Missouri dogs. *J Clin Microbiol* **41:**4617-22.

4405. Lidgren, L., K. Knutson, and A. Stefansdottir. 2003. Infection and arthritis. Infection of prosthetic joints. *Best Pract Res Clin Rheumatol* **17:**209-18.

4406. Lidwell, O. M., E. J. Lowbury, W. Whyte, R. Blowers, S. J. Stanley, and D. Lowe. 1983. Airborne contamination of wounds in joint replacement operations: the relationship to sepsis rates. *J Hosp Infect* **4:**111-31.

4407. Lieb, S., R. A. Gunn, R. Medina, N. Singh, R. D. May, H. T. Janowski, and W. E. Woodward. 1985. Norwalk virus gastroenteritis. An outbreak associated with a cafeteria at a college. *Am J Epidemiol* **121:**259-68.

4408. Liechti, M., H. R. Baur, H. P. Gurtner, and P. W. Straub. 1990. [Cardiac complications of American trypanosomiasis (Chagas disease). Various case reports and general observations]. *Schweiz Med Wochenschr* **120:**1493-6.

4409. Lienhardt, C., R. Ghebray, E. Candolfi, T. Kien, and G. Hedlin. 1990. Malaria in refugee camps in eastern Sudan: a sero-epidemiological approach. *Ann Trop Med Parasitol* **84:**215-22.

4410. Lietzau, S., T. Sturmer, A. Erb, H. Von Baum, R. Marre, and H. Brenner. 2004. Prevalence and determinants of nasal colonization with antibiotic-resistant Staphylococcus aureus among unselected patients attending general practitioners in Germany. *Epidemiol Infect* **132:**655-62.

4411. Lievano, F. A., M. J. Papania, R. F. Helfand, R. Harpaz, L. Walls, R. S. Katz, I. Williams, Y. S. Villamarzo, P. A. Rota, and W. J. Bellini. 2004. Lack of evidence of measles virus shedding in people with inapparent measles virus infections. *J Infect Dis* **189 Suppl 1:**165-70.

4412. Lifson, A. R., and L. L. Halcon. 2001. Substance abuse and high-risk needle-related behaviors among homeless youth in Minneapolis: implications for prevention. *J Urban Health* **78:**690-698.

4413. Lifson, A. R., L. L. Halcon, A. M. Johnston, C. R. Hayman, P. Hannan, C. A. Miller, and S. E. Valway. 1999. Tuberculin skin testing among economically disadvantaged youth in a federally funded job training program. *Am J Epidemiol* **149:**671-9.

4414. Lifson, A. R., D. Thai, A. O'Fallon, W. A. Mills, and K. Hang. 2002. Prevalence of tuberculosis, hepatitis B virus, and intestinal parasitic infections among refugees to Minnesota. *Public Health Rep* **117:**69-77.

4415. Lightburn, E., J. B. Meynard, J. J. Morand, E. Garnotel, P. Kraemer, P. Hovette, S. Banzet, H. Dampierre, J. Lepage, B. Carme, R. Pradinaud, M. Morillon, J. P. Dedet, C. Chouc, and J. P. Boutin. 2002. [Epidemiologic surveillance of cutaneous leishmaniasis in Guiana. Summary of military data collected over 10 years]. *Med Trop (Mars)* **62:**545-53.

4416. Likitnukul, S., N. Prapphal, K. Tatiyakavee, P. Nunthapisud, and S. Chumdermpadetsuk. 1994. Risk factors of streptococcal colonization in school age children. *Southeast Asian J Trop Med Public Health* **25:**664-71.

4417. Lillebaek, T., A. B. Andersen, A. Dirksen, E. Smith, L. T. Skovgaard, and A. Kok-Jensen. 2002. Persistent high incidence of tuberculosis in immigrants in a low-incidence country. *Emerg Infect Dis* **8:**679-84.

4418. Lillibridge, K. M., R. Parsons, Y. Randle, A. P. Travassos Da Rosa, H. Guzman, M. Siirin, T. Wuithiranyagool, C. Hailey, S. Higgs, A. A. Bala, R. Pascua, T. Meyer, D. L. Vanlandingham, and R. B. Tesh. 2004. The 2002 Introduction of West Nile Virus into Harris County, Texas, an Area Historically Endemic for St. Louis Encephalitis. *Am J Trop Med Hyg* **70:**676-681.

4419. Lillington, T., and E. M. Shanahan. 1997. Cutaneous infection in meatworkers. *Occup Med (Lond)* **47:**197-202.

4420. Lim, M. K., E. H. Tan, C. S. Soh, and T. L. Chang. 1997. Burkholderia pseudomallei infection in the Singapore armed forces from 1987 to 1994 — an epidemiological review. *Ann Acad Med Singapore* **26:**13-17.

4421. Lim, P. L., A. Kurup, G. Gopalakrishna, K. P. Chan, C. W. Wong, L. C. Ng, S. Y. Se-Thoe, L. Oon, X. Bai, L. W. Stanton, Y. Ruan, L. D. Miller, V. B. Vega, L. James, P. L. Ooi, C. S. Kai, S. J. Olsen, B. Ang, and Y. S. Leo. 2004. Laboratory-acquired severe acute respiratory syndrome. *N Engl J Med* **350:**1740-5.

4422. Lim-Quizon, M. C., R. M. Benabaye, F. M. White, M. M. Dayrit, and M. E. White. 1994. Cholera transmission in metropolitan Manila: foodborne transmission via street vendors. *Bull WHO* **72:**745-9.

4423. **Limaye, A. P., P. A. Connolly, M. Sagar, T. R. Fritsche, B. T. Cookson, L. J. Wheat, and W. E. Stamm.** 2000. Transmission of Histoplasma capsulatum by organ transplantation. *N Engl J Med* **343:**1163-6.

4424. **Limentani, A. E., L. M. Elliott, N. D. Noah, and J. K. Lamborn.** 1979. An outbreak of hepatitis B from tattooing. *Lancet* **2:**86-8.

4425. **Lin, D. B., W. T. Nieh, H. M. Wang, M. W. Hsiao, U. P. Ling, S. P. Changlai, M. S. Ho, S. L. You, and C. J. Chen.** 1999. Seroepidemiology of Helicobacter pylori infection among preschool children in Taiwan. *Am J Trop Med Hyg* **61:**554-8.

4426. **Lin, F., and R. P. Kitching.** 2000. Swine vesicular disease: an overview. *Vet J* **160:**192-201.

4427. **Lin, F. Y., J. M. Becke, C. Groves, B. P. Lim, E. Israel, E. F. Becker, R. M. Helfrich, D. S. Swetter, T. Cramton, and J. B. Robbins.** 1988. Restaurant-associated outbreak of typhoid fever in Maryland: identification of carrier facilitated by measurement of serum Vi antibodies. *J Clin Microbiol* **26:**1194-7.

4428. **Lin, H. H., J. H. Kao, K. Y. Yeh, D. P. Liu, M. H. Chang, P. J. Chen, and D. S. Chen.** 1998. Mother-to-infant transmission of GB virus C/hepatitis G virus: the role of high-titered maternal viremia and mode of delivery. *J Infect Dis* **177:**1202-6.

4429. **Lin, H. H., S. S. Lin, Y. M. Chiang, L. Y. Wang, L. C. Huang, S. C. Huang, and T. T. Liu.** 2002. Trend of hepatitis B virus infection in freshmen classes at two high schools in Hualien, Taiwan from 1991 to 1999. *J Med Virol* **67:**472-6.

4430. **Lin, S. J., J. Schranz, and S. M. Teutsch.** 2001. Aspergillosis case-fatality rate: systematic review of the literature. *Clin Infect Dis* **32:**358-366.

4431. **Lin, S. K., J. R. Lambert, M. A. Schembri, L. Nicholson, and I. H. Johnson.** 1998. The prevalence of Helicobacter pylori in practising dental staff and dental students. *Aust Dent J* **43:**35-9.

4432. **Lin, T. Y., L. Y. Chang, S. H. Hsia, Y. C. Huang, C. H. Chiu, C. Hsueh, S. R. Shih, C. C. Liu, and M. H. Wu.** 2002. The 1998 enterovirus 71 outbreak in Taiwan: pathogenesis and management. *Clin Infect Dis* **34 (suppl 2):**S52-7.

4433. **Lina, G., J. Etienne, and F. Vandenesch.** 1998. Les syndromes toxiques staphylococciques en France de 1994 à 1997. Données du centre national de référence des staphylocoques. *Bull Epidémiol Hebdomadaire* **17 (28 april):**69-70.

4434. **Linacre, E., and B. Geerts.** 1997. Climates and weather explained. Routledge, London.

4435. **Linardi, P. M., J. M. Barata, P. R. Urbinatti, D. de Souza, J. R. Botelho, and M. De Maria.** 1998. [Infestation by Pediculus humanus (Anoplura: Pediculidae) in a metropolitan area of southeast Brazil]. *Rev Saude Publica* **32:**77-81.

4436. **Lindbäck, H., J. Lindbäck, A. Tegnell, R. Janzon, S. Vene, and K. Ekdahl.** 2003. Dengue fever in travelers to the tropics, 1998 and 1999. *Emerg Infect Dis* **9:**438–42.

4437. **Lindblade, K. A., F. Odhiambo, D. H. Rosen, and K. M. DeCock.** 2003. Health and nutritional status of orphans <6 years old cared for by relatives in western Kenya. *Trop Med Int Health* **8:**67-72.

4438. **Lindblom, A., A. Isa, O. Norbeck, S. Wolf, B. Johansson, K. Broliden, and T. Tolfvenstam.** 2005. Slow clearance of human parvovirus B19 viremia following acute infection. *Clin Infect Dis* **41:**1201-3.

4439. **Lindenmayer, J. M., S. Schoenfeld, R. O'Grady, and J. K. Carney.** 1998. Methicillin-resistant Staphylococcus aureus in a high school wrestling team and the surrounding community. *Arch Intern Med* **158:**895-9.

4440. **Linder, P. E.** 1991. [An interesting incidental finding in a patient with knee injury]. *Schweiz Rundsch Med (Praxis)* **80:**879-82.

4441. **Lindergard, G., D. V. Nydam, S. E. Wade, S. L. Schaaf, and H. O. Mohammed.** 2003. A novel multiplex polymerase chain reaction approach for detection of four human infective Cryptosporidium isolates: Cryptosporidium parvum, types H and C, Cryptosporidium canis, and Cryptosporidium felis in fecal and soil samples. *J Vet Diagn Invest* **15:**262-7.

4442. **Lindo, J. F., C. Waugh, J. Hall, C. Cunningham-Myrie, D. Ashley, M. L. Eberhard, J. J. Sullivan, H. S. Bishop, D. G. Robinson, T. Holtz, and R. D. Robinson.** 2002. Enzootic Angiostrongylus cantonensis in rats and snails after an outbreak of human eosinophilic meningitis, JAMAica. *Emerg Infect Dis* **8:**324-6.

4443. **Lindsay, D. S., J. P. Dubey, and B. L. Blagburn.** 1997. Biology of Isospora spp. from humans, nonhuman primates, and domestic animals. *Clin Microbiol Rev* **10:**19-34.

4444. **Lindsay, S. W.** 1993. 200 years of lice in Glasgow: an index of social deprivation. *Parasitol Today* **9:**412-7.

4445. **Lindsay, S. W., R. Bodker, R. Malima, H. A. Msangeni, and W. Kisinza.** 2000. Effect of 1997-98 El Nino on highland malaria in Tanzania. *Lancet* **355:**989-90.

4446. **Lindsay, S. W., M. Jawara, K. Paine, M. Pinder, G. E. Walraven, and P. M. Emerson.** 2003. Changes in house design reduce exposure to malaria mosquitoes. *Trop Med Int Health* **8:**512-7.

4447. **Ling, M. L., K. T. Goh, G. C. Y. Wang, K. S. Neo, and T. Chua.** 2002. An outbreak of multidrug-resistant Salmonella enterica subsp. enterica serotype Typhimurium, DT104L linked to dried anchovy in Singapore. *Epidemiol Infect* **128:**1-5.

4448. **Linhares, A. C., Y. B. Gabbay, R. B. Freitas, E. S. da Rosa, J. D. Mascarenhas, and E. C. Loureiro.** 1989. Longitudinal study of rotavirus infections among children from Belém, Brazil. *Epidemiol Infect* **102:**129-45.

4449. **Linhares, A. C., F. P. Pinheiro, R. B. Freitas, Y. B. Gabbay, J. A. Shirley, and G. M. Beards.** 1981. An outbreak of rotavirus diarrhea among a nonimmune, isolated South American Indian community. *Am J Epidemiol* **113:**703-10.

4450. **Linhares, I. M., S. S. Witkin, P. Giraldo, I. Sziller, J. Jeremias, J. A. Pinotti, and A. Segurado.** 2000. Ureaplasma urealyticum colonization in the vaginal introitus and cervix of human immunodeficiency virus-infected women. *Int J STD AIDS* **11:**176-9.

4451. **Link, B., J. Phelan, M. Bresnahan, A. Stueve, R. Moore, and E. Susser.** 1995. Lifetime and five-year prevalence of homelessness in the United States: new evidence on an old debate. *Am J Orthopsychiatry* **65:**347-54.

4452. **Linnan, M. J., L. Mascola, X. D. Lou, V. Goulet, S. May, C. Salminen, D. W. Hird, M. L. Yonekura, P. Hayes, R. Weaver, et al.** 1988. Epidemic listeriosis associated with Mexican-style cheese. *N Engl J Med* **319:**823-8.

4453. **Linnane, E., R. J. Roberts, and P. T. Mannion.** 2002. An outbreak of Salmonella enteritidis phage type 34a infection in primary school children: the use of visual aids and food preferences to overcome recall bias in a case control study. *Epidemiol Infect* **129:**35-9.

4454. **Linnemann, C. C., Jr., N. Ramundo, P. H. Perlstein, S. D. Minton, and G. S. Englender.** 1975. Use of pertussis vaccine in an epidemic involving hospital staff. *Lancet* **2:**540-3.

4455. **Lins, Z. C.** 1970. Studies on enteric bacterias in the lower Amazon Region. I. Serotypes of Salmonella isolated from wild forest animals in Para State, Brazil. *Trans R Soc Trop Med Hyg* **64:**439-43.

4456. **Linthicum, K. J., A. Anyamba, C. J. Tucker, P. W. Kelley, M. F. Myers, and C. J. Peters.** 1999. Climate and satellite indicators to forecast Rift Valley fever epidemics in Kenya. *Science* **285:**397-400.

4457. **Lipp, E. K., and J. B. Rose.** 1997. The role of seafood in foodborne diseases in the United States of America. *Rev Sci Tech* **16:**620-40.

4458. **LiPuma, J. J., S. E. Dasen, D. W. Nielson, R. C. Stern, and T. L. Stull.** 1990. Person-to-person transmission of Pseudomonas cepacia between patients with cystic fibrosis. *Lancet* **336:**1094-6.

4459. **LiPuma, J. J., T. Spilker, T. Coenye, and C. F. Gonzalez.** 2002. An epidemic Burkholderia cepacia complex strain identified in soil. *Lancet* **359:**2002-3.

4460. **Little, C. L., I. A. Gillespie, and R. T. Mitchell.** 2001. Microbiological examination of ready-to-eat burgers sampled anonymously at the point of sale in the United Kingdom. *Commun Dis Public Health* **4:**293-9.

4461. **Little, C. L., R. Omotoye, and R. T. Mitchell.** 2003. The microbiological quality of ready-to-eat foods with added spices. *Int J Environ Health Res* **13:**31-42.

4462. **Litwin, C. M.** 2003. Pet-transmitted infections: diagnosis by microbiologic and immunologic methods. *Pediatr Infect Dis J* **22:**768-77.

4463. **Liu, C. J., C. C. Hung, M. Y. Chen, Y. P. Lai, P. J. Chen, S. H. Huang, and D. S. Chen.** 2001. Amebic liver abscess and human immunodeficiency virus infection: a report of three cases. *J Clin Gastroenterol* **33:**64-8.

4464. **Liu, C. P., N. Y. Wang, C. M. Lee, L. C. Weng, H. K. Tseng, C. W. Liu, C. S. Chiang, and F. Y. Huang.** 2004. Nosocomial and community-acquired Enterobacter cloacae bloodstream infection: risk factors for and prevalence of SHV-12 in multiresistant isolates in a medical centre. *J Hosp Infect* **58:**63-77.

4465. **Liu, J. W., L. H. Chao, L. H. Su, J. W. Wang, and C. J. Wang.** 2002. Experience with a bone bank operation and allograft bone infection in recipients at a medical centre in southern Taiwan. *J Hosp Infect* **50:**293-7.

4466. **Liu, W.** 2004. Long-term SARS Coronavirus Excretion from Patient Cohort, China. *Emerg Infect Dis* **10:**1841-3.

4467. **Liu, Y., Z. Zhao, Z. Yang, J. Zhang, J. Xu, Q. Wu, Z. Peng, and Z. Miao.** 2003. Epidemiological studies on host animals of scrub typhus of the autumn-winter type in Shandong province, China. *Southeast Asian J Trop Med Public Health* **34:**826-30.

4468. **Liu, Z., E. Wang, W. Taylor, H. Yu, T. Wu, Y. Wan, Y. Huang, Z. Ni, and D. Sackett.** 1990. Prevalence survey of cytomegalovirus infection in children in Chengdu. *Am J Epidemiol* **131:**143-50.

4469. **Liz, J. S., L. Anderes, J. W. Sumner, R. F. Massung, L. Gern, B. Rutti, and M. Brossard.** 2000. PCR detection of granulocytic ehrlichiae in Ixodes ricinus ticks and wild small mammals in Western Switzerland. *J Clin Microbiol* **38:**1002-7.

4470. **Ljungstrom, I., and B. Castor.** 1992. Immune response to Giardia lamblia in a water-borne outbreak of giardiasis in Sweden. *J Med Microbiol* **36:**347-52.

4471. **Lledó, L., M. I. Gegúndez, J. V. Saz, and M. Beltrán.** 2002. Prevalence of antibodies to Rickettsia typhi in an area of the center of Spain. *Eur J Epidemiol* **17:**927-8.

4472. **Lledo, L., M. I. Gegundez, J. L. Serrano, J. V. Saz, and M. Beltran.** 2003. A sero-epidemiological study of Rickettsia typhi infection in dogs from Soria province, central Spain. *Ann Trop Med Parasitol* **97:**861-4.

4473. **Llewellyn, L. J., M. R. Evans, and S. R. Palmer.** 1998. Use of sequential case-control studies to investigate a community Salmonella outbreak in Wales. *J Epidemiol Community Health* **52:**272-6.

4474. **Llewelyn, C. A., P. E. Hewitt, R. S. G. Knight, K. Amar, S. Cousens, J. Mackenzie, and R. G. Will.** 2004. Possible transmission of variant Creutzfeldt-Jakob disease by blood transfusion. *Lancet* **363:**417-21.

4475. **Lloyd, G., and N. Jones.** 1986. Infection of laboratory workers with hantavirus acquired from immunocytomas propagated in laboratory rats. *J Infect* **12:**117-25.

4476. **Lo Re, V., 3rd, and S. J. Gluckman.** 2001. Eosinophilic meningitis due to Angiostrongylus cantonensis in a returned traveler: case report and review of the literature. *Clin Infect Dis* **33:**e112-5.

4477. **Lo, S. S., J. C. de Andrade, M. L. Condino, M. J. Alves, M. G. Semeghini, and C. Galvao Eda.** 1991. [Malaria in intravenous drug users associated with HIV seropositivity]. *Rev Saude Publica* **25:**17-22.

4478. **Lo, S. V., A. M. Connolly, S. R. Palmer, D. Wright, P. D. Thomas, and D. Joynson.** 1994. The role of the pre-symptomatic food handler in a common source outbreak of foodborne SRSV gastroenteritis in a group of hospitals. *Epidemiol Infect* **113:**513-21.

4479. **Lobato, M. N., D. J. Vugia, and I. J. Frieden.** 1997. Tinea capitis in California children: a population-based study of a growing epidemic. *Pediatrics* **99:**551-4.

4480. **LoBue, P. A., W. Betancourt, L. Cowan, L. Seli, C. Peter, and K. S. Moser.** 2004. Identification of a familial cluster of pulmonary Mycobacterium bovis disease. *Int J Tuberc Lung Dis* **8:**1142-6.

4481. **Lodha, R., N. R. Dash, A. Kapil, and S. K. Kabra.** 2000. Diphtheria in urban slums in north India. *Lancet* **355:**204.

4482. **Lodhi, S., A. R. Sarwari, M. Muzammil, A. Salam, and R. A. Smego.** 2004. Features distinguishing amoebic from pyogenic liver abscess: a review of 577 adult cases. *Trop Med Int Health* **9:**718-23.

4483. **Loeb, M., A. McGeer, B. Henry, M. Ofner, D. Rose, T. Hlywka, J. Levie, J. McQueen, S. Smith, L. Moss, A. Smith, K. Green, and S. D. Walter.** 2004. SARS among critical care nurses, Toronto. *Emerg Infect Dis* **10:**251-5.

4484. **Loeb, M., A. McGeer, M. McArthur, R. W. Peeling, M. Petric, and A. E. Simor.** 2000. Surveillance for outbreaks of respiratory tract infections in nursing homes. *CMAJ* **162:**1133-7.

4485. **Loeb, M., A. E. Simor, L. Mandell, P. Krueger, M. McArthur, M. James, S. Walter, E. Richardson, M. Lingley, J. Stout, D. Stronach, and A. McGeer.** 1999. Two nursing home outbreaks of respiratory infection with Legionella sainthelensi. *J Am Geriatr Soc* **47:**547-52.

4486. **Lofgren, J., B. Whitley, D. Johnson, F. Downes, P. Somsel, B. Robinson-Dunn, J. Massey, G. Stoltman, M. G. Stobierski, S. Bidol, C. Hahn, L. Tengelson, P. Murray, D. L. Sewell, W. Schaffner, D. Stephens, M. Miller, J. Sejvar, T. Popovic, B. Perkins, and N. Rosenstein.** 2002. Laboratory-acquired meningococcal disease - United States, 2000. *MMWR* **51:**141-4.

4487. **Logan, T. M., F. G. Davies, K. J. Linthicum, and T. G. Ksiazek.** 1992. Rift valley fever antibody in human sera collected after an outbreak in domestic animals in Kenya. *Trans R Soc Trop Med Hyg* **86:**202-3.

4488. **Logigian, E. L., R. F. Kaplan, and A. C. Steere.** 1990. Chronic neurologic manifestations of Lyme disease. *N Engl J Med* **323:**1438-44.

4489. **Logue, C. M., J. S. Sherwood, L. M. Elijah, P. A. Olah, and M. R. Dockter.** 2003. The incidence of Campylobacter spp. on processed turkey from processing plants in the midwestern United States. *J Appl Microbiol* **95:**234-41.

4490. **Loh, W., V. V. Ng, and J. Holton.** 2000. Bacterial flora on the white coats of medical students. *J Hosp Infect* **45:**65-8.

4491. **Lohiya, G. S., K. Stewart, K. Perot, and R. Widman.** 1995. Parvovirus B19 outbreak in a developmental center. *Am J Infect Control* **23:**373-6.

4492. **Lohiya, G. S., L. Tan-Figueroa, F. M. Crinella, and S. Lohiya.** 2000. Epidemiology and control of enterobiasis in a developmental center. *West J Med* **172:**305-8.

4493. **Loiez, C., F. Wallet, M. O. Husson, and R. J. Courcol.** 2002. Pasteurella multocida and intrauterine device: a woman and her pets. *Scand J Infect Dis* **34:**473.

4494. **Lokugamage, K., H. Kariwa, D. Hayasaka, B. Z. Cui, T. Iwasaki, N. Lokugamage, L. I. Ivanov, V. I. Volkov, V. A. Demenev, R. Slonova, G. Kompanets, T. Kushnaryova, T. Kurata, K. Maeda, K. Araki, T. Mizutani, K. Yoshimatsu, J. Arikawa, and I. Takashima.** 2002. Genetic Characterization of Hantaviruses Transmitted by the Korean Field Mouse (Apodemus peninsulae), Far East Russia. *Emerg Infect Dis* **8:**768-76.

4495. **Lolekha, S., W. Tanthiphabha, P. Sornchai, P. Kosuwan, S. Sutra, B. Warachit, S. Chup-Upprakarn, Y. Hutagalung, J. Weil, and H. L. Bock.** 2001. Effect of climatic factors and population density on varicella zoster virus epidemiology within a tropical country. *Am J Trop Med Hyg* **64:**131-6.

4496. **Lomar, A. V., D. Diament, and J. R. Torres.** 2000. Leptospirosis in Latin America. *Infect Dis Clin North Am* **14:**23-39.

4497. **Londero, A. T., and C. D. Ramos.** 1976. Chromomycosis: a clinical and mycologic study of thirty-five cases observed in the hinterland of Rio Grande do Sul, Brazil. *Am J Trop Med Hyg* **25:**132-5.

4498. **Long, J., S. Allwright, J. Barry, S. R. Reynolds, L. Thornton, F. Bradley, and J. V. Parry.** 2001. Prevalence of antibodies to hepatitis B, hepatitis C, and HIV and risk factors in entrants to Irish prisons: a national cross sectional survey. *BMJ* **323:**1209.

4499. **Long, S. M., G. K. Adak, S. J. O'Brien, and I. A. Gillespie.** 2002. General outbreaks of infectious intestinal disease linked with salad vegetables and fruit, England and Wales, 1992-2000. *Commun Dis Public Health* **5:**101-5.

4500. **Longfield, J. N., R. E. Winn, R. L. Gibson, S. V. Juchau, and P. V. Hoffman.** 1990. Varicella outbreaks in Army recruits from Puerto Rico. Varicella susceptibility in a population from the tropics. *Arch Intern Med* **150:**970-3.

4501. **Longhurst, A.** 1998. Ecological geography of the sea. Academic Press, San Diego.

4502. **Lopes, J. O., S. H. Alves, C. R. Mari, L. M. Brum, J. B. Westphalen, M. J. Altermann, and F. B. Prates.** 1999. [Epidemiology of sporotrichosis in the central region of Rio Grande do Sul]. *Rev Soc Bras Med Trop* **32:**541-5.

4503. **Lopes, J. O., S. H. Alves, C. R. D. Mari, L. T. O. Oliveira, L. M. Brum, J. B. Westphalen, F. W. Furian, and M. J. Altermann.** 1999. A ten-year survey of tinea pedis in the central region of the Rio Grande do sul, Brazil. *Rev Inst Med Trop Sao Paulo* **41:**75-7.

4504. **Lopez, A., V. J. Dietz, M. S. Wilson, T. R. Navin, and J. L. Jones.** 2000. Preventing congenital toxoplasmosis. *MMWR* **49 (RR-2):**59-68.

4505. **Lopez, A., P. Miranda, E. Tejada, and D. B. Fishbein.** 1992. Outbreak of human rabies in the Peruvian jungle. *Lancet* **339:**408-11.

4506. **Lopez, A. S., J. M. Bendik, J. Y. Alliance, J. M. Roberts, A. J. da Silva, I. N. Moura, M. J. Arrowood, M. L. Eberhard, and B. L. Herwaldt.** 2003. Epidemiology of Cyclospora cayetanensis and other intestinal parasites in a community in Haiti. *J Clin Microbiol* **41:**2047-54.

4507. **Lopez, A. S., D. R. Dodson, M. J. Arrowood, P. A. Orlandi Jr, A. J. da Silva, J. W. Bier, S. D. Hanauer, R. L. Kuster, S. Oltman, M. S. Baldwin, K. Y. Won, E. M. Nace, M. L. Eberhard, and B. L. Herwaldt.** 2001. Outbreak of cyclosporiasis associated with basil in Missouri in 1999. *Clin Infect Dis* **32:**1010-7.

4508. **Lopez, B., M. D. Cima, F. Vazquez, A. Fenoll, J. Gutierrez, C. Fidalgo, M. Caicoya, and F. J. Mendez.** 1999. Epidemiological study of Streptococcus pneumoniae carriers in healthy primary-school children. *Eur J Clin Microbiol Infect Dis* **18:**771-6.

4509. **Lopez, C. E., A. C. Dykes, D. D. Juranek, S. P. Sinclair, J. M. Conn, R. W. Christie, E. C. Lippy, M. G. Schultz, and M. H. Mires.** 1980. Waterborne giardiasis: a communitywide outbreak of disease and a high rate of asymptomatic infection. *Am J Epidemiol* **112:**495-507.

4510. **Lopez, C. E., D. D. Juranek, S. P. Sinclair, and M. G. Schultz.** 1978. Giardiasis in American travelers to Madeira island, Portugal. *Am J Trop Med Hyg* **27:**1128-32.

4511. **Lopez, E., M. Ascher, R. Roberto, and J. Chin.** 1986. Q fever among slaughterhouse workers - California. *MMWR* **35:**223-226.

4512. **Lopez, L., J. Romero, and F. Duarte.** 2003. [Microbiological quality and effect of washing disinfection of pre-cut Chilean vegetables]. *Arch Latinoam Nutr* **53:**383-8.

4513. **Lopez Martinez, R., L. J. Mendez Tovar, P. Lavalle, O. Welsh, A. Saul, and E. Macotela Ruiz.** 1992. [Epidemiology of mycetoma in Mexico: study of 2105 cases]. *Gac Med Mex* **128:**477-81.

4514. **Lopez-Calleja, A. I., M. A. Lezcano, S. Samper, F. de Juan, and M. J. Revillo.** 2004. Mycobacterium malmoense lymphadenitis in Spain: first two cases in immunocompetent patients. *Eur J Clin Microbiol Infect Dis* **23:**567-9.

4515. **Lopez-Cortes, L., F. Lozano de Leon, J. M. Gomez-Mateos, A. Sanchez-Porto, and C. Obrador.** 1989. Tick-borne relapsing fever in intravenous drug abusers. *J Infect Dis* **159:**804.

4516. **López-Vélez, R., H. Huerga, and M. C. Turrientes.** 2003. Infectious diseases in immigrants from the perspective of a tropical medicine referral unit. *Am J Trop Med Hyg* **69:**115-21.

4517. **Lopez-Velez, R., M. C. Turrientes, C. Garron, P. Montilla, R. Navajas, S. Fenoy, and C. del Aguila.** 1999. Microsporidiosis in travelers with diarrhea from the tropics. *J Travel Med* **6:**223-7.

4518. **Lopman, B. A., G. K. Adak, M. H. Reacher, and D. W. Brown.** 2003. Two epidemiologic patterns of norovirus outbreaks: surveillance in England and wales, 1992-2000. *Emerg Infect Dis* **9:**71-7.

4519. **Lopman, B. A., M. H. Reacher, I. B. Vipond, D. Hill, C. Perry, T. Halladay, D. W. Brown, W. J. Edmunds, and J. Sarangi.** 2004. Epidemiology and cost of nosocomial gastroenteritis, Avon, England, 2002-2003. *Emerg Infect Dis* **10:**1827-34.

4520. **Lorca, M., A. Garcia, M. C. Contreras, H. Schenone, and A. Rojas.** 2001. Evaluation of a Triatoma infestans elimination program by the decrease of Trypanosoma cruzi infection frequency in children younger than 10 years, Chile, 1991-1998. *Am J Trop Med Hyg* **65:**861-4.

4521. **Loreille, O., and F. Bouchet.** 2003. Evolution of ascariasis in humans and pigs: a multi-disciplinary approach. *Mem Inst Oswaldo Cruz* **98 Suppl 1:**39-46.

4522. **Lores, B., I. Lopez-Miragaya, C. Arias, S. Fenoy, J. Torres, and C. del Aguila.** 2002. Intestinal microsporidiosis due to Enterocytozoon bieneusi in elderly human immunodeficiency virus—negative patients from Vigo, Spain. *Clin Infect Dis* **34:**918-21.

4523. **Löscher, T., H. D. Nothdurft, H. Taelman, M. Boogaerts, M. Omar, and F. von Sonnenburg.** 1989. Schlafkrankheit bei deutschen Tropenreisenden. *Dtsch Med Wochenschr* **114:**1203-6.

4524. **Lot, F., J. C. Seguier, S. Fegueux, P. Astagneau, P. Simon, M. Aggoune, P. van Amerongen, M. Ruch, M. Cheron, G. Brucker, J. C. Desenclos, and J. Drucker.** 1999. Probable transmission of HIV from an orthopedic surgeon to a patient in France. *Ann Intern Med* **130:**1-6.

4525. **Louie, J. K., S. Yagi, F. A. Nelson, D. Kiang, C. A. Glaser, J. Rosenberg, C. K. Cahill, and D. P. Schnurr.** 2005. Rhinovirus outbreak in a long term care facility for elderly persons associated with unusually high mortality. *Clin Infect Dis* **41:**262-5.

4526. **Louie, K., L. Gustafson, M. Fyfe, I. Gill, L. MacDougall, L. Tom, Q. Wong, and J. Isaac-Renton.** 2004. An outbreak of Cryptosporidium parvum in a Surrey pool with detection in pool water sampling. *Can Commun Dis Rep* **30:**61-6.

4527. **Louis, F. J., J. P. Louis, H. Schill, and F. Parc.** 1987. Ultime offensive de la lèpre dans le Pacifique sud: l'épidémie de Rapa (1922-1950). *Bull Soc Pathol Exot* **80:**306-19.

4528. **Louis, F. J., B. Maubert, J.-Y. Le Hesran, J. Kemmegne, E. Delaporte, and J. P. Louis.** 1994. High prevalence of anti-hepatitis C virus antibodies in a Cameroon rural forest area. *Trans R Soc Trop Med Hyg* **88:**53-4.

4529. **Loukil, C., C. Saizou, C. Doit, P. Bidet, P. Mariani-Kurkdjian, Y. Aujard, F. Beaufils, and E. Bingen.** 2003. Epidemiologic investigation of Burkholderia cepacia acquisition in two pediatric intensive care units. *Infect Control Hosp Epidemiol* **24:**707-10.

4530. **Lounibos, L. P.** 2002. Invasions by insect vectors of human disease. *Annu Rev Entomol* **47:**233-66.

4531. **Lounici, M., M. Lazri, and K. Rahal.** 2005. [Plague in Algeria: about five strains of Yersinia pestis isolated during the outbreak of June 2003.]. *Pathol Biol (Paris)* **53:**15-18.

4532. **Loutan, L.** 1995. [Babesiosis, a little-known zoonosis]. *Schweiz Med Wochenschr* **125:**886-9.

4533. **Loutan, L., M. Bouvier, B. Rojanawisut, H. Stalder, M. C. Rouan, G. Buescher, and A. A. Poltera.** 1989. Single treatment of invasive fascioliasis with triclabendazole. *Lancet* **2 (12 August):**383.

4534. **Love, S. S., X. Jiang, E. Barrett, T. Farkas, and S. Kelly.** 2002. A large hotel outbreak of Norwalk-like virus gastroenteritis among three groups of guests and hotel employees in Virginia. *Epidemiol Infect* **129:**127-32.

4535. **Low, D. E., and A. McGeer.** 2003. SARS - one year later. *N Engl J Med* **349:**2381-2.

4536. **Lowery, C. J., P. Nugent, J. E. Moore, B. C. Millar, X. Xiru, and J. S. Dooley.** 2001. PCR-IMS detection and molecular typing of Cryptosporidium parvum recorded from a recreational river source and an associated mussel (Mytilus edulis) bed in Northern Ireland. *Epidemiol Infect* **127:**545-53.

4537. **Lowhagen, G. B., E. Jansen, E. Nordenfelt, and E. Lycke.** 1990. Epidemiology of genital herpes infections in Sweden. *Acta Derm Venereol* **70:**330-4.

4538. **Lowry, P. W., W. R. Jarvis, A. D. Oberle, L. A. Bland, R. Silberman, J. A. Bocchini, Jr., H. D. Dean, J. M. Swenson, and R. J. Wallace, Jr.** 1988. Mycobacterium chelonae causing otitis media in an ear-nose-and-throat practice. *N Engl J Med* **319:**978-82.

4539. **Lowry, P. W., R. Levine, D. F. Stroup, R. A. Gunn, M. H. Wilder, and C. Konigsberg, Jr.** 1989. Hepatitis A outbreak on a floating restaurant in Florida, 1986. *Am J Epidemiol* **129:**155-64.

4540. **Lowry, P. W., L. M. McFarland, B. H. Peltier, N. C. Roberts, H. B. Bradford, J. L. Herndon, D. F. Stroup, J. B. Mathison, P. A. Blake, and R. A. Gunn.** 1989. Vibrio gastroenteritis in Louisiana: a prospective study among attendees of a scientific congress in New Orleans. *J Infect Dis* **160:**978-84.

4541. **Lowy, F. D., and M. A. Miller.** 2002. New methods to investigate infectious disease transmission and pathogenesis - Staphylococcus aureus disease in drug users. *Lancet Infect Dis* **2:**605-12.

4542. **Lu, Q.** 1990. [A prospective serological epidemiological investigation of hepatitis B virus infection in a prison]. *Zhonghua Liu Xing Bing Xue Za Zhi* **11:**267-70.

4543. **Luby, S.** 2001. Injection safety. *Emerg Infect Dis* **7(3):**535.

4544. **Luby, S., M. Agboatwalla, B. M. Schnell, R. M. Hoekstra, M. H. Rahbar, and B. H. Keswick.** 2002. The effect of antibacterial soap on impetigo incidence, Karachi, Pakistan. *Am J Trop Med Hyg* **67:**430-5.

4545. **Luby, S., J. Jones, H. Dowda, J. Kramer, and J. Horan.** 1993. A large outbreak of gastroenteritis caused by diarrheal toxin-producing Bacillus cereus. *J Infect Dis* **167:**1452-5.

4546. **Luby, S. P., M. Agboatwalla, J. Painter, A. Altaf, W. L. Billhimer, and R. M. Hoekstra.** 2004. Effect of intensive handwashing promotion on childhood diarrhea in high-risk communities in Pakistan: a randomized controlled trial. *JAMA* **291:**2547-54.

4547. **Luby, S. P., M. K. Faizan, S. P. Fisher-Hoch, A. Syed, E. D. Mintz, Z. A. Bhutta, and J. B. McCormick.** 1998. Risk factors for typhoid fever in an endemic setting, Karachi, Pakistan. *Epidemiol Infect* **120:**129-38.

4548. **Luby, S. P., K. Qamruddin, A. A. Shah, A. Omair, O. Pahsa, A. J. Khan, J. B. McCormick, F. Hoodbhouy, and S. Fisher-Hoch.** 1997. The relationship between therapeutic injections and high prevalence of hepatitis C infection in Hafizabad, Pakistan. *Epidemiol Infect* **119:**349-56.

4549. Lucas, C. M., E. D. Franke, M. I. Cachay, A. Tejada, M. E. Cruz, R. D. Kreutzer, D. C. Barker, S. H. McCann, and D. M. Watts. 1998. Geographic distribution and clinical description of leishmaniasis cases in Peru. Am J Trop Med Hyg 59:312-7.

4550. Lucas, R. E., and P. K. Armstrong. 2000. Two cases of mycetoma due to Nocardia brasiliensis in central Australia. Med J Aust 172:167-9.

4551. Lucena, W. A., R. Dhalia, F. G. Abath, L. Nicolas, L. N. Regis, and A. F. Furtado. 1998. Diagnosis of Wuchereria bancrofti infection by the polymerase chain reaction using urine and day blood samples from amicrofilaraemic patients. Trans R Soc Trop Med Hyg 92:290-3.

4552. Lucero, N. E., G. I. Escobar, S. M. Ayala, and N. Jacob. 2005. Diagnosis of human brucellosis caused by Brucella canis. J Med Microbiol 54:457-61.

4553. Lucet, J. C., D. Decre, A. Fichelle, M. L. Joly-Guillou, M. Pernet, C. Deblangy, M. J. Kosmann, and B. Regnier. 1999. Control of a prolonged outbreak of extended-spectrum beta-lactamase-producing enterobacteriaceae in a university hospital. Clin Infect Dis 29:1411-8.

4554. Lucht, E., M. Brytting, L. Bjerregaard, I. Julander, and A. Linde. 1998. Shedding of cytomegalovirus and herpesviruses 6, 7, and 8 in saliva of human immunodeficiency virus type 1-infected patients and healthy controls. Clin Infect Dis 27:137-41.

4555. Lucht, E., B. Evengard, J. Skott, P. Pehrson, and C. E. Nord. 1998. Entamoeba gingivalis in human immunodeficiency virus type 1-infected patients with periodontal disease. Clin Infect Dis 27:471-3.

4556. Luck, P. C., E. Dinger, J. H. Helbig, V. Thurm, H. Keuchel, C. Presch, and M. Ott. 1994. Analysis of Legionella pneumophila strains associated with nosocomial pneumonia in a neonatal intensive care unit. Eur J Clin Microbiol Infect Dis 13:565-71.

4557. Luck, P. C., B. Lau, S. Seidel, and U. Postl. 1992. [Legionellae in dental units—a hygienic risk?]. Dtsch Zahn Mund Kieferheilkd Zentralbl 80:341-6.

4558. Luck, P. C., I. Leupold, M. Hlawitschka, J. H. Helbig, I. Carmienke, L. Jatzwauk, and T. Guderitz. 1993. Prevalence of Legionella species, serogroups, and monoclonal subgroups in hot water systems in south-eastern Germany. Zentralbl Hyg Umweltmed 193:450-60.

4559. Luck, S., M. Torry, K. d'Agapeyeff, A. Pitt, P. Heath, A. Breathnach, and A. B. Russell. 2003. Estimated early-onset group B streptococcal neonatal disease. Lancet 361:1953-4.

4560. Ludlam, H., and B. Cookson. 1986. Scrum kidney: epidemic pyoderma caused by a nephritogenic Streptococcus pyogenes in a rugby team. Lancet 2:331-3.

4561. Luft, B. J., and J. S. Remington. 1984. Acute Toxoplasma infection among family members of patients with acute lymphadenopathic toxoplasmosis. Arch Intern Med 144:53-6.

4562. Lugagne, P. M., J. M. Herve, T. Lebret, F. Gaudez, P. Barre, and H. Botto. 1997. [Infectious risks of outpatient cystoscopy in men with sterile urine]. Prog Urol 7:615-7.

4563. Lui, S. L., W. K. Luk, C. Y. Cheung, T. M. Chan, K. N. Lai, and J. S. Peiris. 2001. Nosocomial outbreak of parvovirus B19 infection in a renal transplant unit. Transplantation 71:59-64.

4564. Luisto, M. 1989. Epidemiology of tetanus in Finland from 1969 to 1985. Scand J Infect Dis 21:655-63.

4565. Luisto, M., and A. M. Seppalainen. 1992. Tetanus caused by occupational accidents. Scand J Work Environ Health 18:323-6.

4566. Lukinmaa, S., E. Takkunen, and A. Siitonen. 2002. Molecular epidemiology of Clostridium perfringens related to foodborne outbreaks of disease in Finland from 1984 to 1999. Appl Environ Microbiol 68:3744-9.

4567. Lumb, R., I. Bastian, D. Dawson, C. Gilpin, F. Haverkort, G. James, and A. Sievers. 2003. Tuberculosis in Australia: bacteriologically confirmed cases and drug resistance, 2001. Commun Dis Intell 27:173-80.

4568. Lumio, J., R. M. Ölander, K. Groundstroem, P. Suomalainen, T. Honkanen, and J. Vuopio-Varkila. 2001. Epidemiology of three cases of severe diphtheria in Finnish patients with low antitoxin antibody levels. Eur J Clin Microbiol Infect Dis 20:705-10.

4569. Lumio, J., P. Suomalainen, R. M. Olander, H. Saxen, and E. Salo. 2003. Fatal case of diphtheria in an unvaccinated infant in Finland. Pediatr Infect Dis J 22:844-6.

4570. Lun, Z. R., R. B. Gasser, D. H. Lai, A. X. Li, X. Q. Zhu, X. B. Yu, and Y. Y. Fang. 2005. Clonorchiasis: a key foodborne zoonosis in China. Lancet Infect Dis 5:31-41.

4571. Luna, E. J. A., N. H. Medina, and M. B. Oliveira. 1992. Epidemiology of trachoma in Bebedouro state of São Paulo, Brazil: prevalence and risk factors. Int J Epidemiol 21:169-77.

4572. Lund, B. M., G. W. Gould, and A. M. Rampling. 2002. Pasteurization of milk and the heat resistance of Mycobacterium avium subsp. paratuberculosis: a critical review of the data. Int J Food Microbiol 77:135-45.

4573. Lunden, J. M., T. J. Autio, and H. J. Korkeala. 2002. Transfer of persistent Listeria monocytogenes contamination between food-processing plants associated with a dicing machine. J Food Prot 65:1129-33.

4574. Lundkvist, A., G. Lindegren, K. B. Sjölander, V. Mavtchoutko, S. Vene, A. Plyusnin, and V. Kalnina. 2002. Hantavirus infections in Latvia. Eur J Clin Microbiol Infect Dis 21:626-9.

4575. Lundstrom, J. O. 1999. Mosquito-borne viruses in western Europe: a review. J Vector Ecol 24:1-39.

4576. Luo, D., W. Zhu, X. Zhang, X. Chen, S. Wang, Z. Wang, G. Liang, H. Sun, and W. Xu. 2000. Molecular epidemiologic study of Mycoplasma genitalium infection in high risk populations of sexually transmitted diseases in China. Chin Med J (Engl) 113:1015-8.

4577. Lurie, P., H. Stafford, P. Tran, C. Teacher, R. Ankeny, M. Barron, J. Bart, K. Bisgard, T. Tiwari, T. Murphy, J. Moran, and P. Cassiday. 2004. Fatal respiratory diphtheria in a U.S. traveler to Haiti - Pennsylvania, 2003. MMWR 52:1285-6.

4578. Lush, D., J. C. Hargrave, and A. Merianos. 1998. Leprosy control in the Northern Territory. Aust N Z J Public Health 22:709-13.

4579. Lutwama, J. J., J. Kayondo, H. M. Savage, T. R. Burkot, and B. R. Miller. 1999. Epidemic O'Nyong-Nyong fever in south-central Uganda, 1996-1997: entomologic studies in Bbaale village, Rakai District. Am J Trop Med Hyg 61:158-62.

4580. Lutwick, L. I. 2001. Brill-Zinsser disease. Lancet 357:1198-200.

4581. Luty, T. 2001. Prevalence of species of Toxocara in dogs, cats and red foxes from the Poznan region, Poland. J Helminthol 75:153-6.

4582. Lutz, B. D., J. Jin, M. G. Rinaldi, B. L. Wickes, and M. M. Huycke. 2003. Outbreak of invasive Aspergillus infection in surgical patients, associated with a contaminated air-handling system. *Clin Infect Dis* **37:**786-93.

4583. Luxemburger, C., M. C. Chau, N. L. Mai, J. Wain, T. H. Tran, J. A. Simpson, H. K. Le, T. T. Nguyen, N. J. White, and J. J. Farrar. 2001. Risk factors for typhoid fever in the Mekong delta, southern Viet Nam: a case-control study. *Trans R Soc Trop Med Hyg* **95:**19-23.

4584. Luz, K. G., V. O. da Silva, E. M. Gomes, F. C. Machado, M. A. Araujo, H. E. Fonseca, T. C. Freire, J. B. d'Almeida, M. Palatnik, and C. B. Palatnik-de Sousa. 1997. Prevalence of anti-Leishmania donovani antibody among Brazilian blood donors and multiply transfused hemodialysis patients. *Am J Trop Med Hyg* **57:**168-71.

4585. Luzzi, G. A., R. Brindle, P. N. Sockett, J. Solera, P. Klenerman, and D. A. Warrell. 1993. Brucellosis: imported and laboratory-acquired cases, and an overview of treatment trials. *Trans R Soc Trop Med Hyg* **87:**138-41.

4586. Lvov, D. K. 1980. Arboviruses in the U.S.S.R., p. 35-46. *In* J. Vesenjak-Hirjan (ed.), Arboviruses in the Mediterranean countries. Gustav Fischer Verlag, Stuttgart.

4587. Lyagoubi, M., A. Datry, R. Mayorga, G. Brucker, I. Hilmarsdottir, P. Gaxotte, D. Neu, M. Danis, and M. Gentilini. 1992. Chronic persistent strongyloidiasis cured by ivermectin. *Trans R Soc Trop Med Hyg* **86:**541.

4588. Lyerla, R., J. G. Rigau-Perez, A. V. Vorndam, P. Reiter, A. M. George, I. M. Potter, and D. J. Gubler. 2000. A dengue outbreak among camp participants in a Caribbean island, 1995. *J Travel Med* **7:**59-63.

4589. Lynn, S., J. Toop, C. Hanger, and N. Millar. 2004. Norovirus outbreaks in a hospital setting: the role of infection control. *N Z Med J* **117:**U771.

4590. Lyon, G. M., A. V. Bravo, A. Espino, M. D. Lindsley, R. E. Gutierrez, I. Rodriguez, A. Corella, F. Carrillo, M. M. McNeil, D. W. Warnock, and R. A. Hajjeh. 2004. Histoplasmosis Associated with Exploring a Bat-Inhabited Cave in Costa Rica, 1998-1999. *Am J Trop Med Hyg* **70:**438-442.

4591. Lyon, G. M., S. Zurita, J. Casquero, W. Holgado, J. Guevara, M. E. Brandt, S. Douglas, K. Shutt, D. W. Warnock, and R. A. Hajjeh. 2003. Population-based surveillance and a case-control study of risk factors for endemic lymphocutaneous sporotrichosis in Peru. *Clin Infect Dis* **36:**34-9.

4592. Lyytikainen, O., T. Autio, R. Maijala, P. Ruutu, T. Honkanen-Buzalski, M. Miettinen, M. Hatakka, J. Mikkola, V. J. Anttila, T. Johansson, L. Rantala, T. Aalto, H. Korkeala, and A. Siitonen. 2000. An outbreak of Listeria monocytogenes serotype 3a infections from butter in Finland. *J Infect Dis* **181:**1838-41.

4593. Lyytikainen, O., E. Hoffmann, H. Timm, B. Schweiger, W. Witte, U. Vieth, A. Ammon, and L. R. Petersen. 1998. Influenza A outbreak among adolescents in a ski hostel. *Eur J Clin Microbiol Infect Dis* **17:**128-30.

4594. Lyytikäinen, O., J. P. Nuorti, E. Halmesmäki, P. Carlson, J. Uotila, R. Vuento, T. Ranta, H. Sarkkinen, M. Ammala, A. Kostiala, and A. L. Jarvenpaa. 2003. Invasive group B streptococcal infections in Finnland: a population-based study. *Emerg Infect Dis* **9:**469-73.

4595. Lyytikainen, O., M. Rautio, P. Carlson, V. J. Anttila, R. Vuento, H. Sarkkinen, A. Kostiala, M. L. Vaisanen, A. Kanervo, and P. Ruutu. 2004. Nosocomial bloodstream infections due to viridans streptococci in haematological and non-haematological patients: species distribution and antimicrobial resistance. *J Antimicrob Chemother* **53:**631-4.

4596. Lyytikainen, O., T. Ziese, B. Schwartlander, P. Matzdorff, C. Kuhnhen, C. Jager, and L. Petersen. 1998. An outbreak of sheep-associated Q fever in a rural community in Germany. *Eur J Epidemiol* **14:**193-9.

4597. Ma, K. C., M. H. Qiu, and Y. L. Rong. 2002. Pathological differentiation of suspected cases of pentastomiasis in China. *Trop Med Int Health* **7:**166-77.

4598. Mabaso, M. L., C. C. Appleton, J. C. Hughes, and E. Gouws. 2004. Hookworm (Necator americanus) transmission in inland areas of sandy soils in KwaZulu-Natal, South Africa. *Trop Med Int Health* **9:**471-6.

4599. Mabey, D. C., A. W. Solomon, and A. Foster. 2003. Trachoma. *Lancet* **362:**223-9.

4600. Mac Kenzie, W. R., N. J. Hoxie, M. E. Proctor, M. S. Gradus, K. A. Blair, D. E. Peterson, J. J. Kazmierczak, D. G. Addiss, K. R. Fox, J. B. Rose, et al. 1994. A massive outbreak in Milwaukee of cryptosporidium infection transmitted through the public water supply. *N Engl J Med* **331:**161-7.

4601. Macaluso, K. R., J. Davis, U. Alam, A. Korman, J. S. Rutherford, R. Rosenberg, and A. F. Azad. 2003. Spotted fever group rickettsiae in ticks from the Masai Mara region of Kenya. *Am J Trop Med Hyg* **68:**551-3.

4602. MacArthur, J. R., T. H. Holtz, J. Jenkins, J. P. Newell, J. E. Koehler, M. E. Parise, and S. P. Kachur. 2001. Probable locally acquired mosquito-transmitted malaria in Georgia, 1999. *Clin Infect Dis* **32:**E124-8.

4603. MacDonald, D. M., M. Fyfe, A. Paccagnella, A. Trinidad, K. Louie, and D. Patrick. 2004. Escherichia coli O157:H7 outbreak linked to salami, British Columbia, Canada, 1999. *Epidemiol Infect* **132:**283-9.

4604. MacDonald, K. L., R. F. Spengler, C. L. Hatheway, N. T. Hargrett, and M. L. Cohen. 1985. Type A botulism from sauteed onions. Clinical and epidemiologic observations. *JAMA* **253:**1275-8.

4605. MacDonald, M., P. Sullivan, A. Locke, A. Wodak, and J. Kaldor. 1998. HIV and HCV prevalence among trawler crew. *Aust N Z J Public Health* **22:**829-31.

4606. MacDonald, P. D., R. E. Whitwam, J. D. Boggs, J. N. MacCormack, K. L. Anderson, J. W. Reardon, J. R. Saah, L. M. Graves, S. B. Hunter, and J. Sobel. 2005. Outbreak of listeriosis among Mexican immigrants as a result of consumption of illicitly produced Mexican-style cheese. *Clin Infect Dis* **40:**677-82.

4607. Mace, J. M., M. Boussinesq, P. Ngoumou, J. Enyegue Oye, A. Koeranga, and C. Godin. 1997. Country-wide rapid epidemiological mapping of onchocerciasis (REMO) in Cameroon. *Ann Trop Med Parasitol* **91:**379-91.

4608. Macedo de Oliveira, A., K. L. White, D. P. Leschinsky, B. D. Beecham, T. M. Vogt, R. L. Moolenaar, J. F. Perz, and T. J. Safranek. 2005. An outbreak of hepatitis C virus infections among outpatients at a hematology/oncology clinic. *Ann Intern Med* **142:**898-902.

4609. MacGowan, A. P., P. H. Cartlidge, F. MacLeod, and J. McLaughlin. 1991. Maternal listeriosis in pregnancy without fetal or neonatal infection. *J Infect* **22:**53-7.

4610. Machuca, A., C. Tuset, V. Soriano, E. Caballero, A. Aguilera, and R. Ortiz de Lejarazu. 2000. Prevalence of HTLV infection in pregnant women in Spain. *Sex Transm Infect* **76:**366-70.

4611. **MacIntyre, C. R., N. Kendig, L. Kummer, S. Birago, and N. M. Graham.** 1997. Impact of tuberculosis control measures and crowding on the incidence of tuberculous infection in Maryland prisons. *Clin Infect Dis* **24:**1060-7.

4612. **MacIntyre, C. R., P. B. McIntyre, and M. Cagney.** 2003. Community-based estimates of incidence and risk factors for childhood pneumonia in Western Sydney. *Epidemiol Infect* **131:**1091-6.

4613. **MacIntyre, C. R., A. J. Plant, J. Hulls, J. A. Streeton, N. M. Graham, and G. J. Rouch.** 1995. High rate of transmission of tuberculosis in an office: impact of delayed diagnosis. *Clin Infect Dis* **21:**1170-4.

4614. **Mackay, I. M., K. C. Jacob, D. Woolhouse, K. Waller, M. W. Syrmis, D. M. Whiley, D. J. Siebert, M. Nissen, and T. P. Sloots.** 2003. Molecular assays for detection of human metapneumovirus. *J Clin Microbiol* **41:**100-5.

4615. **Mackelprang, R., M. D. Dearing, and S. St Jeor.** 2001. High prevalence of sin nombre virus in rodent populations, Central Utah: a consequence of human disturbance? *Emerg Infect Dis* **7:**480-2.

4616. **Mackenzie, J. S., and A. K. Broom.** 1995. Australian X disease, Murray Valley encephalitis and the French connection. *Vet Microbiol* **46:**79-90.

4617. **Mackenzie, J. S., A. K. Broom, R. A. Hall, C. A. Johansen, M. D. Lindsay, D. A. Phillips, S. A. Ritchie, R. C. Russell, and D. W. Smith.** 1998. Arboviruses in the Australian region, 1990 to 1998. *Commun Dis Intell* **22:**93-100.

4618. **Mackenzie, J. S., H. E. Field, and K. J. Guyatt.** 2003. Managing emerging diseases borne by fruit bats (flying foxes), with particular reference to henipaviruses and Australian bat lyssavirus. *J Appl Microbiol* **94 Suppl:**59S-69S.

4619. **Mackenzie, J. S., M. D. Lindsay, R. J. Coelen, A. K. Broom, R. A. Hall, and D. W. Smith.** 1994. Arboviruses causing human disease in the Australasian zoogeographic region. *Arch Virol* **136:**447-67.

4620. **MacKenzie, W. R., J. J. Kazmierczak, and J. P. Davis.** 1995. An outbreak of cryptosporidiosis associated with a resort swimming pool. *Epidemiol Infect* **115:**545-53.

4621. **Mackey, T. A., E. H. Page, K. F. Martinez, T. A. Seitz, B. P. Bernard, et al.** 2002. Suspected cutaneous anthrax in a laboratory worker - Texas, 2002. *MMWR* **51:**279-81.

4622. **Mackiewicz, V., E. Dussaix, M. F. Le Petitcorps, and A. M. Roque-Afonso.** 2004. Detection of hepatitis A virus RNA in saliva. *J Clin Microbiol* **42:**4329-31.

4623. **Mackowiak, P. A., and J. W. Smith.** 1978. Septicemic melioidosis. Occurrence following acute influenza A six years after exposure in Vietnam. *JAMA* **240:**764-6.

4624. **MacLean, J. D., J. R. Arthur, B. J. Ward, T. W. Gyorkos, M. A. Curtis, and E. Kokoskin.** 1996. Common-source outbreak of acute infection due to the North American liver fluke Metorchis conjunctus. *Lancet* **347:**154-8.

4625. **MacLean, J. D., L. Poirier, T. W. Gyorkos, J. F. Proulx, J. Bourgeault, A. Corriveau, S. Illisituk, and M. Staudt.** 1992. Epidemiologic and serologic definition of primary and secondary trichinosis in the Arctic. *J Infect Dis* **165:**908-12.

4626. **Macnish, M. G., U. M. Morgan-Ryan, P. T. Monis, J. M. Behnke, and R. C. Thompson.** 2002. A molecular phylogeny of nuclear and mitochondrial sequences in Hymenolepis nana (Cestoda) supports the existence of a cryptic species. *Parasitology* **125:**567-75.

4627. **Macphail, G. L. P., G. D. Taylor, M. Buchanan-Chell, C. Ross, S. Wilson, and A. Kureishi.** 2002. Epidemiology, treatment and outcome of candidemia: a five year review at three Canadian hospitals. *Mycoses* **45:**141-5.

4628. **Macpherson, C. N., M. Kachani, M. Lyagoubi, M. Berrada, M. Shepherd, P. F. Fields, and M. El Hasnaoui.** 2004. Cystic echinococcosis in the Berber of the Mid Atlas mountains, Morocco: new insights into the natural history of the disease in humans. *Ann Trop Med Parasitol* **98:**481-90.

4629. **Macpherson, C. N. L., P. S. Craig, T. Romig, E. Zeyhle, and H. Watschinger.** 1989. Observations on human echinococcosis (hydatidosis) and evaluation of transmission factors in the Maasai of northern Tanzania. *Ann Trop Med Parasitol* **83:**489-97.

4630. **Macpherson, C. N. L., F. X. Meslin, and A. I. Wandeler.** 2000. Dogs, zoonoses and public health. CABI publishing, Wallingford, U.K., and New York, N.Y.

4631. **Macsween, K. F., and D. H. Crawford.** 2003. Epstein-Barr virus-recent advances. *Lancet Infect Dis* **3:**131-40.

4632. **Madani, T. A., Y. Y. Al-Mazrou, M. H. Al-Jeffri, A. A. Mishkhas, A. M. Al-Rabeah, A. M. Turkistani, M. O. Al-Sayed, A. A. Abodahish, A. S. Khan, T. G. Ksiazek, and O. Shobokshi.** 2003. Rift Valley fever epidemic in Saudi Arabia: epidemiological, clinical, and laboratory characteristics. *Clin Infect Dis* **37:**1084-92.

4633. **Madariaga, M. G., K. Rezai, G. M. Trenholme, and R. A. Weinstein.** 2003. Q fever: a biological weapon in your backyard. *Lancet Infect Dis* **3:**709-21.

4634. **Maeda, H., M. Nakagawa, and M. Yokoyama.** 1996. [Hospital admissions for respiratory diseases in the aftermath of the great Hanshin earthquake]. *Nihon Kyobu Shikkan Gakkai Zasshi* **34:**164-73.

4635. **Maestre, A., J. M. Ramos, M. Elia, and F. Gutierrez.** 2001. [Endocarditis caused by Erysipelothrix rhusiopathiae: a rare professional disease difficult to diagnose]. *Enferm Infecc Microbiol Clin* **19:**456-7.

4636. **Mafojane, N. A., C. C. Appleton, R. C. Krecek, L. M. Michael, and A. L. Willingham, 3rd.** 2003. The current status of neurocysticercosis in Eastern and Southern Africa. *Acta Trop* **87:**25-33.

4637. **Maghazy, S. M.** 2001. Incidence of dermatophytes and cyclohexamide resistant fungi on healthy children hairs and nails in nurseries. *Mycopathologia* **154:**171-5.

4638. **Magill, A. J., M. Grogl, R. A. Gasser, Jr., W. Sun, and C. N. Oster.** 1993. Visceral infection caused by Leishmania tropica in veterans of Operation Desert Storm. *N Engl J Med* **328:**1383-7.

4639. **Magnarelli, L. A., and J. F. Anderson.** 1988. Ticks and biting insects infected with the etiologic agent of Lyme disease, Borrelia burgdorferi. *J Clin Microbiol* **26:**1482-6.

4640. **Magnaval, J. F., P. Marchessau, and G. Larrouy.** 1983. [Ascaridian visceral larva migrans syndromes in the region of the Southern Pyrenees. Apropos of 48 cases]. *Bull Soc Pathol Exot Filiales* **76:**69-75.

4641. **Magruder, C., R. Woodruff, G. Minns, V. Barnett, and P. Baker.** 2001. Cluster of tuberculosis cases among exotic dancers and their close contacts - Kansas, 1994-2000. *MMWR* **50:**291-293.

4642. **Maguire, H., J. Cowden, M. Jacob, B. Rowe, D. Roberts, J. Bruce, and E. Mitchell.** 1992. An outbreak of Salmonella dublin infection in England and Wales associated with a soft unpasteurized cows' milk cheese. *Epidemiol Infect* **109**:389-96.

4643. **Maguire, H. C., P. Atkinson, M. Sharland, and J. Bendig.** 1999. Enterovirus infections in England and Wales: laboratory surveillance data: 1975 to 1994. *Commun Dis Public Health* **2**:122-5.

4644. **Maguire, H. C., C. Seng, S. Chambers, T. Cheasty, G. Double, N. Soltanpoor, and D. Morse.** 1998. Shigella outbreak in a school associated with eating canteen food and person to person spread. *Commun Dis Public Health* **1**:279-80.

4645. **Maguire, J. D., S. Tuti, P. Sismadi, I. Wiady, H. Basri, Krisin, S. Masbar, P. Projodipuro, I. R. Elyazar, A. L. Corwin, and M. J. Bangs.** 2005. Endemic coastal malaria in the Thousand Islands District, near Jakarta, Indonesia. *Trop Med Int Health* **10**:489-96.

4646. **Maguire, T.** 1994. Do Ross river and dengue viruses pose a threat to New Zealand? *N Z Med J* **9 nov**:448-50.

4647. **Mahajan, V. K., N. L. Sharma, R. C. Sharma, M. L. Gupta, G. Garg, and A. K. Kanga.** 2005. Cutaneous sporotrichosis in Himachal Pradesh, India. *Mycoses* **48**:25-31.

4648. **Mahanty, S., and M. Bray.** 2004. Pathogenesis of filoviral haemorrhagic fevers. *Lancet Infect Dis* **4**:487-98.

4649. **Mahara, F.** 1997. Japanese spotted fever: report of 31 cases and review of the literature. *Emerg Infect Dis* **3**:105-11.

4650. **Mahe, A., M. Develoux, C. Lienhardt, S. Keita, and P. Bobin.** 1996. Mycetomas in Mali: causative agents and geographic distribution. *Am J Trop Med Hyg* **54**:77-9.

4651. **Mahe, A., O. Faye, T. N'Diaye H, F. Ly, H. Konare, S. Keita, A. K. Traore, and R. Hay.** 2005. Definition of an algorithm for the management of common skin diseases at primary health care level in sub-Saharan Africa. *Trans R Soc Trop Med Hyg* **99**:39-47.

4652. **Mahgoub, S., J. Ahmed, and A. E. Glatt.** 2002. Underlying characteristics of patients harboring highly resistant Acinetobacter baumannii. *Am J Infect Control* **30**:386-90.

4653. **Mahmoud, A.-L. E.** 2002. A study of dermatophytoses in Sana'a, Yemen republic. *Mycoses* **45**:105-8.

4654. **Mahmoud, A. A. F.** 2001. Schistosomiasis. Imperial College Press, London.

4655. **Mahmud, M. A., C. L. Chappell, M. M. Hossain, D. B. Huang, M. Habib, and H. L. DuPont.** 2001. Impact of breast-feeding on Giardia lamblia infections in Bilbeis, Egypt. *Am J Trop Med Hyg* **65**:257-60.

4656. **Mahon, B. E., E. D. Mintz, K. D. Greene, J. G. Wells, and R. V. Tauxe.** 1996. Reported cholera in the United States, 1992-1994. A reflection of global changes in cholera epidemiology. *JAMA* **276**:307-12.

4657. **Mahon, B. E., A. Ponka, W. N. Hall, K. Komatsu, S. E. Dietrich, A. Siitonen, G. Cage, P. S. Hayes, M. A. Lambert-Fair, N. H. Bean, P. M. Griffin, and L. Slutsker.** 1997. An international outbreak of Salmonella infections caused by alfalfa sprouts grown from contaminated seeds. *J Infect Dis* **175**:876-82.

4658. **Mahoney, F. J., T. A. Farley, D. F. Burbank, N. H. Leslie, and L. M. McFarland.** 1993. Evaluation of an intervention program for the control of an outbreak of shigellosis among institutionalized persons. *J Infect Dis* **168**:1177-80.

4659. **Mahoney, F. J., T. A. Farley, K. Y. Kelso, S. A. Wilson, J. M. Horan, and L. M. McFarland.** 1992. An outbreak of hepatitis A associated with swimming in a public pool. *J Infect Dis* **165**:613-8.

4660. **Mahoney, F. J., T. A. Farley, B. J. Moriniere, D. K. Winsor, R. L. Silberman, and L. M. McFarland.** 1991. Evaluation of an intervention program in the control of an urban outbreak of shigellosis. *Am J Prev Med* **7**:292-7.

4661. **Mahoney, F. J., C. W. Hoge, T. A. Farley, J. M. Barbaree, R. F. Breiman, R. F. Benson, and L. M. McFarland.** 1992. Communitywide outbreak of Legionnaires' disease associated with a grocery store mist machine. *J Infect Dis* **165**:736-9.

4662. **Maia-Herzog, M., A. J. Shelley, J. E. Bradley, A. P. Luna Dias, R. H. Calvao, C. Lowry, M. Camargo, J. M. Rubio, R. J. Post, and G. E. Coelho.** 1999. Discovery of a new focus of human onchocerciasis in central Brazil. *Trans R Soc Trop Med Hyg* **93**:235-9.

4663. **Maibach, R. C., F. Dutly, and M. Altwegg.** 2002. Detection of Tropheryma whipplei DNA in feces by PCR using a target capture method. *J Clin Microbiol* **40**:2466-71.

4664. **Mailles, A., Muna Abu Sin, G. Ducoffre, P. Heyman, J. Koch, and H. Zeller.** 2005. Larger than usual increase in cases of hantavirus infections in Belgium, France and Germany, June 2005. *Eurosurveillance Weekly* **10**:8-14.

4665. **Mairiang, E., and P. Mairiang.** 2003. Clinical manifestation of opisthorchiasis and treatment. *Acta Trop* **88**:221-7.

4666. **Maiti, P. K., A. Ray, and S. Bandyopadhyay.** 2002. Epidemiological aspects of mycetoma from a retrospective study of 264 cases in West Bengal. *Trop Med Int Health* **7**:788-92.

4667. **Maiwald, M., A. von Herbay, D. N. Fredricks, C. C. Ouverney, J. C. Kosek, and D. A. Relman.** 2003. Cultivation of Tropheryma whipplei from cerebrospinal fluid. *J Infect Dis* **188**:801-8.

4668. **Maiztegui, J., M. Feuillade, and A. Briggiler.** 1986. Progressive extension of the endemic area and changing incidence of Argentine Hemorrhagic Fever. *Med Microbiol Immunol* **175**:149-52.

4669. **Maiztegui, J. I.** 1975. Clinical and epidemiological patterns of Argentine haemorrhagic fever. *Bull WHO* **52**:567-75.

4670. **Majowicz, S. E., K. Dore, J. A. Flint, V. L. Edge, S. Read, M. C. Buffett, S. McEwen, W. B. McNab, D. Stacey, P. Sockett, and J. B. Wilson.** 2004. Magnitude and distribution of acute, self-reported gastrointestinal illness in a Canadian community. *Epidemiol Infect* **132**:607-17.

4671. **Mak, D. B., C. D'Arcy, and J. Holman.** 2000. A decision to end a periodic syphilis-screening program in the Kimberley region. *Commun Dis Intell* **24**:386-90.

4672. **Mak, D. B., D. F. Fry, and M. K. Bulsara.** 2003. Prevalence of markers of Q fever exposure in the Kimberley, Western Australia. *Commun Dis Intell* **27**:267-71.

4673. **Mak, D. B., G. H. Johnson, and A. J. Plant.** 2004. A syphilis outbreak in remote Australia: epidemiology and strategies for control. *Epidemiol Infect* **132**:805-12.

4674. **Mak, J. W., W. H. Cheong, P. K. Yen, P. K. Lim, and W. C. Chan.** 1982. Studies on the epidemiology of subperiodic Brugia malayi in Malaysia: problems in its control. *Acta Trop* **39**:237-45.

4675. **Makela, P. H., H. Kayhty, P. Weckstrom, A. Sivonen, and O. V. Renkonen.** 1975. Effect of group-A meningococcal vaccine in army recruits in Finland. *Lancet* **2**:883-6.

4676. **Makhlouf, S. A., M. A. Sarwat, D. M. Mahmoud, and A. A. Mohamad.** 1994. Parasitic infection among children living in two orphanages in Cairo. *J Egypt Soc Parasitol* **24**:137-45.

4677. **Maki, D. G., and W. A. Agger.** 1988. Enterococcal bacteremia: clinical features, the risk of endocarditis, and management. *Medicine (Baltimore)* **67:**248-69.

4678. **Makino, K., K. Oshima, K. Kurokawa, K. Yokoyama, T. Uda, K. Tagomori, Y. Iijima, M. Najima, M. Nakano, A. Yamashita, Y. Kubota, S. Kimura, T. Yasunaga, T. Honda, H. Shinagawa, M. Hattori, and T. Iida.** 2003. Genome sequence of Vibrio parahaemolyticus: a pathogenic mechanism distinct from that of V cholerae. *Lancet* **361:**743-9.

4679. **Makino, S. I., K. Kawamoto, K. Takeshi, Y. Okada, M. Yamasaki, S. Yamamoto, and S. Igimi.** 2005. An outbreak of food-borne listeriosis due to cheese in Japan, during 2001. *Int J Food Microbiol.*

4680. **Makino, S. I., T. Kii, H. Asakura, T. Shirahata, T. Ikeda, K. Takeshi, and K. Itoh.** 2000. Does enterohemorrhagic Escherichia coli O157:H7 enter the viable but nonculturable state in salted salmon roe? *Appl Environ Microbiol* **66:**5536-9.

4681. **Makintubee, S., J. Mallonee, and G. R. Istre.** 1987. Shigellosis outbreak associated with swimming. *Am J Public Health* **77:**166-8.

4682. **Makkai, T., and I. McAllister.** 2001. Prevalence of tattooing and body piercing in the Australian community. *Commun Dis Intell* **25:**67-72.

4683. **Makras, P., S. Alexiou-Daniel, A. Antoniadis, and D. Hatzigeorgiou.** 2001. Outbreak of meningococcal disease after an influenza B epidemic at a Hellenic Air Force recruit training center. *Clin Infect Dis* **33:**e48-50.

4684. **Malaty, H. M., A. El-Kasabany, D. Y. Graham, C. C. Miller, S. G. Reddy, S. R. Srinivasan, Y. Yamaoka, and G. S. Berenson.** 2002. Age at acquisition of Helicobacter pylori infection: a follow-up study from infancy to adulthood. *Lancet* **359:**931-5.

4685. **Malavaud, S., B. Malavaud, K. Sandres, D. Durand, N. Marty, J. Icart, and L. Rostaing.** 2001. Nosocomial outbreak of influenza virus A (H3N2) infection in a solid organ transplant department. *Transplantation* **72:**535-7.

4686. **Male, S.** 1996. Refugees: do not forget the basics. *World Health Stat Q* **49:**221-5.

4687. **Malengreau, M., K. Molima, M. Gillieaux, M. de Feyter, D. Kyele, and N. Mukolo.** 1983. Outbreak of Shigella dysentery in Eastern Zaire, 1980-1982. *Ann Soc Belg Med Trop* **63:**59-67.

4688. **Malesker, M. A., D. Boken, T. A. Ruma, P. J. Vuchetich, P. J. Murphy, and P. W. Smith.** 1999. Rhodesian trypanosomiasis in a splenectomized patient. *Am J Trop Med Hyg* **61:**428-30.

4689. **Maleville, J., M. Geniaux, and A. Basset.** 1994. Ou en sont les tréponématoses endémiques non vénériennes exotiques? *Med Trop* **54:**427-31.

4690. **Malik, G. F.** 1997. A clinical study of brucellosis in adults in the Asir region of southern Saudi Arabia. *Am J Trop Med Hyg* **56:**375-7.

4691. **Malik Peiris, J. S., W.-H. Tang, K.-H. Chan, P. L. Khong, Y. Guan, Y. L. Lau, and S. S. Chiu.** 2003. Children with respiratory disease associated with metapneumovirus in Hong Kong. *Emerg Infect Dis* **9:**628-33.

4692. **Malkinson, M., C. Banet, Y. Weisman, S. Pokamonski, R. King, and V. Deubel.** 2001. Intercontinental transmission of West Nile virus by migrating white storks. *Emerg Infect Dis* **7:**540.

4693. **Malkinson, M., C. Banet, Y. Weisman, S. Pokamunski, R. King, M. T. Drouet, and V. Deubel.** 2002. Introduction of West Nile virus in the Middle East by Migrating White Storks. *Emerg Infect Dis* **8:**392-7.

4694. **Malmberg, E., D. Birkhed, G. Norvenius, J. G. Noren, and G. Dahlen.** 1994. Microorganisms on toothbrushes at day-care centers. *Acta Odontol Scand* **52:**93-8.

4695. **Malonza, I. M., M. W. Tyndall, J. O. Ndinya-Achola, I. Maclean, S. Omar, K. S. MacDonald, J. Perriens, K. Orle, F. A. Plummer, A. R. Ronald, and S. Moses.** 1999. A randomized, double-blind, placebo-controlled trial of single-dose ciprofloxacin versus erythromycin for the treatment of chancroid in Nairobi, Kenya. *J Infect Dis* **180:**1886-93.

4696. **Maltezou, H. C., and M. Drancourt.** 2003. Nosocomial influenza in children. *J Hosp Infect* **55:**83-91.

4697. **Maltz, G., and C. M. Knauer.** 1991. Amebic liver abscess: a 15-year experience. *Am J Gastroenterol* **86:**704-10.

4698. **Malvy, D., F. Djossou, F. X. Weill, P. Chapuis, M. Longy-Boursier, and M. Le Bras.** 2001. [Human African trypanosomiasis from Trypanosoma brucei gambiense with inoculation chancre in a French expatriate]. *Med Trop (Mars)* **61:**323-7.

4699. **Manangan, L. P., M. L. Pearson, J. I. Tokars, E. Miller, and W. R. Jarvis.** 2002. Feasibility of national surveillance of health-care-associated infections in home-care settings. *Emerg Infect Dis* **8:**233-6.

4700. **Mancianti, F., S. Nardoni, and R. Ceccherelli.** 2001. Occurrence of yeasts in psittacines droppings from captive birds in Italy. *Mycopathologia* **153:**121-4.

4701. **Mancianti, F., and R. Papini.** 1996. Isolation of keratinophilic fungi from the floors of private veterinary clinics in Italy. *Vet Res Commun* **20:**161-6.

4702. **Mandal, B., N. K. Mitra, A. K. Mukhopadhyay, H. Mukherjee, and A. K. Hati.** 1998. Emerging Plasmodium falciparum in an endemic area in Calcutta. *J Indian Med Assoc* **96:**328-9.

4703. **Mandelbrot, L., A. Landreau-Mascaro, C. Rekacewicz, A. Berrebi, J. L. Benifla, M. Burgard, E. Lachassine, B. Barret, M. L. Chaix, A. Bongain, N. Ciraru-Vigneron, C. Crenn-Hebert, J. F. Delfraissy, C. Rouzioux, M. J. Mayaux, and S. Blanche.** 2001. Lamivudine-zidovudine combination for prevention of maternal-infant transmission of HIV-1. *JAMA* **285:**2083-93.

4704. **Mandell, L. A., J. G. Bartlett, S. F. Dowell, T. M. File, Jr., D. M. Musher, and C. Whitney.** 2003. Update of practice guidelines for the management of community-acquired pneumonia in immunocompetent adults. *Clin Infect Dis* **37:**1405-33.

4705. **Mandell, L. A., T. J. Marrie, R. F. Grossman, A. W. Chow, and R. H. Hyland.** 2000. Canadian guidelines for the initial management of community-acquired pneumonia: an evidence-based update by the Canadian Infectious Diseases Society and the Canadian Thoracic Society. The Canadian Community-Acquired Pneumonia Working Group. *Clin Infect Dis* **31:**383-421.

4706. **Manfredi, R., A. Nanetti, S. Morelli, M. Ferri, R. Valentini, L. Calza, and F. Chiodo.** 2004. A decade surveillance study of Mycobacterium xenopi disease and antimicrobial susceptibility levels in a reference teaching hospital of northern Italy: HIV-associated versus non-HIV-associated infection. *HIV Clin Trials* **5:**206-15.

4707. **Manfredi Selvaggi, T., G. Rezza, M. Scagnelli, R. Rigoli, M. Rassu, F. De Lalla, G. P. Pellizzer, A. Tramarin, C. Bettini, L. Zampieri, M. Belloni, E. D. Pozza, S. Marangon, N. Marchioretto, G. Togni, M. Giacobbo, A. Todescato, and N.

Binkin. 1996. Investigation of a Q-fever outbreak in northern Italy. *Eur J Epidemiol* **12**:403-8.

4708. Mangili, A., and M. A. Gendreau. 2005. Transmission of infectious diseases during commercial air travel. *Lancet* **365**:989-96.

4709. Mangione, E. J., G. Huitt, D. Lenaway, J. Beebe, A. Bailey, M. Figoski, M. P. Rau, K. D. Albrecht, and M. A. Yakrus. 2001. Nontuberculous mycobacterial disease following hot tub exposure. *Emerg Infect Dis* **7**:1039-1042.

4710. Manhart, L. E., C. W. Critchlow, K. K. Holmes, S. M. Dutro, D. A. Eschenbach, C. E. Stevens, and P. A. Totten. 2003. Mucopurulent cervicitis and Mycoplasma genitalium. *J Infect Dis* **187**:650-7.

4711. Mani, G. G., S. T. Rao, and R. Madhavi. 1993. Estimation of hookworm intensity by anthelmintic expulsion in primary schoolchildren in south India. *Trans R Soc Trop Med Hyg* **87**:634-5.

4712. Manian, F. A. 2003. Asymptomatic nasal carriage of mupirocin-resistant, methicillin-resistant Staphylococcus aureus (MRSA) in a pet dog associated with MRSA infection in household contacts. *Clin Infect Dis* **36**:e26-8.

4713. Manjrekar, R. R., S. K. Partridge, A. K. Korman, R. S. Barwick, and D. D. Juranek. 2000. Efficacy of 1% permethrin for the treatment of head louse infestations among Kosovar refugees. *Mil Med* **165**:698-700.

4714. Manjunath, J. V., D. M. Thappa, and T. J. Jaisankar. 2002. Sexually transmitted diseases and sexual lifestyles of long-distance truck drivers: a clinico-epidemiologic study in south India. *Int J STD AIDS* **13**:612-7.

4715. Mann, J., R. Kropp, T. Wong, S. Venne, and B. Romanowski. 2004. Gonorrhea treatment guidelines in Canada: 2004 update. *CMAJ* **171**:1345-6.

4716. Mannelli, A., G. Boggiatto, E. Grego, M. Cinco, R. Murgia, S. Stefanelli, D. De Meneghi, and S. Rosati. 2003. Acarological risk of exposure to agents of tick-borne zoonoses in the first recognized Italian focus of Lyme disease. *Epidemiol Infect* **131**:1139-47.

4717. Manns, A., M. Hisada, and L. La Grenade. 1999. Human T-lymphotropic virus type I infection. *Lancet* **353**:1951-8.

4718. Manns, B. J., B. W. Baylis, S. J. Urbanski, A. P. Gibb, and H. R. Rabin. 1996. Paracoccidioidomycosis: case report and review. *Clin Infect Dis* **23**:1026-32.

4719. Manock, S. R., P. M. Kelley, K. C. Hyams, R. Douce, R. D. Smalligan, D. M. Watts, T. W. Sharp, J. L. Casey, J. L. Gerin, R. Engle, A. Alava-Alprecht, C. M. Martinez, N. B. Bravo, A. G. Guevara, K. L. Russell, W. Mendoza, and C. Vimos. 2000. An outbreak of fulminant hepatitis delta in the Waorani, an indigenous people of the Amazon basin of Ecuador. *Am J Trop Med Hyg* **63**:209-13.

4720. Manoloff, E. S., P. Francioli, P. Taffe, G. Van Melle, J. Bille, and P. M. Hauser. 2003. Risk for Pneumocystis carinii transmission among patients with pneumonia: a molecular epidemiology study. *Emerg Infect Dis* **9**:132-4.

4721. Manor, Y., R. Handsher, T. Halmut, M. Neuman, A. Bobrov, H. Rudich, A. Vonsover, L. Shulman, O. Kew, and E. Mendelson. 1999. Detection of poliovirus circulation by environmental surveillance in the absence of clinical cases in Israel and the Palestinian authority. *J Clin Microbiol* **37**:1670-5.

4722. Mantel, C. F., C. Klose, S. Scheurer, R. Vogel, A. L. Wesirow, and U. Bienzle. 1995. Plasmodium falciparum malaria acquired in Berlin, Germany. *Lancet* **346**:320-1.

4723. Mao, J. S., P. H. Yu, Z. S. Ding, N. L. Chen, B. Z. Huang, R. Y. Xie, and S. A. Chai. 1980. Patterns of shedding of hepatitis A virus antigen in feces and of antibody responses in patients with naturally acquired type A hepatitis. *J Infect Dis* **142**:654-9.

4724. Maqsudur Rahman, K. M. 1983. Rubella epidemic in the Lauder's infant school, St. Vincent - 1983. *Caribbean Epidemiology Centre (CAREC) Surveillance Report* **9**:1-3.

4725. Maragakis, L. L., S. E. Cosgrove, X. Song, D. Kim, P. Rosenbaum, N. Ciesla, A. Srinivasan, T. Ross, K. Carroll, and T. M. Perl. 2004. An outbreak of multidrug-resistant Acinetobacter baumannii associated with pulsatile lavage wound treatment. *JAMA* **292**:3006-11.

4726. Maraha, B., B. H., H. van Hooff, H. Fiolet, A. G. Buiting, and E. E. Stobberingh. 2001. Infectious complications and antibiotic use in renal transplant recipients during a 1-year follow-up. *Clin Microbiol Infect* **7**:616-625.

4727. Marangi, M., B. Zechini, A. Fileti, G. Quaranta, and A. Aceti. 2003. Hymenolepis diminuta infection in a child living in the urban area of Rome, Italy. *J Clin Microbiol* **41**:3994-5.

4728. Maravi-Poma, E., J. L. Rodriguez-Tudela, J. G. De Jalon, A. Manrique-Larralde, L. Torroba, J. Urtasun, B. Salvador, M. Montes, E. Mellado, F. Rodriguez-Albarran, and A. Pueyo-Royo. 2004. Outbreak of gastric mucormycosis associated with the use of wooden tongue depressors in critically ill patients. *Intensive Care Med* **30**:724-8.

4729. Marchisio, P., S. Esposito, G. C. Schito, A. Marchese, R. Cavagna, and N. Principi. 2002. Nasopharyngeal Carriage of Streptococcus pneumoniae in Healthy Children: Implications for the Use of Heptavalent Pneumococcal Conjugate Vaccine. *Emerg Infect Dis* **8**:479-84.

4730. Marchisio, P., S. Gironi, S. Esposito, G. C. Schito, S. Mannelli, and N. Principi. 2001. Seasonal variations in nasopharyngeal carriage of respiratory pathogens in healthy Italian children attending day-care centres or schools. *J Med Microbiol* **50**:1095-9.

4731. Marcolini, J. A., S. Malik, D. Suki, E. Whimbey, and G. P. Bodey. 2003. Respiratory disease due to parainfluenza virus in adult leukemia patients. *Eur J Clin Microbiol Infect Dis* **22**:79-84.

4732. Marcus, U., P. Zucs, V. Bremer, O. Hamouda, R. Prager, H. Tschaepe, U. Futh, and M. Kramer. 2004. Shigellosis - a re-emerging sexually transmitted infection: outbreak in men having sex with men in Berlin. *Int J STD AIDS* **15**:533-7.

4733. Marcuse, E. K., and M. G. Grand. 1973. Epidemiology of diphtheria in San Antonio, Tex, 1970. *JAMA* **224**:305-10.

4734. Mardh, P. A., M. Arvidson, and D. Hellberg. 1996. Sexually Transmitted Diseases and Reproductive History in Women with Experience of Casual Travel Sex Abroad. *J Travel Med* **3**:138-142.

4735. Mardo, D., R. A. Christensen, N. Nielson, S. Hutt, R. Hyun, J. Shaffer, A. V. Gundlapalli, C. Barton, G. Dowdle, S. Mottice, C. Brokopp, R. Rolfs, and D. Panebaker. 2001. Coccidioidomycosis in workers at an archeologic site - Dinosaur National Monument, Utah, June-July, 2001. *MMWR* **50**:1005-1008.

4736. Marfin, A. A., J. Moore, C. Collins, R. Biellik, U. Kattel, M. J. Toole, and P. S. Moore. 1994. Infectious disease surveillance during emergency releif to Bhutanese refugees in Nepal. *JAMA* **272**:377-81.

4737. Margono, S. S., A. Ito, M. O. Sato, M. Okamoto, R. Subahar, H. Yamasaki, A. Hamid, T. Wandra, W. H. Purba, K. Nakaya,

M. Ito, P. S. Craig, and T. Suroso. 2003. Taenia solium taeniasis/cysticercosis in Papua, Indonesia in 2001: detection of human worm carriers. *J Helminthol* **77**:39-42.

4738. Marie, J., H. Morvan, F. Berthelot-Herault, P. Sanders, I. Kempf, A. V. Gautier-Bouchardon, E. Jouy, and M. Kobisch. 2002. Antimicrobial susceptibility of Streptococcus suis isolated from swine in France and from humans in different countries between 1996 and 2000. *J Antimicrob Chemother* **50**:201-9.

4739. Marinella, M. A., C. Pierson, and C. Chenoweth. 1997. The stethoscope. A potential source of nosocomial infection? *Arch Intern Med* **157**:786-90.

4740. Mariner, J. C., J. Morrill, and T. G. Ksiazek. 1995. Antibodies to hemorrhagic fever viruses in domestic livestock in Niger: Rift Valley fever and Crimean-Congo hemorrhagic fever. *Am J Trop Med Hyg* **53**:217-21.

4741. Markel, S. F., P. T. LoVerde, and E. M. Britt. 1978. Prolonged latent schistosomiasis. *JAMA* **240**:1746-7.

4742. Markell, E. K., R. F. Havens, R. A. Kuritsubo, and J. Wingerd. 1984. Intestinal protozoa in homosexual men of the San Francisco Bay area: prevalence and correlates of infection. *Am J Trop Med Hyg* **33**:239-45.

4743. Marks, J. S., M. K. Serdula, N. A. Halsey, M. V. Gunaratne, R. B. Craven, K. A. Murphy, G. Y. Kobayashi, and N. H. Wiebenga. 1981. Saturday night fever: a common-source outbreak of rubella among adults in Hawaii. *Am J Epidemiol* **114**:574-83.

4744. Marks, P. J., I. B. Vipond, D. Carlisle, D. Deakin, R. E. Fey, and E. O. Caul. 2000. Evidence for airborne transmission of Norwalk-like virus (NLV) in a hotel restaurant. *Epidemiol Infect* **124**:481-7.

4745. Marnell, F., A. Guillet, and C. Holland. 1992. A survey of the intestinal helminths of refugees in Juba, Sudan. *Ann Trop Med Parasitol* **86**:387-93.

4746. Marquez, F. J., M. A. Muniain, J. M. Perez, and J. Pachon. 2002. Presence of Rickettsia felis in the cat flea from southwestern Europe. *Emerg Infect Dis* **8**:89-91.

4747. Marquino, W., J. R. MacArthur, L. M. Barat, F. E. Oblitas, M. Arrunategui, G. Garavito, M. L. Chafloque, B. Pardave, S. Gutierrez, N. Arrospide, C. Carrillo, C. Cabezas, and T. K. Ruebush, 2nd. 2003. Efficacy of chloroquine, sulfadoxine-pyrimethamine, and mefloquine for the treatment of uncomplicated Plasmodium falciparum malaria on the north coast of Peru. *Am J Trop Med Hyg* **68**:120-3.

4748. Marr, J. S. 1999. Typhoid Mary. *Lancet* **353**:1714.

4749. Marr, K. A., R. A. Carter, F. Crippa, A. Wald, and L. Corey. 2002. Epidemiology and outcome of mould infections in hematopoietic stem cell transplant recipients. *Clin Infect Dis* **34**:909-17.

4750. Marrama, L., R. Jambou, I. Rakotoarivony, J. M. Leong Pock Tsi, J. B. Duchemin, S. Laventure, J. Mouchet, and J. Roux. 2004. Malaria transmission in Southern Madagascar: influence of the environment and hydro-agricultural works in sub-arid and humid regions. Part 1. Entomological investigations. *Acta Trop* **89**:193-203.

4751. Marras, T. K., and C. L. Daley. 2002. Epidemiology of human pulmonary infection with nontuberculous mycobacteria. *Clin Chest Med* **23**:553-67.

4752. Marrazzo, J. M., L. A. Koutsky, D. A. Eschenbach, K. Agnew, K. Stine, and S. L. Hillier. 2002. Characterization of vaginal flora and bacterial vaginosis in women who have sex with women. *J Infect Dis* **185**:1307-13.

4753. Marrazzo, J. M., K. Stine, and L. A. Koutsky. 2000. Genital human papillomavirus infection in women who have sex with women: a review. *Am J Obstet Gynecol* **183**:770-4.

4754. Marrie, T. J. 1998. Community-acquired pneumonia: epidemiology, etiology, treatment. *Infect Dis Clin N Am* **12**:723-40.

4755. Marrie, T. J., D. Langille, V. Papukna, and L. Yates. 1989. Truckin' pneumonia - an outbreak of Q fever in a truck repair plant probably due to aerosols from clothing contaminated by contact with newborn kittens. *Epidemiol Infect* **102**:119-127.

4756. Marrie, T. J., S. H. Lee, R. S. Faulkner, J. Ethier, and C. H. Young. 1982. Rotavirus infection in a geriatric population. *Arch Intern Med* **142**:313-6.

4757. Marrie, T. J., A. MacDonald, H. Durant, L. Yates, and L. McCormick. 1988. An outbreak of Q fever probably due to contact with a parturient cat. *Chest* **93**:98-103.

4758. Marrie, T. J., H. Major, M. Gurwith, A. R. Ronald, G. K. Harding, G. Forrest, and W. Forsythe. 1978. Prolonged outbreak of nosocomial urinary tract infection with a single strain of Pseudomonas aeruginosa. *Can Med Assoc J* **119**:593-6.

4759. Marrie, T. J., and M. F. Saron. 1998. Seroprevalence of lymphocytic choriomeningitis virus in Nova Scotia. *Am J Trop Med Hyg* **58**:47-9.

4760. Marrie, T. J., W. F. Schlech, 3rd, J. C. Williams, and L. Yates. 1986. Q fever pneumonia associated with exposure to wild rabbits. *Lancet* **1**:427-9.

4761. Marschang, A., H. D. Nothdurft, S. Kumlien, and F. von Sonnenburg. 1995. Imported rickettsioses in German travelers. *Infection* **23**:94-7.

4762. Marsden, A. G. 2003. Influenza outbreak related to air travel. *Med J Aust* **179**:172-3.

4763. Marsh, R. F., and W. J. Hadlow. 1992. Transmissible mink encephalopathy. *Rev Sci Tech* **11**:539-50.

4764. Marshall, J. A., M. E. Hellard, M. I. Sinclair, C. K. Fairley, B. J. Cox, M. G. Catton, H. Kelly, and P. J. Wright. 2004. Failure to detect norovirus in a large group of asymptomatic individuals. *Public Health* **118**:230-3.

4765. Marshall, J. A., L. K. Yuen, M. G. Catton, I. C. Gunesekere, P. J. Wright, K. A. Bettelheim, J. M. Griffith, D. Lightfoot, G. G. Hogg, J. Gregory, R. Wilby, and J. Gaston. 2001. Multiple outbreaks of Norwalk-like virus gastro-enteritis associated with a Mediterranean-style restaurant. *J Med Microbiol* **50**:143-51.

4766. Marshall, R., L. Barkess-Jones, and S. Sivayoham. 1995. An outbreak of scabies in a school for children with learning disabilities. *Commun Dis Rep CDR Rev* **5**:R90-2.

4767. Marshall, T. M., D. Hlatswayo, and B. Schoub. 2003. Nosocomial outbreaks-a potential threat to the elimination of measles? *J Infect Dis* **187**:S97-S101.

4768. Marston, B. J., M. O. Diallo, C. R. Horsburgh, I. Diomande, M. Z. Saki, J. M. Kanga, G. Patrice, H. B. Lipman, S. M. Ostroff, and R. C. Good. 1995. Emergence of Buruli ulcer disease in the Daloa region of Cote d'Ivoire. *Am J Trop Med Hyg* **52**:219-24.

4769. Martens, H. 2000. [Serologic study of the prevalence and course of Hantavirus infections in Mecklenburg-Vorpommern]. *Gesundheitswesen* **62**:71-7.

4770. **Martin, G., and D. Schimmel.** 2000. [Mycobacterium avium infections in poultry—a risk for human health or not?]. *Dtsch Tierarztl Wochenschr* **107:**53-8.

4771. **Martin, G. S., D. M. Mannino, S. Eaton, and M. Moss.** 2003. The epidemiology of sepsis in the United States from 1979 through 2000. *N Engl J Med* **348:**1546-54.

4772. **Martin, J. M., M. Green, K. A. Barbadora, and E. R. Wald.** 2002. Erythromycin-resistant group S streptococci in schoolchildren in Pittsburgh. *N Engl J Med* **346:**1200-6.

4773. **Martin, J. M., M. Green, K. A. Barbadora, and E. R. Wald.** 2004. Group A streptococci among school-aged children: clinical characteristics and the carrier state. *Pediatrics* **114:**1212-9.

4774. **Martin, M., J. H. Turco, M. E. Zegans, R. R. Facklam, S. Sodha, J. A. Elliott, J. H. Pryor, B. Beall, D. D. Erdman, Y. Y. Baumgartner, P. A. Sanchez, J. D. Schwartzman, J. Montero, A. Schuchat, and C. G. Whitney.** 2003. An outbreak of conjunctivitis due to atypical Streptococcus pneumoniae. *N Engl J Med* **348:**1112-21.

4775. **Martin, T., G. F. Kasian, and S. Stead.** 1982. Family outbreak of yersiniosis. *J Clin Microbiol* **16:**622-6.

4776. **Martin, V., J. A. Cayla, A. Bolea, and J. A. de Paz.** 1998. [Evolution of the prevalence of Mycobacterium tuberculosis infection in a penitentiary population on admission to prison from 1991 to 1996]. *Med Clin (Barc)* **111:**11-6.

4777. **Martinez, A. J., and G. S. Visvesvara.** 1997. Free-living, amphizoic and opportunistic amebas. *Brain Pathol* **7:**583-98.

4778. **Martinez, G., J. Harel, R. Higgins, S. Lacouture, D. Daignault, and M. Gottschalk.** 2000. Characterization of Streptococcus agalactiae isolates of bovine and human origin by randomly amplified polymorphic DNA analysis. *J Clin Microbiol* **38:**71-8.

4779. **Martinez-Campillo, F., J. Lopez, M. Verdu, M. Andreu, and M. V. Rigo.** 2002. [Parvovirus B19 outbreak in a rural community in Alicante]. *Enferm Infecc Microbiol Clin* **20:**376-9.

4780. **Martini, G. A.** 1973. Marburg virus disease. *Postgrad Med J* **49:**542-6.

4781. **Martini, G. A., H. G. Knauff, H. A. Schmidt, G. Mayer, and G. Baltzer.** 1968. [On the hitherto unknown, in monkeys originating infectious disease: Marburg virus disease]. *Dtsch Med Wochenschr* **93:**559-71.

4782. **Martins, D. F., Jr., and M. L. Barreto.** 2003. [Macro-epidemiologic aspects of schistosomiasis mansoni: analysis of the impacts of irrigation systems on the spatial profile of the endemic in Bahia, Brazil]. *Cad Saude Publica* **19:**383-93.

4783. **Martins, R., O. Ciquini Junior, H. Matushita, N. D. Cabral, and J. P. Plese.** 1997. [Infections of cerebrospinal fluid shunts in children. Review of 100 infections in 87 children]. *Arq Neuropsiquiatr* **55:**75-81.

4784. **Martins, R. M. B., S. O. B. Porto, B. O. M. Vanderborght, C. D. Rouzere, D. A. O. Queiroz, D. D. Cardoso, and C. F. Yoshida.** 1995. Short report: prevalence of hepatitis C viral antibody among Brazilian children, adolescents, and street youths. *Am J Trop Med Hyg* **53:**654-5.

4785. **Martinson, F. E. A., K. A. Weigle, R. A. Royce, D. J. Weber, C. M. Suchindran, and S. M. Lemon.** 1998. Risk factors for horizontal transmission of hepatitis B virus in a rural district in Ghana. *Am J Epidemiol* **147:**478-87.

4786. **Martiquet, P.** 1989. Two institutional outbreaks of Norwalk-like gastroenteritis - Ontario. *Can Dis Weekly Rep* **15:**113-116.

4787. **Martone, W. J., L. W. Marshall, A. F. Kaufmann, J. H. Hobbs, and M. E. Levy.** 1979. Tularemia pneumonia in Washington, DC. A report of three cases with possible common-source exposures. *JAMA* **242:**2315-7.

4788. **Martone, W. J., and R. L. Nichols.** 2001. Recognition, prevention, surveillance, and management of surgical site infections: introduction to the problem and symposium overview. *Clin Infect Dis* **33 Suppl 2:**S67-8.

4789. **Marty, P., Y. Le Fichoux, M. A. Izri, M. Mora, B. Mathieu, and P. Vessaud.** 1992. Autochtonous Plasmodium falciparum malaria in southern France. *Trans R Soc Trop Med Hyg* **86:**478.

4790. **Maruyama, S., H. Kabeya, R. Nakao, S. Tanaka, T. Sakai, X. Xuan, Y. Katsube, and T. Mikami.** 2003. Seroprevalence of Bartonella henselae, Toxoplasma gondii, FIV and FeLV infections in domestic cats in Japan. *Microbiol Immunol* **47:**147-53.

4791. **Marzochi, M. C. A., K. B. F. Marzochi, and R. W. Carvalho.** 1994. Visceral leishmaniasis in Rio de Janeiro. *Parasitol Today* **10:**37-40.

4792. **Mas-Coma, M. S., J. G. Esteban, and M. D. Bargues.** 1999. Epidemiology of human fascioliasis: a review and proposed new classification. *Bull WHO* **77:**340-6.

4793. **Mas-Coma, S., R. Angles, J. G. Esteban, M. D. Bargues, P. Buchon, M. Franken, and W. Strauss.** 1999. The Northern Bolivian Altiplano: a region highly endemic for human fascioliasis. *Trop Med Int Health* **4:**454-67.

4794. **Mascher, F., F. F. Reinthaler, W. Sixl, G. Schuhmann, and U. Enayat.** 1989. Aeromonas spp. aus Trinkwasser und Stuhlproben in Südindien: Isolierung, Charakterisierung und Toxinnachweis. *Mitt Österr Ges Tropenmed Parasitol* **11:**189-96.

4795. **Maschmann, J., K. Hamprecht, K. Dietz, G. Jahn, and C. P. Speer.** 2001. Cytomegalovirus infection of extremely low-birth weight infants via breast milk. *Clin Infect Dis* **33:**1998-2003.

4796. **Mashek, H., B. Licznerski, and S. Pincus.** 1997. Tungiasis in New York. *Int J Dermatol* **36:**276-8.

4797. **Masia Canuto, M., F. Gutierrez Rodero, V. Ortiz de la Tabla Ducasse, I. Hernandez Aguado, C. Martin Gonzalez, A. Sanchez Sevillano, and A. Martin Hidalgo.** 2000. Determinants for the development of oropharyngeal colonization or infection by fluconazole-resistant Candida strains in HIV-infected patients. *Eur J Clin Microbiol Infect Dis* **19:**593-601.

4798. **Maskell, N. A., D. J. Waine, A. Lindley, J. C. Pepperell, A. E. Wakefield, R. F. Miller, and R. J. Davies.** 2003. Asymptomatic carriage of Pneumocystis jiroveci in subjects undergoing bronchoscopy: a prospective study. *Thorax* **58:**594-7.

4799. **Maslow, J. N., B. Lee, and E. Lautenbach.** 2005. Fluoroquinolone-resistant Escherichia coli carriage in long-term care facility. *Emerg Infect Dis* **11:**889-94.

4800. **Mason, B. W., N. Williams, R. L. Salmon, A. Lewis, J. Price, K. M. Johnston, and R. M. Trott.** 2001. Outbreak of Salmonella indiana associated with egg mayonnaise sandwiches at an acute NHS hospital. *Commun Dis Public Health* **4:**300-4.

4801. **Mason, J., and P. Cavalie.** 1965. Malaria epidemic in Haiti following a hurricane. *Am J Trop Med Hyg* **1965:**533-539.

4802. **Mason, P. R., L. Gwanzura, S. Gregson, and D. a. Katzenstein.** 2000. Chlamydia trachomatis in symptomatic and asymptomatic men: detection in urine by enzyme immunoassay. *Cent Afr J Med* **46:**62-5.

4803. **Mason, P. R., and B. A. Patterson.** 1987. Epidemiology of Giardia lamblia infection in children: cross-sectional and longitudinal studies in urban and rural communities in Zimbabwe. *Am J Trop Med Hyg* **37:**277-82.

4804. **Mason, P. R., and B. A. Patterson.** 1994. Epidemiology of Hymenolepis nana infections in primary school children in urban and rural communities in Zimbabwe. *J Parasitol* **80:**245-50.

4805. **Mason, W. H., L. A. Ross, J. Lanson, and H. T. Wright, Jr.** 1993. Epidemic measles in the postvaccine era: evaluation of epidemiology, clinical presentation and complications during an urban outbreak. *Pediatr Infect Dis J* **12:**42-8.

4806. **Masoodi, M., and K. Hosseini.** 2003. The respiratory and allergic manifestations of human myiasis caused by larvae of the sheep boot fly (Oestrus ovis): a report of 33 pharyngeal cases from southern Iran. *Ann Trop Med Parasitol* **97:**75-81.

4807. **Massa, S., D. Cesaroni, G. Poda, and L. D. Trovatelli.** 1988. Isolation of Yersinia enterocolitica and related species from river water. *Zentralbl Mikrobiol* **143:**575-81.

4808. **Massad, E., M. Rozman, R. S. Azevedo, A. S. B. Silveira, K. Takey, Y. I. Yamamoto, L. Strazza, M. M. Ferreira, and M. N. Burattini.** 1999. Seroprevalence of HIV, HCV and syphilis in Brazilian prisoners: preponderance of parenteral transmission. *Eur J Epidemiol* **15:**439-45.

4809. **Massara, C. L., S. V. Peixoto, S. Barros Hda, M. J. Enk, S. Carvalho Odos, and V. Schall.** 2004. Factors associated with schistosomiasis mansoni in a population from the municipality of Jaboticatubas, State of Minas Gerais, Brazil. *Mem Inst Oswaldo Cruz* **99 suppl 1:**127-34.

4810. **Massel, B. F.** 1997. Rheumatic fever and streptococcal infection. Unraveling the mysteries of a dread disease. Harvard University Press, Boston.

4811. **Massoudi, M. S., B. P. Bell, V. Paredes, J. Insko, K. Evans, and C. N. Shapiro.** 1999. An outbreak of hepatitis A associated with an infected foodhandler. *Public Health Rep* **114:**157-64.

4812. **Massung, R. F., L. E. Davis, K. Slater, D. B. McKechnie, and M. Puerzer.** 2001. Epidemic typhus meningitis in the southwestern United States. *Clin Infect Dis* **32:**979-82.

4813. **Mastella, G., M. Rainisio, H. K. Harms, M. E. Hodson, C. Koch, J. Navarro, B. Strandvik, and S. G. McKenzie.** 2000. Allergic bronchopulmonary aspergillosis in cystic fibrosis. A European epidemiological study. Epidemiologic Registry of Cystic Fibrosis. *Eur Respir J* **16:**464-71.

4814. **Mastro, T. D., B. S. Fields, R. F. Breiman, J. Campbell, B. D. Plikaytis, and J. S. Spika.** 1991. Nosocomial Legionnaires' disease and use of medication nebulizers. *J Infect Dis* **163:**667-71.

4815. **Mastro, T. D., S. C. Redd, and R. F. Breiman.** 1992. Imported leprosy in the United States, 1978 through 1988: an epidemic without secondary transmission. *Am J Public Health* **82:**1127-30.

4816. **Masuko, K., T. Mitsui, K. Iwano, C. Yamazaki, K. Okuda, T. Meguro, N. Murayama, T. Inoue, F. Tsuda, H. Okamoto, Y. Miyakawa, and M. Mayumi.** 1996. Infection with hepatitis GB virus C in patients on maintenance hemodialysis. *N Engl J Med* **334:**1485-90.

4817. **Masuzawa, T.** 2004. Terrestrial distribution of the Lyme borreliosis agent Borrelia burgdorferi sensu lato in East Asia. *Jpn J Infect Dis* **57:**229-35.

4818. **Mathai, D., R. N. Jones, and M. A. Pfaller.** 2001. Epidemiology and frequency of resistance among pathogens causing urinary tract infections in 1,510 hospitalized patients: a report from the SENTRY Antimicrobial Surveillance Program (North America). *Diagn Microbiol Infect Dis* **40:**129-36.

4819. **Mathema, B., E. Cross, E. Dun, S. Park, J. Bedell, B. Slade, M. Williams, L. Riley, V. Chaturvedi, and D. S. Perlin.** 2001. Prevalence of vaginal colonization by drug-resistant candida species in college-age women with previous exposure to over-the-counter azole antifungals. *Clin Infect Dis* **33:**E23-7.

4820. **Mathieu, E., D. A. Levy, F. Veverka, M. K. Parrish, J. Sarisky, N. Shapiro, S. Johnston, T. Handzel, A. Hightower, L. Xiao, Y. M. Lee, S. York, M. Arrowood, R. Lee, and J. L. Jones.** 2004. Epidemiologic and environmental investigation of a recreational water outbreak caused by two genotypes of Cryptosporidium parvum in Ohio in 2000. *Am J Trop Med Hyg* **71:**582-9.

4821. **Mathiot, C. C., G. Grimaud, P. Garry, J. C. Bouquety, A. Mada, A. M. Daguisy, and A. J. Georges.** 1990. An outbreak of human Semliki Forest virus infections in Central African Republic. *Am J Trop Med Hyg* **42:**386-93.

4822. **Matlow, A. G., A. Harrison, A. Monteath, P. Roach, and J. W. Balfe.** 2000. Nosocomial transmission of tuberculosis (TB) associated with care of an infant with peritoneal TB. *Infect Control Hosp Epidemiol* **21:**222-3.

4823. **Matricardi, P. M., R. D'Amelio, R. Biselli, M. Rapicetta, A. Napoli, P. Chionne, and T. Stroffolini.** 1994. Incidence of hepatitis A virus infection among an Italian military population. *Infection* **22:**51-2.

4824. **Matrician, L., G. Ange, S. Burns, W. L. Fanning, C. Kioski, G. D. Cage, and K. K. Komatsu.** 2000. Outbreak of nosocomial Burkholderia cepacia infection and colonization associated with intrinsically contaminated mouthwash. *Infect Control Hosp Epidemiol* **21:**739-41.

4825. **Matsaniotis, N. S., V. P. Syriopoulou, M. C. Theodoridou, K. G. Tzanetou, and G. I. Mostrou.** 1984. Enterobacter sepsis in infants and children due to contaminated intravenous fluids. *Infect Control* **5:**471-7.

4826. **Matson, D. O., C. Byington, M. Canfield, P. Albrecht, and R. D. Feigin.** 1993. Investigation of a measles outbreak in a fully vaccinated school population including serum studies before and after revaccination. *Pediatr Infect Dis J* **12:**292-9.

4827. **Matsui, T., M. H. Kramer, J. M. Mendlein, K. Osaka, T. Ohyama, H. Takahashi, T. Ono, and N. Okabe.** 2002. Evaluation of National Tsutsugamushi Disease Surveillance—Japan, 2000. *Jpn J Infect Dis* **55:**197-203.

4828. **Matsui, T., S. Suzuki, H. Takahashi, T. Ohyama, J. Kobayashi, H. Izumiya, H. Watanabe, F. Kasuga, H. Kijima, K. Shibata, and N. Okabe.** 2004. Salmonella Enteritidis outbreak associated with a school-lunch dessert: cross-contamination and a long incubation period, Japan, 2001. *Epidemiol Infect* **132:**873-9.

4829. **Matsumoto, C., J. Okuda, M. Ishibashi, M. Iwanaga, P. Garg, T. Rammamurthy, H. C. Wong, A. Depaola, Y. B. Kim, M. J. Albert, and M. Nishibuchi.** 2000. Pandemic spread of an O3:K6 clone of Vibrio parahaemolyticus and emergence of related strains evidenced by arbitrarily primed PCR and toxRS sequence analyses. *J Clin Microbiol* **38:**578-85.

4830. **Matsumoto, J., S. Muth, D. Socheat, and H. Matsuda.** 2002. The first reported cases of canine schistosomiasis mekongi in Cambodia. *Southeast Asian J Trop Med Public Health* **33:**458-61.

4831. **Matsumoto, K., M. Hatano, K. Kobayashi, A. Hasegawa, S. Yamazaki, S. Nakata, S. Chiba, and Y. Kimura.** 1989. An outbreak of gastroenteritis associated with acute rotaviral infection in schoolchildren. *J Infect Dis* **160**:611-5.

4832. **Matsumoto, M., Y. Miwa, H. Matsui, M. Saito, M. Ohta, and Y. Miyazaki.** 1999. An outbreak of pharyngitis caused by food-borne group A Streptococcus. *Jpn J Infect Dis* **52**:127-8.

4833. **Matsumoto, W. K., M. G. Vicente, M. A. Silva, and L. L. de Castro.** 1998. [Epidemiological trends for malaria in the cities of the upper Paraguay River basin, Mato Grosso do Sul, Brazil 1990-1996]. *Cad Saude Publica* **14**:797-802.

4834. **Matsuoka, D. M., S. F. Costa, C. Mangini, G. M. Almeida, C. N. Bento, I. M. Van Der Heijden, R. E. Soares, S. Gobara, L. G. Tavora, and A. S. Levin.** 2004. A nosocomial outbreak of Salmonella enteritidis associated with lyophilized enteral nutrition. *J Hosp Infect* **58**:122-7.

4835. **Matsuoka, M., S. Izumi, T. Budiawan, N. Nakata, and K. Saeki.** 1999. Mycobacterium leprae DNA in daily using water as a possible source of leprosy infection. *Indian J Lepr* **71**:61-7.

4836. **Matteelli, A., and G. Carosi.** 2001. Sexually transmitted diseases in travelers. *Clin Infect Dis* **32**:1063-1067.

4837. **Matteelli, A., F. Castelli, A. Spinetti, F. Bonetti, S. Graifenberghi, and G. Carosi.** 1994. Short report: verruga peruana in an Italian traveler from Peru. *Am J Trop Med Hyg* **50**:143-4.

4838. **Matter, H. C.** 1998. The epidemiology of bite and scratch injuries by vertebrate animals in Switzerland. *Eur J Epidemiol* **14**:483-90.

4839. **Matter, L., P. Hohl, T. Abelin, and K. Schopfer.** 1992. Rötelnepidemiologie in Rekrutenschulen. *Schweiz Med Wochenschr* **122**:1606-13.

4840. **Matthewman, L., P. Kelly, D. Hayter, S. Downie, K. Wray, N. Bryson, A. Rycroft, and D. Raoult.** 1997. Domestic cats as indicators of the presence of spotted fever and typhus group rickettsiae. *Eur J Epidemiol* **13**:109-11.

4841. **Mattick, K. L., and T. J. Donovan.** 1998. The risk to public health of aeromonas in ready-to-eat salad products. *Commun Dis Public Health* **1**:267-70.

4842. **Mattioli, R. C., J. A. Faye, and P. Büscher.** 1999. Susceptibility of N'Dama cattle to experimental challenge and cross-species superchallenges with bloodstream forms of Trypanosoma congolense and T. vivax. *Vet Parasitol* **86**:83-94.

4843. **Matui, T., T. Ono, and Y. Inoue.** 2004. An outbreak of Vibrio vulnificus infection in Kumamoto, Japan, 2001. *Arch Dermatol* **140**:888-9.

4844. **Matuschka, F. R., S. Endepols, D. Richter, A. Ohlenbusch, H. Eiffert, and A. Spielman.** 1996. Risk of urban Lyme disease enhanced by the presence of rats. *J Infect Dis* **174**:1108-11.

4845. **Matuszczyk, I., H. Tarnowska, J. Zabicka, and W. Gut.** 1997. [The outbreak of an epidemic of tick-borne encephalitis in Kielec province induced by milk ingestion]. *Przegl Epidemiol* **51**:381-8.

4846. **Mauclère, P., J.-Y. Le Hesran, R. Mahieux, R. Salla, J. Mfoupouendoun, E. T. Abada, J. Millan, G. de The, and A. Gessain.** 1997. Demographic, ethnic, and geographic differences between human T cell lymphotropic virus (HTLV) type I-seropositive carriers and persons with HTLV-I gag-indeterminate western blots in Central Africa. *J Infect Dis* **176**:505-9.

4847. **Maunula, L., S. Kalso, C. H. Von Bonsdorff, and A. Ponka.** 2004. Wading pool water contaminated with both noroviruses and astroviruses as the source of a gastroenteritis outbreak. *Epidemiol Infect* **132**:737-43.

4848. **Maupin, G. O., D. Fish, J. Zultowsky, E. G. Campos, and J. Piesman.** 1991. Landscape ecology of Lyme disease in a residential area of Westchester county, New York. *Am J Epidemiol* **133**:1105-13.

4849. **Maurer, A. M., and D. Sturchler.** 2000. A waterborne outbreak of small round structured virus, campylobacter and shigella co-infections in La Neuveville, Switzerland, 1998. *Epidemiol Infect* **125**:325-32.

4850. **Maurer, R. L., C. Graeff-Teixeira, J. W. Thome, L. A. Chiaradia, H. Sugaya, and K. Yoshimura.** 2002. Natural infection of Deroceras laeve (Mollusca: Gastropoda) with metastrongylid larvae in a transmission focus of abdominal angiostrongyliasis. *Rev Inst Med Trop Sao Paulo* **44**:53-4.

4851. **Maurin, M., and D. Raoult.** 1996. Bartonella (Rochalimaea) quintana infections. *Clin Microbiol Rev* **9**:273-92.

4852. **Maurin, M., and D. Raoult.** 1999. Q fever. *Clin Microbiol Rev* **12**:518-53.

4853. **Mäusezahl, D., F. Cheng, S. Q. Zhang, and M. Tanner.** 1996. Hepatitis A in a Chinese urban population: the spectrum of social and behavioural risk factors. *Int J Epidemiol* **25**:1271-9.

4854. **Mayer, H. O., D. Stunzner, H. M. Grubbauer, C. Faschinger, E. Wocheslander, and M. Moser.** 1986. [Follow-up of children after toxoplasmosis infection in pregnancy]. *Zentralbl Gynakol* **108**:1482-6.

4855. **Mayer, J., S. Wever, C. Lurz, and E. B. Brocker.** 2000. [Scabies epidemic in a sheltered workshop—what should be done?]. *Hautarzt* **51**:75-8.

4856. **Mayfield, J. L., T. Leet, J. Miller, and L. M. Mundy.** 2000. Environmental control to reduce transmission of Clostridium difficile. *Clin Infect Dis* **31**:995-1000.

4857. **Mayhall, C. G.** 2003. The epidemiology of burn wound infections: then and now. *Clin Infect Dis* **37**:543-50.

4858. **Mayo, D., N. Karabatsos, F. J. Scarano, T. Brennan, D. Buck, T. Fiorentino, J. Mennone, and S. Tran.** 2001. Jamestown Canyon virus: seroprevalence in Connecticut. *Emerg Infect Dis* **7**:911-2.

4859. **Mays, E. E., and E. A. Ricketts.** 1975. Melioidosis: recrudescence associated with bronchogenic carcinoma twenty-six years following initial geographic exposure. *Chest* **68**:261-3.

4860. **Mazick, A., M. Howitz, S. Rex, I. Jensen, N. Weis, T. Katzenstein, J. Haff, and K. Molbak.** 2005. Hepatitis A outbreak among MSM linked to casual sex and gay saunas in Copenhagen, Denmark. *Eurosurveillance* **10**:111-4.

4861. **Mazyad, S. A., and S. A. Khalaf.** 2002. Studies on theileria and babesia infecting live and slaughtered animals in Al Arish and El Hasanah, North Sinai Governorate, Egypt. *J Egypt Soc Parasitol* **32**:601-10.

4862. **Mazza, C., A. Ravaggi, A. Rodella, D. Padula, M. Duse, M. Lomini, M. Puoti, A. Rossini, and E. Cariani.** 1998. Prospective study of mother-to-infant transmission of hepatitis C virus (HCV) infection. Study Group for Vertical Transmission. *J Med Virol* **54**:12-9.

4863. **Mbulamberi, D. B.** 1989. Possible causes leading to an epidemic outbreak of sleeping sickness: facts and hypotheses. *Ann Soc Belg Med Trop* **69 Suppl 1**:173-9; discussion 212-4.

4864. **McAnulty, J. M., D. W. Fleming, and A. H. Gonzalez.** 1994. A community-wide outbreak of cryptosporidiosis associated with swimming at a wave pool. *JAMA* **272**:1597-600.

4865. **McAulay, J. B., M. K. Michelson, A. W. Hightower, S. Engeran, L. A. Wintermeyer, and P. M. Schantz.** 1992. A trichinosis outbreak among Southeast Asian refugees. *Am J Epidemiol* **135**:1404-10.

4866. McAuley, J. B., M. K. Michelson, and P. M. Schantz. 1991. Trichinella infection in travelers. *J Infect Dis* **164**:1013-6.

4867. McBean, M., and S. RaJAMAni. 2001. Increasing rates of hospitalization due to septicemia in the US elderly population, 1986-1997. *J Infect Dis* **183**:596-603.

4868. McBride, W. J., C. T. Taylor, J. A. Pryor, and J. D. Simpson. 1999. Scrub typhus in north Queensland. *Med J Aust* **170**: 318-20.

4869. McBride, W. J. H., H. Mullner, J. T. LaBroody, and J. Wronski. 1998. The 1993 dengue 2 epidemic in north Queensland: a serosurvey and comparison of hemagglutination inhibition with an ELISA. *Am J Trop Med Hyg* **59**:457-461.

4870. McCall, B., R. Stafford, S. Cherian, K. Heel, H. Smith, N. Corones, and S. Gilmore. 2000. An outbreak of multi-resistant Shigella sonnei in a long-stay geriatric nursing centre. *Commun Dis Intell* **24**:272-5.

4871. McCallum, S. J., J. Corkill, M. Gallagher, M. J. Ledson, C. A. Hart, and M. J. Walshaw. 2001. Superinfection with a transmissible strain of Pseudomonas aeruginosa in adults with cystic fibrosis chronically colonised by P aeruginosa. *Lancet* **358**:558-60.

4872. McCarthy, M., M. K. Estes, and K. C. Hyams. 2000. Norwalk-like virus infection in military forces: epidemic potential, sporadic disease, and the future direction of prevention and control efforts. *J Infect Dis* **181 Suppl 2**:S387-91.

4873. McCarthy, M. C., J. He, K. C. Hyams, A. el-Tigani, I. O. Khalid, and M. Carl. 1994. Acute hepatitis E infection during the 1988 floods in Khartoum, Sudan. *Trans R Soc Trop Med Hyg* **88**:177.

4874. McCarthy, S. A., and F. M. Khambaty. 1994. International dissemination of epidemic Vibrio cholerae by cargo ship ballast and other nonpotable waters. *Appl Environ Microbiol* **60**:2597-601.

4875. McCarthy, S. A., R. M. McPhearson, and A. M. Guarino. 1992. Toxigenic Vibrio cholerae O1 and cargo ships entering Gulf of Mexico. *Lancet* **339**:624-5.

4876. McCarthy, V. P., and M. D. Murphy. 1990. Lawnmower tularemia. *Pediatr Infect Dis J* **9**:298-300.

4877. McClelland, G. 2002. The trouble with sealworms (Pseudoterranova decipiens species complex, Nematoda): a review. *Parasitology* **124 supplement**:S183-S203.

4878. McCormick, J. B., P. Hayes, and R. Feldman. 1976. Epidemic streptococcal sore throat following a community picnic. *JAMA* **236**:1039-41.

4879. McCormick, J. B., D. J. Sexton, J. G. McMurray, E. Carey, P. Hayes, and R. A. Feldman. 1975. Human-to-human transmission of Pseudomonas pseudomallei. *Ann Intern Med* **83**:512-3.

4880. McCormick, J. B., P. A. Webb, J. W. Krebs, K. M. Johnson, and E. S. Smith. 1987. A prospective study of the epidemiology and ecology of Lassa fever. *J Infect Dis* **155**:437-44.

4881. McCoy, L., F. Sorvillo, and P. Simon. 2004. Varicella-related mortality in California, 1988-2000. *Pediatr Infect Dis J* **23**:498-503.

4882. McDermott, J. J., and S. M. Arimi. 2002. Brucellosis in sub-Saharan Africa: epidemiology, control and impact. *Vet Microbiol* **90**:111-34.

4883. McDermott, J. M., L. Slutsker, R. W. Steketee, J. J. Wirima, J. G. Breman, and D. L. Heymann. 1996. Prospective assessment of mortality among a cohort of pregnant women in rural Malawi. *Am J Trop Med Hyg* **55(1**:66-70.

4884. McDiarmid, S. V., S. Jordan, G. S. Kim, M. Toyoda, J. A. Goss, J. H. Vargas, M. G. Martin, R. Bahar, A. L. Maxfield, M. E. Ament, R. W. Busuttil, and G. S. Lee. 1998. Prevention and preemptive therapy of postransplant lymphoproliferative disease in pediatric liver recipients. *Transplantation* **66**: 1604-11.

4885. McDonald, J. C., T. W. Gyorkos, B. Alberton, J. D. MacLean, G. Richer, and D. Juranek. 1990. An outbreak of toxoplasmosis in pregnant women in northern Quebec. *J Infect Dis* **161**:769-74.

4886. McDonald, L. C., S. Rossiter, C. Mackinson, Y. Y. Wang, S. Johnson, M. Sullivan, R. Sokolow, E. DeBess, L. Gilbert, J. A. Benson, B. Hill, and F. J. Angulo. 2001. Quinupristin-dalfopristin-resistant Enterococcus faecium on chicken and in human stool specimens. *N Engl J Med* **345**:1155-60.

4887. McDonald, S., D. Cox, R. Allen, W. Staggs, D. Bixler, and G. Steele. 1997. Respiratory diphtheria caused by Corynebacterium ulcerans - Terre Haute, Indiana, 1996. *MMWR* **46**: 330-2.

4888. McDonnell, G., and A. D. Russell. 1999. Antiseptics and disinfectants: activity, action, and resistance. *Clin Microbiol Rev* **12**:147-79.

4889. McDonnell, R. J., P. G. Wall, G. K. Adak, H. S. Evans, J. M. Cowden, and E. O. Caul. 1995. Outbreaks of infectious intestinal disease associated with person to person spread in hotels and restaurants. *Commun Dis Rep CDR Rev* **5**:R150-2.

4890. McEachern, R., and G. D. Campbell. 1998. Hospital-acquired pneumonia: epidemiology, etiology, and treatment. *Inf Dis Clin N Am* **12**:761-79.

4891. McElnay, C., C. Thornley, and R. Armstrong. 2004. A community and workplace outbreak of tuberculosis in Hawke's Bay in 2002. *N Z Med J* **117**:U1019.

4892. McElnea, C. L., and G. M. Cross. 1999. Methods of detection of Chlamydia psittaci in domesticated and wild birds. *Aust Vet J* **77**:516-21.

4893. McElroy, P. D., K. L. Southwick, E. R. Fortenberry, E. C. Levine, L. A. Diem, C. L. Woodley, P. M. Williams, K. D. McCarthy, R. Ridzon, and P. A. Leone. 2003. Outbreak of tuberculosis among homeless persons coinfected with human immunodeficiency virus. *Clin Infect Dis* **36**:1305-12.

4894. McEvoy, M., N. Batchelor, G. Hamilton, A. MacDonald, M. Faiers, A. Sills, J. Lee, and T. Harrison. 2000. A cluster of cases of legionnaires' disease associated with exposure to a spa pool on display. *Commun Dis Public Health* **3**:43-5.

4895. McEvoy, M. B., N. D. Noah, and R. Pilsworth. 1987. Outbreak of fever caused by Streptobacillus moniliformis. *Lancet* **2**:1361-3.

4896. McEwen, S. A., and P. J. Fedorka-Cray. 2002. Antimicrobial use and resistance in animals. *Clin Infect Dis* **34 suppl 3**:S93-106.

4897. McFarland, L. V., M. E. Mulligan, R. Y. Kwok, and W. E. Stamm. 1989. Nosocomial acquisition of Clostridium difficile infection. *N Engl J Med* **320**:204-10.

4898. McGarry, J. W., P. J. McCall, and S. Welby. 2001. Arthropod dermatoses acquired in the UK and overseas. *Lancet* **357**:2105-6.

4899. McGill, S., L. Wesslen, E. Hjelm, M. Holmberg, C. Rolf, and G. Friman. 2001. Serological and epidemiological analysis of the prevalence of Bartonella spp. antibodies in Swedish elite orienteers 1992-93. *Scand J Infect Dis* **33**:423-8.

4900. McGlade, T. R., I. D. Robertson, A. D. Elliot, C. Read, and R. C. Thompson. 2003. Gastrointestinal parasites of domestic cats in Perth, Western Australia. *Vet Parasitol* **117**:251-62.

4901. McGowan, K. L., J. A. Foster, and S. E. Coffin. 2000. Outpatient pediatric blood cultures: time to positivity. *Pediatrics* **106**:251-5.

4902. McGuigan, C. 2005. Cryptosporidium outbreak after a visit to a wildlife centre in northeast Scotland: 62 confirmed cases. *Eurosurveillance* **10**:125.

4903. McHugh, C. P., P. C. Melby, and S. G. LaFon. 1996. Leishmaniasis in Texas: epidemiology and clinical aspects of human cases. *Am J Trop Med Hyg* **55**:547-55.

4904. McIntosh, E. D., M. D. Bek, M. Cardona, K. Goldston, D. Isaacs, M. A. Burgess, and Y. E. Cossart. 1997. Horizontal transmission of hepatitis B in a children's day-care centre: a preventable event. *Aust N Z J Public Health* **21**:791-2.

4905. McIntyre, P. 1997. Epidemiology and prevention of pneumococcal disease. *Commun Dis Intell* **21**:41-6.

4906. McIvor, A., M. Paluzzi, and M. M. Meguid. 1991. Intramuscular injection abscess—past lessons relearned. *N Engl J Med* **324**:1897-8.

4907. McJunkin, J. E., R. R. Khan, and T. F. Tsai. 1998. California-La Crosse encephalitis. *Infect Dis Clin North Am* **12**:83-93.

4908. McKay, L., H. Clery, K. Carrick-Anderson, S. Hollis, and G. Scott. 2003. Genital Chlamydia trachomatis infection in a subgroup of young men in the U.K. *Lancet* **361**:1792.

4909. McKee, K. T., Jr., W. E. Burns, L. K. Russell, P. R. Jenkins, A. E. Johnson, T. L. Wong, and K. B. McLawhorn. 1998. Early syphilis in an active duty military population and the surrounding civilian community, 1985-1993. *Mil Med* **163**:368-76.

4910. McKee, K. T., Jr., P. R. Jenkins, R. Garner, R. A. Jenkins, E. D. Nannis, I. F. Hoffman, J. L. Schmitz, and M. S. Cohen. 2000. Features of urethritis in a cohort of male soldiers. *Clin Infect Dis* **30**:736-41.

4911. McKee, T., L. Davis, P. Blake, L. Kreckman, S. Bialek, M. J. Beach, G. Visvesvara, J. H. Maguire, L. Fox, and J. Amann. 2003. Primary amebic meningoencephalitis - Georgia, 2002. *MMWR* **52**:962-4.

4912. McKelvie, P. 1980. Q fever in a Queensland meatworks. *Med J Aust* **1**:590-3.

4913. McKenzie, F. E., G. M. Jeffery, and W. E. Collins. 2001. Plasmodium malariae blood-stage dynamics. *J Parasitol* **87**:626-37.

4914. McKeown, I., P. Orr, S. Macdonald, A. Kabani, R. Brown, G. Coghlan, M. Dawood, J. Embil, M. Sargent, G. Smart, and C. N. Bernstein. 1999. Helicobacter pylori in the Canadian Arctic: seroprevalence and detection in community water samples. *Am J Gastroenterol* **94**:1823-9.

4915. McLauchlin, J. 1997. Listeria and listeriosis. *Clin Microbiol Infect* **3**:484-92.

4916. McLaughlin, J. B., A. DePaola, C. A. Bopp, K. A. Martinek, N. P. Napolilli, C. G. Allison, S. L. Murray, E. C. Thompson, M. M. Bird, and J. P. Middaugh. 2005. Outbreak of Vibrio parahaemolyticus gastroenteritis associated with Alaskan oysters. *N Engl J Med* **353**:1463-70.

4917. McLaughlin, J. B., B. D. Gessner, and A. M. Bailey. 2005. Gastroenteritis outbreak among mountaineers climbing the West Buttress route of Denali - Denali National Park, Alaska, June 2002. *Wilderness Environ Med* **16**:92-6.

4918. McLaughlin, J. B., B. D. Gessner, T. V. Lynn, E. A. Funk, and J. P. Middaugh. 2004. Association of regulatory issues with an echovirus 18 meningitis outbreak at a children's summer camp in Alaska. *Pediatr Infect Dis J* **23**:875-7.

4919. McLaughlin, S. I., P. Spradling, D. Drociuk, R. Ridzon, C. J. Pozsik, and I. Onorato. 2003. Extensive transmission of Mycobacterium tuberculosis among congregated, HIV-infected prison inmates in south Carolina, United States. *Int J Tuberc Lung Dis* **7**:665-72.

4920. McLean, D. M. 1975. Mosquito-borne arboviruses in arctic America. *Med Biol* **53**:264-70.

4921. McLean, R. G., R. B. Shriner, K. S. Pokorny, and G. S. Bowen. 1989. The ecology of Colorado tick fever in Rocky Mountain National Park in 1974. III. Habitats supporting the virus. *Am J Trop Med Hyg* **40**:86-93.

4922. McLean, R. G., S. R. Ubico, D. Bourne, and N. Komar. 2002. West Nile virus in livestock and wildlife. *Curr Top Microbiol Immunol* **267**:271-308.

4923. McMahon, B. J. 2004. Viral hepatitis in the Arctic. *Int J Circumpolar Health* **63 Suppl 2**:41-8.

4924. McMahon, M. A., and I. G. Wilson. 2001. The occurrence of enteric pathogens and Aeromonas species in organic vegetables. *Int J Food Microbiol* **70**:155-62.

4925. McMichael, A. J., A. Haines, R. Slooff, and S. Kovats. 1996. Climate change and human health. World Health Organization, Geneva.

4926. McMinn, P. C., J. Stewart, and C. J. Burrell. 1991. A community outbreak of epidemic keratoconjunctivitis in central Australia due to adenovirus type 8. *J Infect Dis* **164**:1113-8.

4927. McNeil, M. M., and J. M. Brown. 1994. The medically important aerobic actinomycetes: epidemiology and microbiology. *Clin Microbiol Rev* **7**:357-417.

4928. McNeil, M. M., L. B. Sweat, S. L. Carter, Jr., C. B. Watson, J. T. Holloway, R. Manning, S. F. Altekruse, and P. A. Blake. 1999. A Mexican restaurant-associated outbreak of Salmonella Enteritidis type 34 infections traced to a contaminated egg farm. *Epidemiol Infect* **122**:209-15.

4929. McNeil, S. A., L. Mody, and S. F. Bradley. 2002. Methicillin-resistant Staphylococcus aureus. Management of asymptomatic colonization and outbreaks of infection in long-term care. *Geriatrics* **57**:16-8, 21-4, 27.

4930. McNeill, W. H. 1976. Plagues and peoples. Anchor Press, Garden City, New York.

4931. McQuillan, G. M., D. Kruszon-Moran, A. Deforest, S. Y. Chu, and M. Wharton. 2002. Serologic immunity to diphtheria and tetanus in the United States. *Ann Intern Med* **136**:660-6.

4932. McQuiston, J. H., and J. E. Childs. 2002. Q fever in humans and animals in the United States. *Vector Borne Zoonotic Dis* **2**:179-91.

4933. McQuiston, J. H., J. E. Childs, M. E. Chamberland, and E. Tabor. 2000. Transmission of tick-borne agents of disease by blood transfusion: a review of known and potential risks in the United States. *Transfusion* **40**:274-84.

4934. McVernon, J., A. J. Howard, M. P. Slack, and M. E. Ramsay. 2004. Long-term impact of vaccination on Haemophilus influenzae type b (Hib) carriage in the United Kingdom. *Epidemiol Infect* **132:**765-7.

4935. **McVernon, J., P. Morgan, C. Mallaghan, T. Biswas, M. Natarajan, D. Griffiths, M. Slack, and R. Moxon.** 2004. Outbreak of Haemophilus influenzae type b disease among fully vaccinated children in a day-care center. *Pediatr Infect Dis J* **23:**38-41.

4936. **McVernon, J., C. L. Trotter, M. P. Slack, and M. E. Ramsay.** 2004. Trends in Haemophilus influenzae type b infections in adults in England and Wales: surveillance study. *BMJ* **329:**655-8.

4937. **Mead, J. H., G. P. Lupton, C. L. Dillavou, and R. B. Odom.** 1979. Cutaneous Rhizopus infection. Occurrence as a postoperative complication associated with an elasticized adhesive dressing. *JAMA* **242:**272-4.

4938. **Mead, P. S., L. Finelli, M. A. Lambert-Fair, D. Champ, J. Townes, L. Hutwagner, T. Barrett, K. Spitalny, and E. Mintz.** 1997. Risk factors for sporadic infection with Escherichia coli O157:H7. *Arch Intern Med* **157:**204-8.

4939. **Mead, P. S., L. Slutsker, V. Dietz, L. F. McCaig, J. S. Bresee, C. Shapiro, P. M. Griffin, and R. V. Tauxe.** 1999. Food-related illness and death in the United States. *Emerg Infect Dis* **5:**607-25.

4940. **Meakins, S. M., G. K. Adak, B. A. Lopman, and S. J. O'Brien.** 2003. General outbreaks of infectious intestinal disease (IID) in hospitals, England and Wales, 1992-2000. *J Hosp Infect* **53:**1-5.

4941. **Meals, L. T., and W. P. McKinney.** 1998. Acute pulmonary histoplasmosis: progressive pneumonia resulting from high inoculum exposure. *J KY Med Assoc* **96:**258-60.

4942. **Medema, G., and C. Schets.** 1993. Occurrence of Plesiomonas shigelloides in surface water: relationship with faecal pollution and trophic state. *Zentralbl Hyg Umweltmed* **194:**398-404.

4943. **Medeot, S., S. V. Nates, A. Recalde, S. Gallego, E. Maturano, M. Giordano, H. Serra, J. Reategui, and C. Cabezas.** 1999. Prevalence of antibody to human T cell lymphotropic virus types 1/2 among Aboriginal groups inhabiting northern Argentina and the Amazon region of Peru. *Am J Trop Med Hyg* **60:**623-9.

4944. **Mediannikov, O. Y., Y. Sidelnikov, L. Ivanov, E. Mokretsova, P. E. Fournier, I. Tarasevich, and D. Raoult.** 2004. Acute tick-borne rickettsiosis caused by Rickettsia heilongjiangensis in Russian Far East. *Emerg Infect Dis* **10:**810-7.

4945. **Medrano, F. J., M. Montes-Cano, M. Conde, C. de la Horra, N. Respaldiza, A. Gasch, M. J. Perez-Lozano, J. M. Varela, and E. J. Calderon.** 2005. Pneumocystis jirovecii in general population. *Emerg Infect Dis* **11:**245-50.

4946. **Meehan, P., K. E. Toomey, J. Drinnon, S. Cunningham, N. Anderson, and E. Baker.** 1998. Public health response for the 1996 Olympic Games. *JAMA* **279:**1469-73.

4947. **Meehan, P. J., T. Atkeson, D. E. Kepner, and M. Melton.** 1992. A foodborne outbreak of gastroenteritis involving two different pathogens. *Am J Epidemiol* **136:**611-6.

4948. **Meek, S. R.** 1988. Epidemiology of malaria in displaced Khmers on the Thai-Kampuchean border. *Southeast Asian J Trop Med Public Health* **19:**243-52.

4949. **Meer-Scherrer, L., M. Adelson, E. Mordechai, B. Lottaz, and R. Tilton.** 2004. Babesia microti infection in Europe. *Curr Microbiol* **48:**435-7.

4950. **Meheus, A., and A. De Schryver.** 1991. Sexually transmitted diseases in the third world, p. 201-217. *In* J. R. W. Harris and S. M. Forster (ed.), Recent advances in sexually transmitted diseases and AIDS, vol. 4. Churchill Livingstone, Edinburgh.

4951. **Mehta, S. D., E. J. Erbelding, J. M. Zenilman, and A. M. Rompalo.** 2003. Gonorrhoea reinfection in heterosexual STD clinic attendees: longitudinal analysis of risks for first reinfection. *Sex Transm Infect* **79:**124-8.

4952. **Mehta, S. H., A. Cox, D. R. Hoover, X.-H. Wang, Q. Mao, S. Ray, S. A. Strathdee, D. Vlahov, and D. L. Thomas.** 2002. Protection against persistence of hepatitis C. *Lancet* **359:**1478-83.

4953. **Mehta, S. K., R. J. Cohrs, B. Forghani, G. Zerbe, D. H. Gilden, and D. L. Pierson.** 2004. Stress-induced subclinical reactivation of varicella zoster virus in astronauts. *J Med Virol* **72:**174-9.

4954. **Mehta, S. K., R. P. Stowe, A. H. Feiveson, S. K. Tyring, and D. L. Pierson.** 2000. Reactivation and shedding of cytomegalovirus in astronauts during spaceflight. *J Infect Dis* **182:**1761-4.

4955. **Meier, J., U. Lienicke, E. Tschirch, D. H. Kruger, R. R. Wauer, and S. Prosch.** 2005. Human cytomegalovirus reactivation during lactation and mother-to-child transmission in preterm infants. *J Clin Microbiol* **43:**1318-24.

4956. **Meier, P. A., C. D. Carter, S. E. Wallace, R. J. Hollis, M. A. Pfaller, and L. A. Herwaldt.** 1996. A prolonged outbreak of methicillin-resistant Staphylococcus aureus in the burn unit of a tertiary medical center. *Infect Control Hosp Epidemiol* **17:**798-802.

4957. **Meier, P. A., W. D. Mathers, J. E. Sutphin, R. Folberg, T. Hwang, and R. P. Wenzel.** 1998. An epidemic of presumed Acanthamoeba keratitis that followed regional flooding. Results of a case-control investigation. *Arch Ophthalmol* **116:**1090-4.

4958. **Meiering, C. D., and M. L. Linial.** 2001. Historical perspective of foamy virus epidemiology and infection. *Clin Microbiol Rev* **14:**165-76.

4959. **Meijer, A., A. Brandenburg, J. de Vries, J. Beentjes, P. Roholl, and D. Dercksen.** 2004. Chlamydophila abortus infection in a pregnant woman associated with indirect contact with infected goats. *Eur J Clin Microbiol Infect Dis* **23:**487-90.

4960. **Meijer, A., C. F. Dagnelie, J. C. De Jong, A. De Vries, T. M. Bestebroer, A. M. Van Loon, A. I. Bartelds, and J. M. Ossewaarde.** 2000. Low prevalence of Chlamydia pneumoniae and Mycoplasma pneumoniae among patients with symptoms of respiratory tract infections in Dutch general practices. *Eur J Epidemiol* **16:**1099-106.

4961. **Meiklejohn, G., L. G. Reimer, P. S. Graves, and C. Helmick.** 1981. Cryptic epidemic of Q fever in a medical school. *J Infect Dis* **144:**107-13.

4962. **Meima, A., J. H. Richardus, and J. D. F. Habbema.** 2004. Trends in leprosy case detection worldwide since 1985. *Lepr Rev* **75:**19-33.

4963. **Mein, J. K., C. M. Palmer, M. C. Shand, D. J. Templeton, V. Parekh, M. Mobbs, K. Haig, S. E. Huffam, and L. Young.** 2003. Management of acute adult sexual assault. *Med J Aust* **178:**226-30.

4964. **Meinecke, C. K., J. Schottelius, L. Oskam, and B. Fleischer.** 1999. Congenital transmission of visceral leishmaniasis (Kala Azar) from an asymptomatic mother to her child. *Pediatrics* **104:**e65.

4965. **Meisel, H., A. Reip, B. Faltus, M. Lu, H. Porst, M. Wiese, M. Roggendorf, and D. H. Kruger.** 1995. Transmission of hepatitis C virus to children and husbands by women infected with contaminated anti-D immunoglobulin. *Lancet* **345:**1209-11.

4966. **Mekmullica, J., S. Kritsaneepaiboon, and C. Pancharoen.** 2003. Risk factors for Epstein-Barr virus infection in Thai infants. *Southeast Asian J Trop Med Public Health* **34:**395-7.

4967. **Melby, K., B. Gondrosen, S. Gregusson, H. Ribe, and O. P. Dahl.** 1991. Waterborne campylobacteriosis in northern Norway. *Int J Food Microbiol* **12:**151-6.

4968. **Melby, K. K., J. G. Svendby, T. Eggebo, L. A. Holmen, B. M. Andersen, L. Lind, E. Sjogren, and B. Kaijser.** 2000. Outbreak of Campylobacter infection in a subarctic community. *Eur J Clin Microbiol Infect Dis* **19:**542-4.

4969. **Melbye, M., and R. J. Biggar.** 1994. A profile of HIV-risk behaviours among travellers—a population based study of Danes visiting Greenland. *Scand J Soc Med* **22:**204-8.

4970. **Mele, A., R. Corona, M. E. Tosti, F. Palumbo, A. Moiraghi, F. Novaco, C. Galanti, R. Bernacchia, and P. Ferraro.** 1995. Beauty treatments and risk of parenterally transmitted hepatitis: results from the hepatitis surveillance system in Italy. *Scand J Infect Dis* **27:**441-4.

4971. **Mele, A., P. J. Paterson, H. G. Prentice, P. Leoni, and C. C. Kibbler.** 2002. Toxoplasmosis in bone marrow transplantation: a report of two cases and systematic review of the literature. *Bone Marrow Transplant* **29:**691-8.

4972. **Mele, A., E. Spada, L. Sagliocca, P. Ragni, M. E. Tosti, G. Gallo, A. Moiraghi, E. Balocchini, M. Sangalli, P. L. Lopalco, and T. Stroffoli.** 2001. Risk of parenterally transmitted hepatitis following exposure to surgery or other invasive procedures: results from the hepatitis surveillance system in Italy. *J Hepatol* **35:**284-9.

4973. **Melegaro, A., N. J. Gay, and G. F. Medley.** 2004. Estimating the transmission parameters of pneumococcal carriage in households. *Epidemiol Infect* **132:**433-41.

4974. **Mellinger, A. K., J. D. Cragan, W. L. Atkinson, W. W. Williams, B. Kleger, R. G. Kimber, and D. Tavris.** 1995. High incidence of congenital rubella syndrome after a rubella outbreak. *Pediatr Infect Dis J* **14:**573-8.

4975. **Mellor, P. S., J. Boorman, and M. Baylis.** 2000. Culicoides biting midges: their role as arbovirus vectors. *Annu Rev Entomol* **45:**307-40.

4976. **Melloul, A., O. Amahmid, L. Hassani, and K. Bouhoum.** 2002. Health effect of human wastes use in agriculture in El Azzouzia (the wastewater spreading area of Marrakesh city, Morocco). *Int J Environ Health Res* **12:**17-23.

4977. **Melville, D., and K. Shortridge.** 2004. Influenza: time to come to grips with the avian dimension. *Lancet Infect Dis* **4:**261-262.

4978. **Memish, Z. A., and H. H. Balkhy.** 2004. Brucellosis and international travel. *J Travel Med* **11:**49-55.

4979. **Memon, M. I., and M. A. Memon.** 2002. Hepatitis C: an epidemiological review. *J Viral Hepat* **9:**84-100.

4980. **Mena, L., X. Wang, T. F. Mroczkowski, and D. H. Martin.** 2002. Mycoplasma genitalium infections in asymptomatic men and men with urethritis attending a sexually transmitted diseases clinic in New Orleans. *Clin Infect Dis* **35:**1167-73.

4981. **Ménard, A., G. Dos Santos, P. Dekumyoy, S. Ranque, J. Delmont, M. Danis, F. Bricaire, and E. Caumes.** 2003. Imported cutaneous gnathostomiasis: report of five cases. *Trans R Soc Trop Med Hyg* **97:**200-2.

4982. **Mencarelli, M., A. Zanchi, C. Cellesi, A. Rossolini, R. Rappuoli, and G. M. Rossolini.** 1992. Molecular epidemiology of nasopharyngeal corynebacteria in healthy adults from an area where diphtheria vaccination has been extensively practiced. *Eur J Epidemiol* **8:**560-7.

4983. **Méndez Martínez, C., A. Páez Jiménez, M. Cortés Blanco, E. Salmoral Chamizo, E. Mohedano Mohedano, C. Plata, A. Varo Baena, and F. Martinez Navarro.** 2003. Brucellosis outbreak due to unpasteurized raw goat cheese in Andalucia (Spain), January - March 2002. *Eurosurveillance* **8:**164-8.

4984. **Mendis, K., B. J. Sina, P. Marchesini, and R. Carter.** 2001. The neglected burden of Plasmodium vivax malaria. *Am J Trop Med Hyg* **64:**97-106.

4985. **Meng, X. J., B. Wiseman, F. Elvinger, D. K. Guenette, T. E. Toth, R. E. Engle, S. U. Emerson, and R. H. Purcell.** 2002. Prevalence of antibodies to hepatitis E virus in veterinarians working with swine and in normal blood donors in the United States and other countries. *J Clin Microbiol* **40:**117-22.

4986. **Mensah, P., D. Yeboah-Manu, K. Owusu-Darko, and A. Ablordey.** 2002. Street foods in Accra, Ghana: how safe are they? *Bull WHO* **80:**546-54.

4987. **Mercat, A., J. Nguyen, and B. Dautzenberg.** 1991. An outbreak of pneumococcal pneumonia in two men's shelters. *Chest* **99:**147-51.

4988. **Merchant, J. C., P. J. Kerr, N. G. Simms, and A. J. Robinson.** 2003. Monitoring the spread of myxoma virus in rabbit Oryctolagus cuniculus populations on the southern tablelands of New South Wales, Australia. I. Natural occurrence of myxomatosis. *Epidemiol Infect* **130:**113-21.

4989. **Merien, F., and P. Perolat.** 1996. Public health importance of human leptospirosis in the South Pacific: a five-year study in New Caledonia. *Am J Trop Med Hyg* **55:**174-8.

4990. **Merilahti-Palo, R., R. Lahesmaa, K. Granfors, C. Gripenberg-Lerche, and P. Toivanen.** 1991. Risk of Yersinia infection among butchers. *Scand J Infect Dis* **23:**55-61.

4991. **Merino, F. J., T. Nebreda, J. Luis Serrano, P. Fernandez-Soto, A. Encinas, and R. Perez-Sanchez.** 2005. Tick species and tick-borne infections identified in population from a rural area of Spain. *Epidemiol Infect* **133:**943-9.

4992. **Merle, V., J. M. Germain, H. Bugel, M. Nouvellon, J. F. Lemeland, P. Czernichow, and P. Grise.** 2002. Nosocomial urinary tract infections in urologic patients: assessment of a prospective surveillance program including 10,000 patients. *Eur Urol* **41:**483-9.

4993. **Mermel, L. A., B. M. Farr, R. J. Sherertz, Raad, II, N. O'Grady, J. S. Harris, and D. E. Craven.** 2001. Guidelines for the management of intravascular catheter-related infections. *Clin Infect Dis* **32:**1249-72.

4994. **Mermel, L. A., S. L. Josephson, J. Dempsey, S. Parenteau, C. Perry, and N. Magill.** 1997. Outbreak of Shigella sonnei in a clinical microbiology laboratory. *J Clin Microbiol* **35:**3163-5.

4995. **Mermin, J., L. Hutwagner, D. Vugia, S. Shallow, P. Daily, J. Bender, J. Koehler, R. Marcus, and F. J. Angulo.** 2004. Reptiles, amphibians, and human salmonella infection: a population-based, case-control study. *Clin Infect Dis* **38 Suppl 3:**S253-61.

4996. **Mermin, J. H., J. M. Townes, M. Gerber, N. Dolan, E. D. Mintz, and R. V. Tauxe.** 1998. Typhoid fever in the United

States, 1985-1994: changing risks of international travel and increasing antimicrobial resistance. *Arch Intern Med* **158:** 633-8.

4997. Merrison, A. F. A., K. E. Chidley, J. Dunnett, and K. A. Sieradzan. 2002. Wound botulism associated with subcutaneous drug use. *BMJ* **325:**1020-1.

4998. Merritt, A., D. Ewald, A. F. van den Hurk, S. Stephen, Jr., and J. Langrell. 1998. Malaria acquired in the Torres Strait. *Commun Dis Intell* **22:**1-2.

4999. Merritt, A., R. Miles, and J. Bates. 1999. An outbreak of Campylobacter enteritis on an island resort, north Queensland. *Commun Dis Intell* **23:**215-9.

5000. Merritt, A., D. Symons, and M. Griffiths. 1999. The epidemiology of acute hepatitis A in north Queensland, 1996-1997. *Commun Dis Intell* **23:**120-4.

5001. Merson, M. H., J. H. Tenney, J. D. Meyers, B. T. Wood, J. G. Wells, W. Rymzo, B. Cline, W. E. DeWitt, P. Skaliy, and F. Mallison. 1975. Shigellosis at sea: an outbreak aboard a passenger cruise ship. *Am J Epidemiol* **101:**165-75.

5002. Mert, A., R. Ozaras, F. Tabak, M. Bilir, R. Ozturk, and Y. Aktuglu. 2003. Malaria in Turkey: a review of 33 cases. *Eur J Epidemiol* **18:**579-82.

5003. Mertens, P. L., J. F. Thissen, A. W. Houben, and F. Sturmans. 1999. [An epidemic of Salmonella typhimurium associated with traditional salted, smoked, and dried ham]. *Ned Tijdschr Geneeskd* **143:**1046-9.

5004. Mertz, K. J., G. M. McQuillan, W. C. Levine, D. H. Candal, J. C. Bullard, R. E. Johnson, M. E. St Louis, and C. M. Black. 1998. A pilot study of the prevalence of chlamydial infection in a national household survey. *Sex Transm Dis* **25:**225-8.

5005. Mertz, K. J., J. R. Schwebke, C. A. Gaydos, H. A. Beidinger, S. D. Tulloch, and W. C. Levine. 2002. Screening women in jails for chlamydial and gonococcal infection using urine tests: feasibility, acceptability, prevalence, and treatment rates. *Sex Transm Dis* **29:**271-6.

5006. Mertz, K. J., D. Trees, W. C. Levine, J. S. Lewis, B. Litchfield, K. S. Pettus, S. A. Morse, M. E. St Louis, J. B. Weiss, J. Schwebke, J. Dickes, R. Kee, J. Reynolds, D. Hutcheson, D. Green, I. Dyer, G. A. Richwald, J. Novotny, I. Weisfuse, M. Goldberg, J. A. O'Donnell, and R. Knaup. 1998. Etiology of genital ulcers and prevalence of human immunodeficiency virus coinfection in 10 US cities. The Genital Ulcer Disease Surveillance Group. *J Infect Dis* **178:**1795-8.

5007. Mertz, K. J., J. B. Weiss, R. M. Webb, W. C. Levine, J. S. Lewis, K. A. Orle, P. A. Totten, J. Overbaugh, S. A. Morse, M. M. Currier, M. Fishbein, and M. E. St Louis. 1998. An investigation of genital ulcers in Jackson, Mississippi, with use of a multiplex polymerase chain reaction assay: high prevalence of chancroid and human immunodeficiency virus infection. *J Infect Dis* **178:**1060-6.

5008. Meselson, M., J. Guillemin, M. Hugh-Jones, A. Langmuir, I. Popova, A. Shelokov, and O. Yampolskaya. 1994. The Sverdlovsk anthrax outbreak of 1979. *Science* **266:**1202-8.

5009. Messenger, S. L., J. S. Smith, and C. E. Rupprecht. 2002. Emerging epidemiology of bat-assocaited cryptic cases of rabies in humans in the United States. *Clin Infect Dis* **35:**738-47.

5010. Mets, M. B., L. L. Barton, A. S. Khan, and T. G. Ksiazek. 2000. Lymphocytic choriomeningitis virus: an underdiagnosed cause of congenital chorioretinitis. *Am J Ophthalmol* **130:** 209-15.

5011. Mets, M. B., A. G. Noble, S. Basti, P. Gavin, A. T. Davis, S. T. Shulman, and K. R. Kazacos. 2003. Eye findings of diffuse unilateral subacute neuroretinitis and multiple choroidal infiltrates associated with neural larva migrans due to Baylisascaris procyonis. *Am J Ophthalmol* **135:**888-90.

5012. Metter, K., H. Glöser, and U. v. Gaisberg. 2000. Fascioliasis nach Turkeiaufenthalt. *Dtsch Med Wochenschr* **125:**1160-3.

5013. Meune, C., C. Arnal, C. Hermand, and J. J. Cocheton. 2000. [Infective endocarditis related to pacemaker leads. A review]. *Ann Med Interne (Paris)* **151:**456-64.

5014. Meyer, H. W., H. Wurtz, P. Suadicani, O. Valbjorn, T. Sigsgaard, and F. Gyntelberg. 2004. Molds in floor dust and building-related symptoms in adolescent school children. *Indoor Air* **14:**65-72.

5015. Meyer, W., A. Castañeda, S. Jackson, M. Huynh, and E. Castaneda. 2003. Molecular typing of IberoAmerican Cryptococcus neoformans isolates. *Emerg Infect Dis* **9:**189-95.

5016. Meyers, H., B. A. Brown-Elliott, D. Moore, J. Curry, C. Truong, Y. Zhang, and R. J. Wallace Jr. 2002. An outbreak of Mycobacterium chelonae infection following liposuction. *Clin Infect Dis* **34:**1500-7.

5017. Meyers, J. D., L. L. Pifer, G. E. Sale, and E. D. Thomas. 1979. The value of Pneumocystis carinii antibody and antigen detection for diagnosis of Pneumocystis carinii pneumonia after marrow transplantation. *Am Rev Respir Dis* **120:**1283-7.

5018. Meyers, J. D., F. J. Romm, W. S. Tihen, and J. A. Bryan. 1975. Food-borne hepatitis A in a general hospital. Epidemiologic study of an outbreak attributed to sandwiches. *JAMA* **231:**1049-53.

5019. Meyn, L. A., D. M. Moore, S. L. Hillier, and M. A. Krohn. 2002. Association of sexual activity with colonization and vaginal acquisition of group B Streptococcus in nonpregnant women. *Am J Epidemiol* **155:**949-57.

5020. Meynard, J. B., J. P. Boutin, S. Banzet, R. Michel, F. Pages, X. Deparis, L. Galoisy-Gibal, E. Bertherat, F. Mérouze, A. Spiegel, and D. Baudon. 2001. Epidémies de leishmanioses cutanées dans les armées fraçaises en 1998 et 1999. *Méd Mal Infect* **31 suppl 2:**306s-7s.

5021. Meynard, J. B., L. Ollivier-Gay, X. Deparis, J. P. Durand, R. Michel, F. Pages, T. Matton, J. P. Boutin, H. Tolou, F. Merouze, and D. Baudon. 2001. [Epidemiologic surveillance of dengue fever in the French army from 1996 to 1999]. *Med Trop (Mars)* **61:**481-6.

5022. Mezarina, K. B., A. Huffmire, J. Downing, N. Core, K. Gershman, and R. Hoffman. 2001. Outbreak of community-acquired pneumonia caused by Mycoplasma pneumoniae - Colorado, 2000. *MMWR* **50:**227-30.

5023. Mezzari, A., C. Perin, S. J. S.A., and L. A. G. Bernd. 2002. Airborne fungi in the city of Porto Alegre, Rio Grande do Sul, Brazil. *Rev Inst Med Trop Sao Paulo* **44:**269-72.

5024. Mgone, C. S., T. Lupiwa, and W. Yeka. 2002. High prevalence of Neisseria gonorrhoeae and multiple sexually transmitted diseases among rural women in the Eastern Highlands Province of Papua New Guinea, detected by polymerase chain reaction. *Sex Transm Dis* **29:**775-9.

5025. Mhalu, F. S., F. D. E. Mtango, and A. E. Msengi. 1984. Hospital outbreaks of cholera transmitted through close person-to-person contact. *Lancet* **2 (july 14):**82-4.

5026. Miaka Mia Bilenge, C., V. Kande Betu Ku Meso, F. J. Louis, and P. Lucas. 2001. Trypanosomiase humaine Africaine en milieu urbain: l'exemple de Kinshasa, république démocratique du Congo, en 1998 et 1999. *Med Trop* **61**:445-8.

5027. **Michael, E., D. A. P. Bundy, and B. T. Grenfell.** 1996. Reassessing the global prevalence and distribution of lymphatic filariasis. *Parasitology* **112**:409-28.

5028. **Michel, R., H. Burghardt, and H. Bergmann.** 1995. [Acanthamoeba, naturally intracellularly infected with Pseudomonas aeruginosa, after their isolation from a microbiologically contaminated drinking water system in a hospital]. *Zentralbl Hyg Umweltmed* **196**:532-44.

5029. **Michel, R., E. Garnotel, A. Spiegel, M. Morillon, P. Saliou, and J. P. Boutin.** 2005. Outbreak of typhoid fever in vaccinated members of the French Armed Forces in the Ivory Coast. *Eur J Epidemiol* **20**:635-42.

5030. **Michel, R., R. Rohl, and H. Schneider.** 1982. [Isolation of free-living amoebae from nasal mucosa of healthy individuals]. *Zentralbl Bakteriol Mikrobiol Hyg [B]* **176**:155-9.

5031. **Michino, H., K. Araki, S. Minami, S. Takaya, N. Sakai, M. Miyazaki, A. Ono, and H. Yanagawa.** 1999. Massive outbreak of Escherichia coli O157:H7 infection in schoolchildren in Sakai City, Japan, associated with consumption of white radish sprouts. *Am J Epidemiol* **150**:787-96.

5032. **Midoneck, S. R., and H. W. Murray.** 1994. Colorado tick fever in a resident of New York city. *Arch Fam Med* **3**:731-2.

5033. **Miegeville, M., V. Koubi, L. C. Dan, J. P. Barbier, and P. D. Cam.** 2003. [Cyclospora cayetanensis presence in aquatic surroundings in Hanoi (Vietnam). Environmental study (well water, lakes and rivers)]. *Bull Soc Pathol Exot* **96**:149-52.

5034. **Miettinen, M. K., K. J. Bjorkroth, and H. J. Korkeala.** 1999. Characterization of Listeria monocytogenes from an ice cream plant by serotyping and pulsed-field gel electrophoresis. *Int J Food Microbiol* **46**:187-92.

5035. **Miettinen, M. K., A. Siitonen, P. Heiskanen, H. Haajanen, K. J. Bjorkroth, and H. J. Korkeala.** 1999. Molecular epidemiology of an outbreak of febrile gastroenteritis caused by Listeria monocytogenes in cold-smoked rainbow trout. *J Clin Microbiol* **37**:2358-60.

5036. **Migliani, R., R. Josse, P. Hovette, A. Keundjian, F. Pages, J. B. Meynard, L. Ollivier, K. Sbai Idrissi, K. Tifratene, E. Orlandi, C. Rogier, and J. P. Boutin.** 2003. Le paludisme vu des tranchées: le cas de la Côte d'Ivoire en 2002-2003. *Med Trop* **63**:282-6.

5037. **Mignani, E., F. Palmieri, M. Fontana, and S. Marigo.** 1988. Italian epidemic of waterborne tularaemia. *Lancet* **2**:1423.

5038. **Mihajlovic, L., J. Bockemühl, J. Heesemann, and R. Laufs.** 1982. Importierte Muscheln als Ursache einer Gastroenteritis durch Vibrio parahaemolyticus. *Infection* **10**:285-6.

5039. **Mikami, T., T. Nakagomi, R. Tsutsui, K. Ishikawa, Y. Onodera, K. Arisawa, and O. Nakagomi.** 2004. An outbreak of gastroenteritis during school trip caused by serotype G2 group A rotavirus. *J Med Virol* **73**:460-4.

5040. **Milas, J., D. Ropac, R. Mulic, V. Milas, I. Valek, I. Zoric, and K. Kozul.** 2000. Hepatitis B in the family. *Eur J Epidemiol* **16**:203-8.

5041. **Milazzo, A., and N. Rose.** 2001. An outbreak of Salmonella Typhimurium phage type 126 linked to a cake shop in South Australia. *Commun Dis Intell* **25**:73.

5042. **Miles, J.** 1997. Infectious diseases: colonising the Pacific? University of Otago Press, Wellington.

5043. **Miles, M. A., M. D. Feliciangeli, and A. R. de Arias.** 2003. American trypanosomiasis (Chagas' disease) and the role of molecular epidemiology in guiding control strategies. *BMJ* **326**:1444-8.

5044. **Millán, J. C., R. Mull, S. Freise, and J. Richter.** 2000. The efficacy and tolerability of triclabendazole in Cuban patients with latent and chronic Fasciola hepatica infection. *Am J Trop Med Hyg* **63**:264-9.

5045. **Millar, D., J. Ford, J. Sanderson, S. Withey, M. Tizard, T. Doran, and J. Hermon-Taylor.** 1996. IS900 PCR to detect Mycobacterium paratuberculosis in retail supplies of whole pasteurized cows' milk in England and Wales. *Appl Environ Microbiol* **62**:3446-52.

5046. **Millard, P. S., K. F. Gensheimer, D. G. Addiss, D. M. Sosin, G. A. Beckett, A. Houck-Jankoski, and A. Hudson.** 1994. An outbreak of cryptosporidiosis from fresh-pressed apple cider. *JAMA* **272**:1592-6.

5047. **Miller, B. R., M. S. Godsey, M. B. Crabtree, H. M. Savage, Y. Al-Mazrao, M. H. Al-Jeffri, A. M. Abdoon, S. M. Al-Seghayer, A. M. Al-Shahrani, and T. G. Ksiazek.** 2002. Isolation and genetic characterization of Rift Valley fever virus from Aedes vexans arabiensis, Kingdom of Saudi Arabia. *Emerg Infect Dis* **8**:1492-4.

5048. **Miller, E., J. E. Cradock-Watson, and T. M. Pollock.** 1982. Consequences of confirmed maternal rubella at successive stages of pregnancy. *Lancet* **2**:781-4.

5049. **Miller, E., C. K. Fairley, B. J. Cohen, and C. Seng.** 1998. Immediate and long term outcome of human parvovirus B19 infection in pregnancy. *Br J Obstet Gynaecol* **105**:174-8.

5050. **Miller, J., T. Tam, C. Afif, S. Maloney, M. Cetron, K. Fukata, A. Klimov, H. Hall, D. Kertesz, and J. Hockin.** 1998. Influenza A outbreak on a cruise ship. *Can Commun Dis Rep* **24**:9-11.

5051. **Miller, L. W., J. J. Older, J. Drake, and S. Zimmerman.** 1972. Diphtheria immunization. Effect upon carriers and the control of outbreaks. *Am J Dis Child* **123**:197-9.

5052. **Miller, M., M. Lin, and J. Spencer.** 2002. Tuberculosis notifications in Australia, 2001. *Commun Dis Intell* **26**:525-36.

5053. **Miller, M. A., S. Valway, and I. M. Onorato.** 1996. Tuberculosis risk after exposure on airplanes. *Tuber Lung Dis* **77**:414-9.

5054. **Miller, M. W.** 2004. Environmental sources of prion transmission in mule deer. *Emerg Infect Dis* **10**:1003-6.

5055. **Miller, M. W., and E. S. Williams.** 2003. Prion disease: horizontal prion transmission in mule deer. *Nature* **425**:35-6.

5056. **Miller, R. F., A. D. Grant, and N. M. Foley.** 1992. Seasonal variation in presentation of Pneumocystis carinii pneumonia. *Lancet* **339**:747-8.

5057. **Miller, R. K., J. Y. Baumgardner, C. W. Armstrong, S. R. Jenkins, C. D. Woolard, G. B. Miller, P. E. Rollin, P. B. Jahrling, T. G. Ksiazek, and C. J. Peters.** 1990. Update: filovirus infection in animal handlers. *MMWR* **39**:221.

5058. **Miller, S. A., C. L. Rosario, E. Rojas, and J. V. Scorza.** 2003. Intestinal parasitic infection and associated symptoms in children attending day care centres in Trujillo, Venezuela. *Trop Med Int Health* **8**:342-7.

5059. **Miller, W. C., C. A. Ford, M. Morris, M. S. Handcock, J. L. Schmitz, M. M. Hobbs, M. S. Cohen, K. M. Harris, and J. R. Udry.** 2004. Prevalence of chlamydial and gonococcal infections among young adults in the United States. *JAMA* **291**:2229-36.

5060. **Millet, V., M. J. Spencer, M. Chapin, M. Stewart, J. A. Yatabe, T. Brewer, and L. S. Garcia.** 1983. Dientamoeba fragilis, a protozoan parasite in adult members of a semicommunal group. *Dig Dis Sci* **28**:335-9.

5061. **Mills, J. N., B. A. Ellis, K. T. McKee, Jr., G. E. Calderon, J. I. Maiztegui, G. O. Nelson, T. G. Ksiazek, C. J. Peters, and J. E. Childs.** 1992. A longitudinal study of Junin virus activity in the rodent reservoir of Argentine hemorrhagic fever. *Am J Trop Med Hyg* **47**:749-63.

5062. **Mills, J. N., T. G. Ksiazek, B. A. Ellis, P. E. Rollin, S. T. Nichol, T. L. Yates, W. L. Gannon, C. E. Levy, D. M. Engelthaler, T. Davis, D. T. Tanda, J. W. Frampton, C. R. Nichols, C. J. Peters, and J. E. Childs.** 1997. Patterns of association with host and habitat: antibody reactive with Sin Nombre virus in small mammals in the major biotic communities of the southwestern United States. *Am J Trop Med Hyg* **56**:273-84.

5063. **Mills, J. N., T. L. Yates, T. G. Ksiazek, C. J. Peters, and J. E. Childs.** 1999. Long-term studies of hantavirus reservoir populations in the southwestern United States: rationale, potential, and methods. *Emerg Infect Dis* **5**:95-101.

5064. **Milne, L. M., A. Plom, I. Strudley, G. C. Pritchard, R. Crooks, M. Hall, G. Duckworth, C. Seng, M. D. Susman, J. Kearney, R. J. Wiggins, M. Moulsdale, T. Cheasty, and G. A. Willshaw.** 1999. Escherichia coli O157 incident associated with a farm open to members of the public. *Commun Dis Public Health* **2**:22-6.

5065. **Mimouni, D., M. Gdalevich, F. B. Mimouni, J. Haviv, and I. Ashkenazi.** 1998. The epidemiologic trends of scabies among Israeli soldiers: a 28-year follow-up. *Int J Dermatol* **37**:586-7.

5066. **Mimouni, D., I. Grotto, J. Haviv, M. Gdalevich, M. Huerta, and O. Shpilberg.** 2001. Secular trends in the epidemiology of pediculosis capitis and pubis among Israeli soldiers: a 27-year follow-up. *Int J Dermatol* **40**:637-9.

5067. **Mimura, K., K. Sugita, K. Tabuki, and T. Nishimura.** 1992. [Mycoplasma pneumoniae respiratory tract infection prevailing among infants at a nursery school]. *Kansenshogaku Zasshi* **66**:1566-71.

5068. **Mineshita, M., Y. Nakamori, Y. Seida, and S. Hiwatashi.** 2005. Legionella pneumonia due to exposure to 24-hour bath water contaminated by Legionella pneumophila serogroup-5. *Intern Med* **44**:662-5.

5069. **Minh, T. T., T. Nhan do, G. R. West, T. M. Durant, R. A. Jenkins, P. T. Huong, and R. O. Valdiserri.** 2004. Sex workers in Vietnam: how many, how risky? *AIDS Educ Prev* **16**:389-404.

5070. **Minotto, R., C. D. Bernardi, L. F. Mallmann, M. I. Edelweiss, and M. L. Scroferneker.** 2001. Chromoblastomycosis: a review of 100 cases in the state of Rio Grande do Sul, Brazil. *J Am Acad Dermatol* **44**:585-92.

5071. **Mintz, E. D., M. Hudson-Wragg, P. Mshar, M. L. Cartter, and J. L. Hadler.** 1993. Foodborne giardiasis in a corporate office setting. *J Infect Dis* **167**:250-3.

5072. **Minuk, G. Y., L. X. Ding, C. Hannon, and L. Sekla.** 1994. The risks of transmission of acute hepatitis A and B virus infection in an urban centre. *J Hepatol* **21**:118-21.

5073. **Miquel, P. H., S. Haeghebaert, C. D., C. Campese, C. Guitard, T. Brigaud, M. Thérouanne, G. Panié, S. Jarraud, and D. Ilef.** 2004. Épidémie communautaire de légionellose, Pas-de-Calais, France, novembre 2003-janvier 2004. *Bull Epidémiol Hebdomadaire* **36-37**:179-81.

5074. **Miranda, M. E., T. G. Ksiazek, T. J. Retuya, A. S. Khan, A. Sanchez, C. F. Fulhorst, P. E. Rollin, A. B. Calaor, D. L. Manalo, M. C. Roces, M. M. Dayrit, and C. J. Peters.** 1999. Epidemiology of Ebola (subtype Reston) virus in the Philippines, 1996. *J Infect Dis* **179 Suppl 1**:S115-9.

5075. **Miranda, M. E., M. E. White, M. M. Dayrit, C. G. Hayes, T. G. Ksiazek, and J. P. Burans.** 1991. Seroepidemiological study of filovirus related to Ebola in the Philippines. *Lancet* **337**:425-6.

5076. **Miranda Paniago, A. M., J. I. Albuquerque Aguiar, E. S. Aguiar, R. V. da Cunha, G. R. Pereira, A. T. Londero, and B. Wanke.** 2003. Paracoccidioidomicose: estudo clínico e epidemiológico de 422 casos observados no estado de Mato Grosso do Sul. *Rev Soc Bras Med Trop* **36**:455-9.

5077. **Mirdha, B. R., and J. C. Samantray.** 2002. Hymenolepis nana: a common cause of paediatric diarrhoea in urban slum dwellers in India. *J Trop Pediatr* **48**:331-4.

5078. **Miró, J. M., A. del Río, and C. A. Mestres.** 2002. Infective endocarditis in intravenous drug abusers and HIV-1 infected patients. *Infect Dis Clin North Am* **16**:273-95.

5079. **Mirza, S. A., M. Phelan, and D. Rimland.** 2003. The changing epidemiology of cryptococcosis: an update from population-based active surveillance in 2 large metropolitan areas, 1992-2000. *Clin Infect Dis* **36**:789-94.

5080. **Mishal, J., N. Ben-Israel, Y. Levin, S. Sherf, J. Jafari, E. Embon, and Y. Sherer.** 1999. Brucellosis outbreak: analysis of risk factors and serologic screening. *Int J Mol Med* **4**:655-8.

5081. **Mishin, V. P., M. S. Nedyalkova, F. G. Hayden, and L. V. Gubareva.** 2005. Protection afforded by intranasal immunization with the neuraminidase-lacking mutant of influenza A virus in a ferret model. *Vaccine* **23**:2922-7.

5082. **Mishu, B., J. Koehler, L. A. Lee, D. Rodrigue, F. H. Brenner, P. Blake, and R. V. Tauxe.** 1994. Outbreaks of Salmonella enteritidis infections in the United States, 1985-1991. *J Infect Dis* **169**:547-52.

5083. **Mitakakis, T. Z., M. I. Sinclair, C. K. Fairley, P. K. Lightbody, K. Leder, and M. E. Hellard.** 2004. Food safety in family homes in Melbourne, Australia. *J Food Prot* **67**:818-22.

5084. **Mitchell, C. J., S. D. Lvov, H. M. Savage, C. H. Calisher, G. C. Smith, D. K. Lvov, and D. J. Gubler.** 1993. Vector and host relationships of California serogroup viruses in western Siberia. *Am J Trop Med Hyg* **49**:53-62.

5085. **Mitchell, C. J., T. P. Monath, M. S. Sabattini, J. F. Daffner, C. B. Cropp, C. H. Calisher, R. F. Darsie, Jr., and W. L. Jakob.** 1987. Arbovirus isolations from mosquitoes collected during and after the 1982-1983 epizootic of western equine encephalitis in Argentina. *Am J Trop Med Hyg* **36**:107-13.

5086. **Mitchell, D. K., S. S. Monroe, X. Jiang, D. O. Matson, R. I. Glass, and L. K. Pickering.** 1995. Virologic features of an astrovirus diarrhea outbreak in a day care center revealed by reverse transcriptase-polymerase chain reaction. *J Infect Dis* **172**:1437-44.

5087. **Mitchell, S. J., J. Gray, M. E. I. Morgan, M. D. Hocking, and G. M. Durbin.** 1996. Nosocomial infection with Rhizopus microsporus in preterm infants: association with wooden tongue depressors. *Lancet* **348**:441-443.

5088. **Mitchell, T. G., and J. R. Perfect.** 1995. Cryptococcosis in the era of AIDS - 100 years after the discovery of Cryptococcus neoformans. *Clin Microbiol Rev* **8**:515-48.

5089. **Mitiku, K., and G. Mengistu.** 2002. Relapsing fever in Gondar, Ethiopia. *East Afr Med J* **79**:85-7.

5090. **Mitrova, E., and G. Belay.** 2000. Creutzfeldt-Jakob disease in health professionals in Slovakia. *Eur J Epidemiol* **16**:353-5.

5091. **Mittal, N., D. Nair, N. Gupta, D. Rawat, S. Kabra, S. Kumar, S. K. Prakash, and V. K. Sharma.** 2003. Outbreak of Acinetobacter spp septicemia in a neonatal ICU. *Southeast Asian J Trop Med Public Health* **34**:365-6.

5092. **Mittal, P. K.** 2003. Biolarvicides in vector control: challenges and prospects. *J Vector Borne Dis* **40**:20-32.

5093. **Miwa, N., T. Masuda, K. Terai, A. Kawamura, K. Otani, and H. Miyamoto.** 1999. Bacteriological investigation of an outbreak of Clostridium perfringens food poisoning caused by Japanese food without animal protein. *Int J Food Microbiol* **49**:103-6.

5094. **Miyamoto, K., M. Ogami, Y. Takahashi, T. Mori, S. Akimoto, H. Terashita, and T. Terashita.** 2000. Outbreak of human parvovirus B19 in hospital workers. *J Hosp Infect* **45**:238-41.

5095. **Miyazaki, M., A. Babazono, M. Kato, S. Takagi, H. Chimura, and H. Une.** 2003. Sexually transmitted diseases in Japanese female commercial sex workers working in massage parlors with cell baths. *J Infect Chemother* **9**:248-53.

5096. **Mocroft, A., C. Katlama, A. M. Johnson, C. Pradier, F. Antunes, et al.** 2000. AIDS across Europe, 1994-98: the EuroSIDA study. *Lancet* **356**:291-6.

5097. **Modlin, J. F.** 2004. Poliomyelitis in the United States: the final chapter? *JAMA* **292**:1749-51.

5098. **Mody, L., C. A. Kauffman, S. A. McNeil, A. T. Galecki, and S. F. Bradley.** 2003. Mupirocin-based decolonization of Staphylococcus aureus carriers in residents of 2 long-term care facilities: a randomized, double-blind, placebo-controlled trial. *Clin Infect Dis* **37**:1467-74.

5099. **Moegle, H., W. Heizmann, P. Katz, and K. Botzenhart.** 1985. Bericht über eine Brucella melitensis-Epidemie in Süddeutschland. *Bundesgesundheitsblatt* **28**:69-74.

5100. **MoH.** 1987. Botulism associated with an in-flight meal - England. *Can Dis Weekly Rep* **13**:213.

5101. **MoH.** 1999. Infection control guidelines. Routine practices and additional precautions for preventing the transmission of infection in health care. *Canada Comm Dis Rep* **25S4**:1-142.

5102. **MoH.** 1999. Infectious agents surveillance report. *Jpn J Infect Dis* 52 (**suppl**)1–111.

5103. **MoH.** 2000. Outbreaks of Escherichia coli O157 infection in two prisons. *Commun Dis Rep CDR Wkly* **10**:375.

5104. **MoH.** 2001. Risk factors for the transmission of Campylobacter bacteria infection in Singapore. *Epidemiol News Bull* **27**: 29-31.

5105. **MoH.** 2001. Surveillance, prevention and control of legionellosis in Singapore. *Epidemiol News Bull* **27**:35-9.

5106. **MoH.** 2002. Canadian immunization guide (6th edition). Minister of Health, Population and Public Health Branch, Ottawa: Ontario.

5107. **MoH.** 2002. Classic Creutzfeldt-Jakob disease in Canada. Infection control guidelines. *Can Commun Dis Rep* **28 (S5)**:1-84.

5108. **MoH.** 2002. An outbreak of erythematous eruption caused by parvovirus B19. *Epidemiol News Bull (Singapore)* **28**:7-9.

5109. **MoH.** 2002. Prevention and control of occupational infections in health care. *Can Commun Dis Rep* **28 suppl 1**:1-264.

5110. **MoH.** 2002. A shellfish-borne outbreak of hepatitis A. *Epidemiol News Bull* **28**:55-7.

5111. **MoH.** 2003. The Australian immunisation handbook (8th edition). National Health & Medical Research Council (NHMRC), Canberra.

5112. **MoH.** 2003. Canadian integrated surveillance report. Salmonella, Campylobacter, pathogenic E. coli and Shigella, from 1996 to 1999. *Can Commun Dis Rep* **29 suppl 1**:1-32.

5113. **MoH.** 2004. Healthcare associated infections. *Commun Dis Rep Weekly* **14**:1-5.

5114. **MoH.** 2004. Illness in England, Wales, and Northern Ireland associated with foreign travel: a baseline report to 2002, Health Protection Agency (HPA), London.

5115. **MoH.** 2004. Infection control guidelines, p. 1-519, Canberra, ACT 2601, Australia.

5116. **Mohamed, A. R. E., and V. Mummery.** 1990. Human dicrocoeliasis: report on 208 cases from Saudi Arabia. *Trop Geogr Med* **42**:1-7.

5117. **Mohandas, K., R. Sehgal, A. Sud, and N. Malla.** 2002. Prevalence of intestinal parasitic pathogens in HIV-seropositive individuals in northern India. *Jpn J Infect Dis* **55**:83-4.

5118. **Mohareb, E. W., E. M. Mikhail, and F. G. Youssef.** 1996. Leishmania tropica in Egypt: an undesirable import. *Trop Med Int Health* **1**:251-4.

5119. **Mohd, M. G.** 1989. Brucellosis in the Gezira area, Central Sudan. *J Trop Med Hyg* **92**:86-8.

5120. **Mohindra, A. R., M. W. Lee, G. Visvesvara, H. Moura, R. Parasuraman, G. J. Leitch, L. Xiao, J. Yee, and R. del Busto.** 2002. Disseminated microsporidiosis in a renal transplant recipient. *Transpl Infect Dis* **4**:102-7.

5121. **Mohle-Boetani, J. C., J. A. Farrar, S. B. Werner, D. Minassian, R. Bryant, S. Abbott, L. Slutsker, and D. J. Vugia.** 2001. Escherichia coli O157 and Salmonella infections associated with sprouts in California, 1996-1998. *Ann Intern Med* **135**:239-47.

5122. **Mohle-Boetani, J. C., C. Matkin, M. Pallansch, R. Helfand, M. Fenstersheib, J. A. Blanding, and S. L. Solomon.** 1999. Viral meningitis in child care center staff and parents: an outbreak of echovirus 30 infections. *Public Health Rep* **114**: 249-56.

5123. **Mohle-Boetani, J. C., M. Stapleton, R. Finger, N. H. Bean, J. Poundstone, P. A. Blake, and P. M. Griffin.** 1995. Communitywide shigellosis: control of an outbreak and risk factors in child day-care centers. *Am J Public Health* **85**:812-6.

5124. **Moisa, I., F. Barnaure, C. Parvu, and D. Sirbu.** 1987. [Circulation of parainfluenza viruses and adenoviruses in groups exposed to the action of noxious chemicals or not]. *Virologie* **38**:103-10.

5125. **Moisiuk, S. E., D. Robson, L. Klass, G. Kliewer, W. Wasyliuk, M. Davi, and P. Plourde.** 1998. Outbreak of parainfluenza virus type 3 in an intermediate care neonatal nursery. *Pediatr Infect Dis J* **17**:49-53.

5126. **Mokrani, K., P. E. Fournier, M. Dalichaouche, S. Tebbal, A. Aouati, and D. Raoult.** 2004. Reemerging threat of epidemic typhus in Algeria. *J Clin Microbiol* **42**:3898-900.

5127. **Molbak, K., D. L. Baggesen, F. M. Aarestrup, J. M. Ebbesen, J. Engberg, K. Frydendahl, P. Gerner-Smidt, A. M. Petersen, and H. C. Wegener.** 1999. An outbreak of multidrug-resistant, quinolone-resistant Salmonella enterica serotype typhimurium DT104. *N Engl J Med* **341**:1420-5.

5128. **Molbak, K., and J. Neimann.** 2002. Risk factors for sporadic infection with Salmonella Enteritidis, Denmark, 1997-1999. *Am J Epidemiol* **156**:654-61.

5129. **Molet, B., A. Feki, R. Haag, and M. Kremer.** 1981. [Isolation of free-living amoebae from nasal swabs in 300 healthy persons (author's transl)]. *Rev Otoneuroophtalmol* **53**:121-6.

5130. **Molina, C. P., J. Ogburn, and P. Adegboyega.** 2003. Infection by Dipylidium caninum in an infant. *Arch Pathol Lab Med* **127:**e157-9.

5131. **Molina, O. M., M. C. Morales, I. D. Soto, J. A. Pena, R. S. Haack, D. P. Cardozo, and J. J. Cardozo.** 1999. [Venezuelan equine encephalitis. 1995 outbreak: clinical profile of the case with neurologic involvement]. *Rev Neurol* **29:**296-8.

5132. **Molke Borgbjerg, B., F. Gjerris, M. J. Albeck, and S. E. Borgesen.** 1997. [Frequency of infections after shunting of hydrocephalus. An analysis of 884 shunts]. *Ugeskr Laeger* **159:**2867-71.

5133. **Molla, B., W. Salah, D. Alemayehu, and A. Mohammed.** 2004. Antimicrobial resistance pattern of Salmonella serotypes isolated from apparently healthy slaughtered camels (Camelus dromedarius) in eastern Ethiopia. *Berl Munch Tierarztl Wochenschr* **117:**39-45.

5134. **Moller, L. N., E. Petersen, C. M. Kapel, M. Melbye, and A. Koch.** 2005. Outbreak of trichinellosis associated with consumption of game meat in West Greenland. *Vet Parasitol.* **132:**131–6.

5135. **Monasch, R., A. Reinisch, R. W. Steketee, E. L. Korenromp, D. Alnwick, and Y. Bergevin.** 2004. Child coverage with mosquito nets and malaria treatment from population-based surveys in african countries: a baseline for monitoring progress in roll back malaria. *Am J Trop Med Hyg* **71:**232-8.

5136. **Monath, T. P.** 1975. Lassa fever: review of epidemiology and epizootiology. *Bull WHO* **52:**577-592.

5137. **Monath, T. P.** 1988. Japanese encephalitis - a plague of the orient. *N Engl J Med* **319:**641-3.

5138. **Monath, T. P.** 1999. Ecology of Marburg and Ebola viruses: speculations and directions for future research. *J Infect Dis* **179 suppl 1:**S127-S138.

5139. **Monath, T. P., and M. S. Cetron.** 2002. Prevention of yellow fever in persons traveling to the tropics. *Clin Infect Dis* **34:**1369-78.

5140. **Moncayo, A.** 2003. Chagas, disease: current epidemiological trends after the interruption of vectorial and transfusional transmission in the southern cone countries. *Mem Inst Oswaldo Cruz* **98:**577-91.

5141. **Moncayo, A. C., and J. D. Edman.** 1999. Toward the incrimination of epidemic vectors of eastern equine encephalomyelitis virus in Massachusetts: abundance of mosquito populations at epidemic foci. *J Am Mosq Control Assoc* **15:**479-92.

5142. **Monjour, L., P. Druilhe, A. Fribourg-Blanc, M. Karam, A. Froment, H. Feldmeier, C. Daniel-Ribeiro, J. M. Kyelem, and M. Gentilini.** 1983. General considerations on endemic treponematosis in the rural Sahel region of Upper Volta. *Acta Trop* **40:**375-82.

5143. **Monnet, D. L., J. W. Biddle, J. R. Edwards, D. H. Culver, J. S. Tolson, W. J. Martone, F. C. Tenover, and R. P. Gaynes.** 1997. Evidence of interhospital transmission of extended-spectrum beta-lactam- resistant Klebsiella pneumoniae in the United States, 1986 to 1993. The National Nosocomial Infections Surveillance System. *Infect Control Hosp Epidemiol* **18:**492-8.

5144. **Monroe, S. S., T. Ando, and R. I. Glass.** 2000. Introduction: human enteric caliciviruses - an emerging pathogen whose time has come. *J Infect Dis* **181 suppl 2:**S249-S251.

5145. **Monsuez, J. J., R. Kidouche, B. Le Gueno, and P. Postic.** 1997. Leptospirosis presenting as haemorrhagic fever in visitor to Africa. *Lancet* **349:**254-5.

5146. **Montgomerie, J. Z., and J. W. Morrow.** 1978. Pseudomonas colonization in patients with spinal cord injury. *Am J Epidemiol* **108:**328-36.

5147. **Montgomery, B. L., and S. A. Ritchie.** 2002. Roof gutters: a key container for Aedes aegypti and Ochlerotatus notoscriptus (Diptera: Culicidae) in Australia. *J Trop Med Hyg* **67:**244-6.

5148. **Montmayeur, A., C. Brosset, P. Imbert, and A. Buguet.** 1994. [The sleep-wake cycle during Trypanosoma brucei rhodesiense human African trypanosomiasis in 2 French parachutists]. *Bull Soc Pathol Exot* **87:**368-71.

5149. **Monto, A. S.** 2002. Epidemiology of viral respiratory infections. *Am J Med* **112 (6A):**4S-12S.

5150. **Monto, A. S.** 2002. The seasonality of rhinovirus infections and its implications for clinical recognition. *Clin Ther* **24:**1987-97.

5151. **Monto, A. S., M. E. Pichichero, S. J. Blanckenberg, O. Ruuskanen, C. Cooper, D. M. Fleming, and C. Kerr.** 2002. Zanamivir prophylaxis: an effective strategy for the prevention of influenza types A and B within households. *J Infect Dis* **186:**1582-8.

5152. **Monto, A. S., and H. Ross.** 1977. Acute respiratory illness in the community: effect of family composition, smoking, and chronic symptoms. *Br J Prev Soc Med* **31:**101-8.

5153. **Monto, A. S., J. Rotthoff, E. Teich, M. L. Herlocher, R. Truscon, H. L. Yen, S. Elias, and S. E. Ohmit.** 2004. Detection and control of influenza outbreaks in well-vaccinated nursing home populations. *Clin Infect Dis* **39:**459-64.

5154. **Montoya, J., C. Jaramillo, G. Palma, T. Gomez, I. Segura, and B. Travi.** 1990. Report of an epidemic outbreak of tegumentary leishmaniasis in a coffee-growing area of Colombia. *Mem Inst Oswaldo Cruz* **85:**119-21.

5155. **Montoya, J. G., and O. Liesenfeld.** 2004. Toxoplasmosis. *Lancet* **363:**1965-76.

5156. **Montoya-Lerma, J., H. Cadena, M. Oviedo, P. D. Ready, R. Barazarte, B. L. Travi, and R. P. Lane.** 2003. Comparative vectorial efficiency of Lutzomyia evansi and Lu. longipalpis for transmitting Leishmania chagasi. *Acta Trop* **85:**19-29.

5157. **Montresor, A., S. Awasthi, and D. W. Crompton.** 2003. Use of benzimidazoles in children younger than 24 months for the treatment of soil-transmitted helminthiasis. *Acta Trop* **86:**223-32.

5158. **Moodley, D., J. Moodley, H. Coovadia, G. Gray, J. McIntyre, J. Hofmyer, C. Nikodem, D. Hall, M. Gigliotti, P. Robinson, L. Boshoff, and J. L. Sullivan.** 2003. A multicenter randomized controlled trial of nevirapine versus a combination of zidovudine and lamivudine to reduce intrapartum and early postpartum mother-to-child transmission of human immunodeficiency virus type 1. *J Infect Dis* **187:**725-35.

5159. **Moodley, P., I. M. Martin, C. A. Ison, and A. W. Sturm.** 2002. Typing of Neisseria gonorrhoeae reveals rapid reinfection in rural South Africa. *J Clin Microbiol* **40:**4567-70.

5160. **Moolenaar, R. L., J. M. Crutcher, V. H. San Joaquin, L. V. Sewell, L. C. Hutwagner, L. A. Carson, D. A. Robison, L. M. Smithee, and W. R. Jarvis.** 2000. A prolonged outbreak of Pseudomonas aeruginosa in a neonatal intensive care unit: did staff fingernails play a role in disease transmission? *Infect Control Hosp Epidemiol* **21:**80-5.

5161. **Moore, A., and M. Richer.** 2001. Re-emergence of epidemic sleeping sickness in southern Sudan. *Trop Med Int Health* **6:**342-7.

5162. Moore, A. C., E. T. Ryan, and M. A. Waldron. 2002. Case records of the Massachusetts General Hospital. Weekly clinicopathological exercises. Case 20-2002. A 37-year-old man with fever, hepatosplenomegaly, and a cutaneous foot lesion after a trip to Africa. *N Engl J Med* **346:**2069-76.

5163. Moore, C. G., and C. J. Mitchell. 1997. Aedes albopictus in the United States: ten-year presence and public health implications. *Emerg Infect Dis* **3:**329-34.

5164. Moore, D. A., M. Edwards, R. Escombe, D. Agranoff, J. W. Bailey, S. B. Squire, and P. L. Chiodini. 2002. African trypanosomiasis in travelers returning to the United kingdom. *Emerg Infect Dis* **8:**74-6.

5165. Moore, D. A., and R. S. Hopkins. 1991. Assessment of a school exclusion policy during a chickenpox outbreak. *Am J Epidemiol* **133:**1161-7.

5166. Moore, D. A., L. Lightstone, B. Javid, and J. S. Friedland. 2002. High rates of tuberculosis in end-stage renal failure: the impact of international migration. *Emerg Infect Dis* **8:**77-8.

5167. Moore, D. A., J. McCroddan, P. Dekumyoy, and P. L. Chiodini. 2003. Gnathostomiasis: an emerging imported disease. *Emerg Infect Dis* **9:**647-50.

5168. Moore, J. E. 2004. Always blow your own trumpet! Potential cross-infection hazards through salivary and respiratory secretions in the sharing of brass and woodwind musical instruments during music therapy sessions. *J Hosp Infect* **56:**245.

5169. Moore, J. E., N. Heaney, B. C. Millar, M. Crowe, and J. S. Elborn. 2002. Incidence of Pseudomonas aeruginosa in recreational and hydrotherapy pools. *Commun Dis Publ Health* **5:**23-6.

5170. Moore, M., R. C. Baron, M. R. Filstein, J. P. Lofgren, D. L. Rowley, L. B. Schonberger, and M. H. Hatch. 1983. Aseptic meningitis and high school football players. 1978 and 1980. *JAMA* **249:**2039-42.

5171. Moore, M., J. Schulte, S. E. Valway, B. Stader, V. Kistler, P. Margraf, D. Murray, R. Christman, and I. M. Onorato. 1998. Evaluation of transmission of Mycobacterium tuberculosis in a pediatric setting. *J Pediatr* **133:**108-12.

5172. Moore, M., S. E. Valway, W. Ihle, and I. M. Onorato. 1999. A train passenger with pulmonary tuberculosis: evidence of limited transmission during travel. *Clin Infect Dis* **28:**52-6.

5173. Moore, P. S., M. W. Reeves, B. Schwartz, B. G. Gellin, and C. V. Broome. 1989. Intercontinental spread of an epidemic group A Neisseria meningitidis strain. *Lancet* **2:**260-3.

5174. Moorehead, W. P., R. Guasparini, C. A. Donovan, R. G. Mathias, R. Cottle, and G. Baytalan. 1990. Giardiasis outbreak from a chlorinated community water supply. *Can J Public Health* **81:**358-62.

5175. Moorhouse, D. E. 1982. Toxocariasis. A possible cause of the palm island mystery disease. *Med J Aust* **1:**172-3.

5176. Moraes, L. R. S., J. Azevedo Cancio, and S. Cairncross. 2004. Impact of drainage and sewerage on intestinal nematode infections in poor urban areas in Salvador, Brazil. *Trans R Soc Trop Med Hyg* **98:**197-204.

5177. Moraes, L. R. S., J. Azevedo Cancio, S. Cairncross, and S. Huttly. 2003. Impact of drainage and sewerage on diarrhoea in poor urban areas in Salvador, Brazil. *Trans R Soc Trop Med Hyg* **97:**153-8.

5178. Moraes, M. A., A. J. Shelley, and A. P. Luna Dias. 1985. [Mansonella ozzardi in the Federal Territory of Roraima, Brazil. Distribution and finding of a new vector in the area of Surumu river]. *Mem Inst Oswaldo Cruz* **80:**395-400.

5179. Moral, L., E. M. Rubio, and M. Moya. 2002. A leishmanin skin test survey in the human population of l'Alacanti region (Spain): implications for the epidemiology of Leishmania infantum infection in southern Europe. *Trans R Soc Trop Med Hyg* **96:**129-32.

5180. Morales, A., M. M. Martinez, A. Tasset-Tisseau, E. Rey, F. Baron-Papillon, and A. Follet. 2004. Costs and benefits of influenza vaccination and work productivity in a Colombian company from the employer's perspective. *Value Health* **7:**433-41.

5181. Morales, J. L., L. Huber, S. Gallego, G. Alvarez, J. Diez-Delgado, A. Gonzalez, L. Aguilar, and R. Dal-Re. 1992. A seroepidemiologic study of hepatitis A in Spanish children. Relationship of prevalence to age and socio-environmental factors. *Infection* **20:**194-6.

5182. Mordhorst, C. H., S. P. Wang, and J. T. Grayston. 1992. Outbreak of Chlamydia pneumoniae infection in four farm families. *Eur J Clin Microbiol Infect Dis* **11:**617-20.

5183. Moreillon, P., and Y. A. Que. 2004. Infective endocarditis. *Lancet* **363:**139-49.

5184. Moreira Galvão, M. A., J. S. Dumler, C. Lisias Mafra, S. Berger Calic, C. Buffe Chamone, G. C. Filho, J. P. Olano, and D. A. Walker. 2003. Fatal spotted fever rickettsiosis, Minas Gerais, Brazil. *Emerg Infect Dis* **9:**1402-5.

5185. Morel, P., N. Roubi, X. Bertrand, V. Lapierre, P. Tiberghien, D. Talon, P. Herve, and B. Delbosc. 2003. Bacterial contamination of a cornea tissue bank: implications for the safety of graft engineering. *Cornea* **22:**221-5.

5186. Morelli, R., C. Davoli, P. Vigano, M. C. Perna, and A. Cargnel. 1983. Recente epidemia di malaria da plasmodium falciparum a Milano in tossicodipendenti: un caso di coagulazione intravascolare disseminata. *Giornale di Malattie Infettive e Parassitarie (Siena)* **35:**334-7.

5187. Moren, A., D. Bitar, and I. Navarre. 1991. Epidemiological surveillance among Mozambican refugees in Malawi, 1987-89. *Disasters* **15:**363-72.

5188. Morera, P. 1985. Abdominal angiostrongyliasis: a problem of public health. *Parasitol Today* **1:**173-5.

5189. Morgado, A. F., and J. G. Da Fonte. 1979. An outbreak of hepatitis attributable to inoculation with contaminated gamma globulin. *Bull Pan Am Health Organ* **13:**177-186.

5190. Morgan, D., C. Gunneberg, D. Gunnell, T. D. Healing, S. Lamerton, N. Soltanpoor, D. A. Lewis, and D. G. White. 1994. An outbreak of Campylobacter infection associated with the consumption of unpasteurised milk at a large festival in England. *Eur J Epidemiol* **10:**581-5.

5191. Morgan, D., C. P. Newman, D. N. Hutchinson, A. M. Walker, B. Rowe, and F. Majid. 1993. Verotoxin producing Escherichia coli O 157 infections associated with the consumption of yoghurt. *Epidemiol Infect* **111:**181-7.

5192. Morgan, J., S. L. Bornstein, A. M. Karpati, M. Bruce, C. A. Bolin, C. C. Austin, C. W. Woods, J. Lingappa, C. Langkop, B. Davis, D. R. Graham, M. Proctor, D. A. Ashford, M. Bajani, S. L. Bragg, K. Shutt, B. A. Perkins, and J. W. Tappero. 2002. Outbreak of leptospirosis among triathlon participants and community residents in Springfield, Illinois, 1998. *Clin Infect Dis* **34:**1593-9.

5193. Morgan, J., M. V. Cano, D. R. Feikin, M. Phelan, O. V. Monroy, P. K. Morales, J. Carpenter, A. Weltman, P. G. Spitzer,

H. H. Liu, S. A. Mirza, D. E. Bronstein, D. J. Morgan, L. A. Kirkman, M. E. Brandt, N. Iqbal, M. D. Lindsley, D. W. Warnock, and R. A. Hajjeh. 2003. A large outbreak of histoplasmosis among American travelers associated with a hotel in Acapulco, Mexico, spring 2001. *Am J Trop Med Hyg* **69:**663-9.

5194. Morgan, M. G., H. McKenzie, M. C. Enright, M. Bain, and F. X. Emmanuel. 1992. Use of molecular methods to characterize Moraxella catarrhalis strains in a suspected outbreak of nosocomial infection. *Eur J Clin Microbiol Infect Dis* **11:**305-12.

5195. Morgan, O. 2004. Infectious disease risks from dead bodies following natural disasters. *Rev Panam Salud Publica* **15:**307-12.

5196. Mori, I., K. Matsumoto, K. Sugimoto, M. Kimura, N. Daimon, T. Yokochi, and Y. Kimura. 2002. Prolonged shedding of rotavirus in a geriatric inpatient. *J Med Virol* **67:**613-5.

5197. Mori, S., Y. Hirotsu, A. Mizoguchi, M. Kawabata, F. Nakamura-Uchiyama, Y. Nawa, and M. Osame. 2004. Pulmonary dirofilariasis with serologic study on familial infection with Dirofilaria immitis. *Intern Med* **43:**327-30.

5198. Mori, T., H. Kameda, H. Ogawa, A. Iizuka, N. Sekiguchi, H. Takei, H. Nagasawa, M. Tokuhira, T. Tanaka, Y. Saito, K. Amano, T. Abe, and T. Takeuchi. 2004. Incidence of cytomegalovirus reactivation in patients with inflammatory connective tissue diseases who are under immunosuppressive therapy. *J Rheumatol* **31:**1349-51.

5199. Morissette, I., M. Gourdeau, and J. Francoeur. 1993. CSF shunt infections: a fifteen-year experience with emphasis on management and outcome. *Can J Neurol Sci* **20:**118-22.

5200. Morner, T., and G. Krogh. 1984. An endemic case of tularemia in the mountain hare (Lepus timidus) on the island of Stora Karlso. *Nord Vet Med* **36:**310-3.

5201. Moro, M. L., C. Maffei, E. Manso, G. Morace, L. Polonelli, and F. Biavasco. 1990. Nosocomial outbreak of systemic candidosis associated with parenteral nutrition. *Infect Control Hosp Epidemiol* **11:**27-35.

5202. Moro, M. L., R. Romi, C. Severini, G. P. Casadio, G. Sarta, G. Tampieri, A. Scardovi, and C. Pozzetti. 2002. Patient-to-patient transmission of nosocomial malaria in Italy. *Infect Control Hosp Epidemiol* **23:**338-41.

5203. Moro, P. L., L. Lopera, M. Cabrera, G. Cabrera, B. Silva, R. H. Gilman, and M. H. Moro. 2004. Short report: endemic focus of cystic echinococcosis in a coastal city of Peru. *Am J Trop Med Hyg* **71:**327-9.

5204. Moro, P. L., J. McDonald, R. H. Gilman, B. Silva, M. Verastegui, V. Malqui, G. Lescano, N. Falcon, G. Montes, and H. Bazalar. 1997. Epidemiology of Echinococcus granulosus infection in the central Peruvian Andes. *Bull WHO* **75:**553-61.

5205. Morris, A. 2004. Current epidemiology of pneumocystis pneumonia. *Emerg Infect Dis* **10:**1713-20.

5206. Morris, A., C. B. Beard, and L. Huang. 2002. Update on the epidemiology and transmission of Pneumocystis carinii. *Microbes Infect* **4:**95-103.

5207. Morris, A., M. G. Strickett, and B. G. Barratt-Boyes. 1990. Use of aortic valve allografts from hepatitis B surface antigen-positive donors. *Ann Thorac Surg* **49:**802-5.

5208. Morris, D. O., K. O'Shea, F. S. Shofer, and S. Rankin. 2005. Malassezia pachydermatis carriage in dog owners. *Emerg Infect Dis* **11:**83-8.

5209. Morris, J. G. 2003. Cholera and other types of vibriosis: a story of human pandemics and oysters on the half shell. *Clin Infect Dis* **37:**272-80.

5210. Morris-Cunnington, M. C., W. J. Edmunds, E. Miller, and D. W. Brown. 2004. A population-based seroprevalence study of hepatitis A virus using oral fluid in England and Wales. *Am J Epidemiol* **159:**786-94.

5211. Morrison, A. J. 1984. Epidemiology of infections due to Pseudomonas aeruginosa. *Rev Infect Dis* **6 suppl 3:**S627-S642.

5212. Morrison, C. S., C. Sekadde-Kigondu, S. K. Sinei, D. H. Weiner, C. Kwok, and D. Kokonya. 2001. Is the intrauterine device appropriate contraception for HIV-1-infected women? *BJOG* **108:**784-90.

5213. Morrison, P. 1999. HIV and infant feeding: to breastfeed or not to breastfeed: the dilemma of competing risks. Part 2. *Breastfeed Rev* **7:**11-20.

5214. Morse, D. L., M. A. Gordon, T. Matte, and G. Eadie. 1985. An outbreak of histoplasmosis in a prison. *Am J Epidemiol* **122:**253-61.

5215. Morse, D. L., M. Shayegani, and R. J. Gallo. 1984. Epidemiologic investigation of a Yersinia camp outbreak linked to a food handler. *Am J Public Health* **74:**589-92.

5216. Morse, E. V., P. M. Simon, H. J. Osofsky, P. M. Balson, and H. R. Gaumer. 1991. The male street prostitute: a vector for transmission of HIV infection into the heterosexual world. *Soc Sci Med* **32:**535-9.

5217. Morse, L. J., J. A. Bryan, J. P. Hurley, J. F. Murphy, T. F. O'Brien, and W. E. Wacker. 1972. The Holy Cross college football team hepatitis outbreak. *JAMA* **219:**706-8.

5218. Morsy, T. A., M. A. al Dakhil, and A. F. el Bahrawy. 1997. Characterization of Leishmania aethiopica from rock hyrax, Procavia capensis trapped in Najran, Saudi Arabia. *J Egypt Soc Parasitol* **27:**349-53.

5219. Mortier, E., J. Pouchot, P. Bossi, and V. Molinie. 1995. Maternal-fetal transmission of Pneumocystis carinii in human immunodeficiency virus infection. *N Engl J Med* **332:**825.

5220. Mortimer, P. P. 1999. Mr N the milker, and Dr Koch's concept of the healthy carrier. *Lancet* **353:**1354-6.

5221. Morvan, J. M., E. Nakoune, V. Deubel, and M. Colyn. 2000. [Forest ecosystems and Ebola virus]. *Bull Soc Pathol Exot* **93:**172-5.

5222. Moscicki, A. B., N. Hills, S. Shiboski, K. Powell, N. Jay, E. Hanson, S. Miller, L. Clayton, S. Farhat, J. Broering, T. Darragh, and J. Palefsky. 2001. Risks for incident human papillomavirus infection and low-grade squamous intraepithelial lesion development in young females. *JAMA* **285:**2995-3002.

5223. Moser, M. R., T. R. Bender, H. S. Margolis, G. R. Noble, A. P. Kendal, and D. G. Ritter. 1979. An outbreak of influenza aboard a commercial airliner. *Am J Epidemiol* **110:**1-6.

5224. Moses, J. S., C. Balachandran, S. Sandhanam, N. Ratnasamay, S. Thanappan, J. Rajaswar, and D. Moses. 1990. Ocular rhinosporidiosis in Tamil Nadu, India. *Mycopathologia* **111:**5-8.

5225. Mosley, J. W., M. J. Nowicki, C. K. Kasper, E. Donegan, L. M. Aledort, M. W. Hilgartner, and E. A. Operskalski. 1994. Hepatitis A virus transmission by blood products in the United States. Transfusion Safety Study Group. *Vox Sang* **67 Suppl 1:**24-8.

5226. **Moss, A. R., J. A. Hahn, J. P. Tulsky, C. L. Daley, P. M. Small, and P. C. Hopewell.** 2000. Tuberculosis in the homeless. A prospective study. *Am J Respir Crit Care Med* **162:**460-4.

5227. **Moss, D. M., S. N. Bennett, M. J. Arrowood, S. P. Wahlquist, and P. J. Lammie.** 1998. Enzyme-linked immunoelectrotransfer blot analysis of a cryptosporidiosis outbreak on a United States Coast Guard cutter. *Am J Trop Med Hyg* **58:**110-8.

5228. **Mossong, J., and C. P. Muller.** 2000. Estimation of the basic reproduction number of measles during an outbreak in a partially vaccinated population. *Epidemiol Infect* **124:**273-8.

5229. **Most, H.** 1973. Plasmodium cynomolgi malaria: accidental human infection. *Am J Trop Med Hyg* **22:**157-8.

5230. **Mostad, S. B., J. K. Kreiss, A. Ryncarz, B. Chohan, K. Mandaliya, J. Ndinya-Achola, J. J. Bwayo, and L. Corey.** 2000. Cervical shedding of herpes simplex virus and cytomegalovirus throughout the menstrual cycle in women infected with human immunodeficiency virus type 1. *Am J Obstet Gynecol* **183:**948-55.

5231. **Mothiron, C., M. Alemanni, G. Manigand, P. Bouree, P. Renaudin, and J. Taillandier.** 1990. [Malaria after a stay in Guadeloupe]. *Presse Med* **19:**1504.

5232. **Motiwala, A. S., M. Strother, A. Amonsin, B. Byrum, S. A. Naser, J. R. Stabel, W. P. Shulaw, J. P. Bannantine, V. Kapur, and S. Sreevatsan.** 2003. Molecular epidemiology of Mycobacterium avium subsp. paratuberculosis: evidence for limited strain diversity, strain sharing, and identification of unique targets for diagnosis. *J Clin Microbiol* **41:**2015-26.

5233. **Mouchet, J., T. Giacomini, and J. Julvez.** 1995. [Human diffusion of arthropod disease vectors throughout the world]. *Sante* **5:**293-8.

5234. **Moyou-Somo, R., M. Antoine Ouambe, E. Fon, and J. Bema.** 2003. Enquête sur la filariose lymphatique dans sept villages du district de santé de Bonassama dans l'estuaire du Wouri, province du littoral, Cameroun. *Med Trop* **63:**583-6.

5235. **Moyou-Somo, R., and D. Tagni-Zukam.** 2003. La paragonimose au Cameroun: tableaux radio-cliniques et évolution sous traitement. *Med Trop* **63:**163-7.

5236. **MSF (Médecins Sans Frontières).** 1997. Refugee health. An approach to emergency situations. Macmillan Education Ltd, London.

5237. **Muder, R. R., R. V. Aghababian, M. B. Loeb, J. A. Solot, and M. Higbee.** 2004. Nursing home-acquired pneumonia: an emergency department treatment algorithm. *Curr Med Res Opin* **20:**1309-20.

5238. **Muehlen, M., J. Heukelbach, T. Wilcke, B. Winter, H. Mehlhorn, and H. Feldmeier.** 2003. Investigations on the biology, epidemiology, pathology and control of Tunga penetrans in Brazil II. Prevalence, parasite load and topographic distribution of lesions in the population of a traditional fishing village. *Parasitol Res* **27:**27.

5239. **Mueller, I., P. Namuigi, J. Kundi, R. Ivivi, T. Tandrapah, S. Bjorge, and J. C. Reeder.** 2005. Epidemic Malaria in the Highlands of Papua New Guinea. *Am J Trop Med Hyg* **72:**554-560.

5240. **Muennig, P., D. Pallin, C. Challah, and K. Khan.** 2004. The cost-effectiveness of ivermectin vs. albendazole in the presumptive treatment of strongyloidiasis in immigrants to the United States. *Epidemiol Infect* **132:**1055-63.

5241. **Muhlenberg, W.** 1993. [Fatal travel-associated legionella infection caused by shower aerosols in a German hotel]. *Gesundheitswesen* **55:**653-6.

5242. **Mujica, O. J., R. E. Quick, A. M. Palacios, L. Beingolea, R. Vargas, D. Moreno, T. J. Barrett, N. H. Bean, L. Seminario, and R. V. Tauxe.** 1994. Epidemic cholera in the Amazon: the role of produce in disease risk and prevention. *J Infect Dis* **169:**1381-4.

5243. **Mulhall, B. P.** 1993. Sexually transmissible diseases and travel. *Br Med Bull* **49:**394-411.

5244. **Mulhall, B. P., G. Hart, and C. Harcourt.** 1995. Sexually transmitted diseases in Australia: a decade of change. Epidemiology and surveillance. *Ann Acad Med Singapore* **24:**569-78.

5245. **Mulhall, B. P., M. Hu, M. Thompson, F. Lin, D. Lupton, D. Mills, M. Maund, R. Cass, and D. Millar.** 1993. Planned sexual behaviour of young Australian visitors to Thailand. *Med J Aust* **158:**530-5.

5246. **Mulholland, K.** 1995. Cholera in Sudan: an account of an epidemic in a refugee camp in eastern Sudan, May-June 1985. *Disasters* **9:**247-58.

5247. **Mulin, B., P. Bailly, M. Thouverez, V. Cailleaux, and C. Cornette.** 1999. Clinical and molecular epidemiology of hospital Enterococcus faecalis isolates in eastern France. *Clin Microbiol Infect* **5:**149-157.

5248. **Muller, A., R. Bialek, A. Kamper, G. Fatkenheuer, B. Salzberger, and C. Franzen.** 2001. Detection of microsporidia in travelers with diarrhea. *J Clin Microbiol* **39:**1630-2.

5249. **Muller, H. E.** 1990. Listeria isolations from feces of patients with diarrhea and from healthy food handlers. *Infection* **18:**97-9.

5250. **Muller, H. E.** 1999. [Real and irrelevant risks of infection by swimming in recreational bodies of water]. *Gesundheitswesen* **61:**473-6; discussion 477-9.

5251. **Müller, J., and A. Polak.** 2003. Classification and taxonomy of fungi pathogenic for warm-blooded hosts, p. 1-248. In E. Jucker (ed.), Antifungal agents - advances and problems. Birkhäuser Verlag, Basel.

5252. **Müller-Pebody, B., W. J. Edmunds, M. C. Zambon, N. J. Gay, and N. S. Crowcroft.** 2002. Contribution of RSV to bronchiolitis and pneumonia-associated hospitalizations in English children, April 1995-March 1998. *Epidemiol Infect* **129:**99-106.

5253. **Munckhof, W. J., M. L. Grayson, and J. D. Turnidge.** 1995. Malaria acquired in Bali. *Med J Aust* **162:**223.

5254. **Mundorff, M. B., P. Gesteland, M. Haddad, and R. Rolfs.** 2004. Syndromic surveillance using chief complaints from urgent-care facilities during the Salt Lake 2002 Olympic winter games. *MMWR* **53 (suppl):**254.

5255. **Mungai, M., G. Tegtmeier, M. Chamberland, and M. Parise.** 2001. Transfusion-transmitted malaria in the United States from 1963 through 1999. *N Engl J Med* **344:**1973-8.

5256. **Mungthin, M., R. Suwannasaeng, T. Naaglor, W. Areekul, and S. Leelayoova.** 2001. Asymptomatic intestinal microsporidiosis in Thai orphans and child-care workers. *Trans R Soc Trop Med Hyg* **95:**304-6.

5257. **Münnich, D., and M. Lakatos.** 1979. Clinical, epidemiological and therapeutical experience with human tularaemia. *Infection* **7:**61-3.

5258. **Munnoch, S. A., R. H. Ashbolt, D. J. Coleman, N. Walton, M. Y. Beers-Deeble, and R. Taylor.** 2004. A multi-jurisdictional outbreak of hepatitis A related to a youth camp -

implications for catering operations and mass gatherings. *Commun Dis Intell* **28**:521-7.

5259. **Muñoz, N., F. X. Bosch, S. de Sanjosé, R. Herrero, X. Castellsague, K. V. Shah, P. J. Snijders, and C. J. Meijer.** 2003. Epidemiological classification of human papillomavirus types associated with cervical cancer. *N Engl J Med* **348**:518-27.

5260. **Munoz, P., C. Rodriguez, and E. Bouza.** 2005. Mycobacterium tuberculosis infection in recipients of solid organ transplants. *Clin Infect Dis* **40**:581-7.

5261. **Munoz, R., T. J. Coffey, M. Daniels, C. G. Dowson, G. Laible, J. Casal, R. Hakenbeck, M. Jacobs, J. M. Musser, B. G. Spratt, et al.** 1991. Intercontinental spread of a multiresistant clone of serotype 23F Streptococcus pneumoniae. *J Infect Dis* **164**:302-6.

5262. **Muraca, P. W., J. E. Stout, V. L. Yu, and Y. C. Yee.** 1988. Legionnaires' disease in the work environment: implications for environmental health. *Am Ind Hyg Assoc J* **49**:584-90.

5263. **Murase, T., M. Yamada, T. Muto, A. Matsushima, and S. Yamai.** 2000. Fecal excretion of Salmonella enterica serovar typhimurium following a food-borne outbreak. *J Clin Microbiol* **38**:3495-7.

5264. **Murata, T., T. Iida, Y. Shiomi, K. Tagomori, Y. Akeda, I. Yanagihara, S. Mushiake, F. Ishiguro, and T. Honda.** 2001. A large outbreak of foodborne infection attributed to Providencia alcalifaciens. *J Infect Dis* **184**:1050-5.

5265. **Murdoch, D. R.** 2003. Diagnosis of Legionella infection. *Clin Infect Dis* **36**:64-9.

5266. **Murdoch, M. E., M. C. Asuzu, M. Hagan, W. H. Makunde, P. Ngoumou, K. F. Ogbuagu, D. Okello, G. Ozoh, and J. Remme.** 2002. Onchocerciasis: the clinical and epidemiological burden of skin disease in Africa. *Ann Trop Med Parasitol* **96**:283-96.

5267. **Murgue, B., S. Murri, H. Triki, V. Deubel, and H. G. Zeller.** 2001. West Nile in the Mediterranean basin: 1950-2000. *Ann N Y Acad Sci* **951**:117-26.

5268. **Murhekar, M. V., K. M. Murhekar, V. A. Arankalle, and S. C. Sehgal.** 2005. Hepatitis delta virus infection among the tribes of the Andaman and Nicobar Islands, India. *Trans R Soc Trop Med Hyg* **99**:483-4.

5269. **Muro, A., C. Genchi, M. Cordero, and F. Simon.** 1999. Human dirofilariasis in the European Union. *Parasitol Today* **15**:386-9.

5270. **Murph, J. R., I. E. Souza, J. D. Dawson, P. Benson, S. J. Petheram, D. Pfab, A. Gregg, M. E. O'Neill, B. Zimmerman, and J. F. Bale, Jr.** 1998. Epidemiology of congenital cytomegalovirus infection: maternal risk factors and molecular analysis of cytomegalovirus strains. *Am J Epidemiol* **147**:940-7.

5271. **Murphy, E. L., J. P. Figueroa, W. N. Gibbs, M. Holding-Cobham, B. Cranston, K. Malley, A. J. Bodner, S. S. Alexander, and W. A. Blattner.** 1991. Human T-lymphotropic virus type I (HTLV-I) seroprevalence in JAMAica. I. Demographic determinants. *Am J Epidemiol* **133**:1114-24.

5272. **Murphy, M. F., and D. H. Phamphilon.** 2001. Practical transfusion medicine. Blackwell Science Ltd, Oxford.

5273. **Murray, A. G., C. D. Busby, and D. W. Bruno.** 2003. Infectious pancreatic necrosis virus in Scottish Atlantic salmon farms, 1996-2001. *Emerg Infect Dis* **9**:455-60.

5274. **Murray, D. L.** 1990. International adoptees and hepatitis B virus infection. *Am J Dis Child* **144**:523-4.

5275. **Murray, H. W.** 2002. Kala-azar - Progress against a neglected disease. *N Engl J Med* **347**:1793-4.

5276. **Murray, J., D. A. McFarland, and R. J. Waldman.** 1998. Cost-effectiveness of oral cholera vaccine in a stable refugee population at risk for epidemic cholera and in a population with endemic cholera. *Bull WHO* **76**:343-52.

5277. **Murray, K., P. Selleck, P. Hooper, A. Hyatt, A. Gould, L. Gleeson, H. Westbury, L. Hiley, L. Selvey, and B. Rodwell.** 1995. A morbillivirus that caused fatal disease in horses and humans. *Science* **268**:94-7.

5278. **Murray, K. F., L. P. Richardson, C. Morishima, J. W. Owens, and D. R. Gretch.** 2003. Prevalence of hepatitis C virus infection and risk factors in an incarcerated juvenile population: a pilot study. *Pediatrics* **111**:153-7.

5279. **Murrell, K. D., R. J. Lichtenfels, D. S. Zarlenga, and E. Pozio.** 2000. The systematics of the genus Trichinella with a key to species. *Vet Parasitol* **93**:293-307.

5280. **Murrell, T. G., L. Roth, J. Egerton, J. Samels, and P. D. Walker.** 1966. Pig-bel: enteritis necroticans. A study in diagnosis and management. *Lancet* **1**:217-22.

5281. **Mushatt, D. M., P. Wattanamano, and F. S. Alvarado.** 1998. Lepromatous leprosy in a renal transplant recipient. *Clin Infect Dis* **26**:217-8.

5282. **Musher, D. M.** 2003. How contagious are common respiratory tract infections? *N Engl J Med* **348**:1256-66.

5283. **Musher, D. M., J. E. Groover, M. R. Reichler, F. X. Riedo, B. Schwartz, D. A. Watson, R. E. Baughn, and R. F. Breiman.** 1997. Emergence of antibody to capsular polysaccharides of Streptococcus pneumoniae during outbreaks of pneumonia: association with nasopharyngeal colonization. *Clin Infect Dis* **24**:441-6.

5284. **Mustaffa-Babjee, A., A. L. Ibrahim, and T. S. Khim.** 1976. A case of human infection with Newcastle disease virus. *Southeast Asian J Trop Med Public Health* **7**:622-4.

5285. **Mutalib, A. A., J. M. King, and P. L. McDonough.** 1993. Erysipelas in caged laying chickens and suspected erysipeloid in animal caretakers. *J Vet Diagn Invest* **5**:198-201.

5286. **Mutanda, L. N., and M. A. Mufson.** 1974. Hepatitis B antigenemia in remote tribes of northern Kenya, northern Liberia, and northern Rhodesia. *J Infect Dis* **130**:406-8.

5287. **Mutero, C. M., C. Kabutha, V. Kimani, L. Kabuage, G. Gitau, J. Ssennyonga, J. Githure, L. Muthami, A. Kaida, L. Musyoka, E. Kiarie, and M. Oganda.** 2004. A transdisciplinary perspective on the links between malaria and agroecosystems in Kenya. *Acta Trop* **89**:171-86.

5288. **Muyembe-Tamfum, J. J., M. Kipasa, C. Kiyungu, and R. Colebunders.** 1999. Ebola outbreak in Kikwit, Democratic Republic of the Congo: discovery and control measures. *J Infect Dis* **179 Suppl 1**:S259-62.

5289. **Muyldermans, G., F. de Smet, D. Pierard, L. Steenssens, D. Stevens, A. Bougatef, and S. Lauwers.** 1998. Neonatal infections with Pseudomonas aeruginosa associated with a waterbath used to thaw fresh frozen plasma. *J Hosp Infect* **39**:309-14.

5290. **Mwenye, K. S., S. Siziya, and D. Peterson.** 1996. Factors associated with human anthrax outbreak in the Chikupo and Ngandu villages of Murewa district in Mashonaland East Province, Zimbabwe. *Cent Afr J Med* **42**:312-5.

5291. **Myamba, J., C. A. Maxwell, A. Asidi, and C. F. Curtis.** 2002. Pyrethroid resistance in tropical bedbugs, Cimex hemipterus, associated with use of treated bednets. *Med Vet Entomol* **16:**448-51.

5292. **Myatt, T. A., S. L. Johnston, Z. Zuo, M. Wand, T. Kebadze, S. Rudnick, and D. K. Milton.** 2004. Detection of airborne rhinovirus and its relation to outdoor air supply in office environments. *Am J Respir Crit Care Med* **169:**1187-90.

5293. **Myers, M. G.** 1978. Longitudinal evaluation of neonatal nosocomial infections: association of infection with a blood pressure cuff. *Pediatrics* **61:**42-5.

5294. **Myles, O., G. Wortmann, R. Barthel, C. Ockenhouse, R. Gasser, P. Weina, S. Patel, N. Crum, H. Groff, and B. L. Herwaldt.** 2004. Two cases of visceral leishmaniasis in U.S. military personnel - Afghanistan, 2002-2004. *MMWR* **53:**265-8.

5295. **Mylonakis, E., B. P. Dickinson, M. D. Mileno, T. Flanigan, F. J. Schiffman, A. Mega, and J. D. Rich.** 1999. Persistent parvovirus B19 related anemia of seven years' duration in an HIV-infected patient: complete remission associated with highly active antiretroviral therapy. *Am J Hematol* **60:**164-6.

5296. **Mylonakis, E., N. Goes, R. H. Rubin, A. B. Cosimi, R. B. Colvin, and J. A. Fishman.** 2001. BK virus in solid organ transplant recipients: an emerging syndrome. *Transplantation* **72:**1587-92.

5297. **Mylotte, J. M.** 2002. Nursing home-acquired pneumonia. *Clin Infect Dis* **35:**1205-11.

5298. **Myrvang, B., and B. von der Lippe.** 2002. [African trypanosomiasis—a rare imported disease]. *Tidsskr Nor Laegeforen* **122:**33-4.

5299. **N'Goran, E. K., S. Diabate, J. Utzinger, and B. Sellin.** 1997. Changes in human schistosomiasis levels after the construction of two large hydroelectric dams in central Côte d'Ivoire. *Bull WHO* **75:**541-5.

5300. **Na-Ngam, N., S. Angkititakul, P. Noimay, and V. Thamlikitkul.** 2004. The effect of quicklime (calcium oxide) as an inhibitor of Burkholderia pseudomallei. *Trans R Soc Trop Med Hyg* **98:**337-41.

5301. **Naaber, P., K. Klaus, E. Sepp, B. Bjorksten, and M. Mikelsaar.** 1997. Colonization of infants and hospitalized patients with Clostridium difficile and Lactobacilli. *Clin Infect Dis* **25 Suppl 2:**S189-90.

5302. **Naber, K. G.** 2003. Prudent use of antibiotic therapy in nosocomial urinary tract infections. *Antibiotics Chemotherapy* **7:**10-11.

5303. **Nabeth, P., D. O. Cheikh, B. Lo, O. Faye, I. O. Vall, M. Niang, B. Wague, D. Diop, M. Diallo, B. Diallo, O. M. Diop, and F. Simon.** 2004. Crimean-Congo hemorrhagic fever, Mauritania. *Emerg Infect Dis* **10:**2143-9.

5304. **Nabeth, P., Y. Kane, M. O. Abdalahi, M. Diallo, K. Ndiaye, K. Ba, F. Schneegans, A. A. Sall, and C. Mathiot.** 2001. Rift valley fever outbreak, Mauritania, 1998: seroepidemiologic, virologic, entomologic, and zoologic investigations. *Emerg Infect Dis* **7:**1052-4.

5305. **Nabeth, P., B. Lo, O. Faye, D. Diop, O. Diop, I. Ould Mohammed Vall, A. Ould Abba, F. Simon, and D. Ould Cheikh.** 2003. Urban outbreak of Crimean-Congo haemorrhagic fever in Mauritania: epidemiologic, virologic and acarologic investigations. *Am J Trop Med Hyg* **69 (suppl):**236.

5306. **Nacapunchai, D., H. Kino, C. Ruangsittichai, P. Sriwichai, A. Ishih, and M. Terada.** 2001. A brief survey of free-living amebae in Thailand and Hamamatsu District, Japan. *Southeast Asian J Trop Med Public Health* **32 Suppl 2:**179-82.

5307. **Nadal, D., W. Wunderli, H. Briner, and K. Hansen.** 1989. Prevalence of antibodies to Borrelia burgdorferi in forestry workers and blood donors from the same region in Switzerland. *Eur J Clin Microbiol Infect Dis* **8:**992-5.

5308. **Nadala, D., W. Bossart, F. Zucol, F. Steiner, C. Berger, U. Lips, and M. Altwegg.** 2001. Community-acquired pneumonia in children due to Mycoplasma pneumoniae: diagnostic performance of a seminested 16S rDNA-PCR. *Diagn Microbiol Infect Dis* **39:**15-9.

5309. **Nafziger, D. A., T. Lundstrom, S. Chandra, and R. M. Massanari.** 1997. Infection control in ambulatory care. *Infect Dis Clin North Am* **11:**279-96.

5310. **Nagakura, K., H. Tachibana, Y. Kaneda, and Y. Kato.** 1989. Toxocariasis possibly caused by ingesting raw chicken. *J Infect Dis* **160:**735-6.

5311. **Nagakura, K., H. Tachibana, T. Tanaka, Y. Kaneda, M. Tokunaga, M. Sasao, and T. Takeuchi.** 1989. An outbreak of amebiasis in an institution for the mentally retarded in Japan. *Jpn J Med Sci Biol* **42:**63-76.

5312. **Nagore, E., P. Ramos, R. Botella-Estrada, J. A. Ramos-Niguez, O. Sanmartin, and P. Castejon.** 2001. Cutaneous infection with Mycobacterium fortuitum after localized microinjections (mesotherapy) treated successfully with a triple drug regimen. *Acta Derm Venereol* **81:**291-3.

5313. **Nahimana, A., M. Rabodonirina, G. Zanetti, I. Meneau, P. Francioli, J. Bille, and P. M. Hauser.** 2003. Association between a specific Pneumocystis jiroveci dihydropteroate synthase mutation and failure of pyrimethamine/sulfadoxine prophylaxis in human immunodeficiency virus-positive and -negative patients. *J Infect Dis* **188:**1017-23.

5314. **Nahimana, I., L. Gern, D. S. Blanc, G. Praz, P. Francioli, and O. Peter.** 2004. Risk of Borrelia burgdorferi infection in western Switzerland following a tick bite. *Eur J Clin Microbiol Infect Dis* **23:**603-8.

5315. **Nahmias, A. J., F. K. Lee, and S. Beckman-Nahmias.** 1990. Sero-epidemiological and -sociological patterns of herpes simplex virus infection in the world. *Scand J Infect Dis Suppl* **69:**19-36.

5316. **Naik, S. R., R. Aggarwal, P. N. Salunke, and N. N. Mehrotra.** 1992. A large waterborne viral hepatitis E epidemic in Kanpur, India. *Bull WHO* **70:**597-604.

5317. **Naimi, T. S., J. H. Wicklund, S. J. Olsen, G. Krause, J. G. Wells, J. M. Bartkus, D. J. Boxrud, M. Sullivan, H. Kassenborg, J. M. Besser, E. D. Mintz, M. T. Osterholm, and C. W. Hedberg.** 2003. Concurrent outbreaks of Shigella sonnei and enterotoxigenic Escherichia coli infections associated with parsley: implications for surveillance and control of foodborne illness. *J Food Prot* **66:**535-41.

5318. **Najioullah, F., F. Tissot Guerraz, D. Thouvenot, M. P. Milon, A. Lachaux, and D. Floret.** 2004. [Nosocomial infections due to adenovirus in a paediatric unit]. *Pathol Biol (Paris)* **52:**16-20.

5319. **Nakagawa, J., K. Hashimoto, C. Cordon-Rosales, J. Abraham Juarez, R. Trampe, and L. Marroquin Marroquin.** 2003. The impact of vector control on Triatoma dimidiata in the Guatemalan department of Jutiapa. *Ann Trop Med Parasitol* **97:**288-97.

5320. **Nakagawa, M., S. Izumo, S. Ijichi, H. Kubota, K. Arimura, M. Kawabata, and M. Osame.** 1995. HTLV-I-associated myelopathy: analysis of 213 patients based on clinical features and laboratory findings. *J Neurovirol* **1:**50-61.

5321. **Nakajima, N., T. Matsuda, T. Ono, H. Murakami, T. Tokutake, C. Matsumiya, S. Tateyama, A. Honjo, T. Katsuta, T. Nakayama, and T. Kato.** 2003. Measles outbreak in a suburb of Tokyo, Japan, in 1998-1999. *Scand J Infect Dis* **35**:495-7.

5322. **Nakamura, H., H. Yagyu, K. Kishi, F. Tsuchida, S. Oh-Ishi, K. Yamaguchi, and T. Matsuoka.** 2003. A large outbreak of Legionnaires' disease due to an inadequate circulating and filtration system for bath water—epidemiologic manifestations. *Intern Med* **42**:806-11.

5323. **Nakamura, M. M., K. L. Rohling, M. Shashaty, H. Lu, Y. W. Tang, and K. M. Edwards.** 2002. Prevalence of methicillin-resistant Staphylococcus aureus nasal carriage in the community pediatric population. *Pediatr Infect Dis J* **21**:917-22.

5324. **Nakamura, Y., Y. Obase, N. Suyama, Y. Miyazaki, H. Ohno, M. Oka, M. Takahashi, and S. Kohno.** 2004. A small outbreak of pulmonary tuberculosis in non-close contact patrons of a bar. *Intern Med* **43**:263-7.

5325. **Nakamura, Y., M. Watanabe, K. Nagoshi, T. Kitamoto, T. Sato, M. Yamada, H. Mizusawa, R. Maddox, J. Sejvar, E. Belay, and L. B. Schonberger.** 2003. Update: Creutzfeldt-Jakob disease associated with cadaveric dura mater grafts - Japan, 1979-2003. *MMWR* **52**:1179-81.

5326. **Nakamura-Uchiyama, F., E. Yamasaki, and Y. Nawa.** 2002. One confirmed and six suspected cases of cutaneous larva migrans caused by overseas infection with dog hookworm larvae. *J Dermatol* **29**:104-11.

5327. **Nakanishi, Y., Y. Oyama, M. Takahashi, and T. Mori.** 1997. [A molecular epidemiological analysis of several outbreaks of tuberculosis in public saunas. A problem of tuberculosis among homeless people in the metropolitan area]. *Nippon Koshu Eisei Zasshi* **44**:769-78.

5328. **Nakano, T., T. Ihara, and H. Kamiya.** 2002. Measles outbreak among non-immunized children in a Japanese hospital. *Scand J Infect Dis* **34**:426-9.

5329. **Nakano, T., K. Murata, Y. Ikeda, and H. Hasegawa.** 2003. Growth of Enterobius vermicularis in a chimpanzee after anthelmintic treatment. *J Parasitol* **89**:439-43.

5330. **Nakashima, A. K., M. A. McCarthy, W. J. Martone, and R. L. Anderson.** 1987. Epidemic septic arthritis caused by Serratia marcescens and associated with a benzalkonium chloride antiseptic. *J Clin Microbiol* **25**:1014-8.

5331. **Nakashima, K., S. Kashiwagi, J. Hayashi, A. Noguchi, M. Hirata, W. Kajiyama, K. Urabe, K. Minami, and Y. Maeda.** 1992. Sexual transmission of hepatitis C virus among female prostitutes and patients with sexually transmitted diseases in Fukuoka, Kyushu, Japan. *Am J Epidemiol* **136**:1132-7.

5332. **Nakata, S., S. Honma, K. K. Numata, K. Kogawa, S. Ukae, Y. Morita, N. Adachi, and S. Chiba.** 2000. Members of the family caliciviridae (Norwalk virus and Sapporo virus) are the most prevalent cause of gastroenteritis outbreaks among infants in Japan. *J Infect Dis* **181**:2029-32.

5333. **Nakata, Y., T. Nakayama, Y. Ide, R. Kizu, G. Koinuma, and M. Bamba.** 2002. Measles virus genome detected up to four months in a case of congenital measles. *Acta Paediatr* **91**:1263-5.

5334. **Nakauchi, K.** 1999. The prevalence of Balantidium coli infection in fifty-six mammalian species. *J Vet Med Sci* **61**:63-5.

5335. **Nakelchik, M., and J. E. Mangino.** 2002. Reactivation of histoplasmosis after treatment with infliximab. *Am J Med* **112**:78.

5336. **Nambiar, S., and N. Singh.** 2002. Change in epidemiology of health care-associated infections in a neonatal intensive care unit. *Pediatr Infect Dis J* **21**:839-42.

5337. **Nandi, S., R. Kumar, P. Ray, H. Vohra, and N. K. Ganguly.** 2001. Group A streptococcal sore throat in a periurban population of northern India: a one-year prospective study. *Bull WHO* **79**:528-33.

5338. **Naqvi, S. H., P. Becherer, and S. Gudipati.** 1993. Ketoconazole treatment of a family with zoonotic sporotrichosis. *Scand J Infect Dis* **25**:543-545.

5339. **Narasimham, M. V. V. L., C. K. Rao, M. S. Bendle, R. L. Yadava, Y. C. Johri, and R. S. Pandey.** 1988. Epidemiological investigation on Japanese encephalitis outbreak in Uttar Pradesh during 1988. *J Commun Dis* **20**:263-75.

5340. **Nardi, R., M. Bettini, C. Bozzoli, P. Cenni, F. Ferroni, R. Grimaldi, A. Pezzi, M. Vivoli, D. Salcito, G. Gordini, R. Gambarin, E. Lavezzi, R. Lippi, T. Mazzolani, F. Montecuccoli, D. Prati, N. Simonetti, A. Ugolini, and C. Zen.** 1997. Emergency medical services in mass gatherings: the experience of the Formula 1 Grand Prix 'San Marino' in Imola. *Eur J Emerg Med* **4**:217-23.

5341. **Nardone, A., I. Capek, G. Baranton, C. Campese, D. Postic, V. Vaillant, M. Lienard, and J. C. Desenclos.** 2004. Risk factors for leptospirosis in metropolitan France: results of a national case-control study, 1999-2000. *Clin Infect Dis* **39**:751-3.

5342. **Nasci, R. S., and C. G. Moore.** 1998. Vector-borne disease surveillance and natural disasters. *Emerg Infect Dis* **4**:333-4.

5343. **Nash, B.** 2003. Treating head lice. *BMJ* **326**:1256-7.

5344. **Nash, D., F. Mostashari, A. Fine, J. Miller, D. O'Leary, K. Murray, A. Huang, A. Rosenberg, A. Greenberg, M. Sherman, S. Wong, and M. Layton.** 2001. The outbreak of West Nile virus infection in the New York City area in 1999. *N Engl J Med* **344**:1807-14.

5345. **Nasidi, A., T. P. Monath, K. DeCock, O. Tomori, R. Cordellier, O. D. Olaleye, T. O. Harry, J. A. Adeniyi, A. O. Sorungbe, A. O. Ajose-Coker, et al.** 1989. Urban yellow fever epidemic in western Nigeria, 1987. *Trans R Soc Trop Med Hyg* **83**:401-6.

5346. **Nasser, R. M., A. C. Rahi, M. F. Haddad, Z. Daoud, N. Irani-Hakime, and W. Y. Almawi.** 2004. Outbreak of Burkholderia cepacia bacteremia traced to contaminated hospital water used for dilution of an alcohol skin antiseptic. *Infect Control Hosp Epidemiol* **25**:231-9.

5347. **Nasta, P., A. Donisi, A. Cattane, A. Chiodera, and S. Casari.** 1997. Acute Histoplasmosis in Spelunkers Returning from Mato Grosso, Peru. *J Travel Med* **4**:176-178.

5348. **Natarajaseenivasan, K., M. Boopalan, K. Selvanayaki, S. R. Suresh, and S. Ratnam.** 2002. Leptospirosis among rice mill workers of Salem, South India. *Jpn J Infect Dis* **55**:170-3.

5349. **Nataro, J. P., and J. B. Kaper.** 1998. Diarrheagenic Escherichia coli. *Clin Microbiol Rev* **11**:142-201.

5350. **Naucke, T. J., and C. Schmitt.** 2004. Is leishmaniasis becoming endemic in Germany? *Int J Med Microbiol* **293 Suppl 37**:179-81.

5351. **Navarro Gracia, J. F., M. Pena Fernandez, I. Garcia Abad, M. Gaztambide Ganuza, J. L. Quiles Dura, J. A. Carratala Torregrosa, I. Padilla Navas, and G. Royo Garcia.** 1997. [Tuberculosis outbreak at a public school]. *Rev Clin Esp* **197**:152-7.

5352. **Nawa, Y.** 1991. Historical review and current status of gnathostomiasis in Asia. *Southeast Asian J Trop Med Public Health* **22 Suppl**:217-9.

5353. **Nawa, Y., J. I. Imai, K. Ogata, and K. Otsuka.** 1989. The first record of a confirmed human case of Gnathostoma doloresi infection. *J Parasitol* **75**:166-9.

5354. **Nayak, N., S. K. Gupta, G. V. Murthy, G. Satpathy, and S. Mohanty.** 1996. Community-based investigation of an outbreak of acute viral conjunctivitis in urban slums. *Trop Med Int Health* **1**:667-71.

5355. **Naylor, G. R. E.** 1983. Incubation period and other features of food-borne and water-borne outbreaks of typhoid fever in relation to pathogenesis and genetics of resistance. *Lancet* **1 (April 16)**:864-6.

5356. **Nazarowec-White, M., and J. M. Farber.** 1997. Enterobacter sakazakii: a review. *Int J Food Microbiol* **34**:103-13.

5357. **Nchito, M., P. W. Geissler, L. Mubila, H. Friis, and A. Olsen.** 2004. Effects of iron and multimicronutrient supplementation on geophagy: a two-by-two factorial study among Zambian schoolchildren in Lusaka. *Trans R Soc Trop Med Hyg* **98**:218-27.

5358. **Ndamba, J., N. Makaza, and K. C. Kaondera.** 1991. A cross-sectional study on the prevalence and intensity of schistosomiasis among sugar cane cutters in Zimbabwe. *Cent Afr J Med* **37**:171-5.

5359. **Ndao, M., E. Bandyayera, E. Kokoskin, T. W. Gyorkos, J. D. MacLean, and B. J. Ward.** 2004. Comparison of blood smear, antigen detection, and nested-PCR methods for screening refugees from regions where malaria is endemic after a malaria outbreak in Quebec, Canada. *J Clin Microbiol* **42**:2694-700.

5360. **Ndawula, E. M., and L. Brown.** 1991. Mattresses as reservoirs of epidemic methicillin-resistant Staphylococcus aureus. *Lancet* **337**:488.

5361. **Ndayimirije, N., and M. K. Kindhauser.** 2005. Marburg hemorrhagic fever in Angola—fighting fear and a lethal pathogen. *N Engl J Med* **352**:2155-7.

5362. **Ndiaye, B., M. Develoux, M. A. Langlade, and A. Kane.** 1994. [Actinomycotic mycetoma. Apropos of 27 cases in Dakar; medical treatment with cotrimoxazole]. *Ann Dermatol Venereol* **121**:161-5.

5363. **Ndip, L. M., E. B. Fokam, D. H. Bouyer, R. N. Ndip, V. P. Titanji, D. H. Walker, and J. W. McBride.** 2004. Detection of Rickettsia africae in patients and ticks along the coastal region of Cameroon. *Am J Trop Med Hyg* **71**:363-6.

5364. **Nduati, R., G. John, D. Mbori-Ngacha, B. Richardson, J. Overbaugh, A. Mwatha, J. Ndinya-Achola, J. Bwayo, F. E. Onyango, J. Hughes, and J. Kreiss.** 2000. Effect of breastfeeding and formula feeding on transmission of HIV-1: a randomized clinical trial. *JAMA* **283**:1167-74.

5365. **Nduati, R., B. A. Richardson, G. John, D. Mbori-Ngacha, A. Mwatha, J. Ndinya-Achola, J. Bwayo, F. E. Onyango, and J. Kreiss.** 2001. Effect of breastfeeding on mortality among HIV-1 infected women: a randomised trial. *Lancet* **357**:1651-5.

5366. **Ndyomugyenyi, R., and P. Magnussen.** 2000. Chloroquine prophylaxis, iron/folic-acid supplementation or case management of malaria attacks in primigravidae in western Uganda: effects on congenital malaria and infant haemoglobin concentrations. *Ann Trop Med Parasitol* **94**:759-68; discussion 769-70.

5367. **Neal, K. R., D. J. Irwin, S. Davies, E. B. Kaczmarski, and M. C. Wale.** 1998. Sustained reduction in the carriage of Neisseria meningitidis as a result of a community meningococcal disease control programme. *Epidemiol Infect* **121**:487-93.

5368. **Neal, K. R., J. Nguyen-Van-Tam, P. Monk, S. J. O'Brien, J. Stuart, and M. Ramsay.** 1999. Invasive meningococcal disease among university undergraduates: association with universities providing relatively large amounts of catered hall accommodation. *Epidemiol Infect* **122**:351-7.

5369. **Neal, K. R., J. S. Nguyen-Van-Tam, N. Jeffrey, R. C. Slack, R. J. Madeley, K. Ait-Tahar, K. Job, M. C. Wale, and D. A. Ala'Aldeen.** 2000. Changing carriage rate of Neisseria meningitidis among university students during the first week of term: cross sectional study. *BMJ* **320**:846-9.

5370. **Neal, S., P. Cieslak, K. Hedberg, and D. Fleming.** 1998. African tick-bite fever among international travelers - Oregon, 1998. *MMWR* **47**:950-2.

5371. **Nebreda Mayoral, T., F. J. Merino, J. L. Serrano, P. Fernandez-Soto, A. Encinas, and R. Perez-Sanchez.** 2004. Detection of antibodies to tick salivary antigens among patients from a region of Spain. *Eur J Epidemiol* **19**:79-83.

5372. **Nechwatal, R., W. Ehret, O. J. Klatte, H. J. Zeissler, A. Prull, and H. Lutz.** 1993. Nosocomial outbreak of legionellosis in a rehabilitation center. Demonstration of potable water as a source. *Infection* **21**:235-40.

5373. **Neiger, R., C. Dieterich, A. Burnens, A. Waldvogel, I. Corthesy-Theulaz, F. Halter, B. Lauterburg, and A. Schmassmann.** 1998. Detection and prevalence of Helicobacter infection in pet cats. *J Clin Microbiol* **36**:634-7.

5374. **Neira, P., I. Goecke, and W. González.** 1987. Ectoparasitosis en escolares rurales de la V región - Valparaíso, Chile, 1986. *Bol Chil Parasitol* **42**:87-9.

5375. **Nekpeni, E. B., J. P. Eouzan, and M. Dagnogo.** 1991. [Infection of Glossina palpalis palpalis (Diptera, Glossinidae) by trypanosomes in the forest zone of Gagnoa in the Ivory Coast]. *Trop Med Parasitol* **42**:399-403.

5376. **Nelson, J. D.** 1996. Jails, microbes, and the three-foot barrier. *N Engl J Med* **335**:885-6.

5377. **Neman-Simha, V., H. Renaudin, B. de Barbeyrac, J. J. Leng, J. Horovitz, D. Dallay, C. Billeaud, and C. Bebear.** 1992. Isolation of genital mycoplasms from blood of febrile obstetrical-gynecologic patients and neonates. *Scand J Infect Dis* **24**:317-21.

5378. **Nemes, Z., G. Kiss, E. P. Madarassi, Z. Peterfi, E. Ferenczi, T. Bakonyi, and G. Ternak.** 2004. Nosocomial transmission of dengue. *Emerg Infect Dis* **10**:1880-1.

5379. **Nenoff, P., W. Handrick, and U. F. Haustein.** 2002. [Sports-induced infections—an overview]. *Wien Med Wochenschr* **152**:574-7.

5380. **Neri, M., and R. De Jongh.** 2004. Medical and trauma evacuations. *Clin Occup Environ Med* **4**:85-110, vii.

5381. **Neringer, R., Y. Andersson, and R. Eitrem.** 1987. A waterborne outbreak of giardiasis in Sweden. *Scand J Infect Dis* **19**:85-90.

5382. **Nesbakken, T., K. Eckner, H. K. Hoidal, and O. J. Rotterud.** 2003. Occurrence of Yersinia enterocolitica and Campylobacter spp. in slaughter pigs and consequences for meat inspection, slaughtering, and dressing procedures. *Int J Food Microbiol* **80**:231-4.

5383. **Nessa, K., S. A. Waris, Z. Sultan, S. Monira, M. Hossain, S. Nahar, H. Rahman, M. Alam, P. Baatsen, and M. Rahman.** 2004. Epidemiology and etiology of sexually transmitted infection among hotel-based sex workers in Dhaka, Bangladesh. *J Clin Microbiol* **42**:618-21.

5384. Nesse, L. L., T. Refsum, E. Heir, K. Nordby, T. Vardund, and G. Holstad. 2005. Molecular epidemiology of Salmonella spp. isolated from gulls, fish-meal factories, feed factories, animals and humans in Norway based on pulsed-field gel electrophoresis. *Epidemiol Infect* **133**:53-8.

5385. Neto, E. C. 2004. Newborn screening for congenital infectious diseases. *Emerg Infect Dis* **10**:1068-73.

5386. Neto, E. C., E. Anele, R. Rubim, A. Brites, J. Schulte, D. Becker, and T. Tuuminen. 2000. High prevalence of congenital toxoplasmosis in Brazil estimated in a 3-year prospective neonatal screening study. *Int J Epidemiol* **29**:941-7.

5387. Nett, G., and M. Schar. 1986. [Transmission of Trichomonas vaginalis in swimming pools?]. *Soz Praventivmed* **31**:247-8.

5388. Nettles, R. E., and D. J. Sexton. 1997. Pasteurella multocida prosthetic valve endocarditis: case report and review. *Clin Infect Dis* **25**:920-1.

5389. Nevas, M., S. Hielm, M. Lindstrom, H. Horn, K. Koivulehto, and H. Korkeala. 2002. High prevalence of Clostridium botulinum types A and B in honey samples detected by polymerase chain reaction. *Int J Food Microbiol* **72**:45-52.

5390. Neveling, F. 1988. [Paracoccidioidomycosis infections caused by an adventure vacation in the Amazon]. *Prax Klin Pneumol* **42**:722-5.

5391. Neville, R., J. Stack, and R. D. Gens. 1985. Measles on college campuses - United States, 1985. *MMWR* **34**:445-9.

5392. Newman, B. H. 1997. Donor reactions and injuries from whole blood donation. *Transfus Med Rev* **11**:64-75.

5393. Newman, C. P., S. R. Palmer, F. D. Kirby, and E. O. Caul. 1992. A prolonged outbreak of ornithosis in duck processors. *Epidemiol Infect* **108**:203-10.

5394. Newman, L. M., F. Miguel, B. B. Jemusse, A. C. Macome, and R. D. Newman. 2001. HIV seroprevalence among military blood donors in Manica Province, Mozambique. *Int J STD AIDS* **12**:225-8.

5395. Newman, P. E., R. A. Goodman, G. O. Waring, 3rd, R. J. Finton, L. A. Wilson, J. Wright, and H. D. Cavanagh. 1984. A cluster of cases of Mycobacterium chelonei keratitis associated with outpatient office procedures. *Am J Ophthalmol* **97**:344-8.

5396. Newman, R. D., S. R. Moore, A. A. Lima, J. P. Nataro, R. L. Guerrant, and C. L. Sears. 2001. A longitudinal study of Giardia lamblia infection in north-east Brazilian children. *Trop Med Int Health* **6**:624-34.

5397. Newman, R. D., C. L. Sears, S. R. Moore, J. P. Nataro, T. Wuhib, D. A. Agnew, R. L. Guerrant, and A. A. Lima. 1999. Longitudinal study of Cryptosporidium infection in children in northeastern Brazil. *J Infect Dis* **180**:167-75.

5398. Newman, R. D., T. Wuhib, A. A. Lima, R. L. Guerrant, and C. L. Sears. 1993. Environmental sources of Cryptosporidium in an urban slum in northeastern Brazil. *Am J Trop Med Hyg* **49**:270-5.

5399. Newman, R. D., S. X. Zu, T. Wuhib, A. A. Lima, R. L. Guerrant, and C. L. Sears. 1994. Household epidemiology of Cryptosporidium parvum infection in an urban community in northeast Brazil. *Ann Intern Med* **120**:500-5.

5400. Newman, S. B., M. B. Nelson, C. A. Gaydos, and H. B. Friedman. 2003. Female prisoners' preferences of collection methods for testing for Chlamydia trachomatis and Neisseria gonorrhoeae infection. *Sex Transm Dis* **30**:306-9.

5401. Newsom, D. H., and J. P. Kiwanuka. 2002. Needle-stick injuries in an Ugandan teaching hospital. *Ann Trop Med Parasitol* **96**:517-22.

5402. Newton, J. A., G. A. Schnepf, M. R. Wallace, H. O. Lobel, C. A. Kennedy, and E. C. Oldfield, 3rd. 1994. Malaria in US marines returning from Somalia. *JAMA* **272**:397-9.

5403. Newton, P., S. Proux, M. Green, F. Smithuis, J. Rozendaal, S. Prakongpan, K. Chotivanich, M. Mayxay, S. Looareesuwan, J. Farrar, F. Nosten, and N. J. White. 2001. Fake artesunate in southeast Asia. *Lancet* **357**:1948-50.

5404. Newton, P. N., N. J. White, J. A. Rozendaal, and M. D. Green. 2002. Murder by fake drugs. *BMJ* **324**:800-801.

5405. Ng, D. P., K. T. Goh, M. G. Yeo, and C. L. Poh. 1997. An institutional outbreak of Salmonella enteritidis in Singapore. *Southeast Asian J Trop Med Public Health* **28**:85-90.

5406. Ng, S. K. C. 2003. Possible role of an animal vector in the SARS outbreak at Amoy Gardens. *Lancet* **362**:570-2.

5407. Nguekam, J. P., A. P. Zoli, P. O. Zogo, A. C. Kamga, N. Speybroeck, P. Dorny, J. Brandt, B. Losson, and S. Geerts. 2003. A seroepidemiological study of human cysticercosis in West Cameroon. *Trop Med Int Health* **8**:144-9.

5408. Nguyen, C., and R. G. Lalonde. 1990. Risk of occupational exposure to Herpesvirus simiae (B virus) in Quebec. *CMAJ* **143**:1203-6.

5409. Nguyen, D. M., L. Mascola, and E. Brancoft. 2005. Recurring methicillin-resistant Staphylococcus aureus infections in a football team. *Emerg Infect Dis* **11**:526-32.

5410. Nguyen, T. A., K. Ha Ba, and T. D. Nguyen. 1993. [Typhoid fever in South Vietnam, 1990-1993]. *Bull Soc Pathol Exot* **86(5)**:476-8.

5411. Nguyen, T. V., P. Le Van, C. Le Huy, and A. Weintraub. 2004. Diarrhea caused by rotavirus in children less than 5 years of age in Hanoi, Vietnam. *J Clin Microbiol* **42**:5745-50.

5412. Niang, M., P. Brouqui, and D. Raoult. 1999. Epidemic typhus imported from Algeria. *Emerg Infect Dis* **5**:716-8.

5413. Nichol, K. L., A. Lind, K. L. Margolis, M. Murdoch, R. McFadden, M. Hauge, S. Magnan, and M. Drake. 1995. The effectiveness of vaccination against influenza in healthy, working adults. *N Engl J Med* **333**:889-93.

5414. Nicholls, S., K. Carroll, J. Crofts, E. Ben-Eliezer, J. Paul, M. Zambon, C. A. Joseph, N. Q. Verlander, N. L. Goddard, and J. M. Watson. 2004. Outbreak of influenza A (H3N2) in a highly-vaccinated religious community: a retrospective cohort study. *Commun Dis Public Health* **7**:272-7.

5415. Nichols, G., I. Gillespie, and J. de Louvois. 2000. The microbiological quality of ice used to cool drinks and ready-to-eat food from retail and catering premises in the United Kingdom. *J Food Prot* **63**:78-82.

5416. Nichols, R. A., B. M. Campbell, and H. V. Smith. 2003. Identification of Cryptosporidium spp. oocysts in United Kingdom noncarbonated natural mineral waters and drinking waters by using a modified nested PCR-restriction fragment length polymorphism assay. *Appl Environ Microbiol* **69**:4183-9.

5417. Nichols, W. G., D. D. Erdman, A. Han, C. Zukerman, L. Corey, and M. Boeckh. 2004. Prolonged outbreak of human parainfluenza virus 3 infection in a stem cell transplant outpatient department: insights from molecular epidemiologic analysis. *Biol Blood Marrow Transplant* **10**:58-64.

5418. Nichols, W. G., T. H. Price, T. Gooley, L. Corey, and M. Boeckh. 2003. Transfusion-transmitted cytomegalovirus infection after receipt of leukoreduced blood products. *Blood* **101**:4195-200.

5419. Nicholson, K. G., J. Kent, V. Hammersley, and E. Cancio. 1996. Risk factors for lower respiratory complications of rhinovirus infections in elderly people living in the community: prospective cohort study. *BMJ* **313**:1119-23.

5420. Nicholson, K. G., J. M. Wood, and M. Zambon. 2003. Influenza. *Lancet* **362**:1733-45.

5421. Nickerson, N., J. Linder, D. Friou, K. F. Gensheimer, P. Kuehnert, D. Hubert, S. Gunston, L. Crinion, K. Ijaz, D. Ruggiero, B. Metchock, L. Diem, L. Cowan, H. Dale, L. Simmons, and V. Gammino. 2003. Tuberculosis outbreak in a homeless population - Portland, Maine, 2002-2003. *MMWR* **52**:1184-5.

5422. Nicolas, L., and G. A. Scoles. 1997. Multiplex polymerase chain reaction for detection of Dirofilaria immitis (Filariidea: Onchocercidae) and Wuchereria bancrofti (Filarioidea: Dipetalonematidae) in their common vector Aedes polynesiensis (Diptera: Culicidae). *J Med Entomol* **34**:741-4.

5423. Nicolas, X., F. Nicolas, O. Gorge, J. L. Perret, and J. E. Touze. 1997. [Malaria in expatriates in Africa. 154 cases. Clinical problems and therapeutic difficulties]. *Presse Med* **26**:158-60.

5424. Nicoletti, P. 2002. A short history of brucellosis. *Vet Microbiol* **90**:5-9.

5425. Nicoll, A., B. Evans, N. Asgari, S. Hahne, E. Johnson, B. A. Jinadu, R. Talbot, S. B. Werner, and D. Vugia. 2001. Coccidioidomycosis among persons attending the world championship of model airplane flying - Kern county, California, October 2001. *MMWR* **50**:1106-1107.

5426. Nicoll, A., and O. N. Gill. 1999. The global impact of HIV infection and disease. *Commun Dis Public Health* **2**:85-95.

5427. Nicolle, L. E. 2001. Preventing infections in non-hospital settings: long-term care. *Emerg Infect Dis* **7**:205-7.

5428. Nielsen, B., and H. C. Wegener. 1997. Public health and pork and pork products: regional perspectives of Denmark. *Rev Sci Tech* **16**:513-24.

5429. Nielsen, H. E., V. Siersma, S. Andersen, B. Gahrn-Hansen, C. H. Mordhorst, B. Norgaard-Pedersen, B. Roder, T. L. Sorensen, R. Temme, and B. F. Vestergaard. 2003. Respiratory syncytial virus infection—risk factors for hospital admission: a case-control study. *Acta Paediatr* **92**:1314-21.

5430. Nielsen, N. J., O. Lindhardt, and K. Ulrich. 1987. HIV antibodies in Danish Volunteer Service personnel in Kenya, Tanzania, and Zambia. *Trans R Soc Trop Med Hyg* **81**.

5431. Nifong, T. P., W. C. Ehmann, J. A. Mierski, R. E. Domen, and W. B. Rybka. 2003. Favorable outcome after infusion of coagulase-negative staphylococci- contaminated peripheral blood hematopoietic cells for autologous transplantation. *Arch Pathol Lab Med* **127**:e19-21.

5432. Niizeki, K., O. Kano, and Y. Kondo. 1984. An epidemic study of molluscum contagiosum. Relationship to swimming. *Dermatologica* **169**:197-8.

5433. Niklasson, B., and R. Eitrem. 1985. Sandfly fever among Swedish UN troops in Cyprus. *Lancet* **1**:1212-3.

5434. Niklasson, B., M. Jonsson, I. Widegren, K. Persson, and J. LeDuc. 1992. A study of nephropathia epidemica among military personnel in Sweden. *Res Virol* **143**:211-4.

5435. Niklasson, B., J. M. Meegan, and E. Bengtsson. 1979. Antibodies to Rift Valley fever virus in Swedish U.N. soldiers in Egypt and the Sinai. *Scand J Infect Dis* **11**:313-4.

5436. Nikolic, N., I. Poljak, and B. Troselj-Vukic. 2000. Malaria, a travel health problem in the maritime community. *J Travel Med* **7**:309-13.

5437. Nilsson, K., O. Lindquist, A. J. Liu, T. G. Jaenson, G. Friman, and C. Pahlson. 1999. Rickettsia helvetica in Ixodes ricinus ticks in Sweden. *J Clin Microbiol* **37**:400-3.

5438. Nilsson, P., and M. H. Laurell. 2001. Carriage of penicillin-resistant Streptococcus pneumoniae by children in day-care centers during an intervention program in Malmo, Sweden. *Pediatr Infect Dis J* **20**:1144-9.

5439. Nimri, L. F., and S. Hijazi. 1996. Rotavirus-associated diarrhoea in children in a refugee camp in Jordan. *J Diarrhoeal Dis Res* **14**:1-4.

5440. Nir-Paz, R., J. Strahilevitz, M. Shapiro, N. Keller, A. Goldschmied-Reouven, O. Yarden, C. Block, and I. Polacheck. 2004. Clinical and epidemiological aspects of infections caused by fusarium species: a collaborative study from Israel. *J Clin Microbiol* **42**:3456-61.

5441. Nisalak, A., T. P. Endy, S. Nimmannnitya, S. Kalayanarooj, U. Thisayakorn, R. M. Scott, D. S. Burke, C. H. Hoke, B. L. Innis, and D. W. Vaughn. 2003. Serotype-specific dengue virus circulation and dengue disease in Bangkok, Thailand from 1973 to 1999. *Am J Trop Med Hyg* **68**:191-202.

5442. Nishioka, S. A., S. T. Handa, and R. S. Nunes. 1994. Pig bite in Brazil: a case series from a teaching hospital. *Rev Soc Bras Med Trop* **27**:15-8.

5443. Nishioka, S. d. A., T. W. Gyorkos, L. Joseph, J. P. Collet, and J. D. Maclean. 2002. Tattooing and risk for transfusion-transmitted diseases: the role of the type, number and design of the tattoo, and the conditions in which they were performed. *Epidemiol Infect* **128**:63-71.

5444. Nithikathkul, C., B. Changsap, S. Wannapinyosheep, C. Poister, and P. Boontan. 2001. The prevalence of Enterobius vermicularis among primary school students in Samut Prakan Province, Thailand. *Southeast Asian J Trop Med Public Health* **32 Suppl 2**:133-7.

5445. Nithikathkul, C., P. Polseela, B. Changsap, and S. Leemingsawat. 2002. Ixodid ticks on domestic animals in Samut Prakan province, Thailand. *Southeast Asian J Trop Med Public Health* **33**:41-4.

5446. Nitidandhaprabhas, P., S. Hanchansin, and Y. Vongsloesvidhya. 1975. A case of expectoration of Gnathostoma spinigerum in Thailand. *Am J Trop Med Hyg* **24**:547-8.

5447. Niu, M. T., L. B. Polish, B. H. Robertson, B. K. Khanna, B. A. Woodruff, C. N. Shapiro, M. A. Miller, J. D. Smith, J. K. Gedrose, and M. J. Alter. 1992. Multistate outbreak of hepatitis A associated with frozen strawberries. *J Infect Dis* **166**:518-24.

5448. Njiokou, F., G. Simo, S. W. Nkinin, C. Laveissiere, and S. Herder. 2004. Infection rate of Trypanosoma brucei s.l., T. vivax, T. congolense "forest type", and T. simiae in small wild vertebrates in south Cameroon. *Acta Trop* **92**:139-46.

5449. Njiru, Z. K., K. Ndung'u, G. Matete, J. M. Ndungu, and W. C. Gibson. 2004. Detection of Trypanosoma brucei rhodesiense in animals from sleeping sickness foci in East Africa using the serum resistance associated (SRA) gene. *Acta Trop* **90**:249-54.

5450. NN. 2004. Avian influenza: update on European response. *Eurosurveillance Weekly* **8**:1-2.

5451. NNIS 2003. National Nosocomial Infections Surveillance (NNIS) System Report, data summary from January 1992 through June 2003, issued August 2003. *Am J Infect Control* **31**:481-98.

5452. **Noah, D. L., C. M. Kramer, M. P. Verbsky, J. A. Rooney, K. A. Smith, and J. E. Childs.** 1997. Survey of veterinary professionals and other veterinary conference attendees for antibodies to Bartonella henselae and B quintana. *J Am Vet Med Assoc* **210**:342-4.

5453. **Nobre, V., E. Braga, A. Rayes, J. C. Serufo, P. Godoy, N. Nunes, C. M. Antunes, and J. R. Lambertucci.** 2003. Opportunistic infections in patients with aids admitted to an university hospital of the Southeast of Brazil. *Rev Inst Med Trop Sao Paulo* **45**:69-74.

5454. **Noel, C., F. Dufernez, D. Gerbod, V. P. Edgcomb, P. Delgado-Viscogliosi, L. C. Ho, M. Singh, R. Wintjens, M. L. Sogin, M. Capron, R. Pierce, L. Zenner, and E. Viscogliosi.** 2005. Molecular phylogenies of Blastocystis isolates from different hosts: implications for genetic diversity, identification of species, and zoonosis. *J Clin Microbiol* **43**:348-55.

5455. **Noeske, J., C. Kuaban, S. Rondini, P. Sorlin, L. Ciaffi, J. Mbuagbaw, F. Portaels, and G. Pluschke.** 2004. Buruli ulcer disease in Cameroon rediscovered. *Am J Trop Med Hyg* **70**:520-6.

5456. **Noguchi, S., M. Sata, H. Suzuki, K. Ohba, M. Mizokami, and K. Tanikawa.** 1997. GB virus C (GBV-C)/hepatitis G virus (HGV) infection among intravenous drug users in Japan. *Virus Res* **49**:155-62.

5457. **Nohlmans, M. K., A. E. van den Bogaard, A. A. Blaauw, and C. P. van Boven.** 1991. [Prevalence of Lyme borreliosis in The Netherlands]. *Ned Tijdschr Geneeskd* **135**:2288-92.

5458. **Nohynkova, E., J. Kubek, O. Mest'ankova, P. Chalupa, and Z. Hubalek.** 2003. [A case of Babesia microti imported into the Czech Republic from the USA]. *Cas Lek Cesk* **142**:377-81.

5459. **Noireau, F.** 1992. Infestation by Auchmeromyia senegalensis as a consequence of the adoption of non-nomadic life by Pygmies in the Congo Republic. *Trans R Soc Trop Med Hyg* **86**:329.

5460. **Noireau, F., F. Breniere, J. Ordonez, L. Cardozo, W. Morochi, T. Gutierrez, M. F. Bosseno, S. Garcia, F. Vargas, N. Yaksic, J. P. Dujardin, C. Peredo, and C. Wisnivesky-Colli.** 1997. Low probability of transmission of Trypanosoma cruzi to humans by domiciliary Triatoma sordida in Bolivia. *Trans R Soc Trop Med Hyg* **91**:653-6.

5461. **Noireau, F., M. G. Cortez, F. A. Monteiro, A. M. Jansen, and F. Torrico.** 2005. Can wild Triatoma infestans foci in Bolivia jeopardize Chagas disease control efforts? *Trends Parasitol* **21**:7-10.

5462. **Noireau, F., R. Flores, T. Gutierrez, F. Abad-Franch, E. Flores, and F. Vargas.** 2000. Natural ecotopes of Triatoma infestans dark morph and other sylvatic triatomines in the Bolivian Chaco. *Trans R Soc Trop Med Hyg* **94**:23-7.

5463. **Noireau, F., and J. P. Gouteux.** 1989. Current considerations on a Loa loa simian reservoir in the Congo. *Acta Trop* **46**:69-70.

5464. **Noireau, F., A. Itoua, and B. Carme.** 1990. Epidemiology of Mansonella perstans filariasis in the forest region of south Congo. *Ann Trop Med Parasitol* **84**:251-4.

5465. **Noji, E. K.** 1997. The public health consequences of disasters. Oxford University Press, New York.

5466. **Noji, Y., N. Takada, F. Ishiguro, S. Fujino, T. Aoyama, H. Fujita, Y. Yano, S. Shiomi, I. Mitsuto, K. Takase, T. Haba, and H. Mabuchi.** 2005. The first reported case of spotted fever in Fukui Prefecture, the northern part of central Japan. *Jpn J Infect Dis* **58**:112-4.

5467. **Nolan, C. M., A. M. Elarth, H. Barr, A. M. Saeed, and D. R. Risser.** 1991. An outbreak of tuberculosis in a shelter for homeless men. A description of its evolution and control. *Am Rev Respir Dis* **143**:257-61.

5468. **Nolan, C. M., P. A. Hashisaki, and D. F. Dundas.** 1991. An outbreak of soft-tissue infections due to Mycobacterium fortuitum associated with electromyography. *J Infect Dis* **163**:1150-3.

5469. **Nolte, K. B., R. L. Hanzlick, D. C. Payne, A. T. Kroger, W. R. Oliver, A. M. Baker, D. E. McGowan, J. L. DeJong, M. R. Bell, J. Guarner, W. J. Shieh, and S. R. Zaki.** 2004. Medical examiners, coroners, and biologic terrorism. *MMWR* **53 (RR-8)**:1-36.

5470. **Nomura, Y., K. Nagakura, N. Kagei, Y. Tsutsumi, K. Araki, and M. Sugawara.** 2000. Gnathostomiasis possibly caused by Gnathostoma malaysiae. *Tokai J Exp Clin Med* **25**:1-6.

5471. **Nonnenmacher, C., R. Mutters, and L. F. de Jacoby.** 2001. Microbiological characteristics of subgingival microbiota in adult periodontitis, localized juvenile periodontitis and rapidly progressive periodontitis subjects. *Clin Microbiol Infect* **7**:213-7.

5472. **Nontasut, P., T. V. Thong, J. Waikagul, W. Fungladda, N. Imamee, and N. V. De.** 2003. Social and behavioral factors associated with Clonorchis infection in one commune located in the Red River Delta of Vietnam. *Southeast Asian J Trop Med Public Health* **34**:269-73.

5473. **Nooman, Z. M., A. H. Hasan, Y. Waheeb, A. M. Mishriky, M. Ragheb, A. N. Abu-Saif, S. M. Abaza, A. A. Serwah, A. El-Gohary, A. Saad, M. El-Sayed, and M. Fouad.** 2000. The epidemiology of schistosomiasis in Egypt: Ismailia governorate. *Am J Trop Med Hyg* **62**:35-41.

5474. **Noormahomed, E. V., J. G. Pividal, S. Azzouz, C. Mascaro, M. Delgado-Rodriguez, and A. Osuna.** 2003. Seroprevalence of anti-cysticercus antibodies among the children living in the urban environs of Maputo, Mozambique. *Ann Trop Med Parasitol* **97**:31-5.

5475. **Norazah, A., I. Rahizan, T. Zainuldin, M. Y. Rohani, and A. G. Kamel.** 1998. Enteropathogenic Escherichia coli in raw and cooked food. *Southeast Asian J Trop Med Public Health* **29**:91-3.

5476. **Norberg, A., C. E. Nord, and B. Evengard.** 2003. Dientmoeba fragilis—a protozoal infection which may cause severe bowel distress. *Clin Microbiol Infect* **9**:65-8.

5477. **Noren, T., T. Akerlund, E. Back, L. Sjoberg, I. Persson, I. Alriksson, and L. G. Burman.** 2004. Molecular epidemiology of hospital-associated and community-acquired Clostridium difficile infection in a Swedish county. *J Clin Microbiol* **42**:3635-43.

5478. **Norhayati, M., B. Zainudin, C. G. Mohammod, P. Oothuman, O. Azizi, and M. S. Fatmah.** 1997. The prevalence of Trichuris, Ascaris and hookworm infection in Orang Asli children. *Southeast Asian J Trop Med Public Health* **28**:161-8.

5479. **Norman, J. E., G. W. Beebe, J. H. Hoofnagle, and L. B. Seeff.** 1993. Mortality follow-up of the 1942 epidemic of hepatitis B in the U.S. Army. *Hepatology* **18**:790-7.

5480. **Normand, P., J. Renault, J. M. Becker, J. M. Millea, and J. C. Doury.** 1982. Une affection exotique sexuellement transmise: la donovanose. *Med Trop* **42**:53-7.

5481. Normann, E., J. Gnarpe, H. Gnarpe, and B. Wettergren. 1998. Chlamydia pneumoniae in children attending day-care centers in Gavle, Sweden. *Pediatr infect Dis J* **17**:474-8.

5482. Normile, D. 2005. Avian influenza. Europe scrambles to control deadly H5N1 Strain. *Science* **310**:417.

5483. Norrung, B. 2000. Microbiological criteria for Listeria monocytogenes in foods under special consideration of risk assessment approaches. *Int J Food Microbiol* **62**:217-21.

5484. Norrung, B., J. K. Andersen, and J. Schlundt. 1999. Incidence and control of Listeria monocytogenes in foods in Denmark. *Int J Food Microbiol* **53**:195-203.

5485. Noskin, G. A., R. J. Rubin, J. J. Schentag, J. Kluytmans, E. C. Hedblom, M. Smulders, E. Lapetina, and E. Gemmen. 2005. The burden of Staphylococcus aureus infections on hospitals in the United States: an analysis of the 2000 and 2001 Nationwide Inpatient Sample Database. *Arch Intern Med* **165**:1756-61.

5486. Nosten, F., M. van Vugt, R. Price, C. Luxemburger, K. L. Thway, A. Brockman, R. McGready, F. ter Kuile, S. Looareesuwan, and N. J. White. 2000. Effects of artesunate-mefloquine combination on incidence of Plasmodium falciparum malaria and mefloquine resistance in western Thailand: a prospective study. *Lancet* **356**:297-302.

5487. Nothdurft, H. D., M. Brommer, D. Eichenlaub, and T. Loscher. 1995. [A small outbreak of trichinosis caused by imported smoked ham]. *Dtsch Med Wochenschr* **120**:173-6.

5488. Nothdurft, H. D., T. Jelinek, A. Mai, B. Sigl, F. von Sonnenburg, and T. Loscher. 1995. Epidemiology of alveolar echinococcosis in southern Germany (Bavaria). *Infection* **23**:85-8.

5489. Novelli, V. M., H. Mostafavipour, M. Abulaban, F. Ekteish, J. Milder, and B. Azadeh. 1987. High prevalence of human immunodeficiency virus infection in children with thalassemia exposed to blood imported from the United States. *Pediatr Infect Dis J* **6**:765-6.

5490. Noviello, S. 2004. Laboratory-acquired Brucellosis. *Emerg Infect Dis* **10**:1848-50.

5491. Nowotny, N. 1996. [Serologic studies of domestic cats for potential human pathogenic virus infections from wild rodents]. *Zentralbl Hyg Umweltmed* **198**:452-61.

5492. Nowotny, N., A. Deutz, K. Fuchs, W. Schuller, F. Hinterdorfer, H. Auer, and H. Aspock. 1997. Prevalence of swine influenza and other viral, bacterial, and parasitic zoonoses in veterinarians. *J Infect Dis* **176**:1414-5.

5493. Nowrouzian, F., B. Hesselmar, R. Saalman, I. L. Strannegard, N. Aberg, A. E. Wold, and I. Adlerberth. 2003. Escherichia coli in infants' intestinal microflora: colonization rate, strain turnover, and virulence gene carriage. *Pediatr Res* **54**:8-14.

5494. Noyer, C. M., C. M. Coyle, C. Werner, J. Dupouy-Camet, H. B. Tanowitz, and M. Wiitner. 2002. Hypereosinophilia and liver mass in an immigrant. *Am J Trop Med Hyg* **66**:774-6.

5495. Nubling, C., A. Groner, and J. Lower. 1998. GB virus C/hepatitis G virus and intravenous immunoglobulins. *Vox Sang* **75**:189-92.

5496. Nucci, M., T. Akiti, G. Barreiros, F. Silveira, S. G. Revankar, B. L. Wickes, D. A. Sutton, and T. F. Patterson. 2002. Nosocomial outbreak of Exophiala jeanselmei fungemia associated with contamination of hospital water. *Clin Infect Dis* **34**:1475-80.

5497. Nucci, M., and E. Anaissie. 2002. Cutaneous infection by Fusarium species in healthy and immunocompromised hosts: implications for diagnosis and management. *Clin Infect Dis* **35**:909-20.

5498. Nucci, M., K. A. Marr, F. Queiroz-Telles, C. A. Martins, P. Trabasso, S. Costa, J. C. Voltarelli, A. L. Colombo, A. Imhof, R. Pasquini, A. Maiolino, C. A. Souza, and E. Anaissie. 2004. Fusarium infection in hematopoietic stem cell transplant recipients. *Clin Infect Dis* **38**:1237-42.

5499. Nuchprayoon, T., and T. Chumnijarakij. 1992. Risk factors for hepatitis B carrier status among blood donors of the National Blood Center, Thai Red Cross Society. *Southeast Asian J Trop Med Public Health* **23**:246-53.

5500. Nuesch, R., C. Bellini, and W. Zimmerli. 1999. Pneumocystis carinii pneumonia in human immunodeficiency virus (HIV)-positive and HIV-negative immunocompromised patients. *Clin Infect Dis* **29**:1519-23.

5501. Nuesch, R., E. Cynke, M. C. Jost, and W. Zimmerli. 2000. Thrombocytopenia after kidney transplantation. *Am J Kidney Dis* **35**:537-8.

5502. Nulens, E., and A. Voss. 2002. Laboratory diagnosis and biosafety issues of biological warfare agents. *Clin Microbiol Inf* **8**:455-66.

5503. Nunes, C. M., F. C. Pena, G. B. Negrelli, C. G. Anjo, M. M. Nakano, and N. S. Stobbe. 2000. [Presence of larva migrans in sand boxes of public elementary schools, Aracatuba, Brazil]. *Rev Saude Publica* **34**:656-8.

5504. Nunes-Araujo, F. R., S. D. Nishioka, I. B. Ferreira, A. Suzuki, R. F. Bonito, and M. S. Ferreira. 1999. Absence of interhuman transmission of hantavirus pulmonary syndrome in Minas Gerais, Brazil: evidence from a serological survey. *Clin Infect Dis* **29**:1588-9.

5505. Nunez, F. A., M. Hernandez, and C. M. Finlay. 1996. A longitudinal study of enterobiasis in three day care centers of Havana City. *Rev Inst Med Trop Sao Paulo* **38**:129-32.

5506. Nunez, S., A. Moreno, K. Green, and J. Villar. 2000. The stethoscope in the Emergency Department: a vector of infection? *Epidemiol Infect* **124**:233-7.

5507. Nunoue, T., K. Kusuhara, and T. Hara. 2002. Human fetal infection with parvovirus B19: maternal infection time in gestation, viral persistence and fetal prognosis. *Pediatr Infect Dis J* **21**:1133-6.

5508. Nuorti, J. P., J. C. Butler, J. M. Crutcher, R. Guevara, D. Welch, P. Holder, and J. A. Elliott. 1998. An outbreak of multidrug-resistant pneumococcal pneumonia and bacteremia among unvaccinated nursing home residents. *N Engl J Med* **338**:1861-8.

5509. Nuorti, J. P., T. Niskanen, S. Hallanvuo, J. Mikkola, E. Kela, M. Hatakka, M. Fredriksson-Ahomaa, O. Lyytikainen, A. Siitonen, H. Korkeala, and P. Ruutu. 2004. A Widespread Outbreak of Yersinia pseudotuberculosis O:3 Infection from Iceberg Lettuce. *J Infect Dis* **189**:766-74.

5510. Nur, Y. A., J. Groen, H. Heuvelmans, W. Tuynman, C. Copra, and A. D. Osterhaus. 1999. An outbreak of West Nile fever among migrants in Kisangani, Democratic Republic of Congo. *Am J Trop Med Hyg* **61**:885-8.

5511. Nurgalieva, Z. Z., H. M. Malaty, D. Y. Graham, R. Almuchambetova, A. Machmudova, D. Kapsultanova, M. S. Osato, F. B. Hollinger, and A. Zhangabylov. 2002. Helicobacter pylori infection in Kazakhstan: effect of water source and household hygiene. *Am J Trop Med Hyg* **67**:201-6.

5512. Nuti, M., D. Amaddeo, M. Crovatto, A. Ghionni, D. Polato, E. Lillini, E. Pitzus, and G. F. Santini. 1993. Infections in an

Alpine environment: antibodies to hantaviruses, leptospira, rickettsiae, and Borrelia burgdorferi in defined Italian populations. *Am J Trop Med Hyg* **48:**20-5.

5513. **Nuti, M., D. A. Serafini, D. Bassetti, A. Ghionni, F. Russino, P. Rombola, G. Macri, and E. Lillini.** 1998. Ehrlichia infection in Italy. *Emerg Infect Dis* **4:**663-5.

5514. **Nutman, T. B.** 2000. Lymphatic filariasis. Imperial College Press, London.

5515. **Nutman, T. B., K. D. Miller, M. Mulligan, G. N. Reinhardt, B. J. Currie, C. Steel, and E. A. Ottesen.** 1988. Diethylcarbamazine prophylaxis for human loiasis. Results of a double-blind study. *N Engl J Med* **319:**752-6.

5516. **Nutman, T. B., T. E. Nash, and E. A. Ottesen.** 1987. Ivermectin in the successful treatment of a patient with Mansonella ozzardi infection. *J Infect Dis* **156:**662-5.

5517. **Nwanyanwu, O. C., N. Kumwenda, P. N. Kazembe, S. Jemu, C. Ziba, W. C. Nkhoma, and S. C. Redd.** 1997. Malaria and human immunodeficiency virus infection among male employees of a sugar estate in Malawi. *Trans R Soc Trop Med Hyg* **91:**567-9.

5518. **Nwosu, A. B.** 1981. Human neonatal infections with hookworms in an endemic area of Southern Nigeria. A possible transmammary route. *Trop Geogr Med* **33:**105-11.

5519. **Nygard, K., Y. Andersson, J. A. Rottingen, A. Svensson, J. Lindback, T. Kistemann, and J. Giesecke.** 2004. Association between environmental risk factors and campylobacter infections in Sweden. *Epidemiol Infect* **132:**317-25.

5520. **Nygard, K., L. Vold, E. Halvorsen, E. Bringeland, J. A. Rottingen, and P. Aavitsland.** 2004. Waterborne outbreak of gastroenteritis in a religious summer camp in Norway, 2002. *Epidemiol Infect* **132:**223-9.

5521. **Nyiri, P., T. Leung, and M. A. Zuckerman.** 2004. Sharps discarded in inner city parks and playgrounds - risk of bloodborne virus exposure. *Commun Dis Publ Health* **7:**287-8.

5522. **Nylen, G., F. Dunstan, S. R. Palmer, Y. Andersson, F. Bager, J. Cowden, G. Feierl, Y. Galloway, G. Kapperud, F. Megraud, K. Molbak, L. R. Petersen, and P. Ruutu.** 2002. The seasonal distribution of campylobacter infection in nine European countries and New Zealand. *Epidemiol Infect* **128:**383-90.

5523. **Nylen, G., H. M. Fielder, and S. R. Palmer.** 1999. An international outbreak of Salmonella enteritidis associated with lasagne; lessons on the need for cross-national co-operation in investigating food-borne outbreaks. *Epidemiol Infect* **123:**31-5.

5524. **Nzeyimana, I., M. C. Henry, J. Dossou-Yovo, J. M. Doannio, L. Diawara, and P. Carnevale.** 2002. [The epidemiology of malaria in the southwestern forests of the Ivory Coast (Tai region)]. *Bull Soc Pathol Exot* **95:**89-94.

5525. **O'Brien, K. L., and H. Nohynek.** 2003. Report from a WHO Working Group: standard method for detecting upper respiratory carriage of Streptococcus pneumoniae. *Pediatr Infect Dis J* **22:**e1-11.

5526. **O'Brien, K. L., J. Shaw, R. Weatherholtz, R. Reid, J. Watt, J. Croll, R. Dagan, A. J. Parkinson, and M. Santosham.** 2004. Epidemiology of invasive Streptococcus pneumoniae among Navajo children in the era before use of conjugate pneumococcal vaccines, 1989-1996. *Am J Epidemiol* **160:**270-8.

5527. **O'Brien, S. J., G. K. Adak, and C. Gilham.** 2001. Contact with farming environment as a major risk factor for shiga toxin (vero cytotoxin)-producing Escherichia coli O157 infections in humans. *Emerg Infect Dis* **7:**1049-1051.

5528. **O'Connell, J. J.** 1991. Nontuberculous respiratory infections among the homeless. *Semin Respir Infect* **6:**247-53.

5529. **O'Donnell, J. M., L. Thornton, E. B. McNamara, T. Prendergast, D. Igoe, and C. Cosgrove.** 2002. Outbreak of Vero cytotoxin-producing Escherichia coli O157 in a child day care facility. *Commun Dis Public Health* **5:**54-8.

5530. **O'Donovan, D., R. P. D. Cooke, R. Joce, A. Eastbury, J. Waite, and K. Stene-Johansen.** 2001. An outbreak of hepatitis A amongst injecting drug users. *Epidemiol Infect* **127:**469-73.

5531. **O'Donovan, D., A. Iversen, J. Trounce, and S. Curtis.** 2000. Outbreak of group C meningococcal infection affecting two preschool nurseries. *Commun Dis Public Health* **3:**177-80.

5532. **O'Farrell, N.** 2002. Donovanosis. *Sex Transm Infect* **78:**452-7.

5533. **O'Grady, N. P., M. Alexander, E. P. Dellinger, J. L. Gerberding, S. O. Heard, D. G. Maki, H. Masur, R. D. McCormick, L. A. Mermel, M. L. Pearson, Raad, II, A. Randolph, and R. A. Weinstein.** 2002. Guidelines for the prevention of intravascular catheter-related infections. *MMWR* **51 (RR-10):**1-29.

5534. **O'Hara, C. M., F. W. Brenner, and J. M. Miller.** 2000. Classification, identification, and clinical significance of Proteus, Providencia, and Morganella. *Clin Microbiol Rev* **13:**534-46.

5535. **O'Lorcain, P., and C. V. Holland.** 2000. The public health importance of Ascaris lumbricoides. *Parasitology* **121 Suppl:**S51-71.

5536. **O'Mahony, M., A. Lakhani, A. Stephens, J. G. Wallace, E. R. Youngs, and D. Harper.** 1989. Legionnaires' disease and the sick-building syndrome. *Epidemiol Infect* **103:**285-92.

5537. **O'Mahony, M., E. Mitchell, R. J. Gilbert, D. N. Hutchinson, N. T. Begg, J. C. Rodhouse, and J. E. Morris.** 1990. An outbreak of foodborne botulism associated with contaminated hazelnut yoghurt. *Epidemiol Infect* **104:**389-95.

5538. **O'Mahony, M. C., C. D. Gooch, D. A. Smyth, A. J. Thrussell, C. L. R. Bartlett, and N. D. Noah.** 1983. Epidemic hepatitis from cockles. *Lancet* **1:**518-20.

5539. **O'Mahony, M. C., R. E. Stanwell-Smith, H. E. Tillett, D. Harper, J. G. Hutchison, I. D. Farrell, D. N. Hutchinson, J. V. Lee, P. J. Dennis, H. V. Duggal, et al.** 1990. The Stafford outbreak of Legionnaires' disease. *Epidemiol Infect* **104:**361-80.

5540. **O'Reilly, L. M., and C. J. Daborn.** 1995. The epidemiology of Mycobacterium bovis infections in animals and man: a review. *Tuber Lung Dis* **76 Suppl 1:**1-46.

5541. **O'Rourke, K., K. J. Goodman, M. Grazioplene, T. Redlinger, and R. S. Day.** 2003. Determinants of geographic variation in Helicobacter pylori infection among children on the US-Mexico border. *Am J Epidemiol* **158:**816-24.

5542. **O'Sullivan, B., V. Delpech, G. Pontivivo, T. Karagiannis, D. Marriott, J. Harkness, and J. M. McAnulty.** 2002. Shigellosis linked to sex venues, Australia. *Emerg Infect Dis* **8:**862-4.

5543. **Oakeshott, P., P. Hay, F. Steinke, E. Rink, and S. Kerry.** 2002. Association between bacterial vaginosis or chlamydial infection and miscarriage before 16 weeks' gestation: prospective community based cohort study. *BMJ* **325:**1334-6.

5544. **Obara, A., F. Nakamura-Uchiyama, K. Hiromatsu, and Y. Nawa.** 2004. Paragonimiasis cases recently found among immigrants in Japan. *Intern Med* **43:**388-92.

5545. **Obasanjo, O. O., P. Wu, M. Conlon, L. V. Karanfil, P. Pryor, G. Moler, G. Anhalt, R. E. Chaisson, and T. M. Perl.** 2001. An outbreak of scabies in a teaching hospital: lessons learned. *Infect Control Hosp Epidemiol* **22:**13-8.

5546. Oberhelman, R. A., J. Flores-Abuxapqui, G. Suarez-Hoil, M. Puc-Franco, M. Heredia-Navarrete, M. Vivas-Rosel, R. Mera, and L. Gutierrez-Cogco. 2001. Asymptomatic salmonellosis among children in day-care centers in Mérida, Yucatàn, Mexico. *Pediatr Infect Dis J* **20:**792-7.

5547. Oberhelman, R. A., R. H. Gilman, P. Sheen, J. Cordova, D. N. Taylor, M. Zimic, R. Meza, J. Perez, C. LeBron, L. Cabrera, F. G. Rodgers, D. L. Woodward, and L. J. Price. 2003. Campylobacter transmission in a Peruvian shantytown: a longitudinal study using strain typing of campylobacter isolates from chickens and humans in household clusters. *J Infect Dis* **187:**260-9.

5548. Oberste, M. S., W. A. Nix, D. R. Kilpatrick, M. R. Flemister, and M. A. Pallansch. 2003. Molecular epidemiology and type-specific detection of echovirus 11 isolates from the Americas, Europe, Africa, Australia, southern Asia and the Middle East. *Virus Res* **91:**241-8.

5549. Ochsenfahrt, C., R. Friedl, A. Hannekum, and B. A. Schumacher. 2001. Endocarditis after nipple piercing in a patient with a bicuspid aortic valve. *Ann Thorac Surg* **71:**1365-6.

5550. Ockenhouse, C. F., A. Magill, D. Smith, and W. Milhous. 2005. History of U.S. military contributions to the study of malaria. *Mil Med* **170:**12-6.

5551. Odorico, D. M., S. R. Graves, B. Currie, J. Catmull, Z. Nack, S. Ellis, L. Wang, and D. J. Miller. 1998. New Orienta tsutsugamushi strain from scrub typhus in Australia. *Emerg Infect Dis* **4:**641-4.

5552. Ogata, K., R. Kato, K. Ito, and S. Yamada. 2002. Prevalence of Escherichia coli possessing the eaeA gene of enteropathogenic E. coli (EPEC) or the aggR gene of enteroaggregative E. coli (EAggEC) in traveler's diarrhea diagnosed in those returning from Tama, Tokyo from other Asian countries. *Jpn J Infect Dis* **55:**14-8.

5553. Ogata, K., Y. Nawa, H. Akahane, S. P. Diaz Camacho, R. Lamothe-Argumedo, and A. Cruz-Reyes. 1998. Short report: gnathostomiasis in Mexico. *Am J Trop Med Hyg* **58:**316-8.

5554. Ogden, I. D., N. F. Hepburn, M. MacRae, N. J. Strachan, D. R. Fenlon, S. M. Rusbridge, and T. H. Pennington. 2002. Long-term survival of Escherichia coli O157 on pasture following an outbreak associated with sheep at a scout camp. *Lett Appl Microbiol* **34:**100-4.

5555. Ogden, N. H., K. Bown, B. K. Horrocks, Z. Woldehiwet, and M. Bennett. 1998. Granulocytic Ehrlichia infection in ixodid ticks and mammals in woodlands and uplands of the U.K. *Med Vet Entomol* **12:**423-9.

5556. Oge, H., A. Doganay, S. Oge, and A. Yildirim. 2003. Prevalence and distribution of Dirofilaria immitis in domestic dogs from Ankara and vicinity in Turkey. *Dtsch Tierarztl Wochenschr* **110:**69-72.

5557. Ogilvie, E. L., F. Veit, N. Crofts, and S. C. Thompson. 1999. Hepatitis infection among adolescents resident in Melbourne Juvenile Justice Centre: risk factors and challenges. *J Adolesc Health* **25:**46-51.

5558. Ognjan, A., M. L. Boulton, P. Somsel, M. G. Stobierski, G. Stoltman, f. Downes, K. Smith, L. Chapman, L. Petersen, A. Marfin, G. Campbell, R. Lanciotti, J. T. Roehrig, D. Gubler, M. chamberland, J. Montgomery, and C. A. Arole. 2002. Possible West Nile virus transmisssion to an infant through breast-feeding - Michigan, 2002. *MMWR* **51:**877-8.

5559. Oh, P., R. Granich, J. Scott, B. Sun, M. Joseph, C. Stringfield, S. Thisdell, J. Staley, D. Workman-Malcolm, L. Borenstein, E. Lehnkering, P. Ryan, J. Soukup, A. Nitta, and J. Flood. 2002. Human exposure following Mycobacterium tuberculosis infection of multiple animal species in a Metropolitan Zoo. *Emerg Infect Dis* **8:**1290-3.

5560. Ohara, H., I. Ebisawa, and H. Naruto. 1997. Prophylaxis of acute viral hepatitis by immune serum globulin, hepatitis B vaccine, and health education: a sixteen year study of Japan overseas cooperation volunteers. *Am J Trop Med Hyg* **56:**76-9.

5561. Ohara, Y., T. Sato, H. Fujita, T. Ueno, and M. Homma. 1991. Clinical manifestations of tularemia in Japan—analysis of 1,355 cases observed between 1924 and 1987. *Infection* **19:**14-7.

5562. Ohara, Y., T. Sato, and M. Homma. 1998. Arthropod-borne tularemia in Japan: clinical analysis of 1,374 cases observed between 1924 and 1996. *J Med Entomol* **35:**471-3.

5563. Ohl, M. E., and D. H. Spach. 2000. Bartonella quintana and urban trench fever. *Clin Infect Dis* **31:**131-5.

5564. Ohnishi, K., and Y. Kato. 2003. Single low-dose treatment with praziquantel for Diphyllobothrium nihonkaiense infections. *Intern Med* **42:**41-3.

5565. Ohnishi, K., Y. Kato, A. Imamura, M. Fukayama, T. Tsunoda, Y. Sakaue, M. Sakamoto, and H. Sagara. 2004. Present characteristics of symptomatic Entamoeba histolytica infection in the big cities of Japan. *Epidemiol Infect* **132:**57-60.

5566. Ohshige, K., S. Morio, S. Mizushima, K. Kitamura, K. Tajima, A. Ito, A. Suyama, S. Usuku, V. Saphonn, S. Heng, L. B. Hor, P. Tia, and K. Soda. 2000. Cross-sectional study on risk factors of HIV among female commercial sex workers in Cambodia. *Epidemiol Infect* **124:**143-52.

5567. Ohto, H., S. Terazawa, N. Sasaki, K. Hino, C. Ishiwata, M. Kako, N. Ujiie, C. Endo, A. Matsui, et al. 1994. Transmission of hepatitis C virus from mothers to infants. The Vertical Transmission of Hepatitis C Virus Collaborative Study Group. *N Engl J Med* **330:**744-50.

5568. Oie, S., A. Kamiya, K. Hironaga, and A. Koshiro. 1993. Microbial contamination of enteral feeding solution and its prevention. *Am J Infect Control* **21:**34-8.

5569. Oishi, I., K. Yamazaki, T. Kimoto, Y. Minekawa, E. Utagawa, S. Yamazaki, S. Inouye, G. S. Grohmann, S. S. Monroe, and S. E. Stine. 1994. A large outbreak of acute gastroenteritis associated with astrovirus among students and teachers in Osaka, Japan. *J Infect Dis* **170:**439-43.

5570. Ojukwu, I. C., and C. Christy. 2002. Rat-bite fever in children: case report and review. *Scand J Infect Dis* **34:**474-7.

5571. Ok, U. Z., I. C. Balcioglu, A. Taylan Ozkan, S. Ozensoy, and Y. Ozbel. 2002. Leishmaniasis in Turkey. *Acta Trop* **84:**43-8.

5572. Okabayashi, T., J. Hagiya, M. Tsuji, C. Ishihara, H. Satoh, and C. Morita. 2002. Detection of Babesia microti-like parasite in filter paper-absorbed blood of wild rodents. *J Vet Med Sci* **64:**145-7.

5573. Okada, D. M., A. W. Chow, and V. T. Bruce. 1977. Neonatal scalp abscess and fetal monitoring: factors associated with infection. *Am J Obstet Gynecol* **129:**185-9.

5574. Okafuji, T., N. Yoshida, M. Fujino, Y. Motegi, T. Ihara, Y. Ota, T. Notomi, and T. Nakayama. 2005. Rapid diagnostic method for detection of mumps virus genome by loop-mediated isothermal amplification. *J Clin Microbiol* **43:**1625-31.

5575. Okazaki, M., T. Watanabe, K. Morita, Y. Higurashi, K. Araki, N. Shukuya, S. Baba, N. Watanabe, T. Egami, N. Furuya, M.

Kanamori, S. Shimazaki, and H. Uchimura. 1999. Molecular epidemiological investigation using a randomly amplified polymorphic DNA assay of Burkholderia cepacia isolates from nosocomial outbreaks. *J Clin Microbiol* **37**:3809-14.

5576. **Okeke, I. N., and J. P. Nataro.** 2001. Enteroaggregative Escherichia coli. *Lancet Infect Dis* **1**:304-13.

5577. **Okhuysen, P. C., X. Jiang, L. M. Ye, P. C. Johnson, and M. K. Estes.** 1995. Viral shedding and fecal IgA response after Norwalk virus infection. *J Infect Dis* **171**:566-569.

5578. **Okoli, E. I., and A. B. Odaibo.** 1999. Urinary schistosomiasis among schoolchildren in Ibadan, an urban community in south-western Nigeria. *Trop Med Int Health* **4**:308-15.

5579. **Okutani, A., Y. Okada, S. Yamamoto, and S. Igimi.** 2004. Overview of Listeria monocytogenes contamination in Japan. *Int J Food Microbiol* **93**:131-40.

5580. **Olender, S., M. Saito, J. Apgar, K. Gillenwater, C. T. Bautista, A. G. Lescano, P. Moro, L. Caviedes, E. J. Hsieh, and R. H. Gilman.** 2003. Low prevalence and increased household clustering of Mycobacterium tuberculosis infection in high altitude villages in Peru. *Am J Trop Med Hyg* **68**:721-7.

5581. **Olivan, G.** 2002. The health status of delinquent gipsy youths in Spain. *Eur J Public Health* **12**:308.

5582. **Oliveira, C. C., H. G. Lacerda, D. R. Martins, J. D. Barbosa, G. R. Monteiro, J. W. Queiroz, J. M. Sousa, M. F. Ximenes, and S. M. Jeronimo.** 2004. Changing epidemiology of American cutaneous leishmaniasis (ACL) in Brazil: a disease of the urban-rural interface. *Acta Trop* **90**:155-62.

5583. **Oliveira, J., S. da Cunha, R. Corte-Real, L. Sampaio, N. Dais, and A. Melico-Silvestre.** 1995. [The prevalence of measles, rubella, mumps and chickenpox antibodies in a population of health care workers]. *Acta Med Port* **8**:206-16.

5584. **Oliveira, R. P., M. A. M. Galvao, C. L. Mafra, C. B. Chamone, S. B. Calic, S. U. Silva, and D. H. Walker.** 2002. Rickettsia felis in Ctenocephalides spp. fleas, Brazil. *Emerg Infect Dis* **8**:317-319.

5585. **Oliveira-Neto, M. P., C. Pirmez, E. Rangel, A. Schubach, and G. Grimaldi Junior.** 1988. An outbreak of American cutaneous leishmaniasis (Leishmania braziliensis braziliensis) in a periurban area of Rio de Janeiro city, Brazil: clinical and epidemiological studies. *Mem Inst Oswaldo Cruz* **83**:427-35.

5586. **Oliver, J. D.** 2005. Wound infections caused by Vibrio vulnificus and other marine bacteria. *Epidemiol Infect* **133**:383-91.

5587. **Oliver, S. E., J. Woodhouse, and V. Hollyoak.** 1999. Lessons from patient notification exercises following the identification of hepatitis B e antigen positive surgeons in an English health region. *Commun Dis Public Health* **2**:130-6.

5588. **Olle-Goig, J. E., and J. Canela-Soler.** 1987. An outbreak of Brucella melitensis infection by airborne transmission among laboratory workers. *Am J Public Health* **77**:335-8.

5589. **Ollero, M., E. Pujol, A. Gimeno, A. Gea, P. Marquez, and J. M. Iturriaga.** 1991. [Risky practices associated with HIV infection of seamen who travel in sub-Saharan West Africa]. *Rev Clin Esp* **189**:416-21.

5590. **Ollomo, B., S. Karch, P. Bureau, N. Elissa, A. J. Georges, and P. Millet.** 1997. Lack of malaria parasite transmission between apes and humans in Gabon. *Am J Trop Med Hyg* **56**:440-5.

5591. **Olowu, J. A., A. Sowunmi, and A. E. Abohweyere.** 2000. Congenital malaria in a hyperendemic area: a revisit. *Afr J Med Med Sci* **29**:211-3.

5592. **Olsen, B., S. Bergstrom, D. J. McCafferty, M. Sellin, and G. Wistrom.** 1996. Salmonella enteritidis in Antarctica: zoonosis in man or humanosis in penguins? *Lancet* **348**:1319-20.

5593. **Olsen, B., D. C. Duffy, T. G. Jaenson, A. Gylfe, J. Bonnedahl, and S. Bergstrom.** 1995. Transhemispheric exchange of Lyme disease spirochetes by seabirds. *J Clin Microbiol* **33**:3270-4.

5594. **Olsen, B., K. Persson, and K. A. Broholm.** 1998. PCR detection of Chlamydia psittaci in faecal samples from passerine birds in Sweden. *Epidemiol Infect* **121**:481-4.

5595. **Olsen, C. W., L. Brammer, B. C. Easterday, N. Arden, E. Belay, I. Baker, and N. J. Cox.** 2002. Serologic evidence of h1 Swine influenza virus infection in Swine farm residents and employees. *Emerg Infect Dis* **8**:814-9.

5596. **Olsen, G. W., J. M. Burris, M. M. Burlew, M. E. Steinberg, N. V. Patz, J. A. Stoltzfus, and J. H. Mandel.** 1998. Absenteeism among employees who participated in a workplace influenza immunization program. *J Occup Environ Med* **40**:311-6.

5597. **Olsen, S. J., S. C. Bleasdale, A. R. Magnano, C. Landrigan, B. H. Holland, R. V. Tauxe, E. D. Mintz, and S. Luby.** 2003. Outbreaks of typhoid fever in the United States, 1960-99. *Epidemiol Infect* **130**:13-21.

5598. **Olsen, S. J., H. L. Chang, T. Y. Y. Cheung, A. F. Tang, T. L. Fisk, S. P. Ooi, H. W. Kuo, D. D. Jiang, K. T. Chen, J. Lando, K. H. Hsu, T. J. Chen, and S. F. Dowell.** 2003. Transmission of the severe acute respiratory syndrome on aircraft. *N Engl J Med* **349**:2416-22.

5599. **Olsen, S. J., E. E. DeBess, T. E. McGivern, N. Marano, T. Eby, S. Mauvais, V. K. Balan, G. Zirnstein, P. R. Cieslak, and F. J. Angulo.** 2001. A nosocomial outbreak of fluoroquinolone-resistant salmonella infection. *N Engl J Med* **344**:1572-9.

5600. **Olsen, S. J., G. R. Hansen, L. Bartlett, C. Fitzgerald, A. Sonder, R. Manjrekar, T. Riggs, J. Kim, R. Flahart, G. Pezzino, and D. L. Swerdlow.** 2001. An outbreak of Campylobacter jejuni infections associated with food handler contamination: the use of pulsed-field gel electrophoresis. *J Infect Dis* **183**:164-7.

5601. **Olsen, S. J., B. Kafoa, N. S. S. Win, M. Jose, W. Bibb, S. Luby, G. Waidubu, M. O'Leary, and E. Mintz.** 2001. Restaurant-associated outbreak of Salmonella Typhi in Nauru: an epidemiological and cost analysis. *Epidemiol Infect* **127**:405-12.

5602. **Olsen, S. J., L. C. MacKinnon, J. S. Goulding, N. H. Bean, and L. Slutsker.** 2000. Surveillance for foodborne-disease outbreaks—United States, 1993-1997. *MMWR* **49 (SS-1)**:1-62.

5603. **Olsen, S. J., G. Miller, M. Kennedy, C. Higgins, J. Walford, G. McKee, K. Fox, W. Bibb, and P. Mead.** 2002. A Waterborne Outbreak of Escherichia coli O157:H7 Infections and Hemolytic Uremic Syndrome: Implications for Rural Water Systems. *Emerg Infect Dis* **8**:370-5.

5604. **Olsen, S. J., M. Patrick, S. B. Hunter, V. Reddy, L. Kornstein, W. R. MacKenzie, K. Lane, S. Bidol, G. A. Stoltman, D. M. Frye, I. Lee, S. Hurd, T. F. Jones, T. N. LaPorte, W. Dewitt, L. Graves, M. Wiedmann, D. J. Schoonmaker-Bopp, A. J. Huang, C. Vincent, A. Bugenhagen, J. Corby, E. R. Carloni, M. E. Holcomb, R. F. Woron, S. M. Zansky, G. Dowdle, F. Smith, S. Ahrabi-Fard, A. R. Ong, N. Tucker, N. A. Hynes, and P. Mead.** 2005. Multistate outbreak of Listeria monocytogenes infection linked to delicatessen turkey meat. *Clin Infect Dis* **40**:962-7.

5605. **Olsen, S. J., M. Ying, M. F. Davis, M. Deasy, B. Holland, L. Iampietro, C. M. Baysinger, F. Sassano, L. D. Polk, B. Gormley, M. J. Hung, K. Pilot, M. Orsini, S. Van Duyne, S. Rankin,

C. Genese, E. A. Bresnitz, J. Smucker, M. Moll, and J. Sobel. 2004. Multidrug-resistant Salmonella Typhimurium infection from milk contaminated after pasteurization. *Emerg Infect Dis* **10**:932-5.

5606. Olson, J. G., T. G. Ksiazek, V. H. Lee, R. Tan, and R. E. Shope. 1985. Isolation of Japanese encephalitis virus from Anopheles annularis and Anopheles vagus in Lombok, Indonesia. *Trans R Soc Trop Med Hyg* **79**:845-7.

5607. Olson, M. E., I. Goemans, D. Bolingbroke, and S. Lundberg. 1988. Gangrenous dermatitis caused by Corynebacterium ulcerans in Richardson ground squirrels. *J Am Vet Med Assoc* **193**:367-8.

5608. Olson, M. E., R. M. O'Handley, B. J. Ralston, T. A. McAllister, and R. C. Andrew Thompson. 2004. Update on Cryptosporidium and Giardia infections in cattle. *Trends Parasitol* **20**:185-91.

5609. Olsson, G. E., F. Dalerum, B. Hörnfeldt, F. Elgh, T. R. Palo, P. Juto, and C. Ahlm. 2003. Human hantavirus infections, Sweden. *Emerg Infect Dis* **9**:1395-1401.

5610. Olsson, M., C. Lidman, S. Latouche, A. Bjorkman, P. Roux, E. Linder, and M. Wahlgren. 1998. Identification of Pneumocystis carinii f. sp. hominis gene sequences in filtered air in hospital environments. *J Clin Microbiol* **36**:1737-40.

5611. Olteanu, G. 2001. Trichinellosis in Romania: a short review over the past twenty years. *Parasite* **8**:S98-9.

5612. Olusi, T. A., J. A. Ajaya, and A. A. Makinde. 1994. Antibodies to Toxoplasma gondii in rat-eating population of Benue state, Nigeria. *Ann Trop Med Parasitol* **88**:217-8.

5613. Omar, M. S., and R. E. Abdalla. 1992. Cutaneous myiasis caused by tumbu fly larvae, Cordylobia anthropophaga in southwestern Saudi Arabia. *Trop Med Parasitol* **43**:128-9.

5614. Omar, M. S., A. K. Sheikha, O. M. Al-Amari, S. E. Abdalla, and R. A. Musa. 2000. Field evaluation of two diagnostic antigen tests for Wuchereria bancrofti infection among Indian expatriates in Saudi Arabia. *Southeast Asian J Trop Med Public Health* **31**:415-8.

5615. Omer, M. K., T. Assefaw, E. Skjerve, T. Tekleghiorghis, and Z. Woldehiwet. 2002. Prevalence of antibodies to Brucella spp. and risk factors related to high-risk occupational groups in Eritrea. *Epidemiol Infect* **129**:85-91.

5616. Omumbo, J. A., C. A. Guerra, S. I. Hay, and R. W. Snow. 2005. The influence of urbanisation on measures of Plasmodium falciparum infection prevalence in East Africa. *Acta Trop* **93**:11-21.

5617. Ong, A. K., R. I. Frankel, and M. H. Maruyama. 1999. Cluster of leprosy cases in Kona, Hawaii; impact of the Compact of Free Association. *Int J Lepr Other Mycobact Dis* **67**:13-8.

5618. Ong, C. S., D. L. Eisler, A. Alikhani, V. W. Fung, J. Tomblin, W. R. Bowie, and J. L. Isaac-Renton. 2002. Novel cryptosporidium genotypes in sporadic cryptosporidiosis cases: first report of human infections with a cervine genotype. *Emerg Infect Dis* **8**:263-8.

5619. Ong, S., D. A. Talan, G. J. Moran, W. Mower, M. Newdow, V. C. Tsang, and R. W. Pinner. 2002. Neurocysticercosis in radiographically imaged seizure patients in U.S. Emergency departments. *Emerg Infect Dis* **8**:608-13.

5620. Ono, K., H. Tsuji, S. K. Rai, A. Yamamoto, K. Masuda, T. Endo, H. Hotta, T. Kawamura, and S. Uga. 2001. Contamination of River Water by Cryptosporidium parvum Oocysts in Western Japan. *Appl Environ Microbiol* **67**:3832-6.

5621. Onyango, C. O., A. A. Grobbelaar, G. V. Gibson, R. C. Sang, A. Sow, R. Swaneopel, and F. J. Burt. 2004. Yellow Fever outbreak, southern Sudan, 2003. *Emerg Infect Dis* **10**:1668-70.

5622. Onyemelukwe, N. F. 1993. A serological survey for leptospirosis in the Enugu area of eastern Nigeria among people at occupational risk. *J Trop Med Hyg* **96**:301-4.

5623. Ooi, W. W., J. M. Gawoski, P. O. Yarbough, and G. A. Pankey. 1999. Hepatitis E seroconversion in United States travelers abroad. *Am J Trop Med Hyg* **61**:822-4.

5624. Ooi, W. W., and S. L. Moschella. 2001. Update on leprosy in immigrants in the United States: status in the year 2000. *Clin Infect Dis* **32**:930-7.

5625. Oostburg, B. F. J., J. E. Anijs, G. P. Oehlers, H. O. Hiwat, and S. M. Burke-Hermelijn. 2003. Case report: the first parasitologically confirmed autochthonous case of acute Chagas disease in Suriname. *Trans R Soc Trop Med Hyg* **97**:166-7.

5626. Oosterheert, J. J., A. M. van Loon, R. Schuurman, A. I. Hoepelman, E. Hak, S. Thijsen, G. Nossent, M. M. Schneider, W. M. Hustinx, and M. J. Bonten. 2005. Impact of rapid detection of viral and atypical bacterial pathogens by real-time polymerase chain reaction for patients with lower respiratory tract infection. *Clin Infect Dis* **41**:1438-44.

5627. Oostvogel, P. M., J. K. van Wijngaarden, H. G. van der Avoort, M. N. Mulders, M. A. Conyn-van Spaendonck, H. C. Rumke, G. van Steenis, and A. M. van Loon. 1994. Poliomyelitis outbreak in an unvaccinated community in The Netherlands, 1992-93. *Lancet* **344**:665-70.

5628. Opara, K. N., O. B. Fagbemi, A. Ekwe, and D. M. Okenu. 2005. Status of Forest Onchocerciasis in the Lower Cross River Basin, Nigeria: Entomologic Profile after Five Years of Ivermectin Intervention. *Am J Trop Med Hyg* **73**:371-376.

5629. Oprica, C., and C. E. Nord. 2005. European surveillance study on the antibiotic susceptibility of Propionibacterium acnes. *Clin Microbiol Infect* **11**:204-13.

5630. Oren, I., T. Zuckerman, I. Avivi, R. Finkelstein, M. Yigla, and J. M. Rowe. 2002. Nosocomial outbreak of Legionella pneumophila serogroup 3 pneumonia in a new bone marrow transplant unit: evaluation, treatment and control. *Bone Marrow Transplant* **30**:175-9.

5631. Orenstein, J. M., J. Chiang, W. Steinberg, P. D. Smith, H. Rotterdam, and D. P. Kotler. 1990. Intestinal microsporidiosis as a cause of diarrhea in human immunodeficiency virus-infected patients: a report of 20 cases. *Hum Pathol* **21**:475-81.

5632. Orenstein, W. A., and A. R. Hinman. 1999. The immunization system in the United States - the role of school immunization laws. *Vaccine* **17 Suppl 3**:S19-24.

5633. Orloski, K. A., and S. L. Lathrop. 2003. Plague: a veterinary perspective. *J Am Vet Med Assoc* **222**:444-8.

5634. Orndorff, G. R., and C. Lebron. 1996. Epidemiology of enterotoxigenic Escherichia coli-associated diarrheal disease occurring on board U.S. Navy ships visiting Asian ports. *Mil Med* **161**:475-8.

5635. Orr, H., E. Kaczmarski, J. Sarangi, B. Pankhania, and J. Stuart. 2001. Meningococcal disease outbreak among young people in northern Ireland. *Commun Dis Publ Health* **4**:316-8.

5636. Orr, P., B. Lorencz, R. Brown, R. Kielly, B. Tan, D. Holton, H. Clugstone, L. Lugtig, C. Pim, S. MacDonald, et al. 1994. An outbreak of diarrhea due to verotoxin-producing Escherichia coli in the Canadian Northwest Territories. *Scand J Infect Dis* **26**:675-84.

5637. **Orr, P., D. Milley, D. Colby, and M. Fost.** 1994. Prolonged fecal excretion of verotoxin-producing Escherichia coli following diarrheal illness. *Clin Infect Dis* **19:**796-7.

5638. **Orr, P. H., and R. Brown.** 1998. Incidence of ectopic pregnancy and sexually transmitted disease in the Canadian Central Arctic. *Int J Circumpolar Health* **57 Suppl 1:**127-34.

5639. **Ortega, Y. R., C. R. Roxas, R. H. Gilman, N. J. Miller, L. Cabrera, C. Taquiri, and C. R. Sterling.** 1997. Isolation of Cryptosporidium parvum and Cyclospora cayetanensis from vegetables collected in markets of an endemic region in Peru. *Am J Trop Med Hyg* **57:**683-6.

5640. **Orth, B., R. Frei, P. H. Itin, M. G. Rinaldi, B. Speck, A. Gratwohl, and A. F. Widmer.** 1996. Outbreak of invasive mycoses caused by Paecilomyces lilacinus from a contaminated skin lotion. *Ann Intern Med* **125:**799-806.

5641. **Ortiz, D. I., A. Wozniak, M. W. Tolson, P. E. Turner, and D. R. Vaughan.** 2003. Isolation of EEE virus from Ochlerotatus taeniorhynchus and Culiseta melanura in coastal South Carolina. *J Am Mosq Control Assoc* **19:**33-8.

5642. **Ortiz-Roque, C. M., and T. C. Hazen.** 1987. Abundance and distribution of Legionellaceae in Puerto Rican waters. *Appl Environ Microbiol* **53:**2231-6.

5643. **Orton, S. L., H. Liu, R. Y. Dodd, and A. E. Williams.** 2002. Prevalence of circulating Treponema pallidum DNA and RNA in blood donors with confirmed-positive syphilis tests. *Transfusion* **42:**94-9.

5644. **Oshima, T.** 1987. Anisakiasis - is the sushi bar guilty? *Parasitol Today* **3:**44-8.

5645. **Osmond, D. H., S. Buchbinder, A. Cheng, A. Graves, E. Vittinghoff, C. K. Cossen, B. Forghani, and J. N. Martin.** 2002. Prevalence of Kaposi sarcoma-associated herpesvirus infection in homosexual men at beginning of and during the HIV epidemic. *JAMA* **287:**221-5.

5646. **Osorio, L., J. Todd, and D. J. Bradley.** 2004. Travel histories as risk factors in the analysis of urban malaria in Colombia. *Am J Trop Med Hyg* **71:**380-6.

5647. **Osterholm, M. T.** 2004. Foodborne disease: the more things change, the more they stay the same. *Clin Infect Dis* **39:**8-10.

5648. **Osterholm, M. T., and A. P. Norgan.** 2004. The role of irradiation in food safety. *N Engl J Med* **350:**1898-901.

5649. **Osterman, K. L., and V. A. Rahm.** 2000. Lactation mastitis: bacterial cultivation of breast milk, symptoms, treatment, and outcome. *J Hum Lact* **16:**297-302.

5650. **Ostroff, S. M., G. Kappeerud, J. Lassen, S. Aasen, and R. V. Tauxe.** 1992. Clinical features of sporadic Yersinia enterocolitica infections in Norway. *J Infect Dis* **166:**812-7.

5651. **Ostroff, S. M., G. Kapperud, L. C. Hutwagner, T. Nesbakken, N. H. Bean, J. Lassen, and R. V. Tauxe.** 1994. Sources of sporadic Yersinia enterocolitica infections in Norway: a prospective case-control study. *Epidemiol Infect* **112:**133-41.

5652. **Ostrowsky, B. E., C. Whitener, H. K. Bredenberg, L. A. Carson, S. Holt, L. Hutwagner, M. J. Arduino, and W. R. Jarvis.** 2002. Serratia marcescens bacteremia traced to an infused narcotic. *N Engl J Med* **346:**1529-37.

5653. **Oteo, J. A., V. Ibarra, J. R. Blanco, L. Metola, M. Vallejo, and V. M. De Artola.** 2003. Epidemiological and clinical differences among Rickettsia slovaca rickettsiosis and other tickborne diseases in Spain. *Ann N Y Acad Sci* **990:**355-6.

5654. **Otero, A. C., V. O. da Silva, K. G. Luz, M. Palatnik, C. Pirmez, O. Fernandes, and C. B. Palatnik de Sousa.** 2000. Short report: occurrence of Leishmania donovani DNA in donated blood from seroreactive Brazilian blood donors. *Am J Trop Med Hyg* **62:**128-31.

5655. **Otofuji, T., H. Tokiwa, and K. Takahashi.** 1987. A food-poisoning incident caused by Clostridium botulinum toxin A in Japan. *Epidemiol Infect* **99:**167-72.

5656. **Otranto, D., and D. Traversa.** 2003. Dicrocoeliosis of ruminants: a little known fluke disease. *Trends Parasitol* **19:**12-5.

5657. **Otsu, R.** 1999. Outbreaks of gastroenteritis caused by SRSVs from 1987 to 1992 in Kyushu, Japan: four outbreaks associated with oyster consumption. *Eur J Epidemiol* **15:**175-80.

5658. **Ou, J., Q. Li, G. Zeng, Z. Dun, A. Qin, and R. E. Fontaine.** 2003. Efficiency of quarantine during an epidemic of severe acute respiratory syndrome - Beijing, China, 2003. *MMWR* **52:**1037-40.

5659. **Ouagari, Z., A. Chakib, M. Sodqi, L. Marih, K. Marhoum Filali, A. Benslama, L. Idrissi, S. Moutawakkil, and H. Himmich.** 2002. Le botulisme à Casablanca. (A propos de 11 cas). *Bull Soc Pathol Exot* **95:**272-5.

5660. **Ouzan, D.** 1999. [Risk of transmission of hepatitis C through endoscopy of the digestive tract]. *Presse Med* **28:**1091-4.

5661. **Overgaauw, P. A.** 1997. Aspects of Toxocara epidemiology: human toxocarosis. *Crit Rev Microbiol* **23:**215-31.

5662. **Overgaauw, P. A., and J. H. Boersema.** 1998. Nematode infections in dog breeding kennels in The Netherlands, with special reference to Toxocara. *Vet Q* **20:**12-5.

5663. **Owen, I. L., M. A. Gomez Morales, P. Pezzotti, and E. Pozio.** 2005. Trichinella infection in a hunting population of Papua New Guinea suggests an ancient relationship between Trichinella and human beings. *Trans R Soc Trop Med Hyg* **99:**618-24.

5664. **Oyofo, B. A., R. Soderquist, M. Lesmana, D. Subekti, P. Tjaniadi, D. J. Fryauff, A. L. Corwin, E. Richie, and C. Lebron.** 1999. Norwalk-like virus and bacterial pathogens associated with cases of gastroenteritis onboard a US Navy ship. *Am J Trop Med Hyg* **61:**904-8.

5665. **Ozbonfil, D., D. Cohen, E. Ohad, and I. Sechter.** 1990. An outbreak of enteritis associated with enteroinvasive E. coli in an Israeli military base. *Public Health Rev* **18:**171-7.

5666. **Pabst, W. L., M. Altwegg, C. Kind, S. Mirjanic, D. Hardegger, and D. Nadal.** 2003. Prevalence of enteroaggregative Escherichia coli among children with and without diarrhea in Switzerland. *J Clin Microbiol* **41:**2289-93.

5667. **Pacha, R. E., G. W. Clark, E. A. Williams, A. M. Carter, J. J. Scheffelmaier, and P. Debusschere.** 1987. Small rodents and other mammals associated with mountain meadows as reservoirs of Giardia spp. and Campylobacter spp. *Appl Environ Microbiol* **53:**1574-9.

5668. **Pacheco Schubach, T. M., A. de Oliveira Schubach, R. S. dos Reis, T. Cuzzi-Maya, T. C. Moita Blanco, D. Ferreira Monteiro, M. B. de Lima Barros, R. Brustein, R. M. Zancopé-Oliveira, P. C. Fialho Monteiro, and B. Wanke.** 2001. Sporothrix schenckii isolated from domestic cats with and without sporotrichosis in Rio de Janeiro, Brazil. *Mycopathologia* **153:**83-6.

5669. **Pachucki, C. T., S. A. Pappas, G. F. Fuller, S. L. Krause, J. R. Lentino, and D. M. Schaaff.** 1989. Influenza A among hospital personnel and patients. Implications for recognition, prevention, and control. *Arch Intern Med* **149:**77-80.

5670. **Pacini, D. L., A. M. Collier, and F. W. Henderson.** 1987. Adenovirus infections and respiratory illnesses in children in group day care. *J Infect Dis* **156**:920-7.

5671. **Paddock, C. D., S. R. Zaki, T. Koss, J. Singleton, Jr., J. W. Sumner, J. A. Comer, M. E. Eremeeva, G. A. Dasch, B. Cherry, and J. E. Childs.** 2003. Rickettsialpox in New York City: a persistent urban zoonosis. *Ann N Y Acad Sci* **990**:36-44.

5672. **Padula, P., M. G. Della Valle, M. G. Alai, P. Cortada, M. Villagra, and A. Gianella.** 2002. Andes virus and first case report of Bermejo virus causing fatal pulmonary syndrome. *Emerg Infect Dis* **8**:437-9.

5673. **Padula, P. J., A. Edelstein, S. D. Miguel, N. M. Lopez, C. M. Rossi, and R. D. Rabinovich.** 1998. Hantavirus pulmonary syndrome outbreak in Argentina: molecular evidence for person-to-person transmission of Andes virus. *Virology* **241**:323-30.

5674. **Paez Jimenez, A., R. Pimentel, M. V. Martinez de Aragon, G. Hernandez Pezzi, S. Mateo Ontanon, and J. F. Martinez Navarro.** 2004. Waterborne outbreak among Spanish tourists in a holiday resort in the Dominican Republic, August 2002. *Eurosurveillance* **9**:21-3.

5675. **Pagane, J., A. Chanmugam, T. Kirsch, and G. D. Kelen.** 1996. New York City police officers incidence of transcutaneous exposures. *Occup Med (Lond)* **46**:285-8.

5676. **Page-Shafer, K. A., W. McFarland, R. Kohn, K. J., and M. H. Katz.** 1999. Increases in usafe sex and rectal gonorrhea among men who have sex with men - San Francisco, California, 1994-1997. *MMWR* **48**:45-48.

5677. **Paget, W. J., R. Zbinden, E. Ritzler, M. Zwahlen, C. Lengeler, D. Sturchler, and H. C. Matter.** 2002. National laboratory reports of Chlamydia trachomatis seriously underestimate the frequency of genital chlamydial infections among women in Switzerland. *Sex Transm Dis* **29**:715-20.

5678. **(PAHO), P. A. H. O.** 2003. Status report on malaria programs in the Americas, p. 1-48, Washington, D.C.

5679. **Pai, H. H., Y. C. Ko, and E. R. Chen.** 2003. Cockroaches (Periplaneta americana and Blattella germanica) as potential mechanical disseminators of Entamoeba histolytica. *Acta Trop* **87**:355-9.

5680. **Pai, M., G. Kang, B. S. Ramakrishna, A. Venkataraman, and J. Muliyil.** 1997. An epidemic of diarrhoea in south India caused by enteroaggregative Escherichia coli. *Indian J Med Res* **106**:7-12.

5681. **Pai, R. K., S. A. Pergam, A. Kedia, C. S. Cadman, and L. A. Osborn.** 2004. Pacemaker lead infection secondary to Haemophilus parainfluenzae. *Pacing Clin Electrophysiol* **27**:1008-10.

5682. **Paine, M., S. Davis, and G. Brown.** 1994. Severe forms of infection with Angiostrongylus cantonensis acquired in Australia and Fiji. *Aust N Z J Med* **24**:415-6.

5683. **Pak, S. I., U. Spahr, T. Jemmi, and M. D. Salman.** 2002. Risk factors for L. monocytogenes contamination of dairy products in Switzerland, 1990-1999. *Prev Vet Med* **53**:55-65.

5684. **Pakendorf, U. W., M. S. Bornman, and D. J. Du Plessis.** 1998. Prevalence of human papilloma virus in men attending the infertility clinic. *Andrologia* **30**:11-4.

5685. **Pakianathan, M. R., and A. McMillan.** 1999. Intestinal protozoa in homosexual men in Edinburgh. *Int J STD AIDS* **10**:780-4.

5686. **Palanduz, A., S. Palanduz, K. Guler, and N. Guler.** 2000. Brucellosis in a mother and her young infant: probable transmission by breast milk. *Int J Infect Dis* **4**:55-6.

5687. **Palau, L. A., and G. A. Pankey.** 1997. Mediterranean spotted fever in travelers from the United States. *J Travel Med* **4**:179-82.

5688. **Palau, L. A., and G. A. Pankey.** 1997. Strongyloides hyperinfection in a renal transplant recipient receiving cyclosporine: possible Strongyloides stercoralis transmission by kidney transplant. *Am J Trop Med Hyg* **57**:413-5.

5689. **Palefsky, J. M., E. A. Holly, M. L. Ralston, and N. Jay.** 1998. Prevalence and risk factors for human papillomavirus infection of the anal canal in human immunodeficiency virus (HIV)-positive and HIV- negative homosexual men. *J Infect Dis* **177**:361-7.

5690. **Palmer, A. E.** 1987. B virus, Herpesvirus simiae: historical perspective. *J Med Primatol* **16**:99-130.

5691. **Palmer, C. J., L. Validum, B. Loeffke, H. E. Laubach, C. Mitchell, R. Cummings, and R. R. Cuadrado.** 2002. HIV Prevalence in a Gold Mining Camp in the Amazon Region, Guyana. *Emerg Infect Dis* **8**:330-1.

5692. **Palmer, C. J., L. Xiao, A. Terashima, H. Guerra, E. Gotuzzo, G. Saldias, J. A. Bonilla, L. Zhou, A. Lindquist, and S. J. Upton.** 2003. Cryptosporidium muris, a rodent pathogen, recovered from a human in Peru. *Emerg Infect Dis* **9**:1174-6.

5693. **Palmer, S. R., B. E. Andrews, and R. Major.** 1981. A common-source outbreaks of ornithosis in veterinary surgeons. *Lancet* **2**:798-9.

5694. **Palmer, S. R., Lord Soulsby, and D. I. H. e. Simpson.** 1998. Zoonoses. Biology, clinical practice, and public health control. Oxford University Press, Oxford.

5695. **Palmer, S. R., and B. Rowe.** 1986. Trends in salmonella infections. *Public Health Laboratory Service Microbiology Digest* **3**:3-5.

5696. **Palmer, S. R., J. E. Watkeys, I. Zamiri, P. G. Hutchings, C. H. Howells, and J. F. Skone.** 1990. Outbreak of Salmonella food poisoning amongst delegates at a medical conference. *J R Coll Physicians Lond* **24**:26-9.

5697. **Palomino, M. A., C. Larranaga, and L. F. Avendano.** 2000. Hospital-acquired adenovirus 7h infantile respiratory infection in Chile. *Pediatr Infect Dis J* **19**:527-31.

5698. **Pamphilon, D. H., J. R. Rider, J. A. Barbara, and L. M. Williamson.** 1999. Prevention of transfusion-transmitted cytomegalovirus infection. *Transfus Med* **9**:115-23.

5699. **Pampiglione, S., M. L. Fioravanti, and F. Rivasi.** 2003. Human sparganosis in Italy. Case report and review of the European cases. *APMIS* **111**:349-54.

5700. **Pampiglione, S., R. Peraldi, and J. P. Burelli.** 1999. [Human dirofilariasis in Corsica: a new local case. Review of reported cases]. *Bull Soc Pathol Exot* **92**:305-8.

5701. **Pampiglione, S., and M. L. Ricciardi.** 1971. The presence of Strongyloides fülleborni von Linstow, 1905, in man in central and east Africa. *Parasitologia* **13**:257-68.

5702. **Pampiglione, S., and F. Rivasi.** 2000. Human dirofilariasis due to Dirofilaria (Nochtiella) repens: an update of world literature from 1995 to 2000. *Parasitologia* **42**:231-54.

5703. **Pampiglione, S., F. Rivasi, M. Criscuolo, A. De Benedittis, A. Gentile, S. Russo, M. Testini, and M. Villan.** 2002. Human anisakiasis in Italy: a report of eleven new cases. *Pathol Res Pract* **198**:429-34.

5704. **Pan, E. S., B. A. Diep, H. A. Carleton, E. D. Charlebois, G. F. Sensabaugh, B. L. Haller, and F. Perdreau-Remington.** 2003. Increasing prevalence of methicillin-resistant Staphylococcus aureus infection in California jails. *Clin Infect Dis* **37:**1384-8.

5705. **Pan, L.** 1993. [Actinomyces-like organisms infection in intrauterine devices wearers]. *Zhonghua Fu Chan Ke Za Zhi* **28:**292-4, 315.

5706. **Panackal, A. A., R. A. Hajjeh, M. S. Cetron, and D. W. Warnock.** 2002. Fungal Infections among Returning Travelers. *Clin Infect Dis* **35:**1088-95.

5707. **Panceri, M. L., F. E. Vegni, A. Goglio, A. Manisco, R. Tambini, A. Lizioli, A. D. Porretta, and G. Privitera.** 2004. Aetiology and prognosis of bacteraemia in Italy. *Epidemiol Infect* **132:**647-54.

5708. **Pancharoen, C., U. Thisyakorn, W. Lawtongkum, and H. Wilde.** 2001. Rabies exposures in Thai children. *Wilderness Environ Med* **12:**239-43.

5709. **Pandey, P., D. R. Shlim, W. Cave, and M. F. B. Springer.** 2002. Risk of possible exposure to rabies among tourists and foreign residents in Nepal. *J Travel Med* **9:**127-31.

5710. **Panella, H., A. Plasencia, M. Sanz, and J. A. Cayla.** 1995. [An evaluation of the epidemiological surveillance system for infectious diseases in the Barcelona Olympic Games of 1992]. *Gac Sanit* **9:**84-90.

5711. **Pang, S. C., R. H. Harrison, J. Brearley, V. Jegathesan, and A. S. Clayton.** 2000. Tuberculosis surveillance in immigrants through health undertakings in Western Australia. *Int J Tuberc Lung Dis* **4:**232-6.

5712. **Panlilio, A. L., C. M. Beck-Sague, J. D. Siegel, R. L. Anderson, S. Y. Yetts, N. C. Clark, P. N. Duer, K. A. Thomassen, R. W. Vess, B. C. Hill, et al.** 1992. Infections and pseudoinfections due to povidone-iodine solution contaminated with Pseudomonas cepacia. *Clin Infect Dis* **14:**1078-83.

5713. **Panlilio, A. L., D. R. Burwen, A. B. Curtis, P. U. Srivastava, J. Bernardo, M. T. Catalano, M. H. Mendelson, P. Nicholas, W. Pagano, C. Sulis, I. M. Onorato, and M. E. Chamberland.** 2002. Tuberculin skin testing surveillance of health care personnel. *Clin Infect Dis* **35:**219-27.

5714. **Panlilio, A. L., D. M. Cardo, L. A. Grohskopf, W. Heneine, and C. S. Ross.** 2005. Updated U.S. Public Health Service guidelines for the management of occupational exposures to HIV and recommendations for postexposure prophylaxis. *MMWR Recomm Rep* **54:**1-17.

5715. **Pannekoek, Y., S. M. Westenberg, J. De Vries, S. Repping, L. Spanjaard, P. P. Eijk, A. van der Ende, and J. Dankert.** 2000. PCR assessment of Chlamydia trachomatis infection of semen specimens processed for artificial insemination. *J Clin Microbiol* **38:**3763-7.

5716. **Pantosti, A., M. Del Grosso, S. Tagliabue, A. Macri, and A. Caprioli.** 1999. Decrease of vancomycin-resistant enterococci in poultry meat after avoparcin ban. *Lancet* **354:**741-2.

5717. **Papa, A., B. Bozovic, V. Pavlidou, E. Papadimitriou, M. Pelemis, and A. Antoniadis.** 2002. Genetic detection and isolation of crimean-congo hemorrhagic Fever virus, kosovo, yugoslavia. *Emerg Infect Dis* **8:**852-4.

5718. **Papa, A., I. Christova, E. Papadimitriou, and A. Antoniadis.** 2004. Crimean-Congo hemorrhagic fever in Bulgaria. *Emerg Infect Dis* **10:**1465-7.

5719. **Papapetropoulou, M., and A. C. Vantarakis.** 1998. Detection of adenovirus outbreak at a municipal swimming pool by nested PCR amplification. *J Infect* **36:**101-3.

5720. **Pape, W. J., T. D. Fitzsimmons, and R. E. Hoffman.** 1999. Risk for rabies transmission from encounters with bats, Colorado, 1977-1996. *Emerg Infect Dis* **5:**433-7.

5721. **Pappas, P. G., I. Tellez, A. E. Deep, D. Nolasco, W. Holgado, and B. Bustamante.** 2000. Sporotrichosis in Peru: description of an area of hyperendemicity. *Clin Infect Dis* **30:**65-70.

5722. **Paquet, C., P. Leborgne, A. Sasse, and F. Varaine.** 1995. [An outbreak of Shigella dysenteriae type 1 dysentery in a refugee camp in Rwanda]. *Sante* **5:**181-4.

5723. **Para, M.** 1965. An outbreak of post-vaccinal rabies (rage de laboratoire) in Fortaleza, Brazil, in 1960. Residual fixed virus as the etiological agent. *Bull WHO* **33:**177-82.

5724. **Paradisi, F., G. Corti, and R. Cinelli.** 2001. Streptococcus pneumoniae as an agent of nosocomial infection: treatment in the era of penicillin-resistant strains. *Clin Microbiol Infect* **7 Suppl 4:**34-42.

5725. **Parashar, U. D., L. Dow, R. L. Fankhauser, C. D. Humphrey, J. Miller, T. Ando, K. S. Williams, C. R. Eddy, J. S. Noel, T. Ingram, J. S. Bresee, S. S. Monroe, and R. I. Glass.** 1998. An outbreak of viral gastroenteritis associated with consumption of sandwiches: implications for the control of transmission by food handlers. *Epidemiol Infect* **121:**615-21.

5726. **Parashar, U. D., E. G. Hummelman, J. S. Bresee, M. A. Miller, and R. I. Glass.** 2003. Global illness and deaths caused by rotavirus disease in children. *Emerg Infect Dis* **9:**565-72.

5727. **Parashar, U. D., E. S. Quiroz, A. W. Mounts, S. S. Monroe, R. L. Fankhauser, T. Ando, J. S. Noel, S. N. Bulens, S. R. Beard, J. F. Li, J. S. Bresee, and R. I. Glass.** 2001. "Norwalk-like Viruses". Public health consequences and outbreak management. *MMWR* **50 (RR-9):**1-17.

5728. **Paris, M., E. Gotuzzo, G. Goyzueta, J. Aramburu, C. F. Caceres, D. Crawford, T. Castellano, S. H. Vermund, and E. W. Hook, 3rd.** 2001. Motorcycle taxi drivers and sexually transmitted infections in a Peruvian Amazon City. *Sex Transm Dis* **28:**11-3.

5729. **Parise, M. E., L. S. Lewis, J. G. Ayisi, B. L. Nahlen, L. Slutsker, R. Muga, S. K. Sharif, J. Hill, and R. W. Steketee.** 2003. A rapid assessment approach for public health decision-making related to the prevention of malaria during pregnancy. *Bull WHO* **81:**316-23.

5730. **Parish, W. L., E. O. Laumann, M. S. Cohen, S. Pan, H. Zheng, I. Hoffman, T. Wang, and K. H. Ng.** 2003. Population-based study of chlamydial infection in China. A hidden epidemic. *JAMA* **289:**1265-73.

5731. **Parisi, A., G. Normanno, N. Addante, A. Dambrosio, C. O. Montagna, N. C. Quaglia, G. V. Celano, and D. Chiocco.** 2004. Market survey of Vibrio spp. and other microorganisms in Italian shellfish. *J Food Prot* **67:**2284-7.

5732. **Park, J. W., T. A. Klein, H. C. Lee, L. A. Pacha, S. H. Ryu, J. S. Yeom, S. H. Moon, T. S. Kim, J. Y. Chai, M. D. Oh, and K. W. Choe.** 2003. Vivax malaria: a continuing health threat to the republic of Korea. *Am J Trop Med Hyg* **69:**159-67.

5733. **Park, J. Y., C. J. Peters, P. E. Rollin, T. G. Ksiazek, C. R. Katholi, K. B. Waites, B. Gray, H. M. Maetz, and C. B. Stephensen.** 1997. Age distribution of lymphocytic choriomeningitis virus serum antibody in Birmingham, Alabama: evidence of a decreased risk of infection. *Am J Trop Med Hyg* **57:**37-41.

5734. **Park, S. G., S. H. Oh, S. B. Suh, K. H. Lee, and K. Y. Chung.** 2005. A case of chromoblastomycosis with an unusual clinical manifestation caused by Phialophora verrucosa on an unexposed area: treatment with a combination of amphotericin B and 5-flucytosine. *Br J Dermatol* **152:**560-4.

5735. **Parkin, R. T., J. A. Soller, and A. W. Olivieri.** 2003. Incorporating susceptible subpopulations in microbial risk assessment: pediatric exposures to enteroviruses in river water. *J Expo Anal Environ Epidemiol* **13:**161-8.

5736. **Parmet, A. J.** 1999. Tuberculosis on the flight deck. *Aviat Space Environ Med* **70:**817-8.

5737. **Parola, P., F. Fenollar, S. Badiaga, P. Brouqui, and D. Raoult.** 2001. First documentation of Rickettsia conorii infection (strain Indian tick typhus) in a traveler. *Emerg Infect Dis* **7:**909-10.

5738. **Parola, P., J. Jourdan, and D. Raoult.** 1998. Tick-borne infection caused by Rickettsia africae in the West Indies. *N Engl J Med* **338:**1391.

5739. **Parola, P., and D. Raoult.** 2001. Ticks and tickborne bacterial diseases in humans: an emerging infectious threat. *Clin Infect Dis* **32:**897-928.

5740. **Parola, P., D. Vogelaers, C. Roure, F. Janbon, and D. Raoult.** 1998. Murine typhus in travelers returning from Indonesia. *Emerg Infect Dis* **4:**677-80.

5741. **Parrott, P. L., P. M. Terry, E. N. Whitworth, L. W. Frawley, R. S. Coble, I. K. Wachsmuth, and J. E. McGowan, Jr.** 1982. Pseudomonas aeruginosa peritonitis associated with contaminated poloxamer-iodine solution. *Lancet* **2:**683-5.

5742. **Parry, C. M., T. T. Hien, G. Dougan, N. J. White, and J. J. Farrar.** 2002. Typhoid fever. *N Engl J Med* **347:**1770-82.

5743. **Parry, S. M., and R. L. Salmon.** 1998. Sporadic STEC O157 infection: secondary household transmission in Wales. *Emerg Infect Dis* **4:**657-61.

5744. **Parry, S. M., R. L. Salmon, G. A. Willshaw, and T. Cheasty.** 1998. Risk factors for and prevention of sporadic infections with vero cytotoxin (shiga toxin) producing Escherichia coli O157. *Lancet* **351:**1019-22.

5745. **Parveen, S., M. S. Islam, and A. Huq.** 1995. Abundance of Aeromonas spp. in river and lake waters in and around Dhaka, Bangladesh. *J Diarrhoeal Dis Res* **13:**183-6.

5746. **Pascal, B., D. Baudon, A. Keundjian, T. Fusai, P. Cochet, J. F. Soupault, G. Brault-Noble, G. Martet, T. Matton, R. Stor, J. C. Doury, and R. Laroche.** 1997. [Malaria epidemic during a military-humanitarian mission in Africa]. *Med Trop (Mars)* **57:**253-5.

5747. **Pascual, F. B., E. L. McGinley, L. R. Zanardi, M. M. Cortese, and T. V. Murphy.** 2003. Tetanus surveillance - United States, 1998-2000. *MMWR* **52 (SS-3):**1-8.

5748. **Pasquini, P., A. Mele, E. Franco, G. Ippolito, and B. Svennerholm.** 1988. Prevalence of herpes simplex virus type 2 antibodies in selected population groups in Italy. *Eur J Clin Microbiol Infect Dis* **7:**54-6.

5749. **Pass, R. F.** 2004. HHV6 and HHV7: persistence and vertical transmission. *J Pediatr* **145:**432-5.

5750. **Passoni, L. F., B. Wanke, M. M. Nishikawa, and M. S. Lazera.** 1998. Cryptococcus neoformans isolated from human dwellings in Rio de Janeiro, Brazil: an analysis of the domestic environment of AIDS patients with and without cryptococcosis. *Med Mycol* **36:**305-11.

5751. **Pastuszak, A. L., M. Levy, B. Schick, C. Zuber, M. Feldkamp, J. Gladstone, F. Bar-Levy, E. Jackson, A. Donnenfeld, W. Meschino, et al.** 1994. Outcome after maternal varicella infection in the first 20 weeks of pregnancy. *N Engl J Med* **330:**901-5.

5752. **Patamasucon, P., U. B. Schaad, and J. D. Nelson.** 1982. Melioidosis. *J Pediatr* **100:**175-82.

5753. **Patel, P. A., and M. D. Voigt.** 2002. Prevalence and interaction of hepatitis B and latent tuberculosis in Vietnamese immigrants to the United States. *Am J Gastroenterol* **97:**1198-203.

5754. **Patel, R., and C. V. Paya.** 1997. Infections in solid-organ transplant recipients. *Clin Microbiol Rev* **10:**86-124.

5755. **Paterson, D. L., P. K. Murray, and J. G. McCormack.** 1998. Zoonotic disease in Australia caused by a novel member of the paramyxoviridae. *Clin Infect Dis* **27:**112-8.

5756. **Paton, A. W., R. M. Ratcliff, R. M. Doyle, J. Seymour-Murray, D. Davos, J. A. Lanser, and J. C. Paton.** 1996. Molecular microbiological investigation of an outbreak of hemolytic-uremic syndrome caused by dry fermented sausage contaminated with Shiga-like toxin-producing Escherichia coli. *J Clin Microbiol* **34:**1622-7.

5757. **Paton, N. I., L. Y.S., S. R. Zaki, A. P. Auchus, K. E. Lee, A. E. Ling, S. K. Chew, B. Ang, P. E. Rollin, T. Umapathi, I. Sng, C. C. Lee, E. Lim, and T. G. Ksiazek.** 1999. Outbreak of Nipavirus infection among aattoir workers in Singapore. *Lancet* **354:**1253-1256.

5758. **Patriarca, P. A., R. W. Sutter, and P. M. Oostvogel.** 1997. Outbreaks of paralytic poliomyelitis, 1976-1995. *J Infect Dis* **175 Suppl 1:**S165-72.

5759. **Patriarca, P. A., J. A. Weber, R. A. Parker, W. A. Orenstein, W. N. Hall, A. P. Kendal, and L. B. Schonberger.** 1986. Risk factors for outbreaks of influenza in nursing homes. A case-control study. *Am J Epidemiol* **124:**114-9.

5760. **Patricio Berrios, E.** 2005. [Equine influenza in Chile (1963-1992): A possible human case.]. *Rev Chilena Infectol* **22:**47-50.

5761. **Patrick, D. M., S. Champagne, S. H. Goh, G. Arsenault, E. Thomas, C. Shaw, T. Rahim, F. Taha, M. Bigham, V. Dubenko, D. Skowronski, and R. C. Brunham.** 2003. Neisseria meningitidis carriage during an outbreak of serogroup C disease. *Clin Infect Dis* **37:**1183-8.

5762. **Patrick, D. M., M. L. Rekart, A. Jolly, S. Mak, M. Tyndall, J. Maginley, E. Wong, T. Wong, H. Jones, C. Montgomery, and R. C. Brunham.** 2002. Heterosexual outbreak of infectious syphilis: epidemiological and ethnographic analysis and implications for control. *Sex Transm Infect* **78 Suppl 1:**i164-9.

5763. **Patrick, M. E., P. M. Adcock, T. M. Gomez, S. F. Altekruse, B. H. Holland, R. V. Tauxe, and D. L. Swerdlow.** 2004. Salmonella Enteritidis infections, United States, 1985-1999. *Emerg Infect Dis* **10:**1-7.

5764. **Patten, J. H., and I. Susanti.** 2001. Reproductive health and STDs among clients of a women's health mobile clinic in rural Bali, Indonesia. *Int J STD AIDS* **12:**47-9.

5765. **Patterson, C. R., and P. J. Kersey.** 2003. Cutaneous larva migrans acquired in England. *Clin Exp Dermatol* **28:**671-2.

5766. **Patterson, S., D. Bugenske, C. Pozsik, E. Brenner, and R. Bellew.** 2000. Drug-susceptible tuberculosis outbreak in a state correctional facility housing HIV-infected inmates—South Carolina, 1999-2000. *MMWR* **49:**1041-4.

5767. **Pattison, S. J.** 1998. The emergence of bovine spongiform encephalopathy and related diseases. *Emerg Infect Dis* **4:**390-394.

5768. **Paul, H. M.** 1993. Mass casualty: Pope's Denver visit causes mega MCI (mass casualty incident). *J Emerg Med Serv JEMS* **18:**64-8, 72-5.

5769. **Paul, J., and J. Bates.** 2000. Is infestation with the common bedbug increasing? *BMJ* **320:**1141.

5770. **Paul, K., and S. S. Patel.** 2001. Eikenella corrodens infections in children and adolescents: case reports and review of the literature. *Clin Infect Dis* **33:**54-61.

5771. **Paul, R. E., A. Y. Patel, S. Mirza, S. P. Fisher-Hoch, and S. P. Luby.** 1998. Expansion of epidemic dengue viral infections to Pakistan. *Int J Infect Dis* **2:**197-201.

5772. **Paul, W. S., G. Maupin, A. O. Scott-Wright, R. B. Craven, and D. T. Dennis.** 2002. Outbreak of tick-borne relapsing fever at the north rim of the Grand Canyon: evidence for effectiveness of preventive measures. *Am J Trop Med Hyg* **66:**71-5.

5773. **Paul, W. S., P. S. Moore, N. Karabatsos, S. P. Flood, S. Yamada, T. Jackson, and T. F. Tsai.** 1993. Outbreak of Japanese encephalitis on the island of Saipan, 1990. *J Infect Dis* **167:**1053-8.

5774. **Paulet, R., C. Caussin, J. M. Coudray, D. Selcer, and P. de Rohan Chabot.** 1994. [Visceral form of human anthrax imported from Africa]. *Presse Med* **23:**477-8.

5775. **Paunio, M., R. Pebody, M. Keskimaki, M. Kokki, P. Ruutu, S. Oinonen, V. Vuotari, A. Siitonen, E. Lahti, and P. Leinikki.** 1999. Swimming-associated outbreak of Escherichia coli O157:H7. *Epidemiol Infect* **122:**1-5.

5776. **Paunio, M., H. Peltola, M. Valle, I. Davidkin, M. Virtanen, and O. P. Heinonen.** 1998. Explosive school-based measles outbreak. Intense exposure may have resulted in high risk, even among revaccinees. *Am J Epidemiol* **148:**1103-10.

5777. **Pavia, A. T., C. R. Nichols, D. P. Green, R. V. Tauxe, S. Mottice, K. D. Greene, J. G. Wells, R. L. Siegler, E. D. Brewer, D. Hannon, et al.** 1990. Hemolytic-uremic syndrome during an outbreak of Escherichia coli O157:H7 infections in institutions for mentally retarded persons: clinical and epidemiologic observations. *J Pediatr* **116:**544-51.

5778. **Pavia, A. T., L. Nielsen, L. Armington, D. J. Thurman, E. Tierney, and C. R. Nichols.** 1990. A community-wide outbreak of hepatitis A in a religious community: impact of mass administration of immune globulin. *Am J Epidemiol* **131:**1085-93.

5779. **Pawlowski, Z., and J. Stefaniak.** 2003. The pig strain of Echinococcus granulosus in humans: a neglected issue? *Trends Parasitol* **19:**439.

5780. **Paxton, L. A., L. Slutsker, L. J. Schultz, S. P. Luby, R. Meriwether, P. Matson, and A. J. Sulzer.** 1996. Imported malaria in Montagnard refugees settling in North Carolina: implications for prevention and control. *Am J Trop Med Hyg* **54:**54-7.

5781. **Paya, C. V.** 2001. Prevention of fungal and hepatitis virus infections in liver transplants. *Clin Infect Dis* **33** (**suppl 1**)S47–S52.

5782. **Payne, L. N., and K. Venugopal.** 2000. Neoplastic diseases: Marek's disease, avian leukosis and reticuloendotheliosis. *Rev Sci Tech* **19:**544-64.

5783. **Payne, S. B., E. A. Grilli, A. J. Smith, and T. W. Hoskins.** 1984. Investigation of an outbreak of adenovirus type 3 infection in a boys' boarding school. *J Hyg (Lond)* **93:**277-83.

5784. **Paz-Bailey, G., C. Monroy, A. Rodas, R. Rosales, R. Tabaru, C. Davies, and J. Lines.** 2002. Incidence of Trypanosoma cruzi infection in two Guatemalan communities. *Trans R Soc Trop Med Hyg* **96:**48-52.

5785. **Pead, P. J.** 2003. Benjamin Jesty: new light in the dawn of vaccination. *Lancet* **362:**2104-9.

5786. **Pealer, L. N., A. A. Marfin, L. R. Petersen, R. S. Lanciotti, P. L. Page, S. L. Stramer, M. G. Stobierski, K. Signs, B. Newman, H. Kapoor, J. L. Goodman, and M. E. Chamberland.** 2003. Transmission of West Nile virus through blood transfusion in the United States in 2002. *N Engl J Med* **349:**1236-45.

5787. **Pearce, M. C., J. W. Sheridan, D. M. Jones, G. W. Lawrence, D. M. Murphy, B. Masutti, C. McCosker, V. Douglas, D. George, A. O'Keefe, et al.** 1995. Control of group C meningococcal disease in Australian aboriginal children by mass rifampicin chemoprophylaxis and vaccination. *Lancet* **346:**20-3.

5788. **Pearson, M. L., J. A. Jereb, T. R. Frieden, J. T. Crawford, B. J. Davis, S. W. Dooley, and W. R. Jarvis.** 1992. Nosocomial transmission of multidrug-resistant Mycobacterium tuberculosis. A risk to patients and health care workers. *Ann Intern Med* **117:**191-6.

5789. **Pebody, R. G., C. Furtado, A. Rojas, N. McCarthy, G. Nylen, P. Ruutu, T. Leino, R. Chalmers, B. de Jong, M. Donnelly, I. Fisher, C. Gilham, L. Graverson, T. Cheasty, G. Willshaw, M. Navarro, R. Salmon, P. Leinikki, P. Wall, and C. L. Bartlett.** 1999. An international outbreak of Vero cytotoxin-producing Escherichia coli O157 infection among tourists: a challenge for the European infectious disease surveillance network. *Epidemiol Infect* **123:**217-23.

5790. **Pebody, R. G., T. Leino, P. Ruutu, L. Kinnunen, I. Davidkin, H. Nohynek, and P. Leinikki.** 1998. Foodborne outbreaks of hepatitis A in a low endemic country: an emerging problem? *Epidemiol Infect* **120:**55-9.

5791. **Pebody, R. G., M. J. Ryan, and P. G. Wall.** 1997. Outbreaks of campylobacter infection: rare events for a common pathogen. *Commun Dis Rep CDR Rev* **7:**R33-7.

5792. **Pedalino, B., B. Cotter, M. Ciofi degli Atti, D. Mandolini, S. Parroccini, and S. Salmaso.** 2002. Epidemiology of tetanus in Italy in years 1971-2000. *Eurosurveillance* **7:**103-10.

5793. **Pedalino, B., E. Feely, P. McKeown, B. Foley, B. Smyth, and A. Moren.** 2003. An outbreak of Norwalk-like viral gastroenteritis in holidaymakers travelling to Andorra, January-February 2002. *Eurosurveillance* **8:**1-8.

5794. **Peden, A. H., M. W. Head, D. L. Ritchie, J. E. Bell, and J. W. Ironside.** 2004. Preclinical vCJD after blood transfusion in a PRNP codon 129 heterozygous patient. *Lancet* **364:**527-9.

5795. **Pedersden, K. A., E. C. Sadasiv, P. W. Chang, and V. J. Yates.** 1990. Detection of antibody to avian viruses in human populations. *Epidemiol Infect* **104:**519-25.

5796. **Pedersen, F. K., and N. E. Moller.** 2000. [Diseases among refugee and immigrant children]. *Ugeskr Laeger* **162:**6207-9.

5797. **Pedro-Botet, M. L., J. E. Stout, and V. L. Yu.** 2002. Legionnaires' disease contracted from patient homes: the coming of the third plague? *Eur J Clin Microbiol Infect Dis* **21:**699-705.

5798. **Pedroli, S., M. Kobisch, O. Beauchet, J. P. Chaussinand, and F. Lucht.** 2003. [Streptococcus suis bacteremia]. *Presse Med* **32:**599-601.

5799. **Peduzzi, R., and J. C. Piffaretti.** 1983. Ancylostoma duodenale and the Saint Gothard anaemia. *BMJ* **287:**1942-5.

5800. **Peel, M. M., G. G. Palmer, A. M. Stacpoole, and T. G. Kerr.** 1997. Human lymphadenitis due to Corynebacterium pseudotuberculosis: report of ten cases from Australia and review. *Clin Infect Dis* **24:**185-91.

5801. **Peeling, R. W., and R. C. Brunham.** 1996. Chlamydiae as pathogens: new species and new issues. *Emerg Infect Dis* **2:**307-19.

5802. **Peeling, R. W., and H. Ye.** 2004. Diagnostic tools for preventing and managing maternal and congenital syphilis: an overview. *Bull WHO* **82**:439-46.

5803. **Peerbooms, P. G. H., M. N. Engelen, D. A. J. Stokman, B. H. van Benthem, M. L. van Weert, S. M. Bruisten, A. van Belkum, and R. A. Coutinho.** 2002. Nasopharyngeal carriage of potential bacterial pathogens related to day care attendance, with special reference to the molecular epidemiology of Haemophilus influenzae. *J Clin Microbiol* **40**:2832-6.

5804. **Peerbooms, P. G. H., v. D. G.J.J., H. van Deutekom, R. A. Coutinho, and D. van Soolingen.** 1995. Laboratory-acquired tuberculosis. *Lancet* **345**:1311-2.

5805. **Peeters, M.** 2004. Cross-species transmissions of simian retroviruses in Africa and risk for human health. *Lancet* **363**:911-2.

5806. **Peeters, M., V. Courgnaud, B. Abela, P. Auzel, X. Pourrut, F. Bibollet-Ruche, S. Loul, F. Liegeois, C. Butel, D. Koulagna, E. Mpoudi-Ngole, G. M. Shaw, B. H. Hahn, and E. Delaporte.** 2002. Risk to human health from a plethora of simian immunodeficiency viruses in primate bushmeat. *Emerg Infect Dis* **8**:451-7.

5807. **Peffers, A. S. R., J. Bailey, G. I. Barrow, and B. C. Hobbs.** 1973. Vibrio parahaemolyticus gastroenteritis and international air travel. *Lancet* **Jan 20**:143-5.

5808. **Pegram, R. G., and C. Eddy.** 2002. Progress towards the eradication of Amblyomma variegatum from the Caribbean. *Exp Appl Acarol* **28**:273-81.

5809. **Pegues, C. F., D. A. Pegues, D. S. Ford, P. L. Hibberd, L. A. Carson, C. M. Raine, and D. C. Hooper.** 1996. Burkholderia cepacia respiratory tract acquisition: epidemiology and molecular characterization of a large nosocomial outbreak. *Epidemiol Infect* **116**:309-17.

5810. **Pegues, D. A., L. A. Carson, R. L. Anderson, M. J. Norgard, T. A. Argent, W. R. Jarvis, and C. H. Woernle.** 1993. Outbreak of Pseudomonas cepacia bacteremia in oncology patients. *Clin Infect Dis* **16**:407-11.

5811. **Pegues, D. A., L. A. Carson, O. C. Tablan, S. C. FitzSimmons, S. B. Roman, J. M. Miller, and W. R. Jarvis.** 1994. Acquisition of Pseudomonas cepacia at summer camps for patients with cystic fibrosis. Summer Camp Study Group. *J Pediatr* **124**: 694-702.

5812. **Peipins, L. A., K. A. Highfill, E. Barrett, M. M. Monti, R. Hackler, P. Huang, and X. Jiang.** 2002. A Norwalk-like virus outbreak on the Appalachian Trail. *J Environ Health* **64**:18-23, 32.

5813. **Peiris, J. S., W. C. Yu, C. W. Leung, C. Y. Cheung, W. F. Ng, J. M. Nicholls, T. K. Ng, K. H. Chan, S. T. Lai, W. L. Lim, K. Y. Yuen, and Y. Guan.** 2004. Re-emergence of fatal human influenza A subtype H5N1 disease. *Lancet* **363**:617-9.

5814. **Peiris, J. S. M., F. P. Amerasinghe, C. K. Arunagiri, L. P. Perera, S. H. Karunaratne, C. B. Ratnayake, T. A. Kulatilaka, and M. R. Abeysinghe.** 1993. Japanese encephalitis in Sri Lanka: comparison of vector and virus ecology in different agro-climatic areas. *Trans R Soc Trop Med Hyg* **87**:541-8.

5815. **Peiris, J. S. M., P. H. Amerasinghe, F. P. Amerasinghe, C. H. Calisher, L. P. Perera, C. K. Arunagiri, N. B. Munasingha, and S. H. Karunaratne.** 1994. Viruses isolated from mosquitoes collected in Sri Lanka. *Am J Trop Med Hyg* **51**:154-61.

5816. **Peleman, R., D. Benoit, L. Goossens, F. Bouttens, H. D. Puydt, D. Vogelaers, F. Colardyn, and K. Van de Woude.** 2000. Indigenous malaria in a suburb of Ghent, Belgium. *J Travel Med* **7**:48-9.

5817. **Pelkonen, P. M., K. Tarvainen, A. Hynninen, E. R. Kallio, K. Henttonen, A. Palva, A. Vaheri, and O. Vapalahti.** 2003. Cowpox with severe generalized eruption, Finland. *Emerg Infect Dis* **9**:1458-61.

5818. **Pelletier, L. L., Jr.** 1984. Chronic strongyloidiasis in World War II Far East ex-prisoners of war. *Am J Trop Med Hyg* **33**:55-61.

5819. **Peltola, H.** 1983. Meningococcal disease: still with us. *Rev Infect Dis* **5**:71-91.

5820. **Peltola, H.** 2000. Worldwide Haemophilus influenzae type b disease at the beginning of the 21st century: global analysis of the disease burden 25 years after the use of the polysaccharide vaccine and a decade after the advent of conjugates. *Clin Microbiol Rev* **13**:302-17.

5821. **Pelton, S. I., and J. O. Klein.** 2002. The future of pneumococcal conjugate vaccines for prevention of pneumococcal diseases in infants and children. *Pediatrics* **110**:805-14.

5822. **Pena Gonzalez, P., J. Perez-Rendon Gonzalez, N. Cifuentes Mimoso, and C. Garcia Colodrero.** 1998. [Epidemic outbreak in a home for the aged caused probably by Bacillus cereus]. *Aten Primaria* **22**:649-54.

5823. **Peng, W., and X. Zhou.** 2001. [Epidemiological study on the influence of pig-derived Ascaris to the transmission of human ascariasis]. *Zhonghua Liu Xing Bing Xue Za Zhi* **22**:116-8.

5824. **Penland, R. L., and K. R. Wilhelmus.** 1999. Microbiologic analysis of bottled water: is it safe for use with contact lenses? *Ophthalmology* **106**:1500-3.

5825. **Pennycott, T. W., and J. K. Kirkwood.** 1998. Feeding wild birds. *Vet Rec* **143**:371-2.

5826. **Pepin, J., A. C. Labbe, N. Khonde, S. Deslandes, M. Alary, A. Dzokoto, C. Asamoah-Adu, H. Meda, and E. Frost.** 2005. Mycoplasma genitalium: an organism commonly associated with cervicitis among west African sex workers. *Sex Transm Infect* **81**:67-72.

5827. **Pepin, J., F. Sobela, S. Deslandes, M. Alary, K. Wegner, N. Khonde, F. Kintin, A. Kamuragiye, M. Sylla, P. J. Zerbo, E. Baganizi, A. Kone, F. Kane, B. Masse, P. Viens, and E. Frost.** 2001. Etiology of urethral discharge in West Africa: the role of Mycoplasma genitalium and Trichomonas vaginalis. *Bull WHO* **79**:118-26.

5828. **Peragallo, M. S., A. M. Croft, and S. J. Kitchener.** 2002. Malaria during a multinational military deployment: the comparative experience of the Italian, British and Australian Armed Forces in East Timor. *Trans R Soc Trop Med Hyg* **96**:481-2.

5829. **Peragallo, M. S., L. Nicoletti, F. Lista, and R. D'Amelio.** 2003. Probable dengue virus infection among Italian troops, East Timor, 1999-2000. *Emerg Infect Dis* **9**:876-80.

5830. **Pereira, M. L., L. S. do Carmo, E. J. dos Santos, and M. S. Bergdoll.** 1994. Staphylococcal food poisoning from cream-filled cake in a metropolitan area of south-eastern Brazil. *Rev Saude Publica* **28**:406-9.

5831. **Pereira, R. M., A. T. Tresoldi, M. T. N. da Silva, and F. Bucaretchi.** 2004. Fatal disseminated paracoccidioidomycosis in a two-year-old child. *Rev Inst Med Trop Sao Paulo* **46**:37-9.

5832. **Perez, C., M. J. Pena, L. Molina, G. Trallero, A. Garcia, F. Alamo, and B. Lafarga.** 2003. [Epidemic outbreak of meningitis due to Echovirus type 13 on the island of Gran Canaria (Spain)]. *Enferm Infecc Microbiol Clin* **21**:340-5.

5833. **Perez Garcia, M. D., A. Rodriguez Alonso, A. Nunez Lopez, A. Ojea Calvo, A. Alonso Rodrigo, B. Rodriguez Iglesias, M. Barros Rodriguez, J. Benavente Delgado, J. Gonzalez-Carrero Fojon, and J. L. Nogueira March.** 2000. [Abdominal-pelvic actinomycosis with urinary tract involvement, secondary to gynecologic infection caused by intrauterine device]. *Actas Urol Esp* **24:**197-201.

5834. **Perfect, J. R., G. M. Cox, J. Y. Lee, C. A. Kauffman, L. de Repentigny, S. W. Chapman, V. A. Morrison, P. Pappas, J. W. Hiemenz, and D. A. Stevens.** 2001. The impact of culture isolation of Aspergillus species: a hospital- based survey of aspergillosis. *Clin Infect Dis* **33:**1824-33.

5835. **Perine, P. L., B. P. Chandler, D. K. Krause, P. McCardle, S. Awoke, E. Habte-Gabr, C. L. Wisseman, Jr., and J. E. McDade.** 1992. A clinico-epidemiological study of epidemic typhus in Africa. *Clin Infect Dis* **14:**1149-58.

5836. **Perine, P. L., D. R. Hopkins, P. L. A. Niemel, R. K. St. John, G. Causse, and G. M. Antal.** 1985. Manuel des tréponématoses endémiques. World Health Organization, Geneva.

5837. **Perna, A., S. Di Rosa, V. Intonazzo, A. Sferlazzo, G. Tringali, and G. La Rosa.** 1990. Epidemiology of boutonneuse fever in western Sicily: accidental laboratory infection with a rickettsial agent isolated from a tick. *Microbiologica* **13:**253-6.

5838. **Perni, S. C., S. Vardhana, I. Korneeva, S. L. Tuttle, L. R. Paraskevas, S. T. Chasen, R. B. Kalish, and S. S. Witkin.** 2004. Mycoplasma hominis and Ureaplasma urealyticum in midtrimester amniotic fluid: association with amniotic fluid cytokine levels and pregnancy outcome. *Am J Obstet Gynecol* **191:**1382-6.

5839. **Perola, O., J. Kauppinen, J. Kusnetsov, U. M. Karkkainen, P. C. Luck, and M. L. Katila.** 2005. Persistent Legionella pneumophila colonization of a hospital water supply: efficacy of control methods and a molecular epidemiological analysis. *APMIS* **113:**45-53.

5840. **Perra, A., V. Servas, G. Terrier, D. Postic, G. Baranton, G. Andre-Fontaine, V. Vaillant, and I. Capek.** 2002. Clustered cases of leptospirosis in Rochefort, France, June 2001. *Eur Surveill* **7:**131-6.

5841. **Perraud, M., M. A. Piens, N. Nicoloyannis, J. P. Garin, and M. Sepetjan.** 1985. [Demolition work and the risk of invasive pulmonary aspergillosis]. *Presse Med* **14:**2195.

5842. **Perret, J. L.** 1997. La mélioidose: une "bombe à retardement tropicale" en voie de dissémination? *Med Trop* **57:**195-201.

5843. **Perrin, L., L. Kaiser, and S. Yerly.** 2003. Travel and the spread of HIV-1 genetic variants. *Lancet Infect Dis* **3:**22-7.

5844. **Perry, R. D., and J. D. Fetherston.** 1997. Yersinia pestis - etiologic agent of plague. *Clin Microbiol Rev* **10:**35-66.

5845. **Perry, R. T., and N. A. Halsey.** 2004. The clinical significance of measles: a review. *J Infect Dis* **189 Suppl 1:**4-16.

5846. **Perz, J. F., A. S. Craig, and W. Schaffner.** 2001. Mixed outbreak of parainfluenza type 1 and influenza B associated with tourism and air travel. *Int J Infect Dis* **5:**189-91.

5847. **Peters, C. J., and D. M. Hartley.** 2002. Anthrax inhalation and lethal human infection. *Lancet* **359:**710-1.

5848. **Peters, C. J., P. B. Jahrling, T. G. Ksiazek, E. D. Johnson, and H. W. Lupton.** 1992. Filovirus contamination of cell cultures. *Dev Biol Stand* **76:**267-74.

5849. **Petersen, J. M., M. E. Schriefer, L. G. Carter, Y. Zhou, T. Sealy, D. Bawiec, B. Yockey, S. Urich, N. S. Zeidner, S. Avashia, J. L. Kool, J. Buck, C. Lindley, L. Celeda, J. A. Monteneiri, K. L. Gage, and M. C. Chu.** 2004. Laboratory analysis of tularemia in wild-trapped, commercially traded prarie dogs, Texas, 2002. *Emerg Infect Dis* **10:**419-25.

5850. **Petersen, L. R., M. L. Cartter, and J. L. Hadler.** 1988. A foodborne outbreak of Giardia lamblia. *J Infect Dis* **157:**846-8.

5851. **Petersen, L. R., S. L. Marshall, C. Barton-Dickson, R. A. Hajjeh, M. D. Lindsley, D. W. Warnock, A. A. Panackal, J. B. Shaffer, M. B. Haddad, F. S. Fisher, D. T. Dennis, and J. Morgan.** 2004. Coccidioidomycosis among workers at an archeological site, northeastern Utah. *Emerg Infect Dis* **10:**637-42.

5852. **Petersen, L. R., R. Mshar, G. H. Cooper, A. R. Bruce, and J. L. Hadler.** 1988. A large Clostridium perfringens foodborne outbreak with an unusual attack rate pattern. *Am J Epidemiol* **127:**605-11.

5853. **Petersen, L. R., L. A. Sawyer, D. B. Fishbein, P. W. Kelley, R. J. Thomas, L. A. Magnarelli, M. Redus, and J. E. Dawson.** 1989. An outbreak of ehrlichiosis in members of an army reserve unit exposed to ticks. *J Infect Dis* **159:**562-8.

5854. **Pether, J. V., S. P. Wang, and J. T. Grayston.** 1989. Chlamydia pneumoniae, strain TWAR, as the cause of an outbreak in a boys' school previously called psittacosis. *Epidemiol Infect* **103:**395-400.

5855. **Petri, W. A., Jr., and U. Singh.** 1999. Diagnosis and management of amebiasis. *Clin Infect Dis* **29:**1117-25.

5856. **Petrin, D., K. Delgaty, R. Bhatt, and G. Garber.** 1998. Clinical and microbiological aspects of Trichomonas vaginalis. *Clin Microbiol Rev* **11:**300-17.

5857. **Petrosillo, N., A. Pantosti, E. Bordi, A. Spano, M. Del Grosso, B. Tallarida, and G. Ippolito.** 2002. Prevalence, determinants, and molecular epidemiology of Streptococcus pneumoniae isolates colonizing the nasopharynx of healthy children in Rome. *Eur J Clin Microbiol Infect Dis* **21:**181-8.

5858. **Petrozzi, J. W.** 1980. Verrucae planae spread by electrolysis. *Cutis* **26:**85.

5859. **Petry, F. E.** 2000. Cryptosporidiosis and microsporidiosis. Karger, Basel.

5860. **Petter, F.** 1999. Les rongeurs et la peste en Iran et au Brésil. Nouvelles données. *Bull Soc Pathol Exot* **92:**411-3.

5861. **Pfaller, M. A., and D. J. Diekema.** 2004. Rare and emerging opportunistic fungal pathogens: concern for resistance beyond Candida albicans and Aspergillus fumigatus. *J Clin Microbiol* **42:**4419-31.

5862. **Pfaller, M. A., A. F. Ehrhardt, and R. N. Jones.** 2001. Frequency of pathogen occurrence and antimicrobial susceptibility among community-acquired respiratory tract infections in the respiratory surveillance program study: microbiology from the medical office practice environment. *Am J Med* **111 (suppl 9A):**4S-12S.

5863. **Pfaller, M. A., R. N. Jones, G. V. Doern, H. S. Sader, S. A. Messer, A. Houston, S. Coffman, and R. J. Hollis.** 2000. Bloodstream infections due to Candida species: SENTRY antimicrobial surveillance program in North America and Latin America, 1997-1998. *Antimicrob Agents Chemother* **44:**747-751.

5864. **Pfisterer, R. M.** 1991. [An anthrax epidemic in Switzerland. Clinical, diagnostic and epidemiological aspects of a mostly forgotten disease]. *Schweiz Med Wochenschr* **121:**813-25.

5865. **Pfyffer, G. E., A. Strässle, T. van Gorkum, F. Portaels, L. Rigouts, C. Mathieu, F. Mirzoyev, H. Traore, and J. D. van Embden.** 2001. Multidrug-resistant tuberculosis in prison inmates, Azerbaijan. *Emerg Infect Dis* **7:**855-861.

5866. **Pham, X. D., Y. Otsuka, H. Suzuki, and H. Takaoka.** 2001. Detection of Orientia tsutsugamushi (Rickettsiales: rickettsiaceae) in unengorged chiggers (Acari: Trombiculidae) from Oita Prefecture, Japan, by nested polymerase chain reaction. *J Med Entomol* **38**:308-11.

5867. **Philip, R. N., K. R. Reinhard, and D. B. Lackman.** 1995. Observations on a mumps epidemic in a "virgin" population. *Am J Epidemiol* **142**:233-53.

5868. **Philippe, J. M., L. Caumon, M. Chouaki, S. Dufraise, H. Rimeize, F. Monchard, T. Cueto, J. Beytout, and P. Delort.** 2002. Infestation paludique collective à l'occasion d'une mission humanitaire en Afrique de l'ouest. *Bull Soc Pathol Exot* **95**:71-3.

5869. **Phillips, L., J. Carlile, and D. Smith.** 2004. Epidemiology of a tuberculosis outbreak in a rural Missouri high school. *Pediatrics* **113**:e514-9.

5870. **Phillips, R. S.** 2001. Current status of malaria and potential for control. *Clin Microbiol Rev* **14**:208-26.

5871. **Phillips-Howard, P., B. L. Nahlen, M. S. Kolczak, A. W. Hightower, F. O. ter Kuile, J. A. Alaii, J. E. Gimnig, J. Arudo, J. M. Vulule, A. Odhacha, S. P. Kachur, E. Schoute, D. H. Rosen, J. D. Sexton, A. J. Oloo, and W. A. Hawley.** 2003. Efficacy of permethrin-treated bed nets in the prevention of mortality in young children in an area of high perennial malaria transmission in western Kenya. *Am J Trop Med Hyg* **68** (suppl 4):23-9.

5872. **Phiri, I. K., H. Ngowi, S. Afonso, E. Matenga, M. Boa, S. Mukaratirwa, S. Githigia, M. Saimo, C. Sikasunge, N. Maingi, G. W. Lubega, A. Kassuku, L. Michael, S. Siziya, R. C. Krecek, E. Noormahomed, M. Vilhena, P. Dorny, and A. L. Willingham, 3rd.** 2003. The emergence of Taenia solium cysticercosis in Eastern and Southern Africa as a serious agricultural problem and public health risk. *Acta Trop* **87**:13-23.

5873. **PHLS.** 1982. Anthrax surveillance 1961-80. *BMJ* **284**:204.

5874. **PHLS.** 1989. Food safety. Microbiological quality of airline meals. *Weekly Epidemiologic Record* **64**:324-327.

5875. **PHLS.** 1990. Prospective study of human parvovirus (B19) infection in pregnancy. Public Health Laboratory Service Working Party on Fifth Disease. *BMJ* **300**:1166-70.

5876. **PHLS.** 1997. Needlestick malaria with tragic consequences. *Commun Dis Rep Weekly* **7**:247.

5877. **PHLS.** 1998. Botulism associated with home-preserved mushrooms. *Commun Dis Rep CDR Wkly* **8**:160-2.

5878. **PHLS.** 1998. Diphtheria in visitors to Africa. *Commun Dis Rep Weekly* **8**(33):289.

5879. **PHLS.** 1999. Hospital-acquired malaria in Nottingham. *Commun Dis Rep Weekly* **9**:123.

5880. **PHLS.** 1999. Suspected viral haemorrhagic fever: rapid tests help to exclude dangerous infections. *Commun Dis Rep Weekly* **9**:1,4.

5881. **PHLS.** 2000. Outbreaks of measles in communities with low vaccine coverage. *Commun Dis Rep Weekly* **10**:29, 32.

5882. **PHLS.** 2001. Human anthrax in England and Wales. *Commun Dis Rep CDR Wkly* **11**(41):3.

5883. **PHLS.** 2001. Surveillance of viral infections in donated blood: England and Wales, 2000. *Commun Dis Rep CDR Wkly* **11**(43):7–10.

5884. **PHLS.** 2002. Bactermia. *Commun Dis Rep Weekly* **12**:5-6.

5885. **PHLS.** 2002. Guidelines for public health management of meningococcal disease in the U.K. *Commun Dis Rep Public Health* **5**:185-207.

5886. **PHLS.** 2002. HIV in Vietnamese sex workers. *Commun Dis Rep Weekly* **12**(4):4.

5887. **PHLS.** 2002. Outbreak of legionnaires' disease in Barrow-in-Furness. *Commun Dis Rep Weekly* **12**:1-2.

5888. **PHLS.** 2002. Outbreak of verocytotoxin-producing Escherichia coli (VTEC O157) and Campylobacter spp associated with a campsite in north Wales. *Commun Dis Rep* **12**(34):3–4.

5889. **PHLS.** 2002. Outbreaks of Norwalk-like virus infection. *Commun Dis Rep Weekly* **12**(4):3-4.

5890. **PHLS.** 2002. Surveillance of hospital-acquired bacteremia. *Public Health Laboratory Service*. (http://www.phls.org.uk/publications/NINSS.htm.)

5891. **PHLS.** 2002. Surveillance of surgical site infection in English hospitals, 1997-2000. *Public Health Laboratory Service*. (http://www.phls.org.uk/publications/NINSS.htm.)

5892. **PHLS.** 2003. Candidaemia and polymicrobial bacteraemias: England, Wales, and northern Ireland, 2002. *Commun Dis Rep Weekly* **13**:1-5.

5893. **PHLS.** 2003. Schistosomiasis in travellers. *Commun Dis Rep CDR Wkly* **13**.

5894. **Phraisuwan, P., E. A. Whitney, P. Tharmaphornpilas, S. Guharat, S. Thongkamsamut, S. Aresagig, J. Liangphongphanthu, K. Junthima, A. Sokampang, and D. A. Ashford.** 2002. Leptospirosis: skin wounds and control strategies, Thailand, 1999. *Emerg Infect Dis* **8**:1455-9.

5895. **Phukan, A. C., P. K. Borah, and J. Mahanta.** 2004. Japanese encephalitis in Assam, northeast India. *Southeast Asian J Trop Med Public Health* **35**:618-22.

5896. **Piacentino, J. D., and B. S. Schwartz.** 2001. Occupational risk of Lyme disease: an epidemiological review. *Occup Environ Med* **59**:75-84.

5897. **Pianetti, A., W. Baffone, B. Citterio, A. Casaroli, F. Bruscolini, and L. Salvaggio.** 2000. Presence of enteroviruses and reoviruses in the waters of the Italian coast of the Adriatic Sea. *Epidemiol Infect* **125**:455-62.

5898. **Pianetti, A., L. Sabatini, F. Bruscolini, F. Chiaverini, and G. Cecchetti.** 2004. Faecal contamination indicators, Salmonella, Vibrio and Aeromonas in water used for the irrigation of agricultural products. *Epidemiol Infect* **132**:231-8.

5899. **Piazza, M., L. Sagliocca, G. Tosone, V. Guadagnino, M. A. Stazi, R. Orlando, G. Borgia, D. Rosa, S. Abrignani, F. Palumbo, A. Manzin, and M. Clementi.** 1997. Sexual transmission of the hepatitis C virus and efficacy of prophylaxis with intramuscular immune serum globulin. A randomized controlled trial. *Arch Intern Med* **157**:1537-44.

5900. **Picazo, J. J.** 2004. Management of the febrile neutropenic patient: a consensus conference. *Clin Infect Dis* **39 Suppl 1**:S1-6.

5901. **Pickering, H., and G. Rose.** 1988. Nasal and hand carriage of Streptococcus pneumoniae in children and mothers in the Tari Basin of Papua New Guinea. *Trans R Soc Trop Med Hyg* **82**:911-3.

5902. **Pickering, L. K., A. V. Bartlett, 3rd, R. R. Reves, and A. Morrow.** 1988. Asymptomatic excretion of rotavirus before and after rotavirus diarrhea in children in day care centers. *J Pediatr* **112**:361-5.

5903. **Pickering, L. K., D. G. Evans, H. L. DuPont, J. J. Vollet, 3rd, and D. J. Evans, Jr.** 1981. Diarrhea caused by Shigella, rotavirus, and Giardia in day-care centers: prospective study. *J Pediatr* **99:**51-6.

5904. **Pickering, L. K., W. E. Woodward, H. L. DuPont, and P. Sullivan.** 1984. Occurrence of Giardia lamblia in children in day care centers. *J Pediatr* **104:**522-6.

5905. **Piérard, G.** 2001. Onychomycosis and other superficial fungal infections of the foot in the elderly: a pan-European survey. *Dermatology* **202:**220-4.

5906. **Pierce, P. F., M. Cappello, and K. W. Bernard.** 1990. Subclinical infection with hepatitis A in peace corps volunteers following immune globulin prophylaxis. *Am J Trop Med Hyg* **42:**465-9.

5907. **Piergentili, P., M. Castellani-Pastoris, R. D. Fellini, G. Farisano, C. Bonello, E. Rigoli, and A. Zampieri.** 1984. Transmission of non O group 1 Vibrio cholerae by raw oyster consumption. *Int J Epidemiol* **13:**340-3.

5908. **Pierson, D. L., S. K. Mehta, B. B. Magee, and S. K. Mishra.** 1995. Person-to-person transfer of Candida albicans in the spacecraft environment. *J Med Vet Mycol* **33:**145-50.

5909. **Piesman, J., and L. Gern.** 2004. Lyme borreliosis in Europe and North America. *Parasitology* **129 Suppl:**S191-220.

5910. **Pike, R. M.** 1976. Laboratory-associated infections: summary and analysis of 3921 cases. *Health Lab Sci* **13:**105-14.

5911. **Pile, J. C., E. A. Henchal, G. W. Christopher, K. E. Steele, and J. A. Pavlin.** 1999. Chikungunya in a North American traveler. *J Travel Med* **6:**137-9.

5912. **Pillonel, J., and S. Laperche.** 2001. Surveillance des marqueurs d'une infection par le VIH, l'HTLV et les virus des hépatites B et C chez les donneurs de sang en France. *Bulletin Epidémiologique Hebdomadaire* **46**(13 Nov)**:**1–5.

5913. **Pillonel, J., and S. Laperche.** 2005. Trends in risk of transfusion-transmitted viral infections (HIV, HCV, HBV) in France between 1992 and 2003 and impact of nucleic acid testing (NAT). *Eur Surveill* **10:**5-8.

5914. **Pilon, P. A., and M. Laurin.** 1997. Outbreak of Salmonella enteritidis phage type 8 in a Montreal hotel. *Can Commun Dis Rep* **23:**148-50.

5915. **Pimentel, J. D., J. Low, K. Styles, O. C. Harris, A. Hughes, and E. Athan.** 2005. Control of an outbreak of multi-drug-resistant Acinetobacter baumannii in an intensive care unit and a surgical ward. *J Hosp Infect* **59:**249-53.

5916. **Pincock, S.** 2004. Patient's death from vCJD may be linked to blood transfusion. *Lancet* **363:**43.

5917. **Pinelli, E., M. Mommers, W. Homan, T. van Maanen, and L. M. Kortbeek.** 2004. Imported human trichinellosis: sequential IgG4 antibody response to Trichinella spiralis. *Eur J Clin Microbiol Infect Dis* **23:**57-60.

5918. **Pinheiro, F. P., A. P. Travassos da Rosa, J. F. Travassos da Rosa, R. Ishak, R. B. Freitas, M. L. Gomes, J. W. LeDuc, and O. F. Oliva.** 1981. Oropouche virus. I. A review of clinical, epidemiological, and ecological findings. *Am J Trop Med Hyg* **30:**149-60.

5919. **Pinheiro, V. C. S., and W. P. Tadei.** 2002. Frequency, diversity, and productivity study on the Aedes aegypti most preferred containers in the city of Manaus, Amazonas, Brazil. *Rev Inst Med Trop Sao Paulo* **44:**245-50.

5920. **Pini, G., R. Donato, E. Faggi, and R. Fanci.** 2004. Two years of a fungal aerobiocontamination survey in a Florentine haematology ward. *Eur J Epidemiol* **19:**693-8.

5921. **Pini, G., E. Faggi, R. Donato, and R. Fanci.** 2005. Isolation of Trichosporon in a hematology ward. *Mycoses* **48:**45-9.

5922. **Pini, N., S. Levis, G. Calderón, J. Ramirez, D. Bravo, E. Lozano, C. Ripoll, S. St Jeor, T. G. Ksiazek, R. M. Barquez, and D. Enria.** 2003. Hantavirus infection in humans and rodents, northwestern Argentina. *Emerg Infect Dis* **9:**1070-6.

5923. **Pinsky, R. L., D. B. Fishbein, C. R. Greene, and K. F. Gensheimer.** 1991. An outbreak of cat-associated Q fever in the United States. *J Infect Dis* **164:**202-4.

5924. **Pinto, V., M. Telenti, C. Palomo, and J. F. Bernaldo De Quiros.** 2000. Transfusion-associated sepsis caused by Candida parapsilosis. *Vox Sang* **79:**57-8.

5925. **Piot, P., M. Bartos, P. D. Ghys, N. Walker, and B. Schwartländer.** 2001. The global impact of HIV/AIDS. *Nature* **410:**968-73.

5926. **Pipitgool, V., P. Sithithaworn, P. Pongmuttasaya, and E. Hinz.** 1997. Angiostrongylus infections in rats and snails in northeast Thailand. *Southeast Asian J Trop Med Public Health* **28 Suppl 1:**190-3.

5927. **Pirnay, J. P., C. Vandenvelde, L. Duinslaeger, P. Reper, and A. Vanderkelen.** 1997. HIV transmission by transplantation of allograft skin: a review of the literature. *Burns* **23:**1-5.

5928. **Pirttijarvi, T. S., L. M. Ahonen, L. M. Maunuksela, and M. S. Salkinoja-Salonen.** 1998. Bacillus cereus in a whey process. *Int J Food Microbiol* **44:**31-41.

5929. **Piscitelli, S. C., A. H. Burstein, D. Chaitt, R. M. Alfaro, and J. Falloon.** 2000. Indinavir concentrations and St John's wort. *Lancet* **355:**547-8.

5930. **Pitman, N. C. A., and P. M. Jorgensen.** 2002. Estimating the size of the world's threatened flora. *Science* **298:**989.

5931. **Pitt, S., B. E. Pearcy, R. H. Stevens, A. Sharipov, K. Satarov, and N. Banatvala.** 1998. War in Tajikistan and re-emergence of Plasmodium falciparum. *Lancet* **352:**1279.

5932. **Pitten, F. A., C. M. Kalveram, U. Kruger, G. Muller, and A. Kramer.** 2000. [Reduction of colonization of new mattresses with bacteria, moulds and house dust mites by complete mattress covers]. *Hautarzt* **51:**655-60.

5933. **Pittet, B., D. Montandon, and D. Pittet.** 2005. Infection in breast implants. *Lancet Infect Dis* **5:**94-106.

5934. **Pittet, D., S. Hugonnet, S. Harbarth, P. Mourouga, V. Sauvan, S. Touveneau, and T. V. Perneger.** 2000. Effectiveness of a hospital-wide programme to improve compliance with hand hygiene. Infection Control Programme. *Lancet* **356:**1307-12.

5935. **Pittman, J., and M. Watters.** 1999. Helicobacter pylori: an occupational hazard for anaesthetists. *Anaesthesia* **54:**398.

5936. **Pladson, T. R., M. A. Stiles, and J. N. Kuritsky.** 1984. Pulmonary histoplasmosis. A possible risk in people who cut decayed wood. *Chest* **86:**435-8.

5937. **Plancoulaine, S., L. Abel, M. van Beveren, D. A. Tregouet, M. Joubert, P. Tortevoye, G. de The, and A. Gessain.** 2000. Human herpesvirus 8 transmission from mother to child and between siblings in an endemic population. *Lancet* **356:**1062-5.

5938. **Plate, D. K., B. I. Strassmann, and M. L. Wilson.** 2004. Water sources are associated with childhood diarrhoea prevalence in rural east-central Mali. *Trop Med Int Health* **9:**416-25.

5939. **Platt, K. B., J. A. Mangiafico, O. J. Rocha, M. E. Zaldivar, J. Mora, G. Trueba, and W. A. Rowley.** 2000. Detection of dengue virus neutralizing antibodies in bats from Costa Rica and Ecuador. *J Med Entomol* **37**:965-7.

5940. **Platt, S. D., C. J. Martin, S. M. Hunt, and C. W. Lewis.** 1989. Damp housing, mould growth, and symptomatic health state. *BMJ* **298**:1673-8.

5941. **Plotkin, S. A.** 2001. John Snow learns from Louis Pasteur. *Pediatr Infect Dis J* **20**:1073-8.

5942. **Plotkin, S. A.** 2001. Rubella eradication. *Vaccine* **19**:3311-9.

5943. **Plotkin, S. A.** 2004. Commentary: congenital rubella syndrome should not be a disease of poor countries. *Pediatr Infect Dis J* **23**:1123-4.

5944. **Plotkin, S. A., P. S. Brachman, M. Utell, F. H. Bumford, and M. M. Atchison.** 1960. An epidemic of inhalation anthrax: the first in the twentieth century. I. Clinical fieatures. *Am J Med* **29**:992-1001.

5945. **Plotkin, S. A., and W. A. Orenstein.** 1999. Vaccines, 3rd ed. W.B. Saunders company, Philadelphia, PA.

5946. **Plummer, F. A., L. J. D'Costa, H. Nsanze, J. Dylewski, P. Karasira, and A. R. Ronald.** 1983. Epidemiology of chancroid and Haemophilus ducreyi in Nairobi, Kenya. *Lancet* **2**:1293-5.

5947. **Podgore, J. K., R. R. Abu-Elyazeed, N. S. Mansour, F. G. Youssef, R. G. Hibbs, and J. A. Gere.** 1994. Evaluation of a twice-a-week application of 1% niclosamide lotion in preventing Schistosoma haematobium reinfection. *Am J Trop Med Hyg* **51**:875-9.

5948. **Podschun, R., and U. Ullmann.** 1998. Klebsiella spp. as nosocomial pathogens: epidemiology, taxonomy, typing methods, and pathogenicity factors. *Clin Microbiol Rev* **11**:589-603.

5949. **Poester, F. P., V. S. P. Gonçalves, and A. P. Lage.** 2002. Brucellosis in Brazil. *Vet Microbiol* **90**:55-62.

5950. **Poeta, P., D. Costa, J. Rodrigues, and C. Torres.** 2005. Study of faecal colonization by vanA-containing Enterococcus strains in healthy humans, pets, poultry and wild animals in Portugal. *J Antimicrob Chemother* **55**:278-80.

5951. **Poggensee, G., I. Kiwelu, V. Weger, D. Goppner, T. Diedrich, I. Krantz, and H. Feldmeier.** 2000. Female genital schistosomiasis of the lower genital tract: prevalence and disease-associated morbidity in northern Tanzania. *J Infect Dis* **181**:1210-3.

5952. **Poikonen, E., O. Lyytikäinen, A. Veli-Jukka, and P. Ruutu.** 2003. Candidemia in Finland, 1995-1999. *Emerg Infect Dis* **9**:985-90.

5953. **Poinsignon, Y.** 1999. Accès palustre au retour d'un voyage aux Antilles françaises. Discussion du mode de transmission. *Med Trop* **59**:55-7.

5954. **Pointier, J. P.** 1993. The introduction of Melanoides tuberculata (Mollusca: Thiaridae) to the island of Saint Lucia (West Indies) and its role in the decline of Biomphalaria glabrata, the snail intermediate host of Schistosoma mansoni. *Acta Trop* **54**:13-8.

5955. **Pointier, J. P., and J. Jourdane.** 2000. Biological control of the snail hosts of schistosomiasis in areas of low transmission: the example of the Caribbean area. *Acta Trop* **77**:53-60.

5956. **Poirriez, J., R. Becquet, E. Dutoit, M. Crépin, and J. Cousin.** 1992. Anguillulose autochtone dans le nord de la France. *Bull Soc Pathol Exot* **85**:292-5.

5957. **Poland, G. A., P. H. Axelsen, and M. W. Felz.** 1996. Hepatitis A and B Infections Among Expatriates in Papua New Guinea: A Missed Opportunity for Immunization. *J Travel Med* **3**: 209-213.

5958. **Polderman, A. M.** 1986. Schistosomiasis in a mining area: intersectoral implications. *Trop Med Parasitol* **37**:195-9.

5959. **Polish, L. B., C. N. Shapiro, F. Bauer, P. Klotz, P. Ginier, R. R. Roberto, H. S. Margolis, and M. J. Alter.** 1992. Nosocomial transmission of hepatitis B virus associated with the use of a spring-loaded finger-stick device. *N Engl J Med* **326**:721-5.

5960. **Polk, B. F., J. A. White, P. C. DeGirolami, and J. F. Modlin.** 1980. An outbreak of rubella among hospital personnel. *N Engl J Med* **303**:541-5.

5961. **Pollard, A. J.** 2004. Global epidemiology of meningococcal disease and vaccine efficacy. *Pediatr Infect Dis J* **23**:S274-9.

5962. **Polo, C., J. L. Perez, A. Mielnichuck, C. G. Fedele, J. Niubo, and A. Tenorio.** 2004. Prevalence and patterns of polyomavirus urinary excretion in immunocompetent adults and children. *Clin Microbiol Infect* **10**:640-4.

5963. **Pon, E., K. T. McKee, Jr., B. M. Diniega, B. Merrell, A. Corwin, and T. G. Ksiazek.** 1990. Outbreak of hemorrhagic fever with renal syndrome among U.S. Marines in Korea. *Am J Trop Med Hyg* **42**:612-9.

5964. **Ponka, A., L. Maunula, C. H. Von Bonsdorff, and O. Lyytikainen.** 1999. An outbreak of calicivirus associated with consumption of frozen raspberries. *Epidemiol Infect* **123**:469-474.

5965. **Pons, V. G., J. Canter, and R. Dolin.** 1980. Influenza A/USSR/77 (H1N1) on a university campus. *Am J Epidemiol* **111**:23-30.

5966. **Pontello, M., L. Sodano, A. Nastasi, C. Mammina, M. Astuti, M. Domenichini, G. Belluzzi, E. Soccini, M. G. Silvestri, M. Gatti, E. Gerosa, and A. Montagna.** 1998. A community-based outbreak of Salmonella enterica serotype Typhimurium associated with salami consumption in Northern Italy. *Epidemiol Infect* **120**:209-14.

5967. **Ponticelli, C., and P. Passerini.** 2005. Gastrointestinal complications in renal transplant recipients. *Transpl Int* **18**:643-50.

5968. **Popovic, T., C. Kim, J. Reiss, M. Reeves, H. Nakao, and A. Golaz.** 1999. Use of molecular subtyping to document long-term persistence of Corynebacterium diphtheriae in South Dakota. *J Clin Microbiol* **37**:1092-9.

5969. **Popugailo, V. M., I. A. Podkin, V. B. Gurvich, E. F. Kuperman, and L. N. Zhukova.** 1983. [Erysipeloid as an occupational disease of workers in shoe enterprises]. *Zh Mikrobiol Epidemiol Immunobiol* **Oct**:46-9.

5970. **Portaels, F., L. Realini, L. Bauwens, B. Hirschel, W. M. Meyers, and W. de Meurichy.** 1996. Mycobacteriosis caused by Mycobacterium genavense in birds kept in a zoo: 11-year survey. *J Clin Microbiol* **34**:319-23.

5971. **Porter, J. D., C. Gaffney, D. Heymann, and W. Parkin.** 1990. Food-borne outbreak of Giardia lamblia. *Am J Public Health* **80**:1259-60.

5972. **Porter, J. D., H. P. Ragazzoni, J. D. Buchanon, H. A. Waskin, D. D. Juranek, and W. E. Parkin.** 1988. Giardia transmission in a swimming pool. *Am J Public Health* **78**:659-62.

5973. **Porter, K. R., R. Tan, Y. Istary, W. Suharyono, Sutaryo, S. Widjaja, C. Ma'Roef, E. Listiyaningsih, H. Kosasih, L. Hueston, J. McArdle, and M. Juffrie.** 2004. A serological study of chikungunya virus transmission in Yogyakarta, Indonesia: evidence for the first outbreak since 1982. *Southeast Asian J Trop Med Public Health* **35**:408-15.

5974. **Posavad, C. M., A. Wald, S. Kuntz, M. L. Huang, S. Selke, E. Krantz, and L. Corey.** 2004. Frequent reactivation of herpes simplex virus among HIV-1-infected patients treated with highly active antiretroviral therapy. *J Infect Dis* **190**:693-6.

5975. **Pospischil, A., R. Thoma, M. Hilbe, P. Grest, and J. O. Gebbers.** 2002. Abortion in woman caused by caprine Chlamydophila abortus (Chlamydia psittaci serovar 1). *Swiss Med Wkly* **132**:64-6.

5976. **Post, J. C., and M. C. Goessier.** 2001. Is pacifier use a risk factor for otitis media? *Lancet* **357**:823-4.

5977. **Postel, S.** 1999. Pillar of sand. W.W. Norton & Co. Inc., New York.

5978. **Potasman, I., A. Oren, and I. Srugo.** 1999. Isolation of Ureaplasma urealyticum and Mycoplasma hominis from public toilet bowls. *Infect Control Hosp Epidemiol* **20**:66-8.

5979. **Potasman, I., A. Paz, and M. Odeh.** 2002. Infectious outbreaks associated with bivalve shellfish consumption: a worldwide perspective. *Clin Infect Dis* **35**:921-8.

5980. **Potasman, I., N. Pick, A. Abel, and M. Dan.** 1996. Schistosomiasis acquired in lake Malawi. *J Travel Med* **3**:32-6.

5981. **Potasman, I., S. Rzotkiewicz, N. Pick, and A. Keysary.** 2000. Outbreak of Q fever following a safari trip. *Clin Infect Dis* **30**:214-5.

5982. **Potasman, I., I. Srugo, and E. Schwartz.** 1999. Dengue seroconversion among Israeli travelers to tropical countries. *Emerg Infect Dis* **5**:824-7.

5983. **Potasman, I., and A. Yitzhak.** 1998. Helicobacter pylori serostatus in backpackers following travel to tropical countries. *Am J Trop Med Hyg* **58**:305-8.

5984. **Potasman, I. I., and N. Pick.** 1997. Primary Herpes Labialis Acquired during Scuba Diving Course. *J Travel Med* **4**:144-145.

5985. **Potter, A., D. Stephens, and B. De Keulenaer.** 2003. Strongyloides hyper-infection: a case for awareness. *Ann Trop Med Parasitol* **97**:855-60.

5986. **Potter, J., D. J. Stott, M. A. Roberts, A. G. Elder, B. O'Donnell, P. V. Knight, and W. F. Carman.** 1997. Influenza vaccination of health care workers in long-term-care hospitals reduces the mortality of elderly patients. *J Infect Dis* **175**:1-6.

5987. **Potter, M. E., M. B. Kruse, M. A. Matthews, R. O. Hill, and R. J. Martin.** 1976. A sausage-associated outbreak of trichinosis in Illinois. *Am J Public Health* **66**:1194-6.

5988. **Pötzsch, C. J., T. Müller, and M. Kramer.** 2002. Summarizing the rabies situation in Europe 1990-2002 from the rabies bulletin Europe. *Rabies Bulletin Europe* **26**:11-6.

5989. **Poulsen, A., F. Cabral, J. Nielsen, A. Roth, I. M. Lisse, B. F. Vestergaard, and P. Aaby.** 2005. Varicella zoster in Guinea-Bissau: intensity of exposure and severity of infection. *Pediatr Infect Dis J* **24**:102-7.

5990. **Poulstrup, A., A. T. Nielsen, M. Binder, K. Moller, M. Moller, J. Nielsen, and H. L. Hansen.** 1999. [Botulism caused by a commercially produced product]. *Ugeskr Laeger* **161**:2815-6.

5991. **Povlsen, K., E. Bjornelius, P. Lidbrink, and I. Lind.** 2002. Relationship of Ureaplasma urealyticum biovar 2 to nongonococcal urethritis. *Eur J Clin Microbiol Infect Dis* **21**:97-101.

5992. **Powell, K. E., G. W. Heath, M. J. Kresnow, J. J. Sacks, and C. M. Branche.** 1998. Injury rates from walking, gardening, weightlifting, outdoor bicycling, and aerobics. *Med Sci Sports Exerc* **30**:1246-9.

5993. **Poynard, T., M. F. Yuen, V. Ratziu, and C. L. Lai.** 2003. Viral hepatitis C. *Lancet* **362**:2095-100.

5994. **Pozio, E.** 2001. New patterns of Trichinella infection. *Vet Parasitol* **98**:133-48.

5995. **Pozio, E., G. La Rosa, and M. A. Gomez Morales.** 2001. Epidemiology of human and animal trichinellosis in Italy since its discovery in 1887. *Parasite* **8**:S106-8.

5996. **Pozio, E., and G. Marucci.** 2003. Trichinella-infected pork products: a dangerous gift. *Trends Parasitol* **19**:338.

5997. **Pozzi, G., A. Melon, A. Scarpa, A. Iannucci, S. Rodella, F. Bonetti, and L. Fiore Donati.** 1990. Prevalence of human papillomaviruses in cervical scrapings of unselected women. *Eur J Clin Microbiol Infect Dis* **9**:703-4.

5998. **Pradel, N., V. Livrelli, C. De Champs, J. B. Palcoux, A. Reynaud, F. Scheutz, J. Sirot, B. Joly, and C. Forestier.** 2000. Prevalence and characterization of Shiga toxin-producing Escherichia coli isolated from cattle, food, and children during a one-year prospective study in France. *J Clin Microbiol* **38**:1023-31.

5999. **Pradier, C., O. Keita-Perse, E. Bernard, C. Gisbert, A. Vezolles, A. Armengaud, D. Carles, F. Grimont, J. C. Desenclos, and P. Dellamonica.** 2000. Outbreak of typhoid fever on the French riviera. *Eur J Clin Microbiol Infect Dis* **19**:464-7.

6000. **Prado, M. S., A. Strina, M. L. Barreto, A. M. Oliveira-Assis, L. M. Paz, and S. Cairncross.** 2003. Risk factors for infection with Giardia duodenalis in pre-school children in the city of Salvador, Brazil. *Epidemiol Infect* **131**:899-906.

6001. **Praetorius, F., G. Altrock, N. Blees, N. Schuh, and M. Faulde.** 1999. [Imported Anopheles: in the luggage or from the airplane? A case of severe autochthonous malaria tropica near an airport]. *Dtsch Med Wochenschr* **124**:998-1002.

6002. **Prakash, A., D. R. Bhattacharyya, P. K. Mohapatra, U. Barua, A. Phukan, and J. Mahanta.** 2003. Malaria control in a forest camp in an oil exploration area of Upper Assam. *Natl Med J India* **16**:135-8.

6003. **Prasad, K. N., S. Chawla, D. Jain, C. M. Pandey, L. Pal, S. Pradhan, and R. K. Gupta.** 2002. Human and porcine Taenia solium infection in rural north India. *Trans R Soc Trop Med Hyg* **96**:515-6.

6004. **Pratlong, F., J. A. Rioux, P. Marty, F. Faraut-Gambarelli, J. Dereure, G. Lanotte, and J. P. Dedet.** 2004. Isoenzymatic analysis of 712 strains of Leishmania infantum in the south of France and relationship of enzymatic polymorphism to clinical and epidemiological features. *J Clin Microbiol* **42**:4077-82.

6005. **Prats, G., B. Mirelis, E. Miro, F. Navarro, T. Llovet, J. R. Johnson, N. Camps, A. Dominguez, and L. Salleras.** 2003. Cephalosporin-resistant Escherichia coli among summer camp attendees with salmonellosis. *Emerg Infect Dis* **9**:1273-80.

6006. **Preece, P. M., K. N. Pearl, and C. S. Peckham.** 1984. Congenital cytomegalovirus infection. *Arch Dis Child* **59**:1120-6.

6007. **Preiksaitis, J. K., R. P. Larke, and G. J. Froese.** 1988. Comparative seroepidemiology of cytomegalovirus infection in the Canadian Arctic and an urban center. *J Med Virol* **24**:299-307.

6008. **Prendergast, T., B. Hwang, R. Alexander, T. Charron, and E. Lopez.** 1999. Tuberculosis outbreaks in prison housing units for HIV-infected inmates- -California, 1995-1996. *MMWR Morb Mortal Wkly Rep* **48**:79-82.

6009. **Press, N., M. Fyfe, W. R. Bowie, and M. Kelly.** 2001. Clinical and microbiological follow-up of an outbreak of Yersinia pseudotuberculosis serotype Ib. *Scand J Infect Dis* **33**:523-6.

6010. **Prestrud, P., J. Krogsrud, and I. Gjertz.** 1992. The occurrence of rabies in the Svalbard Islands of Norway. *J Wildl Dis* **28:** 57-63.

6011. **Prestrud, P., G. Stuve, and G. Holt.** 1993. The prevalence of Trichinella sp. in Arctic foxes (Alopex lagopus) in Svalbard. *J Wildl Dis* **29:**337-40.

6012. **Pretorius, A., M. J. Oelofsen, M. S. Smith, and E. Van der Ryst.** 1997. Rift valley fever virus: a seroepidemiologic study of small terrestrial vertebrates in South Africa. *Am J Trop Med Hyg* **57:**693-8.

6013. **Prevots, D. R., R. K. Burr, R. W. Sutter, and T. V. Murphy.** 2000. Poliomyelitis prevention in the United States. *MMWR* **49 (RR-5):**1-22.

6014. **Prevots, D. R., M. L. Ciofi degli Atti, A. Sallabanda, E. Diamante, R. B. Aylward, E. Kakariqqi, L. Fiore, A. Ylli, H. van der Avoort, R. W. Sutter, A. E. Tozzi, P. Panei, N. Schinaia, D. Genovese, G. Oblapenko, D. Greco, and S. G. Wassilak.** 1998. Outbreak of paralytic poliomyelitis in Albania, 1996: high attack rate among adults and apparent interruption of transmission following nationwide mass vaccination. *Clin Infect Dis* **26:**419-25.

6015. **Préziosi, M.-P., A. Yam, S. G. F. Wassilak, L. Chabirand, A. Simaga, M. Ndiaye, M. Dia, F. Dabis, and F. Simondon.** 2002. Epidemiology of pertussis in a West African community before and after introduction of a widespread vaccination program. *Am J Epidemiol* **155:**891-6.

6016. **Priola, S. A., and I. Vorberg.** 2004. Identification of possible animal origins of prion disease in human beings. *Lancet* **363:**2013-4.

6017. **Prociv, P., and M. S. Carlisle.** 2001. The spread of Angiostrongylus cantonensis in Australia. *Southeast Asian J Trop Med Public Health* **32 Suppl 2:**126-8.

6018. **Prociv, P., and J. Croese.** 1996. Human enteric infection with Ancylostoma caninum: hookworms reappraised in the light of a "new" zoonosis. *Acta Trop* **62:**23-44.

6019. **Prociv, P., and R. Luke.** 1993. Observations on strongyloidiasis in Queensland aboriginal communities. *Med J Aust* **158:**160-3.

6020. **Prociv, P., D. M. Spratt, and M. S. Carlisle.** 2000. Neuro-angiostrongyliasis: unresolved issues. *Int J Parasitol* **30:**1295-303.

6021. **Proctor, E. M., J. L. Isaac-Renton, W. B. Robertson, and W. A. Black.** 1985. Strongyloidiasis in Canadian Far East war veterans. *CMAJ* **133:**876-8.

6022. **Proctor, E. M., H. A. Muth, D. L. Proudfoot, A. B. Allen, R. Fisk, J. Isaac-Renton, and W. A. Black.** 1987. Endemic institutional strongyloidiasis in British Columbia. *CMAJ* **136:**1173-6.

6023. **Proctor, M. E., B. S. Klein, J. M. Jones, and J. P. Davis.** 2002. Cluster of pulmonary blastomycosis in a rural community: evidence for multiple high-risk environmental foci following a sustained period of diminished precipitation. *Mycopathologia* **153:**113-20.

6024. **Prodinger, W. M., H. Bonatti, F. Allerberger, G. Wewalka, T. G. Harrison, C. Aichberger, M. P. Dierich, R. Margreiter, and F. Tiefenbrunner.** 1994. Legionella pneumonia in transplant recipients: a cluster of cases of eight years' duration. *J Hosp Infect* **26:**191-202.

6025. **Prokopowicz, D., E. Bobrowska, M. Bobrowski, and A. Grzeszczuk.** 1995. Prevalence of antibodies against tick-borne encephalitis among residents of north-eastern Poland. *Scand J Infect Dis* **27:**15-6.

6026. **Prospero, J. M., and P. J. Lamb.** 2003. African droughts and dust transport to the Caribbean: climate change implications. *Science* **302:**1024-7.

6027. **Proulx, J. F., J. D. MacLean, T. W. Gyorkos, D. Leclair, A. K. Richter, B. Serhir, L. Forbes, and A. A. Gajadhar.** 2002. Novel prevention program for trichinellosis in inuit communities. *Clin Infect Dis* **34:**1508-14.

6028. **Provost, F., F. Laurent, M. V. Blanc, and P. Boiron.** 1997. Transmission of nocardiosis and molecular typing of Nocardia species: a short review. *Eur J Epidemiol* **13:**235-8.

6029. **Prusiner, S. B.** 2001. Sthattuck lecture - neurodegenerative diseases and prions. *N Engl J Med* **344:**1516-1526.

6030. **Pryce, D., R. Behrens, R. Davidson, P. Chiodini, A. Bryceson, and J. McLeod.** 1992. Onchocerciasis in members of an expedition to Cameroon: role of advice before travel and long term follow up. *BMJ* **304:**1285-6.

6031. **Psaroulaki, A., F. Loukaidis, C. Hadjichristodoulou, and Y. Tselentis.** 1999. Detection and identificationof the aetiological agent of Mediterranean spotted fever (MSF) in two genera of ticks in Cyprus. *Trans R Soc Trop Med Hyg* **93:**597-8.

6032. **Puech, M. C., J. M. McAnulty, M. Lesjak, N. Shaw, L. Heron, and J. M. Watson.** 2001. A statewide outbreak of cryptosporidiosis in New South Wales associated with swimming at public pools. *Epidemiol Infect* **126:**389-96.

6033. **Pulverer, G., H. Schutt-Gerowitt, and K. P. Schaal.** 2003. Human cervicofacial actinomycoses: microbiological data for 1997 cases. *Clin Infect Dis* **37:**490-7.

6034. **Pungpak, S., C. Viravan, B. Radomyos, K. Chalermrut, C. Yemput, W. Plooksawasdi, M. Ho, T. Harinasuta, and D. Bunnag.** 1997. Opisthorchis viverrini infection in Thailand: studies on the morbidity of the infection and resolution following praziquantel treatment. *Am J Trop Med Hyg* **56:**311-4.

6035. **Punyagupta, S., T. Sirisanthana, and B. Stapatayavong.** 1989. Melioidosis. Medical Publisher, Bangkok.

6036. **Puranen, M., K. Syrjanen, and S. Syrjanen.** 1996. Transmission of genital human papillomavirus infections is unlikely through the floor and seats of humid dwellings in countries of high-level hygiene. *Scand J Infect Dis* **28:**243-6.

6037. **Purcell, B., S. Samuelsson, S. J. Hahne, I. Ehrhard, S. Heuberger, I. Camaroni, A. Charlett, and J. M. Stuart.** 2004. Effectiveness of antibiotics in preventing meningococcal disease after a case: systematic review. *BMJ* **328:**1339.

6038. **Puro, V., S. Cicalini, G. De Carli, F. Soldani, F. Antunes, U. Balslev, J. Begovac, E. Bernasconi, J. L. Boaventura, M. C. Marti, R. Civljak, B. Evans, P. Francioli, F. Genasi, C. Larsen, F. Lot, S. Lunding, U. Marcus, A. A. Pereira, T. Thomas, S. Schonwald, and G. Ippolito.** 2004. Post-exposure prophylaxis of HIV infection in healthcare workers: recommendations for the European setting. *Eur J Epidemiol* **19:**577-84.

6039. **Pusterla, N., J. B. Pusterla, U. Braun, and H. Lutz.** 1998. Serological, hematologic, and PCR studies of cattle in an area of Switzerland in which tick-borne fever (caused by Ehrlichia phagocytophila) is endemic. *Clin Diagn Lab Immunol* **5:** 325-7.

6040. **Pusterla, N., J. B. Pusterla, P. Deplazes, C. Wolfensberger, W. Muller, A. Horauf, C. Reusch, and H. Lutz.** 1998. Seroprevalence of Ehrlichia canis and of canine granulocytic Ehrlichia infection in dogs in Switzerland. *J Clin Microbiol* **36:**3460-2.

6041. Putkonen, T. 1966. [Chromomycosis in Finland. The possible role of the Finnish sauna in its spreading]. *Hautarzt* **17:**507-9.

6042. Puvimanasinghe, J. P., C. K. Arambepola, N. M. Abeysinghe, L. C. Rajapaksa, and T. A. Kulatilaka. 2003. Measles outbreak in Sri Lanka, 1999-2000. *J Infect Dis* **187 Suppl 1:**S241-5.

6043. Qaqish, A. M., M. A. Nasrieh, K. M. Al-Qaoud, P. S. Craig, and S. K. Abdel-Hafez. 2003. The seroprevalences of cystic echinococcosis, and the associated risk factors, in rural-agricultural, bedouin and semi-bedouin communities in Jordan. *Ann Trop Med Parasitol* **97:**511-20.

6044. Qiu, D. C., A. E. Hubbard, B. Zhong, Y. Zhang, and R. C. Spear. 2005. A matched, case-control study of the association between Schistosoma japonicum and liver and colon cancers, in rural China. *Ann Trop Med Parasitol* **99:**47-52.

6045. Quaglio, G., F. Lugoboni, B. Pajusco, M. Sarti, G. Talamini, A. Lechi, P. Mezzelani, and D. C. Des Jarlais. 2003. Factors associated with hepatitis C virus infection in injection and noninjection drug users in Italy. *Clin Infect Dis* **37:**33-40.

6046. Quaglio, G., F. Lugoboni, G. Talamini, A. Lechi, and P. Mezzelani. 2002. Prevalence of tuberculosis infection and comparison of multiple- puncture liquid tuberculin test and Mantoux test among drug users. *Scand J Infect Dis* **34:**574-6.

6047. Quaglio, G., G. Talamini, F. Lugoboni, A. Lechi, L. Venturini, D. C. Jarlais, and P. Mezzelani. 2002. Compliance with hepatitis B vaccination in 1175 heroin users and risk factors associated with lack of vaccine response. *Addiction* **97:**985-92.

6048. Quale, J. M., D. Landman, P. A. Bradford, M. Visalli, J. Ravishankar, C. Flores, D. Mayorga, K. Vangala, and A. Adedeji. 2002. Molecular Epidemiology of a Citywide Outbreak of Extended-Spectrum beta- Lactamase-Producing Klebsiella pneumoniae Infection. *Clin Infect Dis* **35:**834-41.

6049. Quddus, A., S. Luby, M. Rahbar, and Y. Pervaiz. 2002. Neonatal tetanus: mortality rate and risk factors in Loralai district, Pakistan. *Int J Epidemiol* **31:**648-53.

6050. Quick, M. L., R. W. Sutter, K. Kobaidze, N. Malakmadze, R. Nakashidze, S. Murvanidze, K. G. Wooten, and P. M. Strebel. 2000. Risk factors for diphtheria: a prospective case-control study in the Republic of Georgia, 1995-1996. *J Infect Dis* **181 Suppl 1:**S121-9.

6051. Quick, R., K. Paugh, D. Addiss, J. Kobayashi, and R. Baron. 1992. Restaurant-associated outbreak of giardiasis. *J Infect Dis* **166:**673-6.

6052. Quick, R. E., C. W. Hoge, D. J. Hamilton, C. J. Whitney, M. Borges, and J. M. Kobayashi. 1993. Underutilization of pneumococcal vaccine in nursing home in Washington State: report of a serotype-specific outbreak and a survey. *Am J Med* **94:**149-52.

6053. Quinn, J. P., P. M. Arnow, D. Weil, and J. Rosenbluth. 1984. Outbreak of JK diphtheroid infections associated with environmental contamination. *J Clin Microbiol* **19:**668-71.

6054. Quinn, T. C., C. Gaydos, M. Shepherd, L. Bobo, E. W. Hook, R. Viscidi, and A. Rompalo. 1996. Epidemiologic and microbiologic correlates of Chlamydia trachomatis infection in sexual partnership. *JAMA* **276:**1737-42.

6055. Quinn, T. C., S. E. Goodell, C. Fennell, S. P. Wang, M. D. Schuffler, K. K. Holmes, and W. E. Stamm. 1984. Infections with Campylobacter jejuni and Campylobacter-like organisms in homosexual men. *Ann Intern Med* **101:**187-92.

6056. Quinn, T. C., M. J. Wawer, N. Sewankambo, D. Serwadda, C. Li, F. Wabwire-Mangen, M. O. Meehan, T. Lutalo, and R. H. Gray. 2000. Viral load and heterosexual transmission of human immunodeficiency virus type 1. Rakai Project Study Group. *N Engl J Med* **342:**921-9.

6057. Quiroz, E., N. Moreno, P. H. Peralta, and R. B. Tesh. 1988. A human case of encephalitis associated with vesicular stomatitis virus (Indiana serotype) infection. *Am J Trop Med Hyg* **39:**312-4.

6058. Quiroz, E. S., C. Bern, J. R. MacArthur, L. Xiao, M. Fletcher, M. J. Arrowood, D. K. Shay, M. E. Levy, R. I. Glass, and A. Lal. 2000. An outbreak of cryptosporidiosis linked to a foodhandler. *J Infect Dis* **181:**695-700.

6059. Qureshi, A., L. Mooney, M. Denton, and K. G. Kerr. 2005. Stenotrophomonas maltophilia in salad. *Emerg Infect Dis* **11:**1157-8.

6060. Qureshi, H., B. D. Gessner, R. Leboulleux, H. Hasan, S. E. Alam, and L. H. Moulton. 2000. The incidence of vaccine preventable influenza-like illness and medication use among Pakistani pilgrims to the Haj in Saudi Arabia. *Vaccine* **18:**2956-62.

6061. Qutaishat, S. S., M. E. Stemper, S. K. Spencer, M. A. Borchardt, J. C. Opitz, T. A. Monson, J. L. Anderson, and J. L. Ellingson. 2003. Transmission of Salmonella enterica serotype Typhimurium DT104 to infants through mother's breast milk. *Pediatrics* **111**.

6062. Raad, II, R. J. Sherertz, C. S. Rains, J. L. Cusick, L. L. Fauerbach, P. D. Reuman, and T. R. Belcuore. 1989. The importance of nosocomial transmission of measles in the propagation of a community outbreak. *Infect Control Hosp Epidemiol* **10:**161-6.

6063. Rab, M. A., M. K. Bile, M. M. Mubarik, H. Asghar, Z. Sami, S. Siddiqi, A. S. Dil, M. A. Barzgar, M. A. Chaudhry, and M. I. Burney. 1997. Water-borne hepatitis E virus epidemic in Islamabad, Pakistan: a common source outbreak traced to the malfunction of a modern water treatment plant. *Am J Trop Med Hyg* **57:**151-7.

6064. Rabaud, C., T. May, T. D. H., and P. Canton. 1995. Aspects de pneumopathies de la fièvre Q. *Méd Mal Infect* **25:**955-7.

6065. Rabodonirina, M., P. Vanhems, S. Couray-Targe, R. P. Gillibert, C. Ganne, N. Nizard, C. Colin, J. Fabry, J. L. Touraine, G. van Melle, A. Nahimana, P. Francioli, and P. M. Hauser. 2004. Molecular Evidence of Interhuman Transmission of Pneumocystis Pneumonia among Renal Transplant Recipients Hospitalized with HIV-Infected Patients. *Emerg Infect Dis* **10:**1766-73.

6066. Rabold, J. G., C. W. Hoge, D. R. Shlim, C. Kefford, R. Rajah, and P. Echeverria. 1994. Cyclospora outbreak associated with chlorinated drinking water. *Lancet* **344:**1360-1.

6067. Raboobee, N., J. Aboobaker, and A. K. Peer. 1998. Tinea pedis et unguium in the Muslim community of Durban, South Africa. *Int J Dermatol* **37:**759-65.

6068. Raccurt, C. P. 1999. [Dirofilariasis, an emerging and underestimated zoonoses in France]. *Med Trop (Mars)* **59:**389-400.

6069. Raccurt, C. P. 2000. [Human dirofilariasis in France: new data confirming the human transmission of Dirofilaria repens to the north of the 46 degree north latitude]. *Med Trop (Mars)* **60:**308-9.

6070. Raccurt, C. P., J. Blaise, and M. C. Durette-Desset. 2003. [Presence of Angiostrongylus cantonensis in Haiti.]. *Trop Med Int Health* **8:**423-6.

6071. **Radulovic, S., H. M. Feng, M. Morovic, B. Djelalija, V. Popov, P. Crocquet-Valdes, and D. H. Walker.** 1996. Isolation of Rickettsia akari from a patient in a region where Mediterranean spotted fever is endemic. *Clin Infect Dis* **22**:216-20.

6072. **Radun, D., M. Niedrig, A. Ammon, and K. Stark.** 2003. SARS: retrospective cohort study among German guests of the hotel 'M', Hong Kong. *Eurosurveillance* **8**:228-30.

6073. **Raeber, P. A., S. Winteler, and J. Paget.** 1994. Fever in the returned traveller: remember rickettsial diseases. *Lancet* **344**:331.

6074. **Raffalli, J., K. A. Sepkowitz, and D. Armstrong.** 1996. Community-based outbreaks of tuberculosis. *Arch Intern Med* **156**:1053-60.

6075. **Raffenot, D., O. Rogeaux, B. De Goer, and B. Zerr.** 1999. Plasmodium falciparum malaria acquired by accidental inoculation. *Eur J Clin Microbiol Infect Dis* **18**:680-1.

6076. **Rafila, A., D. Nicolaiciuc, A. Pistol, E. Darstaru, and A. Grigoriu.** 2004. Attack by bear with rabies in Brasov county, Romania. *Eur Surveill* **9**:50.

6077. **Ragan, V. E.** 2002. The animal and health inspection service (APHIS) brucellosis eradication program in the United States. *Vet Microbiol* **90**:11-8.

6078. **Raglio, A., V. Russo, G. Swierczynski, A. Sonzogni, A. Goglio, and L. S. Garcia.** 2002. Acute Schistosoma mansoni infection with progression to chronic lesion in Italian travelers returning from Cameroon, West Africa: a diagnostic and prevention problem. *J Travel Med* **9**:100-2.

6079. **Rahim, Z., and K. M. Aziz.** 1994. Enterotoxigenicity, hemolytic activity and antibiotic resistance of Aeromonas spp. isolated from freshwater prawn marketed in Dhaka, Bangladesh. *Microbiol Immunol* **38**:773-8.

6080. **Rahman, M., A. Alam, K. Nessa, A. Hossain, S. Nahar, D. Datta, S. Alam Khan, R. Amin Mian, and M. J. Albert.** 2000. Etiology of sexually transmitted infections among street-based female sex workers in Dhaka, Bangladesh. *J Clin Microbiol* **38**:1244-6.

6081. **Rahman, W. A., C. R. Adanan, and A. Abu Hassan.** 1998. A study on some aspects of the epidemiology of malaria in an endemic district in northern Peninsular Malaysia near Thailand border. *Southeast Asian J Trop Med Public Health* **29**:537-40.

6082. **Raimundo, O., H. Heussler, J. B. Bruhn, S. Suntrarachun, N. Kelly, M. A. Deighton, and S. M. Garland.** 2002. Molecular epidemiology of coagulase-negative staphylococcal bacteraemia in a newborn intensive care unit. *J Hosp Infect* **51**:33-42.

6083. **Raisanen, S., L. Ruuskanen, and S. Nyman.** 1985. Epidemic ascariasis—evidence of transmission by imported vegetables. *Scand J Prim Health Care* **3**:189-91.

6084. **Rajagopalan, P. K., P. Jambulingam, S. Sabesan, K. Krishnamoorthy, S. Rajendran, K. Gunasekaran, N. P. Kumar, and R. M. Prothero.** 1986. Population movement and malaria persistence in Rameswaram Island. *Soc Sci Med* **22**:879-86.

6085. **Rajpura, A., K. Lamden, S. Forster, S. Clarke, J. Cheesbrough, S. Gornall, and S. Waterworth.** 2003. Large outbreak of infection with Escherichia coli O157 PT21/28 in Eccleston, Lancashire, due to cross contamination at a butcher's counter. *Commun Dis Publ Health* **6**:279-84.

6086. **Rajshekhar, V., D. D. Joshi, N. Q. Doanh, N. van De, and Z. Xiaonong.** 2003. Taenia solium taeniosis/cysticercosis in Asia: epidemiology, impact and issues. *Acta Trop* **87**:53-60.

6087. **Ralph, A., J. McBride, and B. J. Currie.** 2004. Transmission of Burkholderia pseudomallei via breast milk in northern Australia. *Pediatr Infect Dis J* **23**:1169-71.

6088. **Ralph, A., M. Raines, P. Whelan, and B. J. Currie.** 2004. Scrub typhus in the Northern Territory: exceeding the boundaries of Litchfield national park. *Commun Dis Intell* **28**:267-9.

6089. **Ramage, I. J., N. Wilson, and R. B. Thomson.** 1997. Fashion victim: infective endocarditis after nasal piercing. *Arch Dis Child* **77**:187.

6090. **Ramaiah, K. D., P. K. Das, P. Vanamail, and S. P. Pani.** 2003. The impact of six rounds of single-dose mass administration of diethylcarbamazine or ivermectin on the transmission of Wuchereria bancrofti by Culex quinquefasciatus and its implications for lymphatic filariasis elimination programmes. *Trop Med Int Health* **8**:1082-92.

6091. **Ramasamy, I., M. Law, S. Collins, and F. Brooke.** 2003. Organ distribution of prion proteins in variant Creutzfeldt-Jakob disease. *Lancet Infect Dis* **3**:214-22.

6092. **Rambajan, I.** 1994. Highly prevalent falciparum malaria in north west Guyana: its development history and control problems. *Bull Pan Am Health Organ* **28**:193-201.

6093. **Rambo, P. R., A. A. Agostini, and C. Graeff-Teixeira.** 1997. Abdominal angiostrongylosis in southern Brazil—prevalence and parasitic burden in mollusc intermediate hosts from eighteen endemic foci. *Mem Inst Oswaldo Cruz* **92**:9-14.

6094. **Ramelli, G. P., G. D. Simonetti, M. Gorgievski-Hrisoho, C. Aebi, and M. G. Bianchetti.** 2004. Outbreak of coxsackie B5 virus meningitis in a Scout camp. *Pediatr Infect Dis J* **23**:86-7.

6095. **Ramers, C., G. Billman, M. Hartin, S. Ho, and M. H. Sawyer.** 2000. Impact of a diagnostic cerebrospinal fluid enterovirus polymerase chain reaction test on patient management. *JAMA* **283**:2680-5.

6096. **Ramirez, B. L., L. Hernandez, F. F. Alberto, M. Collins, V. Nfonsam, T. Punsalan, and M. A. Kron.** 2004. Contrasting Wuchereria Bancrofti Microfilaria Rates in Two Mangyan-Populated Philippine Villages. *Am J Trop Med Hyg* **71**:17-23.

6097. **Ramis, A., L. Ferrer, A. Aranaz, E. Liebana, A. Mateos, L. Dominguez, C. Pascual, J. Fdez-Garayazabal, and M. D. Collins.** 1996. Mycobacterium genavense infection in canaries. *Avian Dis* **40**:246-51.

6098. **Ramjee, G., and E. E. Gouws a.** 2002. Prevalence of HIV among truck drivers visiting sex workers in KwaZulu-Natal, South Africa. *Sex Transm Dis* **29**:44-9.

6099. **Ramos, J. M., E. Malmierca, F. Reyes, W. Wolde, A. Galata, A. Tesfamariam, and M. Gorgolas.** 2004. Characteristics of louse-borne relapsing fever in Ethiopian children and adults. *Ann Trop Med Parasitol* **98**:191-6.

6100. **Rampersad, F. S., S. Laloo, A. La Borde, K. Maharaj, L. Sookhai, J. Teelucksingh, S. Reid, L. McDougall, and A. A. Adesiyun.** 1999. Microbial quality of oysters sold in Western Trinidad and potential health risk to consumers. *Epidemiol Infect* **123**:241-50.

6101. **Ramsay, C. N., and J. Marsh.** 1990. Giardiasis due to deliberate contamination of water supply. *Lancet* **336**:880-1.

6102. **Ramsay, C. N., and P. A. Upton.** 1989. Hepatitis A and frozen raspberries. *Lancet* **1**:43-4.

6103. **Ramsey, A. H., T. V. Oemig, J. P. Davis, J. P. Massey, and T. J. Török.** 2002. An outbreak of bronchoscopy-related Mycobacterium tuberculosis infections due to lack of bronchoscope leak testing. *Chest* **121**:976-81.

6104. Ranganathan, S., R. Tasker, R. Booy, P. Habibi, S. Nadel, and J. Britto. 1999. Pertussis is increasing in unimmunized infants: is a change in policy needed? *Arch Dis Child* **80:** 297-9.

6105. Rangel, J. M., P. H. Sparling, C. Crowe, P. M. Griffin, and D. L. Swerdlow. 2005. Epidemiology of Escherichia coli O157:H7 outbreaks, United States, 1982-2002. *Emerg Infect Dis* **11:**603-9.

6106. Rank, E. L., L. Brettman, H. Katz-Pollack, D. DeHertogh, and D. Neville. 1992. Chronology of a hospital-wide measles outbreak: lessons learned and shared from an extraordinary week in late March 1989. *Am J Infect Control* **20:**315-8.

6107. Ranque, S., B. Faugere, E. Pozio, G. La Rosa, A. Tamburrini, J. F. Pellissier, and P. Brouqui. 2000. Trichinella pseudospiralis outbreak in France. *Emerg Infect Dis* **6:**543-7.

6108. Rao, B. L., A. Basu, N. S. Wairagkar, M. M. Gore, V. A. Arankalle, J. P. Thakare, R. S. Jadi, K. A. Rao, and A. C. Mishra. 2004. A large outbreak of acute encephalitis with high fatality rate in children in Andhra Pradesh, India, in 2003, associated with Chandipura virus. *Lancet* **364:**869-74.

6109. Rao, J. S., S. P. Misra, S. K. Patanayak, T. V. Rao, R. K. Das Gupta, and B. R. Thapar. 2000. Japanese Encephalitis epidemic in Anantapur district, Andhra Pradesh (October-November, 1999). *J Commun Dis* **32:**306-12.

6110. Rao, M. R., A. B. Naficy, S. J. Savarino, R. Abu-Elyazeed, T. F. Wierzba, L. F. Peruski, I. Abdel-Messih, R. Frenck, and J. D. Clemens. 2001. Pathogenicity and convalescent excretion of Campylobacter in rural Egyptian children. *Am J Epidemiol* **154:**166-73.

6111. Rao, P. S., N. M. Mozhi, and M. V. Thomas. 2000. Leprosy affected beggars as a hidden source for transmission of leprosy. *Indian J Med Res* **112:**52-5.

6112. Rao, V. K., G. P. Krasan, D. R. Hendrixson, S. Dawid, and J. W. St Geme, 3rd. 1999. Molecular determinants of the pathogenesis of disease due to non-typable Haemophilus influenzae. *FEMS Microbiol Rev* **23:**99-129.

6113. Raoul, F., D. Michelat, M. Ordinaire, Y. Decote, M. Aubert, P. Delattre, P. Deplazes, and P. Giraudoux. 2003. Echinococcus multilocularis: secondary poisoning of fox population during a vole outbreak reduces environmental contamination in a high endemicity area. *Int J Parasitol* **33:**945-54.

6114. Raoult, D., R. J. Birtles, M. Montoya, E. Perez, H. Tissot-Dupont, V. Roux, and H. Guerra. 1999. Survey of three bacterial louse-associated diseases among rural Andean communities in Peru: prevalence of epidemic typhus, trench fever, and relapsing fever. *Clin Infect Dis* **29:**434-6.

6115. Raoult, D., C. Foucault, and P. Brouqui. 2001. Infections in the homeless. *Lancet Infect Dis* **1:**77-84.

6116. Raoult, D., P. E. Fournier, F. Fenollar, M. Jensenius, T. Prioe, J. J. de Pina, G. Caruso, N. Jones, H. Laferl, J. E. Rosenblatt, and T. J. Marrie. 2001. Rickettsia africae, a tick-borne pathogen in travelers to sub-Saharan Africa. *N Engl J Med* **344:**1504-10.

6117. Raoult, D., B. La Scola, P. Lecocq, H. Lepidi, and P. E. Fournier. 2001. Culture and immunological detection of Tropheryma whippelii from the duodenum of a patient with Whipple disease. *JAMA* **285:**1039-43.

6118. Raoult, D., A. Lakos, F. Fenollar, J. Beytout, P. Brouqui, and P. E. Fournier. 2002. Spotless rickettsiosis caused by Rickettsia slovaca and associated with Dermacentor ticks. *Clin Infect Dis* **34:**1331-6.

6119. Raoult, D., J. B. Ndihokubwayo, H. Tissot-Dupont, V. Roux, B. Faugere, R. Abegbinni, and R. J. Birtles. 1998. Outbreak of epidemic typhus associated with trench fever in Burundi. *Lancet* **352:**353-8.

6120. Raoult, D., and V. Roux. 1999. The body louse as a vector of reemerging human diseases. *Clin Infect Dis* **29:**888-911.

6121. Raoult, D., H. Tissot-Dupont, C. Foucault, J. Gouvernet, P. E. Fournier, E. Bernit, A. Stein, M. Nesri, J. R. Harle, and P. J. Weiller. 2000. Q fever 1985-1998. Clinical and epidemiologic features of 1,383 infections. *Medicine (Baltimore)* **79:**109-23.

6122. Raper, J., M. P. Portela Molina, M. Redpath, S. Tomlinson, E. Lugli, and H. Green. 2002. Natural immunity to human African trypanosomiasis: trypanosome lytic factors and the blood incubation infectivity test. *Trans R Soc Trop Med Hyg* **96 Suppl 1:**S145-50.

6123. Rappole, J. H., S. R. Derrickson, and Z. Hubalek. 2000. Migratory birds and spread of West Nile virus in the Western Hemisphere. *Emerg Infect Dis* **6:**319-28.

6124. Rasch, G., I. Schöneberg, L. Apitzsch, and U. Menzel. 1997. Brucellose-Erkrankungen in Deutschland. *Bundesgesundheitsblatt* **40:**50-4.

6125. Rasmussen, F., and C. Sundelin. 1990. Use of medical care and antibiotics among preschool children in different day care settings. *Acta Paediatr Scand* **79:**838-46.

6126. Rasmussen-Cruz, B., A. Hidalgo-San Martin, and N. Alfaro-Alfaro. 2003. [STD/AIDS-related practices and occupational risk factors in adolescent hotel workers in Puerto Vallarta, Mexico]. *Salud Publica Mex* **45 Suppl 1:**S81-91.

6127. Rasnake, M. S., N. G. Conger, K. McAllister, K. K. Holmes, and E. C. Tramont. 2005. History of U.S. military contributions to the study of sexually transmitted diseases. *Mil Med* **170:**61-5.

6128. Raso, T. F., K. Werther, E. T. Miranda, and M. J. Mendes-Giannini. 2004. Cryptococcosis outbreak in psittacine birds in Brazil. *Med Mycol* **42:**355-62.

6129. Rasrinaul, L., O. Suthienkul, P. D. Echeverria, D. N. Taylor, J. Seriwatana, A. Bangtrakulnonth, and U. Lexomboon. 1988. Foods as a source of enteropathogens causing childhood diarrhea in Thailand. *Am J Trop Med Hyg* **39:**97-102.

6130. Rastawicki, W., S. Kaluzewski, M. Jagielski, and R. Gierczynski. 2003. Changes in the epidemiological pattern of Mycoplasma pneumoniae infections in Poland. *Eur J Epidemiol* **18:**1163-4.

6131. Rath, P. M., G. Rögler, A. Schönberg, H. D. Pohle, and F. J. Fehrenbach. 1992. Relapsing fever and its serological discrimination from Lyme borreliosis. *Infection* **20:**283-6.

6132. Rathi, S. K., S. Akhtar, M. H. Rahbar, and S. I. Azam. 2002. Prevalence and risk factors associated with tuberculin skin test positivity among household contacts of smear-positive pulmonary tuberculosis cases in Umerkot, Pakistan. *Int J Tuberc Lung Dis* **6:**851-7.

6133. Ratnam, S., K. Hogan, S. B. March, and R. W. Butler. 1986. Whirlpool-associated folliculitis caused by Pseudomonas aeruginosa: report of an outbreak and review. *J Clin Microbiol* **23:**655-9.

6134. Ratnam, S., E. Mercer, B. Picco, S. Parsons, and R. Butler. 1982. A nosocomial outbreak of diarrheal disease due to Yersinia enterocolitica serotype O:5, biotype 1. *J Infect Dis* **145:**242-7.

6135. Ratnam, S., F. Stratton, C. O'Keefe, A. Roberts, R. Coates, M. Yetman, S. Squires, R. Khakhria, and J. Hockin. 1999. Salmonella enteritidis outbreak due to contaminated cheese—Newfoundland. *Can Commun Dis Rep* **25:**17-9; discussion 19-21.

6136. Ratsitorahina, M., S. Chanteau, L. Rahalison, L. Ratsifasoamanana, and P. Boisier. 2000. Epidemiological and diagnostic aspects of the outbreak of pneumonic plague in Madagascar. *Lancet* **355:**111-3.

6137. Rauch, A., M. Rickenbach, R. Weber, B. Hirschel, P. E. Tarr, H. C. Bucher, P. Vernazza, E. Bernasconi, A. S. Zinkernagel, J. Evison, and H. Furrer. 2005. Unsafe sex and increased incidence of hepatitis C virus infection among HIV-infected men who have sex with men: the Swiss HIV Cohort Study. *Clin Infect Dis* **41:**395-402.

6138. Raúl Velázquez, F., D. O. Matson, J. J. Calva, et al. 1996. Rotavirus infection in infants as protection against subsequent infections. *N Engl J Med* **335:**1022-8.

6139. Raupach, J. C., and R. L. Hundy. 2003. An outbreak of Campylobacter jejuni infection among conference delegates. *Commun Dis Intell* **27:**380-3.

6140. Rausch, R. L. 2003. Cystic echinococcosis in the Arctic and Sub-Arctic. *Parasitology* **127 Suppl:**S73-85.

6141. Rausch, R. L., and A. M. Adams. 2000. Natural transfer of helminths of marine origin to freshwater fishes with observations on the development of Diphyllobothrium alascense. *J Parasitol* **86:**319-27.

6142. Rausch, R. L., J. F. Wilson, and P. M. Schantz. 1990. A programme to reduce the risk of infection by Echinococcus multilocularis: the use of praziquantel to control the cestode in a village in the hyperendemic region of Alaska. *Ann Trop Med Parasitol* **84:**239-50.

6143. Rautelin, H., K. Koota, R. von Essen, M. Jahkola, A. Siitonen, and T. U. Kosunen. 1990. Waterborne Campylobacter jejuni epidemic in a Finnish hospital for rheumatic diseases. *Scand J Infect Dis* **22:**321-6.

6144. Rautelin, H., A. Sivonen, A. Kuikka, O. V. Renkonen, V. Valtonen, and T. U. Kosunen. 1995. Enteric Plesiomonas shigelloides infections in Finnish patients. *Scand J Infect Dis* **27:**495-8.

6145. Ravaonindrina, N., R. Rasolomandimby, E. Rajaomiarisoa, R. Rakotoarisoa, L. Andrianantara, N. Rasolofonirina, and J. F. Roux. 1996. [Street-vendor foods: quality of ice creams, sherbets and sorbets sold in the urban agglomeration of Antananarivo]. *Arch Inst Pasteur Madagascar* **63:**67-75.

6146. Ravdin, J. I. 1995. Amebiasis. *Clin Infect Dis* **20:**1453-64; quiz 1465-6.

6147. Ravdin, J. I. e. 2000. Amebiasis. Imperial College Press, London.

6148. Ravn, P., J. D. Lundgren, P. Kjaeldgaard, W. Holten-Anderson, N. Hojlyng, J. O. Nielsen, and J. Gaub. 1991. Nosocomial outbreak of cryptosporidiosis in AIDS patients. *BMJ* **302:**277-80.

6149. Rawlings, J. A., K. A. Hendricks, C. R. Burgess, R. M. Campman, and G. G. Clark. 1998. Dengue surveillance in Texas, 1995. *Am J Trop Med Hyg* **59:**95-99.

6150. Rawlins, S. C., A. Siung-Chang, S. Baboolal, and D. D. Chadee. 2004. Evidence for the interruption of transmission of lymphatic filariasis among schoolchildren in Trinidad and Tobago. *Trans R Soc Trop Med Hyg* **98:**473-7.

6151. Rawlins, S. C., T. Tiwari, D. D. Chadee, L. Validum, H. Alexander, R. Nazeer, and S. R. Rawlins. 2001. American cutaneous leishmaniasis in Guyana, South America. *Ann Trop Med Parasitol* **95:**245-51.

6152. Ray, A. J., C. K. Hoyen, T. F. Taub, E. C. Eckstein, and C. J. Donskey. 2002. Nosocomial transmission of vancomycin-resistant enterococci from surfaces. *JAMA* **287:**1400-1.

6153. Ray, R., R. Aggarwal, P. N. Salunke, N. N. Mehrotra, G. P. Talwar, and S. R. Naik. 1991. Hepatitis E virus genome in stools of hepatitis patients during large epidemic in north India. *Lancet* **338:**783-4.

6154. Ray, S. M., S. D. Ahuja, P. A. Blake, M. M. Farley, M. Samuel, T. Fiorentino, E. Swanson, M. Cassidy, J. C. Lay, and T. Van Gilder. 2004. Population-Based Surveillance for Yersinia enterocolitica Infections in FoodNet Sites, 1996-1999: Higher Risk of Disease in Infants and Minority Populations. *Clin Infect Dis* **38 Suppl 3:**S181-9.

6155. Ray, S. M., D. D. Erdman, J. D. Berschling, J. E. Cooper, T. J. Torok, and H. M. Blumberg. 1997. Nosocomial exposure to parvovirus B19: low risk of transmission to healthcare workers. *Infect Control Hosp Epidemiol* **18:**109-14.

6156. Raymond, J., L. Armand-Lefèvre, F. Moulin, H. Dabernat, A. Commeau, D. Gendrel, and P. Berche. 2001. Nasopharyngeal colonization by Haemophilus influenzae in children living in an orphanage. *Pediatr Infect Dis J* **20:**779-784.

6157. Raz, R., R. Colodner, and C. M. Kunin. 2005. Who are you—Staphylococcus saprophyticus? *Clin Infect Dis* **40:**896-8.

6158. Razmuviene, D. 2004. Death of a child from rabies in Lithuania and update on the Lithuanian rabies situation. *Eurosurveillance* **9:**48-9.

6159. Reacher, M., M. Ramsay, J. White, A. De Zoysa, A. Efstratiou, G. Mann, A. Mackay, and R. C. George. 2000. Nontoxigenic corynebacterium diphtheriae: an emerging pathogen in England and Wales? *Emerg Infect Dis* **6:**640-5.

6160. Read, J. S. 2003. Human milk, breastfeeding, and transmission of human immunodeficiency virus type 1 in the United States. American Academy of Pediatrics Committee on Pediatric AIDS. *Pediatrics* **112:**1196-205.

6161. Read, S. C., C. L. Gyles, R. C. Clarke, H. Lior, and S. McEwen. 1990. Prevalence of verocytotoxigenic Escherichia coli in ground beef, pork, and chicken in southwestern Ontario. *Epidemiol Infect* **105:**11-20.

6162. Reading, F. C., and M. E. Brecher. 2001. Transfusion-related bacterial sepsis. *Curr Opin Hematol* **8:**380-6.

6163. Ready, P. D., R. Lainson, and J. J. Shaw. 1983. Leishmaniasis in Brazil: XX. Prevalence of "enzootic rodent leishmaniasis" (Leishmania mexicana amazonensis), and apparent absence of "pian bois" (Le. braziliensis guyanensis), in plantations of introduced tree species and in other non-climax forests in eastern Amazonia. *Trans R Soc Trop Med Hyg* **77:**775-85.

6164. Reboli, A. C., J. F. John, Jr., C. G. Platt, and J. R. Cantey. 1990. Methicillin-resistant Staphylococcus aureus outbreak at a Veterans' Affairs Medical Center: importance of carriage of the organism by hospital personnel. *Infect Control Hosp Epidemiol* **11:**291-6.

6165. Reboli, A. C., R. Koshinski, K. Arias, K. Marks-Austin, D. Stieritz, and T. L. Stull. 1996. An outbreak of Burkholderia cepacia lower respiratory tract infection associated with contaminated albuterol nebulization solution. *Infect Control Hosp Epidemiol* **17:**741-3.

6166. Reche, M. P., P. A. Jimenez, F. Alvarez, J. E. Garcia de los Rios, A. M. Rojas, and P. de Pedro. 2003. Incidence of salmonellae in captive and wild free-living raptorial birds in central Spain. *J Vet Med B Infect Dis Vet Public Health* **50:**42-4.

6167. **Redd, S. C., F. Y. C. Lin, B. S. Fields, J. Biscoe, B. B. Plikaytis, P. Powers, J. Patel, B. P. Lim, J. M. Joseph, and C. Devadason.** 1990. A rural outbreak of legionnaires' disease linked to visiting a retail store. *Am J Public Health* **80:**431-4.

6168. **Redd, S. C., J. J. Wirima, R. W. Steketee, J. G. Breman, and D. L. Heymann.** 1996. Transplacental transmission of Plasmodium falciparum in rural Malawi. *Am J Trop Med Hyg* **55:**57-60.

6169. **Redjah, A., M. F. Benkortbi, S. Mesbah, and B. Ould Rouis.** 1992. Epidémie de fièvre typhoïde de Dergana (banlieue d'Alger). Aspects cliniques et évolutifs de la maladie chez l'enfant. *Méd Mal Infect* **22:**652-655.

6170. **Redlinger, T., V. Corella-Barud, J. Graham, A. Galindo, R. Avitia, and V. Cardenas.** 2002. Hyperendemic Cryptosporidium and Giardia in households lacking municipal sewer and water on the United States-Mexico border. *Am J Trop Med Hyg* **66:**794-8.

6171. **Redman, J. C.** 1974. Pneumocystis carinii pneumonia in an adopted Vietnamese infant. A case of diffuse, fulminant disease, with recovery. *JAMA* **230:**1561-3.

6172. **Ree, H. I., T. E. Kim, I. Y. Lee, S. H. Jeon, U. W. Hwang, and W. H. Chang.** 2001. Determination and geographical distribution of Orientia tsutsugamushi serotypes in Korea by nested polymerase chain reaction. *Am J Trop Med Hyg* **65:**528-34.

6173. **Reechaipichitkul, W., and P. Tantiwong.** 2002. Clinical features of community-acquired pneumonia treated at Srinagarind hospital, Khon Kaen, Thailand. *Southeast Asian J Trop Med Public Health* **33:**355-61.

6174. **Reed, D. S., C. M. Lind, L. J. Sullivan, W. D. Pratt, and M. D. Parker.** 2004. Aerosol infection of cynomolgus macaques with enzootic strains of venezuelan equine encephalitis viruses. *J Infect Dis* **189:**1013-7.

6175. **Reed, W., J. Carroll, and A. Agramonte.** 1901. The etiology of yellow fever. *JAMA* **36:**431-40.

6176. **Reef, S., T. K. Frey, K. Theall, E. Abernathy, C. L. Burnett, J. Icenogle, M. M. McCauley, and M. Wharton.** 2002. The changing epidemiology of rubella in the 1990s. On the verge of elimination and new challenges for control and prevention. *JAMA* **287:**464-72.

6177. **Reefhuis, J., M. A. Honein, and C. G. Whitney.** 2003. Risk of bacterial meningitis in children with cochlear implants. *N Engl J Med* **349:**435-45.

6178. **Rees, D. H., and J. S. Axford.** 1994. Evidence for Lyme disease in urban park workers: a potential new health hazard for city inhabitants. *Br J Rheumatol* **33:**123-8.

6179. **Rees, J. R., R. W. Pinner, R. A. Hajjeh, M. E. Brandt, and A. L. Reingold.** 1998. The epidemiological features of invasive mycotic infections in the San Francisco Bay area, 1992-1993: results of population-based laboratory active surveillance. *Clin Infect Dis* **27:**1138-47.

6180. **Reeve, G., D. L. Martin, J. Pappas, R. E. Thompson, and K. D. Greene.** 1989. An outbreak of shigellosis associated with the consumption of raw oysters. *N Engl J Med* **321:**224-7.

6181. **Refai, M.** 2002. Incidence and control of brucellosis in the Near East region. *Vet Microbiol* **90:**81-110.

6182. **Refregier-Petton, J., N. Rose, M. Denis, and G. Salvat.** 2001. Risk factors for Campylobacter spp. contamination in French broiler-chicken flocks at the end of the rearing period. *Prev Vet Med* **50:**89-100.

6183. **Refsum, T., T. Vikoren, K. Handeland, G. Kapperud, and G. Holstad.** 2003. Epidemiologic and pathologic aspects of Salmonella typhimurium infection in passerine birds in Norway. *J Wildl Dis* **39:**64-72.

6184. **Regamey, N., M. Tamm, M. Wernli, A. Witschi, G. Thiel, G. Cathomas, and P. Erb.** 1998. Transmission of human herpesvirus 8 infection from renal-transplant donors to recipients. *N Engl J Med* **339:**1358-1363.

6185. **Regan, C. M., F. Johnstone, C. A. Joseph, and M. Urwin.** 2002. Local surveillance of influenza in the United Kingdom: from sentinel general practices to sentinel cities? *Commun Dis Public Health* **5:**17-22.

6186. **Regan, C. M., Q. Syed, and P. J. Tunstall.** 1995. A hospital outbreak of Clostridium perfringens food poisoning—implications for food hygiene review in hospitals. *J Hosp Infect* **29:**69-73.

6187. **Regan, F., and C. Taylor.** 2002. Blood transfusion medicine. *BMJ* **325:**143-7.

6188. **Rehacek, J., and I. V. Tarasevich.** 1991. Ecological questions concerning rickettsiae. *Eur J Epidemiol* **7:**229-36.

6189. **Rehacek, J., J. Urvolgyi, E. Kocianova, Z. Sekeyova, M. Vavrekova, and E. Kovacova.** 1991. Extensive examination of different tick species for infestation with Coxiella burnetii in Slovakia. *Eur J Epidemiol* **7:**299-303.

6190. **Rehmet, S., G. Sinn, O. Robstad, H. David, D. Lesser, K. Noeckler, G. Scherholz, D. Erkrath, D. Pechmann, L. R. Petersen, R. Kundt, G. Oltmans, R. Lange, J. Laumen, U. Nogay, M. Dixius, J. Eichenberg, F. Dinse, D. Stegemann, W. Lotz, D. Franke, P. Hag, and A. Ammon.** 1999. Two outbreaks of trichinellosis in the state of Northrhine-Westfalia, Germany, 1998. *Eur Surveill* **4:**78-81.

6191. **Reichler, M. R., A. Abbas, S. Kharabsheh, A. Mahafzah, J. P. Alexander, Jr., P. Rhodes, S. Faouri, H. Otoum, S. Bloch, M. A. Majid, M. Mulders, R. Aslanian, H. F. Hull, M. A. Pallansch, and P. A. Patriarca.** 1997. Outbreak of paralytic poliomyelitis in a highly immunized population in Jordan. *J Infect Dis* **175 Suppl 1:**S62-70.

6192. **Reid, T. M., and H. G. Robinson.** 1987. Frozen raspberries and hepatitis A. *Epidemiol Infect* **98:**109-12.

6193. **Reida, P., M. Wolff, H. W. Pohls, W. Kuhlmann, A. Lehmacher, S. Aleksic, H. Karch, and J. Bockemuhl.** 1994. An outbreak due to enterohaemorrhagic Escherichia coli O157:H7 in a children day care centre characterized by person-to-person transmission and environmental contamination. *Zentralbl Bakteriol* **281:**534-43.

6194. **Reidl, J., and K. E. Klose.** 2002. Vibrio cholerae and cholera: out of the water and into the host. *FEMS Microbiol Rev* **26:**125-39.

6195. **Reif, J. S., P. A. Webb, T. P. Monath, J. K. Emerson, J. D. Poland, G. E. Kemp, and G. Cholas.** 1987. Epizootic vesicular stomatitis in Colorado, 1982: infection in occupational risk groups. *Am J Trop Med Hyg* **36:**177-82.

6196. **Reij, M. W., and E. D. Den Aantrekker.** 2004. Recontamination as a source of pathogens in processed foods. *Int J Food Microbiol* **91:**1-11.

6197. **Reilly, S., T. A. I. Rees, and R. P. Thomas.** 1984. Fecal carriage of gastrointestinal protozoa and helminths in a home for educationally subnormal. *Commun Dis Rep* **84:**3-4.

6198. **Reindollar, R. W.** 1999. Hepatitis C and the correctional population. *Am J Med* **107 suppl 6B:**100S-103S.

6199. **Reinert, J. F., R. E. Harbach, and I. J. Kitching.** 2004. Phylogeny and classification of Aedini (Diptera:Culicidae), based on morphological characters of all life stages. *Zool J Linn Soc* **142**:289-368.

6200. **Reinthaler, F. F., F. Mascher, and D. Stunzner.** 1988. Serological examinations for antibodies against Legionella species in dental personnel. *J Dent Res* **67**:942-3.

6201. **Reintjes, R., A. Bosman, O. De Zwart, M. Stevens, L. van der Knaap, and K. van den Hoek.** 1999. Outbreak of hepatitis A in Rotterdam associated with visits to 'darkrooms? in gay bars. *Commun Dis Public Health* **2**:43-6.

6202. **Reintjes, R., I. Dedushaj, A. Gjini, T. R. Jorgensen, B. Cotter, A. Lieftucht, F. D'Ancona, D. T. Dennis, M. A. Kosoy, G. Mulliqi-Osmani, R. Grunow, A. Kalaveshi, L. Gashi, and I. Humolli.** 2002. Tularemia outbreak investigation in Kosovo: case control and environmental studies. *Emerg Infect Dis* **8**:69-73.

6203. **Reisberg, B. E., R. Wurtz, D. P., B. Francis, P. Zakowski, S. Fannin, D. Sesline, S. Waterman, R. Sanderson, T. McChesney, R. Boddie, g. Miller, and G. A. Herrera.** 1997. Outbreak of leptospirosis among white-water rafters - Costa Rica, 1996. *MMWR* **46**:577-9.

6204. **Reisen, W. K., and R. E. Chiles.** 1997. Prevalence of antibodies to western equine encephalomyelitis and St. Louis encephalitis viruses in residents of California exposed to sporadic and consistent enzootic transmission. *Am J Trop Med Hyg* **57**:526-9.

6205. **Reisen, W. K., H. D. Lothrop, and R. E. Chiles.** 1998. Ecology of Aedes dorsalis (Diptera: Culicidae) in relation to western equine encephalomyelitis virus in the Coachella Valley of California. *J Med Entomol* **35**:561-6.

6206. **Reisen, W. K., J. O. Lundstrom, T. W. Scott, B. F. Eldridge, R. E. Chiles, R. Cusack, V. M. Martinez, H. D. Lothrop, D. Gutierrez, S. E. Wright, K. Boyce, and B. R. Hill.** 2000. Patterns of avian seroprevalence to western equine encephalomyelitis and Saint Louis encephalitis viruses in California, USA. *J Med Entomol* **37**:507-27.

6207. **Reiss, I., A. Borkhardt, R. Fussle, A. Sziegoleit, and L. Gortner.** 2000. Disinfectant contaminated with Klebsiella oxytoca as a source of sepsis in babies. *Lancet* **356**:310.

6208. **Reiter, P., S. Lathrop, M. Bunning, B. Biggerstaff, D. Singer, T. Tiwari, L. Baber, M. Amador, J. Thirion, J. Hayes, C. Seca, J. Mendez, B. Ramirez, J. Robinson, J. Rawlings, V. Vorndam, S. Waterman, D. Gubler, G. Clark, and E. Hayes.** 2003. Texas lifestyle limits transmission of dengue virus. *Emerg Infect Dis* **9**:86-9.

6209. **Reithinger, R., and C. R. Davies.** 1999. Is the domestic dog (Canis familiaris) a reservoir host of American cutaneous leishmaniasis? A critical review of the current evidence. *Am J Trop Med Hyg* **61**:530-41.

6210. **Reithinger, R., J. C. Espinoza, A. Llanos-Cuentas, and C. R. Davies.** 2003. Domestic dog ownership: a risk factor for human infection with Leishmania (Viannia) species. *Trans R Soc Trop Med Hyg* **97**:141-5.

6211. **Rekart, M. L., D. M. Patrick, B. Chakraborty, J. J. Maginley, H. D. Jones, C. D. Bajdik, B. Pourbohloul, and R. C. Brunham.** 2003. Targeted mass treatment for syphilis with oral azithromycin. *Lancet* **361**:313-4.

6212. **Reller, M. E., C. E. Mendoza, M. B. Lopez, M. Alvarez, R. M. Hoekstra, C. A. Olson, K. G. Baier, B. H. Keswick, and S. P. Luby.** 2003. A randomized controlled trial of household-based flocculant-disinfectant drinking water treatment for diarrhea prevention in rural Guatemala. *Am J Trop Med Hyg* **69**:411-9.

6213. **Reller, M. E., S. J. Olsen, A. B. Kressel, T. D. Moon, K. A. Kubota, M. P. Adcock, S. F. Nowicki, and E. D. Mintz.** 2003. Sexual transmission of typhoid fever: a multistate outbreak among men who have sex with men. *Clin Infect Dis* **37**:141-4.

6214. **Remington, J. S., and J. O. Klein.** 2001. Infectious diseases of the fetus and newborn infant. W.B. Saunders Company, Philadelphia.

6215. **Remington, J. S., P. Thulliez, and J. G. Montoya.** 2004. Minireview. Recent developments for diagnosis of toxoplasmosis. *J Clin Microbiol* **42**:941-5.

6216. **Remington, P. L., T. Shope, and J. Andrews.** 1985. A recommended approach to the evaluation of human rabies exposure in an acute-care hospital. *JAMA* **254**:67-9.

6217. **Renault, P.** 1998. Meningococcal disease in holiday settings: summer 1998. *Eurosurveillance Weekly* **2**:2-3.

6218. **Rendi-Wagner, P.** 2004. Risk and prevention of tick-borne encephalitis in travelers. *J Travel Med* **11**:307-12.

6219. **Rendtorff, R. C.** 1954. The experimental transmission of human intestinal protozoan parasites. II. Giardia lamblia cysts given in capsules. *Am J Hyg* **59**:209-20.

6220. **Renoult, E., E. Georges, M. F. Biava, C. Hulin, L. Frimat, D. Hestin, and M. Kessler.** 1997. Toxoplasmosis in kidney transplant recipients: report of six cases and review. *Clin Infect Dis* **24**:625-34.

6221. **Renston, J. P., J. Morgan, and A. F. DiMarco.** 1992. Disseminated miliary blastomycosis leading to acute respiratory failure in an urban setting. *Chest* **101**:1463-5.

6222. **Rentier, B., and A. A. Gershon.** 2004. Consensus: varicella vaccination of healthy children—a challenge for Europe. *Pediatr Infect Dis J* **23**:379-89.

6223. **Renukaradhya, G. J., S. Isloor, and M. Rajasekhar.** 2002. Epidemiology, zoonotic aspects, vaccination and control/eradication of brucellosis in India. *Vet Microbiol* **90**:183-95.

6224. **Renzi, C., J. M. Douglas, Jr., M. Foster, C. W. Critchlow, R. Ashley-Morrow, S. P. Buchbinder, B. A. Koblin, D. J. McKirnan, K. H. Mayer, and C. L. Celum.** 2003. Herpes simplex virus type 2 infection as a risk factor for human immunodeficiency virus acquisition in men who have sex with men. *J Infect Dis* **187**:19-25.

6225. **Repina, L. P., A. I. Nikulina, and I. A. Kosilov.** 1993. [A case of human infection with brucellosis from a cat]. *Zh Mikrobiol Epidemiol Immunobiol*:66-8.

6226. **Repiso Ortega, A., M. Alcantara Torres, C. Gonzalez de Frutos, T. de Artaza Varasa, R. Rodriguez Merlo, J. Valle Munoz, and J. L. Martinez Potenciano.** 2003. [Gastrointestinal anisakiasis. Study of a series of 25 patients]. *Gastroenterol Hepatol* **26**:341-6.

6227. **Respaldiza, N., F. J. Medrano, A. C. Medrano, J. M. Varela, C. de la Horra, M. Montes-Cano, S. Ferrer, I. Wichmann, D. Gargallo-Viola, and E. J. Calderon.** 2004. High seroprevalence of Pneumocystis infection in Spanish children. *Clin Microbiol Infect* **10**:1029-31.

6228. **Resti, M., C. Azzari, L. Lega, M. E. Rossi, E. Zammarchi, E. Novembre, and A. Vierucci.** 1995. Mother-to-infant transmission of hepatitis C virus. *Acta Paediatr* **84**:251-5.

6229. **Restrepo, A., J. G. McEwen, and E. Castaneda.** 2001. The habitat of Paracoccidioides brasiliensis: how far from solving the riddle? *Med Mycol* **39**:233-41.

6230. Réthy, L., and L. A. Réthy. 1997. Human lethal dose of tetanus toxin. *Lancet* **350**:1518.

6231. Reves, R. R., A. L. Morrow, A. V. Bartlett, 3rd, C. J. Caruso, R. L. Plumb, B. T. Lu, and L. K. Pickering. 1993. Child day care increases the risk of clinic visits for acute diarrhea and diarrhea due to rotavirus. *Am J Epidemiol* **137**:97-107.

6232. Rey, J. L., M. Meyran, and P. Saliou. 1982. Situation épidémiologique de charbon humain en Haute Volta. *Bull Soc Pathol Exot* **75**:249-257.

6233. Reyburn, H., M. Rowland, M. Mohsen, B. Khan, and C. R. Davies. 2003. The prolonged epidemic of anthroponotic cutaneous leishmaniasis in Kabul, Afghanistan: 'bringing down the neighbourhood'. *Trans R Soc Trop Med Hyg* **97**:170-6.

6234. Reynolds, K. A., C. P. Gerba, M. Abbaszadegan, and L. L. Pepper. 2001. ICC/PCR detection of enteroviruses and hepatitis A virus in environmental samples. *Can J Microbiol* **47**:153-7.

6235. Reynolds, M. G., J. W. Krebs, J. A. Comer, J. W. Sumner, T. C. Rushton, C. E. Lopez, W. L. Nicholson, J. A. Rooney, S. E. Lance-Parker, J. H. McQuiston, C. D. Paddock, and J. E. Childs. 2003. Flying squirrel-associated typhus, United States. *Emerg Infect Dis* **9**:1341-3.

6236. Rezza, G., R. T. Danaya, T. M. Wagner, L. Sarmati, and I. L. Owen. 2001. Human herpesvirus-8 and othr viral infections, Papua New Guinea. *Emerg Infect Dis* **7**:893-895.

6237. Riarte, A., C. Luna, R. Sabatiello, A. Sinagra, R. Schiavelli, A. De Rissio, E. Maiolo, M. M. Garcia, N. Jacob, M. Pattin, M. Lauricella, E. L. Segura, and M. Vazquez. 1999. Chagas' disease in patients with kidney transplants: 7 years of experience 1989-1996. *Clin Infect Dis* **29**:561-7.

6238. Ribes, J. A., C. L. Vanover-Sams, and D. J. Baker. 2000. Zygomycetes in human disease. *Clin Microbiol Rev* **13**:236-301.

6239. Rice, P. S., and B. J. Cohen. 1996. A school outbreak of parvovirus B19 infection investigated using salivary antibody assays. *Epidemiol Infect* **116**:331-8.

6240. Rice, R. J., P. L. Roberts, H. H. Handsfield, and K. Holmes. 1991. Sociodemographic distribution of gonorrhea incidence: implications for prevention and behavioral research. *Am J Public Health* **81**:1252-1258.

6241. Rich, J. D., B. P. Dickinson, A. B. Flaxman, and E. Mylonakis. 1999. Local spread of molluscum contagiosum by electrolysis. *Clin Infect Dis* **28**:1171.

6242. Rich, J. D., J. C. Hou, A. Charuvastra, C. W. Towe, M. Lally, A. Spaulding, U. Bandy, E. F. Donnelly, and A. Rompalo. 2001. Risk factors for syphilis among incarcerated women in Rhode Island. *AIDS Patient Care STDS* **15**:581-5.

6243. Richard, J. L., M. Zwahlen, M. Feuz, and H. C. Matter. 2003. Comparison of the effectiveness of two mumps vaccines during an outbreak in Switzerland in 1999 and 2000: a case-cohort study. *Eur J Epidemiol* **18**:569-77.

6244. Richard, M., A. G. Biacabe, A. Perret-Liaudet, L. McCardle, J. W. Ironside, and N. Kopp. 1999. Protection of personnel and environment against Creutzfeldt-Jakob disease in pathology laboratories. *Clin Exp Pathol* **47**:192-200.

6245. Richard-Yegres, N., F. Yegres, and G. Zeppenfeldt. 1992. Cromomicosis: endemia rural, laboral y familiar en Venezuela. *Rev Iberoam Micol* **9**:38-41.

6246. Richards, A. L., D. W. Soeatmadji, M. A. Widodo, T. W. Sardjono, B. Yanuwiadi, T. E. Hernowati, A. D. Baskoro, Roebiyoso, L. Hakim, M. Soendoro, E. Rahardjo, M. P. Putri, J. M. Saragih, D. Strickman, D. J. Kelly, G. A. Dasch, J. G. Olson, C. J. Church, and A. L. Corwin. 1997. Seroepidemiologic evidence for murine and scrub typhus in Malang, Indonesia. *Am J Trop Med Hyg* **57**:91-5.

6247. Richards, F. O., Jr., B. Boatin, M. Sauerbrey, and A. Seketeli. 2001. Control of onchocerciasis today: status and challenges. *Trends Parasitol* **17**:558-63.

6248. Richards, M. J., J. R. Edwards, D. H. Culver, and R. P. Gaynes. 1999. Nosocomial infections in medical intensive care units in the United States. National Nosocomial Infections Surveillance System. *Crit Care Med* **27**:887-92.

6249. Richards, M. J., J. R. Edwards, D. H. Culver, and R. P. Gaynes. 1999. Nosocomial infections in pediatric intensive care units in the United States. National Nosocomial Infections Surveillance System. *Pediatrics* **103**:e39.

6250. Richards, M. J., J. R. Edwards, D. H. Culver, and R. P. Gaynes. 2000. Nosocomial infections in combined medical-surgical intensive care units in the United States. *Infect Control Hosp Epidemiol* **21**:510-5.

6251. Richards, M. S., M. Rittman, T. T. Gilbert, S. M. Opal, B. A. DeBuono, R. J. Neill, and P. Gemski. 1993. Investigation of a staphylococcal food poisoning outbreak in a centralized school lunch program. *Public Health Rep* **108**:765-71.

6252. Richardson, M., D. Elliman, H. Maguire, J. A. Simpson, and A. Nicoll. 2001. Evidence base of incubation periods, periods of infectiousness and exclusion policies for the control of communicable diseases in schools and preschools. *Pediatr Infect Dis J* **20**:380-391.

6253. Richen, D., and P. Lundrie. 1983. Epidemic of shigellosis - Alberta. *Can Dis Weekly Rep* **9**:65-7.

6254. Richet, H., P. Roux, and C. Des Champs. 2002. Candidemia in French hospitals: incidence rates and characteristics. *Clin Microbiol Inf* **8**:405-12.

6255. Richie, E., N. H. Punjabi, A. Corwin, M. Lesmana, I. Rogayah, C. Lebron, P. Echeverria, and C. H. Simanjuntak. 1997. Enterotoxigenic Escherichia coli diarrhea among young children in Jakarta, Indonesia. *Am J Trop Med Hyg* **57**:85-90.

6256. Richmond, J. K., and D. J. Baglole. 2003. Lassa fever: epidemiology, clinical features, and social consequences. *BMJ* **327**:1271-5.

6257. Richt, J. A., I. Pfeuffer, M. Christ, K. Frese, K. Bechter, and S. Herzog. 1997. Borna disease virus infection in animals and humans. *Emerg Infect Dis* **3**:343-52.

6258. Richter, D., D. B. Schlee, and F. R. Matuschka. 2003. Relapsing fever-like spirochetes infecting European vector tick of Lyme disease agent. *Emerg Infect Dis* **9**:697-701.

6259. Richter, D., A. Spielman, N. Komar, and F. R. Matuschka. 2000. Competence of American robins as reservoir hosts for Lyme disease spirochetes. *Emerg Infect Dis* **6**:133-8.

6260. Richter, J., P. E. Fournier, J. Petridou, D. Haussinger, and D. Raoult. 2002. Rickettsia felis infection acquired in Europe and documented by polymerase chain reaction. *Emerg Infect Dis* **8**:207-8.

6261. Rickard, M. D., and A. J. Adolph. 1977. The prevalence of cysticerci of Taenia saginata in cattle reared on sewage-irrigated pasture. *Med J Aust* **1**:525-7.

6262. Ricketts, K., and C. Joseph. 2004. Travel Associated Legionnaires' Disease in Europe : 2003. *Eur Surveill* **9**(10):40–43.

6263. **Ridder, G. J., C. C. Boedeker, K. Technau-Ihling, R. Grunow, and A. Sander.** 2002. Role of cat-scratch disease in lymphadenopathy in the head and neck. *Clin Infect Dis* **35**:643-9.

6264. **Ridgway, E. J., C. H. Tremlett, and K. D. Allen.** 1995. Capsular serotypes and antibiotic sensitivity of Streptococcus pneumoniae isolated from primary-school children. *J Infect* **30**:245-51.

6265. **Ridzon, R., J. H. Kent, S. Valway, P. Weismuller, R. Maxwell, M. Elcock, J. Meador, S. Royce, A. Shefer, P. Smith, C. Woodley, and I. Onorato.** 1997. Outbreak of drug-resistant tuberculosis with second-generation transmission in a high school in California. *J Pediatr* **131**:863-8.

6266. **Rieder, H. L.** 2001. Risk of travel-associated tuberculosis. *Clin Infect Dis* **33**:1393-6.

6267. **Riedo, F. X., R. W. Pinner, and M. de Lourdes.** 1994. A point-source foodborne listeriosis outbreak: documented incubation period and possible mild illness. *J Infect Dis* **170**:693-6.

6268. **Rieger, M. A., M. Nübling, R. M. Kaiser, F. W. Tiller, and F. Hofmann.** 1998. FSME-Infektionen durch Rohmilch - welche Rolle spielt dieser Infektionsweg? Untersuchungen aus dem südwestdeutschen FSME-Endemiegebiet. *Gesundheitswesen* **60**:348-56.

6269. **Ries, A. A., D. J. Vugia, L. Beingolea, A. M. Palacios, E. Vasquez, J. G. Wells, N. Garcia Baca, D. L. Swerdlow, M. Pollack, and N. H. Bean.** 1992. Cholera in Piura, Peru: a modern urban epidemic. *J Infect Dis* **166**:1429-33.

6270. **Rigau-Perez, J. G., D. J. Gubler, A. V. Vorndam, and G. G. Clark.** 1997. Dengue: A Literature Review and Case Study of Travelers from the United States, 1986-1994. *J Travel Med* **4**:65-71.

6271. **Rigau-Perez, J. G., A. V. Vorndam, and G. G. Clark.** 2001. The dengue and dengue hemorrhagic fever epidemic in Puerto Rico, 1994- 1995. *Am J Trop Med Hyg* **64**:67-74.

6272. **Rijnders, B. J., E. Van Wijngaerden, A. Wilmer, and W. E. Peetermans.** 2003. Use of full sterile barrier precautions during insertion of arterial catheters: a randomized trial. *Clin Infect Dis* **36**:743-8.

6273. **Rijpkema, S. G., R. G. Herbes, N. Verbeek-De Kruif, and J. F. Schellekens.** 1996. Detection of four species of Borrelia burgdorferi sensu lato in Ixodes ricinus ticks collected from roe deer (Capreolus capreolus) in The Netherlands. *Epidemiol Infect* **117**:563-6.

6274. **Riley, E. C., G. Murphy, and R. L. Riley.** 1978. Airborne spread of measles in a suburban elementary school. *Am J Epidemiol* **107**:421-32.

6275. **Riley, L. W., R. S. Remis, S. D. Helgerson, H. B. McGee, J. G. Wells, B. R. Davis, R. J. Hebert, E. S. Olcott, L. M. Johnson, N. T. Hargrett, P. A. Blake, and M. L. Cohen.** 1983. Hemorrhagic colitis associated with a rare Escherichia coli serotype. *N Engl J Med* **308**:681-5.

6276. **Riley, T. V.** 2004. Nosocomial diarrhoea due to Clostridium difficile. *Curr Opin Infect Dis* **17**:323-7.

6277. **Riley, T. V., M. Cooper, B. Bell, and C. L. Golledge.** 1995. Community-acquired Clostridium difficile-associated diarrhea. *Clin Infect Dis* **20 Suppl 2**:S263-5.

6278. **Ringot, D., J. P. Durand, H. Tolou, J. P. Boutin, and B. Davoust.** 2004. Rift valley fever in Chad. *Emerg Infect Dis* **10**:945-7.

6279. **Rinne, S., E. J. Rodas, R. Galer-Unti, N. Glickman, and L. T. Glickman.** 2005. Prevalence and risk factors for protozoan and nematode infections among children in an Ecuadorian highland community. *Trans R Soc Trop Med Hyg* **99**:585-92.

6280. **Riordan, T., K. Cartwright, N. Andrews, J. Stuart, A. Burris, A. Fox, R. Borrow, T. Douglas-Riley, J. Gabb, and A. Miller.** 1998. Acquisition and carriage of meningococci in marine commando recruits. *Epidemiol Infect* **121**:495-505.

6281. **Riordan, T., T. J. Humphrey, and A. Fowles.** 1993. A point source outbreak of campylobacter infection related to bird-pecked milk. *Epidemiol Infect* **110**:261-5.

6282. **Ripert, C.** 2003. [Schistosomiasis due to Schistosoma intercalatum and urbanization in central Africa]. *Bull Soc Pathol Exot* **96**:183-6.

6283. **Ripert, C. L., and C. P. Raccurt.** 1987. The impact of small dams on parasitic diseases in Cameroon. *Parasitol Today* **3**:287-9.

6284. **Ripoll, C. M., C. E. Remondegui, G. Ordonez, R. razamendi, H. Fusaro, M. J. Hyman, C. D. Paddock, S. R. Zaki, J. G. Olson, and C. A. Santos-Buch.** 1999. Evidence of rickettsial spotted fever and Ehrlichial infections in a subtropical territory of Jujuy, Argentina. *Am J Trop Med Hyg* **61**:350–4.

6285. **Risser, D., A. Uhl, M. Stichenwirth, S. Honigschnabl, W. Hirz, B. Schneider, C. Stellwag-Carion, N. Klupp, W. Vycudilik, and G. Bauer.** 2000. Quality of heroin and heroin-related deaths from 1987 to 1995 in Vienna, Austria. *Addiction* **95**:375-82.

6286. **Ritacco, V., M. Di Lonardo, A. Reniero, M. Ambroggi, L. Barrera, A. Dambrosi, B. Lopez, N. Isola, and I. N. de Kantor.** 1997. Nosocomial spread of human immunodeficiency virus-related multidrug- resistant tuberculosis in Buenos Aires. *J Infect Dis* **176**:637-42.

6287. **Ritchie, S. A., J. N. Hanna, S. L. Hills, J. P. Piispanen, W. J. H. McBride, A. Pyke, and R. L. Spark.** 2002. Dengue control in North Queensland, Australia: case recognition and selective indoor residual spraying. *Dengue Bull* **26**:7-13.

6288. **Rivas, F., L. A. Diaz, V. M. Cardenas, E. Daza, L. Bruzon, A. Alcala, O. De la Hoz, F. M. Caceres, G. Aristizabal, J. W. Martinez, D. Revelo, F. De la Hoz, J. Boshell, T. Camacho, L. Calderon, V. A. Olano, L. I. Villarreal, D. Roselli, G. Alvarez, G. Ludwig, and T. Tsai.** 1997. Epidemic Venezuelan equine encephalitis in La Guajira, Colombia, 1995. *J Infect Dis* **175**:828-32.

6289. **Rivas, M., M. Gracia Caletti, I. Chinen, S. M. Refi, C. D. Roldan, G. Chillemi, G. Fiorilli, A. Bertolotti, L. Aguerre, and S. S. Estani.** 2003. Home-prepared hamburger and sporadic hemolytic uremic syndrome, Argentina. *Emerg Infect Dis* **9**:1184-6.

6290. **Rizzo, F., N. Morandi, G. Riccio, G. Ghiazza, and P. Garavelli.** 1989. Unusual transmission of falciparum malaria in Italy. *Lancet* **1**:555-6.

6291. **Rizzo, G., and D. De Vito.** 2003. [Typhoid fever and environmental contamination in Apulia Region, Italy]. *Ann Ig* **15**:487-92.

6292. **RKI.** 1997. Fallbericht: Botulismus nach Verzehr von Räucherfleisch. *Epidemiol Bull* **25**:167-9.

6293. **RKI.** 1997. Q-Fieber-Ausbruch durch eine infizierte Damwildherde. *Epidemiol Bull* **36**:249-50.

6294. **RKI.** 1997. Q-Fieber-Ausbruch, ausgehend von einer Lehrund Forschungsstation für Tierzucht in Hessen. *Epidemiol Bull* **49**:347-9.

6295. **RKI.** 1998. Hepatitis-A-Ausbruch in Nordbayern. *Epidemiol Bull* **30**:213-5.

6296. **RKI.** 1998. Ornithose-Erkrankungen im Zusammenhang mit Jungenten-Handel. Erfahrungen bei der Aufklärung eines Ausbruches in Sachsen-Anhalt. *Epidemiol Bull* **38**.

6297. **RKI.** 1998. Shigellose-Ausbruch in einem Zeltlager. *Epidemiol Bull* **39 (2 oct)**:277.

6298. **RKI.** 1999. Fallbericht: Reise-assoziierte Legionella-Pneumonie. *Epidemiol Bull* **25**:187-9.

6299. **RKI.** 1999. Risikoabschätzung für Kontaktpersonen bei Verdacht auf VHF. Erfahrungen aus dem Land Brandenburg. *Epidemiol Bull* **33**:243-5.

6300. **RKI.** 1999. Zur Airport-Malaria und Baggage-Malaria. *Epidemiol Bull* **37**:274.

6301. **RKI.** 2000. Campylobacter-Enteritis nach Genuss von Rohmilch. Regelungen der Milchverordnung werden immer wieder missachtet. *Epidemiol Bull* **26**:207-9.

6302. **RKI.** 2000. Gastroenteritis-Ausbruch durch Clostridium perfringens. *Epidemiol Bull* **41**:327-9.

6303. **RKI.** 2000. Ratgeber Infektionskrankheiten. 14. Folge: Listeriose. *Epidemiol Bull* **16**:127-30.

6304. **RKI.** 2000. Rückfallfieber - selten, aber ernst zu nehmen. *Epidemiol Bull* **44**:349-52.

6305. **RKI.** 2001. Fallbericht: Look-back-Untersuchung bei 2'285 Patientinnen nach einer in einem Krankenhaus erworbenen HCV-Infektion. *Epidemiol Bull* **10**:71-3.

6306. **RKI.** 2001. Hepatitis A bei Urlaubern in einer Ferienanlage auf Ibiza. *Epidemiol Bull* **50**:381-2.

6307. **RKI.** 2002. Anforderungen an die Hygiene bei der Aufbereitung flexibler Endoskope und endoskopischen Zusatzinstrumenten. *Bundesgesundheitsblatt* **45**:395-411.

6308. **RKI.** 2002. Aufklärung eines Q-Fieber-Ausbruchs durch Erkrankungen in einem Film-Team. *Epidemiol Bull* **37**:316-7.

6309. **RKI.** 2002. Ausbruchmanagement und strukturiertes Vorgehen bei gehäuftem Auftreten nosokomialer Infektionen. *Bundesgesundheitsblatt* **45**:180-6.

6310. **RKI.** 2002. Empfehlungen zur HIV-Postexpositionsprophylaxe. *Epidemiol Bull* **30**:256-8.

6311. **RKI.** 2002. Massnahmen der Postexpositionsprophylaxe. *Epidemiol Bull* **30**:253-5.

6312. **RKI.** 2002. Salmonella Oranienburg in Schokolade: Internationaler Ausbruch von Oktober bis Dezember 2001. *Epidemiol Bull* **18 Jan**:17-20.

6313. **RKI.** 2002. Tularämie - zwei Erkrankungen nach Verarbeiten und Verzehr eines Wildhasen. *Epidemiol Bull* **9**:71-2.

6314. **RKI.** 2004. Erkrankungen an Hepatitis A und Hepatitis E in den Jahren 2001 bis 2003. *Epidemiol Bull* **33**:269-72.

6315. **RKI.** 2004. Erkrankungen an Lyme-Borreliose in den sechs östlichen Bundesländern in den Jahren 2002 und 2003. *Epidemiol Bull* **28**:219-22.

6316. **RKI.** 2004. Fallbericht: Wahrscheinliche West-Nil-Virus-Erkrankung - dritter importierter Fall in Deutschland. *Epidemiol Bull* **48**:417.

6317. **RKI.** 2004. Reiseassoziierte Infektionskrankheiten im Jahr 2003. *Epidemiol Bull* **38**:319-26.

6318. **RKI.** 2004. Surveillance nosokomialer Infektionen in Intensivstationen. *Epidemiol Bull* **41**:349-51.

6319. **RKI.** 2004. Tollwut - ein Erkrankungsfall nach Indienaufenthalt. *Epidemiol Bull* **42**:362-3.

6320. **RKI.** 2004. Zu einem lebensmittelassoziierten Hepatitis-A-Ausbruch im südlichen Nordrhein-Westfalen und nördlichen Rheinland-Pfalz im März/April 2004. *Epidemiol Bull* **33**:274-5.

6321. **Roach, R. L., and D. G. Sienko.** 1992. Clostridium perfringens outbreak associated with minestrone soup. *Am J Epidemiol* **136**:1288-91.

6322. **Robain, M., N. Carre, E. Dussaix, D. Salmon-Ceron, and L. Meyer.** 1998. Incidence and sexual risk factors of cytomegalovirus seroconversion in HIV-infected subjects. The SEROCO Study Group. *Sex Transm Dis* **25**:476-80.

6323. **Robays, J., A. Ebeja Kadima, P. Lutumba, C. Miaka mia Bilenge, V. Kande Betu Ku Mesu, R. De Deken, J. Makabuza, M. Deguerry, P. Van der Stuyft, and M. Boelaert.** 2004. Human African trypanosomiasis amongst urban residents in Kinshasa: a case-control study. *Trop Med Int Health* **9**:869-75.

6324. **Roberson, J. R., L. K. Fox, D. D. Hancock, J. M. Gay, and T. E. Besser.** 1994. Ecology of Staphylococcus aureus isolated from various sites on dairy farms. *J Dairy Sci* **77**:3354-64.

6325. **Robert, V., M. Lhuillier, D. Meunier, J. L. Sarthou, N. Monteny, J. P. Digoutte, M. Cornet, M. Germain, and R. Cordellier.** 1993. Virus amaril, dengue 2 et autres arbovirus isolés de moustiques, au Burkina Faso, de 1983 à 1986. Considérations entomologiques et épidémiologiques. *Bull Soc Pathol Exot* **86**:90-100.

6326. **Robert, V., K. Macintyre, J. Keating, J. F. Trape, J. B. Duchemin, M. Warren, and J. C. Beier.** 2003. Malaria transmission in urban sub-Saharan Africa. *Am J Trop Med Hyg* **68**:169-76.

6327. **Roberts, D. R., S. Manguin, and J. Mouchet.** 2000. DDT house spraying and re-emerging malaria. *Lancet* **356**:330-2.

6328. **Roberts, J. A., P. N. Sockett, and O. N. Gill.** 1989. Economic impact of a nationwide outbreak of salmonellosis: cost-benefit of early intervention. *BMJ* **298**:1227-30.

6329. **Roberts, R. J.** 2002. Head lice. *N Engl J Med* **346**:1645-50.

6330. **Roberts, S. A., T. McClelland, and S. D. Lang.** 2000. Queensland tick typhus infection acquired whilst on holiday in Queensland. *N Z Med J* **113**:343.

6331. **Robertson, B., M. I. Sinclair, A. B. Forbes, M. Veitch, M. Kirk, D. Cunliffe, J. Willis, and C. K. Fairley.** 2002. Case-control studies of sporadic cryptosporidiosis in Melbourne and Adelaide, Australia. *Epidemiol Infect* **128**:419-31.

6332. **Robertson, I. D., and D. K. Blackmore.** 1989. Occupational exposure to Streptococcus suis type 2. *Epidemiol Infect* **103**:157-64.

6333. **Robertson, J. N., J. S. Gray, and P. Stewart.** 2000. Tick bite and Lyme borreliosis risk at a recreational site in England. *Eur J Epidemiol* **16**:647-52.

6334. **Robertson, L. J., and B. Gjerde.** 2001. Occurrence of parasites on fruits and vegetables in Norway. *J Food Prot* **64**:1793-8.

6335. **Robertson, S. E., B. P. Hull, O. Tomori, O. Bele, J. W. LeDuc, and K. Esteves.** 1996. Yellow fever. A decade of reemergence. *JAMA* **276**:1157-62.

6336. **Robertson, S. E., L. E. Markowitz, D. A. Berry, E. F. Dini, and W. A. Orenstein.** 1992. A million dollar measles outbreak: epidemiology, risk factors, and a selective revaccination strategy. *Public Health Rep* **107**:24-31.

6337. **Robicsek, F., H. K. Daugherty, J. W. Cook, J. G. Selle, T. N. Masters, P. R. O'Bar, C. R. Fernandez, C. U. Mauney, and D. M. Calhoun.** 1978. Mycobacterium fortuitum epidemics after open-heart surgery. *J Thorac Cardiovasc Surg* **75**:91-6.

6338. **Robins-Browne, R. M.** 2004. Escherichia coli and community-acquired gastroenteritis, Melbourne, Australia. *Emerg Infect Dis* **10**:1797-805.

6339. **Robins-Browne, R. M., and E. L. Hartland.** 2002. Escherichia coli as a cause of diarrhea. *J Gastroenterol Hepatol* **17**:467-75.

6340. **Robinson, A. J., and G. V. Petersen.** 1983. Orf virus infection of workers in the meat industry. *N Z Med J* **96**:81-5.

6341. **Robinson, K. A., G. Rothrock, Q. Phan, B. Sayler, K. Stefonek, C. Van Beneden, and O. S. Levine.** 2003. Risk for severe group A streptococcal disease among patients' household contacts. *Emerg Infect Dis* **9**:443-7.

6342. **Robinson, L. G. E., F. L. Black, F. K. Lee, A. O. Sousa, M. Owens, D. Danielsson, A. J. Nahmias, and B. D. Gold.** 2002. Helicobacter pylori prevalence among indigenous peoples of South America. *J Infect Dis* **186**:1131-7.

6343. **Robinson, P., A. W. Jenney, M. Tachado, A. Yung, J. Manitta, K. Taylor, and B. A. Biggs.** 2001. Imported malaria treated in Melbourne, Australia: epidemiology and clinical features in 246 patients. *J Travel Med* **8**:76-81.

6344. **Robles Garcia, M., J. de la Lama Lopez-Areal, C. Avellaneda Martinez, R. Gimenez Garcia, B. Cortejoso Gonzalo, and J. L. Vaquero Puerta.** 2000. [Nosocomial scabies outbreak]. *Rev Clin Esp* **200**:538-42.

6345. **Robson, J. M. B., R. N. Wood, J. J. Sullivan, N. J. Nicolaides, and B. R. Lewis.** 1995. A probable foodborne outbreak of toxoplasmosis. *Commun Dis Intell* **19**:517-22.

6346. **Robson, S. C., S. Adams, N. Brink, B. Woodruff, and D. Bradley.** 1992. Hospital outbreak of hepatitis E. *Lancet* **339**:1424-5.

6347. **Roca, C., X. Balanzó, J. Gascón, J. L. Fernandez-Roure, T. Vinuesa, M. E. Valls, G. Sauca, and M. Corachan.** 2002. Comparative, clinico-epidemiologic study of Schistosoma mansoni infections in travelers and immigrants in Spain. *Eur J Clin Microbiol Infect Dis* **21**:219-23.

6348. **Roca, C., X. Balanzo, G. Sauca, J. L. Fernandez-Roure, R. Boixeda, and M. Ballester.** 2003. [Imported hookworm infection in African immigrants in Spain: study of 285 patients]. *Med Clin (Barc)* **121**:139-41.

6349. **Rocha, G., A. Verissimo, R. Bowker, N. Bornstein, and M. S. Da Costa.** 1995. Relationship between Legionella spp. and antibody titres at a therapeutic thermal spa in Portugal. *Epidemiol Infect* **115**:79-88.

6350. **Roche, P., L. Halliday, E. O'Brien, and J. Spencer.** 2002. The laboratory virology and serology reporting scheme, 1991 to 2000. *Commun Dis Intell* **26**:323-74.

6351. **Roche, P., and V. Krause.** 2002. Invasive pneumococcal disease in Australia, 2001. *Commun Dis Intell* **26**:505-19.

6352. **Roche, P., A. Merianos, R. Antic, J. Carnie, A. Christensen, J. Waring, A. Konstantinos, V. Krause, M. Hurwitz, A. V. Misrachi, and I. Bastian.** 2001. Tuberculosis notifications in Australia, 1999. *Commun Dis Intell* **25**:254-60.

6353. **Rockx, B., M. de Wit, H. Vennema, J. Vinje, E. De Bruin, Y. Van Duynhoven, and M. Koopmans.** 2002. Natural history of human calicivirus infection: a prospective cohort study. *Clin Infect Dis* **35**:246-53.

6354. **Rocourt, J., and J. Bille.** 1997. Foodborne listeriosis. *World Health Stat Q* **50**:67-73.

6355. **Rocourt, J., C. Jacquet, and A. Reilly.** 2000. Epidemiology of human listeriosis and seafoods. *Int J Food Microbiol* **62**:197-209.

6356. **Rocourt, J., G. Moy, K. Vierk, and J. Schlundt.** 2003. The present state of foodborne disease in OECD countries. WHO, Food Safety Department, Geneva.

6357. **Rodgers, E., P. Masendycz, H. Bugg, and R. Bishop.** 1996. An outbreak of severe gastroenteritis caused by rotavirus in the Solomon islands. *Commun Dis Intell* **20**:352-4.

6358. **Rodier, G. R., B. Couzineau, G. C. Gray, C. S. Omar, E. Fox, J. Bouloumie, and D. Watts.** 1993. Trends of human immunodeficiency virus type-1 infection in female prostitutes and males diagnosed with a sexually transmitted disease in Djibouti, east Africa. *Am J Trop Med Hyg* **48**:682-6.

6359. **Rodrigues, A., A. Sandstrom, T. Ca, H. Steinsland, H. Jensen, and P. Aaby.** 2000. Protection from cholera by adding lime juice to food - results from community and laboratory studies in Guinea-Bissau, West Africa. *Trop Med Int Health* **5**:418-22.

6360. **Rodrigues, L. C., J. M. Cowden, J. G. Wheeler, D. Sethi, P. G. Wall, P. Cumberland, D. S. Tompkins, M. J. Hudson, J. A. Roberts, and P. J. Roderick.** 2001. The study of infectious intestinal disease in England: risk factors for cases of infectious intestinal disease with Campylobacter jejuni infection. *Epidemiol Infect* **127**:185-93.

6361. **Rodriguez Calabuig, D., R. Igual Adell, C. Oltra Alcaraz, P. Sanchez Sanchez, M. Bustamante Balen, F. Parra Godoy, and E. Nagore Enguidanos.** 2001. [Agricultural occupation and strongyloidiasis. A case-control study]. *Rev Clin Esp* **201**:81-4.

6362. **Rodriguez, E., M. Gamboa Mdel, and P. Vargas.** 2002. [Clostridium perfringens in raw and cooked meats and its relation with the environment in Costa Rica]. *Arch Latinoam Nutr* **52**:155-9.

6363. **Rodriguez, J. C., A. Ayelo, M. Ruiz, M. Lopez, and G. Royo.** 2003. [Infection due to Mycobacterium kansasii in Elche, Spain]. *Med Clin (Barc)* **120**:253-4.

6364. **Rodriguez Valin, M. E., A. Pousa Ortega, C. Pons Sanchez, A. Larrosa Montanes, L. P. Sanchez Serrano, and F. Martinez Navarro.** 2001. [Brucellosis as occupational disease: study of an outbreak of air-born transmission at a slaughter house]. *Rev Esp Salud Publica* **75**:159-69.

6365. **Rodriguez-Baez, N., R. O'Brien, S. Q. Qiu, and D. M. Bass.** 2002. Astrovirus, adenovirus, and rotavirus in hospitalized children: prevalence and association with gastroenteritis. *J Pediatr Gastroenterol Nutr* **35**:64-8.

6366. **Rodriguez-Calleja, J. M., J. A. Santos, A. Otero, and M. L. Garcia-Lopez.** 2004. Microbiological quality of rabbit meat. *J Food Prot* **67**:966-71.

6367. **Rodriguez-Hernandez, J., A. Canut-Blasco, and A. M. Martin-Sanchez.** 1996. Seasonal prevalences of Cryptosporidium and Giardia infections in children attending day care centres in Salamanca (Spain) studied for a period of 15 months. *Eur J Epidemiol* **12**:291-5.

6368. **Rodriguez-Perez, M. A., R. Danis-Lozano, M. H. Rodriguez, and J. E. Bradley.** 1999. Comparison of serological and parasitological assessments of Onchocerca volvulus transmission after 7 years of mass ivermectin treatment in Mexico. *Trop Med Int Health* **4**:98-104.

6369. **Roeckel, I. E., and E. T. Lyons.** 1977. Cutaneous larva migrans, an occupational disease. *Ann Clin Lab Sci* **7**:405-10.

6370. **Roels, T. H., P. A. Frazak, J. J. Kazmierczak, W. R. Mackenzie, M. E. Proctor, T. A. Kurzynski, and J. P. Davis.** 1997. Incomplete sanitation of a meat grinder and ingestion of raw ground beef: contributing factors to a large outbreak of Salmonella typhimurium infection. *Epidemiol Infect* **119**:127-34.

6371. **Roels, T. H., B. Wickus, H. H. Bostrom, J. J. Kazmierczak, M. A. Nicholson, T. A. Kurzynski, and J. P. Davis.** 1998. A foodborne outbreak of Campylobacter jejuni (O:33) infection associated with tuna salad: a rare strain in an unusual vehicle. *Epidemiol Infect* **121**:281-7.

6372. **Rogstad, K. E.** 2004. Sex, sun, sea, and STIs: sexually transmitted infections acquired on holiday. *BMJ* **329**:214-7.

6373. **Rogues, A. M., J. Maugein, A. Allery, C. Fleureau, H. Boulestreau, S. Surcin, C. Bebear, G. Janvier, and J. P. Gachie.** 2001. Electronic ventilator temperature sensors as a potential source of respiratory tract colonization with Stenotrophomonas maltophilia. *J Hosp Infect* **49**:289-92.

6374. **Rohde, R. E., B. C. Mayes, J. S. Smith, and S. U. Neill.** 2004. Bat rabies, Texas, 1996-2000. *Emerg Infect Dis* **10**:948-52.

6375. **Rohela, M., I. JAMAiah, K. W. Chan, and W. S. Yusoff.** 2002. Diphyllobothriasis: the first case report from Malaysia. *Southeast Asian J Trop Med Public Health* **33**:229-30.

6376. **Rohner, P., I. Schnyder, B. Ninet, J. Schrenzel, D. Lew, T. Ramla, J. Garbino, and V. Jacomo.** 2004. Severe Mycoplasma hominis infections in two renal transplant patients. *Eur J Clin Microbiol Infect Dis* **23**:203-4.

6377. **Rojas de Arias, A., I. de Guillen, A. Inchausti, M. Samudio, and G. Schmeda-Hirschmann.** 1993. Prevalence of Chagas' disease in Ayoreo communities of the Paraguayan Chaco. *Trop Med Parasitol* **44**:285-8.

6378. **Rojas de Arias, A., E. A. Ferro, M. E. Ferreira, and L. C. Simancas.** 1999. Chagas disease vector control through different intervention modalities in endemic localities of Paraguay. *Bull WHO* **77**:331-9.

6379. **Rojas-Molina, N., S. Pedraza-Sanchez, B. Torres-Bibiano, H. Meza-Martinez, and A. Escobar-Gutierrez.** 1999. Gnathostomosis, an emerging foodborne zoonotic disease in Acapulco, Mexico. *Emerg Infect Dis* **5**:264-6.

6380. **Rojekittikhun, W., J. Waikagul, and T. Chaiyasith.** 2002. Fish as the natural second intermediate host of Gnathostoma spinigerum. *Southeast Asian J Trop Med Public Health* **33 suppl 2**:63-9.

6381. **Rolain, J. M., M. Jensenius, and D. Raoult.** 2004. Rickettsial infections—a threat to travellers? *Curr Opin Infect Dis* **17**:433-7.

6382. **Rolain, J. M., C. Locatelli, L. Chabanne, B. Davoust, and D. Raoult.** 2004. Prevalence of Bartonella clarridgeiae and Bartonella henselae in domestic cats from France and detection of the organisms in erythrocytes by immunofluorescence. *Clin Diagn Lab Immunol* **11**:423-5.

6383. **Rolland, R. M., G. Hausfater, B. Marshall, and S. B. Levy.** 1985. Antibiotic-resistant bacteria in wild primates: increased prevalence in baboons feeding on human refuse. *Appl Environ Microbiol* **49**:791-4.

6384. **Rollin, P. E., R. J. Williams, D. S. Bressler, S. Pearson, M. Cottingham, G. Pucak, A. Sanchez, S. G. Trappier, R. L. Peters, P. W. Greer, S. Zaki, T. Demarcus, K. Hendricks, M. Kelley, D. Simpson, T. W. Geisbert, P. B. Jahrling, C. J. Peters, and T. G. Ksiazek.** 1999. Ebola (subtype Reston) virus among quarantined nonhuman primates recently imported from the Philippines to the United States. *J Infect Dis* **179 Suppl 1**:S108-14.

6385. **Rollins, N. C., M. Dedicoat, S. Danaviah, T. Page, K. Bishop, I. Kleinschmidt, H. M. Coovadia, and S. A. Cassol.** 2002. Prevalence, incidence, and mother-to-child transmission of HIV-1 in rural South Africa. *Lancet* **360**:389-90.

6386. **Rollison, D. E., W. F. Page, H. Crawford, G. Gridley, S. Wacholder, J. Martin, R. Miller, and E. A. Engels.** 2004. Case-control study of cancer among US Army Veterans exposed to Simian virus 40-contaminated adenovirus vaccine. *Am J Epidemiol* **160**:317-24.

6387. **Romalde, J. L., I. Torrado, C. Ribao, and J. L. Barja.** 2001. Global market: shellfish imports as a source of reemerging food-borne hepatitis A virus infections in Spain. *Int Microbiol* **4**:223-6.

6388. **Roman, R. S., J. Smith, M. Walker, S. Byrne, K. Ramotar, B. Dyck, A. Kabani, and L. E. Nicolle.** 1997. Rapid geographic spread of a methicillin-resistant Staphylococcus aureus strain. *Clin Infect Dis* **25**:698-705.

6389. **Roman-Crossland, R., L. Forrester, and G. Zaniewski.** 2004. Sex differences in injecting practices and hepatitis C: a systematic review of the literature. *Can Commun Dis Rep* **30**:125-32.

6390. **Roman-Sanchez, P., A. Pastor-Guzman, S. Moreno-Guillen, R. Igual-Adell, S. Suner-Generoso, and C. Tornero-Estebanez.** 2003. High prevalence of Strongyloides stercoralis among farm workers on the Mediterranean coast of Spain: analysis of the predictive factors of infection in developed countries. *Am J Trop Med Hyg* **69**:336-40.

6391. **Romaña, C. A., D. Brunstein, A. Collin-Delavaud, O. Sousa, and E. Ortega-Barria.** 2003. Public policies of development in Latin America and Chagas' disease. *Lancet* **362**:579.

6392. **Romano, C., C. Gianni, and E. M. Difonzo.** 2005. Retrospective study of onychomycosis in Italy: 1985-2000. *Mycoses* **48**:42-4.

6393. **Rombo, L., E. Bengtsson, and M. Grandien.** 1978. Serum Q fever antibodies in Swedish UN soldiers in Cyprus - reflecting a domestic or foreign disease? *Scand J Infect Dis* **10**:157-8.

6394. **Romeu, J., J. Roig, J. L. Bada, C. Riera, and C. Munoz.** 1991. Adult human toxocariasis acquired by eating raw snails. *J Infect Dis* **164**:438.

6395. **Romi, R., G. Pontuale, M. G. Ciufolini, G. Fiorentini, A. Marchi, L. Nicoletti, M. Cocchi, and A. Tamburro.** 2004. Potential vectors of West Nile Virus following an equine disease outbreak in Italy. *Med Vet Entomol* **18**:14-9.

6396. **Romi, R., G. Sabatinelli, and G. Majori.** 2001. Could malaria reappear in Italy? *Emerg Infect Dis* **7**:915-9.

6397. **Romi, R., G. Sabatinelli, L. G. Savelli, M. Raris, M. Zago, and R. Malatesta.** 1997. Identification of a North American mosquito species, Aedes atropalpus (Diptera: Culicidae), in Italy. *J Am Mosq Control Assoc* **13**:245-6.

6398. **Ronghe, M. D., A. B. Foot, J. M. Cornish, C. G. Steward, D. Carrington, N. Goulden, D. I. Marks, and A. Oakhill.** 2002. The impact of transfusion of leucodepleted platelet concentrates on cytomegalovirus disease after allogeneic stem cell transplantation. *Br J Haematol* **118**:1124-7.

6399. **Ronveaux, O., S. Quoilin, F. Van Loock, P. Lheureux, M. Struelens, and J. P. Butzler.** 2000. A Campylobacter coli foodborne outbreak in Belgium. *Acta Clin Belg* **55**:307-11.

6400. Ronveaux, O., D. Vos, A. Bosman, K. Brandwijk, J. Vinjé, M. Koopmans, and R. Reintjes. 2000. An outbreak of Norwalk-like virus gastroenteritis in a nursing home in Rotterdam. *Eurosurveillance* **5**:54-7.

6401. Rooney, R. M., J. K. Bartram, E. H. Cramer, S. Mantha, G. Nichols, R. Suraj, and E. C. Todd. 2004. A review of outbreaks of waterborne disease associated with ships: evidence for risk management. *Public Health Rep* **119**:435-42.

6402. Rooney, R. M., E. H. Cramer, S. Mantha, G. Nichols, J. K. Bartram, J. M. Farber, and P. K. Benembarek. 2004. A review of outbreaks of foodborne disease associated with passenger ships: evidence for risk management. *Public Health Rep* **119**:427-34.

6403. Roos, B. 1956. [Hepatitis epidemic transmitted by oysters]. *Sven Lakartidn* **53**:989-1003.

6404. Rosci, M. A., M. G. Paglia, A. De Felici, G. Antonucci, O. Armignacco, A. Cardini, L. Rosci, and L. Savioli. 1987. A case of falciparum malaria acquired in Italy. *Trop Geogr Med* **39**:77-9.

6405. Rose, A. M. C., O. Vapalahti, O. Lyytikäinen, and P. Nuorti. 2003. Patterns of Puumala virus infection in Finland. *Eurosurveillance* **8**:9-13.

6406. Rosen, L., D. J. Gubler, and P. H. Bennett. 1981. Epidemic polyarthritis (Ross river) virus infection in the Cook islands. *Am J Trop Med Hyg* **30**:1294-1302.

6407. Rosenbaum, J. R., and K. A. Sepkowitz. 2002. Infectious disease experimentation involving human volunteers. *Clin Infect Dis* **34**:963-71.

6408. Rosenberg, M. L., J. P. Koplan, I. K. Wachsmuth, J. G. Wells, E. J. Gangarosa, R. L. Guerrant, and D. A. Sack. 1977. Epidemic diarrhea at Crater Lake from enterotoxigenic Escherichia coli. A large waterborne outbreak. *Ann Intern Med* **86**:714-8.

6409. Rosenberg, S. D., L. A. Goodman, F. C. Osher, M. S. Swartz, S. M. Essock, M. I. Butterfield, N. T. Constantine, G. L. Wolford, and M. P. Salyers. 2001. Prevalence of HIV, hepatitis B, and hepatitis C in people with severe mental illness. *Am J Public Health* **91**:31-7.

6410. Rosenberg, T., O. Kendall, J. Blanchard, S. Martel, C. Wakelin, and M. Fast. 1997. Shigellosis on Indian reserves in Manitoba, Canada: its relationship to crowded housing, lack of running water, and inadequate sewage disposal. *Am J Public Health* **87**:1547-51.

6411. Rosenblum, L. S., I. R. Mirkin, D. T. Allen, S. Safford, and S. C. Hadler. 1990. A multifocal outbreak of hepatitis A traced to commercially distributed lettuce. *Am J Public Health* **80**:1075-9.

6412. Rosenblum, L. S., M. E. Villarino, O. V. Nainan, M. E. Melish, S. C. Hadler, P. P. Pinsky, W. R. Jarvis, C. E. Ott, and H. S. Margolis. 1991. Hepatitis A outbreak in a neonatal intensive care unit: risk factors for transmission and evidence of prolonged viral excretion among preterm infants. *J Infect Dis* **164**:476-82.

6413. Rosenstein, N. E., K. W. Emery, S. B. Werner, A. Kao, R. Johnson, D. Rogers, D. Vugia, A. Reingold, R. Talbot, B. D. Plikaytis, B. A. Perkins, and R. A. Hajjeh. 2001. Risk factors for severe pulmonary and disseminated coccidioidomycosis: Kern County, California, 1995-1996. *Clin Infect Dis* **32**:708-15.

6414. Rosenstein, N. E., and B. Perkins. 2000. Update on Haemophilus influenzae b and meningococcal vaccines. *Pediatr Clin North Am* **47**:337-52.

6415. Rosenstein, N. E., B. A. Perkins, D. S. Stephens, T. Popovic, and J. M. Hughes. 2001. Meningococcal disease. *N Engl J Med* **344**:1378-88.

6416. Roshanravan, B., E. Kari, R. H. Gilman, L. Cabrera, E. Lee, J. Metcalfe, M. Calderon, A. G. Lescano, S. H. Montenegro, C. Calampa, and J. M. Vinetz. 2003. Endemic malaria in the Peruvian Amazon region of Iquitos. *Am J Trop Med Hyg* **69**:45-52.

6417. Ross, A. G., A. C. Sleigh, Y. Li, G. M. Davis, G. M. Williams, Z. Jiang, Z. Feng, and D. P. McManus. 2001. Schistosomiasis in the People's Republic of China: prospects and challenges for the 21st century. *Clin Microbiol Rev* **14**:270-95.

6418. Ross, D. J., N. M. Cherry, and J. C. McDonald. 1998. Occupationally acquired infectious disease in the United Kingdom: 1996 to 1997. *Commun Dis Publ Health* **1**:98-102.

6419. Ross, R. S., S. Viazov, T. Gross, F. Hofmann, H. M. Seipp, and M. Roggendorf. 2000. Transmission of hepatitis C virus from a patient to an anesthesiology assistant to five patients. *N Engl J Med* **343**:1851-4.

6420. Rossier, P., E. Urfer, A. Burnens, J. Bille, P. Francioli, F. Mean, and A. Zwahlen. 2000. Clinical features and analysis of the duration of colonisation during an outbreak of Salmonella braenderup gastroenteritis. *Schweiz Med Wochenschr* **130**:1185-91.

6421. Rossitto, P. V., L. Ruiz, Y. Kikuchi, K. Glenn, K. Luiz, J. L. Watts, and J. S. Cullor. 2002. Antibiotic susceptibility patterns for environmental streptococci isolated from bovine mastitis in central California dairies. *J Dairy Sci* **85**:132-8.

6422. Rotger, M., T. Serra, M. G. de Cardenas, A. Morey, and M. A. Vicente. 2004. Increasing incidence of imported schistosomiasis in Mallorca, Spain. *Eur J Clin Microbiol Infect Dis* **23**:855-6.

6423. Rothe, J., P. J. McDonald, and A. M. Johnson. 1985. Detection of Toxoplasma cysts and oocysts in an urban environment in a developed country. *Pathology* **17**:497-9.

6424. Rothenbacher, D., G. Bode, and H. Brenner. 2002. History of breastfeeding and Helicobacter pylori infection in preschool children: results of a population-based study from Germany. *Int J Epidemiol* **31**:632-7.

6425. Rothenbacher, D., M. Winkler, T. Gonser, G. Adler, and H. Brenner. 2002. Role of infected parents in transmission of helicobacter pylori to their children. *Pediatr Infect Dis J* **21**:674-9.

6426. Rotily, M., C. Vernay-Vaisse, M. Bourliere, A. Galinier-Pujol, S. Rousseau, and Y. Obadia. 1997. HBV and HIV screening, and hepatitis B immunization programme in the prison of Marseille, France. *Int J STD AIDS* **8**:753-9.

6427. Rotily, M., C. Weilandt, S. M. Bird, K. Käll, H. J. A. Van Haastrecht, E. Iandolo, and S. Rousseau. 2001. Surveillance of HIV infection and related risk behaviour in European prisons. A multicenter pilot study. *Eur J Public Health* **11**:243-250.

6428. Rotivel, Y., M. Goudal, H. Bourhy, and H. Tsiang. 2001. La rage des chiroptères en France. Actualités et importance en santé publique. *Bull Epidémiol Hebdomadaire* **39**:1-9.

6429. Rotz, L., L. Callejas, D. McKechnie, D. Wolfe, E. Gaw, L. Hathcock, and J. Childs. 1998. An epidemiologic and entomologic investigation of a cluster of Rocky Mountain spotted fever cases in Delaware. *Del Med J* **70**:285-91.

6430. **Roudot-Thoraval, F., A. Bastie, J. M. Pawlotsky, and D. Dhumeaux.** 1997. Epidemiological factors affecting the severity of hepatitis C virus-related liver disease: a French survey of 6,664 patients. The Study Group for the Prevalence and the Epidemiology of Hepatitis C Virus. *Hepatology* **26:**485-90.

6431. **Roumeliotou, A., A. Papachristopoulos, D. Alexiou, V. Papaevangelou, G. Stergiou, and G. Papaevangelou.** 1994. Intrafamilial clustering of hepatitis A. *Infection* **22:**96-8.

6432. **Round, A., M. R. Evans, R. L. Salmon, I. K. Hosein, A. K. Mukerjee, R. W. Smith, and S. R. Palmer.** 2001. Public health management of an outbreak of group C meningococcal disease in university campus residents. *Eur J Public Health* **11:**431-6.

6433. **Rousseau, M. C., M. F. Saron, P. Brouqui, and A. Bourgeade.** 1997. Lymphocytic choriomeningitis virus in southern France: four case reports and a review of the literature. *Eur J Epidemiol* **13:**817-23.

6434. **Roussere, G. P., W. J. Murray, C. B. Raudenbush, M. J. Kutilek, D. J. Levee, and K. R. Kazacos.** 2003. Raccoon roundworm eggs near homes and risk for larva migrans disease, California communities. *Emerg Infect Dis* **9:**1516-22.

6435. **Rousset, E., P. Russo, M. Pépin, and D. Raoult.** 2001. Epidémiologie de la fièvre Q animale. Situation en France. *Méd Mal Infect* **31 suppl 2:**233-246.

6436. **Rowbotham, T. J.** 1998. Legionellosis associated with ships: 1977 to 1997. *Commun Dis Public Health* **1:**146-51.

6437. **Rowe, B., N. T. Begg, D. N. Hutchinson, H. C. Dawkins, R. J. Gilbert, M. Jacob, B. H. Hales, F. A. Rae, and M. Jepson.** 1987. Salmonella ealing infections associated with consumption of infant dried milk. *Lancet* **2:**900-3.

6438. **Rowe, S. Y., J. R. Rocourt, B. Shiferaw, H. D. Kassenborg, S. D. Segler, R. Marcus, P. J. Daily, F. P. Hardnett, and L. Slutsker.** 2004. Breast-Feeding Decreases the Risk of Sporadic Salmonellosis among Infants in FoodNet Sites. *Clin Infect Dis* **38 Suppl 3:**S262-70.

6439. **Rowland, M.** 2001. Refugee health in the tropics. Malaria control in Afghan refugee camps: novel solutions. *Trans R Soc Trop Med Hyg* **95:**125-6.

6440. **Rowland, M., N. Mohammed, H. Rehman, S. Hewitt, C. Mendis, M. Ahmad, M. Kamal, and R. Wirtz.** 2002. Anopheline vectors and malaria transmission in eastern Afghanistan. *Trans R Soc Trop Med Hyg* **96:**620-6.

6441. **Rowland, M., A. Munir, N. Durrani, H. Noyes, and H. Reyburn.** 1999. An outbreak of cutaneous leishmaniasis in an Afghan refugee settlement in north-west Pakistan. *Trans R Soc Trop Med Hyg* **93:**133-6.

6442. **Rowland, M., and F. Nosten.** 2001. Malaria epidemiology and control in refugee camps and complex emergencies. *Ann Trop Med Parasitol* **95:**741-54.

6443. **Roy, E., N. Haley, P. Leclerc, J. F. Boivin, L. Cedras, and J. Vincelette.** 2001. Risk factors for hepatitis C virus infection among street youths. *CMAJ* **165:**557-60.

6444. **Roy, E., N. Haley, P. Leclerc, B. Sochanski, J. F. Boudreau, and J. F. Boivin.** 2004. Mortality in a cohort of street youth in Montreal. *JAMA* **292:**569-74.

6445. **Roy, K., G. Hay, R. Andragetti, A. Taylor, D. Goldberg, and L. Wiessing.** 2002. Monitoring hepatitis C virus infection among injecting drug users in the European Union: a review of the literature. *Epidemiol Infect* **129:**577-85.

6446. **Roy, S. L., S. M. DeLong, S. A. Stenzel, B. Shiferaw, J. M. Roberts, A. Khalakdina, R. Marcus, S. D. Segler, D. D. Shah, S. Thomas, D. J. Vugia, S. M. Zansky, V. Dietz, and M. J. Beach.** 2004. Risk factors for sporadic cryptosporidiosis among immunocompetent persons in the United States from 1999 to 2001. *J Clin Microbiol* **42:**2944-51.

6447. **Roy, S. L., A. S. Lopez, and P. Schantz.** 2003. Trichinellosis surveillance - United States, 1997-2001. *MMWR* **52 (SS-6):**1-8.

6448. **Royce, R. A., A. Sena, W. Cates, Jr., and M. S. Cohen.** 1997. Sexual transmission of HIV. *N Engl J Med* **336:**1072-8.

6449. **Rozendaal, J. A.** 1997. Vector control. Methods for use by individuals and communities. World Health Organization, Geneva.

6450. **Rubel, D., G. Zunino, G. Santillan, and C. Wisnivesky.** 2003. Epidemiology of Toxocara canis in the dog population from two areas of different socioeconomic status, Greater Buenos Aires, Argentina. *Vet Parasitol* **115:**275-86.

6451. **Rubertone, M. V., R. F. DeFraites, M. R. Krauss, and C. A. Brandt.** 1993. An outbreak of hepatitis A during a military field training exercise. *Mil Med* **158:**37-41.

6452. **Rubin, R. H.** 1990. Impact of cytomegalovirus infection on organ transplant recipients. *Rev Infect Dis* **12 Suppl 7:**S754-66.

6453. **Rubin, R. H., A. Schaffner, and R. Speich.** 2001. Introduction to the Immunocompromised Host Society consensus conference on epidemiology, prevention, diagnosis, and management of infections in solid-organ transplant patients. *Clin Infect Dis* **33 Suppl 1:**S1-4.

6454. **Rubio, J. M., J. Roche, P. J. Berzosa, E. Moyano, and A. Benito.** 2000. The potential utility of the Semi-Nested Multiplex PCR technique for the diagnosis and investigation of congenital malaria. *Diagn Microbiol Infect Dis* **38:**233-6.

6455. **Rudakov, N. V., S. N. Shpynov, I. E. Samoilenko, and M. A. Tankibaev.** 2003. Ecology and epidemiology of spotted fever group Rickettsiae and new data from their study in Russia and Kazakhstan. *Ann N Y Acad Sci* **990:**12-24.

6456. **Rudan, I., L. Tomaskovic, C. Boschi-Pinto, and H. Campbell.** 2004. Global estimate of the incidence of clinical pneumonia among children under five years of age. *Bull WHO* **82:**895-903.

6457. **Ruddy, M., M. Cummins, and Y. Drabu.** 2001. Hospital hairdresser as a potential source of cross-infection with MRSA. *J Hosp Infect* **49:**225-7.

6458. **Ruden, A. K., A. Jonsson, P. Lidbrink, P. Allebeck, and S. M. Bygdeman.** 1993. Endemic versus non-endemic gonorrhoea in Stockholm: results of contact tracing. *Int J STD AIDS* **4:**284-92.

6459. **Ruebush, T. K., 2nd, D. D. Juranek, A. Spielman, J. Piesman, and G. R. Healy.** 1981. Epidemiology of human babesiosis on Nantucket Island. *Am J Trop Med Hyg* **30:**937-41.

6460. **Ruel, N., M. F. Odelin, J. Jolly, C. Momplot, M. C. Diana, T. Bourlet, R. Gonthier, M. Aymard, and B. Pozzetto.** 2002. [Outbreaks due to respiratory syncytial virus and influenza-virus A/H3N in institutionalized aged. Role of immunological status to influenza vaccine and possible implication of caregivers in the transmission]. *Presse Med* **31:**349-55.

6461. **Ruf, M.** 2005. Should a low prevalence of asymptomatic Chlamydia trachomatis infection in gay men attending HIV clinics discourage from opportunistic screening? *Int J STD AIDS* **16:**622-4.

6462. **Ruff, A. J.** 1994. Breastmilk, breastfeeding, and transmission of viruses to the neonate. *Semin Perinatol* **18:**510-6.

6463. **Ruiz, A.** 2001. Plague in the Americas. *Emerg Infect Dis* **7 (no 3 suppl):**539-40.

6464. **Ruiz, A., and G. S. Bulmer.** 1981. Particle size of airborn Cryptococcus neoformans in a tower. *Appl Environ Microbiol* **1981:**1225-9.

6465. **Ruiz, A., and J. K. Frenkel.** 1980. Intermediate and transport hosts of Toxoplasma gondii in Costa Rica. *Am J Trop Med Hyg* **29:**1161-6.

6466. **Ruiz, G. M., T. K. Rawlings, F. C. Dobbs, L. A. Drake, T. Mullady, A. Huq, and R. R. Colwell.** 2000. Global spread of microorganisms by ships. *Nature* **408:**49-50.

6467. **Ruiz, J. A., P. P. Simarro, and T. Josenando.** 2002. Control of human African trypanosomiasis in the Quicama focus, Angola. *Bull WHO* **80:**738-45.

6468. **Ruiz-Beltran, R., J. I. Herrero-Herrero, A. M. Martin-Sanchez, and J. A. Martin-Gonzalez.** 1990. Prevalence of antibodies to Rickettsia conorii Coxiella burnetii and Rickettsia typhi in Salamanca Province (Spain). Serosurvey in the human population. *Eur J Epidemiol* **6:**293-9.

6469. **Ruppert, J., B. Panzig, L. Guertler, P. Hinz, G. Schwesinger, S. B. Felix, and S. Friesecke.** 2004. Two cases of severe sepsis due to Vibrio vulnificus wound infection acquired in the Baltic Sea. *Eur J Clin Microbiol Infect Dis* **23:**912-5.

6470. **Rupprecht, C. E., C. A. Hanlon, and T. Hemachudha.** 2002. Rabies re-examined. *Lancet Infect Dis* **2:**327-43.

6471. **Rushdy, A. A., R. P. Cooke, A. M. Iversen, and B. J. Pickering.** 1995. Boarding school outbreak of group A streptococcal pharyngitis. *Commun Dis Rep CDR Rev* **5:**R106-8.

6472. **Rushdy, A. A., J. M. White, M. E. Ramsay, and N. S. Crowcroft.** 2003. Tetanus in England and Wales, 1984-2000. *Epidemiol Infect* **130:**71-7.

6473. **Rusnak, J. M., M. G. Kortepeter, J. Aldis, and E. Boudreau.** 2004. Experience in the medical management of potential laboratory exposures to agents of bioterrorism on the basis of risk assessment at the United States Army Medical Research Institute of Infectious Diseases (USAMRIID). *J Occup Environ Med* **46:**801-11.

6474. **Russell, F. M., J. R. Carapetis, O. Mansoor, A. Darcy, T. Fakakovi, A. Metai, N. T. Potoi, N. Wilson, and E. K. Mulholland.** 2003. High incidence of Haemophilus influenzae type b infection in children in Pacific island countries. *Clin Infect Dis* **37:**1593-9.

6475. **Russell, K. L., M. A. Montiel Gonzalez, D. M. Watts, R. C. Lagos-Figueroa, G. Chauca, M. Ore, J. E. Gonzalez, C. Moron, R. B. Tesh, and J. M. Vinetz.** 2003. An outbreak of leptospirosis among Peruvian military recruits. *Am J Trop Med Hyg* **69:**53-7.

6476. **Russell, R. C.** 1987. Survival of insects in the wheel bays of a Boeing 747B aircraft on flights between tropical and temperate airports. *Bull WHO* **65:**659-62.

6477. **Russell, R. C.** 2002. Ross River virus: ecology and distribution. *Annu Rev Entomol* **47:**1-31.

6478. **Russi, J. C., M. Serra, J. Vinoles, M. T. Perez, D. Ruchansky, G. Alonso, J. L. Sanchez, K. L. Russell, S. M. Montano, M. Negrete, and M. Weissenbacher.** 2003. Sexual transmission of hepatitis B virus, hepatitis C virus, and human immunodeficiency virus type 1 infections among male transvestite comercial sex workers in Montevideo, Uruguay. *Am J Trop Med Hyg* **68:**716-20.

6479. **Russomando, G., M. M. de Tomassone, I. de Guillen, N. Acosta, N. Vera, M. Almiron, N. Candia, M. F. Calcena, and A. Figueredo.** 1998. Treatment of congenital Chagas' disease diagnosed and followed up by the polymerase chain reaction. *Am J Trop Med Hyg* **59:**487-91.

6480. **Rusul, G., and N. H. Yaacob.** 1995. Prevalence of Bacillus cereus in selected foods and detection of enterotoxin using TECRA-VIA and BCET-RPLA. *Int J Food Microbiol* **25:**131-9.

6481. **Rutala, W. A., F. A. Sarubi, C. S. Finch, J. N. McCormack, and G. E. Steinkraus.** 1982. Oyster-associated outbreak of diarrhoeal disease possibly caused by Plesiomonas shigelloides. *Lancet* **1:**739.

6482. **Rutala, W. A., and D. J. Weber.** 2001. Creutzfeldt-Jakob disease: recommendations for disinfection and sterilization. *Clin Infect Dis* **32:**1348-56.

6483. **Rutala, W. A., and D. J. Weber.** 2001. A review of single-use and reusable gowns and drapes in health care. *Infect Control Hosp Epidemiol* **22:**248-57.

6484. **Rutala, W. A., D. J. Weber, and C. A. Thomann.** 1987. Outbreak of wound infections following outpatient podiatric surgery due to contaminated bone drills. *Foot Ankle* **7:**350-4.

6485. **Rutar, T., E. J. Baldomar Salgueiro, and J. H. Maguire.** 2004. Introduced Plasmodium vivax malaria in a Bolivian community at an elevation of 2,300 meters. *Am J Trop Med Hyg* **70:**15-9.

6486. **Ruuskanen, O., T. T. Salmi, and P. Halonen.** 1978. Measles vaccination after exposure to natural measles. *J Pediatr* **93:**43-6.

6487. **Ruxrungtham, K., T. Brown, and P. Phanuphak.** 2004. HIV/AIDS in Asia. *Lancet* **364:**69-82.

6488. **Ryan, C. A., M. K. Nickels, N. T. Hargrett-Bean, M. E. Potter, T. Endo, L. Mayer, C. W. Langkop, C. Gibson, R. C. McDonald, R. T. Kenney, et al.** 1987. Massive outbreak of antimicrobial-resistant salmonellosis traced to pasteurized milk. *JAMA* **258:**3269-74.

6489. **Ryan, C. A., O. V. Vathiny, P. M. Gorbach, H. B. Leng, A. Berlioz-Arthaud, W. L. Whittington, and K. K. Holmes.** 1998. Explosive spread of HIV-1 and sexually transmitted diseases in Cambodia. *Lancet* **351:**1175.

6490. **Ryan, M. A., G. C. Gray, B. Smith, J. A. McKeehan, A. W. Hawksworth, and M. D. Malasig.** 2002. Large epidemic of respiratory illness due to adenovirus types 7 and 3 in healthy young adults. *Clin Infect Dis* **34:**577-82.

6491. **Ryan, U. M., B. Samarasinghe, C. Read, J. R. Buddle, I. D. Robertson, and R. C. Thompson.** 2003. Identification of a novel Cryptosporidium genotype in pigs. *Appl Environ Microbiol* **69:**3970-4.

6492. **Ryder, R. W., M. Kamenga, M. Nkusu, V. Batter, and W. L. Heyward.** 1994. AIDS orphans in Kinshasa, Zaire: incidence and socioeconomic consequences. *AIDS* **8:**673-9.

6493. **Rydkina, E., V. Roux, N. Rudakov, M. Gafarova, I. Tarasevich, and D. Raoult.** 1999. New rickettsiae in ticks collected in territories of the former Soviet Union. *Emerg Infect Dis* **5:**811-4.

6494. **Rydkina, E. B., V. Roux, E. M. Gagua, A. B. Predtechenski, I. V. Tarasevich, and D. Raoult.** 1999. Bartonella quintana in body lice collected from homeless persons in Russia. *Emerg Infect Dis* **5:**176-8.

6495. **Rygg, M., and F. Bruun.** 1992. Rat bite fever (Streptobacillus moniliformis) with septicemia in a child. *Scand J Infect Dis* **24:**535-40.

6496. Rysstad, O. G., and F. Gallefoss. 2003. TB status among Kosovar refugees. *Int J Tuberc Lung Dis* **7**:458-63.

6497. Sa-Leao, R., A. Tomasz, I. S. Sanches, A. Brito-Avo, S. E. Vilhelmsson, K. G. Kristinsson, and H. de Lencastre. 2000. Carriage of internationally spread clones of Streptococcus pneumoniae with unusual drug resistance patterns in children attending day care centers in Lisbon, Portugal. *J Infect Dis* **182**:1153-60.

6498. Saal, M. B., J. F. Schemann, B. Saar, M. Faye, G. Momo, S. Mariotti, and A. D. Negrel. 2003. Le trachome au Sénégal: résultats d'une enquête nationale. *Med Trop* **63**:53-9.

6499. Saathoff, E., A. Olsen, J. D. Kvalsvig, and P. W. Geissler. 2002. Geophagy and its association with geohelminth infection in rural schoolchildren from northern KwaZulu-Natal, South Africa. *Trans R Soc Trop Med Hyg* **96**:485-90.

6500. Saathoff, E., A. Olsen, B. Sharp, J. D. Kvalsvig, C. C. Appleton, and I. Kleinschmidt. 2005. Ecologic covariates of hookworm infection and reinfection in rural Kwazulu-natal/south Africa: a geographic information system-based study. *Am J Trop Med Hyg* **72**:384-91.

6501. Saba, R., M. Korkmaz, D. Inan, L. Mamikoglu, O. Turhan, F. Gunseren, C. Cevikol, and A. Kabaalioglu. 2004. Human fascioliasis. *Clin Microbiol Infect* **10**:385-7.

6502. Sabatinelli, G., M. Ejov, and P. Joergensen. 2001. Malaria in the WHO European region (1971-1999). *Eurosurveillance* **6**:61-5.

6503. Sabbuba, N. A., E. Mahenthiralingam, and D. J. Stickler. 2003. Molecular epidemiology of Proteus mirabilis infections of the catheterized urinary tract. *J Clin Microbiol* **41**:4961-5.

6504. Sabin, K. M., R. L. Frey, R. Horsley, and S. M. Greby. 2001. Characteristics and trends of newly identified HIV infections among incarcerated populations: CDC HIV voluntary counseling, testing and referral system, 1992-1998. *J Urban Health* **78**:241-55.

6505. Sachar, D. S., R. Narayan, J. W. Song, H. C. Lee, and T. A. Klein. 2003. Hantavirus infection in an active duty U.S. Army soldier stationed in Seoul, Korea. *Mil Med* **168**:231-3.

6506. Sack, D. A., R. B. Sack, G. B. Nair, and A. K. Siddique. 2004. Cholera. *Lancet* **363**:223-33.

6507. Sacks, J. J., L. Ajello, and L. K. Crockett. 1986. An outbreak and review of cave-associated histoplasmosis capsulati. *J Med Vet Mycol* **24**:313-25.

6508. Sacks, J. J., E. R. Brenner, D. C. Breeden, H. M. Anders, and R. L. Parker. 1985. Epidemiology of a tuberculosis outbreak in a South Carolina junior high school. *Am J Public Health* **75**:361-5.

6509. Sacks, J. J., D. G. Delgado, H. O. Lobel, and R. L. Parker. 1983. Toxoplasmosis infection associated with eating undercooked venison. *Am J Epidemiol* **118**:832-8.

6510. Sacks, J. J., S. Lieb, L. M. Baldy, S. Berta, C. M. Patton, M. C. White, W. J. Bigler, and J. J. Witte. 1986. Epidemic campylobacteriosis associated with a community water supply. *Am J Public Health* **76**:424-8.

6511. Sacks, J. J., R. R. Roberto, and N. F. Brooks. 1982. Toxoplasmosis infection associated with raw goat's milk. *JAMA* **248**:1728-32.

6512. Sacks, S. L. 2004. Famciclovir suppression of asymptomatic and symptomatic recurrent anogenital herpes simplex virus shedding in women: a randomized, double-blind, double-dummy, placebo-controlled, parallel-group, single-center trial. *J Infect Dis* **189**:1341-7.

6513. Sacks, S. L., P. D. Griffiths, L. Corey, C. Cohen, A. Cunningham, G. M. Dusheiko, S. Self, S. Spruance, L. R. Stanberry, A. Wald, and R. J. Whitley. 2004. HSV shedding. *Antiviral Res* **63 Suppl 1**:S19-26.

6514. Sadjjadi, S. M., M. Khosravi, D. Mehrabani, and A. Orya. 2000. Seroprevalence of toxocara infection in school children in Shiraz, southern Iran. *J Trop Pediatr* **46**:327-30.

6515. Saeki, H., H. Masu, H. Yokoi, and M. Yamamoto. 1997. Long-term survey on intestinal nematode and cestode infections in stray puppies Ibaraki Prefecture. *J Vet Med Sci* **59**:725-6.

6516. Saenz, A. C., F. A. Assaad, and W. C. Cockburn. 1969. Outbreak of A2-Hong Kong-68 influenza at an international medical conference. *Lancet* **1**:91-3.

6517. Saez-Alquezar, A., A. M. Ramos, S. M. Di Santi, M. S. Branquinho, K. Kirchgatter, I. A. Cordeiro, M. Murta, J. C. Saraiva, S. G. Oliveira, M. G. Bochetti, J. A. Pirolla, D. Guerzoni, and D. A. Chamone. 1998. [Control of blood transfusion malaria in an endemic and in a non-endemic region in Brazil]. *Rev Soc Bras Med Trop* **31**:27-34.

6518. Sáez-Llorens, X., and G. H. McCracken, Jr. 2003. Bacterial meningitis in children. *Lancet* **361**:2139-48.

6519. Safdar, A., and D. Armstrong. 2003. Listeriosis in patients at a comprehensive cancer center, 1955-1997. *Clin Infect Dis* **37**:359-64.

6520. Safdar, N., R. B. Love, and D. G. Maki. 2002. Severe Ehrlichia chaffeensis Infection in a Lung Transplant Recipient: A Review of Ehrlichiosis in the Immunocompromised Patient. *Emerg Infect Dis* **8**:320-3.

6521. Safdar, N., and D. G. Maki. 2002. The commonality of risk factors for nosocomial colonization and infection with antimicrobial-resistant Staphylococcus aureus, enterococcus, gram-negative bacilli, Clostridium difficile, and Candida. *Ann Intern Med* **136**:834-44.

6522. Safeukui-Noubissi, I., S. Ranque, M. Poudiougou, M. Keita, A. Traore, D. Traore, M. Diakite, M. B. Cisse, M. M. Keita, A. Dessein, and O. K. Doumbo. 2004. Risk factors for severe malaria in Bamako, Mali: a matched case-control study. *Microbes Infect* **6**:572-8.

6523. Safranek, T. J., W. R. Jarvis, L. A. Carson, L. B. Cusick, L. A. Bland, J. M. Swenson, and V. A. Silcox. 1987. Mycobacterium chelonae wound infections after plastic surgery employing contaminated gentian violet skin-marking solution. *N Engl J Med* **317**:197-201.

6524. Sagin, D. D., G. Ismail, L. M. Nasian, J. J. Jok, and E. K. Pang. 2000. Rickettsial infection in five remote Orang Ulu villages in upper Rejang River, Sarawak, Malaysia. *Southeast Asian J Trop Med Public Health* **31**:733-5.

6525. Sagliocca, L., P. Amoroso, T. Stroffolini, B. Adamo, M. E. Tosti, G. Lettieri, C. Esposito, S. Buonocore, P. Pierri, and A. Mele. 1999. Efficacy of hepatitis A vaccine in prevention of secondary hepatitis A infection: a randomised trial. *Lancet* **353**:1136-9.

6526. Sagoo, S. K., C. L. Little, L. Ward, I. A. Gillespie, and R. T. Mitchell. 2003. Microbiological study of ready-to-eat salad vegetables from retail establishments uncovers a national outbreak of salmonellosis. *J Food Prot* **66**:403-9.

6527. Sagrera, X., G. Ginovart, F. Raspall, N. Rabella, P. Sala, M. Sierra, X. Demestre, and C. Vila. 2002. Outbreaks of influenza A virus infection in neonatal intensive care units. *Pediatr Infect Dis J* **21**:196-200.

6528. Saha, S. K., A. H. Baqui, M. Hanif, G. L. Darmstadt, M. Ruhulamin, T. Nagatake, M. Santosham, and R. E. Black. 2001. Typhoid fever in Bangladesh: implications for vaccination policy. *Pediatr Infect Dis J* **20:**521-4.

6529. Sahani, M., U. D. Parashar, R. Ali, P. Das, M. S. Lye, M. M. Isa, M. T. Arif, T. G. Ksiazek, and M. Sivamoorthy. 2001. Nipah virus infection among abattoir workers in Malaysia, 1998-1999. *Int J Epidemiol* **30:**1017-1020.

6530. Sahathevan, M., F. A. Harvey, G. Forbes, J. O'Grady, A. Gimson, S. Bragman, R. Jensen, J. Philpott-Howard, R. Williams, and M. W. Casewell. 1991. Epidemiology, bacteriology and control of an outbreak of Nocardia asteroides infection on a liver unit. *J Hosp Infect* **18 suppl A:**473-80.

6531. Sahlstrom, L. 2003. A review of survival of pathogenic bacteria in organic waste used in biogas plants. *Bioresour Technol* **87:**161-6.

6532. Said, B., F. Wright, G. L. Nichols, M. Reacher, and M. Rutter. 2003. Outbreaks of infectious disease associated with private drinking water supplies in England and Wales 1970-2000. *Epidemiol Infect* **130:**469-79.

6533. Saigal, S., O. Lunyk, R. P. Larke, and M. A. Chernesky. 1982. The outcome in children with congenital cytomegalovirus infection. A longitudinal follow-up study. *Am J Dis Child* **136:**896-901.

6534. Saiman, L., J. Aronson, J. Zhou, C. Gomez-Duarte, P. S. Gabriel, M. Alonso, S. Maloney, and J. Schulte. 2001. Prevalence of infectious diseases among internationally adopted children. *Pediatrics* **108:**608-12.

6535. Saisongkorh, W., M. Chenchittikul, and K. Silpapojakul. 2004. Evaluation of nested PCR for the diagnosis of scrub typhus among patients with acute pyrexia of unknown origin. *Trans R Soc Trop Med Hyg* **98:**360-6.

6536. Saito, M., T. Sunagawa, Y. Makino, M. Tadano, H. Hasegawa, K. Kanemura, Y. Zamami, B. J. Killenbeck, and T. Fukunaga. 1999. Three Japanese encephalitis cases in Okinawa, Japan, 1991. *Southeast Asian J Trop Med Public Health* **30:**277-9.

6537. Sakai, R., H. Kawashima, H. Shibui, K. Kamata, C. Kambara, and H. Matsuoka. 1998. Toxocara cati-induced ocular Toxocariasis. *Arch Ophthalmol* **116:**1686-7.

6538. Sakdisiwasdi, O., S. Achananuparp, A. Limsuwan, P. Nanna, and L. Barnyen. 1982. Salmonella and Shigella carrier rates and environmental sanitation in a rural district, Central Thailand. *Southeast Asian J Trop Med Public Health* **13:**380-4.

6539. Sakhnini, E., A. Weissmann, and I. Oren. 2002. Fulminant Stenotrophomonas maltophilia soft tissue infection in immunocompromised patients: an outbreak transmitted via tap water. *Am J Med Sci* **323:**269-72.

6540. Saksirisampant, W., S. Nuchprayoon, V. Wiwanitkit, K. Kraivichian, and J. Suwansaksri. 2002. Prevalence and intensity of third stage Gnathostoma spinigerum larvae in swamp eels sold in three large markets in Bangkok, Thailand. *Southeast Asian J Trop Med Public Health* **33 suppl 3:**60-2.

6541. Salakova, M., V. Nemecek, J. Konig, and R. Tachezy. 2004. Age-specific prevalence, transmission and phylogeny of TT virus in the Czech Republic. *BMC Infect Dis* **4:**56.

6542. Salama, P., P. Spiegel, L. Talley, and R. Waldman. 2004. Lessons learned from complex emergencies over past decade. *Lancet* **364:**1801-13.

6543. Salamina, G., E. Dalle Donne, A. Niccolini, G. Poda, D. Cesaroni, M. Bucci, R. Fini, M. Maldini, A. Schuchat, B. Swaminathan, W. Bibb, J. Rocourt, N. Binkin, and S. Salmaso. 1996. A foodborne outbreak of gastroenteritis involving Listeria monocytogenes. *Epidemiol Infect* **117:**429-36.

6544. Salas, R. A., N. de Manzione, and R. Tesh. 1998. [Venezuelan hemorrhagic fever: eight years of observation]. *Acta Cient Venez* **49:**46-51.

6545. Salas, R. A., C. Z. Garcia, J. Liria, R. Barrera, J. C. Navarro, G. Medina, C. Vasquez, Z. Fernandez, and S. C. Weaver. 2001. Ecological studies of enzootic Venezuelan equine encephalitis in north-central Venezuela, 1997-1998. *Am J Trop Med Hyg* **64:**84-92.

6546. Salasia, S. I., I. W. Wibawan, F. H. Pasaribu, A. Abdulmawjood, and C. Lammler. 2004. Persistent occurrence of a single Streptococcus equi subsp. zooepidemicus clone in the pig and monkey population in Indonesia. *J Vet Sci* **5:**263-5.

6547. Salazar-Bravo, J., J. W. Dragoo, M. D. Bowen, C. J. Peters, T. G. Ksiazek, and T. L. Yates. 2002. Natural nidality in Bolivian hemorrhagic fever and the systematics of the reservoir species. *Infect Genet Evol* **1:**191-9.

6548. Salem, G., and P. Schantz. 1992. Toxocaral visceral larva migrans after ingestion of raw lamb liver. *Clin Infect Dis* **15:**743-4.

6549. Salgado, C. D., B. M. Farr, and D. P. Calfee. 2003. Community-acquired methicillin-resistant Staphylococcus aureus: a meta- analysis of prevalence and risk factors. *Clin Infect Dis* **36:**131-9.

6550. Salgado, C. D., E. T. Giannetta, F. G. Hayden, and B. M. Farr. 2004. Preventing nosocomial influenza by improving the vaccine acceptance rate of clinicians. *Infect Control Hosp Epidemiol* **25:**923-8.

6551. Salgado, C. G., J. P. da Silva, J. A. Diniz, M. B. da Silva, P. F. da Costa, C. Teixeira, and U. I. Salgado. 2004. Isolation of Fonsecaea pedrosoi from thorns of Mimosa pudica, a probable natural source of chromoblastomycosis. *Rev Inst Med Trop Sao Paulo* **46:**33-6.

6552. Saliba, E. K., M. R. Tawfiq, S. Kharabsheh, and J. Rahamneh. 1997. Urinary schistosomiasis contracted from an irrigation pool in Ramah, the southern Jordan valley, Jordan. *Am J Trop Med Hyg* **57:**158-61.

6553. Saliba, G. S., W. P. Glezen, and T. D. Chin. 1967. Mycoplasma pneumoniae infection in a resident boys' home. *Am J Epidemiol* **86:**408-18.

6554. Saliba, L. J., and R. Helmer. 1990. Health risks associated with pollution of coastal bathing waters. *World Health Stat Q* **43:**177-87.

6555. Salinas-Carmona, M. C. 2000. Nocardia brasiliensis: from microbe to human and experimental infections. *Microbes Infect* **2:**1373-81.

6556. Salleras, L., A. Dominguez, M. Bruguera, N. Cardenosa, J. Batalla, G. Carmona, E. Navas, and J. L. Taberner. 2005. Dramatic decline in acute hepatitis B infection and disease incidence rates among adolescents and young people after 12 years of a mass hepatitis B vaccination programme of pre-adolescents in the schools of Catalonia (Spain). *Vaccine* **23:**2181-4.

6557. Sallon, S., R. el-Shawwa, M. Khalil, G. Ginsburg, J. el Tayib, J. el-Eila, V. Green, and C. A. Hart. 1994. Diarrhoeal disease in children in Gaza. *Ann Trop Med Parasitol* **88:**175-82.

6558. Salmon, M. M., B. Howells, E. J. Glencross, A. D. Evans, and S. R. Palmer. 1982. Q fever in an urban area. *Lancet* **1:**1002-4.

6559. **Salmon, R.** 2004. Preventing person-to-person spread following gastrointestinal infections: guidelines for public health physicians and environmental health officers. *Commun Dis Publ Health* **7:**362-84.

6560. **Salomon, O. D., S. Sosa Estani, G. C. Rossi, and G. R. Spinelli.** 2001. [Lutzomyia longipalpis and Leishmaniasis visceral in Argentina]. *Medicina (B Aires)* **61:**174-8.

6561. **Saloojee, H., S. Velaphi, Y. Goga, N. Afadapa, R. Steen, and O. Lincetto.** 2004. The prevention and management of congenital syphilis: and overview and recommendations. *Bull WHO* **82:**424-30.

6562. **Saltoglu, N., Y. Tasova, D. Midikli, R. Burgut, and I. H. Dundar.** 2004. Prognostic factors affecting deaths from adult tetanus. *Clin Microbiol Infect* **10:**229-33.

6563. **Saluzzo, J. F., J. P. Digoutte, J. L. Camicas, and G. Chauvancy.** 1985. Crimean-Congo haemorrhagic fever and Rift Valley fever in south-eastern Mauritania. *Lancet* **1:**116.

6564. **Samaan, G., P. Roche, and J. Spencer.** 2003. Tuberculosis notifications in Australia, 2002. *Commun Dis Intell* **27:**449-58.

6565. **Samadpour, M., J. E. Ongerth, J. Liston, N. Tran, D. Nguyen, T. S. Whittam, R. A. Wilson, and P. I. Tarr.** 1994. Occurrence of Shiga-like toxin-producing Escherichia coli in retail fresh seafood, beef, lamb, pork, and poultry from grocery stores in Seattle, Washington. *Appl Environ Microbiol* **60:**1038-40.

6566. **Samarawickrema, W. A., E. Kimura, F. Sones, G. S. Paulson, and R. F. Cummings.** 1992. Natural infections of Dirofilaria immitis in Aedes (Stegomyia) polynesiensis and Aedes (Finlaya) samoanus and their implication in human health in Samoa. *Trans R Soc Trop Med Hyg* **86:**187-8.

6567. **Sambola, A., J. M. Miro, M. P. Tornos, B. Almirante, A. Moreno-Torrico, M. Gurgui, E. Martinez, A. Del Rio, M. Azqueta, F. Marco, and J. M. Gatell.** 2002. Streptococcus agalactiae infective endocarditis: analysis of 30 cases and review of the literature, 1962-1998. *Clin Infect Dis* **34:**1576-84.

6568. **Samonis, G., L. Elting, E. Skoulika, S. Maraki, and Y. Tselentis.** 1994. An outbreak of diarrhoeal disease attributed to Shigella sonnei. *Epidemiol Infect* **112:**235-45.

6569. **Sampaio, J. L., V. A. Alves, S. C. Leao, V. D. De Magalhaes, M. D. Martino, C. M. Mendes, A. C. Misiara, K. Miyashiro, J. Pasternak, E. Rodrigues, R. Rozenbaum, C. A. Filho, S. R. Teixeira, A. C. Xavier, M. S. Figueiredo, and J. P. Leite.** 2002. Mycobacterium haemophilum: emerging or underdiagnosed in Brazil? *Emerg Infect Dis* **8:**1359-60.

6570. **Sampaio, J. L. M., V. P. de Andrade, M. da Conceição Lucas, L. Fung, S. M. B. Gagliardi, S. R. P. Santos, C. M. F. Mendes, M. B. de Paula Eduardo, and T. Dick.** 2005. Diphyllobothriasis, Brazil. *Emerg Infect Dis* **11:**1598-1600.

6571. **Sampere, M., B. Font, J. Font, I. Sanfeliu, and F. Segura.** 2003. Q fever in adults: review of 66 clinical cases. *Eur J Clin Microbiol Infect Dis* **22:**108-10.

6572. **Samuel, D.** 2000. [Clinical trials using cell xenografts. Their place in the treatment of fulminant hepatitis]. *Pathol Biol (Paris)* **48:**407-10.

6573. **Samuel, M. C., P. M. Doherty, M. Bulterys, and S. A. Jenison.** 2001. Association between heroin use, needle sharing and tattoos received in prison with hepatitis B and C positivity among street-recruited injecting drug users in New Mexico, USA. *Epidemiol Infect* **127:**475-84.

6574. **Samuel, M. C., D. J. Vugia, S. Shallow, R. Marcus, S. Segler, T. McGivern, H. Kassenborg, K. Reilly, M. Kennedy, F. Angulo, and R. V. Tauxe.** 2004. Epidemiology of Sporadic Campylobacter Infection in the United States and Declining Trend in Incidence, FoodNet 1996-1999. *Clin Infect Dis* **38 Suppl 3:**S165-74.

6575. **Samuel, M. D., D. J. Shadduck, D. R. Goldberg, V. Baranyuk, L. Sileo, and J. I. Price.** 1999. Antibodies against Pasteurella multocida in snow geese in the western Arctic. *J Wildl Dis* **35:**440-9.

6576. **Samuels, L. E., S. Sharma, R. J. Morris, M. P. Solomon, M. S. Granick, C. A. Wood, and S. K. Brockman.** 1996. Mycobacterium fortuitum infection of the sternum. Review of the literature and case illustration. *Arch Surg* **131:**1344-6.

6577. **Sanchez, A., G. Gerhardt, S. Natal, D. Capone, A. Espinola, W. Costa, J. Pires, A. Barreto, E. Biondi, and B. Larouze.** 2005. Prevalence of pulmonary tuberculosis and comparative evaluation of screening strategies in a Brazilian prison. *Int J Tuberc Lung Dis* **9:**633-9.

6578. **Sanchez, A. L., O. Gomez, P. Allebeck, H. Cosenza, and L. Ljungstrom.** 1997. Epidemiological study of Taenia solium infections in a rural village in Honduras. *Ann Trop Med Parasitol* **91:**163-71.

6579. **Sanchez, G., R. M. Pinto, H. Vanaclocha, and A. Bosch.** 2002. Molecular characterization of hepatitis a virus isolates from a transcontinental shellfish-borne outbreak. *J Clin Microbiol* **40:**4148-55.

6580. **Sanchez, J. L., I. Bendet, M. Grogl, J. B. Lima, L. W. Pang, M. F. Guimaraes, C. M. Guedes, W. K. Milhous, M. D. Green, and G. D. Todd.** 2000. Malaria in Brazilian military personnel deployed to Angola. *J Travel Med* **7:**275-82.

6581. **Sanchez, J. L., L. N. Binn, B. L. Innis, R. D. Reynolds, T. Lee, F. Mitchell-Raymundo, S. C. Craig, J. P. Marquez, G. A. Shepherd, C. S. Polyak, J. Conolly, and K. F. Kohlhase.** 2001. Epidemic of adenovirus-induced respiratory illness among US military recruits: epidemiologic and immunologic risk factors in healthy, young adults. *J Med Virol* **65:**710-8.

6582. **Sanchez, J. L., W. H. Candler, D. B. Fishbein, C. R. Greene, T. R. Cote, D. J. Kelly, D. P. Driggers, and B. J. Johnson.** 1992. A cluster of tick-borne infectionsé association with military training and asymptomatic infections due to Rickettsia rickettsii. *Trans R Soc Trop Med Hyg* **86:**321-5.

6583. **Sanchez, J. L., S. C. Craig, S. Kolavic, D. Hastings, B. J. Alsip, G. C. Gray, M. K. Hudspeth, and M. A. Ryan.** 2003. An outbreak of pneumococcal pneumonia among military personnel at high risk: control by low-dose azithromycin postexposure chemoprophylaxis. *Mil Med* **168:**1-6.

6584. **Sanchez, J. L., B. M. Diniega, J. W. Small, R. N. Miller, J. M. Andujar, P. J. Weina, P. G. Lawyer, W. R. Ballou, and J. K. Lovelace.** 1992. Epidemiologic investigation of an outbreak of cutaneous leishmaniasis in a defined geographic focus of transmission. *Am J Trop Med Hyg* **47:**47-54.

6585. **Sanchez, J. L., M. H. Sjogren, J. D. Callahan, D. M. Watts, C. Lucas, M. Abdel-Hamid, N. T. Constantine, K. C. Hyams, S. Hinostroza, R. Figueroa-Barrios, and J. C. Cuthie.** 2000. Hepatitis C in Peru: risk factors for infection, potential iatrogenic transmission, and genotype distribution. *Am J Trop Med Hyg* **63:**242-8.

6586. **Sanchez, J. L., E. T. Takafuji, W. M. Lednar, J. W. LeDuc, F. F. Macasaet, J. A. Mangiafico, R. R. Rosato, D. P. Driggers, and J. C. Haecker.** 1984. Venezuelan equine encephalomyelitis:

report of an outbreak associated with jungle exposure. *Mil Med* **149:**618-21.

6587. **Sanchez, J. L., B. Vasquez, R. E. Begue, R. Meza, G. Castellares, C. Cabezas, D. M. Watts, A. M. Svennerholm, J. C. Sadoff, and D. N. Taylor.** 1994. Protective efficacy of oral whole-cell/recombinant-B-subunit cholera vaccine in Peruvian military recruits. *Lancet* **344:**1273-6.

6588. **Sanchez, M. A., G. F. Lemp, C. Magis-Rodriguez, E. Bravo-Garcia, S. Carter, and J. D. Ruiz.** 2004. The epidemiology of HIV among Mexican migrants and recent immigrants in California and Mexico. *J Acquir Immune Defic Syndr* **37 Suppl 4:**S204-14.

6589. **Sanchez, M. P., D. D. Erdman, T. J. Torok, C. J. Freeman, and B. T. Matyas.** 1997. Outbreak of adenovirus 35 pneumonia among adult residents and staff of a chronic care psychiatric facility. *J Infect Dis* **176:**760-3.

6590. **Sánchez Thevenet, P., A. Nancufil, C. M. Oyarzo, C. Torrecillas, S. Raso, I. Mellado, M. E. Flores, M. G. Cordoba, M. C. Minvielle, and J. A. Basualdo.** 2004. An eco-epidemiological study of contamination of soil with infective forms of intestinal parasites. *Eur J Epidemiol* **19:**481-9.

6591. **Sanchez-Salas, J. L., A. López-Luna, S. Reyna-Tellez, and B. Barroeta.** 2003. Parasites common in blended fruit drinks. *Am J Trop Med Hyg* **69 suppl:**415.

6592. **Sandberg, M., B. Bergsjo, M. Hofshagen, E. Skjerve, and H. Kruse.** 2002. Risk factors for Campylobacter infection in Norwegian cats and dogs. *Prev Vet Med* **55:**241-53.

6593. **Sande, M. A., and J. M. Gwaltney.** 2004. Acute community-acquired bacterial sinusitis: continuing challenges and current management. *Clin Infect Dis* **39 suppl 3:**S151-8.

6594. **Sander, A., M. Posselt, K. Oberle, and W. Bredt.** 1998. Seroprevalence of antibodies to Bartonella henselae in patients with cat scratch disease and in healthy controls: evaluation and comparison of two commercial serological tests. *Clin Diagn Lab Immunol* **5:**486-90.

6595. **Sanders, E. J., J. G. Rigau-Perez, H. L. Smits, C. C. Deseda, V. A. Vorndam, T. Aye, R. A. Spiegel, R. S. Weyant, and S. L. Bragg.** 1999. Increase of leptospirosis in dengue-negative patients after a hurricane in Puerto Rico in 1996. *Am J Trop Med Hyg* **61:**399-404.

6596. **Sanders, E. J., E. B. Rwaguma, J. Kawamata, N. Kiwanuka, J. J. Lutwama, F. P. Ssengooba, M. Lamunu, R. Najjemba, W. A. Were, G. Bagambisa, and G. L. Campbell.** 1999. O'nyong-nyong fever in south-central Uganda, 1996-1997: description of the epidemic and results of a household-based seroprevalence survey. *J Infect Dis* **180:**1436-43.

6597. **Sanders, J. W., D. W. Isenbarger, S. E. Walz, L. W. Pang, D. A. Scott, C. Tamminga, B. A. Oyofo, W. C. Hewitson, J. L. Sanchez, C. Pitarangsi, P. Echeverria, and D. R. Tribble.** 2002. An observational clinic-based study of diarrheal illness in deployed United States military personnel in Thailand: presentation and outcome of Campylobacter infection. *Am J Trop Med Hyg* **67:**533-8.

6598. **Sanders, J. W., S. D. Putnam, P. Gould, J. Kolisnyk, N. Merced, V. Barthel, P. J. Rozmajzl, H. Shaheen, S. Fouad, and R. W. Frenck.** 2005. Diarrheal illness among deployed U.S. military personnel during Operation Bright Star 2001—Egypt. *Diagn Microbiol Infect Dis* **52:**85-90.

6599. **Sandoe, J. A.** 2004. Capnocytophaga canimorsus endocarditis. *J Med Microbiol* **53:**245-8.

6600. **Sands, K. E., D. S. Yokoe, D. C. Hooper, J. L. Tully, T. C. Horan, R. P. Gaynes, S. L. Solomon, and R. Platt.** 2003. Detection of postoperative surgical-site infections: comparison of health plan-based surveillance with hospital-based programs. *Infect Control Hosp Epidemiol* **24:**741-3.

6601. **Sandstrom, P. A., K. O. Phan, W. M. Switzer, T. Fredeking, L. Chapman, W. Heneine, and T. M. Folks.** 2000. Simian foamy virus infection among zoo keepers. *Lancet* **355:**551-2.

6602. **Sanford, M. D., A. F. Widmer, M. J. Bale, R. N. Jones, and R. P. Wenzel.** 1994. Efficient detection and long-term persistence of the carriage of methicillin-resistant Staphylococcus aureus. *Clin Infect Dis* **19:**1123-8.

6603. **Sang, D. K., G. B. Okelo, and M. L. Chance.** 1993. Cutaneous leishmaniasis due to Leishmania aethiopica, on Mount Elgon, Kenya. *Ann Trop Med Parasitol* **87:**349-57.

6604. **Sanghavi, D. M., R. H. Gilman, A. G. Lescano-Guevara, W. Checkley, L. Z. Cabrera, and V. Cardenas.** 1998. Hyperendemic pulmonary tuberculosis in a Peruvian shantytown. *Am J Epidemiol* **148:**384-9.

6605. **Sanogo, Y. O., Z. Zeaiter, G. Caruso, F. Merola, S. Shpynov, P. Brouqui, and D. Raoult.** 2003. Bartonella henselae in Ixodes ricinus Ticks (Acari: Ixodida) Removed from Humans, Belluno Province, Italy. *Emerg Infect Dis* **9:**329-32.

6606. **Santaniello-Newton, A., and P. R. Hunter.** 2000. Management of an outbreak of meningococcal meningitis in a Sudanese refugee camp in Northern Uganda. *Epidemiol Infect* **124:**75-81.

6607. **Santantonio, T., S. Lo Caputo, C. Germinario, S. Squarcione, D. Greco, V. Laddago, and G. Pastore.** 1993. Prevalence of hepatitis virus infections in Albanian refugees. *Eur J Epidemiol* **9:**537-40.

6608. **Santiago, M. L., C. M. Rodenburg, S. Kamenya, F. Bibollet-Ruche, F. Gao, E. Bailes, S. Meleth, S. J. Soong, J. M. Kilby, Z. Moldoveanu, B. Fahey, M. N. Muller, A. Ayouba, E. Nerrienet, H. M. McClure, J. L. Heeney, A. E. Pusey, D. A. Collins, C. Boesch, R. W. Wrangham, J. Goodall, P. M. Sharp, G. M. Shaw, and B. H. Hahn.** 2002. SIVcpz in wild chimpanzees. *Science* **295:**465.

6609. **Santin, M., F. Alcaide, M. A. Benitez, A. Salazar, C. Ardanuy, D. Podzamczer, G. Rufi, J. Dorca, R. Martin, and F. Gudiol.** 2004. Incidence and molecular typing of Mycobacterium kansasii in a defined geographical area in Catalonia, Spain. *Epidemiol Infect* **132:**425-32.

6610. **Santos, A. S., M. M. Santos-Silva, V. C. Almeida, F. Bacellar, and J. S. Dumler.** 2004. Detection of Anaplasma phagocytophilum DNA in Ixodes ticks (Acari: Ixodidae) from Madeira Island and Setubal District, mainland Portugal. *Emerg Infect Dis* **10:**1643-8.

6611. **Santos, E. O., E. C. Loureiro, I. M. Jesus, E. Brabo, R. S. Silva, M. C. Soares, V. M. Camara, M. R. Souza, and F. Branches.** 1995. [Diagnosis of health conditions in a pan-mining community in the Tapajos River Basin, Itaituba, Par , Brazil, 1992]. *Cad Saude Publica* **11:**212-25.

6612. **Sanz, J. C., M. F. Dominguez, M. J. Sagues, M. Fernandez, R. Feito, R. Noguerales, A. Asensio, and K. Fernandez De La Hoz.** 2002. [Diagnosis and epidemiological investigation of an outbreak of Clostridium perfringens food poisoning]. *Enferm Infecc Microbiol Clin* **20:**117-22.

6613. **Saravanakumar, P. S., P. Eslami, and F. A. Zar.** 1996. Lymphocutaneous sporotrichosis associated with a squirrel bite: case report and review. *Clin Infect Dis* **23:**647-8.

6614. **Saravia, N. G., K. Weigle, I. Segura, S. H. Giannini, R. Pacheco, L. A. Labrada, and A. Goncalves.** 1990. Recurrent lesions in human Leishmania braziliensis infection—reactivation or reinfection? *Lancet* **336:**398-402.

6615. **Sargent, S. J., and J. T. Martin.** 1994. Scabies outbreak in a day-care center. *Pediatrics* **94:**1012-3.

6616. **Sarkar, U., S. F. Nascimento, R. Barbosa, R. Martins, H. Nuevo, I. Kalafanos, I. Grunstein, B. Flannery, J. Dias, L. W. Riley, M. G. Reis, and A. I. Ko.** 2002. Population-based case-control investigation of risk factors for leptospirosis during an urban epidemic. *Am J Trop Med Hyg* **66:**605-10.

6617. **Sarti, E., P. M. Schantz, A. Plancarte, M. Wilson, I. O. Gutierrez, A. S. Lopez, J. Roberts, and A. Flisser.** 1992. Prevalence and risk factors for Taenia solium taeniasis and cysticercosis in humans and pigs in a village in Morelos, Mexico. *Am J Trop Med Hyg* **46:**677-85.

6618. **Sartor, C., V. Jacomo, C. Duvivier, H. Tissot-Dupont, R. Sambuc, and M. Drancourt.** 2000. Nosocomial Serratia marcescens infections associated with extrinsic contamination of a liquid nonmedicated soap. *Infect Control Hosp Epidemiol* **21:**196-9.

6619. **Sarwari, A. R., T. Strickland, C. Pena, and T. R. Burkot.** 2005. Tick exposure and Lyme disease at a summer camp in Maryland. *W V Med J* **101:**126-30.

6620. **Sas, D., M. A. Enrione, and R. H. Schwartz.** 2004. Pseudomonas aeruginosa septic shock secondary to "gripe water" ingestion. *Pediatr Infect Dis J* **23:**176-7.

6621. **Sasaki, K., Y. Tajiri, M. Sata, Y. Fujii, F. Matsubara, M. Zhao, S. Shimizu, A. Toyonaga, and K. Tanikawa.** 1999. Helicobacter pylori in the natural environment. *Scand J Infect Dis* **31:**275-9.

6622. **Sateren, W. B., P. O. Renzullo, J. K. Carr, D. L. Birx, and J. G. McNeil.** 2003. HIV-1 infection among civilian applicants for US military service, 1985 to 2000: epidemiology and geography. *J Acquir Immune Defic Syndr* **32:**215-22.

6623. **Sathe, P. V., V. N. Karandikar, M. D. Gupte, K. B. Niphadkar, B. N. Joshi, J. K. Polakhare, P. L. Jahagirdar, and N. S. Deodhar.** 1983. Investigation report of an epidemic of typhoid fever. *Int J Epidemiol* **12:**215-9.

6624. **Sato, H., H. Kamiya, and H. Furuoka.** 2003. Epidemiological aspects of the first outbreak of Baylisascaris procyonis larva migrans in rabbits in Japan. *J Vet Med Sci* **65:**453-7.

6625. **Sato, K., T. Morishita, E. Nobusawa, Y. Suzuki, Y. Miyazaki, Y. Fukui, S. Suzuki, and K. Nakajima.** 2000. Surveillance of influenza viruses isolated from travellers at Nagoya International Airport. *Epidemiol Infect* **124:**507-14.

6626. **Sato, Y., and M. Otsuru.** 1983. Studies on eosinophilic meningitis and meningoencephalitis caused by Angiostrongylus cantonensis in Japan. *Southeast Asian J Trop Med Public Health* **14:**515-24.

6627. **Sattabongkot, J., T. Tsuboi, G. E. Zollner, J. Sirichaisinthop, and L. Cui.** 2004. Plasmodium vivax transmission: chances for control? *Trends Parasitol* **20:**192-8.

6628. **Sattar, S. A., H. Jacobsen, V. S. Springthorpe, T. M. Cusack, and J. R. Rubino.** 1993. Chemical disinfection to interrupt transfer of rhinovirus type 14 from environmental surfaces to hands. *Appl Environ Microbiol* **59:**1579-85.

6629. **Saubolle, M. A., and D. Sussland.** 2003. Nocardiosis: review of clinical and laboratory experience. *J Clin Microbiol* **41:**4497-501.

6630. **Savage, H. M., C. Ceianu, G. Nicolescu, N. Karabatsos, R. Lanciotti, A. Vladimirescu, L. Laiv, A. Ungureanu, C. Romanca, and T. F. Tsai.** 1999. Entomologic and avian investigations of an epidemic of West Nile fever in Romania in 1996, with serologic and molecular characterization of a virus isolate from mosquitoes. *Am J Trop Med Hyg* **61:**600-11.

6631. **Savage, H. M., C. L. Fritz, D. Rutstein, A. Yolwa, V. Vorndam, and D. J. Gubler.** 1998. Epidemic of dengue-4 virus in Yap State, Federated States of Micronesia, and implication of Aedes hensilli as an epidemic vector. *Am J Trop Med Hyg* **58:**519-24.

6632. **Savolainen, C., and T. Hovi.** 2003. Caveat: poliovirus may be hiding under other labels. *Lancet* **361:**1145-6.

6633. **Sawamura, R., I. Machado Fernandes, L. C. Peres, L. C. Galvao, H. A. Goldani, S. M. Jorge, G. de Melo Rocha, and N. M. de Souza.** 1999. Hepatic capillariasis in children: report of 3 cases in Brazil. *Am J Trop Med Hyg* **61:**642-7.

6634. **Sawayama, Y., J. Hayashi, Y. Etoh, H. Urabe, K. Minami, and S. Kashiwagi.** 1999. Heterosexual transmission of GB virus C/hepatitis G virus infection to non-intravenous drug-using female prostitutes in Fukuoka, Japan. *Dig Dis Sci* **44:**1937-43.

6635. **Sawayama, Y., J. Hayashi, K. Kakuda, N. Furusyo, I. Ariyama, Y. Kawakami, N. Kinukawa, and S. Kashiwagi.** 2000. Hepatitis C virus infection in institutionalized psychiatric patients: possible role of transmission by razor sharing. *Dig Dis Sci* **45:**351-6.

6636. **Sax, H., S. Dharan, and D. Pittet.** 2002. Legionnaires' disease in a renal transplant recipient: nosocomial or home-grown? *Transplantation* **74:**890-2.

6637. **Sax, H., C. Ruef, and D. Pittet.** 2004. Resultate der schweizerischen Prävalenzstudie nosokomialer Infektionen 2003 (snip03). *Swiss Noso* **11:**1-5.

6638. **Sax, P. E.** 2001. Opportunistic infections in HIV disease: down but not out. *Infect Dis Clin North Am* **15:**433-55.

6639. **Saxen, H., and M. Virtanen.** 1999. Randomized, placebo-controlled double blind study on the efficacy of influenza immunization on absenteeism of health care workers. *Pediatr Infect Dis J* **18:**779-83.

6640. **Saxena, A. K., B. R. Panhotra, M. Naguib, W. Uzzaman, and M. K. Al.** 2002. Nosocomial transmission of syphilis during haemodialysis in a developing country. *Scand J Infect Dis* **34:**88-92.

6641. **Saygun, I., A. Kubar, A. Ozdemir, and J. Slots.** 2005. Periodontitis lesions are a source of salivary cytomegalovirus and Epstein-Barr virus. *J Periodontal Res* **40:**187-191.

6642. **Scaglia, M., R. Brustia, S. Gatti, A. M. Bernuzzi, M. Strosselli, A. Malfitano, and D. Capelli.** 1984. Autochthonous strongyloidiasis in Italy: an epidemiological and clinical review of 150 cases. *Bull Soc Pathol Exot Filiales* **77:**328-32.

6643. **Scaglia, M., S. Gatti, A. Bruno, C. Cevini, L. Marchi, and P. G. Sargeaunt.** 1991. Autochthonous amoebiasis in institutionalized mentally-retarded patients: preliminary evaluation of isoenzyme patterns in three isolates. *Ann Trop Med Parasitol* **85:**509-13.

6644. **Scales, D., K. Green, A. K. Chan, S. M. Poutanen, D. Foster, K. Nowak, J. M. Raboud, R. Saskin, S. E. Lapinsky, and T. E. Stewart.** 2003. Illness in intensive care staff after brief exposure to severe acute respiratory syndrome. *Emerg Infect Dis* **9:**1205-10.

6645. **Scallan, E., M. Fitzgerald, C. Collins, D. Crowley, L. Daly, M. Devine, D. Igoe, T. Quigley, T. Robinson, and B. Smyth.** 2004. Acute gastroenteritis in northern Ireland and the Republic of Ireland: a telephone survey. *Commun Dis Public Health* **7:**61-7.

6646. **Scandrett, W. B., and A. A. Gajadhar.** 2004. Recovery of putative taeniid eggs from silt in water associated with an outbreak of bovine cysticercosis. *Can Vet J* **45:**758-60.

6647. **Schachter, J., and C. R. Dawson.** 2002. Elimination of blinding trachoma. *Curr Opin Infect Dis* **15:**491-5.

6648. **Schachter, J., M. Grossman, R. L. Sweet, J. Holt, C. Jordan, and E. Bishop.** 1986. Prospective study of perinatal transmission of Chlamydia trachomatis. *JAMA* **255:**3374-3377.

6649. **Schachter, J., and A. O. Osoba.** 1983. Lymphogranuloma venereum. *Br Med Bull* **39:**151-4.

6650. **Schacker, T., J. Zeh, H. L. Hu, E. Hill, and L. Corey.** 1998. Frequency of symptomatic and asymptomatic herpes simplex virus type 2 reactivations among human immunodeficiency virus-infected men. *J Infect Dis* **178:**1616-22.

6651. **Schaffner, A.** 2001. Pretransplant evaluation for infections in donors and recipients of solid organs. *Clin Infect Dis* **33 suppl 1:**S9-14.

6652. **Schantz, P. M., A. C. Moore, J. L. Munoz, B. J. Hartman, J. A. Schaefer, A. M. Aron, D. Persaud, E. Sarti, M. Wilson, and A. Flisser.** 1992. Neurocysticercosis in an Orthodox Jewish community in New York City. *N Engl J Med* **327:**692-5.

6653. **Schaumberg, D. A., K. K. Snow, and M. R. Dana.** 1998. The epidemic of Acanthamoeba keratitis: where do we stand? *Cornea* **17:**3-10.

6654. **Scheil, W., S. Cameron, C. Dalton, C. Murray, and D. Wilson.** 1998. A South Australian Salmonella Mbandaka outbreak investigation using a database to select controls. *Aust N Z J Public Health* **22:**536-9.

6655. **Schelenz, S., and G. French.** 2000. An outbreak of multidrug-resistant Pseudomonas aeruginosa infection associated with contamination of bronchoscopes and an endoscope washer-disinfector. *J Hosp Infect* **46:**23-30.

6656. **Schellekens, J., C. H. von Konig, and P. Gardner.** 2005. Pertussis sources of infection and routes of transmission in the vaccination era. *Pediatr Infect Dis J* **24:**S19-24.

6657. **Schellenberg, R. S., B. J. Tan, J. D. Irvine, D. R. Stockdale, A. A. Gajadhar, B. Serhir, J. Botha, C. A. Armstrong, S. A. Woods, J. M. Blondeau, and T. L. McNab.** 2003. An outbreak of trichinellosis due to consumption of bear meat infected with Trichinella nativa, in 2 northern Saskatchewan communities. *J Infect Dis* **188:**835-43.

6658. **Schelling, E., C. Diguimbaye, S. Daoud, J. Nicolet, P. Boerlin, M. Tanner, and J. Zinsstag.** 2003. Brucellosis and Q-fever seroprevalences of nomadic pastoralists and their livestock in Chad. *Prev Vet Med* **61:**279-93.

6659. **Schémann, J. F., C. Guinot, L. Ilboudo, G. Momo, B. Ko, O. Sanfo, B. Ramde, A. Ouedraogo, and D. Malvy.** 2003. Trachoma, flies and environmental factors in Burkino Faso. *Trans R Soc Trop Med Hyg* **97:**63-8.

6660. **Schémann, J. F., D. Sacko, D. Malvy, G. Momo, L. Traore, O. Bore, S. Coulibaly, and A. Banou.** 2002. Risk factors for trachoma in Mali. *Int J Epidemiol* **31:**194-201.

6661. **Schembre, D. B.** 2000. Infectious complications associated with gastrointestinal endoscopy. *Gastrointest Endosc Clin N Am* **10:**215-32.

6662. **Schets, F. M., G. B. Engels, and E. G. Evers.** 2004. Cryptosporidium and Giardia in swimming pools in the Netherlands. *J Water Health* **2:**191-200.

6663. **Schilling, M., L. Povinelli, P. Krause, M. Gravenstein, A. Ambrozaitis, H. H. Jones, P. Drinka, P. Shult, D. Powers, and S. Gravenstein.** 1998. Efficacy of zanamivir for chemoprophylaxis of nursing home influenza outbreaks. *Vaccine* **16:**1771-4.

6664. **Schlagenhauf, P., R. Steffen, and L. Loutan.** 2003. Migrants as a major risk group for imported malaria in European countries. *J Travel Med* **10:**106-7.

6665. **Schlagenhauf-Lawlor, P.** 2001. Travelers' malaria. BC Decker Inc., Hamilton, Ontario, Canada.

6666. **Schlapfer, G., J. D. Cherry, U. Heininger, M. Uberall, S. Schmitt-Grohe, S. Laussucq, M. Just, and K. Stehr.** 1995. Polymerase chain reaction identification of Bordetella pertussis infections in vaccinees and family members in a pertussis vaccine efficacy trial in Germany. *Pediatr Infect Dis J* **14:**209-14.

6667. **Schlech, W. F., 3rd.** 2000. Foodborne listeriosis. *Clin Infect Dis* **31:**770-5.

6668. **Schlech, W. F., 3rd, G. W. Gorman, M. C. Payne, and C. V. Broome.** 1985. Legionnaires' disease in the Caribbean. An outbreak associated with a resort hotel. *Arch Intern Med* **145:**2076-9.

6669. **Schlech, W. F., 3rd, P. M. Lavigne, R. A. Bortolussi, A. C. Allen, E. V. Haldane, A. J. Wort, A. W. Hightower, S. E. Johnson, S. H. King, E. S. Nicholls, and C. V. Broome.** 1983. Epidemic listeriosis—evidence for transmission by food. *N Engl J Med* **308:**203-6.

6670. **Schlech, W. F., 3rd, L. J. Wheat, J. L. Ho, M. L. French, R. J. Weeks, R. B. Kohler, C. E. Deane, H. E. Eitzen, and J. D. Band.** 1983. Recurrent urban histoplasmosis, Indianapolis, Indiana, 1980-1981. *Am J Epidemiol* **118:**301-12.

6671. **Schlegel, L., F. Grimont, E. Ageron, P. A. Grimont, and A. Bouvet.** 2003. Reappraisal of the taxonomy of the Streptococcus bovis/Streptococcus equinus complex and related species: description of Streptococcus gallolyticus subsp. gallolyticus subsp. nov., S. gallolyticus subsp. macedonicus subsp. nov. and S. gallolyticus subsp. pasteurianus subsp. nov. *Int J Syst Evol Microbiol* **53:**631-45.

6672. **Schleicher, S., A. Normann, M. Gregor, G. Hess, and B. Flehming.** 1997. Hepatitis G virus infection. *Lancet* **349:**954-5.

6673. **Schlemper, B. R., Jr., M. Steindel, E. C. Grisard, C. J. Carvalho-Pinto, O. J. Bernardini, C. V. de Castilho, G. Rosa, S. Kilian, A. A. Guarneri, A. Rocha, Z. Medeiros, and J. A. Ferreira Neto.** 2000. Elimination of bancroftian filariasis (Wuchereria bancrofti) in Santa Catarina state, Brazil. *Trop Med Int Health* **5:**848-54.

6674. **Schliessler, K. H., B. Rozendaal, C. Taal, and S. G. Meawissen.** 1980. Outbreak of Salmonella agona infection after upper intestinal fibreoptic endoscopy. *Lancet* **2:**1246.

6675. **Schlossberg, D.** 2001. Infections from leisure-time activities. *Microbes Infect* **3:**509-14.

6676. **Schlosser, O., D. Grall, and M. N. Laurenceau.** 1999. Intestinal parasite carriage in workers exposed to sewage. *Eur J Epidemiol* **15:**261-5.

6677. **Schlosser, R. L., A. Zubcov, M. Bollinger, M. Kuhnert, and V. Loewenich.** 1993. [Congenital candida infections]. *Monatsschr Kinderheilkd* **141:**864-7.

6678. **Schmid, G., and A. Kaufmann.** 2002. Anthrax in Europe: its epidemiology, clinical characteristics, and role in bioterrorism. *Clin Microbiol Inf* **8**:479-88.

6679. **Schmid, G. P., A. Buve, P. Mugyenyi, G. P. Garnett, R. J. Hayes, B. G. Williams, J. G. Calleja, K. M. De Cock, J. A. Whitworth, S. H. Kapiga, P. D. Ghys, C. Hankins, B. Zaba, R. Heimer, and J. T. Boerma.** 2004. Transmission of HIV-1 infection in sub-Saharan Africa and effect of elimination of unsafe injections. *Lancet* **363**:482-8.

6680. **Schmid, G. P., R. E. Schaefer, B. D. Plikaytis, J. R. Schaefer, J. H. Bryner, L. A. Wintermeyer, and A. F. Kaufmann.** 1987. A one-year study of endemic campylobacteriosis in a midwestern city: associationwith consumption of raw milk. *J Infect Dis* **156**:218-22.

6681. **Schmid, H., and A. Baumgartner.** 2001. Campylobacter and Salmonella - Stand Ende August 2001. *Bull BAG* **52**:1012-14.

6682. **Schmidt, A., C. F. Noldechen, W. Mendling, W. Hatzmann, and M. H. Wolff.** 1997. [Oral contraception and vaginal candida colonization]. *Zentralbl Gynäkol* **119**:545-9.

6683. **Schmidt, K.** 1995. WHO surveillance programme for control of foodborne infections and intoxications in Europe. Federal Institute for health protection of consumers and veterinary medicine (FAO/WHO collaborating centre for research and training in food hygiene and zoonoses), Berlin.

6684. **Schmidt, S. M., C. E. Müller, B. Mahner, and S. K. W. Wiersbitzky.** 2002. Prevalence, rate of persistence and respiratory tract symptoms of Chlamydia pneumoniae infection in 1211 kindergarten and school age children. *Pediatr infect Dis J* **21**:758-62.

6685. **Schmitt, D. L., D. W. Johnson, and F. W. Henderson.** 1991. Herpes simplex type 1 infections in group day care. *Pediatr Infect Dis J* **10**:729-34.

6686. **Schmitt, S. M., D. J. O'Brien, C. S. Bruning-Fann, and S. D. Fitzgerald.** 2002. Bovine tuberculosis in Michigan wildlife and livestock. *Ann N Y Acad Sci* **969**:262-8.

6687. **Schmitz, H., P. Emmerich, and J. ter Meulen.** 1996. Imported tropical virus infections in Germany. *Arch Virol Suppl* **11**:67-74.

6688. **Schmunis, G. A., F. Zicker, J. R. Cruz, and P. Cuchi.** 2001. Safety of blood supply for infectious diseases in Latin American countries, 1994-1997. *Am J Trop Med Hyg* **65**:924-30.

6689. **Schmutzhard, E., G. Stanek, M. Pletschette, A. M. Hirschl, A. Pallua, R. Schmitzberger, and R. Schlogl.** 1988. Infections following tickbites. Tick-borne encephalitis and Lyme borreliosis—a prospective epidemiological study from Tyrol. *Infection* **16**:269-72.

6690. **Schnagl, R. D., K. Belfrage, R. Farrington, K. Hutchinson, V. Lewis, J. Erlich, and F. Morey.** 2002. Incidence of human astrovirus in central Australia (1995 to 1998) and comparison of deduced serotypes detected from 1981 to 1998. *J Clin Microbiol* **40**:4114-20.

6691. **Schneider, E., R. A. Hajjeh, R. A. Spiegel, R. W. Jibson, E. L. Harp, G. A. Marshall, R. A. Gunn, M. M. McNeil, R. W. Pinner, R. C. Baron, R. C. Burger, L. C. Hutwagner, C. Crump, L. Kaufman, S. E. Reef, G. M. Feldman, D. Pappagianis, and S. B. Werner.** 1997. A coccidioidomycosis outbreak following the Northridge, Calif, earthquake. *JAMA* **277**:904-8.

6692. **Schneider, L., R. Geha, and W. G. Magnuson.** 1994. Outbreak of hepatitis C associated with intravenous immunoglobulin administration - United States, October 1993-June 1994. *MMWR* **43**:505-9.

6693. **Schneider, M. C., C. Santos-Burgoa, A. J., B. Munoz, S. Ruiz-Velazco, and W. Uieda.** 1996. Potential force of infection of human rabies transmitted by vampire bats in the Amazonian region of Brazil. *Am J Trop Med Hyg* **55**:680-4.

6694. **Schneider, T., H. U. Jahn, D. Steinhoff, H. M. Guschoreck, O. Liesenfeld, H. Mater-Bohm, A. L. Wesirow, H. Lode, W. D. Ludwig, T. Dissmann, et al.** 1993. [A Q fever epidemic in Berlin. The epidemiological and clinical aspects]. *Dtsch Med Wochenschr* **118**:689-95.

6695. **Schocken-Iturrino, R. P., M. C. Carneiro, E. Kato, J. O. Sorbara, O. D. Rossi, and L. E. Gerbasi.** 1999. Study of the presence of the spores of Clostridium botulinum in honey in Brazil. *FEMS Immunol Med Microbiol* **24**:379-82.

6696. **Schoenbaum, S. C., O. Baker, and Z. Jezek.** 1976. Common-source epidemic of hepatitis due to glazed and iced pastries. *Am J Epidemiol* **104**:74-80.

6697. **Schoenlaub, P., and P. Plantin.** 2000. [Warts and molluscum contagiosum: practical point of view]. *Arch Pediatr* **7**:1103-10.

6698. **Schofield, F.** 1986. Selective primary health care: strategies for control of disease in the developing world. XXII. Tetanus: a preventable problem. *Rev Infect Dis* **8**:144-56.

6699. **Schorr, D., H. Schmid, L. Rieder, A. Baumgartner, H. Vorkauf, and A. Burnens.** 1994. Risk factors for Campylobacter enteritis in Switzerland. *Zbl Hyg* **196**:327-37.

6700. **Schottelius, J., G. D. Burchard, and I. Sobottka.** 2003. [Microsporidiosis in humans: parasitology, clinical features and treatment]. *Dtsch Med Wochenschr* **128**:87-91.

6701. **Schou, S., and A. K. Hansen.** 2000. Marburg and Ebola virus infections in laboratory non-human primates: a literature review. *Comp Med* **50**:108-23.

6702. **Schrag, S., R. Gorwitz, K. Fultz-Butts, and A. Schuchat.** 2002. Prevention of perinatal group B streptococcal disease. Revised guidelines from CDC. *MMWR* **51 (RR-11)**:1-22.

6703. **Schrag, S. J., E. R. Zell, R. Lynfield, A. Roome, K. E. Arnold, A. S. Craig, L. H. Harrison, A. Reingold, K. Stefonek, G. Smith, M. Gamble, and A. Schuchat.** 2002. A population-based comparison of strategies to prevent early-onset group B streptococcal disease in neonates. *N Engl J Med* **347**:233-9.

6704. **Schubach, T. M. P., F. B. Figueiredo, S. A. Pereira, M. F. Madeira, I. B. Santos, M. V. Andrade, T. Cuzzi, M. C. Marzochi, and A. Schubach.** 2004. American cutaneous leishmaniasis in two cats from Rio de Janeiro, Brazil: first report of natural infection with Leishmania (Viannia) braziliensis. *Trans R Soc Trop Med Hyg* **98**:165-7.

6705. **Schubiger, G., J. Munzinger, C. Dudli, and U. Wipfli.** 1986. Meningokokken-Epidemie in einer Internatsschule: Sekundärerkrankungen mit rifampicin-resistentem Erreger unter Chemoprophylaxe. *Schweiz Med Wochenschr* **116**:1172-1175.

6706. **Schuchat, A., T. Hilger, E. Zell, M. M. Farley, A. Reingold, L. Harrison, L. Lefkowitz, R. Danila, K. Stefonek, N. Barrett, D. Morse, and R. Pinner.** 2001. Active bacterial core surveillance of the emerging infections program network. *Emerg Infect Dis* **7**:92-9.

6707. **Schuchat, A., and J. D. Wenger.** 1994. Epidemiology of group B streptococcal disease. Risk factors, prevention strategies, and vaccine development. *Epidemiol Rev* **16**:374-402.

6708. **Schulpen, T. W. J., A. H. J. Van Seventer, H. C. Rümke, and A. M. Van Loon.** 2001. Immunisation status of children adopted from China. *Lancet* **358**:2131-2132.

6709. **Schulte, C., M. Schunk, and B. Krebs.** 2002. Mit Speck fängt man nicht nur Mäuse. Eine atraumatische Behandlungsmethode der kutanen Myiasis. *Dtsch Med Wochenschr* **127:**266-8.

6710. **Schulte, J. M., S. E. Valway, E. McCray, and I. M. Onorato.** 2001. Tuberculosis cases reported among migrant farm workers in the United States, 1993-97. *J Health Care Poor Underserved* **12:**311-22.

6711. **Schultsz, C., H. H. Meester, A. M. Kranenburg, P. H. Savelkoul, L. E. Boeijen-Donkers, A. M. Kaiser, R. de Bree, G. B. Snow, and C. J. Vandenbroucke-Grauls.** 2003. Ultra-sonic nebulizers as a potential source of methicillin-resistant Staphylococcus aureus causing an outbreak in a university tertiary care hospital. *J Hosp Infect* **55:**269-75.

6712. **Schultze, D., A. Lundkvist, U. Blauenstein, and P. Heyman.** 2002. Tula virus infection associated with fever and exanthema after a wild rodent bite. *Eur J Clin Microbiol Infect Dis* **21:**304-6.

6713. **Schulze, K.** 1988. Erkrankungen nach dem Verzehr von massiv mit Sarkosporidien befallenem Rehfleisch. *Fleischwirtschaft* **68:**1139-40.

6714. **Schupp, P., M. Pfeffer, H. Meyer, G. Burck, K. Kolmel, and C. Neumann.** 2001. Cowpox virus in a 12-year-old boy: rapid identification by an orthopoxvirus-specific polymerase chain reaction. *Br J Dermatol* **145:**146-50.

6715. **Schuster, F. L.** 2002. Cultivation of Babesia and Babesia-like blood parasites: agents of an emerging zoonotic disease. *Clin Microbiol Rev* **15:**365-73.

6716. **Schuster, F. L., T. H. Dunnebacke, G. C. Booton, S. Yagi, C. K. Kohlmeier, C. Glaser, D. Vugia, A. Bakardjiev, P. Azimi, M. Maddux-Gonzalez, A. J. Martinez, and G. S. Visvesvara.** 2003. Environmental isolation of Balamuthia mandrillaris associated with a case of amebic encephalitis. *J Clin Microbiol* **41:**3175-80.

6717. **Schuster, R., A. Kaufmann, and S. Hering.** 1997. [Investigations on the endoparasitic fauna of domestic cats in eastern Brandenburg]. *Berl Munch Tierarztl Wochenschr* **110:**48-50.

6718. **Schutt, M., P. Gerke, H. Meisel, R. Ulrich, and D. H. Kruger.** 2001. Clinical characterization of Dobrava hantavirus infections in Germany. *Clin Nephrol* **55:**371-4.

6719. **Schutze, G. E., E. O. Mason, Jr., W. J. Barson, K. S. Kim, E. R. Wald, L. B. Givner, T. Q. Tan, J. S. Bradley, R. Yogev, and S. L. Kaplan.** 2002. Invasive pneumococcal infections in children with asplenia. *Pediatr Infect Dis J* **21:**278-82.

6720. **Schutze, G. E., J. D. Sikes, R. Stefanova, and M. D. Cave.** 1999. The home environment and salmonellosis in children. *Pediatrics* **103:**E1.

6721. **Schuurkamp, G. J., and R. K. Kereu.** 1989. Resistance of Plasmodium falciparum to chemotherapy with 4- aminoquinolines in the Ok Tedi area of Papua New Guinea. *P N G Med J* **32:**33-44.

6722. **Schvarcz, R., B. Johansson, B. Nystrom, and A. Sonnerborg.** 1997. Nosocomial transmission of hepatitis C virus. *Infection* **25:**74-7.

6723. **Schvoerer, C.** 2001. La psittacose: une pathologie émergente en milieu professionnel? *Méd Mal Infect* **31 suppl 2:**S217-25.

6724. **Schvoerer, E., F. Bonnet, V. Dubois, G. Cazaux, R. Serceau, H. J. Fleury, and M. E. Lafon.** 2000. PCR detection of human enteric viruses in bathing areas, waste waters and human stools in Southwestern France. *Res Microbiol* **151:**693-701.

6725. **Schwab, C. J., and D. C. Straus.** 2004. The roles of Penicillium and Aspergillus in sick building syndrome. *Adv Appl Microbiol* **55:**215-38.

6726. **Schwan, T. G., P. F. Policastro, Z. Miller, R. L. Thompson, T. Damrow, and J. E. Keirans.** 2003. Tick-borne relapsing fever caused by Borrelia hermsii, Montana. *Emerg Infect Dis* **9:**1151-4.

6727. **Schwarcz, S., T. Kellogg, W. McFarland, B. Louie, R. Kohn, M. Busch, M. Katz, G. Bolan, J. Klausner, and H. Weinstock.** 2001. Differences in the temporal trends of HIV seroincidence and seroprevalence among sexually transmitted disease clinic patients, 1989- 1998: application of the serologic testing algorithm for recent HIV seroconversion. *Am J Epidemiol* **153:**925-34.

6728. **Schwartz, B., and M. D. Goldstein.** 1990. Lyme disease in outdoor workers: risk factors, preventive measures, and tick removal methods. *Am J Epidemiol* **131:**877-85.

6729. **Schwartz, B., L. H. Harrison, J. S. Motter, R. N. Motter, A. W. Hightower, and C. V. Broome.** 1989. Investigation of an outbreak of Moraxella conjunctivitis at a Navajo boarding school. *Am J Ophthalmol* **107:**341-7.

6730. **Schwartz, E., and H. Gur.** 2002. Dermatobia hominis Myiasis: An Emerging Disease among Travelers to the Amazon Basin of Bolivia. *J Travel Med* **9:**97-9.

6731. **Schwartz, E., N. P. Jenks, P. Van Damme, and E. Galun.** 1999. Hepatitis E virus infection in travelers. *Clin Infect Dis* **29:**1312-4.

6732. **Schwartz, M. A., S. R. Tabet, A. C. Collier, C. K. Wallis, L. C. Carlson, T. T. Nguyen, M. M. Kattar, and M. B. Coyle.** 2002. Central venous catheter-related bacteremia due to Tsukamurella species in the immunocompromised host: a case series and review of the literature. *Clin Infect Dis* **35:**e72-7.

6733. **Schwartz, R. A.** 2004. Superficial fungal infections. *Lancet* **364:**1173-82.

6734. **Schwarz, T. F., G. Jager, S. Gilch, and C. Pauli.** 1995. Serosurvey and laboratory diagnosis of imported sandfly fever virus, serotype Toscana, infection in Germany. *Epidemiol Infect* **114:**501-10.

6735. **Schwebke, J. R., and E. W. Hook, 3rd.** 2003. High rates of Trichomonas vaginalis among men attending a sexually transmitted diseases clinic: implications for screening and urethritis management. *J Infect Dis* **188:**465-8.

6736. **Scieux, C., R. Barnes, A. Bianchi, I. Casin, P. Morel, and Y. Perol.** 1989. Lymphogranuloma venereum: 27 cases in Paris. *J Infect Dis* **160:**662-8.

6737. **Sclar, E. D., P. Garau, and G. Carolini.** 2005. The 21st century health challenge of slums and cities. *Lancet* **365:**901-3.

6738. **Scolari, C., C. Torti, A. Beltrame, A. Matteelli, F. Castelli, M. Gulletta, M. Ribas, S. Morana, and C. Urbani.** 2000. Prevalence and distribution of soil-transmitted helminth (STH) infections in urban and indigenous schoolchildren in Ortigueira, State of Parana, Brasil: implications for control. *Trop Med Int Health* **5:**302-7.

6739. **Scolnik, D., L. Aronson, R. Lovinsky, K. Toledano, R. Glazier, J. Eisenstadt, P. Eisenberg, L. Wilcox, R. Rowsell, and M. Silverman.** 2003. Efficacy of a targeted, oral penicillin-based yaws control program among children living in rural South America. *Clin Infect Dis* **36:**1232-8.

6740. **Scopel, K. K., C. J. Fontes, A. C. Nunes, M. F. Horta, and E. M. Braga.** 2004. High prevalence of Plamodium malariae infections in a Brazilian Amazon endemic area (Apiacas-Mato Grosso State) as detected by polymerase chain reaction. *Acta Trop* **90**:61-4.

6741. **Scott, E.** 2000. Relationship between cross-contamination and the transmission of foodborne pathogens in the home. *Pediatr Infect Dis J* **19**:S111-3.

6742. **Scott, G. A. J.** 1995. Canada's vegetation. A world perspective. McGill-Queen's University Press, Montreal.

6743. **Scott, J. D., K. Fernando, S. N. Banerjee, L. A. Durden, S. K. Byrne, M. Banerjee, R. B. Mann, and M. G. Morshed.** 2001. Birds disperse ixodid (Acari: Ixodidae) and Borrelia burgdorferi-infected ticks in Canada. *J Med Entomol* **38**:493-500.

6744. **Scott, P. T., D. W. Niebuhr, J. B. McGready, and J. C. Gaydos.** 2005. Hepatitis B immunity in United States military recruits. *J Infect Dis* **191**:1835-41.

6745. **Scoular, A., J. Norrie, G. Gillespie, N. Mir, and W. F. Carman.** 2002. Longitudinal study of genital infection by herpes simplex virus type 1 in western Scotland over 15 years. *BMJ* **324**:1366-7.

6746. **Scrimgeour, E. M., A. Zaki, F. R. Mehta, A. K. Abraham, S. Al-Busaidy, H. El-Khatim, S. F. Al-Rawas, A. M. Kamal, and A. J. Mohammed.** 1996. Crimean-Congo haemorrhagic fever in Oman. *Trans R Soc Trop Med Hyg* **90**:290-1.

6747. **Scudamore, J. M., G. M. Trevelyan, M. V. Tas, E. M. Varley, and G. A. Hickman.** 2002. Carcass disposal: lessons from Great Britain following the foot and mouth disease outbreaks of 2001. *Rev Sci Tech* **21**:775-87.

6748. **Seal, D., F. Stapleton, and J. Dart.** 1992. Possible environmental sources of Acanthamoeba spp in contact lens wearers. *Br J Ophthalmol* **76**:424-7.

6749. **Seals, J. E., J. D. Snyder, T. A. Edell, C. L. Hatheway, C. J. Johnson, R. C. Swanson, and J. M. Hughes.** 1981. Restaurant-associated type A botulism: transmission by potato salad. *Am J Epidemiol* **113**:436-44.

6750. **Sebai, Z. A.** 1988. Malaria in Saudi Arabia. *Trop Doct* **18**:183-8.

6751. **Sebert, M. E., M. L. Manning, K. L. McGowan, E. R. Alpern, and L. M. Bell.** 2002. An outbreak of Serratia marcescens bacteremia after general anesthesia. *Infect Control Hosp Epidemiol* **23**:733-9.

6752. **Sedyaningsih-Mamahit, E. R., R. P. Larasati, K. Laras, A. Sidemen, N. Sukri, N. Sabaruddin, S. Didi, J. M. Saragih, K. S. Myint, T. P. Endy, A. Sulaiman, J. R. Campbell, and A. L. Corwin.** 2002. First documented outbreak of hepatitis E virus transmission in Java, Indonesia. *Trans R Soc Trop Med Hyg* **96**:398-404.

6753. **Seepersadsingh, N., A. A. Adesiyun, and R. Seebaransingh.** 2004. Prevalence and antimicrobial resistance of Salmonella spp. in non-diarrhoeic dogs in Trinidad. *J Vet Med B Infect Dis Vet Public Health* **51**:337-42.

6754. **Segura Del Pozo, J., J. C. Sanz Moreno, M. J. Gascon Sancho, E. Ramos Lledo, F. Ory Manchon Fd, and M. Fernandez Diaz.** 2002. [Pertussis outbreak in a poorly immunized community]. *Med Clin (Barc)* **119**:601-4.

6755. **Segura, E. L., E. N. Cura, S. A. Estani, J. Andrade, J. C. Lansetti, A. M. de Rissio, A. Campanini, S. B. Blanco, R. E. Gurtler, and M. Alvarez.** 2000. Long-term effects of a nationwide control program on the seropositivity for Trypanosoma cruzi infection in young men from Argentina. *Am J Trop Med Hyg* **62**:353-62.

6756. **Segura-Porta, F., G. Diestre-Ortin, A. Ortuno-Romero, I. Sanfeliu-Sala, B. Font-Creus, T. Munoz-Espin, E. M. de Antonio, and J. Casal-Fabrega.** 1998. Prevalence of antibodies to spotted fever group rickettsiae in human beings and dogs from and endemic area of mediterranean spotted fever in Catalonia, Spain. *Eur J Epidemiol* **14**:395-8.

6757. **Sehgal, V. N., and A. L. S. Prasad.** 1986. Donovanosis. Current concepts. *Int J Dermatol* **25**:8-16.

6758. **Sehulster, L., and R. Y. Chinn.** 2003. Guidelines for environmental infection control in health-care facilities. Recommendations of CDC and the Healthcare Infection Control Practices Advisory Committee (HICPAC). *MMWR* **52 (RR-10)**:1-42.

6759. **Seidler, A., A. Nienhaus, and R. Diel.** 2005. Review of epidemiological studies on the occupational risk of tuberculosis in low-incidence areas. *Respiration* **72**:431-46.

6760. **Seijo, A., D. Curcio, G. Aviles, B. Cernigoi, B. Deodato, and S. Lloveras.** 2000. Imported dengue in Buenos Aires, Argentina. *Emerg Infect Dis* **6**:655-6.

6761. **Sejvar, J., E. Bancroft, K. Winthrop, J. Bettinger, M. Bajani, S. Bragg, K. Shutt, R. Kaiser, N. Marano, T. Popovic, J. Tappero, D. Ashford, L. Mascola, D. Vugia, B. Perkins, and N. Rosenstein.** 2003. Leptospirosis in "eco-challenge" athletes, Malaysian Borneo, 2000. *Emerg Infect Dis* **9**:702-7.

6762. **Sekla, L., W. Stackiw, S. Dzogan, and D. Sargeant.** 1989. Foodborne gastroenteritis due to Norwalk virus in a Winnipeg hotel. *CMAJ* **140**:1461-4.

6763. **Selik, R. M., M. K. Glynn, and M. T. McKenna.** 2004. Diagnoses of HIV/AIDS—32 States, 2000-2003. *MMWR* **53**:1106-10.

6764. **Sellers, R. F., and S. M. Daggupaty.** 1990. The epidemic of foot-and-mouth disease in Saskatchewan, Canada, 1951-1952. *Can J Vet Res* **54**:457-64.

6765. **Sellers, R. F., and A. R. Maarouf.** 1988. Impact of climate on western equine encephalitis in Manitoba, Minnesota and North Dakota, 1980-1983. *Epidemiol Infect* **101**:511-35.

6766. **Semel, J. D., and G. Trenholme.** 1990. Aeromonas hydrophila water-associated traumatic wound infections: a review. *J Trauma* **30**:324-7.

6767. **Semenas, L., A. Kreiter, and J. Urbanski.** 2001. New cases of human diphyllobothriasis in Patagonia, Argentina. *Rev Saude Publica* **35**:214-6.

6768. **Semret, M., G. Koromihis, J. D. MacLean, M. Libman, and B. J. Ward.** 1999. Mycobacterium ulcerans infection (Buruli ulcer): first reported case in a traveler. *Am J Trop Med Hyg* **61**:689-93.

6769. **Sencan, I., I. Sahin, D. Kaya, S. Oksuz, and A. Yildirim.** 2004. Assessment of HAV and HEV seroprevalence in children living in post-earthquake camps from Düzce, Turkey. *Eur J Epidemiol* **19**:461-5.

6770. **Sendra Gutierrez, J., D. Martin Rios, I. Casas, P. Saez, A. Tovar, and C. Moreno.** 2004. An outbreak of Adenovirus type 8 Keratoconjunctivitis in a nursing home in Madrid. *Eur Surveill* **9(3)**:27–30.

6771. **Senechal, M., R. Dorent, S. T. du Montcel, A. M. Fillet, J. J. Ghossoub, M. Dubois, A. Pavie, and I. Gandjbakhch.** 2003. Monitoring of human cytomegalovirus infections in heart transplant recipients by pp65 antigenemia. *Clin Transplant* **17**:423-7.

6772. Seng, C., P. Watkins, D. Morse, S. P. Barrett, M. Zambon, N. Andrews, M. Atkins, S. Hall, Y. K. Lau, and B. J. Cohen. 1994. Parvovirus B19 outbreak on an adult ward. *Epidemiol Infect* **113**:345-53.

6773. Senol, E., J. DesJardin, P. C. Stark, L. Barefoot, and D. R. Snydman. 2002. Attributable mortality of Stenotrophomonas maltophilia bacteremia. *Clin Infect Dis* **34**:1653-6.

6774. Sentjens, R. E. J. H., Y. Sisay, H. Vrielink, D. Kebede, H. J. Adèr, G. Leckie, and H. W. Reesink. 2002. Prevalence of and risk factors for HIV infection in blood donors and various population subgroups in Ethiopia. *Epidemiol Infect* **128**:221-8.

6775. Sepkowitz, K. A. 1996. How contagious is tuberculosis? *Clin Infect Dis* **23**:954-62.

6776. Sepkowitz, K. A. 2003. How contagious is vaccinia? *N Engl J Med* **348**:439-46.

6777. Seppänen, M., A. Virolainen-Julkunen, I. Kakko, P. Vilkamaa, and S. Meri. 2004. Myiasis during adventure sports race. *Emerg Infect Dis* **10**:137-9.

6778. Serbezov, V. S., J. Kazar, V. Novkirishki, N. Gatcheva, E. Kovacova, and V. Voynova. 1999. Q fever in Bulgaria and Slovakia. *Emerg Infect Dis* **5**:388-94.

6779. Sergiev, V. P., A. M. Baranova, V. S. Orlov, L. G. Mihajlov, R. L. Kouznetsov, N. I. Neujmin, L. P. Arsenieva, M. A. Shahova, L. A. Glagoleva, and M. M. Osipova. 1993. Importation of malaria into the USSR from Afghanistan, 1981-89. *Bull WHO* **71**:385-8.

6780. Serjeant, B. E., I. R. Hambleton, S. Kerr, C. G. Kilty, and G. R. Serjeant. 2001. Haematological response to parvovirus B19 infection in homozygous sickle-cell disease. *Lancet* **358**:1779-80.

6781. Serjeant, G. R., J. M. Topley, K. Mason, B. E. Serjeant, J. R. Pattison, S. E. Jones, and R. Mohamed. 1981. Outbreak of aplastic crises in sickle cell anaemia associated with parvovirus-like agent. *Lancet* **2**:595-7.

6782. Sermet-Gaudelus, I., M. Le Bourgeois, C. Pierre-Audigier, C. Offredo, D. Guillemot, S. Halley, C. Akoua-Koffi, V. Vincent, V. Sivadon-Tardy, A. Ferroni, P. Berche, P. Scheinmann, G. Lenoir, and J. L. Gaillard. 2003. Mycobacterium abscessus and children with cystic fibrosis. *Emerg Infect Dis* **9**:1587-91.

6783. Setasuban, P., W. Punsri, and C. Meunnoo. 1980. Transmammary transmission of Necator americanus larva in the human host. *Southeast Asian J Trop Med Public Health* **11**:535-8.

6784. Sethi, D., P. Cumberland, M. J. Hudson, L. C. Rodrigues, J. G. Wheeler, J. A. Roberts, D. S. Tompkins, J. M. Cowden, and P. J. Roderick. 2001. A study of infectous intestinal disease in England: risk factors associated with group A rotavirus in children. *Epidemiol Infect* **126**:63-70.

6785. Sethi, S., and T. F. Murphy. 2001. Bacterial infection in chronic obstructive pulmonary disease in 2000: a state-of-the-art review. *Clin Microbiol Rev* **14**:336-63.

6786. Sethi, S., M. Sharma, P. Ray, M. Singh, and A. Gupta. 2001. Mycobacterium fortuitum wound infection following laparoscopy. *Indian J Med Res* **113**:83-4.

6787. Seuri, M., J. Koivunen, K. Granfors, and H. Heinonen-Tanski. 2005. Work-related symptoms and Salmonella antibodies among wastewater treatment plant workers. *Epidemiol Infect* **133**:603-9.

6788. Severo, C. A., P. Abensur, Y. Buisson, A. Lafuma, B. Detournay, and M. Pechevis. 1997. An outbreak of hepatitis A in a French day-care center and efforts to combat it. *Eur J Epidemiol* **13**:139-44.

6789. Sevilla-Casas, E. 1993. Human mobility and malaria risk in the Naya river basin of Colombia. *Soc Sci Med* **37**:1155-67.

6790. Seward, J. F., J. X. Zhang, T. J. Maupin, L. Mascola, and A. O. Jumaan. 2004. Contagiousness of varicella in vaccinated cases: a household contact study. *JAMA* **292**:704-8.

6791. Sewell, D. L. 1995. Laboratory-associated infections and biosafety. *Clin Microbiol Rev* **8**:389-405.

6792. Sexton, D. J., G. R. Corey, J. C. Greenfield, Jr., C. S. Burton, and D. Raoult. 1999. Imported African tick bite fever: a case report. *Am J Trop Med Hyg* **60**:865-7.

6793. Sexton, D. J., B. Dwyer, R. Kemp, and S. Graves. 1991. Spotted fever group rickettsial infections in Australia. *Rev Infect Dis* **13**:876-86.

6794. Sexton, D. J., and K. S. Kaye. 2002. Rocky mountain spotted fever. *Med Clin North Am* **86**:351-60, vii-viii.

6795. Sexton, D. J., M. R. Muniz, G. R. Corey, E. B. Breitschwerdt, B. C. Hegarty, S. Dumler, D. H. Walker, P. M. Pecanha, and R. Dietze. 1993. Brazilian spotted fever in Espirito Santo, Brazil: description of a focus of infection in a new endemic region. *Am J Trop Med Hyg* **49**:222-6.

6796. Sexton, D. J., P. E. Rollin, and E. B. Breitschwerdt. 1997. Life-threatening Cache Valley virus infection. *N Engl J Med* **336**:547-49.

6797. Shah, I., M. Rowland, P. Mehmood, C. Mujahid, F. Razique, S. Hewitt, and N. Durrani. 1997. Chloroquine resistance in Pakistan and the upsurge of falciparum malaria in Pakistani and Afghan refugee populations. *Ann Trop Med Parasitol* **91**:591-602.

6798. Shah, K. V. 2004. Simian virus 40 and human disease. *J Infect Dis* **190**:2061-4.

6799. Shah, N., C. Hing, K. Tucker, and R. Crawford. 2002. Infected compartment syndrome after acupuncture. *Acupunct Med* **20**:105-6.

6800. Shah, P. C., S. Krajden, J. Kane, and R. C. Summerbell. 1988. Tinea corporis caused by Microsporum canis: report of a nosocomial outbreak. *Eur J Epidemiol* **4**:33-8.

6801. Shah, S., S. Filler, L. M. Causer, A. K. Rowe, P. B. Bloland, A. M. Barber, J. M. Roberts, M. R. Desai, M. E. Parise, and R. W. Steketee. 2004. Malaria surveillance—United States, 2002. *MMWR Surveill Summ* **53**:21-34.

6802. Shahid, N. S., W. B. Greenough, 3rd, A. R. Samadi, M. I. Huq, and N. Rahman. 1996. Hand washing with soap reduces diarrhoea and spread of bacterial pathogens in a Bangladesh village. *J Diarrhoeal Dis Res* **14**:85-9.

6803. Shaikenov, B. S., T. F. Vaganov, and P. R. Torgerson. 1999. Cystic echinococcosis in Kazakhstan: an emerging disease since independence from the Soviet Union. *Parasitol Today* **15**:172-4.

6804. Shaman, J., J. F. Day, and M. Stieglitz. 2002. Drought-induced amplification of Saint Louis encephalitis virus, Florida. *Emerg Infect Dis* **8**:575-80.

6805. Shaman, J., J. F. Day, and M. Stieglitz. 2003. St. Louis encephalitis virus in wild birds during the 1990 south Florida epidemic: the importance of drought, wetting conditions, and the emergence of Culex nigripalpus (Diptera: Culicidae) to arboviral amplification and transmission. *J Med Entomol* **40**:547-54.

6806. **Shamsul Huq, A. K. M., and F. Huq.** 1987. Diphtheria in Dhaka city. *Bangladesh Med Res Council Bull* **13:**1-7.

6807. **Shane, A. L., N. A. Tucker, J. A. Crump, E. D. Mintz, and J. A. Painter.** 2003. Sharing Shigella: risk factors for a multicommunity outbreak of shigellosis. *Arch Pediatr Adolesc Med* **157:**601-3.

6808. **Shang, D., D. Xiao, and J. Yin.** 2002. Epidemiology and control of brucellosis in China. *Vet Microbiol* **90:**165-82.

6809. **Shanks, G. D., K. Biomndo, S. I. Hay, and R. W. Snow.** 2000. Changing patterns of clinical malaria since 1965 among a tea estate population located in the Kenyan highlands. *Trans R Soc Trop Med Hyg* **94:**253-5.

6810. **Shanson, D. C.** 1980. Outbreaks of Pseudomonas aeruginosa infection in a nursery. *J Hosp Infect* **1:**83-6.

6811. **Shapiro, D. S., and D. R. Schwartz.** 2002. Exposure of laboratory workers to Francisella tularensis despite a bioterrorism procedure. *J Clin Microbiol* **40:**2278-81.

6812. **Shapiro, E. D., and J. I. Ward.** 1991. The epidemiology and prevention of disease caused by Haemophilus influenzae type b. *Epidemiol Rev* **13:**113-42.

6813. **Shapiro, R., M. L. Ackers, S. Lance, M. Rabbani, L. Schaefer, J. Daugherty, C. Thelen, and D. Swerdlow.** 1999. Salmonella Thompson associated with improper handling of roast beef at a restaurant in Sioux Falls, South Dakota. *J Food Prot* **62:**118-22.

6814. **Shapiro, R. L., M. R. Otieno, P. M. Adcock, P. A. Phillips-Howard, W. A. Hawley, L. Kumar, P. Waiyaki, B. L. Nahlen, and L. Slutsker.** 1999. Transmission of epidemic Vibrio cholerae O1 in rural western Kenya associated with drinking water from Lake Victoria: an environmental reservoir for cholera? *Am J Trop Med Hyg* **60:**271-6.

6815. **Sharek, P. J., W. E. Benitz, N. J. Abel, M. J. Freeburn, M. L. Mayer, and D. A. Bergman.** 2002. Effect of an evidence-based hand washing policy on hand washing rates and false-positive coagulase negative staphylococcus blood and cerebrospinal fluid culture rates in a level III NICU. *J Perinatol* **22:**137-43.

6816. **Shariatzadeh, M. R., J. Q. Huang, G. J. Tyrrell, M. M. Johnson, and T. J. Marrie.** 2005. Bacteremic pneumococcal pneumonia: a prospective study in Edmonton and neighboring municipalities. *Medicine (Baltimore)* **84:**147-61.

6817. **Sharma, N. L., R. C. Sharma, P. S. Grover, M. L. Gupta, A. K. Sharma, and V. K. Mahajan.** 1999. Chromoblastomycosis in India. *Int J Dermatol* **38:**846-851.

6818. **Sharma, R. S., R. S. Mishra, D. Pal, J. P. Gupta, M. Dutta, and K. K. Datta.** 1984. An epidemiological study of scabies in a rural community in India. *Ann Trop Med Parasitol* **78:**157-64.

6819. **Sharma, S., M. Sharma, and S. Rathaur.** 1999. Bancroftian filariasis in the Varanasi region of north India: an epidemiological study. *Ann Trop Med Parasitol* **93:**379-87.

6820. **Sharma, S. K., P. Pradhan, and D. M. Padhi.** 2001. Socio-economic factors associated with malaria in a tribal area of Orissa, India. *Indian J Public Health* **45:**93-8.

6821. **Sharma, S. K., P. K. Tyagi, K. Padhan, T. Adak, and S. K. Subbarao.** 2004. Malarial morbidity in tribal communities living in the forest and plain ecotypes of Orissa, India. *Ann Trop Med Parasitol* **98:**459-68.

6822. **Sharp, J. C.** 1987. Infections associated with milk and dairy products in Europe and North America, 1980-85. *Bull WHO* **65:**397-406.

6823. **Sharp, T. W., M. R. Wallace, C. G. Hayes, J. L. Sanchez, R. F. DeFraites, R. R. Arthur, S. A. Thornton, R. A. Batchelor, P. J. Rozmajzl, R. K. Hanson, et al.** 1995. Dengue fever in U.S. troops during Operation Restore Hope, Somalia, 1992-1993. *Am J Trop Med Hyg* **53:**89-94.

6824. **Shaw, P. K., R. E. Brodsky, D. O. Lyman, B. T. Wood, C. P. Hibler, G. R. Healy, K. I. Macleod, W. Stahl, and M. G. Schultz.** 1977. A communitywide outbreak of giardiasis with evidence of transmission by a municipal water supply. *Ann Intern Med* **87:**426-32.

6825. **Shaw, P. K., R. E. Brodsky, and M. G. Schultz.** 1976. Malaria surveillance in the United States, 1974. *J Infect Dis* **133:**95-101.

6826. **Shay, K.** 2002. Infectious complications of dental and periodontal diseases in the elderly population. *Clin Infect Dis* **34:**1215-23.

6827. **Shayegani, M., D. Morse, I. DeForge, T. Root, L. M. Parsons, and P. S. Maupin.** 1983. Microbiology of a major foodborne outbreak of gastroenteritis caused by Yersinia enterocolitica serogroup O:8. *J Clin Microbiol* **17:**35-40.

6828. **Shazberg, G., J. Moise, N. Terespolsky, and H. Hurvitz.** 1999. Family outbreak of Rickettsia conorii infection. *Emerg Infect Dis* **5:**723-4.

6829. **She, S. L., L. Y. Shi, Y. J. Wu, Z. Z. Li, C. Z. Zheng, Y. P. Wu, and X. H. Yu.** 1988. A seroepidemiologic study of hepatitis B virus infection among barbers in Huangshi city, Hubei, China. *Microbiol Immunol* **32:**229-33.

6830. **Shefer, A. M., D. Koo, S. B. Werner, E. D. Mintz, R. Baron, J. G. Wells, T. J. Barrett, M. Ginsberg, R. Bryant, S. Abbott, and P. M. Griffin.** 1996. A cluster of Escherichia coli O157:H7 infections with the hemolytic-uremic syndrome and death in California. A mandate for improved surveillance. *West J Med* **165:**15-9.

6831. **Shehabi, A. A., W. Abu-Al-Soud, A. Mahafzah, N. Khuri-Bulos, I. Abu Khader, I. S. Ouis, and T. Wadstrom.** 2004. Investigation of Burkholderia cepacia nosocomial outbreak with high fatality in patients suffering from diseases other than cystic fibrosis. *Scand J Infect Dis* **36:**174-8.

6832. **Sheik-Mohamed, A., and J. P. Velema.** 1999. Where health care has no access: the nomadic populations of sub-Saharan Africa. *Trop Med Int Health* **4:**695-707.

6833. **Shelby-James, T. M., A. J. Leach, J. R. Carapetis, B. J. Currie, and J. D. Mathews.** 2002. Impact of single dose azithromycin on group A streptococci in the upper respiratory tract and skin of Aboriginal children. *Pediatr Infect Dis J* **21:**375-80.

6834. **Sheldon, C. D., C. S. Probert, H. Cock, K. King, D. S. Rampton, N. C. Barnes, and J. F. Mayberry.** 1993. Incidence of abdominal tuberculosis in Bangladeshi migrants in east London. *Tuber Lung Dis* **74:**12-5.

6835. **Shelley, A. J., and S. Coscaron.** 2001. Simuliid blackflies (Diptera: Simuliidae) and ceratopogonid midges (Diptera: Ceratopogonidae) as vectors of Mansonella ozzardi (Nematoda: Onchocercidae) in northern Argentina. *Mem Inst Oswaldo Cruz* **96:**451-8.

6836. **Shelton, S., S. Haire, and B. Gerard.** 1997. Medical care for mass gatherings at collegiate football games. *South Med J* **90:**1081-3.

6837. **Shen, C. Y., S. F. Chang, M. F. Chao, H. W. Chang, and P. C. Hsu.** 1991. Cytomegalovirus (CMV) in voluntary blood donors in northern Taiwan. *Am J Epidemiol* **134:**782.

6838. **Shen, C. Y., S. F. Chang, H. J. Lin, H. N. Ho, T. S. Yeh, S. L. Yang, E. S. Huang, and C. W. Wu.** 1994. Cervical cytomegalovirus infection in prostitutes and in women attending a sexually transmitted disease clinic. *J Med Virol* **43:**362-6.

6839. **Shen, C. Y., S. F. Chang, S. L. Yang, E. S. Huang, and C. W. Wu.** 1993. Urinary cytomegalovirus shedding profile in children with subclinical infection. *Lancet* **342:**1432.

6840. **Shenep, J. L., S. J. Barenkamp, S. A. Brammeier, and T. D. Gardner.** 1984. An outbreak of toxoplasmosis on an Illinois farm. *Pediatr Infect Dis* **3:**518-22.

6841. **Shenoy, S., G. Wilson, H. V. Prashanth, K. Vidyalakshmi, B. Dhanashree, and R. Bharath.** 2002. Primary meningoencephalitis by Naegleria fowleri: first reported case from Mangalore, south India. *J Clin Microbiol* **40:**309-10.

6842. **Shepherd, A. J., R. Swanepoel, P. A. Leman, and S. P. Shepherd.** 1987. Field and laboratory investigation of Crimean-Congo haemorrhagic fever virus (Nairovirus, family Bunyaviridae) infection in birds. *Trans R Soc Trop Med Hyg* **81:**1004-7.

6843. **Shepherd, A. J., R. Swanepoel, S. P. Shepherd, P. A. Leman, N. K. Blackburn, and A. F. Hallett.** 1985. A nosocomial outbreak of Crimean-Congo haemorrhagic fever at Tygerberg Hospital. Part V. Virological and serological observations. *S Afr Med J* **68:**733-6.

6844. **Shepherd, A. J., R. Swanepoel, S. P. Shepherd, G. M. McGillivray, and L. A. Searle.** 1987. Antibody to Crimean-Congo hemorrhagic fever virus in wild mammals from southern Africa. *Am J Trop Med Hyg* **36:**133-42.

6845. **Sherchand, J. B., J. H. Cross, M. Jimba, S. Sherchand, and M. P. Shrestha.** 1999. Study of Cyclospora cayetanensis in health care facilities, sewage water and green leafy vegetables in Nepal. *Southeast Asian J Trop Med Public Health* **30:**58-63.

6846. **Sherertz, R. J., and M. L. Sullivan.** 1985. An outbreak of infections with Acinetobacter calcoaceticus in burn patients: contamination of patients' mattresses. *J Infect Dis* **151:**252-8.

6847. **Sherrard, J., G. Luzzi, and A. Edwards.** 1997. Imported syphilis and other sexually transmitted infections among UK travellers to Russia and Poland. *Genitourin Med* **73:**75.

6848. **Shi, Z. Y., P. Y. F. Liu, Y.-J. Lau, Y. H. Lin, and B. S. Hu.** 1997. Use of pulsed-field gel electrophoresis to investigate an outbreak of Serratia marcescens. *J Clin Microbiol* **35:**325-7.

6849. **Shidrawi, G. R.** 1990. A WHO global programme for monitoring vector resistance to pesticide. *Bull WHO* **68:**403-8.

6850. **Shieh, Y. C., R. S. Baric, J. W. Woods, and K. R. Calci.** 2003. Molecular surveillance of enterovirus and norwalk-like virus in oysters relocated to a municipal-sewage-impacted gulf estuary. *Appl Environ Microbiol* **69:**7130-6.

6851. **Shieh, Y. S., R. S. Baric, M. D. Sobsey, J. Ticehurst, T. A. Miele, R. DeLeon, and R. Walter.** 1991. Detection of hepatitis A virus and other enteroviruses in water by ssRNA probes. *J Virol Methods* **31:**119-36.

6852. **Shieh, Y. S. C., S. S. Monroe, R. L. Fankhauser, G. W. Langlois, W. Burkhardt, 3rd, and R. S. Baric.** 2000. Detection of norwalk-like virus in shellfish implicated in illness. *J Infect Dis* **181 Suppl 2:**S360-6.

6853. **Shiferaw, B., S. Shallow, R. Marcus, S. Segler, D. Soderlund, F. P. Hardnett, and T. Van Gilder.** 2004. Trends in Population-Based Active Surveillance for Shigellosis and Demographic Variability in FoodNet Sites, 1996-1999. *Clin Infect Dis* **38 Suppl 3:**S175-80.

6854. **Shigematsu, M., M. E. Kaufmann, A. Charlett, Y. Niho, and T. L. Pitt.** 2000. An epidemiological study of Plesiomonas shigelloides diarrhoea among Japanese travellers. *Epidemiol Infect* **125:**523-30.

6855. **Shih, J. Y., P. R. Hsueh, Y. L. Chang, M. T. Chen, P. C. Yang, and K. T. Luh.** 1997. Osteomyelitis and tenosynovitis due to Mycobacterium marinum in a fish dealer. *J Formos Med Assoc* **96:**913-6.

6856. **Shih, Y., and S. Y. Chao.** 1986. Botulism in China. *Rev Infect Dis* **8:**984-90.

6857. **Shihab, K., and M. Sultan.** 1985. Parasitic diseases among Egyptian workers in Bahdad city. *Bull Endem Dis (Baghdad)* **26:**65-70.

6858. **Shililu, J., T. Ghebremeskel, S. Mengistu, H. Fekadu, M. Zerom, C. Mbogo, J. Githure, R. Novak, E. Brantly, and J. C. Beier.** 2003. High seasonal variation in entomologic inoculation rates in Eritrea, a semi-arid region of unstable malaria in Africa. *Am J Trop Med Hyg* **69:**607-13.

6859. **Shim, J. K., S. Johnson, H. Samore, D. Z. Bliss, and D. N. Gerding.** 1998. Primary symptomless colonisation by Clostridium difficile and decreased risk of subsequent diarrhea. *Lancet* **351:**633-6.

6860. **Shimizu, C., S. Nabeshima, K. Kikuchi, N. Furusyo, S. Kashiwagi, and J. Hayashi.** 2002. Prevalence of antibody to Chlamydia pneumoniae in residents of Japan, the Solomon islands, and Nepal. *Am J Trop Med Hyg* **67:**170-5.

6861. **Shimizu, T.** 1993. Prevalence of Toxocara eggs in sandpits in Tokushima city and its outskirts. *J Vet Med Sci* **55:**807-11.

6862. **Shimoyama, R., S. Sekiguchi, M. Suga, S. Sakamoto, and A. Yachi.** 1993. The epidemiology and infection route of asymptomatic HCV carriers detected through blood donations. *Gastroenterol Jpn* **28 Suppl 5:**1-5.

6863. **Shin, H. R., S. Franceschi, S. Vaccarella, J. W. Roh, Y. H. Ju, J. K. Oh, H. J. Kong, S. H. Rha, S. I. Jung, J. I. Kim, K. Y. Jung, L. J. van Doorn, and W. Quint.** 2004. Prevalence and determinants of genital infection with papillomavirus, in female and male university students in Busan, South Korea. *J Infect Dis* **190:**468-76.

6864. **Shin, J. H., S. Chang, and D. H. Kang.** 2004. Application of antimicrobial ice for reduction of foodborne pathogens (Escherichia coli O157:H7, Salmonella Typhimurium, Listeria monocytogenes) on the surface of fish. *J Appl Microbiol* **97:**916-22.

6865. **Shireley, L., T. Dwelle, D. Streitz, and L. Schuler.** 2001. Human anthrax associated with an epizootic among livestock - North Dakota, 2000. *MMWR* **50:**677-680.

6866. **Shlim, D. R., and T. Solomon.** 2002. Japanese encephalitis vaccine for travelers: exploring the limits of risk. *Clin Infect Dis* **35:**183-8.

6867. **Shoda, M., K. Shimizu, M. Nagano, and M. Ishii.** 2001. Malaria infections in crews of Japanese ships. *Int Marit Health* **52:**9-18.

6868. **Shoemaker, T., C. Boulianne, M. J. Vincent, L. Pezzanite, M. M. Al-Qahtani, Y. Al-Mazrou, A. S. Khan, P. E. Rollin, R. Swanepoel, T. G. Ksiazek, and S. T. Nichol.** 2002. Genetic analysis of viruses associated with emergence of rift valley fever in Saudi Arabia and Yemen, 2000-01. *Emerg Infect Dis* **8:**1415-20.

6869. **Shortridge, K. F.** 1999. Poultry and the influenza H5N1 outbreak in Hong Kong, 1997: abridged chronology and virus isolation. *Vaccine* **17 Suppl:**S26-S29.

6870. Shpynov, S., P. Parola, N. Rudakov, I. Samoilenko, M. Tankibaev, I. Tarasevich, and D. Raoult. 2001. Detection and identification of spotted fever group rickettsiae in Dermacentor ticks from Russia and central Kazakhstan. *Eur J Clin Microbiol Infect Dis* **20**:903-5.

6871. Shrestha, S. P., A. Hennig, and S. C. Parija. 1998. Prevalence of rhinosporidiosis of the eye and its adnexa in Nepal. *Am J Trop Med Hyg* **59**:231-4.

6872. Shriram, A. N., K. D. Ramaiah, K. Krishnamoorthy, and S. C. Sehgal. 2005. Diurnal pattern of human-biting activity and transmission of subperiodic wuchereria bancrofti (filariidea: dipetalonematidae) by ochlerotatus niveus (Diptera: culicidae) on the andaman and nicobar islands of India. *Am J Trop Med Hyg* **72**:273-7.

6873. Shugar, R. A., and J. J. Ryan. 1975. Clonorchis sinensis and pancreatitis. Twenty-five years after endemic exposure. *Am J Gastroenterol* **64**:400-3.

6874. Shugars, D. C., L. L. Patton, S. A. Freel, L. R. Gray, R. T. Vollmer, J. J. Eron, Jr., and S. A. Fiscus. 2001. Hyper-excretion of human immunodeficiency virus type 1 RNA in saliva. *J Dent Res* **80**:414-20.

6875. Shvartsblat, S., M. Kochie, P. Harber, and J. Howard. 2004. Fatal rat bite fever in a pet shop employee. *Am J Ind Med* **45**:357-60.

6876. Sibold, C., H. Meisel, A. Lundkvist, A. Schulz, F. Cifire, R. Ulrich, O. Kozuch, M. Labuda, and D. H. Kruger. 1999. Short report: simultaneous occurrence of Dobrava, Puumala, and Tula hantaviruses in Slovakia. *Am J Trop Med Hyg* **61**:409-11.

6877. Sibold, C., R. Ulrich, M. Labuda, A. Lundkvist, H. Martens, M. Schutt, P. Gerke, K. Leitmeyer, H. Meisel, and D. H. Kruger. 2001. Dobrava hantavirus causes hemorrhagic fever with renal syndrome in central Europe and is carried by two different Apodemus mice species. *J Med Virol* **63**:158-67.

6878. Siddique, A. K., Q. Islam, K. Akram, Y. Mazumder, A. Mitra, and A. Eusof. 1989. Cholera epidemic and natural disasters: where is the link. *Trop Geogr Med* **41**:377-82.

6879. Siddiqui, A. A., and S. L. Berk. 2001. Diagnosis of Strongyloides stercoralis infection. *Clin Infect Dis* **33**:1040-7.

6880. Siddiqui, A. H., M. E. Mulligan, E. Mahenthiralingam, J. Hebden, J. Brewrink, S. Qaiyumi, J. A. Johnson, and J. J. LiPuma. 2001. An episodic outbreak of genetically related Burkholderia cepacia among non-cystic fibrosis patients at a university hospital. *Infect Control Hosp Epidemiol* **22**:419-22.

6881. Siebke, J. C., N. Wessel, P. Kvandal, and T. Lie. 1989. The prevalence of hepatitis A and B in Norwegian merchant seamen—a serological study. *Infection* **17**:77-80.

6882. Siegel, J. D., G. H. McCracken, Jr., N. Threlkeld, B. Milvenan, and C. R. Rosenfeld. 1980. Single-dose penicillin prophylaxis against neonatal group B streptococcal infections. A controlled trial in 18,738 newborn infants. *N Engl J Med* **303**:769-75.

6883. Siegman-Igra, Y., H. Golan, D. Schwartz, Y. Cahaner, G. DeMayo, and R. Orni-Wasserlauf. 2000. Epidemiology of vascular catheter-related bloodstream infections in a large university hospital in Israel. *Scand J Infect Dis* **32**:411-5.

6884. Siegman-Igra, Y., R. Levin, M. Weinberger, Y. Golan, D. Schwartz, Z. Samra, H. Konigsberger, A. Yinnon, G. Rahav, N. Keller, N. Bisharat, R. Finkelstein, M. Alkan, Z. Landau, J. Novikov, D. Hassin, C. Rudnicki, R. Kitzes, S. Ovadia, Z. Shimoni, R. Lang, and T. Shohat. 2002. Listeria monocytogenes Infection in Israel and Review of Cases Worldwide. *Emerg Infect Dis* **8**:305-10.

6885. Siegman-Igra, Y., and D. Schwartz. 2003. Streptococcus bovis revisited: a clinical review of 81 bacteremic episodes paying special attention to emerging antibiotic resistance. *Scand J Infect Dis* **35**:90-3.

6886. Sierra-Honigmann, A., and P. R. Krause. 2000. Live oral poliovirus vaccines do not contain detectable simian virus 40 (SV40) DNA. *Biologicals* **28**:1-4.

6887. Sievers, M. L., and J. R. Fisher. 1982. Decreasing incidence of disseminated coccidioidomycosis among Piman and San Carlos Apache indians. *Chest* **82**:455-460.

6888. Sigauke, E., W. E. Beebe, R. M. Gander, D. Cavuoti, and P. M. Southern. 2003. Case report: ophthalmomyiasis externa in Dallas county, Texas. *Am J Trop Med Hyg* **68**:46-7.

6889. Signorini, L., P. Colombini, F. Cristini, A. Matteelli, B. Cadeo, C. Casalini, and P. Viale. 2002. Inappropriate footwear and rat-bite fever in an international traveler. *J Travel Med* **9**:275-6.

6890. Silarug, N., H. M. Foy, S. Kupradinon, S. Rojanasuphot, A. Nisalak, and Y. Pongsuwant. 1990. Epidemic of fever of unknown origin in rural Thailand, caused by influenza A (H1N1) and dengue fever. *Southeast Asian J Trop Med Public Health* **21**:61-7.

6891. Silpapojakul, K. 1997. Scrub typhus in the Western Pacific region. *Ann Acad Med Singapore* **26**:794-800.

6892. Silpapojakul, K., and B. Varachit. 2004. Paediatric scrub typhus in Thailand: a study of 73 confirmed cases. *Trans R Soc Trop Med Hyg* **98**:354-9.

6893. Silva, A. M., E. G. Leite, R. M. Assis, S. Majerowicz, and J. P. Leite. 2001. An outbreak of gastroenteritis associated with astrovirus serotype 1 in a day care center, in Rio de Janeiro, Brazil. *Mem Inst Oswaldo Cruz* **96**:1069-73.

6894. Silva, C. M., R. M. da Rocha, J. S. Moreno, M. R. Branco, R. R. Silva, S. G. Marques, and J. M. Costa. 1995. [The coconut babacu (Orbignya phalerata martins) as a probable risk of human infection by the agent of chromoblastomycosis in the State of Maranhao, Brazil]. *Rev Soc Bras Med Trop* **28**:49-52.

6895. Silva, J. P., W. de Souza, and S. Rozental. 1998. Chromoblastomycosis: a retrospective study of 325 cases on Amazonic Region (Brazil). *Mycopathologia* **143**:171-5.

6896. Silva, L. J., and P. M. Papaiordanou. 2004. Murine (endemic) typhus in Brazil: case report and review. *Rev Inst Med Trop Sao Paulo* **46**:283-5.

6897. Silver, H. M. 1998. Listeriosis during pregnancy. *Obstet Gynecol Surv* **53**:737-40.

6898. Silverman, J., L. A. Thal, M. B. Perri, G. Bostic, and M. J. Zervos. 1998. Epidemiologic evaluation of antimicrobial resistance in community- acquired enterococci. *J Clin Microbiol* **36**:830-2.

6899. Silverman, M. S., L. Aronson, M. Eccles, J. Eisenstat, M. Gottesman, R. Rowsell, M. Ferron, and D. Scolnik. 2004. Leptospirosis in febrile men ingesting Agouti paca in South America. *Ann Trop Med Parasitol* **98**:851-9.

6900. Silvestro, L., M. Caputo, S. Blancato, L. Decastelli, A. Fioravanti, R. Tozzoli, S. Morabito, and A. Caprioli. 2004. Asymptomatic carriage of verocytotoxin-producing Escherichia coli O157 in farm workers in Northern Italy. *Epidemiol Infect* **132**:915-9.

6901. **Simhon, A., G. Rahav, M. Shapiro, and C. Block.** 2001. Skin disease presenting as an outbreak of pseudobacteremia in a laboratory worker. *J Clin Microbiol* **39**:392-3.

6902. **Simitzis, A. M., F. Le Goff, and M. T. L'Azou.** 1979. [Isolation of free-living amoebae from the nasal mucosa of man. Potential risk (author's transl)]. *Ann Parasitol Hum Comp* **54**:121-7.

6903. **Simmons, G., G. Greening, W. Gao, and D. Campbell.** 2001. Raw oyster consumption and outbreaks of viral gastroenteritis in New Zealand: evidence for risk to the public's health. *Aust N Z J Public Health* **25**:234-40.

6904. **Simmons, G., D. Martin, J. Stewart, N. Jones, L. Calder, and D. Bremner.** 2001. Carriage of Neisseria meningitidis among household contacts of patients with meningococcal disease in New Zealand. *Eur J Clin Microbiol Infect Dis* **20**:237-42.

6905. **Simmons, N.** 2002. Honey - the streptomycin story. *Antibiot Chemother* **6**:9.

6906. **Simms, I., K. Eastick, H. Mallinson, K. Thomas, R. Gokhale, P. Hay, A. Herring, and P. A. Rogers.** 2003. Associations between Mycoplasma genitalium, Chlamydia trachomatis, and pelvic inflammatory disease. *Sex Transm Infect* **79**:154-6.

6907. **Simondon, F., and N. Guiso.** 2001. Épidémiologie de la coqueluche dans le monde. *Méd Mal Infect* **31 suppl 1**:5-11.

6908. **Simonsen, L., M. J. Clarke, L. B. Schonberger, N. H. Arden, N. J. Cox, and K. Fukuda.** 1998. Pandemic versus epidemic influenza mortality: a pattern of changing age distribution. *J Infect Dis* **178**:53-60.

6909. **Simonsen, L., A. Kane, J. Lloyd, M. Zaffran, and M. Kane.** 1999. Unsafe injections in the developing world and transmission of bloodborne pathogens: a review. *Bull WHO* **77**:789-800.

6910. **Simonsen, L., D. M. Morens, A. Elixhauser, M. Gerber, M. Van Raden, and W. C. Blackwelder.** 2001. Effect of rotavirus vaccination programme on trends in admission of infants to hospital for intussusception. *Lancet* **358**:1224-9.

6911. **Simonsen, P. E., S. M. Magesa, S. K. Dunyo, M. N. Malecela-Lazaro, and E. Michael.** 2004. The effect of single dose ivermectin alone or in combination with albendazole on Wuchereria bancrofti infection in primary school children in Tanzania. *Trans R Soc Trop Med Hyg* **98**:462-72.

6912. **Simor, A. E., J. L. Brunton, I. E. Salit, H. Vellend, L. Ford-Jones, and L. P. Spence.** 1984. Q fever: hazard from sheep used in research. *Can Med Assoc J* **130**:1013-6.

6913. **Simor, A. E., M. Ofner-Agostini, D. Gravel, M. Varia, S. Paton, A. McGeer, E. Bryce, M. Loeb, and M. Mulvey.** 2005. Surveillance for methicillin-resistant Staphylococcus aureus in Canadian hospitals - a report update from the Canadian nosocomial infection surveillance program. *Can Commun Dis Rep* **31**:33-40.

6914. **Simpson, B. B., and M. C. Ogorzaly.** 2001. Economic botany. Plants in our world, vol. (3rd ed). McGraw-Hill, Boston.

6915. **Sinei, S. K., C. S. Morrison, C. Sekadde-Kigondu, M. Allen, and D. Kokonya.** 1998. Complications of use of intrauterine devices among HIV-1-infected women. *Lancet* **351**:1238-41.

6916. **Singal, M., P. M. Schantz, and S. B. Werner.** 1976. Trichinosis acquired at sea—report of an outbreak. *Am J Trop Med Hyg* **25**:675-81.

6917. **Singh, A. E., and B. Romanowski.** 1999. Syphilis: review with emphasis on clinical, epidemiologic, and some biologic features. *Clin Microbiol Rev* **12**:187-209.

6918. **Singh, B., L. K. Sung, A. Matusop, A. Radhakrishnan, S. S. Shamsul, J. Cox-Singh, A. Thomas, and D. J. Conway.** 2004. A large focus of naturally acquired Plasmodium knowlesi infections in human beings. *Lancet* **363**:1017-24.

6919. **Singh, J., D. C. Jain, R. Bhatia, R. L. Ichhpujani, A. K. Harit, R. C. Panda, K. N. Tewari, and J. Sokhey.** 2001. Epidemiological characteristics of rabies in Delhi and surrounding areas, 1998. *Indian Pediatr* **38**:1354-60.

6920. **Singh, N.** 2001. Changing spectrum of invasive candidiasis and its therapeutic implications. *Clin Microbiol Infect* **7**:1-7.

6921. **Singh, N., O. Belen, M. M. Leger, and J. M. Campos.** 2003. Cluster of Trichosporon mucoides in children associated with a faulty bronchoscope. *Pediatr Infect Dis J* **22**:609-12.

6922. **Singh, N., R. K. Mehra, and V. P. Sharma.** 1999. Malaria and the Narmada-river development in India: a case study of the Bargi dam. *Ann Trop Med Parasitol* **93**:477-88.

6923. **Singh, N., A. C. Nagpal, A. Saxena, and M. P. Singh.** 2004. Changing scenario of malaria in central India, the replacement of Plasmodium vivax by Plasmodium falciparum (1986-2000). *Trop Med Int Health* **9**:364-71.

6924. **Singh, N., C. Wannstedt, L. Keyes, M. M. Wagener, T. Gayowski, and T. V. Cacciarelli.** 2005. Indirect outcomes associated with cytomegalovirus (opportunistic infections, hepatitis C virus sequelae, and mortality) in liver-transplant recipients with the use of preemptive therapy for 13 years. *Transplantation* **79**:1428-34.

6925. **Singh, S.** 2002. Human strongyloidiasis in AIDS era: its zoonotic importance. *J Assoc Physicians India* **50**:415-22.

6926. **Singh-Naz, N., M. Willy, and N. Riggs.** 1990. Outbreak of parainfluenza virus type 3 in a neonatal nursery. *Pediatr Infect Dis J* **9**:31-3.

6927. **Singhal, T., A. Bajpai, V. Kalra, S. K. Kabra, J. C. Samantaray, G. Satpathy, and A. K. Gupta.** 2001. Successful treatment of Acanthamoeba meningitis with combination oral antimicrobials. *Pediatr Infect Dis J* **20**:623-7.

6928. **Singhasivanon, P., K. Thimasarn, S. Yimsamran, K. Linthicum, K. Nualchawee, D. Dawreang, S. Kongrod, N. Premmanisakul, W. Maneeboonyang, and N. Salazar.** 1999. Malaria in tree crop plantations in south-eastern and western provinces of Thailand. *Southeast Asian J Trop Med Public Health* **30**:399-404.

6929. **Sinha, A., C. Grace, W. K. Alston, F. Westenfeld, and J. H. Maguire.** 1999. African trypanosomiasis in two travelers from the United States. *Clin Infect Dis* **29**:840-4.

6930. **Sinha, A., D. Yokoe, and R. Platt.** 2003. Epidemiology of neonatal infections: experience during and after hospitalization. *Pediatr Infect Dis J* **22**:244-50.

6931. **Sinkala, M., M. Makasa, F. Mwanza, P. Mulenga, P. Kalluri, R. Quick, E. Mintz, R. M. Hoekstra, and A. DuBois.** 2004. Cholera epidemic associated with raw vegetables - Lusaka, Zambia, 2003-2004. *MMWR* **53**:783-6.

6932. **Siqueira, J. B., Jr., C. M. Martelli, G. E. Coelho, A. C. Simplicio, and D. L. Hatch.** 2005. Dengue and dengue hemorrhagic fever, Brazil, 1981-2002. *Emerg Infect Dis* **11**:48-53.

6933. **Siqueira, J. B., C. M. Martelli, I. J. Maciel, R. M. Oliveira, M. G. Ribeiro, F. P. Amorim, B. C. Moreira, D. D. Cardoso, W. V. Souza, and A. L. Andrade.** 2004. Household survey of dengue infection in central Brazil: spatial point pattern analysis and risk factors assessment. *Am J Trop Med Hyg* **71**:646-51.

6934. **Sirikulchayanonta, V., and P. Viriyavejakul.** 2001. Various morphologic features of Gnathostoma spinigerum in histologic sections: report of 3 cases with reference to topographic studo of the reference worm. *Southeast Asian J Trop Med Public Health* **32**:302-7.

6935. **Sirinavin, S., P. Nuntnarumit, S. Supapannachart, S. Boonkasidecha, C. Techasaensiri, and S. Yoksarn.** 2004. Vertical dengue infection: case reports and review. *Pediatr Infect Dis J* **23**:1042-7.

6936. **Siringi, S.** 2002. Fake health certificate racket rife in Kenya. *Lancet Infect Dis* **2**:454.

6937. **Sirivichayakul, C., C. Pojjaroen-anant, P. Wisetsing, C. Siripanth, P. Chanthavanich, and K. Pengsaa.** 2003. Prevalence of intestinal parasitic infection among Thai people with mental handicaps. *Southeast Asian J Trop Med Public Health* **34**:259-63.

6938. **Sirivichayakul, C., P. Radomyos, R. Praevanit, C. Pojjaroen-Anant, and P. Wisetsing.** 2000. Hymenolepis nana infection in Thai children. *J Med Assoc Thai* **83**:1035-8.

6939. **Sissoko, M. S., A. Dicko, O. J. Briet, M. Sissoko, I. Sagara, H. D. Keita, M. Sogoba, C. Rogier, Y. T. Toure, and O. K. Doumbo.** 2004. Malaria incidence in relation to rice cultivation in the irrigated Sahel of Mali. *Acta Trop* **89**:161-70.

6940. **Sithithaworn, P., T. Srisawangwong, S. Tesana, W. Daenseekaew, J. Sithithaworn, Y. Fujimaki, and K. Ando.** 2003. Epidemiology of Strongyloides stercoralis in north-east Thailand: application of the agar plate culture technique compared with the enzyme-linked immunosorbent assay. *Trans R Soc Trop Med Hyg* **97**:398-402.

6941. **Sivapalasingam, S., E. Barrett, A. Kimura, S. Van Duyne, W. De Witt, M. Ying, A. Frisch, Q. Phan, E. Gould, P. Shillam, V. Reddy, T. Cooper, M. Hoekstra, C. Higgins, J. P. Sanders, R. V. Tauxe, and L. Slutsker.** 2003. A multistate outbreak of Salmonella enterica Serotype Newport infection linked to mango consumption: impact of water-dip disinfestation technology. *Clin Infect Dis* **37**:1585-90.

6942. **Sivertson, S. E., and A. F. Lincoln.** 1952. Acute phase of Japanese B encephalitis. Two hundred and one cases in American soldiers, Korea 1950. *JAMA* **158**:268-73.

6943. **Sixbey, J. W., S. M. Lemon, and J. S. Pagano.** 1986. A second site for Epstein-Barr virus shedding: the uterine cervix. *Lancet* **2**:1122-4.

6944. **Sjolander, K. B., I. Golovljova, V. Vasilenko, A. Plyusnin, and A. Lundkvist.** 2002. Serological divergence of Dobrava and Saaremaa hantaviruses: evidence for two distinct serotypes. *Epidemiol Infect* **128**:99-103.

6945. **Skarphédinsson, S., P. M. Jensen, and K. Kristiansen.** 2005. Survey of tickborne infections in Denmark. *Emerg Infect Dis* **11**:1055-61.

6946. **Skidmore, S., J. V. Parry, and P. Nottage.** 2001. An investigation of the potential risk of an HAV outbreak in a prison population following the introduction of cases from a community outbreak. *Commun Dis Public Health* **4**:133-5.

6947. **Skidmore, S. J.** 1997. Hepatitis E. *Trans R Soc Trop Med Hyg* **91**:125-6.

6948. **Skidmore, S. J.** 1999. Factors in spread of hepatitis E. *Lancet* **354**:1049-50.

6949. **Skinhoj, P., F. B. Hollinger, K. Hovind-Hougen, and P. Lous.** 1981. Infectious liver diseases in three groups of Copenhagen workers: correlation of hepatitis A infection to sewage exposure. *Arch Environ Health* **36**:139-43.

6950. **Skinner, L. J., A. C. Timperley, D. Wightman, J. M. Chatterton, and D. O. Ho-Yen.** 1990. Simultaneous diagnosis of toxoplasmosis in goats and goatowner's family. *Scand J Infect Dis* **22**:359-61.

6951. **Skjerve, E.** 1999. Possible increase of human Taenia saginata infections through import of beef to Norway from a high prevalence area. *J Food Prot* **62**:1314-9.

6952. **Skoretz, S., G. Zaniewski, and H. J. Goedhuis.** 2004. Hepatitis C virus transmission in the prison / inmate population. *Can Commun Dis Rep* **30**:141-8.

6953. **Skotarczak, B., and A. Cichocka.** 2001. Isolation and amplification by polymerase chain reaction DNA of Babesia microti and Babesia divergens in ticks in Poland. *Ann Agric Environ Med* **8**:187-9.

6954. **Skowronski, D. M., G. De Serres, D. MacDonald, W. Wu, C. Shaw, J. Macnabb, S. Champagne, D. M. Patrick, and S. A. Halperin.** 2002. The changing age and seasonal profile of pertussis in Canada. *J Infect Dis* **185**:1448-53.

6955. **Skull, S. A., and G. Tallis.** 2001. Epidemiology of malaria in Victoria 1999-2000: East Timor emerges as a new source of disease. *Commun Dis Intell* **25**:149-51.

6956. **Sladden, M. J., and G. A. Johnston.** 2004. Common skin infections in children. *BMJ* **329**:95-9.

6957. **Slaten, D. D., R. I. Oropeza, and S. B. Werner.** 1992. An outbreak of Bacillus cereus food poisoning—are caterers supervised sufficiently. *Public Health Rep* **107**:477-80.

6958. **Slater, P. E., D. G. Addiss, A. Cohen, A. Leventhal, G. Chassis, H. Zehavi, A. Bashari, and C. Costin.** 1989. Foodborne botulism: an international outbreak. *Int J Epidemiol* **18**:693-6.

6959. **Slavin, M. A., J. D. Meyers, J. S. Remington, and R. C. Hackman.** 1994. Toxoplasma gondii infection in marrow transplant recipients: a 20 year experience. *Bone Marrow Transplant* **13**:549-57.

6960. **Slesak, G., and P. C. Döller.** 2001. Fieber und Wadenschmerz nach Thailandaufenthalt: murines Fleckfieber und tiefe Beinvenenthrombose. *Dtsch Med Wochenschr* **126**:649-52.

6961. **Slinger, R., A. Giulivi, M. Bodie-Collins, F. Hindieh, R. S. John, G. Sher, M. Goldman, M. Ricketts, and K. C. Kain.** 2001. Transfusion-transmitted malaria in Canada. *CMAJ* **164**:377-9.

6962. **Sloan, D., M. Ramsay, L. Prasad, D. Gelb, and C. G. Teo.** 2005. Prevention of perinatal transmission of hepatitis B to babies at high risk: an evaluation. *Vaccine* **23**:5500-8.

6963. **Slom, T. J., M. M. Cortese, S. I. Gerber, R. C. Jones, T. H. Holtz, A. S. Lopez, C. H. Zambrano, R. L. Sufit, Y. Sakolvaree, W. Chaicumpa, B. L. Herwaldt, and S. Johnson.** 2002. An outbreak of eosinophilic meningitis caused by Angiostrongylus cantonensis in travelers returning from the Caribbean. *N Engl J Med* **346**:668-75.

6964. **Slonim, A., E. S. Walker, E. Mishori, N. Porat, R. Dagan, and P. Yagupsky.** 1998. Person-to-person transmission of Kingella kingae among day care center attendees. *J Infect Dis* **178**:1843-6.

6965. **Sloss, J. M., and D. N. Faithfull-Davies.** 1993. Non-toxigenic Corynebacterium diphtheriae in military personnel. *Lancet* **341**:1021.

6966. **Slowik, T. J., and R. S. Lane.** 2001. Birds and their ticks in northwestern California: minimal contribution to Borrelia burgdorferi enzootiology. *J Parasitol* **87**:755-61.

6967. **Slusarczyk, J.** 2000. Who needs vaccination against hepatitis viruses? *Vaccine* **18 suppl:**S4-S5.

6968. **Smacchia, C., A. Parolin, G. Di Perri, S. Vento, and E. Concia.** 1998. Syphilis in prostitutes from Eastern Europe. *Lancet* **351:**572.

6969. **Small, D., B. Klusaritz, and P. Muller.** 2001. Evaluation of Bacillus anthracis contamination inside the Brentwood mail processing and distribution center - District of Columbia, October 2001. *MMWR* **50:**1129-1133.

6970. **Small, R. G., and J. C. Sharp.** 1979. A milk-borne outbreak due to Salmonella dublin. *J Hyg (Lond)* **82:**95-100.

6971. **Smalligan, R. D., W. R. Lange, J. D. Frame, P. O. Yarbough, D. L. Frankenfield, and K. C. Hyams.** 1995. The risk of viral hepatitis A, B, C, and E among North American missionaries. *Am J Trop Med Hyg* **53:**233-6.

6972. **Smallman-Raynor, M., and A. Cliff.** 1991. The spread of human immunodeficiency virus type 2 into Europe: a geographical analysis. *Int J Epidemiol* **20:**480-9.

6973. **Smallman-Raynor, M. R., and A. D. Cliff.** 2004. Impact of infectious diseases on war. *Infect Dis Clin North Am* **18:**341-68.

6974. **Smego, R. A., J. Frean, and H. J. Koornhof.** 1999. Yeresiniosis I: microbiological and clinicoepidemiological aspects of plague and non-plague Yersinia infections. *Eur J Clin Microbiol Infect Dis* **18:**1-15.

6975. **Smego, R. A., B. Gebrian, and G. Desmangels.** 1998. Cutaneous manifestations of anthrax in rural Haiti. *Clin Infect Dis* **26:**97-102.

6976. **Smego, R. A., A. R. Sarwari, and A. R. Siddiqui.** 2004. Crimean-Congo hemorrhagic fever: prevention and control limitations in a resource-poor country. *Clin Infect Dis* **38:**1731-5.

6977. **Smerdon, W. J., G. K. Adak, S. J. O'Brien, I. A. Gillespie, and M. Reacher.** 2001. General outbreaks of infectious intestinal disease linked with red meat, England and Wales, 1992-1999. *Commun Dis Public Health* **4:**259-67.

6978. **Smith, B., M. A. Ryan, G. C. Gray, J. M. Polonsky, and D. H. Trump.** 2002. Tuberculosis infection among young adults enlisting in the United States Navy. *Int J Epidemiol* **31:**934-9.

6979. **Smith, D. B., E. Lawlor, J. Power, J. O'Riordan, J. McAllister, C. Lycett, F. Davidson, S. Pathirana, J. A. Garson, R. S. Tedder, P. L. Yap, and P. Simmonds.** 1999. A second outbreak of hepatitis C virus infection from anti-D immunoglobulin in Ireland. *Vox Sang* **76:**175-80.

6980. **Smith, D. D., and J. K. Frenkel.** 1995. Prevalence of antibodies to Toxoplasma gondii in wild mammals of Missouri and east central Kansas: biologic and ecologic considerations of transmission. *J Wildl Dis* **31:**15-21.

6981. **Smith, D. K., L. A. Grohskopf, R. J. Black, J. D. Auerbach, F. Veronese, K. A. Struble, L. Cheever, M. Johnson, L. A. Paxton, I. M. Onorato, and A. E. Greenberg.** 2005. Treating Opportunistic Infections Among HIV-Exposed and Infected Children: Recommendations from CDC, the National Institutes of Health, and the Infectious Diseases Society of America. *MMWR* **54 (RR-2):**1-112.

6982. **Smith, G., A. Norman, and J. Banks.** 1997. Management of school leavers given a diphtheria and tetanus vaccine intended for children instead of the intended low dose preparation. *Commun Dis Rep CDR Rev* **7:**R67-9.

6983. **Smith, H. M., R. Reporter, M. P. Rood, A. J. Linscott, L. M. Mascola, W. Hogrefe, and R. H. Purcell.** 2002. Prevalence Study of Antibody to Ratborne Pathogens and Other Agents among Patients Using a Free Clinic in Downtown Los Angeles. *J Infect Dis* **186:**1673-6.

6984. **Smith, H. R., T. Cheasty, and B. Rowe.** 1997. Enteroaggregative Escherichia coli and outbreaks of gastroenteritis in U.K. *Lancet* **350:**814-5.

6985. **Smith, J., L. McElhinney, G. Parsons, N. Brink, T. Doherty, D. Agranoff, M. E. Miranda, and A. R. Fooks.** 2003. Case report: rapid ante-mortem diagnosis of a human case of rabies imported into the UK from the Philippines. *J Med Virol* **69:**150-5.

6986. **Smith, J. L.** 2001. A review of hepatitis E virus. *J Food Prot* **64:**572-86.

6987. **Smith, J. L., and D. M. Fonseca.** 2004. Rapid Assays for Identification of Members of the Culex (Culex) Pipiens Complex, Their Hybrids, and Other Sibling Species (Diptera: Culicidae). *Am J Trop Med Hyg* **70:**339-345.

6988. **Smith, J. P., D. P. Daifas, W. El-Khoury, J. Koukoutsis, and A. El-Khoury.** 2004. Shelf life and safety concerns of bakery products—a review. *Crit Rev Food Sci Nutr* **44:**19-55.

6989. **Smith, J. S., D. B. Fishbein, C. E. Rupprecht, and K. Clark.** 1991. Unexplained rabies in three immigrants in the United States. *N Engl J Med* **324:**205-11.

6990. **Smith, J. S., and N. J. Robinson.** 2002. Age-specific prevalence of infection with herpes simplex virus types 2 and 1: a global review. *J Infect Dis* **186 Suppl 1:**S3-S28.

6991. **Smith, K. E., J. M. Besser, C. W. Hedberg, F. T. Leano, J. B. Bender, J. H. Wicklund, B. P. Johnson, K. A. Moore, and M. T. Osterholm.** 1999. Quinolone-resistant Campylobacter jejuni infections in Minnesota, 1992-1998. *N Engl J Med* **340:**1525 32.

6992. **Smith, K. E., S. A. Stenzel, J. B. Bender, E. Wagstrom, D. Soderlund, F. T. Leano, C. M. Taylor, P. A. Belle-Isle, and R. Danila.** 2004. Outbreaks of enteric infections caused by multiple pathogens associated with calves at a farm day camp. *Pediatr Infect Dis J* **23:**1098-104.

6993. **Smith, K. L., V. DeVos, H. Bryden, L. B. Price, M. E. Hugh-Jones, and P. Keim.** 2000. Bacillus anthracis diversity in Kruger National Park. *J Clin Microbiol* **38:**3780-3784.

6994. **Smith, P., M. Eidson, A. Willsey, B. Wallace, M. Kacica, G. Johnson, M. Frary-Pelletieri, A. Burns, W. J. Stone, J. Narro, C. T. Faulkner, D. Rotstein, L. Sheeler, P. C. Erwin, B. Kirkpatrick, D. S. Zarlenga, P. Schantz, and F. Coronado.** 2004. Trichinellosis associated with bear meat - New York and Tennessee, 2003. *MMWR* **53:**606-10.

6995. **Smith, P. G.** 2003. The epidemics of bovine spongiform encephalopathy and variant Creutzfeldt-Jakob disease: current status and future prospects. *Bull WHO* **81:**123-30.

6996. **Smith, R. M. M., F. Drobniewski, A. Gibson, J. D. Montague, M. N. Logan, D. Hunt, G. Hewinson, R. L. Salmon, and B. O'Neill.** 2004. Mycobacterium bovis infection, United Kingdom. *Emerg Infect Dis* **10:**539-41.

6997. **Smith, W. H., D. Davies, K. D. Mason, and J. P. Onions.** 1982. Intraoral and pulmonary tuberculosis following dental treatment. *Lancet* **1:**842-4.

6998. **Smittle, R. B.** 2000. Microbiological safety of mayonnaise, salad dressings, and sauces produced in the United States: a review. *J Food Prot* **63:**1144-53.

6999. **Smoak, B. L., J. B. McClain, J. F. Brundage, L. Broadhurst, D. J. Kelly, G. A. Dasch, and R. N. Miller.** 1996. An outbreak of spotted fever rickettsiosis in U.S. Army troops deployed to Botswana. *Emerg Infect Dis* **2**:217-21.

7000. **Smolyakov, R., A. Borer, K. Riesenberg, F. Schlaeffer, M. Alkan, A. Porath, D. Rimar, Y. Almog, and J. Gilad.** 2003. Nosocomial multi-drug resistant Acinetobacter baumannii bloodstream infection: risk factors and outcome with ampicillin-sulbactam treatment. *J Hosp Infect* **54**:32-8.

7001. **Smyth, E. T., and A. M. Emmerson.** 2000. Surgical site infection surveillance. *J Hosp Infect* **45**:173-84.

7002. **Sniadack, D. H., S. M. Ostroff, M. A. Karlix, R. W. Smithwick, B. Schwartz, M. A. Sprauer, V. A. Silcox, and R. C. Good.** 1993. A nosocomial pseudo-outbreak of Mycobacterium xenopi due to a contaminated potable water supply: lessons in prevention. *Infect Control Hosp Epidemiol* **14**:636-41.

7003. **Snider, R., S. Landers, and M. L. Levy.** 1993. The ringworm riddle: an outbreak of Microsporum canis in the nursery. *Pediatr Infect Dis J* **12**:145-8.

7004. **Snow, J.** 1855 (2nd ed). On the mode of communication of cholera. John Churchill, London.

7005. **Snow, R. W., C. A. Guerra, A. M. Noor, H. Y. Myint, and S. I. Hay.** 2005. The global distribution of clinical episodes of Plasmodium falciparum malaria. *Nature* **434**:214-7.

7006. **Snowdon, J. A., and D. O. Cliver.** 1996. Microorganisms in honey. *Int J Food Microbiol* **31**:1-26.

7007. **Snyder, J. D., J. G. Wells, J. Yashuk, N. Puhr, and P. A. Blake.** 1984. Outbreak of invasive Escherichia coli gastroenteritis on a cruise ship. *Am J Trop Med Hyg* **33**:281-4.

7008. **Snydman, D. R.** 2001. Epidemiology of infections after solid-organ transplantation. *Clin Infect Dis* **33 Suppl 1**:S5-8.

7009. **Snydman, D. R., N. V. Jacobus, L. A. McDermott, R. Ruthazer, E. J. Goldstein, S. M. Finegold, L. J. Harrell, D. W. Hecht, S. G. Jenkins, C. Pierson, R. Venezia, J. Rihs, and S. L. Gorbach.** 2002. National survey on the susceptibility of Bacteroides fragilis group: report and analysis of trends for 1997-2000. *Clin Infect Dis* **35 suppl 1**:S126-S134.

7010. **Soares, R. P., and S. J. Turco.** 2003. Lutzomyia longipalpis (Diptera: Psychodidae: Phlebotominae): a review. *An Acad Bras Cienc* **75**:301-30.

7011. **Soares, S., K. G. Kristinsson, J. M. Musser, and A. Tomasz.** 1993. Evidence for the introduction of a multiresistant clone of serotype 6B Streptococcus pneumoniae from Spain to Iceland in the late 1980s. *J Infect Dis* **168**:158-63.

7012. **Soave, R.** 2001. Prophylaxis strategies for solid-organ transplantation. *Clin Infect Dis* **33 suppl 1**:S26-31.

7013. **Sobel, J., D. N. Cameron, J. Ismail, N. Strockbine, M. Williams, P. S. Diaz, B. Westley, M. Rittmann, J. DiCristina, H. Ragazzoni, R. V. Tauxe, and E. D. Mintz.** 1998. A prolonged outbreak of Shigella sonnei infections in traditionally observant Jewish communities in North America caused by a molecularly distinct bacterial subtype. *J Infect Dis* **177**:1405-9.

7014. **Sobel, J., N. Tucker, A. Sulka, J. McLaughlin, and S. Maslanka.** 2004. Foodborne botulism in the United States, 1990-2000. *Emerg Infect Dis* **10**:1606-11.

7015. **Sobral, C. A., M. R. Amendoeira, A. Teva, B. N. Patel, and C. H. Klein.** 2005. Seroprevalence of infection with Toxoplasma gondii in indigenous Brazilian populations. *Am J Trop Med Hyg* **72**:37-41.

7016. **Sockett, P. N.** 1991. Communicable disease associated with milk and dairy products: England and Wales 1987-1989. *CDR (Lond Engl Rev)* **1**:R9-12.

7017. **Söderberg, S., W. Temihango, C. Kadete, B. Ekstedt, A. Masawe, A. Vahlne, and P. Horal.** 1994. Prevalence of HIV-1 infection in rural, semi-urban, and urban villages in southwest Tanzania: estimates from a blood-donor study. *AIDS* **8**:971-6.

7018. **Sofianou, D., E. Avgoustinakis, A. Dilopoulou, S. Pournaras, G. Tsirakidis, and A. Tsakris.** 2004. Soft-tissue abscess involving Actinomyces odontolyticus and two Prevotella species in an intravenous drug abuser. *Comp Immunol Microbiol Infect Dis* **27**:75-9.

7019. **Sogayar, M. I., and E. L. Yoshida.** 1995. Giardia survey in live-trapped small domestic and wild mammals in four regions in the southwest region of the state of Sao Paulo, Brazil. *Mem Inst Oswaldo Cruz* **90**:675-8.

7020. **Solarz, K., P. Szilman, and E. Szilman.** 2004. Occupational exposure to allergenic mites in a Polish zoo. *Ann Agric Environ Med* **11**:27-33.

7021. **Solberg, C. O.** 2000. Spread of Staphylococcus aureus in hospitals: causes and prevention. *Scand J Infect Dis* **32**:587-95.

7022. **Soldan, K., M. Ramsay, and M. Collins.** 1999. Acute hepatitis B infection associated with blood transfusion in England and Wales, 1991-7: review of database. *BMJ* **318**:95.

7023. **Soldan, K., M. Ramsay, A. Robinson, H. Harris, N. Anderson, E. Caffrey, C. Chapman, A. Dike, G. Gabra, A. Gorman, A. Herborn, P. Hewitt, N. Hewson, D. A. Jones, C. Llewelyn, E. Love, V. Muddu, V. Martlew, and A. Townley.** 2002. The contribution of transfusion to HCV infection in England. *Epidemiol Infect* **129**:587-91.

7024. **Soledad Fontanarrosa, M., M. Cristina Marinone, S. Fischer, P. W. Orellano, and N. J. Schweigmann.** 2000. Effects of flooding and temperature on Aedes albifasciatus development time and larval density in two rain pools at Buenos Aires university city. *Mem Inst Oswaldo Cruz* **95**:787-93.

7025. **Soledad Gomez, M., M. Gracenea, I. Montoliu, C. Feliu, A. Monleon, J. Fernandez, and C. Ensenat.** 1996. Intestinal parasitism—protozoa and helminths—in primates at the Barcelona Zoo. *J Med Primatol* **25**:419-23.

7026. **Solomon, S. L., R. F. Khabbaz, R. H. Parker, R. L. Anderson, M. A. Geraghty, R. M. Furman, and W. J. Martone.** 1984. An outbreak of Candida parapsilosis bloodstream infections in patients receiving parenteral nutrition. *J Infect Dis* **149**:98-102.

7027. **Solomon, T.** 2004. Flavivirus encephalitis. *N Engl J Med* **351**:370-8.

7028. **Sommers, C., M. Kozempel, X. Fan, and E. R. Radewonuk.** 2002. Use of vacuum-steam-vacuum and ionizing radiation to eliminate Listeria innocua from ham. *J Food Prot* **65**:1981-3.

7029. **Sonder, G. J., L. P. Bovee, R. A. Coutinho, D. Baayen, J. Spaargaren, and A. van den Hoek.** 2005. Occupational exposure to bloodborne viruses in the Amsterdam police force, 2000-2003. *Am J Prev Med* **28**:169-74.

7030. **Song, H. J., C. H. Cho, J. S. Kim, M. H. Choi, and S. T. Hong.** 2003. Prevalence and risk factors for enterobiasis among preschool children in a metropolitan city in Korea. *Parasitol Res* **91**:46-50.

7031. **Song, H. J., S. Y. Seong, M. S. Huh, S. G. Park, W. J. Jang, S. H. Kee, K. H. Kim, S. C. Kim, M. S. Choi, I. S. Kim, and W. H. Chang.** 1998. Molecular and serologic survey of Orientia tsutsugamushi infection among field rodents in southern Cholla province, Korea. *Am J Trop Med Hyg* **58**:513-8.

7032. **Song, M., B. Wang, J. W. Liu, and N. Gratz.** 2003. Insect vectors and rodents arriving in China aboard international transport. *J Travel Med* **10**:241-4.

7033. **Sonnenberg, P., J. Murray, J. R. Glynn, S. Shearer, B. Kambashi, and P. Godfrey-Faussett.** 2001. HIV-1 and recurrence, relapse, and reinfection of tuberculosis after cure: a cohort study in South African mineworkers. *Lancet* **358**:1687-1693.

7034. **Sonnenberg, P., E. Silber, K. C. Ho, and H. J. Koornhof.** 2000. Meningococcal disease in South African goldmines—epidemiology and strategies for control. *S Afr Med J* **90**:513-7.

7035. **Soper, F. L.** 1967. Dynamics of Aedes aegypti distribution and density. Seasonal fluctuations in the Americas. *Bull WHO* **36**:536-8.

7036. **Sorensen, K. K., T. Mork, O. G. Sigurdardottir, K. Asbakk, J. Akerstedt, B. Bergsjo, and E. Fuglei.** 2005. Acute toxoplasmosis in three wild arctic foxes (Alopex lagopus) from Svalbard; one with co-infections of Salmonella Enteritidis PT1 and Yersinia pseudotuberculosis serotype 2b. *Res Vet Sci* **78**:161-7.

7037. **Soriano, V., A. Vallejo, M. Gutiérrez, C. Tuset, G. Cilla, R. Martinez-Zapico, F. Dronda, E. Caballero, E. Calderon, A. Aguilera, A. M. Martin, J. Llibre, J. del Romero, R. Ortiz de Lejarazu, F. Ulloa, J. Eiros, and J. M. Gonzalez-Lahoz.** 1996. Epidemiology of human T-lymphotropic virus type II (HTLV-II) infection in Spain. *Eur J Epidemiol* **12**:625-9.

7038. **Sorin, M., S. Segal-Maurer, N. Mariano, C. Urban, A. Combest, and J. J. Rahal.** 2001. Nosocomial transmission of imipenem-resistant Pseudomonas aeruginosa following bronchoscopy associated with improper connection to the Steris System 1 processor. *Infect Control Hosp Epidemiol* **22**:409-13.

7039. **Sornmani, S.** 1987. Control of opisthorchiasis through community participation. *Parasitol Today* **3**:31-3.

7040. **Sorvillo, F., L. Smith, P. Kerndt, and L. Ash.** 2001. Trichomonas vaginalis, HIV, and African-Americans. *Emerg Infect Dis* **7**:927-32.

7041. **Sorvillo, F. J., K. Fujioka, B. Nahlen, M. P. Tormey, R. Kebabjian, and L. Mascola.** 1992. Swimming-associated cryptosporidiosis. *Am J Public Health* **82**:742-4.

7042. **Sorvillo, F. J., B. Gondo, R. Emmons, P. Ryan, S. H. Waterman, A. Tilzer, E. M. Andersen, R. A. Murray, and R. N. Barr.** 1993. A surburban focus of endemic typhus in Los Angeles county: association with seropositive domestic cats and opossums. *Am J Trop Med Hyg* **48**:269-73.

7043. **Sorvillo, F. J., S. F. Huie, M. A. Strassburg, A. Butsumyo, W. X. Shandera, and S. L. Fannin.** 1984. An outbreak of respiratory syncytial virus pneumonia in a nursing home for the elderly. *J Infect* **9**:252-6.

7044. **Sorvillo, F. J., L. E. Lieb, P. R. Kerndt, and L. R. Ash.** 1994. Epidemiology of cryptosporidiosis among persons with acquired immunodeficiency syndrome in Los Angeles County. *Am J Trop Med Hyg* **51**:326-31.

7045. **Sorvillo, F. J., L. E. Lieb, J. Seidel, P. Kerndt, J. Turner, and L. R. Ash.** 1995. Epidemiology of isosporiasis among persons with acquired immunodeficiency syndrome in Los Angeles County. *Am J Trop Med Hyg* **53**:656-9.

7046. **Sorvillo, F. J., S. H. Waterman, F. O. Richards, and P. M. Schantz.** 1992. Cysticercosis surveillance: locally acquired and travel-related infections and detection of intestinal tapeworm carriers in Los Angeles County. *Am J Trop Med Hyg* **47**:365-71.

7047. **Sosa-Estani, S., D. Rossi, and M. Weissenbacher.** 2003. Epidemiology of human immunodeficiency virus (HIV)/acquired immunodeficiency syndrome in injection drug users in Argentina: high seroprevalence of HIV infection. *Clin Infect Dis* **37 Suppl 5**:S338-42.

7048. **Sosin, D. M., R. A. Gunn, W. L. Ford, and J. W. Skaggs.** 1989. An outbreak of furunculosis among high school athletes. *Am J Sports Med* **17**:828-32.

7049. **Sotiraki, S. T., L. V. Athanasiou, C. A. Himonas, V. J. Kontos, and I. Kyriopoulos.** 2001. Trichinellosis in Greece: a review. *Parasite* **8**:S83-5.

7050. **Soubani, A. O., G. Khanchandani, and H. P. Ahmed.** 2004. Clinical significance of lower respiratory tract Aspergillus culture in elderly hospitalized patients. *Eur J Clin Microbiol Infect Dis* **23**:491-4.

7051. **Soucie, J. M., B. Evatt, and D. Jackson.** 1998. Occurrence of hemophilia in the United States. The Hemophilia Surveillance System Project Investigators. *Am J Hematol* **59**:288-94.

7052. **Soucie, J. M., L. C. Richardson, B. L. Evatt, J. V. Linden, B. M. Ewenstein, S. F. Stein, C. Leissinger, M. Manco-Johnson, and C. L. Sexauer.** 2001. Risk factors for infection with HBV and HCV in a largecohort of hemophiliac males. *Transfusion* **41**:338-43.

7053. **Southgate, V., L. A. Tchuem Tchuente, M. Sene, D. De Clercq, A. Theron, J. Jourdane, B. L. Webster, D. Rollinson, B. Gryseels, and J. Vercruysse.** 2001. Studies on the biology of schistosomiasis with emphasis on the Senegal river basin. *Mem Inst Oswaldo Cruz* **96 Suppl**:75-8.

7054. **Southwick, K. L., S. Blanco, A. Santander, M. Estenssoro, F. Torrico, G. Seoane, W. Brady, M. Fears, J. Lewis, V. Pope, J. Guarner, and W. C. Levine.** 2001. Maternal and congenital syphilis in Bolivia, 1996: prevalence and risk factors. *Bull WHO* **79**:33-42.

7055. **Souza, J. P., M. Boeckh, T. A. Gooley, M. E. Flowers, and S. W. Crawford.** 1999. High rates of Pneumocystis carinii pneumonia in allogeneic blood and marrow transplant recipients receiving dapsone prophylaxis. *Clin Infect Dis* **29**:1467-71.

7056. **Souza, L. S., E. A. Ramos, F. M. Carvalho, V. M. Guedes, C. M. Rocha, A. B. Soares, F. Velloso Lde, I. S. Macedo, F. E. Moura, M. Siqueira, S. Fortes, C. C. de Jesus, C. M. Santiago, A. M. Carvalho, and E. Arruda.** 2003. Viral respiratory infections in young children attending day care in urban Northeast Brazil. *Pediatr Pulmonol* **35**:184-91.

7057. **Sow, S., S. J. de Vlas, D. Engels, and B. Gryseels.** 2002. Water-related disease patterns before and after the construction of the Diama dam in northern Senegal. *Ann Trop Med Parasitol* **96**:575-86.

7058. **Spach, D. H., A. S. Kanter, M. J. Dougherty, A. M. Larson, M. B. Coyle, D. J. Brenner, B. Swaminathan, G. M. Matar, D. F. Welch, R. K. Root, et al.** 1995. Bartonella (Rochalimaea) quintana bacteremia in inner-city patients with chronic alcoholism. *N Engl J Med* **332**:424-8.

7059. **Spach, D. H., F. E. Silverstein, and W. E. Stamm.** 1993. Transmission of infection by gastrointestinal endoscopy and bronchoscopy. *Ann Intern Med* **118**:117-28.

7060. **Spada, E., D. Genovese, M. E. Tosti, A. Mariano, M. Cuccuini, L. Proietti, C. D. Giuli, A. Lavagna, G. E. Crapa, G. Morace, S. Taffon, A. Mele, G. Rezza, and M. Rapicetta.** 2005. An outbreak of hepatitis A virus infection with a high case-fatality rate among injecting drug users. *J Hepatol*.

7061. **Spalding, M. D., C. Ravilious, and E. P. Green.** 2001. World Atlas of Coral Reefs. University of California Press, Berkeley.

7062. **Spear, R. C., B. Zhong, Y. Mao, A. Hubbard, M. Birkner, J. Remais, and D. Qiu.** 2004. Spatial and temporal variability in schistosome cercarial density detected by mouse bioassays in village irrigation ditches in Sichuan, China. *Am J Trop Med Hyg* **71:**554-7.

7063. **Spencer, H. C., Jr., J. J. Gibson, Jr., R. E. Brodsky, and M. G. Schultz.** 1975. Imported African trypanosomiasis in the United States. *Ann Intern Med* **82:**633-8.

7064. **Spencer, H. C., C. Muchnick, D. J. Sexton, P. Dodson, and K. W. Walls.** 1977. Endemic amebiasis in an extended family. *Am J Trop Med Hyg* **26:**628-35.

7065. **Spencer, J. D., J. Azoulas, A. K. Broom, T. D. Buick, B. Currie, P. W. Daniels, S. L. Doggett, G. D. Hapgood, P. J. Jarrett, M. D. Lindsay, G. Lloyd, J. S. Mackenzie, A. Merianos, R. J. Moran, S. A. Ritchie, R. C. Russell, D. W. Smith, F. O. Stenhouse, and P. I. Whelan.** 2001. Murray Valley encephalitis virus surveillance and control initiatives in Australia. National Arbovirus Advisory Committee of the Communicable Diseases Network Australia. *Commun Dis Intell* **25:**33-47.

7066. **Spencer, M.** 1992. The history of malaria control in the southwest Pacific region, with particular reference to Papua New Guinea and the Solomon Islands. *P N G Med J* **35:**33-66.

7067. **Spencer, S., A. D. Grant, J. Piola, K. Tukpo, M. Okia, M. Garcia, P. Salignon, C. Genevier, J. Kiguli, and J. P. Guthmann.** 2004. Malaria in camps for internally-displaced persons in Uganda: evaluation of an insecticide-treated bednet distribution programme. *Trans R Soc Trop Med Hyg* **98:**719-27.

7068. **Spicer, P. E., D. Phillips, A. Pike, C. Johansen, W. Melrose, and R. A. Hall.** 1999. Antibodies to Japanese encephalitis virus in human sera collected from Irian Jaya. Follow-up of a previously reported case of Japanese encephalitis in that region. *Trans R Soc Trop Med Hyg* **93:**511-4.

7069. **Spika, J. S., F. Dabis, N. Hargrett-Bean, J. Salcedo, S. Veillard, and P. A. Blake.** 1987. Shigellosis at a Caribbean resort. Hamburger and North American origin as risk factors. *Am J Epidemiol* **126:**1173-80.

7070. **Spira, A. M.** 2003. Preparing the traveller. *Lancet* **361:**1368-81.

7071. **Splino, M., J. Beran, and R. Chlibek.** 2003. Q fever outbreak during the Czech Army deployment in Bosnia. *Mil Med* **168:**840-2.

7072. **Spotts Whitney, E. A., M. E. Beatty, T. H. Taylor, R. Weyant, J. Sobel, M. J. Arduino, and D. A. Ashford.** 2003. Inactivation of Bacillus anthracis spores. *Emerg Infect Dis* **9:**623-7.

7073. **Sprague, J. B., J. C. Hierholzer, R. W. Currier, 2nd, M. A. Hattwick, and M. D. Smith.** 1973. Epidemic keratoconjunctivitis. A severe industrial outbreak due to adenovirus type 8. *N Engl J Med* **289:**1341-6.

7074. **Sprott, V., C. D. Selby, P. Ispahani, and P. J. Toghill.** 1987. Indigenous strongyloidiasis in Nottingham. *BMJ* **294:**741-2.

7075. **Squarcione, S., A. Prete, and L. Vellucci.** 1999. Botulism surveillance in Italy: 1992-1996. *Eur J Epidemiol* **15:**917-22.

7076. **Squier, C., V. L. Yu, and J. E. Stout.** 2000. Waterborne nosocomial infections. *Curr Inf Dis Rep* **2**.

7077. **Squires, S., and J. Doherty.** 1997. Trends in gonorrhea in Canada, 1990-1995. *Can Commun Dis Rep* **23:**89-95.

7078. **Squires, S. G., S. L. Deeks, and R. S. W. Tsang.** 2004. Enhanced surveillance of invasive meningococcal disease in Canada: 1 January. 1999, through 31 December 2001. *Can Commun Dis Rep* **30:**17-28.

7079. **Sreenivasan, M. A., H. R. Bhat, and P. K. Rajagopalan.** 1986. The epizootics of Kyasanur Forest disease in wild monkeys during 1964 to 1973. *Trans R Soc Trop Med Hyg* **80:**810-4.

7080. **Sreter, T., Z. Sreter-Lancz, Z. Szell, and D. Kalman.** 2004. Anaplasma phagocytophilum: an emerging tick-borne pathogen in Hungary and Central Eastern Europe. *Ann Trop Med Parasitol* **98:**401-5.

7081. **Sriamporn, S., P. Pisani, V. Pipitgool, K. Suwanrungruang, S. Kamsa-Ard, and D. M. Parkin.** 2004. Prevalence of Opisthorchis viverrini infection and incidence of cholangiocarcinoma in Khon Kaen, Northeast Thailand. *Trop Med Int Health* **9:**588-94.

7082. **Srikantiah, P., J. C. Lay, S. Hand, J. A. Crump, J. Campbell, M. S. Van Duyne, R. Bishop, R. Middendor, M. Currier, P. S. Mead, and K. Molbak.** 2004. Salmonella enterica serotype Javiana infections associated with amphibian contact, Mississippi, 2001. *Epidemiol Infect* **132:**273-81.

7083. **Srinivasan, A., C. N. Kraus, D. DeShazer, P. M. Becker, J. D. Dick, L. Spacek, J. G. Bartlett, W. R. Byrne, and D. L. Thomas.** 2001. Glanders in a military research microbiologist. *N Engl J Med* **345:**256-8.

7084. **Srinivasan, A., L. L. Wolfenden, X. Song, K. Mackie, T. L. Hartsell, H. D. Jones, G. B. Diette, J. B. Orens, R. C. Yung, T. L. Ross, W. Merz, P. J. Scheel, E. F. Haponik, and T. M. Perl.** 2003. An outbreak of Pseudomonas aeruginosa infections associated with flexible bronchoscopes. *N Engl J Med* **348:**221-7.

7085. **Sriratanaban, A., and S. Reinprayoon.** 1982. Vibrio parahaemolyticus: a major cause of travelers' diarrhea in Bangkok. *Am J Trop Med Hyg* **31:**128-30.

7086. **Srivastava, G., K. Y. Wong, A. K. Chiang, K. Y. Lam, and Q. Tao.** 2000. Coinfection of multiple strains of Epstein-Barr virus in immunocompetent normal individuals: reassessment of the viral carrier state. *Blood* **95:**2443-5.

7087. **Srugo, I., D. Benilevi, R. Madeb, S. Shapiro, T. Shohat, E. Somekh, Y. Rimmar, V. Gershtein, R. Gershtein, E. Marva, and N. Lahat.** 2000. Pertussis infection in fully vaccinated children in day-care centers, Israel. *Emerg Infect Dis* **6:**526-9.

7088. **St Louis, M. E., S. H. Peck, D. Bowering, G. B. Morgan, J. Blatherwick, S. Banerjee, G. D. Kettyls, W. A. Black, M. E. Milling, and A. H. Hauschild.** 1988. Botulism from chopped garlic: delayed recognition of a major outbreak. *Ann Intern Med* **108:**363-8.

7089. **St Louis, M. E., J. D. Porter, A. Helal, K. Drame, N. Hargrett-Bean, J. G. Wells, and R. V. Tauxe.** 1990. Epidemic cholera in West Africa: the role of food handling and high-risk foods. *Am J Epidemiol* **131:**719-28.

7090. **Staat, M. A.** 2002. Infectious disease issues in internationally adopted children. *Pediatr Infect Dis J* **21:**255-8.

7091. **Staat, M. A., P. H. Azimi, T. Berke, N. Roberts, D. I. Bernstein, R. L. Ward, L. K. Pickering, and D. O. Matson.** 2002. Clinical presentations of rotavirus infection among hospitalized children. *Pediatr Infect Dis J* **21:**221-7.

7092. **Staat, M. A., D. Kruszon-Moran, G. M. McQuillan, and R. A. Kaslow.** 1996. A population-based serologic survey of Helicobacter pylori infection in children and adolescents in the United States. *J Infect Dis* **174:**1120-3.

7093. **Stacey, A., P. Burden, C. Croton, and E. Jones.** 1998. Contamination of television sets by methicillin-resistant Staphylococcus aureus (MRSA). *J Hosp Infect* **39:**243-4.

7094. Stacey, A. R., K. E. Endersby, P. C. Chan, and R. R. Marples. 1998. An outbreak of methicillin resistant Staphylococcus aureus infection in a rugby football team. *Br J Sports Med* **32:**153-4.

7095. Staedke, S. G., E. W. Nottingham, J. Cox, M. R. Kamya, P. J. Rosenthal, and G. Dorsey. 2003. Short report: proximity to mosquito breeding sites as a risk factor for clinical malaria episodes in an urban cohort of Ugandan children. *Am J Trop Med Hyg* **69:**244-6.

7096. Staes, C. J., T. L. Schlenker, I. Risk, K. G. Cannon, H. Harris, A. T. Pavia, C. N. Shapiro, and B. P. Bell. 2000. Sources of infection among persons with acute hepatitis A and no identified risk factors during a sustained community-wide outbreak. *Pediatrics* **106:**E54.

7097. Stafford, K. C., 3rd, M. L. Cartter, L. A. Magnarelli, E. Starr-Hope, and P. A. Mshar. 1998. Temporal correlation between tick abundance and prevalence of ticks infected with Borrelia burgdorferi and increasing incidence of Lyme disease. *J Clin Microbiol* **36:**1240-4.

7098. Stafford, R., G. Neville, C. Towner, and B. McCall. 2000. A community outbreak of Cryptosporidium infection associated with a swimming pool complex. *Commun Dis Intell* **24:**236-9.

7099. Stafford, R., D. Strain, M. Heymer, C. Smith, M. Trent, and J. Beard. 1997. An outbreak of Norwalk virus gastroenteritis following consumption of oysters. *Commun Dis Intell* **21:**317-20.

7100. Stafford, R. J., B. J. McCall, A. S. Neil, D. S. Leon, G. J. Dorricott, C. D. Towner, and G. R. Micalizzi. 2002. A statewide outbreak of Salmonella Bovismorbificans phage type 32 infection in Queensland. *Commun Dis Intell* **26:**568-73.

7101. Stagno, S., A. C. Dykes, C. S. Amos, R. A. Head, D. D. Juranek, and K. Walls. 1980. An outbreak of toxoplasmosis linked to cats. *Pediatrics* **65:**706-12.

7102. Stagno, S., R. F. Pass, G. Cloud, W. J. Britt, R. E. Henderson, P. D. Walton, D. A. Veren, F. Page, and C. A. Alford. 1986. Primary cytomegalovirus infection in pregnancy. Incidence, transmission to fetus, and clinical outcome. *JAMA* **256:**1904-8.

7103. Stagno, S., D. W. Reynolds, R. F. Pass, and C. A. Alford. 1980. Breast milk and the risk of cytomegalovirus infection. *N Engl J Med* **302:**1073-6.

7104. Stalder, H., R. Isler, W. Stutz, M. Salfinger, S. Lauwers, and W. Vischer. 1983. Beitrag zur Epidemiologie von Campylobacter jejuni. Von der asymptomatischen Ausscheidung im Stall zur Erkrankung bei über 500 Personen. *Schweiz Med Wochenschr* **113:**245-9.

7105. Stamm, W. E. 1999. Chlamydia trachomatis infections: progress and problems. *J Infect Dis* **179 suppl 2:**S380-3.

7106. Stanberry, L. R., S. L. Rosenthal, L. Mills, P. A. Succop, F. M. Biro, R. A. Morrow, and D. I. Bernstein. 2004. Longitudinal risk of herpes simplex virus (HSV) type 1, HSV type 2, and cytomegalovirus infections among young adolescent girls. *Clin Infect Dis* **39:**1433-8.

7107. Stanczak, J., R. M. Gabre, W. Kruminis-Lozowska, M. Racewicz, and B. Kubica-Biernat. 2004. Ixodes ricinus as a vector of Borrelia burgdorferi sensu lato, Anaplasma phagocytophilum and Babesia microti in urban and suburban forests. *Ann Agric Environ Med* **11:**109-14.

7108. Standaert, S. M., J. E. Dawson, W. Schaffner, J. E. Childs, K. L. Biggie, J. Singleton, Jr., R. R. Gerhardt, M. L. Knight, and R. H. Hutcheson. 1995. Ehrlichiosis in a golf-oriented retirement community. *N Engl J Med* **333:**420-5.

7109. Standaert, S. M., R. H. Hutcheson, and W. Schaffner. 1994. Nosocomial transmission of Salmonella gastroenteritis to laundry workers in a nursing home. *Infect Control Hosp Epidemiol* **15:**22-6.

7110. Standaert, S. M., W. Schaffner, J. N. Galgiani, R. W. Pinner, L. Kaufman, E. Durry, and R. H. Hutcheson. 1995. Coccidioidomycosis among visitors to a Coccidioides immitis-endemic area: an outbreak in a military reserve unit. *J Infect Dis* **171:**1672-5.

7111. Stanek, G. 1995. Borreliosis and Travel Medicine. *J Travel Med* **2:**244-251.

7112. Stanford, C. F., J. H. Connolly, W. A. Ellis, E. T. Smyth, P. V. Coyle, W. I. Montgomery, and D. I. Simpson. 1990. Zoonotic infections in Northern Ireland farmers. *Epidemiol Infect* **105:**565-70.

7113. Stanghellini, A., R. Josse, P. Cattand, T. Bopang, N. Tirandibaye, P. Emery, J. M. Milleliri, and G. Cordoliani. 1989. [Epidemiological aspects of human African trypanosomiasis in south Chad]. *Med Trop (Mars)* **49:**395-400.

7114. Stanley, S. L., Jr. 2003. Amoebiasis. *Lancet* **361:**1025-34.

7115. Stansfield, R. E., R. G. Masterton, B. A. Dale, and R. J. Fallon. 1994. Primary meningococcal conjunctivitis and the need for prophylaxis in close contacts. *J Infect* **29:**211-4.

7116. Stanwell-Smith, R. E., and L. R. Ward. 1986. An international point source outbreak of typhoid fever: a European collaborative investigation. *Bull WHO* **64:**271-278.

7117. Stapleton, J. T. 2003. GB virus type C/Hepatitis G virus. *Semin Liver Dis* **23:**137-48.

7118. Stark, K., U. Bienzle, R. Vonk, and I. Guggenmoos-Holzmann. 1997. History of syringe sharing in prison and risk of hepatitis B virus, hepatitis C virus, and human immunodeficiency virus infection among injecting drug users in Berlin. *Int J Epidemiol* **26:**1359-66.

7119. Stark, M. E., D. A. Herrington, G. V. Hillyer, and D. B. McGill. 1993. An international traveler with fever, abdominal pain, eosinophilia, and a liver lesion. *Gastroenterology* **105:**1900-8.

7120. Starr, J. R., T. C. White, B. G. Leroux, H. S. Luis, M. Bernardo, J. Leitao, and M. C. Roberts. 2002. Persistence of oral Candida albicans carriage in healthy Portuguese schoolchildren followed for 3 years. *Oral Microbiol Immunol* **17:**304-10.

7121. Staszkiewicz, J., C. M. Lewis, J. Colville, M. Zervos, and J. Band. 1991. Outbreak of Brucella melitensis among microbiology laboratory workers in a community hospital. *J Clin Microbiol* **29:**287-90.

7122. Stauffer, W. M., J. S. Sellman, and P. F. Walker. 2004. Biliary liver flukes (Opisthorchiasis and Clonorchiasis) in immigrants in the United States: often subtle and diagnosed years after arrival. *J Travel Med* **11:**157-60.

7123. Stead, W. W., J. W. Senner, W. T. Reddick, and J. P. Lofgren. 1990. Racial differences in susceptibility to infection by Mycobacterium tuberculosis. *N Engl J Med* **322:**422-427.

7124. Steele, M., S. Unger, and J. Odumeru. 2003. Sensitivity of PCR detection of Cyclospora cayetanensis in raspberries, basil, and mesclun lettuce. *J Microbiol Methods* **54:**277-80.

7125. Steele, T. W., C. V. Moore, and N. Sangster. 1990. Distribution of Legionella longbeachae serogroup 1 and other legionellae in potting soils in Australia. *Appl Environ Microbiol* **56:**2984-8.

7126. **Steen, R.** 2001. Eradicating chancroid. *Bull WHO* **79:**818-26.

7127. **Steen, R., and G. Dallabetta.** 2003. Sexually transmitted infection control with sex workers: regular screening and presumptive treatment augment efforts to reduce risk and vulnerability. *Reprod Health Matters* **11:**74-90.

7128. **Steere, A. C.** 2001. Lyme disease. *N Engl J Med* **345:**115-25.

7129. **Steffen, R.** 1990. Risks of hepatitis B for travellers. *Vaccine* **8 Suppl:**S31-2.

7130. **Steffen, R., C. de Bernardis, and A. Banos.** 2003. Travel epidemiology - a global perspective. *Int J Antimicrob Agents* **21:**89-95.

7131. **Steffen, R., M. Desaules, J. Nagel, F. Vuillet, P. Schubarth, C. H. Jeanmaire, and A. Huber.** 1992. Epidemiological experience in the mission of the United Nations Transition Assistance Group (UNTAG) in Namibia. *Bull WHO* **70:**129-33.

7132. **Steffen, R., H. DuPont, and A. Wilder-Smith.** 2003. Manual of travel medicine and health. BC Decker, Hamilton, Ontario, Canada.

7133. **Steffen, R., H. Kollaritsch, and K. Fleisher.** 2003. Travelers' diarrhea in the new millenium: consensus among experts from German-speaking countries. *J Travel Med* **10:**38-45.

7134. **Steffen, R., B. Somaini, and A. Gubser.** 1985. Sind "epidemiologisch bedeutsame medizinische Notfälle" auf interkontinentalen Flughäfen möglich? *Ther Umsch* **42:**12-6.

7135. **Steffen, T., R. Blattler, F. Gutzwiller, and M. Zwahlen.** 2001. HIV and hepatitis virus infections among injecting drug users in a medically controlled heroin prescription programme. *Eur J Public Health* **11:**425-30.

7136. **Stehr-Green, J. K., L. McCaig, H. M. Remsen, C. S. Rains, M. Fox, and D. D. Juranek.** 1987. Shedding of oocysts in immunocompetent individuals infected with Cryptosporidium. *Am J Trop Med Hyg* **36:**338-42.

7137. **Stehr-Green, J. K., C. Nicholls, A. Payne, and P. Mitchell.** 1991. Waterborne outbreak of Campylobacter jejuni in Christchurch: the importance of a combined epidemiologic and microbiologic investigation. *N Z Med J* **104:**356-8.

7138. **Stein, A., R. Purgus, M. Olmer, and D. Raoult.** 1999. Brill-Zinsser disease in France. *Lancet* **353:**1936.

7139. **Stein, A., and D. Raoult.** 1998. Q fever during pregnancy: a public health problem in southern France. *Clin Infect Dis* **27:**592-6.

7140. **Stein, A., and D. Raoult.** 1999. Pigeon pneumonia in Provence: a bird-borne Q fever outbreak. *Clin Infect Dis* **29:**617-20.

7141. **Stein, H. A.** 1983. Trichinose-Erkrankungen im Bitburger Raum (Eifel). Aus der Sicht der Humanmediziner des öffentlichen Gesundheitsdienstes. *Öff Gesundh-Wes* **45:**532-3.

7142. **Stein, M. D., K. A. Freedberg, L. M. Sullivan, J. Savetsky, S. M. Levenson, R. Hingson, and J. H. Samet.** 1998. Sexual ethics. Disclosure of HIV-positive status to partners. *Arch Intern Med* **158:**253-7.

7143. **Steinbach, W. J., and J. R. Perfect.** 2003. Scedosporium species infections and treatments. *J Chemother* **15 Suppl 2:**16-27.

7144. **Steinberg, E. B., R. Bishop, P. Haber, A. F. Dempsey, R. M. Hoekstra, J. M. Nelson, M. Ackers, A. Calugar, and E. D. Mintz.** 2004. Typhoid fever in travelers: who should be targeted for prevention? *Clin Infect Dis* **39:**186-97.

7145. **Steinberg, E. B., K. D. Greene, C. A. Bopp, D. N. Cameron, J. G. Wells, and E. D. Mintz.** 2001. Cholera in the United States, 1995-2000: trends at the end of the twentieth century. *J Infect Dis* **184:**799-802.

7146. **Steinbrook, R.** 2004. The AIDS epidemic in 2004. *N Engl J Med* **351:**115-7.

7147. **Steinemann, T. L., U. Pinninti, L. B. Szczotka, R. A. Eiferman, and F. W. Price, Jr.** 2003. Ocular complications associated with the use of cosmetic contact lenses from unlicensed vendors. *Eye Contact Lens* **29:**196-200.

7148. **Steiner, H. A., D. Raveh, B. Rudensky, E. Paz, Z. Jerassi, Y. Schlesinger, and A. M. Yinnon.** 2001. Outbreak of Q fever among kitchen employees in an urban hospital. *Eur J Clin Microbiol Infect Dis* **20:**898-900.

7149. **Steinert, M., U. Hentschel, and J. Hacker.** 2002. Legionella pneumophila: an aquatic microbe goes astray. *FEMS Microbiol Rev* **26:**149-62.

7150. **Steinhoff, D., H. Lode, G. Ruckdeschel, B. Heidrich, A. Rolfs, F. J. Fehrenbach, H. Mauch, G. Hoffken, and J. Wagner.** 1996. Chlamydia pneumoniae as a cause of community-acquired pneumonia in hospitalized patients in Berlin. *Clin Infect Dis* **22:**958-64.

7151. **Steininger, C., M. Kundi, G. Jatzko, H. Kiss, A. Lischka, and H. Holzmann.** 2003. Increased risk of mother-to-infant transmission of hepatitis C virus by intrapartum infantile exposure to maternal blood. *J Infect Dis* **187:**345-51.

7152. **Steketee, R. W., M. R. Eckman, E. C. Burgess, J. N. Kuritsky, J. Dickerson, W. L. Schell, M. S. Godsey, Jr., and J. P. Davis.** 1985. Babesiosis in Wisconsin. A new focus of disease transmission. *JAMA* **253:**2675-8.

7153. **Steketee, R. W., B. L. Nahlen, M. E. Parise, and C. Menendez.** 2001. The burden of malaria in pregnancy in malaria-endemic areas. *Am J Trop Med Hyg* **64:**28-35.

7154. **Steketee, R. W., S. Reid, T. Cheng, J. S. Stoebig, R. G. Harrington, and J. P. Davis.** 1989. Recurrent outbreaks of giardiasis in a child day care center, Wisconsin. *Am J Public Health* **79:**485-90.

7155. **Steketee, R. W., S. G. Wassilak, W. N. Adkins, Jr., D. G. Burstyn, C. R. Manclark, J. Berg, D. Hopfensperger, W. L. Schell, and J. P. Davis.** 1988. Evidence for a high attack rate and efficacy of erythromycin prophylaxis in a pertussis outbreak in a facility for the developmentally disabled. *J Infect Dis* **157:**434-40.

7156. **Stensballe, L. G., J. K. Devasundaram, and E. A. F. Simoes.** 2003. Respiratory syncytial virus epidemics: the ups and downs of a seasonal virus. *Pediatr Infect Dis* **22 suppl:**S21-32.

7157. **Stensballe, L. G., S. Trautner, P. E. Kofoed, E. Nante, K. Hedegaard, I. P. Jensen, and P. Aaby.** 2002. Comparison of nasopharyngeal aspirate and nasal swab specimens for detection of respiratory syncytial virus in different settings in a developing country. *Trop Med Int Health* **7:**317-21.

7158. **Stenzel, D. J., and P. F. L. Boreham.** 1996. Blastocystis hominis revisited. *Clin Microbiol Rev* **9:**563-84.

7159. **Stephan, C., K. P. Hunfeld, A. Schonberg, M. G. Ott, M. Hetzenecker, R. Bitzer, and G. Just-Nubling.** 2000. [Leptospirosis after a staff outing]. *Dtsch Med Wochenschr* **125:**623-7.

7160. **Stephan, R., N. Borel, C. Zweifel, M. Blanco, and J. E. Blanco.** 2004. First isolation and further characterization of enteropathogenic Escherichia coli (EPEC) O157:H45 strains from cattle. *BMC Microbiol* **4:**10.

7161. **Stephan, R., S. Ragettli, and F. Untermann.** 2000. Prevalence and characteristics of verotoxin-producing Escherichia coli (VTEC) in stool samples from asymptomatic human carriers working in the meat processing industry in Switzerland. *J Appl Microbiol* **88:**335-41.

7162. **Stephens, R. S. e.** 1999. Chlamydia. Intracellular biology, pathogenesis, and immunity. American Society for Microbiology, Washington, D.C.

7163. **Stephenson, I., K. G. Nicholson, J. M. Wood, M. C. Zambon, and J. M. Katz.** 2004. Confronting the avian influenza threat: vaccine development for a potential pandemic. *Lancet Infect Dis* **4:**499-509.

7164. **Stephenson, J.** 1991. Spring rubella outbreak amongst military apprentices in north-west Sydney. *Commun Dis Intell* **15:**464-.

7165. **Stephenson, L. S., C. V. Holland, and E. S. Cooper.** 2000. The public health significance of Trichuris trichiura. *Parasitology* **121 suppl:**S73-95.

7166. **Steppberger, K., S. Walter, M. C. Claros, F. B. Spencker, W. Kiess, A. C. Rodloff, and C. Vogtmann.** 2002. Nosocomial Neonatal Outbreak of Serratia marcescens - Analysis of Pathogens by Pulsed Field Gel Electrophoresis and Polymerase Chain Reaction. *Infection* **30:**277-81.

7167. **Sterling, T. R., D. S. Pope, W. R. Bishai, S. Harrington, R. R. Gershon, and R. E. Chaisson.** 2000. Transmission of Mycobacterium tuberculosis from a cadaver to an embalmer. *N Engl J Med* **342:**246-8.

7168. **Stern, N. J., K. L. Hiett, G. A. Alfredsson, K. G. Kristinsson, J. Reiersen, H. Hardardottir, H. Briem, E. Gunnarsson, F. Georgsson, R. Lowman, E. Berndtson, A. M. Lammerding, G. M. Paoli, and M. T. Musgrove.** 2003. Campylobacter spp. in Icelandic poultry operations and human disease. *Epidemiol Infect* **130:**23-32.

7169. **Stetler, H. C., P. L. Garbe, D. M. Dwyer, R. R. Facklam, W. A. Orenstein, G. R. West, K. J. Dudley, and A. B. Bloch.** 1985. Outbreaks of group A streptococcal abscesses following diphtheria- tetanus toxoid-pertussis vaccination. *Pediatrics* **75:**299-303.

7170. **Stevens, D. L., and A. E. Bryant.** 2002. The role of clostridial toxins in the pathogenesis of gas gangrene. *Clin Infect Dis* **35 suppl 1:**S93-100.

7171. **Stevens, D. L., and E. L. E. Kaplan.** 2000. Streptococcal infections. Oxford University Press, New York.

7172. **Stevenson, J., G. Murdoch, A. Riley, B. Duncan, M. McWhirter, and P. Christie.** 1998. Implementation and evaluation of a measles/rubella vaccination campaign in a campus university in the UK following an outbreak of rubella. *Epidemiol Infect* **121:**157-64.

7173. **Stevenson, P.** 1979. Toxocara and ascaris infection in British pigs: a serological survey. *Vet Rec* **104:**526-8.

7174. **Stich, A., P. M. Abel, and S. Krishna.** 2002. Human African trypanosomiasis. *BMJ* **325:**203-6.

7175. **Stich, A., H. Meyer, B. Kohler, and K. Fleischer.** 2002. Tanapox: first report in a European traveller and identification by PCR. *Trans R Soc Trop Med Hyg* **96:**178-9.

7176. **Stich, A. H., S. Biays, P. Odermatt, C. Men, C. Saem, K. Sokha, C. S. Ly, P. Legros, M. Philips, J. D. Lormand, and M. Tanner.** 1999. Foci of Schistosomiasis mekongi, Northern Cambodia: II. Distribution of infection and morbidity. *Trop Med Int Health* **4:**674-85.

7177. **Stinebaugh, B. J., F. X. Schloeder, K. M. Johnson, R. B. Mackenzie, G. Entwisle, and E. De Alba.** 1966. Bolivian hemorrhagic fever. A report of four cases. *Am J Med* **40:**217-30.

7178. **Stobierski, M. G., C. J. Hospedales, W. N. Hall, B. Robinson-Dunn, D. Hoch, and D. A. Sheill.** 1996. Outbreak of histoplasmosis among employees in a paper factory— Michigan, 1993. *J Clin Microbiol* **34:**1220-3.

7179. **Stockmann, M., M. Stoffler-Meilicke, A. Schwarz, M. Pohly, and H. Scherubl.** 2002. [Puumala virus infection (nephropathia epidemica) as different diagnosis of acute renal failure]. *Dtsch Med Wochenschr* **127:**557-560.

7180. **Stokes, M. L., M. J. Ferson, and L. C. Young.** 1997. Outbreak of hepatitis A among homosexual men in Sydney. *Am J Public Health* **87:**2039-41.

7181. **Stoller, J. S., H. M. Adam, B. Weiss, and M. Wittner.** 1991. Incidence of intestinal parasitic disease in an acquired immunodeficiency syndrome day-care center. *Pediatr Infect Dis J* **10:**654-8.

7182. **Stone, J. H., K. Dierberg, G. Aram, and J. S. Dumler.** 2004. Human monocytic ehrlichiosis. *JAMA* **292:**2263-70.

7183. **Stoppato, M. C., and A. Bini.** 2003. Deserts. Firefly Books Ltd, Toronto, Ontario.

7184. **Storey, P. A., N. R. Steenhard, L. Van Lieshout, S. Anemana, P. Magnussen, and A. M. Polderman.** 2001. Natural progression of Oesophagostomum bifurcatum pathology and infection in a rural community of northern Ghana. *Trans R Soc Trop Med Hyg* **95:**295-9.

7185. **Stout, J. E., and V. L. Yu.** 1997. Legionellosis. *N Engl J Med* **337:**682-7.

7186. **Stout, J. E., V. L. Yu, Y. C. Yee, S. Vaccarello, W. Diven, and T. C. Lee.** 1992. Legionella pneumophila in residential water supplies: environmental surveillance with clinical assessment for Legionnaires' disease. *Epidemiol Infect* **109:**49-57.

7187. **Strachan, D. P., and D. G. Cook.** 1997. Health effects of passive smoking. 1. Parental smoking and lower respiratory illness in infancy and early childhood. *Thorax* **52:**905-14.

7188. **Strangmann, E., H. Froleke, and K. P. Kohse.** 2002. Septic shock caused by Streptococcus suis: case report and investigation of a risk group. *Int J Hyg Environ Health* **205:**385-92.

7189. **Strassburg, M. A., D. T. Imagawa, S. L. Fannin, J. A. Turner, A. W. Chow, R. A. Murray, and J. D. Cherry.** 1981. Rubella outbreak among hospital employees. *Obstet Gynecol* **57:**283-8.

7190. **Stratigos, A. J., R. Stern, E. Gonzalez, R. A. Johnson, J. O'Connell, and J. S. Dover.** 1999. Prevalence of skin disease in a cohort of shelter-based homeless men. *J Am Acad Dermatol* **41:**197-202.

7191. **Strausbaugh, L. J., C. Jacobson, D. L. Sewell, S. Potter, and T. T. Ward.** 1991. Methicillin-resistant Staphylococcus aureus in extended-care facilities: experiences in a Veterans' Affairs nursing home and a review of the literature. *Infect Control Hosp Epidemiol* **12:**36-45.

7192. **Strausbaugh, L. J., S. R. Sukumar, and C. L. Joseph.** 2003. Infectious disease outbreaks in nursing homes: an unappreciated hazard for frail elderly persons. *Clin Infect Dis* **36:**870-6.

7193. **Strauss, B., M. Fyfe, K. Higo, K. Louie, D. Cross, M. Sisler, A. Paccagnella, A. Trinidad, C. Kurzac, G. Eng, B. Zaharia, and S. Chan.** 2000. An outbreak of Salmonella enteritidis linked to baked goods from a local bakery in lower Mainland, British Columbia. *Can Commun Dis Rep* **26:**173-4.

7194. **Strauss, S., P. Sastry, C. Sonnex, S. Edwards, and J. Gray.** 2002. Contamination of environmental surfaces by genital human papillomaviruses. *Sex Transm Infect* **78**:135-8.

7195. **Streatfield, R., D. Sinclair, G. Bielby, J. Sheridan, and D. Phillips.** 1993. Dengue serotype 2 epidemic, Townsville, 1992-93. *Commun Dis Intell* **17**:330-332.

7196. **Strebel, P., G. Hussey, C. Metcalf, D. Smith, D. Hanslo, and J. Simpson.** 1991. An outbreak of whooping cough in a highly vaccinated urban community. *J Trop Pediatr* **37**:71-6.

7197. **Strebel, P. M., A. Aubert-Combiescu, N. Ion-Nedelcu, S. Biberi-Moroeanu, M. Combiescu, R. W. Sutter, O. M. Kew, M. A. Pallansch, P. A. Patriarca, and S. L. Cochi.** 1994. Paralytic poliomyelitis in Romania, 1984-1992. Evidence for a high risk of vaccine-associated disease and reintroduction of wild-virus infection. *Am J Epidemiol* **140**:1111-24.

7198. **Streeton, C. L., J. N. Hanna, R. D. Messer, and A. Merianos.** 1995. An epidemic of acute post-streptococcal glomerulonephritis among aboriginal children. *J Paediatr Child Health* **31**:245-8.

7199. **Strelkova, M. V., L. N. Eliseev, E. N. Ponirovsky, T. I. Dergacheva, D. K. Annacharyeva, P. I. Erokhin, and D. A. Evans.** 2001. Mixed leishmanial infections in Rhombomys opimus: a key to the persistence of Leishmania major from one transmission season to the next. *Ann Trop Med Parasitol* **95**:811-9.

7200. **Strickler, H. D., P. S. Rosenberg, S. S. Devesa, J. Hertel, J. F. Fraumeni, Jr., and J. J. Goedert.** 1998. Contamination of poliovirus vaccines with simian virus 40 (1955-1963) and subsequent cancer rates. *JAMA* **279**:292-5.

7201. **Strickman, D., R. Sithiprasasna, P. Kittayapong, and B. L. Innis.** 2000. Distribution of dengue and Japanese encephalitis among children in rural and suburban Thai villages. *Am J Trop Med Hyg* **63**:27-35.

7202. **Strickman, D., P. Tanskul, C. Eamsila, and D. J. Kelly.** 1994. Prevalence of antibodies to rickettsiae in the human population of suburban Bangkok. *Am J Trop Med Hyg* **51**:149-53.

7203. **Strle, F.** 2004. Human granulocytic ehrlichiosis in Europe. *Int J Med Microbiol* **293 Suppl 37**:27-35.

7204. **Strle, F., V. Maraspin, S. Furlan-Lotric, and J. Cimperman.** 1996. Epidemiological study of a cohort of adult patients with Erythema migrans registered in Slovenia in 1993. *Eur J Epidemiol* **12**:503-7.

7205. **Strobaek, S., J. Zimakoff, K. F. Kristensen, H. Borgen, and L. Sorensen.** 1997. [Puerperal fever. A survey of an epidemic using a case-controlled study]. *Ugeskr Laeger* **159**:4117-22.

7206. **Strobel, E., J. Heesemann, G. Mayer, J. Peters, S. Muller-Weihrich, and P. Emmerling.** 2000. Bacteriological and serological findings in a further case of transfusion-mediated Yersinia enterocolitica sepsis. *J Clin Microbiol* **38**:2788-90.

7207. **Stroffolini, T., W. Biagini, L. Lorenzoni, G. P. Palazzesi, M. Divizia, and R. Frongillo.** 1990. An outbreak of hepatitis A in young adults in central Italy. *Eur J Epidemiol* **6**:156-9.

7208. **Strom, J.** 1979. A study of infections and illnesses in a day nursery based on inclusion- bearing cells in the urine and infectious agent in faeces, urine and nasal secretion. *Scand J Infect Dis* **11**:265-9.

7209. **Stromdahl, E. Y., S. R. Evans, J. J. O'Brien, and A. G. Gutierrez.** 2001. Prevalence of infection in ticks submitted to the human tick test kit program of the U.S. Army Center for Health Promotion and Preventive Medicine. *J Med Entomol* **38**:67-74.

7210. **Strong, B. S., and S. A. Young.** 1995. Intrauterine coxsackie virus, group B type 1, infection: viral cultivation from amniotic fluid in the third trimester. *Am J Perinatol* **12**:78-9.

7211. **Struve, J., O. Norrbohm, J. Stenbeck, J. Giesecke, and O. Weiland.** 1995. Risk factors for hepatitis A, B and C virus infection among Swedish expatriates. *J Infect* **31**:205-9.

7212. **Stryker, W. S., R. A. Gunn, and D. P. Francis.** 1986. Outbreak of hepatitis B associated with acupuncture. *J Fam Pract* **22**:155-8.

7213. **Stuart, J. M., H. J. Orr, F. G. Warburton, S. Jeyakanth, C. Pugh, I. Morris, J. Sarangi, and G. Nichols.** 2003. Risk factors for sporadic giardiasis: a case-control study in southwestern England. *Emerg Infect Dis* **9**:229-33.

7214. **Study, E. C.** 1992. Risk factors for mother-to-child transmission of HIV-1. *Lancet* **339**:1007-12.

7215. **Stuen, S., I. Van De Pol, K. Bergstrom, and L. M. Schouls.** 2002. Identification of Anaplasma phagocytophila (formerly Ehrlichia phagocytophila) variants in blood from sheep in Norway. *J Clin Microbiol* **40**:3192-7.

7216. **Stürchler, D.** 1988. Endemic areas of tropical infections (2nd ed). Hans Huber Verlag, Toronto - Lewiston N.Y. - Bern - Stuttgart.

7217. **Sturchler, D., R. Berger, and M. Just.** 1987. [Congenital toxoplasmosis in Switzerland. Seroprevalence, risk factors and recommendations for prevention]. *Schweiz Med Wochenschr* **117**:161-7.

7218. **Sturchler, D., and A. Degremont.** 1976. [Filariasis in patients returned from the tropics. Studies on 64 cases]. *Schweiz Med Wochenschr* **106**:682-8.

7219. **Sturchler, D., R. F. DiGiacomo, and L. Rausch.** 1987. Parasitic infections in Yakima Indians. *Ann Trop Med Parasitol* **81**:291-9.

7220. **Sturchler, D., F. Speiser, F. Bogenmann, and G. Delmore.** 1981. [Liver fascioliasis with unusual abscess formation. Case report]. *Schweiz Med Wochenschr* **111**:1578-82.

7221. **Sturchler, D., E. Stahel, K. Saladin, and B. Saladin.** 1980. Intestinal parasitoses in eight Liberian settlements: prevalences and community anthelminthic chemotherapy. *Tropenmed Parasitol* **31**:87-93.

7222. **Sturchler, D., N. Weiss, and M. Gassner.** 1990. Transmission of toxocariasis. *J Infect Dis* **162**:571.

7223. **Sturm, P. D., C. Connolly, N. Khan, S. Ebrahim, and A. W. Sturm.** 2004. Vaginal tampons as specimen collection device for the molecular diagnosis of non-ulcerative sexually transmitted infections in antenatal clinic attendees. *Int J STD AIDS* **15**:94-8.

7224. **Sturm-Ramirez, K., H. Brumblay, K. Diop, A. Gueye-Ndiaye, J. L. Sankale, I. Thior, I. N'Doye, C. C. Hsieh, S. Mboup, and P. J. Kanki.** 2000. Molecular epidemiology of genital Chlamydia trachomatis infection in high-risk women in Senegal, West Africa. *J Clin Microbiol* **38**:138-45.

7225. **Sturrock, R. F.** 2001. Schistosomiasis epidemiology and control: how did we get here and where should we go? *Mem Inst Oswaldo Cruz* **96 suppl**:17-27.

7226. **Su, L. H., J. T. Ou, H. S. Leu, P. C. Chiang, Y. P. Chiu, J. H. Chia, A. J. Kuo, C. H. Chiu, C. Chu, T. L. Wu, C. F. Sun, T. V. Riley, and B. J. Chang.** 2003. Extended epidemic of nosocomial urinary tract infections caused by Serratia marcescens. *J Clin Microbiol* **41**:4726-32.

7227. **Suarez Hernandez, M., C. M. Fernandez Andreu, A. Estrada Ortiz, and E. Cisneros Despaigne.** 1992. [Histoplasmin reactivity in poultry farm workers in the province of Ciego de Avila, Cuba]. *Rev Inst Med Trop Sao Paulo* **34:**329-33.

7228. **Suarez-Estrada, J., J. I. Rodriguez-Barbosa, C. B. Gutierrez-Martin, M. R. Castaneda-Lopez, J. M. Fernandez-Marcos, O. R. Gonzalez-Llamazares, and E. F. Rodriguez-Ferri.** 1996. Seroepidemiological survey of Q fever in Leon province, Spain. *Eur J Epidemiol* **12:**245-50.

7229. **Subekti, D., B. A. Oyofo, P. Tjaniadi, A. L. Corwin, W. Larasati, M. Putri, C. H. Simanjuntak, N. H. Punjabi, J. Taslim, B. Setiawan, A. A. Djelantik, L. Sriwati, A. Sumardiati, E. Putra, J. R. Campbell, and M. Lesmana.** 2001. Shigella spp. surveillance in Indonesia: the emergence or reemergence of S. dysenteriae. *Emerg Infect Dis* **7:**137-40.

7230. **Sucato, G., C. Celum, D. Dithmer, R. Ashley, and A. Wald.** 2001. Demographic rather than behavioral risk factors predict herpes simplex virus type 2 infection in sexually active adolescents. *Pediatr Infect Dis J* **20:**422-6.

7231. **Sudarshi, S., R. Stumpfle, M. Armstrong, T. Ellman, S. Parton, P. Krishnan, P. L. Chiodini, and C. J. Whitty.** 2003. Clinical presentation and diagnostic sensitivity of laboratory tests for Strongyloides stercoralis in travellers compared with immigrants in a non-endemic country. *Trop Med Int Health* **8:**728-32.

7232. **Suess, J., A. Weber, H. Berg, B. Keller, and W. Schmahl.** 2001. Rabies in a vaccinated dog imported from Azerbaijan to Germany. *Rabies Bulletin Europe* **25:**14-15.

7233. **Suggaravetsiri, P., H. Yanai, V. Chongsuvivatwong, O. Naimpasan, and P. Akarasewi.** 2003. Integrated counseling and screening for tuberculosis and HIV among household contacts of tuberculosis patients in an endemic area of HIV infection: Chiang Rai, Thailand. *Int J Tuberc Lung Dis* **7:**S424-31.

7234. **Sugita, T., R. Ikeda, and A. Nishikawa.** 2004. Analysis of Trichosporon isolates obtained from the houses of patients with summer-type hypersensitivity pneumonitis. *J Clin Microbiol* **42:**5467-71.

7235. **Sugiyama, A., Y. Nakano, Y. Iwade, A. Yamauchi, N. Sakurai, O. Nakayama, Y. Yamamoto, M. Nakatsu, Y. Mori, Y. Kishida, T. Oida, N. H. Kumazawa, J. Terajima, and A. Nakamura.** 1999. Epidemiological studies of an outbreak of paratyphoid fever in the Shima area of Mie Prefecture. *Jpn J Infect Dis* **52:**253-5.

7236. **Sugunan, A. P., A. R. Ghosh, S. Roy, M. D. Gupte, and S. C. Sehgal.** 2004. A cholera epidemic among the Nicobarese tribe of Nancowry, Andaman, and Nicobar, India. *Am J Trop Med Hyg* **71:**822-7.

7237. **Sukonthaman, A., J. D. Freeman, M. Ratanavararak, V. Khaoparisuthi, and W. Snidvongs.** 1981. Mycoplasma pneumoniae infections-the first demonstration of an outbreak at a Kampuchean Holding Center in Thailand. *J Med Assoc Thai* **64:**392-400.

7238. **Sukthana, Y., J. Kaewkungwal, C. Jantanavivat, A. Lekkla, R. Chiabchalard, and W. Aumarm.** 2003. Toxoplasma gondii antibody in Thai cats and their owners. *Southeast Asian J Trop Med Public Health* **34:**733-8.

7239. **Sukvirach, S., J. S. Smith, S. Tunsakul, N. Munoz, V. Kesararat, O. Opasatian, S. Chichareon, V. Kaenploy, R. Ashley, C. J. Meijer, P. J. Snijders, P. Coursaget, S. Franceschi, and R. Herrero.** 2003. Population-based human papillomavirus prevalence in Lampang and Songkla, Thailand. *J Infect Dis* **187:**1246-56.

7240. **Sulaiman, H. A., Julitasari, A. Sie, M. Rustam, W. Melani, A. Corwin, and G. B. Jennings.** 1995. Prevalence of hepatitis B and C viruses in healthy Indonesian blood donors. *Trans R Soc Trop Med Hyg* **89:**167-70.

7241. **Sulaiman, I. M., R. Fayer, C. Bern, R. H. Gilman, J. M. Trout, P. M. Schantz, P. Das, A. A. Lal, and L. Xiao.** 2003. Triosephosphate isomerase gene characterization and potential zoonotic transmission of Giardia duodenalis. *Emerg Infect Dis* **9:**1444-52.

7242. **Sulakvelidze, A.** 2000. Yersiniae other than Y. enterocolitica, Y. pseudotuberculosis, and Y. pestis: the ignored species. *Microbes Infect* **2:**497-513.

7243. **Suleiman, M. N., J. M. Muscat-Baron, J. R. Harries, A. G. Satti, G. S. Platt, E. T. Bowen, and D. I. Simpson.** 1980. Congo/Crimean haemorrhagic fever in Dubai. An outbreak at the Rashid Hospital. *Lancet* **2:**939-41.

7244. **Suligoi, B., C. Galli, S. Ciuta, and R. Decker.** 1999. Low seroprevalence of HTLV-I and HTLV-II in patients with a sexually transmitted disease. Study Group for HTLV and STDs. *Eur J Epidemiol* **15:**225-9.

7245. **Sulkowski, M. S., S. C. Ray, and D. L. Thomas.** 2002. Needlestick transmission of hepatitis C. *JAMA* **287:**2406-13.

7246. **Sumaya, C. V., and Y. Ench.** 1986. Epstein-Barr virus infections in families: the role of children with infectious mononucleosis. *J Infect Dis* **154:**842-50.

7247. **Summanen, P. H., D. A. Talan, C. Strong, M. McTeague, R. Bennion, J. E. Thompson, Jr., M. L. Vaisanen, G. Moran, M. Winer, and S. M. Finegold.** 1995. Bacteriology of skin and soft-tissue infections: comparison of infections in intravenous drug users and individuals with no history of intravenous drug use. *Clin Infect Dis* **20 Suppl 2:**S279-82.

7248. **Sun, C. A., D. M. Wu, C. C. Lin, S. N. Lu, S. L. You, L. Y. Wang, M. H. Wu, and C. J. Chen.** 2003. Incidence and cofactors of hepatitis C virus-related hepatocellular carcinoma: a prospective study of 12,008 men in Taiwan. *Am J Epidemiol* **157:**674-82.

7249. **Sun, D. X., F. G. Zhang, Y. Q. Geng, and D. S. Xi.** 1996. Hepatitis C transmission by cosmetic tattooing in women. *Lancet* **347:**541.

7250. **Sundkvist, T., C. Aitken, G. Duckworth, and D. Jeffries.** 1997. Outbreak of acute hepatitis A among homosexual men in East London. *Scand J Infect Dis* **29:**211-2.

7251. **Sundkvist, T., G. R. Hamilton, B. M. Hourihan, and I. J. Hart.** 2000. Outbreak of hepatitis A spread by contaminated drinking glasses in a public house. *Commun Dis Public Health* **3:**60-2.

7252. **Sundnes, K. O., and A. T. Haimanot.** 1993. Epidemic of louse-borne relapsing fever in Ethiopia. *Lancet* **342:**1213-5.

7253. **Sung, J. F., R. S. Lin, K. C. Huang, S. Y. Wang, and Y. J. Lu.** 2001. Pinworm control and risk factors of pinworm infection among primary-school children in Taiwan. *Am J Trop Med Hyg* **65:**558-62.

7254. **Sung, V., D. P. O'Brien, E. Matchett, G. V. Brown, and J. Torresi.** 2003. Dengue Fever in travelers returning from southeast Asia. *J Travel Med* **10:**208-13.

7255. **Sunstrum, J., L. J. Elliott, L. M. Barat, E. D. Walker, and J. R. Zucker.** 2001. Probable autochthonous Plasmodium vivax malaria transmission in Michigan: case report and epidemiological investigation. *Am J Trop Med Hyg* **65:**949-53.

7256. **Supramaniam, V., G. C. Datta, V. Singam, and J. Singh.** 1987. Malaria in the Malaysian army with particular reference to chemosuppressive use. *Med J Malaysia* **42:**44-9.

7257. **Suputtamongkol, Y., W. Chaowagul, P. Chetchotisakd, N. Lertpatanasuwun, S. Intaranongpai, T. Ruchutrakool, D. Budhsarawong, P. Mootsikapun, V. Wuthiekanun, N. Teerawatasook, and A. Lulitanond.** 1999. Risk factors for melioidosis and bacteremic melioidosis. *Clin Infect Dis* **29:**408-13.

7258. **Suputtamongkol, Y., J. M. Rolain, K. Losuwanaruk, K. Niwatayakul, C. Suttinont, W. Chierakul, K. Pimda, and D. Raoult.** 2003. Q fever in Thailand. *Emerg Infect Dis* **9:**1186-8.

7259. **Sur, D., P. Dutta, G. B. Nair, and S. K. Bhattacharya.** 2000. Severe cholera outbreak following floods in a northern district of West Bengal. *Indian J Med Res* **112:**178-82.

7260. **Surmieda, M. R., J. M. Lopez, G. Abad-Viola, M. E. Miranda, I. P. Abellanosa, R. A. Sadang, F. P. Magboo, N. S. Zacarias, R. L. Magpantay, F. M. White, et al.** 1992. Surveillance in evacuation camps after the eruption of Mt. Pinatubo, Philippines. *MMWR CDC Surveill Summ* **41:**9-12.

7261. **Suss, J.** 2003. Epidemiology and ecology of TBE relevant to the production of effective vaccines. *Vaccine* **21 Suppl 1:**S19-35.

7262. **Suss, J., C. Schrader, U. Falk, and N. Wohanka.** 2004. Tick-borne encephalitis (TBE) in Germany—epidemiological data, development of risk areas and virus prevalence in field-collected ticks and in ticks removed from humans. *Int J Med Microbiol* **293 Suppl 37:**69-79.

7263. **Sutmoller, F., R. S. Azeredo, M. D. Lacerda, O. M. Barth, H. G. Pereira, E. Hoffer, and H. G. Schatzmayr.** 1982. An outbreak of gastroenteritis caused by both rotavirus and Shigella sonnei in a private school in Rio de Janeiro. *J Hyg (Lond)* **88:**285-93.

7264. **Sutter, R. W., and E. Haefliger.** 1990. Tuberculosis morbidity and infection in Vietnamese in Southeast Asian refugee camps. *Am Rev Respir Dis* **141:**1483-6.

7265. **Sutter, R. W., L. E. Markowitz, J. M. Bennetch, W. Morris, E. R. Zell, and S. R. Preblud.** 1991. Measles among the Amish: a comparative study of measles severity in primary and secondary cases in households. *J Infect Dis* **163:**12-6.

7266. **Sutton, R. G.** 1974. An outbreak of cholera in Australia due to food served in flight on an international aircraft. *J Hyg (Lond)* **72:**441-51.

7267. **Suwanabun, N., C. Chouriyagune, C. Eamsila, P. Watcharapichat, G. A. Dasch, R. S. Howard, and D. J. Kelly.** 1997. Evaluation of an enzyme-linked immunosorbent assay in Thai scrub typhus patients. *Am J Trop Med Hyg* **56:**38-43.

7268. **Suzuki, A., I. Bisordi, S. Levis, J. Garcia, L. E. Pereira, R. P. Souza, T. K. N. Sugahara, N. Pini, D. Enria, and L. T. M. Souza.** 2004. Identifying rodent hantavirus reservoirs, Brazil. *Emerg Infect Dis* **10:**2127-34.

7269. **Suzuki, K., T. Yoshikawa, A. Tomitaka, K. Matsunaga, and Y. Asano.** 2004. Detection of aerosolized varicella-zoster virus DNA in patients with localized herpes zoster. *J Infect Dis* **189:**1009-12.

7270. **Suzuki, S., K. Nakabayashi, H. Ohkouchi, J. Hatada, S. Kawaguchi, M. Sakai, N. Sasaki, and A. Ito.** 1997. [Tuberculosis in the crew of a submarine]. *Nihon Kyobu Shikkan Gakkai Zasshi* **35:**61-6.

7271. **Suzuki, T., K. Omata, T. Satoh, T. Miyasaka, C. Arai, M. Maeda, T. Matsuno, and T. Miyamura.** 2005. Quantitative Detection of Hepatitis C Virus (HCV) RNA in Saliva and Gingival Crevicular Fluid of HCV-Infected Patients. *J Clin Microbiol* **43:**4413-7.

7272. **Svoboda, T., B. Henry, L. Shulman, E. Kennedy, E. Rea, W. Ng, T. Wallington, B. Yaffe, E. Gournis, E. Vicencio, S. Basrur, and R. H. Glazier.** 2004. Public health measures to control the spread of the severe acute respiratory syndrome during the outbreak in Toronto. *N Engl J Med* **350:**2352-61.

7273. **Svobodova, M., J. Sadlova, K. P. Chang, and P. Volf.** 2003. Short report: distribution and feeding preference of the sand flies Phlebotomus sergenti and P. papatasi in a cutaneous leishmaniasis focus in Sanliurfa, Turkey. *Am J Trop Med Hyg* **68:**6-9.

7274. **Swaddiwudhipong, W., P. Akarasewi, and T. Chayaniyayodhin.** 1990. A cholera outbreak associated with eating uncooked pork in Thailand. *J Diarrhoeal Dis Res* **8:**94-6.

7275. **Swaddiwudhipong, W., and J. Kanlayanaphotporn.** 2001. A common-source water-borne outbreak of multidrug-resistant typhoid fever in a rural Thai community. *J Med Assoc Thai* **84:**1513-7.

7276. **Swaddiwudhipong, W., and P. Kunasol.** 1989. An outbreak of nosocomial cholera in a 755-bed hospital. *Trans R Soc Trop Med Hyg* **83:**279-81.

7277. **Swanepoel, R., A. J. Shepherd, P. A. Leman, S. P. Shepherd, and G. B. Miller.** 1985. A common-source outbreak of Crimean-Congo haemorrhagic fever on a dairy farm. *S Afr Med J* **68:**635-7.

7278. **Swenne, C. L., C. Lindholm, J. Borowiec, and M. Carlsson.** 2004. Surgical-site infections within 60 days of coronary artery by-pass graft surgery. *J Hosp Infect* **57:**14-24.

7279. **Swerdlow, D. L., and P. M. Griffin.** 1997. Duration of faecal shedding of Escherichia coli O157:H7 among children in day-care centres. *Lancet* **349:**745-6.

7280. **Swerdlow, D. L., E. D. Mintz, M. Rodriguez, E. Tejada, C. Ocampo, L. Espejo, K. D. Greene, W. Saldana, L. Seminario, R. V. Tauxe, et al.** 1992. Waterborne transmission of epidemic cholera in Trujillo, Peru: lessons for a continent at risk. *Lancet* **340:**28-33.

7281. **Swerdlow, D. L., B. A. Woodruff, R. C. Brady, P. M. Griffin, S. Tippen, H. D. Donnell, Jr., E. Geldreich, B. J. Payne, A. Meyer, Jr., J. G. Wells, et al.** 1992. A waterborne outbreak in Missouri of Escherichia coli O157:H7 associated with bloody diarrhea and death. *Ann Intern Med* **117:**812-9.

7282. **Swinne, D., H. Taelman, J. Batungwanayo, A. Bigirankana, and J. Bogaerts.** 1994. [Ecology of Cryptococcus neoformans in central Africa]. *Med Trop* **54:**53-5.

7283. **Syrjala, H., P. Kujala, V. Myllyla, and A. Salminen.** 1985. Airborne transmission of tularemia in farmers. *Scand J Infect Dis* **17:**371-5.

7284. **Szmuness, W., I. Much, A. M. Prince, J. H. Hoofnagle, C. E. Cherubin, E. J. Harley, and G. H. Block.** 1975. On the role of sexual behavior in the spread of hepatitis B infection. *Ann Intern Med* **83:**489-95.

7285. **Szmuness, W., R. H. Purcell, J. L. Dienstag, and C. E. Stevens.** 1977. Antibody to hepatitis A antigen in institutionalized mentally retarded patients. *JAMA* **237:**1702-5.

7286. **Tabaqchali, S., S. O'Farrell, J. Q. Nash, and M. Wilks.** 1984. Vaginal carriage and neonatal acquisition of Clostridium difficile. *J Med Microbiol* **18:**47-53.

7287. **Tacket, C. O., J. Ballard, N. Harris, J. Allard, C. Nolan, T. Quan, and M. L. Cohen.** 1985. An outbreak of Yersinia enterocolitica infections caused by contaminated tofu (soybean curd). *Am J Epidemiol* **121**:705-11.

7288. **Tacket, C. O., J. P. Narain, R. Sattin, J. P. Lofgren, C. Konigsberg, Jr., R. C. Rendtorff, A. Rausa, B. R. Davis, and M. L. Cohen.** 1984. A multistate outbreak of infections caused by Yersinia enterocolitica transmitted by pasteurized milk. *JAMA* **251**:483-6.

7289. **Tadei, W. P., B. D. Thatcher, J. M. Santos, V. M. Scarpassa, I. B. Rodrigues, and M. S. Rafael.** 1998. Ecologic observations on anopheline vectors of malaria in the Brazilian Amazon. *Am J Trop Med Hyg* **59**:325-35.

7290. **Taha, T. E., N. I. Kumwenda, A. Gibbons, R. L. Broadhead, S. Fiscus, V. Lema, G. Liomba, C. Nkhoma, P. G. Miotti, and D. R. Hoover.** 2003. Short postexposure prophylaxis in newborn babies to reduce mother-to-child transmission of HIV-1: NVAZ randomised clinical trial. *Lancet* **362**:1171-7.

7291. **Tai, K. S., P. I. Whelan, M. S. Patel, and B. Currie.** 1993. An outbreak of epidemic polyarthritis (Ross river virus disease) in the Northern Territory during the 1990-1991 wet season. *Med J Aust* **158**:522-5.

7292. **Taillard, C., G. Greub, R. Weber, G. E. Pfyffer, T. Bodmer, S. Zimmerli, R. Frei, S. Bassetti, P. Rohner, J. C. Piffaretti, E. Bernasconi, J. Bille, A. Telenti, and G. Prod'hom.** 2003. Clinical Implications of Mycobacterium kansasii Species Heterogeneity: Swiss National Survey. *J Clin Microbiol* **41**:1240-1244.

7293. **Taji, S. S., and A. H. Rogers.** 1998. ADRF Trebitsch Scholarship. The microbial contamination of toothbrushes. A pilot study. *Aust Dent J* **43**:128-30.

7294. **Takabe, K., S. Ohki, O. Kunihiro, T. Sakashita, I. Endo, Y. Ichikawa, H. Sekido, T. Amano, Y. Nakatani, K. Suzuki, and H. Shimada.** 1998. Anisakidosis: a cause of intestinal obstruction from eating sushi. *Am J Gastroenterol* **93**:1172-3.

7295. **Takafuji, E. T., L. D. Hendricks, J. L. Daubek, K. M. McNeil, H. M. Scagliola, and C. L. Diggs.** 1980. Cutaneous leishmaniasis associated with jungle training. *Am J Trop Med Hyg* **29**:516-20.

7296. **Takafuji, E. T., J. W. Kirkpatrick, R. N. Miller, J. J. Karwacki, P. W. Kelley, M. R. Gray, K. M. McNeill, H. L. Timboe, R. E. Kane, and J. L. Sanchez.** 1984. An efficacy trial of doxycycline chemoprophylaxis against leptospirosis. *N Engl J Med* **310**:497-500.

7297. **Takahashi, H., M. H. Kramer, Y. Yasui, H. Fujii, K. Nakase, K. Ikeda, T. Imai, A. Okazawa, T. Tanaka, T. Ohyama, and N. Okabe.** 2004. Nosocomial Serratia marcescens outbreak in Osaka, Japan, from 1999 to 2000. *Infect Control Hosp Epidemiol* **25**:156-61.

7298. **Takahashi, T., M. Goto, T. Endo, T. Nakamura, N. Yusa, N. Sato, and A. Iwamoto.** 2002. Pneumocystis carinii carriage in immunocompromised patients with and without human immunodeficiency virus infection. *J Med Microbiol* **51**:611-4.

7299. **Takahashi, Y., L. Mingyuan, and J. Waikagul.** 2000. Epidemiology of trichinellosis in Asia and the Pacific Rim. *Vet Parasitol* **93**:227-39.

7300. **Takai, S., P. Tharavichitkul, C. Sasaki, S. Onishi, S. Yamano, T. Kakuda, S. Tsubaki, C. Trinarong, S. Rojanasthien, A. Sirimalaisuwan, T. Tesaprateep, N. Maneekarn, T. Sirisanthana, and T. Kirikae.** 2002. Identification of virulence-associated antigens and plasmids in Rhodococcus equi from patients with acquired immune deficiency syndrome and prevalence of virulent R. equi in soil collected from domestic animal farms in Chiang Mai, Thailand. *Am J Trop Med Hyg* **66**:52-5.

7301. **Takala, A. K., J. Eskola, J. Palmgren, P. R. Ronnberg, E. Kela, P. Rekola, and P. H. Makela.** 1989. Risk factors of invasive Haemophilus influenzae type b disease among children in Finland. *J Pediatr* **115**:694-701.

7302. **Takami, T., H. Kawashima, Y. Takei, T. Miyajima, T. Mori, T. Nakayama, K. Takekuma, and A. Hoshika.** 1998. Usefulness of nested PCR and sequence analysis in a nosocomial outbreak of neonatal enterovirus infection. *J Clin Virol* **11**:67-75.

7303. **Takayanagui, O. M., C. D. Oliveira, A. M. Bergamini, D. M. Capuano, M. H. Okino, L. H. Febronio, E. S. A. A. Castro, M. A. Oliveira, E. G. Ribeiro, and A. M. Takayanagui.** 2001. [Monitoring of vegetables sold in Ribeirao Preto, SP, Brazil]. *Rev Soc Bras Med Trop* **34**:37-41.

7304. **Takeda, N., K. Kikuchi, R. Asano, T. Harada, K. Totsuka, T. Sumiyoshi, T. Uchiyama, and S. Hosoda.** 2001. Recurrent septicemia caused by Streptococcus canis after a dog bite. *Scand J Infect Dis* **33**:927-8.

7305. **Takeda, T., T. Ito, M. Osada, K. Takahashi, and I. Takashima.** 1999. Isolation of tick-borne encephalitis virus from wild rodents and a seroepizootiologic survey in Hokkaido, Japan. *Am J Trop Med Hyg* **60**:287-91.

7306. **Takeda, Y.** 1997. Enterohaemorrhagic Escherichia coli. *World Health Stat Q* **50**:74-80.

7307. **Takeuchi, S., K. Matuda, and K. Sasano.** 1995. Protein A in Staphylococcus aureus isolates from pigs. *J Vet Med Sci* **57**:581-2.

7308. **Takimoto, S., E. A. Waldman, R. C. Moreira, F. Kok, P. Pinheiro Fde, S. G. Saes, M. Hatch, D. F. de Souza, C. Carmona Rde, D. Shout, J. C. de Moraes, and A. M. Costa.** 1998. Enterovirus 71 infection and acute neurological disease among children in Brazil (1988-1990). *Trans R Soc Trop Med Hyg* **92**:25-8.

7309. **Takougang, I., M. Meremikwu, S. Wandji, E. V. Yenshu, B. Aripko, S. B. Lamlenn, B. L. Eka, P. Enyong, J. Meli, O. Kale, and J. H. Remme.** 2002. Rapid assessment method for prevalence and intensity of Loa loa infection. *Bull WHO* **80**:852-8.

7310. **Takwale, A., S. Agarwal, S. C. Holmes, and J. Berth-Jones.** 2001. Tinea capitis in two elderly women: transmission at the hairdresser. *Br J Dermatol* **144**:898-900.

7311. **Talan, D. A., F. M. Abrahamian, G. J. Moran, D. M. Citron, J. O. Tan, and E. J. Goldstein.** 2003. Clinical presentation and bacteriologic analysis of infected human bites in patients presenting to emergency departments. *Clin Infect Dis* **37**:1481-9.

7312. **Talan, D. A., D. M. Citron, F. M. Abrahamian, G. J. Moran, and E. J. C. Goldstein.** 1999. Bacteriologic analysis of infected dog and cat bites. *N Engl J Med* **340**:85-92.

7313. **Talarmin, A., L. J. Chandler, M. Kazanji, B. de Thoisy, P. Debon, J. Lelarge, M. Labeau, E. Bourreau, J. C. Vie, R. E. Shope, and J. L. Sarthou.** 1998. Mayaro virus fever in French Guiana: isolation, identification, and seroprevalence. *Am J Trop Med Hyg* **59**:452-6.

7314. **Talarmin, A., E. Nicand, M. Doucet, C. Fermanian, B. P., and Y. Buisson.** 1993. Toxi-infection alimentaire collective à Bacillus cereus. *Bull Epidémiol Hebdomaire* **33**:154-155.

7315. **Talbert, A., A. Nyange, and F. Molteni.** 1998. Spraying tick-infested houses with lambda-cyhalothrin reduces the incidence of tick-borne relapsing fever in children under five years old. *Trans R Soc Trop Med Hyg* **92**:251-3.

7316. **Talbot, E. A., M. Moore, E. McCray, and N. J. Binkin.** 2000. Tuberculosis among foreign-born persons in the United States, 1993-1998. *JAMA* **284:**2894-900.

7317. **Talla, I., A. Kongs, P. Verle, J. Belot, S. Sarr, and A. M. Coll.** 1990. Outbreak of intestinal schistosomiasis in the Senegal River Basin. *Ann Soc Belg Med Trop* **70:**173-80.

7318. **Tallis, G., and J. Gregory.** 1997. An outbreak of hepatitis A associated with a spa pool. *Commun Dis Intell* **21:**353-4.

7319. **Tallis, G., S. Ng, C. Ferreira, A. Tan, and J. Griffith.** 1999. A nursing home outbreak of Clostridium perfringens associated with pureed food. *Aust N Z J Public Health* **23:**421-3.

7320. **Talon, D., P. Menget, M. Thouverez, G. Thiriez, H. Gbaguidi Haore, C. Fromentin, A. Muller, and X. Bertrand.** 2004. Emergence of Enterobacter cloacae as a common pathogen in neonatal units: pulsed-field gel electrophoresis analysis. *J Hosp Infect* **57:**119-25.

7321. **Tan, C. T., and K. S. Tan.** 2001. Nosocomial transmissibility of Nipah virus. *J Infect Dis* **184:**1367.

7322. **Tanaka, T., K. Nakashima, H. Kishimoto, H. Takahashi, T. Ohyama, H. Toshima, N. Tsumura, K. Outi, S. Miwa, and N. Okabe.** 2001. [Field epidemiological investigation on an outbreak of Chlamydia pneumoniae infection—first recognized incidence in a nursing home for elderly in Japan]. *Kansenshogaku Zasshi* **75:**876-82.

7323. **Tanaka, T., H. Takahashi, J. M. Kobayashi, T. Ohyama, and N. Okabe.** 2004. A nosocomial outbreak of febrile bloodstream infection caused by heparinized-saline contaminated with Serratia marcescens, Tokyo, 2002. *Jpn J Infect Dis* **57:**189-92.

7324. **Tangermann, R. H., S. Gordon, P. Wiesner, and L. Kreckman.** 1991. An outbreak of cryptosporidiosis in a day-care center in Georgia. *Am J Epidemiol* **133:**471-6.

7325. **Tangkanakul, W., P. Tharmaphornpil, B. D. Plikaytis, S. Bragg, D. Poonsuksombat, P. Choomkasien, D. Kingnate, and D. A. Ashford.** 2000. Risk factors associated with leptospirosis in northeastern Thailand, 1998. *Am J Trop Med Hyg* **63:**204-8.

7326. **Tangkanakul, W., P. Tharmaphornpilas, D. Datapon, and S. Sutantayawalee.** 2000. Food poisoning outbreak from contaminated fish-balls. *J Med Assoc Thai* **83:**1289-95.

7327. **Tansel, O., G. Ekuklu, M. Otkun, M. T. Otkun, F. Akata, and M. Tugrul.** 2003. A food-borne outbreak caused by Salmonella enteritidis. *Yonsei Med J* **44:**198-202.

7328. **Tanser, F. C., B. Sharp, and D. le Sueur.** 2003. Potential effect of climate change on malaria transmission in Africa. *Lancet* **362:**1792-8.

7329. **Tantawi, H. H., M. O. Shony, and S. K. Al-Tikriti.** 1981. Antibodies to Crimean-Congo haemorrhagic fever virus in domestic animals in Iraq: a seroepidemiological survey. *Int J Zoonoses* **8:**115-20.

7330. **Tanyuksel, M., H. Gun, and L. Doganci.** 1996. Prevalence of Trichomonas vaginalis in prostitutes in Turkey. *Cent Eur J Public Health* **4:**96-7.

7331. **Tanzi, M., E. Bellelli, G. Benaglia, E. Cavatorta, A. Merialdi, E. Mordacci, M. L. Ribero, A. Tagger, C. Verrotti, and A. Volpicelli.** 1997. The prevalence of HCV infection in a cohort of pregnant women, the related risk factors and the possibility of vertical transmission. *Eur J Epidemiol* **13:**517-21.

7332. **Tanzi, M. G., and M. P. Gabay.** 2002. Association between honey consumption and infant botulism. *Pharmacotherapy* **22:**1479-83.

7333. **Taormina, P. J., L. R. Beuchat, and L. Slutsker.** 1999. Infections associated with eating seed sprouts: an international concern. *Emerg Infect Dis* **5:**626-34.

7334. **Tappero, J. W., R. Reporter, J. D. Wenger, B. A. Ward, M. W. Reeves, T. S. Missbach, B. D. Plikaytis, L. Mascola, and A. Schuchat.** 1996. Meningococcal disease in Los Angeles County, California, and among men in the county jails. *N Engl J Med* **335:**833-40.

7335. **Tapsall, J.** 2001. Annual report of the Australian gonococcal surveillance programme, 2000. *Commun Dis Intell* **25:**59-63.

7336. **Tapsell, S.** 2000. Flooding and human health. The dangers posed are not always obvious. *BMJ* **321:**1167-8.

7337. **Taranto, N. J., S. P. Cajal, M. C. De Marzi, M. M. Fernandez, F. M. Frank, A. M. Bru, M. C. Minvielle, J. A. Basualdo, and E. L. Malchiodi.** 2003. Clinical status and parasitic infection in a Wichí Aboriginal community in Salta, Argentina. *Trans R Soc Trop Med Hyg* **97:**554-8.

7338. **Tarantola, A. P., A. C. Rachline, C. Konto, S. Houze, S. Lariven, A. Fichelle, D. Ammar, C. Sabah-Mondan, H. Vrillon, O. Bouchaud, F. Pitard, and E. Bouvet.** 2004. Occupational malaria following needlestick injury. *Emerg Infect Dis* **10:**1878-80.

7339. **Tarasevich, I., E. Rydkina, and D. Raoult.** 1998. Outbreak of epidemic typhus in Russia. *Lancet* **352:**1151.

7340. **Tarasevich, I. V., V. A. Makarova, N. F. Fetisova, A. V. Stepanov, E. D. Miskarova, N. Balayeva, and D. Raoult.** 1991. Astrakhan fever, a spotted-fever rickettsiosis. *Lancet* **337:**172-3.

7341. **Tariq, W. U., M. S. Shafi, S. JAMAl, and M. Ahmad.** 1991. Rabies in man handling infected calf. *Lancet* **337:**1224.

7342. **Tarr, P. E., L. Kuppens, T. C. Jones, B. Ivanoff, P. G. Aparin, and D. L. Heymann.** 1999. Considerations regarding mass vaccination against typhoid fever as an adjunct to sanitation and public health measures: potential use in an epidemic in Tajikistan. *Am J Trop Med Hyg* **61:**163-70.

7343. **Tarradas, C., I. Luque, D. de Andres, Y. E. Abdel-Aziz Shahein, P. Pons, F. Gonzalez, C. Borge, and A. Perea.** 2001. Epidemiological relationship of human and swine Streptococcus suis isolates. *J Vet Med B Infect Dis Vet Public Health* **48:**347-55.

7344. **Tarrago, D., R. Lopez-Velez, C. Turrientes, F. Baquero, and M. L. Mateos.** 2000. Prevalence of hepatitis E antibodies in immigrants from developing countries. *Eur J Clin Microbiol Infect Dis* **19:**309-11.

7345. **Tarry, D. W.** 1986. Progress in warble fly eradication. *Parasitol Today* **2:**111-6.

7346. **Tasbakan, M. I., T. Yamazhan, D. Gokengin, B. Arda, M. Sertpolat, S. Ulusoy, E. Ertem, and S. Demir.** 2003. Brucellosis: a retrospective evaluation. *Trop Doct* **33:**151-3.

7347. **Tasker, S. A., G. A. Schnepf, M. Lim, H. E. Caraviello, A. Armstrong, M. Bavaro, B. K. Agan, J. Delmar, N. Aronson, M. R. Wallace, and J. D. Grabenstein.** 2004. Unintended smallpox vaccination of HIV-1-infected individuals in the United States military. *Clin Infect Dis* **38:**1320-2.

7348. **Tate, D., S. Mawer, and A. Newton.** 2003. Outbreak of Pseudomonas aeruginosa folliculitis associated with a swimming pool inflatable. *Epidemiol Infect* **130:**187-92.

7349. **Tateishi, K., Y. Toh, H. Minagawa, and H. Tashiro.** 1994. Detection of herpes simplex virus (HSV) in the saliva from 1,000 oral surgery outpatients by the polymerase chain reaction (PCR) and virus isolation. *J Oral Pathol Med* **23:**80-4.

7350. Tatem, A. J., and S. I. Hay. 2004. Measuring urbanization pattern and extent for malaria research: a review of remote sensing approaches. *J Urban Health* **81**:363-76.

7351. Tatti, V. 1986. Démonstrations cliniques. *Schweiz Med Wochenschr* **116**:1751-63.

7352. Taubenberger, J. K., A. H. Reid, A. E. Krafft, K. E. Bijwaard, and T. G. Fanning. 1997. Initial genetic characterization of the 1918 "Spanish" influenza virus. *Science* **275**:1793-6.

7353. Tauxe, R. V., N. D. Puhr, J. G. Wells, N. Hargrett-Bean, and P. A. Blake. 1990. Antimicrobial resistance of Shigella isolates in the USA: the importance of international travelers. *J Infect Dis* **162**:1107-11.

7354. Tauxe, R. V., M. P. Tormey, L. Mascola, N. T. Hargrett-Bean, and P. A. Blake. 1987. Salmonellosis outbreak on transatlantic flights; foodborne illness on aircraft: 1947-1984. *Am J Epidemiol* **125**:150-7.

7355. Tavris, D. R., R. P. Murphy, J. W. Jolley, S. M. Harmon, C. Williams, and C. L. Brumback. 1985. Two successive outbreaks of Clostridium perfringens at a state correctional institution. *Am J Public Health* **75**:287-8.

7356. Tay, S. T., M. Kamalanathan, and M. Y. Rohani. 2003. Antibody prevalence of Orienta tsutsugamushi, Rickettsia typhi and TT118 spotted fever group rickettsiae among Malasian blood donors and febrile patients in the urban areas. *Southeast Asian J Trop Med Public Health* **34**:165-70.

7357. Taylor, A., D. Goldberg, J. Emslie, J. Wrench, L. Gruer, S. Cameron, J. Black, B. Davis, J. McGregor, E. Follett, et al. 1995. Outbreak of HIV infection in a Scottish prison. *BMJ* **310**:289-92.

7358. Taylor, D. J., A. Efstratiou, and W. J. Reilly. 2002. Diphtheria toxin production by Corynebacterium ulcerans from cats. *Vet Rec* **150**:355.

7359. Taylor, D. M. 2002. Current perspectives on bovine spongiform encephalopathy and variant Creutzfeldt-Jakob disease. *Clin Microbiol Infect* **8**:332-9.

7360. Taylor, D. N., and M. J. Blaser. 1991. The epidemiology of Helicobacter pylori infections. *Epidemiol Rev* **13**:42-59.

7361. Taylor, D. N., R. Houston, D. R. Shlim, M. Bhaibulaya, B. L. Ungar, and P. Echeverria. 1988. Etiology of diarrhea among travelers and foreign residents in Nepal. *JAMA* **260**:1245-8.

7362. Taylor, D. N., J. Rizzo, R. Meza, J. Perez, and D. Watts. 1996. Cholera among Americans living in Peru. *Clin Infect Dis* **22**:1108-9.

7363. Taylor, D. N., I. K. Wachsmuth, Y. H. Shangkuan, E. V. Schmidt, T. J. Barrett, J. S. Schrader, C. S. Scherach, H. B. McGee, R. A. Feldman, and D. J. Brenner. 1982. Salmonellosis associated with marijuana: a multistate outbreak traced by plasmid fingerprinting. *N Engl J Med* **306**:1249-53.

7364. Taylor, E. W., K. Duffy, K. Lee, A. Noone, A. Leanord, P. M. King, and P. O'Dwyer. 2003. Telephone call contact for postdischarge surveillance of surgical site infections. A pilot, methodological study. *J Hosp Infect* **55**:8-13.

7365. Taylor, G., D. Gravel, L. Johnston, J. Embil, D. Holton, and S. Paton. 2004. Incidence of bloodstream infection in multicenter inception cohorts of hemodialysis patients. *Am J Infect Control* **32**:155-60.

7366. Taylor, G. S., I. B. Vipond, and E. O. Caul. 2001. Molecular epidemiology of outbreak of respiratory syncytial virus within bone marrow transplantation unit. *J Clin Microbiol* **39**:801-3.

7367. Taylor, H. R., F. M. Velasco, and A. Sommer. 1985. The ecology of trachoma: an epidemiological study in southern Mexico. *Bull WHO* **63**:558-67.

7368. Taylor, J. L., J. Tuttle, T. Pramukul, K. O'Brien, T. J. Barrett, B. Jolbitado, Y. L. Lim, D. Vugia, J. G. Morris, Jr., R. V. Tauxe, et al. 1993. An outbreak of cholera in Maryland associated with imported commercial frozen fresh coconut milk. *J Infect Dis* **167**:1330-5.

7369. Taylor, J. P., B. J. Barnett, L. del Rosario, K. Williams, and S. S. Barth. 1998. Prospective investigation of cryptic outbreaks of Salmonella agona salmonellosis. *J Clin Microbiol* **36**:2861-4.

7370. Taylor, J. P., W. X. Shandera, T. G. Betz, K. Schraitle, L. Chaffee, L. Lopez, R. Henley, C. N. Rothe, R. F. Bell, and P. A. Blake. 1984. Typhoid fever in San Antonio, Texas: an outbreak traced to a continuing source. *J Infect Dis* **149**:553-7.

7371. Taylor, L. H., S. M. Latham, and M. E. Woolhouse. 2001. Risk factors for human disease emergence. *Philos Trans R Soc Lond B Biol Sci* **356**:983-9.

7372. Taylor, M. B., N. Cox, M. A. Vrey, and W. O. Grabow. 2001. The occurrence of hepatitis A and astroviruses in selected river and dam waters in South Africa. *Water Res* **35**:2653-60.

7373. Taylor, M. B., F. E. Marx, and W. O. Grabow. 1997. Rotavirus, astrovirus and adenovirus associated with an outbreak of gastroenteritis in a South African child care centre. *Epidemiol Infect* **119**:227-30.

7374. Taylor, M. L., C. B. Chavez-Tapia, R. Vargas-Yanez, G. Rodriguez-Arellanes, G. R. Pena-Sandoval, C. Toriello, A. Perez, and M. R. Reyes-Montes. 1999. Environmental conditions favoring bat infection with Histoplasma capsulatum in Mexican shelters. *Am J Trop Med Hyg* **61**:914-9.

7375. Taylor, M. L., A. Perez-Mejia, J. K. Yamamoto-Furusho, and J. Granados. 1997. Immunologic, genetic and social human risk factors associated to histoplasmosis: studies in the State of Guerrero, Mexico. *Mycopathologia* **138**:137-42.

7376. Taylor, M. M., B. Chohan, L. Lavreys, W. Hassan, M. L. Huang, L. Corey, R. Ashley Morrow, B. A. Richardson, K. Mandaliya, J. Ndinya-Achola, J. Bwayo, and J. Kreiss. 2004. Shedding of human herpesvirus 8 in oral and genital secretions from HIV-1-seropositive and -seronegative Kenyan women. *J Infect Dis* **190**:484-8.

7377. Taylor, N. S., M. A. Ellenberger, P. Y. Wu, and J. G. Fox. 1989. Diversity of serotypes of Campylobacter jejuni and Campylobacter coli isolated in laboratory animals. *Lab Anim Sci* **39**:219-21.

7378. Taylor, P., and S. L. Mutambu. 1986. A review of the malaria situation in Zimbabwe with special reference to the period 1972-1981. *Trans R Soc Trop Med Hyg* **80**:12-9.

7379. Taylor, R., K. King, P. Vodicka, J. Hall, and D. A. Evans. 2003. Screening for leprosy in immigrants - a decision analysis model. *Lepr Rev* **74**:240-8.

7380. Taylor, R., H. Nemaia, C. Tukuitonga, M. Kennett, J. White, S. Rodger, S. Levy, and I. Gust. 1985. An epidemic of influenza in the population of Niue. *J Med Virol* **16**:127-36.

7381. Taylor-Robinson, D., and P. M. Furr. 1998. Update on sexually transmitted mycoplasmas. *Lancet* **351** (**suppl III**):12-5.

7382. Taylor-Wiedeman, J., G. P. Hayhurst, J. G. Sissons, and J. H. Sinclair. 1993. Polymorphonuclear cells are not sites of persistence of human cytomegalovirus in healthy individuals. *J Gen Virol* **74** (**Pt 2**):265-8.

7383. **Tchuem Tchuente, L. A., V. R. Southgate, J. Jourdane, B. L. Webster, and J. Vercruysse.** 2003. Schistosoma intercalatum: an endangered species in Cameroon? *Trends Parasitol* **19**:389-93.

7384. **Te Giffel, M. C., R. R. Beumer, P. E. Granum, and F. M. Rombouts.** 1997. Isolation and characterisation of Bacillus cereus from pasteurised milk in household refrigerators in The Netherlands. *Int J Food Microbiol* **34**:307-18.

7385. **Tea, A., S. Alexiou-Daniel, M. Arvanitidou, E. Diza, and A. Antoniadis.** 2003. Occurrence of Bartonella henselae and Bartonella quintana in a healthy Greek population. *Am J Trop Med Hyg* **68**:554-6.

7386. **Teale, C., D. B. Cundall, and S. B. Pearson.** 1991. Outbreak of tuberculosis in a poor urban community. *J Infect* **23**:327-9.

7387. **team, I. s.** 1978. Ebola haemorrhagic fever in Sudan, 1976. Report of a WHO/International Study Team. *Bull WHO* **56**:247-70.

7388. **Team, P. S.** 2002. Efficacy of three short-course regimens of zidovudine and lamivudine in preventing early and late transmission of HIV-1 from mother to child in Tanzania, South Africa, and Uganda (Petra study): a randomised, double- blind, placebo-controlled trial. *Lancet* **359**:1178-86.

7389. **Tedder, R. S., M. A. Zuckerman, A. H. Goldstone, A. E. Hawkins, A. Fielding, E. M. Briggs, D. Irwin, S. Blair, A. M. Gorman, and K. G. Patterson.** 1995. Hepatitis B transmission from contaminated cryopreservation tank. *Lancet* **346**:137-40.

7390. **Tee, T. S., M. Kamalanathan, K. A. Suan, S. S. Chun, H. T. Ming, R. M. Yasin, and S. Devi.** 1999. Seroepidemiologic survey of Orientia tsutsugamushi, Rickettsia typhi, and TT118 spotted fever group rickettsiae in rubber estate workers in Malaysia. *Am J Trop Med Hyg* **61**:73-7.

7391. **Tegnell, A., B. Saeedi, B. Isaksson, H. Granfeldt, and L. Ohman.** 2002. A clone of coagulase-negative staphylococci among patients with post- cardiac surgery infections. *J Hosp Infect* **52**:37-42.

7392. **Tei, S., N. Kitajima, K. Takahashi, and S. Mishiro.** 2003. Zoonotic transmission of hepatitis E virus from deer to human beings. *Lancet* **362**:371-3.

7393. **Teichmann, D., K. Gobels, J. Simon, M. P. Grobusch, and N. Suttorp.** 2001. A severe case of leptospirosis acquired during an iron man contest. *Eur J Clin Microbiol Infect Dis* **20**:137-8.

7394. **Teitelbaum, P.** 2004. An estimate of the incidence of hepatitis A in unimmunized Canadian travelers to developing countries. *J Travel Med* **11**:102-6.

7395. **Teixeira, A. R., P. S. Monteiro, J. M. Rebelo, E. R. Arganaraz, D. Vieira, L. Lauria-Pires, R. Nascimento, C. A. Vexenat, A. R. Silva, S. K. Ault, and J. M. Costa.** 2001. Emerging Chagas disease: trophic network and cycle of transmission of Trypanosoma cruzi from palm trees in the Amazon. *Emerg Infect Dis* **7**:100-12.

7396. **Teixeira Md, M., M. L. Barreto, M. Costa Md, L. D. Ferreira, P. F. Vasconcelos, and S. Cairncross.** 2002. Dynamics of dengue virus circulation: a silent epidemic in a complex urban area. *Trop Med Int Health* **7**:757-762.

7397. **Teixeira Nunes, M. R., L. C. Martins, S. G. Rodrigues, J. O. Chiang, R. do Socorro da Silva Azevedo, A. P. A. Travassos da Rosa, and P. F. da Costa Vasconcelos.** 2005. Oropouche virus isolation, Southeast Brazil. *Emerg Infect Dis* **11**:1610-3.

7398. **Telander, B., R. Lerner, J. Palmblad, and O. Ringertz.** 1988. Corynebacterium group JK in a hematological ward: infections, colonization and environmental contamination. *Scand J Infect Dis* **20**:55-61.

7399. **Teles, H. M., M. E. de Carvalho, C. Santos Ferreira, F. Zacharias, V. R. de Lima, and M. L. Fadel.** 2002. Schistosomiasis mansoni in Bananal (State of Sao Paulo, Brazil): I. Efficiency of diagnostic and treatment procedures. *Mem Inst Oswaldo Cruz* **97 Suppl 1**:181-6.

7400. **Telzak, E. E., E. P. Bell, D. A. Kautter, L. Crowell, L. D. Budnick, D. L. Morse, and S. Schultz.** 1990. An international outbreak of type E botulism due to uneviscerated fish. *J Infect Dis* **161**:340-2.

7401. **Templeton, G. L., L. A. Illing, L. Young, D. Cave, W. W. Stead, and J. H. Bates.** 1995. The risk for transmission of Mycobacterium tuberculosis at the bedside and during autopsy. *Ann Intern Med* **122**:922-5.

7402. **Templeton, K. E., S. A. Scheltinga, M. F. Beersma, A. C. Kroes, and E. C. Claas.** 2004. Rapid and sensitive method using multiplex real-time PCR for diagnosis of infections by influenza a and influenza B viruses, respiratory syncytial virus, and parainfluenza viruses 1, 2, 3, and 4. *J Clin Microbiol* **42**:1564-9.

7403. **Tenkate, T.** 1994. Clostridium perfringens food poisoning from a wedding reception, Queensland. *Commun Dis Intell* **18**:206-7.

7404. **Tepsumethanon, V., B. Lumlertdacha, C. Mitmoonpitak, V. Sitprija, F. X. Meslin, and H. Wilde.** 2004. Survival of naturally infected rabid dogs and cats. *Clin Infect Dis* **39**:278-80.

7405. **ter Meulen, J., O. Lenz, L. Koivogui, N. Magassouba, S. K. Kaushik, R. Lewis, and W. Aldis.** 2001. Short communication: Lassa fever in Sierra Leone: UN peacekeepers are at risk. *Trop Med Int Health* **6**:83-4.

7406. **Ter Meulen, J., I. Lukashevich, K. Sidibe, A. Inapogui, M. Marx, A. Dorlemann, M. L. Yansane, K. Koulemou, J. Chang-Claude, and H. Schmitz.** 1996. Hunting of peridomestic rodents and consumption of their meat as possible risk factors for rodent-to-human transmission of Lassa virus in the Republic of Guinea. *Am J Trop Med Hyg* **55**:661-6.

7407. **Terashima, A., H. Alvarez, R. Tello, R. Infante, D. O. Freedman, and E. Gotuzzo.** 2002. Treatment failure in intestinal strongyloidiasis: an indicator of HTLV-I infection. *Int J Infect Dis* **6**:28-30.

7408. **Terramocci, R., L. Pagani, P. Brunati, S. Gatti, A. M. Bernuzzi, and M. Scaglia.** 2001. Reappearance of human diphyllobothriasis in a limited area of Lake Como, Italy. *Infection* **29**:93-5.

7409. **Terranova, W., J. G. Breman, R. P. Locey, and S. Speck.** 1978. Botulism type B: epidemiologic aspects of an extensive outbreak. *Am J Epidemiol* **108**:150-6.

7410. **Terry, B. C., F. Kanjah, F. Sahr, S. Kortequee, I. Dukulay, and A. A. Gbakima.** 2001. Sarcoptes scabiei infestation among children in a displacement camp in Sierra Leone. *Public Health* **115**:208-11.

7411. **Terry, J., M. Trent, and M. Bartlett.** 2000. A cluster of leptospirosis among abattoir workers. *Commun Dis Intell* **24**:158-60.

7412. **Tertti, R., R. Vuento, P. Mikkola, K. Granfors, A. L. Makela, and A. Toivanen.** 1989. Clinical manifestations of Yersinia pseudotuberculosis infection in children. *Eur J Clin Microbiol Infect Dis* **8**:587-91.

7413. **Tesh, R., S. Saidi, E. Javadian, and A. Nadim.** 1977. Studies on the epidemiology of sandfly fever in Iran. I. Virus isolates obtained from Phlebotomus. *Am J Trop Med Hyg* **26:**282-7.

7414. **Tesh, R. B.** 1994. The emerging epidemiology of Venezuelan hemorrhagic fever and Oropouche fever in tropical South America. *Ann N Y Acad Sci* **740:**129-37.

7415. **Tesh, R. B.** 1995. Control of zoonotic visceral leishmaniasis: is it time to change strategies? *Am J Trop Med Hyg* **52:**287-92.

7416. **Tesh, R. B., M. L. Wilson, R. Salas, N. M. De Manzione, D. Tovar, T. G. Ksiazek, and C. J. Peters.** 1993. Field studies on the epidemiology of Venezuelan hemorrhagic fever: implication of the cotton rat Sigmodon alstoni as the probable rodent reservoir. *Am J Trop Med Hyg* **49:**227-35.

7417. **Teutsch, S. M., D. D. Juranek, A. Sulzer, J. P. Dubey, and R. K. Sikes.** 1979. Epidemic toxoplasmosis associated with infected cats. *N Engl J Med* **300:**695-9.

7418. **Teutsch, S. M., W. J. Martone, E. W. Brink, M. E. Potter, G. Eliot, R. Hoxsie, R. B. Craven, and A. F. Kaufmann.** 1979. Pneumonic tularemia on Martha's Vineyard. *N Engl J Med* **301:**826-8.

7419. **Tewari, S. C., V. Thenmozhi, C. R. Katholi, R. Manavalan, A. Munirathinam, and A. Gajanana.** 2004. Dengue vector prevalence and virus infection in a rural area in south India. *Trop Med Int Health* **9:**499-507.

7420. **Thacker, S. B., S. Simpson, T. J. Gordon, M. Wolfe, and A. M. Kimball.** 1979. Parasitic disease control in a residential facility for the mentally retarded. *Am J Public Health* **69:**1279-81.

7421. **Thai, K. T., T. Q. Binh, P. T. Giao, H. L. Phuong, Q. Hung le, N. Van Nam, T. T. Nga, J. Groen, N. Nagelkerke, and P. J. de Vries.** 2005. Seroprevalence of dengue antibodies, annual incidence and risk factors among children in southern Vietnam. *Trop Med Int Health* **10:**379-86.

7422. **Thaikruea, L., O. Charearnsook, S. Reanphumkarnkit, P. Dissomboon, R. Phonjan, S. Ratchbud, Y. Kounsang, and D. Buranapiyawong.** 1997. Chikungunya in Thailand: a re-emerging disease? *Southeast Asian J Trop Med Public Health* **28:**359-64.

7423. **Thakur, C. P.** 2000. Socio-economics of visceral leishmaniasis in Bihar (India). *Trans R Soc Trop Med Hyg* **94:**156-7.

7424. **Thakur, S. D., and D. C. Thapliyal.** 2002. Seroprevalence of brucellosis in man. *J Commun Dis* **34:**106-9.

7425. **Thapar, M. K., and E. J. Young.** 1986. Urban outbreak of goat cheese brucellosis. *Pediatr Infect Dis* **5:**640-3.

7426. **Tharmaphornpilas, P., S. Srivanichakorn, and N. Phraesrisakul.** 1994. Recurrence of yaws outbreak in Thailand, 1990. *Southeast Asian J Trop Med Public Health* **25:**152-6.

7427. **Tharmaphornpilas, P., P. Yoocharoan, P. Prempree, S. Youngpairoj, P. Sriprasert, and C. R. Vitek.** 2001. Diphtheria in Thailand in the 1990s. *J Infect Dis* **184:**1035-40.

7428. **Thathaisong, U., J. Worapong, M. Mungthin, P. Tan-Ariya, K. Viputtigul, A. Sudatis, A. Noonai, and S. Leelayoova.** 2003. Blastocystis isolates from a pig and a horse are closely related to Blastocystis hominis. *J Clin Microbiol* **41:**967-75.

7429. **Thayer, J., C. Milat, M. Meier, J. Hadman, S. Paciotti, R. Palmer, C. Story, D. Larson, L. Bjerkness, H. Parker, V. Jensen, R. Rognstad, P. Anderson, J. Lynne, N. Therien, B. Bartleson, L. Kentala, J. Lewis, and J. M. Kobayashi.** 1990. Typhoid fever - Skagit county, Washington. *MMWR* **39:**749-751.

7430. **Theamboonlers, A., T. Hansurabhanon, V. Verachai, V. Chongsrisawat, and Y. Poovorawan.** 2002. Hepatitis D virus infection in Thailand: HDV genotyping by RT-PCR, RFLP and direct sequencing. *Infection* **30:**140-4.

7431. **Theis, J. H., F. Stevens, and M. Law.** 2001. Distribution, prevalence, and relative risk of filariasis in dogs from the State of Washington (1997-1999). *J Am Anim Hosp Assoc* **37:**339-47.

7432. **Thepthai, C., T. Dharakul, S. Smithikarn, S. Trakulsomboon, and S. Songsivilai.** 2001. Differentiation between non-virulent and virulent Burkholderia pseudomallei with monoclonal antibodies to the ara+ or ara- biotypes. *Am J Trop Med Hyg* **65:**10-2.

7433. **Therre, H.** 1999. Botulism in the European Union. *Eurosurveillance* **4:**1-7.

7434. **Thibon, M., V. Villiers, P. Souque, A. Dautry-Varsat, R. Duquesnel, and D. M. Ojcius.** 1996. High incidence of Coxiella burnetii markers in a rural population in France. *Eur J Epidemiol* **12:**509-13.

7435. **Thimothe, J., J. Walker, V. Suvanich, K. L. Gall, M. W. Moody, and M. Wiedmann.** 2002. Detection of Listeria in crawfish processing plants and in raw, whole crawfish and processed crawfish (Procambarus spp.). *J Food Prot* **65:**1735-9.

7436. **Thin, R. N.** 1976. Melioidosis antibodies in Commonwealth soldiers. *Lancet* **1:**31-3.

7437. **Thio, C. L., D. Smith, W. G. Merz, A. J. Streifel, G. Bova, L. Gay, C. B. Miller, and T. M. Perl.** 2000. Refinements of environmental assessment during an outbreak investigation of invasive aspergillosis in a leukemia and bone marrow transplant unit. *Infect Control Hosp Epidemiol* **21:**18-23.

7438. **Thobois, S., E. Broussolle, G. Aimard, and G. Chazot.** 1996. [Ingestion of raw fish: a cause of eosinophilic meningitis caused by Angiostrongylus cantonensis after a trip to Tahiti]. *Presse Med* **25:**508.

7439. **Thomas, C., H. L. Cadwallader, and T. V. Riley.** 2004. Surgical-site infections after orthopaedic surgery: statewide surveillance using linked administrative databases. *J Hosp Infect* **57:**25-30.

7440. **Thomas, C., M. Stevenson, D. J. Williamson, and T. V. Riley.** 2002. Clostridium difficile-associated diarrhea: epidemiological data from Western Australia associated with a modified antibiotic policy. *Clin Infect Dis* **35:**1457-62.

7441. **Thomas, C. F., Jr., and A. H. Limper.** 2004. Pneumocystis pneumonia. *N Engl J Med* **350:**2487-98.

7442. **Thomas, C. J., J. Y. Lee, L. A. Conn, M. E. Bradley, R. W. Gillespie, S. R. Dill, R. W. Pinner, and P. G. Pappas.** 1998. Surveillance of cryptococcosis in Alabama, 1992-1994. *Ann Epidemiol* **8:**212-6.

7443. **Thomas, D. B., R. M. Ray, J. Kuypers, N. Kiviat, A. Koetsawang, R. L. Ashley, Q. Qin, and S. Koetsawang.** 2001. Human papillomaviruses and cervical cancer in Bangkok. III. The role of husbands and commercial sex workers. *Am J Epidemiol* **153:**740-8.

7444. **Thomas, D. L., J. M. Zenilman, H. J. Alter, J. W. Shih, N. Galai, A. V. Carella, and T. C. Quinn.** 1995. Sexual transmission of hepatitis C virus among patients attending sexually transmitted diseases clinics in Baltimore—an analysis of 309 sex partnerships. *J Infect Dis* **171:**768-75.

7445. **Thomas, D. R., M. Sillis, T. J. Coleman, S. M. Kench, N. H. Ogden, R. L. Salmon, P. Morgan-Capner, P. Softley, and D. Meadows.** 1998. Low rates of ehrlichiosis and Lyme borreliosis in English farmworkers. *Epidemiol Infect* **121:**609-614.

7446. Thomas, D. R., L. Treweek, R. L. Salmon, S. M. Kench, T. J. Coleman, D. Meadows, P. Morgan-Capner, and E. O. Caul. 1995. The risk of acquiring Q fever on farms: a seroepidemiological study. *Occup Environ Med* **52**:644-7.

7447. Thomas, M. C., A. Chereshsky, and K. Manning. 1994. An outbreak of leptospirosis on a single farm in east Otago. *N Z Med J* **107**:290-1.

7448. Thomas, P., H. C. Korting, W. Strassl, and T. Ruzicka. 1994. Microsporum canis infection in a 5-year-old boy: transmission from the interior of a second-hand car. *Mycoses* **37**:141-2.

7449. Thompson, C., M. Macdonald, and S. Sutherland. 2001. A family cluster of Chlamydia trachomatis infection. *BMJ* **322**:1473-4.

7450. Thompson, J. M., G. Savoia, G. Powell, E. B. Challis, and P. Law. 1991. Level of medical care required for mass gatherings: the XV Winter Olympic Games in Calgary, Canada. *Ann Emerg Med* **20**:385-90.

7451. Thompson, J. S., F. E. Cahoon, and D. S. Hodge. 1986. Rate of campylobacter ssp. isolation in three regions of Ontario, Canada, from 1978 to 1985. *J Clin Microbiol* **24**:876-8.

7452. Thompson, R. C., and P. T. Monis. 2004. Variation in Giardia: implications for taxonomy and epidemiology. *Adv Parasitol* **58**:69-137.

7453. Thompson, R. C., J. A. Reynoldson, S. C. Garrow, J. S. McCarthy, and J. M. Behnke. 2001. Towards the eradication of hookworm in an isolated Australian community. *Lancet* **357**:770-1.

7454. Thompson, R. C. A., and D. P. McManus. 2002. Towards a taxonomic revision of the genus Echinococcus. *Trends Parasitol* **18**:452-7.

7455. Thompson, R. G., D. S. Karandikar, and J. Leek. 1974. Giardiasis. An unusual cause of epidemic diarrhoea. *Lancet* **1**:615-6.

7456. Thompson, R. S., W. Burgdorfer, R. Russell, and B. J. Francis. 1969. Outbreak of tick-borne relapsing fever in Spokane county, Washington. *JAMA* **210**:1045-50.

7457. Thomson, J. R., N. MacIntyre, L. E. Henderson, and C. S. Meikle. 2001. Detection of Pasteurella multocida in pigs with porcine dermatitis and nephropathy syndrome. *Vet Rec* **149**:412-7.

7458. Thomson, K. J., D. P. Hart, L. Banerjee, K. N. Ward, K. S. Peggs, and S. Mackinnon. 2005. The effect of low-dose aciclovir on reactivation of varicella zoster virus after allogeneic haemopoietic stem cell transplantation. *Bone Marrow Transplant* **35**:1065-9.

7459. Thomson, M. C., D. A. Elnaiem, R. W. Ashford, and S. J. Connor. 1999. Towards a kala azar risk map for Sudan: mapping the potential distribution of Phlebotomus orientalis using digital data of environmental variables. *Trop Med Int Health* **4**:105-13.

7460. Thomson, M. C., V. Obsomer, M. Dunne, S. J. Connor, and D. H. Molyneux. 2000. Satellite mapping of Loa loa prevalence in relation to ivermectin use in west and central Africa. *Lancet* **356**:1077-8.

7461. Thonnon, J., A. Spiegel, M. Diallo, A. Diallo, and F. Fontenille. 1999. [Chikungunya virus outbreak in Senegal in 1996 and 1997]. *Bull Soc Pathol Exot* **92**:79-82.

7462. Thorburn, K. M., R. Bohorques, P. Stepak, L. L. Smith, C. Jobb, and J. P. Smith. 2001. Immunization strategies to control a community-wide hepatitis A epidemic. *Epidemiol Infect* **127**:461-7.

7463. Thornley, C. N., M. G. Baker, P. Weinstein, and E. W. Maas. 2002. Changing epidemiology of human leptospirosis in New Zealand. *Epidemiol Infect* **128**:29-36.

7464. Thornton, A. C., E. M. O'Hara, S. J. Sorensen, T. J. Hiltke, K. Fortney, B. Katz, R. E. Shoup, A. F. Hood, and S. M. Spinola. 1998. Prevention of experimental Haemophilus ducreyi infection: a randomized, controlled clinical trial. *J Infect Dis* **177**:1608-13.

7465. Thornton, S., D. Davies, F. Chapman, T. Farkas, N. Wilton, D. Doggett, and X. Jiang. 2002. Detection of Norwalk-like virus infection aboard two U.S. navy ships. *Mil Med* **167**:826-30.

7466. Thorpe, L. E., K. Laserson, S. Cookson, W. Mills, K. Field, V. R. Koppaka, M. Oxtoby, S. Maloney, and C. Wells. 2004. Infectious tuberculosis among newly arrived refugees in the United States. *N Engl J Med* **350**:2105-6.

7467. Thorpe, L. E., L. J. Ouellet, R. Hershow, S. L. Bailey, I. T. Williams, J. Williamson, E. R. Monterroso, and R. S. Garfein. 2002. Risk of hepatitis C virus infection among young adult injection drug users who share injection equipment. *Am J Epidemiol* **155**:645-53.

7468. Thorsen, S., J. Ronne-Rasmussen, E. Petersen, H. Isager, T. Seefeldt, and L. Mathiesen. 1993. Extra-intestinal amebiasis: clinical presentation in a non-endemic setting. *Scand J Infect Dis* **25**:747-50.

7469. Threlfall, E. J., and L. R. Ward. 2001. Decreased susceptibility to ciprofloxacin in Salmonella enterica serotype typhi, United Kingdom. *Emerg Infect Dis* **7**:448-50.

7470. Threlfall, E. J., L. R. Ward, M. D. Hampton, A. M. Ridley, B. Rowe, D. Roberts, R. J. Gilbert, P. Van Someren, P. G. Wall, and P. Grimont. 1998. Molecular fingerprinting defines a strain of Salmonella enterica serotype Anatum responsible for an international outbreak associated with formula-dried milk. *Epidemiol Infect* **121**:289-93.

7471. Thu, T. P., N. X. Nguyen, T. Lan le, and M. Kuchle. 2002. [Ocular angiostrongylus cantonensis in a female Vietnamese patient: case report]. *Klin Monatsbl Augenheilkd* **219**:892-5.

7472. Thurm, V., and B. Gericke. 1994. Identification of infant food as a vehicle in a nosocomial outbreak of Citrobacter freundii: epidemiological subtyping by allozyme, whole-cell protein and antibiotic resistance. *J Appl Bacteriol* **76**:553-8.

7473. Thurman, H. V., and A. P. Trujillo. 1999 (6th ed). Essentials of oceanography. Prentice Hall, Upper Saddle River, New Jersey.

7474. Thurston, H., J. Stuart, B. McDonnell, S. Nicholas, and T. Cheasty. 1998. Fresh orange juice implicated in an outbreak of Shigella flexneri among visitors to a South African game reserve. *J Infect* **36**:350.

7475. Thwaites, C. L., L. M. Yen, N. T. Nga, J. Parry, N. T. Binh, H. T. Loan, T. T. Thuy, D. Bethell, C. M. Parry, N. J. White, N. P. Day, and J. J. Farrar. 2004. Impact of improved vaccination programme and intensive care facilities on incidence and outcome of tetanus in southern Vietnam, 1993-2002. *Trans R Soc Trop Med Hyg* **98**:671-7.

7476. Tichonova, L., K. Borisenko, H. Ward, A. Meheus, A. Gromyko, and A. Renton. 1997. Epidemics of syphilis in the Russian Federation: trends, origins, and priorities for control. *Lancet* **350**:210-3.

7477. Tierney, R. J., N. Steven, L. S. Young, and A. B. Rickinson. 1994. Epstein-Barr virus latency in blood mononuclear cells: analysis of viral gene transcription during primary infection and in the carrier state. *J Virol* **68:**7374-85.

7478. Tikhomirov, E., M. Santamaria, and K. Esteves. 1997. Meningococcal disease: public health burden and control. *World Health Stat Q* **50:**170-7.

7479. Tilden, J., Jr., W. Young, A. M. McNamara, C. Custer, B. Boesel, M. A. Lambert-Fair, J. Majkowski, D. Vugia, S. B. Werner, J. Hollingsworth, and J. G. Morris, Jr. 1996. A new route of transmission for Escherichia coli: infection from dry fermented salami. *Am J Public Health* **86:**1142-5.

7480. Tilley, P. A., R. Azar, S. Banerjee, and A. Bell. 1994. Three cases of relapsing fever associated with lakeside cabins in Idaho. *Can Commun Dis Rep* **20:**29-31.

7481. Tilley, P. A., R. Azar, S. Banerjee, and A. Bell. 1994. Three cases of relapsing fever associated with lakeside cabins in Idaho. *Can Commun Dis Rep* **20:**29-31.

7482. Tillotson, J. R., D. Axelrod, and D. O. Lyman. 1977. Rabies in a laboratory worker. *MMWR* **26:**183-4, 249-50.

7483. Tindberg, Y., M. Wikman, and S. Sylvan. 1998. [Specimen culture from all children in a day care center because of an outbreak of streptococcal infection]. *Lakartidningen* **95:** 2580-4.

7484. Tissot-Dupont, H., M. A. Amadei, M. Nezri, and D. Raoult. 2004. Wind in November, Q fever in December. *Emerg Infect Dis* **10:**1264-9.

7485. Tissot-Dupont, H., and D. Raoult. 1993. Epidémiologie de la fièvre boutonneuse méditerranéenne en France. *Bull Epidémiol Hebdomadaire* **6 Sep:**164-5.

7486. Tiwari, T. S. P., B. J. Ray, K. C. Jost, Jr., M. K. Rathod, Y. Zhang, B. A. Brown-Elliott, K. Hendricks, and R. J. Wallace, Jr. 2003. Forty years of disinfectant failure: outbreak of postinjection Mycobacterium abscessus infection caused by contamination of bezalkonium chloride. *Clin Infect Dis* **36:**954-62.

7487. Tkatch, L. S., S. Kusne, W. D. Irish, S. Krystofiak, and E. Wing. 1998. Epidemiology of Legionella pneumonia and factors associated with Legionella-related mortality at a tertiarey care center. *Clin Infect Dis* **27:**1479-86.

7488. Tobe, K., K. Matsuura, T. Ogura, Y. Tsuo, Y. Iwasaki, M. Mizuno, K. Yamamoto, T. Higashi, and T. Tsuji. 2000. Horizontal transmission of hepatitis B virus among players of an American football team. *Arch Intern Med* **160:**2541-5.

7489. Tobian, A. A., R. K. Mehlotra, I. Malhotra, A. Wamachi, P. Mungai, D. Koech, J. Ouma, P. Zimmerman, and C. L. King. 2000. Frequent umbilical cord-blood and maternal-blood infections with Plasmodium falciparum, P. malariae, and P. ovale in Kenya. *J Infect Dis* **182:**558-63.

7490. Tobin-D'Angelo, M. J., M. A. Blass, C. del Rio, J. S. Halvosa, H. M. Blumberg, and C. R. Horsburgh, Jr. 2004. Hospital water as a source of Mycobacterium avium complex isolates in respiratory specimens. *J Infect Dis* **189:**98-104.

7491. Todd Faulks, J., P. J. Drinka, and P. Shult. 2000. A serious outbreak of parainfluenza type 3 on a nursing unit. *J Am Geriatr Soc* **48:**1216-8.

7492. Tokars, J. I., M. Frank, M. J. Alter, and M. J. Arduino. 2002. National surveillance of dialysis-associated diseases in the United States, 2000. *Semin Dial* **15:**162-71.

7493. Tokars, J. I., E. R. Miller, and G. Stein. 2002. New national surveillance system for hemodialysis-associated infections: initial results. *Am J Infect Control* **30:**288-95.

7494. Tolfvenstam, T., N. Papadogiannakis, O. Norbeck, K. Petersson, and K. Broliden. 2001. Frequency of human parvovirus B19 infection in intrauterine fetal death. *Lancet* **357:**1494-1497.

7495. Toma, H., J. Kobayashi, B. Vannachone, T. Arakawa, Y. Sato, S. Nambanya, K. Manivong, and S. Inthakone. 2001. A field study on malaria prevalence in southeastern Laos by polymerase chain reaction assay. *Am J Trop Med Hyg* **64:**257-61.

7496. Toma, H., I. Shimabukuro, J. Kobayashi, T. Tasaki, M. Takara, and Y. Sato. 2000. Community control studies on Strongyloides infection in a model island of Okinawa, Japan. *Southeast Asian J Trop Med Public Health* **31:**383-7.

7497. Tomao, P., L. Ciceroni, M. C. D'Ovidio, M. De Rosa, N. Vonesch, S. Iavicoli, S. Signorini, S. Ciarrocchi, M. G. Ciufolini, C. Fiorentini, and B. Papaleo. 2005. Prevalence and incidence of antibodies to Borrelia burgdorferi and to tick-borne encephalitis virus in agricultural and forestry workers from Tuscany, Italy. *Eur J Clin Microbiol Infect Dis* **24:**457-63.

7498. Tomaska, N. A., K. Lalor, J. E. Gregory, H. J. O'Donnell, F. Dawood, and C. M. Williams. 2003. Salmonella Typhimurium U290 outbreak linked to a bakery. *Commun Dis Intell* **27:**514-6.

7499. Tomaso, H., M. P. Dierich, and F. Allerberger. 2001. Helminthic infestations in the Tyrol, Austria. *Clin Microbiol Infect* **7:**639-41.

7500. Tomaszunas, S. 1998. Malaria in seafarers. 2. The status of malaria in large ports of the world. Protective measures against malaria in crews of ships. *Bull Inst Marit Trop Med Gdynia* **49:**63-71.

7501. Tomes, N. 1998. The gospel of germs. Men, women, and the microbe in American life. Harvard University Press, Cambridge, Massachusetts.

7502. Tomford, W. W., J. Thongphasuk, H. J. Mankin, and M. J. Ferraro. 1990. Frozen musculoskeletal allografts. A study of the clinical incidence and causes of infection associated with their use. *J Bone Joint Surg Am* **72:**1137-43.

7503. Tomlinson, P. B. 1999. The botany of mangroves. Cambridge University Press, Cambridge, United Kingdom.

7504. Tompkins, D. S., M. J. Hudson, H. R. Smith, R. P. Eglin, J. G. Wheeler, M. M. Brett, R. J. Owen, J. S. Brazier, P. Cumberland, V. King, and P. E. Cook. 1999. A study of infectious intestinal disease in England: microbiological findings in cases and controls. *Commun Dis Public Health* **2:**108-13.

7505. Tong, T. R., O. W. Chan, T. C. Chow, V. Yu, K. M. Leung, and S. H. To. 2003. Detection of human papillomavirus in sanitary napkins: a new paradigm in cervical cancer screening. *Diagn Cytopathol* **28:**140-1.

7506. Tongyoo, S., P. Sithinamsuwan, N. Apakupakul, and P. Chayakul. 2002. Invasive streptococcal group A infection and toxic shock syndrome in Songklanagarind hospital. *J Med Assoc Thai* **85:**749-56.

7507. Toole, M. J., R. W. Steketee, R. J. Waldman, and P. Nieburg. 1989. Measles prevention and control in emergency settings. *Bull WHO* **67:**381-8.

7508. Toovey, S., A. Jamieson, and M. Holloway. 2004. Travelers' knowledge, attitudes and practices on the prevention of infectious diseases: results from a study at Johannesburg International Airport. *J Travel Med* **11:**16-22.

7509. **Torano, G., D. Quinones, I. Hernandez, T. Hernandez, I. Tamargo, and S. Borroto.** 2001. [Nasal carriers of methicillin-resistant Staphylococcus aureus among cuban children attending day-care centers]. *Enferm Infecc Microbiol Clin* **19**:367-70.

7510. **Torgerson, P. R., B. S. Shaikenov, K. K. Baitursinov, and A. M. Abdybekova.** 2002. The emerging epidemic of echinococcosis in Kazakhstan. *Trans R Soc Trop Med Hyg* **96**:124-8.

7511. **Torkko, P., S. Suomalainen, E. Iivanainen, M. Suutari, E. Tortoli, L. Paulin, and M. L. Katila.** 2000. Mycobacterium xenopi and related organisms isolated from stream waters in Finland and description of Mycobacterium botniense sp. nov. *Int J Syst Evol Microbiol* **50 Pt 1**:283-9.

7512. **Toro, J., J. D. Vega, A. S. Khan, J. N. Mills, P. Padula, W. Terry, Z. Yadon, R. Valderrama, B. A. Ellis, C. Pavletic, R. Cerda, S. Zaki, W. J. Shieh, R. Meyer, M. Tapia, C. Mansilla, M. Baro, J. A. Vergara, M. Concha, G. Calderon, D. Enria, C. J. Peters, and T. G. Ksiazek.** 1998. An outbreak of hantavirus pulmonary syndrome, Chile, 1997. *Emerg Infect Dis* **4**:687-94.

7513. **Torok, T. J., P. E. Kilgore, M. J. Clarke, R. C. Holman, J. S. Bresee, and R. I. Glass.** 1997. Visualizing geographic and temporal trends in rotavirus activity in the United States, 1991 to 1996. National Respiratory and Enteric Virus Surveillance System Collaborating Laboratories. *Pediatr Infect Dis J* **16**:941-6.

7514. **Torok, T. J., R. V. Tauxe, R. P. Wise, J. R. Livengood, R. Sokolow, S. Mauvais, K. A. Birkness, M. R. Skeels, J. M. Horan, and L. R. Foster.** 1997. A large community outbreak of salmonellosis caused by intentional contamination of restaurant salad bars. *JAMA* **278**:389-95.

7515. **Torre, D., C. Sampietro, G. Ferraro, C. Zeroli, and F. Speranza.** 1990. Transmission of HIV-1 infection via sports injury. *Lancet* **335**:1105.

7516. **Torres, F. D., C. Valenca, and G. V. Andrade Filho.** 2005. First record of Desmodus rotundus in urban area from the city of Olinda, Pernambuco, Northeastern Brazil: a case report. *Rev Inst Med Trop Sao Paulo* **47**:107-8.

7517. **Torres, J. R., K. L. Russell, C. Vasquez, R. Barrera, R. B. Tesh, R. Salas, and D. M. Watts.** 2004. Family cluster of Mayaro fever, Venezuela. *Emerg Infect Dis* **10**:1304-6.

7518. **Torres, L., A. I. Lopez, S. Escobar, C. Marne, M. L. Marco, M. Perez, and J. Verhaegen.** 2003. Bacteremia by Streptobacillus moniliformis: first case described in Spain. *Eur J Clin Microbiol Infect Dis* **22**:258-60.

7519. **Torres-Pérez, F., J. Navarrete-Droguett, A. R., T. L. Yates, G. J. Mertz, P. A. Vial, M. Ferres, P. A. Marquet, and R. E. Palma.** 2004. Peridomestic small mammals associated with confirmed cases of human hantavirus disease in southcentral Chile. *Am J Trop Med Hyg* **70**:305-9.

7520. **Torrico, F., C. Alonso-Vega, E. Suarez, P. Rodriguez, M. C. Torrico, M. Dramaix, C. Truyens, and Y. Carlier.** 2004. Maternal Trypanosoma cruzi infection, pregnancy outcome, morbidity, and mortality of congenitally infected and non-infected newborns in Bolivia. *Am J Trop Med Hyg* **70**:201-9.

7521. **Tosato, G., G. Rocchi, and I. Archetti.** 1975. Epidemiological study of an "hand-foot-and-mouth disease" outbreak observed in Rome in the fall of 1973. *Zentralbl Bakteriol [Orig A]* **230**:415-21.

7522. **Toscano, C., Y. S. Hai, P. Nunn, and K. E. Mott.** 1995. Paragonimiasis and tuberculosis, diagnostic confusion: a review of the literature. *Trop Dis Bull* **92**:R1-26.

7523. **Tosh, F. E., I. L. Doto, D. J. D'Alessio, A. A. Medeiros, S. L. Hendricks, and T. D. Chin.** 1966. The second of two epidemics of histoplasmosis resulting from work on the same starling roost. *Am Rev Respir Dis* **94**:406-13.

7524. **Tosin, I., and R. A. Machado.** 1995. [Occurrence of Campylobacter spp among food handlers in hospital kitchens in urban areas of the southern region of Brazil]. *Rev Saude Publica* **29**:472-7.

7525. **Tosswill, J. H. C., G. P. Taylor, R. S. Tedder, and P. P. Mortimer.** 2000. HTLV-I/II associated disease in England and Wales, 1993-7: retrospective review of serology requests. *BMJ* **320**:611-2.

7526. **Totaro, J., C. Tan, V. Reddy, K. Dail, M. Davies, P. A. Jenkins, J. M. Maillard, J. Murphy, A. Beall, E. Mintz, M. Drees, and A. Shane.** 2004. Day care-related outreaks of rhamnose-negative Shigella sonnei - six states, June 2001-March 2003. *MMWR* **53**:60-3.

7527. **Totet, A., S. Latouche, P. Lacube, J. C. Pautard, V. Jounieaux, C. Raccurt, P. Roux, and G. Nevez.** 2004. Pneumocystis jirovecii dihydropteroate synthase genotypes in immunocompetent infants and immunosuppressed adults, Amiens, France. *Emerg Infect Dis* **10**:667-73.

7528. **Toth, E. L., L. R. Boychuk, and P. A. Kirkland.** 1995. Recurrent infection of continuous subcutaneous insulin infusion sites with Mycobacterium fortuitum. *Diabetes Care* **18**:1284-5.

7529. **Totten, P. A., M. A. Schwartz, K. E. Sjostrom, G. E. Kenny, H. H. Handsfield, J. B. Weiss, and W. L. Whittington.** 2001. Association of Mycoplasma genitalium with nongonococcal urethritis in heterosexual men. *J Infect Dis* **183**:269-276.

7530. **Toure, F. S., E. Mavoungou, P. Deloron, and T. G. Egwang.** 1999. [Comparative analysis of 2 diagnostic methods of human loiasis: IgG4 serology and nested PCR]. *Bull Soc Pathol Exot* **92**:167-70.

7531. **Toure, F. S., E. Mavoungou, L. Kassambara, T. Williams, G. Wahl, P. Millet, and T. G. Egwang.** 1998. Human occult loiasis: field evaluation of a nested polymerase chain reaction assay for the detection of occult infection. *Trop Med Int Health* **3**:505-11.

7532. **Toure, Y. T., A. M. Oduola, and C. M. Morel.** 2004. The Anopheles gambiae genome: next steps for malaria vector control. *Trends Parasitol* **20**:142-9.

7533. **Touze, A., S. de Sanjose, P. Coursaget, M. R. Almirall, V. Palacio, C. J. Meijer, J. Kornegay, and F. X. Bosch.** 2001. Prevalence of anti-human papillomavirus type 16, 18, 31, and 58 virus-like particles in women in the general population and in prostitutes. *J Clin Microbiol* **39**:4344-8.

7534. **Townes, J. M., P. R. Cieslak, C. L. Hatheway, H. M. Solomon, J. T. Holloway, M. P. Baker, C. F. Keller, L. M. McCroskey, and P. M. Griffin.** 1996. An outbreak of type A botulism associated with a commercial cheese sauce. *Ann Intern Med* **125**:558-63.

7535. **Toyota, M., and S. Morioka.** 2001. [Tuberculosis outbreak in a junior high school in Kochi City—studies on factors relating to extent of tuberculosis infection and the efficacy of isoniazid chemoprophylaxis]. *Kekkaku* **76**:625-34.

7536. **Trabulsi, L. R., R. Keller, and T. A. Tardelli Gomes.** 2002. Typical and atypical enteropathogenic Escherichia coli. *Emerg Infect Dis* **8**:508-13.

7537. **Tran, H. H., G. Bjune, B. M. Nguyen, J. A. Rottingen, R. F. Grais, and P. J. Guerin.** 2005. Risk factors associated with typhoid fever in Son La province, northern Vietnam. *Trans R Soc Trop Med Hyg* **99**:819-26.

7538. Tran, T., J. D. Druce, M. C. Catton, H. Kelly, and C. J. Birch. 2004. Changing epidemiology of genital herpes simplex virus infection in Melbourne, Australia, between 1980 and 2003. *Sex Transm Infect* **80:**277-9.

7539. Traore, O., V. S. Springthorpe, and S. A. Sattar. 2002. A quantitative study of the survival of two species of Candida on porous and non-porous environmental surfaces and hands. *J Appl Microbiol* **92:**549-55.

7540. Traub, R., C. L. Wisseman, and A. F. Azad. 1978. The ecology of murine typhus - a critical review. *Trop Dis Bull* **75:**237-317.

7541. Traub, R. J., I. D. Robertson, P. Irwin, N. Mencke, and R. C. Andrew Thompson. 2004. The prevalence, intensities and risk factors associated with geohelminth infection in tea-growing communities of Assam, India. *Trop Med Int Health* **9:**688-701.

7542. Traub, R. J., I. D. Robertson, P. Irwin, N. Mencke, and R. C. Thompson. 2002. The role of dogs in transmission of gastrointestinal parasites in a remote tea-growing community in northeastern India. *Am J Trop Med Hyg* **67:**539-45.

7543. Traub-Dargatz, J. L., L. P. Garber, P. J. Fedorka-Cray, S. Ladely, and K. E. Ferris. 2000. Fecal shedding of Salmonella spp by horses in the United States during 1998 and 1999 and detection of Salmonella spp in grain and concentrate sources on equine operations. *J Am Vet Med Assoc* **217:**226-30.

7544. Traverso, H. P., S. Kamil, H. Rahim, A. R. Samadi, J. R. Boring, and J. V. Bennett. 1991. A reassessment of risk factors for neonatal tetanus. *Bull WHO* **69:**573-9.

7545. Treadwell, T. A., R. C. Holman, M. J. Clarke, J. W. Krebs, C. D. Paddock, and J. E. Childs. 2000. Rocky Mountain spotted fever in the United States, 1993-1996. *Am J Trop Med Hyg* **63:**21-6.

7546. Trebucq, A., J. P. Louis, C. Hengy, N. Guelina, and M. Danyod. 1989. Etude des maladies sexuellement transmissibles chez des chauffeurs routiers du Tchad. *Bull Liais Doc OCEAC* **89:**33-5.

7547. Tremblay, A., J. D. MacLean, T. Gyorkos, and D. W. Macpherson. 2000. Outbreak of cutaneous larva migrans in a group of travellers. *Trop Med Int Health* **5:**330-4.

7548. Treml, F., and E. Nesnalova. 1993. [Occurrence of Leptospira antibodies in the blood of game animals]. *Vet Med* **38:**123-7.

7549. Trent, S. C. 1963. Reevaluation of World War Ii Veterans with Filariasis Acquired in the South Pacific. *Am J Trop Med Hyg* **12:**877-87.

7550. Tresoldi, A. T., M. C. Padoveze, P. Trabasso, J. F. Veiga, S. T. Marba, A. von Nowakonski, and M. L. Branchini. 2000. Enterobacter cloacae sepsis outbreak in a newborn unit caused by contaminated total parenteral nutrition solution. *Am J Infect Control* **28:**258-61.

7551. Trevejo, R. T., S. L. Abbott, M. I. Wolfe, J. Meshulam, D. Yong, and G. R. Flores. 1999. An untypeable Shigella flexneri strain associated with an outbreak in California. *J Clin Microbiol* **37:**2352-3.

7552. Trevejo, R. T., J. G. Rigau-Perez, D. A. Ashford, E. M. McClure, C. Jarquin-Gonzalez, J. J. Amador, J. O. de los Reyes, A. Gonzalez, S. R. Zaki, W. J. Shieh, R. G. McLean, R. S. Nasci, R. S. Weyant, C. A. Bolin, S. L. Bragg, B. A. Perkins, and R. A. Spiegel. 1998. Epidemic leptospirosis associated with pulmonary hemorrhage-Nicaragua, 1995. *J Infect Dis* **178:**1457-63.

7553. Trevejo, R. T., M. E. Schriefer, K. L. Gage, T. J. Safranek, K. A. Orloski, W. J. Pape, J. A. Montenieri, and G. L. Campbell. 1998. An interstate outbreak of tick-borne relapsing fever among vacationers at a Rocky Mountain cabin. *Am J Trop Med Hyg* **58:**743-7.

7554. Trevena, W. B., G. A. Willshaw, T. Cheasty, G. Domingue, and C. Wray. 1999. Transmission of Vero cytotoxin producing Escherichia coli O157 infection from farm animals to humans in Cornwall and west Devon. *Commun Dis Public Health* **2:**263-8.

7555. Tribe, I. G., S. Hart, D. Ferrall, and R. Givney. 2003. An outbreak of Salmonella typhimurium phage type 99 linked to contaminated bakery piping bags. *Commun Dis Intell* **27:**389-90.

7556. Trick, W. E., M. J. Kuehnert, S. B. Quirk, M. J. Arduino, S. M. Aguero, L. A. Carson, B. C. Hill, S. N. Banerjee, and W. R. Jarvis. 1999. Regional dissemination of vancomycin-resistant enterococci resulting from interfacility transfer of colonized patients. *J Infect Dis* **180:**391-6.

7557. Trick, W. E., M. O. Vernon, R. A. Hayes, C. Nathan, T. W. Rice, B. J. Peterson, J. Segreti, S. F. Welbel, S. L. Solomon, and R. A. Weinstein. 2003. Impact of ring wearing on hand contamination and comparison of hand hygiene agents in a hospital. *Clin Infect Dis* **36:**1383-90.

7558. Trick, W. E., R. A. Weinstein, P. L. DeMarais, M. J. Kuehnert, W. Tomaska, C. Nathan, T. W. Rice, S. K. McAllister, L. A. Carson, and W. R. Jarvis. 2001. Colonization of skilled-care facility residents with antimicrobial- resistant pathogens. *J Am Geriatr Soc* **49:**270-6.

7559. Triga, M. G., M. B. Anthracopoulos, P. Saikku, and G. A. Syrogiannopoulos. 2002. Chlamydia pneumoniae infection among healthy children and children hospitalized with pneumonia in Greece. *Eur J Clin Microbiol Infect Dis* **21:**300-3.

7560. Tripodi, M. F., L. E. Adinolfi, E. Ragone, E. Durante Mangoni, R. Fortunato, D. Iarussi, G. Ruggiero, and R. Utili. 2004. Streptococcus bovis Endocarditis and Its Association with Chronic Liver Disease: An Underestimated Risk Factor. *Clin Infect Dis* **38:**1394-400.

7561. Trisler, Z., K. Seme, M. Poljak, B. Celan-Lucu, and S. Sakoman. 1999. Prevalence of hepatitis C and G virus infections among intravenous drug users in Slovenia and Croatia. *Scand J Infect Dis* **31:**33-5.

7562. Triteeraprapab, S., I. Nuchprayoon, C. Porksakorn, Y. Poovorawan, and A. L. Scott. 2001. High prevalence of Wuchereria bancrofti infection among Myanmar migrants in Thailand. *Ann Trop Med Parasitol* **95:**535-8.

7563. Trock, S. C., D. A. Senne, M. Gaeta, A. Gonzalez, and B. Lucio. 2003. Low-pathogenicity avian influenza virus in live bird markets—what about the livestock area? *Avian Dis* **47:**1111-3.

7564. Trofa, A. F., R. F. DeFraites, B. L. Smoak, N. Kanesa-thasan, A. D. King, J. M. Burrous, P. O. MacArthy, C. Rossi, and C. H. Hoke, Jr. 1997. Dengue fever in US military personnel in Haiti. *JAMA* **277:**1546-8.

7565. Troillet, N., and G. Praz. 1995. Epidémie de botulisme de type B: Sion, décembre 1993 - janvier 1994. *Schweiz Med Wochenschr* **125:**1805-12.

7566. Trollfors, B. 1991. Invasive Haemophilus influenzae infections in household contacts of patients with Haemophilus influenzae meningitis and epiglottitis. *Acta Paediatr Scand* **80:**795-7.

7567. **Trollfors, B., J. Taranger, T. Lagergard, V. Sundh, D. A. Bryla, R. Schneerson, and J. B. Robbins.** 1998. Immunization of children with pertussis toxoid decreases spread of pertussis within the family. *Pediatr Infect Dis J* **17:**196-9.

7568. **Tronel, H., H. Chaudemanche, N. Pechier, L. Doutrelant, and B. Hoen.** 2001. Endocarditis due to Neisseria mucosa after tongue piercing. *Clin Microbiol Infect* **7:**275-6.

7569. **Trottier, S., K. Stenberg, I. A. Von Rosen, and C. Svanborg.** 1991. Haemophilus influenzae causing conjunctivitis in day-care children. *Pediatr Infect Dis J* **10:**578-84.

7570. **Trouillet, J. L., A. Vuagnat, A. Combes, N. Kassis, J. Chastre, and C. Gibert.** 2002. Pseudomonas aeruginosa ventilator-associated pneumonia: comparison of episodes due to piperacillin-resistant versus piperacillin-susceptible organisms. *Clin Infect Dis* **34:**1047-54.

7571. **Trout, D., T. M. Gomez, B. P. Bernard, C. A. Mueller, C. G. Smith, L. Hunter, and M. Kiefer.** 1995. Outbreak of brucellosis at a United States pork packing plant. *J Occup Environ Med* **37:**697-703.

7572. **Trout, D., C. Mueller, L. Venczel, and A. Krake.** 2000. Evaluation of occupational transmission of hepatitis A virus among wastewater workers. *J Occup Environ Med* **42:**83-7.

7573. **Troutt, H. F., and B. I. Osburn.** 1997. Meat from dairy cows: possible microbiological hazards and risks. *Rev Sci Tech* **16:**405-14.

7574. **Troy, C. J., R. W. Peeling, A. G. Ellis, J. C. Hockin, D. A. Bennett, M. R. Murphy, and J. S. Spika.** 1997. Chlamydia pneumoniae as a new source of infectious outbreaks in nursing homes. *JAMA* **277:**1214-8.

7575. **Trujillo, L., D. Munoz, E. Gotuzzo, A. Yi, and D. M. Watts.** 1999. Sexual practices and prevalence of HIV, HTLV-I/II, and Treponema pallidum among clandestine female sex workers in Lima, Peru. *Sex Transm Dis* **26:**115-8.

7576. **Trung, H. D., W. Van Bortel, T. Sochantha, K. Keokenchanh, N. T. Quang, L. D. Cong, and M. Coosemans.** 2004. Malaria transmission and major malaria vectors in different geographical areas of Southeast Asia. *Trop Med Int Health* **9:**230-7.

7577. **Trunk, G., R. Leavey, and R. B. Byrd.** 1976. Acute histoplasmosis in a military housing area: case reports with pulmonary function studies. *Mil Med* **141:**333-4.

7578. **Tsai, G. J., and S. C. Yu.** 1997. Microbiological evaluation of bottled uncarbonated mineral water in Taiwan. *Int J Food Microbiol* **37:**137-43.

7579. **Tsai, H. C., S. S. Lee, C. K. Huang, C. M. Yen, E. R. Chen, and Y. C. Liu.** 2004. Outbreak of eosinophilic meningitis associated with drinking raw vegetable juice in southern Taiwan. *Am J Trop Med Hyg* **71:**222-6.

7580. **Tsai, H. C., Y. C. Liu, C. M. Kunin, P. H. Lai, S. S. Lee, Y. S. Chen, S. R. Wann, W. R. Lin, C. K. Huang, L. P. Ger, H. H. Lin, and M. Y. Yen.** 2003. Eosinophilic meningitis caused by Angiostrongylus cantonensis associated with eating raw snails: correlation of brain magnetic resonance imaging scans with clinical findings. *Am J Trop Med Hyg* **68:**281-5.

7581. **Tsai, H. C., Y. C. Liu, C. M. Kunin, S. S. Lee, Y. S. Chen, H. H. Lin, T. H. Tsai, W. R. Lin, C. K. Huang, M. Y. Yen, and C. M. Yen.** 2001. Eosinophilic meningitis caused by Angiostrongylus cantonensis: report of 17 cases. *Am J Med* **111:**109-14.

7582. **Tsai, T. F.** 1991. Arboviral infections in the United States. *Infect Dis Clin North Am* **5:**73-102.

7583. **Tsai, T. F., M. A. Canfield, C. M. Reed, V. L. Flannery, K. H. Sullivan, G. R. Reeve, R. E. Bailey, and J. D. Poland.** 1988. Epidemiological aspects of a St. Louis encephalitis outbreak in Harris County, Texas, 1986. *J Infect Dis* **157:**351-6.

7584. **Tsanadis, G., S. N. Kalantaridou, A. Kaponis, E. Paraskevaidis, K. Zikopoulos, E. Gesouli, N. Dalkalitsis, I. Korkontzelos, E. Mouzakioti, and D. E. Lolis.** 2002. Bacteriological cultures of removed intrauterine devices and pelvic inflammatory disease. *Contraception* **65:**339-42.

7585. **Tsang, R. S., L. Kiefer, D. K. Law, J. Stoltz, R. Shahin, S. Brown, and F. Jamieson.** 2003. Outbreak of serogroup C meningococcal disease caused by a variant of Neisseria meningitidis serotype 2a ET-15 in a community of men who have sex with men. *J Clin Microbiol* **41:**4411-4.

7586. **Tsang, S. X., W. M. Switzer, V. Shanmugam, J. A. Johnson, C. Goldsmith, A. Wright, A. Fadly, D. Thea, H. Jaffe, T. M. Folks, and W. Heneine.** 1999. Evidence of avian leukosis virus subgroup E and endogenous avian virus in measles and mumps vaccines derived from chicken cells: investigation of transmission to vaccine recipients. *J Virol* **73:**5843-51.

7587. **Tsay, R. W., L. K. Siu, C. P. Fung, and F. Y. Chang.** 2002. Characteristics of bacteremia between community-acquired and nosocomial Klebsiella pneumoniae infection: risk factor for mortality and the impact of capsular serotypes as a herald for community-acquired infection. *Arch Intern Med* **162:**1021-7.

7588. **Tschopp, R., J. Frey, L. Zimmermann, and M. Giacometti.** 2005. Outbreaks of infectious keratoconjunctivitis in alpine chamois and ibex in Switzerland between 2001 and 2003. *Vet Rec* **157:**13-8.

7589. **Tsega, E., K. Krawczynski, B. G. Hansson, E. Nordenfelt, Y. Negusse, W. Alemu, and Y. Bahru.** 1991. Outbreak of acute hepatitis E virus infection among military personnel in northern Ethiopia. *J Med Virol* **34:**232-6.

7590. **Tselentis, Y., A. Psaroulaki, J. Maniatis, I. Spyridaki, and T. Babalis.** 1996. Genotypic identification of murine typhus rickettsia in rats and their fleas in an endemic area of Greece by the polymerase chain reaction and restriction fragment length polymorphism. *Am J Trop Med Hyg* **54:**413-7.

7591. **Tseng, H. K., C. P. Liu, W. C. Li, S. C. Su, and C. M. Lee.** 2002. Characteristics of Plesiomonas shigelloides infection in Taiwan. *J Microbiol Immunol Infect* **35:**47-52.

7592. **Tshikuka, J. G., M. E. Scott, and K. Gray-Donald.** 1995. Ascaris lumbricoides infection and environmental risk factors in an urban African setting. *Ann Trop Med Parasitol* **89:**505-14.

7593. **Tshimanga, M., D. E. Peterson, and R. A. Dlodlo.** 1997. Using epidemiologic tools to control an outbreak of diarrhoea in a textile factory, Bulawayo, Zimbabwe. *East Afr Med J* **74:**719-22.

7594. **Tsolia, M., S. Drakonaki, A. Messaritaki, T. Farmakakis, M. Kostaki, H. Tsapra, and T. Karpathios.** 2002. Clinical features, complications and treatment outcome of childhood brucellosis in central Greece. *J Infect* **44:**257-62.

7595. **Tsuang, W. M., J. C. Bailar, and J. A. Englund.** 2004. Influenza-like symptoms in the college dormitory environment: a survey taken during the 1999-2000 influenza season. *J Environ Health* **66:**39-42, 44.

7596. **Tsugane, S., S. Watanabe, H. Sugimura, T. Otsu, K. Tobinai, M. Shimoyama, S. Nanri, and H. Ishii.** 1988. Infectious states of human T lymphotropic virus type I and hepatitis B virus among Japanese immigrants in the Republic of Bolivia. *Am J Epidemiol* **128:**1153-61.

7597. Tsuji, H., T. Oshibe, K. Hamada, S. Kawanishi, A. Nakayama, and H. Nakajima. 2002. An outbreak of enterohemorrhagic Escherichia coli O157 caused by ingestion of contaminated beef at grilled meat-restaurant chain stores in the Kinki district in Japan: epidemiological analysis by pulsed-field gel electrophoresis. *Jpn J Infect Dis* **55**:91-2.

7598. Tsukamoto, T., Y. Kinoshita, T. Shimada, and R. Sakazaki. 1978. Two epidemics of diarrhoeal disease possibly caused by Plesiomonas shigelloides. *J Hyg (Lond)* **80**:275-80.

7599. Tsunemi, Y., T. Takahashi, and T. Tamaki. 2003. Penicillium marneffei infection diagnosed by polymerase chain reaction from the skin specimen. *J Am Acad Dermatol* **49**:344-6.

7600. Tsunoe, H., M. Tanaka, H. Nakayama, M. Sano, G. Nakamura, T. Shin, A. Kanayama, I. Kobayashi, O. Mochida, J. Kumazawa, and S. Naito. 2000. High prevalence of Chlamydia trachomatis, Neisseria gonorrhoeae and Mycoplasma genitalium in female commercial sex workers in Japan. *Int J STD AIDS* **11**:790-4.

7601. Tucci, V., and H. D. Isenberg. 1981. Hospital cluster epidemic with Morganella morganii. *J Clin Microbiol* **14**:563-6.

7602. Tuck, J. J., A. D. Green, and K. I. Roberts. 2003. A malaria outbreak following a British military deployment to Sierra Leone. *J Infect* **47**:225-30.

7603. Tucker, G. S., and G. Zerk. 1991. Primary amoebic meningoencephalitis in the Western province. *P N G Med J* **34**.

7604. Tugwell, B. D., L. E. Lee, H. Gillette, E. M. Lorber, K. Hedberg, and P. R. Cieslak. 2004. Chickenpox outbreak in a highly vaccinated school population. *Pediatrics* **113**:455-9.

7605. Tullus, K., B. Aronsson, S. Marcus, and R. Möllby. 1989. Intestinal colonization with Clostridium difficile in infants up to 18 months of age. *Eur J Clin Microbiol Infect Dis* **8**:390-3.

7606. Tumminelli, F., P. Marcellin, S. Rizzo, S. Barbera, G. Corvino, P. Furia, J. P. Benhamou, and S. Erlinger. 1995. Shaving as potential source of hepatitis C virus infection. *Lancet* **345**:658.

7607. Tumwine, J. K., A. Kekitiinwa, N. Nabukeera, D. E. Akiyoshi, M. A. Buckholt, and S. Tzipori. 2002. Enterocytozoon bieneusi among children with diarrhea attending Mulago Hospital in Uganda. *Am J Trop Med Hyg* **67**:299-303.

7608. Tumwine, J. K., A. Kekitinwa, N. Nabukeera, D. E. Akiyoshi, S. M. Rich, G. Widmer, X. Feng, and S. Tzipori. 2003. Cryptosporidium parvum in children with diarrhea in Mulago hospital, Kampala, Uganda. *Am J Trop Med Hyg* **68**:710-5.

7609. Tuppin, P., D. Jeannel, G. Brucker, M. Danis, and M. Gentilini. 1989. Les leishmanioses importées et autochtones. *Bull Epidémiol Hebdomadaire* **22**:90-1.

7610. Turcinov, D., I. Kuzman, and B. Herendic. 2000. Failure of azithromycin in treatment of Brill-Zinsser disease. *Antimicrob Agents Chemother* **44**:1737-8.

7611. Turco, J. H., J. H. Pryor, Y. Y. Baumgartner, M. E. Zegans, P. Sanchez, A. Bashir, J. D. Schwertzman, J. Puffer, J. T. Montero, S. Sodha, J. Elliott, C. G. Whitney, and M. Martin. 2002. Outbreak of bacterial conjunctivitis at a college - New Hampshire, January-March, 2002. *MMWR* **51**:205-7.

7612. Turgeon, N., M. Tucci, D. Deshaies, P. A. Pilon, J. Carsley, L. Valiquette, J. Teitelbaum, A. C. Jackson, A. Wandeler, H. Arruda, and L. Alain. 2000. Human rabies in Montreal, Quebec - October 2000. *Can Commun Dis Rep* **26**:209-10.

7613. Turk, N., Z. Milas, J. Margaletic, V. Staresina, A. Slavica, N. Riquelme-Sertour, E. Bellenger, G. Baranton, and D. Postic. 2003. Molecular characterization of Leptospira spp. strains isolated from small rodents in Croatia. *Epidemiol Infect* **130**:159-66.

7614. Turkeltaub, P. C., and P. J. Gergen. 1989. The risk of adverse reactions from percutaneous prick-puncture allergen skin testing, venipuncture, and body measurements: data from the second National Health and Nutrition Examination Survey 1976-80 (NHANES II). *J Allergy Clin Immunol* **84**:886-90.

7615. Turkmen, A., M. S. Sever, T. Ecder, A. Yildiz, A. E. Aydin, R. Erkoc, H. Eraksoy, U. Eldegez, and E. Ark. 1996. Posttransplant malaria. *Transplantation* **62**:1521-3.

7616. Turner, A. J., J. W. Galvin, R. J. Rubira, R. J. Condron, and T. Bradley. 1999. Experiences with vaccination and epidemiological investigations on an anthrax outbreak in Australia in 1997. *J Appl Microbiol* **87**:294-7.

7617. Turner, C. F., S. M. Rogers, H. G. Miller, W. C. Miller, J. N. Gribble, J. R. Chromy, P. A. Leone, P. C. Cooley, T. C. Quinn, and J. M. Zenilman. 2002. Untreated gonococcal and chlamydial infection in a probability sample of adults. *JAMA* **287**:726-33.

7618. Turner, R. B., K. A. Biedermann, J. M. Morgan, B. Keswick, K. D. Ertel, and M. F. Barker. 2004. Efficacy of organic acids in hand cleansers for prevention of rhinovirus infections. *Antimicrob Agents Chemother* **48**:2595-8.

7619. Turner, S. B., L. M. Kunches, K. F. Gordon, P. H. Travers, and N. E. Mueller. 1989. Occupational exposure to human immunodeficiency virus (HIV) and hepatitis B virus (HBV) among embalmers: a pilot seroprevalence study. *Am J Public Health* **79**:1425-6.

7620. Tuttle, J., T. Gomez, M. P. Doyle, J. G. Wells, T. Zhao, R. V. Tauxe, and P. M. Griffin. 1999. Lessons from a large outbreak of Escherichia coli O157:H7 infections: insights into the infectious dose and method of widespread contamination of hamburger patties. *Epidemiol Infect* **122**:185-92.

7621. Tuyet, D. T., V. D. Thiem, L. von Seidlein, A. Chowdhury, E. Park, G. Canh do, B. T. Chien, T. Van Tung, A. Naficy, M. R. Rao, M. Ali, H. Lee, T. H. Sy, M. Nichibuchi, J. Clemens, and D. D. Trach. 2002. Clinical, epidemiological, and socioeconomic analysis of an outbreak of Vibrio parahaemolyticus in Khanh Hoa Province, Vietnam. *J Infect Dis* **186**:1615-20.

7622. Tweed, S. A., D. M. Skowronski, S. T. David, A. Larder, M. Petric, W. Lees, Y. Li, J. Katz, M. Krajden, R. Tellier, C. Halpert, M. Hirst, C. Astell, D. Lawrence, and A. Mak. 2004. Human illness from avian influenza H7N3, British Columbia. *Emerg Infect Dis* **10**:2196-99.

7623. Tweeten, S. S., and L. S. Rickman. 1998. Infectious complications of body piercing. *Clin Infect Dis* **26**:735-40.

7624. Tyagi, B. K. 2004. A review of the emergence of Plasmodium falciparum-dominated malaria in irrigated areas of the Thar Desert, India. *Acta Trop* **89**:227-39.

7625. Tyagi, B. K., R. C. Chaudhary, and S. P. Yadav. 1995. Epidemic malaria in Thar desert, India. *Lancet* **346**:634-5.

7626. Tyagi, B. K., S. P. Yadav, R. Sachdev, and P. K. Dam. 2001. Malaria outbreak in the Indira Gandhi Nahar Pariyojna command area in Jaisalmer district, Thar Desert, India. *J Commun Dis* **33**:88-95.

7627. Tylewska-Wierzbanowska, S., D. Kruszewska, and T. Chmielewski. 1996. Epidemics of Q fever in Poland in 1992-1994. *Rocz Akad Med Bialymst* **41**:123-8.

7628. Tytgat, G. N. 1995. Endoscopic transmission of Helicobacter pylori. *Aliment Pharmacol Ther* **9**:105-10.

7629. **Uchida, T., T. T. Aye, X. Ma, F. Iida, T. Shikata, M. Ichikawa, T. Rikihisa, and K. M. Win.** 1993. An epidemic outbreak of hepatitis E in Yangon of Myanmar: antibody assay and animal transmission of the virus. *Acta Pathol Jpn* **43**:94-8.

7630. **Uchida, T., Y. Yan, and S. Kitaoka.** 1995. Detection of Rickettsia japonica in Haemaphysalis longicornis ticks by restriction fragment length polymorphism of PCR product. *J Clin Microbiol* **33**:824-8.

7631. **Uchiyama, F., Y. Morimoto, and Y. Nawa.** 1999. Re-emergence of paragonimiasis in Kyushu, Japan. *Southeast Asian J Trop Med Public Health* **30**:686-91.

7632. **Udonsi, J. K.** 1983. Necator americanus infection: a longitudinal study of an urban area in Nigeria. *Ann Trop Med Parasitol* **77**:305-10.

7633. **Udonsi, J. K., and M. I. Amabibi.** 1992. The human environment, occupation, and possible water-borne transmission of the human hookworm, Necator americanus, in endemic coastal communities of the Niger Delta, Nigeria. *Public Health* **106**:63-71.

7634. **Udonsi, J. K., A. B. Nwosu, and A. O. Anya.** 1980. Necator americanus: population structure, distribution, and fluctuations in population densities of infective larvae in contaminated farmlands. *Z Parasitenkd* **63**:251-9.

7635. **Udwadia, F. E.** 1994. Tetanus. Oxford University Press, Bombay.

7636. **Uemura, N., S. Okamoto, S. Yamamoto, N. Matsumura, S. Yamaguchi, M. Yamakido, K. Taniyama, N. Sasaki, and R. J. Schlemper.** 2001. Helicobacter pylori infection and the development of gastric cancer. *N Engl J Med* **345**:784-9.

7637. **Uga, S., and N. Kataoka.** 1995. Measures to control Toxocara egg contamination in sandpits of public parks. *Am J Trop Med Hyg* **52**:21-4.

7638. **Uga, S., T. Minami, and K. Nagata.** 1996. Defecation habits of cats and dogs and contamination by Toxocara eggs in public park sandpits. *Am J Trop Med Hyg* **54**:122-6.

7639. **Uhari, M., and M. Mottonen.** 1999. An open randomized controlled trial of infection prevention in child day-care centers. *Pediatr Infect Dis J* **18**:672-7.

7640. **Ulloa-Gutierrez, R., M. L. Avila-Aguero, M. L. Herrera, J. F. Herrera, and A. Arguedas.** 2003. Invasive pneumococcal disease in Costa Rican children: a seven year survey. *Pediatr Infect Dis J* **22**:1069-74.

7641. **Umenai, T., H. W. Lee, P. W. Lee, T. Saito, T. Toyoda, M. Hongo, K. Yoshinaga, T. Nobunaga, T. Horiuchi, and N. Ishida.** 1979. Korean haemorrhagic fever in staff in an animal laboratory. *Lancet* **1**:1314-6.

7642. **United Nations** 2002. International migration report 2002, vol. ST/ESA/SER.A/220. United Nations, New York.

7643. **UNAIDS (United Nations Program on HIV/AIDS).** 2004. 2004 report on the global AIDS epidemic. 4th global report. UNAIDS, Geneva, Switzerland.

7644. **UNAIDS.** 2000. Report on the global HIV/AIDS epidemic. UNAIDS, Geneva, Switzerland.

7645. **Unal, S., G. Ersoz, F. Demirkan, E. Arslan, N. Tutuncu, and A. Sari.** 2005. Analysis of skin-graft loss due to infection: infection-related graft loss. *Ann Plast Surg* **55**:102-6.

7646. **Unal, S., R. Masterton, and H. Gossens.** 2004. Bacteremia in Europe - antimicrobial susceptibility data from the MYSTIC surveillance programme. *Int J Antimicrob Agents* **23**:155-63.

7647. **United Nations Develpment Program.** 2000. World resources 2000-2001. Elsevier, Amsterdam.

7648. **Ungchusak, K., P. Auewarakul, S. F. Dowell, R. Kitphati, W. Auwanit, P. Puthavathana, M. Uiprasertkul, K. Boonnak, C. Pittayawonganon, N. J. Cox, S. R. Zaki, P. Thawatsupha, M. Chittaganpitch, R. Khontong, J. M. Simmerman, and S. Chunsutthiwat.** 2005. Probable person-to-person transmission of avian influenza A (H5N1). *N Engl J Med* **352**:333-40.

7649. **Ungs, T. J., and S. P. Sangal.** 1990. Flight crews with upper respiratory tract infections: epidemiology and failure to seek aeromedical attention. *Aviat Space Environ Med* **61**:938-41.

7650. **UNICEF, and WHO.** 2004. Meeting the millenium development goals. Drinking water and sanitation target. A mid-term assessment of progress. UNICEF / WHO, New York / Geneva.

7651. **Unicomb, L., P. Bird, and C. Dalton.** 2003. Outbreak of Salmonella Potsdam associated with salad dressing at a restaurant. *Commun Dis Intell* **27**:508-12.

7652. **Upton, P., and J. E. Cola.** 1994. Outbreak of Escherichia coli O157 infection associated with pasteurized milk supply. *Lancet* **344**:1015.

7653. **Urabe, A.** 2004. Clinical features of the neutropenic host: definitions and initial evaluation. *Clin Infect Dis* **39 Suppl 1**:S53-5.

7654. **Urabe, S., S. Yoshida, and Y. Mizuguchi.** 1988. Sexually transmitted diseases among prostitutes in Fukuoka, Japan. *Jpn J Med Sci Biol* **41**:15-20.

7655. **Urbani, C., M. Sinoun, D. Socheat, K. Pholsena, H. Strandgaard, P. Odermatt, and C. Hatz.** 2002. Epidemiology and control of mekongi schistosomiasis. *Acta Trop* **82**:157-68.

7656. **Urfer, E., P. Rossier, F. Mean, M. J. Krending, A. Burnens, J. Bille, P. Francioli, and A. Zwahlen.** 2000. Outbreak of Salmonella braenderup gastroenteritis due to contaminated meat pies: clinical and molecular epidemiology. *Clin Microbiol Infect* **6**:536-42.

7657. **Uribe-Salas, F., C. J. Conde-Glez, L. Juarez-Figueroa, and A. Hernandez-Castellanos.** 2003. Sociodemographic dynamics and sexually transmitted infections in female sex workers at the Mexican-Guatemalan border. *Sex Transm Dis* **30**:266-71.

7658. **Urrea, M., M. Pons, M. Serra, C. Latorre, and A. Palomeque.** 2003. Prospective incidence study of nosocomial infections in a pediatric intensive care unit. *Pediatr Infect Dis J* **22**:490-4.

7659. **Ursi, D., J. P. Ursi, M. Ieven, M. Docx, P. Van Reempts, and S. R. Pattyn.** 1995. Congenital pneumonia due to Mycoplasma pneumoniae. *Arch Dis Child Fetal Neonatal Ed* **72**:F118-20.

7660. **Usera, M. A., A. Aladuena, A. Echeita, E. Amor, J. L. Gomez-Garces, C. Ibanez, I. Mendez, J. C. Sanz, and M. Lopez-Brea.** 1993. Investigation of an outbreak of Salmonella typhi in a public school in Madrid. *Eur J Epidemiol* **9**:251-4.

7661. **Usera, M. A., A. Echeita, A. Aladuena, J. Alvarez, C. Carreno, A. Orcau, and C. Planas.** 1995. [Investigation of an outbreak of water-borne typhoid fever in Catalonia in 1994]. *Enferm Infecc Microbiol Clin* **13**:450-4.

7662. **Usera, M. A., A. Echeita, A. Aladuena, M. C. Blanco, R. Reymundo, M. I. Prieto, O. Tello, R. Cano, D. Herrera, and F. Martinez-Navarro.** 1996. Interregional foodborne salmonellosis outbreak due to powdered infant formula contaminated with lactose-fermenting Salmonella virchow. *Eur J Epidemiol* **12**:377-81.

7663. **Uspensky, I., and I. Ioffe-Uspensky.** 2002. The dog factor in brown dog tick Rhipicephalus sanguineus (Acari: Ixodidae) infestations in and near human dwellings. *Int J Med Microbiol* **291 Suppl 33:**156-63.

7664. **Ussery, X. T., J. A. Bierman, S. E. Valway, T. A. Seitz, G. T. DiFerdinando, Jr., and S. M. Ostroff.** 1995. Transmission of multidrug-resistant Mycobacterium tuberculosis among persons exposed in a medical examiner's office, New York. *Infect Control Hosp Epidemiol* **16:**160-5.

7665. **Uthman, M., A. Satir, and K. Tabbara.** 2005. Clinical and histopathological features of zoonotic cutaneous leishmaniasis in Saudi Arabia. *J Eur Acad Dermatol Venereol* **19:**431-6.

7666. **Utili, R., A. Rambaldi, M. F. Tripodi, and A. Andreana.** 1995. Visceral leishmaniasis during pregnancy treated with meglumine antimoniate. *Infection* **23:**182-3.

7667. **Utsalo, S. J., F. O. Eko, F. Umoh, and A. A. Asindi.** 1999. Faecal excretion of Vibrio cholerae during convalescence of cholera patients in Calabar, Nigeria. *Eur J Epidemiol* **15:**379-81.

7668. **Utsalo, S. J., C. I. Mboto, E. I. Gemade, and M. A. Nwangwa.** 1988. Halophilic Vibrio spp. associated with hard clams (Mercenaria spp.) from the Calabar river estuary. *Trans R Soc Trop Med Hyg* **82:**327-9.

7669. **Uttley, A. H., C. H. Collins, J. Naidoo, and R. C. George.** 1988. Vancomycin-resistant enterococci. *Lancet* **1:**57-8.

7670. **Utzinger, J., R. Bergquist, X. Shu-Hua, B. H. Singer, and M. Tanner.** 2003. Sustainable schistosomiasis control—the way forward. *Lancet* **362:**1932-4.

7671. **Utzinger, J., E. K. N'Goran, M. Tanner, and C. Lengeler.** 2000. Simple anamnestic questions and recalled water-contact patterns for self-diagnosis of Schistosoma mansoni infection among schoolchildren in western Côte d'Ivoire. **62:**649-55.

7672. **Uyeki, T., K. Teates, L. Brammer, A. Klimov, K. Fukuda, and N. Cox.** 2004. Update: influenza activity - United States and worldwide, 2003-04 season, and composition of the 2004-05 influenza vaccine. *MMWR* **53:**547-52.

7673. **Uyeki, T. M., S. B. Zane, U. R. Bodnar, K. L. Fielding, J. A. Buxton, J. M. Miller, J. C. Butler, K. Fukuda, S. A. Maloney, and M. S. Cetron.** 2003. Large summertime influenza A outbreak among tourists in Alaska and Yukon territory. *Clin Infect Dis* **36:**1095-1102.

7674. **Uzel, M., S. Sasmaz, S. Bakaris, E. Cetinus, E. Bilgic, A. Karaoguz, A. Ozkul, and O. Arican.** 2005. A viral infection of the hand commonly seen after the feast of sacrifice: human orf (orf of the hand). *Epidemiol Infect* **133:**653-7.

7675. **Vabres, P., B. Roose, S. Berdah, S. Fraitag, and Y. D. Prost.** 1999. [Bejel: an unusual cause of stomatitis in the child]. *Ann Dermatol Venereol* **126:**49-50.

7676. **Vabret, A., T. Mourez, S. Gouarin, J. Petitjean, and F. Freymuth.** 2003. An Outbreak of Coronavirus OC43 Respiratory Infection in Normandy, France. *Clin Infect Dis* **36:**985-9.

7677. **Vachon, F., C. Katlama, and C. Catinaud.** 1986. Trypanosomiase humaine africaine. Sémiologie et thérapeutique de la phase précoce. A propos de 8 cas européens contractés en Afrique francophone. *Méd Mal Infect* **4:**206-11.

7678. **Vado-Solís, I., M. F. Cárdenas-Marrufo, B. Jiménez-Delgadillo, M. A. Alzina-Lopez, H. Laviada-Molina, V. Suarez-Solis, and J. E. Zavala-Velazquez.** 2002. Clinical-epidemiological study of leptospirosis in humans and reservoirs in Yucatán, México. *Rev Inst Med Trop Sao Paulo* **44:**335-40.

7679. **Vail, G. M., R. S. Young, L. J. Wheat, R. S. Filo, K. Cornetta, and M. Goldman.** 2002. Incidence of histoplasmosis following allogeneic bone marrow transplant or solid organ transplant in a hyperendemic area. *Transpl Infect Dis* **4:**148-51.

7680. **Vaillant, V., E. Espie, I. Fisher, M. Hjertqvist, B. de Jong, C. Kornschober, C. Berghold, I. Gillespie, K. Alpers, H. Schmid, and H. Hächler.** 2005. International outbreak of Salmonella Stourbridge infection in Europe recognised following Enterneg enquiry, June-July 2005. *Eurosurveillance* **10:**1-5.

7681. **Vaillant, V., F. X. Weill, J. M. Thiolet, A. Collignon, D. Salamanca, E. Bouvet, C. Collinet, C. Cosson, C. Gloaguen, and H. de Valk.** 2004. Cas groupés de fièvre typhoïde liés à un établissement de restauration à Paris, 2003. *Bull Epidémiol Hebdomadaire* **21:**85-6.

7682. **Vaissaire, J., M. Mock, C. Le Doujet, and M. Levy.** 2001. Le charbon bactéridien. Epidémiologie de la maladie en France. *Méd Mal Infect* **31 suppl 2:**257-271.

7683. **Vajpayee, A., M. K. Mukherjee, A. K. Chakraborty, and M. S. Chakraborty.** 1991. Investigation of an outbreak of Japanese encephalitis in Rourkela City (Orissa) during 1989. *J Commun Dis* **23:**18-21.

7684. **Valadares De Amorim, G., B. Whittome, B. Shore, and D. B. Levin.** 2001. Identification of Bacillus thuringiensis subsp. kurstaki strain HD1- Like bacteria from environmental and human samples after aerial spraying of Victoria, British Columbia, Canada, with Foray 48B. *Appl Environ Microbiol* **67:**1035-43.

7685. **Valcour, J. E., P. Michel, S. A. McEwen, and J. B. Wilson.** 2002. Associations between Indicators of Livestock Farming Intensity and Incidence of Human Shiga Toxin-Producing Escherichia coli Infection. *Emerg Infect Dis* **8:**252-7.

7686. **Valdez, H., and R. A. Salata.** 1999. Bat-associated histoplasmosis in returning travelers: case presentation and description of a cluster. *J Travel Med* **6:**258-60.

7687. **Valenciano, M., S. Baron, A. Fisch, F. Grimont, and J. C. Desenclos.** 2000. Investigation of concurrent outbreaks of gastroenteritis and typhoid fever following a party on a floating restaurant, France, March 1998. *Am J Epidemiol* **152:**934-9.

7688. **Valenti, W. M., T. A. Clarke, C. B. Hall, M. A. Menegus, and D. L. Shapiro.** 1982. Concurrent outbreaks of rhinovirus and respiratory syncytial virus in an intensive care nursery: epidemiology and associated risk factors. *J Pediatr* **100:**722-6.

7689. **Valentine, C. C., R. J. Hoffner, and S. O. Henderson.** 2001. Three common presentations of ascariasis infection in an urban Emergency Department. *J Emerg Med* **20:**135-9.

7690. **Valentino, M., and V. Rapisarda.** 2001. Tetanus in a central Italian region: scope for more effective prevention among unvaccinated agricultural workers. *Occup Med (Lond)* **51:** 114-7.

7691. **Valenton, M.** 1996. Wound infection after cataract surgery. *Jpn J Ophthalmol* **40:**447-55.

7692. **Valeur-Jensen, A. K., C. B. Pedersen, T. Westergaard, I. P. Jensen, M. Lebech, P. K. Andersen, P. Aaby, B. N. Pedersen, and M. Melbye.** 1999. Risk factors for parvovirus B19 infection in pregnancy. *JAMA* **281:**1099-105.

7693. **Valin, N., F. Antoun, C. Chouaid, M. Renard, B. Dautzenberg, V. Lalande, B. Ayache, P. Morin, W. Sougakoff, J. M. Thiolet, C. Truffot-Pernot, V. Jarlier, and B. Decludt.** 2005. Outbreak of tuberculosis in a migrants' shelter, Paris, France, 2002. *Int J Tuberc Lung Dis* **9:**528-33.

7694. **Vally, H., A. Whittle, S. Cameron, G. K. Dowse, and T. Watson.** 2004. Outbreak of Aeromonas hydrophila wound infections associated with mud football. *Clin Infect Dis* **38:**1084-9.

7695. **Valway, S. E., R. B. Greifinger, M. Papania, J. O. Kilburn, C. Woodley, G. T. DiFerdinando, and S. W. Dooley.** 1994. Multidrug-resistant tuberculosis in the New York State prison system, 1990-1991. *J Infect Dis* **170:**151-6.

7696. **Valway, S. E., S. B. Richards, J. Kovacovich, R. B. Greifinger, J. T. Crawford, and S. W. Dooley.** 1994. Outbreak of multidrug-resistant tuberculosis in a New York State prison, 1991. *Am J Epidemiol* **140:**113-22.

7697. **Valway, S. E., M. P. C. Sanchez, T. F. Shinnick, I. Orme, T. Agerton, D. Hoy, J. S. Jones, H. Westmoreland, and I. M. Onorato.** 1998. An outbreak involving extensive transmission of a virulent strain of Mycobacterium tuberculosis. *N Engl J Med* **338:**633-9.

7698. **van Acker, J., F. de Smet, G. Muyldermans, A. Bougatef, A. Naessens, and S. Lauwers.** 2001. Outbreak of necrotizing enterocolitis associated with Enterobacter sakazakii in powdered milk formula. *J Clin Microbiol* **39:**293-7.

7699. **van Asperen, I. A., C. M. de Rover, J. F. Schijven, S. B. Oetomo, J. F. Schellekens, N. J. van Leeuwen, C. Colle, A. H. Havelaar, D. Kromhout, and M. W. Sprenger.** 1995. Risk of otitis externa after swimming in recreational fresh water lakes containing Pseudomonas aeruginosa. *BMJ* **311:**1407-10.

7700. **Van Asperen, I. A., G. Medema, M. W. Borgdorff, J. W. Sprenger, and A. H. Havelaar.** 1998. Risk of gastroenteritis among triathletes in relation to faecal pollution of fresh waters. *Int J Epidemiol* **27:**309-15.

7701. **van Baarle, D., E. Hovenkamp, N. H. Dukers, N. Renwick, M. J. Kersten, J. Goudsmit, R. A. Coutinho, F. Miedema, and M. H. van Oers.** 2000. High prevalence of Epstein-Barr virus type 2 among homosexual men is caused by sexual transmission. *J Infect Dis* **181:**2045-9.

7702. **van Beers, S. M., M. Hatta, and P. R. Klatser.** 1999. Patient contact is the major determinant in incident leprosy: implications for future control. *Int J Lepr Other Mycobact Dis* **67:**119-28.

7703. **van Belkum, A., W. J. Melchers, C. Ijsseldijk, L. Nohlmans, H. Verbrugh, and J. F. Meis.** 1997. Outbreak of amoxicillin-resistant Haemophilus influenzae type b: variable number of tandem repeats as novel molecular markers. *J Clin Microbiol* **35:**1517-20.

7704. **Van Beneden, C. A., W. E. Keene, R. A. Strang, D. H. Werker, A. S. King, B. Mahon, K. Hedberg, A. Bell, M. T. Kelly, V. K. Balan, W. R. Mac Kenzie, and D. Fleming.** 1999. Multinational outbreak of Salmonella enterica serotype Newport infections due to contaminated alfalfa sprouts. *JAMA* **281:**158-62.

7705. **van Burik, J. A., R. C. Hackman, S. Q. Nadeem, J. W. Hiemenz, M. H. White, M. E. Flowers, and R. A. Bowden.** 1997. Nocardiosis after bone marrow transplantation: a retrospective study. *Clin Infect Dis* **24:**1154-60.

7706. **Van Buynder, P., J. Eccleston, J. Leese, and D. N. J. Lockwood.** 1999. Leprosy in England and Wales. *Commun Dis Publ Health* **2:**119-21.

7707. **Van Crevel, R., P. Speelman, C. Gravekamp, and W. J. Terpstra.** 1994. Leptospirosis in travelers. *Clin Infect Dis* **19:**132-4.

7708. **van Cuyck-Gandre, H., J. D. Caudill, H. Y. Zhang, C. F. Longer, C. Molinie, R. Roue, R. Deloince, P. Coursaget, N. N. Mamouth, and Y. Buisson.** 1996. Short report: polymerase chain reaction detection of hepatitis E virus in north African fecal samples. *Am J Trop Med Hyg* **54:**134-5.

7709. **van de Beek, D., J. de Gans, L. Spanjaard, M. Weisfelt, J. B. Reitsma, and M. Vermeulen.** 2004. Clinical features and prognostic factors in adults with bacterial meningitis. *N Engl J Med* **351:**1849-59.

7710. **van de Laar, M. J. W., H. M. Götz, O. de Zwart, W. I. van der Meijden, J. M. Ossewaarde, H. B. Thio, J. S. A. Fennema, J. Spaargaren, H. J. C. de Vries, S. M. Berman, J. R. Papp, and K. A. Workowski.** 2004. Lymphogranuloma venereum among men who have sex with men - Netherlands, 2003-2004. *MMWR* **53:**985-8.

7711. **van den Berg, R. W., H. L. Claahsen, M. Niessen, H. L. Muytjens, K. Liem, and A. Voss.** 2000. Enterobacter cloacae outbreak in the NICU related to disinfected thermometers. *J Hosp Infect* **45:**29-34.

7712. **van den Bogaard, A. E., L. B. Jensen, and E. E. Stobberingh.** 1997. Vancomycin-resistant enterococci in turkeys and farmers. *N Engl J Med* **337:**1558-9.

7713. **van den Bosch, C. A., B. Cohen, T. Walters, and L. Jin.** 2000. Mumps outbreak confined to a religious community. *Eurosurveillance* **5:**58-60.

7714. **van den Hof, S., C. M. A. Meffre, M. A. E. Conyn-van Spaendonck, F. Woonink, H. E. de Melker, and R. S. van Binnendijk.** 2001. Measles outbreak in a community with very low vaccine coverage, The Netherlands. *Emerg Infect Dis* **7:**593-6.

7715. **van den Hoogen, B. G., D. M. Osterhaus, and R. A. Fouchier.** 2004. Clinical impact and diagnosis of human metapneumovirus infection. *Pediatr Infect Dis J* **23:**S25-32.

7716. **van der Eijk, A. A., H. G. Niesters, H. M. Gotz, H. L. Janssen, S. W. Schalm, A. D. Osterhaus, and R. A. de Man.** 2004. Paired measurements of quantitative hepatitis B virus DNA in saliva and serum of chronic hepatitis B patients: implications for saliva as infectious agent. *J Clin Virol* **29:**92-4.

7717. **van der Hoek, W., N. V. De, F. Konradsen, P. D. Cam, N. T. Hoa, N. D. Toan, and D. Cong le.** 2003. Current status of soil-transmitted helminths in Vietnam. *Southeast Asian J Trop Med Public Health* **34 Suppl 1:**1-11.

7718. **van der Hoek, W., S. G. Feenstra, and F. Konradsen.** 2002. Availability of irrigation water for domestic use in Pakistan: its impact on prevalence of diarrhoea and nutritional status of children. *J Health Popul Nutr* **20:**77-84.

7719. **Van Der Hoek, W., F. Konradsen, P. H. Amerasinghe, D. Perera, M. Piyaratne, and F. P. Amerasinghe.** 2003. Towards a risk map of malaria for Sri Lanka: the importance of house location relative to vector breeding sites. *Int J Epidemiol* **32:**280-285.

7720. **Van Der Kleij, F. G., R. T. Gansevoort, H. G. Kreeftenberg, and W. D. Reitsma.** 1998. Imported rickettsioses: think of murine typhus. *J Intern Med* **243:**177-9.

7721. **van der Vorm, E. R., and C. Woldring-Zwaan.** 2002. Source, carriers, and management of a Serratia marcescens outbreak on a pulmonary unit. *J Hosp Infect* **52:**263-7.

7722. **van der Werf, T. S., T. Stinear, Y. Stienstra, W. T. van der Graaf, and P. L. Small.** 2003. Mycolactones and Mycobacterium ulcerans disease. *Lancet* **362:**1062-4.

7723. **Van Der Zwet, W. C., G. A. Parlevliet, P. H. Savelkoul, J. Stoof, A. M. Kaiser, A. M. Van Furth, and C. M. Vandenbroucke-Grauls.** 2000. Outbreak of Bacillus cereus infections in a neonatal intensive care unit traced to balloons used in manual ventilation. *J Clin Microbiol* **38:**4131-6.

7724. van Dijk, Y., E. M. Bik, S. Hochstenbach-Vernooij, G. J. van der Vlist, P. H. Savelkoul, J. A. Kaan, and R. J. Diepersloot. 2002. Management of an outbreak of Enterobacter cloacae in a neonatal unit using simple preventive measures. *J Hosp Infect* **51**:21-6.

7725. van Ditzhuijsen, T. J. M., E. de Witte-van der Schoot, A. M. van Loon, P. J. M. Rijntjes, and S. H. Yap. 1988. Hepatitis B virus infection in an institution for the mentally retarded. *Am J Epidemiol* **128**:629-38.

7726. van Dobbenburgh, A., A. P. van Dam, and E. Fikrig. 1999. Human granulocytic ehrlichiosis in western Europe. *N Engl J Med* **340**:1214-5.

7727. Van Doornum, G. J., J. A. Van den Hoek, E. J. Van Ameijden, H. J. Van Haastrecht, M. T. Roos, C. J. Henquet, W. G. Quint, and R. A. Coutinho. 1993. Cervical HPV infection among HIV-infected prostitutes addicted to hard drugs. *J Med Virol* **41**:185-90.

7728. van Duijkeren, E., W. J. Wannet, M. E. Heck, W. van Pelt, M. M. Sloet van Oldruitenborgh-Oosterbaan, J. A. Smit, and D. J. Houwers. 2002. Sero types, phage types and antibiotic susceptibilities of Salmonella strains isolated from horses in The Netherlands from 1993 to 2000. *Vet Microbiol* **86**:203-12.

7729. van Duijn, C. M., N. Delasnerie-Laupretre, C. Masullo, I. Zerr, R. de Silva, D. P. Wientjens, J. P. Brandel, T. Weber, V. Bonavita, M. Zeidler, A. Alperovitch, S. Poser, E. Granieri, A. Hofman, and R. G. Will. 1998. Case-control study of risk factors of Creutzfeldt-Jakob disease in Europe during 1993-95. European Union (EU) Collaborative Study Group of Creutzfeldt-Jakob disease (CJD). *Lancet* **351**:1081-5.

7730. Van Gompel, A., E. Van den Enden, J. Van den Ende, and S. Geerts. 1993. Laboratory infection with Schistosoma mansoni. *Trans R Soc Trop Med Hyg* **87**:554.

7731. van Gool, T., C. Biderre, F. Delbac, E. Wentink-Bonnema, R. Peek, and C. P. Vivarès. 2004. Serodiagnostic studies in an immunocompetent individual infected with Encephalitozoon cuniculi. *J Infect Dis* **189**:2243-9.

7732. van Heerden, J., M. M. Ehlers, A. Heim, and W. O. Grabow. 2005. Prevalence, quantification and typing of adenoviruses detected in river and treated drinking water in South Africa. *J Appl Microbiol* **99**:234-42.

7733. Van Herck, K., P. Van Damme, F. Castelli, J. Zuckerman, H. Nothdurft, A. L. Dahlgren, S. Gisler, R. Steffen, P. Gargalianos, R. Lopez-Velez, D. Overbosch, E. Caumes, and E. Walker. 2004. Knowledge, attitudes and practices in travel-related infectious diseases: the European airport survey. *J Travel Med* **11**:3-8.

7734. van Hest, N. A., F. Smit, and J. P. Verhave. 2002. Underreporting of malaria incidence in The Netherlands: results from a capture-recapture study. *Epidemiol Infect* **129**:371-7.

7735. Van Heukelem, H. A., A. De Geus, and L. G. Thijs. 1979. Leptospirosis acquired in Surinam. *Trop Geogr Med* **31**:301-4.

7736. Van Immerseel, F., J. De Buck, F. Pasmans, G. Huyghebaert, F. Haesebrouck, and R. Ducatelle. 2004. Clostridium perfringens in poultry: an emerging threat for animal and public health. *Avian Pathol* **33**:537-49.

7737. Van Immerseel, F., F. Pasmans, J. De Buck, I. Rychlik, H. Hradecka, J. M. Collard, C. Wildemauwe, M. Heyndrickx, R. Ducatelle, and F. Haesebrouck. 2004. Cats as a risk for transmission of antimicrobial drug-resistant Salmonella. *Emerg Infect Dis* **10**:2169-74.

7738. van Keulen, H., P. T. Macechko, S. Wade, S. Schaaf, P. M. Wallis, and S. L. Erlandsen. 2002. Presence of human Giardia in domestic, farm and wild animals, and environmental samples suggests a zoonotic potential for giardiasis. *Vet Parasitol* **108**:97-107.

7739. van Laer, F., D. Raes, P. Vandamme, C. Lammens, J. P. Sion, C. Vrints, J. Snoeck, and H. Goossens. 1998. An outbreak of Burkholderia cepacia with septicemia on a cardiology ward. *Infect Control Hosp Epidemiol* **19**:112-3.

7740. Van Looveren, M., and H. Goossens. 2004. Antimicrobial resistance of Acinetobacter spp. in Europe. *Clin Microbiol Infect* **10**:684-704.

7741. van Middelkoop, A., J. E. van Wyk, H. G. Kustner, I. Windsor, C. Vinsen, B. D. Schoub, S. Johnson, and J. M. McAnerney. 1992. Poliomyelitis outbreak in Natal/KwaZulu, South Africa, 1987-1988. 1. Epidemiology. *Trans R Soc Trop Med Hyg* **86**:80-2.

7742. van Netten, P., J. Leenaerts, G. M. Heikant, and D. A. Mossel. 1986. [A small outbreak of salmonellosis caused by Bologna sausage]. *Tijdschr Diergeneeskd* **111**:1271-5.

7743. van Niekerk, A. B., J. B. Vries, J. Baard, B. D. Schoub, C. Chezzi, and N. K. Blackburn. 1994. Outbreak of paralytic poliomyelitis in Namibia. *Lancet* **344**:661-4.

7744. van Ogtrop, M. L., D. van Zoeren-Grobben, E. M. Verbakel-Salomons, and C. P. van Boven. 1997. Serratia marcescens infections in neonatal departments: description of an outbreak and review of the literature. *J Hosp Infect* **36**:95-103.

7745. van Pelt, W., H. van der Zee, W. J. B. Wannet, A. W. van de Giessen, D. J. Mevius, N. M. Bolder, R. E. Komijn, and Y. T. van Duynhoven. 2003. Explosive increase of Salmonella Java in poultry in the Netherlands: consequences for public health. *Eurosurveillance* **8**:31-5.

7746. Van, R., C. C. Wun, A. L. Morrow, and L. K. Pickering. 1991. The effect of diaper type and overclothing on fecal contamination in day-care centers. *JAMA* **265**:1840-4.

7747. Van, R., C. C. Wun, M. L. O'Ryan, D. O. Matson, L. Jackson, and L. K. Pickering. 1992. Outbreaks of human enteric adenovirus types 40 and 41 in Houston day care centers. *J Pediatr* **120**:516-21.

7748. Van Regenmortel, M. H. V. 2000. Virus taxonomy. Academic Press, San Diego.

7749. Van Steenbergen, J. E., A. G. Kraayeveld, and L. Spanjaard. 1999. Vaccination campaign for meningococcal disease in a rural area in the Netherlands - January 1998. *Eurosurveillance* **4**:18-21.

7750. Van Steenbergen, J. E., S. Van den Hof, M. W. Langendam, J. H. T. C. van de Kerkhof, and W. L. M. Ruijs. 2000. Measles outbreak - Netherlands, April 1999-January 2000. *MMWR* **49**:299-303.

7751. Van Thiel, P. H. 1976. Review. The present state of anisakiasis and its causative worms. *Trop Geogr Med* **28**:75-85.

7752. van Tongeren, H. A. E. 1981. Imported virus diseases in the Netherlands out of tropical areas 1977-1980 (30 months). *Tropenmed Parasitol* **32**:205.

7753. van Valkengoed, I. G., A. J. Boeke, A. J. van den Brule, S. A. Morre, J. H. Dekker, C. J. Meijer, and J. T. van Eijk. 1999. [Systematic home screening for Chlamydia trachomatis infections of asymptomatic men and women in family practice by means of mail-in urine samples]. *Ned Tijdschr Geneeskd* **143**:672-6.

7754. van Vliet, J. A., M. Samsom, and J. E. van Steenbergen. 1998. [Causes of spread and return of scabies in health care institutes; literature analysis of 44 epidemics]. *Ned Tijdschr Geneeskd* **142:**354-7.

7755. van Woerden, H. C., B. W. Mason, L. K. Nehaul, R. Smith, R. L. Salmon, B. Healy, M. Valappil, D. Westmoreland, S. de Martin, M. R. Evans, G. Lloyd, M. Hamilton-Kirkwood, and N. S. Williams. 2004. Q fever outbreak in industrial setting. *Emerg Infect Dis* **10:**1282-9.

7756. Vandelaer, J., M. Birmingham, F. Gasse, M. Kurian, C. Shaw, and S. Garnier. 2003. Tetanus in developing countries: an update on the Maternal and Neonatal Tetanus Elimination Initiative. *Vaccine* **21:**3442-5.

7757. Vandenberg, O. 2004. Arcobacter species in humans. *Emerg Infect Dis* **10:**1863-7.

7758. VandenBergh, M. F., P. E. Verweij, and A. Voss. 1999. Epidemiology of nosocomial fungal infections: invasive aspergillosis and the environment. *Diagn Microbiol Infect Dis* **34:**221-7.

7759. Vandenplas, Y. 1999. Helicobacter pylori infection. *Clin Microbiol Inf* **5:**1-11.

7760. Vandermeulen, C., M. Roelants, M. Vermoere, K. Roseeuw, P. Goubau, and K. Hoppenbrouwers. 2004. Outbreak of mumps in a vaccinated child population: a question of vaccine failure? *Vaccine* **22:**2713-6.

7761. Vanlandingham, D. L., B. S. Davis, D. K. Lvov, E. Samokhvalov, S. D. Lvov, W. C. Black, S. Higgs, and B. J. Beaty. 2002. Molecular characterization of California serogroup viruses isolated in Russi. *Am J Trop Med Hyg* **67:**306-9.

7762. Vanlandingham, D. L., C. Hong, K. Klingler, K. Tsetsarkin, K. L. McElroy, A. M. Powers, M. J. Lehane, and S. Higgs. 2005. Differential Infectivities of O'nyong-Nyong and Chikungunya Virus Isolates in Anopheles Gambiae and Aedes Aegypti Mosquitoes. *Am J Trop Med Hyg* **72:**616-621.

7763. Vanzee, B. E., R. G. Douglas, R. F. Betts, A. W. Bauman, D. W. Fraser, and A. R. Hinman. 1975. Lymphocytic choriomeningitis in university hospital personnel. Clinical features. *Am J Med* **58:**803-9.

7764. Vapalahti, K., M. Paunio, M. Brummer-Korvenkontio, A. Vaheri, and O. Vapalahti. 1999. Puumala virus infections in Finland: increased occupational risk for farmers. *Am J Epidemiol* **149:**1142-51.

7765. Vapalahti, O., A. Lundkvist, V. Fedorov, C. J. Conroy, S. Hirvonen, A. Plyusnina, K. Nemirov, K. Fredga, J. A. Cook, J. Niemimaa, A. Kaikusalo, H. Henttonen, A. Vaheri, and A. Plyusnin. 1999. Isolation and characterization of a hantavirus from Lemmus sibiricus: evidence for host switch during hantavirus evolution. *J Virol* **73:**5586-92.

7766. Varejao, J. B., C. B. Santos, H. R. Rezende, L. C. Bevilacqua, and A. Falqueto. 2005. [Aedes (Stegomyia) aegypti (Linnaeus, 1762) breeding sites in native bromeliads in Vitoria City, ES]. *Rev Soc Bras Med Trop* **38:**238-40.

7767. Varela, J. A., L. Otero, E. Espinosa, C. Sanchez, M. L. Junquera, and F. Vazquez. 2003. Phthirus pubis in a sexually transmitted diseases unit: a study of 14 years. *Sex Transm Dis* **30:**292-6.

7768. Varga, V. 1997. An explosive outbreak of Q-fever in Jedl'ove Kostol'any, Slovakia. *Cent Eur J Public Health* **5:**180-2.

7769. Vargas, M., J. Gascón, F. Gallardo, M. T. Jimenez De Anta, and J. Vila. 1998. Prevalence of diarrheagenic Escherichia coli strains detected by PCR in patients with travelers' diarrhea. *Clin Microbiol Infect* **4:**682-8.

7770. Vargas, S. L., C. A. Ponce, F. Gigliotti, A. V. Ulloa, S. Prieto, M. P. Munoz, and W. T. Hughes. 2000. Transmission of Pneumocystis carinii DNA from a patient with P. carinii pneumonia to immunocompetent contact health care workers. *J Clin Microbiol* **38:**1536-8.

7771. Vargas, S. L., C. A. Ponce, V. Luchsinger, C. Silva, M. Gallo, R. Lopez, J. Belletti, L. Velozo, R. Avila, M. A. Palomino, S. Benveniste, and L. F. Avendano. 2005. Detection of Pneumocystis carinii f. sp. hominis and viruses in presumably immunocompetent infants who died in the hospital or in the community. *J Infect Dis* **191:**122-6.

7772. Vargo, K., and B. A. Cohen. 1993. Prevalence of undetected tinea capitis in household members of children with disease. *Pediatrics* **92:**155-7.

7773. Varma, J. K., K. D. Greene, M. E. Reller, S. M. DeLong, J. Trottier, S. F. Nowicki, M. DiOrio, E. M. Koch, T. L. Bannerman, S. T. York, M. A. Lambert-Fair, J. G. Wells, and P. S. Mead. 2003. An outbreak of Escherichia coli O157 infection following exposure to a contaminated building. *JAMA* **290:**2709-12.

7774. Varma, J. K., G. Katsitadze, M. Moiscrafishvili, T. Zardiashvili, M. Chikheli, N. Tarkashvili, E. Jhorjholiani, M. Chubinidze, T. Kukhalashvili, I. Khmaladze, N. Chakvetadze, P. Imnadze, and J. Sobel. 2004. Foodborne botulism in the Republic of Georgia. *Emerg Infect Dis* **10:**1601-5.

7775. Varon, E., C. Levy, F. De La Rocque, M. Boucherat, D. Deforche, I. Podglajen, M. Navel, and R. Cohen. 2000. Impact of antimicrobial therapy on nasopharyngeal carriage of Streptococcus pneumoniae, Haemophilus influenzae, and Branhamella catarrhalis in children with respiratory tract infections. *Clin Infect Dis* **31:**477-81.

7776. Vas, S. I. 2002. Infections related to prosthetic materials in patients on chronic dialysis. *Clin Microbiol Infect* **8:**705–8.

7777. Vasconcelos, P. F. 2003. [Yellow Fever]. *Rev Soc Bras Med Trop* **36:**275-93.

7778. Vasilakopoulou, A., K. Dimarongona, A. Samakovli, K. Papadimitris, and A. Avlami. 2003. Balantidium coli pneumonia in an immunocompromised patient. *Scand J Infect Dis* **35:**144-6.

7779. Vassiloyanakopoulos, A., G. Spala, E. Mavrou, and C. Hadjichristodoulou. 1999. A case of tuberculosis on a long distance flight: the difficulties of the investigation. *Eurosurveillance* **4:**96-97.

7780. Vaughn, D. W., and C. H. Hoke, Jr. 1992. The epidemiology of Japanese encephalitis: prospects for prevention. *Epidemiol Rev* **14:**197-221.

7781. Vaz, R. G., S. Gloyd, E. Folgosa, and J. Kreiss. 1995. Syphilis and HIV infection among prisoners in Maputo, Mozambique. *Int J STD AIDS* **6:**42-6.

7782. Vazquez Castellanos, J. L. 1991. [Coffee tree cultivation and the social history of onchocerciasis in Soconusco, Chiapas state, Mexico]. *Salud Publica Mex* **33:**124-35.

7783. Vazquez, J. A., L. M. Dembry, V. Sanchez, M. A. Vazquez, J. D. Sobel, C. Dmuchowski, and M. J. Zervos. 1998. Nosocomial Candida glabrata colonization: an epidemiologic study. *J Clin Microbiol* **36:**421-6.

7784. Vazquez, J. A., V. Sanchez, C. Dmuchowski, L. M. Dembry, J. D. Sobel, and M. J. Zervos. 1993. Nosocomial acquisition of

Candida albicans: an epidemiologic study. *J Infect Dis* **168:**195-201.

7785. **Vazquez Tsuji, O., I. Martinez Barbabosa, J. Tay Zavala, A. Ruiz Hernandez, and A. Perez Torres.** 1997. [Vegetables for human consumption as probable source of Toxocara sp. infection in man]. *Bol Chil Parasitol* **52:**47-50.

7786. **Vazquez-Prokopec, G. M., L. A. Ceballos, M. C. Cecere, and R. E. Gurtler.** 2002. Seasonal variations of microclimatic conditions in domestic and peridomestic habitats of Triatoma infestans in rural northwest Argentina. *Acta Trop* **84:**229-38.

7787. **Veeken, H.** 1993. Malaria and gold fever. *BMJ* **307:**433-4.

7788. **Vehmeyer, S. B., R. M. Bloem, and P. L. Petit.** 2001. Microbiological screening of post-mortem bone donors - two case reports. *J Hosp Infect* **47:**193-7.

7789. **Veitch, M. G. K., P. D. R. Johnson, P. E. Flood, D. E. Leslie, A. C. Street, and J. A. Hayman.** 1997. A large localized outbreak of Mycobacterium ulcerans infection on a temperate southern Australian island. *Epidemiol Infect* **119:**313-8.

7790. **Vela, M., N. L. Heredia, P. Feng, and J. Santos Garcia-Alvarado.** 1999. DNA probe analysis for the carriage of enterotoxigenic Clostridium perfringens in feces of a Mexican subpopulation. *Diagn Microbiol Infect Dis* **35:**101-4.

7791. **Velazquez, O., H. C. Stetler, C. Avila, G. Ornelas, C. Alvarez, S. C. Hadler, D. W. Bradley, and J. Sepulveda.** 1990. Epidemic transmission of enterically transmitted non-A, non-B hepatitis in Mexico, 1986-1987. *JAMA* **263:**3281-5.

7792. **Velazquez, R., B. Munoz-Hernandez, R. Arenas, M. L. Taylor, F. Hernandez-Hernandez, M. E. Manjarrez, and R. Lopez-Martinez.** 2003. An imported case of Blastomyces dermatitidis infection in Mexico. *Mycopathologia* **156:**263-7.

7793. **Vélez B, I. D., J. Ortega, M. I. Hurtado M., A. L. Salazar, S. M. Robledo, J. N. Jimenez, and L. E. Velasquez.** 2000. Epidemiology of paragonimiasis in Colombia. *Trans R Soc Trop Med Hyg* **94:**661-3.

7794. **Velho, P. E., A. V. Faria, M. L. Cintra, E. M. de Souza, and A. M. de Moraes.** 2003. Larva migrans: a case report and review. *Rev Inst Med Trop Sao Paulo* **45:**167-71.

7795. **Vellinga, A., and F. Van Loock.** 2002. The dioxin crisis as experiment to determine poultry-related campylobacter enteritis. *Emerg Infect Dis* **8:**19-22.

7796. **Velo, E., S. Bino, M. Kuli-Lito, K. Pano, L. Gradoni, and M. Maroli.** 2003. Recrudescence of visceral leishmaniasis in Albania: retrospective analysis of cases during 1997 to 2001 and results of an entomological survey carried out during 2001 in some districts. *Trans R Soc Trop Med Hyg* **97:**288-90.

7797. **Venkataramana, C. B. S., and P. V. Sarada.** 2001. Extent and speed of spread of HIV infection in India through the commercial sex networks: a perspective. *Trop Med Int Health* **6:**1040-1061.

7798. **Verboon-Maciolek, M. A., M. Nijhuis, A. M. van Loon, N. van Maarssenveen, H. van Wieringen, M. A. Pekelharing-Berghuis, T. G. Krediet, L. J. Gerards, A. Fleer, R. J. Diepersloot, and S. F. Thijsen.** 2003. Diagnosis of enterovirus infection in the first 2 months of life by real-time polymerase chain reaction. *Clin Infect Dis* **37:**1-6.

7799. **Verdier, M., F. Denis, A. Sangaré, F. Barin, G. Gershy-Damet, J. L. Rey, B. Soro, G. Leonard, M. Mounier, and J. Hugon.** 1989. Prevalence of antibody to human T cell leukemia virus type 1 (HTLV-1) in populations of Ivory Coast, West Africa. *J Infect Dis* **160:**363-70.

7800. **Verduin, C. M., C. Hol, A. Fleer, H. van Dijk, and A. van Belkum.** 2002. Moraxella catarrhalis: from emerging to established pathogen. *Clin Microbiol Rev* **15:**125-44.

7801. **Verghese, A., and S. L. Berk.** 1990. Infections in nursing homes and long-term care facilities. Karger, Basel.

7802. **Verhaegen, J., J. Charlier, P. Lemmens, M. Delmee, R. Van Noyen, L. Verbist, and G. Wauters.** 1998. Surveillance of human Yersinia enterocolitica infections in Belgium: 1967-96. *Clin Infect Dis* **27:**59-64.

7803. **Verhamme, M. A., and C. H. Ramboer.** 1988. Anisakiasis caused by herring in vinegar: a little known medical problem. *Gut* **29:**843-7.

7804. **Vernazza, P. L.** 2001. Genital shedding of HIV-1 despite successful antiretroviral therapy. *Lancet* **358:**1564.

7805. **Vernon, A. A., C. Schable, and D. Francis.** 1982. A large outbreak of hepatitis A in a day-care center: association with non-toilet-trained children and persistence of IgM antibody to hepatitis A virus. *Am J Epidemiol* **115:**325-31.

7806. **Verver, S., D. van Soolingen, and M. W. Borgdorff.** 2002. Effect of screening of immigrants on tuberculosis transmission. *Int J Tuberc Lung Dis* **6:**121-9.

7807. **Verver, S., R. M. Warren, Z. Munch, M. Richardson, G. D. van der Spuy, M. W. Borgdorff, M. A. Behr, N. Beyers, and P. D. van Helden.** 2004. Proportion of tuberculosis transmission that takes place in households in a high-incidence area. *Lancet* **363:**212-4.

7808. **Verver, S., R. M. Warren, Z. Munch, E. Vynnycky, P. D. Van Helden, M. Richardson, G. D. Van Der Spuy, D. A. Enarson, M. W. Borgdorff, M. A. Behr, and N. Beyers.** 2004. Transmission of tuberculosis in a high incidence urban community in South Africa. *Int J Epidemiol* **33:**351-7.

7809. **Verville, T. D., M. M. Huycke, R. A. Greenfield, D. P. Fine, T. L. Kuhls, and L. N. Slater.** 1994. Rhodococcus equi infections of humans. 12 cases and a review of the literature. *Medicine (Baltimore)* **73:**119-32.

7810. **Verweij, J. J., J. Vermeer, E. A. Brienen, C. Blotkamp, D. Laeijendecker, L. van Lieshout, and A. M. Polderman.** 2003. Entamoeba histolytica infections in captive primates. *Parasitol Res* **90:**100-3.

7811. **Verweij, P. E., J. F. Meis, V. Christmann, M. Van der Bor, W. J. Melchers, B. G. Hilderink, and A. Voss.** 1998. Nosocomial outbreak of colonization and infection with Stenotrophomonas maltophilia in preterm infants associated with contaminated tap water. *Epidemiol Infect* **120:**251-6.

7812. **Vesley, D., and H. M. Hartmann.** 1988. Laboratory-acquired infections and injuries in clinical laboratories: a 1986 survey. *Am J Public Health* **78:**1213-5.

7813. **Vesper, E., and R. Standke.** 1982. Mykologische Studie zur epidemiologischen Situation in Fusspflegesalons. *Z Gesamte Hyg Grenzgeb* **28:**105-107.

7814. **Veverka, F., N. Shapiro, M. K. Parish, S. York, W. Becker, F. Smith, C. Allensworth, T. Baker, P. Iwen, and T. Safranek.** 2001. Protracted outbreaks of cryptosporidiosis associated with swimming pool use - Ohio and Nebraska, 2000. *MMWR* **50:**406-410.

7815. **Vezzani, D., A. Rubio, S. M. Velazquez, N. Schweigmann, and T. Wiegand.** 2005. Detailed assessment of microhabitat suitability for Aedes aegypti (Diptera: Culicidae) in Buenos Aires, Argentina. *Acta Trop* **95:**123-31.

7816. **Victor, C. R.** 1997. The health of homeless people in Britain. *Eur J Public Health* **7:**398-404.

7817. Vieira, C., I. D. Vélez, M. N. Montoya, et al. 1998. Dirofilaria immitis in Tikuna Indians and their dogs in the Colombian Amazon. *Ann Trop Med Parasitol* **92:**123-5.

7818. Vieira, J. C., H. D. Blankespoor, P. J. Cooper, and R. H. Guderian. 1992. Paragonimiasis in Ecuador: prevalence and geographical distribution of parasitisation of second intermediate hosts with Paragonimus mexicanus in Esmeraldas province. *Trop Med Parasitol* **43:**249-52.

7819. Vieira, J. C., L. Brackenboro, C. H. Porter, M. G. Basanez, and R. C. Collins. 2005. Spatial and temporal variation in biting rates and parasite transmission potentials of onchocerciasis vectors in Ecuador. *Trans R Soc Trop Med Hyg* **99:**178-95.

7820. Vieth, U. C., M. Kunzelmann, S. Diedrich, H. Timm, A. Ammon, O. Lyytikainen, and L. R. Petersen. 1999. An echovirus 30 outbreak with a high meningitis attack rate among children and household members at four day-care centers. *Eur J Epidemiol* **15:**655-8.

7821. Vigeant, P., V. G. Loo, C. Bertrand, C. Dixon, R. Hollis, M. A. Pfaller, A. P. McLean, D. J. Briedis, T. M. Perl, and H. G. Robson. 1998. An outbreak of Serratia marcescens infections related to contaminated chlorhexidine. *Infect Control Hosp Epidemiol* **19:**791-4.

7822. Vijaikumar, M., D. M. Thappa, and K. Karthikeyan. 2002. Cutaneous anthrax: an endemic outbreak in south India. *J Trop Pediatr* **48:**225-6.

7823. Vikerfors, T., M. Grandien, and P. Olcen. 1987. Respiratory syncytial virus infections in adults. *Am Rev Respir Dis* **136:**561-4.

7824. Vila, J., J. Ruiz, F. Gallardo, M. Vargas, L. Soler, M. J. Figueras, and J. Gascon. 2003. Aeromonas spp. and traveler's diarrhea: clinical features and antimicrobial resistance. *Emerg Infect Dis* **9:**552-5.

7825. Vilaichone, R. K., W. Vilaichone, P. Nunthapisud, and H. Wilde. 2002. Streptococcus suis infection in Thailand. *J Med Assoc Thai* **85 Suppl 1:**S109-17.

7826. Vilchez, R. A., C. A. Kozinetz, A. S. Arrington, C. R. Madden, and J. S. Butel. 2003. Simian virus 40 in human cancers. *Am J Med* **114:**675–84.

7827. Viljanen, M. K., T. Peltola, S. Y. Junnila, L. Olkkonen, H. Jarvinen, M. Kuistila, and P. Huovinen. 1990. Outbreak of diarrhoea due to Escherichia coli O111:B4 in schoolchildren and adults: association of Vi antigen-like reactivity. *Lancet* **336:**831-4.

7828. Villagra, M., L. Suarez, R. Arce, and M. G. Moreira. 1994. Bolivian hemorrhagic fever - El Beni department, Bolivia, 1994. *MMWR* **43:**943-946.

7829. Villahermosa, L. G., T. T. Fajardo, Jr., R. M. Abalos, R. V. Cellona, M. V. Balagon, E. C. Dela Cruz, E. V. Tan, G. P. Walsh, and D. S. Walsh. 2004. Parallel assessment of 24 monthly doses of rifampin, ofloxacin, and minocycline versus two years of World Health Organization multi-drug therapy for multi-bacillary leprosy. *Am J Trop Med Hyg* **70:**197-200.

7830. Villar, L. M., M. C. Costa, V. S. Paula, and A. M. Gaspar. 2002. Hepatitis outbreak in a public school in Rio de Janeiro, Brazil. *Mem Inst Oswaldo Cruz* **97:**301-5.

7831. Villar, R. G., M. D. Macek, S. Simons, P. S. Hayes, M. J. Goldoft, J. H. Lewis, L. L. Rowan, D. Hursh, M. Patnode, and P. S. Mead. 1999. Investigation of multidrug-resistant Salmonella serotype typhimurium DT104 infections linked to raw-milk cheese in Washington State. *JAMA* **281:**1811-6.

7832. Villar, R. G., R. L. Shapiro, S. Busto, C. Riva-Posse, G. Verdejo, M. I. Farace, F. Rosetti, J. A. San Juan, C. M. Julia, J. Becher, S. E. Maslanka, and D. L. Swerdlow. 1999. Outbreak of type A botulism and development of a botulism surveillance and antitoxin release system in Argentina. *JAMA* **281:**1334-8, 1340.

7833. Villaseca, P., A. Llanos-Cuentas, E. Perez, and C. R. Davies. 1993. A comparative field study of the relative importance of Lutzomyia peruensis and Lutzomyia verrucarum as vectors of cutaneous leishmaniasis in the Peruvian Andes. *Am J Trop Med Hyg* **49:**260-9.

7834. Villegas-Garcia, J. C., and S. Santillan-Alarcon. 2004. American trypanosomiasis in central Mexico: Trypanosoma cruzi infection in triatomine bugs and mammals from the municipality of Jiutepec in the state of Morelos. *Ann Trop Med Parasitol* **98:**529-32.

7835. Villena, C., R. Gabrieli, R. M. Pinto, S. Guix, D. Donia, E. Buonomo, L. Palombi, F. Cenko, S. Bino, A. Bosch, and M. Divizia. 2003. A large infantile gastroenteritis outbreak in Albania caused by multiple emerging rotavirus genotypes. *Epidemiol Infect* **131:**1105-10.

7836. Vincent, J. L. 2003. Nosocomial infections in adult intensive-care units. *Lancet* **361:**2068-77.

7837. Vincent, J. L., D. J. Bihari, P. M. Suter, H. A. Bruining, J. White, M. H. Nicolas-Chanoin, M. Wolff, R. C. Spencer, and M. Hemmer. 1995. The prevalence of nosocomial infection in intensive care units in Europe. Results of the European Prevalence of Infection in Intensive Care (EPIC) Study. EPIC International Advisory Committee. *JAMA* **274:**639-44.

7838. Vinetz, J. M., G. E. Glass, C. E. Flexner, P. Mueller, and D. C. Kaslow. 1996. Sporadic urban leptospirosis. *Ann Intern Med* **125:**794-8.

7839. Vinetz, J. M., J. Li, T. F. McCuthan, and D. C. Kaslow. 1998. Plasmodium malariae infection in an asymptomatic 74-year-old Greek woman with splenomegaly. *N Engl J Med* **338:**367-371.

7840. Vinje, J., S. A. Altena, and M. P. Koopmans. 1997. The incidence and genetic variability of small round-structured viruses in outbreaks of gastroenteritis in The Netherlands. *J Infect Dis* **176:**1374-8.

7841. Visca, P., G. Cazzola, A. Petrucca, and C. Braggion. 2001. Travel-associated Burkholderia pseudomallei infection (Melioidosis) in a patient with cystic fibrosis: a case report. *Clin Infect Dis* **32:**E15-6.

7842. Vismer, H. F., and P. R. Hull. 1997. Prevalence, epidemiology and geographical distribution of Sporothrix schenckii infections in Gauteng, South Africa. *Mycopathologia* **137:**137-43.

7843. Visser, L. G., A. M. Polderman, and P. C. Stuiver. 1995. Outbreak of schistosomiasis among travelers returning from Mali, West Africa. *Clin Infect Dis* **20:**280-5.

7844. Visvesvara, G. S., and J. K. Stehr-Green. 1990. Epidemiology of free-living ameba infections. *J Protozool* **37:**25S-33S.

7845. Viswanathan, P., and R. Kaur. 2001. Prevalence and growth of pathogens on salad vegetables, fruits and sprouts. *Int J Hyg Environ Health* **203:**205-13.

7846. Vitek, C. R., R. F. Breiman, T. G. Ksiazek, P. E. Rollin, J. C. McLaughlin, E. T. Umland, K. B. Nolte, A. Loera, C. M. Sewell, and C. J. Peters. 1996. Evidence against person-to-person transmission of hantavirus to health care workers. *Clin Infect Dis* **22:**824-6.

7847. Vitek, C. R., T. G. Ksiazek, C. J. Peters, and R. F. Breiman. 1996. Evidence against infection with hantaviruses among forest and park workers in the southwestern United States. *Clin Infect Dis* **23**:283-5.

7848. Vittecoq, D., T. May, R. T. Roue, M. Stern, C. Mayaud, P. Chavanet, F. Borsa, P. Jeantils, M. Armengaud, J. Modai, et al. 1987. Acquired immunodeficiency syndrome after travelling in Africa: an epidemiological study in seventeen Caucasian patients. *Lancet* **1**:612-5.

7849. Vittecoq, D., J. F. Mettetal, C. Rouzioux, J. F. Bach, and J. P. Bouchon. 1989. Acute HIV infection after acupuncture treatments. *N Engl J Med* **320**:250-1.

7850. Vivas-Martinez, S., M. G. Basanez, M. E. Grillet, H. Weiss, C. Botto, M. Garcia, N. J. Villamizar, and D. C. Chavasse. 1998. Onchocerciasis in the Amazonian focus of southern Venezuela: altitude and blackfly species composition as predictors of endemicity to select communities for ivermectin control programmes. *Trans R Soc Trop Med Hyg* **92**:613-20.

7851. Vivier, J. C., M. M. Ehlers, and W. O. Grabow. 2004. Detection of enteroviruses in treated drinking water. *Water Res* **38**:2699-705.

7852. Vlaminckx, B., W. van Pelt, L. Schouls, A. van Silfhout, C. Elzenaar, E. Mascini, J. Verhoef, and J. Schellekens. 2004. Epidemiological features of invasive and noninvasive group A streptococcal disease in the Netherlands, 1992-1996. *Eur J Clin Microbiol Infect Dis* **23**:434-44.

7853. Vlatkovic, V., J. Antonijevic, and S. Nozic. 1967. [Epidemic of tuberculosis of the respiratory tract in a military unit]. *Vojnosanit Pregl* **24**:397-401.

7854. Vochem, M., M. Vogt, and G. Doring. 2001. Sepsis in a newborn due to Pseudomonas aeruginosa from a contaminated tub bath. *N Engl J Med* **345**:378-9.

7855. Voetsch, A. C., F. J. Angulo, T. Rabatsky-Ehr, S. Shallow, M. Cassidy, S. M. Thomas, E. Swanson, S. M. Zansky, M. A. Hawkins, T. F. Jones, P. J. Shillam, T. J. Van Gilder, J. G. Wells, and P. M. Griffin. 2004. Laboratory Practices for Stool-Specimen Culture for Bacterial Pathogens, Including Escherichia coli O157:H7, in the FoodNet Sites, 1995-2000. *Clin Infect Dis* **38 Suppl 3**:S190-7.

7856. Voglino, M. C., G. Donelli, P. Rossi, A. Ludovisi, V. Rinaldi, F. Goffredo, R. Paloscia, and E. Pozio. 1996. Intestinal microsporidiosis in Italian individuals with AIDS. *Ital J Gastroenterol* **28**:381-6.

7857. Vogt, M. 2003. [Diagnosis and treatment of bites by cats, dogs and humans]. *Dtsch Med Wochenschr* **128**:1059-63.

7858. Vogt, R. L., H. E. Sours, T. Barrett, R. A. Feldman, R. J. Dickinson, and L. Witherell. 1982. Campylobacter enteritis associated with contaminated water. *Ann Intern Med* **96**:292-6.

7859. Vollaard, A. M., S. Ali, H. A. van Asten, I. S. Ismid, S. Widjaja, L. G. Visser, C. Surjadi, and J. T. van Dissel. 2004. Risk factors for transmission of foodborne illness in restaurants and street vendors in Jakarta, Indonesia. *Epidemiol Infect* **132**:863-72.

7860. Vollaard, A. M., S. Ali, H. A. van Asten, S. Widjaja, L. G. Visser, C. Surjadi, and J. T. van Dissel. 2004. Risk factors for typhoid and paratyphoid fever in Jakarta, Indonesia. *JAMA* **291**:2607-15.

7861. Volney, B., J. F. Pouliquen, B. De Thoisy, and T. Fandeur. 2002. A sero-epidemiological study of malaria in human and monkey populations in French Guiana. *Acta Trop* **82**:11-23.

7862. Voltz, J. M., C. Drobacheff, C. Derancourt, S. Coumes-Marquet, C. Mougin, and R. Laurent. 1999. [Papillomavirus-induced anogenital lesions in 121 HIV seropositive men. Clinical, histological, viral study, and evolution]. *Ann Dermatol Venereol* **126**:424-9.

7863. Von Dolinger Brito, D., C. Matos, V. V. Abdalla, D. A. Filho, and P. F. Pinto Gontijo. 1999. An Outbreak of Nosocomial Infection Caused by ESBLs Producing Serratia marcescens in a Brazilian Neonatal Unit. *Braz J Infect Dis* **3**:149-155.

7864. von Eiff, C., G. Peters, and C. Heilmann. 2002. Pathogenesis of infections due to coagulase-negative staphylococci. *Lancet Infect Dis* **2**:677-85.

7865. von Hunolstein, C., G. Alfarone, F. Scopetti, M. Pataracchia, R. La Valle, F. Franchi, L. Pacciani, A. Manera, A. Giammanco, S. Farinelli, K. Engler, A. De Zoysa, and A. Efstratiou. 2003. Molecular epidemiology and characteristics of Corynebacterium diphtheriae and Corynebacterium ulcerans strains isolated in Italy during the 1990s. *J Med Microbiol* **52**:181-8.

7866. von Reyn, C. F., R. D. Arbeit, C. R. Horsburgh, M. A. Ristola, R. D. Waddell, S. M. Tvaroha, M. Samore, L. R. Hirschhorn, J. Lumio, A. D. Lein, M. R. Grove, and A. N. Tosteson. 2002. Sources of disseminated Mycobacterium avium infection in AIDS. *J Infect* **44**:166-70.

7867. von Reyn, C. F., A. M. Barnes, N. S. Weber, and U. G. Hodgin. 1976. Bubonic plague from exposure to a rabbit: a documented case, and a review of rabbit-associated plague cases in the United States. *Am J Epidemiol* **104**:81-7.

7868. von Reyn, C. F., J. N. Maslow, T. W. Barber, J. O. Falkinham, 3rd, and R. D. Arbeit. 1994. Persistent colonisation of potable water as a source of Mycobacterium avium infection in AIDS. *Lancet* **343**:1137-41.

7869. von Reyn, C. F., R. D. Waddell, T. Eaton, R. D. Arbeit, J. N. Maslow, T. W. Barber, R. J. Brindle, C. F. Gilks, J. Lumio, J. Lahdevirta, et al. 1993. Isolation of Mycobacterium avium complex from water in the United States, Finland, Zaire, and Kenya. *J Clin Microbiol* **31**:3227-30.

7870. von Sonnenburg, F., N. Tornieporth, P. Waiyaki, B. Lowe, L. F. Peruski, Jr., H. L. DuPont, J. J. Mathewson, and R. Steffen. 2000. Risk and aetiology of diarrhoea at various tourist destinations. *Lancet* **356**:133-4.

7871. von Suzani, C., and P. Hazeghi. 1976. [Infections transmitted in swimming pools]. *Soz Praventivmed* **21**:120-1.

7872. Vong, S., A. E. Fiore, D. O. Haight, J. Li, N. Borgsmiller, W. Kuhnert, F. Pinero, K. Boaz, T. Badsgard, C. Mancini, O. V. Nainan, S. Wiersma, and B. P. Bell. 2005. Vaccination in the county jail as a strategy to reach high risk adults during a community-based hepatitis A outbreak among methamphetamine drug users. *Vaccine* **23**:1021-8.

7873. Vonstille, W. T., W. T. Stille, 3rd, and R. C. Sharer. 1993. Hepatitis A epidemics from utility sewage in Ocoee, Florida. *Arch Environ Health* **48**:120-4.

7874. Vos, K., A. P. Van Dam, H. Kuiper, H. Bruins, L. Spanjaard, and J. Dankert. 1994. Seroconversion for Lyme borreliosis among Dutch military. *Scand J Infect Dis* **26**:427-34.

7875. Vos, M. C., P. E. de Haas, H. A. Verbrugh, N. H. Renders, N. G. Hartwig, P. de Man, A. H. Kolk, H. van Deutekom, J. L. Yntema, A. G. Vulto, M. Messemaker, and D. van Soolingen. 2003. Nosocomial Mycobacterium bovis-bacille Calmette-Guerin infections due to contamination of chemotherapeutics: case finding and route of transmission. *J Infect Dis* **188**:1332-5.

7876. **Voss, L. M., K. H. Rhodes, and K. A. Johnson.** 1992. Musculoskeletal and soft tissue Aeromonas infection: an environmental disease. *Mayo Clin Proc* **67**:422-7.

7877. **Vought, K. J., and S. R. Tatini.** 1998. Salmonella enteritidis contamination of ice cream associated with a 1994 multistate outbreak. *J Food Prot* **61**:5-10.

7878. **Vreden, S. G., L. G. Visser, J. J. Verweij, J. Blotkamp, P. C. Stuiver, A. Aguirre, and A. M. Polderman.** 2000. Outbreak of amebiasis in a family in The Netherlands. *Clin Infect Dis* **31**:1101-4.

7879. **Vrioni, G., C. Gartzonika, A. Kostoula, C. Boboyianni, C. Papadopoulou, and S. Levidiotou.** 2004. Application of a polymerase chain reaction enzyme immunoassay in peripheral whole blood and serum specimens for diagnosis of acute human brucellosis. *Eur J Clin Microbiol Infect Dis* **23**:194-9.

7880. **Vugia, D., J. Hadler, S. Chaves, D. Blythe, K. Smith, D. Morse, P. Cieslak, T. Jones, A. Cronquist, D. Goldman, J. Guzewich, F. Angulo, P. Griffin, and R. Tauxe.** 2003. Preliminary FoodNet data on the incidence of foodborne illnesses - selected sites, United States, 2002. *MMWR* **52**:340-3.

7881. **Vugia, D. J., M. Samuel, M. M. Farley, R. Marcus, B. Shiferaw, S. Shallow, K. Smith, and F. J. Angulo.** 2004. Invasive Salmonella Infections in the United States, FoodNet, 1996-1999: Incidence, Serotype Distribution, and Outcome. *Clin Infect Dis* **38 Suppl 3**:S149-56.

7882. **Vukovic, Z., A. Bobic-Radovanovic, Z. Latkovic, and Z. Radovanovic.** 1995. An epidemiological investigation of the first outbreak of rhinosporidiosis in Europe. *J Trop Med Hyg* **98**:333-337.

7883. **Vukshich Oster, N., R. Harpaz, S. B. Redd, and M. J. Papania.** 2004. International importation of measles virus—United States, 1993-2001. *J Infect Dis* **189 Suppl 1**:48-53.

7884. **Vural, T., C. Ergin, and F. Sayin.** 1998. Investigation of Rickettsia conorii antibodies in the Antalya area. *Infection* **26**:170-2.

7885. **Vyse, A. J., N. J. Gay, L. M. Hesketh, N. J. Andrews, B. Marshall, H. I. Thomas, P. Morgan-Capner, and E. Miller.** 2002. The burden of Helicobacter pylori infection in England and Wales. *Epidemiol Infect* **128**:411-7.

7886. **Vythilingam, I., B. Sidavong, S. T. Chan, T. Phonemixay, V. Vanisaveth, P. Sisoulad, R. Phetsouvanh, S. L. Hakim, and S. Phompida.** 2005. Epidemiology of malaria in Attapeu Province, Lao PDR in relation to entomological parameters. *Trans R Soc Trop Med Hyg* **99**:833-9.

7887. **Wachsmuth, I. K., P. A. Blake, and O. Olsvik.** 1994. Vibrio cholerae and cholera. Molecular to global perspectives. American Society of Microbiology, Washington, D.C.

7888. **Wacker, K., E. Rodriguez, T. Garate, L. Geue, K. Tackmann, T. Selhorst, C. Staubach, and F. J. Conraths.** 1999. Epidemiological analysis of Trichinella spiralis infections of foxes in Brandenburg, Germany. *Epidemiol Infect* **123**:139-47.

7889. **Wade, T., R. Booy, E. L. Teare, and S. Kroll.** 1999. Pasteurella multocida meningitis in infancy - (a lick may be as bad as a bite). *Eur J Pediatr* **158**:875-8.

7890. **Wade, T. J., N. Pai, J. N. Eisenberg, and J. M. Colford, Jr.** 2003. Do U.S. Environmental Protection Agency water quality guidelines for recreational waters prevent gastrointestinal illness? A systematic review and meta-analysis. *Environ Health Perspect* **111**:1102-9.

7891. **Wade, T. J., S. K. Sandhu, D. Levy, S. Lee, M. W. LeChevallier, L. Katz, and J. M. Colford, Jr.** 2004. Did a severe flood in the midwest cause an increase in the incidence of gastrointestinal symptoms? *Am J Epidemiol* **159**:398-405.

7892. **Wadsworth, J. D., S. Joiner, A. F. Hill, T. A. Campbell, M. Desbruslais, P. J. Luthert, and J. Collinge.** 2001. Tissue distribution of protease resistant prion protein in variant Creutzfeldt-Jakob disease using a highly sensitive immunoblotting assay. *Lancet* **358**:171-80.

7893. **Wagenlehner, F. M., and K. G. Naber.** 2004. Emergence of antibiotic resistance and prudent use of antibiotic therapy in nosocomially acquired urinary tract infections. *Int J Antimicrob Agents* **23 Suppl 1**:S24-9.

7894. **Wagenvoort, J. H., H. G. Houben, G. L. Boonstra, and J. Scherpbier.** 1994. Pulmonary superinfection with Strongyloides stercoralis in an immunocompromised retired coal miner. *Eur J Clin Microbiol Infect Dis* **13**:518-9.

7895. **Waggoner-Fountain, L. A., M. W. Walker, R. J. Hollis, M. A. Pfaller, J. E. Ferguson, 2nd, R. P. Wenzel, and L. G. Donowitz.** 1996. Vertical and horizontal transmission of unique Candida species to premature newborns. *Clin Infect Dis* **22**:803-8.

7896. **Wagner, D.** 2004. Nosocomial acquisition of dengue. *Emerg Infect Dis* **10**:1872-3.

7897. **Wagner, J., R. Ignatius, S. Voss, V. Hopfner, S. Ehlers, G. Funke, U. Weber, and H. Hahn.** 2001. Infection of the skin caused by Corynebacterium ulcerans and mimicking classical cutaneous diphtheria. *Clin Infect Dis* **33**:1598-600.

7898. **Wahlberg, P., P. Saikku, and M. Brummer-Korvenkontio.** 1989. Tick-borne viral encephalitis in Finland. The clinical features of Kumlinge disease during 1959-1987. *J Intern Med* **225**:173-7.

7899. **Waiswa, C., and E. Katunguka-Rwakishaya.** 2004. Bovine trypanosomiasis in south-western Uganda: packed-cell volumes and prevalences of infection in the cattle. *Ann Trop Med Parasitol* **98**:21-7.

7900. **Waiswa, C., W. Olaho-Mukani, and E. Katunguka-Rwakishaya.** 2003. Domestic animals as reservoirs for sleeping sickness in three endemic foci in south-eastern Uganda. *Ann Trop Med Parasitol* **97**:149-55.

7901. **Waite, D., P. Beckenhaupt, L. LoBianco, P. Mshar, A. Nepaul, K. Marshall, K. Brennan, J. L. Hadler, W. A. Nix, M. Pallansch, and E. M. Begier.** 2004. Aseptic meningitis outbreak associated with echovirus 9 among recreational vehicle campers - Connecticut, 2003. *MMWR* **53**:710-3.

7902. **Wakayama, M., K. Shibuya, T. Ando, T. Oharaseki, K. Takahashi, S. Naoe, and W. F. Coulson.** 2002. Deep-seated mycosis as a complication in bone marrow transplantation patients. *Mycoses* **45**:146-51.

7903. **Wakefield, A. E.** 1996. DNA sequences identical to Pneumocystis carinii f. sp. carinii and Pneumocystis carinii f. sp. hominis in samples of air spora. *J Clin Microbiol* **34**:1754-9.

7904. **Wakefield, A. E., A. R. Lindley, H. E. Ambrose, C. M. Denis, and R. F. Miller.** 2003. Limited asymptomatic carriage of Pneumocystis jiroveci in human immunodeficiency virus-infected patients. *J Infect Dis* **187**:901-8.

7905. **Wald, A., A. G. Langenberg, K. Link, A. E. Izu, R. Ashley, T. Warren, S. Tyring, J. M. Douglas, Jr., and L. Corey.** 2001. Effect of condoms on reducing the transmission of herpes simplex virus type 2 from men to women. *JAMA* **285**:3100-6.

7906. **Wald, A., W. Leisenring, J. A. van Burik, and R. A. Bowden.** 1997. Epidemiology of Aspergillus infections in a large cohort of patients undergoing bone marrow transplantation. *J Infect Dis* **175**:1459-66.

7907. **Wald, A., J. Zeh, S. Selke, T. Warren, R. Ashley, and L. Corey.** 2002. Genital Shedding of Herpes Simplex Virus among Men. *J Infect Dis* **186 Suppl 1**:S34-9.

7908. **Wald, E. R., B. Dashefsky, C. Byers, N. Guerra, and F. Taylor.** 1988. Frequency and severity of infections in day care. *J Pediatr* **112**:540-6.

7909. **Wald, T. G., P. Shult, P. Krause, B. A. Miller, P. Drinka, and S. Gravenstein.** 1995. A rhinovirus outbreak among residents of a long-term care facility. *Ann Intern Med* **123**:588-93.

7910. **Waldenstrom, J., T. Broman, I. Carlsson, D. Hasselquist, R. P. Achterberg, J. A. Wagenaar, and B. Olsen.** 2002. Prevalence of Campylobacter jejuni, Campylobacter lari, and Campylobacter coli in different ecological guilds and taxa of migrating birds. *Appl Environ Microbiol* **68**:5911-7.

7911. **Walder, R., O. M. Suarez, and C. H. Calisher.** 1984. Arbovirus studies in the Guajira region of Venezuela: activities of eastern equine encephalitis and Venezuelan equine encephalitis viruses during an interepizootic period. *Am J Trop Med Hyg* **33**:699-707.

7912. **Walderich, B., A. Weber, and J. Knobloch.** 1997. Differentiation of Entamoeba histolytica and Entamoeba dispar from German travelers and residents of endemic areas. *Am J Trop Med Hyg* **57**:70-4.

7913. **Waldman, R. J., A. C. England, R. Tauxe, T. Kline, R. J. Weeks, L. Ajello, L. Kaufman, B. Wentworth, and D. W. Fraser.** 1983. A winter outbreak of acute histoplasmosis in northern Michigan. *Am J Epidemiol* **117**:68-75.

7914. **Walia, J. S., and C. L. Chronister.** 2001. Possible iatrogenic transmission of Creutzfeldt-Jakob disease via tonometer tips: a review of the literature. *Optometry* **72**:649-52.

7915. **Walker, D., and D. Campbell.** 1999. A survey of infections in United Kingdom laboratories, 1994-1995. *J Clin Pathol* **52**:415-8.

7916. **Walker, D. G., and G. J. Walker.** 2002. Forgotten but not gone: the continuing scourge of congenital syphilis. *Lancet Infect Dis* **2**:432-6.

7917. **Walker, W.** 1965. The Aberdeen typhoid outbreak of 1964. *Scott Med J* **10**:466-79.

7918. **Wallace, G. D., L. Marshall, and M. Marshall.** 1972. Cats, rats, and toxoplasmosis on a small Pacific island. *Am J Epidemiol* **95**:475-82.

7919. **Wallace, M. R., C. J. Chamberlin, M. H. Sawyer, A. M. Arvin, J. Harkins, A. LaRocco, M. W. Colopy, W. A. Bowler, and E. C. Oldfield, 3rd.** 1996. Treatment of adult varicella with sorivudine: a randomized, placebo-controlled trial. *J Infect Dis* **174**:249-55.

7920. **Wallace, M. R., T. W. Sharp, B. Smoak, C. Iriye, P. Rozmajzl, S. A. Thornton, R. Batchelor, A. J. Magill, H. O. Lobel, C. F. Longer, and J. P. Burans.** 1996. Malaria among United States troops in Somalia. *Am J Med* **100**:49-55.

7921. **Wallach, J. C., L. E. Samartino, A. Efron, and P. C. Baldi.** 1997. Human infection by Brucella melitensis: an outbreak attributed to contact with infected goats. *FEMS Immunol Med Microbiol* **19**:315-21.

7922. **Wallis, P. M., S. L. Erlandsen, J. L. Isaac-Renton, M. E. Olson, W. J. Robertson, and H. van Keulen.** 1996. Prevalence of Giardia cysts and Cryptosporidium oocysts and characterization of Giardia spp. isolated from drinking water in Canada. *Appl Environ Microbiol* **62**:2789-97.

7923. **Wallon, M., L. Kodjikian, C. Binquet, J. Garweg, J. Fleury, C. Quantin, and F. Peyron.** 2004. Long-term ocular prognosis in 327 children with congenital toxoplasmosis. *Pediatrics* **113**:1567-72.

7924. **Walls, T., A. G. Shankar, and D. Shingadia.** 2003. Adenovirus: an increasingly important pathogen in paediatric bone marrow transplant patients. *Lancet Infect Dis* **3**:79-86.

7925. **Walochnik, J., E. Haller-Schober, H. Kolli, O. Picher, A. Obwaller, and H. Aspock.** 2000. Discrimination between clinically relevant and nonrelevant Acanthamoeba strains isolated from contact lens-wearing keratitis patients in Austria. *J Clin Microbiol* **38**:3932-6.

7926. **Walpole, I. R., N. Hodgen, and C. Bower.** 1991. Congenital toxoplasmosis: a large survey in western Australia. *Med J Aust* **154**:720-4.

7927. **Walsh, B., H. Maguire, and D. Carrington.** 1999. Outbreak of hepatitis B in an acupuncture clinic. *Commun Dis Public Health* **2**:137-40.

7928. **Walsh, T. J., A. Groll, J. Hiemenz, R. Fleming, E. Roilides, and E. Anaissie.** 2004. Infections due to emerging and uncommon medically important fungal pathogens. *Clin Microbiol Infect* **10 Suppl 1**:48-66.

7929. **Walter, H., and S. W. Breckle.** 1999 (7th ed). Vegetation und Klimazonen. Eugen Ulmer Verlag, Stuttgart.

7930. **Walter, J. E., and D. K. Mitchell.** 2003. Astrovirus infection in children. *Curr Opin Infect Dis* **16**:247-53.

7931. **Walter, V. A., and A. J. DiMarino, Jr.** 2000. American Society for Gastrointestinal Endoscopy-Society of Gastroenterology Nurses and Associates Endoscope Reprocessing Guidelines. *Gastrointest Endosc Clin N Am* **10**:265-73.

7932. **Walters, L. L., S. J. Tirrell, and R. E. Shope.** 1999. Seroepidemiology of California and Bunyamwera serogroup (Bunyaviridae) virus infections in native populations of Alaska. *Am J Trop Med Hyg* **60**:806-21.

7933. **Walton, S. F., J. L. Choy, A. Bonson, A. Valle, J. McBroom, D. Taplin, L. Arlian, J. D. Mathews, B. Currie, and D. J. Kemp.** 1999. Genetically distinct dog-derived and human-derived Sarcoptes scabiei in scabies-endemic communities in northern Australia. *Am J Trop Med Hyg* **61**:542-7.

7934. **Walton, T. E., F. R. Holbrook, R. Bolivar-Raya, J. Ferrer-Romero, and M. D. Ortega.** 1992. Venezuelan equine encephalomyelitis and African horse sickness. Current status and review. *Ann N Y Acad Sci* **653**:217-27.

7935. **Walzer, P. D., F. N. Judson, K. B. Murphy, G. R. Healy, D. K. English, and M. G. Schultz.** 1973. Balantidiasis outbreak in Truk. *Am J Trop Med Hyg* **22**:33-41.

7936. **Wamola, I. A., N. B. Mirza, J. J. Ombette, and F. E. Onyango.** 1993. Recent epidemic meningococcal meningitis in Nairobi. *East Afr Med J* **70**:195-7.

7937. **Wan, K. S., and W. C. Weng.** 2004. Eosinophilic meningitis in a child raising snails as pets. *Acta Trop* **90**:51-3.

7938. **Wandra, T., A. Ito, H. Yamasaki, T. Suroso, and S. S. Margono.** 2003. Taenia solium cysticercosis, Irian Jaya, Indonesia. *Emerg Infect Dis* **9**:884-5.

7939. **Wang, C. C., D. Mattson, and A. Wald.** 2001. Corynebacterium jeikeium bacteremia in bone marrow transplant patients with Hickman catheters. *Bone Marrow Transplant* **27**:445-9.

7940. **Wang, H. C., Y. S. Liaw, P. C. Yang, S. H. Kuo, and K. T. Luh.** 1995. A pseudoepidemic of Mycobacterium chelonae infection caused by contamination of a fibreoptic bronchoscope suction channel. *Eur Respir J* **8**:1259-62.

7941. **Wang, H. L., and D. Y. Jin.** 1997. Prevalence and genotype of hepatitis G virus in Chinese professional blood donors and hepatitis patients. *J Infect Dis* **175**:1229-33.

7942. **Wang, J. P., K. F. Granlund, S. A. Bozzette, M. J. Botte, and J. Fierer.** 2000. Bursal sporotrichosis: case report and review. *Clin Infect Dis* **31**:615-6.

7943. **Wang, J. T., L. C. McDonald, S. C. Chang, and M. Ho.** 2002. Community-acquired Acinetobacter baumannii bacteremia in adult patients in Taiwan. *J Clin Microbiol* **40**:1526-9.

7944. **Wang, K. W., W. N. Chang, T. Y. Shih, C. R. Huang, N. W. Tsai, C. S. Chang, Y. C. Chuang, P. C. Liliang, T. M. Su, C. S. Rau, Y. D. Tsai, B. C. Cheng, P. L. Hung, C. J. Chang, and C. H. Lu.** 2004. Infection of cerebrospinal fluid shunts: causative pathogens, clinical features, and outcomes. *Jpn J Infect Dis* **57**:44-8.

7945. **Wang, L. C.** 1998. Parasitic infections among Southeast Asian labourers in Taiwan: a long-term study. *Epidemiol Infect* **120**:81-6.

7946. **Wang, Q., S. Fidalgo, B. J. Chang, B. J. Mee, and T. V. Riley.** 2002. The detection and recovery of Erysipelothrix spp. in meat and abattoir samples in Western Australia. *J Appl Microbiol* **92**:844-50.

7947. **Wang, Q., D. A. Vuitton, J. Qiu, P. Giraudoux, Y. Xiao, P. M. Schantz, F. Raoul, T. Li, W. Yang, and P. S. Craig.** 2004. Fenced pasture: a possible risk factor for human alveolar echinococcosis in Tibetan pastoralist communities of Sichuan, China. *Acta Trop* **90**:285-93.

7948. **Wang, S. S., S. C. FitzSimmons, L. A. O'Leary, M. J. Rock, M. L. Gwinn, and M. J. Khoury.** 2001. Early diagnosis of cystic fibrosis in the newborn period and risk of Pseudomonas aeruginosa acquisition in the first 10 years of life: a registry-based longitudinal study. *Pediatrics* **107**:274-9.

7949. **Wang, X., H. Huang, Q. Dong, Y. Lin, Z. Wang, F. Li, Y. Nawa, and K. Yoshimura.** 2002. A clinical study of eosinophilic meningoencephalitis caused by angiostrongyliasis. *Chin Med J (Engl)* **115**:1312-5.

7950. **Wang, Y. H., M. T. Rogan, D. A. Vuitton, H. Wen, B. Bartholomot, C. N. Macpherson, P. F. Zou, Z. X. Ding, H. X. Zhou, X. F. Zhang, J. Luo, H. B. Xiong, Y. Fu, A. McVie, P. Giraudoux, W. G. Yang, and P. S. Craig.** 2001. Cystic echinococcosis in semi-nomadic pastoral communities in north-west China. *Trans R Soc Trop Med Hyg* **95**:153-8.

7951. **Wang, Y. J., E. Vuori-Holopainen, Y. Yang, Y. Wang, Y. Hu, D. Leboulleux, K. Hedman, M. Leinonen, and H. Peltola.** 2002. Relative frequency of Haemophilus influenzae type b pneumonia in Chinese children as evidenced by serology. *Pediatr Infect Dis J* **21**:271-7.

7952. **Wang, Z. Q., and J. Cui.** 2001. The epidemiology of human trichinellosis in China during 1964-1999. *Parasite* **8**:S63-6.

7953. **Wanji, S., N. Tendongfor, M. Esum, S. N. Atanga, and P. Enyong.** 2003. Heterogeneity in the prevalence and intensity of loiasis in five contrasting bioecological zones in Cameroon. *Trans R Soc Trop Med Hyg* **97**:183-7.

7954. **Wanji, S., N. Tendongfor, M. Esum, S. Ndindeng, and P. Enyong.** 2003. Epidemiology of concomitant infections due to Loa loa, Mansonella perstans, and Onchocerca volvulus in rain forest villages of Cameroon. *Med Microbiol Immunol (Berl)* **192**:15-21.

7955. **Wanji, S., N. Tendongfor, M. E. Esum, and P. Enyong.** 2002. Chrysops silacea biting densities and transmission potential in an endemic area of human loiasis in south-west Cameroon. *Trop Med Int Health* **7**:371-7.

7956. **Ward, J., A. Neill, B. McCall, R. Stafford, G. Smith, and R. Davison.** 2000. Three nursing home outbreaks of Norwalk-like virus in Brisbane in 1999. *Commun Dis Intell* **24**:229-233.

7957. **Ward, J. I., D. W. Fraser, L. J. Baraff, and B. D. Plikaytis.** 1979. Haemophilus influenzae meningitis. A national study of secondary spread in household contacts. *N Engl J Med* **301**:122-6.

7958. **Ward, L. R., C. Maguire, M. D. Hampton, E. de Pinna, H. R. Smith, C. L. Little, I. A. Gillespie, S. J. O'Brien, R. T. Mitchell, C. Sharp, R. A. Swann, O. Doyle, and E. J. Threlfall.** 2002. Collaborative investigation of an outbreak of Salmonella enterica serotype Newport in England and Wales in 2001 associated with ready-to- eat salad vegetables. *Commun Dis Public Health* **5**:301-4.

7959. **Ward, R. L., A. M. Dinsmore, G. Goldberg, D. S. Sander, R. S. Rappaport, and E. T. Zito.** 1998. Shedding of rotavirus after administration of the tetravalent rhesus rotavirus vaccine. *Pediatr Infect Dis J* **17**:386-90.

7960. **Waree, P., P. Polseela, S. Pannarunothai, and V. Pipitgool.** 2001. The present situation of paragonimiasis in endemic area in Phitsanulok province. *Southeast Asian J Trop Med Public Health* **32 suppl 2**:51-4.

7961. **Warner, L., D. R. Newman, H. D. Austin, M. L. Kamb, J. M. Douglas, Jr., C. K. Malotte, J. M. Zenilman, J. Rogers, G. Bolan, M. Fishbein, D. G. Kleinbaum, M. Macaluso, and T. A. Peterman.** 2004. Condom effectiveness for reducing transmission of gonorrhea and chlamydia: the importance of assessing partner infection status. *Am J Epidemiol* **159**:242-51.

7962. **Warnock, D. W., B. Dupont, C. A. Kauffman, and T. Sirisanthana.** 1998. Imported mycoses in Europe. *Med Mycol* **36**:87-94.

7963. **Warrell, M. J., and D. A. Warrell.** 2004. Rabies and other lyssavirus diseases. *Lancet* **363**:959-69.

7964. **Warren, J. W.** 1986. Providencia stuartii: a common cause of antibiotic-resistant bacteriuria in patients with long-term indwelling catheters. *Rev Infect Dis* **8**:61-7.

7965. **Warrilow, D., B. Harrower, I. L. Smith, H. Field, R. Taylor, C. Walker, and G. A. Smith.** 2003. Public health surveillance for Australian bat lyssavirus, in Queensland, Australia, 2000-2001. *Emerg Infect Dis* **9**:262-4.

7966. **Warrilow, D., I. L. Smith, B. Harrower, and G. A. Smith.** 2002. Sequence analysis of an isolate from a fatal human infection of Australian bat lyssavirus. *Virology* **297**:109-19.

7967. **Warris, A., C. H. Klaassen, J. F. Meis, M. T. De Ruiter, H. A. De Valk, T. G. Abrahamsen, P. Gaustad, and P. E. Verweij.** 2003. Molecular epidemiology of Aspergillus fumigatus isolates recovered from water, air, and patients shows two clusters of genetically distinct strains. *J Clin Microbiol* **41**:4101-6.

7968. **Watanabe, Y., K. Ozasa, J. H. Mermin, P. M. Griffin, K. Masuda, S. Imashuku, and T. Sawada.** 1999. Factory outbreak of Escherichia coli O157:H7 infection in Japan. *Emerg Infect Dis* **5**:424-8.

7969. **Watanakunakorn, C., and J. Jura.** 1991. Klebsiella bacteremia: a review of 196 episodes during a decade (1980-1989). *Scand J Infect Dis* **23**:399-405.

7970. **Watanakunakorn, C., and S. C. Perni.** 1994. Proteus mirabilis bacteremia: a review of 176 cases during 1980-1992. *Scand J Infect Dis* **26:**361-7.

7971. **Waters, T. D., P. S. Anderson, Jr., G. W. Beebe, and R. W. Miller.** 1972. Yellow fever vaccination, avian leukosis virus, and cancer risk in man. *Science* **177:**76-7.

7972. **Watkin, R. W., N. Baker, S. Lang, and J. Ment.** 2002. Eikenella corrodens infective endocarditis in a previously healthy non-drug user. *Eur J Clin Microbiol Infect Dis* **21:**890-1.

7973. **Watkins, R. E., and A. J. Plant.** 2002. Predicting tuberculosis among migrant groups. *Epidemiol Infect* **129:**623-8.

7974. **Watson, C. R.** 2003. Human infestation with bird mites in Wollongong. *Commun Dis Intell* **27:**259-61.

7975. **Watson-Jones, D., J. Changalucha, B. Gumodoka, H. Weiss, M. Rusizoka, L. Ndeki, A. Whitehouse, R. Balira, J. Todd, D. Ngeleja, D. Ross, A. Buve, R. Hayes, and D. Mabey.** 2002. Syphilis in pregnancy in Tanzania. I. Impact of maternal symphilis on outcome of pregnancy. *J Infect Dis* **186:**940-7.

7976. **Watson-Jones, D. L., P. S. Craig, D. Badamochir, M. T. Rogan, H. Wen, and B. Hind.** 1997. A pilot, serological survey for cystic echinococcosis in north-western Mongolia. *Ann Trop Med Parasitol* **91:**173-7.

7977. **Watt, G., C. Chouriyagune, R. Ruangweerayud, P. Watcharapichat, D. Phulsuksombati, K. Jongsakul, P. Teja-Isavadharm, D. Bhodhidatta, K. D. Corcoran, G. A. Dasch, and D. Strickman.** 1996. Scrub typhus infections poorly responsive to antibiotics in northern Thailand. *Lancet* **348:**86-9.

7978. **Watt, G., K. Jongsakul, and C. Suttinont.** 2003. Possible scrub typhus coinfections in Thai agricultural workers hospitalized with leptospirosis. *Am J Trop Med Hyg* **68:**89-91.

7979. **Watts, C., and C. Zimmerman.** 2002. Violence against women: global scope and magnitude. *Lancet* **359:**1232-7.

7980. **Watts, D. M., J. Callahan, C. Rossi, M. S. Oberste, J. T. Roehrig, M. T. Wooster, J. F. Smith, C. B. Cropp, E. M. Gentrau, N. Karabatsos, D. Gubler, and C. G. Hayes.** 1998. Venezuelan equine encephalitis febrile cases among humans in the Peruvian Amazon river region. *Am J Trop Med Hyg* **58:**35-40.

7981. **Watts, D. M., V. Lavera, J. Callahan, C. Rossi, M. S. Oberste, J. T. Roehrig, C. B. Cropp, N. Karabatsos, J. F. Smith, D. J. Gubler, M. T. Wooster, W. M. Nelson, and C. G. Hayes.** 1997. Venezuelan equine encephalitis and Oropouche virus infections among Peruvian army troops in the Amazon region of Peru. *Am J Trop Med Hyg* **56:**661-7.

7982. **Wawer, M. J., D. Serwadda, S. D. Musgrave, J. K. Konde-Lule, M. Musagara, and N. K. Sewankambo.** 1991. Dynamics of spread of HIV-I infection in a rural district of Uganda. *BMJ* **303:**1303—6.

7983. **Wawer, M. J., N. Sewankambo, D. Serwadda, T. C. Quinn, L. A. Paxton, N. Kiwanuka, F. Wabwire-Mangen, C. Li, T. Lutalo, F. Nalugoda, C. A. Gaydos, L. H. Moulton, M. O. Meehan, S. Ahmed, and R. H. Gray.** 1999. Control of sexually transmitted diseases for AIDS prevention in Uganda: a randomised community trial. *Lancet* **353:**525-35.

7984. **World Bank.** 2004. World development Report 2004. Oxford University Press, Oxford.

7985. **Weaver, S. C., C. Ferro, R. Barrera, J. Boshell, and J. C. Navarro.** 2004. Venezuelan equine encephalitis. *Annu Rev Entomol* **49:**141-74.

7986. **Weaver, S. C., M. Pfeffer, K. Marriott, W. Kang, and R. M. Kinney.** 1999. Genetic evidence for the origins of Venezuelan equine encephalitis virus subtype IAB outbreaks. *Am J Trop Med Hyg* **60:**441-8.

7987. **Webber, J.** 2003. Towards a national surveillance program for antimicrobial resistance in animals and animal-derived food. *Commun Dis Intell* **27 suppl:**S111-6.

7988. **Weber, A. E., K. J. Craib, K. Chan, S. Martindale, M. L. Miller, M. T. Schechter, and R. S. Hogg.** 2001. Sex trade involvement and rates of human immunodeficiency virus positivity among young gay and bisexual men. *Int J Epidemiol* **30:**1449-54; discussion 1455-6.

7989. **Weber, D. J., and A. R. Hansen.** 1991. Infections resulting from animal bites. *Infect Dis Clin N Am* **5:**663-80.

7990. **Weber, D. J., and W. A. Rutala.** 2001. The emerging nosocomial pathogens Cryptosporidium, Escherichia coli O157:H7, Helicobacter pylori, and hepatitis C: epidemiology, environmental survival, efficacy of disinfection, and control measures. *Infect Control Hosp Epidemiol* **22:**306-15.

7991. **Weber, D. J., and W. A. Rutala.** 2001. Lessons from outbreaks associated with bronchoscopy. *Infect Control Hosp Epidemiol* **22:**403-408.

7992. **Weber, G., W. Mohr, K. Fleischer, and P. G. Sargeaunt.** 1990. Entamoeba histolytica infections in flight personnel of an international airline. *Trans R Soc Trop Med Hyg* **84:**803-5.

7993. **Weber, J. T., R. G. Hibbs, Jr., A. Darwish, B. Mishu, A. L. Corwin, M. Rakha, C. L. Hatheway, S. el Sharkawy, S. A. el-Rahim, M. F. al-Hamd, et al.** 1993. A massive outbreak of type E botulism associated with traditional salted fish in Cairo. *J Infect Dis* **167:**451-4.

7994. **Weber, M. W., P. Milligan, M. Sanneh, A. Awemoyi, R. Dakour, G. Schneider, A. Palmer, M. Jallow, A. Oparaogu, H. Whittle, E. K. Mulholland, and B. M. Greenwood.** 2002. An epidemiological study of RSV infection in the Gambia. *Bull WHO* **80:**562-8.

7995. **Webster, G. J., R. Hallett, S. A. Whalley, M. Meltzer, K. Balogun, D. Brown, C. P. Farrington, S. Sharma, G. Hamilton, S. C. Farrow, M. E. Ramsay, C. G. Teo, and G. M. Dusheiko.** 2000. Molecular epidemiology of a large outbreak of hepatitis B linked to autohaemotherapy. *Lancet* **356:**379-84.

7996. **Webster, R. G.** 2004. Wet markets - a continuing source of severe acute respiratory syndrome or influenza? *Lancet* **363:**234-6.

7997. **Weems, J. J., Jr.** 1993. Nosocomial outbreak of Pseudomonas cepacia associated with contamination of reusable electronic ventilator temperature probes. *Infect Control Hosp Epidemiol* **14:**583-6.

7998. **Weems, J. J., Jr.** 2001. The many faces of Staphylococcus aureus infection. Recognizing and managing its life-threatening manifestations. *Postgrad Med* **110:**24-6, 29-31, 35-6.

7999. **Weerasooriya, M. V., M. Itoh, M. P. Mudalige, X. G. Qiu, E. Kimura, N. K. Gunawardena, and Y. Fujimaki.** 2003. Human infection with Wuchereria bancrofti in Matara, Sri Lanka: the use, in parallel, of an ELISA to detect filaria-specific IgG4 in urine and of ICT card tests to detect filarial antigen in whole blood. *Ann Trop Med Parasitol* **97:**179-85.

8000. **Weese, J. S., M. Archambault, B. M. Willey, P. Hearn, B. N. Kreiswirth, B. Said-Salim, A. McGeer, Y. Likhoshvay, J. F. Prescott, and D. E. Low.** 2005. Methicillin-resistant Staphylococcus aureus in horses and horse personnel, 2000-2002. *Emerg Infect Dis* **11:**430-5.

8001. **Wegener, H. C., T. Hald, D. L. F. Wong, M. Madsen, H. Korsgaard, F. Bager, P. Gerner-Smidt, and K. Molbak.** 2003. Salmonella control programs in Denmark. *Emerg Infect Dis* **9**:774–780.

8002. **Wehner, H., R. Morris, M. Logan, D. Hunt, L. Jin, J. Stuart, and K. Cartwright.** 2000. A secondary school outbreak of mumps following the childhood immunization programme in England and Wales. *Epidemiol Infect* **124**:131-6.

8003. **Wehrle, P. F., J. Posch, K. H. Richter, and D. A. Henderson.** 1970. An airborne outbreak of smallpox in a German hospital and its significance with respect to other recent outbreaks in Europe. *Bull WHO* **43**:669-79.

8004. **Wei, G. Z., C. J. Li, J. M. Meng, and M. C. Ding.** 1988. Cysticercosis of the central nervous system. A clinical study of 1 400 cases. *Chin Med J* **101**:493-500.

8005. **Wei, H. L., and C. S. Chiou.** 2002. Molecular subtyping of Staphylococcus aureus from an outbreak associated with a food handler. *Epidemiol Infect* **128**:15-20.

8006. **Wei, Q., M. Tsuji, A. Zamoto, M. Kohsaki, T. Matsui, T. Shiota, S. R. Telford, 3rd, and C. Ishihara.** 2001. Human babesiosis in Japan: isolation of Babesia microti-like parasites from an asymptomatic transfusion donor and from a rodent from an area where babesiosis is endemic. *J Clin Microbiol* **39**:2178-83.

8007. **Weigl, J. A., W. Puppe, B. Grondahl, and H. J. Schmitt.** 2000. Epidemiological investigation of nine respiratory pathogens in hospitalized children in Germany using multiplex reverse-transcriptase polymerase chain reaction. *Eur J Clin Microbiol Infect Dis* **19**:336-43.

8008. **Weigle, K. A., C. Santrich, F. Martinez, L. Valderrama, and N. G. Saravia.** 1993. Epidemiology of cutaneous leishmaniasis in Colombia: a longitudinal study of the natural history, prevalence, and incidence of infection and clinical manifestations. *J Infect Dis* **168**:699-708.

8009. **Weigle, K. A., C. Santrich, F. Martinez, L. Valderrama, and N. G. Saravia.** 1993. Epidemiology of cutaneous leishmaniasis in Colombia: environmental and behavioral risk factors for infection, clinical manifestations, and pathogenicity. *J Infect Dis* **168**:709-14.

8010. **Weina, P. J., R. C. Neafie, G. Wortmann, M. Polhemus, and N. E. Aronson.** 2004. Old world leishmaniasis: an emerging infection among deployed US military and civilian workers. *Clin Infect Dis* **39**:1674-80.

8011. **Weinbaum, C., R. Lyerla, and H. S. Margolis.** 2003. Prevention and control of infections with hepatitis viruses in correctional settings. *MMWR* **52 (RR-1)**:1-44.

8012. **Weinberg, A., M. R. Zamora, S. Li, F. Torres, and T. N. Hodges.** 2002. The value of polymerase chain reaction for the diagnosis of viral respiratory tract infections in lung transplant recipients. *J Clin Virol* **25**:171-5.

8013. **Weinberg, J. B., and R. A. Blackwood.** 2003. Case report of Staphylococcus aureus endocarditis after naval piercing. *Pediatr Infect Dis J* **22**:94-6.

8014. **Weinberg, M., J. Hopkins, L. Farrington, L. Gresham, M. Ginsberg, and B. P. Bell.** 2004. Hepatitis A in Hispanic children who live along the United States-Mexico border: the role of international travel and food-borne exposures. *Pediatrics* **114**:e68-73.

8015. **Weinberg, M., J. Weeks, S. Lance-Parker, M. Traeger, S. Wiersma, Q. Phan, D. Dennison, P. MacDonald, M. Lindsley, J. Guarner, P. Connolly, M. Cetron, and R. Hajjeh.** 2003. Severe histoplasmosis in travelers to Nicaragua. *Emerg Infect Dis* **9**:1322-5.

8016. **Weinke, T., B. Friedrich-Janicke, P. Hopp, and K. Janitschke.** 1990. Prevalence and clinical importance of Entamoeba histolytica in two high-risk groups: travelers returning from the tropics and male homosexuals. *J Infect Dis* **161**:1029-31.

8017. **Weinstein, M. R., M. Litt, D. A. Kertesz, P. Wyper, D. Rose, M. Coulter, A. McGeer, R. Facklam, C. Ostach, B. M. Willey, A. Borczyk, and D. E. Low.** 1997. Invasive infections due to a fish pathogen, Streptococcus iniae. S. iniae Study Group. *N Engl J Med* **337**:589-94.

8018. **Weinstein, P.** 1991. Summary of occupation-related zoonoses in South Australia, 1986-1990. *Commun Dis Intell* **15**:194.

8019. **Weinstein, R. A.** 1998. Nosocomial infection update. *Emerg Infect Dis* **4**:416-20.

8020. **Weinstock, D. M., and A. E. Brown.** 2002. Rhodococcus equi: an emerging pathogen. *Clin Infect Dis* **34**:1379-85.

8021. **Weis, C. P., A. J. Intrepido, A. K. Miller, P. G. Cowin, M. A. Durno, J. S. Gebhardt, and R. Bull.** 2002. Secondary aerosolization of viable Bacillus anthracis spores in a contaminated US Senate Office. *JAMA* **288**:2853-8.

8022. **Weismann, K.** 1973. [An epidemic of molluscum contagiosum originating in an out-door public swimming-pool. An analysis of 125 consecutive cases]. *Ugeskr Laeger* **135**:2151-6.

8023. **Weiss, B. P., L. Mascola, and S. L. Fannin.** 1988. Public health at the 1984 Summer Olympics: the Los Angeles County experience. *Am J Public Health* **78**:686-8.

8024. **Weiss, C. A., 3rd, C. L. Statz, R. A. Dahms, M. J. Remucal, D. L. Dunn, and G. J. Beilman.** 1999. Six years of surgical wound infection surveillance at a tertiary care center: review of the microbiologic and epidemiological aspects of 20,007 wounds. *Arch Surg* **134**:1041-8.

8025. **Weiss, K., M. Laverdiere, M. Lovgren, J. Delorme, L. Poirier, and C. Beliveau.** 1999. Group A Streptococcus carriage among close contacts of patients with invasive infections. *Am J Epidemiol* **149**:863-8.

8026. **Weiss, K., C. Restieri, R. Gauthier, M. Laverdiere, A. McGeer, R. J. Davidson, L. Kilburn, D. J. Bast, J. de Azavedo, and D. E. Low.** 2001. A nosocomial outbreak of fluoroquinolone-resistant Streptococcus pneumoniae. *Clin Infect Dis* **33**:517-22.

8027. **Weissenbacher, M., D. Rossi, G. Radulich, S. Sosa-Estani, M. Vila, E. Vivas, M. M. Avila, P. Cuchi, J. Rey, and L. M. Peralta.** 2003. High seroprevalence of bloodborne viruses among street-recruited injection drug users from Buenos Aires, Argentina. *Clin Infect Dis* **37 Suppl 5**:S348-52.

8028. **Weissenbacher, M. C., E. Edelmuth, M. J. Frigerio, C. E. Coto, and L. B. de Guerrero.** 1980. Serological survey to detect subclinical Junin virus infection in laboratory personnel. *J Med Virol* **6**:223-6.

8029. **Weissenbacher, M. C., M. S. Sabattini, M. M. Avila, P. M. Sangiorgio, M. R. de Sensi, M. S. Contigiani, S. C. Levis, and J. I. Maiztegui.** 1983. Junin virus activity in two rural populations of the Argentine hemorrhagic fever (AHF) endemic area. *J Med Virol* **12**:273-80.

8030. **Weissmann, C., M. Enari, P. C. Klöhn, D. Rossi, and E. Flechsig.** 2002. Transmission of prions. *J Infect Dis* **186 suppl 2**:S157-65.

8031. **Weithaler, K. L.** 1981. Zur epidemiologischen Problematik des Rift Valley Fiebers. *Mitteilungen der Österreichische Gesellschaft für Tropenmedizin und Parasitologie* **3**:9-16.

8032. Wejda, B. U., H. Huchzermeyer, and A. J. Dormann. 2002. Hotel malariain Greece: Mozambique origin, American vector, German victims. *J Travel Med* **9**:277.

8033. Wejstal, R., A. S. Manson, A. Widell, and G. Norkrans. 1999. Perinatal transmission of hepatitis G virus (GB virus type C) and hepatitis C virus infections—a comparison. *Clin Infect Dis* **28**:816-21.

8034. Welch, D. F., K. C. Carroll, E. K. Hofmeister, D. H. Persing, D. A. Robison, A. G. Steigerwalt, and D. J. Brenner. 1999. Isolation of a new subspecies, Bartonella vinsonii subsp. arupensis, from a cattle rancher: identity with isolates found in conjunction with Borrelia burgdorferi and Babesia microti among naturally infected mice. *J Clin Microbiol* **37**:2598-601.

8035. Weldon, M., M. J. VanEgdom, K. A. Hendricks, G. Regner, B. P. Bell, and L. M. Sehulster. 2000. Prevalence of antibody to hepatitis A virus in drinking water workers and wastewater workers in Texas from 1996 to 1997. *J Occup Environ Med* **42**:821-6.

8036. Wells, D. L., D. J. Hopfensperger, N. H. Arden, M. W. Harmon, J. P. Davis, M. A. Tipple, and L. B. Schonberger. 1991. Swine influenza virus infections. Transmission from ill pigs to humans at a Wisconsin agricultural fair and subsequent probable person-to- person transmission. *JAMA* **265**:478-81.

8037. Wells, E. V., M. Boulton, W. Hall, and S. A. Bidol. 2004. Reptile-associated salmonellosis in preschool-aged children in Michigan, January 2001-June 2003. *Clin Infect Dis* **39**:687-91.

8038. Wells, R. M., S. Sosa Estani, Z. E. Yadon, D. Enria, P. Padula, N. Pini, J. N. Mills, C. J. Peters, and E. L. Segura. 1997. An unusual hantavirus outbreak in southern Argentina: person-to-person transmission? Hantavirus Pulmonary Syndrome Study Group for Patagonia. *Emerg Infect Dis* **3**:171-4.

8039. Wells, S. J., S. L. Ott, and A. Hillberg Seitzinger. 1998. Key health issues for dairy cattle - new and old. *J Dairy Sci* **81**:3029-35.

8040. Weltman, A. C., N. M. Bennett, D. A. Ackman, J. H. Misage, J. J. Campana, L. S. Fine, A. S. Doniger, G. J. Balzano, and G. S. Birkhead. 1996. An outbreak of hepatitis A associated with a bakery, New York, 1994: The 1968 'West Branch, Michigan' outbreak repeated. *Epidemiol Infect* **117**:333-41.

8041. Wen, C. P., S. P. Tsai, Y. T. Shih, and W. S. Chung. 2004. Bridging the gap in life expectancy of the aborigines in Taiwan. *Int J Epidemiol* **33**:320-7.

8042. Wendel, K., and A. Rompalo. 2002. Scabies and pediculosis pubis: an update of treatment regimens and general review. *Clin Infect Dis* **35 suppl 2**:S146-51.

8043. Wendel, K. A., E. J. Erbelding, C. A. Gaydos, and A. M. Rompalo. 2003. Use of urine polymerase chain reaction to define the prevalence and clinical presentation of Trichomonas vaginalis in men attending an STD clinic. *Sex Transm Infect* **79**:151-3.

8044. Wendt, C., B. Wiesenthal, E. Dietz, and H. Ruden. 1998. Survival of vancomycin-resistant and vancomycin-susceptible enterococci on dry surfaces. *J Clin Microbiol* **36**:3734-6.

8045. Wenger, J. D., J. S. Spika, R. W. Smithwick, V. Pryor, D. W. Dodson, G. A. Carden, and K. C. Klontz. 1990. Outbreak of Mycobacterium chelonae infection associated with use of jet injectors. *JAMA* **264**:373-6.

8046. Wenger, P. N., J. M. Brown, M. M. McNeil, and W. R. Jarvis. 1998. Nocardia farcinica sternotomy site infections in patients following open heart surgery. *J Infect Dis* **178**:1539-43.

8047. Wenger, P. N., J. Otten, A. Breeden, D. Orfas, C. M. Beck-Sague, and W. R. Jarvis. 1995. Control of nosocomial transmission of multidrug-resistant Mycobacterium tuberculosis among healthcare workers and HIV-infected patients. *Lancet* **345**:235-40.

8048. Weniger, B. G., M. J. Blaser, J. Gedrose, E. C. Lippy, and D. D. Juranek. 1983. An outbreak of waterborne giardiasis associated with heavy water runoff due to warm weather and volcanic ashfall. *Am J Public Health* **73**:868-72.

8049. Wenz, M., B. Gorissen, and S. Wieshammer. 2001. Morbus Weil mit Knochenmarkbefall nach Walnusssammeln. *Dtsch Med Wochenschr* **126**:1132-1135.

8050. Wenzel, R. P., and M. B. Edmond. 2001. The impact of hospital-acquired bloodstream infections. *Emerg Infect Dis* **7**:174-7.

8051. Wenzel, R. P., and M. B. Edmond. 2003. Managing SARS amidst uncertainty. *N Engl J Med* **348**:1947-8.

8052. Werber, D., J. Dreesman, F. Feil, U. van Treeck, and G. Fell. 2002. International outbreak of Salmonella Oranienburg, October-December 2001, Part 1: Germany. *Eurosurveillance Weekly* **6**:020117.

8053. Werchniak, A. E., O. P. Herfort, T. J. Farrell, K. S. Connolly, and R. D. Baughman. 2003. Milker's nodule in a healthy young woman. *J Am Acad Dermatol* **49**:910-1.

8054. Werner, M., P. Nordin, B. Arnholm, B. Elgefors, and I. Krantz. 2001. Borrelia burgdorferi antibodies in outdoor and indoor workers in southwest Sweden. *Scand J Infect Dis* **33**:128-31.

8055. Werner, S. B., D. Pappagianis, I. Heindl, and A. Mickel. 1972. An epidemic of coccidioidomycosis among archeology students in northern California. *N Engl J Med* **286**:507-12.

8056. Werner, S. B., D. Passaro, J. McGee, R. Schechter, and D. J. Vugia. 2000. Wound botulism in California, 1951-1998: recent epidemic in heroin injectors. *Clin Infect Dis* **31**:1018-24.

8057. West, N. S., and F. A. Riordan. 2003. Fever in returned travellers: a prospective review of hospital admissions for a 2(1/2) year period. *Arch Dis Child* **88**:432-4.

8058. West, T. E., J. J. Walshe, C. P. Krol, and D. Amsterdam. 1986. Staphylococcal peritonitis in patients on continuous peritoneal dialysis. *J Clin Microbiol* **23**:809-12.

8059. Westerhuis, J. B., and T. G. Mank. 2002. [Intestinal parasites in African asylum seekers: prevalence and risk factors]. *Ned Tijdschr Geneeskd* **146**:1497-501.

8060. Wetterhall, S. F., D. M. Coulombier, J. M. Herndon, S. Zaza, and J. D. Cantwell. 1998. Medical care delivery at the 1996 Olympic Games. Centers for Disease Control and Prevention Olympics Surveillance Unit. *JAMA* **279**:1463-8.

8061. Wharton, M. 1996. The epidemiology of varicella-zoster virus infections. *Infect Dis Clin North Am* **10**:571-81.

8062. Wharton, M., S. L. Cochi, R. H. Hutcheson, J. M. Bistowish, and W. Schaffner. 1988. A large outbreak of mumps in the postvaccine era. *J Infect Dis* **158**:1253-60.

8063. Wharton, M., S. L. Cochi, R. H. Hutcheson, and W. Schaffner. 1990. Mumps transmission in hospitals. *Arch Intern Med* **150**:47-9.

8064. Wharton, M., R. A. Spiegel, J. M. Horan, R. V. Tauxe, J. G. Wells, N. Barg, J. Herndon, R. A. Meriwether, J. N. MacCormack, and R. H. Levine. 1990. A large outbreak of antibiotic-resistant shigellosis at a mass gathering. *J Infect Dis* **162**:1324-8.

8065. Wheat, L. J. 1992. Histoplasmosis in Indianapolis. *Clin Infect Dis* **14 Suppl 1**:S91-9.

8066. Wheat, L. J., T. G. Slama, H. E. Eitzen, R. B. Kohler, M. L. French, and J. L. Biesecker. 1981. A large urban outbreak of histoplasmosis: clinical features. *Ann Intern Med* **94:**331-7.

8067. Wheeler, J. G., D. Sethi, J. M. Cowden, P. G. Wall, L. C. Rodrigues, D. S. Tompkins, M. J. Hudson, and P. J. Roderick. 1999. Study of infectious intestinal disease in England: rates in the community, presenting to general practice, and reported to national surveillance. The Infectious Intestinal Disease Study Executive. *BMJ* **318:**1046-50.

8068. Wheeler, S. M., and A. R. Morton. 1942. Epidemiologic observations in the Halifax epidemic. *Am J Public Health* **32:**947-56.

8069. Whelan, E. A., C. C. Lawson, B. Grajewski, M. R. Petersen, L. E. Pinkerton, E. M. Ward, and T. M. Schnorr. 2003. Prevalence of respiratory symptoms among female flight attendants and teachers. *Occup Environ Med* **60:**929-34.

8070. Whiley, R. A., and D. Beighton. 1998. Current classification of the oral streptococci. *Oral Microbiol Immunol* **13:**195-216.

8071. White, A. C., and A. Blum. 1994. Taenia Saginata Tapeworm Infection in a Traveler to Mexico. *J Travel Med* **1:**168.

8072. White, J. M., R. D. Barker, J. R. Salisbury, A. J. Fife, S. B. Lucas, D. C. Warhurst, and E. M. Higgins. 2004. Granulomatous amoebic encephalitis. *Lancet* **364:**220.

8073. White Jr, A. C., and R. L. Atmar. 2002. Infections in Hispanic immigrants. *Clin Infect Dis* **34:**1627-32.

8074. White, K. E., C. W. Hedberg, L. M. Edmonson, D. B. Jones, M. T. Osterholm, and K. L. MacDonald. 1989. An outbreak of giardiasis in a nursing home with evidence for multiple modes of transmission. *J Infect Dis* **160:**298-304.

8075. Whitehouse, C. A. 2004. Crimean-Congo hemorrhagic fever. *Antiviral Res* **64:**145-60.

8076. Whitley, R. J. 1995. Herpes simplex virus infections in women and their offspring: implications for a developed society, p. 171-189. *In* B. Roizman (ed.), Infectious diseases in an age of change. The impact of human ecology and behavior on disease transmission. National Academy Press, Washington, D.C.

8077. Whitlock, G., L. Calder, and H. Perry. 2001. A case of infectious tuberculosis on two long-haul aircraft flights: contact investigation. *N Z Med J* **114:**353-5.

8078. Whitney, C. G., and L. K. Pickering. 2002. The potential of pneumococcal conjugate vaccines for children. *Pediatr Infect Dis J* **21:**961-70.

8079. Whittaker, S., T. F. Jackson, V. Gathiram, and L. D. Regensberg. 1994. Control of an amoebiasis outbreak in the Philippi area near Cape Town. *S Afr Med J* **84:**389-93.

8080. Whittington, R. J., and E. S. Sergeant. 2001. Progress towards understanding the spread, detection and control of Mycobacterium avium subsp paratuberculosis in animal populations. *Aust Vet J* **79:**267-78.

8081. Whitty, C. J., B. Carroll, M. Armstrong, C. Dow, D. Snashall, T. Marshall, and P. L. Chiodini. 2000. Utility of history, examination and laboratory tests in screening those returning to Europe from the tropics for parasitic infection. *Trop Med Int Health* **5:**818-23.

8082. Whitty, C. J. M., D. C. Mabey, M. Armstrong, S. G. Wright, and P. L. Chiodini. 2000. Presentation and outcome of 1107 cases of schistosomiasis from Africa diagnosed in a non-endemic country. *Trans R Soc Trop Med Hyg* **94:**531-4.

8083. WHO. 1985. Yellow fever in Presidente Prudente, São Paulo. *WER* **60:**359.

8084. WHO. 1986. WHO expert committee on venereal diseases and treponematoses. *WHO Technical Report Series* **736:**1-141.

8085. WHO. 1991. Cholera in Africa. Summary background: the initial epidemic (1970-1971). *WER* **66:**305-11.

8086. WHO. 1994. Epidemic typhus risk in Rwandan refugee camps. *WER* **69:**259.

8087. WHO. 1995. Onchocerciasis and its control. *WHO Technical Report Series* **852:**1-103.

8088. WHO. 1996. Cholera outbreaks. Ineffective control measures. *WER* **71**.

8089. WHO. 1997. A large outbreak of epidemic louse-borne typhus in Burundi. *WER* **72:**152-3.

8090. WHO. 1998. Control and surveillance of African trypanosomiasis. *WHO Technical Report Series* **881:**1-113.

8091. WHO. 1999. Leptospirosis worldwide. *WER* **74:**237-42.

8092. WHO. 1999. New frontiers in the development of vaccines against enterotoxinogenic (ETEC) and enterohaemorrhagic (EHEC) E. coli infections. Part I. *WER* **74:**98-101.

8093. WHO. 2000. Human plague in 1998 and 1999. *WER* **75:**338-43.

8094. WHO. 2000. Legionnaires' disease, Europe, 1999. *WER* **75:**347-52.

8095. WHO. 2000. Leptospirosis, India. Report of the investigation of a post-cyclone outbreak in Orissa, November 1999. *WER* **75:**217-23.

8096. WHO. 2000. Rubella vaccines. WHO position paper. *WER* **75:**161-169.

8097. WHO. 2001. Mumps virus vaccines. *WER* **76:**346-355.

8098. WHO. 2001. Outbreak of Ebola haemorrhagic fever, Uganda, August 2000-January 2001. *WER* **76:**41-6.

8099. WHO. 2002. Control of Chagas disease. *WHO Technical Report Series* **905:**1-109.

8100. WHO. 2002. Dengue prevention and control. *WER* **77:**41-8.

8101. WHO. 2002. Limited measles outbreak, Tunisia, 2002. *WER* **77:**341-4.

8102. WHO. 2002. Onchocerciasis (river blindness). *WER* **77:**249-53.

8103. WHO. 2002. Prevention and control of schistosomiasis and soil-transmitted helminthiasis. Report of a WHO expert committee. *WHO Technical Report Series* **912:**1-57.

8104. WHO. 2002. Rabies vaccines. WHO position paper. *WER* **77:**109-19.

8105. WHO. 2002. Urbanization: an increasing risk factor for leishmaniasis. *WER* **77:**365-70.

8106. WHO. 2002. World survey of rabies no 35 for the year 1999. *WHO unpubl doc* **WHO/CDS/CSR/EPH/2002.10:**1-25.

8107. WHO. 2003. Buruli ulcer disease. Mycobacterium ulcerans infection. *WER* **78:**163-8.

8108. WHO. 2003. Global situation of the HIV/AIDS pandemic, end 2003. *WER* **78:**417-24.

8109. WHO. 2003. Human plague in 2000 and 2001. *WER* **78:**130-5.

8110. WHO. 2003. Outbreak(s) of Ebola haemorrhagic fever, Congo and Gabon, October 2001-July 2002. *WER* **78:**223-8.

8111. WHO. 2003. Summary table of SARS cases by country, 1 November 2002-7 August 2003. *WER* **78:**310-1.

8112. **WHO.** 2003. Yellow fever vaccine. *WER* **78**:349-59.

8113. **WHO.** 2004. Avian influenza (A(H5N1) in humans and poultry, Viet Nam. *WER* **79**:13-4.

8114. **WHO.** 2004. Cholera, 2003. *WER* **79**:281-8.

8115. **WHO.** 2004. Ebola haemorrhagic fever—fact sheet revised in May 2004. *WER* **79**:435-9.

8116. **WHO.** 2004. Global tuberculosis control. Surveillance, planning, financing. WHO, Geneva.

8117. **WHO.** 2004. Guidelines for drinking-water quality. Third edition. Volume 1 recommendations, vol. 1. WHO, Geneva.

8118. **WHO.** 2004. Human plague in 2002 and 2003. *WER* **79**:301-6.

8119. **WHO.** 2004. Measles vaccines. WHO position paper. *WER* **79**:130-42.

8120. **WHO.** 2004. Progress in reducing global measles deaths: 1999-2002. *WER* **79**:20-1.

8121. **WHO.** 2004. Wild poliovirus importations in west and central Africa, January 2003 - March 2004. *WER* **79**:206-10.

8122. **WHO.** 2005. Dracunculus eradication. Global surveillance summary, 2004. *WER* **80**:165-76.

8123. **WHO.** 2005. Global leprosy situation, 2004. *WER* **80**:118-24.

8124. **WHO.** 2005. Global programme to eliminate lymphatic filariasis. Progress report for 2004. *WER* **80**:202-12.

8125. **WHO.** 2005. Marburg haemorrhagic fever, Angola. *WER* **80**:158-9.

8126. **WHO.** 2005. A new form of human trypanosomiasis in India. Description of the first human case in the world caused by Trypanosoma evansi. *WER* **80**:62-3.

8127. **WHO.** 2005. Outbreak of Ebola haemorrhagic fever in Yambio, south Sudan, April - June 2004. *WER* **80**:370-5.

8128. **WHO.** 2005. Rapid health response, assessment and surveillance after a tsunami, Thailand, 2004-2005. *WER* **80**:55-60.

8129. **WHO.** 2005. Shigellosis: disease burden, epidemiology and case management. *Wkly Epidemiol Rec* **80**:94-9.

8130. **WHO.** 2005. Travel by air: health considerations. *WER* **80**:181-91.

8131. **WHO.** 2005. Update on Lassa fever in West Africa. *WER* **80**:86-8.

8132. **WHO.** 2005. WHO consultation on human papillomavirus vaccines. *WER* **80**:299-302.

8133. **WHO.** 1974. Human anthrax. *WER* **49**:301.

8134. **WHO.** 1984. WHO expert committee on rabies. Seventh report. *WHO Technical Report Series* **709**:1-104.

8135. **WHO.** 1986. Joint FAO/WHO expert committee on brucellosis. *WHO Technical Report Series* **740**:1-132.

8136. **WHO.** 1986. La fièvre jaune aujourd'hui: Mémorandum d'une réunion de l'OPS. *Bull WHO* **64**:821-36.

8137. **WHO.** 1989. Human plague in 1988. *WER* **64**:345-7.

8138. **WHO.** 1996. Crimean-Congo haemorrhagic fever. South Africa. *WER* **71**:381-382.

8139. **WHO.** 1996. Vaccine supply and quality. *WER* **71**:237-242.

8140. **WHO.** 1997. Guidelines for the safe transport of infectious substances and diagnostic specimens, Unpubl doc, Geneva.

8141. **WHO.** 1998. Reverse transcriptase activity in chicken-cell derived vaccine. *WER* **73**:209-216.

8142. **WHO.** 1999. Vibrio parahaemolyticus, Japan, 1996-1998. *WER* **74**:361-3.

8143. **WHO.** 2001. Global prevalence and incidence of selected curable sexually transmitted infections. Overview and estimates. *Unpublished document WHO/CDS/CSR/EDI/2001.10.*

8144. **WHO.** 2003. Pertussis in Bulgaria, 1952-2001: 50 years of surveillance. *WER* **78**:203-7.

8145. **Wibawa, I. D., D. H. Muljono, Mulyanto, I. G. Suryadarma, F. Tsuda, M. Takahashi, T. Nishizawa, and H. Okamoto.** 2004. Prevalence of antibodies to hepatitis E virus among apparently healthy humans and pigs in Bali, Indonesia: Identification of a pig infected with a genotype 4 hepatitis E virus. *J Med Virol* **73**:38-44.

8146. **Wick, R. L., Jr., and L. A. Irvine.** 1995. The microbiological composition of airliner cabin air. *Aviat Space Environ Med* **66**:220-4.

8147. **Wicki, R., P. Sauter, C. Mettler, A. Natsch, T. Enzler, N. Pusterla, P. Kuhnert, G. Egli, M. Bernasconi, R. Lienhard, H. Lutz, and C. M. Leutenegger.** 2000. Swiss Army Survey in Switzerland to determine the prevalence of Francisella tularensis, members of the Ehrlichia phagocytophila genogroup, Borrelia burgdorferi sensu lato, and tick-borne encephalitis virus in ticks. *Eur J Clin Microbiol Infect Dis* **19**:427-32.

8148. **Widdowson, M. A., R. Glass, S. Monroe, R. S. Beard, J. W. Bateman, P. Lurie, and C. Johnson.** 2005. Probable transmission of norovirus on an airplane. *JAMA* **293**:1859-60.

8149. **Widdowson, M. A., G. J. Morales, S. Chaves, and J. McGrane.** 2002. Epidemiology of urban canine rabies, Santa Cruz, Bolivia, 1972-1997. *Emerg Infect Dis* **8**:458-61.

8150. **Widdowson, M. A., A. Sulka, S. N. Bulens, R. S. Beard, S. S. Chaves, R. Hammond, E. D. Salehi, E. Swanson, J. Totaro, R. Woron, P. S. Mead, J. S. Bresee, S. S. Monroe, and R. I. Glass.** 2005. Norovirus and foodborne disease, United States, 1991-2000. *Emerg Infect Dis* **11**:95-102.

8151. **Widdowson, M. A., G. J. van Doornum, W. H. van der Poel, A. S. de Boer, U. Mahdi, and M. Koopmans.** 2000. Emerging group-A rotavirus and a nosocomial outbreak of diarrhoea. *Lancet* **356**:1161-2.

8152. **Widjana, D. P., and P. Sutisna.** 2000. Prevalence of soil-transmitted helminth infections in the rural population of Bali, Indonesia. *Southeast Asian J Trop Med Public Health* **31**:454-9.

8153. **Widmer, A. F.** 2001. New developments in diagnosis and treatment of infection in orthopedic implants. *Clin Infect Dis* **33 suppl 2**:S94-S106.

8154. **Wiener, J., J. P. Quinn, P. A. Bradford, R. V. Goering, C. Nathan, K. Bush, and R. A. Weinstein.** 1999. Multiple antibiotic-resistant Klebsiella and Escherichia coli in nursing homes. *JAMA* **281**:517-23.

8155. **Wientjens, D. P., B. Rikken, J. M. Wit, A. Hofman, and B. H. Stricker.** 2000. A nationwide cohort study on Creutzfeldt-Jakob disease among human growth hormone recipients. *Neuroepidemiology* **19**:201-5.

8156. **Wiese, M., K. Grungreiff, W. Guthoff, M. Lafrenz, U. Oesen, and H. Porst.** 2005. Outcome in a hepatitis C (genotype 1b) single source outbreak in Germany—a 25-year multicenter study. *J Hepatol* **43**:590-8.

8157. **Wiesli, P., M. Flepp, and P. Greminger.** 1997. Fieber und trockener Husten bei einem Bauarbeiter aus Portugal. *Schweiz Rundsch Med Prax* **86**:1215-9.

8158. **Wijnands, S.** 2000. Public health management of fatal case of Lassa fever in the Netherlands. *Eurosurveillance Weekly* **31**:1-2.

8159. Wilde, H., J. Pornsilapatip, T. Sokly, and S. Thee. 1991. Murine and scrub typhus at Thai-Kampuchean border displaced persons camps. *Trop Geogr Med* **43**:363-9.

8160. Wilde, J. A., J. A. McMillan, J. Serwint, J. Butta, M. A. O'Riordan, and M. C. Steinhoff. 1999. Effectiveness of influenza vaccine in health care professionals: a randomized trial. *JAMA* **281**:908-13.

8161. Wilder-Smith, A., A. Earnest, S. Ravindran, and N. I. Paton. 2003. High incidence of pertussis among Hajj pilgrims. *Clin Infect Dis* **37**:1270-2.

8162. Wilder-Smith, A., K. T. Goh, T. Barkham, and N. I. Paton. 2003. Hajj-associated outbreak strain of Neisseria meningitidis serogroup W135: estimates of the attack rate in a defined population and the risk of invasive disease developing in carriers. *Clin Infect Dis* **36**:679-83.

8163. Wilder-Smith, A., N. S. Khairullah, J. H. Song, C. Y. Chen, and J. Torresi. 2004. Travel health knowledge, attitudes and practices among Australasian travelers. *J Travel Med* **11**:9-15.

8164. Wilder-Smith, A., N. I. Paton, and K. T. Goh. 2003. Experience of severe acute respiratory syndrome in Singapore: importation of cases, and defense strategies at the airport. *J Travel Med* **10**:259-62.

8165. Wilder-Smith, A., N. I. Paton, and K. T. Goh. 2003. Low risk of transmission of severe acute respiratory syndrome on airplanes: the Singapore experience. *Trop Med Int Health* **8**:1035-7.

8166. Wiley, D. J., J. Douglas, K. Beutner, T. Cox, K. Fife, A. B. Moscicki, and L. Fukumoto. 2002. External genital warts: diagnosis, treatment, and prevention. *Clin Infect Dis* **35 suppl 2**:S210-24.

8167. Wilfert, C. M., J. N. MacCormack, K. Kleeman, R. N. Philip, E. Austin, V. Dickinson, and L. H. Turner. 1984. Epidemiology of Rocky Mountain spotted fever as determined by active surveillance. *J Infect Dis* **150**:469-79.

8168. Wilhelmi, I., J. C. Bernaldo de Quiros, J. Romero-Vivas, J. Duarte, E. Rojo, and E. Bouza. 1987. Epidemic outbreak of Serratia marcescens infection in a cardiac surgery unit. *J Clin Microbiol* **25**:1298-300.

8169. Wilkins, C. A., M. B. Richter, W. B. Hobbs, M. Whitcomb, N. Bergh, and J. Carstens. 1988. Occurrence of Clostridium tetani in soil and horses. *S Afr Med J* **73**:718-20.

8170. Wilkins, E. 1993. Tres difficile. *J Infect* **26**:1-7.

8171. Wilkins, E., A. Cope, and S. Waitkins. 1988. Rapids, rafts, and rats. *Lancet* **2 (July 30)**:283-4.

8172. Wilkins, J. R., 3rd, and M. E. Bowman. 1997. Needlestick injuries among female veterinarians: frequency, syringe contents and side-effects. *Occup Med (Lond)* **47**:451-7.

8173. Wilkins, M. J., S. A. Bidol, M. L. Boulton, M. G. Stobierski, J. P. Massey, and B. Robinson-Dunn. 2002. Human salmonellosis associated with young poultry from a contaminated hatchery in Michigan and the resulting public health interventions, 1999 and 2000. *Epidemiol Infect* **129**:19-27.

8174. Wilkinson, D., S. S. Abdool Karim, A. Harrison, M. Lurie, M. Colvin, C. Connolly, and A. W. Sturm. 1999. Unrecognized sexually transmitted infections in rural South African women: a hidden epidemic. *Bull WHO* **77**:22-8.

8175. Wilkinson, F. H., and K. G. Kerr. 1998. Bottled water as a source of multi-resistant Stenotrophomonas and Pseudomonas species for neutropenic patients. *Eur J Cancer Care (Engl)* **7**:12-4.

8176. Will, R. G., J. W. Ironside, M. Zeidler, S. N. Cousens, K. Estibeiro, A. Alperovitch, S. Poser, M. Pocchiari, A. Hofman, and P. G. Smith. 1996. A new variant of Creutzfeldt-Jakob disease in the U.K. *Lancet* **347**:921-925.

8177. Will, R. G., and W. B. Matthews. 1982. Evidence for case-to-case transmission of Creutzfeldt-Jakob disease. *J Neurol Neurosurg Psychiatry* **45**:235-8.

8178. Willems, R. J., W. Homan, J. Top, M. van Santen-Verheuvel, D. Tribe, X. Manzioros, C. Gaillard, C. M. Vandenbroucke-Grauls, E. M. Mascini, E. van Kregten, J. D. van Embden, and M. J. Bonten. 2001. Variant esp gene as a marker of a distinct genetic lineage of vancomycin-resistant Enterococcus faecium spreading in hospitals. *Lancet* **357**:853-5.

8179. Williams, B. G., D. Taljaard, C. M. Campbell, E. Gouws, L. Ndhlovu, J. Van Dam, M. Carael, and B. Auvert. 2003. Changing patterns of knowledge, reported behaviour and sexually transmitted infections in a South African gold mining community. *AIDS* **17**:2099-107.

8180. Williams, C. L. 1999. Helicobacter pylori and endoscopy. *J Hosp Infect* **41**:263-8.

8181. Williams, D. R., G. B. Rees, and M. E. Rogers. 1992. Observations on an outbreak of anthrax in pigs in north Wales. *Vet Rec* **131**:363-6.

8182. Williams, E. S., and M. W. Miller. 2003. Transmissible spongiform encephalopathies in non-domestic animals: origin, transmission and risk factors. *Rev Sci Tech* **22**:145-56.

8183. Williams, J., G. Tallis, C. Dalton, S. Ng, M. Beaton, M. Catton, J. Elliott, and J. Carnie. 1998. Community outbreak of psittacosis in a rural Australian town. *Lancet* **351**:1697-99.

8184. Williams, J. L., B. T. Innis, T. R. Burkot, D. E. Hayes, and I. Schneider. 1983. Falciparum malaria: accidental transmission to man by mosquitoes after infection with culture-derived gametocytes. *Am J Trop Med Hyg* **32**:657-9.

8185. Williams, J. V., P. A. Harris, S. J. Tollefson, L. L. Halburnt-Rush, J. M. Pingsterhaus, K. M. Edwards, P. F. Wright, and J. E. Crowe, Jr. 2004. Human metapneumovirus and lower respiratory tract disease in otherwise healthy infants and children. *N Engl J Med* **350**:443-50.

8186. Williams, L. K., A. Reichert, W. R. MacKenzie, A. W. Hightower, and P. A. Blake. 2001. Lice, nits, and school policy. *Pediatrics* **107**:1011-5.

8187. Williams, P. B., and O. Ekundayo. 2001. Study of distribution and factors affecting syphilis epidemic among inner-city minorities of Baltimore. *Public Health* **115**:387-93.

8188. Williams, R. C., S. Isaacs, M. L. Decou, E. A. Richardson, M. C. Buffett, R. W. Slinger, M. H. Brodsky, B. W. Ciebin, A. Ellis, and J. Hockin. 2000. Illness outbreak associated with Escherichia coli O157:H7 in Genoa salami. E. coli O157:H7 Working Group. *CMAJ* **162**:1409-13.

8189. Williams, R. J., S. Al-Busaidy, F. R. Mehta, G. O. Maupin, K. D. Wagoner, S. Al-Awaidy, A. J. Suleiman, A. S. Khan, C. J. Peters, and T. G. Ksiazek. 2000. Crimean-congo haemorrhagic fever: a seroepidemiological and tick survey in the Sultanate of Oman. *Trop Med Int Health* **5**:99-106.

8190. Williams, R. J., R. T. Bryan, J. N. Mills, R. E. Palma, I. Vera, F. De Velasquez, E. Baez, W. E. Schmidt, R. E. Figueroa, C. J. Peters, S. R. Zaki, A. S. Khan, and T. G. Ksiazek. 1997. An outbreak of hantavirus pulmonary syndrome in western Paraguay. *Am J Trop Med Hyg* **57**:274-82.

8191. Williams-Blangero, S., J. Subedi, R. P. Upadhayay, D. B. Manral, D. R. Rai, B. Jha, E. S. Robinson, and J. Blangero.

1999. Genetic analysis of susceptibility to infection with Ascaris lumbricoides. *Am J Trop Med Hyg* **60:**921-6.

8192. **Willingham, A. L., 3rd, N. V. De, N. Q. Doanh, D. Cong le, T. V. Dung, P. Dorny, P. D. Cam, and A. Dalsgaard.** 2003. Current status of cysticercosis in Vietnam. *Southeast Asian J Trop Med Public Health* **34 Suppl 1:**35-50.

8193. **Willingham, F. F., T. L. Schmitz, M. Contreras, S. E. Kalangi, A. M. Vivar, L. Caviedes, E. Schiantarelli, P. M. Neumann, C. Bern, and R. H. Gilman.** 2001. Hospital control and multidrug-resistant pulmonary tuberculosis in female patients, Lima, Peru. *Emerg Infect Dis* **7:**123-7.

8194. **Willis, B. M., and B. S. Levy.** 2002. Child prostitution: global health burden, research needs, and interventions. *Lancet* **359:**1417-22.

8195. **Willshaw, G. A., T. Cheasty, B. Rowe, H. R. Smith, D. N. Faithfull-Davies, and T. G. Brooks.** 1995. Isolation of enterotoxigenic Escherichia coli from British troops in Saudi Arabia. *Epidemiol Infect* **115:**455-63.

8196. **Wilson, A. P.** 1995. The return of Corynebacterium diphtheriae: the rise of non-toxigenic strains. *J Hosp Infect* **30 Suppl:**306-12.

8197. **Wilson, A. P., C. Gibbons, B. C. Reeves, B. Hodgson, M. Liu, D. Plummer, Z. H. Krukowski, J. Bruce, J. Wilson, and A. Pearson.** 2004. Surgical wound infection as a performance indicator: agreement of common definitions of wound infection in 4773 patients. *BMJ* **329:**720.

8198. **Wilson, C. B., J. S. Remington, S. Stagno, and D. W. Reynolds.** 1980. Development of adverse sequelae in children born with subclinical congenital Toxoplasma infection. *Pediatrics* **66:**767-74.

8199. **Wilson, I. G.** 1996. Occurrence of Listeria species in prepacked retail sandwiches. *Epidemiol Infect* **117:**89-93.

8200. **Wilson, I. G.** 2002. Salmonella and campylobacter contaminaton of raw retail chickens from different producers: a six year survey. *Epidemiol Infect* **129:**635-45.

8201. **Wilson, I. G., and J. E. Moore.** 1996. Presence of Salmonella spp. and Campylobacter spp. in shellfish. *Epidemiol Infect* **116:**147-53.

8202. **Wilson, J. B., R. C. Clarke, S. A. Renwick, K. Rahn, R. P. Johnson, M. A. Karmali, H. Lior, D. Alves, C. L. Gyles, K. S. Sandhu, S. A. McEwen, and J. S. Spika.** 1996. Vero cytotoxigenic Escherichia coli infection in dairy farm families. *J Infect Dis* **174:**1021-7.

8203. **Wilson, K., C. Code, and M. N. Ricketts.** 2000. Risk of acquiring Creutzfeldt-Jakob disease from blood transfusions: systematic review of case-control studies. *BMJ* **321:**17-9.

8204. **Wilson, K., and M. N. Ricketts.** 2004. Transfusion transmission of vCJD: a crisis avoided? *Lancet* **364:**477-9.

8205. **Wilson, L. A., R. L. Schlitzer, and D. G. Ahearn.** 1981. Pseudomonas corneal ulcers associated with soft contact-lens wear. *Am J Ophthalmol* **92:**546-54.

8206. **Wilson, M. D., R. A. Cheke, S. P. Flasse, S. Grist, M. Y. Osei-Ateweneboana, A. Tetteh-Kumah, G. K. Fiasorgbor, F. R. Jolliffe, D. A. Boakye, J. M. Hougard, L. Yameogo, and R. J. Post.** 2002. Deforestation and the spatio-temporal distribution of savannah and forest members of the Simulium damnosum complex in southern Ghana and south-western Togo. *Trans R Soc Trop Med Hyg* **96:**632-9.

8207. **Wilson, M. E.** 2003. The traveller and emerging infections: sentinel, courier, transmitter. *J Appl Microbiol* **94 Suppl:**1S-11S.

8208. **Wilson, M. L.** 1994. Rift valley fever virus ecology and the epidemiology of disease emergence. *Ann N Y Acad Sci* **740:**169-80.

8209. **Wilson, M. L., L. E. Chapman, D. B. Hall, E. A. Dykstra, K. Ba, H. G. Zeller, M. Traore-Lamizana, J. P. Hervy, K. J. Linthicum, and C. J. Peters.** 1994. Rift valley fever in rural northern Senegal: human risk factors and potential vectors. *Am J Trop Med Hyg* **50:**663-75.

8210. **Wilson, M. L., and L. Gaido.** 2004. Laboratory diagnosis of urinary tract infections in adult patients. *Clin Infect Dis* **38:**1150-8.

8211. **Wilson, N., M. Baker, D. Martin, D. Lennon, J. O'Hallahan, N. Jones, J. Wenger, O. Mansoor, M. Thomas, and C. Jefferies.** 1995. Meningococcal disease epidemiology and control in New Zealand. *N Z Med J* **108:**437-42.

8212. **Wilton, D. P., and R. A. Cedillos.** 1978. Domestic triatomines (Reduviidae) and insect trypanosome infections in El Salvador, C.A. *Bull Pan Am Health Organ* **12:**116-23.

8213. **Windiyaningsih, C., H. Wilde, F. X. Meslin, T. Suroso, and H. S. Widarso.** 2004. The rabies epidemic on Flores Island, Indonesia (1998-2003). *J Med Assoc Thai* **87:**1389-93.

8214. **Windrantz, P., and M. L. Arias.** 2000. Evaluation of the bacteriological quality of ice cream sold at San Jose, Costa Rica. *Arch Latinoam Nutr* **50:**301-3.

8215. **Windsor, J. J., and E. H. Johnson.** 1999. Dientamoeba fragilis: the unflagellated human flagellate. *Br J Biomed Sci* **56:**293-306.

8216. **Windsor, J. J., L. Macfarlane, G. Hughes-Thapa, S. K. Jones, and T. M. Whiteside.** 2003. Detection of Dientamoeba fragilis by culture. *Br J Biomed Sci* **60:**79-83.

8217. **Winkler, W. G.** 1968. Airborne rabies virus isolation. *Bull Wildl Dis Assoc* **4:**37-40.

8218. **Winkler, W. G., T. R. Fashinell, L. Leffingwell, P. Howard, and P. Conomy.** 1973. Airborne rabies transmission in a laboratory worker. *JAMA* **226:**1219-21.

8219. **Winner, S. J., R. P. Eglin, V. I. M. Moore, and R. T. Mayon-Wite.** 1987. An outbreak of Q fever affecting postal workers in Oxfordshire. *J Infect* **14:**255-261.

8220. **Winthrop, K. L., M. Abrams, M. Yakrus, I. Schwartz, J. Ely, D. Gillies, and D. J. Vugia.** 2002. An outbreak of mycobacterial furunculosis associated with footbaths at a nail salon. *N Engl J Med* **346:**1366-71.

8221. **Winthrop, K. L., K. Albridge, D. South, P. Albrecht, M. Abrams, M. C. Samuel, W. Leonard, J. Wagner, and D. J. Vugia.** 2004. The clinical management and outcome of nail salon-acquired Mycobacterium fortuitum skin infection. *Clin Infect Dis* **38:**38-44.

8222. **Wirsing von Konig, C. H., S. Halperin, M. Riffelmann, and N. Guiso.** 2002. Pertussis of adults and infants. *Lancet Infect Dis* **2:**744-50.

8223. **Wirsing von Konig, C. H., S. Postels-Multani, H. L. Bock, and H. J. Schmitt.** 1995. Pertussis in adults: frequency of transmission after household exposure. *Lancet* **346:**1326-9.

8224. **Wirtz, A., M. Niedrig, and R. Fock.** 2002. Management of patients with suspected viral haemorrhagic fever and other potentially lethal contagious infections in Germany. *Eurosurveillance* **7:**36-42.

8225. **Wishart, M. M., and T. V. Riley.** 1976. Infection with Pseudomonas maltophilia hospital outbreak due to contaminated disinfectant. *Med J Aust* **2:**710-2.

8226. **Wisniewski, H. M., S. Sigurdarson, R. Rubenstein, R. J. Kascsak, and R. I. Carp.** 1996. Mites as vectors for scrapie. *Lancet* **347:**1114.

8227. **Wisplinghoff, H., T. Bischoff, S. M. Tallent, H. Seifert, R. P. Wenzel, and M. B. Edmond.** 2004. Nosocomial bloodstream infections in US hospitals: analysis of 24,179 cases from a prospective nationwide surveillance study. *Clin Infect Dis* **39:**309-17.

8228. **Wisplinghoff, H., H. Seifert, S. M. Tallent, T. Bischoff, R. P. Wenzel, and M. B. Edmond.** 2003. Nosocomial bloodstream infections in pediatric patients in United States hospitals: epidemiology, clinical features and susceptibilities. *Pediatr Infect Dis J* **22:**686-91.

8229. **Wisplinghoff, H., H. Seifert, R. P. Wenzel, and M. B. Edmond.** 2003. Current trends in the epidemiology of nosocomial bloodstream infections in patients with hematological malignancies and solid neoplasms in hospitals in the United States. *Clin Infect Dis* **36:**1103-10.

8230. **Wistrom, J., S. R. Norrby, E. B. Myhre, S. Eriksson, G. Granstrom, L. Lagergren, G. Englund, C. E. Nord, and B. Svenungsson.** 2001. Frequency of antibiotic-associated diarrhoea in 2462 antibiotic-treated hospitalized patients: a prospective study. *J Antimicrob Chemother* **47:**43-50.

8231. **Witt, C., and E. A. Ottesen.** 2001. Lymphatic filariasis: an infection of childhood. *Trop Med Int Health* **6:**582-606.

8232. **Wittes, R., J. D. MacLean, C. Law, and J. O. Lough.** 1984. Three cases of schistosomiasis mekongi from northern Laos. *Am J Trop Med Hyg* **1984:**1159-65.

8233. **Wittesjö, B., R. Eitrem, B. Niklasson, S. Vene, and J. A. Mangiafico.** 1995. Japanese encephalitis after a 10-day holiday in Bali. *Lancet* **345:**856-7.

8234. **Witthuhn, R. C., S. Engelbrecht, E. Joubert, and T. J. Britz.** 2005. Microbial content of commercial South African high-moisture dried fruits. *J Appl Microbiol* **98:**722-6.

8235. **Wittlinger, F., R. Steffen, H. Watanabe, and H. Handszuh.** 1995. Risk of Cholera Among Western and Japanese Travelers. *J Travel Med* **2:**154-158.

8236. **Wiwanitkit, V., S. Nithiuthai, J. Suwansaksri, C. Chongboonprasert, and K. Tangwattakanont.** 2001. Survival of heterophyid metacercariae in uncooked Thai fish dishes. *Ann Trop Med Parasitol* **95:**725-727.

8237. **Wlodaver, C. G., G. J. Palumbo, and J. L. Waner.** 2004. Laboratory-acquired vaccinia infection. *J Clin Virol* **29:**167-70.

8238. **Woessner, R., B. C. Gaertner, M. T. Grauer, K. Weber, N. Mueller-Lantzsch, K. P. Hunfeld, and J. Treib.** 2001. Incidence and prevalence of infection with human granulocytic ehrlichiosis agent in Germany. A prospective study in young healthy subjects. *Infection* **29:**271-3.

8239. **Wohl, A. R., P. Simon, Y. W. Hu, and J. S. Duchin.** 2002. The role of person-to-person transmission in an epidemiologic study of Pneumocystis carinii pneumonia. *AIDS* **16:**1821-5.

8240. **Wolfe, M. I., F. Xu, P. Patel, M. O'Cain, J. A. Schillinger, M. E. St Louis, and L. Finelli.** 2001. An outbreak of syphilis in Alabama prisons: correctional health policy and communicable disease control. *Am J Public Health* **91:**1220-5.

8241. **Wolfe, M. S., C. U. Tuazon, and R. Schultz.** 1999. Bubonic plague - an imported case (abstract no. 182). *Am J Trop Med Hyg* **61 suppl:**227-8.

8242. **Wolfe, N. D., A. M. Kilbourn, W. B. Karesh, H. A. Rahman, E. J. Bosi, B. C. Cropp, M. Andau, A. Spielman, and D. J. Gubler.** 2001. Sylvatic transmission of arboviruses among Bornean orangutans. *Am J Trop Med Hyg* **64:**310-6.

8243. **Wolfe, N. D., W. M. Switzer, J. K. Carr, V. B. Bhullar, V. Shanmugam, U. Tamoufe, A. T. Prosser, J. N. Torimiro, A. Wright, E. Mpoudi-Ngole, F. E. McCutchan, D. L. Birx, T. M. Folks, D. S. Burke, and W. Heneine.** 2004. Naturally acquired simian retrovirus infections in central African hunters. *Lancet* **363:**932-7.

8244. **Wolff, M.** 1999. [Outbreak of acute histoplasmosis in Chilean travelers to the ecuadorian jungle: an example of geographic medicine]. *Rev Med Chil* **127:**1359-64.

8245. **Wolfs, T. F., J. A. Wagenaar, H. G. Niesters, and A. D. Osterhaus.** 2002. Rat-to-Human Transmission of Cowpox Infection. *Emerg Infect Dis* **8:**1495-6.

8246. **Wolstenholm, J.** 1992. Ross river virus: an Australian export? *Med J Aust* **156:**515-6.

8247. **Woltsche-Kahr, I., B. Schmidt, W. Aberer, and E. Aberer.** 1999. Pinta in Austria (or Cuba?): import of an extinct disease? *Arch Dermatol* **135:**685-8.

8248. **Wong, C., and T. Ng.** 1991. A case report. Cuaneous anthrax - British Columbia. *Can Dis Wkly Rep* **17:**31-33.

8249. **Wong, C. S., S. Jelacic, R. L. Habeeb, S. L. Watkins, and P. I. Tarr.** 2000. The risk of the hemolytic-uremic syndrome after antibiotic treatment of Escherichia coli O157:H7 infections. *N Engl J Med* **342:**1930-6.

8250. **Wong, K. T., and R. Pathmanathan.** 1992. High prevalence of human skeletal muscle sarcocystosis in south-east Asia. *Trans R Soc Trop Med Hyg* **86:**631-2.

8251. **Wong, L. C., B. Amega, C. Connors, R. Barker, M. E. Dulla, A. Ninnal, L. Kolumboort, M. M. Cumaiyi, and B. J. Currie.** 2001. Outcome of an interventional program for scabies in an Indigenous community. *Med J Aust* **175:**367-70.

8252. **Wong, M. S., D. A. Bundy, and M. H. Golden.** 1991. The rate of ingestion of Ascaris lumbricoides and Trichuris trichiura eggs in soil and its relationship to infection in two children's homes in JAMAica. *Trans R Soc Trop Med Hyg* **85:**89-91.

8253. **Wong, T. W., Y. C. Chan, E. H. Yap, Y. G. Joo, H. W. Lee, P. W. Lee, R. Yanagihara, C. J. Gibbs, Jr., and D. C. Gajdusek.** 1988. Serological evidence of hantavirus infection in laboratory rats and personnel. *Int J Epidemiol* **17:**887-90.

8254. **Wongwatcharapaiboon, P., L. Thaikruea, K. Ungchusak, S. Wattanasri, P. Sriprasert, S. Nanthavas, T. Visajsuk, S. Chaiupala, K. Tuntisririwit, S. Leksririvili, and A. Thanawong.** 1999. Foodborne botulism associated with home-canned bamboo shoots - Thailand, 1998. *MMWR* **48:**437-9.

8255. **Woo, P. C., J. H. Li, W. Tang, and K. Yuen.** 2001. Acupuncture mycobacteriosis. *N Engl J Med* **345:**842-3.

8256. **Woo, P. C., A. P. To, H. Tse, S. K. Lau, and K. Y. Yuen.** 2003. Clinical and molecular epidemiology of erythromycin-resistant beta-hemolytic lancefield group G streptococci causing bacteremia. *J Clin Microbiol* **41:**5188-91.

8257. **Wood, B., and M. Rademaker.** 1997. Nosocomial Trichophyton tonsurans in a long stay ward. *N Z Med J* **110:**277-8.

8258. **Wood, R. C., K. L. MacDonald, and M. T. Osterholm.** 1992. Campylobacter enteritis outbreaks associated with drinking raw milk during youth activities. A 10-year review of outbreaks in the United States. *JAMA* **268:**3228-30.

8259. **Woodhouse, S., and P. R. Hunter.** 2001. Risk of invasive meningococcal disease among school workers in Cheshire, United Kingdom. *Clin Infect Dis* **32:**1795-7.

8260. **Woodman, C. B., S. Collins, H. Winter, A. Bailey, J. Ellis, P. Prior, M. Yates, T. P. Rollason, and L. S. Young.** 2001. Natural history of cervical human papillomavirus infection in young women: a longitudinal cohort study. *Lancet* **357:**1831-6.

8261. **Woodruff, A. W., E. T. W. Bowen, and G. S. Platt.** 1978. Viral infections in travellers from tropical Africa. *BMJ* **1:**956-8.

8262. **Woodruff, A. W., D. A. Evans, and N. O. Owino.** 1982. A 'healthy' carrier of African trypanosomiasis. *J Infect* **5:**89-92.

8263. **Woods, C. W., A. M. Karpati, T. Grein, N. McCarthy, P. Gaturuku, E. Muchiri, L. Dunster, A. Henderson, A. S. Khan, R. Swanepoel, I. Bonmarin, L. Martin, P. Mann, B. L. Smoak, M. Ryan, T. G. Ksiazek, R. R. Arthur, A. Ndikuyeze, N. N. Agata, and C. J. Peters.** 2002. An outbreak of Rift Valley fever in northeastern Kenya, 1997-98. *Emerg Infect Dis* **8:**138-44.

8264. **Woods, C. W., K. Ospanov, A. Myrzabekov, M. Favorov, B. Plikaytis, and D. A. Ashford.** 2004. Risk Factors for Human anthrax among contacts of anthrax-infected livestock in Kazakhstan. *Am J Trop Med Hyg* **71:**48-52.

8265. **Woolaway, M. C., C. L. Bartlett, A. A. Wieneke, R. J. Gilbert, H. C. Murrell, and P. Aureli.** 1986. International outbreak of staphylococcal food poisoning caused by contaminated lasagne. *J Hyg (Lond)* **96:**67-73.

8266. **Work, K.** 1967. Isolation of Toxoplasma gondii from the flesh of sheep, swine and cattle. *Acta Pathol Microbiol Scand* **71:**296-306.

8267. **Workneh, W., M. Fletcher, and G. Olwit.** 1993. Onchocerciasis in field workers at Baya Farm, Teppi Coffee Plantation Project, southwestern Ethiopia: prevalence and impact on productivity. *Acta Trop* **54:**89-97.

8268. **Workowski, K. A., and W. C. Levine.** 2002. Sexually transmitted diseases. Treatment guidelines 2002. *MMWR* **51 (RR-6):**1-82.

8269. **Worm, H. C., W. H. van der Poel, and G. Brandstatter.** 2002. Hepatitis E: an overview. *Microbes Infect* **4:**657-66.

8270. **Wreghitt, T. G.** 1999. Blood-borne virus infections in dialysis units—a review. *Rev Med Virol* **9:**101-9.

8271. **Wreghitt, T. G., and C. E. Taylor.** 1988. Respiratory tract chlamydial infection and importation of psittacine birds. *Lancet* **2:**743.

8272. **Wreghitt, T. G., E. L. Teare, O. Sule, R. Devi, and P. S. Rice.** 2003. Cytomegalovirus infection in immunocompetent patients. *Clin Infect Dis* **37:**1603-6.

8273. **Wright, J., S. Gundry, and R. Conroy.** 2004. Household drinking water in developing countries: a systematic review of microbiological contamination between source and point-of-use. *Trop Med Int Health* **9:**106-17.

8274. **Wright, S. W., M. D. Decker, and K. M. Edwards.** 1999. Incidence of pertussis infection in healthcare workers. *Infect Control Hosp Epidemiol* **20:**120-3.

8275. **Wu, J. C., W. Y. Sheng, Y. H. Huang, S. J. Hwang, and S. D. Lee.** 1997. Prevalence and risk factor analysis of GBV-C/HGV infection in prostitutes. *J Med Virol* **52:**83-5.

8276. **Wu, J. C., F. Xu, W. Zhou, D. R. Feikin, C. Y. Lin, X. He, Z. Zhu, W. Liang, D. P. Chin, and A. Schuchat.** 2004. Risk factors for SARS among persons without known contact with SARS patients, Beijing, China. *Emerg Infect Dis* **10:**210-6.

8277. **Wu, T. S., C. H. Chiu, L. H. Su, J. H. Chia, M. H. Lee, P. C. Chiang, A. J. Kuo, T. L. Wu, and H. S. Leu.** 2002. Mycobacterium marinum infection in Taiwan. *J Microbiol Immunol Infect* **35:**42-6.

8278. **Wuethrich, B.** 2003. Chasing the fickle swine flu. *Science* **299:**1502-5.

8279. **Wurm, R., G. Dobler, M. Peters, and S. T. Kiessig.** 2000. Serological investigations of red foxes (Vulpes vulpes L.) for determination of the spread of tick-borne encephalitis in Northrhine-Westphalia. *J Vet Med B Infect Dis Vet Public Health* **47:**503-9.

8280. **Wuthe, H. H., and S. Aleksic.** 1997. [Yersinia enterocolitica serovar 2a, wb, 3:b,c biovar 5 in hares and sheep]. *Berl Munch Tierarztl Wochenschr* **110:**176-7.

8281. **Wyatt, G. B., B. A. Boatin, and F. K. Wurapa.** 1985. Risk factors associated with the acquisition of sleeping sickness in north-east Zambia: a case-control study. *Ann Trop Med Parasitol* **79:**385-92.

8282. **Wyatt, H. V.** 1996. Unnecessary injections and poliomyelitis in Pakistan. *Trop Doct* **26:**179-80.

8283. **Wyatt, J. D., W. H. Barker, N. M. Bennett, and C. A. Hanlon.** 1999. Human rabies postexposure prophylaxis during a raccoon rabies epizootic in New York, 1993 and 1994. *Emerg Infect Dis* **5:**415-23.

8284. **Wyler, R., and M. H.** 1984. Zeckenenzephalitis in der Schweiz. *Schweiz Rundsch Med Prax* **73:**601-19.

8285. **Wysoki, R. S., B. Majmudar, and D. Willis.** 1988. Granuloma inguinale (donovanosis) in women. *J Reprod Med* **33:**709-13.

8286. **Wyss, R., H. Sager, N. Muller, F. Inderbitzin, M. Konig, L. Audige, and B. Gottstein.** 2000. [The occurrence of Toxoplasma gondii and Neospora caninum as regards meat hygiene]. *Schweiz Arch Tierheilkd* **142:**95-108.

8287. **Wyszynski, D. F., and M. Kechichian.** 1997. Outbreak of tetanus among elderly women treated with sheep cell therapy. *Clin Infect Dis* **24:**738.

8288. **Xercavins, M., T. Llovet, F. Navarro, M. A. Morera, J. More, F. Bella, N. Freixas, M. Simo, A. Echeita, P. Coll, J. Garau, and G. Prats.** 1997. Epidemiology of an unusually prolonged outbreak of typhoid fever in Terrassa, Spain. *Clin Infect Dis* **24:**506-10.

8289. **Ximenes, R. A., B. Southgate, P. G. Smith, and L. Guimaraes Neto.** 2001. Social environment, behavior, and schistosomiasis in an urban population in the northeast of Brazil. *Rev Panam Salud Publica* **9:**13-22.

8290. **Xu, F., J. A. Schillinger, M. R. Sternberg, R. E. Johnson, F. K. Lee, A. J. Nahmias, and L. E. Markowitz.** 2002. Seroprevalence and coinfection with herpes simplex virus type 1 and type 2 in the United States, 1988-1994. *J Infect Dis* **185:**1019-24.

8291. **Xu, J., and H. Liu.** 1997. Border malaria in Yunnan, China. *Southeast Asian J Trop Med Public Health* **28:**456-9.

8292. **Xu, Y., S. Zhang, X. Huang, C. Bayin, X. Xuan, I. Igarashi, K. Fujisaki, H. Kabeya, S. Maruyama, and T. Mikami.** 2003. Seroepidemiologic studies on Babesia equi and Babesia caballi infections in horses in Jilin province of China. *J Vet Med Sci* **65:**1015-7.

8293. **Xu, Z. Y., C. S. Guo, Y. L. Wu, X. W. Zhang, and K. Liu.** 1985. Epidemiological studies of hemorrhagic fever with renal syndrome: analysis of risk factors and mode of transmission. *J Infect Dis* **152:**137-44.

8294. **Xu, Z. Y., Y. W. Tang, L. Y. Kan, and T. F. Tsai.** 1987. Cats—source of protection or infection? A case-control study of hemorrhagic fever with renal syndrome. *Am J Epidemiol* **126:**942-8.

8295. **Xue, D. Y., Y. Z. Ruan, B. C. Lin, R. Y. Zheng, J. Q. Fang, Q. X. Zhao, M. F. Li, and C. W. Pan.** 2000. [Epidemiological investigation on an outbreak of angiostrongyliasis cantonensis in Wenzhou]. *Zhongguo Ji Sheng Chong Xue Yu Ji Sheng Chong Bing Za Zhi* **18:**176-8.

8296. **Xueref, S., J. Holianjavony, R. Daniel, D. Kerouedan, J. Fabry, and P. Vanhems.** 2003. The absence of HIV seropositivity contrasts with a high prevalence of markers of sexually transmitted infections among registered female sex workers in Toliary, Madagascar. *Trop Med Int Health* **8:**60-6.

8297. **Yabsley, M. J., V. G. Dugan, D. E. Stallknecht, S. E. Little, J. M. Lockhart, J. E. Dawson, and W. R. Davidson.** 2003. Evaluation of a prototype Ehrlichia chaffeensis surveillance system using white-tailed deer (Odocoileus virginianus) as natural sentinels. *Vector Borne Zoonotic Dis* **3:**195-207.

8298. **Yabsley, M. J., A. S. Varela, C. M. Tate, V. G. Dugan, D. E. Stallknecht, S. E. Little, and W. R. Davidson.** 2002. Ehrlichia ewingii infection in white-tailed deer (Odocoileus virginianus). *Emerg Infect Dis* **8:**668-71.

8299. **Yabuuchi, E., M. Mori, A. Saito, T. Kishimoto, S. Yoshizawa, M. Arakawa, R. Kinouchi, L. Wang, K. Furuhata, M. Koide, et al.** 1995. [An outbreak of Pontiac fever due to Legionella pneumophila serogroup 7. II. Epidemiological aspects]. *Kansenshogaku Zasshi* **69:**654-65.

8300. **Yadav, A. S., and A. Kumar.** 2000. Prevalence of enterotoxigenic motile aeromonads in children, fish, milk and ice-cream and their public health significance. *Southeast Asian J Trop Med Public Health* **31 Suppl 1:**153-6.

8301. **Yadav, R. S., R. M. Bhatt, V. K. Kohli, and V. P. Sharma.** 2003. The burden of malaria in Ahmedabad city, India: a retrospective analysis of reported cases and deaths. *Ann Trop Med Parasitol* **97:**793-802.

8302. **Yadav, R. S., S. K. Ghosh, S. K. Chand, and A. Kumar.** 1991. Prevalence of malaria and economic loss in two major iron ore mines in Sundargarh district, Orissa. *Indian J Malariol* **28:**105-13.

8303. **Yadon, Z. E., L. C. Rodrigues, C. R. Davies, and M. A. Quigley.** 2003. Indoor and peridomestic transmission of American cutaneous leishmaniasis in northwestern Argentina: a retrospective case-control study. *Am J Trop Med Hyg* **68:**519-26.

8304. **Yaghoobi-Ershadi, M. R., and E. Javadian.** 1996. Seasonal variation of Leishmania major infection rates in sandflies from rodent burrows in Isfahan province, Iran. *Med Vet Entomol* **10:**181-4.

8305. **Yagita, K., and T. Endo.** 1999. Malaria infections in Japan. *Jpn J Infect Dis* **52:**20.

8306. **Yagupsky, P.** 2004. Kingella kingae: from medical rarity to an emerging paediatric pathogen. *Lancet Infect Dis* **4:**358-67.

8307. **Yagupsky, P., and E. J. Baron.** 2005. Laboratory exposures to brucellae and implications for bioterrorism. *Emerg Infect Dis* **11:**1180-5.

8308. **Yagupsky, P., D. Landau, A. Beck, and R. Dagan.** 1995. Carriage of Streptococcus pyogenes among infants and toddlers attending day-care facilities in closed communities in southern Israel. *Eur J Clin Microbiol Infect Dis* **14:**54-8.

8309. **Yagupsky, P., N. Peled, K. Riesenberg, and M. Banai.** 2000. Exposure of hospital personnel to Brucella melitensis and occurrence of laboratory-acquired disease in an endemic area. *Scand J Infect Dis* **32:**31-5.

8310. **Yagupsky, P., B. Sarov, and I. Sarov.** 1989. A cluster of cases of spotted fever in a kibbutz in southern Israel. *Scand J Infect Dis* **21:**155-60.

8311. **Yahaya, N.** 1991. Review of toxoplasmosis in Malaysia. *Southeast Asian J Trop Med Public Health* **22 Suppl:**102-6.

8312. **Yahnke, C. J., P. L. Meserve, T. G. Ksiazek, and J. N. Mills.** 2001. Patterns of infection with Laguna Negra virus in wild populations of Calomys laucha in the central Paraguayan Chaco. *Am J Trop Med Hyg* **65:**768-76.

8313. **Yajko, D. M., D. P. Chin, P. C. Gonzalez, P. S. Nassos, P. C. Hopewell, A. L. Reingold, C. R. Horsburgh, Jr., M. A. Yakrus, S. M. Ostroff, and W. K. Hadley.** 1995. Mycobacterium avium complex in water, food, and soil samples collected from the environment of HIV-infected individuals. *J Acquir Immune Defic Syndr Hum Retrovirol* **9:**176-82.

8314. **Yamada, K. I., T. Takasaki, M. Nawa, M. Nakayama, Y. T. Arai, S. Yabe, and I. Kurane.** 1999. The features of imported dengue fever cases from 1996 to 1999. *Jpn J Infect Dis* **52:**257-9.

8315. **Yamada, S., S. Matsushita, S. Dejsirilert, and Y. Kudoh.** 1997. Incidence and clinical symptoms of Aeromonas-associated travellers' diarrhoea in Tokyo. *Epidemiol Infect* **119:**121-6.

8316. **Yamada, S., S. Matushita, and Y. Kudoh.** 1999. [Recovery and its evaluation of Shigella bacilli or Salmonella from healthy food handlers in Tokyo (1961-1997)]. *Kansenshogaku Zasshi* **73:**758-65.

8317. **Yamada, S., K. Ogata, R. Kato, K. Morimoto, Y. Hayashi, T. Ito, S. Matushita, N. Konishi, A. Kai, and M. Endoh.** 1999. [Outbreak case caused by different colicin type of Shigella sonnei in a day nursery in Tokyo (1998)]. *Kansenshogaku Zasshi* **73:**1130-9.

8318. **Yamagata, Y., T. Suzuki, and G. A. Garcia Manzo.** 1986. Geographical distribution of the prevalence of nodules of Onchocerca volvulus in Guatemala over the last four decades. *Trop Med Parasitol* **37:**28-34.

8319. **Yamamoto, K., M. Kijima, H. Yoshimura, and T. Takahashi.** 2001. Antimicrobial susceptibilities of Erysipelothrix rhusiopathiae isolated from pigs with swine erysipelas in Japan, 1988-1998. *J Vet Med B Infect Dis Vet Public Health* **48:**115-26.

8320. **Yamamoto, N., R. Kishi, Y. Katakura, and H. Miyake.** 2001. Risk factors for human alveolar echinococcosis: a case-control study in Hokkaido, Japan. *Ann Trop Med Parasitol* **95:**689-96.

8321. **Yamashiro, T., N. Nakasone, N. Higa, M. Iwanaga, S. Insisiengmay, T. Phounane, K. Munnalath, N. Sithivong, L. Sisavath, B. Phanthauamath, K. Chomlasak, P. Sisulath, and P. Vongsanith.** 1998. Etiological study of diarrheal patients in Vientiane, Lao People's Democratic Republic. *J Clin Microbiol* **36:**2195-9.

8322. **Yamashita, H., H. Tsukayama, A. R. White, Y. Tanno, C. Sugishita, and E. Ernst.** 2001. Systematic review of adverse events following acupuncture: the Japanese literature. *Complement Ther Med* **9:**98-104.

8323. **Yamazaki, T., H. Nakada, N. Sakurai, C. C. Kuo, S. P. Wang, and J. T. Grayston.** 1990. Transmission of Chlamydia pneumoniae in young children in a Japanese family. *J Infect Dis* **162:**1390-2.

8324. **Yanagihara, R., C. T. Chin, M. B. Weiss, D. C. Gajdusek, A. R. Diwan, J. B. Poland, K. T. Kleeman, C. M. Wilfert, G. Meiklejohn, and W. P. Glezen.** 1985. Serological evidence of Hantaan virus infection in the United States. *Am J Trop Med Hyg* **34:**396-9.

8325. Yanez Ortega, J. L., J. L. Cobos Lopez, F. J. Martinez Rodriquez, and J. Mingo Lopez. 1994. Outbreak of Q fever in the province of Burgos in 1992. *Boletín Microbiológico Semanal* **6:**17-22.

8326. Yang, C. Y., W. T. Chang, H. Y. Chuang, S. S. Tsai, T. N. Wu, and F. C. Sung. 2001. Adverse health effects among household waste collectors in Taiwan. *Environ Res* **85:**195-9.

8327. Yang, J., and T. Scholten. 1977. Dientamoeba fragilis: a review with notes on its epidemiology, pathogenicity, mode of transmission, and diagnosis. *Am J Trop Med Hyg* **26:**16-22.

8328. Yang, P. Y., C. C. Huang, H. S. Leu, P. C. Chiang, T. L. Wu, and T. C. Tsao. 2001. Klebsiella pneumoniae bacteremia: community-acquired vs. nosocomial infections. *Chang Gung Med J* **24:**688-96.

8329. Yangco, B. G., A. L. Vincent, A. C. Vickery, J. K. Nayar, and D. M. Sauerman. 1984. A survey of filariasis among refugees in south Florida. *Am J Trop Med Hyg* **33:**246-51.

8330. Yano, Y., M. Yokoyama, M. Satomi, H. Oikawa, and S. S. Chen. 2004. Occurrence of Vibrio vulnificus in fish and shellfish available from markets in China. *J Food Prot* **67:**1617-23.

8331. Yapabandara, A. M., and C. F. Curtis. 2004. Vectors and malaria transmission in a gem mining area in Sri Lanka. *J Vector Ecol* **29:**264-76.

8332. Yasuda, A., H. Kimura, M. Hayakawa, M. Ohshiro, Y. Kato, O. Matsuura, C. Suzuki, and T. Morishima. 2003. Evaluation of cytomegalovirus infections transmitted via breastmilk in preterm infants with a real-time polymerase chain reaction assay. *Pediatrics* **111:**1333-6.

8333. Yazaki, Y., H. Mizuo, M. Takahashi, T. Nishizawa, N. Sasaki, Y. Gotanda, and H. Okamoto. 2003. Sporadic acute or fulminant hepatitis E in Hokkaido, Japan, may be food-borne, as suggested by the presence of hepatitis E virus in pig liver as food. *J Gen Virol* **84:**2351-7.

8334. Yazdanpanah, Y., G. De Carli, B. Migueres, F. Lot, M. Campins, C. Colombo, T. Thomas, S. Deuffic-Burban, M. H. Prevot, M. Domart, A. Tarantola, D. Abiteboul, P. Deny, S. Pol, J. C. Desenclos, V. Puro, and E. Bouvet. 2005. Risk factors for hepatitis C virus transmission to health care workers after occupational exposure: a European case-control study. *Clin Infect Dis* **41:**1423-30.

8335. Yeruham, I., D. Elad, S. Friedman, and R. Perl. 2003. Corynebacterium pseudotuberculosis infection in Israeli dairy cattle. *Epidemiol Infect* **131:**947-55.

8336. Yevich, S. J., J. L. Sanchez, R. F. DeFraites, C. C. Rives, J. E. Dawson, I. J. Uhaa, B. J. Johnson, and D. B. Fishbein. 1995. Seroepidemiology of infections due to spotted fever group rickettsiae and Ehrlichia species in military personnel exposed in areas of the United States where such infections are endemic. *J Infect Dis* **171:**1266-73.

8337. Yiannakou, J., J. Croese, L. R. Ashdown, and P. Prociv. 1992. Strongyloidiasis in North Queensland: re-emergence of a forgotten risk group? *Med J Aust* **156:**24-7.

8338. Yildirim, A. O., C. Lammler, R. Weiss, and P. Kopp. 2002. Pheno- and genotypic properties of streptococci of serological group B of canine and feline origin. *FEMS Microbiol Lett* **212:**187-92.

8339. Yilmaz, H., and A. Godekmerdan. 2004. Human fasciolosis in Van province, Turkey. *Acta Trop* **92:**161-2.

8340. Yoder, J. S., B. G. Blackburn, G. F. Craun, V. Hill, D. A. Levy, N. Chen, S. H. Lee, R. L. Calderon, and M. J. Beach. 2004. Surveillance for waterborne-disease outbreaks associated with recreational water—United States, 2001-2002. *MMWR* **53 (SS-8):**1-22.

8341. Yoeli, M., H. Most, J. Hammond, and G. P. Scheinesson. 1972. Parasitic infections in a closed community: results of a 10-year survey in Willowbrook state school. *Trans R Soc Trop Med Hyg* **66:**764-776.

8342. Yohannes, K., P. Roche, C. Blumer, J. Spencer, A. Milton, C. Bunn, H. Gidding, M. Kirk, and T. Della-Porta. 2004. Australia's notifiable diseases status, 2002: Annual report of the National Notifiable Diseases Surveillance System. *Commun Dis Intell* **28:**6-68.

8343. Yoon, J., S. Segal-Maurer, and J. J. Rahal. 2004. An Outbreak of Domestically Acquired Typhoid Fever in Queens, NY. *Arch Intern Med* **164:**565-7.

8344. Yoshida, T., S. I. Maeda, T. Deguchi, T. Miyazawa, and H. Ishiko. 2003. Rapid Detection of Mycoplasma genitalium, Mycoplasma hominis, Ureaplasma parvum, and Ureaplasma urealyticum Organisms in Genitourinary Samples by PCR-Microtiter Plate Hybridization Assay. *J Clin Microbiol* **41:**1850-1855.

8345. Yoshikawa, T., Y. Asano, M. Ihira, K. Suzuki, M. Ohashi, S. Suga, K. Kudo, K. Horibe, S. Kojima, K. Kato, T. Matsuyama, and Y. Nishiyama. 2002. Human herpesvirus 6 viremia in bone marrow transplant recipients: clinical features and risk factors. *J Infect Dis* **185:**847-53.

8346. Yoshimine, H., K. Oishi, F. Mubiru, H. Nalwoga, H. Takahashi, H. Amano, P. Ombasi, K. Watanabe, M. Joloba, T. Aisu, K. Ahmed, M. Shimada, R. Mugerwa, and T. Nagatake. 2001. Community-acquired pneumonia in Ugandan adults: short-term parenteral ampicillin therapy for bacterial pneumonia. *Am J Trop Med Hyg* **64:**172-7.

8347. Yossepowitch, O., T. Gotesman, M. Assous, E. Marva, R. Zimlichman, and M. Dan. 2004. Opisthorchiasis from imported raw fish. *Emerg Infect Dis* **10:**2122-6.

8348. Young, E. J. 1995. An overview of human brucellosis. *Clin Infect Dis* **21:**283-9.

8349. Young, J. C., G. R. Hansen, T. K. Graves, M. P. Deasy, J. G. Humphreys, C. L. Fritz, K. L. Gorham, A. S. Khan, T. G. Ksiazek, K. B. Metzger, and C. J. Peters. 2000. The incubation period of hantavirus pulmonary syndrome. *Am J Trop Med Hyg* **62:**714-7.

8350. Young, L. C., D. E. Dwyer, M. Harris, Z. Guse, V. Noel, and M. H. Levy. 2005. Summer outbreak of respiratory disease in an Australian prison due to an influenza A/Fujian/411/2002(H3N2)-like virus. *Epidemiol Infect* **133:**107-12.

8351. Young, N. S., and K. E. Brown. 2004. Parvovirus B19. *N Engl J Med* **350:**586-97.

8352. Youwang, Y., D. Jianming, X. Yong, and Z. Pong. 1992. Epidemiological features of an outbreak of diphtheria and its control with diphtheria toxoid immunization. *Int J Epidemiol* **21:**807-11.

8353. Yu, D., H. Li, R. Xu, et al. 2003. Prevalence of IgG antibody to SARS-associated coronavirus in animal traders - Guangdong province, China, 2003. *MMWR* **52:**986-7.

8354. Yu, I. T., Y. Li, T. W. Wong, W. Tam, A. T. Chan, J. H. Lee, D. Y. Leung, and T. Ho. 2004. Evidence of airborne transmission of the severe acute respiratory syndrome virus. *N Engl J Med* **350:**1731-9.

8355. Yu, S. H., M. Kawanaka, X. M. Li, L. Q. Xu, C. G. Lan, and L. Rui. 2003. Epidemiological investigation on Clonorchis sinensis in human population in an area of South China. *Jpn J Infect Dis* **56:**168-71.

8356. **Yu, S. H., and K. E. Mott.** 1994. Epidemiology and morbidity of food-borne intestinal trematode infections. *Trop Dis Bull* **91:**R126-R150.

8357. **Yu, W. L., H. S. Cheng, H. C. Lin, C. T. Peng, and C. H. Tsai.** 2000. Outbreak investigation of nosocomial enterobacter cloacae bacteraemia in a neonatal intensive care unit. *Scand J Infect Dis* **32:**293-8.

8358. **Yuen, K. Y., and P. C. Woo.** 2002. Tuberculosis in blood and marrow transplant recipients. *Hematol Oncol* **20:**51-62.

8359. **Yusuf, H. R., C. R. Braden, A. J. Greenberg, A. C. Weltman, I. M. Onorato, and S. E. Valway.** 1997. Tuberculosis transmission among five school bus drivers and students in two New York counties. *Pediatrics* **100:**E9.

8360. **Yutu, J. A., M. Jing, and X. H. Guang.** 1988. Outbreaks of smallpox due to variolation in China, 1962-1965. *Am J Epidemiol* **128:**39-45.

8361. **Zaaijer, H. L., M. H. Koppelman, and C. P. Farrington.** 2004. Parvovirus B19 viraemia in Dutch blood donors. *Epidemiol Infect* **132:**1161-6.

8362. **Zaal, M. J., H. J. Volker-Dieben, M. Wienesen, J. D'Amaro, and A. Kijlstra.** 2001. Longitudinal analysis of varicella-zoster virus DNA on the ocular surface associated with herpes zoster ophthalmicus. *Am J Ophthalmol* **131:**25-9.

8363. **Zachariah, R., A. D. Harries, A. S. Chantulo, A. E. Yadidi, W. Nkhoma, and O. Maganga.** 2002. Sexually transmitted infections amng prison inmates in a rural district of Malawi. *Trans R Soc Trop Med Hyg* **96:**617-9.

8364. **Zachariah, R., M. P. Spielmann, A. D. Harries, P. Gomani, S. M. Graham, E. Bakali, and P. Humblet.** 2003. Passive versus active tuberculosis case finding and isoniazid preventive therapy among household contacts in a rural district of Malawi. *Int J Tuberc Lung Dis* **7:**1033-9.

8365. **Zadoks, R. N., W. B. van Leeuwen, D. Kreft, L. K. Fox, H. W. Barkema, Y. H. Schukken, and A. van Belkum.** 2002. Comparison of Staphylococcus aureus isolates from bovine and human skin, milking equipment, and bovine milk by phage typing, pulsed-field gel electrophoresis, and binary typing. *J Clin Microbiol* **40:**3894-902.

8366. **Zagaria, N., and L. Savioli.** 2002. Elimination of lymphatic filariasis: a public-health challenge. *Ann Trop Med Parasitol* **96 Suppl 2:**S3-13.

8367. **Zaidenberg, M., and A. Segovia.** 1993. [Congenital Chagas disease in the city of Salta, Argentina]. *Rev Inst Med Trop Sao Paulo* **35:**35-43.

8368. **Zaidi, A. M., and R. J. Cryer.** 1997. Case report: holiday-acquired tick-borne encephalitis. *Travel Med Internat* **15:**187-8.

8369. **Zaim, M., and P. Guillet.** 2002. Alternative insecticides: an urgent need. *Trends Parasitol* **18:**161-3.

8370. **Zanelli, G., A. Sansoni, A. Zanchi, S. Cresti, S. Pollini, G. M. Rossolini, and C. Cellesi.** 2002. Staphylococcus aureus nasal carriage in the community: a survey from central Italy. *Epidemiol Infect* **129:**417-20.

8371. **Zanetti, F., G. De Luca, and S. Stampi.** 2000. Recovery of Burkholderia pseudomallei and B. cepacia from drinking water. *Int J Food Microbiol* **59:**67-72.

8372. **Zanetti, F., S. Stampi, G. De Luca, P. Fateh-Moghadam, M. Antonietta, B. Sabattini, and L. Checchi.** 2000. Water characteristics associated with the occurrence of Legionella pneumophila in dental units. *Eur J Oral Sci* **108:**22-8.

8373. **Zanetti, G., P. Francioli, D. Tagan, C. D. Paddock, and S. R. Zaki.** 1998. Imported epidemic typhus. *Lancet* **352:**1709.

8374. **Zangwill, K. M., A. Schuchat, F. X. Riedo, R. W. Pinner, D. T. Koo, M. W. Reeves, and J. D. Wenger.** 1997. School-based clusters of meningococcal disease in the United States. Descriptive epidemiology and a case-control analysis. *JAMA* **277:**389-95.

8375. **Zanini, G. M., and C. Graeff-Teixeira.** 1995. [Abdominal angiostrongyliasis: its prevention by the destruction of infecting larvae in food treated with salt, vinegar or sodium hypochlorite]. *Rev Soc Bras Med Trop* **28:**389-92.

8376. **Zanoni, R.** 2003. Rabies in a puppy in Nyon, Switzerland. *Rabies Bulletin Europe* **27:**5-6.

8377. **Zansky, S., B. Wallace, and M. S. Schoonmaker-Bopp.** 2002. Outbreak of multidrug-resistant Salmonella Newport - United States, January-April 2002. *MMWR* **51:**545-8.

8378. **Zastrow, K. D., and I. Schoneberg.** 1993. [Importation of leprosy into Germany 1981-1992]. *Gesundheitswesen* **55:**414-7.

8379. **Zawacki, A., E. O'Rourke, G. Potter-Bynoe, A. Macone, S. Harbarth, and D. Goldmann.** 2004. An outbreak of Pseudomonas aeruginosa pneumonia and bloodstream infection associated with intermittent otitis externa in a healthcare worker. *Infect Control Hosp Epidemiol* **25:**1083-9.

8380. **Zayas, C. F., C. Perlino, A. Caliendo, D. Jackson, E. J. Martinez, P. Tso, T. G. Heffron, J. L. Logan, B. L. Herwaldt, A. C. Moore, F. J. Steurer, C. Bern, and J. H. Maguire.** 2002. Chagas disease after organ transplantation - United States, 2001. *MMWR* **51:**210-2.

8381. **Zeitz, P. S., J. M. Graber, R. A. Voorhees, C. Kioski, L. A. Shands, T. G. Ksiazek, S. Jenison, and R. F. Khabbaz.** 1997. Assessment of occupational risk for hantavirus infection in Arizona and New Mexico. *J Occup Environ Med* **39:**463-7.

8382. **Zekri, A. R., W. S. Mohamed, M. A. Samra, G. M. Sherif, A. M. El-Shehaby, and M. H. El-Sayed.** 2004. Risk factors for cytomegalovirus, hepatitis B and C virus reactivation after bone marrow transplantation. *Transpl Immunol* **13:**305-11.

8383. **Zeledon, R., G. Solano, L. Burstin, and J. C. Swartzwelder.** 1975. Epidemiological pattern of Chagas' disease in an endemic area of Costa Rica. *Am J Trop Med Hyg* **24:**214-25.

8384. **Zeller, H.** 2000. [Lessons from the Marburg virus epidemic in Durba, Democratic Republic of the Congo (1998-2000)]. *Med Trop (Mars)* **60(2:**23-6.

8385. **Zeller, H. G., J. P. Cornet, A. Diop, and J. L. Camicas.** 1997. Crimean-Congo hemorrhagic fever in ticks (Acari: Ixodidae) and ruminants: field observations of an epizootic in Bandia, Senegal (1989-1992). *J Med Entomol* **34:**511-6.

8386. **Zeller, H. G., and I. Schuffenecker.** 2004. West nile virus: an overview of its spread in Europe and the Mediterranean basin in contrast to its spread in the Americas. *Eur J Clin Microbiol Infect Dis* **23:**147-56.

8387. **Zen-Yoji, H., S. Sakai, T. Terayama, Y. Kudo, T. Ito, M. Benoki, and M. Nagasaki.** 1965. Epidemiology, enteropathogenicity, and classification of Vibrio parahaemolyticus. *J Infect Dis* **116:**436-44.

8388. **Zerr, D. M., A. L. Allpress, J. Heath, R. Bornemann, and E. Bennett.** 2005. Decreasing hospital-associated rotavirus infection: a multidisciplinary hand hygiene campaign in a children's hospital. *Pediatr Infect Dis J* **24:**397-403.

8389. **Zerr, D. M., A. S. Meier, S. S. Selke, L. M. Frenkel, M. L. Huang, A. Wald, M. P. Rhoads, L. Nguy, R. Bornemann, R. A.**

Morrow, and L. Corey. 2005. A population-based study of primary human herpesvirus 6 infection. *N Engl J Med* **352:**768-76.

8390. Zerr, I., J. P. Brandel, C. Masullo, D. Wientjens, R. de Silva, M. Zeidler, E. Granieri, S. Sampaolo, C. van Duijn, N. Delasnerie-Laupretre, R. Will, and S. Poser. 2000. European surveillance on Creutzfeldt-Jakob disease: a case-control study for medical risk factors. *J Clin Epidemiol* **53:**747-54.

8391. Zervos, M. J., M. S. Terpenning, D. R. Schaberg, P. M. Therasse, S. V. Medendorp, and C. A. Kauffman. 1987. High-level aminoglycoside-resistant enterococci. Colonization of nursing home and acute care hospital patients. *Arch Intern Med* **147:**1591-4.

8392. Zhang, K.-L., and S.-J. Ma. 2002. Epidemiology of HIV in China. *BMJ* **324:**803-4.

8393. Zhang, Y., L. B. Mann, R. W. Wilson, B. A. Brown-Elliott, V. Vincent, Y. Iinuma, and R. J. Wallace, Jr. 2004. Molecular analysis of Mycobacterium kansasii isolates from the United States. *J Clin Microbiol* **42:**119-25.

8394. Zhang, Z., and C. Yang. 1996. Application of deltamethrin-impregnated bednets for mosquito and malaria control in Yunnan, China. *Southeast Asian J Trop Med Public Health* **27:**367-71.

8395. Zhang, Z. F. 1996. Epidemiology of trichomonas vaginalis. A prospective study in China. *Sex Transm Dis* **23:**415-24.

8396. Zhao, J. 1992. [An outbreak of rubella with a cinema as source]. *Zhonghua Liu Xing Bing Xue Za Zhi* **13:**359-61.

8397. Zhao, S., A. R. Datta, S. Ayers, S. Friedman, R. D. Walker, and D. G. White. 2003. Antimicrobial-resistant Salmonella serovars isolated from imported foods. *Int J Food Microbiol* **84:**87-92.

8398. Zheng, B. J., Y. Guan, K. H. Wong, J. Zhou, K. L. Wong, B. W. Y. Young, L. W. Lu, and S. S. Lee. 2004. SARS-related virus predating SARS outbreak, Hong Kong. *Emerg Infect Dis* **10:**176-8.

8399. Zheng, J., X. G. Gu, Y. L. Xu, J. H. Ge, X. X. Yang, C. H. He, C. Tang, K. P. Cai, Q. W. Jiang, Y. S. Liang, T. P. Wang, X. J. Xu, J. H. Zhong, H. C. Yuan, and X. N. Zhou. 2002. Relationship between the transmission of schistosomiasis japonica and the construction of the Three Gorge Reservoir. *Acta Trop* **82:**147-56.

8400. Zhibang, Y., Z. BiXia, L. Qishan, C. Lihao, L. Xiangquan, and L. Huaping. 2002. Large-Scale Outbreak of Infection with Mycobacterium chelonae subsp. abscessus after Penicillin Injection. *J Clin Microbiol* **40:**2626-2628.

8401. Zhioua, E., F. Rodhain, P. Binet, and C. Perez-Eid. 1997. Prevalence of antibodies to Borrelia burgdorferi in forestry workers of Ile de France, France. *Eur J Epidemiol* **13:**959-62.

8402. Zhong, N. S., B. J. Zheng, Y. M. Li, Poon, Z. H. Xie, K. H. Chan, P. H. Li, S. Y. Tan, Q. Chang, J. P. Xie, X. Q. Liu, J. Xu, D. X. Li, K. Y. Yuen, Peiris, and Y. Guan. 2003. Epidemiology and cause of severe acute respiratory syndrome (SARS) in Guangdong, People's Republic of China, in February, 2003. *Lancet* **362:**1353-8.

8403. Zhou, G., J. Sirichaisinthop, J. Sattabongkot, J. Jones, O. N. Bjornstad, G. Yan, and L. Cui. 2005. Spatio-Temporal Distribution of Plasmodium Falciparum and P. Vivax Malaria in Thailand. *Am J Trop Med Hyg* **72:**256-262.

8404. Zhou, L., A. Singh, J. Jiang, and L. Xiao. 2003. Molecular surveillance of Cryptosporidium spp. in raw wastewater in Milwaukee: implications for understanding outbreak occurrence and transmission dynamics. *J Clin Microbiol* **41:**5254-7.

8405. Zhu, J. Q., W. L. Wu, Y. Z. Li, G. Liu, and C. M. Wang. 1993. A study on the epidemic patterns and control measures of human plague in Qinghai Province. *Endemic Dis Bull* **8:**1-8.

8406. Zichichi, L., G. Asta, and G. Noto. 2000. Pseudomonas aeruginosa folliculitis after shower/bath exposure. *Int J Dermatol* **39:**270-3.

8407. Ziebold, C., B. Hassenpflug, H. Wegner-Bröse, K. Wegner, and H. J. Schmitt. 2003. An outbreak of rubella aboard a ship of the German navy. *Infection* **31:**136-42.

8408. Zieger, B. 1999. Malaria: zwei Fallberichte als Beispiele unterschiedlichen individuellen Verhaltens. *Epidemiol Bull* **46 (19 Nov):**347-8.

8409. Ziegler, E., C. Roth, and T. Wreghitt. 2003. Prevalence of measles susceptibility among health care workers in a UK hospital. Does the UK need to introduce a measles policy for its health care workers? *Occup Med (Lond)* **53:**398-402.

8410. Ziem, J. B., I. M. Kettenis, A. Bayita, E. A. Brienen, S. Dittoh, J. Horton, A. Olsen, P. Magnussen, and A. M. Polderman. 2004. The short-term impact of albendazole treatment on Oesophagostomum bifurcum and hookworm infections in northern Ghana. *Ann Trop Med Parasitol* **98:**385-90.

8411. Zijlstra, E. E., and A. M. El-Hassan. 2001. Leishmaniasis in Sudan. 3. Visceral leishmaniasis. *Trans R Soc Trop Med Hyg* **95 suppl 1:**S27-S58.

8412. Zimmerli, W., A. F. Widmer, M. Blatter, R. Frei, and P. E. Ochsner. 1998. Role of rifampin for treatment of orthopedic implant-related staphylococcal infections: a randomized controlled trial. Foreign-Body Infection (FBI) Study Group. *JAMA* **279:**1537-41.

8413. Zimmerman, L., and S. E. Reef. 2001. Incidence of congenital rubella syndrome at a hospital serving a predominantly Hispanic population, El Paso, Texas. *Pediatrics* **107:**E40.

8414. Zingg, W., C. Colombo, T. Jucker, W. Bossart, and C. Ruef. 2005. Impact of an outbreak of norovirus infection on hospital resources. *Infect Control Hosp Epidemiol* **26:**263-7.

8415. Zintl, A., G. Mulcahy, H. E. Skerrett, S. M. Taylor, and J. S. Gray. 2003. Babesia divergens, a Bovine Blood Parasite of Veterinary and Zoonotic Importance. *Clin Microbiol Rev* **16:**622-636.

8416. Ziring, D., R. Tran, S. Edelstein, S. V. McDiarmid, N. Gajjar, G. Cortina, J. Vargas, J. F. Renz, J. D. Cherry, P. Krogstad, M. Miller, R. W. Busuttil, and D. G. Farmer. 2005. Infectious enteritis after intestinal transplantation: incidence, timing, and outcome. *Transplantation* **79:**702-9.

8417. Zoguereh, D. D., J. B. Ndihokubwayo, and A. Simboyinuma. 2000. [Epidemic typhus in tropical Africa. A reemerging disease that is severe but curable]. *Sante* **10:**339-44.

8418. Zoli, A., O. Shey-Njila, E. Assana, J. P. Nguekam, P. Dorny, J. Brandt, and S. Geerts. 2003. Regional status, epidemiology and impact of Taenia solium cysticercosis in Western and Central Africa. *Acta Trop* **87:**35-42.

8419. Zolopa, A. R., J. A. Hahn, R. Gorter, J. Miranda, D. Wlodarczyk, J. Peterson, L. Pilote, and A. R. Moss. 1994. HIV and tuberculosis infection in San Francisco's homeless adults. Prevalence and risk factors in a representative sample. *JAMA* **272:**455-61.

8420. Zou, S., R. Y. Dodd, S. L. Stramer, and D. M. Strong. 2004. Probability of viremia with HBV, HCV, HIV, and HTLV among tissue donors in the United States. *N Engl J Med* **351:**751-9.

8421. **Zribi, M., and F. Messadi Akrout.** 1988. La bilharziose en Tunisie de 1970 à 1987. *Bull Soc Fr Parasitol* **6:**201-7.

8422. **Zucker, B. A., S. Trojan, and W. Muller.** 2000. Airborne gram-negative bacterial flora in animal houses. *J Vet Med B Infect Dis Vet Public Health* **47:**37-46.

8423. **Zucker, J. R.** 1996. Changing patterns of autochthonous malaria transmission in the United States: a review of recent outbreaks. *Emerg Infect Dis* **2:**37-43.

8424. **Zuidema, P. J.** 1981. The Katayama syndrome; an outbreak in Dutch tourists to the Omo national park, Ethiopia. *Trop Geogr Med* **33:**30-5.

8425. **Zulkifli, A., A. A. Khairul, A. S. Atiya, B. Abdullah, and A. Yano.** 1999. The prevalence and intensity of soil-transmitted helminthiasis among pre-school children in Orang Asli resettlement villages in Kelantan. *Med J Malaysia* **54:**453-8.

8426. **Zulueta, A. M., E. Villarroel, N. Rodriguez, M. D. Feliciangeli, M. Mazzarri, O. Reyes, V. Rodriguez, M. Centeno, R. M. Barrios, and M. Ulrich.** 1999. Epidemiologic aspects of American visceral leishmaniasis in an endemic focus in Eastern Venezuela. *Am J Trop Med Hyg* **61:**945-50.

8427. **Zumla, A. I., and J. Grange.** 2002. Non-tuberculous mycobacterial pulmonary infections. *Clin Chest Med* **23:**369-76.

8428. **Zurawski, C. A., M. Bardsley, B. Beall, J. A. Elliott, R. Facklam, B. Schwartz, and M. M. Farley.** 1998. Invasive group A streptococcal disease in metropolitan Atlanta: a population-based assessment. *Clin Infect Dis* **27:**150-7.

8429. **Zurita, S., C. Costa, D. Watts, S. Indacochea, P. Campos, J. Sanchez, and E. Gotuzzo.** 1997. Prevalence of human retroviral infection in Quillabamba and Cuzco, Peru: a new endemic area for human T cell lymphotropic virus type 1. *Am J Trop Med Hyg* **56:**561-5.

8430. **Zweighaft, R. M., D. W. Fraser, M. A. Hattwick, W. G. Winkler, W. C. Jordan, M. Alter, M. Wolfe, H. Wulff, and K. M. Johnson.** 1977. Lassa fever: response to an imported case. *N Engl J Med* **297:**803-7.

Index

A

Abdominal infections, acute food-borne, 147
Absidia, 499
Acanthamoeba, 141, 499
Acinetobacter
    antimicrobial resistance, 494
    description of genus, 499, 502
    nosocomial infections, 472
    plant-derived foods and, 180
Acinetobacter baumannii
    drinking water-associated, 197–198
    nosocomial infections, 449, 461, 477
Acinetobacter calcoaceticus-baumannii, 261
Acremonium
    description of genus, 503
    nosocomial infections, 463
Acronyms, 597–600
Actinobacillus, 503
Actinomadura, 503
Actinomyces
    description of genus, 503
    nosocomial infections, 492
Acupuncture, infections from, 469
Adenovirus
    from bowel, 342
    description of genus, 503
    drinking water-associated, 200
    long-term care and, 233
    from nose, mouth, and throat, 339
    on objects, 142
    occupational infections, 251, 254, 285–286
    pools and, 311
    school-associated, 360
Aedes, 73–75, 431–432
Aeromonas
    animal-derived foods and, 167, 169
    community-acquired, 379
    description of genus, 503
    drinking water-associated, 201–202
    freshwater habitats and floods, 96
    long-term care and, 235
    marine habitat, 91
    occupational infections, 274
    outdoor leisure and, 318
    travel-associated, 408
Age groups, 347–353
    adult age, 351–352
    elderly, 352–353
    peaks of infections, 347–349
    preschool age, 349–351
    school age, 351
Air
    in buildings, 128
    in nosohabitats, 458–461
Aircraft and airport travel, 401–404
Alcaligenes, 503
Alkhurma virus, 530–531
Alpaca. *See* Camelids
Alpharetrovirus, 503
Alphavirus
    bats, 54
    description of genus, 503–505
    lagomorphs, 50
    mosquitoes and, 74, 77, 79
    primates, 52
    rodents, 44
Alpine and boreal tundra, 112–115
Alternative care, infections from, 469
Amblyomma, 67
Amebas, free-living
    drinking water-associated, 195, 203
    from nose, mouth, and throat, 342
    nosocomial infections, 463
    occupational infections, 298
    outdoor leisure and, 319
    pools and, 313
    soil and plant-associated, 100
Amphibians, 60–61
Anaplasma, 505
Anaplasma bovis, 429–430
Anaplasma phagocytophilum
    bovids, 24
    camelids, 34
    description, 505
    dogs, 15
    equids, 33
    herbivores, 38
    occupational infections, 259, 270, 291
    outdoor leisure and, 317
    rodents, 46
    seasons and, 122
    terrestrial biomes, 109
    ticks, 69
    urban environment and, 135
Ancylostoma
    description, 505–506
    domicile-associated, human substandard, 221
    marine habitat, 91
    outdoor leisure and, 319
    primates, 52
    soil and plants, 100
Andes virus, 536
Angiostrongylus
    description of genus, 506
Angiostrongylus catonensis
    animal-derived foods and, 169, 172–173
    catering and restaurant-associated, 309
    description, 506
    plant-derived foods and, 181, 184
    rodent hosts, 44
    terrestrial biomes, 108
    transported animals and goods, 429
    travel-associated, 410
Angiostrongylus costaricensis
    animal-derived foods and, 173
    description, 506
    plant-derived foods and, 181
    rodent hosts, 44
Animal bites, 7–11
    Clostridium tetani, 9–10
    fish trauma, agents of, 10–11
    Francisella tularensis, 10
    Pasteurella, 10

870 INDEX

Animal bites *(continued)*
  rabies, 7–9s
  risks, 7
  Sporothrix schenckii, 10
  Streptobacillus moniliformis, 10
  trauma, 7
  wound infection agents, 10
  wound infection risks and managements, 10
Animal-derived foods, 149–173
  eggs and egg products, 156–157
  meat and meat products, 159–166
  milk and dairy products, 149–156
  poultry, 157–159
  seafood, fish, and molluscs, 166–173
Animals, 5–85
  animal bites, 7–11
  antimicrobials, 5–6
  domestic mammals, 13–35
  invertebrates, 65–85
  wild vertebrates, 37–63
  zoonoses, 5
Anisakis
  animal-derived foods and, 168, 173
  catering and restaurant-associated, 309
  description of genus, 506
  fish, 61–62
  nosocomial infections, 451
  travel-associated, 410
Anopheles, 76–78, 432
Antimalarials, fake, 450
Antimicrobial resistance, nosocomial infections and, 457, 494
Aphthovirus, 506
Arboviruses. *See also specific viruses*
  freshwater habitats and floods, 95
Arcobacter, 507
Arenavirus
  description of genus, 506
  nosocomial infections, 464
  occupational infections, 268, 290
  rodents, 44–45
Arid lands, 110–111
Arthropods
  day care-associated, 358
  domicile-associated, human substandard, 223
  homeless persons and, 225
  human travel and, 415, 419, 425
  leisure and lifestyle-associated, 307
  long-term care and, 237
  nosocomial infections, 443
  occupational infections, 264, 276, 296
  in orphans and adoptees, 233
  prisons and, 241
  relief camps and, 229
  school-associated, 365
  from ships and aircraft, 431–432
  wind and, 118
Ascaris
  description of genus, 507–508
  outdoor leisure and, 317
  soil and plants, 99
Ascaris lumbricoides
  description, 507–508

  domicile-associated, human substandard, 217
  drinking water-associated, 204
  occupational infections, 267
  in orphans and adoptees, 232
  plant-derived foods and, 181, 186
  sanitation and, 131
  urban environment and, 134
Ascaris suum, 29–30
Aspergillus
  birds, 56
  description of genus, 508
  dust and, 117
  nosocomial infections, 460, 463, 484
  occupational infections, 249
Aspergillus fumigatus, 452
Astrovirus
  from bowel, 342
  long-term care and, 235
  occupational infections, 256
  school-associated, 362
Australian bat lyssavirus, 54
Avian infectious bronchitis virus (AIBV), 268
Avian leukosis virus (ALV), 60
Avians. *See* Birds
Avipoxvirus
  birds, 60
  description, 508
Avulavirus, 508

B

Babesia
  birds, 60
  bovids, 25
  description of genus, 508–509
  dogs, 16
  domicile-associated, human regular, 213
  equids, 33
  herbivores, 39
  latency, 375
  nosocomial infections, 481
  occupational infections, 274
  outdoor leisure and, 318
  rodents, 47
  terrestrial biomes, 109
  ticks, 70–71
  travel-associated, 413
  urban environment and, 136
Babesia microti, 107
Babesia ovis, 34
Baby care and toys, 141
Bacillus
  description of genus, 509
Bacillus anthracis
  air in buildings and, 128
  animal-derived foods and, 160, 162
  bovids, 24
  camelids, 34
  cats, 20
  clothing and, 142
  description, 509
  dogs, 15
  equids, 33

  flies and, 72
  herbivores, 39
  on objects, 142
  occupational infections, 248, 251, 260, 270–271, 286, 291, 301
  pigs, 30
  terrestrial biomes, 106
  transported animals and goods, 430, 435
  travel-associated, 416
Bacillus cereus
  animal-derived foods and, 152, 153, 161
  catering and restaurant-associated, 308
  description, 509
  drinking water-associated, 196, 198
  food-borne illness and, 145
  injection drug use and, 332
  long-term care and, 235
  nosocomial infections, 452
  plant-derived foods and, 176, 180, 182, 185
  school-associated, 362
Bacillus subtilis, 176
Bacteremia, 471–473
Bacteria. *See also specific bacteria*
  animal-derived foods and, 150–169, 171–172
  avian, 56–60
  bovid, 21–27
  from bowel, 343–344
  from breast milk, 391
  camelid, 34–35
  carnivore, 40–42
  cat, 18–21
  chiropteran, 55
  community-acquired, 377–383, 386–387, 389–391
  dam-related, 126–127
  day care-associated, 354–358
  dog, 13, 14, 15–16, 17, 18
  domicile-associated
    human regular, 209–214
    human substandard, 214–217, 219–222
  drinking water-associated, 195–199, 201–203
  dust, 117
  equid, 31–33
  finished food products and, 188–189
  fish, 61
  flies and, 72
  food-borne illness and, 145–147
  freshwater habitats and floods, 93–94, 96–97
  herbivore, 38–40
  homeless persons and, 223–225
  hotels and, 242–244
  human travel and, 396–400, 402–409, 412–422, 424–425
  intrauterine infections, 386–387
  lagomorph, 49–51
  latent, 374
  leisure and lifestyle-associated, 305–313, 315–325, 327–333

long-term care and, 234–237
marine habitat, 90–91
minorities and, 366–370
mosquitoes and, 75
from nose, mouth, and throat, 340–342
nosocomial infections
    invasive procedures, 468–477, 481, 484–485, 487–494
    noninvasive procedures, 442–443, 446–449, 451–454, 456–464
occupational infections, 248–253, 255–257, 259–263, 265–266, 269–276, 278–281, 286–289, 291–293, 295–301
in orphans and adoptees, 231–232
peripartal infections of neonates, 389–390
plant-derived foods and, 176–180, 182–186
porcine, 28, 30–31
prisons and, 238–241
relief camps and, 226–229
reptile and amphibian, 61
rodent, 43–44, 46–49
sandflies and, 81
sanitation and, 129–131
school-associated, 360–364
seasons and, 120–122, 124
simian, 51–52
from skin, 345
soil and plants, 98–100
taxonomic overview, 497–498
terrestrial biomes, 102, 105–114
ticks and, 69–70
transfusion-associated infections, 481
transported animals and goods, 428–431, 433–435
urban environment and, 132–133, 135, 137–138
from urogenital tract, 346–347
utensils and belongings, 139–142
Bacteriuria, 447
Bacteroides, 509
Balamuthia, 509
Balantidium coli
  description, 509–510
  domicile-associated, human substandard, 217
  freshwater habitats and floods, 95
Balantidium hominis, 28
Barmah forest virus (BFV), 504
Bartonella
  cats, 20
  description of genus, 510
  dogs, 15
  fleas, 71
  herbivores, 39
  homeless persons and, 224
  injection drug use and, 331
  lice and, 85
  occupational infections, 271
  outdoor leisure and, 317
  rodents, 46
  ticks and, 69
  urban environment and, 135

Bartonella alsatica, 50
Bartonella bacilliformis
  description, 510
  sandflies and, 81–82
Bartonella henselae, 510
Bartonella quintana
  description, 510
  latency, 374
  occupational infections, 259
  relief camps and, 228
Basidiobolus, 510
Bats, 53–55
  droplet-air cluster, 54
  environmental cluster, 55
  feces-food cluster, 54
  migrating and transported, 428
  rabies, 9, 54
  zoonoses, 54
  zoonotic cluster, 54–55
Baylisascaris procyonis
  description, 510
  lagomorphs, 50
Bedbugs, 82–83, 140, 432
Bedding, 139–140
Beef meat, 159–160
Bermejo virus, 536
Betaretrovirus, 510
Beverages. *See* Drinking water and beverages
Bioproducts, 455–456
Biosafety levels for laboratory work, 284
Birds, 55–60
  droplet-air cluster, 55–57
  feces-food cluster, 57–58
  migrating and transported, 427–428
  skin-blood cluster, 60
  ticks on, 432
  zoonoses, 55
  zoonotic cluster, 58–60
Bites, human, 320
Bivalves, 170–172
BK virus
  latency, 373
  nosocomial infections, 486
Bladder catheters and UTIs, 447–448
Blastocystis hominis
  bovids, 23
  day care-associated, 357
  description, 510–511
  long-term care and, 236
  in orphans and adoptees, 231
  travel-associated, 409
Blastomyces dermatitidis
  description, 511
  dust and, 117
  freshwater habitats and floods, 93
  latency, 374
  occupational infections, 265, 288
  travel-associated, 417
Blood gas analyzers, 446
Blood samplings, infections from, 470
Boar. *See* Pigs
Body care, 140–141
Bordetella
  description of genus, 511–512

Bordetella bronchiseptica
  description, 511
  nosocomial infections, 456
Bordetella parapertussis
  description, 511
  minority-associated, 366
Bordetella pertussis
  description, 511–512
  domicile-associated, human substandard, 215
  long-term care and, 234
  from nose, mouth, and throat, 340
  nosocomial infections, 459
  occupational infections, 252, 255, 301
  in orphans and adoptees, 231
  school-associated, 360
  travel-associated, 405
  urban environment and, 132
Bornavirus
  camelids, 34
  description, 512
Borrelia. *See also* Louse-borne relapsing fever (LBRF); Tick-borne relapsing fever (TBRF)
  description of genus, 512–513
  latency, 374
Borrelia burgdorferi
  birds, 59
  description, 512
  dogs, 15
  domicile-associated, human regular, 212
  flies and, 72
  herbivores, 39
  latency, 374
  occupational infections, 259, 269–270
  outdoor leisure and, 317–318
  rodents, 46
  seasons and, 122
  terrestrial biomes, 105
  ticks, 69–70
  urban environment and, 135
Borrelia duttoni
  description, 513
  domicile-associated, human substandard, 219
  latency, 374
Borrelia hermsii
  description, 398
  travel-associated, 398
Borrelia recurrentis
  description, 512–513
  homeless persons and, 224–225
  occupational infections, 291
  relief camps and, 228
  travel-associated, 412
Bottled and mineral waters, 194–195
Bovids, domestic, 21–27
  droplet-air cluster, 21–22
  environmental cluster, 26
  feces-food cluster, 22–23
  rabies, 24
  skin-blood cluster, 26–27
  zoonoses, 21
  zoonotic cluster, 23–26

Bovine spongiform encephalopathy (BSE)
    description, 22, 564
    transported animals and goods, 435
Bowel, agents from, 342–344
Breast implants, 492
Breast milk, 390–391
Bronchoscopy, 446–447
Brucella
    animal-derived foods and, 150, 153–154, 160
    bovids, 24–25
    cats, 20
    description of genus, 513
    dogs, 15
    dust and, 117
    equids, 33
    herbivores, 39
    intrauterine infections, 386
    latency, 374
    nosocomial infections, 451, 456
    occupational infections, 260, 271, 291
    pigs, 30
    rodents, 46
    transported animals and goods, 430
    travel-associated, 412, 422
Brucella melitensis
    camelids, 34
    seasons and, 122
Brucella suis, 50
Brugia malayi
    description, 513
    occupational infections, 261, 274
    terrestrial biomes, 104, 110
Bugs, nocturnal, 82–83
Buildings, sanitation, and wastewater, 128–132
Burkholderia
    description of genus, 514
    outdoor leisure and, 318
    seasons and, 124
Burkholderia cepacia
    description, 514
    nosocomial infections, 451, 452–453, 461
Burkholderia mallei
    description, 514
    equids, 33
    occupational infections, 292
Burkholderia pseudomallei
    bovids, 26
    description, 514
    drinking water-associated, 202
    dust and, 117
    freshwater habitats and floods, 96
    latency, 374
    nosocomial infections, 453, 461
    occupational infections, 261–262, 274, 292–293
    soil and plants, 99
    transported animals and goods, 430, 435
    travel-associated, 414, 424

C
Cache Valley virus, 557
Caliciviruses. *See* Norovirus

Camelids
    droplet-air cluster, 34
    environmental cluster, 35
    feces-food cluster, 34
    skin-blood cluster, 35
    zoonoses, 34
    zoonotic cluster, 34–35
Campylobacter
    animal-derived foods and, 150, 153, 158, 160, 161
    birds, 57
    bovids, 22
    from bowel, 343
    catering and restaurant-associated, 308
    cats, 19
    community-acquired, 379
    description of genus, 514
    dogs, 14
    domicile-associated, human regular, 211
    domicile-associated, human sub-standard, 217
    drinking water-associated, 195, 198, 202
    fairs and, 306
    food-borne illness and, 146
    freshwater habitats and floods, 94
    homosexual males and, 327
    hotels and, 244
    indoor leisure and, 322
    long-term care and, 235
    marine habitat, 90
    occupational infections, 256–257, 266, 278–279, 289
    outdoor leisure and, 315
    pigs, 28
    plant-derived foods and, 180
    prisons and, 239
    school-associated, 363
    terrestrial biomes, 108, 114
    travel-associated, 408
Candida
    babies and, 141
    from bowel, 344
    description of genus, 514–515
    long-term care and, 237
    minority-associated, 370
    from nose, mouth, and throat, 342
    nosocomial infections, 455, 464, 472, 473, 474, 486
    occupational infections, 296
    from skin, 345
    travel-associated, 398
    from urogenital tract, 347
Candida albicans
    description, 514–515
    nosocomial infections, 443, 448
    peripartal infections of neonates, 390
Candida parapsilosis, 515
Capillaria
    description of genus, 515
Capillaria hepatica
    description, 515
    occupational infections, 267
Capillaria philippensis
    birds, 58

description, 515
    transported animals and goods, 429
Capnocytophaga, 515
Cardiobacterium, 515
Cardiovascular implants, 490
Cardiovirus, 515
Carnivores, 40–42
    droplet-air cluster, 40
    environmental cluster, 42
    feces-food cluster, 40–41
    rabies, 41
    SARS-CoV, 41
    skin-blood cluster, 42
    zoonoses, 40
    zoonotic cluster, 41–42
Carpets, 142
Carriage. *See* Colonization, carriage, and contact
Catered events and restaurants, 307–310
    droplet-air cluster, 307
    feces-food cluster, 307–309
    skin-blood cluster, 309–310
Catering, 276–281
    droplet-air cluster, 277
    feces-food cluster, 277–280
    skin-blood cluster, 280–281
Cats, 18–21
    droplet-air cluster, 18
    environmental cluster, 20–21
    feces-food cluster, 18–19
    rabies, 9, 19–20
    skin-blood cluster, 21
    zoonoses, 18
    zoonotic cluster, 19–20
Caves, 115–116
Cephalopods, 172–173
Cercarial dermatitis, 97
Cerebrospinal fluid shunts, 491
Cestodes. *See* Helminths
Chagas disease. *See Trypanosoma cruzi*
Chandipura virus, 587
Cheese, 153–155
Chikungunya virus (CHIKV)
    occupational infections, 291
    travel-associated, 418, 422
    urban environment and, 134
Chiropterans. *See* Bats
Chlamydia trachomatis
    clothing and, 142
    community-acquired, 382
    description, 516
    domicile-associated, human sub-standard, 219
    flies and, 72
    homosexual males and, 328, 329
    minority-associated, 369–370
    nosocomial infections, 492
    occupational infections, 263, 295, 301
    peripartal infections of neonates, 389
    pools and, 313
    prisons and, 241
    prostitution and, 324
    terrestrial biomes, 111, 112
    travel-associated, 416, 425

urban environment and, 138
from urogenital tract, 346
Chlamydophila
  bovids, 26
  description of genus, 516–517
Chlamydophila abortus, 516
Chlamydophila pneumoniae
  community-acquired, 378
  description, 516–517
  domicile-associated, human regular, 209
  injection drug use and, 330
  long-term care and, 234
  from nose, mouth, and throat, 340
  occupational infections, 252, 255–256, 287
  outdoor leisure and, 315
  school-associated, 361
Chlamydophila psittaci
  birds, 59–60
  description, 516–517
  domicile-associated, human regular, 212
  occupational infections, 271–272, 291
  transported animals and goods, 430
Chromomycosis
  indoor leisure and, 322
  occupational infections, 275
Chronic wasting disease, 38, 564
Chrysops, 72
Cimex, 82–83
  bedding and, 140
  relief camps and, 229
  transport of, 432
Cities, 132–138
  droplet-air cluster, 132–133
  environmental cluster, 137–138
  feces-food cluster, 133–134
  zoonotic cluster, 134–137
Citrobacter
  from breast milk, 391
  description of genus, 517
Cladophialophora, 517
Cladosporium, 517
Cleaning and waste work, 296–299
  droplet-air cluster, 296–297
  environmental cluster, 298
  feces-food cluster, 297–298
  skin-blood cluster, 298–299
  zoonotic cluster, 298
Clerk, class, and sales work, 300–301
  droplet-air cluster, 300–301
  skin-blood cluster, 301
  zoonotic cluster, 301
Clonorchis
  description of genus, 517
  fish, 62
  travel-associated, 422
Clonorchis sinensis
  animal-derived foods and, 168
  description, 517
  domicile-associated, human substandard, 217
  latency, 375
Clostridium
  birds, 57
  description of genus, 517–519

injection drug use and, 332
long-term care and, 235
nosocomial infections, 477, 487
soil and plants, 98
Clostridium botulinum
  animal-derived foods and, 155, 160, 162, 165, 167, 169, 172
  catering and restaurant-associated, 308
  description, 517–518
  dust and, 117
  finished food products and, 189
  food-borne illness and, 147
  injection drug use and, 332
  marine habitat, 90
  minority-associated, 367
  plant-derived foods and, 178–179, 185–186
  seasons and, 120
  transported animals and goods, 431, 433
  travel-associated, 397, 403
Clostridium difficile
  from bowel, 343
  community-acquired, 379
  description, 518
  nosocomial infections, 442, 457–458, 461, 463–464
  occupational infections, 289
  travel-associated, 397
Clostridium perfringens
  animal-derived foods and, 159, 161, 167
  catering and restaurant-associated, 308
  description, 518
  finished food products and, 189
  food-borne illness and, 146
  minority-associated, 367
  outdoor leisure and, 315–316
  plant-derived foods and, 180
  prisons and, 239
  school-associated, 362–363
Clostridium tetani
  animal bites, 9–10
  bovids, 26
  description, 518–519
  domicile-associated, human regular, 213
  equids, 33
  injection drug use and, 332
  minority-associated, 368
  nosocomial infections, 456, 469, 471
  occupational infections, 250, 274–275, 298
  outdoor leisure and, 318
  peripartal infections of neonates, 389–390
  soil and plants, 99
  travel-associated, 424
Clothes, 142
Coccidioides immitis
  description, 519
  domicile-associated, human regular, 210
  dust and, 118
  occupational infections, 249, 256, 265, 288
  seasons and, 121
  travel-associated, 406
Cochlear implants, 491

Cochliomyia hominivorax, 432
Cold-weather peaks, 119–121
Colonization, carriage, and contact, 335–347
  agents by site, 337–339
    bowel, 342–344
    nose, mouth, and throat, 339–342
    skin, 344–345
    urogenital tract, 345–347
  cohorting, 337
  prevention, 336–337
  quarantine, 337, 339
Colorado tick fever virus (CTFV)
  description, 519
  occupational infections, 290
Coltivirus
  description, 519
  lagomorphs, 50
  rodents, 45
  ticks, 69
Community-acquired syndromes, 376–391
  diarrhea, 378–380
  mother-to-child transmission, 384–391
  pneumonia, 376–378
  sexually transmitted infections, 380–384
Construction and mining, 248–251
  droplet-air cluster, 248–249
  environmental cluster, 250–251
  feces-food cluster, 249
  skin-blood cluster, 251
  zoonotic cluster, 250
Contact. *See* Colonization, carriage, and contact
Cooking utensils, 138–139
Coquillettidia, 80
Cornea, 487
Coronavirus, 519–520
Corynebacterium
  bovids, 26
  description of genus, 520
Corynebacterium diphtheriae
  description, 520
  domicile-associated, human substandard, 215
  homeless persons and, 223
  injection drug use and, 330
  from nose, mouth, and throat, 340
  nosocomial infections, 456
  occupational infections, 255, 286–287
  relief camps and, 226
  school-associated, 360
  from skin, 345
  travel-associated, 399, 405–406, 415, 420
  urban environment and, 133
Corynebacterium jeikeium, 520
Corynebacterium pseudotuberculosis, 520
Corynebacterium ulcerans
  description, 520
  rodents, 49
Cosmetic products, 451–452
Cosmetic procedures, infections from, 467–469
Cowpox virus (CPXV)
  description, 557

Cowpox virus *(continued)*
   occupational infections, 269
   rodents, 48
Coxiella burnetii
   animal-derived foods and, 150–151
   birds, 60
   bovids, 25
   camelids, 34
   cats, 20
   clothing and, 142
   community-acquired, 378
   description, 520–521
   dogs, 15–16
   domicile-associated, human regular, 213
   dust and, 117
   equids, 33
   herbivores, 39
   homeless persons and, 223
   indoor leisure and, 321
   lagomorphs, 50
   occupational infections, 252, 260, 272–273, 291, 301
   outdoor leisure and, 318
   pigs, 30
   rodents, 46
   seasons and, 122
   terrestrial biomes, 106
   ticks, 70
   travel-associated, 398, 412, 422
   urban environment and, 133
Cream, ice cream, yogurt, and butter, 155–156
Creutzfeldt-Jakob disease
   description, 564–565
   latency, 372–373
   nosocomial infections, 475, 478
Crimean-Congo hemorrhagic fever virus (CCHFV)
   birds, 58
   bovids, 15
   camelids, 34
   description, 553
   dogs, 15
   domicile-associated, human sub-standard, 218
   fairs and, 306
   herbivores, 38
   nosocomial infections, 465
   occupational infections, 258, 267, 290
   outdoor leisure and, 317
   transported animals and goods, 429
   urban environment and, 134
Crop-and-herd work, 264–276
   droplet-air cluster, 264–265
   environmental cluster, 274–276
   feces-food cluster, 265–267
   skin-blood cluster, 276
   zoonotic cluster, 267–274
Crustaceans, 169–170
Cryptococcus neoformans
   birds, 56
   description, 521
   domicile-associated, human regular, 210
   dust and, 118
   latency, 374
   nosocomial infections, 484
   occupational infections, 249, 265, 288
   terrestrial biomes, 102
   transported animals and goods, 433
   urban environment and, 133
Cryptosporidium
   animal-derived foods and, 152, 172
   birds, 58
   bovids, 23
   catering and restaurant-associated, 309
   description of genus, 521–522
   domicile-associated, human regular, 212
   domicile-associated, human sub-standard, 217
   drinking water-associated, 195, 196, 199
   fairs and, 306
   freshwater habitats and floods, 95
   hotels and, 244
   marine habitat, 91
   minority-associated, 367
   occupational infections, 257, 266, 280
   in orphans and adoptees, 231
   outdoor leisure and, 316
   pigs, 28–29
   plant-derived foods and, 180–181
   pools and, 312
   school-associated, 363
   soil and plants, 99
   terrestrial biomes, 113
   travel-associated, 409
Cryptosporidium canis, 14
Cryptosporidium felis, 19
Cryptosporidium hominis
   from bowel, 344
   community-acquired, 380
   day care-associated, 357
   homosexual males and, 327–328
Cryptosporidium muris, 44
Cryptosporidium parvum
   animal-derived foods and, 158
   baby care and toys, 141
   drinking water-associated, 203
   herbivores, 38
   long-term care and, 236
   urban environment and, 134
Culex, 78–80, 432
Culicoides (midges), 76
Culiseta, 80
Cunninghamella, 521
Curvularia, 452
Cutaneous larva migrans, 414–415
Cyclospora
   description of genus, 522
   dogs, 14
   occupational infections, 257, 266
   plant-derived foods and, 181
Cyclospora cayetanensis
   description, 522
   drinking water-associated, 199, 203
   occupational infections, 280
   plant-derived foods and, 184
   soil and plants, 99
   transported animals and goods, 434
   travel-associated, 409
Cystoscopy, 447
Cytomegalovirus (CMV)
   from breast milk, 391
   community-acquired, 383
   day care-associated, 357–358
   description, 522
   domicile-associated, human regular, 213
   homosexual males and, 329
   intrauterine infections, 385
   latency, 373
   from nose, mouth, and throat, 339
   nosocomial infections, 485–486, 487
   occupational infections, 294, 300
   in orphans and adoptees, 232
   peripartal infections of neonates, 388
   prisons and, 240
   transfusion-transmitted agents, 479–480
   travel-associated, 415
   from urogenital tract, 345–346

D

Dairy products
   cheese, 153–155
   cream, ice cream, yogurt, and butter, 155–156
   dried and formula milk, 153
   milk chocolate, 156
   pasteurized milk, 152
   raw milk, 149–152
Dams and irrigation, 125–128
Day care, 353–358
   droplet-air cluster, 354–355
   environmental cluster, 357
   feces-food cluster, 355–357
   skin-blood cluster, 357–358
Defibrillators, 490
Deltaretrovirus, 522
Dengue virus (DENV)
   domicile-associated, human sub-standard, 218
   fairs and, 306
   minority-associated, 368
   occupational infections, 250, 258, 290
   outdoor leisure and, 317
   relief camps and, 228
   terrestrial biomes, 108
   travel-associated, 410–411, 418, 422
   urban environment and, 134
Dental care, infections from, 470
Dental instruments, 445
Dermacentor, 67
Dermatophytes
   bovid, 27
   camelid, 35
   domicile-associated, human sub-standard, 222
   equid, 33–34
   homeless persons and, 225
   lagomorph, 51
   nosocomial infections, 443
   occupational infections, 263–264, 276
   pools and, 313
   porcine, 31
   rodent, 49

from skin, 345
travel-associated, 425
Desert oases, 111–112
Deserts, 110–111
Detention facilities, 237–241
 droplet-air cluster, 238–239
 environmental cluster, 240
 feces-food cluster, 239–240
 skin-blood cluster, 240–241
Diagnostic workup, 3–4
Dialysers, 446
Dialysis, 492–494
 hemodialysis, 492–493
 peritoneal dialysis, 493–494
Diarrhea
 acute food-borne, 146–147
 community-acquired, 378–380
 hospital-acquired, 457
 travel-associated, 407
Dicrocoelium, 522
Dientamoeba fragilis
 description, 522–523
 in orphans and adoptees, 231
 travel-associated, 409
Diphyllobothrium
 animal-derived foods and, 168
 carnivores, 40–41
 description of genus, 523
 drinking water-associated, 204
 fish, 62–63
 terrestrial biomes, 114
 transported animals and goods, 434
 travel-associated, 422
Dipylidium caninum
 carnivores, 42
 description, 523
 dogs, 16
Dirofilaria
 carnivores, 42
 description of genus, 523
 dogs, 17
Dirofilaria immitis
 description, 523
 minority-associated, 368
 mosquitoes and, 75
Disposable materials, 443–444
Dobrava virus, 536
Dogs, 13–18
 droplet-air cluster, 13–14
 environmental cluster, 17–18
 feces-food cluster, 14–15
 rabies, 8–9, 15
 skin-blood cluster, 18
 zoonoses, 13
 zoonotic cluster, 15–17
Domestic mammals, 13–35. *See also specific species*
Domiciles
 human regular
  droplet-air cluster, 207–210
  environmental cluster, 213–214
  feces-food cluster, 210–212
  zoonotic cluster, 212–213
 human substandard
  droplet-air cluster, 214–216

environmental cluster, 221–222
feces-food cluster, 216–218
skin-blood cluster, 222–223
zoonotic cluster, 218–221
Donkeys. *See* Equids
Dracunculus, 523
Drinking water and beverages, 193–204
Droplet-air cluster
 adult age and, 351–352
 agents, 2–3
 avian, 55–57
 bovine, 21–22
 camelid, 34
 canine, 13–14
 carnivore, 40
 catering, 277, 307
 chiropteran, 54
 cleaning and waste work, 296–297
 clerk, class, and sales work, 300–301
 cold-weather peaks, 120
 construction and mining, 248–249
 crop-and-herd work, 264–265
 day care, 354–355
 detention facilities, 238–239
 domiciles, human regular, 207–210
 domiciles, human substandard, 214–216
 elderly and, 352
 equine, 31
 fairs, 304–305
 feline, 18
 freshwater habitats and floods, 93
 hands, transmission by, 441–442
 health-and-laboratory work, 282–288
 herbivore, 38
 homeless persons, 223–224
 homosexual men, 327–328
 hotels, 242–243
 indoor leisure, 321–322
 injection drug use, 330–331
 islands, 108
 lagomorph, 49
 long-term care facilities, 233–234
 manufacture and maintenance work, 251–252
 minorities and, 365–367
 orphans and adoptees, 230–231
 outdoor leisure, 314–315
 pools and spas, 311
 porcine, 27–28
 preschool age and, 350
 rainy seasons, 123
 relief camps, 226–227
 rodent, 43
 school age and, 351
 school-associated, 359–362
 simian, 51
 soil and plants, 98
 stem cell recipients and, 488
 transfusion-transmitted agents, 478–479
 transportation work, 299
 transported goods and, 433
 travel-associated, 395–397, 399, 401–402, 405–407, 416–417, 420–421
 uniformed services, 254–256
 urban, 132–133

vertebrates, migrating and transported, 428
 warm-weather peaks, 121
Drug use. *See* Injection drug use
Drugs, 449–458
 antimicrobials and nosocomial diarrhea, 457–458
 bioproducts, 455–456
 cosmetic products, 451–452
 experimental, 452
 fake, 450
 herbal and alternative, 450–451
 illicit, 450
 parenteral nutrition and formula feed, 454–455
 solutions, disinfectants, and multidose vials, 452–454
Dura mater, 487
Dust and winds, 116–118
Dust mites, 140

E

Eastern equine encephalitis virus (EEEV)
 birds, 58
 description, 504
 equids, 32
 occupational infections, 258
Ebola virus
 description, 529–530
 domicile-associated, human substandard, 218
 herbivores, 38
 nosocomial infections, 465
 occupational infections, 250, 268, 298
Echinococcus
 bovids, 26
 camelids, 34–35
 carnivores, 42
 description of genus, 523–524
 dogs, 17
 latency, 376
 occupational infections, 292
 pigs, 29
 plant-derived foods and, 181
 terrestrial biomes, 109–110, 114–115
 urban environment and, 137
Echinococcus granulosus
 description, 524
 domicile-associated, human substandard, 221
 drinking water-associated, 204
 dust and, 118
 fairs and, 306
 latency, 376
 minority-associated, 368
 occupational infections, 274, 298
 terrestrial biomes, 107
 transported animals and goods, 430
 travel-associated, 424
Echinococcus multilocularis
 description, 524
 latency, 376
 occupational infections, 274
 rodents, 48

876 INDEX

Echinococcus multilocularis (continued)
  transported animals and goods, 430
Echinostoma
  animal-derived foods and, 169–170, 173
  description of genus, 524
Ectoparasites, 83–85. *See also specific parasites*
  avian, 60
  bovid, 27
  cat, 21
  dog, 18
  domicile-associated, human substandard, 221
  minorities and, 370
  minority-associated, 370
  rodent, 49
  from skin, 345
  utensils and belongings, 140–142
Eggs and egg products, 156–157
Ehrlichia
  description of genus, 524–525
  dogs, 16
Ehrlichia canis, 16, 524
Ehrlichia chaffeensis
  description, 524–525
  herbivores, 39
  occupational infections, 259, 270
  outdoor leisure and, 318
  seasons and, 122
  ticks, 70
Ehrlichia ewingii, 525
Eikenella, 525
Electrodes, nosocomial infections and, 444
Elevation, limits of human-infective agents, 113
Encephalitozoon cuniculi, 484–485
Encephalomyocarditis virus, 269
Endocarditis, 469, 470, 490
Endogenous viruses, 525
Endoscopy, 446
Entamoeba
  description of genus, 525
  dogs, 14
  plant-derived foods and, 181
Entamoeba histolytica
  description, 525
  domicile-associated, human regular, 212
  drinking water-associated, 199, 204
  homosexual males and, 328
  latency, 375
  occupational infections, 298
  travel-associated, 421–422
Entamoeba histolytica/dispar
  from bowel, 344
  community-acquired, 380
  day care-associated, 357
  domicile-associated, human substandard, 217
  hotels and, 244
  long-term care and, 236
  occupational infections, 257, 280, 299
  in orphans and adoptees, 232
  travel-associated, 409–410
Enteritis, acute food-borne, 146–147

Enterobacter
  antimicrobial resistance, 494
  description of genus, 525–526
Enterobacter agglomerans, 453
Enterobacter cloacae
  description, 525–526
  nosocomial infections, 453
  occupational infections, 289
Enterobacter sakazakii
  animal-derived foods and, 153
  birds, 57
  description, 526
  plant-derived foods and, 176
Enterobius
  description of genus, 526
  domicile-associated, human substandard, 222
Enterobius vermicularis
  day care-associated, 358
  description, 526
  domicile-associated, human regular, 214
  long-term care and, 237
  in orphans and adoptees, 232
  sanitation and, 130
  school-associated, 364
Enterococcus
  animal-derived foods and, 158
  antimicrobial resistance, 494
  birds, 57
  from bowel, 343
  description of genus, 526
  long-term care and, 235
  nosocomial infections, 442, 449, 472
  occupational infections, 289
  travel-associated, 397
  utensils and belongings, 139
Enterovirus
  from breast milk, 391
  description, 526–527
  domicile-associated, human regular, 208–209
  drinking water-associated, 195, 201
  freshwater habitats and floods, 93
  indoor leisure and, 321
  marine habitat, 89
  from nose, mouth, and throat, 340
  occupational infections, 286
  outdoor leisure and, 314–315
  pools and, 311
  school-associated, 360
  seasons and, 121
Environmental cluster
  adult age and, 352
  agents, 3
  bovine, 26
  camelid, 35
  canine, 17–18
  carnivore, 42
  chiropteran, 55
  cleaning and waste work, 298
  construction and mining, 250–251
  crop-and-herd work, 274–276
  dam-related, 127
  day care, 357

  detention facilities, 240
  domiciles, human regular, 213–214
  domiciles, human substandard, 221–222
  elderly and, 352–353
  equine, 33
  feline, 20–21
  freshwater habitats and floods, 96–98
  hands, transmission by, 442
  health-and-laboratory work, 292–293
  herbivore, 40
  hotels, 245
  indoor leisure, 322
  injection drug use, 332
  islands, 110
  lagomorph, 50
  long-term care facilities, 236–237
  manufacture and maintenance work, 253
  minorities and, 368
  orphans and adoptees, 232
  outdoor leisure, 318–320
  pools and spas, 313
  porcine, 30–31
  preschool age and, 351
  rainy seasons, 124
  relief camps, 229–230
  rodent, 48
  school age and, 351
  school-associated, 364
  simian, 52–53
  soil and plants, 99–100
  stem cell recipients and, 488–489
  transportation work, 300
  transported goods and, 435
  travel-associated, 398, 414–415, 419, 424
  uniformed services, 261–262
  urban, 137–138
  vertebrates, migrating and transported, 430
  warm-weather peaks, 122–123
Environments
  exposure, 87–88
  human-made, 125–142
    buildings, sanitation, and wastewater, 128–132
    cities, 132–138
    dams and irrigation, 125–128
    utensils and belongings, 138–142
  natural, 89–124
    dust and winds, 116–118
    freshwater habitats and floods, 92–98
    marine habitats, 89–92
    seasons, 118–124
    soil and plants, 98–100
    terrestrial biomes, 100–116
Epidermophyton, 527
Epstein-Barr virus (EBV)
  domicile-associated, human regular, 209
  latency, 373
  from nose, mouth, and throat, 339
  nosocomial infections, 486
  occupational infections, 254, 286
  school-associated, 360
  terrestrial biomes, 110
  from urogenital tract, 345

Equids, 31–34
  droplet-air cluster, 31
  environmental cluster, 33
  feces-food cluster, 32
  rabies, 32
  skin-blood cluster, 33–34
  zoonoses, 31
  zoonotic cluster, 32–33
Erysipelothrix rhusiopathiae
  animal-derived foods and, 161
  birds, 60
  description, 527
  marine habitat, 91
  occupational infections, 252, 273
  pigs, 31
Erythrovirus, 527–528
Escherichia coli
  animal-derived foods and, 151, 152, 154, 159–160, 161, 162, 163, 165, 169
  baby care and toys, 141
  birds, 57
  bovids, 22
  from bowel, 343
  catering and restaurant-associated, 308
  community-acquired, 379–380
  description, 528–529
  dogs, 14
  domicile-associated, human regular, 211
  domicile-associated, human substandard, 217
  drinking water-associated, 195, 196, 198, 202
  enteroaggregative *E. coli* (EAEC), 528
  enterohemorrhagic *E. coli* (EHEC), 528
  enteroinvasive *E. coli* (EIEC), 528
  enteropathogenic *E. coli* (EPEC), 528–529
  enterotoxigenic *E. coli* (ETEC), 529
  equids, 32
  fairs and, 306
  finished food products and, 188–189
  food-borne illness and, 146
  freshwater habitats and floods, 94
  herbivores, 38
  hotels and, 244
  long-term care and, 235–236
  marine habitat, 90
  occupational infections, 257, 266, 279, 289
  outdoor leisure and, 316
  pigs, 28
  plant-derived foods and, 176, 179, 182, 183, 185
  pools and, 312
  prisons and, 239
  school-associated, 363
  soil and plants, 98
  terrestrial biomes, 108
  transported animals and goods, 433
  travel-associated, 397, 400, 408
  utensils and belongings, 139
European bat lyssavirus, 54
Exophiala
  description of genus, 529
  nosocomial infections, 463

Expatriates, 416–419
Exposure checklist, 593–595
Exposure history
  food, 145
  human community, 336
  nosocomial infections, 438
  travel, 394
Eye care, 140, 141

F

Fairs and mass gatherings, 303–307
  droplet-air cluster, 304–305
  feces-food cluster, 305–306
  skin-blood cluster, 307
  zoonotic cluster, 306–307
Fasciola
  bovids, 23
  description of genus, 529
  terrestrial biomes, 112
Fasciola hepatica
  description, 529
  domicile-associated, human regular, 212
  drinking water-associated, 204
  plant-derived foods and, 181–182
  transported animals and goods, 434
  travel-associated, 397, 410
Fasciolopsis buskii
  description, 529
  drinking water-associated, 204
  occupational infections, 267
  plant-derived foods and, 182
Febrile illness, food-borne, 147–148
Feces-food cluster
  adult age and, 352
  agents, 3
  avian, 57–58
  bovine, 22–23
  camelid, 34
  canine, 14–15
  carnivore, 40–41
  catering, 277–280, 307–309
  chiropteran, 54
  cleaning and waste work, 297–298
  cold-weather peaks, 120
  construction and mining, 249
  crop-and-herd work, 265–267
  dam-related, 126
  day care, 355–357
  detention facilities, 239–240
  domiciles, human regular, 210–212
  domiciles, human substandard, 216–218
  elderly and, 352
  equine, 32
  fairs, 305–306
  feline, 18–19
  freshwater habitats and floods, 93–95
  hands, transmission by, 442
  health-and-laboratory work, 288–290
  herbivore, 38
  homeless persons, 224
  hotels, 243–245
  indoor leisure, 322
  injection drug use, 331

  islands, 108
  lagomorph, 49
  long-term care facilities, 234–236
  manufacture and maintenance work, 252
  marine habitats, 89–91
  minorities and, 367–368
  orphans and adoptees, 231–232
  outdoor leisure, 315–317
  pools and spas, 311–312
  porcine, 28–30
  preschool age and, 350–351
  rainy seasons, 123
  relief camps, 227–228
  rodent, 43–44
  school age and, 351
  school-associated, 362–363
  simian, 51
  soil and plants, 98–99
  stem cell recipients and, 488
  transfusion-transmitted agents, 479
  transportation work, 299
  transported goods and, 433–434
  travel-associated, 397, 399–400, 402–403, 407–410, 417, 421–422
  uniformed services, 256–258
  urban, 133–134
  vertebrates, migrating and transported, 428–429
  warm-weather peaks, 121
Feline retroviruses, 269
Female prostitution, 323–326
Feminine care, 141
Filovirus
  bats, 54
  description, 529–530
  herbivores, 38
  nosocomial infections, 465
  occupational infections, 268, 290
  primates, 52
  rodents, 45
Fish, 61–63
  finished food products and, 189–191
  food-borne illness, 167–169
  migrating and transported, 427
  trauma, agents of, 10–11
Flavivirus
  bats, 54
  description, 530–533
  lagomorphs, 50
  mosquitoes and, 74–75, 77, 79
  nosocomial infections, 466
  occupational infections, 267–268, 290, 293
  outdoor leisure and, 317
  primates, 52
  rodents, 45
  terrestrial biomes, 114
  ticks, 69
Fleas
  overview, 71
  transport from ships and aircraft, 432
Flies
  larvae, 83–84
  overview, 72–73
  transport from ships and aircraft, 432

Fonsecaea pedrosoi
   description, 533
   terrestrial biomes, 102
Foods, 143–204
   acute abdominal infections, 147
   acute and subacute food-borne neurosyndromes, 147
   acute diarrhea and enteritis, 146–147
   acute vomiting, gastritis, and food poisoning, 144–146
   animal-derived, 149–173
      eggs and egg products, 156–157
      meat and meat products, 159–166
      milk and dairy products, 149–156
      poultry, 157–159
      seafood, fish, and molluscs, 166–173
   causality of food-borne illness, 143–144
   drinking water and beverages, 193–204
      bottled and mineral waters, 194–195
      ice cubes, 195–196
      juices, 196
      private and low-income water supplies, 200–204
      soft drinks, 197
      tap water, municipal high-income, 197–200
   exposure history, 145
   finished, 187–191
      African cuisines, 189
      American cuisines, 189–190
      Asian cuisines, 190–191
      European cuisines, 191
      international cuisine, 188–189
      snacks and sandwiches, 187–188
   food-borne febrile illness, 147–148
   impact of food-borne illness, 143
   incubation period, 144
   outbreaks, food-borne, 148
   plant-derived, 175–186
      cereals, pasta, bakery, and sweets, 175–177
      vegetables, salads, fruits, and spices, 177–186
   prevention of food-borne illness, 144
Foot-and-mouth disease virus
   animal-derived foods and, 150
   occupational infections, 298
   transported animals and goods, 429
   travel-associated, 397
Formula milk, 153
Francisella tularensis
   animal bites, 10
   animal-derived foods and, 162
   carnivores, 41
   description, 533
   dogs, 16
   drinking water-associated, 196, 202
   dust and, 117
   flies and, 72
   lagomorphs, 50
   mosquitoes and, 75
   occupational infections, 252–253, 260, 273, 291
   outdoor leisure and, 318
   rodents, 46

   seasons and, 122
   terrestrial biomes, 106, 114
   ticks, 70
   transported animals and goods, 430
Freezers, 446
Freshwater habitats and floods, 92–98
   droplet-air cluster, 93
   environmental cluster, 96–98
   feces-food cluster, 93–95
   risks, 92–93
   zoonotic cluster, 95–96
Fruits, 183–184
Fungi. *See also* Microsporidia; *specific fungal agents*
   animal-derived foods and, 154–155, 168
   avian, 56–58, 60
   bovid, 22, 23, 27
   from bowel, 344
   carnivore, 40
   cat, 18–21
   chiropteran, 54
   community-acquired, 378, 380, 387
   day care-associated, 358
   dog, 14–15, 17, 18
   domicile-associated, human regular, 210
   domicile-associated, human substandard, 222
   drinking water-associated, 199
   dust, 117–118
   equid, 31, 33–34
   flies and, 72
   freshwater habitats and floods, 93–94, 97
   homeless persons and, 225
   hotels and, 243
   human travel and, 397, 398, 406–407, 409, 414, 417, 421, 424–425
   intrauterine infections, 387
   lagomorph, 49, 51
   latent, 374–375
   leisure and lifestyle-associated, 312–315, 319, 322–323, 327
   long-term care and, 237
   minorities and, 367, 370
   from nose, mouth, and throat, 342
   nosocomial infections
      invasive procedures, 473–474, 477, 481, 484–486, 488–489
      noninvasive procedures, 442–443, 448–449, 452, 455, 460–461, 463–464
   occupational infections, 249, 251–252, 256, 263–266, 274–276, 288–289, 293, 296
   in orphans and adoptees, 231
   peripartal infections of neonates, 390
   plant-derived foods and, 184
   porcine, 28, 31
   prisons and, 239, 241
   rodent, 43, 44, 48, 49
   sanitation and, 130
   school-associated, 361–362, 365
   seasons and, 121
   simian, 51, 53
   from skin, 345
   soil and plants, 98, 100

   taxonomic overview, 498
   terrestrial biomes, 102, 105, 111, 116
   transfusion-associated infections, 481
   urban environment and, 133
   from urogenital tract, 347
   utensils and belongings, 140–142
Fusarium
   description, 533
   nosocomial infections, 463
Fusobacterium, 533–534

G

Gardnerella, 534
Gastritis, food-borne illness and, 144–146
Gastrocolonoscopy, 447
Gastropods, 172–173
GBV-C virus
   description, 534
   injection drug use and, 332
   nosocomial infections, 455, 493
   prisons and, 240
   prostitution and, 325
   transfusion-transmitted agents, 480
   from urogenital tract, 346
Genera, description of, 499–590
Geotrichum, 534
Giardia
   animal-derived foods and, 172
   bovids, 23
   from bowel, 344
   catering and restaurant-associated, 309
   cats, 19
   community-acquired, 380
   day care-associated, 357
   description of genus, 534
   dogs, 14
   domicile-associated, human regular, 212
   domicile-associated, human substandard, 217
   drinking water-associated, 199–200, 204
   finished food products and, 188
   freshwater habitats and floods, 95
   homosexual males and, 328
   hotels and, 244–245
   long-term care and, 236
   marine habitat, 91
   minority-associated, 367–368
   occupational infections, 280, 298
   in orphans and adoptees, 232
   outdoor leisure and, 316–317
   plant-derived foods and, 176, 181, 184
   pools and, 312
   rodents, 44
   sanitation and, 131
   school-associated, 363
   soil and plants, 99
   terrestrial biomes, 113
   travel-associated, 400, 410
   urban environment and, 133
Glossary, 601–606
Glossina, 72, 432
Gnathostoma
   animal-derived foods and, 168, 170
   birds, 58

description of genus, 534–535
drinking water-associated, 204
fish, 62
pigs, 29
transported animals and goods, 429
travel-associated, 410
Grasslands, 106–107
Ground beef, hamburgers, and corned beef, 163–164
Guanaco. *See* Camelids
Guanarito virus (GUAV), 268

H

Haemagogus, 80
Haemaphysalis, 67–68
Haemophilus
　description of genus, 535–536
Haemophilus ducreyi
　community-acquired, 383
　description, 535
　domicile-associated, human substandard, 222
　homosexual males and, 328
　prostitution and, 325
　travel-associated, 425
　urban environment and, 138
　from urogenital tract, 346
Haemophilus influenzae
　community-acquired, 378
　description, 535–536
　domicile-associated, human substandard, 215–216
　long-term care and, 234
　minority-associated, 366
　from nose, mouth, and throat, 340–341
　occupational infections, 287
　in orphans and adoptees, 231
　school-associated, 360
　terrestrial biomes, 108
Hair care, 141
Hands, transmission by, 441–443
　droplet-air cluster, 441–442
　environmental cluster, 442
　feces-food cluster, 442
　skin-blood cluster, 442
Hantaan virus, 536
Hantavirus
　cats, 19
　description, 536–537
　domicile-associated, human substandard, 218–219
　herbivores, 38
　homeless persons and, 224
　occupational infections, 258–259, 268, 290, 298
　outdoor leisure and, 317
　rodents, 43, 45
　terrestrial biomes, 106
　urban environment and, 134–135
Hard ticks. *See* Ticks, hard
Hartmannella, 537
Health-and-laboratory work, 281–296
　biosafety levels for laboratory work, 284
　droplet-air cluster, 282–288

environmental cluster, 292–293
feces-food cluster, 288–290
skin-blood cluster, 293–296
suggested measures on entry and after exposure, 283
zoonotic cluster, 290–292
Heart transplant recipients, infections in, 484
Heart valves, 489, 490
Helicobacter
　cats, 19
　description of genus, 537
　dogs, 14
　pigs, 28
Helicobacter pylori
　from bowel, 343
　description, 537
　domicile-associated, human regular, 211
　drinking water-associated, 202
　freshwater habitats and floods, 94
　latency, 374
　long-term care and, 236
　minority-associated, 367
　nosocomial infections, 447
　occupational infections, 257, 289, 297, 299
　terrestrial biomes, 114
　travel-associated, 408
Helminths. *See also specific species*
　animal-derived foods and, 160–164, 166, 168–170, 172–173
　avian, 58
　bovid, 23, 26
　from bowel, 344
　camelid, 34–35
　carnivore, 40–42
　cat, 19, 20
　community-acquired, 380
　dam-related, 126–127
　day care-associated, 357–358
　dog, 15, 16–18
　domicile-associated, human regular, 212, 214
　domicile-associated, human substandard, 217–218, 221–223
　drinking water-associated, 196, 204
　dust, 18
　equid, 32–33
　fish, 61–63
　flies and, 73
　freshwater habitats and floods, 95–98
　herbivore, 40
　human travel and, 397, 400, 410, 414–419, 422–425
　lagomorph, 50
　latent, 375–376
　leisure and lifestyle-associated, 309, 313, 317–320
　long-term care and, 236–237
　marine habitat, 91–92
　minorities and, 368, 370
　mosquitoes and, 78, 79–80
　nosocomial infections, 451, 482, 485, 489
　occupational infections, 249–251, 261–262, 267, 274, 276, 280, 290, 292, 293, 298

in orphans and adoptees, 232–233
plant-derived foods and, 181–182, 184, 186
porcine, 29–31
prisons and, 241
relief camps and, 228–230
rodent, 44, 48, 49
sanitation and, 130–132
school-associated, 363, 365
seasons and, 124
simian, 51–53
soil and plants, 99–100
taxonomic overview, 498
terrestrial biomes, 103–104, 106–110, 112, 114–115
transfusion-associated infections, 482
transported animals and goods, 429–430
urban environment and, 134, 137–138
utensils and belongings, 139–140
Hemodialysis, 492–493
Hemorrhagic fevers
　in hospitals, 464–466
　relief camps and, 228
　travel-associated, 403–404
Hendra virus, 537
Henipavirus
　bats, 55
　description, 537
Hepacivirus, 537
Hepatitis A virus (HAV)
　animal-derived foods and, 150, 164, 170
　from bowel, 342
　catering and restaurant-associated, 307
　community-acquired, 379
　dam-related, 126
　description, 538–539
　domicile-associated, human regular, 211
　domicile-associated, human substandard, 216
　drinking water-associated, 194, 196, 197, 201
　fairs and, 305
　finished food products and, 187
　freshwater habitats and floods, 93
　homosexual males and, 327
　hotels and, 243
　indoor leisure and, 322
　injection drug use and, 331
　long-term care and, 235
　marine habitat, 90
　minority-associated, 367
　nosocomial infections, 479
　occupational infections, 256, 265, 277–278, 288, 297, 299
　in orphans and adoptees, 231
　outdoor leisure and, 315
　plant-derived foods and, 176, 178, 183
　pools and, 311
　prisons and, 239
　relief camps and, 227
　sanitation and, 128
　school-associated, 362
　terrestrial biomes, 114
　transported animals and goods, 433
　travel-associated, 397, 407, 417

Hepatitis B virus (HBV)
  body acre and, 140
  community-acquired, 383
  day care-associated, 358
  description, 556–557
  domicile-associated, human regular, 213
  homeless persons and, 225
  homosexual males and, 329
  indoor leisure and, 322
  injection drug use and, 332
  latency, 373
  long-term care and, 237
  minority-associated, 369
  from nose, mouth, and throat, 339
  nosocomial infections, 452, 455, 456, 468–470, 475, 480, 486, 493
  occupational infections, 251, 262, 293–294, 298–299, 300
  in orphans and adoptees, 232
  outdoor leisure and, 319–320
  peripartal infections of neonates, 388–389
  prisons and, 240
  prostitution and, 325–326
  relief camps and, 229
  school-associated, 364
  terrestrial biomes, 114
  travel-associated, 415, 419, 424–425
Hepatitis C virus (HCV)
  body acre and, 140
  description, 537–538
  domicile-associated, human regular, 213
  homeless persons and, 225
  homosexual males and, 329
  indoor leisure and, 322
  injection drug use and, 332–333
  intrauterine infections, 385
  long-term care and, 237
  minority-associated, 369
  from nose, mouth, and throat, 339
  nosocomial infections, 447, 452, 455, 468–471, 475, 480, 486, 493
  occupational infections, 262–263, 300
  in orphans and adoptees, 232
  peripartal infections of neonates, 389
  prisons and, 240
  prostitution and, 325–326
  relief camps and, 229
  terrestrial biomes, 110, 114
  travel-associated, 419, 425
  from urogenital tract, 346
Hepatitis D virus (HDV)
  domicile-associated, human regular, 213
  domicile-associated, human substandard, 222
  injection drug use and, 333
Hepatitis E virus (HEV), 539
  animal-derived foods and, 150, 162
  from bowel, 342
  domicile-associated, human substandard, 216
  drinking water-associated, 201
  freshwater habitats and floods, 93–94
  long-term care and, 235
  nosocomial infections, 451, 479
  occupational infections, 256, 265–266, 278, 297
  outdoor leisure and, 315
  pigs, 28
  relief camps and, 227
  rodents, 43
  school-associated, 362
  travel-associated, 407, 417
Hepatitis G virus (HGV). *See* GBV-C virus
Hepatovirus, 538–539
Hepevirus, 539
Herbal and alternative drugs, 450–451
Herbivores, wild, 37–40
  droplet-air cluster, 38
  environmental cluster, 40
  feces-food cluster, 38
  zoonotic cluster, 38–40
Herd work. *See* Crop-and-herd work
Herpes simplex virus (HSV)
  community-acquired, 383
  day care-associated, 358
  description, 574
  domicile-associated, human regular, 214
  homosexual males and, 328
  indoor leisure and, 323
  latency, 373
  from nose, mouth, and throat, 340
  nosocomial infections, 486
  on objects, 142
  peripartal infections of neonates, 389
  prostitution and, 325
  school-associated, 364
  from urogenital tract, 346
Heterophyes
  description of genus, 539
  fish, 62
Histoplasma capsulatum
  bats, 54
  birds, 56–57
  description, 539–540
  dust and, 118
  hotels and, 243
  latency, 374
  nosocomial infections, 484
  occupational infections, 249, 256, 265, 288
  outdoor leisure and, 315
  school-associated, 361–362
  terrestrial biomes, 116
  travel-associated, 397, 407
  urban environment and, 133
HIV. *See* Human immunodeficiency virus (HIV)
Hobbies
  indoor sports and hobbies, 320–323
  outdoor sports and hobbies, 314–320
Homeless persons, 223–225
  droplet-air cluster, 223–224
  feces-food cluster, 224
  skin-blood cluster, 225
  zoonotic cluster, 224–225
Homes. *See* Domiciles
Homosexual men, 326–330
  droplet-air cluster, 327–328
  skin-blood cluster, 328–330
Honey, 186
Hookworms
  dogs, 17
  domicile-associated, human substandard, 221
  minority-associated, 368
  occupational infections, 250–251, 262, 276
  in orphans and adoptees, 232
  outdoor leisure and, 319
  plant-derived foods and, 182
  sanitation and, 131
  school-associated, 364
  seasons and, 124
  soil and plants, 100
  travel-associated, 414–415, 419, 424
  urban environment and, 137–138
Horse meat, 162
Horses. *See* Equids
Hospital
  air, 458–461
  viral hemorrhagic fevers, 464–466
  water, 461–464
Hospital-acquired infections. *See* Nosocomial infections
Hotels, 241–245
  droplet-air cluster, 242–243
  environmental cluster, 245
  feces-food cluster, 243–245
  skin-blood cluster, 245
  zoonotic cluster, 245
Human community, 335–391
  age groups, 347–353
  colonization, carriage, and contact, 335–347
  community-acquired syndromes, 376–391
  day care, 353–358
  exposure history, 336
  latency, reactivation, and immune impairment, 370–376
  minorities, 365–370
  schools and training, 358–365
Human coronavirus, 519
Human domiciles, 207–245
  detention facilities, 237–241
  homeless persons, 223–225
  hotels, 241–245
  long-term care, 233–237
  orphans and adoptees, 230–233
  refugees and relief camps, 225–230
  regular, 207–214
  substandard, 214–223
Human granulocytic ehrlichiosis (HGE), 259
Human herpes virus 6 (HHV6)
  description, 569
  intrauterine infections, 385
  nosocomial infections, 486
Human herpes virus 8 (HHV8)
  community-acquired, 383–384
  description, 566
  domicile-associated, human substandard, 222
  homosexual males and, 329

injection drug use and, 333
latency, 373
from nose, mouth, and throat, 339–340
nosocomial infections, 486
occupational infections, 294
prostitution and, 326
Human immunodeficiency virus (HIV)
from breast milk, 391
community-acquired, 383–384
description, 544
domicile-associated, human regular, 213–214
domicile-associated, human sub-standard, 222
homeless persons and, 225
homosexual males and, 329
indoor leisure and, 322–323
injection drug use and, 333
intrauterine infections, 385
long-term care and, 237
from nose, mouth, and throat, 339–340
nosocomial infections, 468–471, 480, 486, 493
occupational infections, 251, 263, 294–295, 299, 300
in orphans and adoptees, 232
outdoor leisure and, 319–320
peripartal infections of neonates, 389
prisons and, 240–241
prostitution and, 326
relief camps and, 229
terrestrial biomes, 111
transported animals and goods, 435
travel-associated, 398, 415, 419, 425
from urogenital tract, 346
Human leisure and lifestyle, 303–333
catered events and restaurants, 307–310
fairs and mass gatherings, 303–307
female prostitution, 323–326
indoor sports and hobbies, 320–323
injection drug use, 330–333
outdoor sports and hobbies, 314–320
sex among men, 326–330
swimming pools and spas, 310–314
Human metapneumovirus (hMPV), 120
Human monocytic ehrlichiosis (HME), 259
Human papillomavirus (HPV)
description, 558–559
domicile-associated, human regular, 214
homosexual males and, 329
indoor leisure and, 323
nosocomial infections, 468
pools and, 313
prostitution and, 325
sanitation and, 129
terrestrial biomes, 110
travel-associated, 415
from urogenital tract, 346
Human T-cell leukemia virus (HTLV)
from breast milk, 391
domicile-associated, human regular, 214
homosexual males and, 329–330
injection drug use and, 333
nosocomial infections, 480–481
occupational infections, 295

prisons and, 241
prostitution and, 326
travel-associated, 425
Human work, 247–301. *See also* Occupational infections
Humans, as sources of infection, 205–391
Hyalomma, 68
Hymenolepis diminuta, 540
Hymenolepis nana
day care-associated, 358
description, 540
domicile-associated, human sub-standard, 223
long-term care and, 237
minority-associated, 370
in orphans and adoptees, 233
relief camps and, 230
rodents, 49
travel-associated, 416

I

Ice cubes, 195–196
Immigrants and migrants, 420–425
Immune impairment, 370–376
Immunoglobulin, contaminated, 455
Implants, 489–492
breast, 492
cardiovascular, 490–491
intrauterine, 491–492
neurosensory, 491
osteosynthetic and orthopedic implants, 491
In vitro fertilization, 487
Incubators, 446
Indoor leisure, 320–323
droplet-air cluster, 321–322
environmental cluster, 322
feces-food cluster, 322
skin-blood cluster, 322–323
Influenzavirus
birds, 56
community-acquired, 377
description, 540–541
domicile-associated, human regular, 209
fairs and, 304–305
hotels and, 242
indoor leisure and, 321
long-term care and, 233–234
minority-associated, 365
from nose, mouth, and throat, 340
nosocomial infections, 458
occupational infections, 251, 254, 264–265, 284, 301
outdoor leisure and, 315
pigs, 27
prisons and, 238
school-associated, 359
seasons and, 120
terrestrial biomes, 108
transported animals and goods, 428
travel-associated, 395–396, 399, 401, 405
Injection drug use, 330–333
droplet-air cluster, 330–331

environmental cluster, 332
feces-food cluster, 331
skin-blood cluster, 332–333
zoonotic cluster, 331
Injections, infections from, 470–471
Inkoo virus
description, 557
herbivores, 38
transported animals and goods, 429
Instruments and machines, 443–446
blood gas analyzers, 446
dental, 445
dialysers, 446
disposable materials, 443–444
freezers, 446
incubators, 446
ophthalmological, 445
otorhinolaryngological, 445
respiratory ventilators, spirometers, and nebulizers, 445
sphygmomanometers, 445
stethoscopes, 445
thermometers, 445
Intensive care, infections associated, 494
International short-term travel, 404–416
Intrauterine devices, 491–492
Intrauterine infections, 384–388
bacterial, 386–387
fungal, 387
protozoal, 387–388
viral, 385–386
Intravascular devices, 471–474
bacteremia, fungemia, and parasitemia, 472–473
bloodstream infection and sepsis, 473–474
local vascular device, 472
Intubation and nosocomial pneumonia, 448–449
Invertebrates, 65–85
bugs, nocturnal, 82–83
ectoparasites, 83–85
fleas, 71
flies, 72–73
hard ticks, 67–71
mosquitoes, diurnal, 73–76
mosquitoes, nocturnal, 76–82
soft ticks, 83
transported, 430–432
vector mites, 71
Islands, 107–110
droplet-air cluster, 108
environmental cluster, 110
feces-food cluster, 108
skin-blood cluster, 110
zoonotic cluster, 108–110
Isospora
description of genus, 541
dogs, 14
drinking water-associated, 204
Isospora belli, 232
Isospora suis, 29
Ixodes, 68
Ixodid ticks. *See* Ticks, hard

J

Jamestown Canyon virus (JCV)
  description, 557
  herbivores, 38
  latency, 373
  nosocomial infections, 486
Japanese encephalitis virus (JEV)
  birds, 58–59
  bovids, 24
  description, 531
  domicile-associated, human sub-standard, 218
  occupational infections, 258, 290
  pigs, 30
  terrestrial biomes, 106
  travel-associated, 411
  urban environment and, 135
Juices, 196
Junin virus, 268, 290

K

Kidney transplant recipients, infections in, 483–484
Kingella, 541
Klebsiella
  description of genus, 541–542
  nosocomial infections, 461, 472
Klebsiella granulomatis
  community-acquired, 383
  description, 541
  travel-associated, 425
  from urogenital tract, 346
Klebsiella oxytoca
  description, 542
  nosocomial infections, 453
Klebsiella pneumoniae
  description, 541–542
  drinking water-associated, 198
  long-term care and, 236
  nosocomial infections, 448, 451, 453, 459
  occupational infections, 263, 287
  travel-associated, 397
Kunjin virus, 531
Kuru, 565
Kyasanur Forest disease virus (KFDV), 531

L

La Crosse encephalitis virus
  description, 557
  outdoor leisure and, 317
Laboratory work. *See* Health-and-laboratory work
Lacazia, 542
Lactobacillus, 542
Lagomorph
  droplet-air cluster, 49
  environmental cluster, 50
  feces-food cluster, 49
  skin-blood cluster, 50–51
  zoonoses, 49
  zoonotic cluster, 49–50
Lagomorphs, 49–51
Laguna Negra virus, 536
Lassa virus
  domicile-associated, human sub-standard, 219
  nosocomial infections, 464
  occupational infections, 259
  travel-associated, 403, 411
Latency, 370–376
  bacteria, 374
  fungi, 374–375
  helminths, 375–376
  prions, 372–373
  protozoa, 375
  viruses, 373–374
Latitude, limits of human-infective agents, 115
Legionella
  catering and restaurant-associated, 307
  community-acquired, 378
  description of genus, 542
  freshwater habitats and floods, 93
  hotels and, 242–243
  indoor leisure and, 321
  long-term care and, 234
  nosocomial infections, 461–462, 484
  occupational infections, 252, 265, 287–288, 297
  pools and, 311
  travel-associated, 396, 399, 406
Legionella pneumophila
  description, 542
  fairs and, 305
  occupational infections, 301
  sanitation and, 129–130
  urban environment and, 133
Leishmania
  carnivores, 41–42
  dam-related, 126
  description of genus, 542–544
  dogs, 16
  domicile-associated, human sub-standard, 220
  herbivores, 39
  intrauterine infections, 387
  latency, 375
  nosocomial infections, 481–482, 485
  occupational infections, 250, 260–261, 274, 292
  relief camps and, 228–229
  rodents, 47–48
  sandflies and, 81–82
  seasons and, 122
  from skin, 345
  terrestrial biomes, 102–103, 105, 107, 109, 111, 112, 113
  travel-associated, 398, 413, 418, 422–423
  urban environment and, 136
Leisure. *See* Human leisure and lifestyle
Lentivirus, 544
Leptosphaeria, 544
Leptospira
  bats, 55
  bovids, 26
  dam-related, 127
  description of genus, 544–545
  dogs, 17
  domicile-associated, human sub-standard, 221
  drinking water-associated, 202
  equids, 33
  freshwater habitats and floods, 96
  occupational infections, 250, 253, 262, 275, 292, 298, 300
  outdoor leisure and, 319
  pigs, 30
  rodents, 48
  seasons and, 122, 124
  terrestrial biomes, 102, 110
  travel-associated, 414, 424
Leptotrombidium, 71
Lice, 84–85, 140–142
  day care-associated, 358
  domicile-associated, human sub-standard, 223
  homeless persons and, 225
  occupational infections, 296
  in orphans and adoptees, 233
  prisons and, 241
  relief camps and, 230
  school-associated, 364
Lifestyle. *See* Human leisure and lifestyle
Liponyssoides, 71
Listeria monocytogenes
  animal-derived foods and, 151, 152, 154, 155, 158, 160, 163–164, 165, 167–168, 169, 172
  bovids, 22
  from bowel, 343
  description, 545
  domicile-associated, human regular, 211
  finished food products and, 188
  food-borne illness and, 147
  intrauterine infections, 386
  nosocomial infections, 484
  occupational infections, 266
  peripartal infections of neonates, 390
  pigs, 28
  plant-derived foods and, 179, 186
Liver transplant recipients, infections in, 484
Llama. *See* Camelids
Loa loa
  description, 545
  fly transmission, 73
  occupational infections, 274
  terrestrial biomes, 104
  travel-associated, 418, 424
Long-term care facilities, 233–237
  droplet-air cluster, 233–234
  environmental cluster, 236–237
  feces-food cluster, 234–236
  skin-blood cluster, 237
Louping ill virus, 531
Louse-borne relapsing fever (LBRF)
  description, 512
  latency, 374
  travel-associated, 412
Lung transplant recipients, infections in, 484
Lutzomyia, 80–81
Lyme disease. *See* *Borrelia burgdorferi*

Lymphocryptovirus, 545
Lymphocytic choriomeningitis virus (LCMV)
    domicile-associated, human substandard, 219
    nosocomial infections, 485
    occupational infections, 268, 290
Lyssavirus
    bats, 54
    description, 545–546
    rodents, 45
    transported animals and goods, 429

M

Machupo virus, 219
Madurella, 546
Malassezia
    description of genus, 546
    nosocomial infections, 455
Mamastrovirus, 546–547
Mansonella
    camelids, 34–35
    description of genus, 547
    occupational infections, 250
    travel-associated, 424
    vectors of, 75, 76
Mansonia, 80
Manufacture and maintenance work, 251–253
    droplet-air cluster, 251–252
    environmental cluster, 253
    feces-food cluster, 252
    zoonotic cluster, 252–253
Marburg virus (MARV)
    description, 530
    domicile-associated, human substandard, 219
    nosocomial infections, 465
    occupational infections, 250, 268
    primates, 52
Marek's disease virus (MDV)
    birds, 60
    description, 547
Marine habitats, 89–92
    environmental cluster, 91–92
    feces-food cluster, 89–91
    zoonotic cluster, 91
Mayaro virus (MAYV)
    description, 504
    occupational infections, 291
Measles virus
    community-acquired, 377
    description, 549
    domicile-associated, human substandard, 214
    fairs and, 305
    indoor leisure and, 321
    minority-associated, 365–366
    from nose, mouth, and throat, 340
    nosocomial infections, 458–459
    occupational infections, 254, 284–285
    in orphans and adoptees, 230–231
    prisons and, 238
    relief camps and, 226

school-associated, 359
    terrestrial biomes, 108
    travel-associated, 396, 402, 405
Meat and meat products, 159–166
    beef meat, 159–160
    finished food products and, 189–191
    ground beef, hamburgers, and corned beef, 163–164
    horse meat, 162
    mutton, lamb, and goat meats, 161–162
    pork meat, 160–161
    rabbit meat, 162
    sausages, deli, and ham, 164–166
    venison and game, 162–163
Mediterranean, temperate and boreal forests, 104–106
Metagonimus, 547
Metapneumovirus, 547
Metorchis, 547
Microbacterium, 548
Microorganisms, transported from ships, 430–431
Microsporidia
    bovids, 23
    community-acquired, 380
    description, 548
    drinking water-associated, 199
    freshwater habitats and floods, 94
    homosexual males and, 327
    occupational infections, 289
    pools and, 312
    terrestrial biomes, 114
    travel-associated, 409
Microsporidium
    description of genus, 548
    in orphans and adoptees, 231
Microsporum canis, 142
Military, police, and guards, 253–264. *See also* Uniformed services
Milk, breast, 390–391
Milk and dairy products, 149–156
Milk chocolate, 156
Mining. *See* Construction and mining
Minorities, 365–370
    droplet-air cluster, 365–367
    environmental cluster, 368
    feces-food cluster, 367–368
    skin-blood cluster, 369–370
    zoonotic cluster, 368
Mites, 71, 140
Modes of spread, 2–3
Molluscipoxvirus
    description, 548
    indoor leisure and, 323
    pools and, 313
Molluscum contagiosum virus, 468
Monkeypox virus (MPXV)
    description, 557–558
    occupational infections, 294
    primates, 53
    rodents, 48
    transported animals and goods, 429
Moraxella
    description of genus, 548
    school-associated, 361

Morbillivirus, 548–549
Morganella, 549
Mosquitoes
    diurnal, 73–76
        Aedes, 73–75, 431–432
        Culicoides (midges), 76
        Simulium (blackflies), 75
    nocturnal, 76–82
        Anopheles, 76–78, 432
        Coquillettidia, 80
        Culex, 78–80, 432
        Culiseta, 80
        Haemagogus, 80
        Mansonia, 80
    transport from ships and aircraft, 431–432
Mother-to-child transmission, 384–391
    intrauterine infections, 384–388
    peripartal infections of neonates, 388–390
    postpartal infections of neonates, 390–391
    prevention, 384
Mouth, agents from, 339–342
Mucor, 549
Mumps virus
    description, 549–550
    domicile-associated, human substandard, 214–215
    minority-associated, 366
    from nose, mouth, and throat, 340
    occupational infections, 254, 285, 301
    school-associated, 359
    terrestrial biomes, 108
Murray Valley encephalitis virus (MVEV)
    birds, 59
    description, 531
Musca, 72
Mushrooms, 186
Mutton, lamb, and goat meats, 161–162
Mycetoma, 275
Mycobacterium
    animal-derived foods and, 151
    birds, 56
    bovids, 25
    dam-related, 127
    description of genus, 550–552
    drinking water-associated, 195, 198
    freshwater habitats and floods, 96
    herbivores, 39
    minority-associated, 366–367
    nosocomial infections, 451, 453, 462, 468–469, 471, 477, 485, 487
    occupational infections, 250, 252
    pigs, 30–31
    sanitation and, 130
    soil and plants, 99
    terrestrial biomes, 110, 112–113
Mycobacterium abscessus
    description, 550
    nosocomial infections, 451, 453
Mycobacterium avium complex
    description, 550
    nosocomial infections, 462
    pools and, 313

Mycobacterium avium paratuberculosis (MAP), 152
Mycobacterium bovis
  carnivores, 41
  description, 550
  nosocomial infections, 452
  occupational infections, 273
  pigs, 30
  transported animals and goods, 430
Mycobacterium chelonae
  description, 550
  nosocomial infections, 453, 469
Mycobacterium fortuitum
  description, 550
  nosocomial infections, 462
Mycobacterium genavense, 550
Mycobacterium haemophilum, 551
Mycobacterium kansasii
  description, 551
  occupational infections, 249
Mycobacterium leprae
  description, 551
  domicile-associated, human sub-standard, 222
  fairs and, 306
  from nose, mouth, and throat, 341
  travel-associated, 415, 425
Mycobacterium malmoense, 551
Mycobacterium marinum
  description, 551
  fish trauma and, 11
  marine habitat, 91
  occupational infections, 275
  pools and, 313
Mycobacterium microti, 34
Mycobacterium tuberculosis
  catering and restaurant-associated, 307
  community-acquired, 378
  description, 551–552
  domicile-associated, human regular, 209–210
  domicile-associated, human sub-standard, 215–216
  fairs and, 305
  homeless persons and, 223–224
  indoor leisure and, 321
  injection drug use and, 330–331
  latency, 374
  long-term care and, 234
  nosocomial infections, 446–447, 449, 456, 459–460, 484
  occupational infections, 249, 252, 255, 265, 287, 297, 301
  in orphans and adoptees, 231
  outdoor leisure and, 315
  primates, 51
  prisons and, 238–239
  relief camps and, 226–227
  school-associated, 361
  terrestrial biomes, 108
  travel-associated, 396–397, 399, 402, 406, 416–417, 420–421
  urban environment and, 133
Mycobacterium ulcerans
  description, 552
  occupational infections, 275
  travel-associated, 414
Mycobacterium xenopi, 552
Mycoplasma
  community-acquired, 382
  description of genus, 552–553
  peripartal infections of neonates, 390
  from urogenital tract, 346–347
Mycoplasma genitalium
  community-acquired, 382
  description, 552
Mycoplasma hominis
  community-acquired, 382
  description, 552–553
  sanitation and, 130
Mycoplasma pneumoniae
  community-acquired, 378
  description, 553
  domicile-associated, human regular, 210
  long-term care and, 234
  from nose, mouth, and throat, 341
  nosocomial infections, 460
  occupational infections, 256, 288
  in orphans and adoptees, 231
  outdoor leisure and, 315
  relief camps and, 227
  school-associated, 361
  seasons and, 121
Myiasis
  bovids, 27
  overview, 83–84

N

Naegleria, 553
Nairovirus
  description, 553
  herbivores, 38
  lagomorphs, 50
  rodents, 45
  ticks, 69
Naucoris cimicoides, 83
Necator
  description, 505–506
  domicile-associated, human sub-standard, 221
  soil and plants, 100
Neisseria gonorrhoeae
  community-acquired, 382
  description, 554
  homosexual males and, 328
  occupational infections, 263, 300, 301
  peripartal infections of neonates, 390
  prisons and, 241
  prostitution and, 324
  travel-associated, 416, 425
  urban environment and, 138
  from urogenital tract, 347
Neisseria meningitidis
  catering and restaurant-associated, 307
  description, 554
  domicile-associated, human regular, 210
  fairs and, 305
  homosexual males and, 327
  hotels and, 243
  indoor leisure and, 321–322
  long-term care and, 234
  minority-associated, 367
  from nose, mouth, and throat, 341
  occupational infections, 249, 255, 287, 301
  outdoor leisure and, 315
  pools and, 311
  prisons and, 238
  relief camps and, 227
  school-associated, 360–361
  seasons and, 120
  terrestrial biomes, 111
  travel-associated, 397, 399, 402, 406
Nematodes. *See* Helminths
Neonates
  peripartal infections of, 388–390
  postpartal infections of, 390–391
Neorickettsia risticii
  description, 554–555
  equids, 32
Neospora, 555
Neurosensory implants, 491
Neurosyndromes, acute and subacute food-borne, 147
Newcastle disease virus
  birds, 56
  occupational infections, 269, 290
Nipah virus
  description, 537
  occupational infections, 259, 269
  pigs, 30
Nocardia
  description of genus, 555
  nosocomial infections, 477, 485
  soil and plants, 100
Nocardia asteroides, 117
Nocardia farcinica, 477
Norovirus
  animal-derived foods and, 164–165, 170–171
  from bowel, 342–343
  carpets and, 142
  catering and restaurant-associated, 308
  community-acquired, 379
  description, 555
  domicile-associated, human regular, 211
  drinking water-associated, 194–195, 197, 201
  fairs and, 306
  finished food products and, 188, 189
  freshwater habitats and floods, 94
  hotels and, 243–244
  long-term care and, 235
  marine habitat, 90
  occupational infections, 256, 278, 288
  outdoor leisure and, 315
  plant-derived foods and, 176, 178, 183
  pools and, 311–312
  prisons and, 239
  sanitation and, 128–129
  school-associated, 362
  seasons and, 120
  terrestrial biomes, 108
  transported animals and goods, 431, 433
  travel-associated, 400, 403, 407
Nose, agents from, 339–342
Nosocomial infections, 437–494
  agents, 438–439

exposure history, 438
impact, 438–439
invasive procedures, 467–494
    dialysis, 492–494
    implants, 489–492
    instant, 467–471
    intensive care, 494
    intravascular devices, 471–474
    surgical site and wound infections, 474–477
    transfusions, 477–482
    transplants, 482–489
modes of acquisition, 438
non-invasive procedures, 441–466
    bladder catheters and UTI, 447–448
    drugs, bioproducts and nosocomial diarrhea, 449–458
    endoscopy, 446–447
    hands, 441–443
    hospital air, water, and surfaces, 458–464
    instruments and machines, 443–446
    intubation and nosocomial pneumonia, 448–449
    viral hemorrhagic fevers in hospitals, 464–466
prevention, 439
rates of acquisition, 438
sites, 437
Nursery equipment, nosocomial infections and, 444
Nuts, 184–185

O

Oases, desert, 111–112
Occupational infections, 247–301
    catering, 276–281
    cleaning and waste work, 296–299
    clerk, class, and sales work, 300–301
    construction and mining, 248–251
    crop-and-herd work, 264–276
    health-and-laboratory work, 281–296
    manufacture and maintenance, 251–253
    military, police, and guards, 253–264
    transportation work, 299–300
Oesophagostomum, 555
Omsk hemorrhagic fever virus (OHFV)
    description, 531
    transported animals and goods, 429
Onchocerca
    bovids, 26
    description of genus, 555–556
    occupational infections, 250
    vectors of, 75, 76
Onchocerca volvulus
    description, 555–556
    domicile-associated, human substandard, 221
    freshwater habitats and floods, 96
    minority-associated, 368
    occupational infections, 274
    terrestrial biomes, 104, 107
    travel-associated, 419, 424
    wind and, 118
O'nyong-nyong virus (ONNV), 504

Opisthorchis
    animal-derived foods and, 168–169
    description of genus, 517, 556
    fish, 62
    travel-associated, 422
Opisthorchis felineus
    description, 556
    transported animals and goods, 434
Opisthorchis viverrini
    description, 556
    occupational infections, 267
Ophthalmological instruments, 445
Oral care, 140–141
Oran virus, 536
Orbivirus, 556
Orf virus, 269
Orientia tsutsugamushi
    description, 556
    occupational infections, 259, 270
    outdoor leisure and, 318
    relief camps and, 228
    rodents, 46
    seasons and, 122
    terrestrial biomes, 102, 109
    travel-associated, 412
Ornithodoros, 83
Oropouche virus, 557
Orphans and adoptees, 230–233
    droplet-air cluster, 230–231
    environmental cluster, 232
    feces-food cluster, 231–232
    skin-blood cluster, 232–233
Orthobunyavirus
    description, 557
    herbivores, 38
    lagomorphs, 50
    mosquitoes and, 75, 77
    occupational infections, 267
    primates, 52
    rodents, 45
    terrestrial biomes, 114
Orthohepadnavirus, 556–557
Orthopedic implants, 491
Orthopoxvirus, 557–558
Osteosynthetic implants, 491
Otorhinolaryngological instruments, 445
Outdoor leisure, 314–320
    droplet-air cluster, 314–315
    environmental cluster, 318–320
    feces-food cluster, 315–317
    skin-blood cluster, 320
    zoonotic cluster, 317–318

P

Pacemakers, 490
Paecilomyces, 558
Pantoea, 558
Papillomavirus. *See also* Human papillomavirus (HPV)
    description, 558–559
    primates, 53
Parachlamydia, 559
Paracoccidioides
    description of genus, 559
    travel-associated, 407, 417

Paracoccidioides brasiliensis
    description, 559
    latency, 375
    occupational infections, 265, 288
    terrestrial biomes, 102
Paragonimus
    animal-derived foods and, 169
    description of genus, 559
    nosocomial infections, 451
    pigs, 29
Parainfluenza virus (PIV)
    baby care and toys, 141
    community-acquired, 377
    description, 559
    domicile-associated, human regular, 209
    long-term care and, 234
    from nose, mouth, and throat, 340
    occupational infections, 286
    in orphans and adoptees, 231
    seasons and, 121
Parapoxvirus, 560
Parasites, from breast milk, 391
Parenteral nutrition and formula feed, 454–455
Parvovirus B19
    description, 527–528
    domicile-associated, human regular, 209
    intrauterine infections, 385–386
    latency, 373–374
    minority-associated, 366
    nosocomial infections, 459, 478–479
    occupational infections, 286, 301
    school-associated, 360
Pasta and cereals, 176
Pasteurella
    animal bites, 10
    description of genus, 560
    occupational infections, 273
Pasteurella aerogenes, 273
Pasteurella multocida
    birds, 60
    occupational infections, 273, 292
    pigs, 30
Pasteurized milk, 152
Pastry and bakery foods, 176–177
Pediculosis, 84–85, 140–142
    day care-associated, 358
    domicile-associated, human substandard, 223
    homeless persons and, 225
    occupational infections, 296
    in orphans and adoptees, 233
    prisons and, 241
    relief camps and, 230
    school-associated, 364
Penicillium marneffei
    description, 560
    travel-associated, 414
Pentastomida, 560
Peptostreptococcus, 560
Peripartal infections of neonates, 388–390
    bacteria, 389–390
    fungi, 390
    protozoa, 390
    viruses, 388–389
Peritoneal dialysis, 493–494

Phialophora, 560
Phlebotomus, 81
Phlebovirus
    bats, 55
    description, 560–561
    mosquitoes and, 75, 79
    rodents, 45–46
    sandflies and, 81–82
Phytotherapy, 450–451
PID (pelvic inflammatory disease), 492
Pigs, 27–31
    droplet-air cluster, 27–28
    environmental cluster, 30–31
    feces-food cluster, 28–30
    rabies, 30
    skin-blood cluster, 31
    zoonoses, 27
    zoonotic cluster, 30
Plasmodium
    birds, 60
    dam-related, 126–127
    description of genus, 561–562
    domicile-associated, human substandard, 220
    freshwater habitats and floods, 95–96
    injection drug use and, 331
    intrauterine infections, 387
    latency, 375
    minority-associated, 368
    nosocomial infections, 482, 485
    occupational infections, 250, 261, 274, 292, 299–300
    outdoor leisure and, 318
    primates, 52
    relief camps and, 229
    seasons and, 123–124
    terrestrial biomes, 103, 106, 109, 112, 113–114
    transported animals and goods, 435
    travel-associated, 398, 400, 404, 413–414, 418, 423
    urban environment and, 136–137
    wind and, 118
Plesiomonas shigelloides
    animal-derived foods and, 172
    description, 562–563
    dogs, 14
    drinking water-associated, 202
    fish, 61
    freshwater habitats and floods, 96–97
    marine habitat, 90
    plant-derived foods and, 180
    travel-associated, 408
Pneumocystis jirovecii
    description, 563
    domicile-associated, human regular, 210
    dust and, 118
    intrauterine infections, 387
    latency, 374
    from nose, mouth, and throat, 342
    nosocomial infections, 460–461, 484
    occupational infections, 288
    in orphans and adoptees, 231
Pneumonia
    community-acquired, 376–378

    intubation and nosocomial pneumonia, 448–449
Pneumovirus, 563
Poliomyelitis virus
    description, 527
    domicile-associated, human substandard, 216
    drinking water-associated, 201
    freshwater habitats and floods, 94
    minority-associated, 366
    occupational infections, 289
    relief camps and, 227
    travel-associated, 396, 420
Polyomavirus
    description, 563–564
    latency, 373
    from urogenital tract, 346
Pools and spas
    droplet-air cluster, 311
    environmental cluster, 313
    feces-food cluster, 311–312
    skin-blood cluster, 313–314
Pork meat, 160–161
Porphyromonas, 564
Postpartal infections of neonates, 390–391
Poultry, 157–159
Powassan virus
    carnivores, 41
    description, 531
    dogs, 15
    outdoor leisure and, 317
Prevotella, 564
Primates, 51–53
    droplet-air cluster, 51
    environmental cluster, 52–53
    feces-food cluster, 51
    skin-blood cluster, 53
    zoonoses, 51
    zoonotic cluster, 52
Prions
    animal-derived foods and, 150, 159, 164
    bovid, 22
    carnivore, 40
    cat, 19
    description, 564–565
    herbivore, 38
    latent, 372–373
    minorities and, 367
    nosocomial infections, 455, 470, 475, 478, 487
    occupational infections, 267, 276, 293
    taxonomic overview, 497
    transfusion-associated infections, 478
Prisons. *See* Detention facilities
Propionibacterium, 565
Prosthetic valve endocarditis (PVE), 490
Prostitution
    female, 323–326
    male, 326
    skin-blood cluster, 324–326
Proteus, 565
Proteus mirabilis, 469
Protists, 498. *See also* Protozoa

Protozoa. *See also specific species*
    animal-derived foods and, 152, 156, 158–164, 166, 172
    avian, 58, 60
    bovid, 23, 25–26
    from bowel, 344
    camelid, 34
    carnivore, 40–42
    cat, 19, 20
    chiropteran, 55
    community-acquired, 380, 382, 387–388, 390
    dam-related, 126–127
    day care-associated, 357
    dog, 14, 16
    domicile-associated, human regular, 212–213
    domicile-associated, human substandard, 217, 220–221
    drinking water-associated, 195, 196, 199–200, 203–204
    dust, 18
    equid, 32–33
    finished food products and, 188
    flies and, 72–73
    food-borne illness and, 145–147
    freshwater habitats and floods, 94–97
    herbivore, 38–40
    hotels and, 243–244
    human travel and, 398, 400–401, 404, 409–410, 413–414, 417–418, 421–425
    intrauterine infections, 387–388
    lagomorph, 49–50
    latent, 375
    leisure and lifestyle-associated, 306, 309, 312–313, 316, 318, 325, 327–328, 331
    long-term care and, 236
    marine habitat, 90–91
    minorities and, 367–368
    mosquitoes and, 77–78, 79
    from nose, mouth, and throat, 342
    nosocomial infections, 461, 463, 471, 473, 481–482
    occupational infections, 249–250, 257, 260–261, 266–267, 274, 280, 289–290, 292–293, 298
    in orphans and adoptees, 231–232
    peripartal infections of neonates, 390
    plant-derived foods and, 180–181, 182, 184, 186
    porcine, 28, 29
    prisons and, 241
    relief camps and, 228–229
    rodent, 44, 47–48
    sandflies and, 81–82
    sanitation and, 130–131
    school-associated, 363
    seasons and, 121–124
    simian, 51, 52
    from skin, 345
    soil and plants, 99
    taxonomic overview, 498

terrestrial biomes, 102–103, 105–109, 111–114
ticks and, 70–71
transfusion-associated infections, 481–482
transported animals and goods, 430, 434–435
urban environment and, 133–134, 136–137
from urogenital tract, 347
utensils and belongings, 139, 141
Providencia
description of genus, 565
occupational infections, 257
plant-derived foods and, 176
Providencia alcalifaciens, 257, 279
Pseudocowpox virus, 269
Pseudomonas aeruginosa
baby care and toys, 141
from bowel, 343
description, 565
eye care and, 140
freshwater habitats and floods, 97
nosocomial infections, 448, 449, 451, 453–454, 462, 469, 472
outdoor leisure and, 319
pools and, 313
sanitation and, 130
Pseudoterranova
animal-derived foods and, 168
description of genus, 506
fish, 61–62
Puumala virus, 536

Q
Q fever, travel-associated, 403

R
Rabbit meat, 162
Rabies, 7–9
bats, 9, 54
bovids, 24
carnivores, 41
cats, 9, 19–20
dogs, 8–9, 15
equids, 32
human risks, 8
in international travelers, 8
latency, 374
nosocomial infections, 466, 485, 487
occupational infections, 259, 269, 290
outdoor leisure and, 317
pigs, 30
rabid mammals, 7–8
terrestrial biomes, 108–109, 114, 116
travel-associated, 418, 422
urban environment and, 135
Rainy seasons, 123–124
Ralstonia
description of genus, 565
nosocomial infections, 454
Reactivation, 370–376
Refugees and relief camps, 225–230

Relief camps
droplet-air cluster, 226–227
environmental cluster, 229–230
feces-food cluster, 227–228
zoonotic cluster, 228–229
Reovirus, 566
Reptiles, 60–61
ticks on, 432
Respiratory syncytial virus (RSV)
baby care and toys, 141
community-acquired, 377
description, 563
domicile-associated, human regular, 209
long-term care and, 234
minority-associated, 366
from nose, mouth, and throat, 340
occupational infections, 286
seasons and, 120
Respiratory ventilators, spirometers, and nebulizers, 445
Retroviruses
avian, 456
minority-associated, 369
occupational infections, 269, 294–295
primates, 53
Rhadinovirus, 566
Rhinosporidium seeberi
description, 566
freshwater habitats and floods, 97
outdoor leisure and, 319
Rhinovirus
baby care and toys, 141
description, 566
domicile-associated, human regular, 209
long-term care and, 234
seasons and, 120
Rhipicephalus, 68
Rhizopus, 566
Rhodococcus equi
description, 566
equids, 33
soil and plants, 100
Rhodotorula, 566
Rickettsia
cats, 20
description of genus, 566–569
dogs, 16
domicile-associated, human regular, 213
fleas, 71
homeless persons and, 225
lagomorphs, 50
lice and, 85
occupational infections, 259–260, 270, 292
outdoor leisure and, 318
pigs, 30
rodents, 46–47
seasons and, 122
terrestrial biomes, 105
ticks, 70
urban environment and, 135
Rickettsia africae
description, 567
occupational infections, 270

transported animals and goods, 430
travel-associated, 412
Rickettsia akari, 331
Rickettsia australis, 567
Rickettsia conorii
description, 567–568
occupational infections, 270, 292
travel-associated, 412
Rickettsia felis, 568
Rickettsia heilongjiangensis, 568
Rickettsia helvetica
description, 568
occupational infections, 270
Rickettsia japonica, 568
Rickettsia prowazekii
description, 568
latency, 374
occupational infections, 259–260, 292
relief camps and, 228
terrestrial biomes, 113
travel-associated, 412–413
Rickettsia rickettsii
description, 568
domicile-associated, human sub-standard, 219
Rickettsia sibirica
description, 568–569
terrestrial biomes, 106
travel-associated, 413
Rickettsia typhi
description, 569
domicile-associated, human sub-standard, 219
occupational infections, 260, 270, 299
relief camps and, 228
terrestrial biomes, 109
travel-associated, 412
Rift Valley fever virus (RVFV)
bovids, 24
camelids, 34
description, 560–561
herbivores, 38
occupational infections, 258, 267, 290
transported animals and goods, 429
Ritual procedures, infections from, 467–469
Rodents, 42–49
cold-weather clusters from, 120
droplet-air cluster, 43
environmental cluster, 48
exposure, 42
feces-food cluster, 43–44
skin-blood cluster, 48–49
zoonoses, 42–43
zoonotic cluster, 44–48
Roseolovirus, 569
Ross River virus (RRV)
description, 504
domicile-associated, human sub-standard, 218
occupational infections, 258
seasons and, 123
terrestrial biomes, 109
travel-associated, 411
Rotavirus
from bowel, 343

Rotavirus *(continued)*
  from breast milk, 391
  community-acquired, 379
  description, 569–570
  domicile-associated, human regular, 211
  domicile-associated, human sub-
    standard, 216
  drinking water-associated, 197, 201
  finished food products and, 188
  freshwater habitats and floods, 94
  hotels and, 244
  long-term care and, 235
  minority-associated, 367
  occupational infections, 256, 278, 288
  relief camps and, 227
  rodents, 43
  sanitation and, 129
  school-associated, 362
  seasons and, 120
  terrestrial biomes, 108
  travel-associated, 407
Rubella virus
  description, 570
  domicile-associated, human sub-
    standard, 214–215
  fairs and, 305
  indoor leisure and, 321
  intrauterine infections, 386
  minority-associated, 366
  from nose, mouth, and throat, 340
  nosocomial infections, 459
  occupational infections, 254, 265, 285, 301
  prisons and, 238
  school-associated, 359–360
  travel-associated, 399, 405, 420
Rubivirus, 570
Rubulavirus, 55

S

Saaremaa virus, 536
Saccharomyces, 570
Saint Louis encephalitis virus (SLEV)
  birds, 59
  description, 531–532
  domicile-associated, human sub-
    standard, 218
  occupational infections, 267
  urban environment and, 135
Salmonella
  animal-derived foods and, 151, 152, 153,
    154, 155–157, 158, 160, 162, 164,
    165–166, 169, 171
  birds, 57–58
  bovids, 22–23
  from bowel, 344
  catering and restaurant-associated,
    308–309
  cats, 19
  community-acquired, 380
  description of genus, 570–571
  dogs, 14
  domicile-associated, human regular,
    211–212

  domicile-associated, human sub-
    standard, 217
  drinking water-associated, 195, 196,
    198–199, 202–203
  equids, 32
  fairs and, 306
  finished food products and, 188, 189
  food-borne illness and, 146
  homosexual males and, 327
  hotels and, 244
  long-term care and, 236
  marine habitat, 90
  nosocomial infections, 447, 450, 451, 484
  occupational infections, 257, 266, 279,
    289, 297–298
  in orphans and adoptees, 231
  outdoor leisure and, 316
  pigs, 28
  plant-derived foods and, 176–177,
    179–180, 182, 184, 185, 186
  prisons and, 239
  reptile and amphibian, 61
  sanitation and, 130
  school-associated, 363
  terrestrial biomes, 114
  transported animals and goods, 428,
    433–434
  travel-associated, 397, 403, 408
  utensils and belongings, 139–140
Sandfleas, 84
Sandflies, 80–82
Sandfly fever virus
  description, 561
  occupational infections, 258
Sanitary installations in buildings, 128–130
Sapovirus, 571
Sarcocystis
  animal-derived foods and, 160, 161, 163
  birds, 58
  bovids, 23
  camelids, 34
  carnivores, 40
  description of genus, 571
  occupational infections, 257
  pigs, 29
Sarcoptes scabiei, 85, 140, 142
  day care-associated, 358
  domicile-associated, human sub-
    standard, 223
  homeless persons and, 225
  long-term care and, 237
  minority-associated, 370
  nosocomial infections, 443
  occupational infections, 296
  in orphans and adoptees, 233
  prisons and, 241
  relief camps and, 230
  school-associated, 364
SARS-CoV
  animal-derived foods and, 162
  carnivores, 41
  carpets and, 142
  description, 519520
  domicile-associated, human regular, 209

  fairs and, 305
  hotels and, 242
  nosocomial infections, 459
  occupational infections, 265, 286
  travel-associated, 396, 402, 405
Saucer bugs, 83
Sausages, deli, and ham, 164–166
Scabies
  bedding and, 140
  clothing-associated, 142
  day care-associated, 358
  domicile-associated, human sub-
    standard, 223
  homeless persons and, 225
  island habitats, 110
  long-term care and, 237
  minority-associated, 370
  nosocomial infections, 443
  occupational infections, 296
  overview, 85
  prisons and, 241
  relief camps and, 230
  school-associated, 364
Scedosporium
  description of genus, 571–572
  nosocomial infections, 461
Schistosoma
  dam-related, 127
  description of genus, 572–573
  dogs, 17
  domicile-associated, human sub-
    standard, 222
  freshwater habitats and floods, 97–
    98
  latency, 376
  marine habitat, 91
  occupational infections, 251, 262, 276,
    293, 298, 300
  outdoor leisure and, 319
  pools and, 313
  rodents, 48
  seasons and, 124
  terrestrial biomes, 110, 112
  travel-associated, 415, 419, 424
  urban environment and, 138
Schistosoma fuelleborni, 104
Schistosoma haematobium, 572
Schistosoma intercalatum, 572
Schistosoma japonicum
  bovids, 26
  description, 572
Schistosoma malayensis, 572
Schistosoma mansoni
  description, 572–573
  primates, 52
Schistosoma mekongi, 573
Schools, 358–365
  droplet-air cluster, 359–362
  environmental cluster, 364
  feces-food cluster, 362–363
  skin-blood cluster, 364–365
  zoonotic cluster, 363–364
Scrapie, 22, 565
Scrub typhus. *See Orientia tsutsugamushi*

Seafood, fish, and molluscs, 166–173
  finished food products and, 189–191
Seasons, 118–124
  cold-weather peaks, 119–121
  rainy seasons, 123–124
  warm-weather peaks, 121–123
Seed sprouts, 182
Semliki Forest virus, 504
Seoul virus, 536–537
Sepsis, 471, 473–474
Serratia marcescens
  baby care and toys, 141
  description, 573
  nosocomial infections, 454, 462–463, 469
  travel-associated, 398
Sewage, waste, 130–132
Sex among men, 326–330
Sexually transmitted infections. *See* STIs (sexually transmitted infections)
Shigella
  animal-derived foods and, 154, 164, 172
  from bowel, 344
  catering and restaurant-associated, 309
  community-acquired, 380
  description, 573–574
  domicile-associated, human regular, 212
  domicile-associated, human sub-standard, 217
  drinking water-associated, 196, 199, 203
  fairs and, 306
  finished food products and, 188
  food-borne illness and, 146
  freshwater habitats and floods, 94
  homosexual males and, 327
  hotels and, 244
  indoor leisure and, 322
  long-term care and, 236
  minority-associated, 367
  occupational infections, 257, 266, 279, 289
  in orphans and adoptees, 231
  outdoor leisure and, 316
  plant-derived foods and, 177, 180, 184
  pools and, 312
  prisons and, 239
  relief camps and, 227
  school-associated, 363
  transported animals and goods, 434
  travel-associated, 400, 403, 409
Ships and seaports, travel and, 398–401
Simian foamy virus, 295
Simian herpes virus (SHV)
  description, 574–575
  nosocomial infections, 451
  occupational infections, 295
  primates, 53
Simian retrovirus D
  description, 510
  occupational infections, 295
Simian retroviruses, 269
Simian virus 40 (SV40)
  description, 564
  latency, 373
  nosocomial infections, 452
  primates, 53
Simians. *See* Primates
Simplexvirus, 574–575
Simulium (blackflies), 75, 432
Sin Nombre virus, 537
Sindbisvirus, 504–505
Skin, agents from, 344–345
Skin grafts, 489
Skin-blood cluster
  adult age and, 352
  agents, 3
  avian, 60
  bovine, 26–27
  camelid, 35
  carnivore, 42
  catering, 280–281, 309–310
  cleaning and waste work, 298–299
  clerk, class, and sales work, 301
  cold-weather peaks, 121
  construction and mining, 251
  crop-and-herd work, 276
  day care, 357–358
  detention facilities, 240–241
  dogs, 18
  domiciles, human substandard, 222–223
  elderly and, 353
  equine, 33–34
  fairs, 307
  feline, 21
  hands, transmission by, 442
  health-and-laboratory work, 293–296
  homeless persons, 225
  homosexual men, 328–330
  hotels, 245
  indoor leisure, 322–323
  injection drug use, 332–333
  islands, 110
  lagomorph, 50–51
  long-term care facilities, 237
  minorities and, 369–370
  orphans and adoptees, 232–233
  outdoor leisure, 320
  pools and spas, 313–314
  porcine, 31
  preschool age and, 351
  prostitution, 324–326
  rodent, 48–49
  school age and, 351
  school-associated, 364–365
  simian, 53
  soil and plants, 100
  stem cell recipients and, 489
  transfusion-transmitted agents, 479–481
  transportation work, 300
  transported goods and, 435
  travel-associated, 398, 401, 415–416, 419, 424–425
  uniformed services, 262–264
Snowshoe hare virus, 557
Soft drinks, 197
Soft ticks. *See* Ticks, soft
Soil and plants, 98–100
  droplet-air cluster, 98
  environmental cluster, 99–100
  feces-food cluster, 98–99
  skin-blood cluster, 100
  zoonotic cluster, 99
Solutions, disinfectants, and multidose vials, 452–454
Speleological agents, 116
Sphygmomanometers, 445
Spices, 185–186
Spirillum, 575
Spirometra
  description of genus, 575
  outdoor leisure and, 317
  pigs, 29
Sporothrix
  description of genus, 575
  domicile-associated, human sub-standard, 221
  occupational infections, 249, 293
  travel-associated, 398
Sporothrix schenckii
  animal bites, 10
  description of genus, 575
  nosocomial infections, 469
  occupational infections, 275–276
  soil and plants, 100
  travel-associated, 414
Sports
  indoor sports and hobbies, 320–323
  outdoor sports and hobbies, 314–320
Spumavirus, 575
Staphylococcus
  antimicrobial resistance, 494
  bovids, 26
  description of genus, 575–576
  fairs and, 306
  nosocomial infections, 443, 460, 472, 474
Staphylococcus aureus
  animal-derived foods and, 151, 153, 156, 166
  catering and restaurant-associated, 309–310
  community-acquired, 378
  day care-associated, 358
  description, 575–576
  domicile-associated, human sub-standard, 222
  equids, 33
  finished food products and, 188, 189
  food-borne illness and, 145
  indoor leisure and, 323
  injection drug use and, 333
  long-term care and, 236, 237
  from nose, mouth, and throat, 341
  nosocomial infections, 449, 454, 469, 476–477
  occupational infections, 263, 280, 295
  peripartal infections of neonates, 390
  pigs, 31
  plant-derived foods and, 177, 184, 186
  prisons and, 240, 241
  school-associated, 364
  from skin, 345
  toxic shock syndrome, 141

Staphylococcus aureus (continued)
    transported animals and goods, 434
    travel-associated, 398, 403, 416
Stem cells, 487–489
Stenotrophomonas maltophilia
    animal-derived foods and, 151
    description, 576
    nosocomial infections, 462–463
    plant-derived foods and, 180
Stents, 490–491
Stethoscopes, 445
STI (sexually transmitted infections)
    community-acquired, 380–384
    genitoanal discharge, 381–382
    genitoanal granulomas, 383
    genitoanal ulcers, 383
    injection drug use and, 333
    from microtrauma, 383–384
    minority-associated, 369–370
    prostitution and, 324–326
    sex tourism and, 415
    travel-associated, 415, 416, 425
Stomoxys, 72
Streptobacillus moniliformis
    animal bites, 10
    description, 576
    drinking water-associated, 203
    occupational infections, 273, 292
    rodents, 47
Streptococcus
    animal-derived foods and, 151–152, 154
    bovids, 26
    description of genus, 576–578
    equids, 33
    occupational infections, 257
    pigs, 31
Streptococcus agalactiae
    description, 576–577
    peripartal infections of neonates, 390
    from urogenital tract, 347
Streptococcus dysgalactiae, 577
Streptococcus equi, 577
Streptococcus iniae, 11
Streptococcus pneumoniae
    community-acquired, 378
    description, 577–578
    domicile-associated, human regular, 210
    homeless persons and, 224
    long-term care and, 234
    minority-associated, 367
    from nose, mouth, and throat, 342
    occupational infections, 255
    prisons and, 239
    school-associated, 361
    travel-associated, 406
Streptococcus pyogenes
    animal-derived foods and, 169, 172
    catering and restaurant-associated, 310
    day care-associated, 358
    description, 578
    domicile-associated, human regular, 214
    domicile-associated, human substandard, 222
    finished food products and, 188
    indoor leisure and, 323
    long-term care and, 237
    from nose, mouth, and throat, 342
    nosocomial infections, 477
    occupational infections, 257, 263, 280–281, 296
    peripartal infections of neonates, 390
    plant-derived foods and, 176, 177, 180
    prisons and, 240
    school-associated, 364
    seasons and, 121
    from skin, 345
Streptococcus suis
    description, 578
    occupational infections, 273, 299
Streptomyces
    description of genus, 578
    nosocomial infections, 451
Strongyloides
    description of genus, 578–579
    domicile-associated, human substandard, 222
    marine habitat, 92
    minority-associated, 368
    nosocomial infections, 485
    occupational infections, 251, 293
    primates, 53
    soil and plants, 100
    urban environment and, 138
Strongyloides fuelleborni, 579
Strongyloides stercoralis
    description, 579
    dogs, 17
    latency, 376
    long-term care and, 236–237
    minority-associated, 368
    occupational infections, 262, 276, 298
    in orphans and adoptees, 232
    outdoor leisure and, 319
    pools and, 313
    terrestrial biomes, 110
    travel-associated, 419, 424
Suctioning and tubing, nosocomial infections and, 444
Suidae. *See* Pigs
Suipoxvirus, 579
Surgical site infections, 474–477
    bacteria, 475–477
    fungi, 477
    prions, 475
    viruses, 475
Swimmer's itch, 97
Swimming pools and spas, 310–314
Swine vesicular disease virus, 527
Systemic inflammatory response syndromes (SIRS), 471

T

Tabanus, 72
Taenia
    animal-derived foods and, 161
    bovids, 23
    description of genus, 579–580
    sanitation and, 132
Taenia asiatica, 579
Taenia saginata
    description, 579
    drinking water-associated, 204
    travel-associated, 417, 422
Taenia solium
    from bowel, 344
    description, 579–580
    domicile-associated, human regular, 212
    domicile-associated, human substandard, 217–218
    latency, 376
    nosocomial infections, 451
    occupational infections, 267, 280
    pigs, 29
    transported animals and goods, 429
    travel-associated, 417, 422
Tahyna virus, 557
Taxonomy, 497–498, 500–502
Terrestrial biomes, 100–116
    alpine and boreal tundra, 112–115
    arid lands, 110–111
    caves, 115–116
    desert oases, 111–112
    grasslands, 106–107
    islands, 107–110
    Mediterranean, temperate and boreal forests, 104–106
    tropical forests and savannas, 100–104
Theileria, 580
Theileria ovis, 34
Thermometers, 445
Throat, agents from, 339–342
Tick-borne encephalitis virus (TBEV)
    animal-derived foods and, 150
    birds, 59
    bovids, 24
    description, 532
    dogs, 15
    domicile-associated, human regular, 212
    herbivores, 38
    occupational infections, 258, 267–268, 290
    outdoor leisure and, 317
    terrestrial biomes, 109
    transported animals and goods, 429
    urban environment and, 135
Tick-borne relapsing fever (TBRF). *See also Borrelia*
    description, 512
    domicile-associated, human substandard, 219
    injection drug use and, 331
    latency, 374
    occupational infections, 269
    outdoor leisure and, 318
    terrestrial biomes, 105
    travel-associated, 412
Ticks
    bedding and, 140
    cold-weather clusters from, 121
    hard, 66–71
        Amblyomma, 67
        Dermacentor, 67
        Haemaphysalis, 67–68
        Hyalomma, 68

Ixodes, 68
Rhipicephalus, 68
soft, 83
transport of, 432
Tinea corporis
  indoor leisure and, 323
Tinea pedis
  indoor leisure and, 323
Tinea tonsurans
  indoor leisure and, 323
  minority-associated, 370
  occupational infections, 296
  school-associated, 364
Toxocara
  animal-derived foods and, 160
  description of genus, 580
  domicile-associated, human substandard, 222
  long-term care and, 236–237
  minority-associated, 368
  nosocomial infections, 451
  occupational infections, 276
  outdoor leisure and, 319–320
  plant-derived foods and, 182, 184
  school-associated, 364
  seasons and, 124
  soil and plants, 100
  terrestrial biomes, 115
  urban environment and, 138
Toxocara canis
  description, 580
  dogs, 17–18
  dust and, 118
  marine habitat, 92
  rodents, 48
Toxocara cati, 580
Toxocara pteropodis, 55
Toxocara vitulorum, 26
Toxoplasma gondii
  animal-derived foods and, 152, 159, 160, 161, 162, 163
  birds, 58
  bovids, 23
  camelids, 34
  carnivores, 40
  cats, 19
  description, 580–581
  dogs, 14
  domicile-associated, human regular, 212
  domicile-associated, human substandard, 217
  drinking water-associated, 200, 204
  dust and, 118
  food-borne illness and, 147
  herbivores, 38
  intrauterine infections, 387–388
  lagomorphs, 49
  latency, 375
  minority-associated, 368
  nosocomial infections, 485
  occupational infections, 257, 266–267
  outdoor leisure and, 317
  pigs, 29
  plant-derived foods and, 181
  rodents, 44

soil and plants, 99
terrestrial biomes, 108
Toys, 141
Training. *See* Schools
Transfusion-associated infections, 477–482
  bacteria, 481
  fungi, 481
  helminths, 482
  prions, 478
  protozoa, 481–482
  viruses, 478–481
Transplants, 482–489
  partial organ, tissue, and cell transplants, 486
  solid organ, 483–486
Transport
  of goods, 432–435
  of invertebrates, 430–432
  of vertebrates, 427–430
Transportation work, 299–300
  droplet-air cluster, 299
  environmental cluster, 300
  feces-food cluster, 299
  skin-blood cluster, 300
  zoonotic cluster, 299–300
Travel, 393–425
  aircraft and airports, 401–404
  expatriates, 416–419
  exposure history, 394
  immigrants and migrants, 420–425
  international short-term, 404–416
  local, 395–398
  ships and seaports, 398–401
Trematodes. *See* Helminths
Treponema
  description of genus, 581–582
  minority-associated, 370
  occupational infections, 296
Treponema carateum, 581
Treponema pallidum
  indoor leisure and, 323
  occupational infections, 263, 300
  in orphans and adoptees, 232
  prisons and, 241
  travel-associated, 425
Treponema pallidum endemicum
  description, 581
  minority-associated, 370
  terrestrial biomes, 111
Treponema pallidum pallidum
  community-acquired, 383
  description, 581–582
  homosexual males and, 328
  intrauterine infections, 386–387
  latency, 374
  nosocomial infections, 481, 493
  prostitution and, 325
  relief camps and, 229
  travel-associated, 398, 416
  urban environment and, 138
  from urogenital tract, 347
Treponema pallidum pertenue
  description, 582
  terrestrial biomes, 102

Treponema pertenue
  domicile-associated, human substandard, 222
  minority-associated, 370
Triatomine bugs, 82
Trichinella
  animal-derived foods and, 160, 161, 162, 163
  carnivores, 41
  catering and restaurant-associated, 309
  description of genus, 582–583
  equids, 32
  occupational infections, 267
  pigs, 29
  rodents, 44
  terrestrial biomes, 115
  transported animals and goods, 434
  travel-associated, 400, 410
Trichinella britovi
  animal-derived foods and, 166
  description, 583
Trichinella nativa
  description, 583
  terrestrial biomes, 104
Trichinella nelsoni, 583
Trichinella papuae, 583
Trichinella pseudospiralis, 583
Trichinella spiralis
  animal-derived foods and, 166
  birds, 58
  bovids, 23
  description, 583
Trichomonas vaginalis
  community-acquired, 382
  description, 583
  homosexual males and, 328
  peripartal infections of neonates, 390
  pools and, 313
  prisons and, 241
  prostitution and, 325
  from urogenital tract, 347
Trichophyton, 583
Trichosporon, 583–584
Trichostrongylus, 584
Trichuris
  description of genus, 584
  plant-derived foods and, 182
  soil and plants, 99
Trichuris trichiura
  description, 584
  domicile-associated, human substandard, 218
  drinking water-associated, 204
  occupational infections, 267
  in orphans and adoptees, 232
  sanitation and, 131–132
  urban environment and, 134
Tropheryma, 584–585
Tropical forests and savannas, 100–104
Trypanosoma
  bovids, 26
  carnivores, 42
  description of genus, 585
  dogs, 16
  equids, 33

Trypanosoma (continued)
flies and, 72–73
freshwater habitats and floods, 96
herbivores, 39–40
occupational infections, 261
pigs, 30
primates, 52
relief camps and, 229
rodents, 48
terrestrial biomes, 103, 107
urban environment and, 137
Trypanosoma brucei gambiense
description, 585
domicile-associated, human substandard, 221
occupational infections, 274, 292
terrestrial biomes, 109
travel-associated, 414
Trypanosoma brucei rhodesiense
description, 585
occupational infections, 274, 292
transported animals and goods, 430
travel-associated, 414, 418, 423
Trypanosoma cruzi
description, 585–586
domicile-associated, human substandard, 221
drinking water-associated, 196
intrauterine infections, 388
latency, 375
minority-associated, 368
nosocomial infections, 482, 485
occupational infections, 250, 261, 274, 292
seasons and, 124
terrestrial biomes, 111, 114
travel-associated, 414, 418, 423
Trypanosoma evansi
camelids, 34
description, 586
transported animals and goods, 430
Trypanosoma rangeli, 586
Trypanosoma vivax, 430
Tsukamurella paurometabola
description, 586
drinking water-associated, 199
TTV, 586
Tula virus, 537
Tundra
alpine, 112–114
boreal, 114–115
Tunga penetrans
fleas from ships and, 432
in orphans and adoptees, 232
overview, 84
travel-associated, 424

U

Uniformed services, 253–264
droplet-air cluster, 254–256
environmental cluster, 261–262
feces-food cluster, 256–258
skin-blood cluster, 262–264
zoonotic cluster, 258–261

Urban environment. *See* Cities
Ureaplasma urealyticum
community-acquired, 382
description, 586
occupational infections, 263
Urine bags, nosocomial infections and, 444
Urogenital tract, agents from, 345–347
Utensils and belongings, 138–142
UTIs, bladder catheters and, 447–448

V

Vaccine
attenuated, 456
contamination, 456
errors of administration, 456
fake, 450
Vaccinia virus, 558
Vahlkampfia, 586
Variant Creutzfeldt-Jakob disease
description, 22, 564–565
nosocomial infections, 475, 478
transported animals and goods, 435
Varicella-zoster virus (VZV)
description, 586–587
domicile-associated, human substandard, 215
indoor leisure and, 321
intrauterine infections, 386
latency, 373
long-term care and, 234
from nose, mouth, and throat, 340
nosocomial infections, 486
occupational infections, 254, 285
prisons and, 238
school-associated, 360
Variola virus
description, 558
fairs and, 306
occupational infections, 294
Vascular grafts, 489
Vascular implants, 490–491
Vegetables and salads, 177–182
Veillonella, 587
Venezuelan equine encephalitis virus (VEEV)
description, 505
equids, 32
occupational infections, 258, 291
Venison and game, 162–163
Vertebrates, migrating and transported, 427–430
droplet-air cluster, 428
environmental cluster, 430
feces-food cluster, 428–429
zoonotic cluster, 429–430
Vertebrates, wild, 37–63
bats, 53–55
birds, 55–60
carnivores, 40–42
fish, 61–63
herbivores, wild, 37–40
lagomorphs, 49–51
primates, 51–53

reptiles and amphibians, 60–61
rodents, 42–49
Vesicular stomatitis virus (VSV)
description, 587
equids, 32
occupational infections, 269, 290
Vesiculovirus, 587
Vibrio
animal-derived foods and, 169, 171–172
community-acquired, 380
description of genus, 587–588
fairs and, 306
fish, 61
food-borne illness and, 146
freshwater habitats and floods, 94
marine habitat, 90–91
occupational infections, 273–274
Vibrio alginolyticus
animal-derived foods and, 169
description, 587
Vibrio cholerae
animal-derived foods and, 168, 169, 171
from bowel, 344
catering and restaurant-associated, 309
description, 587–588
domicile-associated, human substandard, 217
drinking water-associated, 195, 196, 199, 203
long-term care and, 236
nosocomial infections, 442
occupational infections, 257, 279–280, 289, 298, 299
plant-derived foods and, 180, 184, 185
relief camps and, 227–228
terrestrial biomes, 106, 108
transported animals and goods, 431, 434
travel-associated, 397, 400, 403, 409
urban environment and, 133
Vibrio mimicus, 169
Vibrio parahaemolyticus
animal-derived foods and, 161, 168, 169.171–172
from bowel, 344
catering and restaurant-associated, 309
description, 588
hotels and, 244
occupational infections, 257, 280
plant-derived foods and, 180
school-associated, 363
transported animals and goods, 431, 434
travel-associated, 400, 403, 409
Vibrio vulnificus
animal bites, 11
animal-derived foods and, 168, 169, 171
description, 588
Viral hemorrhagic fevers
relief camps and, 228
travel-associated, 403–404
Viruses. *See also specific viral agents*
animal-derived foods and, 150, 155, 158, 159–161, 164, 170–171
avian, 55–60
bovid, 21–24, 26
from bowel, 342–343

from breast milk, 391
camelid, 34–35
carnivore, 41
cat, 18–21
chiropteran, 54–55
community-acquired, 377, 379, 383–386, 388–389, 391
dam-related, 126
day care-associated, 354, 356, 357–358
dog, 13, 14, 15
domicile-associated, human regular, 208–209, 211–214
domicile-associated, human substandard, 214–216, 218–219, 222
drinking water-associated, 194–197, 200–201
dust, 116–117
equid, 31–33
finished food products and, 187–189
fish, 61
flies and, 72
food-borne illness and, 144–145
freshwater habitats and floods, 93–95
herbivore, 38
homeless persons and, 223–225
hotels and, 242–244
human travel and, 395–397, 399–405, 407, 410–411, 415, 417–422, 424–425
intrauterine infections, 385–386
lagomorph, 49–51
latent, 373–374
leisure and lifestyle-associated, 304–308, 311–315, 317, 320–323, 325–329, 331–333
long-term care and, 233–235, 237
marine habitat, 89–91
minorities and, 365–368
mosquitoes and, 74–75, 77, 79–81
from nose, mouth, and throat, 339–340
nosocomial infections, 468–471, 475, 478–481, 484–489, 493–494
noninvasive procedures, 441–443, 447–449, 451, 455–456, 458–459, 461, 463–466
occupational infections, 250–251, 254, 256, 258–259, 262–269, 277–278, 284–286, 288, 290–291, 293–295, 297–301
in orphans and adoptees, 230–232
peripartal infections of neonates, 388–389
plant-derived foods and, 176, 178, 183
porcine, 27–28, 30–31
prisons and, 238–241
relief camps and, 226–229
rodent, 43–46, 48
sandflies and, 81
sanitation and, 128–129, 131
school-associated, 359–360, 362, 364
seasons and, 120–123
simian, 51–53
from skin, 344–345
taxonomic overview, 497
terrestrial biomes, 101–102, 104–106, 108–110, 112, 116

ticks and, 68–69
transfusion-associated infections, 478–481
transported animals and goods, 428–429, 431, 433, 435
urban environment and, 132–135
from urogenital tract, 345–346
utensils and belongings, 139–142
Vomiting, food-borne illness and, 144–146
VRE (vancomycin-resistant *Enterococcus*)
nosocomial infections, 442, 464
travel-associated, 397

W

Wangiella, 588
Warm-weather peaks, 121–123
Waste, 130–132
Waste work. *See* Cleaning and waste work
Water and beverages, 193–204
bottled and mineral waters, 194–195
hospital, 461–464
ice cubes, 195–196
juices, 196
private and low-income water supplies, 200–204
soft drinks, 197
tap water, municipal high-income, 197–200
Weaponized bacteria, 117, 128
Wesselbron virus, 532
West Nile virus (WNV)
birds, 59
from breast milk, 391
description, 532
dogs, 15
domicile-associated, human substandard, 218
equids, 32–33
nosocomial infections, 485
occupational infections, 258, 268, 290
transfusion-transmitted agents, 479
travel-associated, 400, 411, 422
urban environment and, 135
Western equine encephalitis virus (WEEV)
birds, 59
description, 505
domicile-associated, human substandard, 218
equids, 32
occupational infections, 258, 268
wind and, 118
Winds, arthropods and, 118
Wolbachia, 588
Work-related infections. *See* Occupational infections
Wound infections, 475
Wuchereria bancrofti
description, 588–589
latency, 376
mosquitoes and, 75, 79–80
terrestrial biomes, 104, 110
travel-associated, 419, 424
urban environment and, 137

Y

Yatapoxvirus, 589
Yellow fever virus (YFV)
description, 532–533
occupational infections, 258, 268, 290
travel-associated, 397, 411
urban environment and, 135
Yersinia
birds, 58
from bowel, 344
cats, 19
description of genus, 589–590
dogs, 14
fleas, 71
food-borne illness and, 146
pigs, 28
school-associated, 363
Yersinia enterocolitica
animal-derived foods and, 152, 154, 160–161, 164, 172
description, 589
domicile-associated, human regular, 212
drinking water-associated, 199
freshwater habitats and floods, 94
nosocomial infections, 442, 481
occupational infections, 266, 280
outdoor leisure and, 316
plant-derived foods and, 180
school-associated, 363
terrestrial biomes, 114
travel-associated, 400, 409
Yersinia pestis
camelids, 34
cats, 20
description, 589–590
dogs, 16
domicile-associated, human substandard, 219–220
fleas from ships and, 432
lagomorphs, 50
occupational infections, 259–260, 270, 292
rodents, 47
seasons and, 122
terrestrial biomes, 106–107, 111
transported animals and goods, 430
travel-associated, 413
Yersinia pseudotuberculosis
animal-derived foods and, 152
description, 590
plant-derived foods and, 180
school-associated, 363
soil and plants, 98

Z

Zika virus, 533
Zoonoses
avian, 55
bovine, 21
camelid, 34
canine, 13
carnivore, 40
chiropterans, 54
equine, 31

Zoonoses (continued)
    feline, 18
    fish, 61
    lagomorph, 49
    porcine, 27
    rodent, 42–43
Zoonotic cluster
    adult age and, 352
    agents, 3
    avian, 58–60
    bovine, 23–26
    camelid, 34–35
    canine, 15–17
    carnivore, 41–42
    chiropteran, 54–55
    cleaning and waste work, 298
    clerk, class, and sales work, 301
    cold-weather peaks, 120–121
    construction and mining, 250
    crop-and-herd work, 267–274
    dam-related, 126–127
    domiciles, human regular, 212–213
    domiciles, human substandard, 218–221
    elderly and, 352
    equine, 32–33
    fairs, 306–307
    feline, 19–20
    freshwater habitats and floods, 95–96
    health-and-laboratory work, 290–292
    herbivore, 38–40
    homeless persons, 224–225
    hotels, 245
    injection drug use, 331
    islands, 108–110
    lagomorph, 49–50
    manufacture and maintenance work, 252–253
    marine habitats, 91
    minorities and, 368
    outdoor leisure, 317–318
    porcine, 30
    preschool age and, 351
    rainy seasons, 123–124
    relief camps, 228–229
    rodent, 44–48
    school age and, 351
    school-associated, 363–364
    simian, 52
    soil and plants, 99
    stem cell recipients and, 488
    transfusion-transmitted agents, 479
    transportation work, 299–300
    transported goods and, 435
    travel-associated, 397–398, 400–401, 403–404, 410–414, 417–419, 422–424
    uniformed services, 258–261
    urban, 134–137
    vertebrates, migrating and transported, 429–430
    warm-weather peaks, 122

About the Author

Dieter A. Stürchler (M.D., M.P.H.) graduated from Basel University in Switzerland in 1970 with a thesis in experimental microbiology. He gained experience in internal medicine, surgery, obstetrics and gynecology, and tropical medicine, including in West and Central Africa and Taiwan. He worked at the Swiss Tropical Institute from 1977-1983, with responsibilities in the clinical, vaccination, and diagnostic departments. With support by the National Science Foundation, he and his family lived in Seattle from 1983-1985, where he obtained an M.P.H. from the University of Washington and did a field investigation among Yakima Indians. He joined the Infectious Disease Department of an international pharmaceutical company in 1986 and was promoted head of the tropical disease unit in 1993, assuming responsibility for tropical disease research and development and marketing worldwide. When the company discontinued activities in this area, he moved to the Federal Office of Public Health where from 1996-2001 he headed the Swiss Infectious Disease Notification System. In 2002 he became a freelance epidemiology consultant to government and industry. He holds board-approved titles in tropical medicine and public health and has been extraordinarius professor for epidemiology at Basel University since 1996. In his leisure time, he and his wife share a passion for pristine lands and plants of arid lands.